# KOCHAR'S CONCISE TEXTBOOK OF MEDICINE

*Fourth Edition*

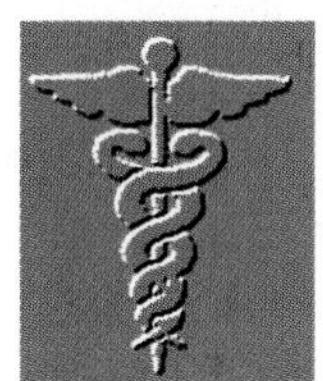

# KOCHAR'S CONCISE TEXTBOOK OF MEDICINE

*Fourth Edition*

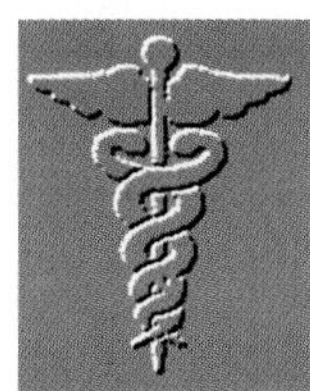


**Editor-in-Chief**
**Kesavan Kutty, MD, FACP, FCCP**
Professor of Medicine
Medical College of Wisconsin
Chairman of Medicine
St. Joseph Regional Medical Center
Milwaukee, Wisconsin

**Editors**
**Ralph M. Schapira, MD, FACP, FCCP**
Professor and Vice-Chairman of Medicine
Medical College of Wisconsin
Chief of Medicine
Zablocki VA Medical Center
Milwaukee, Wisconsin

**Jerome Van Ruiswyk, MD, MS, FACP**
Associate Professor of Medicine
Medical College of Wisconsin
Associate Chief of Staff for Clinical Affairs
Zablocki VA Medical Center
Milwaukee, Wisconsin

**Consulting Editor**
**Mahendr S. Kochar, MD, FACP, FRCP (London & Canada)**
Professor of Medicine
Senior Associate Dean, Graduate Medical Education
Medical College of Wisconsin
Milwaukee, Wisconsin



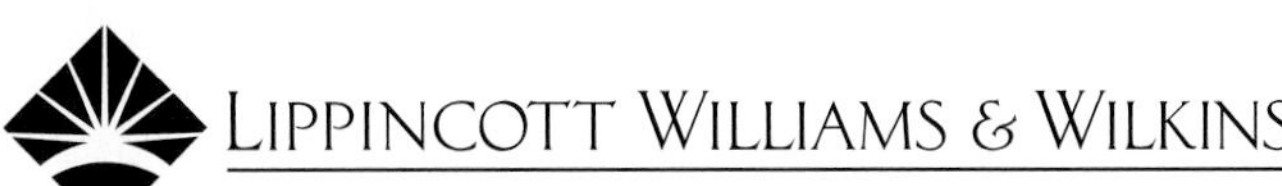

*Editor:* Neil Marquardt
*Managing Editor:* Daniel Pepper
*Marketing Manager:* Scott Lavine
*Production Editor:* Christina Remsberg
*Compositor:* Graphic World
*Printer:* Quebecor World



351 West Camden Street
Baltimore, Maryland 21201-2436 USA

530 Walnut Street
Philadelphia, PA 19106



*Printed in the United States of America*

First Edition, 1982    Second Edition, 1990    Third Edition, 1998

**Library of Congress Cataloging-in-Publication Data**

Kochar's concise textbook of medicine / editor-in-chief, Kesavan Kutty ; editors, Mahendr S. Kochar, Ralph Schapira, Jerome Van Ruiswyk.—4th ed.
p. ; cm.
Includes bibliographical references and index.
ISBN 0-7817-2942-4
1. Internal medicine. I. Title: Concise textbook of medicine. II. Kutty, Kesavan.
[DNLM: 1. Internal Medicine. 2. Primary Health Care. WB 115 K76 2002]
RC46 .T328 2002
616—dc21

2002030016

*The publishers have made every effort to trace the copyright holders for borrowed material. If they have inadvertently overlooked any, they will be pleased to make the necessary arrangements at the first opportunity.*

To purchase additional copies of this book, call our customer service department at **(800) 638-3030** or fax orders to **(301) 824-7390.** International customers should call **(301) 714-2324.**

***Visit Lippincott Williams & Wilkins on the Internet: http://www.LWW.com.*** Lippincott Williams & Wilkins customer service representatives are available from 8:30 am to 6:00 pm, EST.

03 04 05 06 07

1 2 3 4 5 6 7 8 9 10

# Foreword

It is a distinct pleasure to write the foreword for the fourth edition of *Kochar's Concise Textbook of Medicine.* This edition, as with its forbearers, is almost entirely written by the faculty of the Department of Medicine at the Medical College of Wisconsin and it reflects their deep commitment to education and patient care.

The book is designed for medical students and residents, but the key to its ongoing success can be found in its title: concise. It contains the essential information on most clinical problems in Internal Medicine without being exhaustive and redundant. I was given a copy of the third edition by Dr. Kochar upon my arrival here at the Medical College and I often turn to it to resolve an interesting point raised on rounds or during resident morning report. It is written by master teachers and reflects not only years of experience, but also a skilled presentation of the fundamentals.

This textbook has been significantly updated since its last edition in 1998. The "Art and Science of Medicine" section has been rewritten. New sections on genetics, the role of hospitalists, palliative care and cost effectiveness of care have been added. The events of September 11, 2001 have resulted in a new section on biological, radioactive and chemical terror. In addition, essentially all the chapters and references have been updated.

A special comment is warranted for this textbook's creator, Dr. Mahendr Kochar. Dr. Kochar served as editor and co-editor for the first two editions. As one of the senior statesmen of our Department, he continues as this textbook's guiding influence. Dr. Kochar is the quintessential teacher and role model and serves as the Medical College's Senior Associate Dean for Graduate Medical Education.

Dr. Kesavan Kutty was the Co-Editor of the second edition and Editor-in-Chief of the third edition. He is a Professor of Medicine at the Medical College of Wisconsin as well as the Chairman of Medicine and Director of the Transitional Year Residency Program at St. Joseph Regional Medical Center in Milwaukee. Dr. Kutty is also the Governor of the Wisconsin Chapter of the American College of Physicians; he is clearly a master teacher.

Two new editors have been added for this edition. Dr. Ralph Schapira is Professor of Medicine, Chief of Medicine at the Zablocki VA Medical Center in Milwaukee, and Program Director for the Medical College of Wisconsin's Internal Medicine residency program. Dr. Jerome Van Ruiswyk is Associate Professor of Medicine and Associate Chief of Staff for Clinical Affairs at the Zablocki VA Medical Center. Drs. Schapira (pulmonary and critical care specialist) and Van Ruiswyk (general internist) are outstanding teachers and role models. They have also added their own perspectives to this updated edition.

Finally, I would like to acknowledge each of the authors in this text. Their sustained commitment to teaching of the medical students and housestaff creates a legacy of excellence for the future.

**G. Richard Olds, MD, FACP**
The John and Linda Mellowes Professor and Chairman,
Department of Medicine
The Medical College of Wisconsin

# Preface to the Fourth Edition

Presenting the Fourth Edition of our Concise Textbook of Medicine represents a proud moment for all of us. Dr. Kochar edited the First Edition in 1983 and has remained a consulting editor for the Third Edition and the current one. Two new senior faculty members from the Department of Medicine at the Medical College of Wisconsin (Drs. Ralph M. Schapira and Jerome Van Ruiswyk) have joined as editors.

The highly favorable response to the Third Edition together with the information explosion of the late 1990s prompted the birth of the Fourth Edition. It became very clear to us that the Third Edition found its niche soon after its publication. The readers found its simplicity and focused nature very appealing—in other words, it lived up to its title of being concise. Its easy-to-read layout, consistent use of simple language to convey complex ideas and an excellent index that afforded "easy lookups" were other strengths, not to mention the complementary Tables and Figures and a large number of representative radiographs and other images. The few criticisms we received were taken seriously and we effected appropriate changes to accommodate those concerns. We are blessed with a highly skilled and acclaimed group of teachers among our colleagues at the Medical College of Wisconsin and almost all authors are from this institution.

Despite our obvious bias, we feel very comfortable extolling the virtues of Internal Medicine—that it is the basis of all interactions with patients; it forms the very essence of a code that all physicians use in diagnosing and treating all disorders. It is all about detail; it is about interactions of information and about distilling down the essence from a morass of information. What we have provided here is an organized, albeit concise way of integrating this information into tangible medical entities: how to recognize them, how to evaluate them and what principles one should embrace in treating them. Finally, our objective continues to be to present this information in a manner that a student in a 2-3 month clerkship can easily comprehend and assimilate into his/her information base.

Concepts are the main theme of any textbook; however, concepts need reinforcing. A proven method is to utilize examples. Students generally have to take an examination at the end of their clerkships. We combined these two needs into a second component of this book, which is presented in an accompanying CD-ROM where we provide multiple-choice questions related to each specialty. The answers are given with appropriate annotations in order to drive the concepts home and to reinforce the information from the book. Finally, with over 1000 pages of text and almost 560 questions, the book really gives you more than your money's worth.

As we have emphasized before, change remains the driving force behind this work of ours. We embrace change when it is for the better, even when it involves some inconvenience. The ideal mind should view change with a dual attitude: one, a healthy and immediate skepticism; and the other, one of acceptance as the skepticism abates. These are unique lessons learned in a Medicine clerkship. When new concepts are contrasted against one's accumulated knowledge and experience, they evolve into clinical wisdom. For such wisdom to evolve, all new concepts have to be contrasted against one's knowledge, but also get reshaped on the anvil of one's own experience.

It has been our pleasure to work with a fine group of professionals at Lippincott Williams & Wilkins. We also thank our families and friends for the encouragement and consideration they gave us in making this publication a success.

**Kesavan Kutty, M.D.**
**Ralph M. Schapira, M.D.**
**Jerome Van Ruiswyk, M.D.**

# Preface to the Third Edition

It has been said, with some degree of seriousness that, the more things change, the more they remain the same. The face of medicine, in as short a spell as within the last decade, has been beset with series of changes. Irrespective of whether or not one considers it consoling that medicine was not singled out for the change, things have hardly remained the same; in fact, these changes will fundamentally alter the practice of medicine for generations to come.

In a sense, besides death and taxes, change remains the only other certainty because change is the "mother's milk" of progress. However, not all change is for the better, and every change involves some inconvenience—even when it is for the better. A healthy attitude toward change revolves around two concepts: one, of exercising a sufficient degree of healthy skepticism toward it; the other, one of accepting it after one's skepticism is resolved. Both are lessons learned during a clerkship in Internal medicine. However, one also needs to pit a new concept or a new approach against the backdrop of one's fundamental concepts and understanding; such a basis is required for furthering one's learning. With the passage of time and gaining of practical experience, new concepts not only get contrasted against one's knowledge, but also get reshaped on the anvil of one's own experience through contemplation and reflection.

Medical students decide their future career(s) rather early during their medical education. Although inherent pros and cons to this early decision making do exist, a thorough basis in internal medicine is essential to the practice of any specialty. The recent "discovery" of primary care underscores this even more, regardless of one's concepts as to the origins of this discovery. It is the essential underpinning of all medical specialties. It teaches the concept of getting the facts straight, assembling the possibilities, and getting a match, generating a hypothesis, and finally, employing a minimum number of specific tests to confirm or refute one's hypothesis. The integration of physiology and pathophysiology are essential components of this process. The scenes and actors change, but the principles remain the same.

That the medical student need not learn a "standard" textbook of medicine cover to cover during a medicine clerkship or more importantly, fails predictably in that mission, was known to us a long time ago; it formed the impetus for the first edition of this textbook. The manner in which it was accepted by both students and critics made us confident of our assessment; the appearance of similar books in the marketplace merely conferred accuracy on our assessment. The doubling of editors through these three editions also signifies our own appreciation of both the length and breadth of internal medicine, and reflects the courage of our conviction that despite our constant involvement with undergraduate education, an optimum number of editors is a prerequisite to conveying our thoughts and concepts in a balanced manner.

In this edition, a number of changes have been made. Although the authors have maintained the emphasis of conciseness in conveying their ideas, they have added a large complement of tables, figures, and line diagrams to convey their ideas effectively and to make the product visually appealing. Almost three-fourths of the authors are new and belong to various divisions of internal medicine and departments of the Medical College of Wisconsin. They are both accomplished teachers and fine clinicians, who have been "in the trenches." Much of the text has been rewritten and where it was only revised, every effort has been made to incorporate current concepts and information. A number of new multiple-choice questions have been provided at the end of every part to help drive the concepts home. Some of these questions involve pictorial material representing actual situations that have confronted many house officers. A completely revised list of references follow as a guide to further reading.

The work on this has been exhilarating as we found our own concepts challenged and consolidated during its development and as we saw the horizons of our own knowledge widening. While we appreciate the help and support of the editorial staff at Williams & Wilkins in making this publication a reality, we also wish to take this opportunity to thank our senior colleague, Dr. Mahendr Kochar, for the confidence and trust he placed in us to continue a project and a fine tradition that he both founded and nurtured.

Samuel Johnson wrote: "The greatest part of a writer's time is spent in reading, in order to write; a man will turn over half a library to make one book." As this textbook made its way from concept to reality, we authors and editors have come to appreciate the enormity of and the truth behind this statement. As we burned our midnight oil "turning over" our libraries, our families and colleagues watched us and encouraged us, which only confirmed we were doing the right thing.

**Kesavan Kutty**
**James Sebastian**
**Beth Mewis**
**Dale Berg**
***June 1998***

# Preface to the Second Edition

Conventional wisdom tells us that the clinician arrives at a bedside diagnosis by careful history taking, thorough clinical examination, assimilation of the available information, and finally, by reflective reshaping of the resultant product on the anvil of prior experience. However, as stated by Dr. Roman Yanda, experience alone is a poor teacher: by the time one has enough, success or failure no longer matters. The background of organizing learning—theoretical knowledge—should supplement experience if one were to succeed. Providing that necessary supplementation is the prime function of a textbook. As was the case with the first edition, published as *Textbook of General Medicine,* our objective in writing and editing this second edition is to provide the student with a course in internal medicine that could be read cover to cover during a 12-week rotation in medicine and to acquire knowledge in that field considered essential to graduation from medical school. Even though the book is directed to medical students, it will also serve as a quick reference source for internal medicine and family practice residents as well as nurses and other health professionals. The success of the first edition indicated that we had attained our objective. Its reviews in peer reviewed journals were extremely favorable, and we came to the inescapable conclusion that a second edition was in order.

Once again each chapter begins with an outline that defines the scope of the subject matter presented and ends with multiple choice questions meant to assist in self-evaluation. Liberal use of headings and use of simple, yet precise, language should make it easier to read. Almost half the contributors to the second edition are new. As was the case with the first edition, they are among today's leading teachers of medicine, all being board certified in their specialties and, where applicable, in the respective subspecialties as well.

Two new chapters, Psychiatry and Medical Genetics, have been added, and a whole section on alcoholism and substance abuse has been added to the chapter on clinical toxicology.

To say that medical practice is being reshaped is perhaps an understatement. At times it is hard to discern whether technology is driving medicine or vice versa. Medicine has made tremendous strides and seen new developments since 1983 when the first edition was published—the advent of magnetic resonance imaging, proliferation of antibiotics, calcium channel blockers, entry of AIDS as the greatest scourge of humankind, refinements in critical care and fibrinolytic therapy, just to name a few. To reflect the current advances, every chapter in the book has been thoroughly revised to reflect the current understanding of the subject, yet at the same time the book has been kept concise and the price affordable to the student.

The use of detailed references has been deliberately avoided, but a selected bibliography is provided at the end of each chapter for further reading. If the reader wishes to study a subject in greater detail, after studying the relevant portion from Concise Textbook of Medicine, he or she is encouraged to seek from a medical library an up-to-date computer printout of recent literature on the subject and then to read the most recent review articles on the subject.

**Mahendr S. Kochar**
**Kesavan Kutty**
***October 1989***

# Preface to the First Edition

"To study the phenomenon of disease without books is to sail an uncharted sea; while to study books without patients is not to go to sea at all," wrote Sir Williams Osler in 1901.[1]

There is only one way to learn clinical medicine, and that is at the bedside participating in diagnosis and treatment of the patient's illness; however no one can expect to acquire even the essential knowledge of internal medicine without books. With intensive biomedical research, there has been a knowledge explosion in medicine in the last three decades; there is too much to learn in a limited amount of time. It is impossible for a medical student to read the standard textbooks of medicine from beginning to end, but the student must acquire knowledge of the essentials of internal medicine in order to become a Doctor of Medicine.

The purpose of this book is to provide the student with a course in internal medicine that can be read from cover to cover during an 8- to 12-week rotation in medicine; it contains the essentials of internal medicine that the student must know before graduating. The book will also serve as a source of concise information for family practice and internal medicine residents desiring a rapid review of internal medicine. Allied health professionals, particularly nurse practitioners and physicians' assistants, will find the book readable and understandable.

Each chapter begins with an outline that defines the scope of the subject matter that one needs to learn and ends with multiple-choice questions, which should help in recapitulating what has been learned. Liberal use of headings and use of simple yet precise language should make the reading of this book an enjoyable experience.

This text has been written by specialists who are among today's leading teachers of internal medicine. All of the authors are board certified in both internal medicine and their subspecialties and have written their chapters with the objective of presenting all relevant information in the most lucid manner. The use of references has been deliberately avoided, but a selected bibliography is provided at the end of each chapter for further reading.

I would like to take this opportunity to thank Daniel J. McCarty, MD, Professor and Chairman of the Department of Medicine at the Medical College of Wisconsin, Milwaukee, for writing the foreword to this book.

**Mahendr S. Kochar**
***September 1982***

[1]Olsen W. Books and men. Boston Med Surg J 1901: 144:60–62.

# Acknowledgments

To the extent that it is almost impossible to list the names and contributions of all those who have assisted in the preparation and publication of this book, this summation of acknowledgments is only a partial list. However, the names and roles of some clearly outstanding professionals come to our mind.

We express our appreciation to the contributors and their office staff who have worked diligently and patiently in getting their literary contributions into our hands on time. The Editorial Staff at Lippincott Williams & Wilkins, including Elizabeth Nieginski, Neil Marquardt, Amy Dinkel, Dan Pepper, and Christina Remsberg, deserve our accolades and thanks for their undivided attention toward bringing out this Fourth Edition. We would also like to take this opportunity to thank Dr. G. Richard Olds, The John and Linda Mellowes Professor and Chairman, Department of Medicine, Medical College of Wisconsin for reviewing the manuscript and writing the Foreword to our textbook. We gratefully acknowledge the gentle encouragement, constructive criticism, and timely suggestions we have received from our friend, colleague, and Consulting editor, Dr. Mahendr Kochar, whose name this textbook bears and without whose help and adherence to the editorial timelines this edition may not have materialized by this time.

We are also indebted to our families for their selfless devotion and love.

**Kesavan Kutty**
**Ralph M. Schapira**
**Jerome Van Ruiswyk**

# Acknowledgments

# Contributors

**Robert T. Adlam, MD**
Clinical Associate Professor of Medicine
Medical College of Wisconsin
St. Joseph Regional Medical Center
Medical Director, Fire Department, City of Milwaukee
Milwaukee, Wisconsin

**Zia Agha, MD, MS**
Assistant Professor of Medicine
Medical College of Wisconsin
Section of General Internal Medicine
Zablocki VA Medical Center
Milwaukee, Wisconsin

**Tom Anderson, MD**
Hematology-Oncology Centers of the Northern Rockies
St. Vincent Healthcare
Billings, Montana

**William Anderson, MD**
Staff Psychiatrist
Mental Health Division
Zablocki VA Medical Center
Milwaukee, Wisconsin

**Rebekah Wang-Cheng, MD, FACP**
Professor of Medicine
Medical College of Wisconsin
Froedtert Hospital
Milwaukee, Wisconsin

**Virinderjit S. Bamrah, MD, FACC**
Professor of Medicine
Division of Cardiovascular Medicine
Medical College of Wisconsin
Zablocki VA Medical Center
Milwaukee, Wisconsin

**Rajesh Bhargava, MD, FACP, FAAP**
Clinical Assistant Professor of Medicine
Medical College of Wisconsin
Professional Internal Medicine Services, SC
St. Joseph Regional Medical Center
Milwaukee, Wisconsin

**David G. Binion, MD**
Associate Professor of Medicine
Division of Gastroenterology and Hepatology
Medical College of Wisconsin
Froedtert Hospital
Milwaukee, Wisconsin

**Peter D. Chapman, MD, FACC**
Associate Clinical Professor of Medicine
Medical College of Wisconsin
Director of Electrophysiology
St. Joseph Regional Medical Center
Milwaukee, Wisconsin

**Christopher R. Chitambar, MD, FACP**
Professor of Medicine
Division of Neoplastic and Related Disorders
Medical College of Wisconsin
Froedtert Hospital
Milwaukee, Wisconsin

**Asriani M. Chiu, MD**
Assistant Professor of Pediatrics and Medicine
Division of Allergy and Immunology
Medical College of Wisconsin
Chief, Section of Allergy
Zablocki VA Medical Center
Milwaukee, Wisconsin

**Mary E. Cohan, MD**
Assistant Professor of Medicine
Division of Geriatrics and Gerontology
Medical College of Wisconsin
Froedtert Hospital
Milwaukee, Wisconsin

**Eric P. Cohen, MD**
Professor of Medicine
Division of Nephrology
Medical College of Wisconsin
Froedtert Hospital
Milwaukee, Wisconsin

**Thomas Driscoll, MD, FACP**
Associate Clinical Professor of Medicine
Medical College of Wisconsin
Harwood Medical Clinic and St. Joseph Regional Medical Center
Milwaukee, Wisconsin

**Kulwinder S. Dua, MD, FACP, FRCP (Edin)**
Associate Professor of Medicine
Division of Gastroenterology and Hepatology
Medical College of Wisconsin
Director, Therapeutic Endoscopy
Froedtert Hospital
Chief, Section of Gastroenterology
Zablocki VA Medical Center
Milwaukee, Wisconsin

**Edmund H. Duthie, Jr., MD**
Professor of Medicine
Chief, Geriatrics and Gerontology
Medical College of Wisconsin
Froedtert Hospital
Zablocki VA Medical Center
Milwaukee, Wisconsin

**Janet A. Fairley, MD**
Professor of Dermatology
The Medical College of Wisconsin
Chief, Section of Dermatology
Zablocki VA Medical Center
Milwaukee, Wisconsin

**Jerome L. Gottschall, MD**
Professor of Medicine
Medical College of Wisconsin
Vice President—Medical Services
The Blood Center of Southeastern Wisconsin, Inc.
Milwaukee, Wisconsin

**Paul B. Halverson, MD, FACP**
Professor of Medicine
Division of Rheumatology
Medical College of Wisconsin
St. Joseph Regional Medical Center
Froedtert Hospital
Milwaukee, Wisconsin

**Janet R. Hosenpud, MD**
Assistant Professor of Medicine
Division of Neoplastic and Related Disorders
Medical College of Wisconsin
Froedtert Hospital
Milwaukee, Wisconsin

**Howard J. Jacob, PhD**
Warren P. Knowles Professor of Human and Molecular Genetics and Physiology
Director, Human and Molecular Genetics Center
Medical College of Wisconsin
Milwaukee, Wisconsin

**Safwan S. Jaradeh, MD**
Professor and Chairman, Department of Neurology
Medical College of Wisconsin
Froedtert Hospital
Milwaukee, Wisconsin

**Albert L. Jochen, MD**
Associate Professor of Medicine
Division of Endocrinology, Metabolism and Clinical Nutrition
Medical College of Wisconsin
Chief, Section of Endocrinology
Zablocki VA Medical Center
Milwaukee, Wisconsin

**Charles L. Junkerman, MD**
Emeritus Professor of Medicine
Center for the Study of Bioethics
Medical College of Wisconsin
Milwaukee, Wisconsin

**Gail A. Kallas, MD**
Assistant Professor of Medicine
Section of General Internal Medicine
Medical College of Wisconsin
Zablocki VA Medical Center
Milwaukee, Wisconsin

**Mahendr S. Kochar, MD, FACP, FRCP (London & Canada)**
Professor of Medicine and Pharmacology/Toxicology
Senior Associate Dean, Graduate Medical Education
Medical College of Wisconsin
Executive Director
Medical College of Wisconsin Affiliated Hospitals
Milwaukee, Wisconsin

**Kesavan Kutty, MD, FACP, FCCP**
Professor of Medicine
Medical College of Wisconsin
Chairman of Medicine
St. Joseph Regional Medical Center
Milwaukee, Wisconsin

**Jon A. Lehrmann, MD**
Assistant Professor of Psychiatry
Associate Director, Psychiatry Residency
Medical College of Wisconsin
Manager, Acute Program
Mental Health Division
Zablocki VA Medical Center
Milwaukee, Wisconsin

**Albert Liebman, MD**
Assistant Clinical Professor of Medicine and Psychiatry
Medical College of Wisconsin
Milwaukee, Wisconsin

**Diana L. Maas, MD**
Associate Professor of Medicine
Division of Endocrinology Metabolism and Clinical Nutrition
Medical College of Wisconsin
Zablocki VA Medical Center
Froedtert Hospital
Milwaukee, Wisconsin

**Marcos L. Montagnini, MD**
Assistant Professor of Medicine
Division of Geriatrics and Gerontology
Medical College of Wisconsin
Director, Palliative Care Program
Zablocki VA Medical Center
Milwaukee, Wisconsin

**G. Richard Olds, MD, FACP**
The Linda and John Mellowes Professor and Chairman
Department of Medicine
Medical College of Wisconsin
Froedtert Hospital
Milwaukee, Wisconsin

**Irene M. O'Shaughnessy, MD**
Associate Professor of Medicine
Division of Endocrinology Metabolism and Clinical Nutrition
Medical College of Wisconsin
Froedtert Hospital
Zablocki VA Medical Center
Milwaukee, Wisconsin

**Walter F. Piering, MD, FACP**
Professor of Medicine
Division of Nephrology
Medical College of Wisconsin
Froedtert Hospital
Milwaukee, Wisconsin

**Lynn F. Reinke, RN, MSN**
Adult Nurse Practitioner
Pulmonary/Critical Care Section
Zablocki VA Medical Center
Milwaukee, Wisconsin

**Kia Saeian, MD, MSc (Epi)**
Assistant Professor of Medicine
Division of Gastroenterology and Hepatology
Medical College of Wisconsin
Froedtert Hospital
Milwaukee, Wisconsin

**Marilyn M. Schapira, MD, MPH, FACP**
Associate Professor of Medicine
Division of General Internal Medicine
Medical College of Wisconsin
Zablocki VA Medical Center
Milwaukee, Wisconsin

**Ralph M. Schapira, MD, FACP, FCCP**
Professor and Vice-Chairman of Medicine
Program Director, Internal Medicine Residency
Medical College of Wisconsin
Chief of Medicine
Zablocki VA Medical Center
Milwaukee, Wisconsin

**David Schiedermayer, MD**
Professor of Medicine
Division of General Internal Medicine
Medical College of Wisconsin
Froedtert Hospital
Milwaukee, Wisconsin

**Bonnie J. Tesch, MD, FACP**
Clinical Associate Professor of Medicine
Medical College of Wisconsin
Falls Medical Clinic—Advanced Health SC
Menomonee Falls, Wisconsin

**Jerome Van Ruiswyk, MD, MS, FACP**
Associate Professor of Medicine
Medical College of Wisconsin
Associate Chief of Staff for Clinical Affairs
Zablocki VA Medical Center
Milwaukee, Wisconsin

**Basil Varkey, MD, FCCP**
Professor of Medicine
Division of Pulmonary and Critical Care Medicine
Medical College of Wisconsin
Froedtert Hospital
Milwaukee, Wisconsin

**David K. Wagner, MD**
Associate Professor of Medicine
Division of Infectious Diseases
Medical College of Wisconsin
Zablocki VA Medical Center
Milwaukee, Wisconsin

# Contents

## XV RHEUMATIC DISEASES

PART I

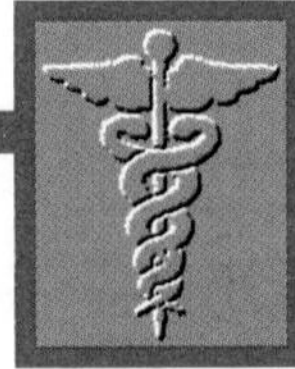

# THE ART AND SCIENCE OF MEDICINE

# CHAPTER 1 ROLE OF THE PRIMARY CARE PHYSICIAN

Medicine is both an art and a science. The diagnosis of illness is based on clinical methods and laboratory tests, supplemented when necessary by the application of the most modern technology. Eliciting a good history, performing a thorough physical examination, and selecting the most crucial laboratory tests without subjecting the patient to undue risk or expense—and then synthesizing the resulting information—require skill. Laboratory tests, diagnostic imaging, endoscopic studies, and electrophysiologic tests are all examples of the application of science in medicine. However, extracting the relevant information from a mass of conflicting physical signs and laboratory data to arrive at the correct diagnosis is an art that requires experience and judgment. Similarly, whereas pharmaceutical modalities and surgical procedures are a highly developed science, knowing when and how to use them is an art.

## The Changing Face of Medicine

Changing population demographics are driving significant changes in medical practice and primary care. The higher prevalence of chronic illnesses in our aging U.S. population and the rapid development of new technologies have required primary care physicians to coordinate increasingly complex, interdependent, interdisciplinary care and also have led to increasing per capita utilization of medical care and increasing costs. New models of health care financing and reimbursement, such as diagnosis-related groups (DRGs) and capitated care, have emerged in response to these increasing costs (see Chapter 2). Utilization management has expanded over the last decade to include critical pathways (care maps) for episodes of inpatient care and disease-specific clinical guidelines for acute and chronic care for a variety of common diagnoses. This attempt to reduce variations in medical practice must be balanced against the individual needs and circumstances of each patient. Because no two patients are alike, this emphasis on cost-cutting, stating what is permitted, sometimes is at odds with what is appropriate or necessary in a particular patient. The rational application of medical art and science, combined with adherence to the principle that the patient's best interest should always guide decisions, should lead the physician to the right choice in such situations.

Purchasers of health care have also fostered the shift of acute care from the hospital to less costly outpatient settings. This transition to earlier and more comprehensive outpatient management has resulted in the burgeoning growth of home care programs. To reduce costs even further, many capitated health care systems are espousing demand-management programs that encourage self-care at home for self-limited illnesses and disease management programs for chronic illnesses; these programs often are based on telephone triage systems and protocol-driven telephone care by physician extenders and allied health care personnel. A corollary of the shift from inpatient to outpatient care settings is that those patients who are hospitalized are more ill, on average, and require more attention from physicians, nurses, and other hospital personnel. The resulting time compression and higher intensity of inpatient interventions has led to the growth of hospital-based internists, who are known as hospitalists (see Chapter 3).

At the same time that purchasers of health care have been trying to control costs, patient expectations for quality and access of care have been increasing. Both patients and purchasers are beginning to demand profiling—i.e., tracking of health care outcomes such as rates of implementing preventive care recommendations—for health care systems and individual care providers. Patients and society also are demanding increased emphasis on and efforts to enhance safety mechanisms in medical care systems. In response to these patient expectations, health care systems are beginning to routinely measure key outcome indicators of health care quality, as well as patient satisfaction with systems and providers of care. These surveys consistently show that patients expect their physicians to be competent; in addition, patients value accessible physicians who are skilled at the art of communication. Physicians who fit this description routinely elicit their patient's preferences after advising them about the major issues surrounding their important health care decisions.

Changes in medical knowledge and practice also have been driven by the explosive growth of medical information. Information science has facilitated storage and sharing of this information, but analysis of the data requires investigators skilled in the art of research. In addition to stimulating new research, the medical information explosion also has spotlighted the need for physicians to develop the skills needed to sift and winnow the resulting vast amounts of data efficiently. Successful clinicians are able to reformulate the clinical conundrums that they encounter into specific, relevant questions before querying medical data bases for evidence-based answers. (See Chapter 4 for more information on evidence-based medicine.)

Many of the recent and ongoing changes in medical care significantly impact the delivery of primary care.

The Institute of Medicine, a branch of National Academy of Science, has defined primary care as "the provision of integrated, accessible health care services by clinicians who are accountable for addressing a large majority of personal health care needs, developing a sustained partnership with patients, and practicing in the context of family and community." However, some targeted evaluations suggest that primary care practitioners and systems need to improve their performance on many of these factors, including access, chronic disease management, preventive care (including vaccinations and screening), and psychosocial aspects of care. Clearly, primary care faces many challenges, but its interpersonal rewards can sustain physicians through the necessary changes.

## Approach to the Patient

In practicing the art of medicine, physicians must approach patients with empathy and tact. The patient should never be regarded as a "case" with a collection of symptoms, signs, physical examination findings, and abnormal laboratory and diagnostic results, but, rather, as an individual who is seeking relief and reassurance. The physician is expected to be knowledgeable, courteous, and wise. In addition, patients want a physician who can assist them in decision-making by clearly communicating the diagnosis, treatment options, and potential outcomes. This can help allay the patient's fear of dependence, disability, or death resulting from the illness. The patient groups described in the following sections may require additional attention and skills.

### Adolescent patients

Adolescent patients often receive primary care from a general internist. These patients tend to be healthy and usually present to the physician for a required physical examination or a minor illness. In adolescence, prevention can have a significant impact on lifelong health, but teenagers often are reluctant to discuss their lifestyle. Adolescent health care visits should ideally include time for the physician to meet with both adolescents and their parents together, and each party separately. Physicians should encourage and welcome questions with the assurance of confidentiality, using this office time as an opportunity to discuss the risks associated with driving, smoking, alcohol and drug use, and, for sexually active adolescents, sex education, birth control, and the risks and prevention of sexually transmitted diseases (STDs).

### Alcohol- and drug-dependent patients

Alcohol and drug abuse (i.e., substance abuse) are common problems in the United States. Because such problems eventually lead to physical and emotional problems, primary care physicians ultimately will see these patients in their practices. Denial is a common component of substance abuse problems, and few patients come forward on their own to request help. If they do, the physician can be most helpful by assisting referral to a detoxification and rehabilitation program. If the physician suspects substance abuse, it should be discussed with the patient in an understanding and nonaccusatory manner, helping the patient to realize that the abuse problem is real and requires intervention. When intervention is unsuccessful, the physician must set limits with the patient regarding prescription writing, frequency of office visits, and accepting phone calls. This firmness eventually may help the patient to realize the severity of his or her problem. (Alcoholism and substance abuse are further discussed in Chapter 28.)

### Geriatric patients

Old age often is associated with illness, frailty, and greater dependency, but the physician's attitude toward elderly patients should be respectful and supportive. The effects of aging on the body must be differentiated from those of illness (see Chapter 122). The patient's capacity and views, not his or her age, should be the deciding factors in determining the extent of diagnostic evaluation and treatment.

### Terminally ill patients

Diagnosing and then caring for a terminally ill patient can be stressful, yet satisfying, for the physician. A supportive relationship among the patient, family, and physician can be sustaining for all during this difficult time. The physician should counsel the patient and the family about the terminal nature of the disease, thus allowing them to prepare themselves for the inevitable. (See Chapter 13, Medical Ethics, for a discussion of cardiopulmonary resuscitation, and the withdrawal of artificial life-support in this setting; and Chapter 14, Palliative Care for a discussion of pain control.) In instances when death is imminent as a result of an accident, the idea of organ donation should be carefully broached with the patient's next-of-kin.

## Approach to the Patient's Family and Significant Others

The patient's well-being is directly related to his or her relationships with others. Therefore, the primary care physician should know about the significant individuals in each patient's life. With the patient's agreement, the physician should include significant others in communications with the patient, seeking their support in restoring the patient to health and comforting them when the patient is seriously ill. When a patient dies, the physician's responsibility is to inform the loved ones gently, offering support when possible. Finally, if an autopsy is contemplated, the physician should seek the family's permission, tactfully explaining the reasons for the autopsy.

### Maintenance of Health and Prevention of Disease: Health Education

The physician who merely diagnoses and treats established illnesses is ignoring the "art" of medicine and is, therefore, only partially effective. A good clinician can foster behavioral change in asymptomatic persons when necessary and help them overcome the social, economic, and geographic barriers that stand in the way of disease prevention. Few aspects of medicine benefit any one person or the community more than maintaining health and preventing illness. A family's participation often is necessary in obtaining the maximum benefit from counseling the patient (see Chapter 7).

### Physician as Healer: Iatrogenic Disorders

With advances in therapeutics, potent medications have become available for the treatment of many illnesses that could only be treated symptomatically in the past. These drugs, however, are potentially harmful and can cause disease (i.e., iatrogenic disorders); therefore, the physician must take precautions to minimize such dangers. Drugs or surgery alone—the "science" of medicine—seldom provide maximal benefit. Physicians must learn to treat the patient, not the illness. Ideally, patients should feel that their individuality is respected and appreciated. The caring attitude of the physician should supplement and complement the drugs or surgical procedures used in restoring the patient to health and happiness. The patient's spouse, family, or significant other often can help provide information on the prescribed and over-the-counter drugs and herbs the patient is taking.

### Consultants

Physicians who are unsure of a diagnosis or prognosis should be honest about their uncertainty and consult with a specialist. No physician loses respect or confidence by admitting ignorance and seeking help. The physician should make use of this opportunity to learn from the consultant the latest advances in diagnosis, prognosis and treatment of the illness in question. If the patient wants another opinion, the physician should respect that wish and assist in obtaining a second opinion without hesitation. Such requests do not necessarily imply that the patient lacks confidence in the physician.

The role of the consultant includes determining the specific question being addressed (which may not be obvious); establishing the urgency of the consultation; gathering appropriate data; making specific recommendations; providing contingency plans; offering educational information; communicating directly, briefly, and succinctly with the referring physician; and discussing with the patient the essence of the consultation, detailing specific areas at the patient's request. Communication with the patient must be in clear and understandable lay terms.

Consulting physicians should serve both the primary physician and the patient. Consultants should be both honest and tactful, and they must be confident without conveying superiority over the primary physician. They should answer all questions from the patient that relate to the issue at hand. If the primary care physician has made errors in diagnosis and treatment, the consultant must courteously and tactfully point these out to the primary care physician and suggest corrective measures. If the patient asks questions whose answers might embarrass the primary care physician, the consultant should answer them honestly and tactfully, keeping the primary care physician fully informed. A consultant should continue to conduct follow-up consultations with the patient for as long as the referring physician and the patient desire.

# CHAPTER 2 THE PHYSICIAN AND THE MEDICAL ENVIRONMENT

### The Larger Environment of Medicine

Change occurs rapidly in medical practice, fueled by technological advances, new medical knowledge, and changing societal demands and constraints. As the medical environment continues to change, some basic premises will assist the physician to deal with the changes, if he or she adheres to them:

- Always strive to provide the most ethical care—i.e., always keep the patient's interest and well-being first.
- Never, for whatever reason, fear searching for answers or asking for help in a clinical or business matter.
- Constantly maintain your own competence and surround yourself with competence.
- Always remain aware that you work *with* people—i.e., they are not working *for* you—to serve the patient.

These four premises are the "platform" for a well-tuned team that, if adhered to, will always provide steady direction as change occurs.

## Allied Health Care Professionals in Medical Practice

In response to the increasing complexity of medical care and societal demands to make care more economical while also increasing patient access to care, a variety of trained professionals other than physicians and nurses have become involved in health care. These professionals include physician assistants, nurse practitioners, clinical pharmacists, dietitians, physical therapists, respiratory therapists, and psychologists, among others. Both the patient and the primary care physician can benefit greatly from such collaboration, but the physician must maintain responsibility as the team leader; must be familiar with the techniques, skills, and objectives of the allied health care professionals with whom he or she is working; and must oversee the total care delivered to the patient. Even if patient care is given in a clinic setting, the physician who is primarily and continuously responsible for each patient must be clearly identified. The primary care physician is responsible for overseeing the patient's total care.

## Group Practice Models

Increasingly, patients are being cared for by groups of physicians, clinics, hospitals, and health maintenance organizations (HMOs) rather than by solo practitioners. There currently exist four types of physician group practice (with the term "group" meaning two or more physicians). These types run the range from single specialty (including primary care specialties) to multispecialty (with variable numbers of specialties represented). The types include (1) physician-owned and operated groups; (2) hospital or health care system–owned groups; (3) payer-owned groups; and (4) corporate-owned groups.

The physician-owned group is owned, governed, and managed by physicians, an arrangement that is appealing to many physicians. Depending on the size of such a group, it may find itself in a weak position (i.e., if it consists of a small number of physician owners) when negotiating or when contracting with payers and health care systems. This is mitigated if the group becomes big enough to be a "significant market player," or if a smaller group (or solo physician) establishes membership in an independent physician association (IPA). An IPA is an association (a formal legal entity) of independent physicians who join together to contract with payers and health care systems. This arrangement provides the ability to compete with larger groups while maintaining autonomy (with this autonomy varying depending on the contract entered into between the physician and the IPA).

In the hospital-owned or health care system–owned group, physicians become employees of the health care entity. Strategically, this allows the health care entity to "direct the business" of these physicians into their system-owned facilities. The physicians enjoy the benefits of being employees of a large parent corporation, but must relinquish a certain degree of independence. Their contracts are in accordance with the parent corporation. In this model, physicians are compensated in varying ways; many are based on a physician productivity formula.

Payer-owned groups employ physicians to care for patients enrolled in a plan owned by the payer. Financial ownership of such plans may be constructed in several different ways. One common example of this type of group is the "closed panel" health maintenance organization (HMO). In this model, the physicians are salaried and care only for patients enrolled in the plan. These physicians enjoy the benefit of employment in a large organization, but, as in the health care entity model, relinquish a degree of independence.

Corporate-owned groups are, generally speaking, large groups spread across multiple geographic market areas. They usually form through the acquisition of various groups by a national corporate entity. The physician's status is an employee of the group. The business case for this type of entity is to establish significant market strength in a number of markets. There are both success and failure stories with this model (as there are, for all of the models discussed), but any failure or success that occurs with the corporate model is amplified in the media simply because of the large size of these entities.

## Reimbursement and Managed Care

Traditionally, hospitals and physicians in the United States had been reimbursed for use or provision of services (the "fee for service" system). This system implicitly provides hospitals and physicians with a monetary incentive to perform as many services as possible. Because such a payment system provides this incentive and there is no incentive to control the patient's cost, the insurance industry and the government entitlement programs have evolved since the early 1970s to address this issue.

Years ago, the method of payment for services was traditional indemnity insurance. A patient (or the patient's employer) purchased a policy that paid for the majority of costs no matter what the number of services, with a small part of the cost being the responsibility of the patient. With expensive technologic advances and a gradually aging population, payers writing indemnity policies started passing on more of the cost of care to the patient. They also began to charge the patient or employer a larger premium. Subsequently, payers attempted to define "usual and customary" costs for care in an area and reimbursed only this amount for the various services provided, with the patient covering the remainder. As the proportion of the population over the age of 65 years grew, reimbursement became even more problematic. This population group was found to use the majority of health services because of age-related illnesses. In addition, this population was, for the most part, retired, and difficulties occurred with employers covering the costs of retirees. This cascade of events (among others) led to the development of Medicare and the beginning of managed care.

Medicare began on January 1, 1966, governed by Title XVIII of the Social Security Act. It initially began as a payer system for the elderly, and later evolved to become the payer for the disabled and patients with end-stage renal disease. It consisted of two parts: part A covered hospital costs, and part B covered supplementary medical costs (primarily physician costs). Regulatory agencies were put in place to monitor the plan. Initially both parts A and B used the "usual and customary" cost methodology based on geographic regions. The amount paid to providers was always less than their actual charges, and, going forward, amounts reimbursed often were less than the provider's actual costs. In essence, it functioned as a discounted fee for service. In spite of regulatory attempts to make Medicare function more efficiently, the cost of the program continued to rise.

In the mid-1980s, Medicare modified the way part A functioned with the establishment of diagnosis-related groups (DRGs). A set fee was paid to hospitals based on the final diagnosis at the time of the patient's discharge from the facility. In essence, what was occurring as this system was implemented was a form of "capitation." A set amount of money was given to a hospital for inpatient episodes of care for patients within a disease group, and the hospital was to use cost-effective measures to maximize the difference between that reimbursement and their total costs of providing that inpatient care. The DRG mechanism continues to exist, but it no longer is used to define just an acute care hospital cost. The mechanism is applied to the entire spectrum of care for the disease (e.g., hospital care, extended care, home care).

The DRG methodology applies only to part A. Other providers in the part B category continue performing in a modified discounted fee-for-service mode. This creates conflicting goals between part A providers and part B providers. For example, physicians are paid more the longer their patient stays in a hospital, but the hospital (having received a fixed fee) loses. This is one of many reasons why hospitals and physicians must collaborate regarding patient care. A team approach using "case management" has become the most effective method for coordinating this collaborative effort.

As the 1990s approached, Medicare modified part B payments, motivated by the fact that a disproportionate amount of physician fees appeared to be directed to physicians who were performing procedures. The thinking was to allocate more to physicians working in the cognitive areas of medicine. One of the hopes was that more preventive care might be encouraged so that costly procedures might be avoided later. The system designed to do this was the resource-based relative value scale (RBRVS).

Many of the processes enabled by Medicare (including DRGs and RBRVS) have been adopted in various forms by the private insurance sector for its use.

As Medicare evolved, so did Medicaid, governed by Title XIX of the federal Social Security Act. Medicaid is jointly sponsored by the federal and state governments. It pays part of the cost of care for certain poor patients and is a major source of payment for nursing home care for elderly patients.

As the government entitlement programs evolved, payer mechanisms in the private sector also were evolving. A major factor in this evolution was the rising costs employers were incurring to provide health coverage to their employees and dependents. Not only were the costs rising, but they also were often unpredictable. Paying a set rate for a period of time (usually 1 year) presented itself as a better business case. The creation of health maintenance organizations (HMOs) followed. The concept of HMOs, in simplified terms, is as follows: the HMO contracts with "patient groups" (usually a group of employees) for a set fee for a set time. The HMO then tries to manage the care of its patients (provide efficient care to cut costs) so that at the end of the set time a profit is made. Needless to say, the processes for doing this are complex.

From the physician's perspective, there are essentially two types of HMOs: open and closed models. In the open model, groups of physicians or IPAs negotiate with the HMO for a fee schedule or a lump sum (capitated amount) for a specific time period. In this model, the physicians may participate in other HMOs as well. In the closed model (also called a staff model), physicians are employed by the HMO and their work is restricted within that HMO. A staff model is somewhat easier to manage, but it does restrict choices for both physicians and patients. In both types the HMO establishes and runs the financial mechanisms.

Other managed care models evolved along with HMOs. Preferred Provider Organizations (PPOs), which are essentially a hybrid of HMOs, have become popular. In this type of organization, a group of providers (physicians and hospitals) agree to provide care to subscribers for a discounted fee and agree to utilization review. The PPO does not establish or run the financing mechanism. A variation of the PPO is the point-of-service (POS) plan, in which enrollees can use the services of either participating or nonparticipating providers. The enrollee is encouraged to choose participating providers because enrollees pay more "out of pocket" costs if a nonparticipating provider is used. Utilization and cost are, in effect, managed to a large degree by patient choice.

## Doctors and Hospitals

The physicians and other independent practitioners who take care of patients at a hospital constitute the medical staff of that hospital. In the traditional model, the medical staff is an entity separate from the hospital. The hospital (health care organization) has its own corporate bylaws and, with the organized medical staff, collaborates in the delivery of health care. The medical staff structure and functions are documented in the medical staff bylaws as well as the medical staff rules and regulations.

The clinical leaders of the medical staff, including medical staff officers, medical department chairpersons, and other appointed physicians in leadership positions, interact formally with hospital leadership at meetings of the medical executive committee (MEC). The medical staff president chairs the MEC meetings. Typically, hospital administration attends the MEC in an "ex officio" capacity, with the hospital president and the president's chosen management personnel in attendance. Any matters involving the hospital and medical staff might be discussed at the MEC meetings. A consistent agenda item is a review of the report of the credentials committee.

## Credentialing and Privileging

Credentialing and privileging are separate processes. Physician credentialing is the process whereby a physician declares on an application his or her demographic data, education, training, and experience. A trained medical staff office must then verify all of this information. The verification process must occur via primary verification for each item (e.g., an original document from a training program, not a copy). In another aspect of this process, an inquiry about the applying physician is made to the National Practitioner Data Bank (NPDB), a federal data repository that contains information on physician disciplinary data and malpractice actions.

When a physician applies to a medical staff, he or she must first be accurately credentialed, as outlined in the preceding paragraph. Then the privileging process begins. Privileging is, in almost all instances, done by the chairperson of a medical staff department and his or her associates. The applying physician completes a form requesting the right (privilege) to perform certain functions or procedures. The physician's department chairperson, by review of this form, the applicant's credentials, and a personal interview, grants whichever of these rights (privileges) he or she believes the physician applicant is properly trained to perform. Each institution grants privileges separately, so physicians must go through this same process at each hospital to which they apply.

The Credentials Committee is a medical staff committee that serves as the end point of the credentialing and privileging process. The Credential Committee analyzes information from the process and interviews applicants for initial appointment or reappointment to the medical staff. Its recommendations are sent to the hospital medical executive committee and then to the hospital board of directors for final approvals.

A variety of trained health professionals other than physicians are involved in the hospital clinical environment. Most of these professionals are hospital employees. The hospital's human resource department implements their employment. There are some nonphysician professionals who are not hospital employees. These may be dependent practitioners (e.g., physician assistants) or independent practitioners (e.g., independent nurse practitioners). These non-employee practitioners may gain entry to the hospital clinical environment via the credentials committee, hospital management, or a combination of both.

## Assessing Health Care Organizations

Reputation and quality are inseparable in evaluating a health care entity. In addition, in this era of managed care, the evaluation of the link between quality and health care utilization becomes important. It is important for a physician, before considering application, to make inquiries about the quality improvement, case management, utilization review, and outcomes programs for a facility.

Another method of evaluating an institution's reputation is to inquire about usage of the facility. If census data on a hospital show high usage, that implies that both physicians and patients consider it to be of high quality. This information also is one of many factors that give preliminary knowledge about the financial viability of a facility, an important factor when deciding on a long-term affiliation.

Strong residency programs and solid continuing medical education programs enhance the quality of a facility as well. An affiliation with a reputable academic center adds deeper value to physicians in training and members of the medical staff.

In addition to researching the reputation of an institution, it is important for physicians to evaluate "service lines" and the spectrum of care provided by a hospital. Particularly important in the case of a specialty-trained physician, but important for other physicians as well, is a strong presence of specialty services. It is important to know that programs, equipment, and staff are in place to cover the entire spectrum of various specialties. When evaluating potential affiliations with health care systems, it is important to know that patients can be cared for from the acute episode, through extended and home care, and on to ambulatory follow-up (vertical integration).

Physicians also should ascertain that the health care organization has received accreditation from relevant organizations (e.g., JCAHO, HCFA, CARF). It is perfectly reasonable for a physician to inquire about the results of the most recent surveys. In addition to surveys by formal organizations, much can be learned about health care entities from "local knowledge" sources (both clinical and nonclinical).

Finally, physicians often view the governance of a health care system or hospital with which they will affiliate in just a cursory way. It is important, however, to know the core values, the mission, and the vision of the health care entity. These numerous personal, professional, and business factors enter into a physician's final decision about whether to affiliate with a given health care organization.

## Specific Aspects of the Medical Environment

### Medical records

The medical record describes the patient's medical condition over time. It is of the utmost importance for physicians and other health care providers to maintain the record in an accurate, legible, and timely manner. In this age of high technology, litigation, and complex care, such a record is an absolute necessity. It is also important for the record to be complete, with all data and signatures in place, because these are required by most payers for appropriate reimbursement to occur.

### Accountability in medical practice

Increasingly, physicians are being held accountable for their actions regarding the quality and cost-effectiveness of care. Review of medical records, mandatory continuing education for relicensing, and recertification by examination are examples of regulatory measures by lawmakers and voluntary efforts by physicians, to ensure and demonstrate competence. For the patient, reducing costly hospital admissions as much as possible and keeping the cost of medical care affordable have become essential. In the final analysis, the medical profession must guide the public in matters of health-related legislation. While maintaining concern for the welfare of their patients, physicians also must make every possible effort to alleviate the socioeconomic problems of health care delivery through civic activism and political awareness.

### Human research

If the science of medicine is to progress, research must be done on human beings. Physicians engaged in research on humans must explain to each patient, in clear and understandable language, the nature, risks, and benefits of all diagnostic and therapeutic procedures that are not well established or are considered experimental, and obtain the patient's informed consent. When conducting research, the physician must take extraordinary precautions to protect the patient's interests and to minimize risks. Only by using these safeguards can human research be undertaken for the progress of medicine without jeopardizing the patient's health.

### Physicians' responsibilities to themselves, their families, and the community

The conflict between meeting one's personal and family responsibilities and addressing the needs of one's patients is a perennial one. This conflict and the rapid pace of the practice of medicine impose tremendous stress on physicians; the suicide rate among physicians is one of the highest compared with that of other professionals. To relieve stress, every physician must devote time to recreation and family and engage regularly in physical exercise.

Physicians also have a responsibility to the community. As is true for all citizens, regular participation in civic affairs and public elections is important, requiring the intelligent prioritization of professional and leisure time. Physicians who work all the time are not serving their patients well.

# CHAPTER 3 THE ROLE OF THE HOSPITALIST

The hospitalist is a physician who spends more than 25% of his or her clinical activity in the inpatient setting. Although physicians who restrict their practice to hospitals have long provided hospital care in Europe and Canada, the hospitalist model is a novel concept in the United States.

Several factors ushered in the hospitalist model in the U.S. The main one was the progress in technology that shifted most patient care to the outpatient setting, thus reserving hospitalization mainly for older or sicker patients and those with more complicated illnesses. With hospital-based care accounting for one third of health care expenditures, the need was felt for more efficient practice models, especially in the managed care environment. The hospitalist participates in one such model, in which a designated group of physicians assumes the care of hospitalized patients, and, upon discharge from the hospital, returns the patients to their primary care physicians for their continuing care. Success of these programs requires good physician-to-physician communication and trust in the professional competence of hospitalists on the part of the primary care physician.

Currently, hospitalist models vary, from private solo and group practices to staff care HMOs, hospital-employed groups, and academic institutions. Hospitalists can fulfill a variety of hospital-based functions, offering inpatient care in general wards and intensive care units (ICUs), consultations with the Emergency Department and surgical services, and pre- and postoperative assessments; performing medical procedures; staffing observation units; developing practice guidelines; and supervising residents and medical students.

The hospitalist model is most highly evolved in the managed care setting. In some large practices and managed care organizations, availability of a hospitalist can free primary care physicians from hospital-based care, thereby improving their efficiency and allowing them to spend more time with ambulatory patients. This arrangement could improve patient satisfaction and generate cost savings. Because hospitalizations often occur without prior warning, the obligation to provide hospital care to his or her patients can add uncertainty—and hours—to a physician's schedule; having a hospitalist available can render the office-based physician's lifestyle and work hours more predictable. The hospitalist is in a unique position that enables him or her to coordinate and expedite inpatient care; enhance communication with primary physicians, patients, families, and specialists; and optimize utilization of resources through development and implementation of practice guidelines. It is estimated that almost 19,000 hospitalists are needed to meet these needs; in 2001 there were only about 4000 internists, pediatricians, family practitioners, and nurse practitioners serving in this capacity.

## Beneficiaries of the Hospitalist Model

### Primary care physicians

The timing, duration, and intensity of hospital rounds often are unpredictable; unexpected delays often keep the physician from beginning office hours as scheduled. Carrying on hospital care in the midst of a busy office schedule also leads to interruptions during office hours. Interposition of a hospitalist frees up primary physicians from such delays and interruptions and increases the office availability and efficiency of the primary physician. Efficient communication allows for better coordination of care in the hospital and office settings and in post-discharge follow-ups.

### Patients

When a patient is hospitalized, a hospitalist can see the patient immediately, initiate treatment plans, re-evaluate the patient repeatedly during the day, and be more available to communicate with patients and their families. Hospitalists are adept at utilization management and at formulating effective discharge plans. Effective hospitalists enhance patient satisfaction by decreasing variability in care, producing better outcomes, shortening the length of stay, and improving the quality of care. Although patients like to see a familiar physician when they are hospitalized, it appears that they are willing to forego this preference in favor of physician availability.

### Hospitals

Management of medical care by an on-site hospitalist not only avoids delays in care, but also fosters timely communication and interventions. The physical presence of a hospitalist makes it possible to perform repeat patient assessments, thus promoting the quality and timeliness of interventions.

In a capitated system in which hospitals are paid according to diagnosis-related group (DRG) codes or managed care contracts, hospitals save costs through better utilization of resources and decreased length of stay. When the hospitalist implements clinical pathways and practice guidelines, the result is less variability of care, fewer medical errors, and better outcomes. The hospitalist's evidence-based approach to problem solving, availability to carry out multiple assessments, and timeliness of care throughout the day improve patient safety and outcomes.

In teaching hospitals, the presence of hospitalist faculty virtually guarantees adequate supervision of trainees by well-rounded experts in hospital care rather than by faculty with varied interests and availability, thereby bringing consistency, accountability and professionalism to the teaching process. Several academic medical centers, including UCSF, Oregon Health Sciences University, Emory University/Grady Memorial Hospital, Cleveland Clinic, and Mayo Clinic have established their own hospitalist groups from their generalist faculty members. Several good research studies from these centers have been published that relate to cost, quality, and outcomes.

#### Managed care organizations

HMOs, the primary goal of which is to reduce health care costs, have realized that hospitalists improve quality and save costs considerably by reducing the patient's length of stay, and by lowering the utilization of ICU, ancillary services, and specialists. Vertical integration of these systems provides for seamless transitions from inpatient to outpatient settings.

### Effect of Hospitalists on Cost and Quality of Care

Although the trigger for the hospitalist movement was the desire to lower costs, quality-of-care issues continue to drive the process. Several large studies involving hospitalists at community hospitals, academic centers, rural health systems, and managed care organizations have shown consistent benefits in both cost and quality of care, regardless of the setting. Besides decreasing length of stay and overall cost of care by $500 to $600, readmission rates are lowered. Studies consistently indicate higher patient satisfaction and better outcomes.

### Hospitalists in the Intensive Care Unit

Recent debates surround the ability and training of hospitalists to care for patients in the intensive care unit (ICU). However, practical experience and expertise gained through training and continuing medical education have allowed most hospitalists to provide high quality care in this setting, and, when necessary, in conjunction with other specialists. This allows continuity of care to be maintained before and after admission to ICU. Hospitalists can perform many invasive procedures, such as insertion of central lines, arterial catheters, and Swan–Ganz catheters; endotracheal intubations; and cardioversion. These skills help hospitalists avoid delays in initiating treatment and enable appropriate utilization of specialists such as intensivists, cardiologists, and pulmonologists.

### Disadvantages of the Hospitalist Model

In most communities, the hospitalist model has been well received, and most primary care physicians tend to view the effect of hospitalists on their patients and their own efficiency quite favorably. However, many perceive possible risks in the implementation of this model. Some fear that it will lead to a decline in the internist's clinical skills and an inability to make shared medical decisions. Some primary physicians consider the surrender of their patients to a hospitalist a breach in the continuity of patient care, whereas others fear a loss of revenue and of professional stimulation and challenge from the discontinuation of hospital work. Still others feel guilty about "abandoning" their patients at a vulnerable period in their lives, when the care by and attention of the physician could mean the most to them. Specialist physicians might feel threatened by the prospects of being underutilized, because utilization of specialists drops significantly when there are experienced hospitalists on staff.

Resident trainees in teaching hospitals fear that the presence of hospitalists could lead to a loss of autonomy for them; however, many also acknowledge that this prospect is more than compensated for by the improved learning experience that the hospitalist can provide.

### Challenges

Although clinical work as a hospitalist is professionally fulfilling, it does take a toll on the energy of physicians, in a manner quite similar to that felt by emergency and critical care physicians. The stress is primarily due to unpredictable workloads, high patient acuities, and if the hospitalist schedule doesn't function on shifts, prolonged workdays caused by unexpected exigencies. Creative scheduling of work hours that includes protected blocks of time off can be extremely helpful in mitigating some of the stress.

Hospitalists must manage their time well and work efficiently with other members of the hospital team. Standardization and automation of repetitive tasks through use of information technology and practice guidelines can improve time management and system performance. Employing better communication systems can also enhance system functioning and teamwork. Hospitalists can effect major system improvements by disseminating these changes throughout the hospital. Appropriate availability of support services, and a supportive administration that helps facilitate these efficiencies all lead to a pleasant and efficient work environment, thus lowering the risk of attrition and turnover due to "burn out" in hospitalist physicians.

## Conclusion

The hospitalist model is being instituted throughout the United States and is living up to its promise to improve efficiency and quality of care in hospitals. Concerns regarding organizational issues linger, but those are to be expected with the evolution of any new system or concept. Several well-designed studies show that the hospitalist model fulfills its stated objectives. Ongoing research and analysis should address the lingering concerns about this model in the near future. Most importantly, this model addresses several urgent needs of the health care system and expands the opportunities for internists.

# CHAPTER 4 EVIDENCE-BASED MEDICINE

## Why Do We Need Evidence-Based Medicine?

Clinicians are entrusted with making difficult clinical decisions to provide the best care for their patients. Yet medical practice is constantly changing, and new information is becoming available at an exponential rate. Most physicians find themselves overwhelmed by this information explosion. Furthermore, new data are not always valid or applicable to clinical practice. Without the means to evaluate medical information critically, physicians cannot decide which interventions to incorporate into their practices.

Clinical decisions are based on information from two principal sources—patient care and clinical research. To provide effective care, both types of information should be considered. Decisions based on patient care rely on knowledge gathered about the individual patient. This involves a careful history, a physical examination, and other similar investigations. In addition, the prior odds of disease, based on the patient's history and demographics, help guide diagnosis and treatment. The ways in which clinicians obtain an understanding of clinical research is more complex.

Clinicians rely on a number of sources to keep them informed, including textbooks, review articles, practice guidelines, consensus statements, lectures by experts in the field, seminars and courses put together by medical societies and universities, advertisements in medical journals, conversations with representatives from pharmaceutical companies, and original articles in medical journals. The diversity of these sources, and the biases inherent in many of them, often leave clinicians with conflicting, and sometimes unsubstantiated, views about a single medical question.

As a result, there is variation in clinical practice, even among the experts; and health services research on actual practices has demonstrated that expert opinion often lags far behind, and often is inconsistent with, evidence-based "best practices." For these reasons, it is important for physicians to develop the skills needed to search, locate, and critically evaluate new information. This is where the principles and skills of evidence-based medicine (EBM) become crucial.

## Definition

Evidence-based medicine (EBM) refers to the incorporation of the best evidence available via systematic research in conjunction with clinical expertise to guide the practice of medicine. Rosenberg and Donald have described four steps in EBM: (1) formulating a concise clinical question that addresses specific uncertainties in patient management; (2) searching the available literature to identify potentially relevant studies; (3) conducting a critical appraisal of these studies to identify the best evidence; and (4) applying this evidence to guide patient management.

### Formulating a concise clinical question

According to Oxman, Sackett and Guyatt, most clinical questions can be formulated in terms of a simple relationship among the patient, some exposure (e.g., to a treatment, a diagnostic test, or a potentially harmful agent), and specific outcomes of interest. An example of a concise question about a specific new therapy would be "Does the use of *intra-articular steroid injections* [exposure] reduce the *severity of knee pain* [outcome] in a *patient with severe osteoarthritis* [patient]?"

A concise question about prevention through early diagnosis would ask "Does a *screening mammogram* [diagnostic test] for breast cancer, if performed in a *40-year-old woman* [patient], decrease her risk of *dying from breast cancer* [outcome]?"

And a concise question regarding patient prognosis or risk of developing a disease might be: "Does *high blood cholesterol level* [potentially harmful exposure] in a *30-year-old man* [patient] increase his likelihood of developing *heart disease* [outcome] later in life?"

Finally, an example of a concise question regarding harm would be: "Will the use of *Warfarin* [potentially harmful agent] during pregnancy increase the risk of *miscarriage* [outcome] in a *pregnant woman* [patient]?"

Questions that are clearly related to a clinical decision such as detailed above, are most likely to be asked during clinical practice. By asking a precise and specific question, it is possible to narrow the literature search.

**Searching the literature for relevant clinical information**

After formulating a concise and pertinent clinical question, the physician needs to obtain the best available evidence. There are five routes for doing this: (1) asking someone; (2) checking reference lists in a textbook; (3) finding a relevant article from available journals; (4) using a bibliographic database such as MEDLINE; and (5) searching online evidence-based medicine data bases. Asking a colleague or consultant is highly efficient but may provide you with an incorrect or incomplete answer. If a recent textbook is at hand, the appropriate information and any pertinent references cited by the author can be located there. Because it can take up to 2 to 3 years to write, edit, and publish a textbook, however, most textbooks refer to articles that are already 3 to 5 years old; as a result, all textbooks are at least partly out-of-date even before they are published. Furthermore, textbooks do not ensure that the conclusions of the clinical experts writing the chapters are based on the best available evidence. Searching for an article at the library or in the physician's personal reprint file or collection of medical journals is another option. Because maintaining an up-to-date file of clinical articles requires a formidable amount of time, and manually searching through a pile of medical journals can be a daunting task, the physician may well give up, and even if he or she persists, the key article to answer the question at hand may not be found.

The fourth route, conducting electronic searches of medical literature data bases, is fast becoming the preferred method to gather relevant clinical information. There are two major types of electronic databases that are excellent starting points for EBM queries. One database, MEDLINE, is bibliographic and retrieves relevant citations in the form of abstracts or full article texts. Electronic access to MEDLINE is readily available in North America in a variety of on-line and CD-ROM formats (Table 4.1). The second type of electronic database provides direct access to select articles that have been appraised and are considered to represent publications of clinical importance. These databases make the task of retrieving information from the medical literature even easier. They include the American College of Physicians Journal Club (a bimonthly supplement of the

**TABLE 4.1. Evidence-Based Medicine Resources**

| Source | Description |
|---|---|
| MEDLINE, PREMEDLINE | National Library Of Medicine; available from 1966 onwards. Available online at http://www.nlm.nih.gov, which offers links to PubMed Central & Medline/PubMed, two free systems to search MEDLINE. Both provide an easy way to search the 11 million references and abstracts in the MEDLINE database. PubMed's retrieval engine provides links to over 700 journals for full article texts (some publishers may require a subscription). Available online at http://www.ncbi.nlm.nih.gov/pubMed/ |
| Best Evidence | The Best Evidence Collection consists of two journals: *ACP Journal Club*, a publication of the American College of Physicians, and *Evidence-Based Medicine*, a joint publication with the British Medical Journal Group. The databases date back to 1991. The editors screen the top clinical journals on a regular basis to identify studies that are both methodologically sound and clinically relevant. An enhanced abstract of the chosen articles and a commentary on the value of the articles for clinical practice are provided. Using this source, clinicians can efficiently understand and apply to their practice important changes in medical knowledge without having to read and synthesize for themselves thousands of journal articles. Available at http://www.acpjc.org |
| The Cochrane Database of Systematic Reviews (COCH) | COCH is produced by the Cochrane Collaboration—an international network of individuals and institutions committed to preparing, maintaining, and disseminating systematic reviews of the effects of health care. Each issue contains new and updated reviews and protocols. COCH is updated and amended regularly as new evidence becomes available and errors are identified. Available online at http://cochrane.co.uk/ |
| Center For Evidence Based Medicine | An excellent online source for publications available in the field of EBM. This resource provides specialized resources for medical students interested in EBM. It also has a searchable database of appraised clinical questions, the CATbank (Critical Appraisals of Topics bank). Available online at http://cebm.jr2.ox.ac.uk/index.html |

*Annals of Internal Medicine*), *Evidence-Based Medicine* (a publication of the British Medical Journal Group), POEMs (Patient Oriented Evidence-based Medicine), formerly the *Journal of Family Practice* Journal Club, and the Cochrane Database of Systematic Reviews. All of these databases can be accessed on the Internet and are outlined in Table 4.1.

The fifth and last option is to subscribe to and search commercial evidence-based data bases such as 'Up To Date'. This reference tool provides access to topic reviews that are evidence-based and regularly updated.

When performing a literature search, the elements of the precise clinical question must be converted to specific MESH headings or short text–word strings. To increase the specificity of the search, Boolean logic can be used to combine search terms; and applying additional restrictions (e.g., English language only; human studies; specific age groups) can further narrow the search results. Once the literature search is completed, it is then necessary to screen the titles and abstracts of the retrieved articles to assess their relevance. Only those articles that address the clinical question at hand and meet some preliminary pre-established screening criteria are selected for further review.

**Appraising the evidence for validity**

Medical researchers use several types of study designs, each of which has certain advantages and disadvantages for answering a specific type of medical question. For example, randomized clinical trials are better suited for answering questions related to a new therapy or preventive measure (e.g., Is drug A better than drug B for treating patients with high blood pressure?), whereas cohort studies are more suited to answer questions related to harm (e.g., Is smoking associated with increased risk for lung cancer?). Both randomized trials and cohort studies are appropriate for answering questions related to prognosis (e.g., What is the 5-year survival of patients who are on chronic hemodialysis?). Each of these study designs has unique validity criteria that must be evaluated by the reader. Table 4.2 presents a quick reference guide to assess the validity of major types of primary and secondary studies (e.g., reviews, practice guidelines). These criteria can be used to screen an abstract; this enables the physician to determine whether it warrants the additional time required to read the article in detail. In particular, if these "validity" criteria are met, then a more detailed appraisal of the article can be conducted according to more detailed guidelines published in the literature.

**Applying the evidence to patients and practice**

The physician must ask whether the article addresses a patient-oriented outcome versus a disease-oriented outcome. Examples of patient-oriented outcomes are studies that evaluate a clinical outcome such as mortality (increased survival), morbidity (better quality of life), or some other clinical aspect of care such as patient satisfaction. Studies that use disease-oriented outcomes report differences in a biochemical (e.g., decreased cholesterol level), physiologic (e.g., decreased heart rate or blood pressure), or anatomic (e.g., decreased inflammation on liver biopsy slides) finding. Such disease-oriented outcomes also are called intermediate outcomes because they are thought to represent an intermediate step between the underlying exposure and final patient-oriented outcomes, or surrogate outcome measures, because they are felt to be expedient substitutes for patient-oriented outcomes. Often, however, the type of association between these intermediate or surrogate outcomes and important clinical outcomes is not as expected, i.e., an improvement in a disease-oriented outcome does not always lead to an improvement in a patient-oriented outcome. For example, patients who had increased numbers of asymptomatic premature ventricular beats (an example of a disease-oriented or intermediate outcome) were thought to be at an increased risk of sudden cardiac death (a patient-oriented outcome). A new drug, Flecainide, was found to be very effective in reducing the frequency of premature ventricular beats. Subsequent research studies, however, found that patients who took Flecainide actually had an increased rate of sudden cardiac death. As a general rule of thumb, studies that evaluate a patient-oriented outcome provide better evidence for guiding clinical care than do studies that report changes in a disease-oriented outcome.

## Conclusion

To be an effective and well-informed clinician, it is no longer sufficient for a doctor simply to practice medicine based on past knowledge transmitted via textbooks and expert opinions. And simply reading the literature without a thorough review and critique of the information also is inadequate. The skilled practitioner needs to apply and master the skills of evidence-based medicine in an active and continuous manner in order to provide the highest level of care to patients.

**TABLE 4.2. Critical Appraisal Criteria for Assessing Study Validity**

| Study Type | |
|---|---|
| Evaluation of new treatment | Were patients randomly assigned to treatment and comparison groups?<br>Is the loss of study participants reported, and are any differences between participants who completed the study vs. those who dropped out explained? |
| Evaluation of new diagnostic test | Was an independent and blind comparison of the new diagnostic test made with a previously established gold standard test?<br>Did each patient receive both the gold standard test and the new diagnostic test to assess both false-negative and false-positive results?<br>Did the spectrum of patients in the study accurately reflect the range of patients who will receive the diagnostic test in clinical practice? |
| Evaluation of harm | Were there clearly identified comparison groups (cohorts) that were similar with respect to other risk factors (other than the risk factor under study)?<br>Were outcomes and risk factors measured in the same way across all groups? |
| Evaluation of prognosis | Were there clearly defined categories for different stages of the disease over the course of the study?<br>Were there representative samples of participants for each of these defined stages in the course of the disease?<br>Was follow-up of the patient's health status sufficiently long and complete over the course of the disease? |
| Literature review | Did the review address a clearly focused question?<br>Were appropriate inclusion criteria used to select articles?<br>Was each study evaluated against a preexisting standard of criteria used to assess study validity? |
| Practice guideline | Were the clinical options available in the practice guideline regarding patient care clearly specified?<br>Were the potential outcomes related to each clinical option clearly specified?<br>Did the practice guideline use an explicit process to identify, select, and combine evidence from research and clinical practice? |
| Clinical decision analysis | Did the decision analysis model accurately represent the scope and range of ethical and clinically important decision pathways?<br>Were the probabilities assigned to each pathway in the model based on valid evidence?<br>Were the outcomes/benefits calculated for each pathway in the model based on valid evidence? |

Adapted from User's Guides to the Medical Literature. How to get started. Oxman et al JAMA, 1993;270:2093–2095.

# CHAPTER 5 BEDSIDE TECHNIQUES

Clinical information comes from the patient's history, physical examination findings, and investigations, including laboratory tests, imaging studies, and other applicable procedures. Information thus obtained enables the physician to make a diagnosis, to decide on the best therapy, and to give a prognosis. The term "clinical methods" encompasses all the ways of obtaining clinical information, and "bedside methods"—history-taking and physical examination—represent the cornerstone of this process. They are inexpensive, but extremely productive, ways to obtain relevant information about the patient's illness, while also providing a way to interact with the patient.

The physician should be meticulous when taking a history and conducting a physical examination, and should devote adequate time to analyzing and reflecting on all the information obtained prior to ordering tests that often are expensive, may pose a hazard to the patient, and may be unnecessary. A focused history and physical examination are crucial to be able to selectively apply the endless number of available studies and tests within the context of the patient's illness; tests should never be ordered based on a "knee-jerk" reaction. Despite such technological marvels as computed tomographic (CT) scanning and magnetic resonance imaging (MRI), the bedside evaluation remains the most important and cost-effective way to diagnose illnesses.

## History

The key to diagnosis is an accurate and comprehensive medical history; its importance cannot be overemphasized. The history summarizes the evolution of the patient's illness and describes symptoms; it should suggest certain diagnostic possibilities, aid in excluding others, and help in determining the necessary studies. At times, it may be the only clue to a diagnosis. It is essential that the physician adopt a standard form and style for the medical history, adhering to this pattern until it becomes a habit. The advantages of establishing such a regimen are that no analytical effort is then needed for the act of history-taking itself, no topic is overlooked, and full attention can be directed toward interpreting the meaning of each response. The information to be gathered in a history, as often used by most physicians, is provided in the sections that follow. In many cases it may be necessary to go back and obtain a more detailed history after the physical examination and laboratory tests are performed, if unexpected findings are detected.

### Demographic information

Demographic information includes the patient's name, age, race, gender, marital status, address, phone number, hospital (medical record) number, date of examination, and source and reliability of the informant.

### Chief complaint or principal reason for seeking care

It is important to identify the major reason for the patient's clinic visit, hospitalization, or visit to the emergency department. The term "chief complaint" is a misnomer, because it implies that the patient complained about something and it presupposes that all patients are capable of expressing their reasons for seeking medical attention. This often is not the case, and it is up to the physician to determine the reason for the visit. In other cases, hospitalization is necessitated by a finding (e.g., thrombocytopenia or a massive pleural effusion) that might have been detected during a work-up of the patient's symptoms and may or may not explain the patient's initial concerns. Perhaps a better term would be "principal reason" for seeking medical care or for consulting a physician. Traditional teaching emphasizes identification of the chief complaint first, but, in practice, it is best to conduct the full interview and synthesize all the issues, at which point the principal reason for the visit may become apparent. Identifying the principal reason for a medical visit is very important, because this not only addresses the patient's concerns but also provides a framework for a plan, essential in today's practice of medicine.

Other symptoms and complaints also must be elicited, because they need to be addressed as well. The presence or absence of symptoms that are relevant to the principal reason for seeking medical care are included in the recorded description of the history of present illness; other symptoms elicited during a comprehensive medical history are recorded in the review of systems.

### History of present illness

Information on the patient's present illness should be recorded as an orderly and chronological account. This account should be lucid and succinct, elaborating on and taking off from the chief complaint. If the patient is not sure when the illness began, the physician should ask, "When did you last feel well or normal?" Each symptom should be described in detail (e.g., pain), including specifics about intensity and location, accompanying symptoms, factors that relieve or aggravate the symptom, and the course (progression or regression). When a symptom suggests several conditions, statements about the lack of concomitant symptoms that often accompany the original symptom should be included.

If the present illness has progressed in attacks separated by symptom-free intervals, a typical attack should be described in terms of onset, duration, and associated symptoms. (Constitutional symptoms such as chills, fever, night sweats, and weight loss should be noted. Mention should be made of the patient's level of activity at work and during leisure time.) In both acute and chronic illnesses, the date that the patient stopped work or assumed bed rest should be noted.

When there is a conspicuous disturbance of a particular organ or system, direct questions should be asked about all possible symptoms referable to the particular organ system. Specific inquiry should be made regarding any past affliction of the specific organ system that is implicated in the present illness.

Finally, the patient's previous treatment should be noted, including over-the-counter medications that the patient may have taken. Current medications and their dosage ideally are listed at the end of the history of the present illness, which fulfills a dual role: (1) if medication is causing the present illness, it will be easier to diagnose an iatrogenic illness, and (2) the evolution of the present illness might necessitate an adjustment of medication dose and frequency.

### Past medical history

The patient's past history includes a description of previous illnesses, general health, operations, injuries, hospitalizations, and allergies, all unrelated to the present illness. They should be listed chronologically.

### Family history

The family history includes a statement on any similar illness or symptoms in the family or the lack thereof; it notes the age and state of health of parents, siblings, and children, or the cause of their death and the age at death. It also includes the family history of common heritable diseases such as diabetes, hypertension, heart disease, kidney disease, cancer, allergy, and mental illness. A family tree is helpful if several members of the family have had the same illness.

#### Personal and social history

Personal and social history includes information on diet and nutrition, smoking, alcohol consumption, use of illicit drugs (e.g., cocaine, marijuana, amphetamines), sleep and exercise habits, education and occupation, marital status and sex life, and home and environmental conditions. An occupational history, chronologically arranged starting with the first job held, sometimes is useful.

#### Review of systems

The patient should be asked about salient symptoms pertaining to each organ system. All of the symptoms reported by the patient should be described and the lack of significant symptoms noted.

### Physical Examination

The physical examination is conducted by means of the four basic methods of **inspection, palpation, percussion,** and **auscultation.** Often, some aspects of the patient's illness are revealed only by physical examination. Thoroughness is, therefore, essential. Physical examination is indispensable in obtaining the following information about a patient: general appearance, including mental status; vital signs (temperature, pulse rate, respiratory rate, blood pressure); visible lesions on the body; palpable lesions, such as masses, local tenderness, deformities, and pulsations; signs of respiratory difficulty; auscultatory findings, such as murmurs, friction rubs, and alteration in breath and/or bowel sounds; and neurologic signs.

The environment in which the patient is examined should be quiet and well-lighted, preferably by daylight. The physician should be considerate when examining the patient, respecting the patient's need for privacy and avoiding provoking discomfort to the patient as much as possible. A systematic approach is essential. The physician's aim when performing the examination is to maintain objectivity and record observations, not to interpret them. For the routine physical examination, a full complement of equipment includes stethoscope, penlight, tongue blades, otoscope and ophthalmoscope, reflex hammer, sphygmomanometer, tuning fork, gloves, lubricating jelly, guaiac test reagents (e.g., Hemoccult), and a pelvic speculum. Infection control precautions—use of gloves, gowns, masks—should be used as appropriate. Hand washing is essential following hand contact with the patient, patient's fomites, or effects. An outline for performing the physical examination and recording the findings appears in Table 5.1.

**TABLE 5.1. Outline of a Physical Examination**

General appearance
Vital signs (pulse, temperature, blood pressure, respirations, height, weight)
Skin
Lymph nodes
Head and neck:
- Head
- Eyes
- Ears
- Nose
- Mouth and throat
- Neck

Back
Thorax
- Chest cage
- Lungs
- Breasts

Heart
Abdomen
Genitalia
Rectum
Limbs and musculoskeletal system
Neurologic system

# CHAPTER 6 DIAGNOSTIC STUDIES

### Laboratory Diagnosis

Laboratory tests cannot supplant a careful history and physical examination, but tests do provide diagnostic information that cannot be obtained by other means. Skills in making effective use of the laboratory are developed through training and experience. Physicians must acquire the ability to integrate laboratory data with other clinical information.

Laboratory data can be useful for a number of purposes, as follows:

- **Screening**. Application of laboratory tests for screening is discussed in Chapter 7.
- **Diagnosis**. The most common and important use of laboratory tests is diagnostic. Physicians use them as aids in selecting the most likely diagnosis from a list of several possibilities that may

have been suggested by the history and physical examination—that is, in making the **differential diagnosis**. Further laboratory testing can help the physician reach a precise diagnosis or limit the differential diagnosis.

- **Selection of therapy**. Results of laboratory studies can be useful in selecting the appropriate mode of therapy. Antimicrobial susceptibility tests used in selecting the most effective antibiotic for bacterial infections are a prime example. Other examples are blood grouping and crossmatching before blood transfusion, and tissue typing before tissue transplantation.
- **Follow-up**. Because laboratory tests are much more objective than the history and physical examination, and because they provide quantitative information, they have proved useful in following the course of a disease and determining the effectiveness of the therapy.
- **Prevention**. Tests used in genetic counseling to detect carrier states are an excellent example of using the laboratory in the prevention of diseases.
- **Medicolegal uses**. Legal evidence is collected, for example, by examining fingerprints or dried blood on clothing, by examining body fluids of rape victims, and by performing autopsies. Other applications include detection of DNA of the accused or assailants in crime scenes or crime-related evidence, and drug screens of urine and serum.
- **Environmental protection**. Environmental protection specialists commonly use microbiologic and toxicologic surveillance.
- **Therapeutic drug monitoring**. Serum levels of drugs such as gentamicin, phenytoin, aminophylline, and procainamide commonly are used to ensure adequate therapy.

The following considerations apply in various applications of laboratory data:

- **Qualitative versus quantitative testing**. Qualitative data are descriptive and include information on the presence or absence of a particular finding. For example, qualitative data would include a statement on the presence or absence of sugar in the urine. Qualitative data often are expressed in semiquantitative terms. Quantitative data are expressed only in numbers, such as blood sugar levels and blood counts.
- **Sensitivity versus specificity.** Sensitivity indicates that the result of the test is positive in the presence of the disease, whereas specificity indicates that it is negative in healthy persons or persons who do not have that particular disease. An ideally sensitive test is one in which all patients with the disease show positive results. A highly sensitive test is used to exclude a diagnosis, whereas a specific test is used to confirm it. For example, a perfusion lung scan is highly sensitive, and it is positive in all patients with clinically significant pulmonary embolism. A normal perfusion scan in a patient suspected of pulmonary embolism excludes this diagnosis. However, a positive scan does not automatically mean pulmonary embolism. On the other hand, positive findings on a pulmonary angiogram are highly specific for pulmonary embolism and confirm the diagnosis. In general, as the specificity of the test rises, the sensitivity diminishes, and as the sensitivity rises, the specificity declines.
- **Precision versus accuracy (reliability versus validity)**. A *precise, reliable* test is one that is highly reproducible. An *accurate, valid* test is one that gives a true measurement of the tested variable. A precise test is not necessarily accurate. Accuracy and precision in clinical laboratories are continually monitored by in-house, regional, and national laboratory proficiency surveys.
- **Normal ranges for laboratory values**. Normal ranges for quantitative test results allow for both the biologic variability in the normal population and the analytic imprecision of the method. Imprecise methods produce wider normal ranges. Nearly all clinical laboratories have a list of normal values that are established by doing the tests on a large number of healthy persons.
- **Errors in laboratory testing.** Errors can occur in clinical laboratories during the collection of specimens, during performance of the test, and in the interpretation of the test results. The physician must appreciate the inherent limitations of laboratory tests and must be aware that misleading or diagnostically useless information may be obtained if inappropriate tests are ordered. Incorrect handling of the specimen often leads to errors—one example would be incorrect use of anticoagulants in tubes used for collecting blood. Improperly handled or inadequate specimens are not an uncommon problem. Technical and clerical errors in the laboratory are additional sources of errors. Cross-contamination of specimens is a well-known source of error in tests that involve DNA amplification. Although laboratory errors do occur, they are not common; therefore, one should not routinely attribute any unanticipated result to laboratory error. When the physician suspects a laboratory error, the test should be repeated and, if the results are the same as before, those results

should not be ignored. Medications can interfere with laboratory tests; however, this is not common, despite combination drug therapy. The ultimate value of the laboratory test depends on the physician's appreciation of the limitations and capabilities of the clinical laboratory.

## Diagnostic Imaging

Imaging using x-rays, sound waves, radioactive isotopes, and magnetic resonance has an increasingly important role in diagnosis today.

### Diagnostic roentgenography

Diagnostic roentgenography supplements the physical examination. The chest radiograph (CXR) is the most common radiographic study. A peripheral lung cancer can be detected in its early stages by CXR. Plain radiographs (taken without the use of radiopaque contrast material) also are widely used in evaluating bones and detecting radiodensities in soft tissues. Contrast radiography is used to delineate soft tissue organs, to study the function of certain organs such as the kidneys, and to observe blood-flow patterns using angiography. The most commonly employed contrast agents are compounds of iodine and barium, which absorb more x-rays than do soft tissues. Iodine-containing contrast materials usually are injected intravenously; when ingested orally, they are absorbed into the bloodstream through the gastrointestinal tract. Barium, on the other hand, is used only for gastrointestinal examinations and is not absorbed through the gastrointestinal tract. Contrast materials can be used to study almost all the organ systems of the body.

A brief clinical summary and the reason for requesting the procedure should always accompany the request for a radiographic imaging study. If more than one procedure is available to accomplish the objective, the radiologist might use this information to determine the best procedure to provide the required information; the information is integrated into the interpretation of the imaging studies. In many instances, direct communication between the clinician and the radiologist before the radiographic study not only helps the radiologist provide the maximum information but also helps minimize the radiation exposure to the patient, because the radiologist would then perform only the necessary procedures. The clinician must review the radiographs personally and must not be satisfied simply by reading the radiologist's report. Consultation with a radiologist in interpreting the films often is beneficial in patient care, and the exchange of information is educational for both the clinician and the radiologist. Because prolonged or frequent exposure to x-rays can be a health hazard, only essential diagnostic radiographic examinations should be performed.

### Computed tomography

Computed (axial) tomography (CAT or CT scanning) is one of the most remarkable applications of computers in medicine. When x-ray beams pass through the body, they are subject to different degrees of attenuation as they pass through organs of varying tissue density. By analyzing such attenuations, and reconstructing an image of the various organs based on this analysis, a computer provides an image of a transverse slice of the body, of variable thicknesses. The examination is done at multiple levels, and images generated after administration of radiographic contrast media help distinguish vascular from nonvascular structures. Valuable information may be obtained about the density of a particular organ or tissue—for example, solid, cystic, and metallic (calcification). Organs that previously could not be visualized on radiographic examination can now be studied using this technique. CT scanning with or without contrast enhancement can help in making an early diagnosis with minimal discomfort and risk to the patient. CT scanning is invaluable in the evaluation and staging of neoplasms and in the diagnosis of intracranial and intra-abdominal lesions. Its availability has greatly reduced the need for angiographic examinations and exploratory surgery.

Because of its cost and the radiation exposure involved, CT should be reserved for conditions in which plain radiographs and routine contrast studies do not provide sufficient information for a diagnosis. As with many such procedures, before ordering them, one should consider both the expense involved and how the information so gained would facilitate decision-making.

### Diagnostic ultrasound

Ultrasonography is a noninvasive, painless technique that has no known harmful effects. A pulse of high-frequency sound waves (1 to 20 million Hz, well above 20,000 Hz, the upper limit of human hearing) is emitted from a transducer placed on the body surface over the organs to be studied. The sound waves are reflected in the form of echoes that are converted electronically into a display on a cathode ray oscilloscope. Acoustic interfaces occur whenever a substance changes in acoustic density. Larger reflections occur when the acoustic density difference is greater. Because the sound is well transmitted through fluid, a large reflection occurs when sound passes from fluid to soft tissues. Ultrasound examination has widespread clinical applications (Table 6.1).

### Radionuclide imaging

A wide range of applications of radionuclide imaging is summarized in Table 6.2. Single photon emission computed tomography (SPECT) imaging uses radioisotopes to obtain information regarding organ blood flow and metabolic function.

**TABLE 6.1. Applications of Ultrasonography**

| Technique | Use or Application |
|---|---|
| Intravascular ultrasound | To obtain high-resolution images of blood vessel lumen, walls, and mural lesions |
| Ultrasound in body cavities | *Transvaginal:* management of women with recurrent miscarriages; detection of early fetal anomalies<br>*Transrectal:* location of appropriate areas for prostate biopsy<br>*Transesophageal or endoscopic:* imaging of focal lesions and direction of the biopsy instruments<br>*Intraoperative:* better delineation of areas for biopsy or resection |
| Portable ultrasound | Used increasingly in physicians' offices to augment the clinical diagnosis of aortic aneurysms, gallstones, and even echocardiography |
| Abdominal ultrasound | Detection of fluid (pancreatic pseudocysts, renal cysts, hydronephrosis and ascites)<br>Diagnosis of gallstones, or help in determining the diameter of the biliary ducts (bile duct obstruction) or the size of kidneys (workup of renal failure) and abdominal aortic aneurysms. |
| Echocardiography | Stress testing, detection of wall motion anomalies, measurement of ejection fraction and various pressures<br>Detection of valvular abnormalities, diagnosis of pericardial effusion, and intracardiac shunts |

**TABLE 6.2. Clinical Applications of Radionuclide Imaging**

| Type | Purpose | Clinical Setting |
|---|---|---|
| Perfusion (Q) scan | Diagnosis | Pulmonary embolism |
| Ventilation (V) lung scan | Diagnosis | Sometimes combined with Q scans |
| Bone scan | Diagnosis | Osteomyelitis and bony metastases from cancer |
| Cardiac imaging | Diagnosis | Myocardial ischemia or infarction |
| | Evaluation | Ventricular performance |
| Tagged RBC scan | Localization | Intestinal bleeding |
| Tagged WBC scan | Diagnosis and localization | Localized pus collections (abscess) |
| Brain SPECT imaging | Diagnosis | Workup of dementia, epilepsy, and psychiatric disorders |

SPECT = single photon emission computed tomography

#### Positron Emission Tomographic (PET) Scans

Using positron emitters, which are special radioisotopes, one can generate images that depict the inner structure and function of various organs. PET scanning is highly reliable in detecting mediastinal metastases from lung cancer, locating epiletogenic foci, and diagnosing coronary artery disease. However, it is extremely expensive.

#### Magnetic resonance imaging

Magnetic resonance imaging (MRI) is a powerful diagnostic technique with widespread clinical applications. Radiofrequency (RF) signals applied to protons situated in a strong external magnetic field "energize" the protons, and they emit weak RF signals. Thus, the MRI uses nuclear resonance induced by RF signals rather than ionizing radiation to detect contrast and spatial resolutions between tissues. Because it uses no ionizing radiation, MRI offers a major advantage in the work-up of pelvic disorders in pregnant women and children. There are no known radiation hazards, but it is contraindicated in patients with pacemakers, surgical clips, and metallic prostheses. The application of MRI will gain further ground in functional brain imaging, spectroscopic imaging, and high-resolution imaging.

### Other Diagnostic Modalities

Since the early 1970s, numerous other diagnostic modalities have emerged. **Fiberoptic endoscopy,** for example, permits visualization of areas of the gastrointestinal tract and bronchi that previously were inaccessible for inspection. Using endoscopes, it is now possible to take biopsy specimens for histopathologic evaluation. **Electrocardiography** and **electroencephalography** are examples of diagnostic electrophysiologic procedures that have been used for decades. **Radioimmunoassay** techniques, which were the first to permit measurement of hormone levels in picogram quantities, have been supplanted by newer, more precise techniques, such as **polymerase chain reaction** (PCR). These techniques have been immensely helpful in clarifying the normal milieu and physiology of various organs, which often aids in diagnosis.

### The Art of Diagnosis

Experienced clinicians use the following six steps, in the order listed, to arrive at a diagnosis: (1) aggregating groups of findings into patterns; (2) selecting a "pivot" or key finding; (3) generating a list of causes; (4) pruning the cause list; (5) selecting a diagnosis; and (6) validating the diagnosis. The etiology is almost invariably one of the following: infection/infestation; physical/traumatic; immunologic; neoplastic; genetic/metabolic; iatrogenic; psychosomatic; or idiopathic. (These etiologic categories are perhaps best remembered using the following mnemonic, based on the first letter of each one: I-PING I-PI.)

# PREVENTION OF DISEASE

### Basic Definitions and Tenets

Prevention consists of evaluation, intervention, or lifestyle modification to prevent or delay the onset of pathologic processes or illnesses or to modify the course of established disease in an individual.

When specific measures are adopted to prevent the development of a specific disorder—for example, vaccination against poliomyelitis—the process is called **primary prevention.** The course of a disease that is present without manifestations might be modified through early detection. Early detection of disease in asymptomatic individuals is termed **screening** and is synonymous with **secondary prevention**—for example, mammograms to detect breast cancer and fecal occult blood testing to detect colon carcinoma. Finally, the disease may already be clinically evident and treated (but not cured), in which case an attempt must be made to delay its progression. This is **tertiary prevention**—for example, the patient who recently underwent coronary artery bypass surgery and is now asymptomatic but needs to modify lifestyle and risk factors to prevent new disease.

In situations in which a given intervention could be applied in any of the three modes of prevention, primary prevention has a greater public health impact than either secondary or tertiary preventive measures. Providing immunizations to prevent infectious diseases, and motivating individuals to avoid exposures or reduce risk factors by changing their lifestyle or health habits can prevent morbidity and mortality in far more individuals than efforts to detect undiagnosed disease in asymptomatic individuals or efforts to prevent progression of established disease. Therefore, the effective preventive health clinician must be skilled at assessing individuals' health risks, motivating them to change their health-related behaviors, and giving them the knowledge and skills they need to successfully change.

### Strategies for Prevention

The practicing physician can implement prevention during specific prevention-focused visits or during any patient encounter. The periodic health examination is a comprehensive prevention-focused history and physical examination, accompanied in the same visit by counseling, if unhealthy behaviors are detected; immunizations, if required; and indicated screening procedures (e.g., cervical Papanicolaou smear, breast examination, and flexible sigmoidoscopy). Alternatively, clinicians can perform many preventive interventions during any encounter for either acute illnesses or routine follow-up of chronic conditions. This strategy helps reduce the number of missed prevention opportunities in patients whose only physician visits are for injuries or acute illnesses.

Physicians practicing in primary care specialties have the unique opportunity to implement systems that facilitate primary, secondary, and tertiary preventive interventions targeted to the population they serve. Primary care practitioners can improve the efficiency of prevention and screening efforts within their practice by involving all team members in improvement efforts to achieve prevention benchmarks such as the Healthy People 2010 goals. Surveys and other case-finding tools can be used to reach out to and identify populations that could benefit from preventive care. Patient recall systems or computerized reminder systems can be used to prompt patients to seek, and clinicians to complete, indicated preventive measures. Tracking rates of completion of indicated preventive care is becoming an accepted indicator of the quality of primary care.

## Specific Preventive Care Recommendations

Preventive health guidelines have been issued by several groups, including government agencies, task forces, health-related organizations, and subspecialty societies. The website for the Centers for Disease Control and Prevention (CDC) (www.phppo.cdc.gov/CDC recommends/AdvSearchV.asp) has a searchable database of prevention guidelines on a large number of topics. Some guidelines are targeted toward the general population, whereas others focus on prevention in patients with various underlying diseases (e.g., individuals with HIV infection). Three commonly quoted sets of preventive recommendations for the general population of adults are those of the Canadian Task Force on the Periodic Health Examination, the United States Preventive Services Task Force, and the American College of Physicians-American Society of Internal Medicine. These guidelines are updated periodically to reflect evolving information about the effectiveness of preventive measures.

As the patient's care director, the physician must know the benefits, risks and limitations of each measure recommended for the prevention or early detection of disease. Some measures have been found definitely effective in well-designed studies, whereas other measures have not been shown conclusively to reduce morbidity or mortality when applied to either individuals or populations. Some preventive measures, while proven effective in populations, are not without risks in individual patients. Under these circumstances, physicians should educate patients about these key factors and allow them to make an informed decision about whether to accept recommended measures.

The set of preventive procedures the physician recommends to patients should be based on the most common causes of premature morbidity and mortality that he or she encounters in practice. Illnesses or risk factors that often go undetected (e.g., substance abuse, domestic violence, and depression) should prompt screening surveys or inquiries. To reap their full benefits, positive screens should receive prompt and thorough follow-up. General and specific recommendations about many of the preventive measures that apply to adults are discussed in the following sections.

**TABLE 7.1. Adult Immunizations for the General Population: Current Recommendations**

| Vaccine | Indications and Comments |
|---|---|
| Influenza vaccine | All individuals > age 65.<br>Patients at high risk for significant morbidity and mortality (e.g., those with diabetes mellitus, heart disease, pulmonary disease, renal disease, and those who are immunocompromised)<br>Health care personnel<br>Residents of chronic care facilities<br>Contraindicated in persons with a history of allergy to egg yolk<br>Vaccine usually is available in the autumn and should be given yearly. |
| Pneumococcal vaccine | Similar to those for influenza vaccine. Other indications are asplenia (anatomic or functional), alcoholism, sickle cell disease, Hodgkin disease, and nephrotic syndrome.<br>Vaccine may be administered year-round but is needed only once in the lifetime. |
| Tetanus toxoid | All adults once every 10 years. |
| Measles vaccine | For individuals born after 1956 who lack evidence of immunity |
| Rubella vaccine | Women of childbearing age who lack proof of immunity. CDC recommends for health care workers, military recruits, and college students.<br>Recipient has to agree not to become pregnant in the 3 months to follow. Pregnancy is an absolute contraindication |
| Hepatitis B vaccine | Individuals with high risk of exposure (e.g., health care workers, individuals at biomedical research laboratories, homosexually active men, intravenous drug abusers, hemodialysis patients)<br>Recombinant, inactivated vaccine. Over 95% of healthy individuals given vaccine develop immunity. Duration of immunity has not been clearly defined. |
| Hepatitis A vaccine | Persons living in or traveling to areas where the disease is endemic, homosexually active men, intravenous drug abusers, military recruits |
| Varicella vaccine | Healthy adults with no history of varicella infection, susceptible health care workers, day care workers, family contacts of immunocompromised individuals |

**Primary prevention**

A prerequisite to prevention is knowledge of the pathophysiology of the disease and the risk factors for development of the disease. An understanding of the pathophysiology of a disease enables the physician to intervene and block the activity of specific, disease-causing agents before they lead to disease development; an understanding of the risk factors of disease is required to modify their influence and thereby decrease the risk of disease development.

*Immunizations*

Vaccinations and immunizations best exemplify the primary prevention of infectious diseases. When administered to an individual, a vaccine, which is a derivative from protein components of a microbe, stimulates the individual's immune system to form antibodies against that microbe, providing protection from disease caused by infection with that microbe. The process is effective in preventing specific infectious diseases (e.g., influenza, pneumococcal pneumonia from certain strains, mumps, measles, rubella, hepatitis B, tetanus, and rabies).

Table 7.1 describes the recommendations for routine booster and primary immunizations in general populations of adults. Many of the primary immunizations are given early in life—that is, when the person is younger than age 6. However, adults who have not received primary immunizations need them, and adults who have been immunized previously sometimes require booster immunization (e.g., to prevent tetanus and hepatitis). Several different vaccines may be given at the same visit. The currently recommended immunizations fulfill the basic tenets of preventive medicine: efficacy, safety, and cost-effectiveness.

*Modification of risk factors*

Modification of risk factors is another exciting example of primary prevention. By working with the patient to modify a lifestyle habit or effectively treat a risk factor, the physician can positively intervene to

**TABLE 7.2. Risk Factors for Atherosclerosis**

| |
|---|
| *Modifiable factors* |
| Cigarette smoking |
| Hypertension |
| Hypercholesterolemia |
| Reduced high-density lipoprotein (HDL) cholesterol level |
| *Nonmodifiable factors* |
| Old age |
| Male gender |
| Family history of premature coronary artery disease |
| Diabetes mellitus |

**TABLE 7.3. Counseling Recommendations to Prevent Injury or Illness in the General Population**

| Setting | Recommendations |
|---|---|
| General | Advise patient regarding:<br>practice of safe sex<br>use of contraceptives<br>preventive dental care<br>use and abuse of drugs, including alcohol, caffeine, tobacco, illicit drugs.<br>Help patient manage stress. |
| Home | Teach firearm safety.<br>Advise against smoking in bed.<br>Advise use of smoke detectors.<br>Advise patient to monitor hot water temperature (especially when there are elderly persons and toddlers in the household).<br>Educate patient to prevent falls (elderly). |
| Outdoors | Advise patient to use seat belts while driving.<br>Advise use of bicycle and motorcycle helmets.<br>Advocate regular physical activity.<br>Encourage prevention of skin cancer through sun protection. |
| Work environment | Review safety precautions commensurate with patient's occupation. |
| Nutrition | Educate patient regarding:<br>balanced diet<br>fiber content of foods<br>vitamin supplements<br>calcium supplements<br>adequate folate intake before pregnancy. |

prevent or delay the development of disease. For example, several risk factors for atherosclerosis have been identified (Table 7.2). Counseling to stop cigarette smoking and intervention to detect and control hypercholesterolemia have been shown to be effective in both primary and tertiary prevention of coronary artery disease. Other examples of generally recommended counseling or lifestyle modification suggestions to prevent illness and injury are listed in Table 7.3.

The effectiveness of patient counseling can be improved by framing benefits of the change from the patient's perspective; engaging the patient in setting jointly agreed upon, specific, attainable goals; teaching them the specific skills or behaviors they will need to succeed in the changes; involving other health care staff in counseling for change or compliance along with physician reinforcement of the message, because physician recommendations carry the greatest weight and often are the primary reasons patients give for accepting preventive measures; monitoring progress through follow-up contacts; or any combination of these strategies.

### Secondary prevention

A **screening intervention** enables the discovery of undetected disorders or detection of disorders in their asymptomatic stage. To be effective against any targeted disease, the screening intervention should satisfy all the following conditions:

1. The disorder is relatively prevalent.
2. The test is reasonably safe, inexpensive, and acceptable to the patient.
3. The test recognizes most patients with the disorder (high sensitivity) while mislabeling few normal patients as having the disorder (high specificity).
4. Follow-up confirmation tests are safe and, ideally, noninvasive and affordable.
5. Treatment of the disorder in its asymptomatic stage will improve the patient's prognosis compared with those patients who have a similar disorder and are treated only when the disease becomes symptomatic.
6. The ultimate outcome of the disorder has grave consequences for the patient's well-being, in terms of either morbidity or mortality.

Of these conditions, the two that are most difficult to evaluate and quantify are the sensitivity/specificity of the screening test, and the enhanced efficacy of treating disease diagnosed in its asymptomatic stage. Ideally, screening tests should have perfect sensitivity so that no opportunities for early intervention are missed; in reality, all screening tests have less than perfect sensitivity. Imperfect sensitivity of a screening test can lead to inappropriate security when false-negative results are obtained in individuals with the underlying disease; conversely, imperfect specificity can lead to the negative consequences of labeling and unnecessary follow-up tests in normal patients with false-positive results. Overall accuracy and efficiency of screening tests, particularly the positive predictive value, can be improved by targeting their use towards higher risk individuals.

There are two main errors that can complicate estimates of the true efficacy of screening strategies that involve treatment of early stage disease. Both of these may be illustrated by potential pitfalls of prostate cancer screening in elderly men. Whereas proponents argue that earlier detection of cancer will lead to its cure, opponents argue that cancers have their own finite prognosis that is unaffected by the time of detection, and that the improvement in survival time after diagnosis is merely a reflection of the cancer being detected early (lead-time bias). The second potential error, when estimating the effectiveness of screening is related to the fact that cancers have their own intrinsic growth rate. Given that premise, periodic screening is more likely to detect asymptomatic cancers that are inherently slower-growing, because faster-growing tumors cause symptoms that lead to their detection before the next screening episode. In other words, the probability that screening will detect prostate cancer before it causes symptoms (i.e., in the preclinical phase) is inversely related to its rate of progression. Therefore, comparisons of screened to unscreened populations that are not adjusted for rate of cancer growth are biased in favor of screening (length bias). Randomized trials of screening followed by early treatment, and adjustment for rates of disease progression, are the best ways to avoid these biases.

Many screening interventions in adults involve the early detection of cancer. Because cancers detected at early stages have a better prognosis and often can be treated using less radical methods, screening attempts to diagnose occult cancers at the earliest possible stage. However, early cancer diagnosis also depends on targeting more intensive evaluation to higher risk individuals and the prompt evaluation of patients with possible cancer-related symptoms or signs. A detailed list of screening recommendations for many neoplasms is shown in Table 7.4.

TABLE 7.4. Recommendations for Cancer Screening

| Type of Cancer | General Recommendations | Additional Screening Recommended by Special Societies/ Panels of Experts |
|---|---|---|
| Breast cancer[a] | Breast examination by a physician every 1–2 yrs from age 40. Yearly mammography, from age 50–75. Monthly breast self-examination at midcycle. | ACS, ACOG: annual or biannual mammography and annual breast examination by a clinician from age 40–50 |
| Colorectal cancer[a] | Annual fecal occult blood testing and flexible sigmoidoscopy every 3–5 years starting at age 50. | ACP: flexible sigmoidoscopy, colonoscopy or barium enema every 10 years from age 50–70. ACS: annual digital rectal examination starting at age 40 |
| Cervical cancer[a] | Papanicolaou smear every 1–3 years, from commencement of sexual activity in all women with a cervix. Screening can be stopped by age 65 if the examinations are consistently normal | More frequent screening for patients with risk factors including early onset of sexual activity; multiple sex partners; low socioeconomic status; or HIV infection. |
| Prostate cancer[b] | Annual counseling about potential risks and benefits of screening with prostate-specific antigen and digital rectal examination so patient can make informed decision. | USPTF: Digital rectal examination and PSA are not recommended in asymptomatic men. ACS; AUA: yearly DRE and PSA starting at age 50; or age 40 in African American men or men with positive family history of prostate cancer |
| Lung cancer | Screening with chest radiograph or sputum cytology is ineffective. | |
| Skin cancer[a] | Complete skin inspection only for patients at high risk, patients with a family or personal history of skin cancer, or patients with a precursor lesion (e.g., dysplastic nevi). | ACS; AAD: periodic complete examination by clinician for all patients as well as monthly self-examination. |
| Ovarian cancer[b] | Careful examination of the uterine adnexa during pelvic examination. | ACP: Counsel high risk patients about the potential risks and benefits of screening with CA-125 and ultrasound. |
| Testicular cancer | Routine examination only in high-risk patients: those with testicular atrophy, cryptorchidism, or orchiopexy. | ACS: testicular exam as part of the periodic health examination. |

[a]Interventions are effective in changing natural history.
[b]Effectiveness of interventions in changing natural history is unknown.
AAD = American Academy of Dermatology; ACOG = American College of Obstetricians and Gynecologists; ACP = American College of Physicians; ACS = American Cancer Society; AUA = American Urological Association; USPTF = United States Preventive Task Force.

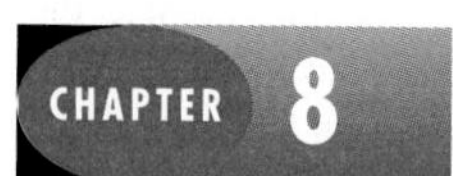

# CHAPTER 8 WOMEN'S HEALTH

## Women's Health Issues

The practice of women's health within the field of internal medicine can be highly stimulating and rewarding. It incorporates many aspects of general and specialized internal medicine, with the addition of gender-specific areas of medicine and gender-specific presentation and natural history of disease. Many areas of reproductive health, including contraception, preconception counseling, and the transition through menopause can be managed by the general internist, with consultation by specialists in related fields if necessary. The care of women is challenging and rewarding because of the broad range of clinical entities involved.

An awareness of gender differences in the practice of medicine can enhance the physician's skills and effectiveness as a clinician. In recent decades, increased efforts have been made to include women in research protocols, thereby enhancing knowledge about the natural history of disease processes among women. Gender-specific differences exist not only in the area of reproductive health but also in the clinical presentation and therapeutic response to a range of disease processes.

Increased initiatives to include female subjects in research studies of common diseases will improve our knowledge regarding differences in presentation, diagnosis, and response to therapy between women and men.

## Cancer Screening and Prevention Among Women

Cancer is the second leading cause of death among women, following cardiovascular disease. The three most prevalent types of cancer among women are breast cancer (30%), lung and bronchial cancer (12%), and colorectal cancer (11%). Viewed another way, the lifetime risk of breast cancer for women is 12.6% (or 1 in 8), for lung and bronchus cancer 5.7% (1 in 18), and for colon and rectal cancer 5.5% (1 in 18). Although cervical cancer represents only 2% of cancer deaths in developed countries, it is the leading cause of cancer death in some underdeveloped countries. Early detection of premalignant lesions by Papanicolaou smears has prevented an estimated 70% of cervical cancers. Adhering to recommendations for breast, colorectal, and cervical cancer screening is an important component of preventive care in women. (See Chapter 7 Prevention of Disease for recommended guidelines.) Although screening for lung cancer is not currently recommended, physicians can promote prevention of lung cancer through identification of cigarette use and by offering smoking cessation counseling or a referral to a smoking cessation program. Smoking rates have declined more slowly among women than among men.

## Contraception

Periodic counseling about contraception is recommended for both men and women who are at risk for unwanted pregnancy. The most widely used contraceptive method worldwide is combined oral contraceptive pills (OCPs), which contain estrogen and progesterone. Physicians should be aware of the risks and benefits of OCPs, common drug interactions, and the appropriate management of women on OCPs. Current use of OCPs is associated with an increased risk of venous thrombosis. Oral contraceptives should not be used by women who have a history of deep vein thrombosis or pulmonary embolism, cardiovascular disease (stroke or coronary heart disease), structural heart disease, diabetes for more than 20 years or with end-organ complications, breast cancer, liver disease, or headaches with focal neurologic symptoms, or who are 35 years or older and smoke, or are pregnant or lactating, or have poorly controlled hypertension. Several medications, including antiseizure medications and antibiotics, can decrease the effectiveness of OCPs. Alternatives to combined oral contraceptive pills can be considered if OCPs are contraindicated or not tolerated. These alternatives include progestin-only pills, injectable hormonal contraception, implantable hormonal contraceptives, intrauterine devices (IUDs), and barrier methods. Barrier methods offer the advantage of protection from STDs and a decreased risk of cervical cancer. Male and female condoms protect against human immunodeficiency virus (HIV) transmission.

### Preconception counseling and pregnancy

Medical care of the pregnant woman includes preconception counseling, diagnosis of pregnancy, management of chronic disease in the pregnant woman, and treatment of the medical complications of pregnancy. Preconception counseling includes identifying high-risk behaviors such as smoking, alcohol use, and illegal drug use, and providing information about nutrition, which includes ensuring that the patient's intake of folic acid is adequate. Preconception counseling should address optimizing control of chronic diseases, including hypertension and diabetes, and screening for infectious diseases including HIV, rubella, and hepatitis B. Patients at risk also may require screening for tuberculosis, cytomegalovirus, and toxoplasmosis. Certain medications, including Accutane and Coumadin, must be avoided in the preconception period. Patients also should be screened for domestic violence. Genetic counseling should be offered if the woman is of advanced maternal age, has a family history of a genetic disease, or has had a previous child or pregnancy affected by a genetic disease.

Hypertension and diabetes mellitus require careful treatment and monitoring during pregnancy. In pregnant women, chronic hypertension is defined as an elevated blood pressure occurring before pregnancy. Pregnant women with chronic hypertension are at increased risk for preeclampsia and abruptio placentae, and the risk of fetal and prenatal death is increased 2- to 4-fold compared to the general population. Patients are considered to have low-risk chronic hypertension if they have mild hypertension without any organ involvement; these patients do not necessarily require antihypertensive therapy. Patients with severe hypertension or mild hypertension complicated by end-organ involvement should be managed with pharmacological treatment. Methyldopa has the best safety record for treatment of pregnant women. Beta-blockers also have been well studied and are thought to be safe and effective in the third trimester of pregnancy, but not earlier in pregnancy. Angiotensin-converting enzyme inhibitors are contraindicated because of associations with neonatal renal failure, renal dysgenesis, and fetal growth restriction. Patients who have diabetes or develop gestational diabetes require tight control of their glucose levels. The risk to the fetus increases in a direct relationship with the level of maternal hyperglycemia.

Drugs for use in pregnant women are classified into five general categories: A, B, C, D, and X. These categories reflect the level of evidence demonstrating safety or potential harm to the fetus of medications used during pregnancy. Category A indicates that controlled studies have shown no risk to the fetus. Category B indicates that there are some human or animal studies that demonstrate no risk to the fetus. Category C indicates that human studies are not available and animal studies are either not available or indicate possible fetal risk. Category D indicates positive evidence of risk to the fetus. Category X indicates that the drug is contraindicated in pregnancy due to studies in humans or animals that indicate the risks clearly outweigh potential benefits. Only about 40% of drugs currently are assigned a pregnancy classification. When possible, medications used during pregnancy should be limited to those in category A or B.

## Menopause

### Definition and diagnosis

The World Health Organization defines menopause as the permanent cessation of menstruation resulting from the loss of ovarian follicular activity when the ovaries are depleted of primordial follicles, resulting in decreasing estrogen secretion. Clinically, this diagnosis is made in retrospect following 12 months of amenorrhea. The term *climacteric*, or *perimenopause*, refers to the 2 to 8 years preceding menopause and the first year of amenorrhea following menopause. Hormonal changes that occur with menopause include a decrease in estradiol levels, a decrease in ovarian androgens, and an increase in follicle-stimulating hormone (FSH >40 mIU/ml) and luteinizing hormone (LH). The median age of menopause in the United States is 51 years. Women who smoke may have an earlier menopause. The menopause offers a time for the patient and physician to reassess health risks and consider a course of management to optimize health and quality of life over the anticipated 30 years that most women live after menopause.

### Decision-making at menopause

At the time of menopause, a woman and her physician should consider both short- and long-term health issues. In the short term, women may have significant symptoms of estrogen deficiency, which may need treatment. The most common symptoms at menopause include vasomotor (such as hot flashes and night sweats) and urogenital (such as vaginal dryness, urinary frequency, or incontinence) symptoms. A wide range of other symptoms, including mood swings, fatigue, decreased sexual desire, and insomnia also are reported. Women within and between cultures vary significantly with respect to the types and severity of symptoms reported in the perimenopausal period.

At the time of menopause, women face changes in their risk factors for long-term health. The incidence of cardiovascular disease (stroke and coronary artery disease) increases with age in both men and women. However, women's risk of coronary artery disease increases significantly after menopause. The lifetime risk of a 50-year-old white woman dying from coronary artery disease is estimated to be 31%. After menopause, women experience a change in their lipid profile that has an adverse effect on CAD risk. Specifically, total cholesterol levels and low-density lipoprotein levels increase, while high density lipoprotein levels decrease. Estradiol is thought to have beneficial effects on vascular function and repair. These protective effects are attenuated with the decline in estradiol levels after menopause.

Osteoporosis is another long-term health concern for women at the time of menopause. Declining levels of estrogen after menopause are thought to play a role in the development of postmenopausal osteoporosis. Bone mass begins to decrease after age 35 in both sexes, but this process accelerates rapidly in women at menopause. A 50-year-old woman's lifetime risk of having a hip fracture is estimated to be 15.6%, her risk of a Colles fracture of the forearm to be 15.0%, and her risk of a vertebral fracture to be 32%. Black women have a lower risk of fractures. Osteoporotic fractures, primarily of the hip and vertebrae, often lead to a decline in independence and quality of life and an increase in mortality.

### Hormone replacement therapy

One of the complex decisions women must consider with their physicians at menopause is whether or not to use hormone replacement therapy (HRT). In HRT, exogenous estrogen is used to partially replace the endogenous estrogen levels the woman had before menopause. Hormone replacement therapy is contraindicated in women with estrogen-dependent tumors, genital bleeding from unknown causes, active liver disease, active thromboembolic disorders, porphyria, and pregnancy. In women who have not had a hysterectomy, it is necessary to partially replace the hormone progestin to protect the uterus from endometrial hyperplasia and endometrial cancer. Most clinicians use a cyclic or continuous regimen. In a cyclic regimen, the estrogen is given every day of the month and the progestin is given for 12 to 14 days. In a continuous regimen, estrogen and progestin are both given every day of the month. In patients who receive continuous combined estrogen and progesterone therapy, endometrial atrophy with absence of bleeding eventually occurs. This state usually is reached in about 6 months. These women sometimes experience unpredictable intermittent bleeding, which may lead to the need for an endometrial biopsy to rule out any pathologic cause for the bleeding. Side effects of HRT can include breast tenderness, bloating, weight gain, and depression.

A number of risks and benefits must be considered individually for each patient regarding the use of HRT. The major known benefits include effective treatment of menopausal vasomotor symptoms, and effective prevention of postmenopausal osteoporosis with long-term use. Evidence is emerging that HRT may reduce colon cancer risk. The major known risks are increased risk of breast cancer with use for more than 5 years, increased risk of thromboembolic disease, and increased risk of gallbladder disease. The use of estrogen replacement therapy (ERT) was thought from earlier observational studies to reduce the risk of coronary artery disease by 35% to 50%. However, the Heart Estrogen/Progestin Replacement Study (HERS) did not show any benefit of HRT over placebo in women with established cardiovascular disease, and showed a possible increase in the risk of myocardial events in the first year of therapy when HRT was used for secondary prevention of coronary heart disease. Subsequently, the Women's Health Initiative (WHI) reported an increased risk of CAD and stroke in a primary prevention trial of combined estrogen and progestin versus placebo in postmenopausal women. This important study also found HRT increased risk of breast cancer and pulmonary embolus, but decreased risks of hip fracture and colon cancer. The combined HRT arm of the study was stopped early due to the increased harm from breast cancer, but an estrogen-only arm of the WHI trial is ongoing.

Symptoms of menopause usually last no more than 5 years. However, for long-term benefits HRT must be continued indefinitely. Patients and physicians must balance the risks and benefits of treatment before making a decision. Whether or not HRT is used, other interventions to reduce the risk of coronary artery disease and osteoporosis are indicated. Interventions to reduce risk for coronary artery disease in postmenopausal women include smoking cessation, controlling hypertension and hyperlipidemia, weight reduction, and exercise. Interventions to decrease the risk of osteoporosis include calcium supplementation, encouragement of weight-bearing exercise, and smoking cessation. Postmenopausal women who have had a nontraumatic fracture or are 65 years or older and are not on a preventive agent for osteoporosis should have a screening bone mineral density test to help guide future therapy. Alternative pharmacologic interventions that are effective in the prevention of osteoporotic fractures include the bisphosphates alendronate and risedronate and the selective estrogen receptor modulator raloxifene.

### Cardiovascular Disease in Women

The epidemiology, diagnostic evaluation, and outcomes of coronary artery disease are different in women than in men. Women develop coronary artery disease approximately 10 years later than men, although the difference in age-specific incidence decreases as age increases. The major risk factors for CAD are similar for men and women and include hypercholesterolemia, hypertension, diabetes, electrocardiographic (EKG) evidence of left ventricular hypertrophy, and cigarette smoking. However, some risk factors are more prognostic in women than in men. A low level of high-density lipoprotein (HDL-C) is a stronger predictor of cardiovascular mortality in women than in men. Diabetes and evidence of left ventricular hypertrophy (LVH) also are stronger risk factors for women than for men. Chest pain is the most common presenting symptom in both men and women with a new diagnosis of coronary artery disease. However, women more commonly have atypical chest pain because of the higher prevalence of less common causes of ischemia such as vasospastic and microvascular angina. Syndrome X—defined as exertional angina, a positive response to exercise testing, and angiographically normal coronary arteries—is most common in postmenopausal women. Diagnostic studies including exercise electrocardiograms and exercise thallium scans are less discriminating of CAD in women than men. Furthermore, it has been found that women are less likely to undergo invasive diagnostic testing and treatment than men in the evaluation of chest pain. For unclear reasons, the prognosis is worse for women than for men who present with acute myocardial infarction or after bypass surgery. In summary, CAD is a major cause of morbidity and mortality among women. However, its presentation, evaluation, treatment, and outcomes may differ from that in men. An appreciation for such differences can help to enhance the prevention and treatment of CAD in women.

# CHAPTER 9 COMPLEMENTARY MEDICINE

The National Center for Complementary and Alternative Medicine has defined complementary medicine as the "broad domain of healing resources that encompasses all health systems, modalities and practices and their accompanying theories and beliefs, other than those intrinsic to the politically dominant health system of a particular society or culture in a given historical period." An operational definition of complementary medicine is that it is every available approach to healing that does not fall into the realm of conventional medicine. The word "alternative" refers to therapies used in place of conventional therapies; "complementary" refers to therapies used in conjunction with conventional therapies; and "integrative" represents a synthesis of both conventional and alternative methodologies. Many complementary medicine practitioners espouse the "holistic" philosophy that any therapeutic treatment affects the emotional, mental, and spiritual, as well as physical, aspects of the patient's life.

American patients spent $18 billion out-of-pocket on complementary therapies in 1998 (see Table 9.1 for list of complementary therapies). Increasingly, insurance companies are paying for these therapies. It is estimated that in 1997 patients paid approximately 1.6 times as many visits to unconventional practitioners as there were to primary care physicians. Academic centers around the country are opening integrative medicine clinics. Many medical schools are offering electives in complementary therapies or include these topics in required courses.

Some complementary therapies are known to be helpful; others may not be helpful but are not harmful; and a few are known to be harmful. Each therapy needs to be evaluated individually, ideally within controlled scientific trials. In 1992 the National Institutes of Health recognized the popularity of unconventional medicine and created the Office of Alternative Medicine (OAM). In 1998, the OAM was upgraded to the National Center for Complementary and Alternative Medicine (NCCAM). At that time, the center's budget was increased from $20 million to $50 million each year to fund studies of the alternative therapies that our patients are using.

## Categories of the Therapies and Underlying Rationales

The NCCAM has divided complementary medicine treatment into seven categories (Table 9.1).

Complementary medicine consists of an unregulated assortment of techniques, philosophies, and cultures of healing, but there are some basic underlying themes.

First, these therapies are vitalistic. Practitioners believe that the body, mind, and emotions are maintained by an underlying vital or life force. In traditional Chinese medicine it is called "chi"; in chiropractic it is referred

**TABLE 9.1. Guide to Alternative Medicine and Complementary Therapies**

1. *Therapeutic Systems*
   a. Acupuncture
   b. Ayurveda
   c. Chinese medicine, traditional
   d. Homeopathy
   e. Native American healing
   f. Naturopathic medicine
2. *Dietary and Herbal Remedies*
   a. Dietary supplements
   b. Flower remedies
   c. Herbal medicine
   d. Vegetarianism
3. *Mind-Body Medicine*
   a. Biofeedback
   b. Hypnosis
   c. Imagery and visualization
   d. Kirlian photography
   e. Meditation
   f. Placebo effect
   g. Qigong
4. *Alternative Biological Treatments*
   a. Biological cancer treatments
   b. Chelation therapy
   c. Colon/detoxification therapies
   d. Enzyme therapy
   e. Metabolic therapies
   f. Oxygen therapies
   g. Shark and bovine cartilage therapies
5. *Bodywork*
   a. Acupressure
   b. Alexander technique
   c. Chiropractic
   d. Craniosacral therapy
   e. Hydrotherapy
   f. Massage
   g. Reflexology
   h. Rolfing
   i. Tai chi
   j. Yoga
6. *Sense Therapy*
   a. Aromatherapy
   b. Art therapy
   c. Dance therapy
   d. Humor therapy
   e. Light therapy
   f. Music therapy
   g. Sound therapy
7. *External Energy Healing*
   a. Crystal health
   b. Electromagnetic therapies
   c. Faith healing
   d. Prayer and spirituality
   e. Shamanism
   f. Therapeutic touch

Adapted with permission from Cassileth BR, The Alternative Medicine Handbook: The Complete Reference Guide to Alternative and Complementary Therapies. New York: WW Norton, 1998.

to as "innate intelligence"; in ayurveda it is called "prana." Within these systems, health and disease reflect balance and imbalance, respectively. Wellness is a state in which the energy of life flourishes; disease is a condition in which vitality is blocked.

Second, the body is believed to be self-healing, and the practitioner's task is to assist the body in the healing process. According to Dr. Andrew Weil, orthodox physicians worship the male god of medicine, Aesculapius, who wages war on disease, whereas complementary practitioners worship Hygeia, the female goddess of healing. These complementary therapies do not attempt to suppress symptoms, eradicate harmful organisms, or eliminate diseased tissue, but, rather, try to correct deficiencies in the body's homeostatic mechanisms.

Third, complementary therapies tend to have a single, all-encompassing theory of disease.

Fourth, complementary therapies often are holistic. The patient is viewed as a physical, spiritual, and emotional whole. Each aspect of a person's life affects all the other aspects. Complementary systems have a view of health that goes beyond the simple absence of symptoms. They promote "wellness."

Finally, many complementary therapies have been used for centuries, but have not been tested scientifically.

## Users of Complementary Medicine

In 1998, Eisenberg reported on a national telephone survey of 20,955 English-speaking patients. Of these, 42% reported using unconventional therapies. The people who used these therapies were more likely to be female, Caucasian, and middle-aged (39-49 years of age); to have some college education; and to live in the western part of the United States. Forty-eight percent of users had annual incomes above $50,000. In 1999, Druss and coworkers published the results of a written survey taken on 16,068 adults who were participating in the Medical Expenditures Panel Survey. Overall, only 8% admitted to using unconventional therapies. Users of these therapies had significantly more visits to alternative practitioners than to traditional practitioners—7.9 vs 5.4 visits annually ($p < .001$). They were more likely to be female, white, and well-educated, and to live in the western part of the United States. Users of both complementary and alternative therapies had poorer self-perceived health status than those who used only conventional therapies. Astin's report on 1035 adults who were part of the 1997 National Family Opinion surveys found that 69% had used unconventional therapies, but only 4% used them exclusively. Users had more education, poorer self-perceived health status, and more chronic medical conditions than non-users.

Most complementary medicine users seek unconventional therapy for chronic, non–life-threatening, medical conditions. But many users receive treatment for serious chronic, or degenerative illnesses (Table 9.2). Among those who use unconventional therapy for serious medical conditions, 72% did not inform their medical doctors that they had done so. Another subset of users consists of patients who try unconventional therapies for conditions for which there are no known effective conventional therapies (e.g., fibromyalgia) or when conventional therapies have been exhausted (e.g., for AIDS or cancer).

**TABLE 9.2. Conditions Treated by Unconventional Therapies in Two Recent Studies**

| Condition | Percent Using Alternative Therapies for Condition in Past 12 Months[a] | Percent Using Alternative Therapies for Condition in Past 12 Months[b] |
|---|---|---|
| Addictive problems | | 25 |
| Allergies | 17 | |
| Anxiety | 43 | 31 |
| Arthritis | 27 | 25 |
| Back problems | 48 | |
| Chronic pain | | 37 |
| Depression | 41 | |
| Digestive problems | 27 | |
| Fatigue | 27 | 31 |
| Headache | 32 | 24 |
| Hypertension | 12 | |
| Insomnia | 26 | |
| Lung problems | 13 | |
| Neck problems | 57 | |
| Skin problems | 7 | |
| Sprain/Strains | 24 | 26 |

[a] Data from Eisenberg DM, David RB, Ettner SL, et al. Trends in alternative medicine use in the United States, 1990-1997. JAMA 1998;280:1569-1575.

[b] Data from Astin JA. Why patients use alternative medicine: results of a national study. JAMA 1998;279:1548-1553.

## Reasons for Using Complementary Therapies

Eisenberg has summarized the diverse reasons why patients seek alternative therapies as follows:

1. They are looking for health promotion and disease prevention.
2. Conventional therapies have been exhausted.
3. Conventional therapies are of indeterminate effectiveness or are associated with significant risk.
4. No conventional therapy is available.
5. The conventional approach is believed to be emotionally or spiritually without benefit.

The philosophies of complementary medicine appeal to some patients. Astin found that National Family Opinion respondents who had used unconventional therapies were more likely to be "cultural creatives," with a commitment to environmentalism, feminism, esoteric forms of spirituality, personal growth psychology, self-actualization, and self-experience that changed their world view. They felt that unconventional medicine was "more congruent with their own values, beliefs and philosophical orientations toward health and life." Kaptchuk and Eisenberg also have explored the "persuasive appeal of alternative medicine." They believe the attraction is related to the power of its underlying beliefs and cultural assumptions. The fundamental premises of unconventional medicine are an advocacy of nature, vitalism (connection with a benevolent power), semiscientific nature, and spirituality. The quest for health becomes a sacred journey. Unconventional medicine is fundamentally more hopeful, viewing the body as self-healing and offering the possibility of cure. Kaptchuk and Eisenberg conclude by saying "it may be that biomedicine, when it is honest, is less optimistic and more realistically accepts the limitations and finitudes of the human condition."

## The Doctor-Patient Relationship in Unconventional Medicine

What can we learn about patient-doctor communication from unconventional practitioners? In a recent study, authors questioned 256 patients of general practitioners, osteopaths, homeopaths, and acupuncturists. All groups felt complementary practitioners were more sympathetic, had more time to listen, were more sensitive to emotional issues, and were better at explaining treatment and explaining why the patient is ill. Also, unconventional providers do not differentiate between "physical" and "psychosomatic" illness. Patients often are offended by the term "psychosomatic," feeling that physicians believe their illness is "all in my head." Physicians often are frustrated because there are no effective therapies for certain disorders. Complementary practitioners do not differentiate the body from the mind and spirit. The practitioner listens to the patient and prescribes a remedy. The clinician-patient encounter itself is healing.

Unconventional providers acknowledge the existence of and use the "placebo effect," which was first described as a modern biomedical concept in 1955 in Beecher's classic article "The Powerful Placebo." He used a meta-analytic method to aggregate the percentage of patients helped by placebo across 15 clinical trials. Of 1082 patients, 35% experienced benefits. Herbert Benson, among others, explored this concept further by renaming it "remembered wellness," and teaching clients the relaxation response, meditation, and prayer to help in recovery. Ultimately, Benson found that faith is central to human life and health and that faith in an infallible force is the most healing.

Post and coworkers recently have stated that "more attention to patient spirituality in the context of standard medical care could attract more patients to proven interventions. The keys to emotional coping with serious illness and disability are frequently found within the matrix of patient spirituality." Physicians, however, rarely ask patients about their religious beliefs. A recent study by King and Bushwick found that 77% of patients said physicians should consider patients' spiritual needs, but 68% said their physician had never discussed religious beliefs with them. Matthews and coworkers suggest that physicians integrate two questions into their initial interviews with patients: "Is your religion (or faith) helpful to you in coping with your illness?" If the answer is yes, then the physician should ask, "What can I do to support your faith (or religious belief)?"

## Physicians Response to Alternative Medicine

Physicians should learn more about alternative therapies, understand what they are, and apply scientific methods to test them. According to Relman, there is no such thing as alternative medicine—only medicine that has been proven to work and medicine that has not. Unconventional medicine may work, but we will not know that it does until we have better evidence.

Physicians should promote open communication with patients who seek help from these alternative methods, and they should always ask patients about their use of unconventional therapy when obtaining medical histories. When examining a new patient or evaluating a new condition, it is important to ask the patient if he or she is using any unconventional therapies. The physician should ask if they are using any herbs, vitamins, or supplements; if they have tried using other therapies; what benefits they hope for when using these therapies; and whether these therapies are helping. The physician needs to be aware of any possible interactions between the complementary therapy and the prescribed conventional regimen. It also is very helpful to ask the patient what he or she believes is wrong and how the problem can be alleviated by using these therapies. With new patients, it can be very helpful to take a religious history and seek help from clergy when needed. Conventional providers can improve communication with patients by listening carefully with special attention to emotional issues and religious beliefs. In today's frantic and increasingly impersonal world, many patients seek simplicity, clarity, attention, and a human touch from their doctors. Physicians should welcome this demand from their patients and spend more time with them. Physicians must remain their patients' advocates and make time for their patients.

# CHAPTER 10 MEDICAL ASPECTS OF TERRORISM

## General Background

The Federal Bureau of Investigation defines terrorism as the unlawful use of force or violence against persons or property for the purpose of intimidating or coercing a government, the civilian population or any segment thereof, because of intolerance of political and social objectives. Until the events of September 11, 2001, many people believed the U.S. was largely immune to terrorist attack. However, at present, the U.S. is a target for over 32% of all terrorist attacks worldwide, second only to Israel. Terrorist attacks in this country are expected to increase roughly at the rate of 15% per year.

Nuclear, biological, and chemical weapons of mass destruction can be used to kill or injure significant numbers of people, decimate livestock, and destroy crops. The goal of the clinician in regards to nuclear, biological and chemical (NBC) terrorism is early recognition of covert attacks; implementation of appropriate general and specific public health measures to minimize morbidity and mortality for the public, first responders, and health care workers; treatment of affected persons; and timely, effective communication and education of the public about related health risks and preventive measures. The initial management for victims of nuclear, biological, or chemical terrorism should include treatment of life-threatening medical conditions, decontamination, and proper exposure-specific treatment. Medical providers should be vigilant, identifying clusters of specific symptoms in terms of geographic location and timing, as well as concomitant outbreaks of disease in human and animal populations.

## Nuclear Terrorism

The killing and destructive power of ionizing radiation was proven by the destruction of Hiroshima and Nagasaki by atomic bombs.

Terrorists could disseminate ionizing radiation either overtly via nuclear detonation or radiation dispersal devices (RDD) using conventional explosives, or covertly through low-grade exposures (e.g., environmental, water, or food pollution). A nuclear detonation results in extremely high dose rates in the first minute (prompt radiation); additional radiation results from the products of fission in fallout. If nuclear material forms a critical mass, the resultant nuclear reaction may release gamma and neutron radiation even without a nuclear explosion. A radiation dispersal device can also emit a high enough dose to cause acute cellular damage.

### Ionizing Radiation

Radiation interacting with atoms causes ionization (electron excitation). Biochemical changes from ionizing radiation include free-radical formation (including toxic hyperoxide molecules) and the breaking and reforming of chemical bonds, including intrastrand and interstrand bond formation in DNA. Cellular changes include disrupted cell growth and motility, increased cellular permeability, and delays in the mitotic cycle. Cells that are either rapidly dividing or else relatively undifferentiated are most affected.

The hazardous effects of ionizing energy vary with the type of radiation and the method of exposure. Radiation-associated injury and illness can be associated with high-energy waves (gamma rays) and with three major kinds of particles. In general order of increasing hazard, they are the following:

1. Alpha particles are charged, massive particles that are unable to penetrate the skin or clothing due to their size. They are a negligible external hazard, but when emitted from an internalized radionuclide source they can cause significant local cell damage.
2. Beta particles are light, charged particles found primarily in radiation fallout. They can travel short distances in tissue and reach the skin's "germinal layer." Persons exposed to large quantities of beta radiation can develop beta burns (similar to thermal burns). Beta radiation is both an external hazard (primarily to the skin and to the lens of the eye) and an internal hazard.
3. Gamma rays are energetic waves (waves have no charge) that are similar to, but of higher energy than, X-rays. They are emitted during nuclear detonation and occur in fallout. They easily penetrate tissue to expose all tissues and organs of the body (whole-body exposure). They are both an external and an internal hazard and frequently accompany the emission of alpha and beta radiation.
4. Neutrons are uncharged particles from atomic nuclei and are emitted primarily from unstable nuclei formed during certain kinds of nuclear detonations. Even though they do not constitute a fallout hazard, they cause twenty times more tissue damage than gamma rays and are an external hazard.

### Acute radiation syndrome

Acute radiation syndrome (ARS) is a sequence of signs and symptoms that vary depending on the type of radiation and dose absorbed but follow a predictable course. Radiation dose is directly correlated with the severity of symptoms and inversely related to the lengths of the prodromal and latent phases (Table 10.1).

- *Initial or Prodromal phase.* Early onset of nausea, vomiting, malaise, and anorexia within minutes to hours after exposure suggests a large radiation dose. This may also be confused with psychogenic vomiting resulting from stress or fear. Use of oral prophylactic antiemetics such as granisetron (Kytril) or ondansetron (Zofran) may be indicated.
- *Latent phase.* This is a relatively symptom-free period following recovery from the prodromal phase. The length of this phase varies inversely with the radiation dose. During this phase, critical cell populations such as white cells and platelets decrease because of bone-marrow insult. Because of the extreme time variability of this phase, it may not always be practical to hospitalize all persons suspected of having radiation injury.
- *Illness phase.* During this phase the person manifests the overt clinical symptoms. Although blood- and lymph-forming bone marrow is the most radiosensitive tissue, followed by cells of the reproductive system, the most prominent acute effects from radiation involve the bone marrow and the gastrointestinal system. The illnesses can be characterized by infection, electrolyte imbalances, diarrhea, bleeding, cardiovascular collapse, and sometimes periods of unconsciousness. Death or a period of recovery follows.

### High-dose radiation: acute effects

Bone-marrow depression leading to pancytopenia occurs when a patient receives radiation doses between 0.7 and 4 Gray (Gy). (A Gray is a unit used to measure absorbed doses of radiation.) The peripheral blood profile may change as early as 24 hours after radiation. Lymphocytes will be depressed most rapidly; a 50% drop in lymphocytes within 24 hours indicates significant radiation injury. The effect of radiation damage to the bone marrow myelopoietic cells is seen in the peripheral blood neutrophil count within two to four days. Although platelets and megakaryocytes are fairly radioresistant, moderate doses of radiation kill thrombopoietic cells and lead to thrombocytopenia three to four weeks after exposure. Erythropoietic cells are the least radiosensitive and recover earliest; thrombopoietic regeneration lags behind both erythropoiesis and myelopoiesis; and lymphopoiesis regeneration after sublethal exposures is usually complete within weeks to months. In general, problems with bleeding, anemia, and decreased resistance to infection are seen on an average at two to three weeks.

Prevention and management of infection is the primary goal when a patient is neutropenic. Patients with profound neutropenia (absolute neutrophil counts [ANC] less than 100 cells per microliter) are the group at greatest risk of developing infections and should be considered for broad-spectrum antibiotic prophylaxis even when afebrile. Life-threatening Gram-negative bacterial infections are common, but the prevalence of life-threatening gram positive infections vary among institutions. As the duration of neutropenia increases, the risk of secondary infections such as invasive mycoses increases. Adjuvant therapy with cytokines is therefore invaluable. Hematopoietic growth factors such as G-CSF and GM-CSF are potent stimulators of hematopoiesis and shorten the neutrophil recovery time. For maximum clinical response, these growth factors should be started 24 to 72 hours after radiation exposure. When an established or suspected infection (with neutropenia and fever) exists, high doses of broad-spectrum antibiotics should be given. Therapy should continue till the patient is afebrile for 24 hours and the ANC is greater than 500 cells per microliter.

Higher radiation doses (6–8 Gy) result in the gastrointestinal syndrome and is almost always accompanied by bone marrow suppression. The small intestine is extremely vulnerable to radiation effects due to the rapidly dividing and migratory cells within the villi. The loss of intestinal cell production in the background of continued cell loss results in denuded intestinal mucosa. In a few days to weeks, the patient will have severe fluid losses, hemorrhage, and diarrhea. Due to the bone-marrow suppression, this degree of radiation may not stimulate an inflammatory response.

The neurovascular syndrome occurs only at very high doses (20–40 Gy) of radiation. The patient develops edema from microvascular leaks from radiation damage. Cerebral edema results in steadily deteriorating consciousness beginning one hour to three days after exposure, with eventual coma and death. There may be convulsions but little or no indication of increased intracranial pressure.

### High-dose radiation: chronic effects

Other long-term medical concerns after radiation exposure include carcinogenesis, cataract formation, infertility, and congenital malformations (from exposure *in utero*). Psychological concerns often result from uncertainty about one's own ultimate fate after radiation exposure. Phobias, general depression, anxiety, and posttraumatic stress syndrome may occur.

### Management of acute radiation syndrome

Almost all radiation injuries are treatable, and survivability is significantly improved with good medical care. Without appropriate medical care for severe

**TABLE 10.1. Phases of Acute Radiation Syndrome**

| Phase of Syndrome | Feature | Whole body radiation dose from external radiation or internal absorption (cGy = centiGray) | | | | | |
|---|---|---|---|---|---|---|---|
| | | Subclinical Range | | Sublethal Range | | Lethal Range | |
| | | 0–100 | 100–200 | 200–600 | 600–800 | 800–3000 | >3000 |
| Initial or prodromal | Nausea, vomiting (%) | 0 | 5–50 | 50–100 | 75–100 | 90–100 | 100 |
| | Time of onset (hours) | | 3–6 | 2–4 | 1–2 | <1 | <1 |
| | Duration (hours) | | <24 | <24 | <48 | <48 | <48 |
| | Lymphocyte count | | | <1000 at 24 h | <500 at 24 h | | |
| | CNS impairment level | None | None | Routine task performance | Simple and routine task performance | Progressive incapacitation | |
| | Duration (hours) | | | 6–20 | >24 | | |
| Latent | Duration (days) | >14 | 7–15 | 0–7 | 0–2 | None | |
| "Manifest illness" (obvious illness) | Organ system | None | | Hematopoietic and respiratory (mucosal) systems | | GI tract mucosal systems | CNS |
| | Signs and symptoms | None | Moderate leukopenia | Severe leukopenia, purpura, hemorrhage<br>Pneumonia<br>Hair loss (>300 cGy doses) | | Diarrhea, fever, electrolyte disturbance | Convulsions, ataxia, tremor, lethargy |
| | Time of onset (days) | | >14 | 2–14 | | 2–3 | |
| | Critical period (days) | | None | 28–42 | | 5–14 | 0–2 |
| | Hospitalization (%) | 0 | <5 | 90 | 100 | 100 | 100 |
| | Duration (days) | | 45–60 | 60–90 | 90+ | 14 | 2 |
| | Fatality (%) | 0 | 0 | 0–80 | 90–100 | 90–100 | |
| | Time to death | | | 3 wks–3 months | | 1–2 wks | 1–2 days |

radiation sickness, the median lethal dose of radiation, the $LD_{50/60}$ (the dose that will kill 50% of an exposed group within 60 days), is 3.5 Gy. Victims of supralethal doses of radiation are usually severely injured by the blast and heat from the nuclear detonation and die within hours to days from the combination of their traumatic injuries and radiation dose (the two act synergistically).

*External radiation contamination*

The most common exposures involve beta-particle skin burns (with subsequent scarring) and whole-body irradiation from gamma radiation. Skin changes are related to dose of radiation. Acute radiation doses of 6–20 Sieverts (Sv is a unit used to measure the biological effects of radiation) typically cause erythema only, doses of 20–40 Sv cause skin breakdown in 2 weeks, and doses greater than 3000 Sv cause acute blistering.

Decontamination helps prevent beta skin damage (so-called beta burns). Simple removal of clothing may decrease the patient's contamination by as much as 90%. The patient should then be decontaminated with soap and water. The radioactive hazard to medical personnel is negligible when dealing with a contaminated patient and life-saving medical and surgical care should therefore not be delayed.

*Internal radiation contamination*

Routes of internal contamination include inhalation, ingestion, and skin absorption of radioactive material as well as wound contamination by radioactive material. Internal contamination can be subsequently confirmed via 24-hour urine or stool collections.

The goal of treatment of internal contamination is to reduce the absorbed radiation dose in order to decrease morbidity. Gastric lavage helps to empty the stomach contents, and cathartics and enemas help reduce the time the radioactive materials are in the colon. Ion-exchange resins decrease radionuclide uptake from ingested or inhaled material. Blocking agents such as iodide compounds (supersaturated potassium iodide [SSKI], or Lugol's solution) need to be given soon (within about two hours of exposure to radioactive iodine) in order to block uptake into thyroid tissue. Mobilizing agents such as propylthiouracil or methimazole can reduce retention of radioactive iodine in the thyroid. Chelating agents can facilitate removal of many metals, but they should be used with extreme caution in patients with pre-existing renal disease (Table 10.2).

## Summary

After radiation exposure, medical personnel should first treat life-threatening injuries. The length of the prodromal and latent periods; the presence and severity of the early signs and symptoms of nausea, vomiting, diarrhea, mental status changes, and shock; and changes in lymphocyte count in the first 48 hours are the most reliable indicators of the radiation dose and the patient's prognosis. Treatment of a patient after radiation exposure is primarily supportive unless high-dose irradiation or specific internal contaminants are present.

**TABLE 10.2. Treatment for Selected Internal Radiation Contaminants**

| Radionuclide | Medication | For Ingestion/Inhalation | Principle of Action |
|---|---|---|---|
| Iodine | KI (potassium iodide) | 130 mg (po) stat, followed by 130 mg q.d.×7 if indicated | Blocks thyroid deposition |
| Rare earths<br>Plutonium<br>Transplutonics<br>Yttrium | Zn-DTPA<br>Ca-DTPA | 1 gm Ca-DTPA (Zn-DTPA) in 150–250 ml 5% D/W IV over 60 minutes | Chelation |
| Uranium | Bicarbonate | 2 ampules sodium bicarbonate (44.3 mEq each; 7.5%) in 1000 cc half-normal saline @ 125 cc/hr; alternately, oral administration of two bicarbonate tablets every 4 hrs until the urine reaches a pH of 8–9 | Alkalinization of urine; reduces chance of acute tubular necrosis |
| Cesium<br>Rubidium<br>Thallium | Prussian Blue | 1 gm with 100–200 ml water p.o. t.i.d. for several days | Blocks absorption from GI tract and prevents recycling |
| Tritium | Water | Force fluids | Isotopic dilution |

DTPA = diethylenetriamine pentaacetic acid; Prussian Blue = ferric hexacyanoferrate

## Biological Terrorism

Several aspects of biological terrorism make it an attractive option for extremists. First of all, it can be highly lethal. Second, obtaining and delivering the agents is not difficult. They are generally far cheaper and easier to produce than nuclear weapons. The agents themselves can be obtained from medical supply companies, and delivery systems are available from industrial supply houses. The agents can be disseminated by several means, including aerial bombs, spray tanks, and ballistic missiles. Third, the long lag time between dispersal and an identifiable death allows time for terrorists to escape and cover their tracks. Fourth, in contrast to nuclear and chemical weapons, the terrorists can often use either vaccines or prophylactic antibiotics to try to protect themselves. Finally, because of the risks of possible unapparent spread of infection, a biological attack may generate more "terror" than chemical or even radiologic terrorism. However, the rapid recognition of a bioterrorist attack could save literally thousands of lives.

The list of potential bioterrorism agents is long and includes a variety of "exotic" and well-known infections. The conditions associated with the agents that appear the most likely to be used in a bioterrorism attack are 1) anthrax (a bacterial infection by *Bacillus anthracis*), 2) plague (a bacterial infection by *Yersinia pestis*), 3) smallpox (a viral infection, *variola major*, from exposure to smallpox virus), 4) tularemia (a bacterial infection from *Francisella tularensis*), and 5) viral hemorrhagic fevers (VHF, a group of viral infections from exposure to viruses such as Ebola and Marburg viruses). We need to become familiar with these pathogens because most U.S. physicians, our first line of medical defense, have never seen a case. As mentioned, botulinum toxin is strictly speaking a chemical rather than a living biological agent and will therefore be discussed specifically in the chemical terrorism section of this chapter.

### Anthrax

Anthrax is the most likely bioterrorism agent. It has been used in warfare since World War I, when German agents allegedly tried to infect horses and mules in American ports with anthrax and glanders. Japan developed anthrax as a biological weapon before and during World War II and used it on at least two Chinese cities. The U.S., along with almost all of the other major powers at the time, developed anthrax bombs during World War II; however, the U.S. refrained from using them and in the 1970s destroyed them. However, the Soviet Union continued the clandestine development of anthrax, as evidenced by the accident in 1979 in Sverdlovsk where over 60 workers and local residents died of inhalation anthrax after a leak from a secret biological-weapons plant. Iraq used anthrax on Iran and deployed anthrax-filled SCUD missiles during the Second Persian Gulf War (Operation Desert Storm). Anthrax was also used in the recent U.S. postal attacks.

Aerosolized anthrax, used as a bioweapon, induces inhalational anthrax, in which the inhaled organism is taken up by macrophages and rapidly infects mediastinal lymph nodes. Replicating bacteria produce several toxins, which are primarily responsible for the hemorrhage, edema, tissue necrosis, and ultimately death. Fatal sequelae can and do occur even after appropriate antibiotics are given.

Clinically, inhalation anthrax is a two-stage disease. Classically, nonspecific flu-like symptoms first develop one to two days after inhalation but may then temporarily improve. However, a few days later, the patient returns extremely ill with high fever, dyspnea, diaphoresis, and chest pain. The chest radiograph may show an enlarged mediastinum, and chest CT can confirm enlarged mediastinal lymph nodes. Up to half of the cases may develop hemorrhagic meningitis. Shock and death occur rapidly. Sputum is often blood streaked, and Gram staining reveals gram-positive rods. A buffy coat of the blood is often positive, and the organism often grows rapidly in culture, where, however, it may be mistaken for a contaminant. Gram stains of cerebrospinal fluid from meningitic patients are also likely to show gram-positive organisms.

Unfortunately, because of the rarity of the natural disease in the U.S., a low index of suspicion, and the nonspecific early signs and symptoms, anthrax may not be recognized early enough to prevent the death of the index case or cases. The first cases will be those with high-inoculum inhalations; the rest will present over the next few days. The smaller the inoculum, the longer is the latent period and thus the later the clinical presentation. Ciprofloxacin is the drug of choice, with amoxicillin and doxycycline reasonable alternatives. Other fluoroquinolones are likely effective but not yet extensively tested. More important than saving the index case will be recognition of what is happening and initiation of early treatment of Stage I patients as well as institution of prophylaxis for asymptomatic exposed individuals. The same drugs are used for prophylaxis, but for 60 days. Although an anthrax vaccine has been developed and has been used to vaccinate members of the U.S. Armed Forces since 1998, the vaccine is not currently available in large enough quantities for postexposure prophylaxis of the public.

Anthrax can also cause cutaneous disease and intestinal disease. Cutaneous anthrax skin lesions usually develop within a week after exposure, in contrast to inhalation anthrax, which can develop weeks or months after exposure. Pruritic vesicles progress to round ulcerating lesions. Development of a coal-like (anthracotic) black eschar is characteristic. Patients respond slowly to antibiotics, but treatment protects against dissemination and is associated with a good outcome. Gram stains of the discharge can be positive, but a biopsy is often necessary to make the diagnosis. Intestinal anthrax occurs following oral ingestion. Initial symptoms include nausea, vomiting, abdominal pain, and bloody diarrhea. Antibiotic treatment is the same as for inhalation anthrax, but the diagnosis is often not suspected until the patient is *in extremis*.

No person-to-person transmission occurs with any form of anthrax, but anthrax spores live on for decades in the environment. Secondary aerosolization, for some time thought to be uncharacteristic of anthrax, depends on factors such as strain, culture medium, and processing (e.g., milling); moreover, estimates of the infective dose, once thought to be in the range of thousands of spores, also depend partially on physical characteristics of the aerosol agent and may need to be revised downward for particular preparations of anthrax. Factors such as these could require the eventual immunization of those living in contaminated environments.

## Plague

Plague, an infection caused by the gram-negative bacterium *Yersinia pestis*, is also a likely bioterrorist agent. Plague is the oldest known biowarfare agent. In 1346, the Tatars catapulted plague corpses into the besieged city of Kaffa in an apparent attempt to induce plague in its defenders. During World War II, the Japanese raised millions of plague-infected human fleas, placed them in clay, and dropped them onto the Chinese cities of Changteh and Chuhsien. There were indeed temporally related outbreaks of bubonic plague, but through proper identification and quarantine, larger outbreaks did not occur.

Today's terrorists might choose to employ clandestine spraying of the organism to induce widespread pneumonic plague. Although less common than bubonic or lymphatic plague (so-called "Black Death"), it is rapidly fatal. Person-to-person spread and the image of the Black Death could make its immediate terror value greater than that of anthrax.

Pneumonic plague presents after a two- to three-day incubation period, after which hospitals are eventually flooded with cases of fulminant pneumonia. Patients present with high fever, headache, and myalgias. Chest radiographs show patchy or consolidated bronchopneumonia. Sputum is blood-tinged, and many patients rapidly develop shock and die. The sputum shows bipolar (safety-pin-shaped) gram-negative coccobacillary forms. Pneumonic plague is easily transmissible person-to-person via relatively large respiratory droplets. Therefore, if the organism is not suspected and if droplet precautions are not taken, panic could ensue among hospital personnel.

Streptomycin is the drug of choice but will probably not be available in large quantities and requires injections. Tetracycline, chloramphenicol, and gentamicin can be used. Hospital personnel should be put on prophylaxis with doxycycline or trimethoprim/sulfamethoxasole. Fluoroquinolones could be used and should be available from national stockpiles maintained for use in the event of bioterrorism. Post-exposure vaccination is recommended for those at continued risk, but the vaccine is not widely available at the present time.

## Smallpox

Smallpox virus causes several varieties of smallpox, the major clinical form of which is called *variola major*. The first use of smallpox as a biological weapon came during the French and Indian Wars, when the British distributed smallpox-contaminated blankets to the Indians. Universal smallpox immunization of civilian and military populations during the 19$^{th}$ century significantly decreased its potential use as a weapon, but with the global eradication of smallpox in 1980, countries stopped routine vaccination. U.S. military personnel continued routine vaccination for a short time thereafter, because the former Soviet Union produced large quantities of smallpox during the 1980s and 1990s. Almost half the U.S. population has now never been vaccinated against smallpox, and those that have received the vaccine in their youth are likely no longer immune. Current stockpiles of vaccine and hyper-immune sera are small.

If smallpox were used as a bioweapon, it would likely be aerosolized, probably inside a building. The incubation period is long (a typical range is 12 to 14 days). The initial cases present with the sudden onset of high fever, malaise, headache, myalgia, abdominal pain, and delirium. Initial symptoms are much like influenza but more severe. A deep-seated maculopapular rash appears shortly, seen first on the face and including the pharynx and oral mucosa. The rash progresses to vesicles and then deep pustules within days. These spread to the upper arms, and then to the legs and trunk. Unlike the rash in chickenpox, the macules, papules, and vesicles in smallpox are generally at approximately the same stage of development at the same time. The rash progresses from the extremities toward the trunk, but the *density* of the lesions is greater on the face and the extremities. Thus, the *progression* is centripetal but the *distribution* is centrifugal. Encephalitis can occur, as can a hemorrhagic fever presentation; both presentations carry a grave prognosis.

The virus can be isolated from the skin lesions, but the diagnosis is generally suspected on clinical grounds. Smallpox is most commonly mistaken for chickenpox, but the rash of chickenpox generally starts on the trunk, rather than on the face, has shallower ulcers, and progresses asynchronously, with macules, papules, and vesicles of different stages of development at the same time. Also, the exanthema in chickenpox is denser on covered parts of the body; that is, it is centripetal in distribution compared with the centrifugally distributed rash of smallpox. Serologic tests for smallpox turn positive only after a week. From approximately the time of onset of fever and of the first mouth and skin lesions until the sloughing of the scabs (about three weeks), the disease is extremely efficiently spread person-to-person (and often throughout buildings unless special ventilation is in place) by much smaller aerosolized droplets than those of plague. Thus, respiratory precautions (not just droplet precautions) are mandated for smallpox patients. Mortality rates for non-immune patients are about 30%, with death generally occurring during the second week of illness from overwhelming systemic toxicity.

Treatment is largely supportive and includes antibiotics for bacterial superinfections. No antiviral therapy has proven efficacious, although cidofovir is effective in tissue culture. The major efforts of the professional staff are isolation of the index case and vaccination of all known face-to-face contacts, and containment of infection by respiratory isolation and quarantine as indicated. The virus itself cannot exist in the environment for more than a few days. Experience from outbreaks of imported smallpox from the 1960s and 1970s in Europe suggests high nosocomial transmission. In the event of an attack, a specific hospital may be designated for all suspected smallpox cases.

The current vaccines, even if they were to be made more widely available, have significant toxicity, making the risk-benefit decision difficult. Clearly, all exposed individuals should be vaccinated within four days of exposure. However, post-vaccination encephalitis with a 25% mortality rate occurs once in every 300,000 vaccinations. Cutaneous complications are more common but less likely to be fatal. Most reactions occur in primary immunizations rather than revaccinations. As a result, universal vaccination is unlikely to be instituted, and when vaccines become more widely available, pre-exposure vaccination will likely be limited to medical personnel.

## Tularemia

Tularemia in humans is an uncommon zoonotic illness of rural North America, Europe, and Northern Asia. The causative organism, *Francisella tularensis*, is a bacterial infection of small mammals including rabbits and squirrels. Humans become infected through the bite of infected arthropods (ticks, flies, and mosquitoes) or from direct contact with infected animals. Tularemia was first developed by the Japanese during World War II as a biological weapon, and tularemia outbreaks among both the German and Russian troops during the war may have been intentionally started. The U.S. studied tularemia extensively as a bioweapon during the 1950s and 1960s because of its ability to incapacitate an enemy without killing large numbers of people. A live attenuated vaccine was also developed.

If *F. tularensis* were used as a bioweapon, it would likely be aerosolized. Thus, like anthrax and plague, inhalational tularemia would be the likely presenting disease. The incubation period can be up to two weeks, but generally the patient becomes ill three to five days after exposure. There is a nonspecific flu-like illness characterized by fever, severe headache, low back pain, sore throat, and respiratory symptoms. Disease progression is slower than with anthrax or plague. A pulse-temperature dissociation, as seen with typhoid, is characteristic, as is the production of prominent watery sputum. Fatal cases develop sepsis, respiratory failure, and shock. Chest radiographs typically show multilobar bronchial pneumonia. Pleural effusions and hilar adenopathy are common. Sputum shows small gram-negative coccobacillary organisms easily confused on a stain with *Haemophilus influenzae*. The diagnosis is confirmed with positive blood, sputum, and pharnygeal cultures. Mortality approaches 50% without treatment but is less than 2% in adequately treated patients.

Streptomycin is the drug of choice for tularemia, but other aminoglycosides (gentamicin) are likely to be used in an attack because of their readier availability. Doxycycline is an effective oral agent but is associated with more frequent treatment failures. Treatment is for 10 days with systemic drugs or 14 days with oral treatment. Fluoroquinolones are effective in both *in vitro* and also animal studies; a few successful trials in humans exist in the literature. Both β-lactam and macrolide antibiotics may have some efficacy and are the mainstays of current treatment of community-acquired pneumonia, but neither is considered a first-line drug, and patients should be switched to aminoglycosides when the bacterial diagnosis is made.

## Viral Hemorrhagic Fevers

The viral hemorrhagic fevers (VHF) include a wide range of infections that are characterized by structural damage to capillaries. Viruses from a variety of families, including filoviridae, bunyaviridae, flaviviridae, and arenaviridae can cause viral hemorrhagic fever syndromes.

Although acquiring these viruses could present a major challenge to terrorists, once acquired, they can be grown in cell cultures in sufficient quantities to allow weaponization. They are also highly infectious by aerosol delivery, although unstable after aerosolization. They produce organ-system involvement and clinical syndromes that vary among the different types of VHFs. There is a bleeding component to each hemorrhagic fever, but the bleeding usually presents as petechiae or ecchymoses rather than frank bleeding from bodily orifices. Fever, myalgia, and prostration are also common; and specific agents have predilections for certain organ systems (for example, the pulmonary system or the liver).

The mainstay of treatment is supportive care concentrating on the affected organ systems. Internal or external bleeding with or without hypotension and shock must be addressed. The antiviral compound ribavirin is effective treatment for certain of these conditions and should probably be tried in most if not all kinds of hemorrhagic fevers. The VHFs are not transmissible from person to person via the respiratory route, but standard precautions would nevertheless apply because of the possibility of transmission by contact with blood or blood-containing body fluids.

### Summary

Bioterrorism should be suspected when there is unusual temporal or geographic clustering of illness in previously healthy individuals or when there are simultaneous outbreaks in both animals and humans. Decontamination of affected patients is usually not required beyond removal and biosafety bagging of clothing and skin washing with soap and water. Equipment used in the care of affected patients should be handled according to standard infection-control practices.

## Chemical Terrorism

The massive use of chemical-warfare agents in modern times dates from April 1915, when an estimated 168 tons of chlorine gas released from emplaced cylinders by German units near Ypres, Belgium killed over 800 French and Algerian soldiers. Subsequently, the U.S. Army formed a chemical-warfare service, which later became the U.S. Army Chemical Corps and was assigned the development of and defense against chemical-warfare agents. Later, the U.S. renounced all use of chemical and biological weapons and restricted its research to defensive programs. Iraq developed stockpiles of chemical, biological, and toxin weapons and in the 1980s used both nerve agents and vesicants against Iranian soldiers. At the end of the Gulf War, the Iraqi military was found to have 100 bombs and 13 SCUD missiles containing botulinum toxin.

Development of the binary concept of chemical weapons in the 1960s has made it more practical for terrorists and militaries to store large quantities of chemical agents. This concept allows two less toxic chemical-agent precursors to be stored separately and then mixed at the time of deployment to form the desired chemical agent.

**TABLE 10.3. Signs Suggestive of a Chemical Terrorism Attack**

- Geographic clusters of dead plants, insects, fish, birds, or other animals
- Mass casualties with numerous individuals exhibiting unexplained serious health problems, especially when affected individuals all have similar symptoms or physical findings
- Unusual liquid drops of an oily or film-like nature on numerous surfaces
- Unexplained odors
- Low-flying clouds or a fog-like condition that is not explained by surrounding weather conditions
- Unusual metal debris from bomb or munitions-like material used to deliver these agents

The identification of a possible chemical terrorism attack is not as easy as one would expect. If the agent is a slow-reacting agent and if it has been disseminated over a wide area, it is very likely that the effects will not be readily apparent at one particular treatment facility. So individuals should be on the alert for signs that are very suggestive of a recent chemical attack (Table 10.3)

### The Nature of Chemical Agents

Chemical agents can kill, seriously injure, or incapacitate people. Lethal agents are those capable of causing death within seconds or hours after exposure. The amount (dose) of liquid agent expected to kill 50% of a group is referred to as the $LD_{50}$, and the amount of liquid agent required to incapacitate half of a group is called the $ID_{50}$. External doses of agents existing as gases or vapors are estimated by multiplying concentration (C) by duration of exposure (time, t) to obtain a so-called Ct product, and with this concept, $LCt_{50}$ and $ICt_{50}$ correspond to $LD_{50}$ and $ID_{50}$, respectively. The North Atlantic Treaty Organization (NATO) has assigned one- or two-letter NATO codes to most of the chemical agents.

Chemical agents can also be classified by their tendency to remain in the environment. Thus, nonpersistent agents remain in target areas for a relatively short period of time, generally less than a day. Agents that remain in the environment longer than a day are considered to be persistent. However, persistence is affected not only by chemical structure but also by environmental factors such as temperature, humidity, and the nature of terrain and of environmental surfaces.

Some chemical agent exposures can be verified by

specific testing protocols, but treatment should be initiated based on symptoms and signs. Therefore, classification of agents by physiologic effects is emphasized to facilitate recognition, management, and treatment of exposures to different types of agents (Table 10.4).

Chemical agents can be classified as:

- Lung agents which effect pulmonary structures of oxygen transport systems,
- Vesicant agents which effect skin or mucous membrane integrity,
- Nerve agents which effect neural transmission,
- Botulinum toxin which also effects neural transmission and is sometimes grouped with the "living-organism" biological agents, and
- Incapacitating agents which produce only temporary disabling effects usually by altering consciousness and perception.

## Lung Agents

Poisons that involve the respiratory tract can be grouped into three categories: Type I agents (usually highly water-soluble or highly chemical reactive) affect the part of the airway (down to the level of the terminal bronchioles) that moves air by bulk flow. Type I agents cause necrosis and sloughing (often as pseudomembranes) of tracheal and bronchial respiratory epithelium. Type II agents (less soluble or less chemically reactive) damage the gas-exchange region distal to the terminal bronchioles. After a latent period inversely correlated with dose, Type II agents lead to noncardiogenic pulmonary edema. It is important to realize that a massive dose of either a Type I or Type II agent will affect both the central airways and peripheral gas exchange regions. Type III agents, general asphyxiants such as cyanide and hydrogen sulfide, use the respiratory tract only as a means to enter the general circulation and reach cells throughout the body.

### "Choking" and "pulmonary" agents

Exposure to choking and pulmonary agents, which at room temperature exist generally as gases, is by inhalation; and except in extremely massive exposures, the site of clinical effects is the respiratory tract. The odor of sulfur mustard has been described as that of mustard, garlic, onions, or horseradish; that of phosgene has classically been compared to newly mown hay.

Type I agents in low to moderate doses cause eye and throat irritation, coughing, sneezing, hoarseness, inspiratory stridor, wheezing, and upper airway obstruction; laryngospasm from irritation at the level of the vocal folds is also common. Type II agents initially

**TABLE 10.4. Physiologic Effects of Chemical Agents**

| Agent Class | Specific Agents | Physiologic Effects | Recommended Protection* |
|---|---|---|---|
| Lung agents | | | |
| Type I 'Choking' | Mineral acids/bases<br>Sulfur mustard | Pseudomembranes of upper airway; laryngospasm | Inhalation hazard mask |
| Type II 'Pulmonary' | Phosgene<br>Diphosgene | Noncardiogenic pulmonary edema | Inhalation hazard mask |
| Type III 'Blood' | Hydrogen cyanide<br>Cyanogen chloride | Asphyxiant | Inhalation hazard mask |
| | Arsine | Intravascular hemolysis | |
| Vesicants | Mustards<br>Arsenical vesicants | Blistering resembling burns; pseudomembranes of upper airway | Level A protective suit |
| | Phosgene oxime | Hives, rather than blisters | |
| Nerve agents | Tabun, sarin, cyclosarin, soman, VX | Cholinergic crisis | Level A protective suit |
| Botulinum toxin | | Descending paralysis | Inhalation hazard mask |
| Incapacitating agents | BZ | Anticholinergic crisis | Level C protective suit with respirator |

**Level A* requires a completely encapsulating, gas/vapor proof chemical resistant suit; a self-contained breathing apparatus (SCBA) or positive pressure supplied air respirator with escape SCBA; both outer and inner chemical resistant gloves; and chemical resistant boots, with steel toe and shank. *Level B* differs from level A gear in that it requires only hooded chemical resistant clothing, rather than the completely encapsulated suit. *Level C* only requires a NIOSH-approved full-face or half mask air purifying respirator, rather than a self-contained breathing apparatus.

cause dyspnea without associated clinical signs; dyspnea within four hours of exposure portends a grave outcome.

Treatment of Type I exposures includes administration of warm, moist air, bronchoscopic removal of pseudomembranes and other necrotic debris, and surveillance for secondary bacterial pneumonia. With Type II exposures, a suitable acronym is TROT: Trust the patient (i.e., accept that dyspnea without signs may indicate incipient pulmonary edema); Rest the patient (exertion, even that from walking, may precipitate a crisis); Observe the patient (because of the latent period); and Transfer the patient as needed to pulmonary intensive-care unit where empirical treatment for pulmonary edema can be instituted. Corticosteroids for the prevention or treatment of pulmonary edema are not indicated unless there is accompanying bronchospasm (as in asthmatics), or unless the Type II agent is either an oxide of nitrogen or HC smoke (a standard military obscurant smoke), neither of which is likely to be used as the primary agent in a terrorist scenario.

### "Blood" agents

*Cyanides*

The cyanides hydrogen cyanide (AC) and cyanogen chloride (CK) are designated "blood agents." They are Type III agents, which are absorbed via the respiratory tract and then systemically distributed in the blood. However, the chief actions of the cyanides are in cells throughout the body, where they bind to an enzyme (cytochrome $aa_3$) within mitochondria, thus impairing cellular utilization of oxygen and cellular generation of energy as ATP (hydrogen sulfide has the same mechanism of action).

At usual ambient temperatures, the cyanides exist either as gases or as volatile liquids producing toxic vapor. Hydrogen cyanide has an almond-like odor, but the ability to detect this odor is conferred by a gene absent in half the population. Cyanogen chloride is pungent and irritating because of its partial dissociation to chlorine.

Symptom onset depends in part upon concentration, but high concentrations of the cyanides act within a few seconds. Prominent gasping (tachypnea with hyperpnea) is quickly followed by loss of consciousness, convulsions, tetanus-like rigidity (including trismus and opisthotonus), decerebrate posture, and central apnea. The skin classically appears pink because of the decreased arteriovenous oxygen extraction. A high-anion-gap acidemia is also common. Exposure to relatively low concentrations is associated with nonspecific symptoms such as headache and nausea.

Antidotal treatment first involves administration of a nitrite (amyl nitrite via inhalation if the patient is breathing, but intravenous sodium nitrite in any case) to convert oxyhemoglobin to methemoglobin, which reversibly combines with cyanide to form cyanmethemoglobin. The next antidote, given intravenously after the nitrite, is sodium thiosulfate, which irreversibly converts cyanide to thiocyanate, which is excreted by the kidneys. General supportive care, including ventilatory support and (paradoxically) oxygen administration may be life-saving even in the absence of specific antidotes.

*Arsine*

Arsine is another Type III agent, absorbed via the respiratory tract but distributed systemically in the blood. Although it is generally not referred to as a "blood agent," its chief action is in fact to bind to circulating hemoglobin, reducing glutathione concentrations within erythrocytes and leading to massive intravascular hemolysis with resulting renal failure. It is also carcinogenic, but in high-dose situations recognition and management of the acute toxicity is the immediate priority.

At room temperature, it is a gas that in low concentrations may elude olfactory detection but that in higher concentrations has a disagreeable garlic-like odor from its arsenic moiety.

After a latent period of 2–24 hours, arsine-induced hemolysis leads to headache, weakness, and chills and eventually to abdominal pain and tenderness. Abdominal pain, hemoglobinuria, and bronze-tinted skin form the classical triad of severe arsine toxicity. The skin bronzing and also reddish discoloration of the conjunctivae represent deposition of extravasated hemoglobin and are relatively late signs, occurring 12–26 hours after exposure. Dyspnea, nausea, and vomiting are also commonly noted, as is jaundice in survivors.

Following removal from exposure and external decontamination with soap and water, the patient should receive general supportive care (including oxygen and cardiac monitoring) en route to an intensive-care unit. Monitoring of serum electrolytes and of serum and urine hemoglobin is essential. With acute hemolysis, the urine should be alkalinized with sodium bicarbonate, and urine output should be maintained with furosemide or mannitol, with careful avoidance of fluid overload. Exchange transfusion may be necessary, and renal failure may mandate dialysis. Neither British anti-Lewisite (BAL, dimercaprol) nor other chelating agents are effective in arsine poisoning.

## Vesicants (blister agents)

Blister agents or vesicants include sulfur mustard (H, HD), the nitrogen mustards ($HN_{1-3}$), arsenical vesicants such as Lewisite (L), and phosgene oxime (CG), an obscure Russian agent that is technically an urticant, producing hives rather than blisters.

### Mustards

Both sulfur mustard (H, for crude mustard; and HD, for distilled mustard) and the nitrogen mustards ($HN_1$, $HN_2$, and $HN_3$) have been stockpiled as chemical-warfare agents, but the most battlefield use by far has been of sulfur mustard, an oily amber to brown liquid (depending upon its purity) with the odor of mustard, garlic, onions, or horseradish (nitrogen mustards range from fishy in smell to odorless). They act by a variety of mechanisms, including rapid alkylation of DNA and other cellular constituents. They act locally on skin, eyes, and the respiratory tract; and in lethal doses (the $LD_{50}$ for mustard is 3 to 7 grams, or about a teaspoon) also affect the body as a whole.

Although sulfur mustard and nitrogen mustards damage cells within the first few minutes after exposure, latent periods (as usual, inversely correlated with dose) range from hours to a day and a half (nitrogen mustards have shorter latent periods compared to sulfur mustard). The skin develops small vesicles that coalesce to form large bullae; with large doses, necrosis and skin sloughing occur instead of vesication. The eyes exhibit reddening (from mustard conjunctivitis) and blepharospasm. At low to moderate doses, mustards are Type I agents, acting in the central pulmonary compartment to cause necrosis and sloughing of respiratory mucosa with associated coughing, wheezing, and partial to total obstruction; in higher doses, they can also cause pulmonary edema. Lethal doses are radiomimetic and kill rapidly dividing or poorly differentiated cells; the subsequent leukopenia can lead to a septic death from secondary bacterial pneumonia. Mustards are also carcinogenic and possibly teratogenic.

Victims must be removed from exposure and decontaminated as soon as possible with water, or with soap and water (bleach makes mustard burns worse) to prevent continuing absorption. There is no specific antidote, and treatment is symptomatic. Skin lesions from mustard are treated as thermal burns, with the exception that there is less fluid loss from mustard burns, and strict use of the Brooke or Parkland fluid-resuscitation guidelines may lead to overhydration. Large blisters may be drained without fear of chemical contamination because blister fluid contains no active mustard.

### Arsenical vesicants

The arsenical vesicants include Lewisite (L), the most important member of the class; methyldichloroarsine (MD), ethyldichloroarsine (ED), and phenyldichloroarsine (PD). Their mechanism of action is unclear but may involve DNA alkylation or effects on enzyme systems. All are oily colorless liquids that also release vapor; however, liquid contact generally produces more severe effects than does vapor exposure. Lewisite has a geranium-like odor; MD and ED may smell like rotting fruit.

The clinical effects of the arsenical vesicants are similar to those of the mustards with two prominent exceptions: 1) Pain occurs in 10 to 20 seconds or less and is followed by grayish necrosis (including graying of the cornea) in about five minutes and painful blisters in several hours; 2) They increase capillary permeability throughout the body, with the important consequences that pulmonary edema is more likely with these agents than with mustard and that more fluid will be required than in mustard patients.

Decontamination with water (or soap and water) at the earliest possible opportunity is critical. An antidote, British anti-Lewisite, or BAL (dimercaprol) exists and should be applied over affected skin areas. However, since it also chelates silver, it should not be applied over silver sulfadiazine.

### Urticants

Phosgene oxime (CG) is a Russian agent that causes corrosive acid-like skin burns and internal bleeding. It exists as a crystalline solid (below 104°F), and as a liquid (between 104° and 129°F) productive of a musty, peppery, prickling vapor. Because it produces urticaria (hives) rather than vesicles, it is technically an urticant; but because of its immediate severe stinging pain, it is also called a nettle agent. Its mechanism of action is not known.

Even very low concentrations of vapor are extremely irritating to the eyes and mucous membranes. Immediate pain on skin exposure is followed 30 seconds later by blanching ringed by erythema; a wheal forms during the next half-hour and eventually develops into a brown eschar with a long healing phase characterized by intense itching. Respiratory effects would be expected to be similar to those of Lewisite. In large doses, phosgene oxime is also associated with gastrointestinal hemorrhage, hypotension, and shock.

There is no specific antidote, and decontamination with water (or soap and water) at the earliest possible moment is vital, even though by the time pain is produced much agent has already penetrated the skin. Ulcers will require supportive care and possible debridement or even excision.

## Nerve agents

Nerve agents are organophosphorus-ester cholinesterase inhibitors that affect the process of cholinergic neurotransmission. In normal cholinergic transmission, the neurotransmitter acetylcholine released from neurons binds to: 1) muscarinic receptors in the central nervous system, exocrine glands, and smooth muscle; and 2) nicotinic receptors in autonomic ganglia and skeletal muscle. Once it has activated the end organ, acetylcholine is hydrolyzed by acetylcholinesterase present on the postsynaptic or postjunctional membrane.

Nerve agents bind essentially irreversibly to acetylcholinesterase, which is then unable to break down acetylcholine. Acetylcholine builds up in the synapse of the neuroglandular or neuromuscular junction and continues to stimulate the end organ. The result is cholinergic crisis, with hyperstimulation of the end organ, followed eventually by end-organ fatigue and failure.

There are two main kinds of nerve agents: 1) the G agents and 2) VX.

The G agents, which include tabun (GA), sarin (GB), soman (GD), and cyclosarin (GF), exist at room temperature as watery, colorless, nearly odorless, and nonirritating nonpersistent liquids (occasionally a sweet fruity odor is present) that also evaporate to produce toxic vapor. Liquid can be absorbed through the skin and from wounds and can cause clinical effects after a latent period of minutes to hours, representing time needed for transit through the skin. Absorption of inhaled vapor, however, is very rapid and can produce effects within seconds.

VX is a colorless, odorless, and nonirritating persistent liquid of approximately the consistency of motor oil. A drop the size of a bead of sweat represents the $LD_{50}$ of 10 mg for this compound. It is absorbed primarily through the skin and wounds. As with the G agents, there is a minutes-to-hours long latent period while the agent penetrates the skin. Once skin absorption has occurred, however, the effects of a massive dose may be just as sudden and precipitous as those of a massive dose of inhaled vapor.

Signs and symptoms may vary somewhat with the route of exposure. Common symptoms include dimness of vision associated with miosis, runny nose, and localized sweating; and then breathing difficulty, chest tightness, nausea, vomiting, abdominal cramps, twitching, staggering, confusion, convulsions, and coma.

Treatment consists of prompt removal from exposure, removal of contaminated clothing, and immediate decontamination to prevent continued absorption through the skin. Self-decontamination can be accomplished by using any kind of field-expedient blotting agent (flour, bread, talc, or special decontamination pads) and then rinsing with large amounts of water, which dilutes and hydrolyzes the agent. Water alone or with soap is faster and less damaging to the skin than are chemicals such as 0.5% hypochlorite solutions. Flushing with water is sufficient for the eyes.

Treatment involves removal from the agent and the use of a nerve-agent antidote kit, usually in the form of auto-injectors. The first antidote is atropine, which counteracts the muscarinic effects of nerve agents and which should be administered at intervals of ten minutes until airway resistance (difficulty breathing) and secretions decrease. The second antidote is an oxime (generally 2-pralidoxime chloride, or 2-PAM chloride), which counteracts nicotinic effects such as twitching and muscle weakness. Up to three autoinjectors of the oxime can be given concomitantly with atropine; additional doses are spaced farther apart. Severe poisonings will also require a benzodiazepine for seizure prevention or control. Assisted ventilation and secretion management may also be needed

### Botulinum toxin

The bacterium *Clostridium botulinum* produces at least seven neurotoxic proteins (serotypes A through G). The most toxic serotype for humans is botulinum toxin A, which gram for gram is the most lethal poison known, with an $LD_{50}$ of about 3 ng/kg by inhalation (1 ng/kg parenterally). Botulinum toxin prevents release of acetylcholine from neurons; the resulting decrease in cholinergic end-organ stimulation leads to descending weakness and eventually paralysis of the diaphragm. Exposure would most likely be from inhalation of aerosolized toxin.

Symptoms begin 24 to 36 hours after inhalation. Initial symptoms include diplopia, dysphagia, dysarthria, and descending weakness, with difficulty breathing as the muscles of respiration become affected. Associated signs include ptosis, dilated or unreactive pupils, and flaccid paralysis in patients without fever, sensory dysfunction, or mental-status changes.

Patients require mechanical ventilatory support, which if instituted early enough may reduce the mortality rate from 100% to less than 5% but which may need to be continued for up to several weeks. An antitoxin available from state health departments and the CDC is effective when given during the latent period; a toxoid vaccine for pre-exposure immunization is also available. Decontamination involves simple removal of clothing and showering with soap or water or with water alone.

### Incapacitating agents

A variety of compounds can result in temporary physiologic or mental incapacitation, but these agents are generally considered to refer principally to glycolate compounds used as anticholinergic agents. The U.S. developed and stockpiled the incapacitating agent 3-quinuclidinyl benzilate, or QNB (NATO code BZ), which is a component of chemical-agent stockpiles of several other nations. BZ is a white crystalline powder that is odorless, tasteless, and nonirritating, and can be dispersed either as a solid aerosol or in organic solution. At the time of the Second Persian Gulf War (1990), Iraq apparently possessed large quantities of an incapacitating agent called Agent 15, which may be identical to BZ or a close analog.

Anticholinergic glycolates include familiar drugs such as atropine and scopolamine as well as certain plant alkaloids such as hyoscine and hyoscyamine. As dose-dependent competitive inhibitors of acetylcholine at postsynaptic and postjunctional muscarinic receptors in both the peripheral and central nervous systems, they reduce the amount of cholinergic stimulation to end organs. The results in the periphery are clinical effects essentially opposite to the muscarinic effects of nerve agents; effects from cholinergic shortage in the central nervous system (CNS) include changes in consciousness and the appearance of illusions and hallucinations.

There is a latent period of 30 minutes to a few hours before the onset of signs and symptoms. In the peripheral nervous system, insufficient cholinergic stimulation results in the peripheral limb of the classical anticholinergic syndrome: patients that are a) "blind as a bat" (from mydriasis and paralysis of accommodation), b) "dry as a bone" (from decreased secretions), c) "hot as a hare" (from heat retention secondary to decreased sweating), and d) "red as a beet" (from cutaneous vasodilatation in an attempt to lose heat). CNS effects from anticholinergic agents include progressive decrease (eventually to coma) in level of consciousness; characteristic hallucinations (vivid, distinct, "Lilliputian" [that is, decreasing in size over time], and capable of being shared among victims), social disinhibition, semiautonomous picking or plucking motions ("woolgathering"), and disrobing; blurred speech; general emotional flatness (but with some lability), and paranoia. The safety ratio of BZ and, presumably, Agent 15, is high; and deaths, when they occur, are usually either from heat stress or from inadvertently dangerous acts undertaken under the influence of hallucinations.

When faced with patients affected by these agents, the important logistical and medical priorities will be patient control (physical restraints will likely be needed) and attention to core temperature. Most cases will recover after several days without pharmacological treatment, but an antidote, the carbamate anticholinesterase drug physostigmine, is available. Although it will not shorten the clinical course of the intoxication, it can control the signs and symptoms when given in repeated doses or as a slow intravenous infusion. Removal of clothing and skin washing with soap or water will suffice for decontamination.

## Responding to Terrorism Incidents

First responders may be firefighters, police officers, or EMS personnel, but can also be emergency-department personnel, including physicians and nurses. It is therefore important for all first responders to follow those portions of a standard NBC-terrorism First Responder Action protocol that are reasonable for the situation and location of the responder:

*Recognition*: Actions to determine the nature of the incident

- On-scene indicators would include two or more victims with the same symptoms; grouping of casualties in the same areas; possible dissemination devices; a credible communicated threat; statements of victims; dead animals, birds, fish, or insects; unexplained smells; and unexplained liquids, clouds, mists, or other aerosols.

*Isolation*: Actions to physically isolate and secure the incident scene

- Stage at a safe distance (chemical/biological: 300 ft.; explosion: 1000 ft.; nuclear/radiologic: upgrade and upwind from the incident); establish a perimeter and secure zone with the help of police; and establish an area for decontamination and for Haz-Mat and EMS ingress and egress.

*Protection*: Actions to protect the public and responders

- Direct victims who can walk to move upgrade and upwind; don personal protective equipment; perform emergency decontamination; initiate public protection by evacuating people downwind or by instituting effective protective measures so that they do not have to move.

*Notification*: Actions to inform and request assistance

- Notify authorities to report the location, number of casualties, signs and symptoms, and to request assistance.

Regional Hazardous Materials Response Teams have developed procedures for dealing with nuclear (radiologic), biological, and chemical agents and have been equipped with monitoring devices, appropriate entry clothing, portable decontamination facilities, and the means to minimize and/or clean up environmental contamination from these agents. All states have regions with level A capability (see Table 10.4 footnote).

Two additional precautions should be kept in mind for those at the scene of an incident. Terrorists often place secondary devices, usually explosives, at the scene for the purpose of injuring first responders. The best action in that regard is to note "ordinary objects out of place". It should also be kept in mind that the scene of an incident is a crime scene and that evidence needs to be preserved.

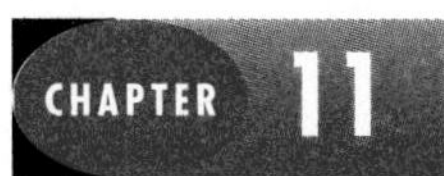

# INFORMATICS AND TELEMEDICINE

Informatics and telemedicine are rapidly evolving disciplines and areas of medical practice, each of which offers tools that have great potential to improve medical care by supporting both individual practitioners and medical systems. Both informatics and telemedicine are tightly interfaced with technological infrastructure and advances. Consequently, they share similar opportunities and threats. This chapter provides a brief introduction to informatics and telemedicine applications in health care, discusses how and why these fields have suddenly emerged from relative obscurity, and outlines the pitfalls that may develop along the way toward their further development, use, and dissemination.

## Medical Informatics

Medical informatics is the scientific field that deals with the storage, retrieval, sharing, and optimal use of biomedical information, data, and knowledge for problem-solving and decision-making. It is closely related to modern information technologies, including computing and communication networks. The emergence of medical informatics as a new discipline can be related to three factors. First, the knowledge base of biomedicine has become tremendously large and continues to expand so rapidly that it has become unmanageable by traditional paper-based methods. Second, improved medical decision-making is as important to modern biomedicine as the discovery of new clinical or research facts. Third, leaders in the medical industry are rapidly adopting advancing computing and communications technologies.

## Current Informatics Applications for Health Care

Informatics and information technology is a very diverse field that has numerous applications in clinical medicine, research, and industry. This chapter provides a brief list of the informatics applications that are most commonly used in health care (see Table 11.1).

**Personal productivity tools**

Hand-held computers, sometimes called Personal Digital Assistants (PDAs), have found numerous uses in medicine. They are commonly used as a reference tool (e.g., for electronic drug databases, medical texts, and medical formulae). They also may be used for taking and maintaining notes and tracking information on interactions with patients, as long as identifying patient information is removed, and managing appointment schedules.

The use of standard or pager e-mail to enhance communication also has become widespread. Common medical applications include basic message communication, information dissemination, and online problem-solving dialogues. Some practices also use e-mail for

**TABLE 11.1. Current Telemedicine Applications**

| Application | Mode of Interaction | Types of Information | Examples |
|---|---|---|---|
| Diagnostic services | Real time; store-and-forward | Digital images (radiographs, tissue slides, cardiac ECHO) | Teleradiology, telepathology, telecardiology |
| Consultation and treatment | Real-time videoconferencing | High-quality audio and motion video; store and forward images | Telepsychiatry, telepulmonary, teledermatology |
| Telementoring | Real-time videoconferencing | Full motion video | Telelaparoscopic surgery, telenurse triage |
| In-home monitoring | Real-time videoconferencing and data acquired and transmitted for later review | Full motion video, electronic data, email/text messages, alerts and reminders | Telehomecare, chronic disease care (e.g., diabetes care, vital signs monitoring, pacemaker monitoring, fall/gait monitors) |
| Medical education | Real-time videoconferencing, Internet-based interactive learning modules | Audio, full motion video, still images, text and graphics | Online virtual universities, medical information hubs (WebMD), conferences and talks transmitted via satellite |

patient–physician communication. E-mail can improve efficiency of communication for the sender, because the message receiver does not have to be online at the same time, but the same feature makes it ineffective in time-sensitive situations that require significant dialogue. Establishing guidelines for its appropriate use is essential.

### Reference data bases

The ability to perform rapid computer searches of the medical literature and reference data bases has provided physicians with one of the tools necessary to make use of the vast quantity of medical knowledge now available. The ability to formulate specific yet sensitive Boolean searches of medical reference data bases, external data repositories such as the Internet or various networked data stores within organizations (e.g., Department of Veterans Affairs intranet) intranets, has become a necessary skill for physicians.

### Computerized medical records

The electronic or computerized medical record is becoming a fact of life for many institutions, although only a few hospitals have adopted a completely paperless medical record. The advantages of such computerized medical records are numerous, including ease of data retrieval from any location; possibility of simultaneous access by several providers, including providers at both local and remote locations; availability of complete and legible records; ability to search and sort components of the record; rapid access to digitized images (e.g., radiographs, pathology slides, pictures of a physical finding, and even streaming video of procedures, such as a cardiac catheterization or an endoscopy); and fewer medical errors due to smart systems that alert prescribers to drug allergies, medication interactions, or improper dosages.

One major drawback of a computerized medical record is that data entry can be time-consuming. However, the use of an automated data collection system and structured data entry templates that automatically insert patient demographics, a list of prior medical conditions, current medicines, recent test results, and vital signs data into the medical note significantly ease progress note entry. Handwriting and speech recognition software also is available to aid data entry. Another data entry system that is being applied to medical settings is barcode technology. Some hospitals have begun using barcode systems to track medication dispensing, blood administration, and laboratory sample collection.

### Decision support systems

Decision support is an important area of medical informatics. Computer-based decision support systems are designed to assist physicians in making medical diagnoses and managing patients. It is important to understand that these systems "support" physicians in making diagnosis or management decisions; they do not take over the decision-making process. A computer-based decision support system draws from the large amount of medical and clinical knowledge that is already stored in its database. For instance, a computerized diagnostic system uses an individual patient's clinical information (symptoms, signs, laboratory data), along with knowledge of disease prevalence in similar patients to come up with the probable diagnosis and a list of less likely possible diagnoses. The Quick Medical Reference (QMR), DxPLAIN, ILIAD, pediatric emergency medicine (PEM-DXP), and MEDITEL are examples of currently available diagnostic decision support systems.

Similarly, therapy-oriented systems provide information regarding optimal treatment plans for patients with specific presenting complaints or previously diagnosed problems. Common examples include computerized clinical pathways, guidelines, and automated reminder tools. These systems work in conjunction with the computerized medical record and offer some of the most powerful and clinically useful tools that are available to physicians as a result of informatics research. Management support systems can be used to generate health reminders on patients tracked in a data base. For example, the system could send a clinical reminder to a physician or to a patient when that patient is due for a mammogram. Similarly, a physician could generate reports of all patients in his practice who have poorly controlled diabetes, or all patients with heart disease who are not on a lipid-lowering drug. Such reports help the physician measure and improve his or her performance against criteria set by practice guidelines.

## Telemedicine

The Greek word *tele* means "far off." Telemedicine can be defined as "medicine from a distance." The Institute of Medicine defines telemedicine as the use of electronic information and communications technologies to provide and support health care when distance separates the participants.

By far the biggest advantage of telemedicine is its ability to provide improved access to medical care and medical knowledge for remote patient populations. In addition to improved access, other benefits of telemedicine include its potential for cost savings, improvement of health outcomes by better monitoring of patients, and more effective utilization of health care resources. Another plus of telemedicine is that it can provide continuous medical education and mentoring opportunities for providers located at small rural institutions by linking them with health professionals at large academic medical centers.

### Background

Modern telemedicine can trace its roots back to the use of the telephone for medical consultation. Perhaps the first documented telemedicine consultation was a telephone call made by Alexander Graham Bell in 1897, seeking help from a physician for an acid burn. Early examples of modern telemedicine, e.g., live interactive video and image transmission, date back to the use of interactive video consultations by physicians at Nebraska Psychiatric Institute for patients 112 miles away at the Norfolk State Hospital in Norfolk, Nebraska in 1964.

As telecommunication technologies have advanced, telemedicine also has grown. There has been a large increase in telemedicine activity over the last 10 years; clinical telemedicine programs are now in place in every state of the U.S., and it is estimated that more than 70 large electronic medical networks currently are under construction. Telemedicine is practiced around the globe. Developed countries such as Australia, the United Kingdom, France, and Canada are in the forefront of telemedicine research and applications. Because of telemedicine's ability to serve remote populations, this method of providing medical care has also expanded to developing nations such as India and Brazil. Currently, telemedicine is far from being a day-to-day activity in most physicians' practices; nevertheless, it is an exciting new area of medicine that should not be ignored.

### Key telemedicine technologies

Telemedicine includes a range of technologies, including the telephone, facsimile, modem, and video. Telemedicine may be conducted in real time, as with interactive video, or asynchronously, for the transmission of text or graphic data, auditory and verbal information, still images, short video clips, and full-motion video. Although robotics and virtual reality interfaces have been introduced into some experimental applications, they are not widely used. The telemedicine technologies listed may be applied in various ways, including management of chronic conditions, routine consultation, preventive medicine, public health, and patient education.

Telemedicine also uses various terrestrial (e.g., telephone lines or high-speed ISDN and T1 lines) and space-based (i.e., satellite) transmission media. The medium that is used to transmit information is important in part because its bandwidth or bit rate (the amount of information sent per unit of time) limits the type of technology that may be used. For instance, full-motion video conferencing requires the ability to transmit very large amounts of data at a very rapid rate, whereas the transmission of still images involves smaller quantities of data transmitted at slower rates. Newer telemedicine systems also use personal computer-based multimedia medical records to share images and conduct video consultations over the inexpensive Internet platform.

### Current telemedicine applications

*Clinical telemedicine*

The clinical applications of telemedicine are varied. Attention has been focused largely on the use of interactive video for specialty and subspecialty consultation in rural areas. The generic interactive video telemedicine system typically uses fixed videoconferencing equipment to link a rural or "remote site" facility with the urban tertiary care center or "hub site." Consultants from the hub site communicate with patients, and often with the primary care providers, at the remote site using videoconferencing technology. The hub site physician is able to conduct a medical interview and perform a limited physical examination via telemedicine. Auscultation of heart and lung sounds is conducted using a special electronic stethoscope. A detailed inspection of skin lesions is performed with a special camera known as a "dermascope." Ear and eye examinations are conducted with electronic otoscope and ophthalmoscope cameras, respectively.

Although telemedicine has been used in almost all major clinical specialties, some specialties use it more than others. Radiologists, for example, have embraced the technology on a large scale. Telemedicine is well suited to transmitting radiology images from a remote site for interpretation by a radiologist at a hub site, thereby eliminating the need for travel. Similarly, in the specialties of telepathology and dermatology, diagnosis can be made via telemedicine based on a "store-and-forward" method in which the image is photographed and later transmitted to a consultant. A diagnosis also can be made by transmitting live images of pathology slides or skin lesions to the consultant at the hub site. Clinical consultations in other fields in which a complete, detailed physical examination is not an important factor, such as psychiatry, also are well suited to telemedicine, where the consultant psychiatrist can interview patients at remote sites and provide diagnoses and treatment plans.

Telemedicine technology also can be used to provide home care for patients. Nurses or physicians conduct scheduled virtual or video home visits with the patient and family with the use of portable videoconferencing equipment installed in the patient's home. For example, a postoperative wound can be monitored at home, so the patient does not have to make repeated long trips to see the doctor in person. Virtual home care visits also have been used for chronic management of patients with advanced heart failure. By close monitoring of vital signs and medications via telemedicine, these patients can be managed more effectively at home, and the number of costly (and stressful) emergency room visits is reduced.

*Patient education and monitoring*

The Internet has become a very powerful tool for providing online medical information for patients and families. Patients are able to explore and gather information about their diagnosis and treatment independently. However, internet surfers should beware because a significant amount of erroneous information is posted on the internet. It is safest to use only websites that are affiliated with well established medical organizations.

Another capability of telemedicine is remote monitoring of a patient's heart rate, blood pressure, blood oxygen saturation, medication compliance, and gait monitoring via small wireless devices that the patient can be hooked up to at home. Interactive patient monitoring, such as pacemaker monitoring and home blood sugar readings, also can be done via telemedicine. Some of these devices, such as an electronic medication dispensing device or an electronic blood sugar monitor, have wireless modems that allow two-way transmission of data between the patient's home and the physician's office or hospital. This technology enables physicians to communicate with and instruct their patients immediately when necessary.

*Distance education and telementoring*

The use of telemedicine technologies such as live videoconferences, satellite conferences, and the Internet to provide continuing medical education has been demonstrated at various sites across the country. The range of educational activities includes transmissions of lecture series, grand rounds, and online courses for physicians, as well as educational programs for patients.

Remote supervision or mentoring of health care providers also has been demonstrated. One of the best examples of telementoring is an ongoing project at Yale University that provides an intensive laparoscopic general surgery course at Yale for physicians located at small rural hospitals throughout Connecticut. After teaching this course, the Yale physicians use telemedicine technology (live video feed from a camera attached to a laparoscope and a videoconferencing camera in the operating room) to supervise student surgeons while they perform laparoscopic procedures at their rural hospitals.

## Legal and Ethical Issues

The risk for breach of patient confidentiality remains an important concern. Because of relatively easier access via computer networks, there is a higher risk that the privacy of electronic records may be violated by unauthorized persons. Furthermore, unauthorized access to a computerized medical record implies access to all patient records in that particular database. Certain types of disclosure, such as the sale of computerized lists of patients with a specific diagnosis to marketers, mailing list brokers, or insurance companies, may be facilitated by the use of electronic databases. Another confidentiality problem may arise when an authorized user neglects to prevent unauthorized viewing or manipulation of the record (such as leaving the room while patient data is displayed on the computer). The electronic transmission of patient data provides another potential window for breach of confidentiality regarding private medical information. Obviously, access to electronic records must be carefully restricted to those who need and are entitled to have access to provide care.

Another major issue in the use of informatics and telemedicine is the lack of well-defined quality standards for these applications and of policies regarding medical malpractice issues. Both informatics and telemedicine are highly reliant on technology and therefore are susceptible to interruption in services from technology failure. Some providers are concerned that the use of telemedicine could increase their liability risk (for example, a technical failure could lead to an adverse patient outcome, or telemedicine could provide an image of inferior quality that interferes with the physician's ability to make an accurate diagnosis). Other physicians are concerned that if these technologies permit high-quality care, they might be found liable for failure to use them. Most experts agree that practice standards need to be developed for these burgeoning areas of medical practice.

Several additional unresolved issues have arisen in the field of telemedicine. For example, medical licensure for physicians is regulated by individual states, which would limit the interstate practice of medicine through telemedicine. Lack of reimbursement is another significant drawback of telemedicine. Currently, neither private nor government-funded medical insurance plans reimburse for telemedicine services. This situation is likely to change in the near future, however, because legislation is already underway to require insurance companies to reimburse certain telemedicine services. Furthermore, there are inadequate research data in this area to guide practitioners. Although the technologic performance of telemedicine has been evaluated positively, and patient satisfaction with telemedicine has been high, little research has been conducted to determine its impact on the doctor–patient relationship or its larger impact on health outcomes or improvements in the provision of health care.

## Conclusion

Technology trends suggest that within the next few years a large proportion of health care providers will be able to "see" patients at remote sites by using a desktop workstation or laptop computer in a mobile, wireless configuration. Clinicians will be able to select interactive video and store-and-forward modes to provide care as needed. Simple, intuitive software shells already allow seamless access to pertinent patient records, radiographs, pathology slides, pharmacy information, and billing records. Instant access to on-line libraries of medical information, decision and management support systems, and patient instructional materials is becoming available. In some practices, scheduling and referrals to specialists and allied health personnel are already computer-based. It is conceivable that in the near future we will have networks that will store and provide patient information that can be accessed by authorized medical personnel anywhere in the world. Encryption of data and restriction of user access by means of passwords will ensure privacy and security. Thus, the hands-on world of the traditional doctor is rapidly transforming into new-age cyberspace medicine, where computers are used to help improve health care.

# CHAPTER 12 MEDICAL GENETICS

The field of human genetics continues to expand rapidly as new technological advances in molecular biology accelerate the mapping and sequencing of the human genome. (Brief definitions of frequently used genetic terms can be found in Table 12.1). The ability to apply structural genomics (sequencing) advances will facilitate the identification of susceptibility loci for common complex diseases, such as heart disease, obesity, and diabetes mellitus. The study of functional genomics (i.e., how genes work) will allow for a further understanding of the molecular basis of disease. Pharmacogenetics (interactions between therapeutic agents and genes) will aid in predicting an individual's probable response to pharmacologic treatments.

This chapter gives a brief overview of those topics and two new genetic techniques, single nucleotide polymorphism (SNP) mapping and expression profiling, and the impact they will have on the practice of clinical medicine. It also touches on the ethical and legal concerns being raised by the genetics revolution.

## The Human Genome Project

The first draft of the human genome sequence, published on February 15, 2001, covered 94% of the human genome. The initial sequencing and analysis of the human genome predicted that there would be 30,000 to 40,000 protein-coding genes in the human genome. Despite this major accomplishment in human genome sequencing, a great deal more work is still needed to elicit a complete list of all human genes and their encoded proteins. Furthermore, discovering how certain genes contribute to the pathogenesis of disease will require understanding of both gene function and the regulation of gene expression.

### Identification of genes involved in monogenic diseases

Since the early 1990s, positional cloning has been the standard approach for determining which diseases are caused by a single gene. Positional cloning involves a series of steps that are used to determine the identity of the causal gene. First, investigators map the region of the genome by genotype-phenotype correlations using linkage analysis within families. Genetic mapping (see Table 12.1), depending on the pedigrees used in the linkage analysis, locates the gene to within several million bases. All genes within the genetically mapped position are positional candidate genes. The second step is to build a physical map. Now that the draft sequence of the human genome is available, it is becoming increasingly easier to identify the genes within a region of interest. Once the physical map is completed, the investigator returns to the families or pedigrees in the study and searches for the affected family member who has the smallest region identical to that of all affected people in the study. The final step is to search for a sequence variation that can be linked causally to a molecular mechanism. A simple example is a sequence variant that produces a stop codon in the middle of the gene, which produces a premature termination. Some monogenic diseases that have been identified using this technique include cystic fibrosis, Marfan's Syndrome, Huntington's Chorea, and Fragile X Syndrome.

### Identification of genes involved in polygenic diseases

Many common complex disorders, such as obesity, depression, heart disease, diabetes mellitus (types 1 and 2), hypertension, metabolic syndrome, Alzheimer's

**TABLE 12.1. Definition of Terms Used in Genetics**

| Term | Definition |
|---|---|
| Allele | One member of a pair of homologous genes in a diploid cell. |
| Genetic marker | A variation in DNA that can distinguish one person from another. An identifiable physical location of a chromosome whose inheritance can be monitored. Markers can be expressed regions of DNA (genes) or a segment of DNA with no known coding function but whose pattern of inheritance can be determined. |
| Candidate genes | Genes whose biological properties make them logical objects of study for a particular disease. |
| Positional candidate genes | All genes within a genetically mapped position. |
| Haplotype | A particular combination of alleles in a specific region of a chromosome. |
| Genetic map | Genetic markers that are ordered on the chromosome based upon genetic recombination. |
| Linkage map | A description of a genome in which many phenotypes are screened to determine the frequency with which genes occur together; these can then be placed in appropriate proximity to one another. |
| Physical map | A goal of the human genome project. A map of the locations of identifiable landmarks, sequence-tagged sites and contigs. The highest resolution map is the complete nucleotide sequence of chromosomes. |
| Linkage disequilibrium | In genetics, the more-frequent-than-random occurrence of two alleles together due to selective pressure or to their close proximity on the same chromosome. The likelihood of a recombination event separating the two traits decreases with their increasing proximity on the chromosome. |
| Single nucleotide polymorphisms (SNPs) | Variations of one nucleotide between the DNA sequence of individuals. |
| Expressed sequence tag (EST) | A small segment of sequence in a DNA coding region generated by random sequencing of complementary DNA (cDNA) libraries that can be used to identify a particular gene or gene family. |
| Sequence tagged site (STS) | Short (200–500 base pairs) DNA sequence that has a single occurrence in the human genome and whose location and base sequence is known. STSs are used for identification and mapping of coding and sequences, for discovery of new genes, and for discovery of identities with other genes. |
| Orthologue | Homologous gene, which has been conserved across species, evolving from the same ancestral gene. |
| Congenic | Moving one small region of the genome of one strain onto the genetic background of another by breeding. |
| Consomic | Moving one chromosome of one strain onto the genetic background of another by breeding. |

disease and end-stage renal disease have evidence of genetic involvement, and show a pattern of inheritance, but they do not conform to simple Mendelian patterns of inheritance (i.e., additive, dominant, recessive) consistent with a single gene. These disorders usually are multifactorial, resulting from a complex interaction between environmental factors and susceptibility alleles of multiple genes, each of which most likely exerts only a small effect and, in some cases, only when a threshold of susceptibility is reached. Therefore, most susceptibility genes are neither necessary nor sufficient to cause disease and confer only a modest increase in risk. For example, the presence of the susceptibility gene, APOE4 (an allele for apolipoprotein E), is a risk factor for Alzheimer's disease. In addition, these complex diseases often result from combinations of unfavorable intermediate phenotypes, many of which are under distinct genetic control. An example is the interaction of variation in plasma LDL, HDL, triglycerides, fibrinogen, blood pressure, insulin levels, and central obesity in the pathogenesis of ischemic heart disease. In this case, the number of susceptibility loci may be so high that it may be preferable to study the intermediate traits, rather than the disease end point. Consequently, the task of identifying genes contributing to complex diseases is daunting.

The first step in identifying the genes contributing to complex diseases is to determine what percentage of the disease can be attributed to genes. The best way to do this in humans is to contrast the expressions of disease in mono- and dizygotic twins. If the trait is highly heritable, the percentage of both monozygotic twins showing the phenotype should be much greater than that of both dizygotic twins expressing the phenotype. However, if development of the trait is highly influenced by environmental factors, the percentage of both dizygotic twins showing the trait will be high. For example, if one monozygotic twin has type II diabetes, the second has an 85% chance of developing the same disease. This means that only 15% of type II diabetes is due to the environment.

Multifactorial diseases also can be studied using linkage analysis; the design of these studies tends to be different, however. In general, an affected sib pair approach is used to study complex disease. The rationale for using affected sib pairs is to avoid including people in the study who carry the disease gene but have not yet developed the disease. Once the sib pairs (usually numbering > 400) are collected, the entire genome is screened using a panel of genetic markers. Typically, significant linkage is defined by a log of odds ratio (lod) score of 3 (which is equivalent to a 1000 : 1 probability in favor of linkage). The identified genetic interval area, usually large, to which the gene or genes contribute a quantitative trait, such as hypertension or body mass index, is called a quantitative trait locus (QTL). Once a QTL is defined, the next step is to identify the gene. Unfortunately, this has proved to be an arduous task, so new strategies are being developed.

One new approach is to revert to association studies (case/control) for complex disease. The principle is based on conserved haplotypes or linkage disequilibrium (see Table 12.1). The term *haplotype* refers to a particular combination of alleles traveling on the same chromosome, whereas the term *conserved haplotypes* implies that a particular combination of alleles has remained essentially unchanged throughout evolution. In genetics, linkage disequilibrium means the nonrandom association or occurrence of two traits or alleles together due to their close proximity on the same chromosome. The likelihood of a recombination event separating the two alleles usually decreases as their proximity on the chromosome increases; in other words, the chance of recombination is a function of the distance between genes or markers. However, over time there is a chance that recombination will occur at every site in the genome; therefore, the age and size of populations must also be considered. The probability of specific alleles at different loci occurring together is based on the frequency of those alleles. However, when alleles at linked loci are associated or conserved, the alleles are in disequilibrium, in other words traveling together as a unit. The link between alleles at the neighboring loci and the mutation will be conserved until recombination has occurred often enough to deplete or break the association.

In humans, as in all other species, recombination is the major force that eliminates linkage and association over generations. When a functional mutation occurs, it does so on a haplotype of preexisting DNA variants. Because linkage analysis focuses on recent generations within a family, there has not been enough time for recombination to occur, and the disease gene regions identified by linkage tend to be large. In contrast, association studies allow for greater opportunity for recombination, which causes the disease mutation to be separated from its original haplotype, ultimately narrowing the disease-associated region. However, particular DNA variants and disease-causing mutations can remain together on the same haplotype for many generations, providing the genetic basis for most association studies.

Association study designs require significant numbers of carefully chosen cases and controls, as well as a high-density genetic map, to give them sufficient power to study genetic disorders. It has been shown that association studies can be more powerful for investigation of multifactorial diseases. However, there is an increased risk that the association is a false-positive based on how the people in the study were collected. Typically, association studies are used for testing candidate genes; however, with the large number of single nucleotide polymorphisms (a type of genetic marker), people are beginning to consider using these studies to search the genome for disease genes.

## New Genetic Technologies

Single nucleotide polymorphisms, microarray expression profiling, and comparative mapping are developing and gaining popularity rapidly as important technological advances for the study of complex genetic diseases.

### SNP technology

Single nucleotide polymorphisms (SNPs) are the most abundant type of DNA sequence variation or mutation in the human genome (see Table 12.1). Specifically, a SNP is a site at which a single base pair varies from person to person. The human genome project identified more than 1.4 million SNPs within the human genome. They are distributed relatively evenly every 300 to 1000 bases and can serve as physical landmarks on the 3 billion–base pair human genome. If this single nucleotide variation is found within a unique segment of DNA, it can serve as a physical landmark and as a genetic marker that can be followed in its transmission from parent to child or in cases versus controls.

These SNPs are projected to play a valuable role in sequence comparison and may become the genetic markers of choice for the study of common complex genetic traits. The SNP Consortium, formed by multiple pharmaceutical companies and academic centers, is working on producing a high-density SNP map of the human genome. It may become possible to use genomic association studies to detect genetic effects that are too weak to identify by standard linkage analysis once the SNP map is complete. This high-density SNP map will provide a greater ability to identify haplotypes linked to genes associated with specific diseases or responses to medicines reliably.

*SNPs and disease prevalences*

Despite the phenotypic diversity across ethnic groups and the diversity of disease propensity in the human population, and the large number of SNPs already identified by the human genome project, 99.9% of the human genome is identical from one person to the next. This means that, on average, only 1 out of every 1000 bases is different between any two individuals, independent of ethnicity. This limited diversity reflects the fact that modern humans are descended from a relatively small population—the proposed "out of Africa" theory. The African origin hypothesis states that modern humans originated in Africa 100,000 to 200,000 years ago and subsequently spread to the rest of the world via a series of migrations.

Evidence from linkage disequilibrium analysis of common single nucleotide polymorphisms between Northern European and Nigerian populations suggests that the human population experienced an extreme founder effect, or bottleneck. This severe bottleneck probably occurred about 27,000 to 53,000 years ago (800–1600 generations ago). This was a period when the population was so small that only a few ancestral haplotypes (see Table 12.1) gave rise to most of the haplotypes that exist today. One potential cause for this bottleneck effect is the Last Glacial Maximum, which substantially depopulated Northern Europe. The major genetic distinctions that we see today among humans occurred within rather than between major continental populations. Additionally, common population variants tend to be of ancient origin and are distributed in all ethnic groups, but a substantially greater diversity of rare variants appears to have developed within recent times, corresponding to major population expansions. The difference in disease prevalences that exist today between ethnic groups may simply be due to differences in allele frequency rather than differences in the diseases.

**Microarray expression profiling**

Expression profiling analysis has become one of the most widely used tools in the attempt to decipher gene function. A variety of profiling techniques have been developed, including serial analysis of gene expression (SAGE), differential display, and oligonucleotide and cDNA microarrays, which allow for the parallel assessment of gene expression for hundreds to thousands of genes in a single experiment. Currently, the microarray system of screening for differences in gene expression is the most powerful mechanism used to characterize the differences in amounts of mRNA between different tissue or cell types, identical tissues subjected to different stimuli, identical tissues from two populations, or different tissue phenotypes or developmental stages. It is the tissue-specific abundance of mRNA that contributes in part to cellular phenotype and function, and until protein arrays are available, mRNA arrays offer the best way to monitor large numbers of genes in parallel.

The microarrays (Figure 12.1) can be used for at least two different expression profiling strategies. The first is gene "hunting," or global arrays in which differential expression is assessed in parallel on a chip that contains the entire genome. Current arrays, however, typically contain on the order of 20,000 genes and expressed sequence tags (ESTs; see Table 12.1) to look for all possible candidate genes for certain phenotypes. For example, if one of the positional candidate genes from the linkage analysis also shows expression differences, then the gene becomes an even more attractive candidate. A second approach would be the identification of gene pathways to implicate causal genes.

*Expression profiling to elucidate cancer pathophysiology*

Expression profiling techniques such as SAGE and cDNA oligonucleotide microarrays have been used for the analysis of various types of cancer, with the aims of discovering pathways involved in tumorigenesis and identifying novel diagnostic tools, prognostic markers, and potential therapeutic targets. Cancer is a complex genetic disease, but the cancer phenotype probably is an accumulation of changes in the expression patterns of hundreds or even thousands of genes that occur as a consequence of the primary mutation of an oncogene or a tumor suppressor gene. The National Cancer Institute has developed the Cancer Genome Anatomy Project (CGAP) to create a Tumor Gene Index; SAGE has been used as a strategic analytic technique. Several interesting patterns have emerged from these initial tumor data. First, cancerous and normal cells derived from the same tissue type are very similar, with only a small percentage of genes demonstrating significant differences in mRNA expression levels. Second, cultured cancer cell lines may lose some or most of the gene expression profile characteristics of their tissue of origin, resulting in difficulties with their analysis. Third, tumors of the same tissue origin but of different histologic type or grade have distinct gene expression patterns. Finally, cancer cells

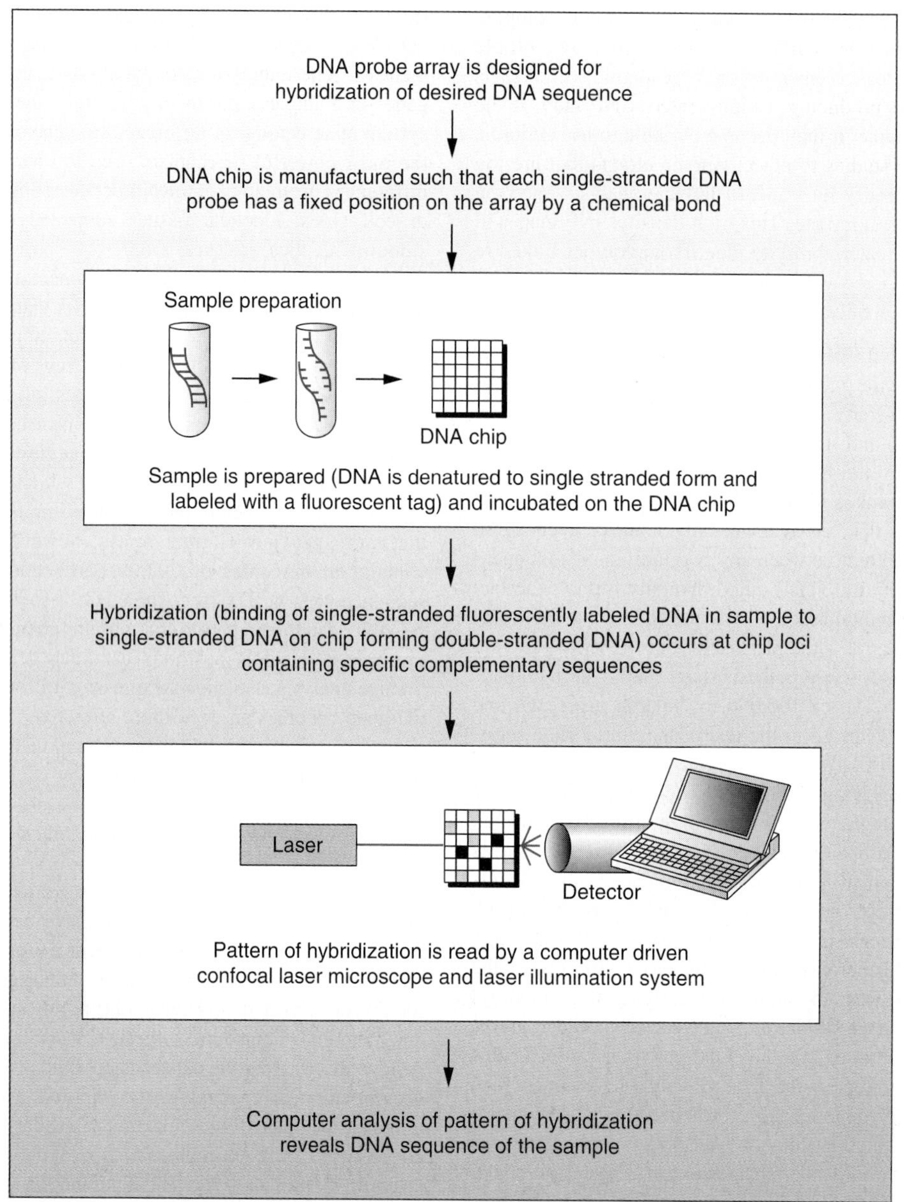

DNA probe array is designed for hybridization of desired DNA sequence
DNA chip is manufactured such that each single-stranded DNA probe has a fixed position on the array by a chemical bond
Sample preparation
DNA chip
Sample is prepared (DNA is denatured to single stranded form and labeled with a fluorescent tag) and incubated on the DNA chip
Hybridization (binding of single-stranded fluorescently labeled DNA in sample to single-stranded DNA on chip forming double-stranded DNA) occurs at chip loci containing specific complementary sequences
Laser
Detector
Pattern of hybridization is read by a computer driven confocal laser microscope and laser illumination system
Computer analysis of pattern of hybridization reveals DNA sequence of the sample


**FIGURE 12.1. Example of DNA probe array developed for the detection of single nucleotide polymorphisms (SNPs).** (Adapted with permission from Rusnak J, Kisabeth R. Mayo Clinic Proceedings 2001; 76: 305, figure 2.)

usually show an increase in the expression of genes associated with proliferation and survival and a decrease in the expression of genes involved in differentiation.

In the past few years, SAGE analysis has been performed in patients harboring tumors of the lung, bladder, ovary, colon, pancreas, and breast, as well as glioblastomas and medulloblastomas. In breast cancer, SAGE and custom array analysis have been combined to decipher pathways that mediate breast cancer progression and to find targets for potential therapeutic interventions. One study, which compared two well-characterized breast tumor cell lines, 21PT and 21MT, with two normal mammary epithelial cell cultures, identified more than 200 transcripts that were differentially expressed by at least 10-fold between cancer and normal cells. Comprehensive gene expression analysis is likely to accelerate knowledge of the molecular pathogenesis dramatically and will revolutionize the way cancer patients are diagnosed. It also is likely to lead to the development of new therapeutic strategies.

## Comparative Mapping of Complex Traits

Comparative gene mapping is based on the fact that genes that are closely linked in one species tend to be closely linked or conserved in other species. Specifically, it identifies regions of a genome that are evolutionarily conserved between species. The probabilities that linkage is conserved or disrupted depend on rearrangements and mutations that have accumulated since the divergence of the lineages leading to the two species. Closely related species tend to have more conserved segments than do distantly related species. These tendencies do have exceptions, with some phylogenetic lineages showing remarkable conservation and others showing extensive rearrangement. Orthologous genes (see Table 12.1) are landmarks needed to relate corresponding chromosome segments between species; they are one of the key elements in comparative mapping.

Attention has focused on the genetic dissection of complex traits in animal models as a way to overcome, at least partially, the restrictions and difficulties of mapping complex diseases in humans. Both the mouse and rat were selected as animal models to study human diseases. Once the loci contributing to a complex phenotype are linked to the genome of the rodent, they can be transferred to the human genome via comparative mapping.

The mouse is the key animal model for gene discovery because of its large number of mutant models and its use in transgenic and knockout studies, whereas the rat is the model of choice for biomedical, physiologic, and pharmacologic research. Fortunately, over the last decade, the genomic resources for the rat and mouse have increased dramatically, increasing their roles for functional genomic studies and pathway identification. The rat is used extensively in the quantitative genetics of complex, polygenic disease. There already are more than 200 inbred rat strains, most of which serve as multigenic models of human diseases such as hypertension, diabetes mellitus, renal failure, and cancer. By selectively breeding inbred rat strains, congenic (see Table 12.1) and consomic (see Table 12.1) rats are easily generated. The rat also remains a major model for drug development.

The ability to cross genetically well-defined, inbred strains of mice or rats that differ in disease susceptibility has permitted the mapping of genes that modify complex phenotypes in rodents in a way that is not feasible in humans. Through the use of congenic strains, different loci contributing to a complex phenotype can be isolated. Because it is not possible to do selective breeding and experimental interventions in humans to characterize the detailed pathobiology, the physiology can be linked to the genome of the mouse and rat. Once linked to the genome of the rodent, it can be transferred to humans via comparative mapping. This strategy will play a major role in annotating gene function. Obviously, results will have to be confirmed in each species.

## Impact of Genetic Discoveries on Clinical Medicine

As functional genomics is refined and extended into the clinical setting, gene identification will have major implications for the treatment of patients. In the new field of pharmacogenomics, drug therapy is customized based on the genotype of a particular patient. Ultimately, this customization will offer the potential for optimal safety and efficacy in each individual patient. A classic example of how understanding the genetic basis of diseases affects the treatment strategy is seen with Alzheimer's disease. Using an association study design, the apolipoprotein E type 4 gene was found to be important in the development of late-onset Alzheimer's disease. Although different drugs are now available to delay the decline in mental agility, some patients do not benefit from this treatment. Patients who are homozygous for the ApoE4 allele respond less well to certain drug therapies, such as the acetylcholinesterase inhibitors.

Knowledge of specific genetic mutations also has proved to be useful in patients with chronic myelogenous leukemia (CML). Chronic myelogenous leukemia is a clonal hematopoietic stem-cell disorder characterized by the swapping of genetic material between chromosomes 9 and 22—Philadelphia chromosome (9:22) translocation. This translocation is present in 95% of CML cases throughout the course of the disease and results in the production of an abnormal enzyme, bcr-abl tyrosine kinase. Chronic myelogenous leukemia is characterized clinically by marked myeloid proliferation, and, if left untreated, it invariably transforms into an acute leukemia or blast crisis. It is the deregulated tyrosine kinase activity that is essential for leukemic transformation. Conventional treatments have included interferon-based regimens and stem-cell transplantation, with stem-cell transplantation offering the only hope for a cure. Because the bcr-abl tyrosine kinase activity is essential to the transforming function of bcr-abl, a potent and selective inhibitor of this kinase called signal transduction inhibitor number 571 (STI571) was deliberately developed specifically to treat CML. In preclinical studies, STI571 was found to selectively kill bcr-abl–expressing cells in vitro and in vivo. Early clinical trials, using STI571 in patients who had CML in the chronic phase and in blast crisis and in CML patients who failed interferon-based therapy, revealed that STI571 is well tolerated and has significant antileukemic activity. These results provide evidence of the essential role of bcr-abl tyrosine kinase activity in CML transformation and demonstrate the potential for the development of anticancer drugs based on the specific molecular abnormality present in a specific cancer. STI571 has emerged as a paradigm for gene product targeted therapy and offers expanded therapeutic options for patients with CML.

Pharmacogenomics uses the genetic approach in the general population, not only to identify patients likely to benefit from new medications but also to identify those likely to suffer adverse side effects. For example, one genetic variability in N-acetyltransferase, NAT-2, is associated with a high incidence of development of peripheral neuropathy from the antituberculosis drug isoniazid. Another example is patients with a variation in the core promoter of the gene ALOX5, who have a decreased clinical response to treatment with a drug that targets the 5-lipoxygenase pathway. Pharmaceutical companies hope to identify which patients are likely to benefit from certain medications and which are more likely to suffer adverse medication side effects. Advances in this field are likely to have a profound impact on clinical medicine.

### Ethical and Legal Concerns Raised by Genetic Discovery

The ultimate goal of structural and functional genomics is to improve the quality of human life; however, this body of knowledge will have profound effects on the health care system. The crucial concerns include proper patient education and consent for genetic testing, proper genetic counseling once results are available, maintenance of confidentiality, and the patient's right to access health insurance. Improper use of genetic tests could lead to genetic discrimination. For example, new gene mapping techniques might eventually allow a person's entire genetic profile to be determined and placed on a computer chip. Although the availability of such detailed genetic information represents a tremendous opportunity for clinical medicine, it also has potential for abuse. Instances of discriminatory uses of genetic tests by insurance companies and employers already have been reported. This risk may cause many people to choose not to be tested for genetic conditions or predisposition to disease, thereby depriving themselves of potential timely treatment.

In 1990, the Ethical, Legal, and Social Implications (ELSI) Project was developed as a subprogram of the Human Genome Project to address the ethical, legal, and social issues brought about by the genetic revolution. The ELSI focuses on four major areas: (1) privacy and fair use of genetic information; (2) responsible clinical integration of new genetic technologies; (3) ethical issues surrounding the conduct of genetic research; and (4) professional and public education. In 1991, the ELSI formed the National Task Force on Genetic Information and Insurance to deal with the growing issues related to genetic testing and insurance.

Unless appropriate legislative protections are developed and enforced, breach of patient confidentiality related to genetic testing results may put individuals at significant risk for losing employment opportunities and for losing their health insurance. Solutions to this problem require continuing research and debate and the creation of new policies and laws that protect patients and uphold the high ethical standards of patient care. It is also critical to determine how to meet the genetic counseling needs that arise with genetic testing.

Although completion of the sequencing of the human genome was a major event in the history of science, we are still left with the task of identifying the 30,000 to 40,000 genes that lie within the 3.2 billion base pairs that make up the human genome. We must then determine the functional role played by each gene. The most important consequence resulting from gene identification and function will be a better understanding of biology and disease. Gene products are the building blocks of all biological processes, so decoding genes will offer a shortcut to understanding the fundamental chemistry of living organisms and their diseases. This knowledge can then be coupled with the development of new robust technologies such as SNP-typing, microarray expression profiling, and comparative mapping to meticulously dissect disease pathways, to provide targeted therapeutic strategies, and to minimize complications or side effects from therapies.

# CHAPTER 13 MEDICAL ETHICS

The medical profession has long subscribed to a body of ethical statements developed primarily for the benefit of the patient. As medical historian Lester King said, "Members of a profession thus found themselves in a position of authority that rested on trust." This dual relationship imposed on the members of a profession a particular moral obligation, which was made explicit by a code of ethics. The American Medical Association (AMA) has summarized these principles, which define the essentials of honorable behavior and expected standards of conduct among physicians (Table 13.1).

**TABLE 13.1. American Medical Association Principles of Medical Ethics**

I. A physician shall be dedicated to providing competent medical service with compassion and respect for human dignity.
II. A physician shall deal honestly with patients and colleagues, and strive to expose those physicians deficient in character or competence, or who engage in fraud or deception.
III. A physician shall respect the law and also recognize a responsibility to seek changes in those requirements which are contrary to the best interests of the patient.
IV. A physician shall respect the rights of patients, of colleagues, and of other health professionals, and shall safeguard patient confidences within the constraints of the law.
V. A physician shall continue to study, apply, and advance scientific knowledge, make relevant information available to patients, colleagues, and the public, obtain consultation, and use the talents of other health professionals when indicated.
VI. A physician shall, in the provision of appropriate patient care except in emergencies, be free to choose whom to serve, with whom to associate, and the environment in which to provide medical services.
VII. A physician shall recognize a responsibility to participate in activities contributing to an improved community.

## Physician and Profession

Clinicians are responsible for reaching a decision that is not only clinically and technically sound but also morally appropriate—one that is suitable for the specific problems of the particular patient they are treating.

Medicine has no single goal. In the encounter between patient and clinician, many appropriate goals are pursued simultaneously (Table 13.2). A realistic understanding of the goals of treatment by both the physician and the patient is essential to sound decision-making. The physician's task is to inform the patient about which goals are attainable. In defining the goals of the encounter, according to Jonsen and coworkers, the clinician should consider the nature of the disease; the preferences of the patient; and social, cultural, political, and economic realities.

### Nature of disease

In determining the nature of a patient's disease and how to manage it, the physician must ask the following questions:

- What is the patient's current medical status, diagnosis, and prognosis?
- What is the recommended treatment?
- What are the reasonable alternative treatments, and what would be the effect of no treatment?
- What goals are attainable for this particular patient with this specific condition?
- What trade-offs must be made among the possible goals—for example, between relief of suffering and maximal preservation of function?

Of course, any such determination in medicine must be expressed in probabilities rather than in certainties.

### Preferences of the patient

The physician should pay attention to the patient's personal goals in this encounter. He or she should make sure the patient is fully informed and has had time to consider the reasonable options, and explore whether the probable outcomes of the suggested course of action are consistent with the patient's value system and life plan. Although the patient's goals usually are the same as the clinician's, occasionally they differ from those of the clinician for personal or psychological reasons, and some accommodations must be made.

### Social, cultural, political, and economic realities

Any goals sought by clinicians and patients must be pursued within the context of religious, social, cultural, political, and economic realities. Access to scarce resources, the mandates of the current health care system, the wealth or poverty of individuals and communities, religious and cultural beliefs, and family pressures will facilitate the attainment of some goals and render the achievement of others unlikely.

**TABLE 13.2. Goals for Physicians in Patient Encounters**

*Always*
Avoidance of harm to the patient in the course of care (*primum non nocere*).
Palliation (relief of pain and suffering) and comfort care *in all situations.*

*Before disease is established*
Prevention of disease and untimely death.

*When disease is established*
Cure of disease and restoration of health, *when possible.*
Improvement or maintenance of functional status *when cure is not possible.*
Education and counseling regarding the condition and its prognosis.

## Basic Concepts in Medical Ethics

### Informed consent

Informed consent is rooted in the English common law on battery, which forbids harmful or offensive nonconsensual touching. No special exceptions were made for medical care, except in emergency situations. The modern American judicial definition of consent is that made by Justice Cardozo in 1914: "Every human being of adult years and sound mind has a right to determine what shall be done with his [or her] own body; and a surgeon who performs an operation without his [or her] patient's consent commits an assault for which he [or she] is liable for damages." In the latter half of the 20th century, the courts began merging the physician's traditional duty to secure consent with an obligation of disclosure, perhaps best understood as a duty to warn patients of potential side effects or consequences of medical treatment, resulting in the legal concept of "informed consent."

The purpose of informed consent is to provide the patient with the information necessary to allow a reasonable person to make a prudent treatment choice. According to the President's Commission, adequate informed consent involves more than just a signature on the bottom of a list of possible complications; it requires effort on the part of the physician to ensure the patient's comprehension. "Such recitations can be so overwhelming that patients are unable to distinguish truly significant information and to make sound decisions." Rather, informed consent attempts to foster a conversational partnership between doctor and patients in the clinical setting.

The elements incorporated into the current doctrine of informed consent require the physician to ensure that the patient has a clear understanding of the following subjects:

- The disease process (diagnosis in understandable terms)
- The prognosis (probable course of this patient's specific disease)
- The benefits and burdens of the recommended treatment
- The benefits and burdens of reasonable alternative treatments
- The probable effect of no treatment (which is always an option).

The consent that follows this disclosure entails the patient's voluntary, autonomous authorization to proceed with the proposed intervention.

### Patient's right to refuse treatment

Adult patients of sound mind have the right to refuse any treatment on their own behalf, and courts have increasingly granted surrogate decision makers the right to withdraw treatment as well. This right extends even to the withdrawal of treatment from patients who are not judged to be terminal. The *Bartling* decision in California states that "competent adult patients with serious illnesses which are probably incurable but have not been diagnosed as terminal have the right over the objections of their physicians and the hospital to have life support equipment disconnected, despite the fact that withdrawal of such devices will surely hasten death."

Since the Bartling decision, there have been no legal cases challenging the right of the "decisional patient" (i.e., one who is capable of making a decision) to refuse any treatment, including fluid and nutrition.

### Confidentiality and the patient's right to privacy

The basis for the principle of confidentiality is respect for an individual's privacy and the special relationship of trust in the doctor–patient encounter. Because confidentiality is considered necessary for the good of society and to prevent harm to the patient, it is not to be breached without a compelling reason.

Legal exceptions exist to the patient's right to confidentiality. Physicians may breach confidentiality to testify in court; to report communicable disease; to report child, spouse, or elder abuse; and to report gunshot or suspicious wounds if there is reasonable cause to believe that the wound occurred as the result of a crime. Aside from these specific situations, breach of confidentiality rarely can be justified ethically; such a breach can be justified only when all of a few specific conditions are met (Table 13.3).

### Decision–making capacity

"Competence" and "incompetence" are legal terms. Technically, a patient remains competent until a court decides otherwise; however, the determination of decision-making capacity can be made by medical personnel and does not require a court hearing.

**TABLE 13.3. Breach of Patient Confidentiality by Physician**

| |
|---|
| Breach of privacy is permissible when all of the following conditions are met: |
| A high probability exists of serious physical harm to an identifiable, specific person. |
| A benefit will result from breaking the confidence (i.e., the harm can be prevented). |
| The breach is a last resort; persuasion and other approaches have failed. |
| The breach is generalizable; it would be reasonable for doctors, in general, to breach such confidence. |

The assessment of a patient's ability to make autonomous judgments requires the evaluation of the following three distinct aspects of his or her decision-making capacity:

**Understanding:** The ability to comprehend the given information about diagnosis and treatment and to appreciate the impact of the disease and its consequences

**Evaluating:** The ability to deliberate in accordance with one's own values, to manipulate information rationally, and to compare the risks and benefits of the options

**Communicating:** The ability to communicate choices to persons providing medical care.

#### Incapacitated (nondecisional) patients

When a surrogate acts for an incapacitated patient, the basis for his or her decision is either "substituted judgment" or the "best interest" standard. Substituted judgment is the guideline the surrogate uses if the patient has expressed a preference before becoming incapacitated or if the surrogate knows the patient well enough to determine what the patient would choose if he or she were still decisional.

The "best interests" standard is what the surrogate must use when he or she is unsure of what the patient might choose or if the patient never has been decisional. It is what a reasonable person might choose in the same context and is based on what is ultimately best for the particular patient in his or her particular circumstances. When a patient has a legal guardian, the guardian has the right to make decisions, including the refusal of life-sustaining treatment, based on the patient's best interests considering the diagnosis, prognosis, and medical goals of treatment.

#### Advance directives

Medical advances have widened the range of options a patient has for the treatment of many diseases, but also have resulted in increased patient concerns about invasive, expensive, and unwanted treatment. An advance directive (AD) provides valuable written evidence of an individual patient's desires, to both physician and family. An AD is a statement a patient makes while he or she still is capable of deciding how treatment decisions should be made if at some future time he or she losses the capacity to make such decisions. There are two types of ADs: the Living Will (LW) and the Power of Attorney for Health Care (PAHC).

Most statutory forms of LW are documents stating the desire of the signer to die a natural death and not to be kept alive by medical treatment and machines. In many states, the principal also may stipulate that fluid and nutrition are to be discontinued in the event that the signer is left in a persistent vegetative state. Usually, the LW becomes effective on the determination of a "terminal" illness or "imminent" death (death expected within 6 months) or when two physicians make the diagnosis of a persistent, vegetative state. Usually, there is no provision for adding a personal statement with specific instructions.

Power of Attorney for Health Care documents allow the signer to appoint a person to act as health care agent, or proxy, to make health care decisions in the event that the signer becomes nondecisional. The PAHC allows the principal to add specific directions; often, the agent may be given authority to have feeding tubes withheld or withdrawn, even in the absence of a persistent vegetative state. The PAHC typically becomes effective when two physicians determine that the principal is no longer decisional.

Patients may ask for advice about advance directives. The statutory form of PAHC has the advantage of allowing all the options of an LW plus the advantage of allowing for the insertion of specific instructions and, most important, of providing an agent—someone who knows the principal well and can take an active role in the decision-making process on the patient's behalf. There is no advantage to filling out both forms. Because the specific laws regarding LW and PAHC vary from state to state, it is wise for patients to check the provision and activating clauses in their own jurisdiction.

## Specific Issues in Medical Ethics

#### "Do-not-resuscitate" orders

The issue of cardiopulmonary resuscitation (CPR) should be addressed early in the treatment of a seriously ill patient in whom cardiac or pulmonary arrest is likely to occur. The subject should be approached sensitively, as part of the overall therapeutic plan. The comfort and therapeutic measures that will remain in effect should be discussed first. The legal authority for the decision to write a do-not-resuscitate (DNR) order may emanate from the specific request of a decisional patient, from the dictates of an advance directive, or from the judgment of a guardian.

In some states, surrogate laws establish a hierarchy of decision-making authority for the nondecisional patient; in others, moral authority but no legal authority exists for others, in the following order: spouse, adult children, parents, siblings. If no relatives or friends are available for consultation, the decision should be based on medical indications, taking into consideration whether CPR would further the reasonable personal medical goals of the patient in his or her current particular circumstances.

Ordinarily, DNR simply means no CPR. A DNR order may have no other significance and may permit all other modalities of treatment, including intensive care.

On the other hand, a DNR order may be the first step in the withdrawal of other treatment; thus, specific orders detailing what may remain in use must be written to avoid misunderstandings. The rationale and specific orders need to be discussed fully with the nursing staff and the patient's other caregivers so there are no uncertainties about care plans. Sometimes, patients or their families fear abandonment by health care professionals when a DNR order is written; therefore, physicians and nurses alike should remain attentive to both the patient and the family and aware of comfort measures. The patient and family must know from the outset that "no code" does not mean "no care."

**Withdrawal versus withholding of treatment**

For the physician, refraining from starting treatment is easier psychologically than discontinuing it. A moment's reflection demonstrates that this is illogical; the decision to omit treatment is just as much a willful judgment as the decision to withdraw it. The decision to withhold a specific treatment may create an "up-front" barrier, denying from the outset a treatment that might be effective. Thus, a decision to withhold treatment must actually have more substantial reasons than a decision to discontinue, or withdraw, treatment that has clearly failed. When the effectiveness of a treatment is uncertain, the bias clearly must be in favor of a time-limited trial. If the treatment proves to be ineffective for a particular patient in a given circumstance, it can be stopped. This way the patient has a reasonable chance of attaining the goals of the specific therapy.

**Futility**

Occasionally, patients demand or request treatment modalities that the physician believes to be ineffective or even medically contraindicated because they are futile. *Futility* has been defined as any effort to achieve a result that is possible but that experience suggests is highly improbable. Some further consider futility a disproportionate burden including treatment that will not serve any useful purpose, that may cause needless pain and suffering, and that will not achieve the goal of restoring the patient to an acceptable quality of life (as defined by the patient).

Professional integrity requires the ethical physician to refuse requests for futile interventions. The President's Commission stated the following: "The well-being principle circumscribes the range of alternatives offered to patients: informed consent does not mean that patients can insist upon anything they might want. Rather, it is a choice among medically accepted and available options, all of which are believed to have some possibility of promoting the patient's welfare." And the Council on Ethical and Judicial Affairs of the AMA stated that "the right of the patient to choose does not imply the right to demand care beyond appropriate options based on medical judgment and accepted standards of care, nor are physicians required to provide care in ways that in their personal judgment violate the principles of medical ethics."

Resolution of this sort of impasse requires a dialogue with the patient to elicit the reasons behind the request for a medically futile intervention. Often, such a conversation will solve the dilemma; if not, the physician may need to transfer the patient to the care of another. Many physicians unreasonably fear liability for not "doing everything," such as using every available technology if the patient requests it, but the law rarely dictates the particulars of clinical practice and does not require that physicians do everything requested by a patient, agent, or guardian.

**Euthanasia and assisted suicide**

The important aspect of agency marks the difference between euthanasia and assisted suicide. Euthanasia, in which the physician is the agent, is an intentional act to cause the immediate death of a person with a terminal, incurable, or painful disease by the medical administration of a lethal drug. In assisted suicide, the physician provides the lethal drug with instructions for its use, but the patient is the agent who decides when and if to use the drug.

Euthanasia is illegal in all states. All states but Oregon now have some sort of legal prohibition against assisted suicide. Thirty-one states have a specific law against assisting a suicide; in the remaining states, prosecution is possible under other existing statutes.

Official medical organizations are uniform in their stance that these actions are unethical. The American College of Physicians Ethics Manual states, "Although a patient may refuse a medical intervention and the physician may comply with this refusal, the physician must never intentionally and directly cause death or assist a patient to commit suicide."

In several recent surveys, the majority of the public has expressed support for some form of physician-assisted death under some circumstances. In 1994 the voters of Oregon authorized controlled physician-assisted suicide. Court challenges delayed implementation until October 1997. In November 1997, another vote failed to repeal the 1994 initiative; thus, Oregon is the only state in which physician-assisted suicide is legal under stipulated safeguards. The "Laboratory of the States" will test this issue.

Analyzing the stimulus for these initiatives, which have such widespread public support, and attempting to change those factors that are amenable to change, is the responsibility of physicians. Prominent among the fears of the public, which fuel this debate, are the concerns that terminal pain will not be controlled adequately and that medical technology might be used inappropriately, thus delaying a timely or natural death. The public is also concerned about loss of control and the indignity of dependence during the final stages of illness and, thus, seeks possible remedies.

Assurance of adequate pain control, which must be given without fear of inducing addiction or respiratory depression in the terminally ill, will help assuage the first fear. Use of appropriate palliative measures and increased reliance on hospice care will relieve many of the other concerns. A resolute recommendation for the use of advance directives by a physician and his or her willingness to discuss these issues will help allay patient worries about end-of-life decisions.

If all of the physician interventions discussed in this chapter are carried out successfully, the stimulus for state initiatives should decrease. Nonetheless, despite good pain control and hospice care, a patient may request aid in dying because, for him or her, there is no acceptable alternative to immediate death. Each physician will have to decide for him or herself how to respond when a patient makes such a request.

#### Ethics consultation

Advances in medicine have resulted in new ethical dilemmas. Questions now concern not only what can be done for this patient but also what *should* be done. In most hospitals today, ethics consultation is available to physicians and patients to help resolve the vexing problems that sometimes arise in patient care. Institutional ethics committees (ECs) have many different configurations. Many are standing committees comprised of members of the professional staff that report to the medical executive committees or governing staff of the hospital. Most meet monthly or more often, as occasion demands. Typically, ECs have three tasks: (1) education, of committee members first, and of staff and community later; (2) formulation of policy at the request of the medical staff or institutional administration (ordinarily the EC is not a policy-making body); and (3) specific case consultation on request.

The attending physician might want an ethics consultation for any of the following reasons: (1) to clarify issues regarding decisional capacity, informed consent, or advance directives; (2) to provide counsel on the ethical aspects of withdrawal of treatment in specific cases; and (3) to help resolve conflicts regarding ethical issues that might arise between patients and caregivers, or between family and caregivers, or among staff members.

No single ethical principle suffices in any case consultation. Cases vary too much to allow for such generalizations. The consultant usually allows the details of the case to frame the issues; the consultation process allows the patient, family, and others to identify the important factors and values at stake. This medical casuistry—solving issues by considering the clinical circumstances that surround and affect the cases instead of applying a set of rules or principles to them—characterizes the consultant's ethical analysis.

After analysis of the issues, the EC, or the ethics consultant acting on behalf of the EC, must ensure that the information is complete and that the ethical problem is delineated clearly. In clarifying the possible options, the EC must ensure that the patient will have as much autonomy as possible. The recommendations should be consistent with the patient's preferences or best interests and with ethical and, if possible, legal principles. Recommendations should be made as recommendations only; the attending physician and the patient must decide whether to take or reject them, as is true of all consultations.

# CHAPTER 14 PALLIATIVE CARE

The World Health Organization defines palliative care as the active total care of patients whose disease is not responsive to curative treatment. Patients with advanced cancer, end-stage cardiac or renal disease, advanced chronic obstructive pulmonary disease, AIDS, end-stage liver disease, or advanced neurologic disease (e.g., dementia, Parkinson disease, cerebrovascular disease, amyotrophic lateral sclerosis, multiple sclerosis) are all candidates for palliative care.

Palliative care makes control of pain and other symptoms, and of psychological, social and spiritual problems, paramount. Palliative care affirms life and regards dying as a normal process, neither hastens nor postpones death, provides relief from pain and other distressing symptoms, integrates the psychological and spiritual aspects of patient care, and offers a support system to help the family cope during the patient's illness and their own bereavement. The goal of palliative care is achievement of the best possible quality of life for patients and their families.

## History

Palliative care has its roots in hospice care. *Hospitium*—the Latin word for hospice—means hospitality. Early hospices, such as those run by the Sisters of Charity founded by Saint Vincent de Paul in the 17th century in France, were always connected to religious organizations. Like current hospices, they provided physical, emotional, and spiritual support to dying patients. The modern hospice movement began in 1967 when Dr. Cicely Saunders founded a formal hospice program at Saint Christopher's in London. The first hospice program in the United States was started in 1974. Currently, there are more than 2000 hospice programs throughout the U.S.

## Palliative Care Versus Hospice Care

Palliative care and hospice care share the same philosophy: to provide physical, emotional, social, and spiritual care to patients whose disease is not responsive to curative treatment. However, palliative care treats symptoms more aggressively and earlier in the disease, whereas hospice care is reserved for the final stages of a terminal disease. Palliative care usually is provided in inpatient settings or in regular home care programs, and is covered under traditional methods of payment for medical illnesses. But hospice care usually is provided where the patient lives—nursing home, assisted living, prison, or residential home—and is covered under the Medicare Hospice Benefit, which requires documentation that the patient's life expectancy is 6 months or less. Finally, in palliative care, a multidisciplinary team of professionals and volunteers works together to address the needs of the dying patient, whereas in hospice care the primary caregiver often is a family member. In palliative care, each member of the team, which can include physicians, nurses, social workers, psychologists, chaplains, rehabilitation professionals, pharmacists, and dietitians, has a unique and important role. The team members meet regularly and follow the patient closely to ensure that the physical, psychosocial, and spiritual domains of care are being attended to.

## The Specific Tasks of Palliative Care

### Symptom relief

#### *Pain*

Pain is a very common symptom in palliative care patients, affecting up to 75% of terminal cancer patients, for example. Nociceptive pain is the most common type of pain experienced by cancer patients. It is generated from direct stimulation of mechanical, chemical, or thermal sensory receptors, and can be somatic or visceral. Somatic pain is the result of direct stimulation of nociceptors in the skin, soft tissues, muscle, and bone. Patients typically describe this kind of pain as sharp, aching, or throbbing, and it is very well localized. Pain due to metastatic bone disease is an example of somatic pain. Visceral pain originates in organs such as the heart, lung, liver, or gastrointestinal or genitourinary tracts, and it is the result of autonomic nervous system stimulation. Visceral pain tends to be vague and poorly localized, and often is referred to distant cutaneous areas. Neuropathic pain is associated with cancer progression and is believed to be caused by dysfunction of the peripheral or central nervous system. Neuropathic pain usually is described as "burning" or "shooting" and may be accompanied by sensations of numbness or tingling. Tumor involvement of the cervical, brachial, or lumbosacral plexus can originate neuropathic pain.

Effective treatment of pain requires a very thorough history and physical examination looking for different sources of pain. Evaluation of the pain complaint should include characteristics of the pain, such as intensity, character, frequency, temporal pattern, location, duration, and precipitating and alleviating factors. Pain also must be quantified by a pain assessment scale such as a numeric pain scale or a visual analog scale. The physician should be aware that pain also may be exacerbated by psychosocial and spiritual distress experienced by the dying patient. Oral administration of opioid analgesics should always be preferred because of convenience and low cost. The intramuscular route should be avoided because of pain and unreliable drug absorption. Intravenous and subcutaneous opioid administration is indicated in patients who have severe pain and intolerance to the oral route, in patients who need rapid titration of opioid analgesics, and in patients who are taking large doses of oral opioids. An opioid equivalence table should always be used when switching opioid administration from the oral to the parenteral route (Table 14.1). The transdermal fentanyl patch is ideal for patients who cannot tolerate oral analgesics or prefer transdermal systems. The most common adverse effects of opioid use are nausea, constipation, sedation, respiratory depression, pruritus, urinary retention, and myoclonus.

Adjuvant analgesics are drugs from different classes that enhance the analgesic efficacy of opioids. The drugs most commonly used in adjuvant therapy for the treatment of cancer pain are NSAIDs, bisphosphonates, and radioisotopes for metastatic bone pain; tricyclic antidepressants and anticonvulsants for neuropathic pain; corticosteroids for raised intracranial pressure; and anticholinergics for visceral or colicky pain.

Fear of causing addiction in patients with chronic pain or terminal situations in which large doses must be continued for long periods can lead to substandard pain control. Studies have shown that addiction is rare in patients who receive opioids for pain, even if the drug

TABLE 14.1. Oral and Parenteral Dose Equivalents of Commonly Used Opioid Analgesic Drugs

| Drug | Dosage | | Dosing Interval |
|---|---|---|---|
| | Oral | Parenteral | |
| Morphine | 30 mg | 10 mg | q 3–4 hr |
| Hydromorphone | 7.5 mg | 1.5 mg | q 3–4 hr |
| Oxycodone | 30 mg | Not available | q 3–4 hr |
| Hydrocodone | 30 mg | Not available | q 3–4 hr |
| Codeine | 180 mg | 130 mg | q 3–4 hr |

must be continued for protracted periods. If the patient is receiving morphine for the pain of terminal malignancy, the question of addiction is irrelevant. Underdosing of a narcotic in terminal patients for fear of producing respiratory depression is another common mistake. The experiences of hospices and oncology services show that respiratory depression is uncommon in patients who are receiving opioids for pain control. The physician must balance the issue of pain control against the rare, undesired effect of respiratory depression.

One ethics panel has addressed the issue as follows: "In the patient whose dying process is irreversible, the balance between minimizing pain and suffering and potentially hastening death should be struck clearly in favor of pain relief. Narcotics and other pain medications should be given in whatever dose and by whatever route is necessary for relief." Most ethicists would agree that it is morally permissible to "increase the dose of narcotics to whatever dose is needed," even though the medication may contribute to the depression of respiration or blood pressure, the dulling of consciousness, or even death—providing the primary goal of the physician is to relieve suffering. The proper dose of pain medication is the dose that is sufficient to relive pain and suffering—even if it causes unconsciousness.

*Dyspnea*

Dyspnea is common in dying patients; up to one half of terminally ill patients may experience severe dyspnea. Dyspnea in terminally ill patients can be caused by neuromuscular disease, restriction of movement of the chest or abdominal walls, pneumonia, pulmonary embolism, pleural effusion, bronchospasm, tracheal obstruction, congestive heart failure, pericardial effusion, cardiac ischemia, lymphangitis carcinomatosa, superior vena cava syndrome, bronchial obstruction by a tumor, and severe anemia. Assessment includes a thorough history and physical examination to try to identify the underlying cause. Investigations should be appropriate to the stage of the disease. Simple tests such as a complete blood cell count, chest radiograph, electrocardiogram, and pulse oximetry may be helpful. More complex tests such as a pulmonary function test, arterial blood gas level, echocardiogram, and ventilation-perfusion scan should be avoided in patients at a very advanced stage of their illness. Treatment is directed to the underlying cause. Thus measures such as antibiotics, therapeutic thoracentesis, bronchodilators, or anticoagulants are very effective in some cases.

Opioids are the drugs of choice for treating unrelieved dyspnea. Immediate-release morphine treats dyspnea effectively and at doses lower than would be necessary for relief of pain. Nebulized opioids also have been used for palliation of dyspnea in chronic lung disease, chronic heart disease, and cancer. Corticosteroids can be used to relieve dyspnea in patients with end-stage chronic obstructive pulmonary disease, lymphangitis carcinomatosa, bronchial obstruction by a tumor, or superior vena cava syndrome. Nonpharmacologic interventions for management of terminal dyspnea include use of supplemental oxygen, adequate positioning in bed, use of a fan, relaxation techniques, and distraction. Anxiolytics can be helpful when a patient's dyspnea is aggravated by feelings of anxiety.

*Nausea and vomiting*

Nausea and vomiting are common symptoms in terminally ill patients. The vomiting center is located in the midbrain and receives input from the cerebral cortex, the inner ear, the gastrointestinal tract, and the chemoreceptor trigger zone. Causes of nausea and vomiting often are multifactorial and may include fluid and electrolyte imbalances (e.g., hyponatremia, hypokalemia, and hypercalcemia), gastrointestinal problems (e.g., candidiasis of the oral or esophageal mucosa, gastric cancer, liver metastases, peptic ulcer disease, pancreatic cancer, constipation, bowel obstruction), central nervous system metastases, tumor toxins, drugs (e.g., opioids, chemotherapy agents), or anxiety.

Evaluation of nausea and vomiting requires a thorough history and physical examination. The volume, content, and timing of emesis should be noted. A rectal digital examination should always be performed to assess

TABLE 14.2. Common Antiemetics

| Drug Class | Route |
|---|---|
| *Serotonin 5-HT3 antagonists* | |
| Ondansetron | po, iv |
| Granisetron | iv |
| Dolasetron | po, iv |
| *Dopamine antagonists* | |
| Prochlorperazine | po, im, pr |
| Promethazine | po, im, pr |
| Droperidol | iv |
| Metoclopramide | po, iv |
| *Antihistamine and anticholinergics* | |
| Diphenhydramine | po, im, iv |
| Scopolamine patch | patch |
| Meclizine | po |
| *Corticosteroids* | |
| Dexamethasone | po, iv |
| *Benzodiazepines* | |
| Diazepam | po, iv |
| Lorazepam | po, iv |
| *Cannabioids* | |
| Dronabinol | po |

for fecal impaction. Abdominal films also may be ordered when there is a suspicion of bowel obstruction or atonic ileus.

Treatment should address the underlying cause. Drugs commonly used to treat terminal nausea and vomiting are listed in Table 14.2. Patients should be encouraged to eat small, frequent meals; avoid disagreeable foods and odors, as well as fatty and fried foods; and take most medications after eating (except antiemetics).

*Constipation*

Constipation is a common problem among dying patients, mostly because of opioid use, poor dietary intake, and physical inactivity. Other causes include bowel obstruction, hypercalcemia, drugs (anticholinergics, antacids, anticonvulsants, iron, and antihypertensives), tumor invasion of the lumbosacral spinal cord, cauda equina or pelvic plexus, systemic diseases (e.g., diabetes, hypothyroidism), and hemorrhoids.

It is important to clarify a complaint of constipation with a careful history and physical examination that includes a digital rectal examination. Abdominal radiographs are useful if there is a suspicion of bowel obstruction or fecal impaction. Blood tests can be performed if the clinical picture is suggestive of either hypercalcemia or hypothyroidism.

Laxatives should be given prophylactically when opioid therapy is begun. Generally, a stool softener (e.g., docusate) and a stimulant laxative (e.g., bisacodyl, senna, cascara sagrada) should be given first. Osmotic laxatives (e.g., lactulose, sorbitol, magnesium citrate) and enemas can be added as needed.

**Nutrition and hydration**

Anorexia is a common problem in patients receiving palliative care. It can be related to endogenous cytokines, metabolic disturbances, infections, chronic pain, nausea, oral candidiasis, xerostomia, constipation, bowel obstruction, and drugs. Assessment requires a thorough history and physical examination, with special emphasis on treatable causes. Some patients may benefit from appetite stimulants such as prednisone, megestrol acetate, and dronabinol.

Patients should always be involved in menu planning and offered easy-to-swallow foods, such as semiliquids, puddings, or soft pureed foods.

Food and fluid administration may play a minimal role in providing comfort to terminally ill patients and should only be given at the specific requests of patients. Nutritional support for dying patients has been shown to provide little benefit in terms of morbidity and mortality; in fact, aggressive nutritional therapy may decrease survival because of complications of dietary therapy and enhanced tumor growth. Nasogastric and gastrostomy tube feeding, as well as total parenteral nutrition, are associated with complications such as infection, epistaxis, pneumothorax, electrolyte imbalance, and aspiration.

Artificial hydration also is a controversial issue in palliative care. Supplemental hydration can adversely affect the quality of life of a terminal patient by increasing oral and airway secretions or by leading to the development or worsening of ascites, pleural effusions, and peripheral and pulmonary edema.

**Delirium and agitation**

Many terminally ill patients develop delirium when death is approaching. Delirium is a an acute confusional state characterized by cognitive loss, impaired attention, hallucinations, illusions, psychomotor agitation or retardation, disturbances of the sleep-wake cycle (e.g., sundowning), fear, and anxiety.

Common causes of delirium can be remembered using the mnemonic DELIRIUM:

**D**rugs (especially psychotropics)
**E**lectrolyte or glucose abnormality
**L**iver failure
**I**schemia or hypoxia
**R**enal failure
**I**mpaction of stool
**U**rinary tract or other infection
**M**etastases to the brain.

Assessment of delirium requires a careful history and physical examination. Blood tests for glucose, electrolytes, blood urea nitrogen, creatinine, calcium, magnesium, and ammonia, and chest radiographs also can be obtained. Appropriate management of delirium involves addressing the underlying cause. General measures include placing the patient in a well-lighted room with family members, familiar objects, and a visible calendar or clock. When the cause of delirium cannot be identified or treated, drugs such as neuroleptics (e.g., haloperidol, thioridazine, risperidone) or benzodiazepines (e.g., lorazepam, diazepam, and midazolam) should be used. When delirium is refractory to these treatments, sedation may be required with the use of barbiturates.

## Psychosocial Care

Patients experience profound psychological, interpersonal, and existential changes as they go through the dying process. The patient with a terminal disease is frequently distressed by increasing losses: of health, physical appearance, job, social role, and relationships, and even loss of control over where and by whom care will be provided. These losses are devastating in many ways, and patients often respond with anger outbursts. Feelings of depression, anxiety, abandonment, and fear of the unknown are frequently experienced by the dying patient.

Pain, advanced illness, and a high level of disability are risk factors for depression in patients receiving palliative care. The somatic symptoms of depression, such as fatigue, anorexia, and insomnia, are common in dying patients, which limits the diagnostic usefulness of those symptoms. Thus, the psychological symptoms such as dysphoric mood, hopelessness, worthlessness, guilt, and suicidal ideation have a greater diagnostic value. Depression in terminally ill patients is managed optimally using a combination of supportive psychotherapy, cognitive-behavioral therapy, and antidepressant medications.

Terminally ill patients usually experience high levels of anxiety, generally described as an unpleasant feeling of helplessness or fear. It can be precipitated by medical complications such as uncontrolled pain, dyspnea, delirium, infection, and withdrawal of opioids and benzodiazepines. Feelings of uncertainty, isolation, fear, anger, guilt, and financial stress, and concern about family members are factors that can contribute to anxiety in terminally ill patients. Management includes brief psychotherapy and use of anxiolytic drugs.

Psychosocial intervention is based on a full assessment of the needs and wishes of the patient and family. Active listening, reassurance, and support may help patients and families deal with psychological challenges. Psychosocial care also involves assessment of the patient's support system within the family and the community, the domestic needs of the patient, and the financial resources available to the patient.

## Spiritual Care

Care in terminal illnesses must include an assessment of the patient's spiritual beliefs and needs. Spirituality is the inner desire to understand or accept the underlying meaning of life, one's relationships to oneself and other people, one's place in the universe, and the possibility of a "higher power" in the universe. Spirituality is considered a universal human concern. Spiritual needs commonly seen in dying patients are the need for belonging and relationships; the need to explore the meaning of life, suffering and death; and the need for reconciliation.

Physicians always should ask their patients about spiritual concerns. For example, asking, "How are you within yourself?," "What does your illness/dying mean to you?," "What do you hope for?," or "What is your source of strength, help or hope?" allows patients an opportunity to share their spiritual beliefs.

## Bereavement Care

Bereavement is a series of reactions, both internal and external, to the loss of a close relationship. Bereavement services are offered to every family after the patient's death.

The goal for the bereaved family members is to learn to accept life and to reorganize, reengage, and redefine themselves apart from the person who has died. A bereavement program can include individual and family counseling, support group, educational materials that describe normal grief, spiritual counseling, friendly visiting, and telephone support.

## Ethical Issues

Palliative care of the terminally ill patient often involves complex medical dilemmas for the patient and family. The physician should know the basic ethical principles that underlie issues such as decision-making capacity, informed consent and shared decision-making, advance directives, withholding or withdrawing medical treatment, medical futility, euthanasia, and physician-assisted suicide (see Chapter 13).

# ■ Questions

**Instructions:** For each question below, select only **one** lettered answer that is the **best** for that question.

1. Primary care is best defined as:
   A. Patient-centered care
   B. Health maintenance
   C. Both high-tech and high-touch care

D. Coordinated, convenient, comprehensive, and continuous care
E. State-of-the-art care

Refer to items A through E below for questions 2 through 5:

A. Medicare part A
B. Medicare part B
C. Medicaid
D. Out-of-pocket expense
E. Usual commercial insurance

2. For patients over the age of 65 years, the appropriate payer mechanism for nursing home care is:

3. For patients over the age of 65 years, the appropriate payer mechanism for physician services is:

4. For patients over the age of 65 years, the appropriate payer mechanism for hospital care is:

5. For patients over the age of 65 years, the appropriate payer mechanism for prescription drugs is:

6. You are taking care of a patient who has had an episode of fainting due to ventricular tachycardia. Recommendations from the cardiology staff are that your patient needs to have an implantable cardiac defibrillator placed or to be placed on amiodarone, a medication he will need to take daily to reduce his risk from sudden death due to ventricular tachycardia. Your patient is undecided about which option he should choose. He has asked you to help him with this decision. How should you help your patient?
   A. Reassure your patient that the cardiologist is an expert so we have asked him to recommend the best option.
   B. Look up the benefits and risks of implantable defibrillators versus amiodarone in a textbook of cardiology.
   C. Read a review article on management of ventricular tachycardia and make a decision based on the author's recommendations.
   D. Conduct a focused literature search looking for randomized clinical trials that compare the effectiveness of defibrillators with amiodarone in human subjects and evaluate clinical outcomes (mortality and morbidity) between the two treatments.

7. Which of the following factors is, in most instances, the most important one in making a diagnosis?
   A. History and physical examination
   B. Blood and urine tests
   C. Electrophysiologic tests
   D. Radiographic imaging of the affected area
   E. Endoscopy

8. Which of the following statements best defines laboratory tests?
   A. They are quantitative and always give the exact diagnosis.
   B. They are part of a complete diagnostic examination and must be performed in every patient.
   C. They are inexpensive when fully automated.
   D. They are most helpful only when combined with a good history and physical examination.
   E. Results often are wrong due to laboratory errors.

9. All of the following are basic tenets of effective screening efforts EXCEPT:
   A. The condition that can be diagnosed by the screening test is prevalent and causes significant morbidity.
   B. Effective treatment of screening-diagnosed cases in presymptomatic patients improves morbidity.
   C. Available screening tests are specific, but not sensitive.
   D. The screening test and any follow-up tests are safe.

10. Which of the following statements regarding health education is TRUE?
   A. The physician should leave it up to the patient to seek it.
   B. It should only be performed by allied health professionals, who have more time.
   C. If the patient is intelligent and well-informed, there is little need to educate him or her in matters of health.
   D. It can be effective in preventing illness and prolonging life.

11. A 28-year-old woman presents to your clinic after testing positive on a home pregnancy test. She wants to know if she should discontinue any of her medications because of the pregnancy. The patient has a history of essential hypertension and is on lisinopril. What should you advise?
   A. Have the patient stay on the lisinopril until she sees her obstetrician because the priority is to control her blood pressure.
   B. Discontinue the lisinopril and begin pharmacologic treatment only if her systolic blood pressure is above 155.
   C. Discontinue the lisinopril and begin a beta-blocker.
   D. Discontinue the lisinopril and begin methyldopa.

12. Which one of the following statements would not promote open communication with patients?
   A. What vitamins or herbal supplements have you tried for this condition?
   B. What benefits do you hope to obtain?

C. I don't believe in that therapy. There is no scientific evidence to prove that it helps.
D. I know you've been trying that therapy. Is it helping?
E. I have not heard much about that therapy, but I am willing to look into it. Do you have any evidence I can review?

13. Jim is a medical student and has been asked by his resident to enter a discharge summary for their patient, Mr. Jaundice, into the computerized medical records system. Because Jim has not yet received his computer password, the resident lets him use his password to gain access to the records. In this situation, which one response is the correct answer?
    A. The senior resident should not have shared his password. Instead, he should have logged on to the system and then let Jim work on it.
    B. Sharing of passwords within the medical community is common and acceptable, as long as they are shared between medical colleagues.
    C. Patient confidentiality and privacy are placed at risk whenever a person shares his password with any other person. This practice is not acceptable.

14. Which of the following is an example of a polygenic or complex genetic disorder?
    A. Diabetes mellitus
    B. Obesity
    C. Hypertension
    D. Alzheimer disease
    E. All of the above

15. An 80-year-old man is hospitalized for palliative treatment of carcinoma of the prostate, which has metastasized widely. His bone pain has been difficult to control, necessitating large doses of morphine. A nurse, concerned because his respiratory rate is 5 per minute 20 minutes after the last dose of morphine, calls the intern, who orders Narcan. The patient awakens in excruciating pain and curses all those in earshot. The resident arrives on the scene, and re-sedates the patient, even though the exact dose of morphine required again results in some respiratory depression. The patient dies 5 hours later. Which of the following statements is correct?
    A. This action is legally and ethically permissible provided the intention is only the relief of pain.
    B. Because of the likelihood of respiratory depression, this action is actually an instance of euthanasia.
    C. The resident physician's action makes him liable to a lawsuit from the family.
    D. A smaller dose of morphine, which would not entirely control his pain but would not cause respiratory depression, is in order.

16. A 92-year-old man is admitted for nausea and vomiting, which was attributed to medication and soon subsided. An Ethics Committee consultation was triggered by his refusal to eat adequate amounts of food—he had lost 40 pounds in the previous 6 months. When confronted with the problem, he said that he knew he would die if he did not eat enough and that was his wish. He repeatedly and vehemently refused the suggestion of a feeding tube. Psychiatric consultation found him to be fully decisional. The appropriate response would be:
    A. To attempt to convince him to eat by threatening to use a nasogastric tube if he did not.
    B. To ignore his requests and place a nasogastric tube for his welfare.
    C. To feed him whatever he will take and use medication to control his symptoms.
    D. To start him on total parenteral nutrition.

17. Which of the following classes of drugs can be used as adjuvant therapy to morphine when treating cancer pain?
    A. Anticholinergics
    B. Tricyclic antidepressants
    C. Anticonvulsants
    D. Corticosteroids
    E. All of the above

18. AB is a 54-year-old woman who works in the regional post office. She reports a 4-day history of flu-like symptoms that have gotten progressively worse. She presents today with high fever, headache, chest pain, and hemoptysis. Chest x-ray shows an enlarged mediastinum, which chest CT confirmed was due to mediastinal lymphadenopathy. Her last chest x-ray from 3 weeks ago was within normal limits. Which of the following agents might be the cause of this illness?
    A. *Francisella tularensis*
    B. *Yersinia pestis*
    C. *Bacillus anthracis*
    D. *Mycobacterium tuberculosis*
    E. Influenza A

## Answers

| | | | | |
|---|---|---|---|---|
| 1. D | 2. C | 3. B | 4. A | 5. D |
| 6. D | 7. A | 8. D | 9. C | 10. D |
| 11. D | 12. C | 13. C | 14. E | 15. A |
| 16. C | 17. E | 18. C | | |

## SUGGESTED READING

### *General*

*Books and Monographs*

Bennett JC, Goldman L, (eds). Cecil Textbook of Medicine. 21st ed. Philadelphia: WB Saunders, 2000.

Braunwald E, Fauci A, Hansen S, et al (eds). Harrison's Principles of Internal Medicine. 15th ed. New York: McGraw-Hill, 2001.

Ahyg, (eds). Manual of Medical Therapeutics. 30th ed. Boston: Little, Brown & Co., 2001.

Stein JH (ed). Internal Medicine. 5th ed. St. Louis: CV Mosby, 1998.

*Articles*

Frisse ME, Florence V. A library for internists IX. Recommended by the American College of Physicians. Ann Intern Med 1997;120:836–846.

### *Primary Care*

*Books and Monographs*

Donaldson M, Yordy K, Vanselow N (eds). Defining Primary Care. IOM Committee on the Future of Primary Care National Academy Press, 1994.

*Articles*

Bodenheimer T, Lo B, Casalino L. Primary care physicians should be coordinators, not gatekeepers. JAMA 1999;281: 2045–2049.

Grumbach K, Selby J, Damberg C, et al. Resolving the gatekeeper conundrum. JAMA 1999;282:261–266.

Mottur-Pilson C. Primary care as form or content? Am J Med Quality 1995;10:177–182.

Yano E, Fink A, Hirsch S, et al. Helping practices reach primary care goals. Arch Intern Med 1995;155:1146–1156.

### *The Physician and the Medical Environment*

*Books and Monographs*

Kovnier A, Jones S. Health Care Delivery in the United States. Springer Publishing, 1998.

Nash D. The Physicians Guide to Managed Care. Aspen Publishing, 1994.

Liebler J, McConnell C. Management Principles for Health Professionals. Aspen Publishing, 1999.

J.C.A.H.O. Accreditation Manuals (published annually)

### *The Role of the Hospitalist*

Diamond HS, Goldberg E, Janosky JE. The effect of full-time faculty hospitalists on the efficiency of care at a community teaching hospital. Ann Intern Med 1998;129:197–203.

Diane E, Craig MD, et al. Implementation of a hospitalist system in a large HMO: The Kaiser Permanente experience. Ann Intern Med 1999;130:355–359.

Goldman, L The impact of hospitalists on medical education and the academic health system. Ann Intern Med 1999;130: 364–367.

Sox HC. The hospitalist model: perspectives of the patient, the internist, and internal medicine. Ann Intern Med 1999;130: 368–72.

Wachter R, Goldman L. The emerging role of "Hospitalists" in the American Health Care System. NEJM. 1996;335:514–7.

Wachter RM. The hospitalist movement: ten issues to consider. Hospital Practice 1999; Feb 15:95–111.

### *Evidence-Based Medicine*

Evidence-based medicine: A new approach to teaching the practice of medicine. Evidence-Based Medicine Working Group. JAMA 1992;268:2420–2425.

Greenhalgh J. How to read a paper. The MEDLINE database. BMJ 1997;315:180–183.

Guyatt GH, Sackett DI, Cook DJ. Users' guides to the medical literature. II. How to use an article about therapy or prevention. A. Are the results of the study valid? The Evidence Based Medicine Working Group. JAMA 1993;270:2598–2601.

Haynes RB, Wilczynski N, McKibbon KA, Walker CJ, Sinclair JC. Developing optimal search strategies for detecting clinically sound studies in MEDLINE. J Am Med Inform Assoc 1994;1:447–458.

Jaeschke R, Guyatt GH, Sackett DI. Users' guides to the medical literature. III. How to use an article about a diagnostic test. A. Are the results of the study valid? The Evidence Based Medicine Working Group. JAMA 1994;271:389–391.

Jaeschke R, Guyatt GH, Sackett DI. Users' guides to the medical literature. IV. How to use an article about harm. Evidence Based Medicine Working Group. JAMA 1994;271:1615–1619.

Laupacis A, Wells G, Richardson WS. Users' guides to the medical literature. V. How to use an article about prognosis. Evidence Based Medicine Working Group. JAMA 1994;272: 234–237.

Oxman AD, Cook DJ, Guyatt GH. Users' guides to the medical literature. VI. How to use an overview. The Evidence Based Medicine Working Group. JAMA 1994;272:1367–1371.

Oxman AD, Sackett DL, Guyatt GH. Users' guides to the medical literature. I. How to get started. The Evidence Based Medicine Working Group. JAMA 1993;270:2093–2095.

Rosenberg W, Donald A. Evidence-based medicine: an approach to clinical problem-solving. BMJ 1995;310:1122–1126.

Shaughnessy AF, Slawson DC, Bennett JH. Becoming an information master: a guidebook to the medical information jungle. J Fam Pract 1994;39:489–99.

### *Bedside Techniques*

*Books and Monographs*

Bickley L, Hoekelman RA. A Guide to Physical Examination. 7th ed. Philadelphia: JB Lippincott, 1999.

DeGowin RL, Brown D. DeGowin's Diagnostic Examination. 7th ed. New York: McGraw-Hill, 2000.

Swash M. Hutchinson's Clinical Methods. 20th ed. Philadelphia: WB Saunders, 1995.

*Articles*

Eddy DM, Clanton CH. The art of diagnosis. N Engl J Med 1982;306:1263–1268.

### *Diagnostic Studies*

*Books & Monographs*

Black E, et al. Diagnostic Strategies for Common Medical Problems. 2nd ed. Philadelphia: American College of Physicians, 1999.

Sutton D. Radiology and Imaging for Medical Students. Edinburgh; New York: Churchill Livingstone, 1998.

Sox H. Common diagnostic tests: use and interpretation. Philadelphia: American College of Physicians, 1990.

Wallach J. Handbook of Interpretation of Diagnostic Tests. 7th ed. Baltimore: Lippincott, Williams and Wilkins, 2000.

### *Prevention of Disease*

*Books and Monographs*

U.S. Preventive Services Task Force. Guide to Clinical Preventive Services. 2nd ed. Alexandria, VA: International Medical Publishing, 1996.

*Articles*

Black W, Welch HG. Advances in diagnostic imaging and overestimations of disease prevalence and the benefits of therapy. N Engl J Med 1993;328:1237–1243.

Gardner P, Eickhoff T, Poland G, et al. Adult immunizations. Ann Intern Med 1996;124:35–40.

Smith R, Mettlin C, Davis KJ, Eyre H. American Cancer Society guidelines for the early detection of cancer. CA Cancer J Clin 2000;50:34–49.

Welch HG, Black W. Evaluating randomized trials of screening. J Gen Intern Med 1997;12:118–124.

### *Women's Health*

Douglas PS, Ginsburg GS. The evaluation of chest pain in women. N Engl J Med 1996;334:1311–1315.

Haddad B, Sibai BM. Chronic hypertension in pregnancy. Ann Med 1999;31:246–252.

Heath CB, Sulik SM. Contraception and preconception counseling. Women's Health 1997;24:123–133.

Kjos SL, Buchanan TA. Gestational diabetes mellitus. N Engl J Med 1999;341:1749–1756.

Mosca L, Manson JE, Suterland SE, Langer RD, Manolia T, Barrett-Connor E. Cardiovascular disease in women: A statement for health care professionals from the American Heart Association. Circulation 1997;96:2468–2482.

NIH Consensus Development Panel on Osteoporosis Prevention, Diagnosis, and Therapy. Osteoporosis Prevention, Diagnosis, and Therapy. JAMA 2001;285:785–793.

Sannerstaedt R, Lundborg P, Danielsson BR, et al. Drugs during pregnancy: An issue of risk classification and information to prescribers. Drug Safety 1996;14:69–77.

Hulley S, Grady P, Bush T, et al. Randomized trial of estrogen plus progestin for secondary prevention of coronary heart disease in postmenopausal women. HERS Research Group. JAMA 280:605–13, 1998.

Writing Group for the Women's Health Initiative Investigators. Risks and benefits of estrogen plus progestin in healthy postmenopausal women: principle results from the Women's Health Initiative randomized controlled trial. JAMA 288:321–33, 2002.

### *Complementary Medicine*

#### *Books and Monographs*

Benson H. Timeless Healing: The Power and Biology of Belief. New York: Scribner, 1996.

Bratman S. The Alternative Medicine Sourcebook: A Realistic Evaluation of Healing Methods. Los Angeles: Lowell House, 1998.

Cassileth BR. The Alternative Medicine Handbook: The Complete Reference Guide to Alternative and Complementary Therapies. New York: WW Norton, 1998.

Weil A. Spontaneous Healing. New York: Alfred A. Knopf, 1995.

#### *Articles*

Defining and Describing Complementary and Alternative Medicine. Panel on Definition and Description, CAM Research Methodology Conference, April 1995. *Alternative Therapies* 1997;3(2):49–57.

Astin JA. Why patients use alternative medicine: results of a national study. JAMA 1998;279:1548–1553.

Beecher HK. The powerful placebo. JAMA 1955;159:1602–1606.

Druss BG, Rosenheck RA. Association between use of unconventional therapies and conventional medical services. JAMA 1999;282:651–656.

Eisenberg DM, David RB, Ettner SL, et al. Trends in alternative medicine use in the United States, 1990–1997. JAMA 1998;280:1569–1575.

Furnham A, Vincent C, Woods R. The health beliefs and behaviours of three groups of complementary medicine and a general practice group of patients. J Altern Complement Med 1995;1:347–359.

Kaptchuk TJ, Eisenberg DM. The persuasive appeal of alternative medicine. Ann Intern Med 1998;129:1061–1065.

King DE, Bushwick B. Beliefs and attitudes of hospital inpatients about faith healing and prayer. J Fam Pract 1994;39:349–352.

Matthews DA, McCullough ME, Larson DB, Koenig HG, et al. Religious commitment and health status: a review of the research and implications for family medicine. Arch Fam Med 1998;7:118–124.

Post SG, Puchalski CM, Larson DB. Physicians and patient spirituality: professional boundaries, competency, and ethics. Ann Intern Med 2000;132:578–583.

### *Nuclear Terrorism*

#### *Books and Monographs*

Domestic Preparedness. Defense Against Weapons of Mass Destruction. US Army SBCCOM. Compton B, Stewart-Craig E, Doak M (eds). Booz-Allen & Hamilton, Inc. 1999. McLean, Virginia.

Duns RF, Cerveny TJ. Triage and Treatment of Radiation-injured mass casualties. In Textbook of Military Medicine, Part 1 and Part 2. DA Office of the Surgeon General and Center of Excellence in Military Medical Research. Washington, D.C. 1989.

Markovchick V. Radiation Injuries. A comprehensive study guide. 4th ed. Tintinalli JB, et al (eds). New York: McGraw-Hill Companies, Inc. 1996.

Medical Management of Radiological Casualties Handbook. Armed Forces Radiobiology Research Institute, 1st ed. December 1999. Bethesda, Maryland.

Weapons of Mass Destruction Terms Reference Handbook (DTRA-AR-40H), Alexandria, Va. Defense Threat Reduction Agency, 2001.

### *Bioterrorism*

#### *Books and Monographs*

Medical Management of Biological Casualties Handbook. Medical Research Institute of Infectious Defense, 4th ed, February 2001.

Textbook of Military Medicine Part I, Medical Aspects of Chemical and Biological Warfare. Office of the Surgeon General, Department of the Army, United States of America. 1997.

#### *Articles*

Dennis DT, Inglesby TV, Henderson DA, et al. Tularemia as a Biological Weapon, Medical and Public Health Management. JAMA 2001; 285(21):2763–2773.

Henderson DA, Inglesby TV, Bartlett JG, et al. Smallpox as a Biological Weapon, Medical and Public Health Management. JAMA 1999; 281(22):2127–2137.

Inglesby TV, Dennis DT, Henderson DA, et al. Plague as a Biological Weapon, Medical and Public Health Management. JAMA 2000; 283(17): 2281–2290.

Inglesby TV, Henderson DA, Bartlett JG, et al. Anthrax as a Biological Weapon, Medical and Public Health Management. JAMA 1999; 281(18):1735–1745.

Khan AS, Sage MJ, et al. Biological and chemical terrorism: Strategic plan for preparedness and response. Recommendations of the CDC Strategic Planning Workgroup. MMWR 2000; 29(RR04):1–14.

### *Chemical Terrorism*

*Books and Monographs*

Center for Disease Control, Interim Recommendations for Firefighter and Other First Responders Protection Against Chemical and Biological Agents. October 2001. www.cdc-gov/niosh/unp-intrecppe.htm

Handbook of Chemical Hazard Analysis Procedures. Federal Emergency Management Agency, Publications Office, 500 C Street, S.W., Washington, D.C. 20472. www.epa.gov/cgi-bin/claritgw

Hazardous Materials: Managing the Incident. Noll G, Hildebrand M, Yvorra J. Oklahoma State University Press, 1995. Stillwater, Oklahoma.

Medical Management of Chemical Casualties Handbook. Medical Research Institute of Chemical Defense, 3rd ed. July 2000. Aberdeen Proving Ground, Maryland.

### *Telemedicine*

*Books and Monographs*

Institute of Medicine. Telemedicine: A Guide to Assessing Telecommunications in Health Care. Washington, DC: National Academy Press, 1996.

*Articles*

Alusi GH, Tan AC, Campos JC, Linney A, Wright A. Tele-education: the virtual medical laboratory. J Telemed Telecare 1997;3(Suppl 1):79–81.

Bai J, Zhang Y, Shen D, et al. A portable ECG and blood pressure telemonitoring system. IEEE Engineering in Medicine & Biology 1999;18(4):63–70.

Boland GW. Teleradiology: another revolution in radiology? Clin Radiol 1998;53:547–553.

Buntic RF, Siko PP, Buncke GM, Ruebeck D, Kind GM, Buncke HJ. Using the Internet for rapid exchange of photographs and X-ray images to evaluate potential extremity replantation candidates. Journal of Trauma—Injury, Infection, & Critical Care 1997;43:342–344.

Callahan EJ, Hilty DM, Nesbitt TS. Patient satisfaction with telemedicine consultation in primary care: comparison of ratings of medical and mental health applications. Telemed J 1998;4:363–369.

Coiera E. Recent advances: Medical informatics. BMJ 1995; 310:1381–1387.

Cubano M, Poulose BK, Talamini MA, et al. Long distance telementoring. A novel tool for laparoscopy aboard the USS Abraham Lincoln. Surg Endosc 1999;13:673–678.

Epstein MA, Pasieka MS, Lord WP, Wong ST, Mankovich NJ. Security for the digital information age of medicine: issues, applications, and implementation. J Digit Imaging 1998;11: 33–44.

Miller RA. Medical diagnostic decision support systems-past present and future: a threaded bibliography and brief commentary. J Am Med Inform Assoc 1994;1:8–27.

### *Genetics*

Boehm T. Positional cloning and gene identification. Methods 1998;14:152–158.

Cardon LR, Bell JI. Association study designs for complex diseases. Nat Rev Genet 2001; 2(2):91–99.

Cunningham GC. The genetics revolution. Ethical, legal, and insurance concerns. Postgrad Med 2000;108:193–196, 199–200, 202.

Emilien G, Ponchon M, Caldas C, Isacson O, Maloteaux JM. Impact of genomics on drug discovery and clinical medicine. QJM 2000;93:391–423.

Hedge P, Qi R, Abernathy K, et al. A concise guide to cDNA microarray analysis. Biotechniques 2000;29:548–562.

International Human Genome Sequencing Consortium. Initial sequencing and analysis of the human genome. Nature 2000;409:860–921.

Nadeau JH, Sankoff D. Counting on comparative maps. Trends Genet 1998;14:495–501.

Polyak K, Riggins GJ. Gene discovery using the serial analysis of gene expression technique: Implications for cancer research. J Clin Oncol 2001;19:2948–2958.

Reich D, Cargill M, Bolk S, et al. Linkage disequilibrium in the human genome. Nature 2000;411:119–204.

Roth MT, Painter RB. Genetic discrimination in health insurance: an overview and analysis of the issues. Nurs Clin North Am 2000;35:731–756.

Rusnak J, Kisabeth R, Herbert D, McNeil D. Pharmacogenomics: a clinician's primer on emerging technologies for improved patient care. Mayo Clin Proc 2001;76:299–309.

### *Medical Ethics*

*Books*

Arras J, Steinbock B. Ethical Issues in Modern Medicine. 5th ed. Mountain View, California: Mayfield, 1999.

Jonsen AR, Siegler M, Winslade WJ. Clinical Ethics. 4th ed. New York: MacMillan, 1998.

Junkerman C, Schiedermayer D. Practical Ethics for Students, Interns and Residents. 2nd ed. Frederick, Maryland: University Publishing Group 1998.

Lo B. Resolving Ethical Dilemmas—A Guide for Clinicians. 2nd ed. Philadelphia: Lippincott Williams & Wilkins, 2000.

President's Commission for the Study of Ethical Problems in Medicine and Biomedical and Behavioral Research. Washington, DC, 1982.

*Articles*

Benson JA. The burdens of professionalism: patients' rights and social justice. The Pharos 2000;Winter:4–9.

Brody H, Campbell ML, Faber-Langendoen K, Ogle KS. Withdrawing intensive life-sustaining treatment—Recommendations for compassionate clinical management. N Engl J Med 1997;336:652–657.

Council on Ethical and Judicial Affairs of the AMA. Medical futility in end-of-life care. JAMA 1999;281:937–941.

Quill TE, Brody H. Physician recommendations and patient autonomy: finding a balance between physician power and patient choice. Ann Intern Med 1996;125:763–769.

Quill TE, Lo B, Brock DW. Palliative options of last resort: a comparison of voluntarily stopping eating and drinking, terminal sedation, physician-assisted suicide and voluntary active euthanasia. JAMA 1997;278:2099–2104.

Singer PA, Martin DK, Kelner M. Quality end-of-life care: patient's perspectives. JAMA 1999;281:163–168.

Specifying the goals of medicine. Special Supplement. Hastings Center Report 1996;November–December.

### *Palliative Care*

*Books*

Doyle D, Hanks GWC, MacDonald N (eds). Oxford Textbook of Palliative Medicine. 2nd ed. Oxford, England: Oxford University Press, 1999.

*Articles*

Barraclough J. ABC of palliative care: depression, anxiety and confusion. BMJ 1997;315:1365–1368.

Bruera E, Neumann CM. Management of specific symptom complexes in patients receiving palliative care. Can Med Assoc J 1998;158:1717–1726.

Byock IR. The nature of suffering and the nature of opportunity at the end of life. Clin Geriatr Med 1996;12:237–251.

Hamilton DG. Believing in patients' beliefs: physician attunement to the terminal spiritual dimension as a positive factor in patient healing and health. Am J Hosp Palliat Care 1998;5:276–279.

Levy MH. Pharmacological treatment of cancer pain. N Engl J Med 1996;335:1124–1132.

O'Neill B, Fallon M. ABC of palliative care: principles of palliative care and pain control. BMJ 1997;315:801–804.

Rousseau P. Hospice and palliative care. Dis Mon 1995;41: 779–842.

Zeppetella G. The palliation of dyspnea in terminal diseases. Am J Hosp Palliat Care 1998;6:322–330.

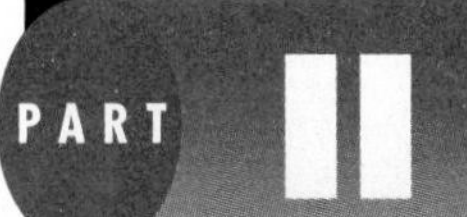

PART II

Asriani M. Chiu

# ALLERGY AND CLINICAL IMMUNOLOGY

# CHAPTER 15 BASIC MECHANISMS

The immune system plays a critical role in the body's defense against pathogens. Both defects and overactivity (generally termed **hypersensitivity**) of the immune response can cause disease. Hypersensitivity results in symptoms through inflammatory mediators, antibodies, complement, and cells. The term **allergy,** derived from the Greek words *allo* and *ergo*, implies "other" or "bad" work by the body's immune system.

**Lymphocytes** and **macrophages** are the key cells in immune defense. The lymphocytes may be derived from the thymus (**T cells**) or bone marrow (**B cells**). T cells, which may be helper or suppressor types, provide cellular immunity, and B cells produce antibodies. As shown in Figure 15.1, the macrophage can serve as an antigen-processing cell (APC). Foreign antigens from pathogens are first internalized and then presented as peptides on the surface of the APC. The peptides are bound to other surface proteins called histocompatibility proteins, which provide cell markers called the major histocompatibility complex (MHC). Aside from enabling T cells to determine whether cells are foreign, MHC also serves as binding sites for T cells. T suppressor cells (TS cells) can recognize and bind the MHC complex, termed MHC I, which is present on nearly all cells in the body. T helper cells (TH cells) recognize a separate MHC protein, called MHC II, which is generally limited to cells that are APCs. The protein on the T cell that binds to MHC II is called CD4 (cluster of differentiation antigen 4). These interactions cause the macrophage to produce interleukin (IL)-1, which stimulates the T cell and helps uncommitted TH cells to differentiate into $TH_1$ or $TH_2$ cells. $TH_1$ cells promote cell-mediated defenses against viruses, fungi, and bacteria; $TH_2$ cells defend against parasites and produce additional IL-4 and IL-5, which activate the eosinophils. Most individuals produce predominantly $TH_1$ cells. Allergic patients usually have an overabundance of $TH_2$ cells.

The proteins that $TH_2$ cells secrete (called cytokines) promote the clinical expression of allergies. IL-4 and IL-5 result in increased amounts of immunoglobulin E (IgE) and tissue eosinophilia, respectively. Eosinophils release toxic substances, such as major basic protein (MBP), that can exacerbate asthma. IL-4 also may promote inflammation by increasing expression of adhesion proteins on blood vessels to which eosinophils bind, thus allowing egress into tissues. Cytokines produced by $TH_1$ and $TH_2$ cells are summarized in Table 15.1. To counteract the allergic response, the macrophage produces IL-12. Interferon-gamma (IFN-$\gamma$) is also produced by pre-existing $TH_1$ cells. Both of these help uncommitted TH ($TH_0$) cells differentiate into $TH_1$. IFN-$\gamma$ also inhibits the ability of $TH_2$ cells to produce IL-4.

An immature form of antibody, immunoglobulin M (IgM), is found on B cell surfaces. IgM serves as an antigen receptor. After antigen-binding by the IgM, the B cells initially produce and secrete additional IgM, followed by production of other antibody classes such as immunoglobulin G (IgG), A (IgA), or E (IgE). Antibody production is enhanced by the binding of B cells to T cells, which express a protein called the CD40 ligand. Lack of T cell help or abnormal CD40 binding can impair antibody production or the switch from IgM to IgG. If $TH_2$ cells predominate, IgM is replaced by IgE, allowing the increased likelihood of a later immediate-type allergy.

During T cell development, those cells that recognize self-antigens are destroyed in the thymus, and those with receptors that recognize foreign antigens survive; however, the depletion of self-reactive cells is thwarted if infection or other toxic effects cause self-antigens to mimic foreign antigens. In such situations, macrophages may produce increased amounts of IL-1. In excess, IL-1 can cause fever, leukocytosis, thrombocytosis, and an elevated sedimentation rate—all signs of inflammation. Some autoimmune reactions may occur when $TH_1$ cells mistake the body's own cells as foreign. Gel and Coombs have classified hypersensitivity reactions into four types (Table 15.2), providing a framework for understanding these reactions.

## Type I Reactions

Type I (**immediate hypersensitivity**) reactions have a rapid onset, appearing within minutes. **Anaphylaxis** (a serious, life-threatening allergic reaction with rapid onset) after a bee sting or penicillin injection is one such example. These reactions involve inflammatory mediator release from tissue mast cells or blood basophils (Figure 15.2). Macrophages, platelets, and eosinophils also may be activated by allergens or pathogens. IgE antibodies made by B cells bind to receptors on mast cells and basophils. When the IgE on these cells comes in contact with allergen, intracellular signals are triggered. Basophils and mast cells then release preformed mediators, such as histamine, from their granules. They also produce de novo (newly formed) mediators when phospholipase $A_2$ acts on the membrane lipids, releasing arachidonic acid.

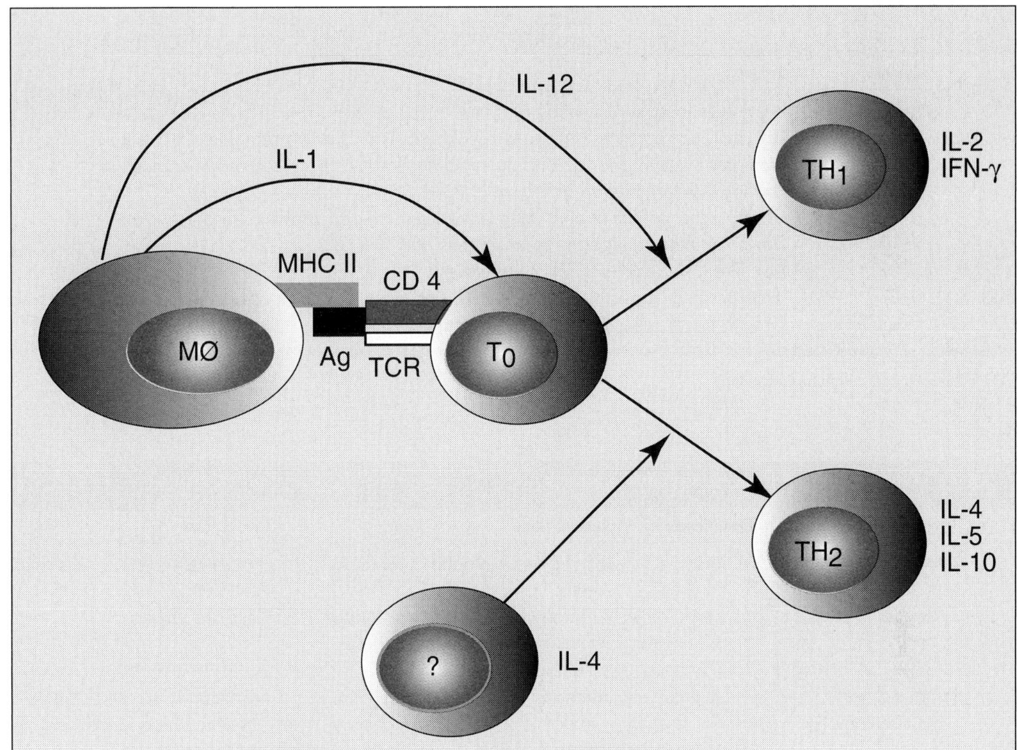


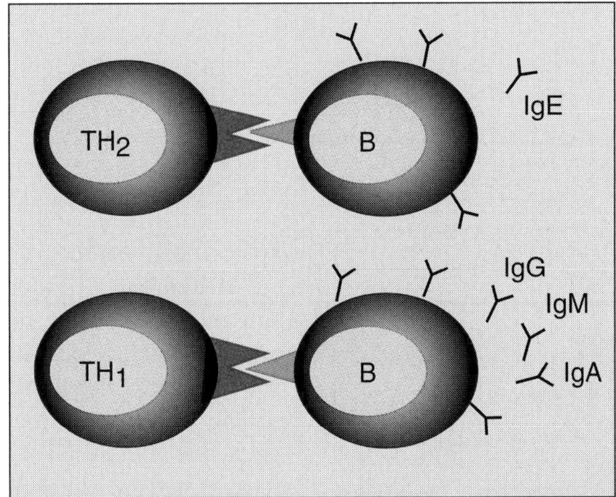


**FIGURE 15.1.** **A.** Macrophage (MØ) processes foreign antigens and presents them as peptides on its surface in association with the major histocompatibility complex (MHC). TH cells recognize these peptides by the T cell receptor because of interactions with the T cell's CD4 antigen. Suppressor/cytotoxic T cells recognize the major histocompatibility complex class I antigens because of interactions with CD8. The MØ then produces IL-1, which stimulates the T cell, and IL-8 (not shown), which activates neutrophils. $TH_0$ cells then differentiate into $TH_1$ cells, which promote cell-mediated defenses against viruses, fungi, and bacteria, or $TH_2$ cells, which promote defense against parasites. IL-12 from the MØ, and IFN-γ from pre-existing $TH_1$ cells, help $T_2$ cells differentiate into $TH_2$, and IL-4 locally helps differentiation into $TH_2$ cells. The cytokines from $TH_2$ cells are associated with atopic conditions, including asthma. **B.** When $TH_2$ cells interact with B lymphocytes, the B cells preferentially produce IgE antibodies. $TH_1$ interactions promote the production of some IgG subclasses, IgM, and IgA.

**TABLE 15.1. $TH_1$ and $TH_2$ Cytokines and Their Actions**

| Group | Cytokine | Actions |
|---|---|---|
| $TH_1$ | IL-2 | Promotes clonal proliferation of T cells. |
| | IFN-γ | Antiviral, up-regulates antigen-presenting cells and down-regulates $TH_2$ cells. |
| $TH_2$ | IL-4 | Promotes switching to IgE and up-regulates VCAM* expression on endothelium. Promotes differentiation of $TH_1$ cells to $TH_2$. |
| | IL-5 | Chemotactic for eosinophils, also activates them and prolongs their survival. |
| | IL-10 | Down-regulates antigen-presenting cells and $TH_1$ cells. |
| | IL-13 | Acts like IL-4, promotes $TH_2$ differentiation. |
| Shared | IL-3 | Growth factor especially for mast cells and basophils; primes basophils to respond to stimuli. |
| | GM-CSF | Growth factor, also promotes eosinophil growth. |

*VCAM = vascular cell adhesion molecule.

**TABLE 15.2. Classification of Hypersensitivity Reactions**

| Type | Synonym | Time/Course | Antibody Role | Cellular Role |
|---|---|---|---|---|
| I | Immediate | Minutes | IgE triggers basophils and mast cells. | Basophils and mast cells release mediators. |
| II | Cytotoxic | <1 hour | Antibody binds to cells or tissues, fixes complement, and causes damage. | Cells are targets. |
| III | Serum sickness; immune complex | 7–14 days | Antibody forms complexes with antigen; complex fixes complement and settles into blood vessels. | Neutrophils are attracted by complex in blood vessel and cause further damage. |
| IV | Delayed | 2–3 days | | Macrophage produces IL-1 and IL-12, promoting $TH_1$ response. $TH_1$ produces IL-2 and IFN-γ, resulting in cellular infiltrate. |

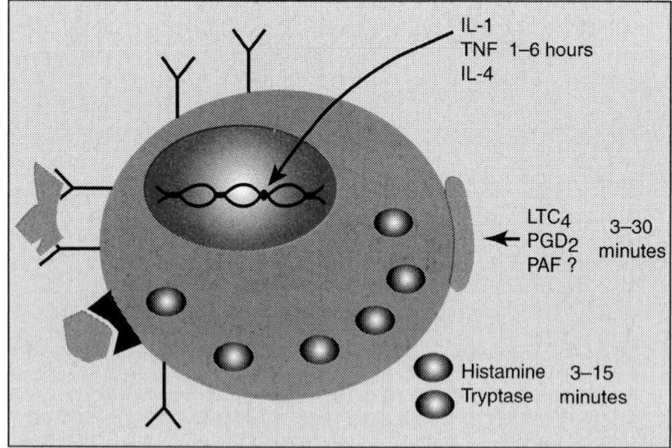


**FIGURE 15.2.** Mast cells (and basophils) express the high-affinity IgE receptor on their surfaces, to which allergen-induced IgE binds. A mast cell activates when two IgE molecules are cross-linked. Histamine and tryptase stored in granules are then rapidly released. Arachidonic acid is generated by the effect of phospholipase $A_2$ on cell membrane; production of leukotriene $C_4$, $PGD_2$, and PAF follows. IL-1 and TNF stored in granules also may be released, but additional amounts are later generated by gene transcription.

## Preformed Mediators

**Histamine,** a preformed mediator, stored almost entirely in mast cells and basophils, is rapidly released after cellular activation and causes vascular leak and venodilation. After local release in the skin, erythema, itching, and wheal formation occur. Thus, itching is predictive of mast cell or basophil activation. On a larger scale, histamine can evoke vasopermeability with resultant loss of vascular fluid into tissues—a process termed third spacing of fluid—leading to hypotension, abdominal pain, and **urticaria** (hives; see Chapter 20). Nasal vasodilatation causes nasal congestion. Type I reactions lead to pruritus and sneezing because histamine binds to type 1 receptors ($H_1$) that are also present on afferent nerves. Histamine binding to type 2 ($H_2$) receptors causes flushing, hypotension, and headache because $H_2$ receptors are located on blood vessels. Pulmonary symptoms include chest tightness and wheezing.

Although elevated blood histamine level is a good indication of a type I reaction, the rapid metabolism of histamine makes this test impractical. Given the stability of mast cell–derived tryptase in the blood for several hours, serum tryptase levels can retrospectively confirm a type I reaction.

## De Novo Mediators

De novo mediators—leukotrienes, prostaglandin $D_2$ ($PGD_2$), and platelet-activating factor (PAF), which are derived from cell membrane phospholipids of mast cells or basophils, cause bronchoconstriction and stimulate mucus secretion (Figure 15.3). Corticosteroids can inhibit the production of these agents by inhibiting phospholipase $A_2$. Nonsteroidal anti-inflammatory drugs (NSAIDs)—aspirin, for example—may shunt more arachidonic acid into the lipoxygenase pathway and cause more leukotriene synthesis in susceptible individuals. Drugs that block binding of leukotrienes to their receptors (e.g., zafirlukast) and those that block production of leukotrienes (e.g., Zileuton, a lipoxygenase inhibitor) can benefit some asthmatics.

## Cytokines and the Late-Phase Reaction

Release of preformed and de novo mediators is rapid. Mast cells and basophils also begin to produce new protein cytokines several hours after IgE-mediated stimulation. Gene regulatory factors migrate from the cytoplasm to the nuclei of mast cells and basophils and enhance gene transcription of cytokines such as tumor necrosis factor (TNF) and IL-4 (Figure 15.4). The local release of IL-4 will selectively enhance the migration of eosinophils and basophils to sites of allergic inflammation. After migration into the tissues, basophils can release additional IL-4, leukotrienes, and histamine. It is now known that "immediate" type I reactions often evoke a late-phase reaction (LPR) within 4-8 hours, probably due to cellular inflammation and tissue damage by chemotactic and pro-adhesive cytokines. Corticosteroids and drugs capable of stabilizing mast cells (such as sodium cromolyn or nedocromil) inhibit the LPR.

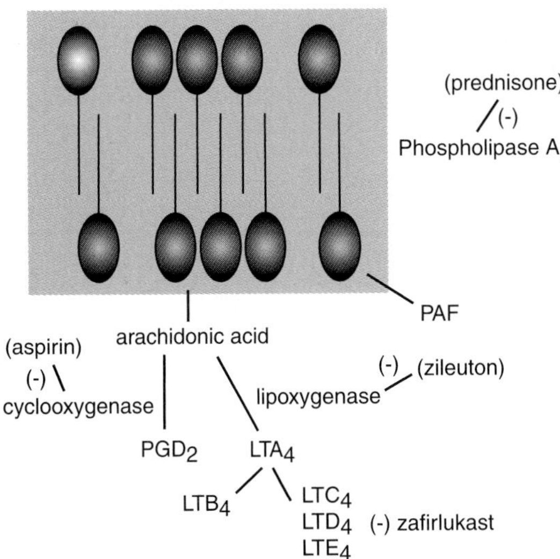


**FIGURE 15.3.** **Phospholipase $A_2$ acts on membrane phospholipids to produce arachidonic acid and PAF; prostaglandins and leukotrienes are produced from arachidonic acid. Cyclooxygenase inhibitors (aspirin) block prostaglandin production, but also may cause increased leukotriene production. Lipoxygenase inhibitors (zileuton) inhibit leukotriene synthesis. Phospholipase $A_2$ is inhibited by corticosteroids, which can inhibit production of inflammatory mediators at all levels.**

## Anaphylactoid Reactions

These reactions, which mimic a type I reaction, follow non–IgE-dependent degranulation of mast cells or basophils and are often induced by certain drugs (morphine and codeine), contrast dye, bacterial peptides, and anaphylatoxins of the complement system (C3a, C5a). These systemic reactions mimic anaphylaxis but are termed **anaphylactoid** to indicate that they bypass the usual IgE-dependent mechanism.

## Diagnosis of Type I Reactions

The clinical identification of a specific sensitivity to an allergen enables avoidance of that allergen, verification of a type I allergy diagnosis, and initiation of immunotherapy or desensitization. Immunotherapy increases the level of blocking IgG antibodies, blunts seasonal changes in IgE, depresses basophil histamine release, and shifts TH cell profiles from $TH_2$ to $TH_1$ by raising IFN-$\gamma$ levels. An elevated total IgE level is rarely helpful clinically. Allergen testing relies on the presence of specific IgE antibodies either in serum or on skin mast cells or basophils. The most common, accurate, and least expensive test is skin testing for allergens.

### Skin testing

The most commonly performed skin test for allergens is the **epicutaneous** or **prick test,** which involves pricking the skin with a small needle or lancet having a drop of stock allergen on it. Such testing correlates well with actual nasal or lung challenge with allergen and is 90% sensitive and 95% specific for identifying allergens. Only the prick test should be performed for diagnosing food allergies, and, because it is safer, it should always precede intradermal skin testing in the evaluation of other allergies. The **intradermal test** involves an injection of 0.02–0.03 ml of diluted allergen (usually about 1:100–1:500) through a 27-gauge needle, which raises an intradermal wheal. By introducing nearly 1000 times more allergen than the prick test, it is more sensitive (95–98%) but less specific (85%). Both the prick test and the intradermal test can be read within 15 minutes (Figure 15.5) of testing. A positive control using histamine and a

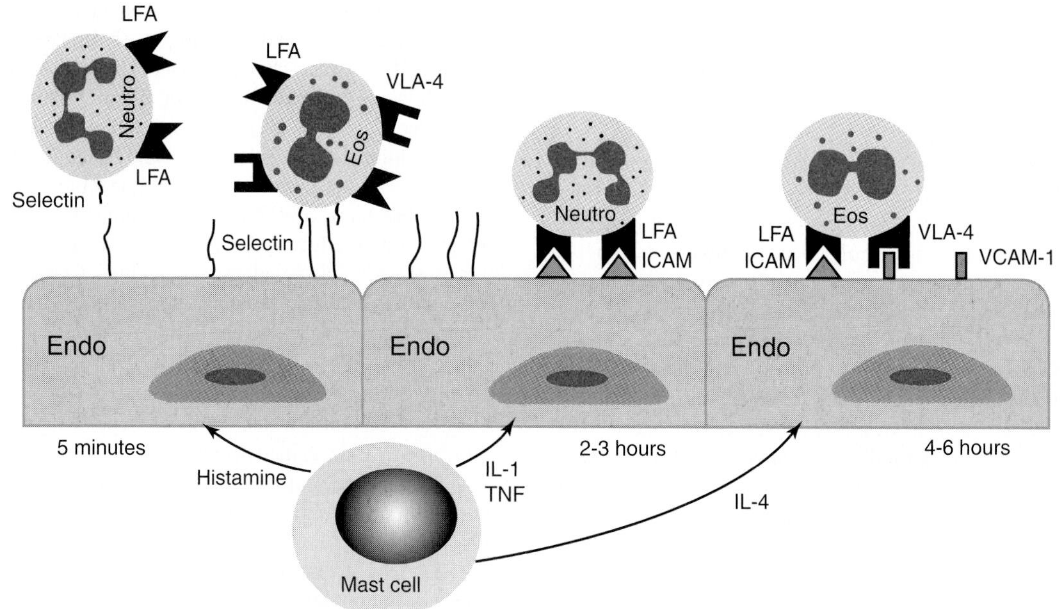


**FIGURE 15.4.** Tissue mast cells resting near vascular endothelium (Endo)-release histamine and cytokines. Histamine promotes weak attachment and rolling of leukocytes along the endothelium. Both neutrophils (Neutro) and eosinophils (Eos) interact with endothelium. Subsequent release of IL-1 and TNF by the mast cell causes increased expression of intercellular adhesion molecules by the endothelial cells, and neutrophils and eosinophils are anchored to the endothelium. IL-4 produced during the late phase by mast cells causes selective enhancement (upregulation) of vascular cell adhesion molecule-1 on the endothelium. Vascular cell adhesion molecule-1 is recognized by very late antigen-4, which is present on eosinophils and basophils but not on neutrophils, resulting in selective recruitment of these cells.

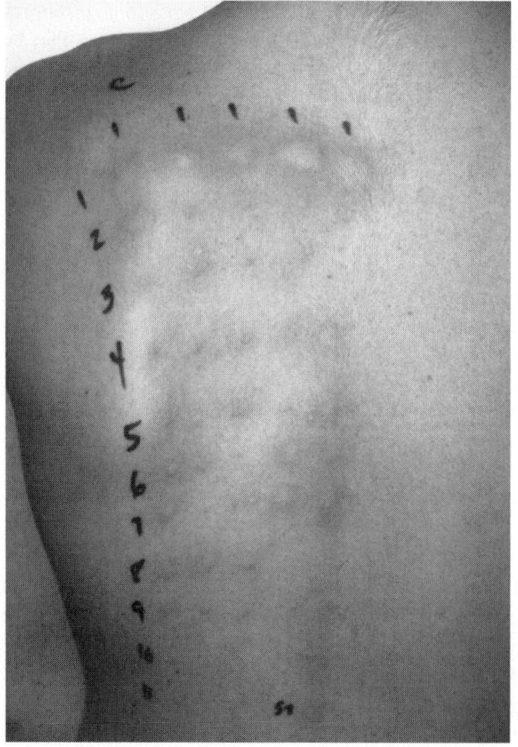

**FIGURE 15.5.** Results of a prick test on an allergic patient. The patient has strongly positive wheal and flare reactions to several grass allergens (row 1) but not to other allergens (such as trees, row 9). A saline control also is found to be negative.

negative saline control are always performed concurrently. Antihistamines must be stopped (generally 3–5 half-lives of the agent) prior to skin testing.

**Radioallergosorbent test**

The **radioallergosorbent test (RAST)** measures specific serum IgE. The allergen is linked to a disk in a test tube or microtiter well and incubated in the patient's serum. If IgE is present against that allergen, it will adhere and remain attached to the disk. The disk is then washed and incubated with an antibody against human IgE (such as goat antihuman IgE). The second antibody is linked to radioactive iodine. After rewashing the disk, the amount of bound IgE is noted by the amount of radioactivity in the tube or well. The RAST is almost as sensitive as the prick test for most common allergens but has several limitations, such as poor binding by some allergens, false-positives with high total IgE levels (>500 ng/ml), and its limited availability (only through special laboratories). When severe eczema, dermatographism, or the use of tricyclic antidepressants preclude skin testing (1–3% of patients), alternate diagnostic tests, such as RAST, are useful. However, because skin tests are more sensitive than RASTs, skin tests should always be used to detect potentially life-threatening allergens such as Hymenoptera venom (bee stings) or type I penicillin allergy.

## Type II Reactions

Also known as **cytotoxic reactions,** type II reactions are mediated by antibodies directed against cells and can use complement to help **cell lysis** or rupture cells. The ABO mismatch-type transfusion reaction best exemplifies them. Because complement fixation is common, IgG and IgM antibodies, which have the ability to bind complement, are the most important. The antigen recognized as foreign can truly be foreign (e.g., transfusion or early rapid graft rejections) or may be neoantigens on a host's own cells. α-Methyldopa (Aldomet), an antihypertensive, can cause **hemolysis** by inducing the cells to express neoantigens on their surface. A cell also can be lysed as an "innocent bystander" when a drug (penicillin or quinidine) binds to its surface. Hemolytic antibody on cells can be detected using the **Coombs test.**

Type II reactions also can occur because of chronic pathologic antibody production. Autoantibody production occurs in systemic lupus erythematosus and is directed against nuclear material. Autoantibodies can cause illness without cellular damage. Long-acting thyroid-stimulating antibodies can cause hyperthyroidism; antibodies against C1 esterase inhibitor (C1 INH) can accelerate clearance of C1 INH, precipitating **angioedema** (see Chapter 20).

## Type III Reactions

In a type III reaction—also called **serum sickness**—a foreign antigen is bound by the patient's own antibodies, forming immune complexes that subsequently fix complement. Immune complexes may enhance IL-1 production, resulting in fever. Complexes, depending on the ratios of antigen and antibody, could settle into blood vessels, leading to **vasculitis** (vascular inflammation). Vasculitis causes leukocyte infiltration, nuclear damage of the endothelial cells, and extravasation of red blood cells. Cutaneous vasculitis can sometimes present as an atypical **urticaria** (see Chapter 20) or palpable purpura. Vasculitis elsewhere is associated with respective organ dysfunction. Typical characteristics of type III reactions are fever, joint pains, proteinuria, lymphadenopathy, consumption of complement factor 4, eosinophilia, and a high sedimentation rate, occurring 7–14 days after exposure. Antinuclear antibodies and anti–double-stranded DNA antibodies are seen in drug-induced lupus.

## Type IV Reactions

In type IV reactions, an antigen triggers macrophages to produce cytokines, which in turn activate local lymphocytes. Macrophage IL-1 and IL-8 enhance leukocyte infiltration. Local IFN-γ production of T cells increases MHC II expression on APCs and enhances defense against viruses, mycobacteria, and intracellular bacteria. Type IV responses can be inhibited by corticosteroids. They are known also as **delayed hypersensitivity** because the clinical onset is delayed by 24–72 hours. The tuberculin skin test embodies a type IV reaction.

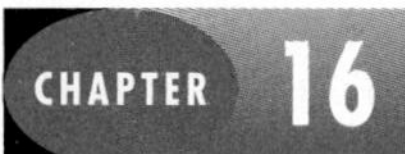

# RHINITIS, SINUSITIS, AND CONJUNCTIVITIS

## Rhinitis

### Definition and Etiology

Rhinitis, or nasal inflammation, may be allergic or nonallergic; the cause must be determined by the history, physical examination, and selected studies. Allergic rhinitis can be perennial or seasonal. Commonly, **acute rhinitis** is viral and **chronic rhinitis** is allergic.

### Epidemiology

Rhinitis is a leading problem in primary care, with an estimated 15% incidence in the United States population younger than 30 years old. Like other atopic diseases (e.g., asthma), allergic rhinitis also has a genetic basis, with almost two thirds of subjects having an affected first-degree relative. Because IgE levels peak around age 11, allergic rhinitis—especially perennial—is more prevalent in children and young adults. Seasonal symptoms (brought on, for example, by ragweed in the early fall, mold in the late fall, tree pollens in the spring, and grasses in the summer) suggest an allergic component; however, some allergens are perennial (such as dust mites, indoor pets, and certain molds). Worldwide, the most common allergen is the *Dermatophagoides* mite species. Because human dander is the food source for these mites, they accumulate in bedding, carpeting, and feather pillows, harboring the main allergenic protein in their feces. Aeroallergies most often result from wind-driven pollen grains. Because some viral infections may be seasonal, nonallergic rhinitis also may be seasonal.

### Pathophysiology

When the nose fails to warm and humidify air, bronchospasm can result, and failure to filter (mouth breathing) results in a predisposition to lower respiratory tract infections. The nasal turbinates, being covered with ciliated epithelium, increase the epithelial surface area for warming, humidifying, and filtering. Excess airflow over these areas can lead to **mucosal hypertrophy,** which, if pronounced, presents as nasal congestion. In **septal deviation,** this effect may arise from shunting airflow to the unobstructed nostril or from breathing air with very low humidity. Similarly, conditions that cause increased blood volume (e.g., pregnancy) or vasodilatation (medications) will produce congestion.

In allergic rhinitis, the allergen activates mucosal mast cells and triggers mediator release (see Chapter 15). A cholinergic reflex causes additional rhinorrhea with mucus secretion. Histamine appears to play a role in sneezing as newer, selective H1 antagonists effectively treat this symptom. LPRs mediated by cytokines may explain the chronicity of rhinitis symptoms. Edema around the eustachian tube opening can cause partial obstruction and concomitant dysfunction.

### Clinical Features

Patients with rhinitis report a variable degree of nasal congestion, rhinorrhea, postnasal drainage, and sneezing. Sneezing is very common in seasonal allergic rhinitis and, when absent, should suggest nonallergic causes. In perennial allergic rhinitis, nasal congestion and thick secretions are reported with less prominent sneezing. In all forms of rhinitis, increased mouth breathing of relatively cool, dry air can exacerbate associated asthma. Nasal congestion can provoke **sleep-disordered breathing** and cause chronic fatigue. Eye and throat itching and irritation are common. "Ear popping" and serous otitis follow eustachian tube dysfunction. The nasal mucosa is often pale and edematous (versus reddened in nonallergic rhinitis), and "allergic shiners" (dark circles under the eyes) are frequent. A lumpy appearance of the pharyngeal mucosa **(posterior pharyngeal lymphoid hyperplasia)** and **anterior cervical adenopathy** are other findings. In children, the "allergic salute" (rubbing or wiping the nose with the back of the hands to allay pruritus) along with nasal creases are striking. With eustachian tube dysfunction, the tympanic membrane may be retracted.

### Diagnosis

Figure 16.1 illustrates the differential diagnosis of rhinitis. The patient's history is critical and should include information about exposure to potential allergens at home and work, drug use, and family history. In the common cold, the most frequent form of nonallergic rhinitis, constitutional symptoms are common, and nasal smear shows no eosinophils. Nonallergic rhinitis with eosinophilia (NARES) features perennial nasal congestion, nasal polyps, and slight pruritus, but skin testing shows no allergies. Aside from being associated with nonallergic asthma, polyps also may block sinus drainage, causing recurrent sinusitis. NSAIDs should be avoided in asthmatics with nasal polyps because such medications may induce asthmatic attacks.

**Rhinitis medicamentosa** is inflammation of the nasal mucosa caused by excessive use of medication such as vasoconstrictor nasal sprays, which temporarily reduce nasal congestion but cause rebound congestion. Rhinitis often follows habitual cocaine snorting; septal ulcers and perforation also may be noted. A subset of

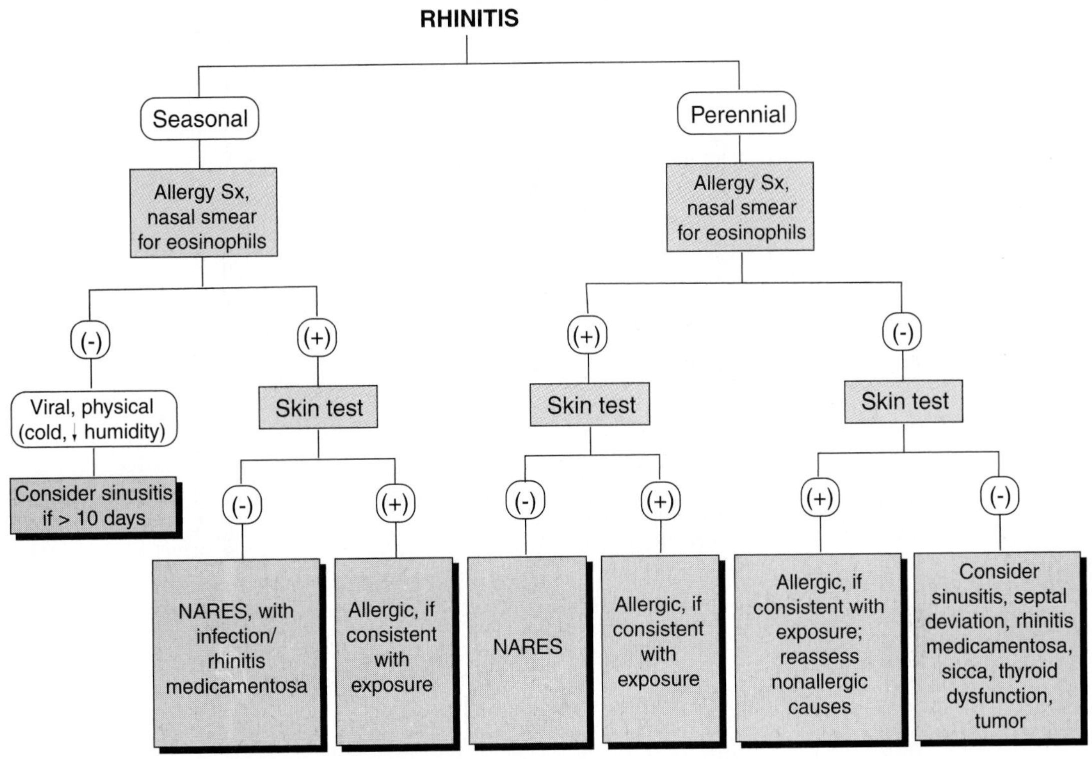


**FIGURE 16.1. Differential diagnosis of rhinitis.**
Sx = symptoms; (+) = positive; (−) = negative; NARES = nonallergic rhinitis with eosinophilia.

patients with nonallergic rhinitis have **vasomotor rhinitis,** with an abnormal cholinergic reflex response to physical stimuli (bright lights; odors; and cold, dry air). Often middle-aged or older, these patients may have a history of rhinorrhea and sneezing when walking barefoot on a cold floor or when eating certain foods—for example, soup (gustatory rhinitis).

Other conditions can mimic rhinitis by causing congestion or apparent rhinorrhea. Normal blood flow to the nostrils cycles periodically, with a mild unilateral increase in resistance, especially on recumbency. This may worsen with high cardiac output (stress), increased blood volume (pregnancy), vasodilatation (β blockers and central α-agonists), or hormonal changes (birth control pills, hypothyroidism). Anatomic obstruction (polyps, septal deviation, intranasal malignancy) may cause constant congestion that responds poorly to therapy. Unilateral obstruction with infection in a child may be caused by a foreign body; when a nasal polyp is the cause, cystic fibrosis should be considered. Profuse rhinorrhea after head trauma or surgery may be caused by cerebrospinal fluid leakage, which can be confirmed quickly using a glucose dipstick (value over 40 mg/dl is nearly diagnostic). With excessive mucosal dryness **(Sjögren's syndrome),** patients often report nasal congestion and associated sinus discomfort. In both allergic rhinitis and NARES, the nasal smear shows eosinophils. Although this implies allergies, skin testing or RAST to show specific IgE is necessary for diagnosis. Chronic nasal congestion without positive skin tests or eosinophilia could suggest the need for a work-up to rule out chronic sinusitis and should direct attention to other nonallergic causes for congestion (listed previously in this chapter).

## Management

Table 16.1 outlines the management of rhinitis. For allergic rhinitis, avoidance of allergens is the first choice (Table 16.2); however, it is difficult to avoid outdoor aeroallergens. Medical management routinely includes the use of nasal saline washes (to reduce inflammatory cells and mediators), anti-inflammatory nasal sprays (corticosteroid sprays and sodium cromolyn), and oral antihistamine-decongestants. The steroid sprays are used once or twice per day, and cromolyn is used several times per day. Both corticosteroids and cromolyn should be

**TABLE 16.1. Medical Management of Rhinitis**

| Therapeutic | Examples | Frequency | Useful for S/I | Useful for C | Useful for PRN | Useful for NA | Comments | Cost/Day |
|---|---|---|---|---|---|---|---|---|
| Avoidance | pillow, mattress cover, air filters | – | S | + | – | – | Usually reduces but does not eliminate symptoms. Only an adjunct to management. | 20–30¢ |
| First-generation antihistamine | diphenhydramine, clemastine, chlorpheniramine, hydroxyzine | BID TID | ++ | +/– | ++ | +/– | Fairly rapid onset; drying effect sometimes useful. Can be sedating and can cause urinary retention in men. | $1 |
| Second-generation antihistamine | fexofenadine, loratadine, cetirizine | QD BID | ++ | +/– | + | – | Usually nonsedating and little tachyphylaxis. | $2–3 |
| Decongestant | pseudoephedrine | BID TID | – | + | + | – | Nonsedating but can cause agitation and insomnia, and may worsen hypertension. Often given with an antihistamine. | 20–30¢ |
| Cromolyn | Nasalcrom | TID | + | + | – | – | Given as topical spray, relatively free of systemic effects. | $2–3 |
| Topical corticosteroid | beclomethasone, triamcinolone, budesonide, fluticasone, mometasone | QD BID | + | ++ | – | + | Topical spray, few systemic effects. Rarely causes nose bleed. Can be effective for NARES, vasomotor. | $2–3 |
| Saline | Ocean, Ayre | TID QID | +/– | + | +/– | +/– | Safe. Often an adjunct to medications. | 5–10¢ |
| Immunotherapy | | Q wk | ++ | + | – | – | Must determine allergens and correlate with symptoms. Effective but takes months to year to begin; occasional reaction. Can work when medications fail. | $1–2 |

BID = twice per day; C = congestion; NA = nonallergic; NARES = nonallergic rhinitis with eosinophilia; PRN = as needed; Q wk = once per week; QD = once per day; QID = 4 times per day; S/I = sneeze/itch; TID = three times per day.

TABLE 16.2. Methods for Reducing Allergen Exposure

| Allergen Type | Methods |
|---|---|
| Outdoor allergens | Close windows, use central air conditioning or window unit. Wear face mask (trees, grasses, molds) when exposed to cut grass or moldy areas such as compost piles. |
| Indoor allergens | |
| Mite | Provide adequate ventilation.<br>Remove feather pillows, down comforters.<br>Cover pillow, mattress, and box spring with airtight covering.<br>Have no carpeting in bedrooms or use only machine-washable area rugs.<br>Wash bedding in hot water (>140°F) every 2 weeks.<br>Maintain humidity <50% and temperature <70°F.<br>Use acaricide (tannic and benzoic acid) on carpet and stuffed furniture every 2–4 months.<br>Minimize knickknacks; frequently dust with damp cloth.<br>Vacuum rugs, mattress, and drapes using multilayered collection bag every 2 weeks.<br>Replace dust filters in furnace/central air conditioning unit regularly.<br>Place cheese cloth across forced air vents. |
| Molds | Maintain humidity <40%.<br>Treat areas containing mildew and bathroom tiles with mold-killing cleansers.<br>Add mold inhibitors to wall and ceiling paint.<br>Empty water pans (e.g., from under refrigerator).<br>Store firewood outside. |
| Animals | Minimize exposure, or at least keep pets out of bedroom and off furniture.<br>Bathe cat or dog weekly.<br>Wash hands thoroughly after touching all animals.<br>Use a high-energy particulate air filter. |

used regularly and prophylactically; the clinical response may take several days. For patients with nasal polyps or severe allergic rhinitis, a course of oral steroids may reduce polyp size and lessen symptoms; topical steroid sprays can be used afterward. Other than cessation of topical decongestant, rhinitis medicamentosa often requires concurrent topical steroids, oral antihistamine-decongestants, and brief oral corticosteroid therapy. Ipratropium bromide nasal spray is effective in treating vasomotor rhinitis.

Several classes of first-generation antihistamines have variable anticholinergic and antiserotoninergic properties, which are sometimes desirable (to "dry up" secretions or provide mild sedation). Besides being effective H1 antagonists, the newer generation of antihistamines causes very little sedation and possesses relatively little anticholinergic activity. Unmetabolized terfenadine and astemizole, in clinical states of impaired hepatic metabolism (from cirrhosis or concomitant use of macrolide antibiotics or azole antifungals), can prolong the QT interval in the electrocardiogram, with rare instances of conduction abnormalities and arrhythmias, including the torsade de pointes form of ventricular tachycardia, and are currently off the market.

Patients with hypertension should be monitored for worsening symptoms while receiving oral decongestants (e.g., pseudoephedrine or phenylephrine). Topical decongestants are occasionally useful, especially with underlying sinusitis. However, because they can cause rebound nasal congestion, they should be given for no more than three consecutive days. Immunotherapy with allergen extracts is quite effective for controlling allergic rhinitis symptoms if the allergens are clearly identified and adequate doses can be tolerated. Immunotherapy may be effective because it can (1) blunt basophil histamine release, (2) inhibit seasonal rises in specific IgE, and (3) produce blocking IgG antibodies. Indicated for patients with symptoms present at least 6 months per year, immunotherapy is also effective for patients with seasonal symptoms who respond poorly to drugs. On its cessation, approximately one third of patients will continue to benefit from immunotherapy, one-third will gradually worsen over the years, and the remainder will relapse more quickly. Given the rare fatalities, such therapy should be initiated only by trained allergists. Because of the increased risk for life-threatening anaphylaxis, immunotherapy is contraindicated in patients using β blockers. Clinical trials are now underway with humanized monoclonal antibody against IgE to block the antibody from binding to sensitized cells, thus preventing the degranulation of those cells, and inhibiting the allergic reactions in patients with allergic asthma and allergic rhinitis. Preliminary data have shown anti-IgE to be safe and effective.

### Complications and Prognosis

Although rhinitis is not lethal, it does add to the morbidity and perhaps mortality of other illnesses. It increases the likelihood of developing sinusitis caused by obstruction of the sinus ostia and exacerbates pre-existing asthma. The use of first-generation antihistamines by patients with rhinitis can impair work performance and/or driving ability, and in a recent study, diphenhydramine was found to cause impairment of driving ability more even than alcohol, without the subjects' realization of their impairment. Most patients with rhinitis, especially allergic rhinitis, have an excellent prognosis with a regimen of allergen or irritant avoidance, topical corticosteroids, or oral antihistamines.

## ■ Sinusitis

### Definition

Although sinusitis is most commonly viral, the term often implies documented bacterial or fungal overgrowth in the sinuses with greater than 10,000 infectious units/ml. Diagnosed clinically and/or radiographically, sinusitis may be acute (<30 days), subacute (1–2 months), or chronic (>2 months).

### Epidemiology

Nearly one in eight adults will experience chronic sinusitis. **Maxillary sinusitis** accounts for 90% of all cases of sinusitis, followed by **ethmoidal sinusitis** in 5–10% of the cases. Thus, maxillary sinusitis is used as a prototype for this discussion. **Acute sinusitis** is very common in children, with 5–10% of upper respiratory infections becoming complicated by acute sinusitis. Although this rate seems to be lower among adults, exact figures are unavailable. Typical bacterial isolates are *Streptococcus pneumoniae*, *Haemophilus influenzae*, and *Moraxella (Branhamella) catarrhalis*. Groups A and C streptococci and *S. viridans* are less frequent. Anaerobic gram-positive organisms such as *Peptococcus* and *Peptostreptococcus* can be found in cases of chronic sinusitis along with *Bacteroides* species. β-Lactamase–producing bacteria, resistant to ampicillin and amoxicillin, are present 20% of the time.

### Pathophysiology

Among the four paranasal sinuses (maxillary, ethmoid, sphenoid, and frontal), the first two develop soon after birth; development of the others may lag until age 3–6. The posterior ethmoid cells and sphenoid sinuses drain by gravity into the superior meatus between the superior and middle turbinates, and the anterior ethmoid cells and maxillary sinuses drain into the middle meatus (Figure 16.2). This region, the **osteomeatal complex,** is readily obstructed by mucosal edema or polyps. Bacteria can enter the sinuses through the ostia or by contiguous spread, as in a dental abscess. The pathogenesis is summarized in Figure 16.3.

The cross-sectional areas of the sinus ostia largely determine gas exchange and mucus clearance, and, thus, even modest obstruction, as in rhinitis, will increase the risk for sinusitis. A low $Pao_2$ also causes vasodilatation, leading to transudation and mucosal congestion. Because the maxillary ostia are located high on the medial wall, ciliary action is required to clear the secretions against gravity. Thus, increased mucus viscosity (cystic fibrosis), reduced ciliary function (smoking, ciliary dyskinesia, viruses, hypoxia), or low $Pao_2$ (smoking) increases the likelihood of maxillary sinusitis.

### Clinical Features

*Acute sinusitis* often follows upper-respiratory viral infections. Its features are persistent symptoms of viral rhinitis lasting more than 10 days: pain in the cheeks radiating into the incisor teeth; fever; bad breath; purulent rhinorrhea; nasal congestion; or, occasionally, a nocturnal cough from postnasal drip of sinus secretions. Untreated sinusitis can lead to more serious complications, including cavernous sinus thrombosis, intracranial abscess, or subperiosteal abscess of the orbit. Eye swelling, exophthalmos, or focal neurologic changes after an unresolved upper respiratory infection suggest such a sequence.

*Chronic sinusitis*, which follows prolonged osteomeatal obstruction, manifests with chronic rhinorrhea, nasal congestion, decreased sense of smell, chronic cough from postnasal drip, or headaches. Asthmatics often report worsening asthma symptoms when a sinus infection develops; the majority of these patients report improved control of asthma after treatment of the sinusitis. **Allergic fungal sinusitis** is rare, most frequently caused by *Aspergillus,* and occurs in highly allergic patients.

### Diagnosis

The history and a clinical suspicion are key to diagnosing sinusitis. In acute sinusitis, sinus tenderness may be demonstrable, and the nasal smear often shows numerous neutrophils. Incisor toothache, poor response to decongestants or antihistamines, or discolored nasal discharge seen by the patient or on physical examination increase the likelihood of bacterial sinusitis twofold to threefold. These factors, combined with the overall clinical impression by the primary care physician, can effectively stratify patients into categories of high or low risk for sinusitis.

Although some studies suggest that transillumination might be useful in diagnosis, others dispute its diagnostic value as an isolated test. The vast majority of patients (>85% of children) with 10 consecutive days of symp-

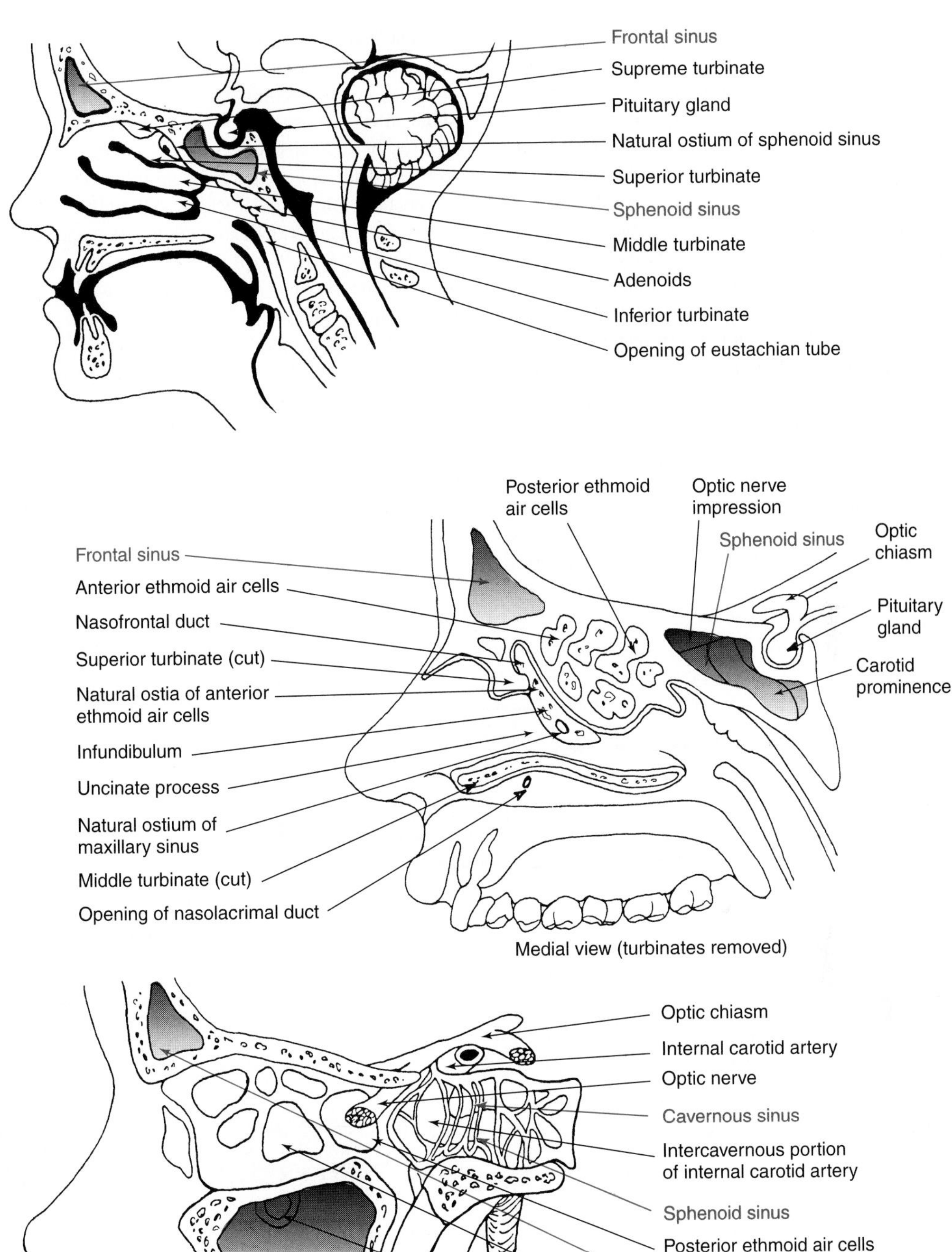


**FIGURE 16.2. Anatomy of the nasal cavity and the sinuses showing the osteomeatal complex.** (Reproduced with permission from: Josephson JS, Rosenberg, SI. Clinical Symposia 1994; 46:5. 8 1994) [Ciba Pharmaceuticals Division, Novartis Corporation, all rights reserved]

toms will have radiographic evidence for sinusitis. Computed tomography (CT) scans are more sensitive than standard radiographs in showing sinusitis; given the ready availability of CT, the cost for limited cuts of the sinuses compares favorably with that for conventional sinus films, making limited CT the first study of choice. In allergic sinusitis caused by *Aspergillus*, a mass effect can be seen in sinus CT. In skilled hands, flexible rhinoscopy also aids diagnosis when a purulent discharge can be visualized below the middle turbinate in the area of the maxillary ostium. Sinus aspiration is generally reserved for those patients who do not respond to a full course (more than 4 weeks) of appropriate management, including antibiotics, or for those with a rapidly progressive course while taking antibiotics.

## Management

Promoting drainage and treating the bacterial infection are the dual goals in treating sinusitis. Because most children and adults with recurrent sinusitis have allergies, allergy treatment also is critical.

The bacteriology of sinusitis is discussed in Chapter 154. Anaerobic bacteria more often play a role in chronic sinusitis. Treatment options are listed in Table 16.3. Some sinus infections resolve spontaneously. Oral and short courses of topical decongestants may be helpful. Oral steroids and topical steroid sprays may reduce osteomeatal complex obstruction, especially when polyps are present. Appropriate antibiotics (amoxicillin, 500 mg three times per day, being the most common first-line agent used) should be given for at least 3 weeks. If the response is not adequate in 10–14 days, β-lactamase–resistant drugs should be used. The initial choice of a β-lactamase–resistant drug such as clarithromycin (500 mg twice daily) or amoxicillin/clavulanate (500 mg/125 mg three times per day) is appropriate for smokers and childcare workers because they are more likely to harbor β-lactamase–producing *Haemophilus influenzae*. In β-lactam allergy, a macrolide or trimethoprim-sulfamethoxazole also can be used as a first-line therapy.

Documented anatomic obstruction or failure of sinusitis to resolve after 2–3 months of therapy with a

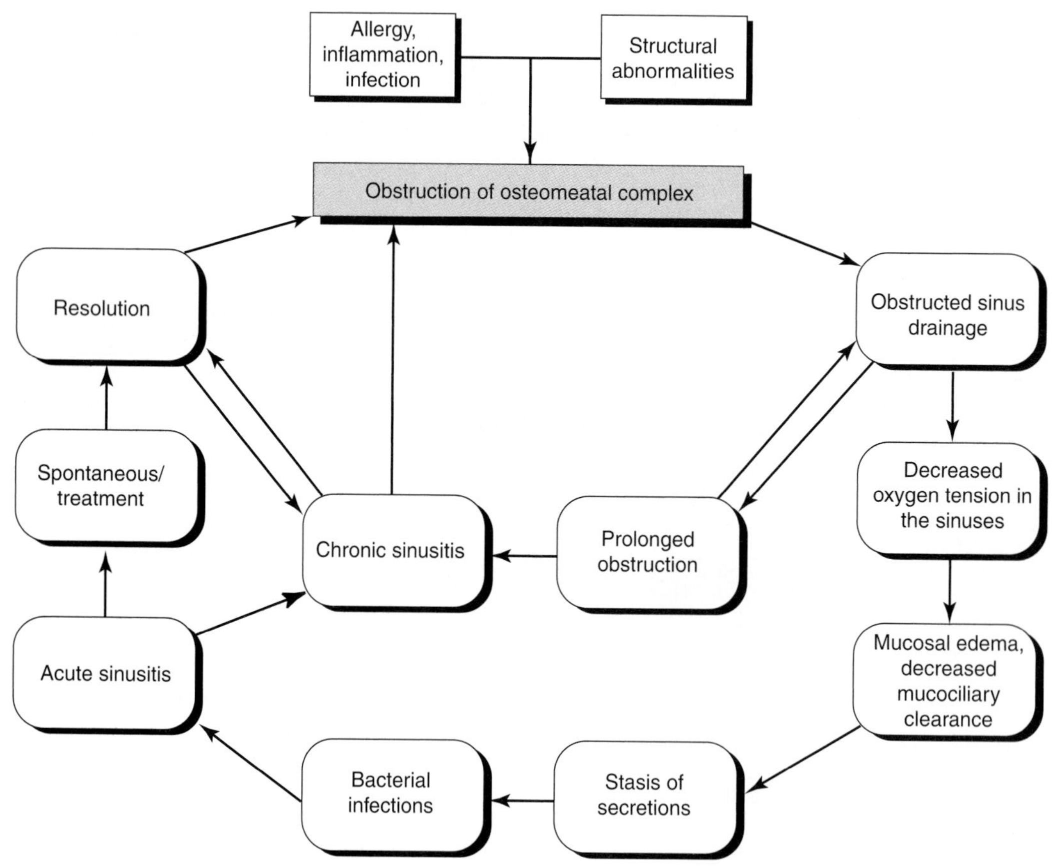


**FIGURE 16.3.** The pathogenesis of acute and chronic sinusitis.

TABLE 16.3. Treatment Options for Sinusitis

| Treatment | Frequency | Cost | Comments |
|---|---|---|---|
| Steam | BID–TID | +/– | May relieve symptoms. |
| Oral decongestant | BID–TID | + | May improve drainage. |
| Topical decongestant | QD–BID | + | May improve drainage but risk of rebound. Usually avoided. |
| Topical corticosteroid | QD–BID | ++ | May shorten clinical course and improve drainage. |
| Oral corticosteroid | QD | + | Can improve symptoms when severe and improve drainage. Limit to 4–7 day taper (start at 0.5–1 mg/kg). |
| Antibiotics | | | |
| *1st line* | | | (All courses for 3 weeks) |
| Amoxicillin | TID | + | Usually effective at 500 mg/dose. 15–20% β lactamase resistance. |
| Erythromycin | TID–QID | + | Suitable in penicillin allergy at 1–1.5 g/day. |
| TMP/SMX | BID | + | Suitable in penicillin allergy at 160/800 mg/dose. |
| *2nd line* | | | |
| Amoxicillin/clavulanate | TID | +++ | Effective at 500 mg/dose for 3 weeks. |
| Cephalosporin | BID–TID | ++ | Cefuroxime 250 mg 2 times per day for 3 weeks or cefaclor 500 mg 3 times per day. |
| Macrolide | QD–BID | ++ | Clarithromycin 500 mg 2 times per day for 3 weeks. |

+/– = trivial; BID = twice per day; QD = once per day; QID = 4 times per day; TID = three times per day; TMP/SMX = trimethoprim/sulfamethoxazole.

course of oral steroids and antibiotics against *H. influenzae* and anaerobic bacteria warrants surgical drainage. Endoscopic sinus surgery, designed to improve osteomeatal drainage, is highly successful also (80% of cases).

IgG subclasses, immunoglobulin responses to encapsulated bacteria, and ciliary function should be evaluated in patients with recurrent episodes (3 or more in 6 months or 4 in 1 year) who have been appropriately treated (see Chapter 21).

### Complications and Prognosis

Sinusitis can exacerbate asthma. If untreated, the infection can spread to adjacent bone and vascular structures, causing osteomyelitis or thrombosis, and into the intracranial cavity, resulting in meningitis. With appropriate antibiotic therapy, the prognosis is excellent for most patients. Those with recurrent sinusitis and an underlying immunodeficiency generally respond well to prophylactic antibiotics, but they might require immunoglobulin replacement. Anatomic obstruction of the sinus ostia generally responds to surgical intervention.

## Conjunctivitis

Allergic conjunctivitis often complicates allergic rhinitis and may be the most bothersome symptom for some patients. Ocular allergy commonly manifests with seasonal allergic conjunctivitis characterized by a mild conjunctivitis with photophobia, moderate itching, gritty sensation in the eyes, tearing, a slight discharge, and mild conjunctival injection. Oral antihistamines and topical agents such as antihistamines (naphazoline, levocabastine), NSAIDs (ketorolac), mast cell stabilizers (lodoxamide, tromethamine), and artificial tears are all helpful.

Other conditions encountered in atopic individuals include atopic keratoconjunctivitis, vernal conjunctivitis, and giant papillary conjunctivitis. Atopic keratoconjunctivitis coexists with atopic dermatitis. Vernal conjunctivitis is usually seasonal, causing conjunctival interstitial inflammation and flat-topped papules. The patient, usually a child, complains of extreme ocular pruritus with mucus strands. Giant papillary conjunctivitis, with giant papillae under the lids and corneal abrasions related to friction of the papillae on the cornea, may follow the use of gas-permeable contact lenses. Frequent lens cleaning sometimes can reduce symptoms.

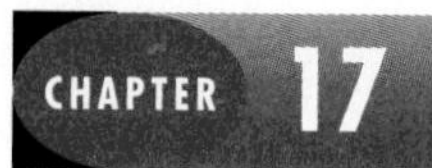

# BRONCHIAL ASTHMA

## Definition

Bronchial asthma (commonly termed "asthma") is a common disease, characterized by reversible bronchial obstruction and nonspecific **bronchial hyperresponsiveness** (BHR). Airway inflammation, another hallmark, correlates with the severity of chronic symptoms. Asthma is sometimes subcategorized into *extrinsic* (when allergens trigger an allergic response) and *intrinsic* (when no allergic trigger can be identified).

## Epidemiology and Pathogenesis

Asthma affects 5.6% of the population (i.e., 14.6 million Americans) and is the prime cause of absenteeism from school and a frequent cause of work absences. During the 1980s, yearly deaths from asthma doubled from 2000 to approximately 4000. The overall mortality rate now is 1 in every 3000 patients, but this rate is at least five times higher for African Americans. Lack of access to medical care and inappropriate medication use both contribute significantly to the rising morbidity and mortality caused by asthma.

Most asthmatics have allergies. Seasonal or perennial rhinitis coexists with asthma in about 75% of children and 50–60% of adults. In these persons, asthma exacerbations frequently follow allergen exposure. Occupational exposure to allergens and sensitizing agents can cause **occupational asthma.** Occupational exposure generally involves isocyanates (in urethane foam) and organic acids (for electronic solders) or chemicals and proteins that induce IgE responses—such as acid anhydrides (used as plasticizers), nickel salts, and cereal proteins. These agents may cause epithelial damage with only modest obstruction early in the disease. Exposure may evoke immediate symptoms, but symptoms commonly are delayed for several hours. Continued exposure progressively worsens BHR and asthma, both of which can become severe and irreversible if the affected person does not leave the offending environment. In **reactive airways dysfunction syndrome**, a subset of occupational asthma, patients develop BHR and symptoms after an acute toxic exposure. Prior asthma is absent; only lymphocytic infiltrates and relatively little inflammation are seen histologically.

Asthma attacks also may follow drug use or preservative exposure. Metabisulfites, used as preservatives in salad bars, beers, sauerkraut, and many other foods, may cause severe symptoms in some asthmatics. Aspirin, which causes asthma attacks in 10% of patients, similarly affects one third of asthmatics with nasal polyps.

A subset of asthma is **exercise-induced asthma** (EIA). Patients with EIA generally develop bronchoconstriction during the cool-down period after strenuous exercise in a cool, dry environment. A high level of ventilation during exercise and the temperature and relative humidity of the ambient air are critical to its genesis.

Respiratory tract inflammation can exacerbate asthma. Viruses, most commonly rhinovirus, influenza, and the respiratory syncytial virus, impede ciliary clearance of mucus and may promote adhesion molecule expression and mediator release. Therapy of sinusitis improves asthma symptoms in many asthmatics; thus, bacterial sinusitis seems to play a role in asthma. In a small subset of highly allergic asthmatics, type I reactions may follow fungal colonization of the bronchi by *Aspergillus* (allergic bronchopulmonary aspergillosis; see Chapter 224).

## Pathophysiology

Despite the overlapping aspects in their clinical expression, the key features of asthma are bronchial obstruction, BHR, and inflammation.

### Bronchial obstruction

Bronchial obstruction is clinically measured indirectly by assessing airflow. Because airflow resistance is proportionate to the fourth power of the airway radius, even small changes in the lumen can cause major airflow changes. Reversible bronchial obstruction can follow smooth muscle contraction, mucosal edema, or intraluminal debris, such as mucus. Collectively, the contribution of each determines the rate of reversibility. Smooth muscle contraction can be induced by cold, dry air (exercise), histamine, $PGD_2$, and leukotriene $C_4$ , as well as vagally by acetylcholine release. Bronchoconstriction thus produced is transient and frequently resolves spontaneously or after bronchodilator use.

### BHR

Nonspecific BHR, determined through bronchoprovocation testing (Chapter 218), is an important criterion for asthma. Asthmatics are many times more sensitive to irritants such as smoke, cold air, and air pollution than those without asthma, and the degree of BHR roughly correlates with asthma severity. Although the mechanism of BHR in asthma is still undefined, it is believed that epithelial damage affords the allergens or irritants greater access to afferent nerve endings. The degree of BHR correlates with eosinophilic inflammation. Baseline obstruction caused by inflammation also may evoke BHR by causing uneven deposition of inhaled irritants throughout the lung, resulting in proximal deposition of more concentrated solutions.

### Inflammation

Most, if not all, asthmatics manifest airway inflammation, including basement membrane thickening, epithelial damage, cellular infiltrates, and excess mucus production. These changes not only limit bronchodilator responsiveness, but also take days or weeks to reverse. Eosinophils play a very important role in asthmatic inflammation, and their toxic granule contents probably cause much of the epithelial damage observed in asthma. Pathologists refer to the disease as **chronic desquamative eosinophilic bronchitis.**

After exposure to stimuli (e.g., an allergen), asthmatics can have an isolated "early" bronchial obstruction, most often with bronchospasm and edema, that generally occurs within 10–15 minutes and resolves in 1 hour. Nearly half of those displaying such an early response also show a late response, occurring spontaneously 4–8 hours after exposure and resolving in a day or two. This late phase, believed to be caused by inflammation, is relatively refractory to bronchodilators compared with the early phase. Development of LPRs contributes to BHR. The cellular events in early-phase and late-phase inflammation are depicted in Figure 17.1. Drugs that inhibit mast cell activation (e.g., cromolyn or nedocromil) and drugs that block cytokine production (e.g., corticosteroids) can block the late phase.

Airflow obstruction produces disturbances in gas exchange. With worsening airflow obstruction, the ventilation-perfusion mismatch worsens, and progressive **hypoxemia** (a low $Pao_2$) results. Respiratory muscles work and their oxygen demand **(work of breathing)** increases as well, which necessitates diversion of an increasing proportion of the cardiac output to the respiratory muscles, a process that seriously imperils the cerebral and coronary blood flow. Declining perfusion of these vital organs, in the face of deteriorating systemic oxygenation, predisposes them to cellular hypoxia and subsequent dysfunction (see Chapter 255). Hyperventilation during acute attacks leads to a low $Paco_2$ **(hypocapnia)** and a high pH (respiratory alkalosis). With worsening obstruction, the 1-second forced expiratory volume ($FEV_{1.0}$) progressively decreases and the $Paco_2$ drops linearly with the $FEV_{1.0}$. When the $FEV_{1.0}$ decreases to 20–30% of normal (<1.0 L), the $Paco_2$ begins to increase **(hypercapnia),** which generally follows an $FEV_{1.0}$ lesser than 0.75 L.

## Clinical Features

Asthma is a chronic illness with episodic exacerbations and a wide spectrum of clinical severity. At one extreme is **episodic asthma,** characterized by very infrequent attacks of bronchospasm with interspersed normal periods; on the other extreme is **chronic asthma,** characterized by persistent airflow obstruction that paroxysmally worsens. The intensity of airflow obstruction in the individual episode determines the severity of the acute event, and the frequency and severity of exacerbations and the severity of airflow obstruction between episodes determines the severity of chronic asthma. Chronic asthma can be mild, moderate, or severe (Table 17.1). Most patients have mild to moderate illness, and, between attacks, many patients function normally with minimal or no symptoms; however, during acute exacerbations, even patients with otherwise mild disease can experience moderate to severe symptoms.

Asthmatics commonly report shortness of breath, wheezing, and chest tightness. Nearly all asthmatics have at least some symptoms (dyspnea, in addition to wheezing and cough or both) when exercising in cool, dry air. Irrespective of daytime symptoms, almost all chronic asthmatics experience nocturnal symptoms, highlighting the need for the treating physician to inquire about both daytime and nocturnal symptoms. A mild form of asthma may present with only a recurrent cough **(cough-variant asthma).**

Classically, asthmatic attacks occur in paroxysms, in which the patient swiftly exhibits an intense sense of air hunger. Acute episodes feature **tachypnea** and **tachycardia.** Fever is absent unless infection is associated. Wheezing, the sine qua non of asthma, manifests as a high-pitched, expiratory, continuous, musical sound, best heard at the mouth and without using a stethoscope. Chest-wall movements may be diminished, and chest percussion generally reveals increased resonance. Breath sounds may be decreased and, aside from the wheeze, some middle to late inspiratory crackles may be heard; confusion with heart failure **(cardiac asthma)** is then possible. As the attack becomes more severe, inability to recline, accessory muscle use, pulsus paradoxus, diaphoresis, and impaired mentation and judgment follow. The attack may terminate spontaneously or after the use of a bronchodilator.

The degree of airflow obstruction roughly correlates with the severity of asthma symptoms and many of the associated physical findings. Whereas wheezing may be noted on examination, symptoms of airflow limitation are not generally apparent until the peak expiratory flow rate (PEFR) or the $FEV_{1.0}$ declines to less than 60% of the predicted values (predicted values are obtained from nomograms). Most patients have acute symptoms as the PEFR falls below 60%, with wheezing and a prolonged expiration being universal beyond this point.

As the PEFR decreases to less than 50% of that predicted, symptoms become severe, especially in those

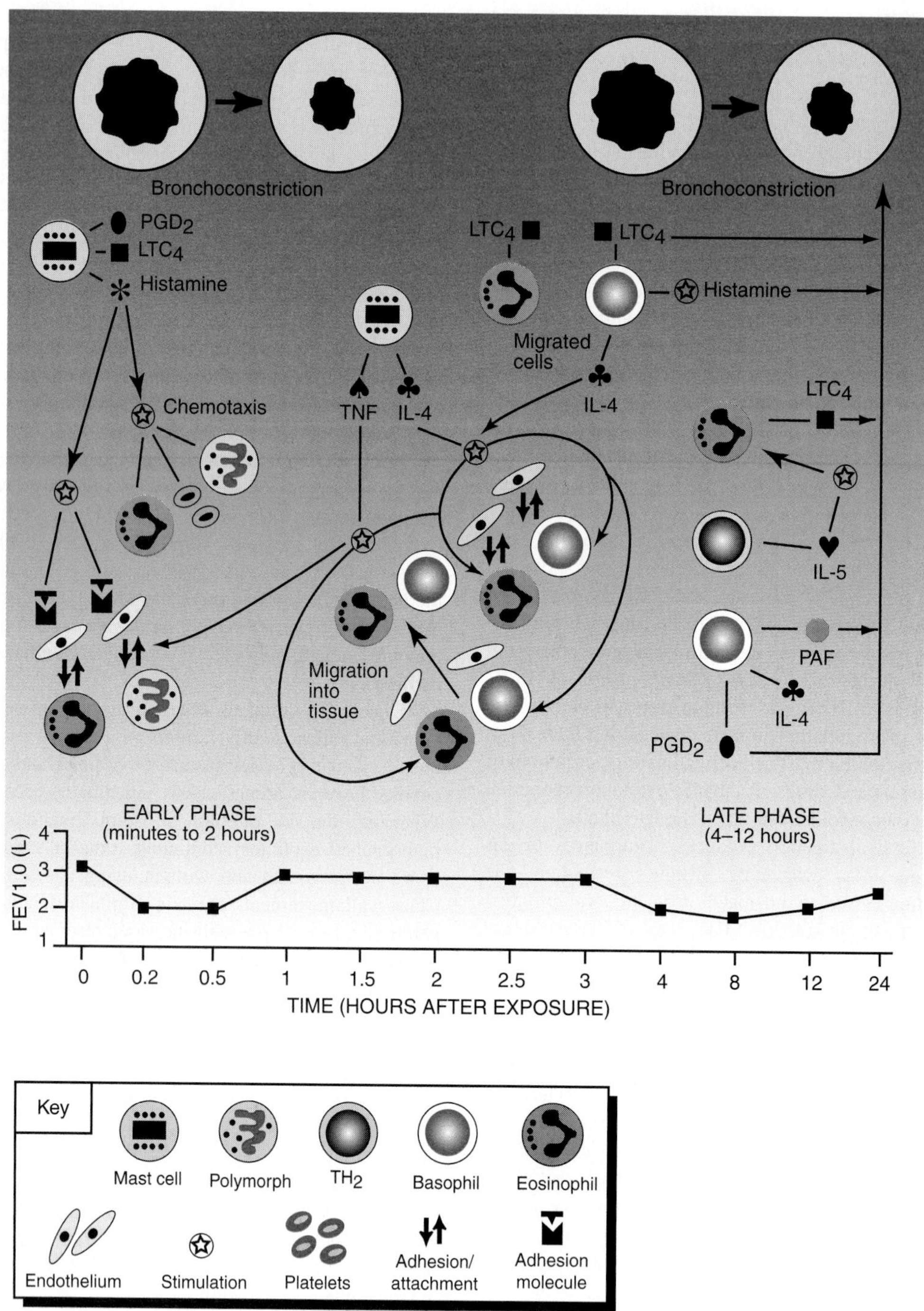


**FIGURE 17.1.** Early-phase and LPR in asthma.

whose illness is normally mild. In addition to chest tightness and dyspnea at rest, patients may report generalized fatigue from the extra work required to breathe. A severe asthmatic attack nearly always causes inability to recline, and this finding in a diaphoretic patient unequivocally indicates very severe airflow obstruction. Conversation consists of short or fragmented sentences (shortened word-strings). The hallmarks of a severe degree of airflow obstruction are accessory muscle use and pulsus paradoxus (see Tables 17.2 and 17.3). With further reductions in airflow, wheezing disappears and, in conjunction with the generalized decrease in breath sounds, causes the so-called **silent chest.** Accessory muscle use becomes evident when the $FEV_{1.0}$ has fallen to about 1.25 L. Pulsus paradoxus, [>12 mm Hg decrease in systolic blood pressure (BP) on inspiration] appears when the $FEV_1$ decreases to less than 1.0–0.75 L. A PEFR of 30–40% of that predicted is a harbinger of impending respiratory muscle fatigue and respiratory arrest. **Status asthmaticus**—which is largely preventable—is a clinical state of acute, severe asthma for which this threat looms large. Although this state of severe obstruction evolves over a few days in most patients, in a minority, an explosive start rapidly progresses to severe obstruction with a high risk of death **(acute asphyctic asthma** or **acute explosive asthma).** As the cerebral and/or coronary blood flow diminish, impaired mentation, confusion, tachycardia, ventricular irritability, and lethal arrhythmias follow.

Oximetry or arterial blood gases are often obtained when the PEFR is less than 40%. Because oximetry reflects only oxygenation and not $Paco_2$, exclusive reliance on oximetry should be avoided. As the asthma attack worsens, the $Pao_2$ and $Paco_2$ decrease; with worsening airflow obstruction, $Paco_2$ normalizes first and hypercapnia may ensue. An asthmatic with a normal or elevated $Paco_2$ during an acute attack is in serious trouble.

## Differential Diagnosis

Accurate diagnosis requires history and physical examination, supplemented by spirometric evidence of reversible obstruction or BHR. Spirometry between attacks may be normal or may show airflow obstruction (see Chapter 218). Airflow obstruction in itself does not prove asthma. Because asthmatics also have BHR, response to histamine or methacholine can assist diagnosis. Although the illness is typical in most patients (history, findings, and spirometry), a few with relatively normal spirometry may manifest only cough or episodic chest tightness. Although bronchoprovocation testing can be useful in this setting (see Chapter 218), it is superfluous in patients who demonstrate airflow obstruction and not indicated when the $FEV_{1.0}$ is less than 70% of that predicted.

Asthma, emphysema, and bronchitis all share the feature of airflow obstruction, and it can be difficult to distinguish between them, especially when a history of smoking is present. Airflow obstruction in the asthmatic shows reversibility, which may be seen on treatment (especially in chronic asthma after initiating corticosteroid therapy) or, more commonly, on spirometry, as an improvement in $FEV_{1.0}$ by 15–20% over baseline after inhalation of a β agonist. Extrathoracic airway obstruction (tumor or granuloma) may present with wheezing. Careful auscultation over the area of the trachea and flow-volume loop (see Chapter 231) may be useful. Peribronchial tumors and foreign bodies, other causes of obstruction, may be suggested by localized wheezing and confirmed by imaging.

Congestive heart failure, cystic fibrosis, pulmonary embolism, carcinoid syndrome, mastocytosis, and mycoplasma infection also can mimic asthma. Angina or esophageal spasm may present with chest tightness. Vocal cord dysfunction (intentional or unconscious apposition of the vocal cords during inspiration) can mimic severe asthma. In these patients, wheezing is loudest over the larynx, and diagnosis is made by laryngoscopy. Counseling and speech therapy can be

**TABLE 17.1. Chronic Asthma: A Suggested Severity Classification**

| Measure | Mild (green zone) | Moderate (yellow zone) | Severe (red zone) |
|---|---|---|---|
| PEFR | | | |
| %pred (post-bronchodilator) | ≥80% | 60–80% | ≤60% |
| intraday variability* | <20% | 20–30% | >30% |
| BDR† | ≤80% | ≥80% | Chronically ≤80% |
| Nocturnal episodes | ≤2/month | >2/month | Almost daily |
| prn β agonist use | ≤3/week | >3/week | Daily |
| Clinical | | | |
| Symptoms | ±/0 | Almost daily | Continuous |
| Activity limitation | None | Almost none | Limited despite optimal medication |
| Hospitalizations | – | – | (+) in the preceding year |
| Prior life-threatening episodes | – | – | + |

**Note:** Zones refer to peak expiratory flow rate (PEFR) monitoring system. Yellow and red zones generally correlate with a PEFR of 60–80% and <80% of personal best, respectively. Otherwise, clinical correlates are similar.
*Variability of PEFR throughout the day.
†BDR = Restoration of PEFR to predicted after bronchodilator administration.

**TABLE 17.2. Clinical Pharmacology of Commonly Used Agent in Asthma**

| Class | Agent | Effect | Mechanism of Action | Use | Route | Side Effects/Comments |
|---|---|---|---|---|---|---|
| β-2 agonists | Albuterol, R-albuterol, metaproterenol, pirbuterol, terbutaline | ↓ vascular permeability, bronchodilation. | ↑ c-AMP, inhibits histamine release from basophils. | Isolated early phase reactions, EIA, for immediate relief of bronchospasm. | Oral/MDI/ nebulizer; use as needed only. | Tachycardia, tremor, nervousness, ?may increase mortality with excessive use. |
| β-2 selective | Salmeterol | Same as above. | Same as above, but lipophilic, thus longer half-life. | May be used to reduce frequency of use of β agonists; may be used to decrease amount of steroid used; EIA | MDI or DPI | Same as above. Not effective for acute attacks. |
| Phosphodiesterase inhibitor | Theophylline | Acts as a bronchodilator. | Inhibits histamine release from basophils. | As a secondary agent in asthma. | Oral/IV | Narrow therapeutic index; drug levels vulnerable to many factors; GI side effects, agitation, potassium wasting, seizures. |
| Mediator release inhibitor | Cromolyn/ nedocromil | Affects early and late phase response; ↓ BHR. | Stabilizes mast cells; inhibits neuropeptide release; ↓ eosinophil chemotaxis. | EIA; allergic asthma, especially cat-induced asthma; prophylactic use. | MDI (Cromolyn and Nedocromil) MDI and nebulizer (cromolyn only) | Slow onset of action. |
| Corticosteroids (oral/IV) | Prednisone and methylprednisolone | Prevents late-phase response; ↓ BHR; potentiates action of β-2 agents. | Down-regulates TH2 cytokines in lung, inhibits adhesion molecule expression. | Antiinflammatory agent; pivotal in acute asthma to produce clinical improvement and prevent relapse. | IV/Oral | May alter mental status, cause fluid retention, potassium wasting, hyperglycemia, and hypertension. Long-term use may lead to osteoporosis, aseptic necrosis, and cataracts. |

*Continued*

TABLE 17.2. Clinical Pharmacology of Commonly Used Agent in Asthma *(continued)*

| Class | Agent | Effect | Mechanism of Action | Use | Route | Side Effects/Comments |
|---|---|---|---|---|---|---|
| Corticosteroids (inhaled) | Beclomethasone, flunisolide; fluticasone, triamcinolone, budesonide | Same as above. | Same as above. | Prophylactic use in chronic asthma. | MDI or DPI or nebulizer (budesonide only) | Variable absorption from tracheobronchial tree; long-term effects on pituitary-adrenal function unknown; may cause oral thrush. |
| Combined inhaled steroid and long-acting β-2 selective | Fluticasone (250 μg) and salmeterol (50 μg) | Same as effects above. | Same as effects above. | Prophylactic use in chronic asthma. | DPI | Same effects as each component separately above. |
| Leukotriene blocker/ inhibitor | Zileuton, zafirlukast, montelukast | Prevents bronchospasm. | Inhibits leukotriene synthesis/ blocks leukotriene receptor. | Prophylactic use in chronic asthma; EIA | Oral | Diarrhea, headache, liver function impairment. Zafirlukast is cleared through hepatic P450CYP3A4 system. |

↓ = decreases/reduces; ↑ = increases/raises; EIA = exercise-induced asthma; DPI = dry powder inhaler.

**TABLE 17.3. Acute Asthma: Evaluating the Severity**

| Severity Category | PEFR L/min | Wheeze | Accessory Muscle Use | Chest Wall Retraction | $Paco_2$ | Pulsus Paradoxus | Mentation |
|---|---|---|---|---|---|---|---|
| Mild | >200 | ± | None | None | ↓ | Absent | Normal |
| Moderate | 100–200 | – | Present | None | ↓ | ± | Normal |
| Severe | 80–100 | ++ | ++ | ± | Normal | ++ | Normal |
| Very severe | <80 | May be absent | +++ | Present | ↑ | ++ | Confusion, loss of judgment |

↓ = decreased; ↑ = increased; ± = may or may not be present.

beneficial. Some drugs (β blockers and NSAIDs) can precipitate asthma, and angiotensin-converting enzyme (ACE) inhibitors can cause coughing. Cough without wheezing or tightness can be caused by rhinitis, sinusitis, gastroesophageal reflux, or cough-variant asthma.

## Management

### Management of the ambulatory asthmatic

The therapy for asthma depends on its type, attack frequency, and severity. Allergic or occupational asthma is best treated by avoidance of the causative agent. Air filtration units with high-energy particulate air filters may help supplement animal dander control measures. Because many asthmatics (75% of children, 50% of adults) have an allergic component to their illness, a screening allergy evaluation is prudent, particularly for those younger than 40. Identification and avoidance of potential allergens and allergy immunotherapy can reduce BHR and the frequency of exacerbations. A careful history of home and work exposures also is important—especially in asthma of new onset in an adult.

Objective follow-up of an asthmatic's progress is best conducted using a peak flow meter, because the perception of symptoms is highly variable. The patient should monitor the PEFR regularly over a course of time to determine his or her best levels ("personal best"), which may then be used as a guide for management. Medication adjustment is required if the PEFR values consistently decrease from the personal best by 20%. Patients should see their physician if β agonist inhalation fails to improve the PEFR to above 80% of their personal best or if their pretreatment PEFR decreases to 50% below the personal best. Frequent interruption of sleep by asthmatic attacks calls for medication adjustment, with a prime goal of therapy being minimization, if not complete elimination, of the nocturnal attacks. Adequate control of asthma implies a normal lifestyle during day and night.

EIA is treated prophylactically with inhaled cromolyn, nedocromil, or β agonists. If no other symptoms exist, this will usually suffice. If episodic asthma symptoms occur at rest, the attacks may be terminated by use of inhaled β agonist. However, if episodes (especially if nocturnal) occur more than two to three times per week, a prophylactic anti-inflammatory drug should be used.

Patients who continue to have symptoms should be treated in a stepwise fashion (Figure 17.2): (1) maximization of an inhaled anti-inflammatory agent, (2) as-needed (PRN) β agonists, (3) addition of a long-acting selective β agonist or theophylline, and (4) PRN use of oral corticosteroids. Steroid-sparing approaches (e.g., use of methotrexate) are as yet somewhat controversial. When patients routinely require a β agonist more frequently than twice per day, the addition of a long-acting selective β agonist such as salmeterol should be considered; however, both salmeterol's delayed onset of action and the need to carry a more rapid-acting agent for acute attacks should be emphasized to the patient.

### Pharmacologic therapy

The clinical pharmacology of commonly used agents in ambulatory asthma is shown in Table 17.2. β-2 agonists offer immediate relief from bronchospasm; many physicians now endorse only their PRN use, instructing patients to contact their physicians when they are used more than four times per day. Aside from concerns that the regular use of β-2 agonists increases the risk of mortality, some believe they may offset the effects of topical corticosteroids on BHR. Inhaled steroids are safe, but can occasionally cause oral candidiasis or hoarseness, which are preventable by gargling after use and by use of a spacer. Allergy shots reduce the late-phase response and BHR when allergens are properly identified, but may take months to work. They may improve BHR and symptom scores and reduce the need for medication.

### Delivery devices

Metered-dose inhalers (MDIs) are effective and generally preferable to oral medications because the drug is delivered to the lung, causing minimal systemic effects; however, only 10–20% of the drug actually enters the lung when using typical MDIs. Much of the spray impacts the tongue and throat and is swallowed. Many patients, particularly children, the elderly, and those with arthritis, have trouble coordinating inspiration with actuation of the MDI. Spacer devices, which differ in their mechanism of operation, may address these problems. Because MDIs currently use fluorocarbon propellants, inhalers are available that deliver powder driven by the patient's inspiratory flow to the lungs (dry powder inhalers, or DPIs).

Nebulizers often are more convenient to use in young children. Clinically, some patients with bronchospasm respond better to nebulized β agonist solutions than to MDIs administered with spacers. Better distribution of the drug was considered the cause, but the greater dispersion of drug may be likely. Thus, if 5-10 puffs from an MDI with a spacer are used, a comparable response might occur.

**Scope of therapy**

With proper, well-supervised medical care, most asthmatics can avoid emergency department (ED) visits (emergent care) or hospitalizations; however, a heavy allergen burden or infection might precipitate rapid deterioration in asthmatics, necessitating emergent care. Relative to careful outpatient management, the cost of such care is much greater. The annual

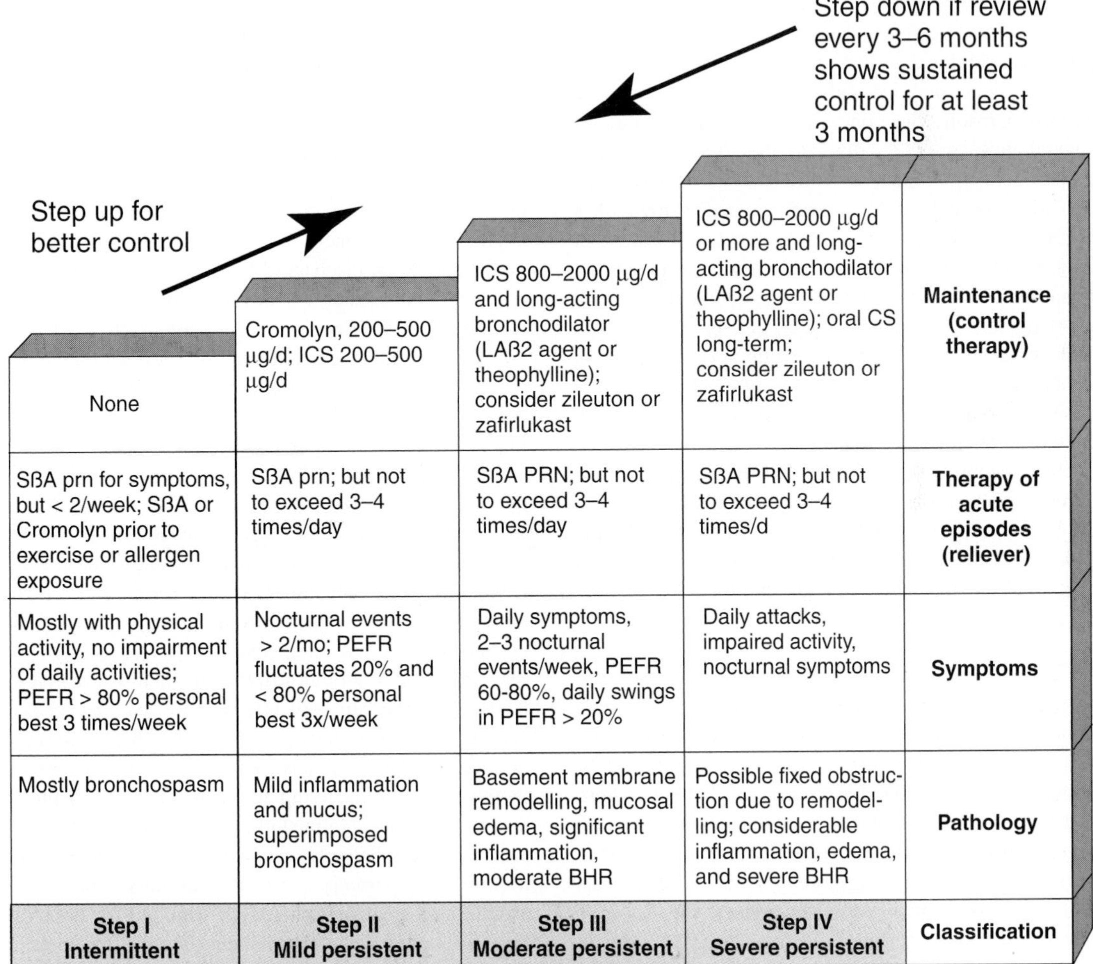
Step down if review every 3–6 months shows sustained control for at least 3 months
Step up for better control

| Step I Intermittent | Step II Mild persistent | Step III Moderate persistent | Step IV Severe persistent | Classification |
|---|---|---|---|---|
| None | Cromolyn, 200–500 µg/d; ICS 200–500 µg/d | ICS 800–2000 µg/d and long-acting bronchodilator (LAß2 agent or theophylline); consider zileuton or zafirlukast | ICS 800–2000 µg/d or more and long-acting bronchodilator (LAß2 agent or theophylline); oral CS long-term; consider zileuton or zafirlukast | **Maintenance (control therapy)** |
| SßA prn for symptoms, but < 2/week; SßA or Cromolyn prior to exercise or allergen exposure | SßA prn; but not to exceed 3–4 times/day | SßA PRN; but not to exceed 3–4 times/day | SßA PRN; but not to exceed 3–4 times/d | **Therapy of acute episodes (reliever)** |
| Mostly with physical activity, no impairment of daily activities; PEFR > 80% personal best 3 times/week | Nocturnal events > 2/mo; PEFR fluctuates 20% and < 80% personal best 3x/week | Daily symptoms, 2–3 nocturnal events/week, PEFR 60-80%, daily swings in PEFR > 20% | Daily attacks, impaired activity, nocturnal symptoms | **Symptoms** |
| Mostly bronchospasm | Mild inflammation and mucus; superimposed bronchospasm | Basement membrane remodelling, mucosal edema, significant inflammation, moderate BHR | Possible fixed obstruction due to remodelling; considerable inflammation, edema, and severe BHR | **Pathology** |

**FIGURE 17.2. Stepwise care in asthma.**
BHR = bronchial hyperreactivity; CS = corticosteroid; ICS = inhaled corticosteroid; $LA\beta_2$ = long-acting $\beta_2$ agent; PRN = as needed; $SA\beta_2$ = short-acting $\beta_2$ agent.

medical cost of asthma care can be reduced substantially by enrolling patients in programs that provide asthma education, routine outpatient visits, and 24-hour telephone access to physicians. The need for emergent care can be further reduced by regular use of inhaled corticosteroids and early initiation of oral corticosteroids as needed. Corticosteroids given to those who are discharged after emergent care can reduce the need for later hospitalization.

Guidelines for outpatient asthma management established by an international consensus are outlined in Table 17.3. Patients should contact their physicians (1) if their asthma symptoms worsen, (2) if the PEFR decreases by 20% from their personal best, or (3) if the PEFR diurnal variation is 20% or more (a drop from the "green zone" to the "yellow zone"). They are evaluated for exposures and infection(s), are advised to increase the frequency of use of β agonist (PRN) or alter its delivery, may be advised to increase their dose of inhaled steroid, or are given an additional medication (such as theophylline). Those whose condition fails to respond acutely to β agonist aerosol, who continue to be symptomatic for several days, or who drop into the "red zone" with greater than 40% reduction in PEFR should be evaluated for infection and, unless contraindicated, started on a regimen of oral prednisone (0.5–0.75 mg/kg for the first 2 days, followed by a taper over the next several days by about 20% less each day; an average course for an adult is 40 mg, 40 mg, 30 mg, 20 mg, 10 mg, and stop). Those with more severe asthma who require frequent steroid intervention may benefit from a slightly higher initial dose and longer taper. A single morning dose is often adequate. Divided doses may provide better relief of nocturnal symptoms, but they also can evoke more severe adrenal suppression. Current clinical trials have shown the benefit of anti-IgE therapy in the treatment of allergic asthma, and in the future this may be one way to control or perhaps even suppress allergic disease.

### Management of acute asthma

In treating acute asthma, β-2 agonists are of prime importance, the objectives being rapid symptom relief and prevention of status asthmaticus (Figure 17.3). Albuterol is administered as an aerosol. Patients whose PEFR is less than 50% of their personal best or those with severe obstruction (PEFR <100 L/min) that fails to respond readily by 10% or more to nebulized β agonists in the outpatient setting require emergency care. Racemic albuterol has both R and S isomers in a 1:1 ratio. S isomers actually have been shown to enhance bronchial hyperreactivity and β adrenergic side effects. There is now a single R isomer form of albuterol available as well. (Xopenex)

In emergency management of asthma, supplemental oxygen is started first to maintain the $O_2$ saturation greater than 90%. Rapid evaluation can then follow, and PEFR is measured. If the history and examination support a diagnosis of asthma, nebulized albuterol is administered, with 2.5 mg (0.5 ml) in 2.5 ml of saline. This dose is repeated at 20-minute intervals for three doses and hourly thereafter until side effects (tremor and tachycardia) appear or the attack begins to subside. Deceptively enough, tachycardia is often caused by the airflow obstruction in the acutely ill asthmatic. If patients are unable to participate in nebulization or if the exacerbation is part of a systemic allergic reaction, 0.3 ml of 1:1000 epinephrine can be given subcutaneously. Use of parenteral epinephrine must be weighed against the potential for cardiac side effects in patients with risk factors for coronary disease and in those older than 50. A common mistake is failure to administer epinephrine in critically ill patients, given concerns about hypertension or coronary artery disease. Routine use of aerosolized anticholinergic agents confers no additional benefits in acute, severe asthma, although studies have shown its benefit in the pediatric population.

Those with mild or moderate attacks could be observed after administration of a β-2 agent. Those who attain a posttreatment PEFR greater than 70% of predicted can be discharged from the ED on a tapering regimen of corticosteroids. Given their high likelihood of relapse, those who attain a posttreatment PEFR of only 40–70% of that predicted require observation before discharge. Some EDs with appropriate facilities might elect to observe these patients for several hours, because improvement often occurs within that time.

All patients presenting to an ED with severe asthma or who are at risk for complications (Table 17.4) should receive corticosteroids initially (prednisone at 30–40 mg every 6 hours). A severe asthmatic attack that has an explosive onset accompanied by respiratory arrest, inability to speak, confusion, complications (pneumothorax, pneumonia, pneumomediastinum), angina, myocardial infarction, or serious arrhythmias should be managed in the intensive care unit after therapy with oxygen, β agonist, and intravenous (IV) corticosteroids is initiated in the ED. Others with a severe episode can be observed in the ED after receiving the same therapy. PEFR is measured before administering treatment and 30 minutes thereafter. Patients who worsen despite therapy or improve only partially and those with persistent, severe asthma after treatment should be admitted for observation. If significant improvement ensues, the patient could be observed further and then discharged on an appropriate regimen of bronchodilators, close follow-up with a primary physician, and a tapering course of corticosteroids.

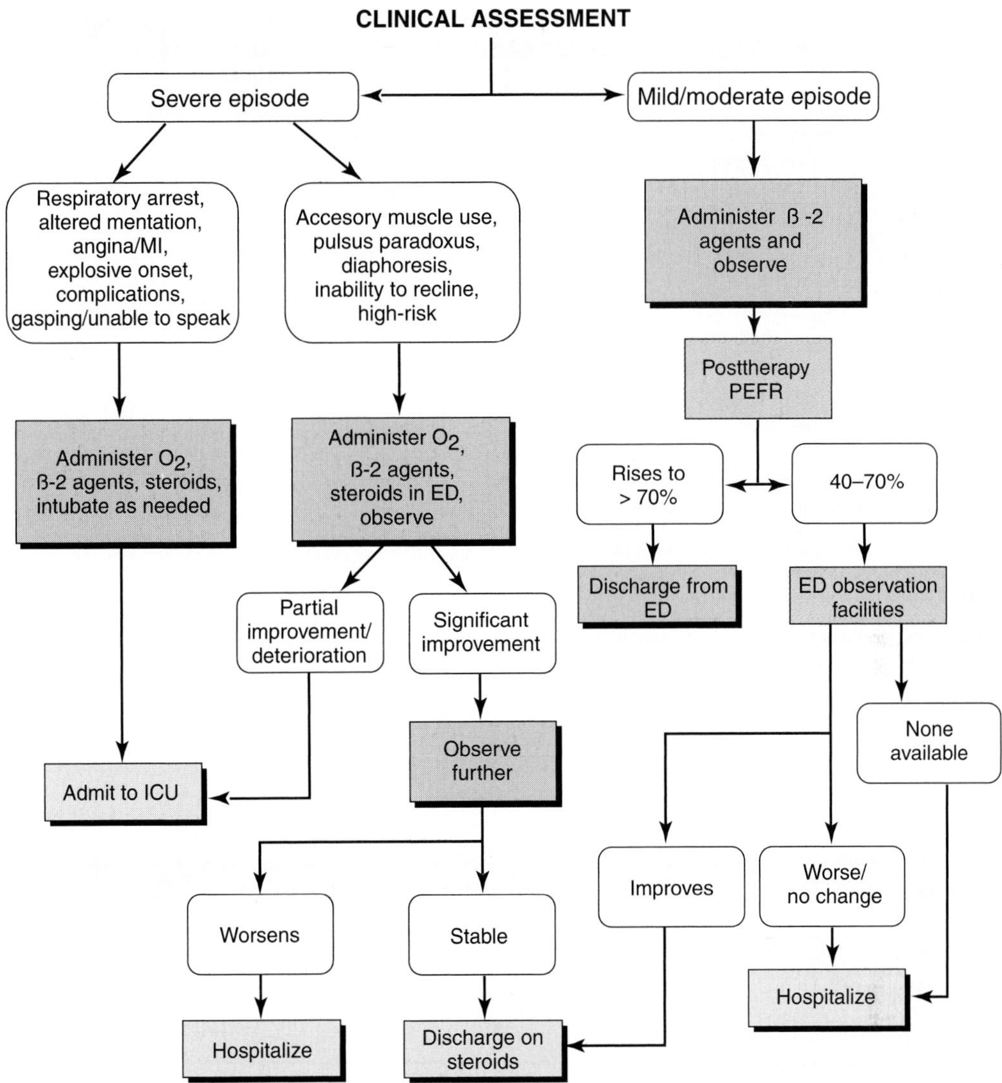


**FIGURE 17.3.** **Management of acute asthma.**

**Management of the patient hospitalized for asthma**

Hospitalized patients should have a complete blood count (CBC), differential count, electrolyte measurement, electrocardiogram (for patients older than 40 or at high risk for coronary disease), and arterial blood-gas study if the initial PEFR is less than 40% of predicted. Chest radiographs contribute little in the absence of a priori suspicion of pneumonia or barotrauma (pneumothorax or pneumomediastinum). Abundant eosinophils in the sputum Gram stain may help confirm allergic exacerbation; excess neutrophils may suggest infection.

As summarized in Table 17.5, pharmacologic management of the asthmatic hospitalized for acute, severe asthma (status asthmaticus) consists of oxygen, nebulized bronchodilators (given either hourly or by continuous nebulization until bronchospasm begins to abate or side effects emerge), and corticosteroids (at first IV and later by mouth, as soon as stability is attained). Corticosteroids are gradually tapered as the patient improves. Concomitant use of an H2 blocker may reduce the occurrence of steroid-related gastric stress ulcers; however, cimetidine reduces theophylline clearance, thereby raising the serum theophylline level.

**TABLE 17.4. Recommended Guidelines for Outpatient Management of Chronic Asthma**

| Asthma Severity | Inhaled β-2 Agonist | Cromolyn Sodium | Nedocromil | Inhaled Corticosteroid | Others |
|---|---|---|---|---|---|
| Mild | PRN, no more than 3 times per week* | Before exercise or before antigen exposure† | Before exercise or before antigen exposure | | |
| Moderate without nocturnal symptoms | prn ≤3–4 times per day | Daily | Daily | 200–500 μg/day | |
| With nocturnal symptoms (e.g., ≥ weekly) | Salmeterol; Albuterol ≤3–4 times per day | | | 800–1,000 μg/day‡ | ThSR++, βA++ |
| Severe§ | Same as moderate with nocturnal symptoms | | | | OCS QD or QOD |

**Note:** Patient should be evaluated for possible allergy component and follow avoidance. If indicated, undergo immunotherapy for improved symptomatic control.

++ = useful; generally necessary; ßA = oral $ß_2$ agonist; OCS = oral corticosteroid; QD = single daily dose; QOD = every other (alternate) day dose; ThSR = sustained release theophylline.

*Use either ß-agonist or cromolyn or nedocromil.

†Use either cromolyn or nedocromil.

‡Use inhaled corticosteroid with Theophylline SR or oral ß-2 agonist or long-acting ß-agonist. Daily dose above 1000 μg requires specialist supervision.

§Evaluate and treat underlying illness such as sinusitis.

**TABLE 17.5. Evaluating Acute Asthma: Harbingers of Trouble**

**History**

1. Prior hospitalization for asthma.
2. Prior endotracheal intubation and mechanical ventilation for asthma.
3. Chronic steroid dependence.
4. Prior explosive or near-fatal asthma.
5. Noncompliance with medications.
6. Overuse/abuse of bronchodilators.
7. Extremes in evolution of current illness: an extremely short one and a very protracted course.
8. Absence of perception of dyspnea in the face of severe airflow obstruction.
9. Associated systemic illnesses, for example, diabetes mellitus, coronary artery disease, and so forth.

**Physical findings**

1. Confusion, lethargy, and/or altered mental status.
2. Accessory muscle use and retraction.
3. Inability to recline, diaphoresis.
4. Ability to recline in the face of very severe obstruction.
5. Respiratory rate >30; heart rate >120; pulsus paradoxus (>12 mm Hg).
6. Silent chest.
7. PEFR ("peak flow") <100 L/min (or <40% of predicted).
8. Hypercapnia.

**Response to therapy**

1. PEFR <70% of predicted at the end of 2 hours, after aggressive bronchodilator treatment.
2. Untoward progression of the following findings: posture, diaphoresis, accessory muscle use, breath sounds, PEFR.

Another potentially useful measure includes theophylline. Monitoring the serum levels of theophylline is critical because it is potentially toxic. In the spontaneously breathing patient, sedation must be avoided. Because the illness often evolves over many days and may involve compromised fluid intake, rehydration is important; however, overhydration to "liquefy tenacious mucus" is without merit.

Endotracheal intubation and mechanical ventilation might become necessary because of worsening asthma, with the usual indications being respiratory arrest, unconsciousness, progressive fatigue, development or progression of hypercapnia (or both), and significant mental obtundation or progressive confusion. In general, the asthmatic requires these measures when (1) the possibility of maintaining spontaneous ventilation until achieving an effective bronchodilator/corticosteroid regimen is dubious, or (2) when the patient's general appearance and the course, despite comprehensive therapy, attests to progressive respiratory failure (worsening inability to recline, combativeness, confusion, dull sensorium, escalating tachypnea, and compromised accessory muscle use). Hypercapnia alone should not be a reason for intubation. A regimen of noninvasive ventilation with a tight-fitting face mask, continuous positive airway pressure, and IV bicarbonate when required to offset acidosis, offers an alternative to be used in selected situations when the need to intubate is less urgent.

### Preventing relapse

Early intervention using corticosteroid therapy is pivotal in preventing relapse, and both the patient and the physician must be properly educated regarding this therapy (Table 17.6). Careful management of chronic asthma—with an emphasis on anti-inflammatory

**TABLE 17.6. Medications in the Treatment of Acute Severe Asthma**

| Agent | Dose | Route | Comments |
|---|---|---|---|
| Albuterol | 2.5 mg in 2.5 ml saline | Nebulizer, initially for three doses at 20-minute intervals, then hourly. May also be given by continuous nebulization. | May cause tachycardia, tremor, and nervousness. |
| Methylprednisolone | 40–125 mg every 6 hours | IV | Start treatment in ED; higher doses do not show any additional benefit, but lower doses may not be as effective. |
| Prednisone | 40–60 mg every 6 hours | Oral administration. | |
| Epinephrine | 0.3 ml (1 : 1000 solution) | Subcutaneous administration. | May cause angina with prior CAD. Drug of choice for asthma with anaphylaxis. Patients with a history of explosive asthma should carry preloaded epinephrine syringe (EpiPen™) to use when such attacks recur. |
| Ipratropium bromide | 0.5 mg | Nebulizer, given every hour for 3–4 doses. | Not a standard regimen in acute asthma, but may be useful when the response to β-2 agents and steroids is suboptimal. |
| Theophylline | 5–6 mg/kg (Loading dose)<br>0.5–0.7 mg/kg/h maintenance | IV infusion in about 20 minutes for loading.<br>IV infusion | Toxicity generally related to serum level.<br>Therapeutic level 10–20 μg/ml, but a level of 9–12 μg/ml may be safer. |
| Magnesium sulfate | 2.0 g (total dose) | Two doses of 1.0 g each, infused IV in 20 minutes, given 20 minutes apart. | Not a standard regimen. If serum levels are low, correct the deficiency. |

**TABLE 17.7. Status Asthmaticus: Keys to Preventing Relapse**

| Patient Education | Physician Education |
|---|---|
| Identify triggers of attacks. | Intervene early and decisively when disease is out of control. |
| Control and avoid triggers. | Give antiinflammatory therapy. |
| Know when to call the physician. | Use reliable methods to monitor control of disease. |
| Recognize early warning signs of loss of disease control. | Overcome fear of using corticosteroids. |
| Be compliant with medications. | |
| Control the environment. | |
| Learn side effects of medications. | |
| Have an emergency care plan. | |

agents—is key to preventing relapses and status asthmaticus (Table 17.7). The physician should remember the adage that "the time to treat status asthmaticus is three days before it happens."

## Complications and Prognosis

Many physicians believe that untreated asthma can progress to an obstructive form of the illness with only partial reversibility because of airway remodeling. Patients with poorly controlled asthma who are undergoing surgery are also at greater risk for postoperative complications and are at higher risk for developing complications associated with radiocontrast studies. Without adequate *and* timely treatment, the mortality rate is several times higher than the previously mentioned 1 for 3000 cases. Although asthma is a chronic illness, most patients should be able to lead normal lives, especially if they receive proper care.

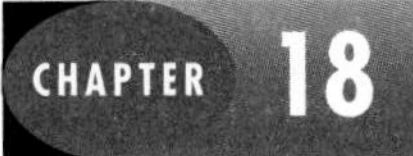

# CHAPTER 18 ANAPHYLAXIS

## Definition

It long has been known that "protective" immunizations with toxins could unexpectedly produce severe and often fatal reactions on re-exposure. Anaphylaxis is a constellation of allergic responses with features dependent on organ involvement, dose, and route of exposure. Symptoms can range from mild, generalized urticaria (see Chapter 20) to respiratory and circulatory collapse. Anaphylactic reactions are mediated through IgE; anaphylactoid reactions, which resemble anaphylaxis, do not require IgE recognition.

## Etiology and Epidemiology

The annual incidence of anaphylaxis in the general population is 3 per 100,000, accounting for 500–700 deaths yearly in the United States. Seen once for every 3000 inpatient admissions, anaphylaxis is most commonly caused by drug allergy, followed by Hymenoptera (bee) stings and food allergies. First reported in 1979, latex allergy became an important cause of anaphylaxis during the 1990s, and several fatalities have occurred. Three high-risk groups are known for latex allergy: spina bifida patients, employees of rubber manufacturers, and health care workers. Latex allergy seems to develop either from occupational exposure or by recurrent intraoperative contact. In adults, most anaphylaxis deaths are caused by a combination of hypoxia, cardiac arrhythmias, and laryngeal edema. Anaphylactoid reactions also cause more than 500 deaths each year, with the majority caused by radiocontrast media.

## Pathogenesis

Several mechanisms have been proposed for anaphylaxis. A type I IgE-dependent reaction is a common mechanism and is typically seen with reactions to proteins (e.g., venoms, insulin, foods) and smaller-weight haptens (penicillin, sulfa). These reactions involve vascular leak, vasodilatation, and bronchospasm caused by the release of platelet-activating factor, histamine, leukotriene $C_4$, and prostaglandin D. Released by mast cells, tryptase can be measured in serum 1–8 hours after the onset of anaphylaxis. Also, mast cells may produce nitric oxide, which acts as a vasodilator and could prolong hypotension.

At least two well-described anaphylactoid reactions do not require IgE. One such mechanism is immune complex anaphylatoxin–induced mast cell degranulation. Patients reacting to some drug infusions form IgG complexes that activate complement, which, in turn, activates mast cells and basophils. In patients undergoing hemodialysis, anaphylatoxin can be produced directly by reaction with the dialysis membrane. Direct cell activation is a third type of reaction, but it is poorly understood. Agents such as morphine, codeine, and contrast media cause mediator release from the cells of certain individuals. Ironically, atopic individuals are at no greater risk for IgE-mediated reactions, but they are four to five times more likely to have an adverse response to direct degranulation reactions. It is believed that their cells are relatively unstable—perhaps because of unique features of the bound IgE.

Regardless of the mechanism, patients with a prior anaphylactic reaction are at increased risk of its repetition on re-exposure. Penicillin, the most frequent cause of anaphylaxis, causes mild reactions in 0.5–1% of persons. Repeat exposure will cause a recurrent reaction in about 10–20% of these patients. Similar rates of recurrence are seen for other hapten drugs. In the United States population, 20% of persons produce IgE against Hymenoptera venoms, but reactions are seen in only 0.5%. However, patients with a prior systemic reaction have a 40–50% risk of another systemic reaction when re-stung. Because IgE levels gradually wane over time, the severity and likelihood of repeat reaction depends partly on the time elapsed since the last exposure. Non–IgE-dependent reactions are also highly recurrent (30–40% risk for radiocontrast), but whether avoidance influences this rate is uncertain.

Other forms of anaphylaxis may be idiopathic or may be induced by NSAIDs or exercise. Although NSAIDs inhibit cyclo-oxygenase and may shunt arachidonic acid into the leukotriene pathway, whether they activate mast cells or basophils is not known. The rate of NSAID anaphylaxis, 1 : 1000 in the general population, is higher among asthmatics with nasal polyps.

## Clinical Features

The presentation varies in severity and with organ system. Often, patients report a vague sense of impending doom as a **prodrome.** Manifestations may be cutaneous (pruritus, flushing, urticaria, and angioedema), upper respiratory with laryngeal edema (stridor, dysphagia, and respiratory distress), respiratory (sneezing, congestion, or initial ocular itch with later bronchospasm), gastrointestinal (nausea, vomiting, diarrhea, and cramping), and cardiovascular (vasodilatation causing skin flushing and vascular leak with associated hypotension and compensatory tachycardia). Histamine-induced coronary artery spasm may cause ischemia in patients with previous coronary artery disease. Patients receiving β blockers are especially prone to severe cardiovascular compromise because they are unable to develop tachycardia and are relatively resistant to epinephrine. Uterine contraction during anaphylaxis could cause miscarriage.

Anaphylaxis caused by percutaneous allergen challenge (e.g., injection or insect sting) has a rapid onset (within minutes) and is complete in 30 minutes. Life-threatening anaphylaxis after allergy injections almost always follows within 20 minutes. Because of its slower absorption rate, oral allergen exposure evokes less severe, delayed symptoms (less than 1 hour); however, reactions to peanuts, tree nuts, or shellfish can be rapid and lethal.

## Differential Diagnosis

When evaluating a patient with possible anaphylaxis, rapid decision-making and initiation of life-saving therapy are essential. Further evaluation can follow stabilization. When anaphylaxis cannot be excluded in the acute setting, assuming this diagnosis is generally the safest course of action. A brief history and physical examination are helpful. If a patient is known to be allergic to certain medications, Hymenoptera, or foods, a presumptive diagnosis is easy if exposure has occurred. Prior history of asthma, cardiovascular disease, MedicAlert bracelets proclaiming anaphylaxis, β-blocker use, or "reactions to needles" should be noted. At least some of the following typical signs and symptoms should be present: urticaria, rhinorrhea, wheeze, abdominal cramps, or hypotension. Unless there has been β-blocker use, tachycardia is usual. Elevated plasma tryptase with attacks can confirm anaphylaxis. By definition, the diagnosis of idiopathic anaphylaxis is one of exclusion.

The differential diagnosis includes anaphylactoid reactions (such as contrast, transfusion, and dialysis reactions)—which are treated as anaphylaxis—and asthma and urticaria. Vasovagal episodes and anxiety are other imitators, usually elicited by a fear of procedures. Patients with vasovagal episodes can experience hypotension and nausea, as in anaphylaxis, but have bradycardia and are usually pale (not flushed), diaphoretic, and without wheezing or urticaria. Patients with anxiety may have a rapid pulse, paresthesias, and light-headedness, but no other signs of anaphylaxis.

Side effects such as hypotension (overdose or increased sensitivity to an antihypertensive) or flushing (rapid infusion of vancomycin) from medications can mimic anaphylaxis. Carcinoid syndrome, aspiration of a foreign body, pulmonary embolism, myocardial infarction, and adrenal insufficiency also may be confused occasionally with anaphylaxis. A lack of precipitators and atypical features help determine the diagnosis. When in doubt, measurement of serum tryptase 1–4 hours after the onset of an attack might help establish or exclude anaphylaxis.

## Management

Acute intervention (Table 18.1) must be quick and decisive, including the use of epinephrine. Adverse outcomes including fatality are more likely caused by slow recognition and undertreatment than by complica-

**TABLE 18.1. Treatment of Anaphylaxis**

| Medication | Route | Dose |
|---|---|---|
| Epinephrine | Subcutaneous | 0.3 ml of 1:1000 every 10–20 minutes |
| Albuterol | Nebulized | 0.5–1.0 ml of 0.5% nebulized every 20 minutes up to three times |
| Oxygen | Nasal/mask | 40–100% to maintain $Pa_{O_2}$ >60 mm Hg, $Sa_{O_2}$ >90% |
| H1 antihistamine | IM | 25–50 mg of hydroxyzine or diphenhydramine every 6–8 hours |
| H2 antihistamine | IV | Cimetidine 300 mg IV every 6 hours |
| Corticosteroid | IV | 250 mg hydrocortisone or 50 mg methylprednisolone every 6 hours for 2–4 doses |
| Aminophylline | IV | For persistent bronchospasm, and if not currently using the drug, load with 5–6 mg/kg over 30 minutes, then maintenance of 0.3–0.5 mg/kg per hour |
| **For cardiovascular collapse** | | |
| Saline | IV | Infuse rapidly 1–2 L over 20–30 minutes until systolic BP is ≥80 mm Hg, then use sufficient fluid to maintain BP |
| Epinephrine | IV[a] | After the initial dose, continuously infuse a 4 μg/ml solution starting at 1 μg/min under careful cardiac monitoring, to keep systolic BP ≥80 mm Hg |
| Dopamine | IV | 200 mg in 500 ml D5W (0.4 mg/ml) starting at 5 μg/kg/min, increase rate by 5–10 μg/kg/min as necessary up to a rate of 20–50 μg/kg/min |
| Levarterenol | IV | 4–8 mg in 1 L of D5W or saline, to infuse at a maximal rate of 2 ml/min |
| Glucagon | IV | 1 mg in 1 L D5W 5–15 ml/min for refractory hypotension |

[a]If no contraindication.

tions from therapy. Early subcutaneous administration of epinephrine might head off more severe reactions. If anaphylaxis is caused by a sting or injection in an extremity, a tourniquet should be applied proximally and epinephrine can be injected directly into the sting site (if on an arm or leg) to delay absorption. For severe cardiovascular collapse unresponsive to subcutaneous injection, some physicians advocate a slow IV infusion of epinephrine. IV epinephrine infusion may induce myocardial damage in adults with risk factors for coronary disease and should thus be reserved for patients in extremis.

A team approach to address *airway, breathing,* and *circulation* is helpful. A patent airway must be maintained by repositioning the head, endotracheal intubation, or emergency cricothyroidotomy, if necessary. Give supplemental oxygen to maintain oxygen saturation above 90%. Endotracheal intubation may be necessary for respiratory failure that is refractory to the measures in Table 18.1. Circulation is assessed by pulse rate, blood pressure, and capillary filling of the nail beds. The patient is placed in the Trendelenburg position. A large-bore IV catheter (16–18 g) should be used to establish access for fluids. Hypotension is treated by rapid infusion of normal saline, followed, if necessary, by an infusion of dopamine or levarterenol bitartrate. Corticosteroids should be infused as soon as IV access has been achieved. Patients who use β blockers and are refractory to these interventions may benefit from glucagon infusion. IV diphenhydramine will reduce cutaneous manifestations but not respiratory, gastrointestinal, or cardiovascular complications. Some physicians find IV cimetidine, which blocks H2 effects of histamine, useful for treating hypotension and flushing, but it needs to be infused slowly, because rapid infusion may cause a decrease in blood pressure.

**TABLE 18.2. A Strategy for Preventing Anaphylaxis**

- Wear MedicAlert™ bracelet to indicate prior adverse reactions.
- Document prior adverse drug reactions in the medical record.
- Patients should wait in office 30 minutes after parenteral drug administration.
- Avoid causative or cross-reacting medications (e.g., cephalosporins with penicillin allergy; an NSAID when drug reactions to another have occurred).
- Use lower ionic contrast media and premedicate when a history of prior reaction exists.
- Substitute β blockers with other antihypertensives for patients at risk.
- Patients with prior anaphylaxis should undergo desensitization to Hymenoptera venom.
- Appropriate patients at risk should carry injectable epinephrine.
- If reaction has formed due to sting or injection in extremity, place tourniquet proximal to sting.

## Prevention

Although anaphylaxis is not always avoidable, its frequency and severity can be reduced for most patients. Many common-sense measures often are overlooked (Table 18.2). Patients with venom sensitivity should adopt additional measures such as avoiding wearing clothes with light-colored floral patterns and staying away from trash cans and open soda and juice containers when outdoors to reduce the likelihood of stings. Patients with a suspected food allergy should undergo skin testing by an allergist to confirm the diagnosis. They should carry a preloaded epinephrine syringe when dining out and carefully read the ingredients on all food labels.

Premedication regimens are available for patients at risk for anaphylactoid reactions to radiocontrast dyes. Use of low ionic strength agents reduces the risk, as does premedication with prednisone (50 mg or 1 mg/kg every 6 hours for 3 doses) and diphenhydramine (1.5 mg/kg, up to 50 mg) IM 30–60 minutes before study. Ephedrine (25 mg), which also has been added to this regimen, is not recommended for patients at high risk for heart disease. Finally, in a patient known to be allergic to a drug (e.g., a β lactam antibiotic) that is essential for his or her care, desensitization before administering a therapeutic dose greatly diminishes the risk of anaphylaxis.

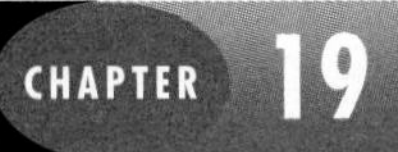


# DRUG ALLERGY

## Definition

Drug allergy is an adverse reaction based on immune recognition, expressed as a hypersensitivity reaction (Table 19.1). Although allergic reactions form a minority (10%) of adverse reactions to drugs, they are often severe. Prior exposure to the drug is usually required to develop immune recognition; however, the reaction is often unforeseen because the prior exposure may have been uneventful, the patient might have been exposed to a cross-reacting drug, or the exposure might have been occult or forgotten. Type II–IV reactions have delayed onset compared with most expected toxic or metabolic drug side effects.

## Etiology and Epidemiology

The high frequency of all adverse drug reactions parallels the frequent use of medications, particularly in the elderly. The average outpatient will consume three over-the-counter medications containing nine active ingredients per month. Drug reactions cause 5% of hospitalizations in the elderly (Table 19.2). A serious drug reaction occurs in 5% of patients hospitalized for 6 days or less but in 40% hospitalized more than 2 weeks.

Nonallergic reactions may be predictable or unpredictable (Table 19.3). Rather than memorizing long lists of medications and their possible adverse effects and interactions, the physician should do the following: (1) review the profile of each drug in the *Physician's Desk Reference* or similar guide before prescribing, (2) use available software for drug interactions (e.g., the HyperCard-based Drug Interaction Software program published by *The Medical Letter*), and (3) be familiar with several broad categories of agents. A small group of seven drug types (aspirin/NSAIDs, digoxin, anticoagulants, antibiotics, diuretics, steroids, and hypoglycemic agents) cause most drug reactions. Antibiotics are the group most likely to cause unpredictable allergic reactions.

Despite overlaps and exceptions, classifying allergic reactions along the type I–IV hypersensitivity scheme is helpful. Because immune recognition is involved, clues for the diagnosis of drug allergy include the following: (1) no reaction on prior exposure, (2) reaction after several days (for types II–IV), (3) reactions after exposure to doses well below the therapeutic norm, (4) a small proportion of the population affected, and (5) unusual presentation with recognized allergic syndromes. It is worth remembering that some patients are prone to multiple drug allergies. A patient with a proven allergy to

**TABLE 19.1. Types of Allergic Reactions**

| Reaction Type | Common Causative Agents | Clinical Presentations |
|---|---|---|
| Type I | | |
| Anaphylactic | Penicillin, chymopapain, insulin, sulfonamides | Urticaria, anaphylaxis |
| Anaphylactoid | Contrast media, morphine, codeine | Urticaria, hypotension |
| Type II | Transfusion reaction, quinidine, methicillin | Hemolysis, thrombocytopenia, nephritis |
| Type III | Penicillin, hydralazine, procainamide, antithymocyte globulin, sulfonamides | Serum sickness (fever, arthralgias, purpuric rash, proteinuria) hypersensitivity angiitis |
| Type IV | Parabens, nitrofurantoin, neomycin, topical antihistamines, ethylenediamine, sulfonamides | Contact dermatitis, pulmonary fibrosis, photosensitivity, toxic epidermal necrolysis |

penicillin is 10 times more likely to experience an IgE-mediated allergic reaction to another antibiotic. A familial trait for increased drug allergy may exist. Allergy to penicillin (and its derivatives) is the most common drug allergy; because penicillin can cause any of the type I–IV reactions, it is a prototype for the pathophysiology and presentations described in the following.

## Type I Reactions

A type I reaction involves mast cell or basophil activation. Classic, IgE-dependent mediator release is seen with complete antigens, such as proteins (serum, insulin), or haptens, such as penicillin or sulfa drugs, bound to proteins. Pseudoallergic reactions cause mediator release without immune recognition by IgE. This form of release can be seen (1) with agents that directly degranulate mast cells such as morphine, codeine, and radiocontrast; (2) as a result of bacterial contamination, which activates cells directly or indirectly by generating anaphylatoxins; and (3) when immune complexes plus complement are generated, which then activate mast cells. This last case may be a mechanism for protamine-induced reactions.

The most common type I reaction arises from penicillin and its derivatives. IgE antibodies are usually directed against the β lactam ring, which is shared with the cephalosporins (Figure 19.1). Occasionally, IgE is directed against the side chains, but such IgE antibodies are less clinically important. Reactive metabolites of penicillin can bind proteins and thus cross-link IgE on cells. Penicilloyl and penicilloate are two prominent metabolites. Penicilloyl is the "major determinant," because 85% of patients with type I penicillin allergy make IgE antibodies to it. Penicilloate and penilloate are "minor determinants." However, these terms are misleading because they do not correlate with the severity of reactions caused by these metabolites. Corresponding cephalosporin metabolites are less stable,

**TABLE 19.2. Determinants/Causes of Drug Reaction(s) in Hospitalized Patients**

- Drug allergy
- Idiosyncrasy
- Drug interactions
- Wrong dose
- Wrong dosing interval
- Wrong patient
- Polypharmacy (multiple drugs)
- Length of stay

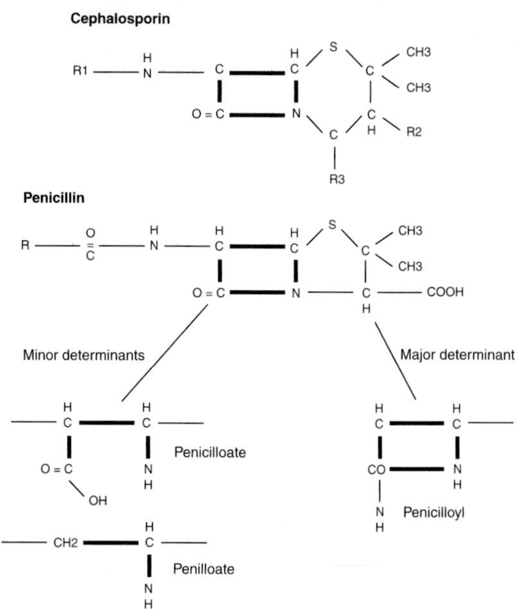


**FIGURE 19.1.** Penicillin and cephalosporins share the β lactam ring (in bold). Penicillin determinants include penicilloyl (major determinant), penicilloate, and penilloate (minor determinants). Most patients allergic to penicillin react to major determinant although the most severe reactions are usually against the minor determinants.

**TABLE 19.3. Examples of Predictable and Unpredictable Drug Reactions**

| Forms | Examples |
|---|---|
| Predictable forms | |
| Toxic side effects | Drowsiness from antihistamines. |
| Toxic supratherapeutic | Heart block from digoxin; CNS dysfunction from lidocaine. |
| Drug interactions | Theophylline toxicity when a macrolide antibiotic is added. |
| Unpredictable forms | |
| Drug intolerance | Hypotension at low dose of antihypertensive; hyponatremia on starting dose of diuretic. |
| Secondary effects | Fever and chills due to Jarisch-Herxheimer reaction when treating syphilis. |
| Idiosyncratic | Hemolysis in glucose-6-phosphate dehydrogenase deficiency; anaphylaxis in response to penicillin; aspirin-induced bronchospasm. |

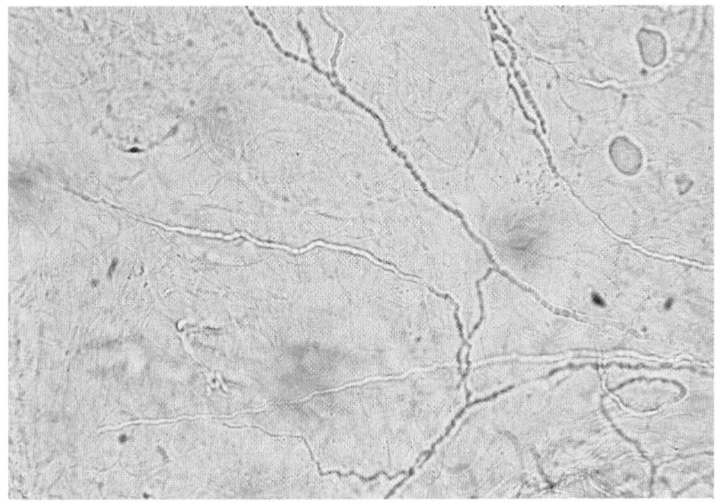

COLOR PLATE **1. Positive potassium hydroxide mount.** These thin, branched, septate hyphae are characteristic of a dermatophyte infection.

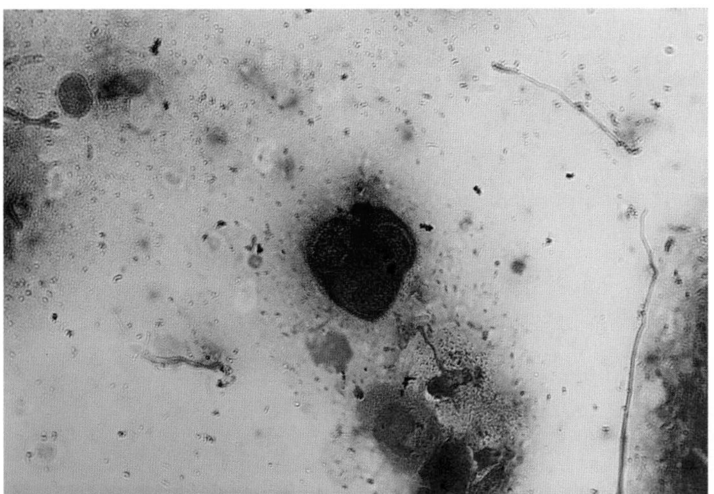

COLOR PLATE **2. Tzanck smear.** The presence of multinucleated giant cells is diagnostic of a herpes virus infection.

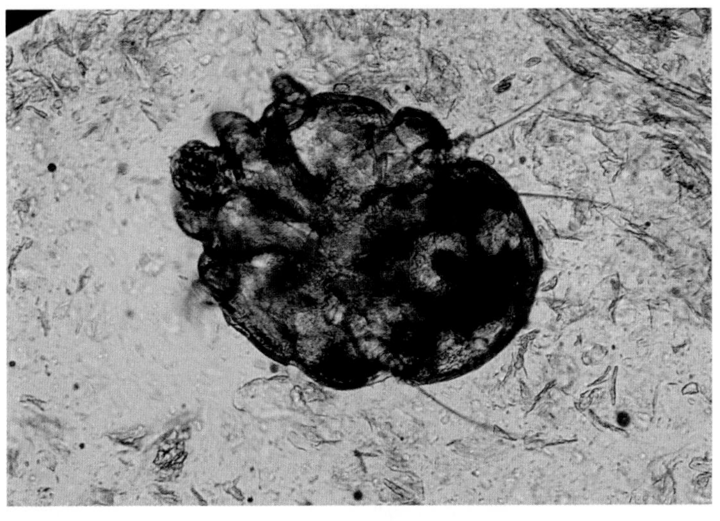

COLOR PLATE **3. Scabies prep.** A female mite is readily visible in this skin scraping. Ova and feces (not shown in this mount) are also diagnostic.

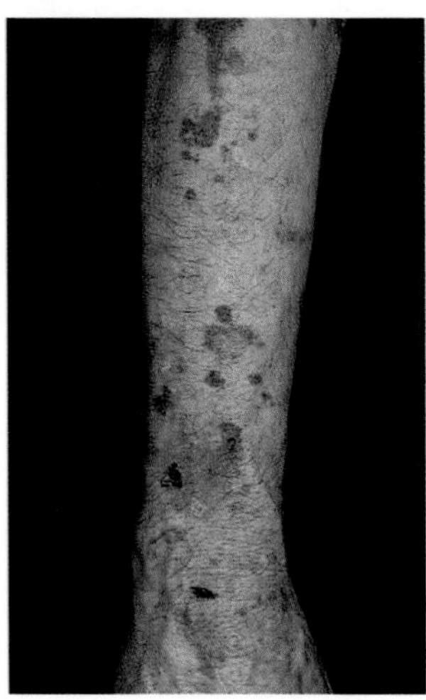

**COLOR PLATE 4. Purpura secondary to topical steroid use.** This complication is most often seen in sun-exposed areas on the hands and forearms of elderly patients.

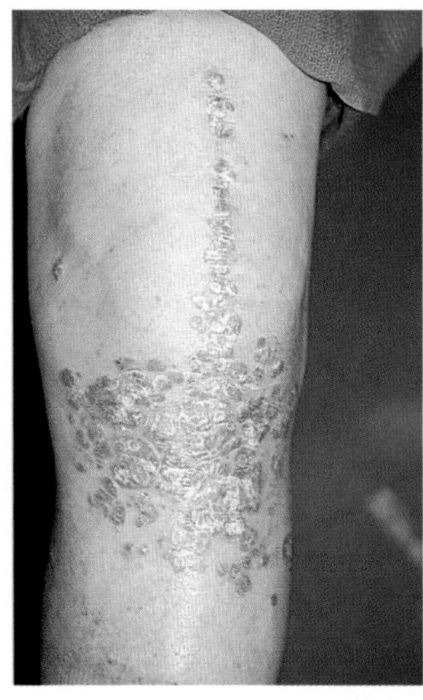

**COLOR PLATE 5. Psoriasis.** A typical erythematous plaque over the knee. Koebner phenomenon, as the linear extension of the lesion above the knee, is seen in the site of a previous knee surgery.

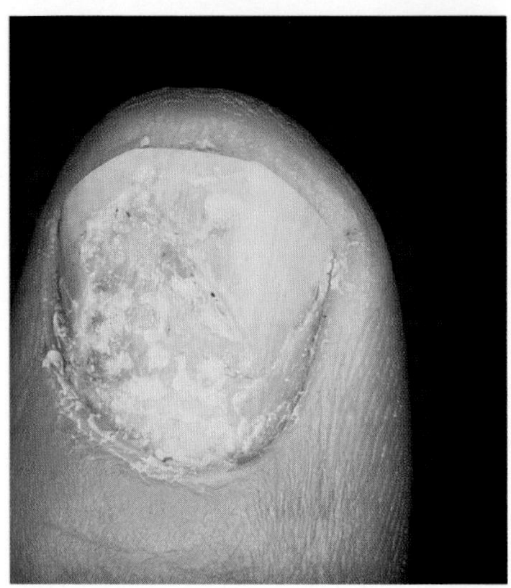

**COLOR PLATE 6. Psoriasis of the nails.** Whitish discoloration of the nail with pits. Lifting of the nail from the plate (onycholysis) and subungual debris are also common findings in psoriatic nails.

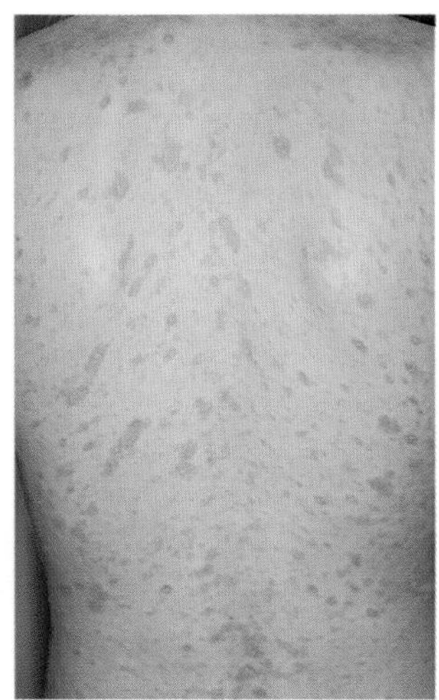

**COLOR PLATE 7. Pityriasis rosea.**

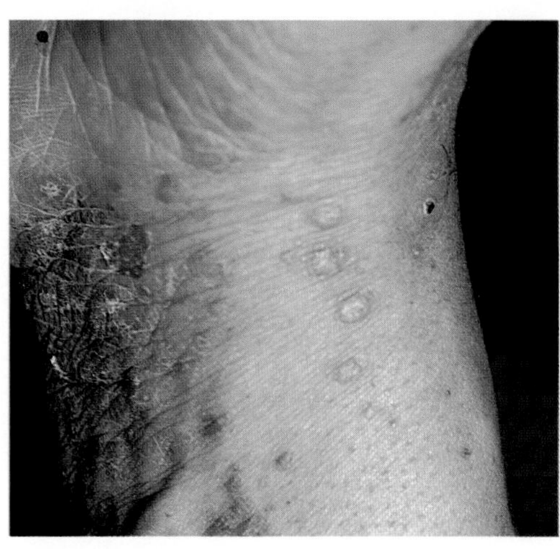

**COLOR PLATE 8. Lichen planus.**

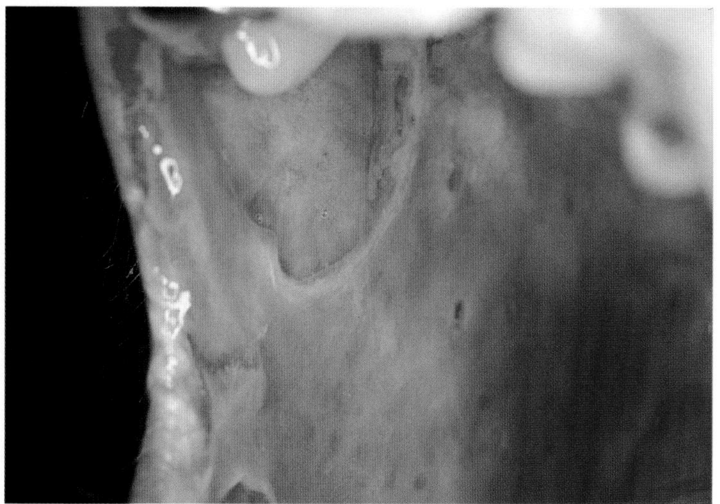

**COLOR PLATE 9. Oral lichen planus.**

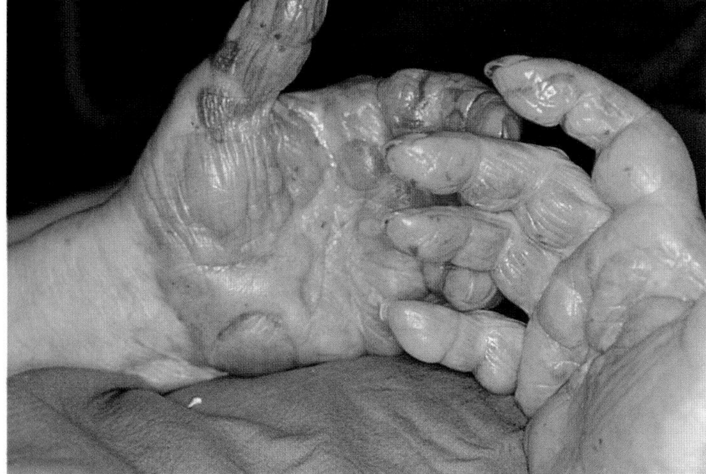

**COLOR PLATE 10. Bullous pemphigoid.** Tense bullae arising on the inflamed skin of the hands of a 74-year-old woman.

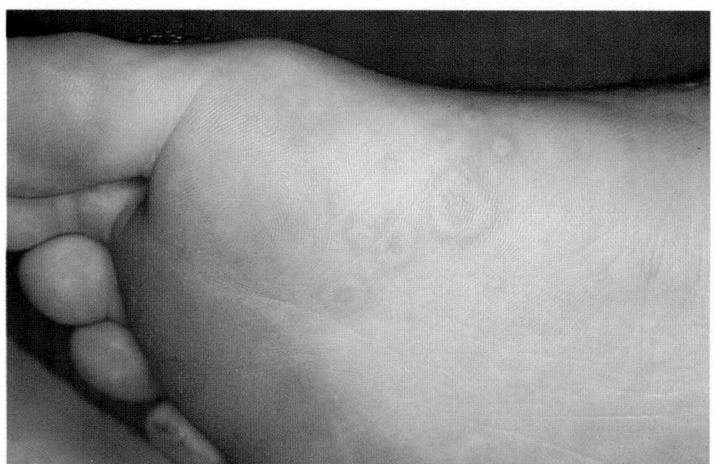

**COLOR PLATE 11. Erythema multiforme.** Typical target lesions are seen on the plantar aspect of the foot.

**COLOR PLATE 12. Vasculitis.** Raised, purpuric lesions are seen in this patient with leukocytoclastic vasculitis secondary to lupus erythematosus.

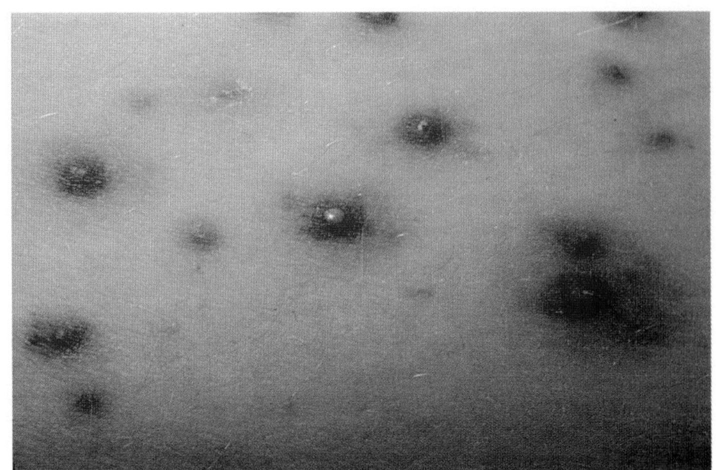

**COLOR PLATE 13. Contact dermatitis secondary to poison ivy.** An acutely inflamed lesion with vesicles in a linear distribution corresponding to contact area with the plant are clues to the correct diagnosis in this patient.

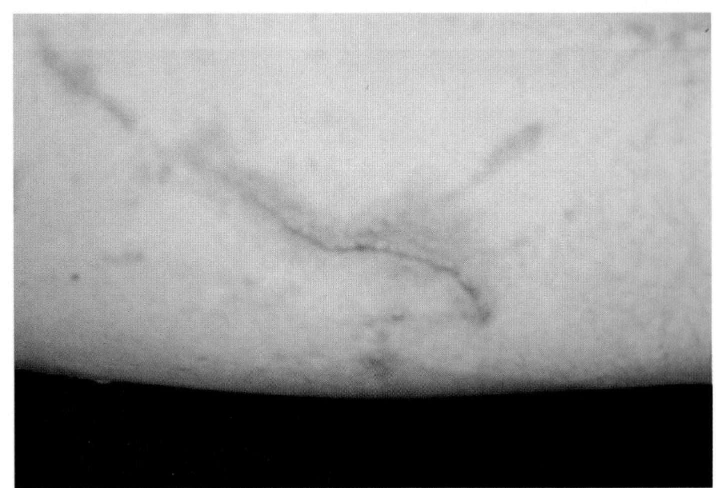

**COLOR PLATE 14. Malignant melanoma, superficial spreading type.**

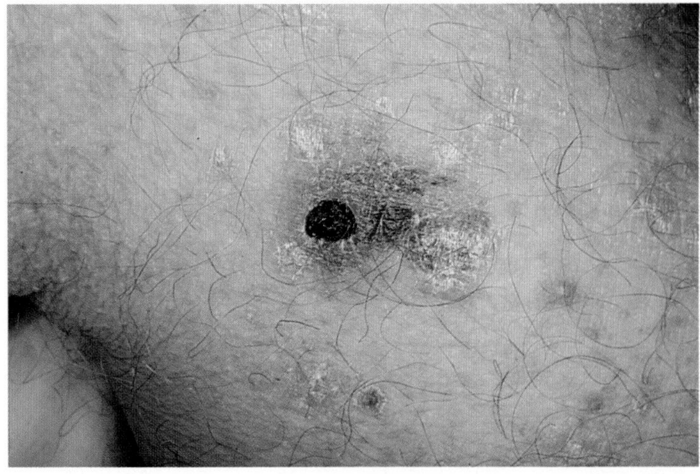

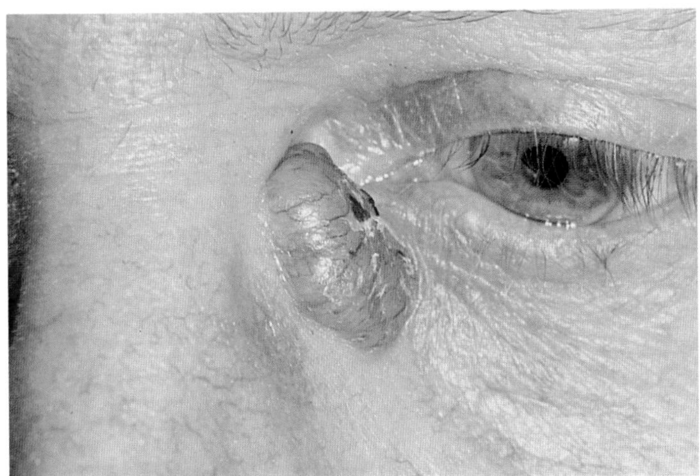

**COLOR PLATE 15. Basal cell carcinoma.** The pearly quality of the lesion, telangiectases, and central ulceration are typical features of basal cell carcinoma of the skin.

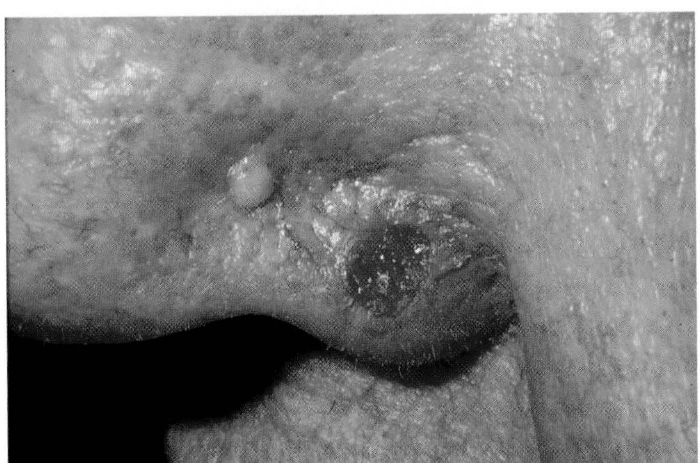

**COLOR PLATE 16. Squamous cell carcinoma.**

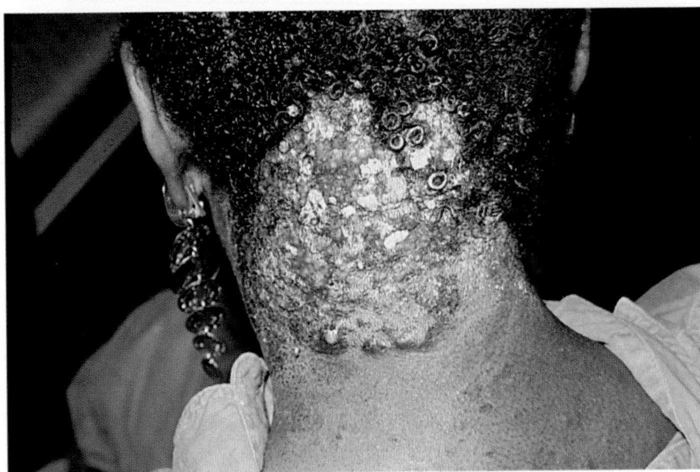

**COLOR PLATE 17. Tinea capitis with kerion formation owing to *Trichophyton tonsurans*.**

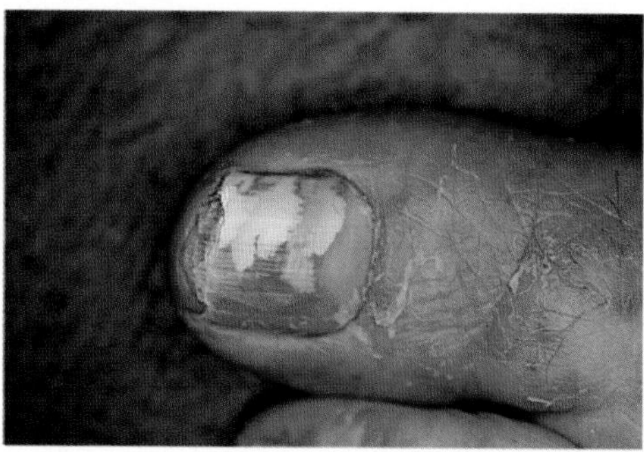

**COLOR PLATE 18. Onychomycosis due to Trichophyton rubrum.** Brownish-white discoloration of the nail plate, with accumulation of subungual debris. The findings can sometimes be difficult to differentiate from those of psoriasis, and a fungal culture may be needed.

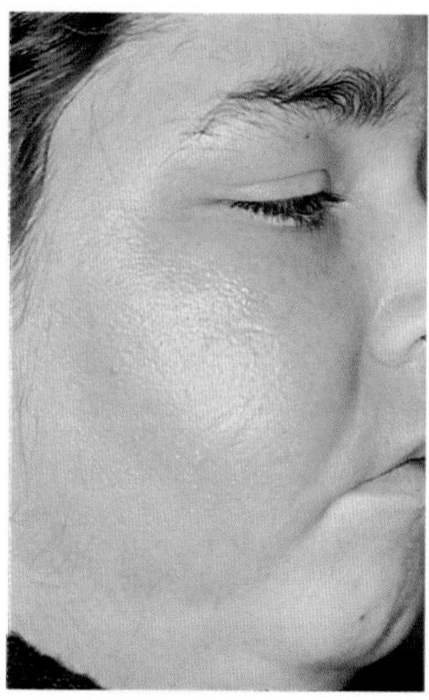

**COLOR PLATE 19. Erysipelas.** Facial cellulitis, with a well-demarcated border, due to group A β-hemolytic streptococci.

**COLOR PLATE 20. Secondary syphilis.** Papulosquamous lesions of secondary syphilis, showing typical involvement of the palms of the hands.

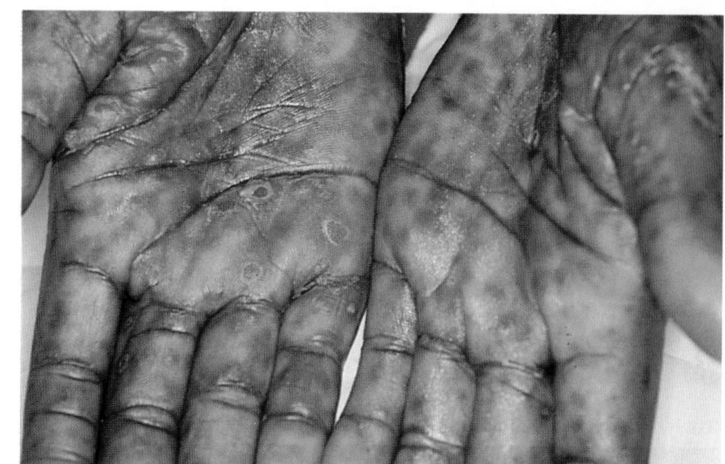

**COLOR PLATE 21. Herpes simplex: Grouped vesicles with surrounding erythema.**

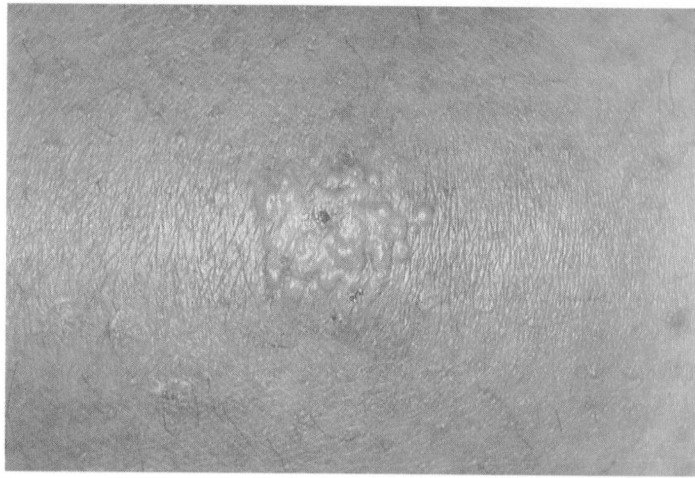

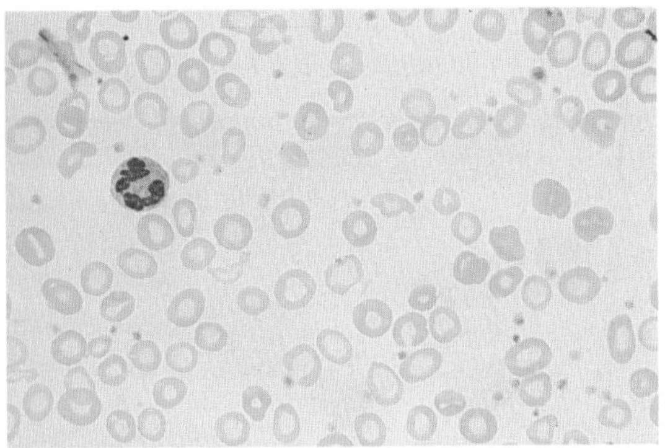

**COLOR PLATE 22.** The peripheral blood smear in iron deficiency anemia.

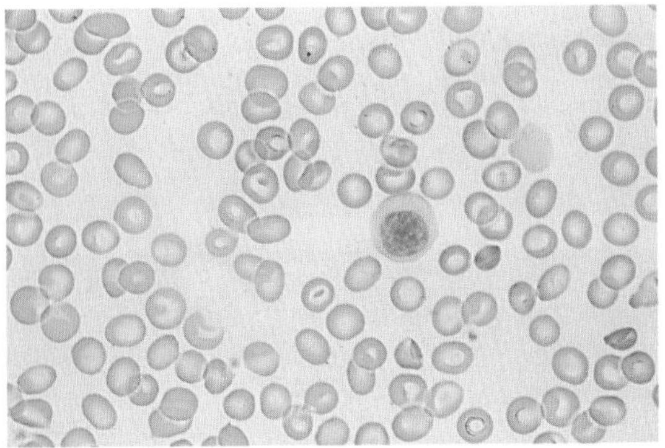

**COLOR PLATE 23.** Ringed sideroblasts.

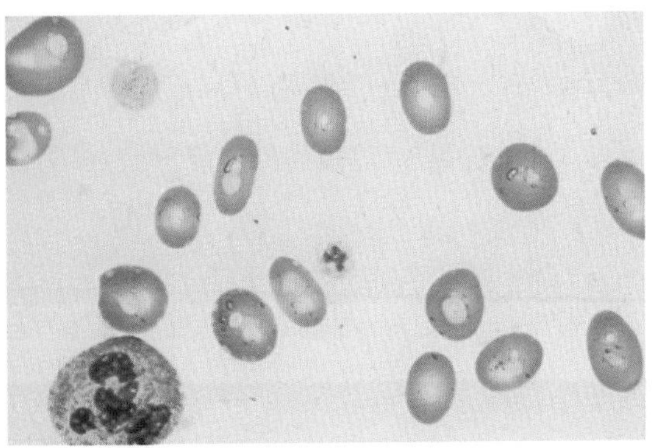

**COLOR PLATE 24.** Pernicious anemia: The PMN has hypersegmented nuclei.

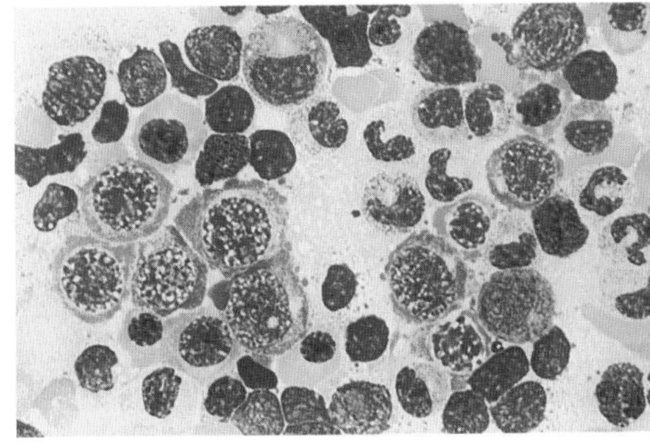

**COLOR PLATE 25.** Bone marrow in $B_{12}$ deficiency showing megaloblasts.

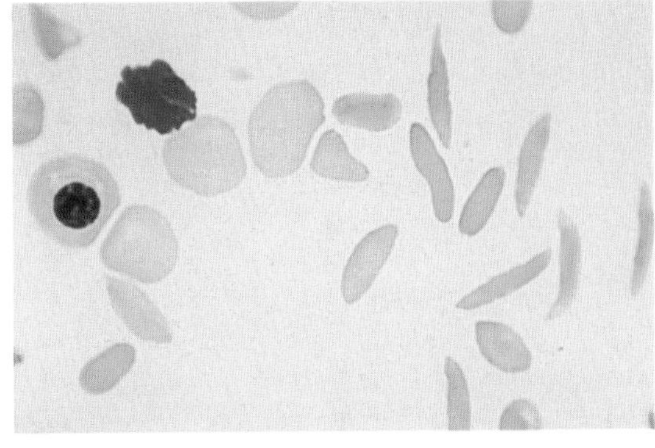

**COLOR PLATE 26.** Sickle cell anemia showing the characteristic sickle cells.

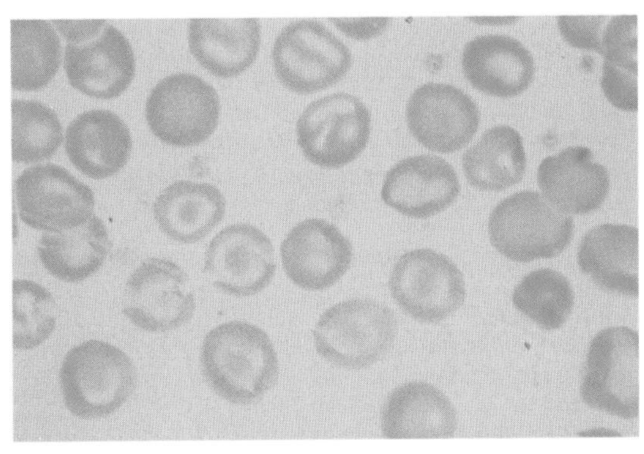

**COLOR PLATE 27.** Hemoglobin C disease: many target cells.

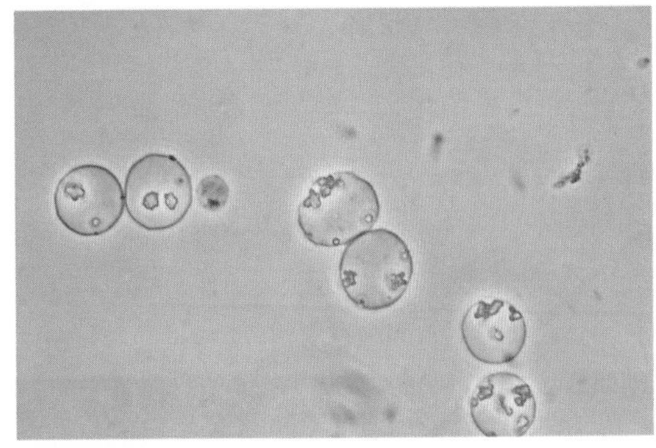

**COLOR PLATE 28.** Heinz bodies.

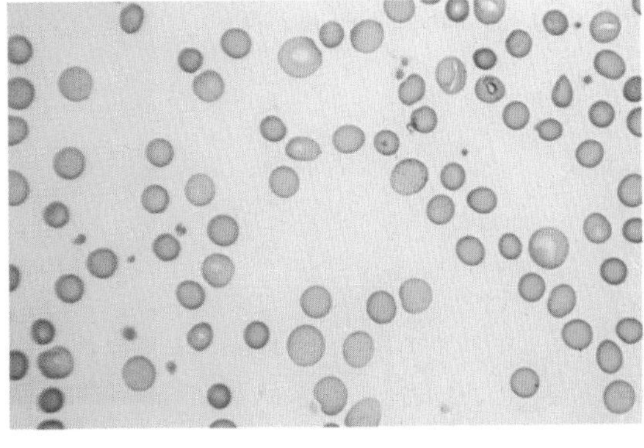

**COLOR PLATE 29.** Peripheral blood smear in auto-immune hemolytic anemia.

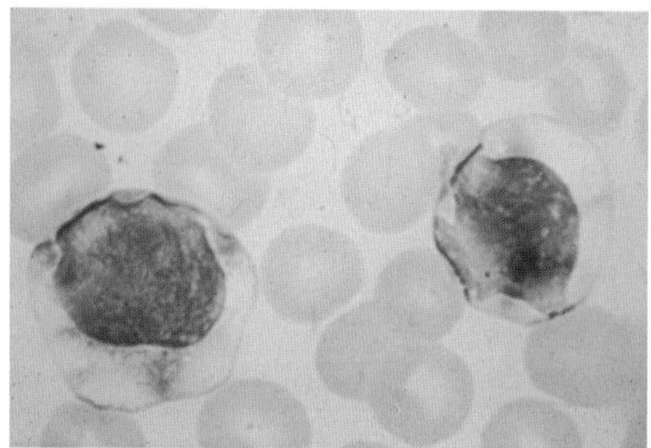

**COLOR PLATE 30.** **Infectious mononucleosis with atypical lymphocytes. Note the delicate cell walls easily indented by the adjacent red cells.**
(Courtesy of Lawrence S. Hurwitz, MD, Milwaukee, Wisconsin.)

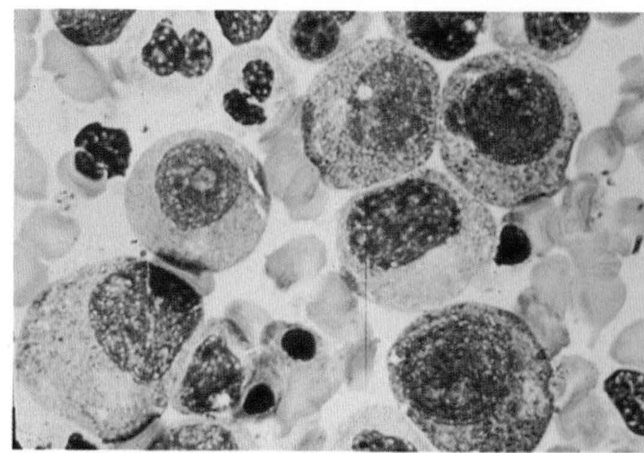

**COLOR PLATE 31.** **Bone marrow examination in acute myelogenous leukemia.**
(Courtesy of Lawrence S. Hurwitz, MD, Milwaukee, Wisconsin.)

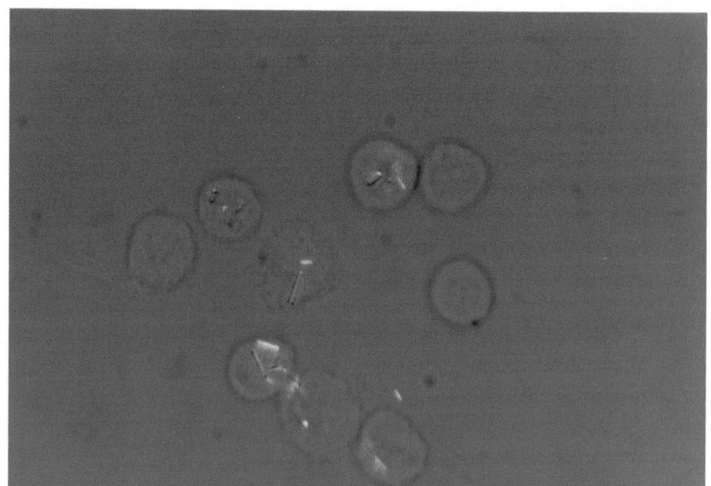

**COLOR PLATE 32.** **Needle-shaped negatively birefringent crystals of monosodium urate in polymorphonuclear leukocytes seen by compensated polarized microscopy.**
(Courtesy of L. Daft, Medical College of Wisconsin, Milwaukee, Wisconsin.)

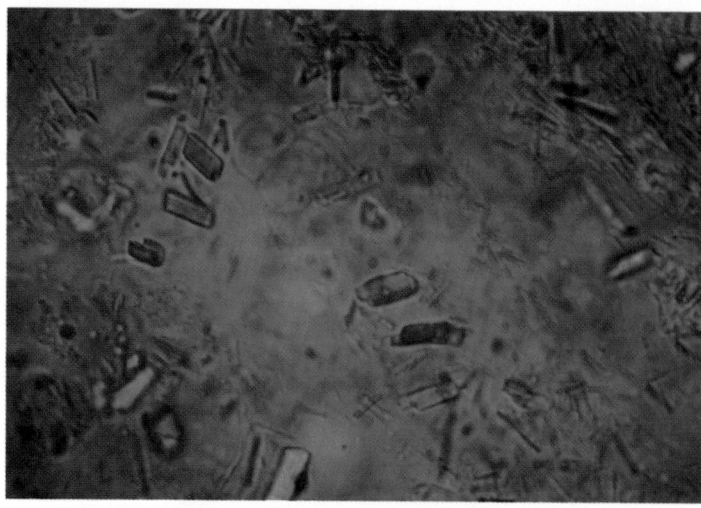

**COLOR PLATE 33.** **Rhomboid-shaped positively birefringent crystals, characteristic of calcium pyrophosphate dihydrate crystals, seen by compensated polarized microscopy. This specimen was obtained from a cartilage deposit of crystals.**
(Courtesy of L. Daft, Medical College of Wisconsin, Milwaukee, Wisconsin.)

perhaps accounting for the lower allergenicity of cephalosporins.

Although patients with rhinitis and asthma are no more likely to have IgE-mediated drug reactions than the general population, they are more likely to have anaphylactoid reactions to contrast dyes, and these reactions are more severe.

Some drug reactions resemble type I reactions, but the mechanism is not clear. Local anesthetics evoke wheal and flare reactions in susceptible persons. Aspirin-sensitive patients, especially those with the aspirin triad (nasal polyps and asthma), can experience asthma attacks, urticaria, or nasal/ocular symptoms. Almost 10% of asthmatics experience worsening airflow after aspirin ingestion, but when asthma is associated with nasal polyps, this incidence increases.

## Clinical Features of Type I Reactions

Reactions can be subdivided by onset as immediate, accelerated, and delayed. *Immediate reactions* (e.g., anaphylaxis or isolated hives) usually occur within 30 minutes. *Accelerated reactions* (usually pruritus only, with or without hives and erythema) occur between 2 hours and 3 days. *Delayed reactions*, which simulate a **morbilliform** (measles-like) **rash,** typically present after 5–10 days of drug use and may not involve IgE antibodies.

The route, rate of administration, and dose play an important role in the clinical presentation. Oral medications are more slowly absorbed than parenteral ones and thus are less likely to elicit serious type I reactions. Minute doses (<1 g) cause partial degranulation with mild to minimal symptoms. This is the principle underlying drug desensitization regimens. Greater exposure may lead to localized hives, pruritus, or cough, usually within minutes. This can be followed by hypotension, gastrointestinal symptoms, and respiratory compromise. Many patients report an eerie sense of impending doom prior to the reactions. Although anaphylactoid reactions also cause symptoms within minutes, warmth or flushing commonly precedes them.

## Diagnosis of Type I Reactions

Drugs that cause allergic reactions are listed in Table 19.4. Diagnosing drug allergy is often a process of deduction in cases in which the patient is using multiple medications. Almost any drug can cause almost any form of reaction, and reactions may occur days, weeks, or even months after initiating use. Skin testing, when available, is the preferred method for diagnosing type I reactions. Ideally, patients with true type I reactions to drugs should be amenable to testing for IgE antibody through skin tests or RAST. Unfortunately, this often is not true for low-molecular-weight drugs. Proteins,

**TABLE 19.4. Common and Uncommon Causes of Allergic Drug Reactions**

| Common (>1%) | Uncommon (<0.1%) |
|---|---|
| Amoxicillin | Potassium chloride |
| Trimethoprim-sulfamethoxazole | Diazepam |
| Ampicillin | Furosemide |
| Whole blood | Tetracycline |
| Cephalosporins | Digoxin |
| Penicillin | Allopurinol |
| Quinidine | Anticoagulants |

such as insulin, being large enough to cross-link IgE, can be used for skin tests. Reagents for penicillin skin testing are available, but not for most other drugs. Skin tests for other agents also are not as reliable as that for penicillin—a possible exception being skin testing for topical anesthetics. Because contrast agents directly degranulate cells, they lack any test; avoidance or premedication are the only ways to reduce the risk of reactions to them. Without reliable skin testing, a presumptive diagnosis is made by history, clinical presentation, onset of reaction, and established knowledge that the suspected drug has evoked allergic reactions. Other clues are prior reactivity to a similar or cross-reacting medication (e.g., sulfonamide-allergic patients using a thiazide diuretic), discontinuation followed by re-exposure to a drug, and rapid improvement when a drug is discontinued.

Pre-Pen™ is commercially available for penicillin testing. This will detect patients with IgE directed against the major determinant but will miss those (about 10%) who are allergic only to the minor determinants—an unfortunate omission, because patients who make IgE to minor determinants more often have severe anaphylactic reactions to penicillin. The likelihood of missing minor-determinant sensitivity can be minimized by prick testing with 100,000 U/ml penicillin G and intradermal tests with 1000 U/ml. However, testing with preparations of minor determinant mixes, which are usually available at referral centers, is preferable. Patients without prior histories of penicillin reaction have a 1–2% chance of a systemic IgE-mediated reaction, which increases to 5–20% in those with prior histories and 40% in those with prior histories of severe anaphylaxis. When a skin test is performed using both Pre-Pen™ and a minor determinant, the result is positive in 2% of patients without positive histories. Those with negative skin tests and positive histories have only a 2% risk of an IgE-mediated reaction, and such reactions usually are mild (pruritus with or without urticaria). However, a positive skin test and positive history increase the risk of a serious reaction to 50–70%.

Most reactions to topical anesthetics are vasovagal, toxic, or trauma-related. Group I local anesthetics are *p*-amino benzoic derivatives and include procaine benzocaine. IgE against these can cross-react with paraben preservatives, which are commonly found in lotions and some injectable medications. Group II includes lidocaine and mepivacaine. Cross-reactivity is rare between groups I and II. Skin testing is conducted with anesthetics lacking preservatives or epinephrine to provide a less ambiguous study. When a positive skin test is found, patients frequently have a negative test for an appropriate substitute.

### Management of Type I Reactions

Mild to moderate reactions (pruritus with or without urticaria) can be treated symptomatically with antihistamines such as hydroxyzine (25 mg every 8 hours) or cetirizine (10 mg, once daily). When possible, the drug should be discontinued. The patient is watched closely for development of **erythema multiforme major** (Stevens-Johnson syndrome) or serum sickness. More serious anaphylactoid or anaphylactic reactions should be treated as outlined in Chapter 18.

Avoidance is the best therapy. In most cases of infection, other classes of antibiotics can be used. Patients with penicillin sensitivity are much more likely than the general population to have a reaction to cephalosporins; thus, cephalosporins should be avoided as a substitute for penicillin, especially if the prior reaction was systemic. Aztreonam, a monobactam, reportedly has little or no cross-reactivity with penicillin. When penicillin or a related β lactam antibiotic is clearly indicated in an allergic patient (e.g., endocarditis, syphilis with pregnancy, or listeria meningitis), skin testing should precede administration of the drug. Patients with positive histamine tests and negative penicillin tests are able to use β lactam antibiotics, although many physicians will first administer a test dose of 1/1000 the therapeutic dose to confirm safety. If pruritus or mild urticaria develops, an antihistamine such as diphenhydramine or hydroxyzine can be given. Patients with positive skin testing to penicillin require desensitization, but only if, after reconsideration, the need to give the drug still clearly outweighs the risk. Desensitization should be performed in an intensive care unit with careful monitoring and epinephrine at bedside. Similar desensitizations can be carried out for other drugs, such as sulfa drugs or insulin.

Insulin allergy, although fairly common, is almost always mild and transient. Immune responses to insulin can include IgE-mediated local reactions with swelling and itching or more severe generalized pruritus and urticaria. Patients sensitized to beef or pork insulin can display cross-reactive IgE to recombinant human insulin also. Desensitization is not useful for contrast media. These patients have a 30% risk for recurrent reactions. When diagnostic procedures with these agents are necessary, the risk for reaction can be reduced by using newer nonionic agents and premedicating patients.

## Type II Reactions

The classic type II reaction is an ABO transfusion mismatch. Low-molecular-weight drugs also may evoke such reactions and, depending on the location in which the drug settles, cause hemolysis or organ damage. Penicillin can coat red cells or platelets, and **thrombocytopenia** or hemolysis results when IgG or IgM antipenicillin antibodies attach to cells with fixation of complement. Type II hematologic reactions also may result from phenacetin, quinidine, heparin, and sulfonamides. Methyldopa may induce red cells to express new antigens that bind cytotoxic antibody and cause hemolysis. Interstitial nephritis may follow nafcillin and phenytoin-induced linear antibody and complement deposition on the renal tubular basement membrane. History and evidence of antibody deposition on red cells (direct Coombs test) or in affected organs are key to diagnosing these reactions. Stopping the drug is essential; corticosteroids are not always beneficial.

## Type III Reactions

A type III reaction (also called serum sickness) involves immune complex deposition, complement fixation, and vasculitis. Such reactions may follow use of antithymocyte globulin, penicillin, and hydralazine. Cutaneous symptoms often begin with erythema around the sides of the fingers, palms, and feet. Drug-induced hypersensitivity angiitis, most often caused by sulfonamides, can also affect the kidneys and lungs. Propylthiouracil can induce vasculitis initially involving the face and ear lobes. Biopsy of affected skin shows fibrinoid necrosis of small, dermal vessels with polymorphonuclear infiltration and C3 and IgM deposition on direct immunofluorescent staining.

Pruritus generally responds to antihistamines, which may, theoretically, reduce vascular changes and immune complex deposition. Gradual spontaneous improvement occurs over 7–14 days, although corticosteroids may hasten recovery.

## Type IV Reactions

Type IV reactions follow the topical use of drugs such as topical anesthetics or coingredients such as methylparaben and ethylenediamine. Oral medications rarely cause a diffuse eczematoid response. A photosensitive cutaneous rash, which characteristically occurs in sun-exposed areas, may follow oral or parenteral use of tetracyclines. A fibrotic lung reaction may follow nitrofurantoin. A component of type IV hypersensitivity has been alleged in some cases of drug-induced interstitial nephritis or hepatitis. In **fixed drug eruption,** a probable example of type IV sensitivity, a delayed, localized pruritic rash occurs in the same location on the skin each time certain drugs are systemically used.

These rashes usually abate spontaneously with the cessation of the drug or the offending agent. Antihistamines may allay pruritus. Topical corticosteroids may ease symptoms, but application over a large area requires care.

# CHAPTER 20 URTICARIA AND ANGIOEDEMA

Urticaria (hives), a symptom complex arising from a variety of causes, consists of raised, usually pruritic cutaneous lesions that vary in size from several millimeters to several centimeters. The term is from the *Urtica urens* nettle, which causes stinging and itching. Key categories of urticaria are listed in Table 20.1.

## Urticaria

### Epidemiology and Etiology

Urticaria can occur at any age, but is most frequent in young adults. Nearly 15% of the general population has had at least one bout of urticaria at some time, and on any given day, 1 of every 1000 people experience it. Patients can have isolated urticaria or urticaria with coexisting angioedema (see the second portions of this chapter). Urticaria will spontaneously resolve within 6 months in most patients. Causes of urticaria are listed in Table 20.1. Because urticaria usually occurs within 30–90 minutes of exposure, many patients are able to associate the onset of urticaria with these exposures and thus limit the duration of the urticaria. Use of a food-and-activity diary is sometimes helpful in determining when the urticaria is delayed in onset. Chronic urticaria (by definition, occurring for more than 6 weeks) is more of a diagnostic challenge, and in 80% of patients, the cause is never clearly established.

### Pathology

Approximately 2–3% of patients will have evidence for leukocytoclastic vasculitis in biopsy specimens, including immunoglobulin and complement deposition in vascular walls. Rarely, in physical urticaria (e.g., delayed pressure urticaria), a polymorphonuclear infil-

**TABLE 20.1. Key Categories of Urticaria**

| Type | Clinical Considerations |
|---|---|
| Acute (<6 weeks) | |
| Etiology known | Bacterial or viral infections.<br>Ingestion of foods or drugs.<br>Topical exposure (soaps, shampoos, detergents, and lotions).<br>Occasionally aeroallergens. |
| Etiology unknown | Idiopathic. |
| Chronic (>6 weeks) | |
| Nonphysical | |
| Underlying disease | Examples: bacterial infection, thyroid disease, parasitic infestation, hepatitis, autoimmune—usually typical hives, but persist >24 hours with autoimmune. |
| Contact urticaria | Due to contact with IgE-mediated allergen (e.g., cat saliva). |
| Cholinergic | Coalescing papular due to cholinergic nerve activation with heating. |
| Adrenergic | Papular-like cholinergic, but with white zones around wheal, provoked with stress. |
| Physical | |
| Dermatographism | Streaks of wheal and flare due to mechanical trauma, often excoriated. |
| Pressure urticaria | Immediate, <30 minutes, or delayed; burning wheals for immediate; induration for delayed at sites of pressure. |
| Cold | Induration at cold exposed sites. |
| Vibratory | Urticaria (or angioedema in hands or feet) due to vibratory stimuli. |
| Aquagenic | Due to tepid water exposure. |
| Solar | Sun-exposed areas, depends on wave length. |

TABLE 20.2. Clinical Diagnosis and Treatment of Common Chronic Urticarias

| Classification | Diagnosis | First-line Treatment |
|---|---|---|
| Nonphysical | | |
| Bacterial infection | CBC and differential, sedimentation rate, chest x-ray, sinus x-rays as appropriate. | Appropriate antibiotic. |
| Contact urticaria | Prick skin test to confirm IgE antibodies. | Avoidance, careful washing after contact, possibly allergy immunotherapy. |
| Cholinergic | Typical rash, occurs with body warming, methacholine skin test positive in <50% of cases. | Antihistamines with anticholinergic properties (e.g., doxepin 10 mg 1–3 times per day); gradual warm-up and cool-down with exercise. |
| Physical | | |
| Dermatographism | Lightly stroke with broken tongue blade to produce linear wheals. | Daily antihistamine (e.g., loratadine, fexofenadine, or cetirizine). |
| Pressure | Apply 15 pounds to 1 square inch area for 10–15 minutes. | Prophylactic antihistamine for immediate type; colchicine or nonsteroidal anti-inflammatory agents for delayed type. |
| Cold | Apply plastic-wrapped ice cube to skin for 5 minutes, remove and observe for induration for 10 minutes. | Warm garments, cyproheptadine, or doxepin prior to exposure. |
| Vibratory | Place extremity on vortexer or reproduce exposure for 5–10 minutes. | Avoidance, antihistamine prior to exposure. |

trate can be seen. Mast cell degranulation is considered central to most urticarias. Histamine release has been shown both in locally draining veins in several forms of urticaria and in biopsy specimens of cold urticaria (urticaria brought on by exposure to cold). Some afferent nerve fibers in the skin release substance P, a neuropeptide that can degranulate mast cells. Histamine from mast cells activates these afferent fibers, causing the release of additional substance P in a feed-forward amplification reaction.

Mediators not associated with mast cell activation also are important in urticaria. Many antihistamines can act as serotonin antagonists, and those most useful for cold urticaria are potent serotonin antagonists. Patients with cholinergic urticaria (prickly heat) may have an abnormality of acetylcholine release from nerves in the skin. Intradermal injection of methacholine causes abnormal wheal responses in one third to one half of these patients. Interestingly, many of the effective antihistamines also have anticholinergic activity.

Some patients with chronic urticaria produce autoantibodies against the IgE high-affinity receptor. Excess cutaneous blood flow or vascular leakage might exacerbate urticaria in these patients, thus explaining how vasodilators such as alcohol and heat or factors that increase cardiac output such as hyperthyroidism and stress occasionally precipitate urticaria. The C1q complement component has amino acid homology with collagen, and, in some patients with collagen vascular disease and autoantibodies against C1q, hypocomplementemic urticarial vasculitis may develop.

## Clinical Features

The clinical presentation (Table 20.2) depends on the form of urticaria and its cause. Although it has many alleged precipitants, it is frequently spontaneous. *Typical urticaria* is one to several centimeters in size, circular, and pruritic. The lesions blanch and resolve within 6 hours. Lesions that do not blanch and take more than a day to resolve, or that leave bruising, should be considered atypical and make an underlying vasculitis suspect. *Cholinergic urticaria* consists of 2–3-mm red papules that coalesce into large areas and follows warming of the corresponding body area. If the core body temperature is raised 1°C, more generalized constitutional symptoms such as hypotension and wheezing can occur. Physical urticarias are fairly rare and can be brought on by exposure to vibration, pressure, or certain ultraviolet wavelengths. For some of these forms, urticaria is a misnomer because the lesions swell and burn, and rarely can fever and arthralgias coexist.

Urticarias caused by an underlying primary disorder reflect the symptoms of the primary condition, such as weight loss and fatigue (hyperthyroidism); weight loss, fatigue, and fever (malignancies or infection); hair loss, Raynaud phenomenon and arthralgias (systemic lupus erythematosus); or anorexia and high-colored (dark) urine (hepatitis).

## Diagnosis

The history and physical findings are the most helpful elements of the work-up and are usually sufficient for diagnosis. Extensive laboratory studies are not helpful. If chronic urticaria is not easily controlled with nonsedating antihistamines, a CBC, differential count, and sedimentation rate are appropriate studies. In suspected vasculitis—particularly with constitutional symptoms such as arthralgias or fatigue—antinuclear antibodies, urinalysis, C3, C4, and $CH_{50}$ are warranted. Poor response to therapy or abnormal laboratory tests suggest the need for skin biopsy to check for **urticarial vasculitis.** Exercise anaphylaxis occurs only with exercise, in contrast to cholinergic urticaria. Given the occasional association of urticaria with hyperthyroidism, the thyroid-stimulating hormone level should be checked. In women with postpartum urticaria, postpartum hyperthyroidism should be excluded. Recent travel or gastrointestinal symptoms should prompt stool examination for ova and parasites. Chest radiograph, liver function tests, stool test for occult blood, cryoglobulin, and cryofibrinogen tests are occasionally helpful.

Several illnesses may mimic urticaria. *Erythema chronicum migrans* in Lyme disease may be mistaken for urticaria. In systemic mastocytosis, urticaria may be associated with hypotension, gastrointestinal symptoms, stomach ulcers, and flushing. In *urticaria pigmentosa*, the skin often has hyperpigmented lesions, and stroking it causes **Darier sign**—linear wheals with larger beady hives. In ***dermatographism,*** a benign condition, figures can be drawn (urticaria with whealing) on the skin by lightly stroking with a sharp object. Patients often have linear wheals with flare owing to scratching. Although pruritic, these lesions usually do not occur spontaneously. *Papular urticaria* consists of crops of small pruritic papules, usually near the ankles and wrists and caused by local reactions to insect bites, especially fleas. *Erythema multiforme* is often associated with bacterial or viral infections and can present with mucus membrane lesions and cutaneous "iris" lesions. These have pale centers with erythematous rims.

## Management

Urticaria is typically episodic and mostly self-limited. Although uncomfortable, urticaria without associated angioedema is rarely life-threatening. A stepwise treatment plan with the fewest adverse reactions should be adopted (Figure 20.1). In cases in which a stimulus can be identified, avoidance is the first choice. Drugs that immunologically cross-react with offending agents (such as cephalosporins in β lactam allergy) or ones with similar mechanisms of action (such as NSAIDs) should be avoided. Physical urticarias can be improved by prudent measures such as using sunblock and wearing protective clothing for solar urticaria, gradual warming of oneself with tepid showers or mild warm-up sessions for cholinergic urticaria, avoiding sudden cold exposure or ice-cold foods and liquids for cold urticaria, and so on. Patients with cold urticaria should be warned not to jump into cool lakes or swimming pools; they also need special premedication when undergoing surgery for coronary artery bypass grafts, because ice-cold saline is used to produce cardioplegia.

The mainstay of drug therapy for the urticarias has been antihistamines. Those with significant anticholinergic or antiserotoninergic effects often have worked best in the past. The newer, nonsedating antihistamines such as cetirizine and fexofenadine work well in mild, uncomplicated urticaria or dermatographism. Some studies suggest that a combination of hydroxyzine plus cyproheptadine is more effective than either drug alone, but cyproheptadine can be very sedating and promotes weight gain. Occasionally, a combination of an H1 antagonist plus an H2 blocker such as cimetidine, 300 mg twice daily, will work better than H1 inhibition alone. One of the most potent antihistamines is doxepin, which is a tricyclic antidepressant with antiserotoninergic, anticholinergic, and H2 blocking effects. Because its H1 inhibition is 1000 times that of diphenhydramine (Benadryl™), relatively low starting doses of 10 mg at bedtime or twice per day can be used.

Although most patients respond well to antihistamines, 10–20% may not. Frequently, a short course of oral corticosteroids will help break the cycle of recurrent hives, and antihistamines often then will suffice to maintain the patients symptom-free. When urticaria persists, the physician must weigh the morbidity of the urticaria against potential side effects of corticosteroids. If corticosteroid maintenance is required, the lowest possible dose should be given. Corticosteroid-dependent patients may be able to taper or stop the steroid dose when stanozolol (an anabolic steroid with potential androgenergic side effects) is added. Anecdotally, colchicine, calcium channel blockers, and oral β adrenergic agonists are occasionally successful.

Aside from avoidance, the physical urticarias are treated similarly to common urticaria. All urticaria patients should be advised to contact their physicians if they experience angioedema.

# Angioedema

Angioedema presents as indurated areas of swelling that often feel numb or burn. Occurring most often in areas of loose tissue, such as the lips and eyelids, angioedema histologically resembles typical urticaria, but the edema and vasodilatation occur deeper in the subcutaneous tissue where few afferent nerve endings

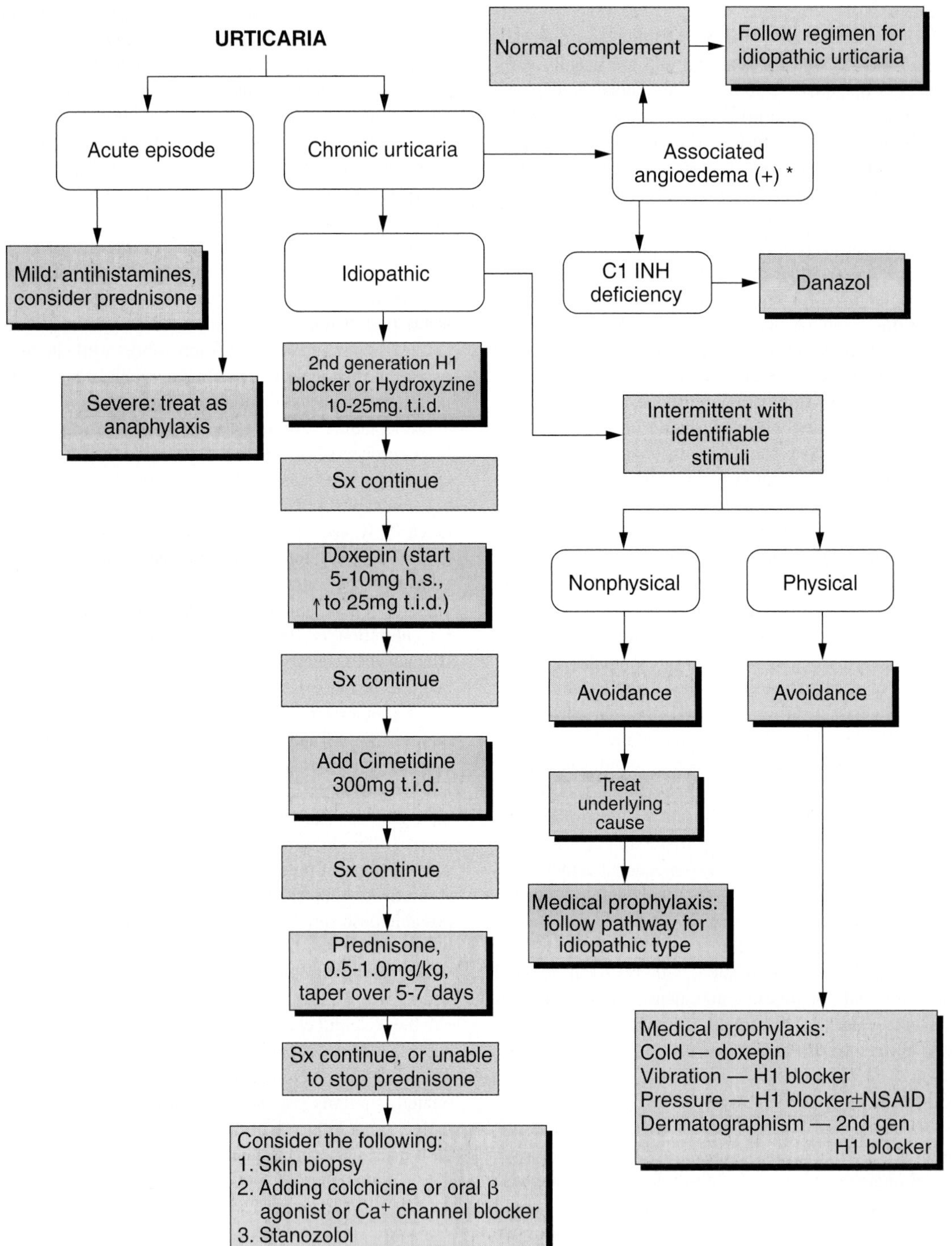


**FIGURE 20.1.** Treatment of urticaria. For mild episodes less frequent than once per week, treatment may be given as needed; for more frequent episodes, preventive treatment is needed.

*Patients with associated angioedema also should be evaluated for a complement disorder and treated more aggressively with prophylactic medications outlined in the idiopathic column.

exist. Urticaria may be associated in about 80–90% of cases. The cause may mimic that of urticaria, but several other causes should be considered for isolated angioedema. ACE inhibitors can cause angioedema alone, and this can occur months after starting the drug. ACE inhibitors may permit activation of the bradykinin system.

Life-threatening, isolated angioedema can also be caused by C1 INH deficiency, which can be genetic or acquired. The genetic form, also termed **hereditary angioedema,** presents during the teen years, but can occur at any age. A history of trauma may be present. Most patients have low levels of C1 INH, usually attributable to reduced transcription of the gene, but in 15% of patients the levels are normal and consist of poorly functioning protein. The acquired form is associated with malignancies or autoimmune diseases. These patients make autoantibodies, which can either accelerate the breakdown of C1 INH or directly bind to it and cause its removal. Both the genetic and acquired forms have low functional amounts of C1 INH and low C4 levels, but patients with the acquired form also have low serum C1 levels.

Angioedema in the gastrointestinal tract or larynx evokes nausea, cramping, or throat tightness. Its potential for laryngeal involvement makes it a more serious issue than isolated urticaria. Although nearly all of the fatalities occurred in patients with isolated angioedema from C1 INH deficiency, all urticaria patients should be questioned carefully for any history of tongue or lip swelling, throat discomfort, or gastrointestinal symptoms. If such symptoms are present, the patient should be instructed in self-administration of epinephrine and provided with a self-administration kit (EpiPen™ or Anakit™). These patients also may be more aggressively treated with potent antihistamines such as doxepin. Patients with C1 INH deficiency are successfully treated with danazol or stanozolol. Virilization (severe masculine somatic characteristics) is a problem with stanozolol.

During acute attacks, especially with impending respiratory compromise, adults should be given 0.3 ml of 1:1000 epinephrine subcutaneously and sent immediately by ambulance to the nearest emergency facility. Injection can be repeated after 15 minutes. The protective effects of epinephrine can wear off in 15–20 minutes; a tapering course of corticosteroids and an additional dose of antihistamine should be started within this time. Epinephrine is not always effective in C1 INH deficiency. Fresh frozen plasma to replace the C1 INH may be used, but it also supplies substrate for activated complement and bradykinins. These patients may require intubation or tracheostomy for respiratory impairment.

# CHAPTER 21 IMMUNODEFICIENCY

Host defenses against microbes and the various deficiencies thereof that predispose to infection are discussed in Chapter 148. This chapter discusses the adult immunodeficiency disorders other than acquired immune deficiency syndrome (AIDS). Despite their relative rarity in adults, these other immunodeficiencies deserve attention because appropriate intervention can limit the potentially serious infectious complications.

Although the immune system can be divided into the *humoral* (antibodies and complement) and *cellular* [T cells, natural killer (NK) cells, macrophages, and neutrophils] components, interplay between these two groups (as in T cell cytokine production to promote B cell antibody production) is very important. Patients with humoral deficiencies suffer recurrent infections with encapsulated bacteria and occasionally enteric viruses and *Giardia*, whereas with T cell defects and normal humoral immunity, recurrent infections with *Pneumocystis carinii,* fungi, viruses, and mycobacteria predominate. (See Tables 21.1 and Table 21.2.)

## Humoral Defects

Defects in humoral response can occur because of a lack of production or inadequate production/dysfunction of antibodies, and antibody consumption.

### Lack of antibody production

This was first described in **X-linked hypogammaglobulinemia.** The immature B cells in affected boys produce only very small quantities of all the immunoglobulins. Resistance to fungi, mycobacteria, most viruses, and parasites is generally adequate, but enteroviral and *Giardia* infections can occur. Although all classes of immunoglobulins are lacking in **common variable immunodeficiency** (CVI), an idiopathic disorder, the infectious complications are not as severe as in X-linked hypogammaglobulinemia. In CVI, antibody production is normal in childhood, but the disease manifests in adults of either gender. Usual initial features are recurrent sinusitis and respiratory infections. Because antibody deficiency impairs the ability to fight encapsulated bacteria (pneumococcus and *Haemophilus influenzae*), it

**TABLE 21.1. Representative Features of Cellular and Humoral Immunodeficiency**

| Type | Clinical Features | Initial Diagnostic Tests |
|---|---|---|
| Cellular | | |
| Neutrophils | Recurrent pyodermic cutaneous infections, especially staphylococcus. | CBC with differential, nitroblue tetrazolium reduction. |
| T-lymphocytes | Opportunistic infections (mycobacterial, fungal, pneumocystis). | Delayed hypersensitivity skin tests (mumps, *Candida*, trichophyton), lymphocyte count, possibly helper/suppressor (CD4/CD8) enumeration by flow cytometry. |
| Humoral | | |
| B cell/ Immunoglobulin | Recurrent infections with encapsulated bacterial organisms resulting in pneumonia, sinusitis, otitis. May have chronic diarrhea due to *Giardia lamblia*. | Lymphocyte count, quantitative IgG, IgA, and IgM and pre-existing antibody titers to tetanus, rubella, *H. influenzae*. If normal but high suspicion, check IgG subclasses and response to pneumococcal and *H. influenzae* immunization. |
| Complement | Infections with encapsulated bacteria, especially *Neisseria*. Possible collagen-vascular symptoms. | CH50, C3, C4 |
| Secondary | May be due to underlying illness such as diabetes mellitus, nephrotic syndrome, drug effect, or absent spleen. | Appropriate screening test such as glucose, urine for protein. |

**TABLE 21.2. Immunodeficiency Treatment**

| Deficiency | Treatment |
|---|---|
| General | Maintain good nutrition; treat any underlying illness; avoid live virus vaccines; treat acute infections rapidly with appropriate antibiotic. |
| Chronic granulomatous disease | Possible prophylaxis with antistaphylococcal antibiotic. Interferon-$\gamma$-1b (Actimmune) may be beneficial. |
| T lymphocytes | If due to genetic defect, may be appropriate for transplantation; patients with adenosine deaminase (ADA) deficiency may benefit from ADA-polyethylene glycol replacement, gene therapy, or bone marrow transplant. |
| Complement | Immunize against *H. influenzae* and pneumococci to boost antibody protection; may require daily prophylactic antibiotic on rotating schedule (such as alternating sulfonamide, clarithromycin, amoxicillin-clavulanate every 2 months). |
| Immunoglobulin | For subclass deficiency, prophylactic antibiotic such as for complement may suffice; for common variable, may require IVIG replacement; start at 300–400 mg/kg/month, adjust dose subsequently to maintain 4-week trough at ≥400 mg/day. |

should be suspected in any adult with two or more proven pneumonias in a year. Chronic diarrhea is common, caused by *Giardia lamblia, Campylobacter,* or nodular lymphoid hyperplasia with features that mimic sprue. Pernicious anemia, hypothyroidism, and hemolytic anemia may coexist.

Most patients with CVI have normal peripheral B cell numbers but no plasma cells in their bone marrow; however, B cells or T cells may be defective. In some, B cells do not respond to T cell cytokines; in others, B cells produce but cannot secrete antibody. Defective TH cell activity may create vulnerability to mycobacterial and fungal infections. The risk for gastrointestinal malignancies and lymphoma is greatly (100 times) enhanced, necessitating close follow-up of these patients.

#### Inadequate antibody production

Among the four subclasses of IgG antibodies, $IgG_1$ is the most plentiful; failure to produce $IgG_1$ leads to a low total IgG level. However, patients with isolated $IgG_2$ or $IgG_3$ deficiencies may have low–normal total IgG. $IgG_1$ and $IgG_3$ preferentially bind proteins, and $IgG_2$ and $IgG_4$ recognize carbohydrate antigens. $IgG_4$ levels are naturally quite low, and its value in host resistance is unclear. Although an abnormally low IgG subclass level may cause recurrent infection, immunodeficiency should be confirmed by measuring a patient's response to immunization. Thus, baseline titers to *Haemophilus influenzae* B, pneumococci, and tetanus toxoid should be measured and retested several weeks after immunization.

IgA deficiency (<5 mg/dl) is fairly common (1 : 500–600 adults), but it does not always cause disease. Phenytoin, carbamazepine, *d*-penicillamine, sulfasalazine, and chloroquine can induce reversible IgA deficiency. Some patients with recurrent respiratory infections have coexisting IgG subclass deficiencies or poor IgG antibody response to immunization.

**Antibody consumption**

Patients with protein-losing enteropathies or the nephrotic syndrome can lose antibody in sufficient amounts to impair immunity. Typically presenting with edema and low-serum albumin, these patients can develop recurrent respiratory infections with pyogenic organisms.

## Complement Deficiency

The complement system amplifies immune response by helping lyse antibody-bound bacteria or by coating pathogens (opsonization), allowing their clearance by phagocytic cells and the reticuloendothelial system. Resistance to some bacteria, particularly encapsulated ones, is defective in complement deficiency. Susceptibility to **Neisserial infections** (e.g., meningococci) is especially enhanced in terminal complement component deficiency. Although the $CH_{50}$ can screen for complement dysfunction, C3 and C4 measurement can indicate affected pathways.

## Cellular Responses

Immune dysfunction can follow altered activity of any of the cell types (T cell, macrophage, neutrophil, or NK) that provide cellular protection, although the most common natural abnormalities are associated with T cell dysfunction. **NK** cells have a low-affinity IgG receptor that allows them to bind antibody-coated cells and participate in antibody-directed cytotoxicity. They also may provide natural resistance to virally infected cells. Altered NK activity may predispose persons to recurrent herpes virus infections. The T cell is critical in amplifying immune surveillance. T cell defects are frequently associated with other abnormalities and defective antibody responses. TH cells (CD4+) recognize antigen presented by APCs and subsequently secrete cytokines in the proximity of B cells that have bound this antigen to positively select those cells and magnify the immune response. $TH_1$ cells further augment the immune response against viruses by producing IFN-$\gamma$. T suppressor cells (CD8+) carry out antibody-directed lysis of virally infected cells and tumor cells and also suppress abnormal autoimmune responses. Infants lack functional T cells because of absent thymic precursor tissue in **DiGeorge syndrome;** they suffer recurrent *Candida* and viral infections.

The macrophage, with its receptors for immunoglobulin and complement, is important for clearing antibody-coated or complement-coated pathogens. Alcoholics with cirrhosis have defective macrophage IgG receptor processing, and life-threatening bacterial infections are most likely to occur in those with the most severely impaired immunoglobulin handling. Defects or loss of the macrophage could impair one's ability to recognize foreign pathogens and mount a response. Asplenic patients (surgical splenectomy or autosplenectomy from sickle cell disease) also lack activated macrophages and are prone to sepsis from encapsulated bacteria.

The neutrophil is usually the first cell to migrate to a site of pathogen invasion. Neutrophils accumulate in response to local trauma and on a true immunologic basis. Once neutrophils arrive at sites of infection, they provide protection by phagocytosis and killing by the production of hydrogen peroxide in their granules. If neutrophils have defective phagocytosis or lack the ability to produce hydrogen peroxide, affected individuals experience chronic granulomatous disease manifested by recurrent infections with gram-positive and gram-negative bacteria, usually involving skin, mucous membranes, and the respiratory tract.

## Diagnosis

The more severe immunodeficiency states (e.g., severe combined, Wiskott-Aldrich, hyper-IgE syndrome) are diagnosed in infancy or early childhood. In others, a high index of suspicion and thorough medical history are very important. Chronic diarrhea, recurrent sinusitis or pneumonia, recurrent infections, and failure to clear infections readily despite appropriate therapy for opportunistic infections should raise a suspicion of immunodeficiency. Recurrent infections can also be attributable to diabetes mellitus, renal failure, and alcoholism; control of these conditions can improve the immune status.

Patients with humoral defects will typically experience recurrent infections (sinusitis, otitis, or meningitis) with encapsulated organisms. Laboratory studies should include a CBC with differential, quantitative immunoglobulin levels, and, if this is normal, IgG subclasses and antibody titers to tetanus toxoid and encapsulated organisms. Low titers should be reassessed by titers 3–5 weeks after immunization. Determination of isohemagglutinin titers to measure IgM antibody function and $CH_{50}$ should be performed. Delayed hypersensitivity skin tests for mumps, *Candida*, and trichophyton can help determine whether the cellular arm of immunity is functional.

Patients with atypical viral or mycobacterial infections or chronic fungal infections should be investigated for cellular immunity. A good initial screening test for macrophage and T cell function is skin testing for delayed hypersensitivity. Constitutional symptoms should suggest tuberculosis, thymoma, or lymphoma. Flow cytometry for elucidating helper, suppressor, and killer cells is useful. When patients have adequate T cell numbers but questionable function, T cell response to mitogens (phytohemagglutinin) should be studied. In patients with cutaneous abscesses, the pus should be examined for neutrophils, and neutrophil studies should include nitro blue tetrazolium dye reduction.

### Management

Treatment varies according to the underlying cause of the immunodeficiency (Table 20.2). Use of prophylactic antibiotics directed against causative bacteria is used for many immunodeficiencies. Patients with complement or splenic dysfunction may respond to immunization. If patients with documented IgG deficiencies or CVI continue to experience recurrent infections despite antibiotic prophylaxis, IV immunoglobulin (IVIG) replacement can be given. However, patients with selective IgA deficiency should not receive IVIG and, in fact, must be treated carefully with IgA-depleted blood products because they may have antibodies to IgA in their serum, which may potentially cause anaphylactic reactions. Patients with immunodeficiency should not be exposed to live attenuated viral vaccines because disseminated disease can follow.

## Questions

**Instructions:** For each question below, select only **one** lettered answer that is the **best** for that question.

1. A 30-year-old man complains of increasing perennial rhinoconjunctivitis symptoms for 2 years. He has had persistent nasal congestion and rhinorrhea, along with sneezing and nasal pruritus, that is worse when he is at home. He smokes 1 pack of cigarettes per day, and he got a dog 3 years ago. Among these, which symptom suggests an allergic etiology?
   A. Nasal congestion
   B. Rhinorrhea
   C. Ear popping
   D. Sneezing and itching

2. Because the symptoms are perennial, which of the following allergens is not expected to be a possible cause?
   A. *Dermatophagoides* mite
   B. Mold
   C. Dog dander
   D. Tree pollen

3. He develops greenish nasal drainage, headaches, and facial pain that is not relieved with his usual antihistamine and nasal steroid spray. Appropriate first-line treatment includes:
   A. Amoxicillin 500 mg three times per day for 3 weeks
   B. Prednisone 30 mg once daily for 2 weeks
   C. Fluconazole 200 mg twice per day for 3 weeks
   D. Amoxicillin/clavulanate 500 mg three times per day for 6 weeks

4. A 45-year-old woman comes into your office complaining of dyspnea and chest tightness related only to aerobics 3 times per week. Appropriate treatment options for her include all of the following except:
   A. Pretreatment albuterol 2 puffs 15 minutes before exercise
   B. Pretreatment cromolyn sodium 2 puffs 15 minutes before exercise
   C. A 2-week course of oral steroids
   D. A leukotriene modifier

5. She returns for follow-up 1 year later and now complains of prolonged cough and wheezing after URIs. She uses her albuterol inhaler every day, and she wakes up coughing 1-2 times per week. She had to go to an emergency department for acute symptoms last week. An appropriate treatment plan for her now would be:
   A. Budesonide 2 puffs twice per day along with sustained-release β-2 agent (salmeterol) 2 puffs twice per day and albuterol MDI 2 puffs PRN for episodes of bronchospasm
   B. Cromolyn sodium MDI 2 puffs 4 times per day
   C. Prednisone 20 mg once daily and albuterol MDI 2 puffs PRN for episodes of bronchospasm
   D. Albuterol MDI 2 puffs scheduled 4 times daily

6. What other things would you discuss and recommend for this patient?
   A. Avoid nonspecific and specific triggers
   B. Use of a spacer device with her inhalers
   C. How to use a peak flow meter
   D. Emergency care plan of action
   E. All of the above

7. A 65-year-old man with a history of asthma and hypertension is undergoing cardiac catheterization when he acutely develops urticaria, respiratory distress, and hypotension. Which answer is true?

A. Radiocontrast media reactions are IgE-mediated.
B. The next time he needs a contrast study, he should be given a less hypertonic agent along with premedication.
C. He should avoid shellfish lifelong.
D. Having a past history of asthma does not put him at a higher risk for developing a reaction to the contrast.

8. Which antihypertensive medications should he now avoid?
A. ACE inhibitors
B. β blockers
C. Calcium channel blockers
D. Diuretics

9. Which of the following is the first-line treatment of choice for this patient's systemic reaction?
A. An oral antihistamine
B. Prednisone 10 mg by mouth
C. Epinephrine 0.3 ml 1 : 1000 subcutaneously
D. Albuterol 0.5 cc by nebulization

10. A 21-year-old student, who was told in the past to avoid penicillin because she had a "reaction" as a child, now comes into your office with symptoms and a physical exam consistent with acute sinusitis. What is the most appropriate next step?
A. Go ahead and give penicillin because the reaction was several years ago.
B. Do standardized skin testing to other antibiotics to make sure she does not have a reaction to those agents.
C. Use TMP/SMX 160/800 mg twice per day for 20 days.
D. Send her to an otolaryngologist.

11. After she finishes the course of antibiotics, she complains of rash, fever, and joint aches. All the answers are true except:
A. This is a type III hypersensitivity reaction and involves immune complex deposition, fixation, and vasculitis.
B. She should get better within the next few weeks.
C. Desensitization to sulfa should help her tolerate the drug next time.
D. She should never take sulfa-containing antibiotics again.

12. A 33-year-old woman presents with a raised, itchy rash and swelling that typically occurs after spending a prolonged period of time outside in the cold air (such as skiing or snow shoveling). The best management approach for her includes:
A. She should go outside in the cold more often to build up tolerance.
B. An antihistamine such as cyproheptadine 8 mg per day or cetirizine 10 mg per day should be used to help control her symptoms.
C. The ice cube test is diagnostic 100% of the time.
D. The size of her lesions are typically small and papular.

13. If her urticaria lasts longer than 48 hours, she should:
A. Increase the dose of her antihistamine.
B. Add an H2 blocker.
C. Undergo skin biopsy.
D. Stay indoors and wear warm clothing.

14. A 19-year-old college student comes in with acute complaints of neck stiffness, photophobia, and fevers. Cerebrospinal fluid (CSF) and blood cultures reveal gram-negative cocci. History reveals that this is the patient's second episode in 2 years. Which of the following laboratory studies would be the most useful?
A. Neutrophil reduction test
B. $CH_{50}$,C3,C4
C. Total serum IgE level
D. Delayed hypersensitivity tests

15. After treatment of the acute infection, chronic maintenance treatment should include:
A. IVIG
B. Prophylactic antibiotics
C. Infusion of complement proteins
D. Stanozolol

## Answers

| | | | | |
|---|---|---|---|---|
| 1. D | 2. D | 3. A | 4. C | 5. A |
| 6. E | 7. B | 8. B | 9. C | 10. C |
| 11. D | 12. B | 13. C | 14. B | 15. B |

## SUGGESTED READING

### *Textbooks and Monographs*

Baker JR Jr, Zylke JW. Primer on allergic and immunologic Diseases. JAMA 1997;278:1799–2034.
Bierman CW, Pearlman D, Shapiro G, et al. Allergy, Asthma and Immunology from Infancy to Adulthood. 3rd ed. Philadelphia: W.B. Saunders Co., 1996.
Busse W, Holgate S. Asthma and Rhinitis. Oxford: Blackwell Scientific, 1995.
Expert Panel Report 2. Guidelines for the Diagnosis and Management of Asthma. Publication No. 97–4051. Bethesda, MD: National Asthma Education Program, Office of Prevention, Education and Control, National Heart, Lung and Blood Institute, National Institutes of Health, April 1997.
International Consensus Report on Diagnosis and Management of Asthma. Publication No. 92–3091. Bethesda, MD: U.S. Department of Health and Human Services, National Heart, Lung and Blood Institute, National Institutes of Health, 1991.
Patterson R, Grammer L, Greenberger P. Allergic Diseases: Diagnosis and Management. 4th ed. New York: Lippincott-Raven, 1997.

*Stites DP, Terr AI, Parslow TG. Medical Immunology. 9th ed. Stamford,CT: Appleton-Lange, 1997.*

### *Articles*

#### *Basic Mechanisms*

Costa JJ, Weller PF, Galli SJ. The cells of the allergic response. JAMA 1997;278:1815–1822.

Fleisher TA, Tomar RH. Introduction to diagnostic laboratory immunology. JAMA 1997;278:1823–1834.

Huston DP. The biology of the immune system. JAMA 1997;278:1804–1814.

#### *Rhinitis, Sinusitis, and Conjunctivitis*

Bernstein IL, Storms WW. Summary statements of practice parameters for allergy diagnostic tests. Ann Allergy Asthma Immunol 1995;75:543–552.

Durham SR, Walker SM, et al. Long-term clinical efficacy of grass-pollen immunotherapy. N Engl J Med 1999;341: 468–475.

Dykewicz MS, Fireman S. Diagnosis and management of rhinitis: Parameter documents of the Joint Task Force on Practice Parameters. Ann Allergy Asthma Immunol 1998;81; 5:463–518.

Levenson T, Greenberger PA. Pathophysiology and therapy for allergic and nonallergic rhinitis: An updated review. Allergy Asthma Proc 1997;18:213–220.

Liebowitz HM. The red eye. N Engl J Med 2000;343;5:345–351.

Low DE, Desrosiers M, McSherry J, et al. A practical guide for the diagnosis and treatment of acute sinusitis. CMAJ 1997;156 (suppl 6):S1–S14.

Patterson R. The role of immunotherapy in respiratory diseases. J Allergy Clin Immunol 1998;101:S403–S404.

Naclerio R, Solomon W. Rhinitis and inhalant allergens. JAMA 1997;278:1842–1848.

Senior BA, Kennedy DW. Management of sinusitis in the asthmatic patient. Ann Allergy Asthma Immunol 1996; 77:6–15.

Weiler JM, Bloomfiedl JR, et al. Effects of fexofenadine, diphenhydramine, and alcohol on driving performance: A randomized, placebo-controlled trial in the Iowa driving simulator. Ann Intern Med 2000;132:354–363.

Williams JW, Simel DLT. The rational clinical examination: Does this patient have sinusitis? JAMA 1993;270:1242–1246.

#### *Bronchial Asthma*

Abramson MJ, Puy RM, Weiner JM. Is allergen immunotherapy effective in asthma? Am J Resp Crit Care Med 1995;151: 969–974.

Bernstein D. Occupational asthma. Med Clin North Am 1992;76:917–934.

Corbridge TC, Hall JT. The assessment and management of adults with status asthmaticus. Am J Resp Crit Care Med 1995;151:1296–1316.

Leff JA, Busse WW, et al. Montelukast, a leukotriene-receptor antagonist, for the treatment of mild asthma and exercise-induced bronchoconstriction. N Engl J Med 1998;339: 147–152.

McFadden ER, Gilbert I. Asthma. N Engl J Med 1992;327: 1928–1937.

McFadden ER, Gilbert I. Exercise-induced asthma. N Engl J Med 1994;330:1362–1367.

Nelson J, Strauss L, et al. Effect of long-term salmeterol treatment on exercise-induced asthma. N Engl J Med 1998; 339:141–146.

Milgrom H, Fick RB, et al. Treatment of allergic asthma with monoclonal anti-IgE antibody. N Engl J Med 1999;341: 1966–1973.

Qureshi F, Pestian J, et al. Effect of nebulized ipratropium on the hospitalization rates of children with asthma. N Engl J Med 1998;339:1030–1035.

#### *Anaphylaxis*

Greenberger P, Patterson R. The prevention of immediate generalized reaction to radiocontrast media in high-risk patients. J Allergy Clin Immunol 1991;87:867–872.

Heffner D. Anaphylaxis. Prim Care 1997;1:220–223.

Poley GE, Slater JE. Latex allergy. J Allergy Clin Immunol 2000;105:1054–1062.

Winbery SL, Lieberman P: Anaphylaxis. In: Virant FS (ed.). Immunology and Allergy Clinics of North America. Philadelphia: WB Saunders Co. August 1995: 447–476.

#### *Drug Allergy*

deShazo RD, Kemp SF. Allergic reactions to drugs and biologic agents. JAMA 1997;278:1895–1906.

Patterson R, DeSwarte RD. Drug allergy and protocols for management of drug allergies. Allergy Proc 1994;15(5): 239–264.

#### *Urticaria and Angioedema*

Greaves M. Chronic urticaria. J Allergy Clin Immunol 2000; 105:664–672.

Maher J. Urticaria and angioedema. A simple approach to a complex problem. Prim Care 1997;1:172–182.

Volcheck GW, Li JT. Exercise-induced urticaria and anaphylaxis. Mayo Clin Proc 1997;72:140–147.

#### *Immunodeficiency*

Puck JM. Primary immunodeficiency diseases. JAMA 1997; 278:1835–1841.

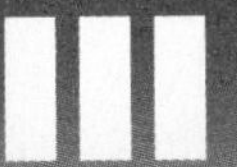

PART III

Rebekah Wang-Cheng
Albert Liebman
Jon Lehrmann
William Anderson
Gail Kallas

# BEHAVIORAL MEDICINE

# CHAPTER 22 A BIOPSYCHOSOCIAL APPROACH TO PATIENT CARE

The medical interview is a dialogue between patient and physician in which information is gathered and a narrative developed, elucidating the patient's condition. Careful observation of the patient can often disclose nonverbal behaviors that may provide significant clues to diagnosis and facilitate communication with the patient. (Table 22.1).

A well-conducted interview is crucial not only for establishing a diagnosis but also for dealing with emotions and building a trusting, open relationship with the patient. The physician may use a variety of cognitive, affective, behavioral, and social strategies to enhance the process (Table 22.2).

A medical interview that interweaves the various elements in the psychological, social, and cultural aspects of the patient's life presents the opportunity for both the physician and the patient to gain awareness of any psychological symptoms and stresses in the patient's life. Disorders in which insight is impaired, such as psychosis, delirium, and dementia, necessitate history taking from both the patient and other observers. Table 22.3 summarizes key areas to explore in the psychiatric interview.

## Role of the Psychiatrist in Medical Care

Most psychiatric conditions cannot be diagnosed by any specific biologic tests. Diagnosis depends on information about the patient's subjective experience and his or her behavior. For guidance in diagnosing mental disorders, the American Psychiatric Association has developed *The Diagnostic and Statistical Manual of Mental Disorders,* currently in its fourth edition with text revision (DSM IV-TR). It uses a multiaxial classification set (Table 22.4). The editors caution against the assumption "that each category of mental disorder therein discussed is a completely described entity with absolute boundaries dividing it from other mental disorders or from no mental disorder." However, the clusters of symptoms of the DSM IV-TR are useful aids in diagnosis, prognosis and psychopharmacologic management. For adequate diagnosis and treatment, it is essential to obtain the vital social, cultural, and developmental information that reveals the particularity of the patient's life experience.

The need for a psychiatric consultation depends on the severity and complexity of the problem and the primary care physician's degree of expertise in dealing with the problems. Timely psychiatric consultation in both inpatient and outpatient settings often may serve to assist the medical diagnostic process by a sensitive sorting out of the variety of factors acting as promoters or direct causes of the patient's illness. In recent years, psychiatric consultative services have developed in

**TABLE 22.1. Nonverbal Behavior that Should Be Observed in the Psychiatric Interview**

1. Dress and demeanor.
2. Posture and carriage.
3. Body movements, including presence of unusual posturing.
4. Gaze, particularly unusual staring or averted gaze.
5. Facial display of happiness, sadness, surprise, fear, anger, interest, disgust.
6. Vocal quality, which can reflect mood as well as the pattern of engaging others.
7. Nonverbal utterances, such as screams, cries, and laughter.
8. Tears, which are not unusual and may represent anger as well as sadness.

**TABLE 22.2. Therapeutic Strategies in the Physician–Patient Encounter**

**Cognitive**
Negotiation of priorities and expectations
Explanation of illness
Suggestion for treatment
Patient education

**Affective**
Empathy
Encouragement of emotional expression
Encouragement and hope
Reassurance

**Behavioral**
Encouragement of patient to take an active role in his or her own recovery
Praise of desired behaviors
Attention to compliance issues

**Social**
Use of family and social supports
Use of community agencies or other health care providers

Adapted with permission from Novack J. Gen Intern Med 1987; 2:346–355.

medical outpatient settings. In the medical clinic, the psychiatrist can serve in a collaborative role with the physician, providing on-site diagnostic evaluation and therapeutic recommendations. In addition to recognizing the variety of psychiatric syndromes in medical patients, the psychiatrist may aid in the management of patients with somatic distress syndromes and patients with difficult behavioral problems interfering with medical care.

**TABLE 22.3. Key Areas to be Explored in the Psychiatric Interview**

1. What symptoms prompted the patient to seek medical care?
2. What is the patient's present life situation? Seeking psychiatric attention generally presupposes a life predicament.
3. What is the developmental life history (childhood, school, occupational, marriage and relationship history, and salient life events)?
4. Have there been any past episodes of mental distress? If so, what was the treatment?
5. Is there a family history of any mental illness, alcoholism, or drug abuse? What are family members' personalities, and their adaptation, particularly in education, occupation, marriage, parenthood, and relationships?
6. What are the current medications?
7. What are the current stresses and the support system of the patient? What is the patient's ability to function in the current situation and the patient's past display of "hardiness"?

**TABLE 22.4. Multiaxial Classification of the Diagnostic and Statistical Manual of Mental Disorders—IV with Text Revision (DSM IV-TR)**

**Axis I**
Clinical disorders
Other conditions that may be a focus of clinical attention

**Axis II**
Personality disorders
Mental retardation

**Axis III**
General medical conditions

**Axis IV**
Psychosocial and environmental problems ("stressors")

**Axis V**
Global assessment of functioning

## Psychiatric Emergencies

An individual observed to have a sudden, acute change in behavior might present in a variety of clinical settings, but often in the emergency room. This situation requires a prompt, concurrent medical and psychiatric diagnostic assessment. A broad variety of diagnoses is possible, ranging from structural brain abnormalities and medical diseases presenting as delirium to behavioral changes attributable to psychiatric syndromes, particularly psychoses. A careful and complete medical evaluation is the first priority. In addition to a careful physical examination, a mental status examination and appropriate laboratory and imaging studies should be performed. A careful history of the events leading to the crisis is crucial. Not infrequently, a history from observers other than the patient also is essential. Observers such as family, police, and other medical facilities must be contacted promptly for information.

Answers to the following questions are critical:

- Has the patient suffered a recent injury, particularly to the head?
- Has there been acute use or withdrawal of a drug (or drugs), alcohol, or both?
- Has the patient been taking any prescription, over-the-counter drugs, or herbal remedies, or been exposed to toxic substances at home or at work?
- Does the patient have a history of previous psychiatric treatment? If so, what was the diagnosis, treatment recommended, and nature of follow-up care?
- Has there been an immediate personal or social crisis in the person's life, such as a separation, divorce, a traumatic event, or a death of a family member or friend?
- Has the patient had a recent hospitalization or emergency room visit?

The treatment process of the patient in a psychiatric emergency requires two stages: the first stage consists of the immediate medical or psychiatric treatment or both, and the second stage requires a determination of the optimal site for further definitive treatment and care. Some situations might require a civil commitment process, if a danger to the patient or others exists and if the patient refuses necessary treatment. A follow-up plan is always necessary in the management of a psychiatric emergency, and a team approach, which includes internists, psychiatrists, social workers, and other personnel, is essential. See Chapter 26 for treatment of acute psychosis.

### Imaging Techniques in Psychiatry

Clinically useful neuroimaging techniques consist of anatomic scans, such as computed tomography (CT) and magnetic resonance imaging (MRI); and functional brain modalities using radionuclides, such as positron-emission tomography (PET), and single-photon emission CT (SPECT). CT and MRI reveal structural brain changes. Anatomic images are of particular use in patients with acute behavioral changes, delirium, and puzzling psychiatric syndromes such as catatonia and amnesia, in which the differential diagnosis includes brain lesions. Although PET and SPECT techniques reveal interesting information on brain function, direct clinical usefulness is limited at present to the diagnosis of structural brain diseases including Alzheimer disease. A characteristic pattern of decreased brain activity in theposterior parietal and temporal areas is seen on PET and SPECT scans in Alzheimer disease, providing increased sensitivity and specificity in the diagnosis of this disease. Imaging abnormalities in other psychiatric syndromes have not yet been consistent enough to be of routine diagnostic use. The recent development of fused-image technology (FIT), which provides accurate anatomic information aligned with PET images, might lead to increased diagnostic capabilities of these modalities. In addition, functional neuroimaging techniques are yielding information that correlates brain functioning on the molecular level with mind and behavior activity. This information may lead to pharmacotherapy that is more finely targeted than that with drugs available today.

# CHAPTER 23 SOMATIC DISTRESS SYNDROMES

It is estimated that in 20-40% of primary care physician visits, the patient's symptoms cannot be explained by or attributed to biologic changes detectable by the medical measures used in the diagnostic process. In these situations, the physician must clearly keep in mind the difference between illness and disease. The hallmark of disease is cellular injury manifested by aberrations in physiology and structure, which can be shown by the variety of modalities available to the scientifically trained physician. On the other hand, illness is a subjective experience of distress that might be caused by disease or experienced by the patient in the absence of a discoverable disease process. When a patient continues to present with symptoms over time without evidence of disease, the diagnosis of a *somatic distress syndrome* or *multiple unexplained physical symptoms* (MUPS) should be considered. Because there is no specific biologic abnormality to treat, the physician is faced with the management of a patient with considerable persistent distress that often produces marked social and occupational dysfunction. Unfortunately, the absence of disease indicators after diagnostic testing does not usually provide sustained relief of the patient's symptoms. It is in one or more diagnostic interviews that incorporates a biopsychosocial perspective that the physician might elicit the needed information to make an appropriate diagnosis. A sensitive interview frequently will enable the patient to make connections between his life predicaments, dysfunctional behavior patterns, and the bodily distress for which he has consulted his doctor.

Psychiatric referral becomes possible when the primary care physician has obtained a comprehensive psychosocial history that reveals underlying stressors for the patient. If psychological factors are not addressed, the patient might seek out more and more specialists and tests, and some patients eventually choose other forms of therapy in the area of alternative medicine. These patients often will become socially withdrawn, and a minority will become completely incapacitated.

The DSM IV-TR lists a number of syndromes under the term *somatoform disorders.* The term somatoform disorders includes somatization disorder, undifferentiated somatoform disorder, conversion disorder, pain disorder, hypochondriasis, body dysmorphic disorder, and somatoform disorder NOS (not otherwise specified). Although some of these disorders have a predominant feature, such as the prominence of pain in pain disorder, pseudoneurologic symptoms in conversion disorder, and a focus on a body feature in body dysmorphic disorder, in general, the somatoform disorders listed in the DSM IV-TR manifest more similarities than differences.

## Somatization Disorder

The estimated prevalence rate of somatoform disorder is 3–4% among primary care patients. The care of somatoform disorder patients entails higher costs, nine times the United States per capita cost. These patients are often frequent users of outpatient and inpatient services. Somatoform disorder often begins in adolescence and usually before age 25. Table 23.1 lists the complete diagnostic criteria. Its chronic course with remissions and exacerbations significantly impairs daily functioning. These patients report multiple symptoms, described in

**TABLE 23.1. Criteria for Somatization Disorder**

1. Usual onset before age 30.
2. Multiple unexplained physical complaints.
3. Symptoms must include the following:
   - Pain in four different sites (e.g., head, joints, chest, abdomen).
   - Two GI symptoms without pain (e.g., constipation, bloating).
   - One sexual symptom without pain (e.g., anorgasmia, decreased libido).
   - One pseudoneurological symptom without pain (e.g., paresthesias, syncope).

Adapted from DSM IV-TR.

meticulous detail, often supported by lists or daily logs. These patients have a higher incidence of major depression and anxiety disorders than seen in the population as a whole. The diagnosis is rarely made in men in the United States, but is reported with higher frequency in men in some other cultures. Commonly, a parent or other family member suffered from a disabling illness or an anxiety disorder. Patients with somatoform disorder frequently give a history of childhood sexual and physical abuse and often have a history of growing up in a socially dysfunctional family.

## Hypochondriasis

Hypochondriacs have a recurring, persistent belief that they are, or will become, afflicted with a serious disease. The patient usually has a focus of somatic distress in a particular location that serves as the nidus for the hypochondriacal fears. The particular bodily distress focus often will rotate among the organ systems. Serious organic disease should be excluded before making this diagnosis. The DSM IV-TR criteria for the diagnosis require that symptoms have lasted for 6 months. The belief that one is suffering from a serious disease is common to all of the somatic distress syndromes, but it also can be a part of a depressive disorder and is commonly seen in panic disorder or other anxiety states. This preoccupation with the body also can result from a form of delusion in schizophrenia. Hidden by the multiplicity of somatic symptoms is the pervasive fear of loss of any kind in the hydochondriac.

### Treatment of Somatic Distress Syndromes/ Multiple Unexplained Physical Symptoms

The patients in this category tax the therapeutic ingenuity of the primary care physician because of the lack of specific curative measures. Typically, it has been recommended that the patient be given scheduled brief appointments with his or her physician at frequent, regular intervals to provide psychological support and monitoring. The treatment effectiveness of this intuitive practice has not been proven. In fact, perpetuation of dysfunctional patterns can be an outcome of well-meaning empathy and frequent supportive doctor visits unless constructive measures are undertaken. Patients with somatic distress syndrome might have other concurrent psychiatric syndromes that require careful psychiatric evaluation. Patients with persistent somatic distress syndromes with prominent anxiety and depressive symptoms will experience some relief of these symptoms when treated with appropriate medication; however, they might not experience a change in their fixed beliefs regarding their bodily symptoms.

A comprehensive program that addresses issues of exercise, appropriate nutrition, and sleep hygiene measures, which moves the patient to an improved sense of physical fitness, is helpful. A graded exercise program has been shown to be therapeutic. The patient often is benefited by joint interviews with involved family members. Information from family members is helpful in providing some treatment directions, as is enlisting family members as allies in the recovery process of the patient. Individual cognitive behavioral therapy has been shown to be most helpful in a recovery process. The patient must be informed that incremental improvement is the goal and that no single therapeutic intervention will alleviate the condition. Patients are drawn to self-help groups that might be a positive influence or merely perpetuate their chronic state of "patienthood". The physician is at risk of becoming resentful of the patient's resistance to recovery or might become an unwitting facilitator of continued illness by prescribing fruitless diagnostic adventures, ineffective medications, and repeated hospitalizations. These risks can be avoided if collaborative cognitive-behavioral treatment with a psychiatrist is carried out.

## Conversion Disorder

Formerly known as hysteria, conversion disorder presents with symptoms that simulate a neurological disorder, such as anesthetic limbs; loss of motor function; aphonia; visual disturbance, including blindness; and behavior suggesting seizures. A common malady in this category is that of pseudoseizures. Symptoms have a sudden onset and usually are precipitated by a threatening social or interpersonal occurrence. A pre-existing personality disorder usually is present. A careful medical and neurological examination is necessary to validate the absence of a disease process.

Treatment necessitates a collaboration of psychiatry with medicine and neurology. The patient also might have a history of a somatic distress disorder. The pseudoneurologic symptoms usually remit in a relatively short period of time with appropriate diagnosis. When the acute symptoms subside, the underlying anxious diathesis of the patient must be addressed. Pharmacologic treatment of accompanying anxiety disorder syndromes and depressive disorders is important. Psychiatric referral to address an underlying personality disorder might be indicated.

## Factitious Disorders

Factitious disorders are the intentional feigning of physical symptoms, psychological symptoms, or both. The full-blown form is known as Munchausen syndrome. The confusing nature of these patients' symptoms leads to emergency department visits, hospitalizations, and even multiple surgeries. The motivations behind such behavior are not usually obvious to the physician, and the patient does not reveal them. An underlying personality disorder exists, often a borderline personality disorder. Many of these patients are associated with the health care field and are adept at simulating illnesses (e.g., hypoglycemia as a result of surreptitious insulin use). However, the patient universally assumes a sick role to gain respite from life predicaments that he or she is unable to resolve. The disorder is more common in women, although it can be seen in men, particularly in restrictive circumstances, such as prison.

In Munchausen syndrome *by proxy,* a sick role is constructed by care-giving persons for someone in their care, and the dependent one assumes the sick role. This is most commonly seen in a mother-child relationship. The child is an unwitting accomplice participating in a folie à deux. The perpetrator repeatedly presents a child for medical care. Genuine illness is absent, but in some circumstances the perpetuator produces physiologic dysfunction by administering substances.

Psychiatric consultation is essential when this diagnosis is suspected. Such a consultation might reveal the nature of the aggressor's social or psychological predicament, or both, and the person then can be confronted before more harm occurs. Unfortunately, physicians can be deceived and enter into unwise therapeutic adventures before the diagnosis is made. Patients frequently flee the hospital or outpatient setting after confrontation and often reappear in other medical care facilities. When the diagnosis is suspected, medical records from other institutions can help to establish the diagnosis of Munchausen syndrome by proxy.

## Chronic Pain Syndromes

Persistent pain, unresponsive to medical treatment and not reasonably explained by demonstrable disease processes, is an increasingly frequent and costly medical and social problem. Chronic pain greatly affects the patient's personal and work life, with attendant social and economic disruption. The knowledge of biologic mechanisms underlying acute pain generated by peripheral nociceptor irritation is insufficient for the understanding of the patient with chronic pain. Neural imaging studies suggest that the neuronal network underlying the cerebral processing of chronic pain might differ from that of acute pain. The experience of pain clearly invokes emotions and cognition, both of which exist to serve the evolutionary survival system of human beings. By evoking emotions and cognition over time, chronic pain establishes a cue-sensitive behavior pattern. Consequently, learning plays a role in establishing chronicity. This contrasts sharply with the simple reflex processes of acute nociceptor-generated pain, which is time limited so that a learned cue-dependent behavior pattern has less chance of evolving. The simple principle of acute pain relief with adequate opiates is an inadequate strategy for the management of chronic pain syndromes.

In general, questionnaires for self-reported psychological distress that survey for indicators of psychopathology fail to differentiate chronic pain patients from other nonpsychiatric general populations. The putative absence of psychological distress detected by these measures may be misleading. Repeated and futile attempts by physicians to establish unequivocal biologic pathology to explain the prolonged pain tends to perpetuate a persistent preoccupation of the patient with the pain. Chronic pain comes to assume the characteristics of an idée fixe and, as such, dominates the mental experience of the sufferer. The domination of the patient's consciousness by the all-consuming chronic pain experience may suppress the awareness of distressing emotions and past and present life predicaments.

### Treatment

The chronic pain pattern usually follows a medical illness, surgery, or a traumatic injury when medical intervention has occurred. Cause and effect become intertwined in chronic pain situations, and a biopsychosocial approach to chronic pain patients is essential. Information regarding the patient's premorbid social and psychological adaptation can provide necessary information to give direction to a comprehensive therapeutic program. The reliance on analgesics alone by the physician is a problematic strategy. The use of opiates alone generally does not lead to either social or occupational rehabilitation of the chronic pain patient and might establish a cue-dependent behavior pattern involving the drugs. Clearly, the consequences of a pain disorder that results in economic hardship, social limitations, and damaged self-esteem profoundly affect the cognitive and affective spheres. A common problem is a corrosive anger often accompanied by a sense of victimhood. Anger and shame often are commingled.

Patients with a chronic pain disorder often are referred finally to a pain clinic after conventional medical treatment fails. Such a clinic usually operates as a multidisciplinary team with a multimodal therapeutic approach. Each patient presents with a unique situation that requires an individual assessment of biologic, psychological, and social factors. It also is essential to treat other medical conditions that contribute to distress and limit function. The emphasis in the pain clinic is on improvement of the patient's ability to function and address economic, social, and psychological issues. The use of fewer addicting pain medications and carefully selected psychotropic drugs are beneficial adjuncts in a comprehensive treatment program. Physical interventions, such as nerve blocks, intraspinal injections, and so on, based on peripheral nociceptor–generated theory have limited usefulness, or even worse, confound the picture with temporary placebo responses. Effective therapeutic strategies in a comprehensive program may involve biofeedback, relaxation training, graduated exercise programs, group therapy, medication for anxiety and depression, and individual psychotherapy where applicable. Group participation in a comprehensive program is particularly beneficial because patients with chronic pain tend to isolate themselves from interpersonal and social contacts.

# CHAPTER 24 ANXIETY DISORDERS

Anxiety is a ubiquitous human experience. It is likely a basic underlying experience in all psychiatric disorders, including the psychoses. A precise definition of anxiety is somewhat elusive. Anxiety might best be characterized as a proto-emotion (primary or early) from which more readily describable emotions derive. Søren Kierkegaard, the Danish philosopher, characterized fear as fear of "some-thing" and dread (a derived emotion of anxiety) as fear of "no-thing." In other words, fear has an intentional object, whereas anxiety does not. The limbic system activation in anxiety disorders is similar to that in fear reactions.

The onset of anxiety syndromes often occurs at a time of life in which individuation is taking place, in the teens and twenties. The person is experiencing a loss of the usual supports that made him or her feel a sense of security. In situations of acute anxiety, the individual experiences an overwhelming sense of a lack of control. It is the fear of loss of control, a loss of a sense of predictability, that leads the anxious person to say that he is under stress. Kirkegaard refers to anxiety as "the dizziness of freedom."

Each anxiety syndrome presents with a unique set of manifestations. In general, fear is the way in which one responds to a sense of being threatened physically. Anxiety is more of a threat to one's sense of conscious mental control. In free-floating anxiety, there is no distinguishable threatening stimulus, external or internal. The anxiety disorders, as defined in the DSM IV-TR, differ from each other in the acuteness of symptoms, the pattern of autonomic nervous system arousal, the nature of somatic symptoms experienced, the predominant social preoccupations of the patient, and the presence of cue precipitation. As in the somatic distress syndromes, the similarities in the underlying structure of the disorders may exceed their apparent symptomatic differences.

## Panic Disorder

Panic disorder is characterized by sudden, recurrent attacks of intense anxiety occurring without warning and causing a terrifying sense of imminent disaster. In the United States, its prevalence rate is 1%, with a lifetime incidence of 2–3%. Onset is usually in adolescence and young adulthood. The long-term course is highly variable and characterized by remissions and exacerbations. Association with major depression is noteworthy, and substance abuse, especially alcohol, and personality disorders may complicate treatment and outcomes. There is usually a history of an anxiety disorder in other family members.

Panic attacks usually have an abrupt onset of intense somatic symptoms (Table 24.1) that often result in visits to hospital emergency departments. Frequent emergency room visits occur before the diagnosis is made. Even those with an established diagnosis might still visit the emergency room during an attack, driven by the severity of symptoms and panic. Without prompt and effective treatment, agoraphobia (a fear of leaving the home or venturing into the open) can develop in the patient who begins to anticipate the return of a panic attack in settings away from home.

### Management

Because patients usually fear that they have a serious physical malady, therapy begins with a clear presentation of the nature of the disorder. Benzodiazepines and selective serotonin reuptake inhibitors (SSRIs) are treatments of choice in management of panic disorder. In the past, tricyclic antidepressants (TCAs) and monoamine oxidase inhibitors (MAOIs) also have been useful in treatment. The side effects of these drugs and inconvenient dietary restrictions of the MAOIs make them less desirable in treatment and rarely necessary. Selective SSRIs are effective in most patients in preventing panic attacks.

Of the benzodiazepines, alprazolam (Xanax) is the most widely studied and used. It is clearly an effective drug in reducing anticipatory anxiety and preventing panic attacks. The longer acting benzodiazepine, clonazepam, has also demonstrated efficacy, perhaps with less addiction potential. When the diagnosis is first made, the benzodiazepines are particularly useful for establishing prompt control of the episodes because SSRI effectiveness might be delayed. Because the benzodiazepines have an addiction potential, the physician should use the lowest effective dose. However, long-term studies of patients who have used benzodiazepines for panic attacks over long periods of time (years) usually report reduction in the required dose over time. The benzodiazepines present an addiction hazard mainly in patients with addiction potential, such as alcoholics, drug abusers, and patients with personality disorders. The principal side effects of sedation, ataxia, and incoordination may limit the dosage.

Given the multitude of available agents, physicians should become familiar with a few anxiolytics that they find most efficacious. The dosages and half-lives of anxiolytic drugs are shown in Table 24.2. Withdrawal symptoms, such as restlessness, nervous feelings, tremor, insomnia, and, in extreme situations, convulsions, can occur with benzodiazepine therapy, commensurate with dosage and length of treatment. Withdrawal symptoms can be avoided by dose tapering, reducing the daily dose by 0.5-1.0 mg each week.

Behavior therapy consisting of graded exposure to situations that have assumed a phobic nature can be a useful supplement to pharmacologic treatment in selected patients. This approach can be particularly useful in treating agoraphobic symptoms.

**TABLE 24.1. Common Features of Panic Disorder**

| |
|---|
| **Somatic symptoms** |
| Palpitations and rapid heart rate |
| Trembling and shaking |
| Chest pain |
| Difficulty breathing |
| Sensation of choking |
| Hyperventilation |
| Dizziness and feeling of faintness |
| Sensation of heat and sweating |
| Paresthesias, particularly of the face |
| **Interpretations of imminent disasters (examples)** |
| Having a heart attack |
| Sense of suffocation |
| Losing control of oneself |
| Going crazy |

## Generalized Anxiety Disorder

In 1894, Freud described two forms of anxiety: (1) free-floating anxiety, now termed generalized anxiety disorder (GAD), which can coexist with or occur separately from (2) panic disorder, a pattern of acute anxiety attacks that can erupt suddenly into consciousness. This delineation of GAD and panic disorder remains valid to this day. Because anxiety is a symptom in other disorders, a careful differential diagnosis is mandatory. The following disorders require consideration in the differential diagnosis of GAD: schizophrenia,

**TABLE 24.2. Dosages and Half-Lives of Anxiolytic Drugs**

| Drug | Daily Dosage Range (mg) | Half-Life |
|---|---|---|
| **Benzodiazepines** | | |
| Alprazolam | 0.75–4 (anxiety)<br>1.5–8 (panic) | Short-intermediate |
| Chlordiazepoxide | 15–100 | Long* |
| Clonazepam | 0.5–2 | Long* |
| Diazepam | 6–30 | Long* |
| Lorazepam | 1–6 | Short-intermediate |
| Oxazepam | 30–60 | Short |
| **Azaspirone** | | |
| Buspirone | 15–60 | Short (delayed onset of action over days) |

**Note:** Other anxiolytic drugs, including SSRI's and venlafaxine are detailed in Table 24.4.
*Benzodiazepines with long half-lives have active metabolites.

bipolar disorder, somatization disorder, borderline personality disorder, obsessive-compulsive disorder, phobic disorders, and medical illnesses such as hyperthyroidism and pheochromocytoma. Alcohol withdrawal syndrome, particularly if the patient conceals his or her alcohol consumption from the physician, and psychoactive drugs, especially amphetamines, can simulate a primary anxiety state. Within the anxiety disorders group, GAD needs to be differentiated from those anxiety disorders that have more clear-cut cue precipitants. The diagnosis of such disorders as social anxiety (social phobia), anger attack syndrome, acute stress reactions, and posttraumatic stress disorders (PTSDs) is made by the elucidation of precipitating cue factors.

### Clinical Features

Common symptoms of GAD include a feeling of inner tension and difficulty concentrating, often with a feeling of one's mind going blank. The patients usually have a significant sleep disorder with difficulty falling asleep and maintaining sleep. Fatigue, muscle tension, and often autonomic symptoms such as palpitations, trembling, and breathlessness are present. The symptomatology might be variable, and all patients do not present with noradrenergic arousal symptoms. Social and occupational functioning and interpersonal relations often are disrupted significantly.

### Management

The severity of anxiety symptoms in patients with an anxious diathesis waxes and wanes in response to perceived social stressors. Treatment with medication frequently may be limited to times of exacerbations of symptoms in response to feelings of personal stress. For that reason, medication must be tailored to the particularity of the anxious patient. Because of a favorable side-effect profile and absence of addiction potential, the SSRIs are a preferred mode of treatment. Venlafaxine also has shown efficacy. The benzodiazepines and buspirone also are useful drugs, generally used for limited periods of time. The benzodiazepines are anxiolytic and sedating with some addiction potential. Buspirone—the only currently available azaspirone—is anxiolytic but not sedating; it modulates serotoninergic neurotransmission via the 5 HT-1A receptor.

## Posttraumatic Stress Disorder

PTSD is precipitated by a threat to one's life or physical integrity, and has been recognized as a formal psychiatric diagnosis since 1980. The onset may be acute, occurring immediately or within days of the event, or delayed. Often the acute form resolves only to be followed by subsequent symptoms, which then assume the form of a characteristic PTSD. Extreme situations such as war, violent crime, and natural disasters are the most common causative factors. Observation of Vietnam War veterans resulted in a more complete characterization and description of PTSD. A prevalence rate of 15% in Vietnam veterans has been noted, with an incidence of 2% approximately 20 years after wartime service.

### Clinical Features

Symptoms occurring in acute stress reactions range from a sensation of being in a daze to feeling a sense of detachment and depersonalization and various conversion symptoms. Varying manifestations are amnesia of the event, prominent agitation and restlessness, hyperarousal symptoms of vigilance, increased scanning, irritability, sleeplessness, difficulty concentrating, and autonomic nervous system lability. Similar symptoms occur in the succeeding chronic illness, the posttraumatic stress reaction. A re-experiencing of the traumatic event or events by thought, images, and intense affect is a prominent symptom. Flashback episodes may vary in intensity and provoke dissociative experiences. The patient attempts to avoid situations that might evoke the intense symptoms. Significantly impaired social and occupational functioning and disruption of marital and other interpersonal relationships are common. Depression and anhedonia (loss of pleasure in one's normal pursuits) may be prominent. Impulse control is impaired; alcohol and drug abuse is frequent. Suicide is a definite risk. Chronic PTSD can lead to significant morbidity and mortality, as exemplified by the observed experience of Vietnam veterans with the disorder.

### Management

Pharmacologic treatment usually is combined with a variety of psychological techniques, including behavioral conditioning and support groups. Sertraline has been approved by the United States Food and Drug Administration (FDA) for use in this disorder, but other SSRIs also are effective. Buspirone and trazodone, because of antiaggressive and anti-irritability features without addiction potential, may have a unique place in long-term treatment. Neuromodulators in the anticonvulsant class of drugs may be useful in selected patients in the chronic phase. Prolonged pharmacological and cognitive-behavioral therapy may be necessary.

In the acute phase, sleep is grossly disturbed and control of racing thoughts and uncontrolled emotions of terror require prompt treatment. When a suicidal hazard is present or severe symptoms prevail, inpatient psychiatric care may be necessary. Although pharmacologic therapy has been better studied in chronic PTSD than in the acute stress forms, psychotropic drugs used in the chronic disorder may be effective in the acute form. In this situation, benzodiazepines are indicated because the effect of SSRIs is delayed. β-blocking drugs such as propranolol may be necessary to blunt excessive noradrenergic peripheral effects. Early pharmacologic treatment in the acute stress phase may prevent chronicity, although this has not been established in controlled studies.

## Obsessive-Compulsive Disorders

Community surveys estimate a 1.5–2.1% incidence of obsessive-compulsive disorder (OCD) in the United States population. The presence of intrusive, compelling thoughts, images, or ideas involving impulsive acts constitute the obsessions. Their theme, although variable in different individuals, is repetitive and remarkably constant in any one individual. The themes usually involve harm to one's self or to others resulting from some act on the part of the afflicted. The compulsions consist of repetitive actions designed to ward off some dreaded consequence. Lady Macbeth's hand-washing compulsion is an obvious famous example for compulsive behavior. The obsessive thoughts are regarded by the patient as alien, and this insight distinguishes this disorder from psychosis.

Despite the established association between obsessions and compulsions in Tourette syndrome, it has only recently become obvious that patients with either OCD or Tourette syndrome have a significant number of family members with the other disorder. Thus, a common gene may exist, containing a phenotype of either OCD or Tourette syndrome.

Effective drug therapy is through agents that affect primarily the serotoninergic neurotransmitter system (Table 24.3). Clomipramine, a TCA; and two SSRIs, fluoxetine and fluvoxamine; are currently the drugs of choice: all three are apparently equally effective. Clomipramine is a tricyclic compound, but it possesses a specific inhibitory effect on serotonin reuptake in presynaptic terminals. It may decrease libido and the ability to achieve orgasm. Fluoxetine and fluvoxamine are SSRIs that may have side effects of anxiety, restlessness, insomnia, and inhibition of orgasm. Paroxetine and sertraline can also be used. Duration of treatment is uncertain, and treatment effects may only become apparent after several months. A 6-month trial is necessary to gauge drug effectiveness. Adjunctive behavioral therapy may be useful.

**TABLE 24.3. Drugs for the Treatment of Obsessive-Compulsive Disorder**

| Drug | Initial Dose (mg) | Maintenance Daily Dose (mg) | Half-Life (h) |
|---|---|---|---|
| Clomipramine | 25 | 100–250 | 32 |
| Fluoxetine | 10 | 20–80 | 160 |
| Fluvoxamine | 50 | 100–300 | 16 |
| Paroxetine | 20 | 20–60 | 24 |
| Sertraline | 50 | 50–200 | 24 |

## Specific Phobias

A specific phobia is a persistent, invariable, inappropriate fear reaction to a specific object, creature, activity, or situation. Symptoms include shakiness, trembling, palpitations, dry mouth, breathlessness, lightheadedness (which can progress to a vasovagal faint), and sometimes a choking sensation. Some provoking agents are certain animals or insects, heights, enclosed spaces such as elevators, airplanes, bridges, and in medical situations, needles and blood. Cognitive-behavioral therapy involving exposure can be an appropriate measure. Benzodiazepines can be effective in blocking symptom response when taken prior to exposure to the phobic cues.

### Agoraphobia

Agoraphobia is a term referring to a phobic reaction to open spaces. Agoraphobia almost always occurs in patients with a history of panic disorder and commonly begins shortly after the initial panic attack. These individuals fear that the panic attack will recur in a public place from which they cannot exit quickly or easily, such as freeways, shopping malls, bridges, and movie theaters. The patient fears leaving home, and if untreated, may become homebound. The prompt and effective treatment of the accompanying panic disorder is the key to successful management. Intensive cognitive-behavioral therapy is indicated for the impaired agoraphobic patient.

### Social Phobia

Also known as social anxiety disorder, social phobia is characterized by a conditioned fear, and consequent avoidance, of social situations in which the person would be exposed to the possible scorn of others. The anticipation of such an event provokes the characteristic somatic accompaniments of anxiety. Social phobia is clearly cue driven. The severity of the disorder is highly variable, but shy children, behaviorally inhibited at age 20–30 months, are at increased risk to develop this disorder. The peak age of onset is between 11 and 15 years, but may begin in childhood. Relatives of social phobic patients have a higher incidence of the disorder than do relatives of normal controls. This disorder is often the hidden cause for school dropout and other social and occupational failures. Patients with social phobia are at increased risk of abusing alcohol because they often discover the calming effect of alcohol when facing social situations.

Pharmacologic therapy has shown efficacy in clinical trials. The SSRIs are drugs of choice. Benzodiazepines are also useful, particularly when used prophylactically on social occasions. Benzodiazepines can be reserved for more chronic use in patients who have not responded or cannot tolerate SSRIs. Clonazepam (0.25–3 mg daily) and Alprazolam (0.5-6 mg daily) are effective. Cognitive-behavioral treatment is frequently useful.

# CHAPTER 25 DEPRESSIVE DISORDERS

The term depression is an "umbrella term" that encompasses a variety of emotions that have an unpleasant, distressing subjective feel. Common emotions experienced in this state are sadness, hopelessness, grief, regret, sorrow, and often despondency and despair. Although emotions are generally thought to have a sudden onset and to be of brief duration, emotions that are persistent may then be characterized as a mood state. Because the presence of these distressing emotions may be subtle and pervasive over a long period of time, it is not unusual to encounter a person who is experiencing and displaying the manifestations of a depression but does not acknowledge the depressive state. This situation requires information by others in the patient's milieu. Facilitating treatment requires that the physician is able to lead the patient to a degree of insight regarding his or her distress.

The DSM IV-TR lists the following depressive disorders: major depressive disorder, dysthymic disorder, and depressive disorder NOS. Indeed, a spectrum of depressive manifestations exists, and the awareness of this helps the physician recognize and treat depressed patients, even when manifestations are not typical. These disorders are characterized by a significant, often profound change in an individual wherein the person becomes dysphoric and despondent. A depressive disorder may begin at any age from childhood to late life. A frequent age of onset is in late adolescence and in the 20s to 40s. Onset may be fairly acute, or the depression may have been present for years in a low-grade form. Chronic, low-grade depression is intimately related to personality.

## Major Depressive Disorder

The 12-month prevalence of major depressive disorder is 10%, with a lifetime prevalence of 17%. For women, the lifetime prevalence is 10–25%, compared with 5–12% for men. The patient with a depressive disorder becomes dysfunctional in family, social, and occupational roles. The economic burden is also profound, with direct and indirect costs exceeding $40 billion per year in 1990. Primary care physicians currently treat some two thirds of patients with depression. Unfortunately depression remains both underdiagnosed by some primary care physicians and overdiagnosed by others. Treatment effectiveness is increased when there is collaborative treatment by the primary care physician and a psychiatrist.

The cause of depression is unclear, but interplay between biologic factors and social/psychological stress is likely. A dysregulation of neurotransmitter function has been postulated. Impaired availability of norepinephrine and/or serotonin at synapses is a possible biochemical mechanism and is the basis for the pharmacological treatment of depression. Although some depressed patients show changes in brain function on functional brain imaging, these changes are not consistent enough for diagnostic use. Individuals with a first-degree blood relative with a mood disorder are at increased risk of developing clinical depression. A family history or prior episode doubles the personal risk for a depressive episode. The familial risk seems to be even higher in patients with bipolar disorder.

### Clinical Features

Depressed patients describe their mood as "depressed," "blue," or "down in the dumps," and often report feeling hopeless. They have lost interest in their usual pursuits and are unable to feel pleasure in life. A dispirited mood and anhedonia are the two major features of depression (Table 25.1 lists other criteria.) Often

**TABLE 25.1. Diagnostic Criteria for Depression**

A. Five (or more) symptoms for at least 2 weeks
- Depressed mood*
- Anhedonia*
- Weight change
- Sleep disturbance
- Psychomotor agitation or retardation
- Fatigue
- Feelings of worthlessness/guilt
- Poor concentration
- Recurrent thoughts of death or suicide

B. Symptoms cause significant functional impairment.

C. Symptoms not accounted for by the following:
- Substance abuse
- Medical condition
- Bereavement

*Must include at least one of these.
Adapted from DSM IV-TR.

**TABLE 25.2. Factors Associated with Suicide**

| |
|---|
| Caucasian |
| Masculine gender |
| Advanced age |
| Adolescence |
| Previous attempts |
| Detailed plan |
| Hopelessness |
| Living alone |
| General medical illness |
| Substance abuse |
| Psychosis |
| Depression |
| Bipolar state |
| Personality disorder |
| Family history of suicide |

cognitive function is affected, resulting in poor concentration, slower mental processes, and a decreased ability to perform complex mental tasks. A common manifestation is unusual irritability, which may be most striking in adolescents and the elderly and is evident to family members but often unnoticed by the patient.

In addition to changes in mood and thought processes, physical well-being is also affected, causing decreased energy, fatigue and lethargy, and a loss of usual motivations. Psychomotor agitation or retardation and apathy may exist. Anorexia and weight loss is common. Sleep is characteristically disturbed, usually with a middle (inability to maintain sleep) or terminal (early morning awakening) insomnia. Terminal insomnia is often immediately accompanied by anxiety. Severely depressed patients often report some relief of symptoms as evening falls, constituting a diurnal variation in mood.

Patients suffering from major depression often become preoccupied with thoughts of death, and suicide is a serious risk. As many as 15% of severely depressed patients commit suicide, and 60% of all suicides result from depression. Overdose with drugs is the most common method, but hanging or shooting are also used. Risk factors for suicide are listed in Table 25.2. All patients with suspected depression should be directly questioned about previous suicide attempts and current thoughts ("Have you considered ending your life?"). Any expressed wish, threat, or gesture should be taken very seriously. One should specifically ask if any definite plans are being considered. Most patients are relieved to express such thoughts. Ascertaining what the precipitant might be for considering suicide is imperative. If the situation is not resolved, the suicidal ideation will likely persist. Psychiatric evaluation should be obtained as soon as suicidal intent is expressed. The patient should be hospitalized for close observation, if the safety of the patient is in jeopardy. Psychotic manifestations are present in some patients (see Chapter 26).

## Diagnosis

A number of scales are available for screening for depression. The Beck, Zung, and Hamilton-D scales may be used. The Patient Health Questionnaire is another screening tool (Figure 25.1), developed especially for use by primary care physicians. No biologic or imaging tests are available to confirm the clinical diagnosis of a depressive disorder. An associated dysregulation of the hypothalamic-pituitary-adrenal axis has been postulated, and some depressed patients show elevated cortisol levels that are not suppressed by dexamethasone. In most studies, a dexamethasone suppression test shows a sensitivity of 40–50% and a specificity of 70–90% for detecting depression. Pharmacological treatment that results in a clinical remission will often show a reversal of the hyper-cortisolism. Persistent nonsuppression of cortisol after dexamethasone following therapy for depression indicates a high risk of early relapse and poor outcome, which might reflect insufficient treatment.

The depressive syndrome may be caused by a number of diseases, drugs, and medications. Substance abuse, including alcohol, cocaine, and other drugs, is a common cause of depression, and the mood disturbance contributes to the cycle of drug abuse. Strokes, especially left hemispheric, Parkinson's disease, endocrine and autoimmune disorders, and certain cancers, may contribute to depression. Adjustment reactions and seasonal affective disorder (SAD) usually cause less functional impairment and are of shorter duration. Dysthymia by definition must be present for 2 years or more and is typically less severe than major depression, with less social and occupational dysfunction. Dysthymic patients present with a history of chronic dysphoria that often dates back to childhood. Bipolar affective disorder (see Chapter 26) is suggested by a strong family history, prior episodes of hypomania, and onset typically in the late teens into the thirties.

## Treatment of Depression

Drug therapy is the primary treatment of depressive disorders (Table 25.3). Initial antidepressant therapy, in appropriately diagnosed cases, leads to a remission rate of approximately 50-60%. Controlled double-blind studies of the treatment of depression yields a placebo response rate in the range of 30-35%. Generally, a response to a drug begins within 3-6 weeks into administration, though 6-8 weeks is required for the full response. If there is no decrease in symptoms in 2-4 weeks, a dosage change or drug change may be indicated. Drug treatment may induce a complete remission, but not

PATIENT HEALTH QUESTIONNAIRE (PHQ-9)

Name: ______________________ Date: ________

Over the last 2 weeks, how often have you been bothered by any of the following problems? (use "√" to indicate your answer)

| | Not at all | Several days | More than half the days | Nearly every day |
|---|---|---|---|---|
| 1. Little interest or pleasure in doing things | | | | |
| 2. Feeling down, depressed, or hopeless | | | | |
| 3. Trouble falling or staying asleep, or sleeping too much | | | | |
| 4. Feeling tired or having little energy | | | | |
| 5. Poor appetite or overeating | | | | |
| 6. Feeling bad about yourself—or that you are a failure or have let yourself or your family down | | | | |
| 7. Trouble concentrating on things, such as reading the newspaper or watching television | | | | |
| 8. Moving or speaking so slowly that other people could have noticed. Or the opposite—being so fidgety or restless that you have been moving around a lot more than usual | | | | |
| 9. Thoughts that you would be better off dead, or of hurting yourself in some way | | | | |

Add columns: [ ] + [ ] + [ ]

*(Healthcare professional: For interpretation of TOTAL, please refer to accompanying scoring card)* TOTAL: [ ]

| 10. If you checked off *any* problems, how *difficult* have these problems made it for you to do your work, take care of things at home, or get along with other people? | Not difficult at all ____<br>Somewhat difficult ____<br>Very difficult ____<br>Extremely difficult ____ |
|---|---|

PHQ-9 SCORING CARD FOR SEVERITY DETERMINATION
*for healthcare professional use only*

Scoring—add up all checked boxes on PHQ-9
For every √: Not at all = 0; Several days = 1; More than half the days = 2; Nearly every day = 3

Interpretation of Total Score

| **Total Score** | **Depression Severity** |
|---|---|
| 1-4 | Minimal depression |
| 5-9 | Mild depression |
| 10-14 | Moderate depression |
| 15-19 | Moderately severe depression |
| 20-27 | Severe depression |

**FIGURE 25.1. PRIME-MD.**

**TABLE 25.3. Principles of Antidepressant Therapy**

1. Early, close monitoring for side effects and clinical response
2. Titration to appropriate dosage
3. Adequate trial of 3–10 weeks to reach clinical efficacy
4. Monitoring of drug-drug interactions (e.g., cytochrome P-450 induction)
5. Treatment for minimum of 4–6 months after complete remission
6. Change of drug regimen if lack of response
7. Maintenance treatment required for recurrent episodes
8. Supportive physician contact essential

infrequently there is only a partial response. In these circumstances, a dose change, augmentation, or a change to another drug may prove effective. Drugs that may be added for augmentation include bupropion, buspirone, lithium, and methylphenidate. The presence of significant anxiety tends to diminish the complete response rate.

Drug treatment of depression is best accomplished by balancing side effects of the drugs with the effectiveness of the selected drug in the individual patient. Monotherapy is preferred to avoid drug–drug interactions. Patients who fail to respond to the first drug trial in adequate dosage may well respond to a drug in the same biochemical class or another biochemical class, or to augmentation treatment with other drugs. Because antidepressants may precipitate mania in patients with bipolar disorder, a careful family and past history must be obtained. A bipolar disorder patient may require a mood stabilizer in addition to the antidepressant to diminish the risk of precipitating a manic episode. Once remission is obtained, maintenance treatment is recommended to prevent recurrence.

**Pharmacologic agents for depression**

There are three phases in the treatment of depression: *acute,* which lasts 6–12 weeks until symptom abatement or remission; *continuation,* which usually lasts 6-9 months, to prevent relapses; and *maintenance therapy,* for preventing recurrence. Fifty percent of patients have a relapse after one episode, 70% after two, and 90% after three. Long-term treatment has been recommended for patients who have had recurrent episodes. Such therapy for 2–3 years has yielded favorable results and is indicated for patients who have had three major episodes, onset before age 20, a life-threatening episode in the past 3 years, recurrence within 1 year after medication was discontinued, or two episodes plus a first-degree relative with depression. For those with a bipolar disorder who are at risk for frequent recurrence, therapy may be lifelong.

Table 25.4 lists pharmacologic agents that can be used to treat depression.

*Selective serotonin reuptake inhibitors*

SSRIs have become first-line treatment for depression. In contrast to TCAs, there is a low incidence of limiting side effects and less need for dose titration. Most studies with direct comparison of treatment with TCA and SSRI reveal equivalent efficacy of SSRIs and TCAs; however, the dropout rate is much higher for the group treated with TCAs because of drug side effects. In addition, quinidine-like cardiac conduction effects and the potential lethal toxicity of the TCAs in overdoses make the SSRIs a safer drug choice. Citalopram, paroxetine, sertraline, and fluoxetine are the first-choice drugs among the SSRIs.

The inhibition of cytochrome P-450 isoenzymes by SSRIs may increase serum levels of other drugs, such as phenytoin, carbamazepine, clozapine, benzodiazepines, and TCAs, increasing the risk of toxicity. Because combination with a MAOI may provoke a potentially lethal toxic serotonin syndrome, an SSRI should not be administered together with an MAOI or within 2 weeks of each other.

These drugs should be tapered slowly over a period of several weeks because untoward symptoms have been observed on withdrawal of SSRIs. The symptoms include dizziness, lightheadedness, insomnia, fatigue, anxiety and agitation, nausea, headache, blurring of vision, and paresthesias. Hypomania, suicidal ideation, aggression, and worsening of mood have been observed less commonly. Symptoms begin 2–5 days after the last dose of medication and subside within 1 or 2 days after the medication is re-introduced. No or few withdrawal reactions have been associated with fluoxetine and sertraline. Approximate frequency of withdrawal reactions is: clomipramine, 30%; paroxetine and fluvoxamine, 20%; sertraline, 3%. However, withdrawal symptoms seldom occur in patients treated for fewer than 6 weeks.

*Tricyclic antidepressants*

The TCAs may be indicated when trials with SSRIs have been ineffective or if side effects of the SSRIs are not tolerable. The noradrenergic properties of the TCAs may be particularly advantageous when severe anergy and anhedonia are present. Patients with severe depression, particularly the hospitalized, may require a drug with prominent noradrenergic activity. However, some newer drugs such as venlafaxine and mirtazapine, which affect both serotonin and norepinephrine receptors, may be effective alternatives in patients with these features.

The side effects of the TCAs result from their actions

on a number of neurochemical receptors: histamine H-1, muscarinic, and alpha-1 adrenergic receptors (Table 25.5). Many psychiatrists prefer nortriptyline and desipramine to the other compounds in this class because of a better side effect profile. An adequate therapeutic trial of TCAs requires a full dosage for at least 4–8 weeks. Serum levels afford an accurate gauge for adequate TCA dosing. Although combinations of an SSRI and TCA are sometimes prescribed, the effects of SSRIs on the cytochrome P-450 system in the liver can cause an increase in TCA levels with consequent serious side effects.

*Monoamine oxidase inhibitors*

MAOIs have rarely been used since the introduction of the new antidepressants. Patients receiving MAOIs need to avoid tyramine-containing foods and sympathomimetic agents because the diet-drug or drug-drug

**TABLE 25.4. Antidepressant Drugs**

| Biological Action | Drug | Daily Dose Range (mg) | Major Side Effects |
|---|---|---|---|
| Predominantly norepinephrine reuptake inhibitors | Amitriptyline | 75–300 | Anticholinergic<br>Sedation<br>Weight gain<br>Postural hypotension |
| | Doxepin | 75–300 | As above |
| | Imipramine | 75–300 | As above |
| | Desipramine | 75–300 | As above but less severe |
| | Nortriptyline | 50–200 | As for desipramine |
| SSRIs | Fluoxetine | 20–60 | GI upset<br>Agitation<br>Akathisia<br>Sexual dysfunction |
| | Paroxetine | 20–50 | Sedation<br>Sexual dysfunction<br>SIADH<br>Withdrawal syndrome |
| | Sertraline | 50–200 | Diarrhea<br>Sexual dysfunction |
| | Citalopram | 20–40 | GI upset<br>Less sexual dysfunction |
| | Fluvoxamine* | 50–300 | GI upset<br>Sedation<br>Sexual dysfunction |
| Norepinephrine and dopamine reuptake inhibitors | Bupropion | 200–450 | Anticholinergic<br>Anxiety |
| Serotonin and norepinephrine reuptake inhibitors | Venlafaxine | 75–300 | Hypertension<br>Withdrawal syndrome<br>Sexual dysfunction |
| Serotonin antagonist and reuptake inhibitor | Trazodone | 200–500 | Sedation<br>Weight gain<br>Anticholinergic—mild |
| | Nefazodone | 200–600 | As for trazodone |
| Noradrenergic and serotonin antagonist | Mirtazapine | 15–45 | Sedation<br>Anticholinergic<br>Increased appetite |
| Monoamine oxidase inhibitors | Phenelzine | 15–60 | Toxic reactions to sympathomimetic drugs and tyramine containing foods<br>Orthostatic hypotension<br>Weight gain |
| | Tranylcypromine | 20–40 | As for phenelzine |

SIADH.
*Used mainly for treatment of obsessive-comulsive disorder.

**TABLE 25.5. Physiologic Effects of Tricyclic Antidepressants**

| |
|---|
| Histamine H-1 receptor blockade |
| Sedation |
| Weight gain |
| Hypotension |
| Potentiation of central depressant drugs |
| Muscarinic receptor blockade |
| Blurred vision |
| Constipation |
| Urinary retention |
| Dry mouth |
| Sinus tachycardia |
| Alpha-1 adrenergic receptor blockade |
| Dizziness |
| Postural hypotension |
| Reflex tachycardia |
| Potentiation of antihypertensive medications ($\alpha$-1 blockers) |

interaction can produce a hypertensive crisis. Other adverse effects are orthostatic hypotension, weight gain, edema, insomnia, and sexual dysfunction. Patients should be instructed to discontinue the drug 2 weeks before a surgical or dental procedure or use another drug because of the risk of drug interactions. A toxic drug-drug interaction also can occur with SSRIs and MAOIs, and at least 2 weeks must elapse between the administrations of drugs from these classes. Because of the range of new antidepressants and the serious MAOI toxic side effects, there is little necessity for these drugs at this time.

*Additional antidepressant drugs*

Effectiveness of treatment of depression is optimal when the treating physician has had experience with a wide variety of the available drugs. Mirtazapine and venlafaxine may be used as first-line treatment or withheld for use when SSRIs are ineffective. Side effects are more frequent with these drugs than with the SSRIs. Bupropion is an atypical antidepressant with effects on norepinephrine and dopamine systems. Nefazodone and trazodone, which have primarily serotoninergic effects, are also available. The predominant mode of action of these drugs and major side effects are listed in Table 25.4.

MIRTAZAPINE

This noradrenergic and serotoninergic modulator may produce side effects of weight gain, sedation, fatigue, and increased appetite. In comparative studies, its effectiveness in the treatment of depression has been shown to be equivalent to that of amitriptyline.

VENLAFAXINE

In addition to its indication for the treatment of depression, venlafaxine has also been approved by the FDA for the treatment of generalized anxiety disorder. It may be particularly useful in severe depression and treatment-resistant depression. It is thought to have a more rapid demonstrable effect than other antidepressants. There is a significant toxic withdrawal syndrome somewhat similar to that seen with withdrawal of some SSRIs. There is a dose-dependent increase in blood pressure, and the drug may provoke hypertension in previously normotensive persons. This effect is believed to subside when the drug is withdrawn.

BUPROPION

This drug has also been used for smoking cessation. It does not carry a risk of sexual dysfunction, as do the SSRIs. There is a risk of seizures at high doses in patients with a history of seizures or head trauma. It is available as a second- or third-line drug in the treatment of depression.

NEFAZODONE

This drug is less sedating than trazodone, yet still has that propensity. Some studies have shown a response in patients in whom an SSRI trial failed when nefazodone was used in doses of 400–600 mg. A carefully designed study found monotherapy with nefazodone and cognitive-behavioral treatment to be equally effective. However, the combination of the two modalities raised the response rate significantly.

TRAZODONE

This drug is not commonly used in the treatment of depression. It is highly sedating and has found use in medical practice as an adjunct in the treatment of some sleep disorders.

**Psychotherapy**

The optimal treatment of patients with depression is a combination of psychotherapy and medication. Despite efforts to standardize forms of psychotherapy, particularly cognitive-behavioral, psychotherapy by its nature will continue to be highly dependent on the experience and skill of the therapist. A match of temperament between psychotherapist and patient facilitates the effectiveness of the process. In general, medication alone is more consistently effective than psychotherapy alone. The role of psychotherapy alone in the treatment of depression is controversial; however, selected patients with mild chronic depression may do well with psychotherapy alone. Patients with a contraindication to antidepressants or who have had an inadequate drug response after a thorough trial are also candidates. Patients who are suicidal require both medication and psychotherapy, and are placed at great risk if antidepressant medication is withheld.

## Seasonal Affective Disorder (Winter Depression)

SAD is a clinical syndrome of depression that occurs in the autumn and winter seasons and remits in the spring. The syndrome is characterized by the presence of a depressed mood, lack of energy, and a tendency to sleep excessively. The patients tend to overeat, crave carbohydrates, and gain weight. Surveys conducted in East Coast cities of the United States suggest a 16–20% incidence. The prevalence is greater at higher latitudes. The syndrome appears to be most common in women and young adults. To be diagnostic, the symptoms must occur yearly during the same time period. The application of bright-light therapy has achieved a good response in approximately 70% of patients. Improvement is seen 4–5 days after initiation of light therapy. A daily exposure for 1 hour to a light intensity of 10,000 lux is required. Some patients are well-treated with antidepressant medication. Careful consideration should be given to the possibility of a bipolar disorder type II manifesting a seasonal pattern.

# CHAPTER 26 PSYCHOTIC DISORDERS

A psychosis is characterized by bizarre subjective mental experiences, and is manifested by behavior that deviates grossly from the ordinary. Although the phenomena of delusions and/or hallucinations are common identifying features of a psychotic process, cognition is markedly impaired, perceptions are misinterpreted, and emotions and mood become inappropriate to the life context. The presumed altered brain physiology in the psychosis results in a profound disruption of the individual's processing of social/cultural signals and their meanings. As a result, the world around them becomes unfamiliar. The previously understood ordinary social signals are deciphered in an idiosyncratic fashion that lacks connection to their socially accepted meanings. Under these circumstances, cognition is severely disrupted and the patient loses the capacity to function in a coherent, socially congruent manner.

It has been postulated that in a psychosis, neural systems become "heated up." In such a state, each neuron behaves in a more random fashion—that is, the neurons become less precise in responding to the excitatory and inhibitory inputs from the other neurons in the system. This theory would suggest a common mechanism of neural network perturbations provoked by a variety of pathologic inciting agents and processes, all leading to a common final pathway of altered neurophysiology resulting in the clinical psychotic state. Common psychotic disorders are listed in Table 26.1.

## Schizophrenia

Schizophrenia is regarded as the quintessential psychotic disorder, in which the patient presents with florid, bizarre manifestations. Reported worldwide, schizophrenia has a lifetime morbidity risk of approximately 8 per 1000. The onset is most often abrupt, beginning during adolescence and in the early 20s in men but allegedly later in women, although still usually by the fourth decade of life. There has been, and continues to be, an unfortunate tendency to conflate psychosis and schizophrenia. As a result, psychoses of other types may be labeled as schizophrenia, resulting in inappropriate treatment.

### Etiology

The etiology and pathogenesis of schizophrenia continue to be elusive. Although genetic factors are

**TABLE 26.1. The Psychotic Disorders**

| Disorder | Age of Onset | External Precipitant | Chronicity | Need for Maintenance Treatment |
|---|---|---|---|---|
| Schizophrenia | Late teens, 20s | No | Yes | Yes |
| Bipolar I—manic | 20s–40s | First episode | Yes | Yes |
| Bipolar II—depressed | 20s–30s | First episode | Yes | Often |
| Delirium | >60 | Yes | No | No |
| Psychosis of dementia | >60 | Sometimes | Yes | Often |
| Psychoactive drug abuse | Teens–35 | Yes | No | No |
| Medication induced | Any age | Yes | No | No |
| Brief psychotic disorder | Teens–35 | Yes | No | No |

thought to play a role, most cases of schizophrenia are sporadic. Post-mortem morphometric studies using new techniques have failed to reveal precise and consistent abnormalities in schizophrenia. A variety of anatomic deviations have been reported on brain imaging, such as increased ventricular volume, reduced gray matter volume, and other abnormalities. The search for the "final theory" of schizophrenia pathogenesis continues, with the neurodevelopment theory currently holding sway. This theory contends that schizophrenics harbor brain lesions that originated very early in life, in the intrauterine period or in the perinatal period, perhaps due to infection (viral), perinatal trauma, or abnormal patterns of neural migration. A genetic defect may render the fetal brain susceptible to early viral infection or associated immune response mechanisms or both. One theoretical model hypothesizes an "over-pruning" of axon–dendrite connections. It is postulated that immature neural circuitry exposed to the synaptic pruning process of late childhood and adolescence suffers an over-pruning with resultant brain dysfunction and the schizophrenic psychosis. The nature of the schizophrenic symptoms suggests a disturbance in neuronal signaling in the circuits that connect the cerebral cortex and limbic system with some involvement of cerebellar and thalamic connections. Glutamate, the brain's principal excitatory neurotransmitter, and its regulator of release, N-methyl-D-aspartate (NMDA), are suspected to be dysfunctional in schizophrenia.

## Clinical Features

Schizophrenia presents as an acute psychosis with a dramatic onset. As a rule, someone notices the patient's inappropriate behavior. A characteristic of an individual in a psychotic state is impaired insight regarding their condition. Hallucinations are usually auditory, although visual perception may be distorted. Memories appear de novo without relation to real events and evolve into delusions, which are impervious to modification by persuasion. Hallucinations are felt as alien, originating from the outside. Delusions and hallucinations are felt by the patient to be imposed by some external force (paranoia). Delusions have varying content and may be somatic (e.g., "I know I have brain cancer"), persecutory (e.g., "My father is trying to poison me"), or grandiose (e.g., "I control the universe"). In the acute phase, the patient is highly excitable, and because a psychosis precludes insight, the patient usually does not believe treatment is necessary, and more often than not, resists it. Hospitalization is essential in the acute psychotic episode because of the hazards of self-harm and aggressive behavior. A commitment process is sometimes required in order to treat the patient.

## Pharmacologic Treatment of Schizophrenia

The antipsychotic drugs exert two principal beneficial roles in the treatment of psychoses. The first and most immediate is a calming or tranquilizing effect that relieves the agitation of the patient, preventing aggressive acts and enabling the patient to carry out his vital life functions. The tranquilizing action is an immediate one and is dependent on careful dose titration. The second clinical effect is to reduce the intensity of, and perhaps eliminate, the florid psychotic symptoms of hallucinations, delusions, thought disorder, and distressed mood.

Tables 26.2 and 26.3 present drugs used in treating schizophrenia.

The treatment of schizophrenia and, indeed, all psychoses was dramatically changed by the introduction of chlorpromazine in the 1950s. It was the first in a series of drugs called neuroleptics (antipsychotic drugs), whose main efficacy is in the treatment of psychotic disorders. The first-generation neuroleptics were presumed to exert their therapeutic effect by blocking dopamine postsynaptic receptors. Beginning with clozapine (1989), a number of antipsychotic drugs emerged with predominant effects on the serotoninergic neurotransmitter systems and less effect on the dopamine systems, particularly the D2 receptors. The action of the new antipsychotic drugs, which do not exert their principal effect on the dopaminergic system, opens to question the unitary theory of dopamine neurotransmitter dysfunction in schizophrenia. The advent of the second-generation anti-psychotic drugs, which have a more favorable side effect profile and a beneficial effect on the so-called "negative symptoms" of schizophrenia, has altered the treatment landscape of this illness.

## Treatment of the Acute Psychosis

The introduction of second-generation antipsychotic drugs has resulted in a reassessment of optimum treatment of the psychoses in both the acute and chronic stages. Up until the introduction of these new drugs, the gold standard of emergency treatment of the agitated psychotic patient was the use of haloperidol in an initial dose of 2–5 mg intramuscularly (IM) combined with lorazepam 2 mg IM. This regimen carries a risk of acute dystonic reactions; diphenhydramine can be used to treat this untoward reaction. Recent studies have validated an equivalent efficacy with a regimen of risperidone 2 mg of liquid concentrate with lorazepam 2 mg orally or 1–2 mg IM. The initial dose of risperidone–lorazepam can be repeated in the first 24 hours as needed. This regimen requires acceptance of the oral route by the patient. Because most second-generation antipsychotics are not currently available in parenteral form, haloperidol is available when necessary and in the event of an inadequate response to a risperidone–lorazepam combination. A particularly strong case can be made for the avoidance of the first-generation antipsychotic drugs in the elderly, patients with a history of cardiac disease, and patients with a history of extrapyramidal effects or tardive dyskinesia.

After the emergency management of the agitated psychotic patient, the treatment of the acute psychosis can proceed with the use of a second-generation antipsychotic drug for pharmacologic management. The use of second-generation drugs enables the physician to avoid the acute dystonias and akathisia produced by the first-generation drugs. The high-potency drugs, risperidone and olanzapine, are preferred over the low-potency drugs, clozapine and quetiapine. Optimal titration of these drugs can usually be effected within 3 days.

The optimal stabilizing doses of antipsychotic drugs may be higher than those used for long-term chronic treatment. The recommended optimal daily dose of risperidone is 6 mg (extrapyramidal symptoms have been reported with risperidone at doses over 6 mg/day), and for olanzapine is 10–20 mg, in the acute phase of the psychosis. Quetiapine is thought to have a slower onset of effectiveness, but if used, an optimal daily dose is 300 mg. If haldol (first-generation drug) is used, it should also be noted that there are few clinical or pharmacologic data to support the use of doses of haloperidol higher than 5–10 mg per day in the management of acute psychosis.

## Treatment in the Chronic Phase

The goals of pharmacologic intervention in schizophrenia are the reduction and control of hallucinations, delusions, cognitive disorganization, and agitation. In addition, the amelioration of negative symptoms can facilitate improved social functioning and promote the well-being of the patient. These negative symptoms are emotional flattening, lack of initiative, depressive symptoms, and cognitive sluggishness. Although these negative symptoms are generally ascribed to the schizophrenic process itself, the first-generation antipsychotic drugs likely contribute to them. The second-generation antipsychotic drugs have efficacy in relieving the negative symptoms seen in schizophrenia. The early use of

**TABLE 26.2. Typical (First-Generation) Antipsychotic Drugs**

| Predominant mode of action: dopamine-2 receptor blockade | | |
|---|---|---|
| **Class** | **Drug** | **Daily Dose (mg)*** |
| **Phenothiazines** | Chlorpromazine | 50–200 |
| | Thioridazine | 25–100 |
| | Fluphenazine | 2–15 |
| | Perphenazine | 4–32 |
| | Trifluoperazine | 2–15 |
| **Thioxanthenes** | Thiothixene | 2–15 |
| **Dibenzapines** | Loxapine | 5–25 |
| **Indoles** | Molindone | 15–100 |
| **Butyrophenones** | Haloperidol | 2–12 |

| **Major Side Effects†** | |
|---|---|
| **Cardiac** | Prolongation QTc interval |
| | Torsades de pointes |
| **Neurologic** | Seizure lability |
| | Neuroleptic malignant syndrome |
| | Akathisia |
| | Extrapyramidal (Parkinson-like) symptoms |
| | Tardive dyskinesia |
| | Anticholinergic symptoms |
| **Histamine 1 blockade** | Somnolence |
| | Weight gain |
| **α-2 blockade** | Orthostatic hypotension |
| | CNS depression |
| | Lethargy |
| | Hyperprolactinemia |

*Higher doses may be required in acute psychosis and selected chronic schizophrenia patients
†Severity of side effects may vary for individual drugs and may depend on the patient's pharmacogenetics.

TABLE 26.3. Atypical (Second-Generation) Antipsychotic Drugs

| Biochemistry | Daily Dose (mg) | Major Side Effects |
|---|---|---|
| **Clozapine*** | | |
| High serotonin 5HT/dopamine binding ratio<br>Less dopamine-2 binding than first-generation drugs<br>Hepatic metabolism via P-450 [CYP1A2] enzymes | 300–900 | Agranulocytosis<br>Weight gain<br>Sedation<br>Orthostatic hypotension<br>Salivation<br>Eosinophilia<br>Seizures (dose related)<br>P-450–related drug-drug interactions |
| **Olanzapine** | | |
| High serotonin 5HT/dopamine binding ratio<br>Hepatic metabolism via P-450 [CYP1A2] enzymes and N-glucuronidation | 5–20† | Weight gain<br>New-onset diabetes reported<br>P-450–related drug-drug interactions |
| **Risperidone** | | |
| Antagonizes dopamine-2 and serotonin—5HT-2 receptors<br>Hepatic metabolism via P-450 [CYP2D6] enzymes to active hydroxylated metabolite | 2–8‡ | Orthostatic hypotension<br>Somnolence<br>Extrapyramidal symptoms at higher doses<br>Weight gain |
| **Quetiapine** | | |
| High serotonin 5HT/dopamine binding ratio<br>Hepatic metabolism via P-450 [CYP3A4] enzymes is slower in elderly | 300–400 | Orthostatic hypotension<br>Somnolence<br>Weight gain<br>Lipid and LFT elevations |

*Available only for patients and providers who submit data to registry, and medication dispensed must only be enough to last until next scheduled blood test.
†Therapeutic level: 0.09–0.023 μg/ml.
‡ Dose adjust for renal impairment and elderly patients.

clozapine in treatment-refractory cases of schizophrenia disclosed an improvement in the negative symptoms of the patients. Risperidone, olanzapine, quetiapine, and ziprasidone have been observed to have similar beneficial effects.

The efficacy of antipsychotic drugs in the acute phase is well established. The successful treatment of the chronic phase is more difficult. It is not uncommon for auditory hallucinations to continue despite best efforts with antipsychotic drugs. Approximately 40% of patients presumed to be under adequate therapy and two thirds of patients not receiving treatment will suffer a psychotic relapse within 1 year. Rehospitalization frequently is caused by noncompliance with prescribed medication and/or an excessive use of alcohol or addicting street drugs. For some noncompliant patients, the administration of injectable depot haloperidol has been necessary to ensure adequate pharmacologic treatment. Anticonvulsants have been prescribed empirically for their mood-stabilizing properties for some chronic schizophrenic patients.

Compliance with medication is improved when the side effects are kept at a minimum. Common side effects of the first-generation drugs such as extrapyramidal Parkinson-like symptoms, persistent akathisia, hyperprolactinemia, autonomic dysfunction, weight gain, and potential tardive dyskinesia cause impaired function of the patient and also frequently result in noncompliance. Life-threatening neuroleptic malignant syndrome is also a risk in administration of first-generation antipsychotics. These symptoms are less common with second-generation drugs; however, other side effects are unique to some of the second-generation neuroleptics. Early on, agranulocytosis was reported in a small number of patients receiving clozapine; as a result, weekly monitoring of white blood cell counts is recommended. An increased incidence of diabetes mellitus has been observed in patients treated with antipsychotics, particularly the second-generation drugs. See Tables 26.2 and 26.3 for more detailed information on neuroleptic side effect profiles and recommended dosages.

The chronicity of the schizophrenic process results in serious social and occupational dysfunction of the patient, entailing much hardship on the patient, family, and society. An active rehabilitative, socially supportive program combined with careful psychiatric monitoring is most desirable. Programs that include active on-site visits and monitoring by a professional team can reduce relapses and hospitalizations and enhance social functioning of the patient.

## Bipolar Disorder

The former diagnosis of manic-depressive disorder has been replaced in DSM IV-TR nomenclature by the term bipolar disorder. This is further subdivided into bipolar I and bipolar II. The essential feature of bipolar I is a clinical course characterized by one or more manic episodes, or mixed manic/depressive episodes; often the individual has had one or more major depressive episodes. Bipolar II is characterized by the occurrence of one or more major depressive episodes accompanied by at least one hypomanic episode.

The manic psychosis is characterized by gross disturbance in mood, behavior, and thought. The typical manic symptoms include euphoric expansiveness with agitation, high energy level, and sleeplessness. Grandiose delusions may lead to self-destructive behavior. Associated irritability occurs, especially if the person senses that he or she will be thwarted. Euphoria usually leads to unrealistic behavior in the occupational, interpersonal, and sexual spheres. Excessive buying and attempts at inappropriate business deals are common. The patient manifests little need for sleep and may be awake for days at a time in the manic state. Hyperactivity and a thought pattern of rapid, loose associations prompting pressured speech often occur. The psychosis may be severe, with persecutory delusions and auditory hallucinations. Despite the euphoria and mania, suicide risk is quite high. Co-morbid substance abuse, particularly of alcohol, is not uncommon in bipolar disorders. As in other psychoses, insight is lacking. Family members or others usually must intervene to obtain treatment for the patient. Hospitalization is almost always necessary in the manic state.

More than 90% of individuals who have a primary manic episode will suffer future episodes. First episodes of mania and depression in bipolar patients are usually precipitated by social or interpersonal stress. Bipolar disorder patients are particularly vulnerable to stressful life events. Major depressive episodes may alternate with manic episodes. In some patients, the episodes of mania and depression may alternate in a matter of weeks, producing the clinical picture known as "rapid cycling". Indeed, the manic state, contrary to popular belief, is not a happy one, and "rapid cyclers" particularly have a significant dysphoria bordering on outright depression in the midst of the mania. As in the manic state, the suicide risk is high. The illness most commonly begins in late adolescence and into the thirties; however, a second peak may occur in women around the menopause, and onset in the elderly, particularly men, has been described. In recent years, the diagnosis of bipolar disorder has been made with increasing frequency by the psychiatric profession.

A secondary manic psychosis may be caused by medications, some medical disorders, neurological diseases, infections, or metabolic derangement. Prednisone has been known to precipitate a manic psychosis. Elderly patients are particularly at risk for secondary mania. Although less frequent than primary manic psychosis, this diagnosis should be considered in hospitalized patients, in whom the symptoms may resemble a delirium. The onset of this type of secondary manic psychosis is usually sudden. The precipitating causes need to be identified and addressed. Treatment may require antimanic drugs for a short period of time.

### Treatment of Acute Mania

Manic episodes frequently require hospitalization. Lithium carbonate has been the mainstay in the treatment of acute manic episodes since its introduction some 50 years ago. As monotherapy, it is effective in controlling the manic episode in about 50% of patients. The usual lithium doses are 900–1500 mg/day to secure a serum level at the high end of the therapeutic range, 1.0–1.5 mEq/L. The anticonvulsant divalproex sodium has also established efficacy equivalent to lithium in the treatment of acute mania. An oral loading dose of 20–30 mg/kg/day may be given for 3 days to effect a serum level above 50 μg/ml. Carbamazepine and other anticonvulsants are available if neither lithium nor divalproex is tolerated, however the efficacy of other anticonvulsants for this disorder has not been well established by controlled trials. The concomitant administration of lorazepam orally or IM may be desirable for its anxiolytic and sedative effects. Patients with gross delusions, hallucinations, and inadequate response to the mood stabilizing drugs will benefit from the addition of an antipsychotic drug to the regimen. Risperidone in a dose of 2–4 mg/day or olanzapine in a dose of 5–10 mg/day are appropriate additions. Haloperidol can be reserved for refractory patients. Outpatients may be maintained at the lower end of the lithium therapeutic range, at 0.6–0.7mEq/L. Lithium therapy, which can have significant medical complications (Table 26.4), requires close monitoring. Lithium and divalproex can be monitored with serum levels.

### Long-Term Management of Bipolar Disorder

The long-term management of the patient with bipolar disorder is a challenging one. Remissions and exacerbations are characteristic, and many of the patients function well when in remission. The phenomena of mixed mania (manic manifestations with dysphoria) and rapid cycling between depression and mania present particular challenges. Divalproex may be preferable in these states, particularly if lithium has failed or produced

TABLE 26.4. Side Effects of Lithium and Valproate*

| Lithium | Valproate |
|---|---|
| **Neuropsychiatric**<br>Ataxia, tremor, confusion, somnolence, delirium, tinnitus, blurred vision | **Neuropsychiatric**<br>Dose-related ataxia, fine resting tremor, drowsiness |
| **Renal**<br>Nephrogenic diabetes insipidus<br>Late development of nephritis | **Endocrine**<br>Hyponatremia due to SIADH |
| **Cardiac**<br>Sinoatrial block<br>T-wave changes | **Gastrointestinal**<br>Liver enzyme elevations<br>Hepatotoxicity (rare) |
| **Endocrine**<br>Goiter and/or hypothyroidism<br>Hyperglycemia | **Dermatologic**<br>Rash |
| **Gastrointestinal**<br>Dose-related nausea<br>Diarrhea | **Hematologic**<br>Thrombocytopenia |
| **Others**<br>Weight gain<br>Lower extremity edema<br>Leukocytosis | **Other**<br>Hyperammonemia |
| **Drug-drug interactions**<br>Some examples are: tetracycline, carbamazepine, NSAIDs, thiazide, SSRIs, ACE-Is. | **Drug-drug interactions**<br>Some examples are: anticonvulsants, anticoagulants, CNS depressants, hepatotoxins |

*The side-effects of Valproate tend to be milder and less frequent than those of lithium.
Syndrome of Inappropriate Antidiuretic Hormone (SIADH); ACE-I = Angiotensin-converting enzyme inhibitor.

untoward side effects. The management of the depression in bipolar disorder is difficult because the classic antidepressant drugs may provoke mania during administration or on cessation. For this reason, it is usually desirable to administer a mood-stabilizing drug with an antidepressant when antidepressant treatment is needed. Patients who have an inadequate response to one mood-stabilizing drug may improve with the addition of a second mood stabilizer. Anticonvulsants such as carbamazepine, lamotrigine, gabapentin, and topiramate have been prescribed empirically for this purpose. Some refractory patients have been maintained on antipsychotic drugs after the acute manic episode. Many of these patients are maintained on multiple drugs. In view of their exquisite vulnerability to stressful life events, psychotherapy and attention to psychosocial stressors should be included in the treatment program.

## Major Depressive Disorder with Psychosis

Psychotic symptoms may occur in some patients with a depressive illness. Although most commonly seen after age 45, this delusional depression may be seen in younger patients as well. The diagnosis is particularly difficult in the elderly, who may have cognitive deficits secondary to dementia. Agitation accompanied by somatic, persecutory, or paranoid delusions and marked withdrawal are the features of a psychotic depression. Auditory hallucinations occur in 20% and visual hallucinations in 7% of these patients. Delusions are characteristic and involve a preoccupation with one's guilt, a need for self-punishment, and suicidal ideation. The psychotic, depressed patient, particularly a man living alone, is at great risk of suicide. Given the high suicide risk, difficulty in treatment, and profound self-neglect of the delusional patient, hospitalization is usually needed.

Approximately 30–40% of these patients will respond to antidepressant therapy, but the response rate increases to 60–70% with the addition of an antipsychotic drug. The TCAs, particularly desipramine and nortriptyline, have the advantage of long-established efficacy, although comparison studies suggest that the SSRIs and the atypical antidepressants (bupropion, mirtazepine and venlafaxine) may be equally effective with fewer side effects. Because venlafaxine may have a more rapid onset of effect, it deserves serious consideration as a first-line choice. Risperidone and olanzapine are antipsychotics of choice in this situation because of their favorable side effect profile. Electroconvulsive treatment (ECT) is available for drug nonresponse or as primary treatment in selected patients. ECT produces a faster clinical response than drug therapy, and when the severity of illness demands urgent treatment, ECT may be appropriate initial therapy. Relapse after remission following ECT may necessitate follow-up ECT and/or maintenance ECT. Antidepressant medication is usually prescribed after ECT.

## Brief Psychotic Disorder (Brief Reactive Psychosis)

The criteria for diagnosing this disorder, previously termed brief reactive psychosis, include the following: the appearance of psychotic symptoms shortly after a traumatic event that is clearly stressful, mental confusion, disorganized speech, rapid shifts of intense affects, and delusions and hallucinations accompanied by disorganized thought processes and behavior. The duration of the psychosis is usually a matter of days but no longer than 2–4 weeks, and full recovery with no residual effects should occur. Other types of psychotic disorders are excluded by careful history taking and by noting the bizarre nature of the shifting symptoms. Patients can often be managed with anxiolytics. If antipsychotic drugs are used, the second-generation drugs in low doses are preferred. If the diagnosis is accurate, they may only be needed for a few days. After the patient recovers from the psychosis, vulnerability factors can be determined. An underlying personality disorder and an anxiety diathesis are often present.

## Psychosis in the Course of Medical Illness

Psychosis in the course of a medical illness is manifested as delirium. This is an acute disorder of brain function characterized by acute onset with the predominant symptoms of fluctuating consciousness, disorientation, perceptual distortions, profound restlessness and agitation, disturbance of the sleep–wake cycle, visual hallucinations, and fragmented, rambling speech. Both recent and remote memory are impaired and distorted. Symptoms tend to fluctuate during a 24-hour period. Autonomic nervous system dysregulation is present with sweating, tachycardia, and flushed appearance. Electroencephalograms reveal generalized cortical slowing.

Delirium in the elderly may be the first manifestation of an underlying medical illness. The delirious patient requires a prompt, complete medical examination and hospitalization for safety reasons because of associated combativeness. Elderly hospitalized patients are particularly prone to delirium, often caused by infections, organ failure, metabolic derangements, dehydration, postoperative states, and neurological events including stroke. Prescribed drugs, particularly when patients are receiving multiple drugs, are frequent precipitants of delirium. The more severe the illness, the greater the risk of delirium. Determining the cause is of primary importance because recovery from the delirium depends on treatment of the underlying illness. Delirium increases length of hospital stay and increases mortality significantly. Delirium must be differentiated from other psychoses, particularly alcohol and drug withdrawal, manic psychosis, agitation in a demented patient, and brain lesions.

Physicians need to be alert to early mental changes in hospitalized patients, particularly the elderly. Usually nurses are the first persons to detect mental status changes in the patients. Prompt measures are desirable to limit the course of the delirium. Treatment requires attention to the environment, limiting stimulation as much as possible. Nursing attention is crucial, as are safety measures. Supportive medical and nursing care is critical. Antipsychotic drugs can effectively control the agitation and decrease the severity of the thought disturbance, delusions, and hallucinations. Because many of the patients are elderly and sensitive to the extrapyramidal side effects of drugs, the second-generation antipsychotic drugs are preferred for initial treatment. Risperidone in doses of 2–4 mg or olanzapine in doses of 5–10 mg can be effective in controlling symptoms. Haloperidol has a longer demonstrated clinical effectiveness and may be used; doses of 1–4 mg initially may be given parenterally and further dose titration should be based on clinical response. If the dose is not controlled, haloperidol may produce delayed excessive sedation, stupor, and extrapyramidal effects. The course of recovery varies, but persistent delirium requires further diagnostic evaluation for brain diseases, particularly dementia.

## Psychosis of Dementia

Deficits in memory, aphasia (deterioration of language function), agnosia (impaired ability to recognize various sensory stimuli), and apraxia (impaired performance of skilled or purposeful movements), which then result in global intellectual impairment, are characteristic of dementia. Psychosis can occur in the course of dementia. Delusions (frequently of theft and infidelity) complicate Alzheimer disease in as many as 30% of patients. These delusions may sometimes precede the cognitive symptoms as the disease advances. Hallucinations, most often visual, have been reported in approximately 25% of patients. Patients with Alzheimer disease often display irritability, agitation, and aggressive behavior. Psychosis should be suspected when such symptoms develop or when behavior changes suddenly in the course of dementia.

As a general rule, antipsychotic drugs for disrupting delusions and hallucinations appearing in the course of dementia may be useful. Second-generation antipsychotics such as risperidone, olanzapine, and quetiapine in small doses are preferred. Low-dose clozapine has been shown to be effective in psychosis in the course of Parkinson disease. Short-term use of the drugs is preferred when possible. Benzodiazepines for agitation are useful in some patients when used cautiously and in small doses. Buspirone may be preferable because of the lack of risk of respiratory depression. Trazodone is a useful sedating drug. SSRIs have sometimes improved mood and increased interest in surroundings. Long-term neuroleptic therapy can be avoided by carefully watching for any reappearance of psychotic symptoms, providing good nursing care, and using anxiolytics (e.g., lorazepam, buspirone). Some Alzheimer disease patients may benefit from treatment of depression with an SSRI.

## Psychosis Caused by Pharmacologic Agents

Many commonly used drugs may cause psychosis, often from an idiosyncratic reaction, a toxic overdose, or withdrawal. The proliferation of new drugs has increased the hazard of drug-drug interactions, producing a psychosis. The differential diagnosis usually involves the exclusion of a toxic delirium, manic state, or direct brain involvement by the disease process. Hallucinations, paranoid delusions, and agitation are presenting symptoms. The list of drugs that reportedly produce psychotic states is long, and one should be alert to this possibility in hospitalized patients and patients on multiple drugs. The risk of adverse drug events increases with the number of drugs taken by the patient. Treatment consists of withdrawal of the drug (psychosis usually remits promptly after this) and treatment with an anxiolytic such as lorazepam and a second-generation antipsychotic agent when necessary.

## Psychosis Caused by Psychoactive Substance Abuse

Cocaine and amphetamines may produce acute toxic states with psychotic manifestations. Amphetamines trigger a release of catecholamines from storage sites in the central and peripheral nervous systems. The action of cocaine is somewhat similar to amphetamines because it inhibits the reuptake of catecholamines both peripherally and centrally. Accordingly, in the acute toxic phase, the patient manifests evidence of sympathetic system hyperactivity as well as a variety of psychiatric and neurological symptoms and signs. Bizarre behavior, agitation, panic, tachycardia, hypertension, and hyperthermia may be seen. The toxic psychosis of chronic amphetamine or cocaine use is manifested by visual, auditory, and sometimes tactile hallucinations. Paranoid ideation with panic is characteristic. The presentation to the emergency department of a young person with sudden, recent onset of a psychosis should arouse suspicion of substance abuse.

The administration of diazepam or lorazepam is an appropriate measure in treating the acute psychosis caused by psychoactive drug abuse. Sympathomimetic blocking agents, administered parenterally, may be useful in blocking peripheral sympathetic effects. If prolonged, the treatment of the psychosis may require the short-term use of an antipsychotic drug.

The hallucinogens lysergic acid diethylamide (LSD) and methylenedioxymethamphetamine (MDMA) can also provoke psychotic episodes. The effects of these agents are believed to be mediated via 5-HT receptors in the brain. The most constant effect of these agents is to produce visual hallucinations and perceptual distortions. The effects on mood are variable, ranging from euphoria to panic to depression, and may provoke suicidal ideation and action. Rage reactions and paranoid delusions may also occur. Sympathomimetic effects may be manifest with hypertension, tachycardia, tremor, and sweating. Hypothermia due to MDMA is life threatening, and supportive medical care is critical. The best acute treatment of toxic psychosis is to provide a protective, tranquil environment and to administer benzodiazepines, either diazepam or lorazepam, and supportive medical and nursing care.

### Toxic States Caused by Psychopharmacologic Drugs

Three life-threatening syndromes caused by psychopharmacologic agents have been described. These are the toxic serotonin syndrome, neuroleptic malignant syndrome, and central anticholinergic syndrome (Table 26.5).

The serotonin syndrome is a potentially lethal condition of serotonin hyperstimulation usually brought on by the prescription of two or more drugs with serotonergic effects together. It may occur with single agents in sensitive patients. It may also present in the context of overdose. Symptoms usually present within 24 hours but can also develop over days to weeks. They include mental status changes (confusion, agitation, lethargy, coma), autonomic instability (fever, tachycardia, sweating, nausea, vomiting, diarrhea), and neuromuscular changes (myoclonus, hyperreflexia, rigidity). Treatment consists of removal of the offending agent and supportive care. Benzodiazepines, particularly clonazepam (Klonopin), are recommended for myoclonus. The use of serotonin antagonists such as cyproheptadine has been recommended, although systematic data regarding its efficacy are lacking. Lorazepam is useful to control agitation. This syn-

TABLE 26.5. Psychotropic Drug-Induced Toxic Syndromes

| Toxic Serotonin Syndrome | Neuroleptic Malignant Syndrome | Central Anticholinergic Syndrome |
|---|---|---|
| Confusion/agitation<br>Lethargy/coma<br>Fever<br>Tachycardia<br>Diaphoresis<br>Hyperreflexia<br>Myoclonus<br>Vomiting/diarrhea | Confusion<br>Possible coma<br>Fever<br>Blood pressure changes<br>Diaphoresis<br>Muscle rigidity<br>Rhabdomyolysis<br>Elevated creatine kinase<br>Leukocytosis | Confusion<br>Hallucinations<br>Fever<br>Tachycardia<br>Hot, dry skin<br>Seizures<br>Dilated pupils |
| | **Offending Drugs** | |
| SSRIs<br>Clomipramine<br>SSRIs in combination with MAOIs or atypical antipsychotics | First-generation antipsychotics<br>Second-generation antipsychotics (rare) | Tricyclic antidepressants<br>Antipsychotic drugs<br>Other anticholinergic drugs<br>Multiple drugs increase risk |
| | **Treatment** | |
| | Remove offending drug(s)<br>Appropriate supportive care | |
| Cyproheptadine<br>Lorazepam<br>Consider Propranolol | Bromocriptine<br>Amantadine<br>Dantrolene<br>Lorazepam | Consider Physostigmine |

drome can be difficult to distinguish from the neuroleptic malignant syndrome (NMS).

The NMS is a potentially fatal complication of the routine prescription of antipsychotic medication. The etiology is related to a dysregulation of the dopaminergic system. The incidence of NMS has been estimated as 1% of patients treated with antipsychotics. It is usually associated with the high-potency agents but has been known to occur with all antipsychotics, including the newer atypical agents. It usually occurs within the first 3–9 days of therapy but can occur any time in the course of therapy. Ambient heat and dehydration are predisposing factors. NMS is similar in presentation to the serotonin syndrome with mental status changes, autonomic instability, and neuromuscular changes. However, NMS tends to have higher fevers and more pronounced muscle rigidity, whereas serotonin syndrome tends to have more gastrointestinal (GI) dysfunction (nausea, diarrhea) and myoclonus. Laboratory evaluation usually reveals increased creatine kinase, myoglobinuria, and leukocytosis. Mortality has been estimated at 12–20%, usually due to renal failure or respiratory failure. Treatment consists of removal of the agent and intensive supportive care, including aggressive hydration and cooling blankets. Dantrolene sodium (Dantrium) and bromocriptine (Parlodel) are often administered to decrease skeletal muscle rigidity, although there have been some questions raised about their efficacy.

The central cholinergic syndrome is a hazard when two or more drugs with anti-cholinergic action are used. (see Table 26.5)

Drug-drug interactions are occurring with increased frequency as the prescription of multiple psychotropic drugs in a single individual has increased. The induction or inhibition of the cytochrome P-450 system by some agents, particularly the SSRIs and the atypical antipsychotics, is an example of the potential hazard of interaction of psychopharmacologic agents with other medications. Consequently, the physician needs to exercise care in differentiating symptoms of the illness from side effects of the drugs.

# CHAPTER 27 EATING DISORDERS

The manifestations of eating disorders vary from severe restriction of food intake and emaciation in anorexia nervosa to compulsive overeating and obesity, but an underlying theme is a preoccupation with external appearance. Although anorexia nervosa, bulimia nervosa, and compulsive overeating are identified as discrete disorders, they exist on a continuum and share some common features.

The vast majority (>90%) of eating disorders in the United States occur in women, with women between the ages 14 and 40 having the highest incidence. A history of sexual abuse prior to age 18 is a common thread in as many as 50% of women with eating disorders. Many of these women also suffer from depression, dysthymia, or OCD. Estimates of prevalence rates in the United States range from 1% to 10%, but the overall prevalence is probably 1%.

Although public awareness about eating disorders has become more widespread, the disorder remains somewhat hidden. Diagnosis may be delayed until serious medical complications arise because the patient conceals the problem even from close family members. Because most of these young women are seen initially by a gynecologist or primary care physician, these physicians must be aware of clues to early diagnosis.

## Anorexia Nervosa

Anorexia nervosa usually has its onset in adolescence and is characterized by extreme weight loss, an intense fear of gaining weight, and a distorted body-image concept. The DSM IV-TR criteria are listed in Table 27.1. The typical patient is a teenage girl, with average or above-average intelligence from a white, middle-class family, in which parental overcontrol or perfectionism may exist. Commonly, the girl is involved in athletic pursuits such as gymnastics or ballet. Obsessive-compulsive personality features may be present. A break-up with a boyfriend or remarks about her weight by other family members or peers may be cited as a precipitant for the weight loss. The weight loss arises from severe restriction of food intake and/or compulsive exercise; it is not unusual for these girls to exercise for 2 or 3 hours per day. They maintain energy by drinking large amounts of caffeinated diet soda. Besides weight loss, the other major symptom is secondary amenorrhea or, in the case of the prepubertal patient, primary amenorrhea. Cold intolerance, lightheadedness, palpitations, or peripheral edema may be noted.

**TABLE 27.1. Diagnostic Criteria for Anorexia Nervosa**

1. Failure to maintain body weight at 85% of normal for age and height.
2. Intense fear of gaining weight or becoming fat.
3. Distorted body concept and undue influence of weight on self-evaluation.
4. Amenorrhea as defined by the absence of at least three consecutive menstrual cycles.

Adapted from DSM IV-TR.

The most obvious physical sign is cachexia (general weight loss and wasting). The skin may be dry, and lanugo hair—a fine growth that is normally present in newborn babies—may be noted on the face or upper extremities. Bradycardia, with pulse rates as low as 30 or 40 beats per minute, and hypotension, with systolic pressures less than 90 mm Hg, are fairly common. In anorexia nervosa, medical complications can arise in many systems, as listed in Table 27.2.

**TABLE 27.2. Medical Complications of Anorexia Nervosa**

| | |
|---|---|
| Hematologic | Bone marrow hypoplasia with leukopenia and anemia |
| Cardiac | Bradycardia, hypotension, arrhythmias, rarely cardiomyopathy |
| Metabolic | Volume depletion, hypochloremic metabolic alkalosis, increased serum carotene |
| Endocrine | Low or normal thyroxine ($T_4$) levels, osteoporosis |
| Gynecologic | Amenorrhea, low LH, FSH, and estrogen levels |

LH = luteinizing hormone; FSH = follicle-stimulating hormone.

### Laboratory Studies

Blood test results may be within normal limits. Electrolyte levels should be obtained because potassium, sodium, and magnesium may be decreased. Marrow hypoplasia may result from malnutrition and be reflected in anemia, leukopenia, and thrombocytopenia. Thyroid function studies may show a low $T_4$, but the thyroid-stimulating hormone is normal (euthyroid sick pattern). Estrogen, luteinizing hormone, and follicle-stimulating hormone are at low pubertal levels, which results in the amenorrhea. Liver function test results may be abnormal.

The serum carotene level is usually elevated and may even cause a yellowish-orange tint to the skin in some patients.

An electrocardiogram (ECG) should be obtained in every patient. Sinus bradycardia, T-wave inversion, ST depression, and QT prolongation may be noted. QT prolongation may be ominous because it has been associated with sudden death.

### Management

Medical and psychiatric care of patients with anorexia nervosa is a challenge. The physician must be aware of potential complications because the long-term mortality rate is between 5% and 15%. About 40% of anorectic patients will recover completely, another 30% improve somewhat, and the remaining 25% have a chronic course throughout their lives. Early referral to a mental health professional with experience in treating eating disorders, regular counseling with a dietitian to evaluate and monitor nutritional intake, and family therapy are all critical. Outpatient care is preferable, but hospitalization is indicated when body weight is extremely low, metabolic abnormalities or dehydration are present, or psychosis is evident.

Because no medication consistently induces weight gain or prevents further loss, cognitive-behavioral therapy remains the mainstay of treatment. This usually involves 10–20 sessions over 3–6 months in which cognitive restructuring of the patient's extreme concerns about shape and weight takes place. In addition, education of the patient in the use of self-control measures and the introduction of regular patterns of eating are essential. This approach has been more effective than treatment with antidepressant drugs.

Drug treatment may be helpful if concurrent depression exists. The TCAs are somewhat effective. Because of their potential for cardiac side effects and the underlying bradycardia and QT prolongation often seen in anorexia nervosa, they must be used with caution. More recently, fluoxetine, an SSRI, has been used with some success. However, because fluoxetine might suppress appetite, food intake must be carefully monitored. Cyproheptadine, an antihistamine that stimulates appetite, has been helpful in severe cases of anorexia resistant to previous treatment. Because some patients have delayed gastric emptying or a sensation of bloating, metoclopramide may be of benefit.

Given the prolonged, extremely low estrogen levels, the risk of osteoporosis is high. About 50% of anorectics will have bone mineral density (BMD) two standard deviations below normal. Although bone density may increase after normal weight is achieved and menses resume, it is not known if BMD ever returns to baseline. Use of hormone replacement or oral contraceptives may increase BMD, but clear evidence from clinical trials is not available as yet. Bisphosphonates have not been studied in conjunction with anorexia. Adequate calcium intake or supplementation and vitamin and protein supplementation is indicated for most patients.

## Bulimia Nervosa

Patients with bulimia nervosa engage in recurrent episodes of binge eating followed by purging through vomiting, laxative use, diuretics, or enemas (Table 27.3). The average binge consists of 4000 calories, eaten rapidly, followed by quick vomiting. The patient has no self-control over the eating binge and usually feels very guilty afterward.

Anorexia nervosa and bulimia overlap considerably. Bulimia occurs predominantly in older (20–40 years) white women (Table 27.4). Bulimic persons are usually of normal weight or obese. They tend to be very well groomed and concerned with external appearance. Although "bingeing and purging" are the primary characteristics, bulimic persons also might restrict their food intake, go on periodic diets, and compulsively exercise. Low self-esteem and depression are very common. Substance abuse, particularly with alcohol, occurs in approximately one-third. Shoplifting and sexual promiscuity are also common. Anxiety and personality disorders (especially borderline personality) may be present.

Usual symptoms are nonspecific symptoms such as weakness; edema of the hands and feet; fainting spells; GI symptoms such as abdominal bloating, pain, or constipation; and menstrual irregularities. Persons with bulimia are even more secretive than those with anorexia. Because cachexia is uncommon, the disorder may escape detection for years.

### Laboratory Studies

Blood counts and protein levels are usually normal. Even in cases of recent, active purging, electrolyte

**TABLE 27.3. Diagnostic Criteria for Bulimia Nervosa**

1. Recurrent episodes of binge eating of a large amount of food within a 2-hour period characterized by a lack of control.
2. Recurrent inappropriate behavior to prevent weight gain such as use of vomiting, laxatives, diuretics, enemas, fasting, or excessive exercise.
3. These behaviors occur at least twice a week for 3 months.
4. Self-evaluation is unduly influenced by body shape and weight.

Adapted from DSM IV-TR.

**TABLE 27.4. Physical Findings in Bulimia Nervosa**

| | |
|---|---|
| Face | Bilateral painless parotid enlargement |
| Teeth | Loss of enamel, many cavities (from contact with gastric acid) |
| Throat | Petechial hemorrhages from vomiting |
| Abdomen | Bloating, distention, hyperactive bowel sounds |
| Fingers | Callus on dorsal surface from inducing vomiting (Russell's sign) |

abnormalities are rare. Cardiac examination is normal; an ECG is necessary to detect any abnormalities such as prolonged QT interval or flattened T waves. Aspiration pneumonia, a Mallory-Weiss tear, or even gastric rupture can follow the vomiting, and pancreatitis has also been reported. Chronic use of syrup of ipecac can lead to a cardiomyopathy or skeletal myopathies.

### Management

Bulimia nervosa is a chronic disorder with frequent remissions and relapses. Relapses are common (50–60% after 1 year), especially at stressful times throughout the person's life. A multidisciplinary approach is important because of the medical, psychiatric, and underlying personality disorders. Collaboration with a mental health professional is usually very helpful. Treatment options include individual psychotherapy, group therapy, family therapy, behavioral therapy, ECT, and pharmacotherapy. The relapse rate remains high regardless of which method is used.

TCAs, especially imipramine and desipramine, have had approximately a 50–75% response rate. More recently, encouraging results have been noted with the use of trazodone and fluoxetine. Anticonvulsants such as phenytoin and carbamazepine, MAOIs, and lithium have also been used, but their high potential for adverse side effects makes them less desirable.

# CHAPTER 28 SUBSTANCE ABUSE AND DEPENDENCE

Alcohol is the most commonly abused substance in the United States, but addiction also occurs with some prescription drugs and illicit drugs. Direct and indirect losses to society from substance abuse include thousands of lives and billions of dollars every year.

Most people who drink or take drugs on occasion do not become addicted. Predicting accurately who will eventually develop dependence is not possible because many factors, such as family influences, genetics, personality, psychiatric disorders, and the addictive properties of the substance, determine the development of addiction. The DSM IV-TR defines two types of substance use disorders: abuse, which is characterized by a pathologic use of the substance that has personal and social consequences in a 12-month period (Table 28.1); and dependence, which has three specific features: preoccupation, compulsive use, and loss of control. Tolerance and withdrawal are often present but are not required for diagnosis (Table 28.2).

Substance abuse is often a chronic relapsing condition. Abusers may have to repeatedly attempt to quit before they are successful. Six stages in the process of behavior change have been identified: precontemplation, contemplation, preparation, action, maintenance, and termination (Table 28.3). Tailoring interventions with this in mind is more effective in moving the patient toward eventual change.

**TABLE 28.1. Criteria for Diagnosis of Substance Abuse**

Recurrent substance use (only one or more of the following needs to occur within a 12-month period)*
- resulting in a failure to fulfill major role obligations at home, work, or school
- in situations in which it is physically hazardous (e.g., driving an automobile)
- causing recurrent related legal problems
- despite persistent social/interpersonal problems

Adapted from DSM IV-TR.
*Criteria can apply to any substance, such as alcohol, cocaine, or narcotics.

## Disease Concept

Most research points to addiction being a neurobiochemical/psychosocial disorder. Educating the patient can be particularly effective in minimizing denial and assisting the patient in accepting responsibility for the treatment of his illness. When taking this approach, the clinician evaluates and educates the patient about the genetic factors in addiction. Subsequent to a thorough physical examination and laboratory screening, the care provider points out all of the negative physical sequelae and then educates the patient about other potential negative effects caused by their "disease."

## Role of the Family

To accommodate a chemically dependent member, most families develop coping strategies that are often unhealthy and may even perpetuate the dependence. Such family members are termed codependent. Because of this dysfunctional family process, family treatment should be integral to rehabilitation. Children in these homes may need specialized counseling and peer-support groups (e.g., Alateen or Adult Children of Alcoholics [ACOA] self-help groups). Al-Anon is a group for family members and friends of alcoholics from which they learn about codependence and addiction as diseases characterized by certain symptoms and reactions. Al-Anon additionally supports family members in healing from the effects of this illness. Family support is very important to the potential success of achieving sobriety. Lacking this, some patients may need referral to a halfway house or transitional living arrangements to enable the development of new social structures that promote sobriety.

**TABLE 28.2. Criteria for Diagnosis of Substance Dependence**

Presence of three or more of the following at any time in a 12-month period:

1. Tolerance: either need for markedly increased (>50%) amounts of substance to achieve effect or markedly diminished effect with same amounts of substance
2. Withdrawal: either at least two characteristic symptoms within hours to days after reduction/cessation of substance or substance taken often to relieve or avoid symptoms
3. Substance is taken in larger amounts over a longer period than person intended
4. Desire but unsuccessful efforts to cut down intake
5. Much time is spent in obtaining and using substance and recovering from its effects
6. Important activities are reduced or given up because of substance use
7. Continued use despite persistent or recurrent problems likely caused by the substance

Adapted from DSM IV-TR.

**TABLE 28.3. Stages of Behavior Change in Addicted Personalities**

| Stage | Behavior |
|---|---|
| Precontemplation | No intention of changing and denies problem, lacks information, intends to remain ignorant |
| Contemplation | Acknowledges the problem; serious thoughts about solving it |
| Preparation | Committed to action, but not necessarily ready; needs to plan detailed action scheme |
| Action | Expends most time and energy (of all stages) modifying behavior and surroundings |
| Maintenance | Can be in this stage for a few months or a lifetime; is at risk for relapse if not committed |
| Termination | Has confidence that addiction no longer presents a threat without any continuing effort |

## Role of the Self-Help Group

Nonprofessional, 12-step support programs modeled after Alcoholics Anonymous (AA) are available virtually everywhere. Traditionally, the only requirement for membership is contemplation (Table 28.3). Groups exist for almost any behavior: Narcotics Anonymous, Overeaters Anonymous, Gamblers Anonymous, and so on. Family members may find 12-step groups for significant others helpful, such as Al-Anon, NarAnon, and Alateen, regardless of the addict's stage of change.

## Prevention and Intervention

The individual physician can do much to diminish alcohol and chemical dependency by identifying high-risk individuals, such as children of alcoholics. The biggest challenge for the physician is managing his or her own negative countertransference feelings that can develop in dealing with the addicted person. It is helpful to remember that the patient did not choose to be vulnerable to addiction and is suffering from a potentially deadly disease whose cardinal symptoms are denial and loss of control. Physicians should routinely inquire about a personal or family history of substance abuse before prescribing any potentially addictive substances. In every clinical encounter, physicians should promote healthful lifestyle changes. Early referral to appropriate counseling settings is also a responsibility of the primary care physician. Physicians should involve themselves in general public health initiatives and educational measures for children, discouraging the use of mood-altering drugs, alcohol, and tobacco.

# ■ Tobacco Abuse

Despite widespread use of tobacco, the overall smoking rate in the United States has declined dramatically from 42% of the population in 1965 to 26% in 1991. Nearly 90% of lung cancer deaths and 20% of all deaths in the United States are caused by tobacco abuse. Smoking is heavily implicated in deaths from arteriosclerotic cardiovascular disease, chronic obstructive pulmonary disease, and cancers of the head, neck, and pancreas. Smoking is also the most important modifiable cause of poor pregnancy outcome. Environmental tobacco smoke may cause lung cancer in nonsmoking adults and respiratory infections and asthma in children, and may be a risk factor for sudden infant death syndrome.

Approximately 87% of successful quitters have used self-help techniques, such as quitting "cold turkey." Assisted methods include clinics, hypnosis, acupuncture, and nicotine adjuncts, e.g., nicotine chewing gum, transdermal patches, or nasal spray. The patches are available in several dosage strengths, thus enabling gradual nicotine withdrawal in patients who have nicotine tolerance. (Table 28.4). Smoking while wearing the nicotine patch can cause cardiac ischemia or even lethal myocardial infarction. Bupropion, an atypical antidepressant, was approved in 1997 for use in smoking cessation. Given as a sustained-release preparation, it may be used in daily doses of 150–300 mg, either alone or in conjunction with the nicotine patch or gum.

**TABLE 28.4. Fagerström Test for Nicotine Dependence**

| | |
|---|---|
| 1. How soon after you wake up do you smoke your first cigarette? | |
| within 5 min | 3 points |
| 5–30 min | 2 points |
| 31–60 min | 1 point |
| after 60 min | 0 points |
| 2. Do you find it hard not to smoke in places that you shouldn't smoke, such as in church, in school, in a movie, on the bus, in court or in a hospital? | |
| Yes | 1 point |
| No | 0 points |
| 3. Which cigarette would you hate most to have to give up? | |
| The first one in the morning | 1 point |
| Any other one | 0 points |
| 4. How many cigarettes do you smoke each day? | |
| 10–fewer | 0 points |
| 11–20 | 1 point |
| 21–30 | 2 points |
| 31 or more | 3 points |
| 5. Do you smoke more in the first few hours after waking up than you do during the rest of the day? | |
| Yes | 1 point |
| No | 0 points |
| 6. Do you still smoke, even if you are so sick that you are in bed most of the day, or if you have the flu or a severe cough? | |
| Yes | 1 point |
| No | 0 points |
| Total ............................................ | ________ points |

| Fagerström Score | Start with |
|---|---|
| 7–10 | 21 mg patch |
| 4–6 | 14 mg patch |
| <4 | 7 mg patch |

Adapted with permission from Fagerstrom KO, Schneider NG. Behav Med 1988;12:159–182.

Pharmacological adjuncts are most effective if used in conjunction with a formal counseling program. Many employers have on-site smoking cessation programs or pay for employees to participate in outside programs. Free group programs, sponsored by local voluntary agencies, hospitals, or churches, exist in many areas. State branches of the American Lung Association and American Cancer Society also offer programs. Quit rates range from 15–40% at 1-year follow-up. Recidivism is high, but most who keep trying are eventually successful.

Physician counseling is an important factor in smoking cessation and does not have to be lengthy or involved. The physician should provide advice, encourage the patient to set a quit date, refer to formal programs, and prescribe adjunctive medication, if indicated. Physicians must be especially attentive to high-risk groups, such as adolescents and pregnant women, but counseling about smoking cessation should be a part of routine practice.

## Alcohol Abuse/Dependence

Three out of four adults in the United States use alcohol. Alcohol remains the most costly substance of abuse with an annual cost to society of over $100 billion. Over 100,000 deaths annually are related to alcohol. The National Comorbidity Survey completed in 1990–1992 based on DSM-IIIR criteria yielded lifetime prevalence rates for alcohol dependency of 20.1% for men and 8.2% for women. Twelve-month prevalence estimates for DSM IV-TR alcohol dependence provided by the 1990 United States National Alcohol Survey yielded 5.7% for men, and 2.2% for women. A diagnosis of alcohol dependency shortens one's life expectancy by 17 years.

The American Medical Association defines alcoholism as "an illness characterized by significant impairment that is directly associated with persistent and excessive use of alcohol. Impairment may involve physiological, psychological or social dysfunction." Simply stated, alcoholism is present when a person experiences repeated harm from drinking.

Alcoholism is regularly underdiagnosed in medical practices. The diagnosis is less likely to be made in patients with higher income, higher education, and private insurance, but in reality only approximately 5% of alcoholics fit the "skid row" stereotype.

Alcoholism is a complex disorder in which genetic, environmental, and personality factors interact. Male gender and a family history appear to be the two major

TABLE 28.5. CAGE Screening Test for Alcoholism

| Have you ever . . . | |
|---|---|
| • felt a need to | **C**ut down on drinking? |
| • felt | **A**nnoyed by criticism of your drinking? |
| • felt | **G**uilty about drinking? |
| • taken an | **E**ye-opener? |

risk factors for alcoholism. No biologic marker has yet been identified, but the risk among sons of alcoholic fathers may be as much as fourfold. Other possible risk factors include tobacco use, history of hyperactivity, unemployment, being reared in a broken home, or being of Irish, Scandinavian, or Native American descent.

## Clinical Features and Diagnosis

Medical history taking should routinely include inquiries about alcohol use. Questions such as: "How often do you use alcohol?" or "When was your last drink?" asked in a matter-of-fact, nonjudgmental way are not offensive and are more likely to elicit an honest response than questions regarding quantity of alcohol consumed. Use of a short screening questionnaire such as the CAGE test (Table 28.5) is another aid to diagnosis. A positive response to two or more questions implies that the person is more likely than not to be alcoholic, and further evaluation is needed.

Any of the following behavioral clues should arouse concern: emotional lability, loss of friends, difficulty with work, divorce or other family problems, sleep disturbance, self-medication, history of trauma (especially unexplained rib fractures), defensiveness or evasiveness when asked about alcohol, and driving while intoxicated or having other clashes with the law. Obviously, symptoms of liver disease, pancreatitis, or gastritis should alert one to surreptitious alcohol abuse. Other clues are insomnia, anxiety, depression, dyspepsia, headache, palpitations, or recurring minor trauma.

In early alcoholism, abnormal physical findings are sparse. Odor of alcohol on the breath or excessive use of mouthwash may be warning signs. Hypertension, tachycardia, or other cardiac arrhythmias are occasionally related to alcoholism. A plethoric face and bilateral parotid enlargement may be seen, on occasion.

No diagnostic laboratory markers exist. With heavy alcohol consumption, γ-glutamyl transferase levels increase and return to normal after weeks of abstinence. Obesity, medications (e.g., anticonvulsants), and liver disease not related to alcohol use can also elevate γ-glutamyl transferase levels. Macrocytosis with a mean corpuscular volume above 90 is another finding. Alkaline phosphatase, aspartate aminotransferase, uric acid, cholesterol, and triglyceride levels may be elevated as well.

To diagnose alcoholism, the patient must meet the criteria for either alcohol abuse or dependence as noted in Tables 28.1 or 28.2. Alcohol dependence is a more severe degree of alcoholism, but alcohol abuse at times can be just as problematic. When a patient presents with withdrawal symptoms, they clearly have become physically dependent on alcohol. This patient meets criteria for alcohol dependence under the DSM IV-TR criteria. However, the patient does not have to have withdrawal symptoms to meet criteria for alcohol dependence. A patient may have developed tolerance, in other words, patient is finding a need to increase the amount or the potency of the alcoholic product they take, or they have begun to notice that they have a markedly diminished effect with the same amount and potency of alcohol. Other criteria for alcohol dependence would include unsuccessful efforts to cut down intake, spending a great deal of time in getting and using alcohol as well as in recovering from its effects, and giving up important activities because of their alcohol use. When alcohol dependence is diagnosed, the physician should pay particular attention to monitoring and managing withdrawal symptoms as they present.

One of the biggest obstacles in treating the alcoholic patient is overcoming the denial. It may take persistence over several encounters to make, and get the patient to accept, the diagnosis. Arguing with the patient serves no useful purpose and engenders more defensiveness and denial. The physician should continue to maintain a positive relationship with the patient without participating in the denial, explaining firmly but sympathetically why an alcohol problem might be present. Adverse medical effects already noted should be shared with the patient in a straightforward manner without using scare tactics or threats. The physician should show concern, convey a clear message of hope, and spend time educating the patient about the disease process and the long course of recovery.

## Medical Complications

Medical complications as a result of alcohol abuse are varied and diffuse. Gastrointestinal problems include decreased salivary production with resultant dental problems; gastritis and upper Gl bleeding; and acute pancreatitis, eventually leading to chronic pancreatitis with malabsorption, diarrhea, and even secondary diabetes mellitus. Approximately 30% of alcoholics have evidence of cirrhosis at autopsy.

Malnutrition and vitamin deficiencies are frequent in alcoholics, causing neurological problems such as peripheral neuropathy. Other neurological problems of alcoholism include Wernicke-Korsakoff syndrome, cerebellar degeneration, alcoholic dementia, alcohol-related seizures, and alcohol-induced depression and hallucinosis.

Miscellaneous complications include hypertension, arrhythmias, hypothermia, hypogonadism, increased susceptibility to pulmonary infections, and increased risk for cancer of the GI tract, urinary tract, bladder, and liver. Alcohol is directly toxic to bone marrow, causing thrombocytopenia, leukopenia, anemia, and macrocytosis.

## Managing Acute Alcohol Withdrawal

The severity of the withdrawal symptoms varies depending on the duration and amount of alcohol intake. Symptoms, which usually peak in approximately 24–72 hours, are of three main types: autonomic hyperactivity, neuronal excitation, and sensory distortion. Tremulousness, fever, diaphoresis, tachycardia, and hypertension result from autonomic hyperactivity. Seizures tend to occur within the first 48 hours after abstinence and are usually generalized, tonic-clonic, and limited to one or two episodes. The withdrawal may progress to delirium tremens (DTs). DTs involve a general clouding of the sensorium with waxing and waning of level of consciousness, and perceptual disturbances, such as formication (tactile hallucinations as if small insects are creeping under the skin) or auditory or visual hallucinations in addition to the nondelirium alcohol withdrawal signs. DTs usually develop 72–96 hours after cessation of alcohol consumption, and can lead to death if untreated.

The severity of symptoms can be quantified with alcohol withdrawal instruments such as the Selective Severity Assessment (SSA) score. Cross-tolerant sedatives such as benzodiazepines are titrated based on SSA scores to an end point of neutrality (i.e., the patient is neither sedated nor in withdrawal). Aggressive treatment with benzodiazepines to match the degree of withdrawal leads to quicker relief of symptoms and prevention of complications such as arrhythmias, seizures, and DTs. Dosing chlordiazepoxide based on symptoms, rather than on a fixed schedule, also reduced the total drug dose and duration of therapy.

Safe withdrawal/detoxification from alcohol is the first step in treatment. Benzodiazepines (Table 28.6) are the pharmacologic agent of choice and are effective in both inpatient and outpatient settings. For patients with possible hepatic dysfunction, lorazepam may be the preferred agent. Also, unlike chlordiazepoxide, it can be given intramuscular and sublingual. If a patient has developed DTs, benzodiazepines should be given on an hourly basis until the patient is able to sleep. Mild to moderate symptoms of alcohol withdrawal can be treated with benzodiazepines on an outpatient basis. Given the risk of cross-addiction, benzodiazepines should be weaned when withdrawal is completed.

Hospitalization is recommended when metabolic or nutritional interventions are indicated, when the patient is also physically dependent on other drugs including sedatives that are complicating the picture, and when comorbid medical conditions warrant admission. Ongoing supportive care during alcohol withdrawal includes routine thiamine replacement (preferably delivered parenterally), seizure precautions, and close monitoring of the patient's oral intake to prevent dehydration and further complications. Management of DTs often requires transfer to the intensive care unit, provision of intravenous fluids, and when indicated, restraint to control agitation until the DTs are resolved.

Adjunctive agents such as carbamazepine, phenytoin, divalproex, or gabapentin are gaining favor as additions to benzodiazepines and may have an advantage of preventing kindling of subsequent withdrawal episode severity. Kindling refers to increasing severity of withdrawal symptoms with each subsequent episode of

**TABLE 28.6. Management of Alcohol Withdrawal**

**General**

Thiamine 100 mg IM or IV immediately and PO daily*
Hydration usually not necessary unless there is vomiting or poor intake
Folic acid and multivitamins
Magnesium sulfate 2.0 g IV every 6 hours if there is hypomagnesemia and normal renal function

**Withdrawal symptoms**

Benzodiazepines (oral route preferred; if IV, should be given slowly over 2–3 minutes)
- Lorazepam 2–4 mg PO/IM/IV every 6 hours

OR

- Chlordiazepoxide 50–100 mg PO or 12.5 mg IV every 2–4 hours

OR

- Diazepam 10–20 mg PO or 5–10 mg slow IV every 2–4 hours

β-blockers
- Atenolol 50–100 mg PO qd

α-2 receptor agonist
- Clonidine 0.2 mg PO three times daily

**Delirium/Hallucinations**

Haloperidol 0.5–5.0 mg IM or 5–10 mg PO every 2 hours until controlled

**Seizures**

Phenytoin (therapeutic value is uncertain)
- Loading dose: 10 mg/kg IV at 50 mg/min
- Maintenance dose: 100 mg PO every 8 hours

PO = orally; qd = every day.
*Deficiency in 30–80% of alcoholics.

withdrawal. Clonidine, an α-2 adrenergic agonist, can control autonomic hyperactivity in alcohol withdrawal, probably by reducing catecholamine levels, but it should not be used alone because it does not prevent seizures. Similarly, β-blockers (e.g., atenolol), given with benzodiazepines, decrease symptoms and reduce benzodiazepine requirements.

### Long-term Management of Alcoholism

The optimal treatment program for rehabilitation and recovery from alcoholism is still unclear. Although even brief interventions by the physician encouraging a patient to abstain from alcohol can be effective, pharmacologic treatment for alcohol abuse with disulfiram alone is of limited use and is most helpful for the impulsive drinker. Disulfiram is an aversive drug that interacts with ingested alcohol to cause severe headache, flushing, and hypotension. Liver enzymes must be checked before starting disulfiram. It may cause hepatotoxicity, neuropathy, and cardiotoxicity. Patients should be made aware of alcohol-disulfiram reactions and cautioned to avoid alcohol, even in mouthwashes, colognes, and cooking wines.

Naltrexone, an opioid-receptor antagonist approved for the treatment of alcoholism, has reduced craving in abstinent patients and prevented relapse. Naltrexone is not habit-forming, and its side effects include nausea, headache, dizziness, and arthralgia. The usual dose is 50 mg per day. Because studies to date have only been of short duration, long-term (>3–6 months) naltrexone therapy is not recommended. For relapse prevention, psychological intervention should occur for those taking naltrexone.

Because inpatient programs lack proven superiority and their cost-effectiveness is of concern, residential programs are probably not essential in all instances. Those in whom outpatient programs have failed, those with serious medical or psychiatric problems, or those with cross-addictions to cocaine, narcotics, or benzodiazepines may benefit from residential programs.

AA groups have existed for 50 years, and consistent attendance at meetings correlates with abstinence. These groups offer support, help participants resist the compulsions, and provide strategies for dealing with the pressures that prompt the return to drinking. AA is also excellent for eliminating the denial of the alcoholic patient.

Efficacy of rehabilitation varies widely depending on the population being studied. Early intervention is more likely to be effective because more personal resources are remaining to apply to the problem; health complications can also be thus prevented. Physicians should routinely assess alcoholic patients for suicidal ideation because the lifetime suicide risk for alcoholics is approximately 10%.

## Sedative-Hypnotics

Abuse of sedative-hypnotics, which are prescription drugs, often begins as an iatrogenic problem. These drugs exert alcohol-like effects on mood and consciousness and reduce anxiety and inhibitions.

Use does not necessarily correlate with abuse, but the potential for inducing tolerance and escalating drug use is constant. Dependence can occur even with appropriate therapeutic doses. As the daily dose and duration of treatment increase, the probability of physical dependence rises. Addiction potential is greatest in patients with a history of alcohol abuse, and it correlates with the intensity and rapidity of action of the addictive drug. The rapid-acting lipophilic drugs—secobarbital, pentobarbital, diazepam (Valium), lorazepam (Ativan), and alprazolam (Xanax)—probably have the highest abuse potential.

### Clinical Features

The person with acute sedative intoxication may exhibit coarse lateral nystagmus, general slowing of mental functions, slurred speech, ataxia, general drowsiness, and impaired judgment. Although benzodiazepines are relatively safe if taken alone, given the inhibitory effect on the arousal and respiratory centers of the brain stem, higher doses, particularly with nonbenzodiazepine sedatives or combined depressants, can produce stupor, coma, and respiratory depression. Anterograde amnesia is also a consequence, which results from a partial or complete failure to acquire or store information after taking the drug.

### Management of Withdrawal Syndrome

Anxiety, tearfulness, and insomnia may follow discontinuation of these drugs. Usually, the withdrawal syndrome is self-limited, and recovery is complete several days or weeks after the drug is eliminated. Abrupt discontinuation of benzodiazepines with short half-lives (oxazepam, lorazepam, alprazolam, etc.) and barbiturates carries a significant potential for seizures, delirium, and hallucinosis. Tremors, diaphoresis, and restlessness similar to that of alcohol withdrawal may develop. Even long-acting drugs such as chlordiazepoxide and diazepam can produce a significant abstinence syndrome with a more extended time course.

Besides delirium, hallucinations, and disorientation, barbiturate withdrawal may be associated with fever, usually within 36–72 hours after barbiturate termination. Withdrawal from barbiturates should be very gradual, and phenobarbital is ideal for detoxification because of its wider safety range. Total daily dose of sedatives should be converted to "sedative equivalent" doses of a long-acting sedative such as clonazepam or phenobarbital. This dose then can be tapered over 7–21 days depending on the duration of the abused drug half-life. A slower detoxification schedule may be preferred for an outpatient.

If accurate intake is unknown, sedative tolerance can be determined by a sedative tolerance test. This should be started only when the patient is at a neutral point (not intoxicated any longer but not in withdrawal yet). Begin with pentobarbital loading with 200 mg. If after 1 hour the withdrawal symptoms are not controlled, 100 mg is given orally hourly until early signs of intoxication develop or a total of 800 mg is reached. The total pentobarbital dose is converted to phenobarbital equivalents (100 mg pentobarbital = 30 mg phenobarbital), which is given in divided doses three or four times per day, tapering by 5–10% daily. Alternatively, give 200 mg pentobarbital and observe after 1 hour. If the patient is asleep, but arousable, he has no tolerance. If the patient is drowsy and has slurred speech, ataxia, coarse nystagmus, and intoxication, the tolerance is comparable to pentobarbital 400–600 mg/24 hours. If the patient is comfortable and the only sign of intoxication is fine lateral nystagmus, then pentobarbital needs are 800 mg/24 hours. If no drug effect is observed, then the dose required would be 1000–1200 mg/24 hours. In this case, give an additional 300 mg pentobarbital and observe 3 hours later. If there is still no response, then the patient's needs are >1600 mg/24 hours. Consultation with an individual who is experienced in sedative detoxification is recommended. Again, conversion to phenobarbital (to allow tapering as described above) is preferable because of smoothness of clearance.

## Opioids

Because much opiate abuse is parenteral, many patients present with medical complications, including skin infections, endocarditis, nephropathy, hepatitis, overdose, and AIDS, which is the fastest growing cause of all illicit drug–related deaths. Many of these complications are related to the sharing and use of contaminated needles. Heroin or cocaine is involved in two thirds of all drug deaths. Nearly 40% of illicit drug deaths occur in the 30- to 39-year-old age group. Rates are increasing, particularly for men, and even more so for African-American men.

Opiates cause euphoria or dysphoria, drowsiness, diaphoresis, constipation, pruritus, miosis, pulmonary edema, and respiratory depression. Physical dependence can develop quite rapidly, especially with the recurrent intravenous (IV) user. To treat patients for whom opiates have had an acutely toxic effect with respiratory depression, naloxone, an opiate antagonist, should be administered IV (0.4 mg) every 3–5 minutes up to three doses. However, this may precipitate acute withdrawal symptoms.

Intense fear of withdrawal, drug craving, abdominal and muscle cramps, nausea, vomiting, diarrhea, lacrimation, and frequent yawning characterize opiate abstinence symptoms. Mild to moderate autonomic hyperactivity is seen with tremor, restlessness, rhinorrhea, mydriasis, and piloerection, seen commonly on the chest. Although terribly unpleasant, this syndrome is rarely life-threatening.

Opiate withdrawal can frequently be controlled with clonidine. Transdermal patches are better tolerated, although oral dosing is required for the first few days. Doses may be titrated upward until withdrawal is controlled or limited by development of symptomatic hypotension. The withdrawal symptoms of insomnia and bone aches are not well treated with clonidine, and use of nonsteroidal anti-inflammatory drugs (NSAIDs) and temporary hypnotic medication may be warranted.

If the patient's opiate withdrawal is poorly controlled with clonidine, methadone may be considered. Methadone, 5 mg, is given orally initially; if objective signs of withdrawal do not improve, the dose may be increased, usually by no more than 5 mg per dose every 4–6 hours. In general, 20–40 mg of methadone in four divided daily doses is adequate for most patients; later, a single daily dose may suffice. The dose should be tapered by 5–20% per day, depending on the severity of the habit. Opiate withdrawal from high-dose methadone maintenance (75–100 mg/day) carries a high failure rate, and should be conducted only by experts in this area.

Detoxification may be followed by highly structured, behaviorally oriented, residential treatment programs, lasting from 6–24 months. Those who are strongly pressured (either legally or socially) to remain in treatment do best. In highly motivated patients, naltrexone may be instituted in a monitored program. Methadone maintenance should be reserved for those who have failed or refused such programs or for those with very severe psychopathology. It may be the treatment of choice for those consistently physically tolerant for longer than the previous year.

All high-risk patients should be screened for HIV, counseled on reducing their risks of acquiring HIV, and educated about "safe sex" and the risks of using contaminated drug paraphernalia. Needle and syringe exchange programs and education regarding safer injection practices are part of a harm-reduction approach.

## Cocaine and Other Stimulants

Stimulants include decongestants (e.g., phenylpropanolamine and ephedrine); anorectics (e.g., phentermine, phenmetrazine, and fenfluramine); methylphenidate (Ritalin) used for attention deficit disorder and narcolepsy; agents such as d-1 amphetamine (Benzedrine), d-amphetamine (Dexedrine), methamphetamine (Desoxyn); and cocaine. Among these, cocaine is presently the most widely abused. Toxic reactions to all of these drugs are similar.

### Pathophysiology

Cocaine and amphetamines share similar neurochemical and clinical effects. They act by blocking reuptake of norepinephrine, dopamine, and serotonin at synaptic junctions, which results in increased energy, a sense of well-being, and decreased appetite. Cocaine has a shorter plasma half-life (90 minutes; amphetamines, 6–12 hours). With both agents, euphoria rapidly declines despite the presence of the stimulant in the plasma.

### Clinical Features

Abusers engage in intensive binges alternating with a few days of abstinence, compared with alcoholic or opiate abusers, who use daily. Impaired judgment, impulsiveness, hypersexuality, compulsively repeated actions, and hyperactivity may occur with acute intoxication, along with euphoria. Anxiety bordering on panic, paranoia, and delusions may occur—even in persons with no premorbid psychiatric conditions. The most common acute presentations (Table 28.7) are psychiatric (altered mental state or behavior), cardiac (chest pain, palpitations, or syncope), or neurological (seizures) symptoms.

### Withdrawal Syndrome

Abstinence from stimulants has three sequential phases: crash, withdrawal, and extinction. The crash immediately follows a binge and may last a day or a week. Features are depression, agitation, and insomnia followed by a craving for sleep. Withdrawal symptoms are decreased energy and anhedonia that fluctuate with near-normal moods, lasting for 6–18 weeks. Periods of intense craving for the drug occur within this time. The extinction phase lasts indefinitely, but craving for the drug may be induced by conditioned cues.

### Management

Treatment of cocaine abuse is often modeled after alcohol programs. Inpatient treatment was previously considered necessary for cocaine withdrawal, but because of the expense and lack of controlled studies demonstrating the superiority of the approach, daily outpatient programs are being used more. Long-term treatment often involves a 12-step group, such as Cocaine Anonymous. Such treatment is imperative because the risk of relapse may persist for years. Success rates appear to be less than for other substances, at least for the first few months. Conditioned craving cues, present with most addictions, are particularly problematic with cocaine. Various pharmacological approaches to reduce cocaine craving have been tried with equivocal success. Most of these are aimed at rectifying presumed depletions of dopamine.

**TABLE 28.7. Common Presentations/Complications of Cocaine Abuse**

**General**
Sudden death
Malnutrition (Vitamin B and C deficiencies)
Rhabdomyolysis with acute renal failure

**Head and neck**
Perforated nasal septum
Chronic rhinitis

**Cardiac**
Chest pain
Myocardial infarction
Ventricular arrhythmias
Cardiomyopathy

**Pulmonary**
Pulmonary edema
"Crack lung"
Pneumothorax
Pneumomediastinum

**Psychiatric**
Depression/suicide
Psychosis
Anxiety

**Neurologic**
Seizures
Headaches
Cerebral hemorrhage/infarctions

## Marijuana

Men are twice as likely as women to be frequent users of marijuana. Smoking or ingestion creates a sense of euphoria, and both stimulation and, later, sedation may occur. The sense of passage of time is slowed, appetite is stimulated, and the user's sense of humor may be heightened or inappropriate. Paranoid ideation, depersonalization reactions, and, rarely, a toxic psychosis may occur. Reassurance is usually effective in mild cases; sometimes a low dose of benzodiazepine is useful, and a neuroleptic may rarely be required.

Chronic use may cause amotivational syndromes with apathy, social withdrawal, and school or work dysfunction. Bronchitis and other pulmonary effects may also occur in heavy users.

## Hallucinogens

LSD and similar drugs may cause transient psychotic episodes, the management of which is similar to marijuana. Organic hallucinogens (Jimson weed, mescaline, psilocybin) and similar plant alkaloids (belladonna) may cause anticholinergic toxicity. One of the most concerning hallucinogens is phencyclidine (PCP), known as angel dust, which may result in toxic psychosis, coma, myoclonic seizures, rhabdomyolysis, and renal failure. Although intoxication with most other hallucinogens only requires reassurance or mild sedation, PCP can cause violent outbursts requiring restraints and neuroleptics (e.g., haloperidol).

## Anabolic Steroids

As many as 5–10% of high school boys use anabolic steroids at some time, and their use is most prevalent among football players. Anabolic steroids are considered a class III controlled substance. Adverse effects include increased secondary sex characteristics, risk for infectious disease if used intravenously, dangerously aggressive behavior, mood derangements, and true dependency manifest by preoccupation, compulsive use, and loss of control.

## Inhalants

Another form of substance abuse that is fairly common among adolescents is the use of inhalants. Some of the substances most frequently used as inhalants include spray paint, gasoline, freon, butane lighter fluid, glue, and nitric oxide. Inhalants are defined as volatile organic substances and often are found in common household and commercial products that are easily accessible, inexpensive, and legally obtained. Because of these factors, inhalants may be some of the first substances of abuse in the development of more severe addictions. Inhalant abuse has been associated with numerous acute and chronic medical problems including confusion, respiratory depression, hypoxia, hypotension, death from arrhythmia, and long-standing brain dysfunction. Irreversible damage to the liver, kidney, and other organs can also occur. Volatile solvents cannot be detected in the urine routinely.

## Impaired Health Professionals

Physicians, dentists, podiatrists, nurses, pharmacists, and veterinarians all have increased access to medicinal mood-altering drugs and the ability to self-prescribe without easily being detected. The level of denial, rationalization, and manipulative behavior is high, and the drug use may be overlooked by colleagues. "Impaired professional" programs, in which confidentiality is preserved, make it easier for the impaired colleague to receive help.

Physicians have a responsibility to each other and to society to be alert to the signs of functional impairment in their peers caused by substance abuse or other disorders. Most state medical societies have supportive impaired physician programs. Although this varies from state to state, licensure for someone getting help usually need not be an issue. Clinicians who suspect that a colleague is impaired should seek the guidance of a local expert to effect appropriate referral and therapy. Individual and group counseling and randomized urine drug screens for at least 2 years are usually part of such a program. Exceptionally high success rates of up to 90% are common.

# CHAPTER 29 CLINICAL TOXICOLOGY

Accidental or intentional overdoses are medical emergencies comprising approximately 10–15% of all emergency department visits. Almost any substance may be ingested, including household poisons, prescribed drugs, over-the-counter preparations, and illicit drugs. Any unexplained or unusual illness, especially involving changes of consciousness, should prompt suspicion of toxic ingestion.

## Basic Management

### Initial stabilization

The ABCs of resuscitation—airway, breathing, and circulation— are the most urgent considerations. An open airway is established, and supplemental oxygen begun. If a gag reflex is absent, an endotracheal tube must be inserted to protect the airway. Cardiopulmonary resuscitation should commence if spontaneous respiration or pulse is absent. IV access is gained with a large-bore (18 gauge or larger) peripheral or central catheter. If blood pressure is low (<90 mm Hg systolic) or if perfusion is compromised, the patient is placed in the Trendelenburg position and appropriate amounts of IV crystalloid infused. Care must be taken to avoid fluid overload. Central monitoring may be warranted, especially if no response to fluid resuscitation occurs. Electrocardiographic monitoring is particularly important with TCAs and cocaine.

All unconscious patients should be given dextrose (50 ml of 50% glucose IV over 3–4 minutes), naloxone (2.0 mg IV and repeated three or four times if narcotic overdose is suspected), and oxygen. Lower doses of naloxone (0.2–0.4 mg) may be necessary to avoid precipitating withdrawal in a suspected narcotic addict. Thiamine (100 mg IV or IM) should precede glucose in all alcoholics to prevent precipitation of Wernicke encephalopathy.

#### Specific antidotes

Antidotes are available for a few poisonings (Table 29.1). The correct use of antidotes requires knowledge of the pharmacology of both the poison and the antidote. Antidotes could be harmful, and in an asymptomatic patient, supportive, watchful care may avoid iatrogenic toxic complications.

### General Principles of Evaluation

After basic management (ABCs), the clinician should consider several key questions in a suspected toxic emergency. Does the patient's current presentation or history indicate any offending substance? What are specific physical findings? Do the clinical features and laboratory tests support one diagnosis? Is a unique therapy available that will make a difference?

#### History

A complete history of recent medication use, both prescription and over-the-counter; intake of alcohol and other drugs; and occupational or other exposures is important. If the patient is unable to give a reliable history, efforts should be made to contact friends, family, co-workers, or neighbors. One should inquire whether any pill bottles or drug paraphernalia were found at the scene where the patient was found. Prior medical and psychiatric history (prior ingestion, overdose, or underlying depression) should be ascertained. Although a complete history is helpful, diagnostic and therapeutic efforts may have to be initiated without it.

#### Key physical findings

Vital signs should be obtained when the patient arrives in the emergency department and, if unstable, should be stabilized and frequently monitored. Hypertension may follow use of amphetamines, cocaine, and

**TABLE 29.1. Common Antidotes for Poisonings**

| Poison | Antidote | Dose/Comment |
|---|---|---|
| Acetaminophen | Acetylcysteine | 140 mg/kg load, then 70 mg/kg every 4 hours X 17 doses |
| Anticholinergics | Physostigmine | 1–2 mg IV over 5 minutes |
| Benzodiazepines | Flumazenil | 0.2 mg IV, then 0.3–0.5 mg every 1 min to 3.0 mg total |
| β-Blockers | Glucagon | 5–10 mg IV. Titrate 2–10 mg/h until response |
| Calcuim channel blockers | Calcium | 1 g calcium chloride over 5 minutes IV with cardiac monitoring |
| Carbon monoxide | Oxygen | 100% by mask |
| Cyanide | Sodium nitrite | 300 mg IV |
| | then sodium thiosulfate | 12.5 g IV over 10 min |
| Digoxin | Digoxin fab | Number of milligrams ingested divided by 0.6 = vials required; if unknown, 10–20 vials IV |
| Ethylene glycol and methanol | Fomepizole, | 15 mg/kg IV load, then 10 mg/kg every 12 hours |
| | or Ethanol | 10% IV: 7.5 ml/kg load, then 1 ml/kg/h maintenance |
| Opiates | Naloxone | 2–4 mg IV |
| Organophosphates | Atropine, or | 2 mg IV |
| | Pralidoxime | 1 g IV |

anticholinergic drugs. Hypotension may indicate poisoning with sedative-hypnotics, antihypertensives, narcotics, or TCAs. Hyperpnea could be from salicylates or other drugs causing metabolic acidosis.

During the initial examination, the physician should concentrate on assessing the level of consciousness; almost half of all cases of coma are due to toxins. In comatose patients, physicians should check for head and neck trauma and stabilize the neck before moving the patient. A focused neurological examination should ensue. Muscle tone will be increased with amphetamines, phencyclidine, and antipsychotics, and decreased with sedative-hypnotics and narcotics. Fasciculations may indicate lithium or organophosphorus toxicity. Tremor is common with lithium or amphetamine overdose and withdrawal from alcohol or sedative-hypnotics. Seizures may occur from the use of alcohol, theophylline, TCAs, cocaine, and phencyclidine. The skin should be inspected carefully for cyanosis, flushing, rash, injury, or signs of skin popping or IV drug use. Breath odors can also provide diagnostic clues. Some odors, such as ethanol, ammonia, and glue, may be obvious. Cyanide can produce a bitter almond odor; methyl salicylate, a wintergreen smell. The eyes should be carefully inspected for miosis (narcotics, phenothiazines, and organophosphorus), mydriasis (anticholinergics, amphetamines, and cocaine), nystagmus (phenytoin, phencyclidine, and many sedative-hypnotics), and optic neuritis (methanol). Cardiopulmonary and abdominal examination should be performed as the diagnostic studies and treatment progress.

General diagnostic tests are listed in Table 29.2. In most cases, because toxicology data may be delayed, treatment should begin based on the clinical impression. Negative toxicology screens are falsely reassuring, and excessive reliance on quantitative data can be dangerous. The history, physical examination, and routine laboratory test results will lead to the correct diagnosis in most cases. Contact with a local poison control center is quite useful.

**TABLE 29.2. Diagnostic Studies in Suspected Poisonings**

| |
|---|
| Blood tests |
| Glucose |
| Electrolytes, blood urea nitrogen, creatinine |
| Calculate osmolality and anion gap; measure osmolality in selected cases |
| Complete blood count, including platelets and differential |
| Liver function, calcium, phosphate |
| Coagulation studies |
| Arterial blood gas analysis, especially if obtundation or respiratory compromise is present |
| Electrocardiogram for QRS or QT prolongation, arrhythmias, ischemia |
| Radiographs |
| Chest radiograph |
| Abdominal radiograph to look for radiopaque drugs/toxins |
| Cross-table cervical spine radiograph if trauma is suspected |
| Toxicology screens |
| Save 30 ml of serum, 60 ml of urine, 60 ml of gastric aspirate for analysis |
| Quantitative assays for specific drugs or toxins (e.g., acetaminophen, phenytoin, phenobarbital, aspirin, methanol, ethylene glycol) |

## Removal of the Offending Substance

### Topical decontamination

Some toxins, such as organophosphorus insecticides, may cause intoxication via cutaneous absorption. Skin-to-skin contact with patients should be avoided; if it occurs, the skin should be flushed immediately with copious amounts of water and dilute soap solution. In patients with skin contamination, the clothing should be decontaminated or destroyed.

If the eyes are involved, they must be irrigated immediately with plain water or normal saline for at least 30 minutes, facilitated by a local anesthetic, such as 0.5% tetracaine. Long-term use of the anesthetic should only be with ophthalmological consultation. For acidic/basic contaminants, pH paper may be used to ensure that all toxic material was removed by washing. Early referral to an eye specialist is urged.

### Methods of enhanced drug removal

Aside from lack of demonstrated usefulness in most cases, forced diuresis is potentially hazardous. Usually, small amounts of drugs are removed and both pulmonary and cerebral edema may occur. Toxin removal may be enhanced by a variety of methods. In the case of ingestions, the stomach can be decontaminated by gastric lavage. Absorption of drug within the gastrointestinal tract by activated charcoal, followed by catharsis with sorbitol (0.5 to 2.0 g/kg) or saline cathartics ($MgSO_4$, magnesium citrate, or disodium phosphate) can remove unabsorbed orally ingested toxins. Activated charcoal is not effective for preventing the absorption of iron, lithium, fluoride, alcohols, or caustic acids or bases. Hemodialysis is effective for water-soluble substances that are not highly protein-bound and is recommended in severe poisonings with salicylate, ethylene glycol, methanol, bromide, lithium, or isopropyl alcohol. In hemoperfusion, toxin is removed from the blood by direct contact with an adsorbent resin such as charcoal, and then the blood is returned to the body. Selected instances of possible benefit from hemoperfusion/dialysis are listed in Table 29.3.

## Aspirin

Both intentional and accidental aspirin overdose is common because it is present in many medications. Salicylate poisoning affects the central nervous system (CNS) and Krebs cycle enzymes, and uncouples oxidative phosphorylation. Because aspirin is a weak acid, acidemia increases its penetration into the CNS. The minimum acute toxic dose is usually 150 mg/kg; severe toxicity occurs at doses greater than 300 mg/kg. Levels must be interpreted with an estimate of the time elapsed since ingestion (Figure 29.1). Levels of more than 50 mg/dl usually require treatment. With concomitant acidosis, toxicity occurs at lower blood levels.

Early symptoms are nausea, vomiting, tinnitus, and hyperventilation. Initial respiratory alkalosis is followed by severe metabolic acidosis. Increased agitation and irritability may progress to seizures and coma. Hypoglycemia and pulmonary edema may also be present. Serum salicylate level should be obtained rapidly and repeated every 4–6 hours, especially if a sustained-release or enteric preparation was the culprit.

Salicylates delay gastric emptying; therefore, measures to decrease GI absorption should be considered. Ipecac-induced vomiting has been found to be of little value. Gastric lavage, as well as the administration of activated charcoal, will help reduce the amount of salicylate load. Dehydration occurs early, and circulating fluid volume and renal perfusion need to be maintained taking care to avoid overhydration which could potentiate cerebral and pulmonary edema. Forced alkaline diuresis is used with sodium bicarbonate (1 mEq/kg/h) to promote urinary excretion and combat acidosis. A urine pH of at least 7.5 should be attained, and deficits of fluid, glucose, and potassium should be corrected. In severe cases with persistent seizures or acidosis, hemodialysis is recommended, especially with serum levels more than 100 mg/dl.

**TABLE 29.3. Methods for Enhanced Toxin Removal in Severe Cases of Poisonings**

| Method | Indication |
|---|---|
| Hemodialysis | Lithium, salicylate, methanol, ethylene glycol |
| Hemoperfusion | Paraquat, theophylline, phenobarbital, salicylate |
| Peritoneal dialysis | Same indications, much less efficient than hemodialysis |

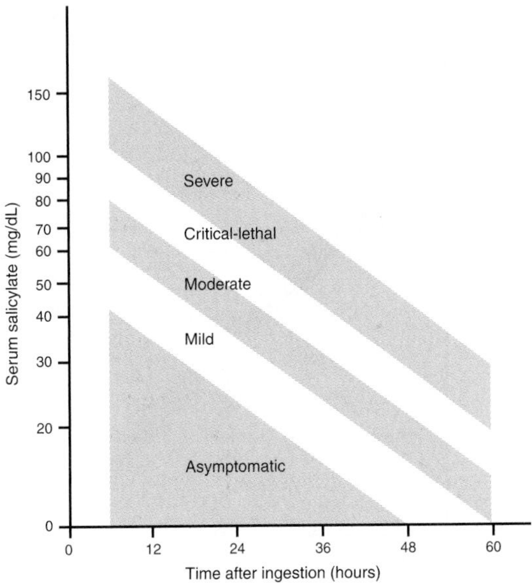


**FIGURE 29.1. Nomogram for determining salicylate toxicity.** (Adapted with permission from: Done AK. Pediatrics. 1960; 26:800.)

## Acetaminophen

Acetaminophen is one of the 10 most commonly used drugs for intentional self-poisoning. Mortality after toxic ingestion is only 0.4% in the United States due to available protective therapies. With ingestion of large amounts of acetaminophen, an intermediate metabolite accumulates, which, by rapid glutathione depletion, causes oxidative liver injury (see Figure 109.1 and chapter 109). Acute tubular necrosis may also occur. Doses exceeding 7.5 g (or >150 mg/kg) may be toxic, but usually 15 g or more must be ingested at one time to produce liver toxicity.

### Clinical Features

Untreated patients progress through four clinical stages. In stage 1 (12–24 hours), mild GI symptoms occur. A transient improvement (stage 2) occurs 24–48 hours after ingestion; the patient feels well, but liver enzymes begin to rise. Increasing serum creatinine at 48 hours reflects the onset of renal dysfunction that occurs in 25% of cases with documented hepatotoxicity. Stage 3 occurs 3–4 days postingestion, with jaundice, coagulopathy, and signs of hepatic encephalopathy. Stage 4 is the recovery period, which begins approximately 5 days postingestion, when normalization of liver function tests begins. Although most treated patients suffer no residual liver damage, mortality exceeds 75% in untreated cases.

Serial acetaminophen levels can predict toxicity from

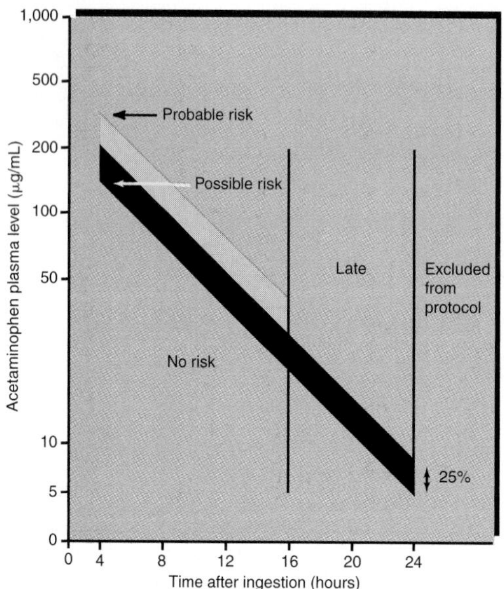


**FIGURE 29.2. Rumack-Matthew nomogram for acetaminophen poisoning.**
(Adapted with permission from: Hall, AH, Rumack BH. American Family Physician 1986; 33: 109, figure 3.)

the Rumack-Matthew nomogram (Figure 29.2). In general, levels of 200 g/ml at 4 hours after ingestion, or 50 g/ml at 12 hours, indicate the likelihood of hepatotoxicity. Prolongation of acetaminophen half-life from the normal 2–4 hours, hyperbilirubinemia, and prolongation of prothrombin time are all indicators of serious liver injury.

### Management

Patients presenting within 1 hour of ingestion should receive activated charcoal and a cathartic (i.e., sorbitol). Acetaminophen is rapidly absorbed; lavage, charcoal, or cathartics are not likely to be effective several hours after ingestion.

Acetylcysteine, a glutathione precursor that prevents accumulation of the toxic intermediary, is the treatment of choice. Between 4 and 24 hours postingestion, acetylcysteine therapy should be initiated based on the nomogram treatment line. If the amount ingested is unknown, or if the known ingestion is >140 mg/kg and at least 8 hours have passed since ingestion, acetylcysteine is given pending the serum acetaminophen levels. A loading dose of 140 mg/kg is given initially, followed by 70 mg/kg every 4 hours for 17 doses. There is some evidence to suggest that patients without hepatotoxicity can be safely treated with oral acetylcysteine for a course of 24 hours or less when acetaminophen levels become undetectable. With prompt treatment, the outcome is very favorable. Once hepatic toxicity has occurred, exchange transfusions and resin hemoperfusion may be tried. The taste of acetylcysteine is poorly tolerated. It may be given as a 1:3 dilution in a drink or as a 5% solution by nasogastric tube. Masking the taste with soft drinks is unsuccessful. If a patient vomits a dose within 1 hour of ingestion, it should be repeated. Ondansetron (or other selective 5HT3 receptor antagonist) given 30 minutes prior to oral acetylcysteine can prevent nausea and vomiting.

## Nonsteroidal Anti-Inflammatory Drugs

NSAIDs can be classified based on their selectivity for inhibition of cyclo-oxygenase isoforms 1 and 2 (COX-1 and COX-2). Inhibition of COX-1 is not necessary for anti-inflammatory or analgesic effects, but is thought to account for the majority of toxicity of traditional NSAIDs.

Nonselective NSAIDs include carboxylic acids (e.g., ibuprofen) and enolic acids (e.g., phenylbutazone, piroxicam). Both classes have similar pharmacologic properties, but overdose with enolic acids may be more serious than with carboxylic acids. The major symptoms seen in overdose greater than 100 mg/kg are mild CNS depression and GI upset, which usually respond to supportive care. More serious effects may follow ingestion of more than 400 mg/kg but are rare (Table 29.4). Figure 29.3 shows the correlation of plasma ibuprofen levels with symptomatic toxicity. This nomogram may help identify those patients who are initially asymptomatic and later develop complications (although this correlation has been controversial). Overdose with mefenamic acid results in a high incidence of seizures 2–7 hours after ingestion; treatment is with IV benzodiazepines.

The relatively selective COX-2 NSAIDs (etodolac

**TABLE 29.4. Complications of Overdose with Nonsteroidal Anti-inflammatory Agents**

| | |
|---|---|
| Gastrointestinal | Nausea, vomiting, ulceration |
| Neurologic | Drowsiness, disorientation, coma, convulsions |
| Renal | Metabolic acidosis, acute renal failure (especially in elderly) |
| Respiratory | Apnea, cyanosis |
| Allergic | Bronchospasm, urticaria in sensitive patients, anaphylactic shock (sulindac, tolmetin) |
| Cardiovascular | Hypotension, bradycardia, tachycardia |
| Hepatic | Hepatitis (sulindac), necrosis (phenylbutazone) |
| Hematologic | Aplastic anemia, hemolytic anemia |

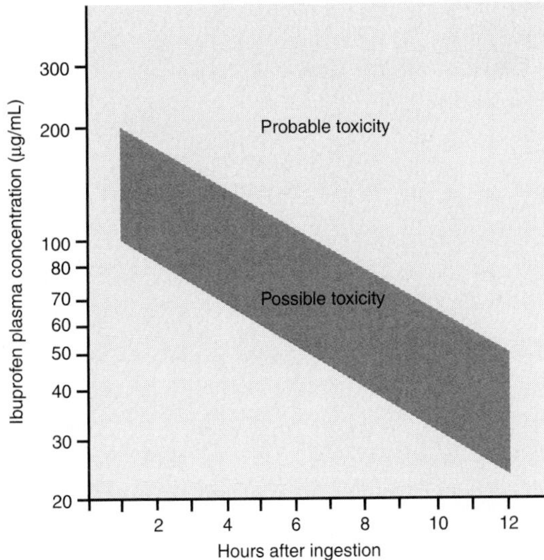


**FIGURE 29.3. Nomogram for determining ibuprofen toxicity in ibuprofen overdose.**
(Adapted with permission from: Hall AH, et al. Ann Emerg Med 1986; 15: 1309.)

and meloxicam) and the highly selective COX-2 inhibitors (celecoxib and rofecoxib) have side effect profiles similar to that of traditional NSAIDs but with fewer GI ulcers. Celecoxib is metabolized hepatically via the P-450–2C9 system, and therefore can increase levels of other drugs metabolized in this way that may be taken concomitantly. These include TCAs, SSRIs, antipsychotics, venlafaxine, some β-blockers, codeine, and dextromethorphan. Rofecoxib is primarily metabolized via cytosolic liver enzymes. There is minimal experience in overdose with COX-2 inhibitors.

Induction of emesis is not recommended in NSAID overdose and is definitely contraindicated for mefenamic acid ingestion. Gastric lavage may be of benefit if the patient presents within 1 hour of ingestion. If presentation is within 4 hours after ingestion, activated charcoal and a cathartic will help decrease absorption. Treatment is usually supportive with airway control, fluids, correction of acidosis, aggressive management of hypotension for renal perfusion, and treatment of bradycardia. Because of high protein binding, hemodialysis or hemoperfusion are not effective. No antidotes are available.

## Ethylene Glycol / Methanol

Ethylene glycol deserves special mention because of a newly marketed antidote, fomepizole (4-methylpyrazole). Ethylene glycol itself is nontoxic but is converted via the enzyme alcohol dehydrogenase to toxic metabolites including glycolic and oxalic acids. The metabolites cause metabolic acidosis, renal failure, hypocalcemia, oxaluria, CNS damage, and cardiovascular instability. A minimum of 60 ml has been reported to be lethal to an adult. Fomepizole inhibits alcohol dehydrogenase and has been shown to prevent renal injury when administered early in an acute intoxication. It is generally well tolerated, but there have been case reports of rash, transient high serum transaminases, and eosinophilia. Until recently, the standard treatment for ethylene glycol poisoning has been IV ethanol and hemodialysis. Prolonged ethanol therapy carries the risk of mental status changes, hepatotoxicity, and hypoglycemia. Kinetics are unpredictable, and frequent blood ethanol concentrations need to be measured. Fomepizole does not cause inebriation or hypoglycemia, and it is not difficult to maintain at therapeutic plasma levels.

Treatment with fomepizole should begin immediately on suspicion of ethylene glycol ingestion or with a confirmed plasma ethylene glycol level >20 mg/dl. Suspicion should arise when the patient appears intoxicated but the breath lacks an alcohol odor, there is anion gap metabolic acidosis, increased osmolar gap, or urine oxalate crystals. Dosing starts at 15 mg/kg IV load, then continues at 10 mg/kg every 12 hours until plasma levels of ethylene glycol are <20 mg/dl. The cofactors, thiamine and pyridoxine, should be administered in doses of 100 mg each to help minimize oxalic acid production. Hemodialysis may be required for significant or worsening metabolic acidosis or to lower the ethylene glycol plasma concentration below 50 mg/dl.

Methanol poisoning is also treated with fomepizole. Methanol is converted by alcohol dehydrogenase to formaldehyde, which in turn becomes formic acid and causes a metabolic acidosis. All patients should also receive folate, 50 mg IV every 4 hours, to increase the metabolism of formic acid.

## Tricyclic Antidepressants

TCA overdose is one of the most common causes of death from overdose in the United States. The death rate for those patients who reach the emergency department is about 2%. Death usually occurs from cardiac complications. The majority of deaths occur within the first 6 hours of admission. TCAs have a narrow therapeutic index: ingestion of 10 mg/kg may be toxic, and more than 20 mg/kg may be lethal. All of the tricyclic compounds and the tetracyclic, maprotiline, have virtually identical toxicity.

### Clinical Features

Symptoms and signs, primarily of the nervous and cardiovascular systems, usually appear within a few hours of overdose. Mild symptoms are anticholinergic effects, which include blurred vision, dry mouth, urinary and stool retention, and dizziness. Some cases may rapidly progress to delirium, hallucinations, seizures, and coma. Hyperthermia may be initially present; later in the course, hypothermia may be severe. Respiratory depression may be severe, and aspiration pneumonia and adult respiratory distress syndrome may occur.

Sinus tachycardia is the earliest and most common cardiac manifestation. It reflects anticholinergic effects and does not, by itself, indicate serious cardiac abnormality. Other ECG changes correlate with higher drug levels. Early evidence of toxicity includes a terminal R wave in the QRS complex in lead aVR. QRS widening over 100 msec is considered a sign of severe toxicity, although serious toxicity may occur in the absence of QRS widening. QRS durations over 160 msec were found in one study to be predictive of both seizures and ventricular arrhythmias.

Hypertension may occur initially after ingestion due to the blockade of norepinephrine uptake, but hypotension eventually develops in approximately 14% of patients. Hypotension is mediated through inhibition of fast sodium channels, which suppress cardiac contractility; peripheral α-blockade, which produces vasodilation; and eventual exhaustion of norepinephrine reserves. Hypotension has been associated with life-threatening arrhythmias, pulmonary edema, and cardiac arrest. Cardiac arrest occurs in 4–12% of TCA overdoses.

**TABLE 29.5. Summary of Treatment of Tricyclic Overdose**

| Symptom/Sign | Treatment* |
|---|---|
| Convulsions | Diazepam 0.1 mg/kg IV per dose as needed<br>Phenobarbital 3 mg/kg IV per dose as needed<br>Alkalinization |
| Coma | Airway support |
| Hypotension | Crystalloid infusion<br>Alkalinization<br>Vasopressors: norepinephrine, phenylephrine† |
| Ventricular arrhythmias‡ | Alkalinization<br>Lidocaine<br>Phenytoin, 15 mg/kg IV over 30 minutes |
| Prolonged QRS (≥0.10 seconds) | Alkalinization |
| Bradyarrhythmia/ heart block§ | Isoproterenol<br>Pacemaker |

*Basic and advanced cardiac support is initiated first, when indicated.
†Preferred agents.
‡Any arrhythmia that compromises hemodynamic status should be treated by cardioversion. Quinidine, procainamide, and disopyramide are contraindicated for any tricyclic overdose.
§Mobitz II second-degree or third-degree heart block.
(Adapted from: Frommer DA, Kulig RW, Marx JA, et al. JAMA 1987;257:525.)

## Management

A summary of treatment options in tricyclic overdose is provided in Table 29.5. When the patient arrives in the emergency department, basic management should be initiated. Gastric lavage is essential, and may be useful up to 12 hours after ingestion because anticholinergic effects slow gastric motility and emptying. Induced vomiting should be avoided because of the potential for rapid fluctuations in level of consciousness and, thus, the risk of aspiration. Activated charcoal, 50–100 g, very effectively binds TCAs. Sorbitol is useful as a cathartic. Because enterohepatic circulation occurs, repeated use of charcoal is indicated as long as GI motility is present. It can be given every 4–8 hours until the patient is improving. Hemodialysis, peritoneal dialysis, and exchange transfusion are ineffective.

Coma, which usually resolves in 24 hours, is treated with respiratory support and meticulous medical management. Seizures need to be treated aggressively because the resulting lactic acidosis can worsen cardiovascular complications. The treatment of choice for seizures is IV diazepam, with phenobarbital as a second choice. Hypotension is treated with fluids, usually normal saline, and bicarbonate. If the patient remains hypotensive after volume loading, hemodynamic monitoring and pressors should be initiated. Norepinephrine and phenylephrine are preferred. Alkalinization, by hyperventilation or sodium bicarbonate, may decrease QRS widening, help correct hypotension, and reduce arrhythmias. Thus, the indications for sodium bicarbonate include marked acidosis, refractory hypotension, prolonged cardiac conduction, ventricular dysrhythmias, and cardiac arrest. In addition, serum pH should be maintained above 7.45 to increase protein binding of TCAs. Lidocaine is the standard therapy for ventricular dysrhythmias if sodium bicarbonate fails. In the past, phenytoin was advocated as the antiarrhythmic of choice, but its efficacy has not been demonstrated in the overdose setting and its use is currently controversial. Supraventricular tachycardias may be cautiously treated with β-blockers, but at the risk of inducing bradycardia or hypotension. Isoproterenol can be used for significant bradyarrhythmias and torsades de pointes until overdrive pacing can be established. Physostigmine, once considered an antidote for anticholinergic effects, is now rarely used because of serious complications.

Serum levels of TCAs are unreliable indicators of the severity of the intoxication or prognosis and should not be used to guide clinical management.

TCA toxicity can occur with the routine prescription of a TCA and SSRI in combination. SSRIs can inhibit cytochrome P-450–2D6 metabolism of TCAs and lead to toxic levels. When a patient is taking this combination of medication and there are mental status changes or other signs of toxicity, the TCA should be discontinued until TCA levels can be obtained.

## Second-Generation Antidepressants

SSRIs are currently the most commonly prescribed antidepressants in the United States. This group includes fluoxetine (Prozac), sertraline (Zoloft), paroxetine (Paxil), citalopram (Celexa), and fluvoxamine (Luvox). SSRIs are rarely fatal when ingested alone, although a large ingestion (usually over 75 times the daily dose) can lead to confusion, agitation, arrhythmias, and seizures. Treatment is supportive and symptomatic, including gastric lavage, activated charcoal, maintaining an adequate airway and ventilation, monitoring vital signs and ECG, and IV diazepam for ongoing seizures. There do not appear to be any differences in overdose toxicity among the SSRIs.

Other second-generation antidepressants include bupropion (Wellbutrin), venlafaxine (Effexor), nefazodone (Serzone), and mirtazapine (Remeron). As with the SSRIs, overdose toxicity is much less than with TCAs. However, fatalities have been reported with bupropion (ongoing seizures) and venlafaxine (cardiac and neurological toxicity). Treatment is again supportive and symptomatic.

## Antipsychotics

High-potency antipsychotics include haloperidol (Haldol), fluphenazine (Prolixin), and thiothixene (Navane) (See Table 26.2). Overdose fatalities are rare in this group, although complications include CNS depression, rigidity, tremor, seizures, and impaired thermoregulation. Arrhythmias are relatively rare. Treatment is supportive and symptomatic. Antiparkinson medication such as benztropine (Cogentin) or diphenhydramine (Benadryl) may be useful for rigidity or tremor.

Low-potency antipsychotics include chlorpromazine (Thorazine), thioridazine (Mellaril), and mesoridazine (Serentil) (See Table 26.2). Overdose on these compounds can lead to sedation, hypotension, confusion, and seizures. Because these compounds can prolong QT intervals, arrhythmias are possible. Treatment again consists of symptomatic and supportive care.

Newer ("atypical") antipsychotics include clozapine (Clozaril), risperidone (Risperdal), olanzapine (Zyprexa), and quetiapine (Seroquel) (See Table 26.3). Symptoms in clozapine overdose include hypotension, delirium, coma, respiratory depression, seizures, arrhythmias, and hypersalivation. Treatment is supportive and symptomatic. Patients should be observed for several days because of a possible delayed effect. There are case reports of overdose fatalities with risperidone, olanzapine, and quetiapine, although the vast majority of patients recover with symptomatic and supportive care. Symptoms can include CNS depression, dystonias, hypertension, and tachycardia. Many of these newer compounds have been associated with QT prolongation, and thus cardiac monitoring should be routine.

## Mood-Stabilizing Agents

Overdose on valproate (Depakote) usually leads to mild and reversible CNS depression, although coma, seizures, impaired liver function (including hyperammonemia), and electrolyte disturbance are possible. Supportive measures are used. Multiple doses of activated charcoal are the mainstay of treatment. Because of rapid absorption, gastric lavage may be of limited value unless delayed release preparations are taken. Naloxone has been reported to reverse the CNS depressant effects of valproate overdose, but could theoretically reverse antiepilepsy effects and should be used with caution. Hemodialysis is sometimes recommended in massive overdose to remove the unbound fraction of valproate.

Overdose on lithium is a serious situation because of the narrow therapeutic index of this medication. Therapeutic levels are between 0.4 and 1.0 mEq/L. Signs of toxicity can start above 1.5 mEq/L, and death can occur over 3.0 mEq/L. Early signs of toxicity include vomiting, diarrhea, confusion, apathy, and ataxia and fine tremor. These can progress to coma, seizures, coarse tremor, dysarthria, hypertonia, myoclonus, and cardiovascular collapse. Treatment is supportive and includes normal saline given IV if the patient is dehydrated or shows signs of infection. Dialysis is used if there is no response to supportive measures. Serial lithium levels are usually monitored, although they do not always correlate with clinical status or prognosis.

## Benzodiazepines

Benzodiazepines are the most popular class of sedative-hypnotics in the United States. They are commonly prescribed for insomnia, anxiety and panic disorders, perioperative sedation, muscle strain, and seizure disorders (see Table 24.2 for dosages and half-lives). Because of their wide therapeutic index, serious toxic reactions seldom occur; nonetheless, they are often implicated in intentional or iatrogenic overdose.

### Clinical Features

Mild manifestations of toxicity include disinhibition, slurred speech, ataxia, and sedation. These can progress to respiratory depression, stupor, and coma, which predispose the patient to pulmonary aspiration of gastric contents. In particular, if other drugs such as alcohol, narcotics, or TCAs have been ingested, hypoventilation may occur.

### Management

Previously, treatment of benzodiazepine overdose was limited to supportive management. The usual measures of lavage, charcoal, cathartics, and mechanical ventilation, if necessary, were successful in the majority of cases. However, flumazenil (Mazicon), the first specific benzodiazepine antagonist, can be used for both diagnosis and treatment of benzodiazepine overdose. An initial bolus of 0.2 mg of flumazenil is given IV over 30 seconds. Within 1–2 minutes, sedation and respiratory depression are usually reversed. A dose of 0.3–0.5 mg may be repeated after 3–5 minutes if an adequate response is not noted. Most patients will respond to cumulative doses of 0.2–1.0 mg; however, in severe overdose, as much as 5.0 mg may be required. Because the half-life of flumazenil is short (approximately 50 minutes), patients must be observed closely for recurrence of sedation or hypoventilation.

Nausea, dizziness, agitation, hot flushes, headache, and sweating are among the adverse effects of flumazenil. Seizures may occur if the patient has been taking benzodiazepines for seizure control or if the patient has ingested both a benzodiazepine and a TCA. If the seizure warrants pharmacologic control, a nonbenzodiazepine anticonvulsant, such as phenytoin, should be used.

## Miscellaneous Drugs

All medicinal agents can be taken in overdose, either deliberately or accidentally, and treatment is usually supportive. Treatment advances in the management of poisoning occur regularly. If the clinician is not familiar with the treatment of a specific substance, prescribing information, a poison control center, and the Poisindex should be consulted.

## Questions

**Instructions:** For each question below, select **one** lettered answer that is the **best** for each question.

1. An 18 year old senior high school student is brought to the emergency room by a friend. The patient is having visual hallucinations, is restless, pulse of 130/min., responds to questions in a tangential manner, keeps insisting that she wants to go home and needs to be restrained from leaving the area. What is your next step?
   A. Administer 5 mg haloperidol intravenously
   B. Call social service to begin commitment proceedings
   C. Obtain recent history from friend and do a physical exam
   D. Have psychologist do a detailed psychological interview

2. A psychiatric consultation is requested on an elderly hospitalized man with diabetes who presents with delirium. Under which axis will the diabetes fall in the *Diagnostic and Statistical Manual on Mental Disorders* classification?
   A. Axis I
   B. Axis II
   C. Axis III
   D. Axis IV
   E. Axis V

3. In a normal-weight, 20 year old college student, which of the following physical signs would be most suggestive of bulimia?
   A. Bilateral parotid enlargement
   B. Cheilosis
   C. Abdominal bloating
   D. Lower extremity edema

4. A 22-year-old female presents with her third bout of sinusitis in the past year. She has no history of allergies and is on no medications. She smokes 1 pack per day for 5 years. Which of the following interventions is likely to have the least impact on her long-term health?
   A. Advice to stop smoking
   B. Referral to a smoking cessation program
   C. Antibiotics for her sinusitis
   D. Bupropion or nicotine replacement therapy

5. Antipsychotics may cause which of the following acute side effects:
   A. Dystonic reaction
   B. QT prolongation
   C. Seizure
   D. Extrapyramidal symptoms
   E. All of the above

6. All of the following are risk factors for suicide except:
   A. substance abuse
   B. personality disorder
   C. female gender

D. advanced age
E. living alone

7. A 52-year-old man is admitted for alcohol withdrawal. He is tremulous and diaphoretic and his heart rate is 110. What is the most appropriate initial treatment?
   A. Naltrexone
   B. Lorazepam
   C. Haloperidol
   D. Phenytoin

8. A 30-year-old man is brought to the emergency department by his roommate. He complains of chest pain and appears somewhat agitated. His roommate suspects that he is using drugs. Which of the following drugs is most likely?
   A. Alcohol
   B. Heroin
   C. Cocaine
   D. Marijuana

9. To prevent liver damage with acetaminophen overdose, the treatment of choice is which of the following?
   A. exchange transfusions
   B. hemodialysis
   C. activated charcoal
   D. N-acetylcysteine

## Answers

| | | | | |
|---|---|---|---|---|
| 1. C | 2. C | 3. A | 4. C | 5. E |
| 6. C | 7. B | 8. C | 9. D | |

## SUGGESTED READING

### *Books and Monographs*

American Psychiatric Association: Diagnostic and Statistical Manual of Mental Disorders. 4th ed. Text Revision. Washington, DC: American Psychiatric Association, 2000.

Sullivan JT, Sykora K, Schneiderman J, et al. Assessment of alcohol withdrawal: the revised Clinical Institute Withdrawal Assessment for Alcohol scale. British Journal of Addiction 1989;84:1353–1357.

Elster J. Strong Feelings. Emotion, Addiction and Human Behavior. Cambridge: MIT Press, 1999.

Hacking I. The Social Construction of What? Cambridge: Harvard University Press, 1999.

Rosen P, Barkin R (eds). Emergency Medicine: Concepts and Clinical Practice. 4th ed. St. Louis: Mosby-Year Book, 1998.

Sadock BJ, Sadock VA (eds). Kaplan & Sadock's Comprehensive Textbook of Psychiatry. ed VII. Philadelphia, PA: Lippincott Williams & Wilkins, 2000.

### *Articles*

*Biopsychosocial Approach*

Engel GL. The need for a new medical model: a challenge for biomedicine. Science 1977;196:129–135.

Leon AC, Olfson M, Broadhead WE. Prevalence of mental disorders in primary care. Arch Fam Med 1995;4:857–861.

Novack DH. Therapeutic aspects of the clinical encounter. J Gen Intern Med 1987;2:346–355.

*Somatic Distress Disorders*

Gamsa A. The role of psychological factors in chronic pain. 1. A half century of study. Pain 1994;57:5.

Noyes R, Kathol RG, Fisher MM, et al. Psychiatric comorbidity among patients with hypochondriasis. Gen Hosp Psychiatry 1994;16:78–87.

Ross SE. "Memes" as infectious agents in psychosomatic illness. Ann Intern Med 1999;131:867–871.

Smith GR. The course of somatization and its effects on utilization of health care resources. Psychosomatics 1994;35: 263–267.

Taylor DC. Hysteria: play-acting and courage. Br J Psychiatry 1986;149:37–41.

Wesselly S. New wine in old bottles: Neurasthenia and ME. Psychological Med 1990;20:35–53.

*Anxiety Disorders*

Brunello N, et al. Social phobia: diagnosis and epidemiology, neurobiology and pharmacology, co-morbidity and treatment. J Affect Disord 2000;60:61–74.

Fleet RP, Dupuis G, Marchand A, et al. Panic disorder in emergency department chest pain patients: prevalence, comorbidity, suicidal ideation, and physician recognition. Am J Med 1996;101:371–380.

Hidalgo RB, Davidson JR. Selective serotonin reuptake inhibitors in post–traumatic stress disorder. J Psychopharmacol 2000;14:70–76.

Moreno FA, Delgado PL. Living with anxiety disorders: As good as it gets . . .? Bull. of Menninger Clinic 2000;64:3 Suppl A: A4–21.

Shader RI, Greenblatt DJ. Use of benzodiazepines in anxiety disorders. N Engl J Med 1993;328:1398–1405.

Simon NM, Pollack MH. Treatment-refractory panic disorder. Psychiatr Clin North Am 1999;6:115–140.

*The Depressive Disorders*

Brown C, Schulberg HC, Madonia MJ, et al. Treatment outcomes for primary care patients with major depression and lifetime anxiety disorders. Am J Psychiatry 1996;153:1293–1300.

Guscott R, Taylor L. Lithium prophylaxis in recurrent affective illness: efficacy, effectiveness, and efficiency. Br J Psychiatry 1994;164:741–746.

Keller MB, et al. A comparison of nefazodone, the cognitive behavioral analysis system of psychotherapy, and their combination for the treatment of chronic depression. N Engl J Med 2000;342:1462–70.

Nemeroff CB. Psychopharmacology of affective disorders in the 21st century. Biol Psychiatry 1998;44:517–525.

Post RM, Weiss SRB. The neurobiology of treatment-resistant mood disorders. Bloom FF, Kupfer DJ. eds. Psychopharmacology: the fourth generation of progress. 1995. Pp. 155–170. Raven Press, NY, NY.

Rosenthal NE. Diagnosis and treatment of seasonal affective disorder. JAMA 1993;270:2717–2720.

Whooley MA, Simon GE. Primary care: managing depression in medical outpatients. N Engl J Med 2000;343:1942–1950.

*Psychotic Disorders*

Allen MH. Managing the agitated psychotic patient: a reappraisal of the evidence. J Clin Psychiatry 2000;61(suppl 14):11–20.

Compton MT, Nemeroff CB. The treatment of bipolar depression. J Clin Psychiatry 2000;61(suppl 9):57–67.

Feifel D. Rationale and guidelines for the inpatient treatment of acute psychosis. J Clin Psychiatry 2000;61(suppl 14): 27–32.

Fujii DE, Ahmed I, Jokumsen M, et al. The effects of clozapine on cognitive functioning in treatment-resistant schizophrenic patients. J Neuropsychiatry Clin Neurosci 1997;9:240–245.

Inouye SK, Schlesinger MJ, Lydon TJ. Delirium: a symptom of how hospital care is failing older persons and a window to improve quality of hospital care. Am J Med 1999;106: 565–573.

Meltzer HY. Treatment of schizophrenia and spectrum disorders: pharmacotherapy, psychosocial treatments, and neurotransmitter interactions. Biol Psychiatry 1999;46:1321–327.

Post RM. Transduction of psychosocial stress into the neurobiology of recurrent affective disorder. Am J Psychiatry 1992;149:999–1010.

Rosenheck R, Cramer J, Xu W, et al. A comparison of clozapine and haloperidol in hospitalized patients with refractory schizophrenia. N Engl J Med 1997:337;809–815.

Tueth MJ. Emergencies caused by side effects of psychiatric medications. Am J Emerg Med 1994;23:212–216.

### *Eating Disorders*

Becker AE, Grinspoon SK, Klibanski A, et al. Eating disorders. N Engl J Med 1999:340;1092–8.

Jimerson DC, Wolfe BE, Brotman AW, et al. Medications in the treatment of eating disorders. Psychiatr Clin North Am 1996;19:739–754.

Mehler P. Diagnosis and care of patients with anorexia nervosa in primary care settings. Ann Intern Med 2001;134: 1048–59.

Walsh JM, Wheat ME, Freund K. Detection, evaluation, and treatment of eating disorders: The role of the primary care physician. J Gen Intern Med 2000:15;577–90.

Warren MP. Anorexia, bulimia, and exercise-induced amenorrhea: medical approach. Curr Ther Endocrinol Metab 1997; 6:13–17.

### *Substance Abuse*

Benzer DG. Quantification of the alcohol withdrawal syndrome in 487 alcoholic patients. J Subst Abuse Treat 1990;7:117–123

Cherubin CE, Sapiera JD. The medical complications of drug addiction and the medical assessment of the intravenous drug user: 25 years later. Ann Intern Med 1993;119:1017–1028.

Hurt RD, Sachs DP, Glover ED, et al. A comparison of sustained-release bupropion and placebo for smoking cessation. N Engl J Med 1997;337:1995–2202.

Lieber CS. Medical disorders of alcoholism. N Engl J Med 1995;333:1058–1065.

Rustin T. Management of nicotine withdrawal; principles of addiction medicine. American Society of Addiction Medicine, Inc. 1998;6:487–495.

Saitz R, Mayo-Smith MF, Roberts MS, et al. Individualized treatment for alcohol withdrawal. A randomized double-blind controlled trial. JAMA 1994;272:519–523.

Wadler GI. Drug use update. Med Clin North Am 1994;2: 439–455.

### *Clinical Toxicology*

Barceloux DG, Krenzelok EP, Olson K, et al. American Academy of Clinical Toxicology Practice Guidelines on the Treatment of Ethylene Glycol Poisoning. J Toxicol Clin Toxicol 1999;37:537–560.

Bolgiano EB, Barish RA. Use of new and established antidotes. Emerg Med Clin North Am 1994;12:317–334.

Brent J, McMartin K, Phillips S, et al. Fomepizole for the treatment of methanol poisoning. N Engl J Med 2001;344: 424–9.

Kulig K. Initial management of ingestions of toxic substances. N Engl J Med 1992;326:1677–1681.

McClain CJ, Holtzman J, Allen J, et al. Clinical features of acetaminophen toxicity. J Clin Gastroenterol 1988;10:76–80.

Pimentel L, Trommer L. Cyclic antidepressant overdoses. A review. Emerg Med Clin North Am 1994;12:533–547.

Vernon DD, Gleich MC. Poisoning and drug overdose. Crit Care Clin 1997;13:647–667.

Yip L, Dart RC, Gabow PA. Concepts and controversies in salicylate toxicity. Emerg Med Clin North Am 1994;12: 351–364.

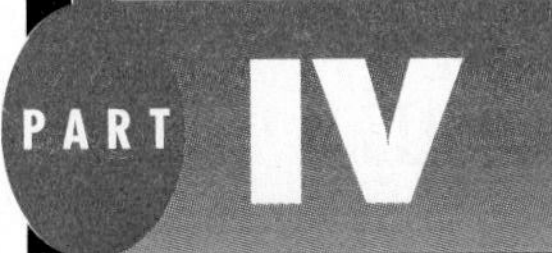

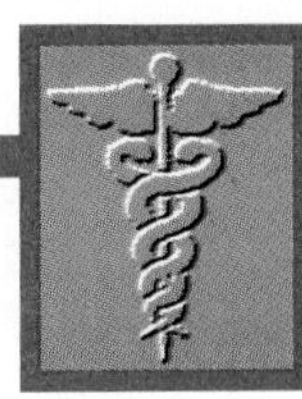

PART IV

Virinderjit S. Bamrah
Peter D. Chapman

# CARDIOVASCULAR DISEASES

# CHAPTER 30 COMMON PRESENTATIONS OF HEART DISEASE IN ADULTS

## Chest Pain/Discomfort

Chest pain or discomfort, an exceedingly common symptom, should be fully characterized by asking the appropriate questions, which may be recalled with the mnemonic PQRST (Table 30.1). The history is the most useful tool for elucidating its cause (Table 30.2).

## Dyspnea

Dyspnea, or shortness of breath, in patients with chronic heart failure results from pulmonary venous hypertension. Mild heart failure may cause dyspnea only on exertion. With progressive heart failure, the threshold for dyspnea decreases, and patients may report orthopnea, paroxysmal nocturnal dyspnea, or episodic acute pulmonary edema.

**Orthopnea** is dyspnea occurring in recumbency and is promptly relieved by sitting the patient up or elevating his or her head. When caused by cardiac disease, orthopnea signifies a high left ventricular (LV) filling pressure. It may also occur in patients with asthma, chronic obstructive lung disease (COPD), massive ascites, or bilateral diaphragmatic paralysis. **Paroxysmal nocturnal dyspnea** (PND) is slightly more specific for left heart failure, but it also occurs in patients with chronic obstructive pulmonary disease and asthma. Usually, the patient awakens gasping for breath and feeling suffocated 2–5 hours after falling asleep. Dyspnea and the associated cough and wheezing ("cardiac asthma") abate in 15–30 minutes, usually by sitting up, walking, or opening a window. Coughing up mucus relieves PND in COPD.

**TABLE 30.1. Important Chest Pain Characteristics**

| | | |
|---|---|---|
| P | – | Provocative (what activities precipitate pain?)<br>Palliative (what alleviates pain?) |
| Q | – | Quality (describe pain and any associated symptoms) |
| R | – | Region (describe location of pain)<br>Radiation (does pain radiate and, if so, where?) |
| S | – | Severity (describe intensity of pain) |
| T | – | Timing (describe usual duration of each episode)<br>Time (how long since episodes first began?) |

## Edema

Peripheral edema develops when fluid volume expands by about 5 L (a 10-lb weight gain) caused by sodium and water retention. Edema owing to heart disease reflects **right heart failure;** it is gravity-dependent and, thus, is first noted in the feet and ankles of ambulatory persons. Right heart failure and edema usually develop late in heart disease.

## Fatigue

Commonly reported by patients with heart disease, fatigue is subjective and nonspecific and is often due to noncardiac causes. When seen in patients with heart failure, fatigue signifies a low cardiac output. Sometimes, it is iatrogenic—following use of β-blockers or excessive use of diuretics.

## Palpitations

Palpitations can be described as experiencing an unpleasant awareness of one's heartbeat, often caused by changes in cardiac rhythm or contraction force. Palpitations do not necessarily indicate the presence of heart disease or arrhythmia; normal persons may report them under conditions such as exercise, acute anxiety, or excessive use of caffeine or other stimulants.

Palpitations may also be caused by arrhythmias, particularly extrasystoles. The patient often senses the forceful beat after the extrasystole occurs, not the extrasystole itself.

All forms of tachycardia, hyperkinetic or high cardiac output states, and volume overload of the heart may evoke palpitations. The onset of rapid heart action (whether it starts and ends suddenly or gradually) and its regularity should be determined.

## Other Symptoms

Many other symptoms may occur in patients with heart disease and should be inquired about and recorded. For example, **hemoptysis,** or bloody expectoration, may be seen in mitral stenosis, pulmonary infarction, or pulmonary hypertension or with an aortic aneurysm eroding the tracheobronchial tree. A dry, nonproductive **cough,** often worse when supine, is seen in pulmonary congestion caused by heart failure. **Nocturia**—large volumes of urine at night rather than simply increased frequency—is common in patients with heart failure. Anorexia, abdominal fullness, and weight loss (cardiac cachexia) may occur in patients with advanced heart

**TABLE 30.2. Frequent Causes of Chest Pain and Their Characteristics**

| Condition | Provocative Factors (P) | Palliative Factors (P) | Quality (Q) | Region (R) | Timing (T) |
|---|---|---|---|---|---|
| Stable angina | Emotion, exercise, meals, cold | Rest, nitroglycerin | Pressure, tightness, ache, heaviness | Variable—see text | <10 min |
| Unstable angina | Same as stable angina, but may be present at rest | Nitroglycerin, sometimes | Same as stable angina | Same as stable angina | >10 min |
| Myocardial infarction | — | Relief of coronary obstruction | Same as stable angina | Same as stable angina | >30 min |
| Pericarditis | Breathing, supine position | Sitting upright | Sharp, pleuritic | Left precordial | Hours/days |
| Dissecting aortic aneurysm | — | None | Severe, tearing | Substernal, interscapular | Abrupt onset, hours |
| Anxiety | Emotion | Removal of stimulus | Sharp, stabbing | Left breast, pinpoint area | Variable |
| Pneumonia, pulmonary embolism/infarction | Deep inspiration | Analgesics | Generally sharp | Substernal, site of pulmonary infarction | Abrupt onset minutes/hours |
| Chest wall pain | Chest wall movement, palpation | Rest, salicylates | Sharp | Variable | Seconds/hours |
| Esophageal reflux | Supine position, empty stomach | Antacids, meals | Burning | Substernal, epigastric | <1 hour |

**TABLE 30.3. Functional Classification of Heart Disease: A Comparison of New York Heart Association (NYHA) and the Canadian Cardiovascular Society (CCS) Criteria**

| Class | NYHA | CCS |
|---|---|---|
| | Evaluates overall functional capacity. | Evaluates functional capacity in angina. |
| I | No limitation of physical activity. | No limitation of activity. Angina does not follow ordinary physical activity. |
| II | Slight limitation of physical activity. Ordinary physical activity results in fatigue, palpitations, dyspnea, or anginal pain. | Slight limitation of ordinary activity. Angina may be provoked by walking >2 blocks on level ground or climbing >1 flight of stairs at a normal pace and under normal conditions. |
| III | Marked limitation of physical activity. Ordinary physical activity causes fatigue, palpitations, dyspnea, or anginal pain. | Marked limitation of ordinary activity. Angina provoked by walking 1–2 blocks on ground or climbing 1 flight of stairs under normal conditions. |
| IV | Unable to carry on any physical activity without discomfort. Symptoms of cardiac insufficiency or angina may be present even at rest and increase with any physical activity. | Severe limitation of activity. Inability to carry on any physical activity without angina. Angina may occur at rest. |

failure; fever and chills in infective endocarditis; epistaxis in hypertension; and recurrent pneumonias in large left-to-right shunts. Syncope is another manifestation of heart disease and may signify aortic stenosis, neurocardiogenic syncope, or arrhythmias.

## Functional Classification of Heart Disease

Functional capacity is an important prognostic indicator in heart disease. The most widely used method is the New York Heart Association (NYHA) Functional Classification, which measures disability in heart failure (see chapter 37, Table 37.5). This system is a fairly subjective measure of disability but more realistically estimates a patient's functional improvement or decline over time and also the effects of therapy. A similar system, the Canadian Cardiovascular Society Criteria, rates disability from angina (Table 30.3).

# CHAPTER 31 CARDIOVASCULAR EXAMINATION

## Arterial Pulse

Arterial pulse (Figure 31.1) is best evaluated by palpating the brachial or, less preferably, the radial artery to determine the rate and rhythm. All accessible arterial pulses should be felt and compared bilaterally; normal arterial pulses are symmetric. As the closest accessible arteries to the aortic valve, the carotids should be palpated, one at a time, for assessing pulse volume and contour, which accurately reflect LV ejection velocity, stroke volume, and aortic valve function. The normal carotid, felt as a gentle tap, has a rapid upstroke. Distal pulses, with their greater amplitude and velocity of flow, can mask diagnostic clues.

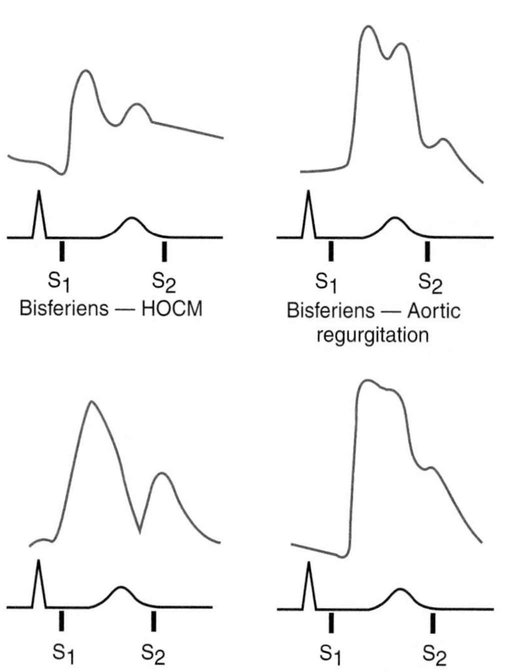


**FIGURE 31.1.** Carotid pulse tracings. The **bisferiens pulse** contains two systolic peaks that occur in conditions with rapid ejection of blood through the aortic valve. In the **dicrotic pulse,** the second palpable wave is diastolic and is due to an exaggerated dicrotic wave following the dicrotic notch (aortic valve closure). A normal carotid pulse is shown for comparison. HOCM = hypertrophic (obstructive) cardiomyopathy.

A **high-volume (amplitude) pulse,** or bounding pulse, corresponds to increased pulse pressure (systolic minus diastolic pressure) that follows rapid ejection of a large stroke volume into the aorta against a low systemic vascular resistance. It occurs in hyperkinetic states (anxiety, fever, thyrotoxicosis, anemia), aortic regurgitation, patent ductus arteriosus, arteriovenous fistula, bradycardia, and arteriosclerosis. A **small-volume pulse** corresponds to decreased pulse pressure that follows slow ejection of a normal or low stroke volume; it may also occur when the systemic vascular resistance is high. The pulse is weak and thready in left heart failure and shock. In severe aortic valvular stenosis, the pulse is typically low volume, with a slowly rising upstroke and a delayed peak (***pulsus parvus et tardus***; *parvus* means "slow rising" and *tardus* means "late"). In the elderly with aortic valve stenosis and hypertension or arteriosclerosis, these features may be absent.

In **pulsus bisferiens** (*bis* means "twice" and *feriens* means "beating"), the pulse has two strong systolic peaks; the percussion and tidal waves occur before the dicrotic notch. Pulsus bisferiens is seen in severe aortic regurgitation, aortic regurgitation with stenosis, and hypertrophic obstructive cardiomyopathy.

In a **dicrotic pulse,** the second palpable peak occurs in diastole and is an exaggerated dicrotic wave following the dicrotic notch (aortic valve closure). Associated with a low cardiac output and low peripheral resistance, dicrotic pulse is typically seen in heart failure, hypovolemic shock, and young patients with fever. It is **rare** in patients older than 45 years.

Pulsus alternans indicates alternately strong and weak pulses, occurring at regular intervals or sometimes detected in the brachial or radial pulses by palpation, it usually requires a blood pressure cuff for detection (manifesting as a sudden doubling of rate as the blood pressure cuff is slowly deflated). Pulsus alternans is produced when high and low stroke volumes are ejected alternately from larger and smaller end-diastolic volumes of the LV. Its presence always indicates severe LV dysfunction.

Pulsus paradoxus is an excessive drop (>10 mm Hg) in systolic pressure during inspiration. In normal subjects, systolic pressure (measured with a blood pressure cuff) falls 3–10 mm Hg during inspiration. When the paradox exceeds 20 mm Hg, it is usually specific for cardiac tamponade due to pericardial effusion. In pericardial tamponade, right ventricular (RV) filling increases during inspiration, causing a larger RV volume and a raised intrapericardial pressure; this lowers inspiratory LV filling and leads to a diminished inspiratory LV stroke volume and pulse amplitude. Pulsus paradoxus may be noted in other conditions such as acute severe asthma, severe cardiomegaly, marked obesity, and massive pulmonary embolism.

## Venous (Jugular) Pulse

### Bedside evaluation

Bedside examination of the jugular venous pulse allows evaluation of the right atrial pressure and the morphology of the venous pulse waveforms. Examining the right internal jugular vein is preferred to the external jugular vein for pulse wave analysis because the right vein is in a direct line with the superior vena cava and, thus, better reflects right atrial events.

The patient should rest quietly in bed with his or her neck muscles relaxed and trunk elevated to a sufficient angle—usually 30–45 degrees—to allow the venous pulse to be visible. Venous pulses are often best seen with tangential lighting. To estimate jugular venous pressure, the vertical distance from the sternal angle to the top of the oscillating venous column is measured (Figure 31.2). This distance is ordinarily less than 3 cm. Because the sternal angle is approximately 5 cm above the mid-right atrium, regardless of body position, the jugular venous pressure would equal 5 cm plus 3 cm (the height of the oscillating venous column), or 8 cm $H_2O$. This value can be converted to mm Hg by dividing it by 1.3 (1 mm Hg = 1.3 cm of blood); thus, the upper limit of normal jugular venous pressure is 6 mm Hg.

Jugular venous pressure reflects the mean right atrial or central venous pressure. The most common cause of an elevated right atrial pressure is **RV failure.** Other causes include tricuspid regurgitation and abnormalities of RV filling (pericardial tamponade, constrictive pericarditis, or rarely, tricuspid stenosis) (Figure 31.3). The normal jugular venous pressure decreases with inspiration and increases with expiration. In superior vena cava obstruction, the venous pressure is elevated but the venous waves and respiratory fluctuation are absent.

### Hepatojugular reflux

In incipient or early right heart failure when the venous pressure is normal, a positive **hepatojugular reflux** may be elicited. When steady pressure is applied to the abdomen (liver) for 15–20 seconds (ensuring that the patient does not perform a Valsalva maneuver) in normal individuals, the venous column rises transiently but returns to normal, despite continued abdominal compression. A positive hepatojugular reflux is one where the venous column increases more than 1 cm and remains high throughout the period of compression and gradually declines only after compression is relieved. The hepatojugular reflux occurs as the abnormal RV is unable to handle the increased venous return during abdominal compression.

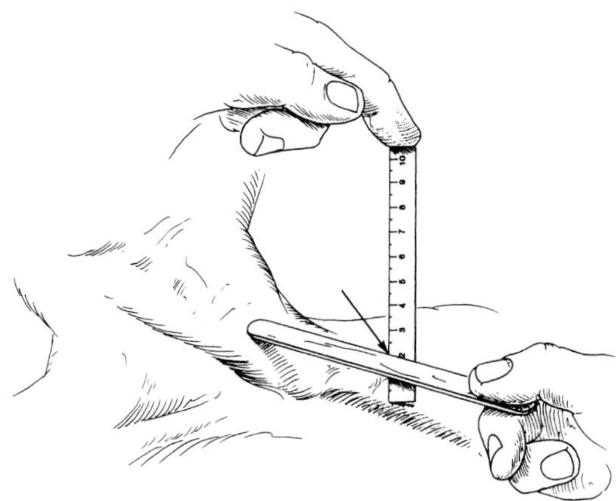

**FIGURE 31.2. Measuring the jugular venous pressure.** (From: Adair OV, Havranck EP (eds.). Cardiology Secrets. Philadelphia: Henley & Belfus, Inc., 1995, p. 17. Used with permission.)

### Jugular venous pulse waves

The normal jugular venous pulse has two visible peaks (the *a* and *v* waves) and two troughs (the *x* and *y* descents) (see Figure 31.3). Another positive deflection after the *a* wave, the *c* wave, is not palpable but can be recorded; however, it is of little clinical importance.

- The ***a wave*** is produced by retrograde blood flow in the jugular veins caused by right atrial contraction. The *a* wave immediately precedes the carotid upstroke and the first heart sound, $S_1$.
- The ***x descent*** reflects a fall in right atrial pressure that occurs with right atrial relaxation and the downward movement of the tricuspid valve ring owing to RV systole. The *x* descent is often the most easily detected motion in the jugular pulse; it occurs during systole and ends just prior to $S_2$.
- The ***v wave*** results from venous inflow to the right atrium during ventricular systole while the tricuspid valve is closed. It occurs roughly coincident with the carotid pulse and the $S_2$.
- The ***y descent*** results from the fall in atrial pressure that occurs as the tricuspid valve opens.

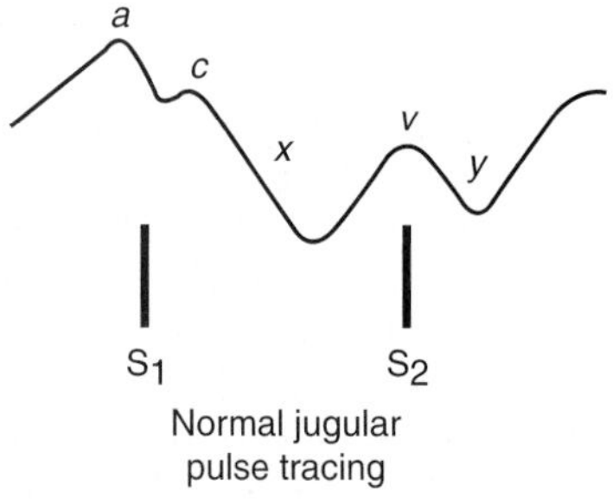


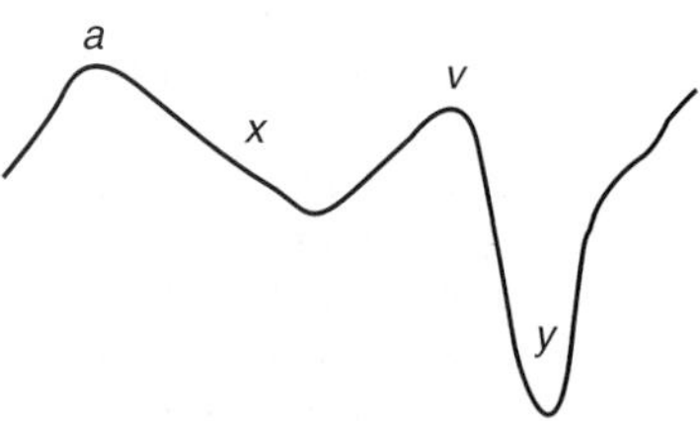


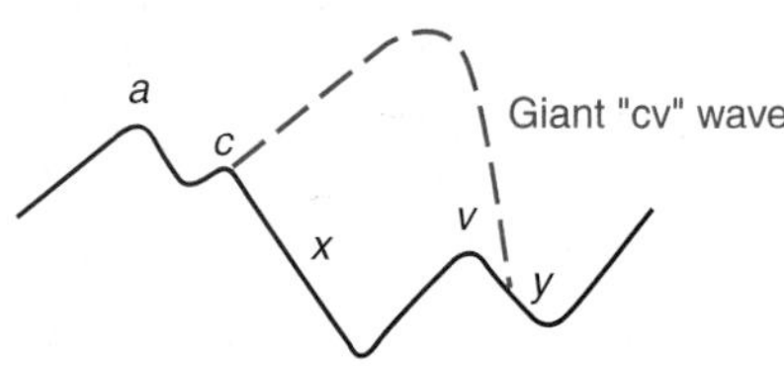


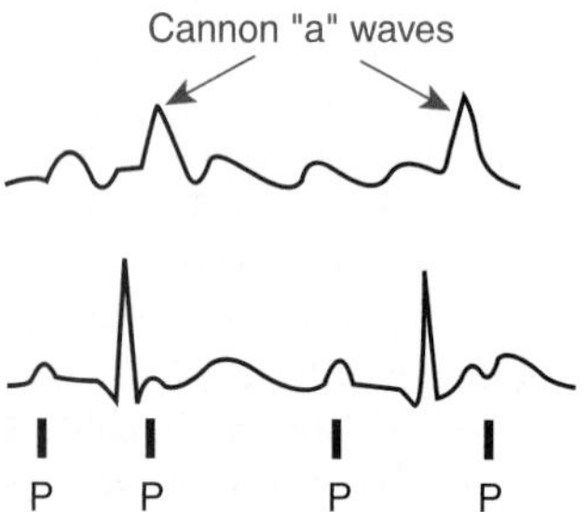


**FIGURE 31.3.** Jugular venous pulse tracings. **Normal jugular venous pressure**—The a wave and x descent are normally more prominent than the v wave and y descent. The c wave may be recorded but is not palpable on examination. **Constrictive pericarditis**—The steep y descent (diastolic ventricular filling) results from elevated venous pressures and rapid early diastolic filling. As the rigid pericardium suddenly limits further inflow, the pressure rapidly rises. **Severe tricuspid regurgitation**—A giant cv wave of tricuspid regurgitation is shown. **Cannon a waves** in complete heart block—Note the large *a* waves in the venous pulse, which occur due to atrial contraction against a closed tricuspid valve during ventricular systole.

Normally, the *a* wave is more visible than the *v* wave, and the *x* descent is more prominent than the *y* descent. In fact, the *v* wave and *y* descent are often not visible in healthy adults owing to the very compliant normal right atrium.

**Abnormalities of jugular venous pulse waves**

The ***a wave*** is increased in RV hypertrophy, tricuspid or pulmonic stenosis, or contraction of the atrium against a closed tricuspid valve (so-called cannon *a* wave, see Figure 31.3). Cannon waves occur regularly in junctional rhythm and irregularly in atrioventricular dissociation. The normal *a* wave is absent and the *x* descent less prominent in atrial fibrillation.

The ***x descent*** becomes deeper in pericardial tamponade and constrictive pericarditis. It is attenuated or disappears with tricuspid regurgitation (being replaced by a cv wave) and is attenuated in atrial fibrillation.

The classic cause of an enlarged ***v*** wave is tricuspid regurgitation. An enlarged ***v wave*** may also be seen in mitral regurgitation, but only when left atrial pressure recordings are made from a wedged pulmonary artery catheter.

A rapid, deep ***y descent*** is seen in tricuspid regurgitation, constrictive pericarditis, and severe right heart failure. The *y* descent becomes dominant in atrial fibrillation. A slow *y* descent suggests impeded RV filling and may be seen in tricuspid stenosis or pericardial tamponade.

## Cyanosis

Cyanosis is a bluish discoloration of the skin and mucous membranes. It is conventionally divided into central and peripheral types. **Central cyanosis** reflects arterial desaturation and is recognized as a blue tinge of the tongue, conjunctivae, lips, nose, ears, and nail beds. It occurs in lung diseases, and congenital heart diseases with right-to-left shunt. In **peripheral cyanosis** the arterial oxygenation is normal; however, an increased extraction of oxygen peripherally by the tissues, due to sluggish blood flow, leads to an excess of reduced hemoglobin. Seen in the ears, nose, lips, nails, and fingertips but not in the tongue or conjunctivae, peripheral cyanosis occurs with low cardiac output states, exposure to cold, and arterial and venous obstruction.

The absolute requirement for cyanosis is only the presence of at least 5 g/dl of reduced hemoglobin in the capillary blood. Thus, in a person with a hemoglobin of 15 g/dl, it reflects an oxygen saturation of 66% or less. However, cyanosis in an anemic patient indicates severe desaturation of hemoglobin (e.g., 50% in a patient with a hemoglobin of 10 g/dl). For the same reasons, cyanosis may appear even with less ominous levels of desaturation in polycythemic states; smaller concentrations of methemoglobin and sulfmethemoglobin (1.5 and 0.5 g/dL, respectively) may also evoke central cyanosis.

## Palpation of the Precordium

The **apical impulse** is located normally in the fourth or fifth left intercostal space, at or inside the midclavicular line. It can best be felt with the fingertips and is normally produced by the left ventricle. The apical impulse occupies a maximal area of 2–3 cm and should be located no more than 10 cm to the left of the midsternal line. If the apical impulse is not felt with the patient supine (which is common in patients older than 50), one should palpate for it in the left lateral position.

Besides location, one should note the duration, force, and contour of the apical impulse (Table 31.1). Normally, the apical impulse is felt as a brief, gentle tapping motion that ends before midsystole.

Simultaneous auscultation of $S_1$ and $S_2$ during precordial palpation allows one to estimate the duration of the apical impulse (Figure 31.4). A **sustained** apical impulse is one that maintains its peak into the second half of systole. It is caused by LV hypertrophy.

**TABLE 31.1. Causes of Abnormal Apical Impulse**

| Hyperkinetic | Sustained |
|---|---|
| Hyperdynamic states | Normal location (suggests normal LVEF) |
| Exercise | Hypertension |
| Excitement | Aortic stenosis |
| Thyrotoxicosis | HOCM |
| Severe anemia | Lateral displacement |
| Volume overload | Chronic volume overload states |
| Aortic regurgitation | LV dilation with decreased LVEF |
| Mitral regurgitation | |
| Ventricular septal defect | |

LV = left ventricle; LVEF = left ventricular ejection fraction; HOCM = hypertrophic cardiomyopathy.

The force of the apical impulse, although subjective, should be determined. A normal impulse is felt as a gentle tap whereas a **hyperkinetic** impulse (exaggeration of the normal contour) may be found in volume overload and other hyperdynamic states.

Other palpable cardiovascular events and structures may be found on examination. Rapid LV distension during early and late diastole may produce distinctly visible and palpable impulses—corresponding in timing to ventricular ($S_3$) and atrial ($S_4$) gallops, respectively. A systolic bulge, medial to the apical impulse, can be produced by an LV aneurysm. An apical tap in mitral stenosis is a palpable first heart sound. A palpable $S_2$ in the second left interspace may occur in pulmonary hypertension. **Thrills** are merely murmurs loud enough to be palpable; these are usually low-frequency murmurs. A left parasternal pansystolic impulse (lift) indicates RV dilation and/or hypertrophy. Severe mitral regurgitation may be associated with a late systolic parasternal lift owing to expansion of the left atrium beneath the RV.

## Cardiac Auscultation

Examination and auscultation are usually best done from the patient's right side and ideally in quiet surroundings. A good-quality stethoscope, having both a diaphragm and bell, is essential. The diaphragm detects higher frequency sounds (>300 Hz) and is applied with moderate pressure. The bell detects lower frequency sounds (30–150 Hz) and is applied with the least pressure necessary to create a skin seal; excess pressure lessens the transmission of low-frequency sounds.

Auscultation should be done with the patient supine, but also when the patient is sitting and lying on the left side. At times, other positions (e.g., standing and squatting) and maneuvers (e.g., isometric exercise or Valsalva maneuver) that alter loading conditions may provide additional diagnostic information.

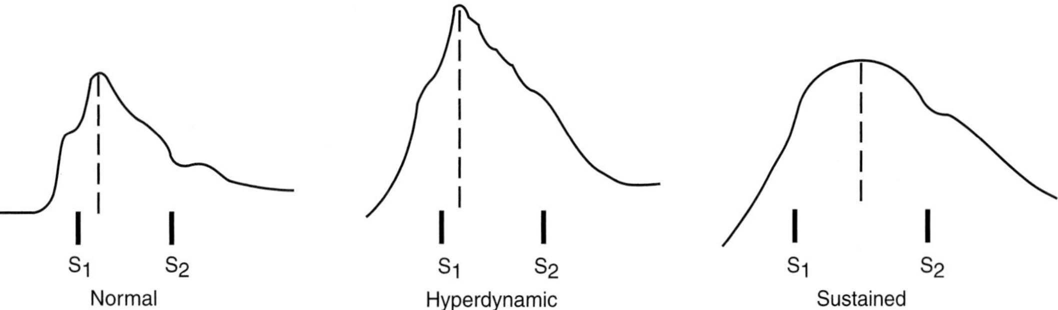


**FIGURE 31.4.** Major types of apical impulses. The **normal** apical impulse is felt as a brief tapping sensation, which clearly peaks before mid-systole (simultaneous auscultation of $S_1$ and $S_2$ is required). A **hyperdynamic** apical impulse is an exaggerated form of a normal impulse contour; it is not sustained or late-peaking but simply more forceful. A **sustained** apical impulse is prolonged and late-peaking; the peak of the impulse may still be felt in the latter half of systole.

Four primary precordial areas for cardiac auscultation are as follows:

- Aortic area—the 2nd right and 3rd left intercostal spaces (ICS)
- Pulmonic area—the 2nd left ICS
- Tricuspid area—the 4th and 5th left ICS adjacent to the left sternal border
- Mitral area—the cardiac apex

Each physician should adopt a systematic method of listening, but it is imperative to focus attention on one auscultatory event in the cardiac cycle at a time. Many cardiac and noncardiac variables can affect the intensity of heart sounds and murmurs (Table 31.2).

### First heart sound ($S_1$)

The first heart sound, $S_1$, signals the beginning of ventricular systole and is generated by mitral and tricuspid valve closure (Figure 31.5). Although audible over the entire precordium, it is loudest over the apex and left lower sternal border. Its pitch, although relatively high, is lower than $S_2$; therefore, it is heard best by using the diaphragm of the stethoscope.

The intensity of $S_1$ is determined primarily by valve mobility, force of ventricular contraction, and most important, the velocity of valve closure (Table 31.3). $S_1$ is louder when atrioventricular valves are widely separated at the onset of ventricular contraction, such as in mitral stenosis with pliable leaflets, a short PR interval, tachycardias, and increased diastolic flow rates. Alternatively, a soft $S_1$ occurs when the atrioventricular valves are partially closed at the onset of ventricular contraction, as with a long PR interval, acute aortic regurgitation, and decreased flow rates (low cardiac output). Finally, the $S_1$ may vary in intensity from beat to beat in atrial fibrillation, reflecting variable ventricular filling and thus contractility.

**TABLE 31.2. Conditions Affecting Intensity of Heart Sounds and Murmurs**

| | Noncardiac Conditions | Cardiac Conditions |
|---|---|---|
| Decreased intensity | Emphysema<br>Obesity<br>Muscular chest wall<br>Pericardial fibrosis<br>Pericardial effusion | Low cardiac output |
| Increased Intensity | Thin chest<br>Anemia | Hyperdynamic states |

### Second heart sound ($S_2$)

Evaluation of $S_2$ is a key component of the cardiac physical examination. $S_2$ is best heard over the base of the heart, especially at the left upper sternal border. The closure of the aortic ($A_2$) and pulmonic ($P_2$) valves at end-systole generates $S_2$ (see Figure 31.5). Abnormalities of $S_2$ relate primarily to alterations in intensity or timing (Table 31.4).

$A_2$ is the louder component and is audible at all locations on the chest wall. In normal subjects, $P_2$ is heard

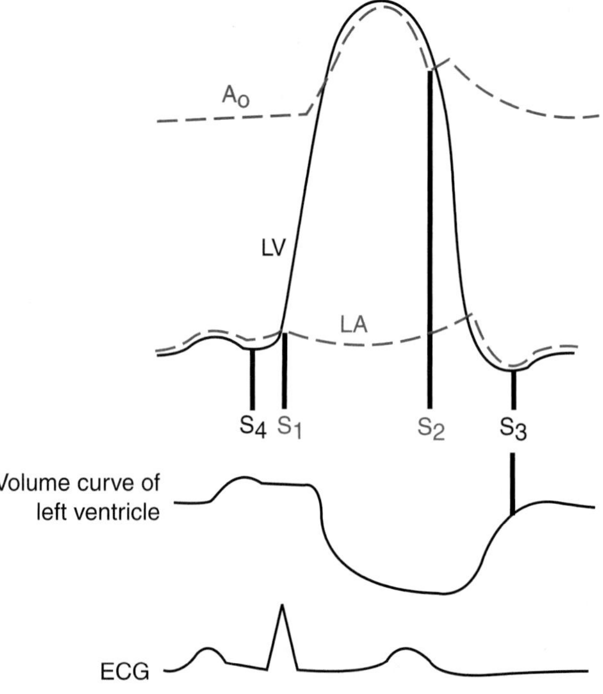


**FIGURE 31.5.** The cardiac cycle and related hemodynamic events. The relationship of intracardiac pressures to the timing and sequence of heart sounds is shown. $S_4$ is a late diastolic event occurring after atrial contraction, and $S_3$ is an early diastolic event occurring during the rapid-filling phase of the left ventricular volume curve. Ao=aortic pressure; LV=left ventricular pressure; LA=left atrial pressure.

**TABLE 31.3. Factors Affecting Intensity of First and Second Heart Sounds**

| | $S_1$ | $S_2$ | |
|---|---|---|---|
| | | $A_2$ | $P_2$ |
| Increased | PR <160 ms<br>Mitral stenosis with pliable valve<br>Hyperdynamic states<br>Holosystolic MVP<br>Rapid heart rates | Systemic HTN<br>Hyperdynamic states<br>Aortic dilation | Pulmonary HTN<br>Atrial septal defect |
| Decreased | PR >200 ms<br>Poor LV systolic function<br>Mitral stenosis with rigid valve<br>LBBB<br>Acute aortic regurgitation | Calcific aortic stenosis<br>Aortic regurgitation | Pulmonic stenosis |

$A_2$ = aortic component of second heart sound; HTN = hypertension; LBBB = left bundle branch block; LV = left ventricle; MVP = mitral valve prolapse; PR = PR interval; $P_2$ = pulmonic component of second heart sound.

**TABLE 31.4. Alterations in the Second Heart Sound and Their Causes**

| Single $S_2$ | Fixed Splitting | Paradoxical Splitting | Wide Splitting |
|---|---|---|---|
| Aging<br>Severe AS<br>Pulmonic stenosis | ASD<br>Right heart failure | Complete LBBB<br>RV pacing<br>Ischemic heart disease | Complete RBBB<br>Atrial septal defect<br>Pulmonary HTN with right heart failure |
| Any cause of delayed $A_2$ | | Aortic stenosis<br>HCM | LV pacing<br>Pulmonic stenosis<br>Severe MR<br>VSD |

AS = aortic stenosis; ASD = atrial septal defect; HCM = hypertrophic cardiomyopathy; HTN = hypertension; LBBB = left bundle branch block; LV = left ventricular; MR = mitral regurgitation; RBBB = right bundle branch block; RV = right ventricular; VSD = ventricular septal defect.

only at the upper left sternal border and is always less audible than $A_2$ at this location. An audible $P_2$ at the apex is an abnormal finding and strongly suggests pulmonary hypertension or atrial septal defect (apical impulse is caused by an enlarged RV).

A **single** $S_2$ results from attenuation of either $A_2$ or $P_2$. A single $S_2$, a common finding in older adults, arises from an inaudible $P_2$ caused by increased anteroposterior chest diameter.

The timing, or **splitting,** of $S_2$ varies with the phases of respiration. Normally, the split widens during inspiration and narrows during expiration. Slow, regular respirations are best for auscultating $S_2$.

- Wide splitting of $S_2$ during expiration with further widening during inspiration, i.e., a widely split $S_2$ having normal respiratory variation occurs when $P_2$ is delayed (e.g., right bundle branch block) or with early $A_2$ (e.g., mitral regurgitation).
- Fixed splitting of $S_2$ occurs when the RV cannot augment its stroke volume (e.g., in right heart failure) or when respiration-induced changes in filling, and hence stroke volumes, are similar in both ventricles (e.g., in atrial septal defect).
- Paradoxical splitting of $S_2$ occurs typically in conditions that delay the onset of LV depolarization and, thus, LV ejection (e.g., in left bundle branch block) or those that delay aortic valve closure (e.g., in severe aortic stenosis). In paradoxical splitting of $S_2$, $A_2$ follows $P_2$ during expiration and coincides with $P_2$ during inspiration.

### Diastolic sounds

A **ventricular gallop** ($S_3$) sound occurs in early diastole, 140–160 ms after $S_2$ as the active ventricular relaxation ends. It corresponds to the end of the rapid filling phase on the LV volume curve (see Figure 31.5). It is a low-frequency sound, best heard with the bell of the stethoscope lightly applied to the apex (LV $S_3$) or left lower sternal border (RV $S_3$). Often, gallops are heard only in the left lateral position.

The $S_3$ is caused by an interplay between ventricular filling and ventricular compliance (Table 31.5). An $S_3$ will be intensified by maneuvers that enhance ventricular filling and lessened by maneuvers that diminish venous return. Although an $S_3$ occurs in many conditions, most commonly, a nonphysiologic $S_3$ is associated with

TABLE 31.5. Causes of Left Ventricular $S_3$ and $S_4$ Gallops

| | $S_3$ | $S_4$ |
|---|---|---|
| Physiological | Children and young adults<br>Common during pregnancy<br>Hyperkinetic states<br>Rare after age 40 years | Rarely a normal finding |
| Pathological | High diastolic flow<br>Mitral regurgitation<br>Ventricular septal defect<br>Aortic regurgitation<br>Systolic dysfunction<br>Diastolic dysfunction<br>Hypertrophic cardiomyopathy<br>Restrictive cardiomyopathy<br>Constrictive pericarditis (knock) | Coronary artery disease<br>Hypertension<br>Aortic stenosis<br>Hypertrophic cardiomyopathy<br>Acute mitral regurgitation<br>Dilated cardiomyopathies<br>Hyperkinetic states |

abnormally high LV filling pressures, low cardiac output, and a dilated, poorly contractile LV. An $S_3$ is not heard when significant mitral stenosis is present. A "pericardial knock," a higher pitched diastolic sound that occurs earlier (closer to $A_2$) than the usual $S_3$, is heard in patients with constrictive pericarditis.

**Atrial gallop** ($S_4$) is a dull, low frequency sound that precedes $S_1$and is best heard over the apical impulse (left-sided $S_4$) or left lower sternal border (right-sided $S_4$). The techniques used to elicit an $S_3$ sound also apply for the $S_4$. The $S_4$ is attributed to forceful atrial contraction to fill a noncompliant or stiff ventricle (see Table 31.5). An $S_4$, although abnormal, is quite common in older adults. It implies a less serious alteration of overall LV function and better prognosis than a pathologic $S_3$. The $S_4$ disappears in atrial fibrillation.

A **summation** gallop occurs in the presence of tachycardia in a patient who has both an $S_3$ and an $S_4$. During tachycardia, the shortened diastole forces the $S_4$ and $S_3$ into a loud, single diastolic sound.

Mitral **opening snap** (OS) is a sharp, high-frequency sound heard best over the left lower sternal border in patients with mitral valve stenosis. It is attributed to the sudden arrest of a rapidly opening mitral valve that is stenotic but pliable. Immobility or calcification of the mitral leaflets causes softening or disappearance of the OS. The $A_2$-OS interval correlates inversely with the severity of the mitral stenosis; because left atrial pressure increases with the progression of severe mitral stenosis, the OS occurs earlier, resulting in a narrow $A_2$-OS interval.

### Systolic sounds

**Ejection click** (EC) is a sharp, high-frequency sound audible immediately after $S_1$. They occur in aortic and pulmonary valvular stenoses as well as in dilation of the ascending aorta and pulmonary artery. An aortic EC is audible over the entire precordium and varies little with respiration. A pulmonary EC is most audible along the left upper sternal border, becoming louder during expiration and less audible or absent during inspiration. ECs occur owing to abrupt cessation of the systolic motion of the dome-shaped, stenotic aortic and pulmonary valves. As the valves become stiff and calcified in aortic and pulmonary valvular stenosis, the EC disappears.

Nonejection clicks are associated with mitral valve prolapse. They are high-frequency sharp clicks occurring over the apex or left lower sternal border. These may occur as isolated findings or be followed by late systolic murmurs. Maneuvers such as squatting and gripping one's hand move a midsystolic click toward $S_2$ whereas standing and performing the Valsalva maneuver move the click toward $S_1$. A midsystolic click arises from the sudden tension on the chordae tendineae or from the sudden halt of the prolapsing mitral valve leaflet during ventricular systole.

### Prosthetic valve sounds

A ball-in-cage prosthesis (Starr-Edwards) has loud, metallic opening and closing sounds. Disc valves produce distinct closing sounds but usually no audible opening sounds. Porcine valves in the aortic position usually generate no abnormal sounds, but when placed in the mitral position, they may produce an opening snap followed by a diastolic rumble.

A pressure gradient exists across all prosthetic valves because the valve area of a prosthesis is typically smaller than that of a normal native valve. This causes a barely audible systolic murmur across prosthetic aortic valves and a soft diastolic rumble across prosthetic mitral valves.

### Heart murmurs

A prolonged series of audible vibrations constitute a heart murmur. Heart murmurs are traditionally classified as systolic, diastolic, or continuous (Table 31.6). During auscultation of a murmur, its timing in the cardiac cycle in relation to $S_1$ and $S_2$, intensity, quality (e.g., blowing, harsh, rumbling), duration, and radiation (e.g., to the neck, axilla, or back) should be defined. Additionally, if a patient with a systolic murmur has a coexistent arrhythmia, the effect of varying diastolic filling periods on the intensity of the murmur should be noted. Commonly, the intensity of outflow murmurs (e.g., aortic sclerosis or stenosis) will clearly increase in intensity in the beat following a longer diastole whereas murmurs owing to mitral regurgitation will remain unchanged.

The grading system for murmur intensity is described in Table 31.7. Most innocent murmurs are grades I or II. With a grade III murmur, one should initiate a search for pathology. Grade IV to VI murmurs are uncommon to rare. Whereas some systolic murmurs may be innocent, all diastolic and continuous murmurs are abnormal and pathological.

*Systolic murmurs*

Systolic murmurs are categorized according to their duration and relationship to $S_1$ and $S_2$. The most important point to ascertain is whether the systolic murmur extends to $S_2$. Ejection murmurs usually are crescendo-decrescendo in shape and end prior to $S_2$. Regurgitant or pansystolic murmurs are usually of more uniform intensity and extend to or even through $S_2$.

A midsystolic **ejection** murmur occupies only the ejection portion of systole. Ejection (and thus the murmur) begins at the time of semilunar valve opening, following $S_1$. Because the pressure gradient and blood flow markedly diminish before semilunar valve closure ($S_2$), these murmurs usually end prior to $S_2$. These murmurs are classically diamond-shaped (crescendo-decrescendo). However, determining whether a systolic murmur extends to $S_2$ is more important than determining its shape.

The most common type of midsystolic ejection murmur is the flow murmur, which arises owing to the normal turbulence of aortic blood flow during systolic ejection. Most pathologic midsystolic ejection murmurs originate at the semilunar valve; the classic example is aortic stenosis (Figure 31.6).

**Regurgitant** or **pansystolic** murmurs begin with $S_1$ and extend to $S_2$. A truly pansystolic murmur implies a large and continuous pressure differential between two chambers, causing a high-velocity stream of flow throughout systole. The resulting murmur is classically high-frequency, blowing in quality (not harsh), and relatively uniform in intensity (Figure 31.7). All pansystolic murmurs are pathologic.

**Late systolic** murmurs occur in the latter part of systole, well after $S_1$ and end in or after $A_2$. If caused by mitral valve prolapse, a midsystolic click may precede the murmur. All late systolic murmurs are pathologic.

*Diastolic murmurs*

**Early diastolic** regurgitant murmurs are heard with aortic and pulmonic regurgitation. Because the pressure difference and thus regurgitant flow between the aorta and left ventricle (or pulmonary artery and right ventricle) decrease throughout diastole, these murmurs are classically decrescendo (Figure 31.8). Unless it is specifically sought, the murmur of aortic regurgitation can be easily missed on auscultation. It is best heard with

**TABLE 31.6. Classification and Causes of Heart Murmurs**

INNOCENT MURMURS
SYSTOLIC MURMURS
- Ejection (midsystolic; crescendo–decrescendo)
  - Subvalvular, valvular, and supravalvular aortic or pulmonic stenosis
  - Malformed but nonstenotic aortic valve (aortic sclerosis)
  - Dilation of aortic or pulmonary artery
  - Increased systolic flow—e.g., aortic regurgitation, atrial septal defect
  - Regurgitant (pansystolic; constant amplitude)
    - Mitral and tricuspid regurgitation
    - Ventricular septal defect
  - Late systolic (onset well after $S_1$; end in $A_2$)
    - Mitral regurgitation—papillary muscle dysfunction or mitral valve prolapse

DIASTOLIC MURMURS
- EARLY (onset with $A_2$ or $P_2$; decrescendo; high-pitched)
  - Aortic and pulmonic regurgitation
- MID-DIASTOLIC (begin after $S_2$; low-pitched rumble)
  - Mitral or tricuspid stenosis
  - Increased atrioventricular valve flow without stenosis—mitral and tricuspid regurgitation, atrial and ventricular septal defects, aortic regurgitation (Austin Flint)

CONTINUOUS MURMURS (systolic/early diastolic; peak late systole)
- Patent ductus arteriosus
- Ruptured aneurysm of sinus of Valsalva
- Coronary arteriovenous fistula

**TABLE 31.7. Grading System for Murmur Intensity**

| Grade | Description |
|---|---|
| I/VI | Very faint; barely audible |
| II/VI | Soft but readily audible |
| III/VI | Moderately loud; no thrill |
| IV/VI | Very loud; thrill present |
| V/VI | Louder; thrill present; still requires a stethoscope on the chest to be heard |
| VI/VI | Audible with stethoscope close to, but not touching, chest; thrill present |

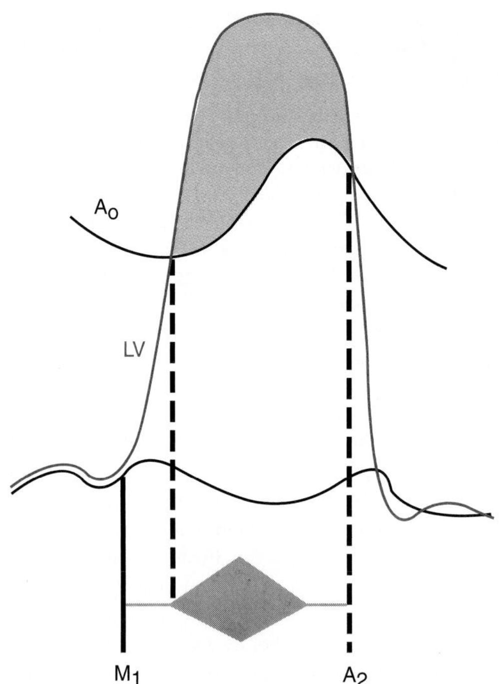


**FIGURE 31.6.** Midsystolic murmur in aortic stenosis. Left ventricular (LV) and aortic (Ao) pressure tracings are shown. The hatched area is the LV-Ao pressure gradient across the stenosis. The diamond-shaped midsystolic murmur begins after the mitral component of the first heart sound ($M_1$), as the aortic valve is not yet open. The murmur ends before aortic valve closure ($A_2$).

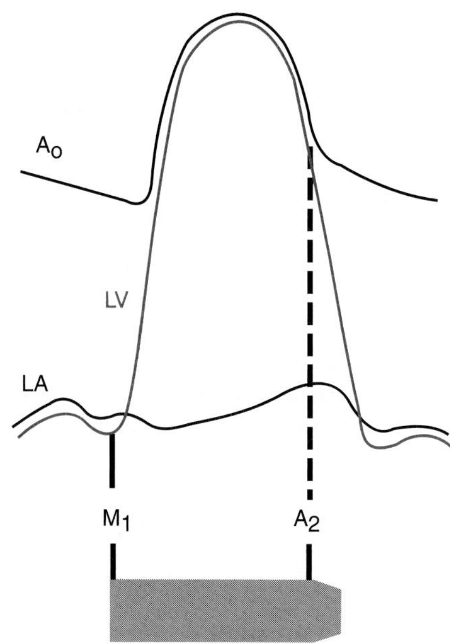


**FIGURE 31.7.** Pansystolic murmur in mitral regurgitation. Left ventricular (LV), aortic (Ao), and left atrial (LA) pressure tracings in typical mitral regurgitation are shown. The classic holosystolic murmur of mitral regurgitation begins with and may replace the first heart sound ($M_1$). The murmur continues up to and even through the second heart sound ($A_2$) since, at that time, left ventricular pressure still exceeds left atrial pressure and thus the pressure gradient causing the regurgitant flow continues to exist.

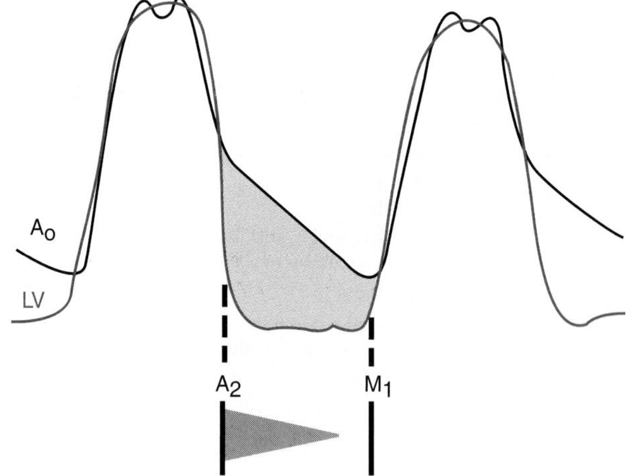


**FIGURE 31.8.** Early diastolic murmur in chronic aortic regurgitation. Left ventricular (LV) and aortic (Ao) pressure curves in chronic aortic regurgitation are shown. Note the low aortic diastolic pressure. The hatched area is the LV-Ao diastolic pressure gradient driving the AR flow. The murmur of aortic regurgitation begins with the second heart sound ($A_2$). Since the gradient between the aorta and LV is maximal almost instantaneously and then slowly decreases, the murmur has a high-pitched, slow-decrescendo character.

the patient sitting up and leaning forward, with breath held in expiration. The murmur of pulmonary regurgitation owing to pulmonary hypertension is termed a Graham Steell murmur.

**Mid-diastolic** murmurs are caused by increased diastolic flow across normal mitral and tricuspid valves or normal diastolic flow across stenosed or distorted mitral and tricuspid valves. Classically, the murmur of mitral stenosis follows the opening snap of the mitral valve and then diminishes in intensity, only to increase again at the end of diastole (presystolic accentuation, Figure 31.9). These murmurs are of low frequency, heard best with the bell of the stethoscope with the patient in the left lateral position. They too can be easily missed unless carefully sought.

A diastolic rumbling murmur may also be heard in patients with severe aortic regurgitation (Austin Flint murmur). This murmur has been ascribed to vibrations of the anterior mitral leaflet sandwiched between the aortic regurgitant stream on one side and blood across the mitral orifice on the other.

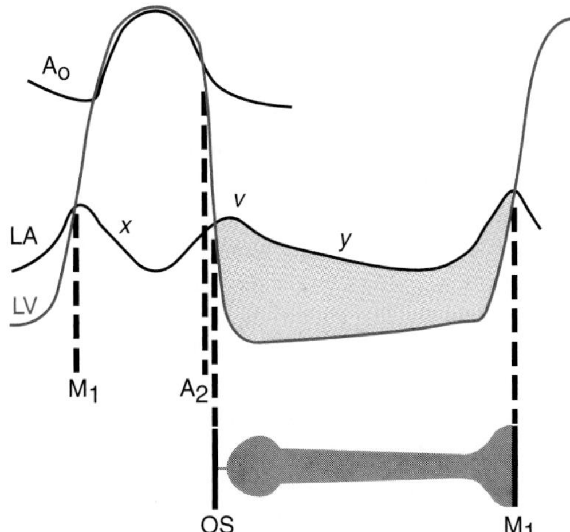


**FIGURE 31.9.** Mid-diastolic murmur in mitral stenosis. Left ventricular (LV), left atrial (LA), and aortic (Ao) pressure curves in mitral stenosis are shown. Note the elevated LA pressure. The pink-shaded area represents the LA-LV diastolic pressure gradient, showing the late diastolic rise in gradient associated with atrial contraction. The low-pitched diastolic rumble of mitral stenosis is immediately preceded by the high-pitched mitral opening snap (OS).

*Continuous murmurs*

Continuous murmurs occur when a large and persistent pressure difference throughout the cardiac cycle exists. This may occur between two communicating chambers or vessels with no intervening valve or across a severely stenosed segment of an artery. Typically, a continuous murmur begins in systole and continues without interruption or change into diastole. These murmurs usually peak at $S_2$.

*Pericardial friction rub*

A pericardial friction rub is a superficial scratching sound heard over the precordium in acute pericarditis. Faint rubs are best heard with the patient sitting up and leaning forward; they are notorious for their evanescence. Friction rubs may be triphasic with systolic, diastolic, and presystolic components. The systolic component is loudest and virtually always present. All three components are present in only about 50% of cases.

*Effects of physical maneuvers on murmurs*

Certain physical maneuvers can profoundly affect murmur intensity by acutely changing loading conditions (Table 31.8). These maneuvers can augment the intensity of soft murmurs or gallops and aid in the differential diagnosis of various murmurs.

**TABLE 31.8. Effects of Physical Maneuvers on Heart Sounds and Murmurs**

| Maneuver | Technique | Pathophysiology | Effect |
|---|---|---|---|
| Valsalva | Place hand on patient's abdomen and exert downward pressure as patient exerts outward pressure | During strain phase: ↓ venous return/ cardiac output; ↓ LV chamber size | ↓ Most heart sounds and murmurs except: • ↑ in HCM • MVP, earlier click and/or murmur |
| Rapid standing | Abrupt assumption of upright posture | Abrupt ↓ in venous return | Augments in HCM and MVP<br>↓ in aortic stenosis, mitral and tricuspid insufficiency |
| Respiration | Normal respiration | Inspiration: ↑ venous return | Inspiration ↑ right heart murmurs and gallops |
| Isometric handgrip | Sustained handgrip for 20–30 sec | ↑ systemic resistance and arterial pressure | Augments aortic and mitral insufficiency, ventricular septal defect<br>Decreases HCM and MVP |
| Post PVC or prolonged RR interval | Auscultate murmur in beat following a longer RR interval | ↑ ventricular filling<br>↑ contractility | Augments aortic stenosis<br>No change in mitral insufficiency |

HCM = hypertrophic cardiomyopathy; LV = left ventricle; MVP = mitral valve prolapse; PVC = premature ventricular contraction.

# CHAPTER 32 ELECTROCARDIOGRAPHY

## Anatomy of the Conduction System

The **sinus node** is located in the right atrium near its junction with the superior vena cava, and the **atrioventricular (AV) node** is located in the right atrium between the opening of the coronary sinus and attachment of the septal leaflet of the tricuspid valve. The AV node is continuous with the **His bundle** that is present on the right side of the membranous ventricular septum. As it reaches the muscular portion of the ventricular septum, the His bundle continues as a slender **right bundle** on the right side of the ventricular septum to the apex of the RV and then enters the moderator band. Numerous branches from the His bundle penetrate the membranous ventricular septum below the aortic ring to enter the LV, where they are grouped into anterior and posterior fascicles of the **left bundle.** All three fascicles, i.e., the right-bundle and the anterior and posterior left-bundle branches, break into numerous Purkinje fibers that spread over the endocardial surfaces of the two ventricles.

## Basic Electrophysiology

In the resting or polarized state, there is a 20-fold greater concentration of $NA^+$ intracellularly than extracellularly, making the inside of the myocardial cell electrically negative by $-90$ mV as compared to the outside (Figure 32.1). On **depolarization** (phase 0), a sudden influx of $Na^+$ into the cell through specific $Na^+$ channels (fast channels) in the cell membrane causes the inside of the cell to become rapidly positive (+20 mV). Phase 1 **(initial repolarization)** ensues, during which the potential falls from +20 to 0 mV. In turn, this phase is followed by phase 2, or the **plateau** phase, which indicates slow repolarization caused predominantly by $Ca^{++}$ influx. In phase 3, **rapid repolarization** occurs owing to the efflux of $NA^+$ from the cell, enabling the membrane potential to return to the resting level. During phase 4, the $Na^+$ efflux and $K^+$ influx maintain the cell in its **resting,** or polarized, state.

Cells that can spontaneously generate an electrical impulse are present in the sinus node and AV junction. These pacemaker cells show a spontaneous diastolic depolarization; i.e., the resting membrane potential drifts slowly upward during phase 4 until the threshold is reached, and then another action potential results. The normal cardiac impulse arises in the sinus node and travels through the anterior, middle, and posterior internodal tracts to the AV node. Upon reaching the AV node, the impulse suddenly slows (decremental conduction, 50 mm/sec) and, after about 60–100 ms, enters the His-Purkinje system. From the AV node, the impulse travels rapidly (2000–3000 mm/sec) over the His-Purkinje system. Thereafter, conduction from the endocardium to the epicardium is relatively slow (200–500 mm/sec).

The midportion of the ventricular septum is activated from left to right, followed sequentially by the lower septum, RV apex, RV free wall, LV free wall, and bases of both ventricles. The RV outflow tract, or crista supraventricularis, is activated last. Repolarization follows the same pathway as depolarization, with the exception of the ventricular wall, which repolarizes from the epicardium to the endocardium.

The normal rate of impulse formation in the sinus node is 60–100 beats per minute. The sinus node is controlled by the sympathetic and parasympathetic nervous system. If the sinus node fails, the AV junction depolarizes the heart at a rate of 40–60 beats per minute. If both the sinus node and AV junction fail, the His-Purkinje system will drive the heart at 20–40 beats per minute.

## Electrocardiographic Leads

A graphic recording of changes in cardiac electrical potential as detected by an electrocardiograph is called an electrocardiogram (ECG) (Figure 32.2). Three standard bipolar ECG leads are commonly placed on the extremities. Lead I records the potential difference between the left arm and right arm; lead II, between the left leg and right arm; and lead III, between the left leg and left arm. The positive and negative sides of all leads are configured to record upright complexes in all three leads in normal persons. Three additional leads are placed on the extremities (the augmented leads aVR, aVL, and aVF) and, together with the three standard limb leads, make a hexaxial system that provides frontal plane representation on the ECG. The six precordial leads, $V_1$ through $V_6$, provide a horizontal (transverse) representation on the ECG.

The direction and spatial orientation of the electrical force profoundly affect the ECG waveform configuration in a given lead. By convention, a lead records an electrical force coming toward it as positive and one directed away from it as negative. If the electrical force is parallel to the lead, the recorded wave will show maximal amplitude whereas an electrical force perpendicular to the lead may show little voltage deflection.

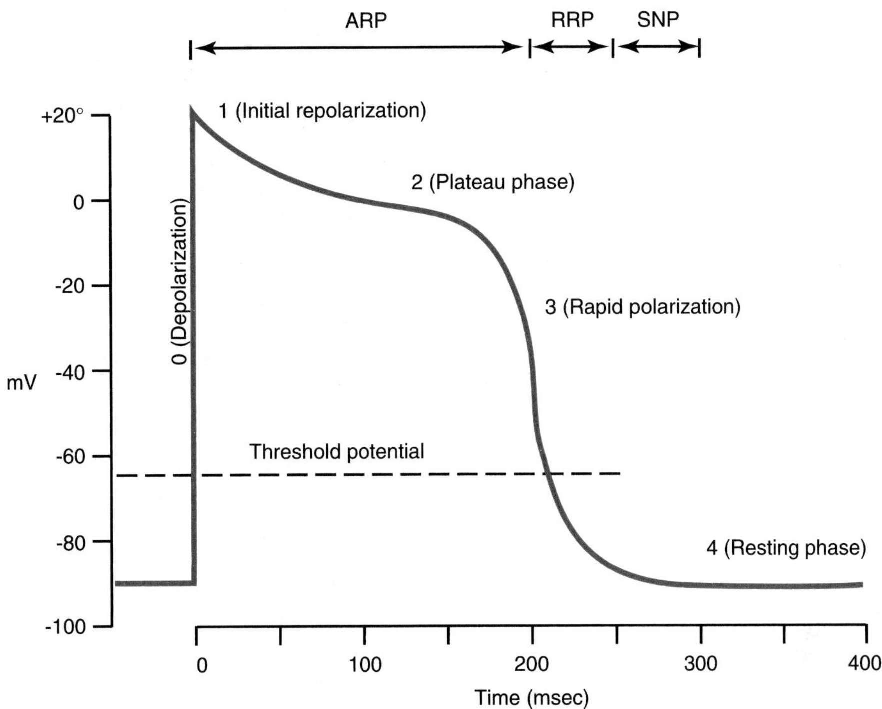


**FIGURE 32.1.** Action potential of the normal myocardial cell. The myocardial cell has a resting transmembrane potential (phase 4) of −90 mV. On excitation, the transmembrane potential is lowered to threshold potential, causing depolarization (phase 0), followed by three phases of repolarization, which return the cell to resting transmembrane potential (phase 4). During phases 1,2, and early phase 3, the cell is completely inexcitable (ARP, absolute refractory period). During the late phase 3, the cell is excitable by a strong stimulus (RRP, relative refractory period). During the last portion of phase 3, even a subthreshold stimulus can excite the cell. SNP=supernormal period.

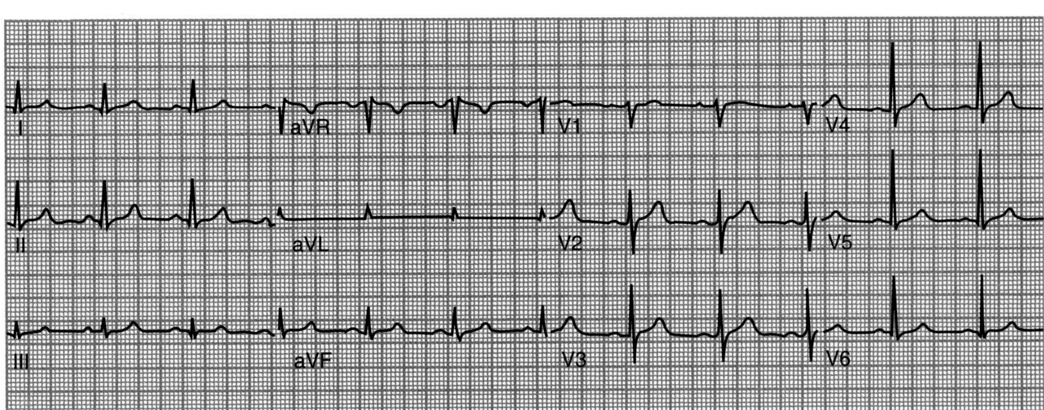


**FIGURE 32.2.** Normal ECG. A normal ECG shows, in sequence, P, QRS and T waves. It is recorded on graph paper for rapid measurement of time intervals and amplitudes. At a standard speed of 25 mm/s, the interval between vertical thin lines is 0.04 s. At standard calibration, a 1-mm height equals 0.1 mV.

## Normal Electrocardiogram

### Electrical axis on the ECG

The ECG is recorded on graph paper for rapid measurements of time intervals and amplitudes. At a standard speed of 25 mm/sec, the interval between vertical thin lines is 0.04 second. At standard calibration, a 1 mm height equals 0.1 mV. A normal ECG shows, in sequence, P, QRS, and T waves (see Figure 32.2). The surface ECG records only the net resultant electrical force. Given the depolarization of the entire heart in sequence, the direction (axis) of depolarization changes from moment to moment. The mean axis of the total depolarization of atria (mean P axis), ventricles (mean QRS axis), and ventricular repolarization (mean T axis) in the frontal plane can be calculated from the six limb leads, i.e., I, II, III, aVR, aVL, and aVF. In clinical practice, the mean QRS axis is more important than the other two axes (Figure 32.3).

In normal persons, the mean QRS axis is between −30° and +110° (see Figure 32.3). An axis in the −30° to −90° range is abnormally deviated to the left, and an axis between +110° and +180° is abnormally deviated to the right; the axis in the right upper quadrant (−90° to +180°) could be an abnormal right or left axis deviation. A left axis deviation occurs in patients with inferior wall myocardial infarction and left anterior hemiblock. A right axis deviation is found in patients with RV hypertrophy, lateral wall infarction, and left posterior hemiblock. In infancy, the mean QRS axis is usually between +90° and +150° but shifts leftward with age.

### P wave

Depolarization of the atria results in a P wave. As the impulse from the sinus node travels inferiorly and leftward, limb leads I, II, III, aVL, and aVF usually record an upright P wave, and aVR records a negative P wave because the impulse is traveling away from this lead. All precordial leads show a positive P wave, except $V_1$, which may show a positive, negative, or biphasic P wave.

A normal P wave is less than 2.5 mm high and less than 0.10 sec wide. Its initial portion represents right atrial depolarization and the terminal portion reflects left atrial depolarization.

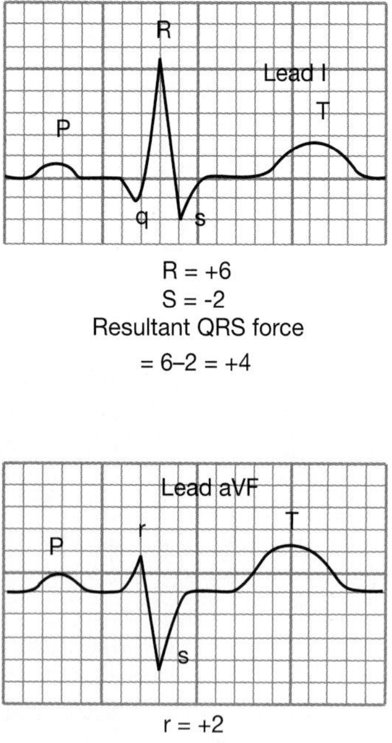


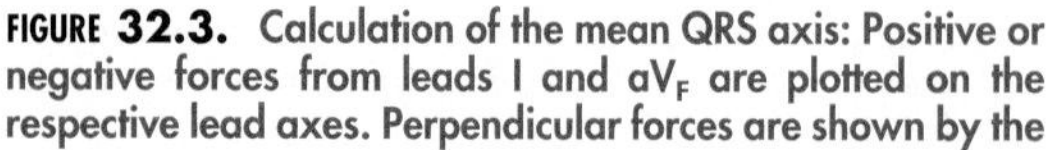


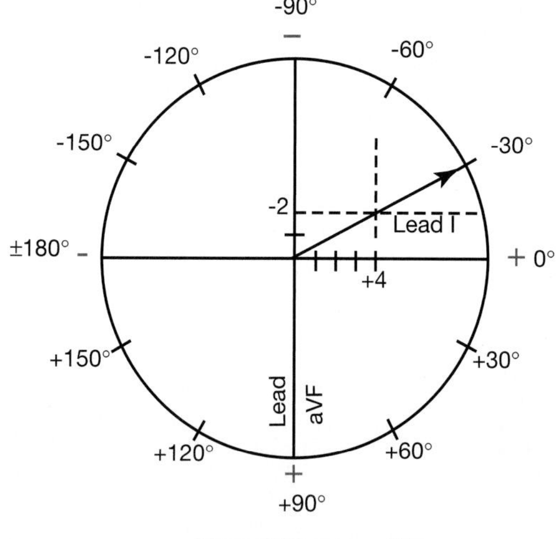


**FIGURE 32.3.** Calculation of the mean QRS axis: Positive or negative forces from leads I and $aV_F$ are plotted on the respective lead axes. Perpendicular forces are shown by the dotted lines. The line connecting the center with the point of intersection of perpendiculars represents the mean QRS axis.

### P-R interval

The P-R interval, measured from the start of the P wave to the beginning of the QRS complex, indicates the time from the start of atrial depolarization to the beginning of ventricular activation. Normally 0.12 to 0.20 sec, this interval is inversely related to the heart rate. Most of the conduction delay occurs in the AV node.

### QRS complex

The Q wave is the first negative wave and the R wave the first positive wave after a P wave. The S wave is the first negative wave after the R wave. The QRS complex reflects depolarization of the ventricles. The initial **Q wave,** an electrical force directed to the right and anteriorly, reflects depolarization of the left midseptum and is recorded as a small r (<5 mm) in lead $V_1$ and a small q (<2 mm) in leads I, aVL, $V_5$, and $V_6$. The main QRS represents depolarization of the free ventricular walls. Because the LV muscle mass exceeds the RV muscle mass, the main depolarization force, which is oriented leftward and posteriorly, appears as an **R wave** in leads I, aVL, $V_5$, and $V_6$, and as an S in aVR, $V_1$, and $V_2$. The terminal **S wave** reflects activation of the base of the heart and RV outflow tract.

The QRS duration, normally 0.06 to 0.10 second, is the time period between initiation and completion of ventricular depolarization. Ventricular activation time (intrinsicoid deflection), measured from the onset of QRS to the peak of R, is the amount of time the electrical force takes to travel from the endocardium to the epicardium (normally <0.035 sec in $V_1$ or $V_2$ and <0.045 sec in $V_5$ or $V_6$).

### ST segment

The ST segment is the isoelectric portion between the S and T waves. This segment denotes the time that the ventricles are partially repolarized, corresponding to phase 2 of the action potential.

### T and U waves

The T wave reflects rapid repolarization of the ventricles. After the T wave, another positive wave, U, is sometimes seen, especially in the midprecordial leads. This wave is usually attributed to repolarization of the papillary muscles. The atrial repolarization produces a negative T wave that is difficult to identify because it is hidden by the QRS complex.

## ECG Changes in Specific Diseases

### Myocardial ischemia, injury, and infarction

With severe and prolonged hypoperfusion, the affected myocardium progresses from a stage of reversible **ischemia,** to a stage of reversible **injury,** and finally to irreversible **infarction.** As ischemia persists, the area most deprived of blood supply—usually the subendocardial region—becomes necrotic. This necrotic region is surrounded by injured tissue that in turn is surrounded by ischemic tissue.

In **Q-wave infarction** (previously termed transmural infarction), the earliest ECG change is a tall and spiked T wave, followed by ST-segment elevation in leads facing the infarcted region and reciprocal ST-segment depression in the opposite leads. ST-segment elevation becomes isoelectric within the first few days. This regression unmasks a symmetrically inverted T wave, reflecting transmural ischemia. A few hours to a few days after the onset of ST-segment elevation, a pathologic Q wave appears in the same leads, which persists for months, years, or indefinitely and serves as an ECG sign of an old scar. Thus, the only ECG sign of acute myocardial injury is ST-segment elevation, which along with a new Q wave, indicates an acute Q-wave infarction (Figure 32.4). During the first few hours of an infarction, the ECG may be entirely normal.

**Non–Q-wave infarction** (previously termed subendocardial infarction) produces ST-segment depression and T-wave inversion without pathologic Q waves.

In some young, healthy subjects, a normal variant of repolarization occurs (Figure 32.5) with ST-segment elevation, primarily in leads I, aVL, and $V_4$ through $V_6$. The ST segment is concave upward and starts from the descending limb of the R wave before it reaches the baseline. No T-wave abnormalities are noted. This pattern may occasionally be confused for an infarct. An elevated ST segment in myocardial injury tends to be convex upward.

### Cardiac hypertrophy

In **left atrial enlargement** (P-mitrale), the P wave is wider (>2.5 mm) and double-peaked, with the second peak representing left atrial depolarization. Since the P axis shifts leftward (–30° to +45°), the double-peaked P wave is best seen in leads I, II, aVL, and $V_4$ through $V_6$. In $V_1$, the P wave is biphasic and the terminal negative component is deep and wide (>0.04 sec). Left atrial enlargement is commonly seen in aortic stenosis, cardiomyopathy, hypertension, coronary artery disease, and mitral valve disease.

With **right atrial enlargement** (P-pulmonale), the P waves are tall (>2.5 mm) and spiked, usually in leads II, III, aVF, and $V_1$. The P axis shifts to the right (> +75°). Right atrial enlargement occurs in pulmonary stenosis, pulmonary hypertension, cor pulmonale, and tricuspid stenosis.

Increased LV mass results in greater amplitude of QRS (Figure 32.6). Because voltage criteria alone may falsely suggest **LV hypertrophy,** especially in thin-chested individuals, the point scoring system described by Estes is more specific for diagnosis (Table 32.1).

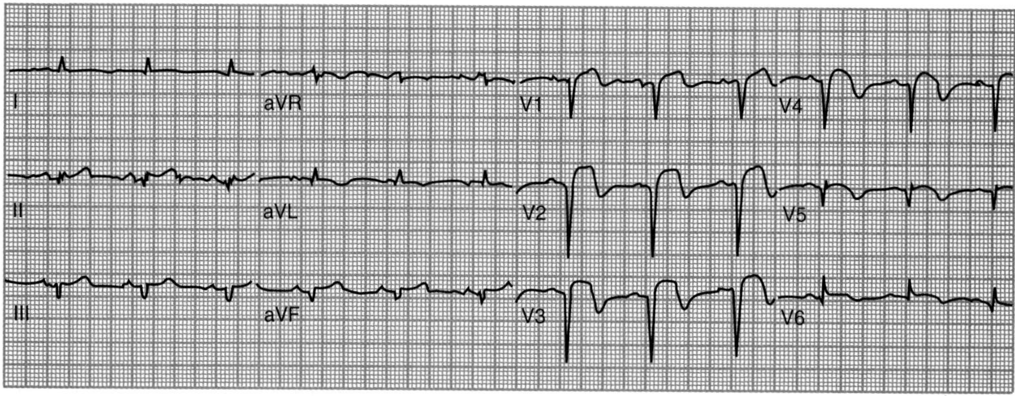


**FIGURE 32.4.** ECG changes in extensive, acute anterior myocardial infarction. ST-segment elevation, T-wave inversions, and Q waves can be seen in leads $V_1$ through $V_6$. The Q waves in leads II, III and $aV_F$ are the residua of an old inferior wall myocardial infarction.

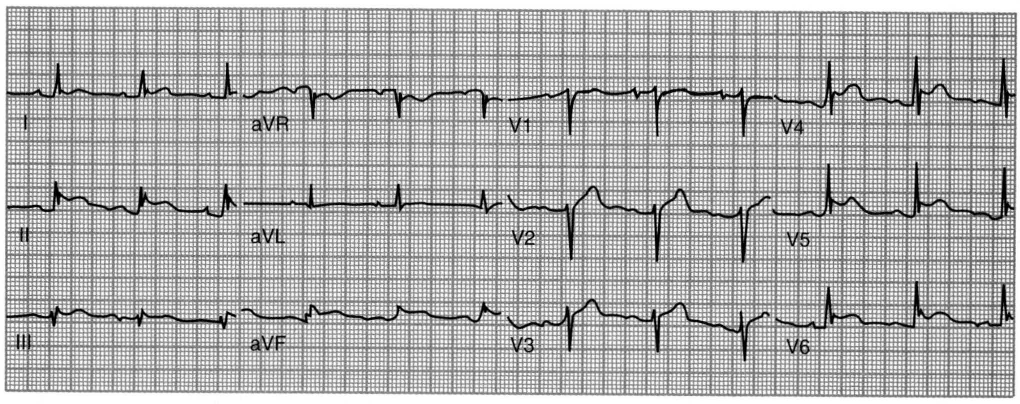


**FIGURE 32.5.** ECG showing early repolarization. ST-segment elevation with upward concavity is seen in leads I, II, $aV_F$, and $V_3$ through $V_6$. Persistence of this pattern over months and years is highly suggestive of early repolarization.

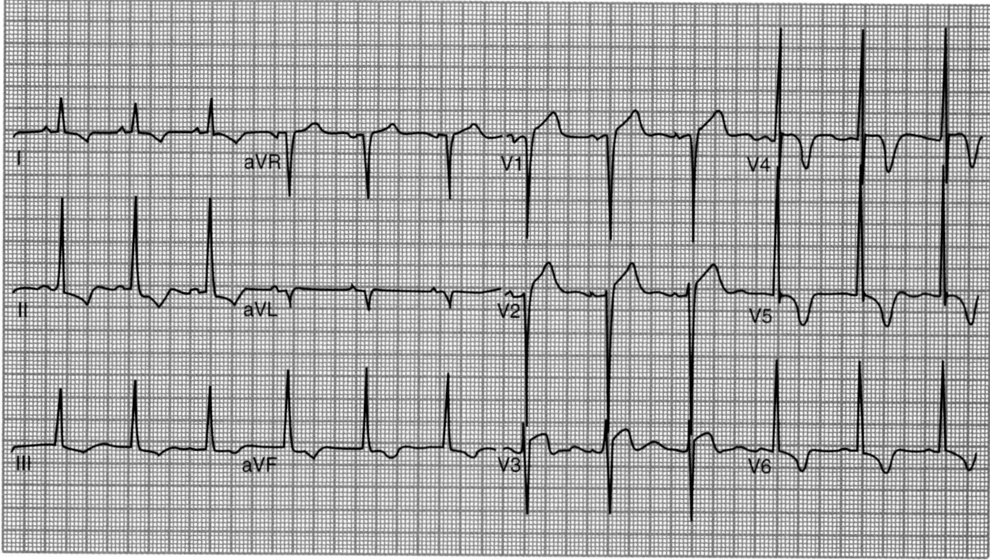


**FIGURE 32.6.** ECG changes in left ventricular hypertrophy. Note increased QRS voltage and secondary ST-T changes.

Similar diagnostic criteria are used for **RV hypertrophy** (Table 32.2, Figure 32.7).

### Acute pericarditis

In acute pericarditis, virtually all the leads except aVR and $V_1$ record ST-segment elevation, indicating diffuse injury. As the inflammation subsides several days later, the ST segments become gradually isoelectric, and the T waves then become inverted.

### Electrolyte disturbances and drug effects

In **hyperkalemia,** the T waves become tall and spiked (Figure 32.8). With an increasing degree of hyperkalemia, the P waves become less distinct and may totally disappear, the QRS complex widens, and ultimately, QRS-T assumes a sine-wave configuration. **Hypokalemia** produces ST-segment depression, T-wave flattening, and prominence of U and P waves. A progressively less distinct T wave merges into the U wave, causing prolongation of the Q-T (actually Q-U) interval. In severe hypokalemia, the QRS also widens. **Hypocalcemia** prolongs the ST segment, and **hypercalcemia** shortens the ST segment.

Digitalis produces a sagging or "hammock-shaped" ST depression, flat or inverted T waves, and shortened Q-T interval. These changes may follow even a therapeutic dose and, thus, constitute the "digitalis effect." Procainamide and quinidine prolong the Q-T interval, flatten or invert T waves, and widen the QRS.

### Neurologic conditions

In neurologic conditions such as head trauma and subarachnoid hemorrhage, an ECG may show bizarre, wide and tall, or deeply inverted T waves with Q-T prolongation.

**TABLE 32.1. Estes Criteria for Left Ventricular Hypertrophy (LVH)**

| Criteria | Points |
|---|---|
| 1. Voltage | 3 |
| R and/or S >20 mm in any one or more of the six limb leads, OR | |
| S >25 mm in $V_1$, $V_2$ or $V_3$, OR | |
| R >25 mm in $V_4$, $V_5$ or $V_6$ | |
| 2. ST-segment deviation opposite to the main QRS complex | |
| In the absence of digitalis therapy | 3 |
| In the presence of digitalis therapy | 1 |
| 3. Left axis deviation (QRS axis to the left of −15°) | 2 |
| 4. QRS duration >0.09 s | 1 |
| 5. Ventricular activation time >0.04 s | 1 |

A sum of 4 points indicates probable LVH and ≥5 points indicates definite LVH.

**TABLE 32.2. Diagnostic Criteria for Right Ventricular Hypertrophy**

Right axis deviation (QRS axis to the right of +110°)
R/S ratio in lead $V_1$ >1, provided R in $V_1$ is >5 mm
R in $V_2$ >7 mm
R in $V_1$ or S in $V_5$ or $V_6$ >10.5 mm
Secondary ST-segment depression and T-wave inversion in leads $V_1$ and $V_2$
Persistence of prominent S wave in leads $V_4$ through $V_6$

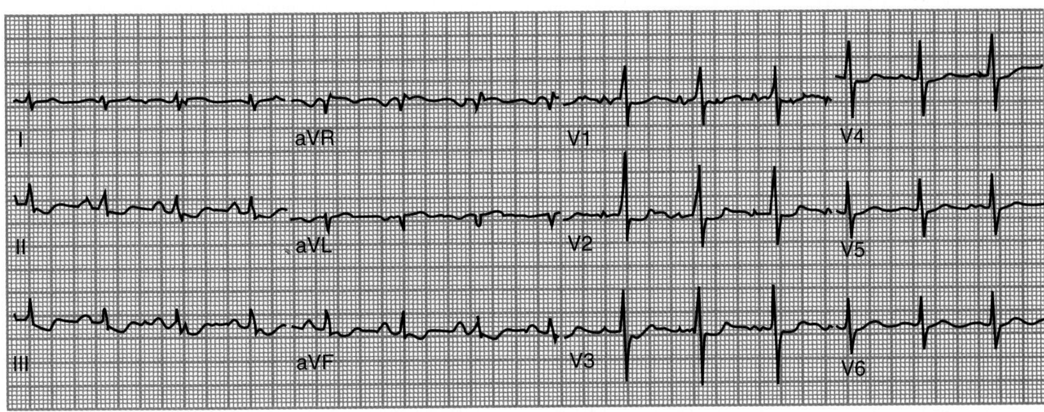


**FIGURE 32.7.** ECG changes in right ventricular hypertrophy. Note the rightward mean QRS axis, prominent R wave in $V_1$ with R/S ratio of >1, and persistence of S waves in leads $V_5$ and $V_6$.

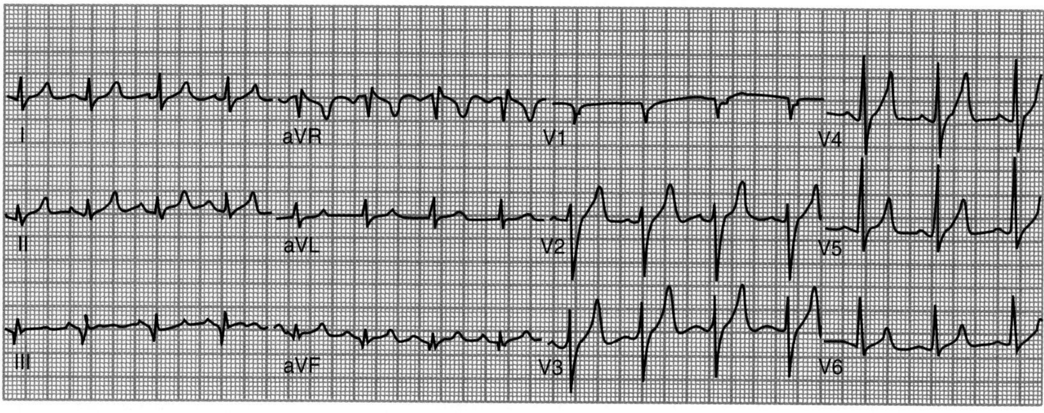


FIGURE 32.8. ECG changes in hyperkalemia. Note the tall and spiky T waves in most leads, especially $V_2$ through $V_6$.

# CHAPTER 33 NONINVASIVE CARDIAC IMAGING

## Roentgenography

Chest radiography permits an assessment of the size and configuration of the heart and great vessels, the pulmonary vascularity, and calcification of cardiac valves and other structures.

### Cardiac silhouette

The **cardiothoracic ratio,** which is an index of cardiac size (normal is <0.5), can be determined on standard chest radiographs by dividing the maximal transverse width of the heart by the maximal internal width of the thorax above the diaphragm. On posteroanterior (PA) and special oblique views, chest radiograph is useful in screening for enlargement of specific heart chambers; however, this technique is only moderately reliable, and echocardiography is the preferred method of assessing chamber sizes.

### Great vessels

A dilated **pulmonary artery** accentuates the shadow of the pulmonary artery segment seen on the left heart border and occurs in conditions of increased pulmonary blood flow (e.g., left-to-right shunts), pulmonary arterial hypertension, and poststenotic dilatation in pulmonary valvular stenosis. An attenuated pulmonary artery segment occurs in the tetralogy of Fallot, tricuspid atresia, and Ebstein's anomaly.

In a PA projection, dilatation of the **ascending aorta** (as in aortic valvular stenosis and aneurysms of the ascending aorta) causes a prominent convexity of the right upper cardiac shadow. Dilatation, elongation, and tortuosity of the **aortic arch** cause a prominent aortic knob. Hypertension, arteriosclerosis, and aortic insufficiency produce aortic dilatation.

### Pulmonary vascularity

A careful examination of the lung fields in a chest radiograph discloses the pulmonary vascularity. Differentiating pulmonary arteries from veins on chest radiographs is difficult; it is, however, easier in the right lung field. In general, upper lobe veins are vertical and remain lateral to the corresponding arteries. The lower lobe veins are more horizontal, remain medial to the arteries, and are usually more prominent than those in the upper lung fields.

In left heart failure and mitral stenosis, as pulmonary venous pressure increases, the veins in the upper lung fields become more prominent than those in the lower lung fields (redistribution of the pulmonary blood flow). When the pulmonary wedge pressure approaches 25–30 mm Hg, it exceeds the capillary oncotic pressure and fluid accumulates in the lung interstitium. The lung fields appear hazy and the small pulmonary vessels indistinct. **Kerley's B lines,** attributed to thickened interlobular septa owing to edema, appear as 1–2-cm horizontal lines in the lower lung fields near the costophrenic angles (Figure 33.1). Worsening of heart disease prompts further fluid transudation into the alveoli, causing **pulmonary edema** (which appears on chest radiographs as confluent opacities in the central lung fields resembling butterfly or bat wings) or interlobar and/or **pleural effusions.**

Pulmonary arteries gradually taper as they proceed peripherally. Enlarged central pulmonary arteries that abruptly taper peripherally indicate pulmonary arterial hypertension (cor pulmonale, Eisenmenger's syndrome, or primary pulmonary hypertension). In severe pulmonary hypertension that follows left heart disease, both pulmonary veins and arteries become prominent. In large left-to-right shunts, the central and peripheral arteries also become enlarged without any sudden peripheral tapering.

### Calcification

Calcification of various cardiac structures is visible on PA chest radiographs but is more easily detected using fluoroscopy or on computed tomography. Mitral valvular calcification indicates prior rheumatic disease. A congenitally bicuspid aortic valve, the pericardium in constrictive pericarditis, atrial myxomas, ventricular aneurysms, intracardiac blood clots, and the coronary artery walls may all undergo calcification.

## Echocardiography

Echocardiography uses ultrasound, generated by a piezoelectric crystal held against the chest wall, to image cardiac structures. It is used in three types of studies. **Motion mode (M-mode) tracings,** which show motion within a single beam of sound, lack spatial orientation, but the resulting high-resolution record of the cardiac cycle helps to *time* events and measure chamber diameters easily.

**Two-dimensional (2D) echocardiography** provides a two-dimensional image by steering the sound beam 30 times/sec through an arc of up to 90°. The images obtained from several transducer positions on the chest wall or upper abdomen (transthoracic 2D echo) provide superior *spatial* resolution, allowing assessment of structural movement in real time. **Transesophageal echocardiography,** obtained by placing a transducer in the esophagus, provides excellent two-dimensional images of the posterior cardiac chambers and aorta.

**Doppler echocardiography** can provide information on blood flow within the heart. The sound reflected by red cells moving within the heart changes frequency (Doppler shift) in proportion to the cells' velocity, allowing one to measure the direction and velocity of blood flow through the cardiac valves and to detect abnormal flow patterns.

Echocardiography is useful in imaging structural abnormalities that underlie numerous heart diseases. It can detect mitral valve prolapse, mitral and aortic stenosis, valvular vegetations, congenital diseases, and intracardiac tumors. Transesophageal echocardiography is superior to transthoracic echo for evaluating the function of prosthetic valves; investigating atrial masses, atrial septal defects, and aortic dissection; and monitoring ventricular function during cardiac surgery. In addition to determining blood-flow velocity across stenotic valves, Doppler echocardiography can be used to calculate transvalvular pressure gradient and to detect and quantify regurgitant lesions. Echocardiography is the test of choice for detecting, quantifying, and locating pericardial effusion and tamponade.

Echocardiography, in conjunction with exercise or pharmacologic stress **(stress echocardiography),** is also useful in detecting coronary artery disease. Echocardiography allows evaluation of LV function, detecting abnormal LV segmental wall motion and the complications of myocardial infarction. With two-dimensional

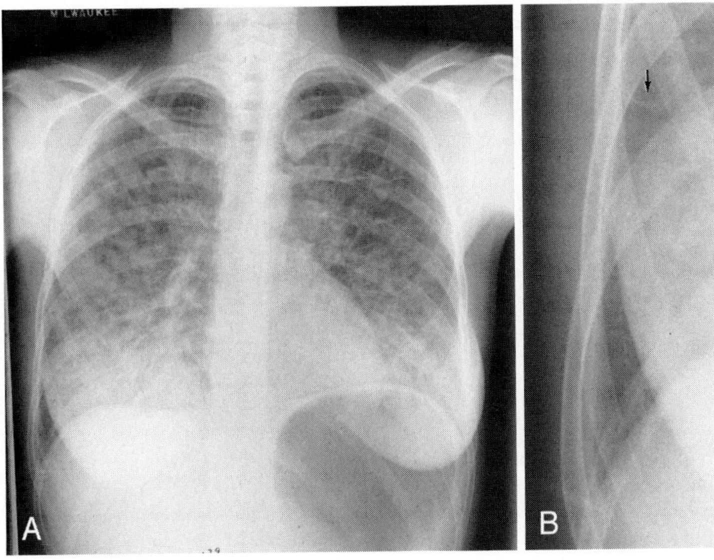


**FIGURE 33.1.** Chest radiograph showing left heart failure with diffuse lung infiltration **(panel A).** Kerley B lines, seen in the periphery of the right lung, are better seen in the magnified view **(panel B).**
(Courtesy, Radiology Museum, St. Joseph's Regional Medical Center, Milwaukee, Wisconsin.)

echocardiography, LV volumes and ejection fraction can be measured, and cardiac output can be measured on a beat-by-beat basis using Doppler echocardiography.

## Radionuclide Imaging

Three types of radionuclide imaging procedures are clinically useful in cardiac diagnosis: radionuclide angiocardiography, myocardial perfusion imaging, and infarct imaging.

### Angiocardiography

The most commonly used radionuclide for cardiac angiography is **technetium 99m** ($^{99m}$Tc), which is tagged to the patient's own red blood cells. This technique helps determine systolic and diastolic ventricular function and intracardiac shunts.

In the **first-pass method,** a scintillation camera records the activity of a peripherally injected radionuclide bolus as it travels for the first time through the cardiac chambers and blood vessels. In the **equilibrium method** (multigated acquisition, MUGA), images of the heart are recorded over several hundred cardiac cycles for several minutes after the radionuclide has equilibrated throughout the vasculature. A computer generates a single, composite cycle. The resulting ventricular images, displayed in a cine format throughout the cardiac cycle, greatly facilitate the detection of segmental wall motion abnormalities.

With either method, the ejection fraction and absolute end-diastolic and end-systolic volumes of the ventricles can be calculated. Radionuclide angiocardiography has many clinical applications (Table 33.1).

### Myocardial perfusion imaging

The imaging stress test enhances the accuracy of the standard electrocardiographic treadmill stress test by nearly 10–20% in detecting coronary artery disease.

**Thallium-201** ($^{201}$Tl) and $^{99m}$Tc-Sesta MIBI are the most suitable radionuclides for myocardial perfusion imaging. As a biological substitute for ionic $K^+$, $^{201}$Tl is rapidly extracted from the bloodstream by normally functioning myocardial cells. Ischemic or infarcted areas accumulate little $^{201}$Tl and appear "cold." Following initial uptake by myocardial cells, $^{201}$Tl undergoes exchange with the systemic pool and gradual equilibration so that transiently ischemic areas show reversible defects (i.e., perfusion defects in the initial scans return to near-normal perfusion in the delayed images) (Figure 33.2). However, infarcted areas show fixed defects. In severe coronary disease owing to exercise-induced left ventricular (LV) failure, initial images may show LV dilatation and increased lung uptake of $^{201}$Tl.

Intravenous dipyridamole or adenosine may be used in patients unable to exercise **(pharmacologic stress).** These agents greatly augment blood flow through the

**TABLE 33.1. Clinical Applications of Radionuclide Angiocardiography**

| Objective | Setting | Comments |
|---|---|---|
| Determine/monitor LV function | Chest pain and abnormal baseline ECG, or Asymptomatic patients with a positive exercise ECG | May detect coronary artery disease, which can be confirmed by coronary angiography |
| | Recent myocardial infarction | Significant reduction in LVEF (<40%) indicates poor prognosis |
| | During or following therapy with cardiotoxic drugs (e.g., doxorubicin) | May detect myocardial damage from drugs |
| | Aortic regurgitation | May help determine optimal timing for intervention |
| | Congestive heart failure | May detect an etiology (LV aneurysm or global LV dysfunction) |
| Detect RV dysfunction | Acute inferior wall myocardial infarction | RV dysfunction may cause a low output state in inferior wall myocardial infarction |
| Detect RV and LV dysfunction | Chronic obstructive lung disease | Long term oxygen therapy may be needed with RV dysfunction; overall management may be altered by LV dysfunction |
| Detect and quantitate intracardiac shunts | Unexplained hypoxemia and/or erythrocytosis | |

LV = left ventricular; ECG = electrocardiography; LVEF = left ventricular ejection fraction; RV = right ventricular.

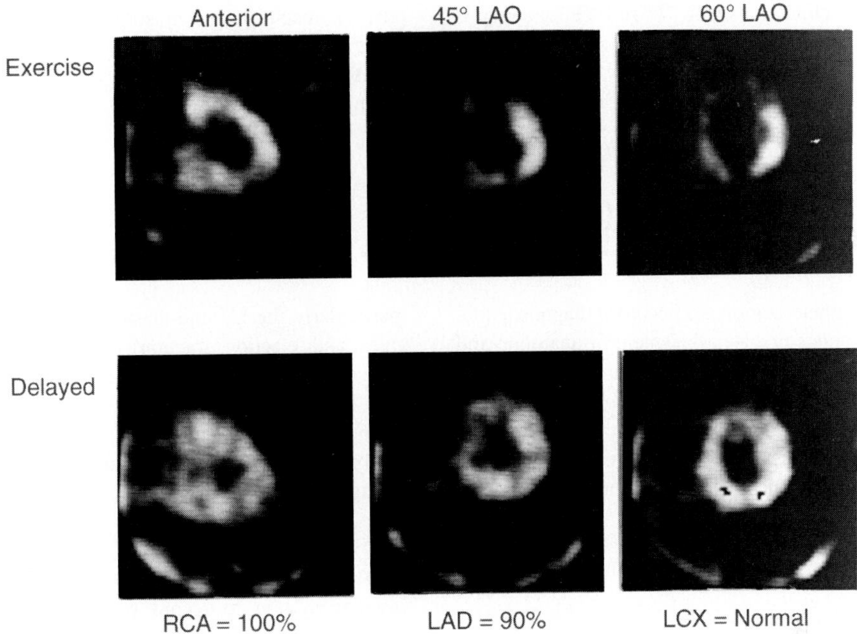


**FIGURE 33.2.** Exercise thallium-201 perfusion imaging. **Exercise** images *(top panels)* show perfusion immediately after exercise in anterior, 45° left anterior oblique (LAO), and 60° LAO views. Perfusion defects are evident in the septal and inferior segments. **Delayed images** *(bottom panels)*, repeated 4 hours after exercise, show that the perfusion defects have "filled in," indicating reversible myocardial ischemia in the septal and inferior segments. Coronary angiography (not shown) revealed total occlusion of the right coronary artery (RCA), 90% stenosis of left anterior descending (LAD) artery, and normal left circumflex (LCX) artery.

normal—but not stenotic—coronary vessels resulting in heterogeneity of blood flow among different myocardial regions. The accuracy of pharmacologic stress tests is similar to that of exercise imaging tests.

Myocardial perfusion imaging is clinically useful in patients with resting abnormal ECGs in whom an exercise ECG would be unreliable and in patients who cannot achieve near-maximal heart rates during exercise stress tests. Current clinical applications are summarized in Table 33.2.

### Infarct imaging

**Technetium-99m stannous pyrophosphate** ($^{99m}$Tc-PYP) binds to calcium and organic macromolecules in the acutely damaged myocardium and appears as a "hot spot" on perfusion imaging. Unlike the fixed defects of $^{201}$Tl imaging, which cannot distinguish acute from old infarctions, $^{99m}$Tc-PYP delineates only the acutely infarcted myocardium. $^{99m}$Tc-PYP imaging becomes positive 48 hours after acute myocardial infarction and remains positive for 6 days. The sensitivity and specificity are excellent for Q-wave infarction but less accurate for non–Q-wave infarction.

**TABLE 33.2. Clinical Applications of Myocardial Perfusion Imaging**

- Diagnosis of coronary artery disease
  - Patients with an intermediate pre-test likelihood of disease
  - Asymptomatic patients with positive exercise ECG test
  - Non-anginal chest pain in middle-aged or elderly men
  - Non-anginal chest pain in patients with positive or inconclusive exercise ECG test
  - Patients with atypical angina
  - Typical angina in men <40 years and in women <60 years
  - Typical angina in patients with negative exercise ECG test.
- Evaluation for multi-vessel disease
  - Perfusion defects in multivessel territories
  - Exercise-induced LV dilatation
  - Increased lung uptake of $^{201}$Tl
- Assess myocardial viability in hypokinetic areas of LV
- Assessment of efficacy of angioplasty/detection of restenosis
  - Serial $^{201}$Tl imaging before and after coronary angioplasty

The main clinical use of $^{99m}$Tc-PYP imaging is to confirm, localize, and evaluate the size of an acute myocardial infarction in patients in whom serial ECGs are inconclusive or difficult to interpret. False-positive results occur in some cases of unstable angina, myocardial contusion, ventricular aneurysms, and calcified heart valves and also after electrical defibrillation.

# CHAPTER 34 CARDIAC CATHETERIZATION

Cardiac catheterization is a powerful diagnostic tool that provides precise assessment of anatomic and physiologic changes in many cardiovascular diseases. Because this technique provides direct and definitive information, it is considered the gold standard against which various noninvasive tests are judged. In general, this technique permits measurements of the following:

1. Pressures in various cardiac chambers and blood vessels
2. Pressure gradients across stenotic cardiac valves
3. Cardiac output
4. Systemic and pulmonary vascular resistances
5. Hemodynamic changes during stress (e.g., supine exercise)
6. Shunts between systemic and pulmonary vessels

Selective injection of contrast material during catheterization helps define the coronary anatomy, quantify valvular regurgitation, and calculate the chamber volume (particularly the LV end-diastolic and end-systolic volumes and ejection fraction). This technique permits cardiac pacing and electrophysiologic studies. In addition, several therapeutic modalities, such as coronary angioplasty, atherectomy, stent placement, and selective administration of thrombolytic agents, can be performed during the procedure (chapters 38 and 39).

## Measurement of Intravascular Pressures

A fluid-filled catheter is routinely introduced into the vascular system to record pressure curves from the cardiac chambers and great vessels. Phasic and mean (electronically measured) pressures are usually recorded from the right atrium, pulmonary artery, pulmonary capillary wedge position, and aorta, but only phasic pressures are recorded from the right and left ventricles (Figure 34.1). The mean pressure is calculated as the diastolic pressure plus one-third of the pulse pressure. Tables 34.1 and 34.2 list the normal values for various hemodynamic measurements obtained by cardiac catheterization.

Normally, the pulmonary artery diastolic, mean pulmonary capillary wedge, mean left atrial, and LV

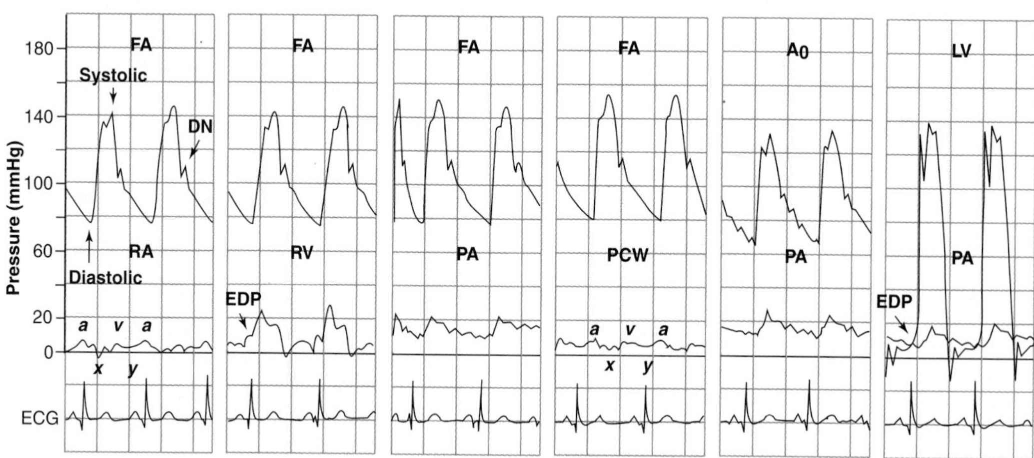


**FIGURE 34.1.** Phasic pressure curves obtained from different cardiac chambers and vessels during right and left heart catheterization. FA = femoral artery; Ao = aorta; LV = left ventricle; RA = right atrium; RV = right ventricle; PA = pulmonary artery; PCW = pulmonary capillary wedge; DN = dicrotic notch; EDP = end-diastolic pressure.

**TABLE 34.1. Normal Values for Intravascular Pressure Measurements**

| Site | Systolic Pressure (mm Hg) | End-Diastolic Pressure (mm Hg) | *a* wave (mm Hg) | *v* wave (mm Hg) | Mean Pressure (mm Hg) |
|---|---|---|---|---|---|
| Right atrium | | | 2.5–9 | 2–7 | 1–5 |
| Right ventricle | 15–30 | 0–8 | | | |
| Pulmonary artery | 15–30 | 3–12 | | | 9–20 |
| Pulmonary capillary wedge | | | 4–6 | 6–20 | 3–12 |
| Left ventricle | 90–140 | 4–14 | | | |
| Aorta | 90–140 | 60–90 | | | 70–105 |

**TABLE 34.2. Normal Values for Hemodynamic and Flow Measurements**

| Measurement | Normal Values |
|---|---|
| Cardiac index | 2.5–4.2 L/min/$m^2$ |
| Stroke index | 40–70 ml/$m^2$ |
| Stroke work index | 40–80 g-m/$m^2$ |
| Pulmonary vascular resistance | 0.2–3 Wood units |
| Systemic vascular resistance | 10–20 Wood units |
| Oxygen consumption | 110–150 ml/min/$m^2$ |
| Arterio-venous oxygen Difference | 30–50 ml/L blood |
| LV end-diastolic volume | 50–90 ml/$m^2$ |
| LV end-systolic volume | 14–34 ml/$m^2$ |
| LV ejection fraction | 50–75% |

LV = left ventricular; Wood units = pressure difference (mm Hg)/Flow (L/min).

diastolic pressures *prior to atrial contraction* are similar. Thus, pulmonary artery diastolic or pulmonary artery wedge pressure accurately reflects the LV filling pressure and can be readily monitored at bedside by a *pulmonary artery* (Swan-Ganz) catheter.

## Measurement of Cardiac Output

Cardiac output (systemic blood flow) is usually expressed as the cardiac index (L/min/$m^2$) after correction for body surface area. It can be measured by three methods:

- In the **Fick** method, cardiac output is calculated by dividing the oxygen consumption ($VO_2$, in ml/min) by the arteriovenous oxygen difference (in ml/L).
- In the **indicator-dilution** method, a bolus of indocyanine green dye is injected into the pulmonary artery, and its concentration in the systemic circulation (LV, aorta, or peripheral artery) is continuously recorded; cardiac output is calculated from the time-concentration curve.
- In the **thermodilution** method, a bolus of cold saline is injected into the right atrium through a multilumen catheter. The thermistor at the catheter tip, positioned in the pulmonary artery, senses an initial decrease in temperature followed by a progressive rise, and the time-temperature curve thus obtained helps compute the cardiac output.

## Other Studies

**Vascular resistance,** or resistance to blood flow, is calculated separately for the systemic and pulmonary circulations. The functional **orifice area** of stenotic valves can be calculated by measuring the pressure gradient and blood flow across the valve. The angiographic stroke volume minus the Fick stroke volume indicates the amount of blood regurgitating across the incompetent valve.

The presence of an abnormal communication between the systemic and pulmonary circulations allows **shunting** of blood from one to the other without traversing the capillary bed. The magnitude of the shunts can be calculated by oximetry or the indicator-dilution method. Cineangiocardiography, following selective injection of contrast material, is helpful in localizing the shunt.

## Indications for Cardiac Catheterization

The primary role of cardiac catheterization is to provide precise anatomic and physiologic information about cardiac abnormality in patients in whom surgical intervention is being contemplated. The recent availability of pulmonary artery catheters has made bedside hemodynamic monitoring practical and extended its use to coronary and intensive care units (Table 34.3).

The incidence of complications of cardiac catheterization relates to the underlying heart disease and experience of the operator. Right heart catheterization is associated with minimal morbidity and no mortality in adults. In most cardiac catheterization laboratories and with experienced operators, the risk of death with coronary catheterization is less than 0.1% and the incidence of arterial complications is 1.0% or less.

**TABLE 34.3. Indications for Bedside Pulmonary Artery Catheterization**

| | |
|---|---|
| Acute myocardial infarction complicated by:<br>Moderate or severe heart failure<br>Hypotension not easily corrected by volume infusion<br>Suspected right ventricular infarction<br>Mechanical complications<br>Ventricular septal rupture<br>Papillary muscle rupture<br>Ventricular free wall rupture with cardiac tamponade<br>Intractable postinfarction ischemia | Intractable heart failure, before inotropic and vasodilator therapy<br>Confirmation and management of cardiac tamponade<br>Differentiation between cardiogenic and noncardiogenic pulmonary edema<br>Perioperative monitoring in high-risk cardiac patients<br>Management of sepsis and/or multisystem organ dysfunction |

# CHAPTER 35 DISORDERS OF CARDIAC RHYTHM AND CONDUCTION

## Basic Electrophysiologic Principles and Applied Pharmacology of Antiarrhythmic Agents

The cardiac transmembrane potential, as outlined in chapter 32, consists of five phases resulting from ion fluxes (see Figure 32.1). Because these ionic currents define the myocardial cells into "fast" and "slow" response types (see Glossary), various ion-channels are inhibited by specific blockers; a fact that assumes critical significance in antiarrythmic drug therapy.

### The role of the nervous system

The **autonomic nervous system** exerts little direct effect on fast-response cell types but profoundly alters conduction velocity and the rate of automaticity in slow-response cell types. **Sympathetic** stimulation enhances calcium influx, causing an increase in both conduction velocity and the slope of phase 4 diastolic depolarization in slow-response cell types, thus increasing the rate of firing. **Parasympathetic** stimulation causes enhanced potassium efflux, causing cell hyperpolarization and a decrease in the slope of phase 4 diastolic depolarization with a reduction in cell firing rate. Parasympathetic stimulation also provokes a reduction in conduction velocity of AV nodal cells and lowers fibrillation thresholds.

### Mechanisms of cardiac arrhythmias

Cardiac arrhythmias can be broadly divided according to their mechanisms into abnormalities of impulse formation (automaticity, see Glossary), impulse conduction (see Glossary), or both. Although the precise mechanism of most clinical arrhythmias remains elusive, one can contend that a given arrhythmia is most likely caused by one electrophysiological mechanism or another. Additionally, many variables—myocardial ischemia, hypoxia, heart failure, electrolyte imbalance, scarred myocardium, drug toxicity, or antiarrhythmic drug use—can provoke or exacerbate arrhythmias.

#### *Abnormalities of automaticity*

Abnormalities of automaticity include **inappropriate rates of discharge** of the sinus node, which is the normal cardiac pacemaker (e.g., inappropriate sinus bradycardia or tachycardia), or of an ectopic pacemaker, which gains control of the atrial or ventricular rhythm (e.g., ectopic atrial tachycardia, accelerated idioventricular rhythm, and nonparoxysmal junctional tachycardia).

A second category of abnormalities of automaticity includes **triggered activity**. Triggered activity is caused by afterdepolarizations (see Glossary) that may occur singly or initiate other afterdepolarizations. **Torsades de pointes**, a unique type of polymorphic ventricular tachycardia, is one such example.

#### *Abnormalities of conduction*

Abnormalities of impulse conduction include **conduction delay** or **block** with or without **reentry**. A bradyarrhythmia may occur in the absence of reentry (e.g., AV block, bundle-branch blocks). In the presence of reentry, tachyarrhythmias may occur if reentry causes a self-perpetuating tachycardia. Most forms of ventricular tachycardia and many supraventricular tachycardias occur on the basis of a reentrant mechanism.

##### MECHANISMS OF REENTRY

Reentry can occur in all portions of the cardiac electrical system. Reentry requires 1) an area of depressed conduction with unidirectional block (i.e., retrograde but not antegrade conduction occurs at the depressed site) and 2) slow impulse propagation in the retrograde direction at the depressed site (Figure 35.1). As mentioned, reentry in the ventricular muscle may prompt ventricular tachycardia. Other reentrant loops may involve atrial muscle fibers (atrial fibrillation and flutter), the AV node region (AV nodal reentrant tachycardia), and large reentrant loops comprised of the atria and the ventricles linked not only by the AV node but also by specialized conducting tissue known as **accessory pathways** (Wolff-Parkinson-White syndrome).

Any factor that causes a local alteration of conduction and/or refractoriness may contribute to reentrant rhythms. Examples are localized myocardial fibrosis, premature stimuli (such as premature atrial or ventricular complexes), or acute myocardial ischemia.

#### Halting Reentrant Rhythms

Interventions that disrupt the reentrant circuit can interrupt reentrant arrhythmias. Such disruption may be realized via mechanical intervention, such as catheter-based radiofrequency ablation (destruction) of accessory pathways, or pharmacologically with antiarrhythmic agents. Antiarrhythmic agents prevent tachyarrhythmias in multiple ways. They may disrupt a reentrant circuit by either producing bidirectional block at the former site of unidirectional block in a Purkinje fiber or by prolonging the refractory period (see Glossary) of tissue in the region proximal to the site of unidirectional block, making this tissue unexcitable (see Figure 35.1). These agents may also preempt reentrant rhythms by preventing the formation of premature stimuli.

### Antiarrhythmic agents

The Vaughan-Williams classification (Table 35.1) groups antiarrhythmic agents into several classes. This scheme enhances communication concerning these agents, despite its many limitations and despite the significant variation of agents within a given class in their electrophysiological, hemodynamic, or myocardial depressant effects. The safe use of any antiarrhythmic drug depends on a thorough knowledge of its pharmacology, dose range, metabolism, drug interactions, and side-effect profile (Table 35.2).

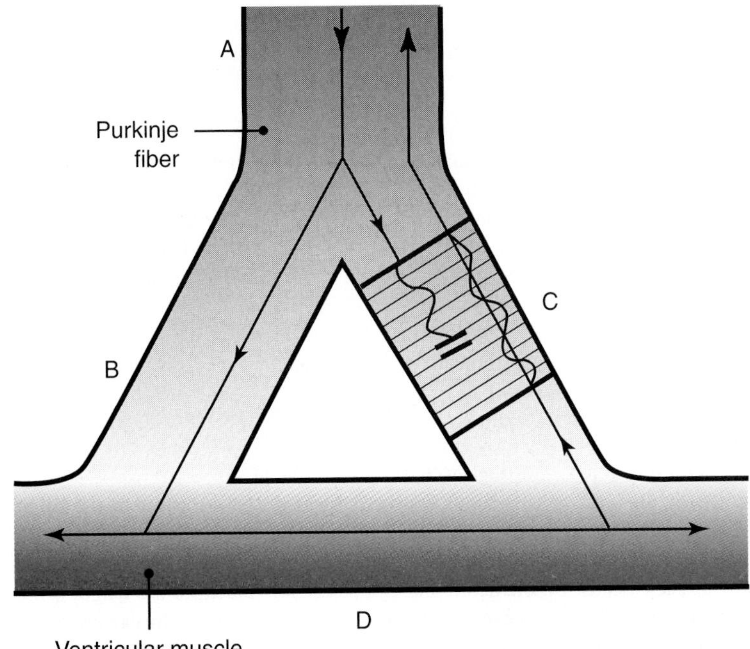


**FIGURE 35.1.** Mechanism of reentry in a branched terminal of the Purkinje system contacting ventricular muscle. An impulse traveling antegrade in Purkinje fiber A is blocked by a unidirectional block in Purkinje fiber C. However, the initial impulse from fiber A is able to conduct normally through Purkinje fiber B to ventricular muscle D. This impulse then travels retrograde to the distal branch of fiber C (which has not yet been depolarized) and through the site of the unidirectional block to again reach fiber A. If retrograde conduction through the site of unidirectional block is slow enough for the cells of fiber A to have regained excitability, then a self-perpetuating circuit or reentrant loop is formed. In this example, ventricular tachycardia would result.

TABLE 35.1. Vaughan Williams Classification of Antiarrhythmic Drugs

| Class | Category | Subclass | Agent(s) | Primary Electrophysiological Effects |
|---|---|---|---|---|
| I | Sodium-channel blockers | A | Procainamide<br>Disopyramide<br>Quinidine | Moderate inhibition of phase 0 depolarization<br>Slows conduction<br>Prolongs action potential duration, and thus refractory period |
| | | B | Lidocaine<br>Tocainide<br>Mexiletine | Mild/moderate inhibition of phase 0 depolarization<br>Minimal effect on conduction<br>Shortens action potential duration and thus refractory period |
| | | C | Flecainide<br>Propafenone<br>Ethmozine | Marked inhibition of phase 0 depolarization<br>Marked slowing of conduction<br>Little effect on action potential duration |
| II | Beta-adrenergic receptor blockers | — | Propranolol<br>Atenolol<br>Metoprolol<br>Others | In absence of catecholamines, no electrophysiologic effect; in presence of catecholamines, slows SA nodal discharge rate and slows conduction through AV node |
| III | Potassium-channel blockers | — | Amiodarone<br>Bretylium<br>Dofetilide<br>Ibutilide<br>Sotalol | Prolongs repolarization |
| IV | Calcium-channel blockers | — | Verapamil<br>Diltiazem | Activates in slow-response cells<br>Slows SA nodal discharge rate; slows conduction and increases refractory period of AV node |

## Specific Arrhythmias

### Sinus Nodal and Atrial Rhythm Disturbances

#### Sinus Tachycardia

Sinus rhythm (see Glossary) with a heart rate exceeding 100 beats per minute is termed **sinus tachycardia.** Numerous stresses—anxiety or excitement, fever, hyperthyroidism, congestive heart failure, and sympathomimetic (e.g., albuterol) and vagolytic drugs (e.g., atropine)—may cause sinus tachycardia.

#### Sinus Bradycardia

Sinus bradycardia is sinus rhythm, but below 60 beats/min. Physiologic **sinus bradycardia** occurs in well-conditioned athletes with enhanced vagal tone and in the elderly. Pharmacologic agents (e.g., digoxin, β-blockers, calcium channel blockers), maneuvers (e.g., eyeball manipulation, carotid sinus massage), and various disease states (e.g., hypothyroidism, sick sinus syndrome) may prompt sinus bradycardia. Usually, augmented stroke volume compensates for the bradycardia; thus, cardiac output remains adequate. The only current long-term solution to symptomatic sinus bradycardia is electrical pacing.

#### Sinus Arrhythmia

Sinus arrhythmia is a common, normal event. Sinus rhythm in most individuals is characterized by varying P-P intervals. When the difference between the longest and shortest P-P intervals exceeds 0.12 seconds, it is referred to as sinus arrhythmia. Neither the P-wave morphology nor P-R interval changes. Sinus arrhythmia is **phasic** when the rate is faster during inspiration or **nonphasic** when the rate change is unrelated to the respiratory cycle.

#### Sinus Arrest

Sinus arrest is defined as a pause caused by the failure of the sinus node to initiate an impulse. Usually, the pause is terminated promptly by a secondary pacemaker site in the heart, and symptoms are related to the length of the pause (unusual for pauses $< 3$ seconds). In a symptomatic patient, permanent pacing may be required.

Sinus arrest is seen in sick sinus syndrome, ischemic

**TABLE 35.2. An Overview of Antiarrhythmic Drugs**

| Drug | Direct Electrophysiologic Actions | Effect on ECG | Clinical Indications | Dose | Major Route of Elimination | Inverse Effects/Drug Interactions |
|---|---|---|---|---|---|---|
| **Class I A**<br>**Quinidine** | Reduces conduction velocity and prolongs refractoriness in most cardiac tissues<br>Suppresses automaticity from ectopic sites<br>Mild alpha-blocker and vagolytic agent, thus may enhance AV conduction | Prolongs the QT interval, mildly prolongs QRS complex | SV/ventr arrhythmias<br>Slows the intrinsic (atrial) rate of atrial arrhythmias, but may raise ventr rate by vagolytic effect<br>Administer other rate-slowing drugs (digitalis, β-blockers, etc) before quinidine for SV arrhythmias | Oral: 300–600 mg q 6 h | Liver | Cause drug discontinuation in 30% of patients<br>Cardiac: proarrhythmia, including torsades de pointes<br>GI: diarrhea, nausea, vomiting, anorexia<br>CNS: cinchonism (tinnitus, visual changes, hearing loss, confusion)<br>Blood: thrombocytopenia<br>Increased serum digoxin levels 2x |
| Procainamide | Same as quinidine; insignificant vagolytic properties | Same as quinidine | SV/ventr arrhythmias, same as for quinidine | Oral: 2–6 g/d; q3–4h doses (procainamide) and q6 or 12h doses for sustained-release forms<br>IV: 100 mg q5 min until arrhythmia controlled or up to a total of 1g, then infuse at 2–6mg/min | Kidneys<br>Metabolites: N-acetylprocainamide (NAPA), which has Class III actions<br>Therapeutic levels: 8–20μg/ml (including NAPA) | Limit long-term use<br>Cardiac: same as quinidine<br>Other: systemic lupus-like syndrome (15–20%)<br>GI: nausea, vomiting |
| Disopyramide | Same as quinidine; prominent vagolytic properties | Same as quinidine | SV/ventr arrhythmias | Oral: 100–300mg q 6–8h | Kidneys | Cardiac: same as quinidine; may also cause/worsen CHF<br>Other: blurred vision, urinary retention, closed-angle glaucoma, dry mouth |
| **Class 1 B**<br>**Lidocaine**<br>**Mexiletine**<br>**Tocainide** | Weak $Na^{++}$ channel blockers. Shortens phase 3 & action potential duration at normal heart rates and in normally polarized tissue.<br>Minimally affect conduction velocity and reduce refractory period | May shorten QT interval | Ventr arrhythmias | Lidocaine: IV: load with 1–2 mg/kg; repeat 50 mg bolus in 10 min; then infuse 1–4 mg /min. Therapeutic levels 2–5 μg/ml .<br>Tocainide: Oral : 400–600 mg q8h<br>Mexiletine: Oral: 150–300 mg q8h | Liver | Lidocaine: primary toxicity CNS, with confusion, coma, seizures<br>Mexiletine: GI: anorexia, nausea, vomiting; CNS: tremor, dysarthria, nystagmus<br>Tocainide: same as Mexiletine (GI and CNS); agranulocytosis (0.2%) and pulmonary fibrosis |
| Moricizine | Does not neatly fit into the classification schema<br>Similar $Na^{++}$ channel blocking properties as class IA drugs but mildly shortens phase 3 | Usually no change | SV and ventr arrhythmias | Oral 100–400 mg q8h | ? Liver | Cardiac: proarrhythmia<br>GI: nausea, vomiting, diarrhea<br>CNS: dizziness, headache |

Abbreviations: AVNRT = AV nodal reentrant tachycardia; BID = twice daily; CHF = congestive heart failure; CNS = central nervous system; GI = gastrointestinal; IV = intravenous; qd = once daily; RBC = red blood cells; SN = sinus node; SV = supraventricular; ventr = ventricular; VT = ventricular tachycardia.

*Continued*

TABLE 35.2. An Overview of Antiarrhythmic Drugs *(continued)*

| Drug | Direct Electrophysiologic Actions | Effect on ECG | Clinical Indications | Dose | Major Route of Elimination | Inverse Effects/Drug Interactions |
|---|---|---|---|---|---|---|
| **Class I C Flecainide** | Potent $Na^{++}$ channel blockade but minimal effect on action potential duration<br>Markedly depressed conduction in all cardiac fibers<br>Mildly prolongs refractory period | Decreases sinus rate<br>Moderately prolongs QRS interval<br>May increase PR interval | SV arrhythmias without organic heart disease<br>Avoid in patients with ventr arrhythmias (especially sustained) and poor systolic function (high risk of proarrhythmia) | Oral 50–200 mg q12h | Liver | Cardiac: proarrhythmia in certain subgroups; heart block; may cause/worsen CHF<br>Other: blurred vision |
| Propafenone | Similar to flecainide except for mild β-blocking properties | Same as flecainide | SV and ventr arrhythmias; may have proarrhythmic potential (use with caution) | Oral: 150–200 mg q8–12h | Liver | Cardiac: proarrhythmia and heart block; may cause/worsen CHF<br>Other: bronchospasm, dizziness, taste disturbance |
| **Class II Propranolol** | Prototypical β-blocker<br>Primarily affects slow-channel dependent tissue (SN and AV nodes)<br>Decreases SN firing rate and prolongs AV nodal conduction | Decreases sinus rate<br>Prolongs PR interval | Slowing ventr rate in SV arrhythmias<br>Prevention of exercise-induced arrhythmias<br>Prevent sudden death in post-MI patients | Oral: 10–200 mg q6–8h<br>IV: 0.25–0.5 mg, q 5 min for< 0.15 to 0.20 mg/kg | Liver | Cardiac: severe bradycardia, heart block; may cause/worsen CHF<br>Other: bronchospasm, lethargy, impotence |
| **Class III Amiodarone** | Lengthens repolarization by blocking outward $K^+$ currents<br>Prolongs action potential duration and refractoriness of all cardiac tissues<br>Blocks $Na^{++}$ channels<br>Slows conduction by reducing phase 0 upstroke velocity<br>Blocks $Ca^{++}$ channels (reducing SN discharge rates and prolonging AV conduction) and non-competitively inhibits β-receptors | Prolongs QRS, PR, and QT<br>Slows sinus rate | SV and ventr arrhythmias<br>Use IV in life-threatening ventr arrhythmias not responsive to lidocaine | Oral: loading: 800–1600 mg qd for 1–3 wk; Maintenance: 200–400mg qd<br>Therapeutic drug level: 1–2.5 μg/ml<br>IV: 150 mg over 10 min; then 0.5–1.0 mg per min IV | Liver<br>Concentrated in lung, liver, heart, and fatty tissue<br>Half-life: 45 days | Cardiac: proarrhythmia, severe bradycardia, heart block<br>Other: pulmonary fibrosis, hepatitis, hyper- and hypothyroidism, peripheral neuropathy, skin: photosensitivity, and discoloration and corneal microdeposits<br>Increases digoxin levels and potentiates warfarin effect |
| Bretylium | Causes initial release of, but then prevents further release of norepinephrine from adrenergic nerve terminals | Prolongs QT interval | Life-threatening ventr arrhythmias not responsive to other drugs | IV only: loading 5–10 mg/kg at 1–2 mg/kg/min; Maintenance: 0.5–2mg/min | Liver | Cardiac: proarrhythmia, orthostatic hypotension |

| | | | | | | |
|---|---|---|---|---|---|---|
| Ibutilide | Prolongs repolarization | Prolongs PR interval<br>Prolongs QT interval | Acute IV conversion of atrial fibrillation/flutter | 1 mg IV over 10 min. (repeat x 1) | Kidney | Cardiac: proarrhythmia; torsades de pointes |
| Dofetilide | Prolongs repolarization | Prolongs PR interval<br>Prolongs QT interval | Conversion/prevention of atrial fibrillation/ flutter | Oral: 125–500 mg BID based on creatinine clearance | Kidney | Cardiac: proarrhythmia; torsades de pointes |
| Sotalol | Nonselective β-blocker; blocks outward potassium current<br>Does not block $Na^{++}$ channels | Decreases sinus rate, prolongs PR and QT intervals | SV and ventr arrhythmias | Oral: 80–240 mg q12h based on creatinine clearance | Kidneys | Cardiac: proarrythmias including torsades de pointes, severe bradycardia, heart block, may cause/ worsen CHF<br>Other: fatigue |
| **Class IV**<br>**Verapamil** | Antagonizes $Ca^{++}$ influx in slow- channel dependent tissue<br>Does not block $Na^{++}$ channels<br>Reduces firing rate by decreasing the slope of phase 4 depolarization in SN<br>Decreases the maximum upstroke velocity of phase 0 depolarization and prolongs AV nodal conduction time and refractory period | Decreases sinus rate and prolongs PR | Rate slowing/termination of SV arrhythmias | Oral: 80–120 mg q6–8h | | Cardiac: hypotension, severe bradycardia, heart block, may cause/worsen CHF<br>Other: elevated liver enzymes, peripheral edema |
| **Other**<br>**Adenosine** | Increases outward $K^+$ conductance similar to acetylcholine<br>Produces marked, brief slowing of AV node conduction and SN discharge rate | | AVNRT or AV reentrant tachycardia utilizing an accessory pathway | IV: 6 mg bolus; use 12 mg IV if ineffective | Metabolized by RBC and vascular endothelium; effects potentiated by dipyridamole and competitively antagonized by methylxanthines<br>Half-life <10 seconds | Fleeting dyspnea, flushing and chest pain; may precipitate asthma |

Abbreviations: AVNRT = AV nodal reentrant tachycardia; BID = twice daily; CHF = congestive heart failure; CNS = central nervous system; GI = gastrointestinal; IV = intravenous; qd = once daily; RBC = red blood cells; SN = sinus node; SV = supraventricular; ventr = ventricular; VT = ventricular tachycardia.

syndromes, digitalis toxicity, or conditions of excess vagal tone (Figure 35.2 A).

## Wandering Atrial Pacemaker

Wandering atrial pacemaker involves transient shifts in location of the dominant pacemaker. Locations may vary among different portions of the SA node, atria, or the AV junction. A continual change in the P-wave morphology occurs with varying P-R and R-R intervals. Treatment is rarely needed.

## Premature Atrial Complexes

A premature atrial complex (PAC) appears on the ECG as a premature, morphologically abnormal P wave. Depending on the degree of prematurity, the PAC may be *nonconducted* (no subsequent QRS complex), *aberrantly conducted* (widened QRS complex), or *normally conducted.* The P-R interval of a PAC lengthens with increasing degrees of prematurity: the more premature the PAC, the longer the P-R; the later the PAC, the more normal the P-R.

PACs are common, benign events that may be produced by use of tobacco, caffeine, or alcohol; emotional stress; or by myocardial ischemia, atrial distension, or hypoxia. They usually cause no symptoms but may cause palpitations or trigger other atrial or A-V nodal reentrant tachycardias (Figure 35.2 B, C).

## Atrial Flutter

Atrial flutter is a common arrhythmia, thought to be due to a macroreentrant mechanism (Figure 35.3 A) that occurs either in a short-lived, paroxysmal form or a sustained, chronic form. Brief episodes of atrial flutter may occur in many acute illnesses (e.g., thyrotoxicosis, acute pulmonary embolism, alcohol intoxication) and are especially common soon after open-heart surgery. In a few patients, no organic heart disease is evident. Atrial flutter commonly occurs in ischemic

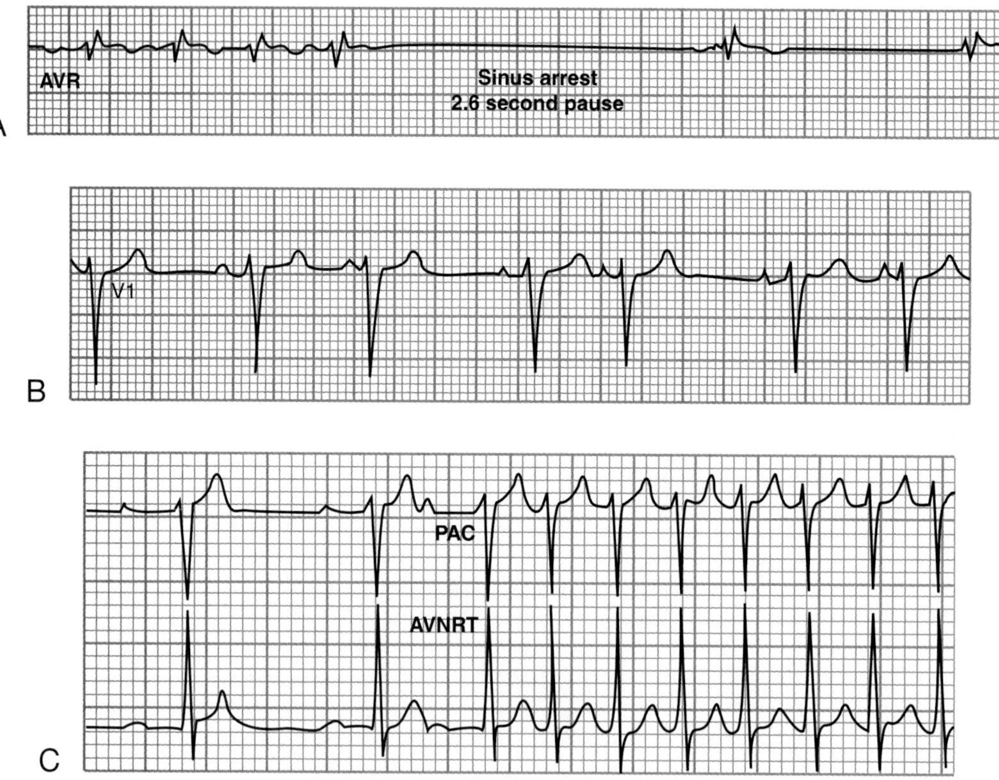


**FIGURE 35.2. A. Sinus arrest.** Following a run of supraventricular tachycardia at a rate of 110 beats/min, sinus arrest occurs, resulting in a 2.6-sec pause, followed by a slow junctional escape rhythm at a rate of 30 beats/min. This type of alteration, between a tachyarrhythmia and a bradyarrhythmia, is characteristic of the sick-sinus syndrome. **B. Premature atrial complexes.** In this strip, PACs are conducted without aberration. C. **AV nodal reentrant tachycardia (AVNRT).** A PAC is found to initiate a run of AVNRT at a rate of 170 beats/min. No P waves are evident because they are obscured in the QRS complexes.

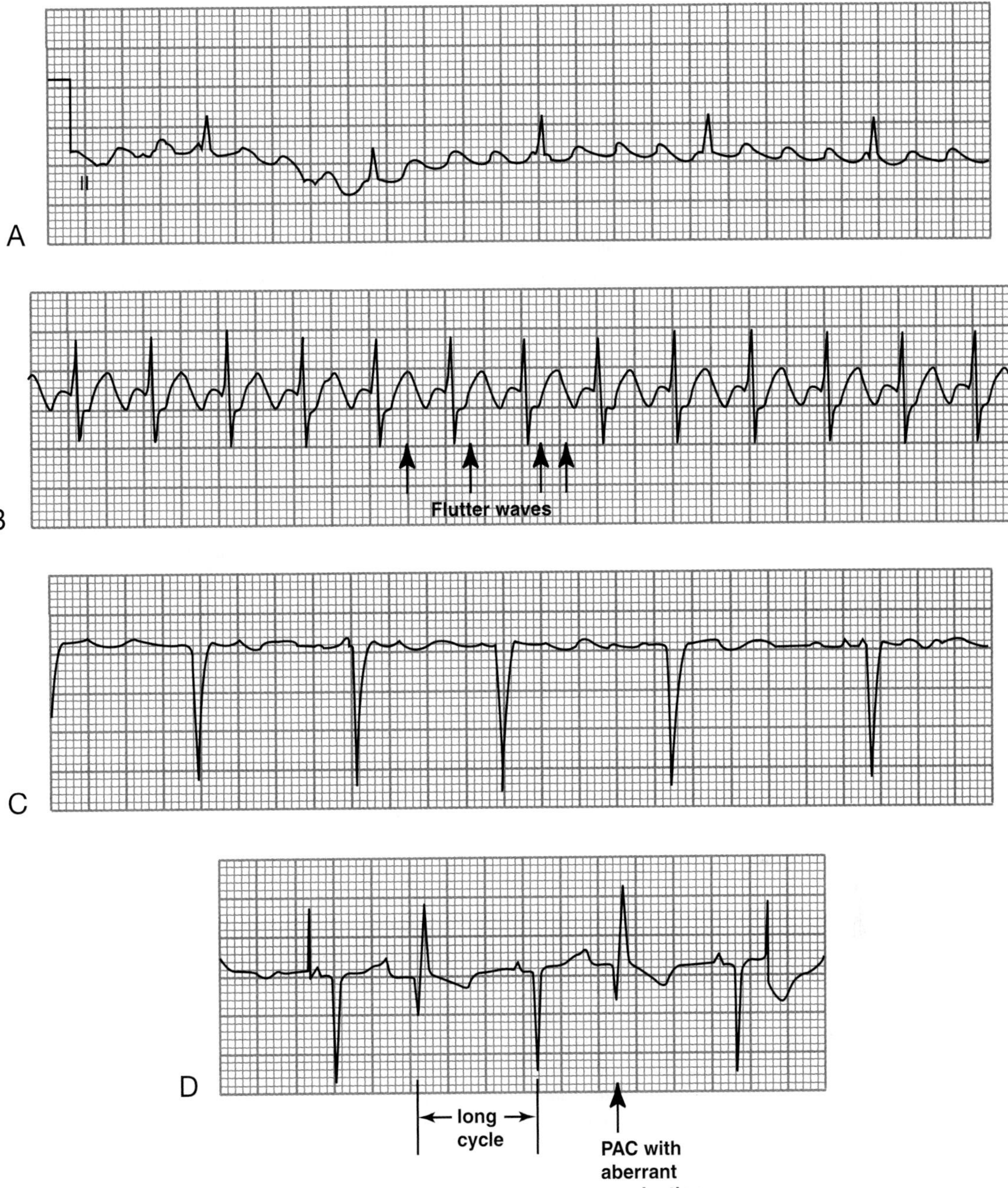


**FIGURE 35.3.** **A. Atrial flutter** with 4:1 AV block. The atrial deflections consist of rapid, sawtooth-shaped regular undulations (F waves). B. **Atrial flutter** with 2:1 AV conduction. The diagnosis of atrial flutter may be missed in 2:1 AV conduction. The F waves may be made more obvious by briefly increasing the degree of AV block (in this case, with IV adenosine). C. **Atrial fibrillation**. The P waves are replaced by fine, undulating fibrillatory waves (f waves). In the absence of complete AV block, the R-R intervals are irregular. D. **Ashman's phenomenon**. Aberrant conduction occurs when a premature atrial impulse(s) occurs after a long preceding cycle length. Aberrant conduction of supraventricular impulses may mimic ventricular tachycardia.

heart disease but is not usually caused by acute myocardial ischemia.

The **ECG** in atrial flutter demonstrates "saw-tooth" flutter (F) waves occurring regularly at 250–350 beats/min. The undulating F waves are best appreciated in leads II, III, and aVF, with an absence of isoelectric baseline between the F waves. Most commonly, a 2 : 1 AV conduction exists, resulting in a ventricular rate of 125–175 beats/min, although higher-grade, variable AV conduction may occur. With 2 : 1 AV conduction, the QRS or T waves may obscure the alternate flutter waves. In these instances, carotid sinus massage or intravenous adenosine may help by increasing the degree of AV block, thus unmasking the otherwise obscured F waves.

The **treatment** of atrial flutter is directed at its conversion into sinus rhythm. Treating the underlying cause (e.g., congestive heart failure) often evokes the spontaneous resumption of sinus rhythm. Cardioversion at low energies (25–50 joules) also usually restores sinus rhythm and is the method of choice when spontaneous reversion does not occur, or when hemodynamic instability or acute myocardial ischemia exists. Rapid atrial pacing may also be in order, especially after open heart surgery when epicardial pacing leads are already in place. Simple rate control can be achieved with a variety of drugs—verapamil, β-blockers, or digitalis. Rate control is important to achieve before instituting Type IA agents such as quinidine, procainamide, or disopyramide because these drugs slow the atrial rate while enhancing AV conduction, thus *actually increasing* ventricular response. Catheter ablation can provide curative therapy in patients not easily treated with medications.

## Atrial Fibrillation

In atrial fibrillation, there is complete disorganization of atrial electrical activity. The atria, if viewed directly, display only a writhing motion with total loss of effective contraction.

The **ECG manifestations** include 1) fibrillatory (f) waves that vary in amplitude, causing random oscillations of the baseline, and 2) an irregular ventricular response, usually between 100 and 160 beats/min in the untreated patient (Figure 35.3 C). QRS complexes are usually normal but may be widened from aberrancy (**Ashman's phenomenon**). This aberrancy is suggested by a relatively long R-R cycle immediately preceding a relatively short R-R cycle, which is terminated by the aberrant QRS complex resembling right bundle branch block. These aberrant beats may occur singly or in multiples and thus may mimic ventricular tachycardia (Figure 35.3 B).

### Clinical manifestations

As with atrial flutter, atrial fibrillation may occur in paroxysmal or persistent forms. Usually seen in patients with hypertension, ischemic heart disease, mitral valvular disease, or chronic lung disease, atrial fibrillation may also occur in many other conditions, for example, pericarditis, thyrotoxicosis, pulmonary embolism, or alcohol intoxication. Its occurrence in structurally normal hearts, albeit uncommon, is called **lone atrial fibrillation**.

Acutely, atrial fibrillation may cause **adverse consequences** because of rapid ventricular rate, loss of the atrial contribution—"atrial kick"—to ventricular filling, or peripheral emboli. The onset of atrial fibrillation is especially poorly tolerated in patients with noncompliant LV chambers such as those with aortic stenosis or hypertrophic cardiomyopathies and in patients who poorly tolerate tachycardias such as those with mitral stenosis.

### Management

As with all arrhythmias, the correction of the underlying cause is paramount. The main treatment objectives are to control the ventricular rate, restore sinus rhythm, and prevent systemic emboli. Rapid ventricular rates should be controlled by β-blockers or calcium channel blockers. Intravenous administration of diltiazem is sometimes needed. Digoxin tends to slow resting rate and not rate with activity. Digoxin should be reserved for use in the setting of significant heart failure or as an adjunct when β-blockers or calcium blockers alone are insufficient. A goal is to achieve a resting heart rate of 70–80 beats/min and a rate below 110–120 beats/min after mild exertion.

Atrial fibrillation can revert spontaneously to sinus rhythm. If not, either chemical or electrical **cardioversion** is needed. Atrial fibrillation associated with hemodynamic compromise warrants immediate synchronized DC cardioversion (100–300 joules). Electrical cardioversion is associated with a 1–3% risk of systemic embolism; thus, full **anticoagulation** with warfarin is warranted in all patients who have had atrial fibrillation for longer than 2 days. Heparin should be used followed by warfarin if immediate cardioversion is required. Anticoagulation should be maintained for 3 weeks before and 2–4 weeks after cardioversion. No anticoagulation is needed for atrial fibrillation less than 2 days' duration. Transesophageal echocardiography, to rule out thrombi in the left atrial appendage, is useful if urgent cardioversion is contemplated in patients with atrial fibrillation of greater than 48 hours duration who have not received appropriate anticoagulation.

Type IA, IC, and III antiarrhythmic agents may be used in an attempt to convert atrial fibrillation to sinus rhythm, but with a typically low success rate. More often, these agents are used to prevent recurrences following electrical cardioversion. Amiodarone is the most efficacious agent for maintaining sinus rhythm following cardioversion but has significant toxicity.

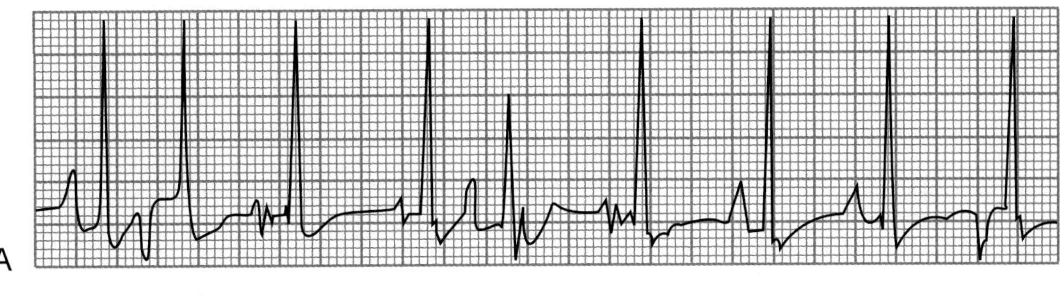


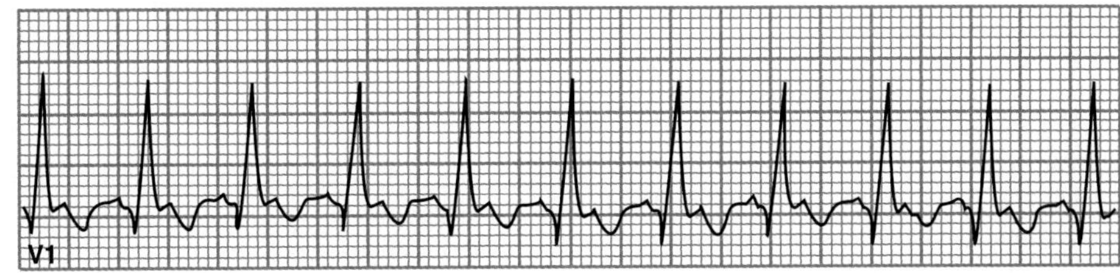


**FIGURE 35.4. A. Multifocal atrial tachycardia.** At least three different P-wave morphologies and varying P-R and R-R intervals are evident in this tracing. **B. Paroxysmal atrial tachycardia** with 2:1 AV block. The P waves occur regularly at 250/min, resulting in a regular ventricular rate of 125 beats/min. PAT with AV block is often caused by digitalis intoxication. This patient had a preexisting complete right bundle branch block.

All antiarrhythmic agents can themselves induce arrhythmias (proarrhythmia), and their potential adverse effects also need to be considered. Despite continued antiarrhythmic therapy in patients successfully converted from atrial fibrillation, the **recurrence rate** after 1 year is high—20–40%.

Catheter ablation aimed at foci in pulmonary veins has shown preliminary promise for patients with normal hearts and paroxysmal atrial fibrillation.

#### Prophylactic anticoagulation

Chronic atrial fibrillation carries a substantial risk of embolization causing 15% of all ischemic strokes. Furthermore, more than one-third of affected patients will experience an ischemic stroke within their lifetime. Long-term anticoagulation with warfarin to maintain an International Normalized Ratio (INR) between 2.0–3.0 reduces thromboembolic risk by 50–75%. Aspirin is far less efficacious and confers only a small reduction in risk of stroke. Patients in chronic atrial fibrillation who have mitral stenosis, a prior history of thromboembolism, recent (prior 3 months) history of congestive heart failure, or history of hypertension (with no contraindications for full anticoagulation) are candidates for chronic warfarin therapy. Patients younger than age 60 with none of these risk factors are considered to be at low risk for thromboembolism and can be treated with aspirin alone.

### Multifocal Atrial Tachycardia

Multifocal atrial tachycardia is characterized by an atrial rate higher than 100 beats/min; at least three different P-wave morphologies in any one lead; and variable P-P, P-R, and R-R intervals (Figure 35.4 A). Caused by enhanced automaticity in the atria, multifocal atrial tachycardia is usually found in the elderly, particularly those with severe obstructive lung disease, coronary artery disease, or diabetes mellitus. Verapamil, which reduces abnormal atrial automaticity, may prove effective as treatment. Vigorous efforts also should be aimed at improving the underlying cardiac or pulmonary status.

### Paroxysmal Atrial Tachycardia with AV Block

Paroxysmal atrial tachycardia (PAT) results from enhanced atrial automaticity combined with evidence of conduction (AV) block. Digitalis toxicity is responsible for most cases (Figure 35.4 B). The ECG demonstrates abnormal P waves with an atrial rate from 150–250 beats/min; the ventricular rate depends on the degree of AV block.

In a patient receiving digitalis, it should be assumed that PAT is caused by digitalis toxicity, and potassium supplements should be given instead of digitalis. In a patient not receiving digitalis, digitalis can be given to slow the ventricular response; if PAT persists, then class IA, IC, or III drugs may be added to restore sinus rhythm.

## *Atrioventricular Junctional Rhythm Disturbances*

### Premature Junctional Beats

Premature junctional beats arise in the AV junction and are transmitted in an antegrade fashion to the ventricles, producing a premature, but normal-appearing, QRS complex. The impulse also conducts to the atria in a retrograde fashion, producing a retrograde P wave that may occur before, during, or after the QRS complex. Treatment is usually not necessary.

### AV Junctional Escape Beats and Junctional Rhythm

If suprajunctional pacemaker sites fail to discharge, then latent pacemaker cells of the AV junction will discharge at a rate of 40–60 beats/min to prevent ventricular asystole. These **escape beats** may occur singly; however, if the normally dominant pacemaker (usually the SA node) continues to fail to discharge, then the escape beats can occur sequentially, termed a **junctional escape rhythm** (Figure 35.5 A). The escape interval is greater than the basic P-P interval. Retrograde P waves may be present, but the QRS is normal.

Therapy is directed at increasing the discharge rate of the normal suprajunctional pacemaker. Occasionally, a pacemaker may be required.

### Nonparoxysmal AV Junctional Tachycardia

In nonparoxysmal AV junctional tachycardia, the AV junction, rather than remaining the default pacemaker, usurps control from the SA node owing to its enhanced automaticity and usually discharges at a rate of 100–130 beats/min. Retrograde P waves may be present, but AV dissociation may also occur.

Digitalis toxicity is most often responsible; however, acute myocardial infarction and myocarditis are other causes. Treatment is directed at the underlying cause (Figure 35.5 B).

### Paroxysmal Supraventricular Tachycardia

An abrupt onset and termination are characteristic of the paroxysmal supraventricular tachycardias (PSVT). Approximately 60% of PSVT occur from reentry involving the AV node, 30% are caused by a concealed accessory pathway, and the remainder are due to sinus node reentry, intra-atrial reentry, or an ectopic focus (atrial tachycardia).

#### AV nodal reentry tachycardia

AV nodal reentry tachycardia (AVNRT) is characterized by a regular, narrow-complex tachycardia at a rate

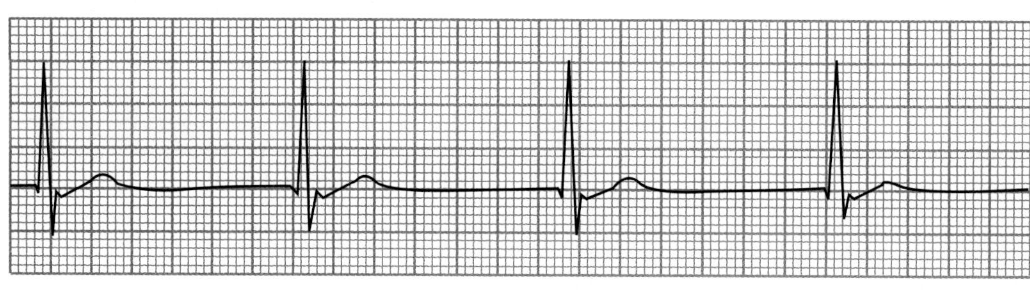


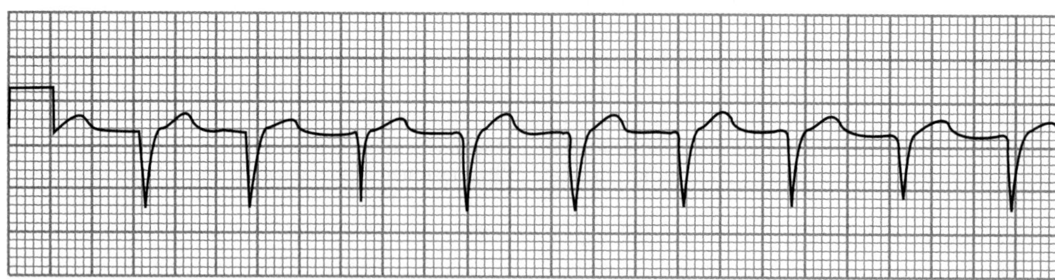


**FIGURE 35.5. A. Junctional rhythm.** There is a regular, narrow-complex rhythm at a rate of 52 beats/min. No P waves are visible. In this instance, the junctional rhythm serves as a passive escape mechanism. B. **Nonparoxysmal junctional tachycardia.** There is a regular, narrow-complex rhythm at a rate of 125 beats/min. No P waves are visible. This rhythm results from abnormal enhancement of impulse formation at the AV junction, commonly from digitalis toxicity.

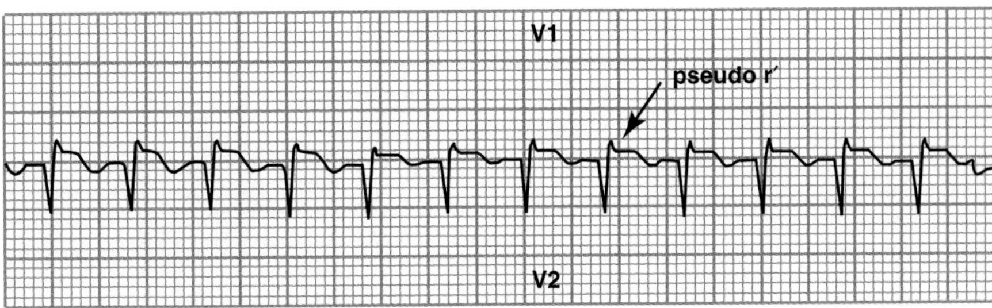


**FIGURE 35.6. AV Nodal Reentrant Tachycardia** **AVNRT** is shown here as a narrow-complex tachycardia at a rate of 150–250 beats/min. In this "slow antegrade-fast retrograde" reentrant circuit (**type I variety**), because of the fast retrograde conduction to the atria, the P wave is most often buried in the QRS complex and not seen. When seen, it distorts the terminal portion of the QRS complex producing a pseudo r′ pattern.

of 150–250 beats/min. Dual AV nodal pathways—α and β pathways—exist in patients with AVNRT. The α pathway is slower-conducting and has a shorter refractory period than the faster-conducting, longer-refractory β pathway. Premature atrial impulses are blocked in the slow-to-recover β pathway but are conducted slowly down the α pathway; thus, the β pathway is able to conduct them retrograde. This "slow antegrade–fast retrograde" reentrant circuit, termed the **type I variety,** accounts for 90% of AVNRT cases. Because of the fast retrograde conduction to the atria, the P wave is most often buried in the QRS complex and not seen. When seen, it distorts the terminal portion of the QRS complex producing a pseudo r′ pattern (Figure 35.6).

In the uncommon **type II variety** of AVNRT, the slow α pathway has the longer refractory period, and the premature impulse travels down the fast β pathway and retrograde up the slow α pathway. In this instance, inverted P waves appear shortly before each ensuing QRS.

#### Concealed accessory pathway tachycardia

A concealed bypass tract, consisting of aberrant muscle fibers connecting the atrium and the ventricle, may provide the necessary substrate for a reentrant tachycardia. Most commonly, the reentrant circuit consists of normal antegrade conduction through the AV node (resulting in a normal-appearing QRS complex) and retrograde conduction from the ventricle to the atria via the accessory pathway (orthodromic tachycardia). In this instance, the retrograde P wave usually distorts the ST segment (Figure 35.7 A). The resting ECG of these patients will not show preexcitation since conduction only occurs in a retrograde manner.

Frequently, PSVT occurs in young patients with normal hearts. The symptoms caused by these PSVTs depend on the rate of the tachycardia and the underlying heart disease.

*Management*

With reentrant forms of PSVT, the tachycardia is terminated by blocking one of the limbs of the circuits. Vagal maneuvers, such as carotid sinus massage, gagging, or Valsalva maneuver, may be successful in this way and should be tried initially. If these maneuvers fail, adenosine (6–12 mg by rapid IV bolus) is 95% successful in restoring sinus rhythm. Verapamil (5–10 mg IV) may also be used. If hemodynamic compromise complicates the arrhythmia, then synchronized DC cardioversion is necessary.

For chronic drug therapy, β-blockers, verapamil, or diltiazem are initially given, with class IC antiarrhythmic agents being reserved for recalcitrant cases. Recently, catheter ablation has become the preferred therapy for both AVNRT and concealed accessory pathway tachycardia, obviating long-term drug therapy.

### Preexcitation Syndromes

Preexcitation syndromes include the **Wolff-Parkinson-White (WPW) syndrome** and its variants. On the ECG, features of the WPW pattern consist of a short P-R interval (<0.12 sec), prolonged QRS duration (>0.11 sec, owing to the addition of a delta wave), and secondary ST-T wave changes (Figure 35.7 B).

In these patients, the existence of anomalous or accessory fibers bridging the AV groove has been demonstrated. The impulse from the sinus node conducts rapidly through the accessory pathway and activates a portion of the ventricle, resulting in a delta wave. The remainder of the sinus impulse travels normally through the AV node and depolarizes the remaining portion of the ventricles. Thus, the QRS complex in the WPW pattern represents a fusion complex owing to activation of the ventricles through two different pathways.

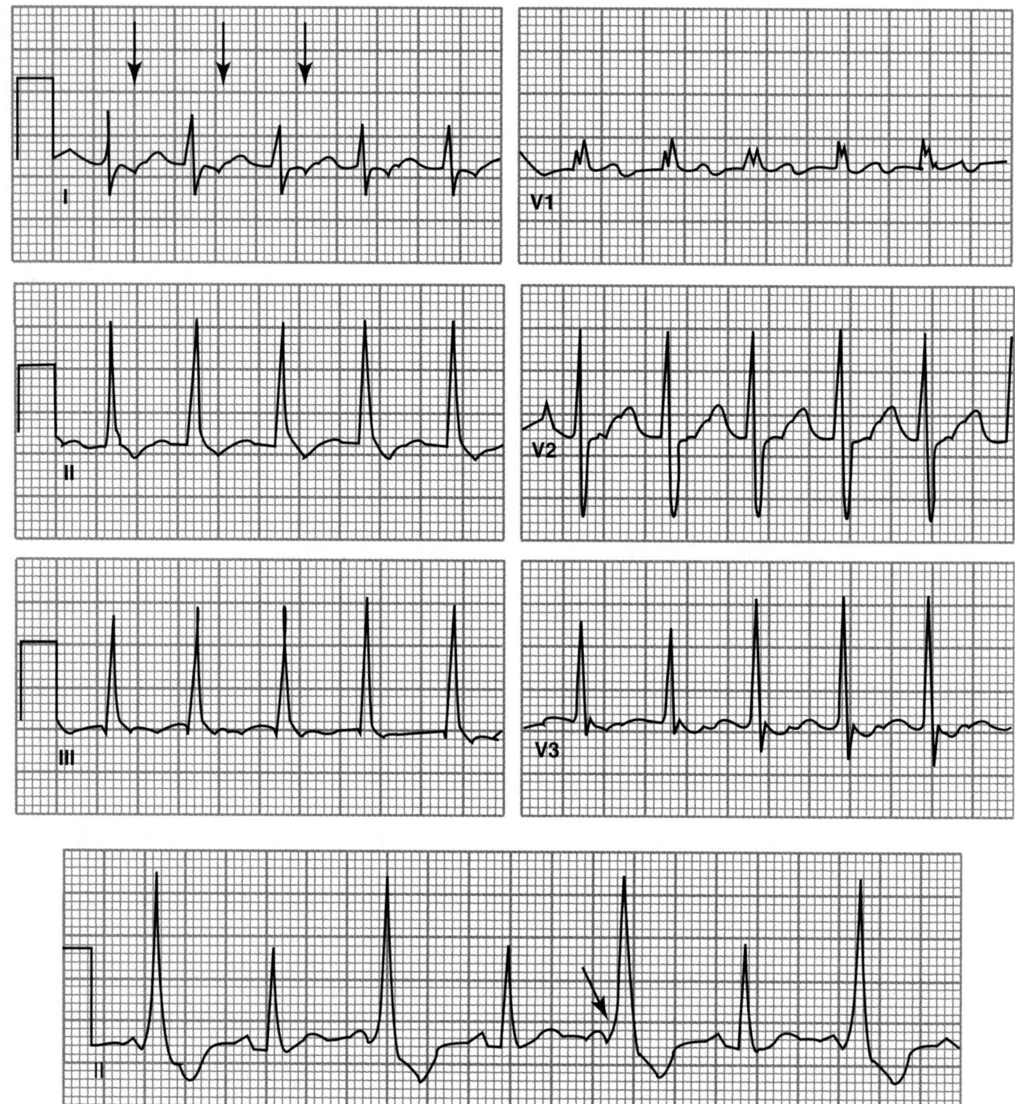


**FIGURE 35.7. A.** Wolff-Parkinson-White syndrome **with orthodromic conduction.** This six-lead strip shows a tachycardia at 135 beats/min in which the supraventricular impulses conduct antegrade down the AV node and retrograde to the atrium via the accessory pathway. In lead I, the arrows point to retrograde P waves deforming the upslope of the T waves. Each P wave is causally related to the prior QRS. The QRS complex is narrow because the ventricles are activated via the normal conduction pathway (AV node and His-Purkinje system). **B. WPW with antidromic conduction.** This strip demonstrates intermittent preexcitation. The arrow points to a "preexcited" ventricular complex. Note the short PR interval (100 ms) and the slurred QRS upstroke (the delta wave, arrow). The preexcited complexes are a result of antegrade conduction down the accessory pathway.

### Clinical manifestations

The prevalence of WPW syndrome in the general population is about 0.15%, with a 2 : 1 preponderance for men. This anomaly is considered to be congenital but not inherited, and it may be associated with other cardiac anomalies (e.g., Ebstein's anomaly).

Approximately 40–60% of patients develop tachyarrhythmias, with the most common variety being paroxysmal supraventricular tachycardia that occurs on a reentrant basis. Usually, the impulse transmits antegrade through the AV node in the usual fashion and retrograde through the accessory pathway back to the atria (**orthodromic tachycardia**) (figure 35.7 A). Less commonly, the impulse conducts antegrade through the accessory pathway and retrograde through the His bundle and AV node (**antidromic tachycardia**) (Figure 35.7 B).

Because the accessory pathway may have the potential to conduct impulses rapidly, patients with WPW are at risk for developing very fast ventricular rates, if atrial arrhythmias, such as atrial fibrillation or flutter were to occur. In general, rapid ventricular rates faster than 200 beats/min during atrial fibrillation are characteristic of WPW syndrome. Chest pain, heart failure, or syncope may occur during these rapid tachycardias. There is a small risk of sudden cardiac death from atrial fibrillation degenerating to ventricular fibrillation.

**Management**

Treatment is not necessary for patients with asymptomatic preexcitation or for patients with a history of infrequent, asymptomatic tachycardias. Treatment options for symptomatic tachycardias consist of 1) lifelong drug therapy with agents that delay conduction in the AV node, accessory pathway, or both, or 2) destruction of the accessory pathway by surgery or radiofrequency catheter ablation. Because it offers a permanent cure and obviates the need for drug therapy, catheter ablation is the preferred treatment. Patients with hemodynamic compromise require immediate, synchronized DC cardioversion.

In patients with antegrade conduction over the AV node (orthodromic tachycardia), acute drug treatment is similar to that of AV nodal reentrant rhythms (e.g., IV adenosine or verapamil). In patients with atrial fibrillation or flutter and antegrade conduction over the accessory pathway (antidromic tachycardia), IV procainamide or electrical cardioversion should be the initial treatment. Digitalis, adenosine, or verapamil are contraindicated because of their propensity to increase the ventricular response by blocking the AV node and lead to ventricular fibrillation.

**Diagnosis of narrow-complex tachycardia**

Narrow QRS tachycardias arise from supraventricular structures, i.e., sinus node, atria, and AV junction. By definition, they imply fast heart rate with normal width and configuration of the QRS complex. Narrow QRS complexes occur in a range of tachycardias. The general approach to these entities is summarized in Figure 35.8. Some key considerations are summarized as follows:

1. 12-lead ECG tracings, rather than a single-lead, are preferable for the analysis of an arrhythmia.
2. The location of the P wave relative to the QRS complex (before, within, or after) should be determined, and the presence of 1 : 1 AV conduction should be noted. The presence of AV block would terminate AV-dependent rhythms and so exclude conditions such as AV nodal reentrant tachycardias or AV reciprocating tachycardias using an accessory pathway. If there is AV block, the differential diagnosis is that of an atrial arrhythmia—either an ectopic atrial focus or reentry in the SA node or atrial tissue.
3. If there is 1 : 1 AV conduction, the relative timing of atrial and ventricular activation—the R-P and P-R intervals—should be noted. The R-P interval is the duration between the start of the QRS and the following P wave. The P-R interval is the duration between the onset of the P wave and the start of the QRS. If a P wave is identifiable, determining whether the R-P exceeds P-R or the P-R exceeds the R-P can suggest other differential diagnoses.
4. The morphology of the P wave should be determined.
5. Esophageal ECG recordings—which requires intraesophageal placement of an electrode for recording—can help demonstrate atrial activity when P waves are not visible on the surface ECG.
6. Carotid sinus massage can help in the differential diagnosis of tachyarrhythmias. By increasing vagal tone, carotid sinus massage causes 1) a slight transient decrease of sinus tachycardia rate; 2) no effect or abrupt termination of AV nodal reentrant tachycardia or supraventricular tachycardia using an accessory pathway, or 3) AV block with continuation (at a slower ventricular rate) of atrial flutter, or atrial fibrillation. Carotid massage should be avoided in patients with known carotid disease, carotid bruits, or prior stroke.
7. Adenosine can be used to produce brief, high-grade block of the AV node, which will terminate supraventricular tachycardias such as AV node reentry or those using accessory pathways. By producing transient AV nodal block, adenosine may aid in the diagnosis of atrial fibrillation, atrial flutter, and other atrial tachycardias, as well as wide QRS tachycardias. Adenosine only rarely terminates ventricular tachycardia. Caution must be exercised when antegrade conduction over an accessory pathway exists, because adenosine may favor conduction over the accessory pathway (by blocking the AV node) and thus increase the ventricular rate.

## *Ventricular Arrhythmias*

### Premature Ventricular Complexes

Premature ventricular complexes (PVCs) are the most common ventricular rhythm disturbance. On the ECG, PVCs produce a wide-complex QRS owing to their abnormal ventricular origin and anomalous conduction pattern. The T wave is oriented opposite to the major QRS deflection. Commonly, the atria and sinus node are

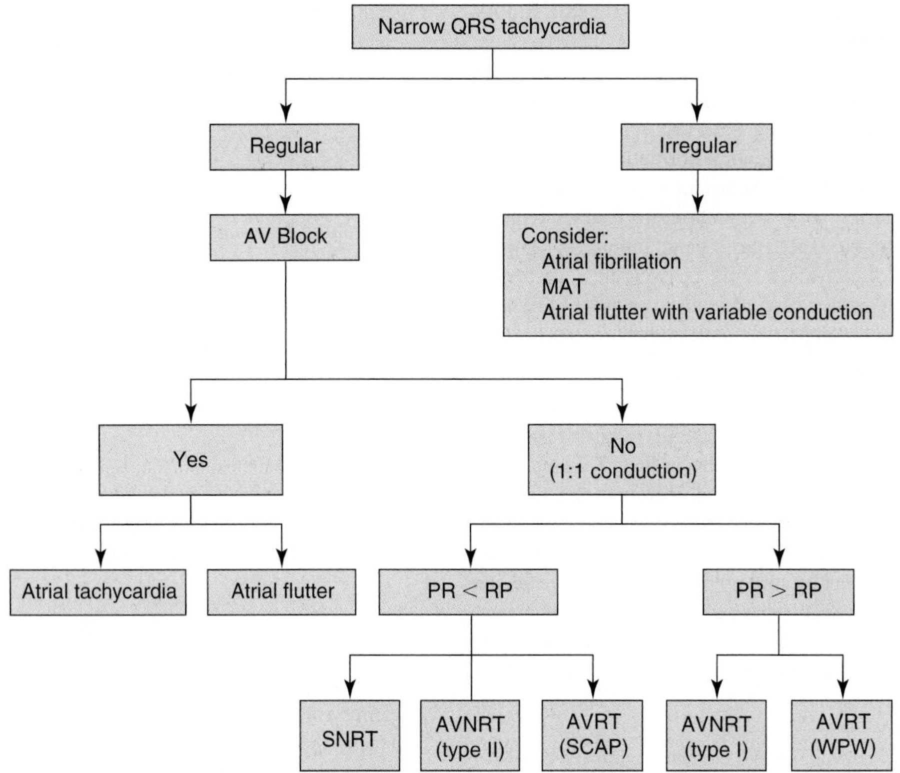


**FIGURE 35.8. Differential diagnosis of tachycardia with a narrow QRS.** This schema excludes atrial fibrillation, multifocal atrial tachycardia, and nonparoxysmal atrial tachycardia and assumes an identifiable P wave is present. It should be noted that AVNRT is most commonly not associated with an identifiable P wave but, rather, the P wave is "obscured" in the QRS. AVNRT = AV nodal reentrant tachycardia; AVRT = AV nodal reciprocating tachycardia; MAT = multifocal atrial tachycardia; SCAP = slow-conducting accessory pathway; SNRT = sinus node reentrant tachycardia; WPW = Wolff-Parkinson-White syndrome.

not depolarized retrograde, thus causing, a **compensatory pause**—that is, the R-R interval containing the PVC is twice the duration of the preexisting basic R-R interval. If there is no compensatory pause, then the PVC is termed **interpolated**.

PVCs arising from the same focus usually maintain a fixed coupling interval to the preceding impulse and thus a reentrant mechanism. If the coupling interval varies by more than 0.08 sec, then **ventricular parasystole** should be considered. In ventricular parasystole, an ectopic ventricular focus, presumably with increased automaticity, activates the ventricles concurrently with, but independent of, the impulse of the basic rhythm.

Two successive PVCs are termed a **couplet**, and three successive PVCs, at a rate of >100 beats/min or similar morphology are **ventricular tachycardia**. PVCs of similar morphology are termed **unifocal**, but if the morphology varies in the same lead, they are **multifocal** or **polymorphic**. If PVCs successively alternate with a sinus beat, the rhythm is termed **bigeminy** (Figure 35.9).

PVCs may be associated with structurally normal hearts and, in the absence of significant symptoms, require no therapy. PVCs may become manifest or exacerbated with excess caffeine, alcohol, emotional stress, sympathomimetic agents, hypoxia, or other conditions, including any type of heart disease. Their prognostic importance depends on the type and severity of the underlying heart disease. When associated with coronary artery disease and, particularly, poor LV systolic function, PVCs portend an increased risk of cardiac death.

Nevertheless, eradication of PVCs with antiarrhythmic therapy has not been proven to improve outcome (except for β-blockers in patients following myocardial infarction), and it may in fact increase mortality owing to proarrhythmic mechanisms. Thus, in patients with PVCs reversible factors should be sought and corrected when possible. If drug therapy is chosen, β-blockers should be tried first. Other antiarrhythmic agents should be used with great caution and preferably under guidance of electrophysiologic testing.

## Ventricular Tachycardia

Ventricular tachycardia (VT) arises from impulses generated from the His-Purkinje system, ventricular myocardium, or both, and can arise from abnormalities of impulse formation (automaticity, triggered activity) or conduction, (e.g., reentry).

In VT, the QRS complex is more than 0.12 sec, with T-wave vectors directed opposite to the main QRS deflection. The R-R intervals are usually regular. Because the atria are controlled by the sinus node, AV dissociation is usually present (Figure 35.10 A); however, retrograde activation of the atria from the ventricles (ventriculoatrial association) may occur. If, in the same lead the QRS complexes do not vary in contour, VT is termed **monomorphic** (Figure 35.10 B); if contours vary, VT is **polymorphic** (Figure 35.11). VT is further subdivided into two types: **sustained** (lasting >30 sec or associated with hemodynamic compromise) and **nonsustained** (>3 consecutive beats lasting <30 sec) (Figure 35.10 C).

The spectrum of manifestations of VT ranges from none to the hemodynamic collapse. VT usually implies a diseased heart. Occurring in all forms of ischemic heart disease, cardiomyopathies, and valvular disease, VT may also result from proarrhythmia caused by many drugs and in patients with long Q-T intervals.

The main differential diagnosis of a wide QRS complex tachycardia is between VT and supraventricular tachycardia (SVT) with aberrancy. Certain historical, clinical, and ECG variables, as described in Table 35.3, may help differentiate between these two conditions. VT is much more common than SVT with aberrancy, and any wide QRS complex tachycardia should be considered VT until proven otherwise. In the presence of known structural heart disease—particularly a prior myocardial infarction—a diagnosis of VT is overwhelmingly likely. Also, VT usually has more profound hemodynamic effects than SVT, but normal hemodynamics do not rule out VT. Intravenous verapamil must be avoided in these patients unless the diagnosis of SVT with aberrancy is an absolute certainty, because verapamil may cause profound hypotension in a patient with VT.

### Management of VT

Steps in the management of VT consist of terminating the VT, identifying underlying causes, and eliminating reversible factors (e.g., hypokalemia, ischemia, bradycardia, fluid overload), thus preventing recurrence. VT associated with hemodynamic compromise requires urgent synchronized DC cardioversion.

For acute treatment, IV lidocaine is usually the initial agent of choice, followed by procainamide or amiodarone. Patients having recurrent sustained VT or symptomatic nonsustained VT require chronic treatment. Those with hemodynamically significant VT should undergo electrophysiologic testing, and many will require both chronic antiarrhythmic therapy and an implantable cardioverter-defibrillator (ICD). In others, endocardial resection, aneurysmectomy, or catheter ablation techniques may be successful.

The treatment of patients with asymptomatic nonsustained VT (a common clinical problem) is controversial. While β-adrenergic-blocking agents may be given empirically, empiric amiodarone or drug therapy selected on the basis of the electrophysiologic testing are other options. As with PVCs, it is not clear whether eradication of asymptomatic nonsustained ventricular arrhythmias actually improves prognosis, and treatment with class I drugs may, in fact, be harmful. There is an increasing emphasis on implantation of ICD in patients with coexistent LV dysfunction.

### Torsades de pointes

Torsades de pointes (twisting of points) refers to a type of polymorphic VT occurring in the presence of a long Q-T interval. Morphologically, this VT is characterized by the gradual oscillation of the peaks of successive QRS complexes around the baseline (Figure 35.11). Torsades de pointes occurs at a rapid rate in

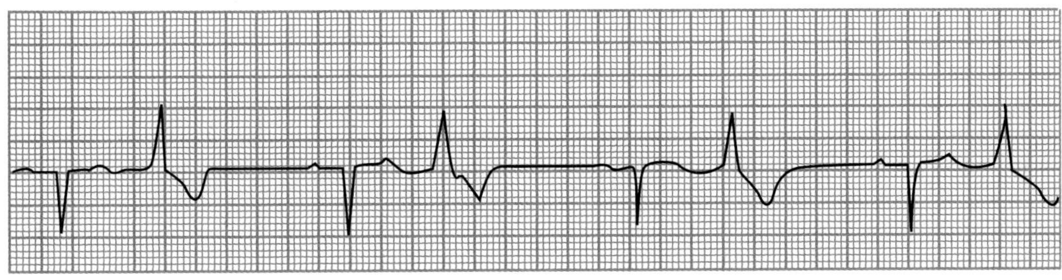

FIGURE **35.9. Bigeminy.** Every other QRS represents a premature ventricular complex (PVC).

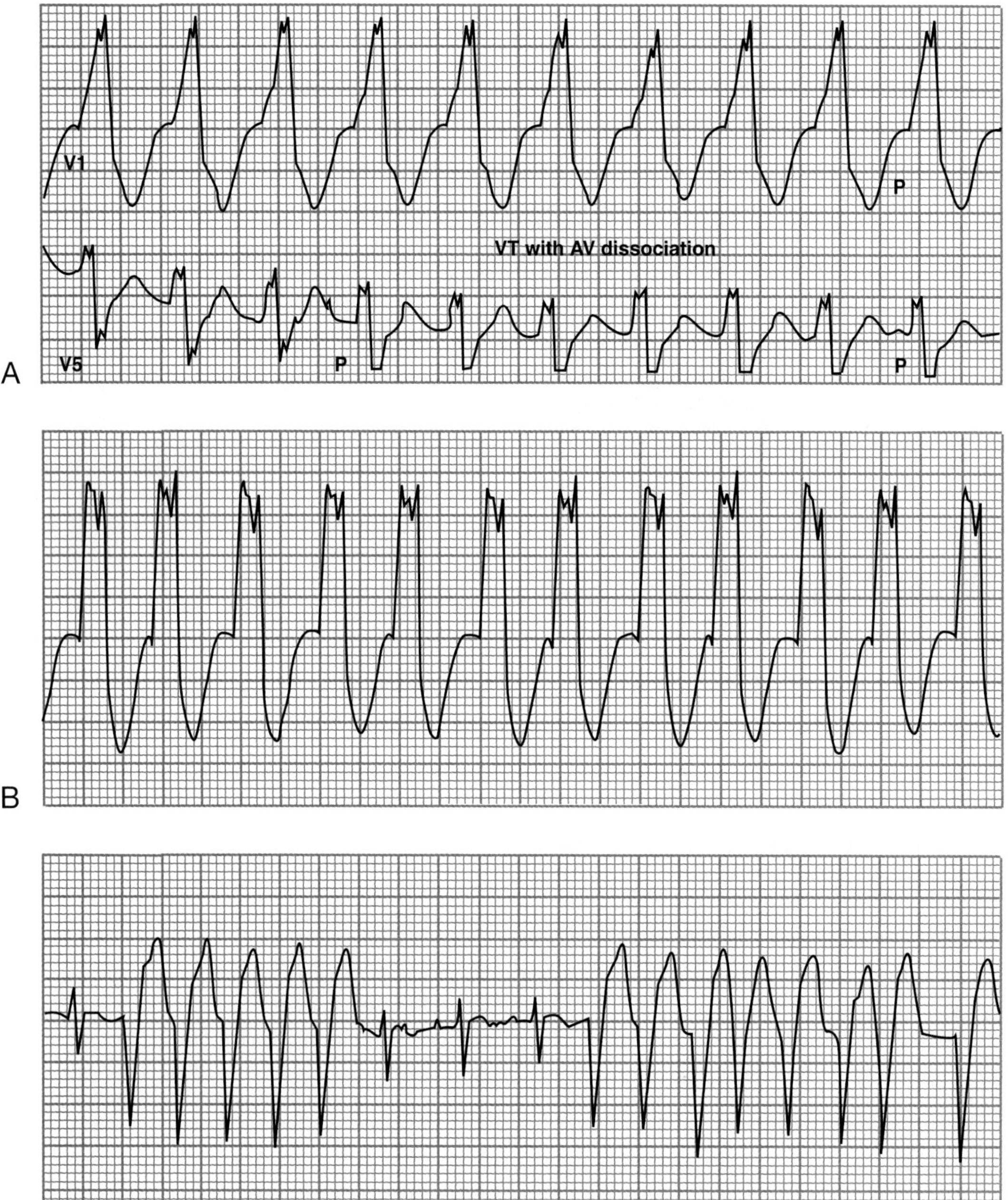


**FIGURE 35.10.** Ventricular **tachycardias** (VT). A. **VT with AV dissociation.** This strip demonstrates VT at 130 beats/min with evidence of dissociated P waves (P). AV dissociation during a wide QRS tachycardia is strong evidence that the tachycardia is of ventricular origin. B. **Monomorphic VT.** The monotony of each complex contrast with the pattern of polymorphic VT (see Fig. 35.11). C, **Nonsustained VT.** Five- and eight-beat runs of nonsustained VT are demonstrated. In this strip, the eight-beat run is irregular, demonstrating that VT need not be absolutely regular.

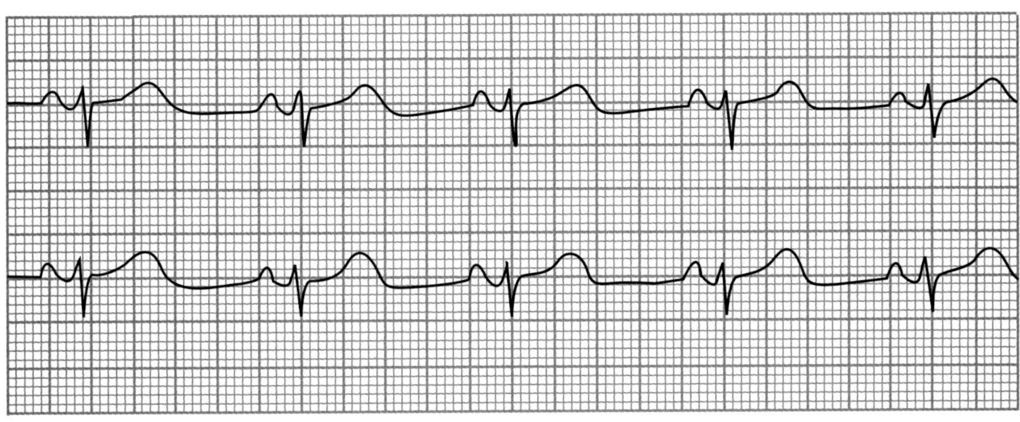

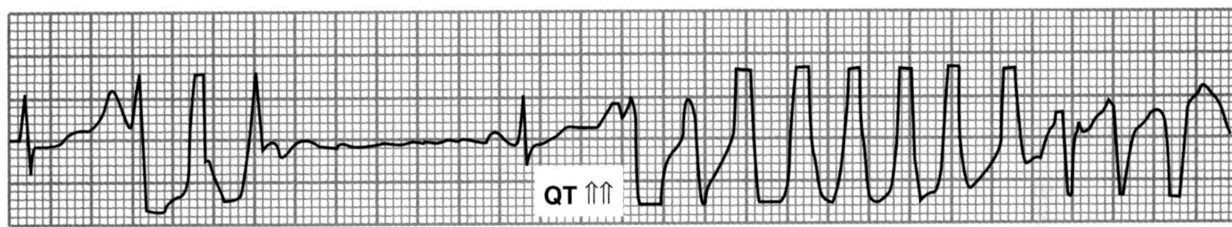


**FIGURE 35.11. Torsades de pointes.** The upper strip demonstrates sinus bradycardia with a mildly prolonged Q-T interval (480 msec, corrected). The lower strip, recorded minutes later, demonstrates an episode of torsades de pointes with marked prolongation of the Q-T interval (>600 msec). The prolonged Q-T interval resulted from the long pause immediately preceding the VT.

**TABLE 35.3. Differential Diagnosis of Wide-QRS-Complex Tachycardia on the 12-Lead ECG**

| | Ventricular Tachycardia | Supraventricular Tachycardia |
|---|---|---|
| AV dissociation | Present | Absent |
| QRS duration | >140 msec if RBBB | <140 msec if RBBB |
| | >160 msec if LBBB | <160 msec if LBBB |
| Axis deviation | −90 to ±180° | All other axes |
| QRS configuration | | |
| RBBB | | |
| Lead V1 | Mono or biphasic | Triphasic (rSR′) |
| Lead V6 | R/S <1 | R/S >1 |
| LBBB | | |
| Lead $V_1$ † | Slurred S wave (Q-S [nadir] >70 ms) | Absence of same (Q-S [nadir] <70 ms) |
| Precordial Leads | | |
| (+) concordance* | present | absent |
| (−) concordance | present | absent |
| If baseline bundle-branch block present | QRS morphology different | QRS morphology same |

LBBB = left bundle branch block; RBBB = right bundle branch block;
* (+) concordance indicates that QRS complexes in leads V1-V6 are all upright; (−) concordance indicates that QRS complexes in leads V1–V6 are all inverted; † QS nadir refers to duration of QRS onset to S wave nadir.

clusters and is self-terminating. Patients present with recurrent dizziness and syncope, and ventricular fibrillation and sudden death are common. Early afterdepolarizations, rather than re-entry, are thought to cause this arrhythmia.

The syndrome may be congenital or acquired. The *acquired form* may be caused by a variety of medications (Table 35.4). Treatment of this arrhythmia involves removing causative drug, if present, and vigorously correcting electrolyte deficiencies. Any agent that may prolong the Q-T interval is contraindicated. Intravenous magnesium (regardless of actual serum magnesium levels) may terminate the arrhythmia. Alternative acute therapies include overdrive atrial or ventricular pacing and isoproterenol administration. Chronic treatment may involve oral β-blockers at maximally tolerated doses. If the arrhythmia recurs despite drug therapy, left-sided cervicothoracic sympathetic ganglionectomy has proven helpful, as has dual chamber permanent pacing. Select patients with congenital long QT syndrome and recurrent syncope may also require ICD implantation.

#### Ventricular escape beats

If the SA node and AV junction fail or conduction defects block the impulses from reaching the ventricles, then the ventricular Purkinje network will activate the ventricles and prevent ventricular asystole. These beats may occur singly or in succession. This escape usually occurs at a rate of 20–40 beats/min.

#### Accelerated idioventricular rhythm

Three or more ventricular complexes occurring at a rate of 60–100 beats/min constitute an accelerated idioventricular rhythm (AIVR), and this arrhythmia

**TABLE 35.4. Medications and Agents that Can Prolong the QT Interval**

Antiarrhythmic agents
- Group IA
  - Ajmaline
  - Disopyramide (Norpace)
  - Procainamide (Procan)
  - Quinidine
- Group IC
  - Flecainide (Tambacor)
  - Propafenone (Rythmol)
- Group III
  - Amiodarone (Cordarone)
  - N-acetylprocainamide
  - Sotalol (Betapace)
  - Ibutilide (Corvert)
  - Dofetilide (Tikosyn)
- Group IV
  - Diltiazem (Cardizem)
  - Nifedipine (Procardia)

Vasodilators
- Bepridil
- Lidoflazine
- Penoxidil
- Prenylamine

Psychotropics
- Amitriptyline (Elavil)
- Chloral hydrate
- Chlorpromazine
- Doxepin
- Haloperidol
- Maprotilene
- Phenothiazines
- Tricyclic antidepressants (All)
- Thioridazine

Antibiotics/antifungals
- Erythromycin
- Erythromycin & ketoconazole
- IV (intravenous) erythromycin
- Fluconazole
- Intraconazole
- Ketoconazole
- IV Miconazole
- Any "-azole" antibiotics with Propulsid (Cisapride)
- Tetracycline
- Troleandomycin capsules

Antihistamines
- Astemizole (Hismanal) alone or with erythromycin +/−ketoconazole
- Terfenadine (Seldane) with pseudoephedrine
- Fexofenadine (Allegra)
- Any combinations of the above antihistamines & erythromycin or any "-zole" agents

Toxins
- Arsenic

Liquid protein diets

Organophosphate insecticides

Miscellaneous drugs
- Amantadine
- Atropine
- Chloroquine
- Tonic water, more than 1 glass per day (contains quinine)
- Corticosteroids (e.g., Prednisone)
- Diruetics (e.g., Furosemide)
- Isoprenaline (Isoproterenol)
- Pentamidine
- Probucol
- Propulsid (cisapride) with any "-azole" antibiotics
- Suxamethonium
- Vasopressin

Miscellaneous
- Grapefruit juice

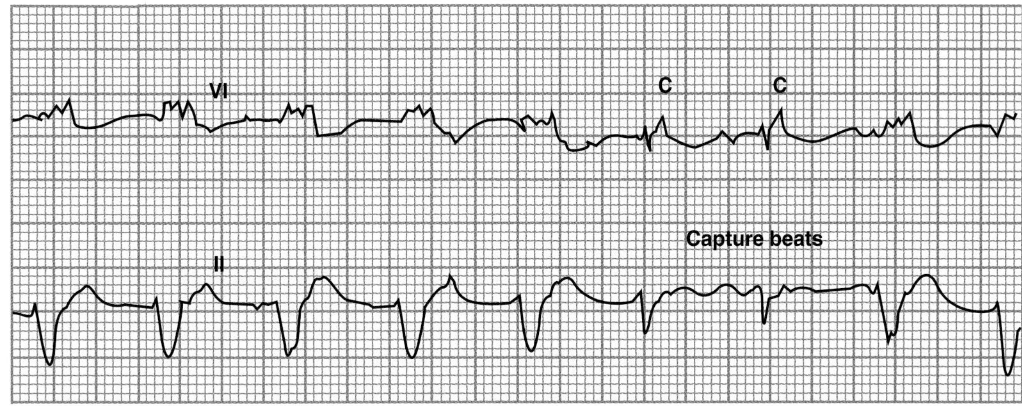


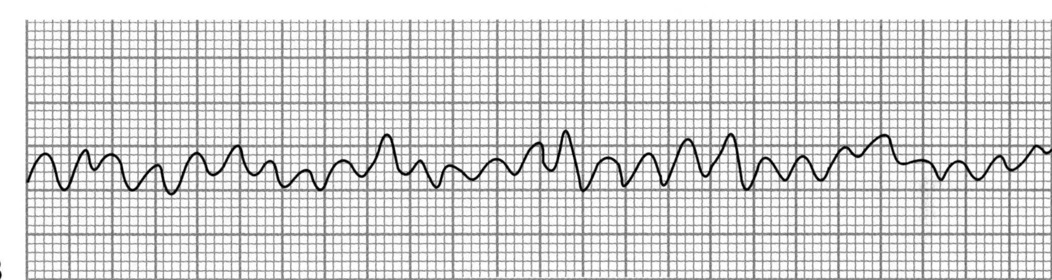


**FIGURE 35.12. A. Accelerated idioventricular rhythm** (AIVR) with capture beats. The basic rhythm is ventricular tachycardia at a rate of 95 beats/min. Capture beats (C) result from capture of the ventricles by sinus impulses. (This patient had an underlying right bundle branch block, and thus the capture beats are conducted accordingly.) The presence of capture beats provides strong evidence that the prevailing rhythm is of ventricular origin. **B. Ventricular fibrillation.** Broad complexes are seen occurring rapidly and at irregular intervals. There are no discrete QRS complexes.

characteristically begins with a ventricular escape complex (Figure 35.12 A). Enhanced automaticity of ventricular tissue causes AIVR. This arrhythmia is commonly observed in acute myocardial infarction and only rarely causes ventricular fibrillation. Because episodes of AIVR are brief and commonly asymptomatic, treatment is not needed. If symptoms occur, atropine or pacing may be required.

### Ventricular Fibrillation

Ventricular fibrillation (VF) is characterized electrocardiographically by baseline undulations with variable amplitude and periodicity (Figure 35.12 B). No QRS complexes or T waves are evident. Because no effective cardiac contraction occurs, VF is a catastrophic event in which pulse and blood pressure are absent. Loss of consciousness ensues, followed by death within 3–5 minutes unless electric countershock is promptly instituted. Frequent causes of VF include acute myocardial infarction, advanced coronary disease with LV systolic dysfunction, marked electrolyte disturbances (e.g., hypokalemia), drug toxicity or proarrhythmia, hypothermia, and electrocution.

## Conduction Disorders

### Heart Block

Optimal cardiac performance depends on an orderly sequence of events occurring in the cardiac conduction system: pacemaker impulses arising in the SA node initially depolarize the atrial myocardium, propagate slowly through the AV node, and finally spread through the His-Purkinje network to the ventricular myocardium. Failure of the conduction can occur anywhere in this electrophysiological chain but is most readily recognized in the AV node, His bundle, and the bundle branches.

#### First-degree AV block

First-degree AV block is defined as a delay in conduction from the sinus node to the ventricles with a resultant P-R interval longer than 0.20 sec (Figure 35.13 A). It is most commonly caused by abnormally slow conduction through the AV node although all impulses are conducted.

#### Second-degree AV block

Second-degree AV block is characterized by intermittent failure of the AV conduction.

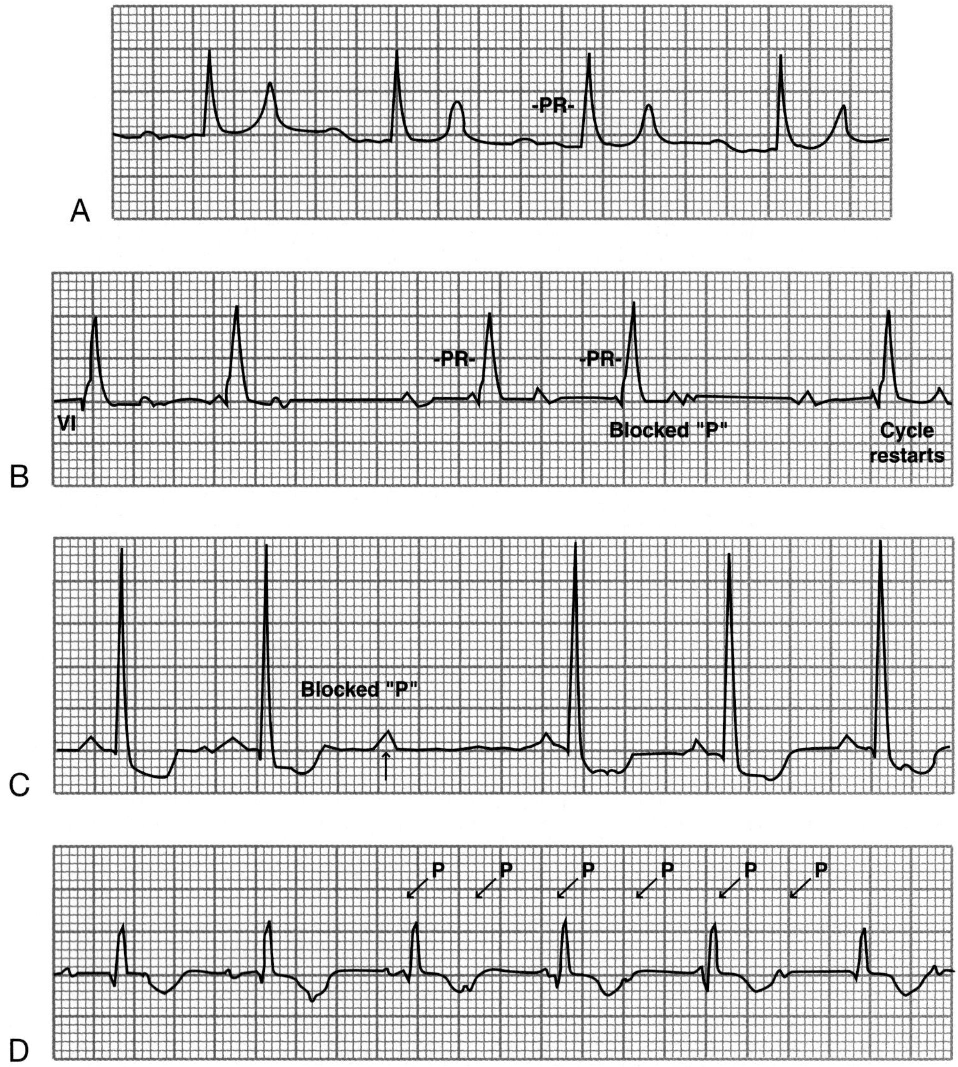


**FIGURE 35.13.** Heart block. A. Normal sinus rhythm with **first-degree AV block.** The P-R interval is 360 msec. B. **Type I second-degree AV block.** There is progressive prolongation of the P-R interval until a P wave is blocked, following which the cycle restarts. C. **Type-II second- degree AV block.** P-R intervals are constant until the third P wave is suddenly blocked. D. **Third-degree or complete AV block.** Regularly occurring P waves at a rate of 115 /min and regularly occurring QRS complexes at a rate of 80/min are evident. There is no relationship between the P waves and the QRS complexes.

**Type I second-degree AV block** (also termed **Mobitz type I** and **Wenckebach**) is the more common type. Characterized by a progressive lengthening of the P-R interval and shortening of the R-R interval until a P wave fails to conduct, second-degree AV block causes an increased R-R interval (Figure 35.13 B). Typically, the beat following the nonconducted P wave has the shortest P-R interval.

The most common site of type I second-degree AV block is the AV node. In such patients, the QRS complex is narrow and the prognosis is benign. Type I block may occur in normal individuals as a manifestation of enhanced vagal tone, but it also occurs in a wide variety of medical conditions, such as acute inferior-wall myocardial infarction and congenital or acquired diseases of the AV node, or with medications that slow AV conduction. Less commonly, type I AV block is caused by conduction disease below the AV node—in the His bundle or its branches. In these patients, the QRS is usually widened.

In most cases, type I AV block requires no specific therapy. However, in patients who develop type I block in the absence of an identifiable acute process, particularly the elderly with severe coronary artery disease or calcific aortic disease, electrophysiologic testing should be considered to identify the site of the block. If the block is within or below the His bundle, particularly if the patient has had prior dizziness or syncope, then permanent pacing is indicated.

**Type II second-degree AV block** (also termed **Mobitz type II** AV block) differs from type I block in that abrupt failure of AV conduction occurs without the preceding gradual P-R prolongation (Figure 35.13 C). The location of the type II block is always within or below the His bundle.

Most patients with type II block have broad QRS complexes indicative of conduction system disease, and are commonly symptomatic (dizziness or syncope). Causes include sclerodegenerative diseases of the conduction system, anterior wall myocardial infarction, calcific aortic valve disease, hypertensive heart disease, and cardiomyopathy. Permanent pacing is indicated in all symptomatic patients with type II block and should be strongly considered even in asymptomatic patients.

In a third type of second-degree AV block, the ratio of P waves to QRS complexes is 2:1 or higher. These cases ("high-degree blocks") cannot be accurately categorized as either type I or type II. If the QRS is narrow, the block is likely in the AV node; but if the QRS is wide, then the block may be in the AV node or His-Purkinje system.

### Complete AV block

Complete or **third-degree AV block** features total independence of the atria and ventricles, due to the complete failure of the atrial impulses to be conducted to the ventricles. When there is sinus rhythm, third-degree AV block exhibits total dissociation between P waves and QRS complexes, with the ventricles being controlled by a subsidiary pacemaker site (Figure 35.13 D). The site of the conduction defect may be at the AV node or infranodal (within or below the His bundle).

The site of the block has prognostic value. If the QRS complexes are narrow and the ventricular rate exceeds 50 beats/min, then the block is likely at the AV node, with a usually favorable prognosis. These patients are usually asymptomatic, and their heart rate can increase with exercise. Causes include congenital complete heart block, in which the block is permanent, as well as acute inferior wall myocardial infarction, drug intoxication, or myocarditis, in which the block is transient.

If the QRS complexes are wide and the ventricular rate is 30–40 beats/min, then the site of the block is likely infranodal. Such blocks account for the vast majority of episodes of complete heart block, causing slow heart rates that are unresponsive to autonomic influence. Symptoms are frequent. Reversible causes being infrequent, permanent pacing is usually indicated.

### Atrioventricular dissociation

AV dissociation is defined as activation of the atria and ventricles by two independent foci (Figure 35.14). Conduction block may or may not exist.

AV dissociation is usually due to one of three general causes:

1. With failure of the normal dominant pacemaker (as in sinus bradycardia), normally latent pacemaker cells in the AV junction gain control of the cardiac rhythm. The atria are under the abnormally slow control of the SA node, and the ventricles are under the control of the AV junction. In this type of AV dissociation, the ventricular rate is faster than the atrial rate, and heart block is not present.

2. Latent pacemakers may gain control, not through failure of higher pacemakers, but rather through abnormal acceleration of their normally slow discharge rate. These pathologic latent pacemakers actively take over from a normally functioning SA node. An example is accelerated junctional or ventricular tachycardia. Again, the ventricular rate exceeds the atrial rate, and heart block is not present.

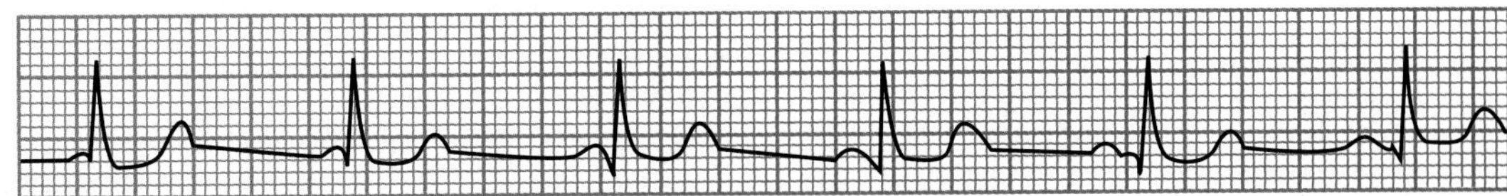

**FIGURE 35.14. Atrioventricular dissociation.** There are regular atrial and ventricular rates of 65 beats/min, but no relationship between P waves and QRS complexes. In this instance, there is a slow sinus rhythm and a junctional rhythm in competition with one another. The junctional impulses fail to be conducted retrogradely to "capture" the atria. Thus, the sinus node and AV junction discharge at similar rates but independent of one another. This strip is an example of isorhythmic AV dissociation.

3. In conduction block, the ventricles are under the control of a slower-discharging, normally latent pacemaker (e.g., complete heart block with a ventricular escape rhythm). This type of AV dissociation features a slower ventricular rate than the atrial rate, and conduction block is present.

*Bundle branch blocks*

Conduction of an impulse may be slowed or totally interrupted in the right bundle, main left bundle, or anterior and posterior fascicles of the left bundle.

*Right bundle branch block*

In right bundle branch block (RBBB) RV activation is delayed. On auscultation, $S_2$ is widely split owing to delayed closure of the pulmonic valve but maintains its respiratory variation. RBBB occurs in sclerodegenerative disease of the conduction system, acute pulmonary embolism, chronic coronary disease, septal trauma (such as during right heart catheterization), and occasionally in otherwise healthy persons.

The clinical significance of RBBB depends on the type and severity of underlying heart disease, if any. As an isolated finding, it is usually harmless, and progression of RBBB to complete AV block is rare. Delayed RV activation generates a secondary R wave (R´) in the right precordial leads (rsR´) and wide S waves in leads I, $V_5$, and $V_6$. The QRS duration exceeds 0.12 sec in complete RBBB, and the T wave is directed opposite to the terminal portion of the QRS. Because RBBB does not affect the initial portion of the QRS, Q waves retain their usual significance.

*Left bundle branch block*

Left bundle branch block (LBBB) results from slow conduction in the main left bundle or, rarely, simultaneous slow conduction in its anterior and posterior fascicles. Delayed closure of the aortic valve results in a reversed or paradoxical splitting of $S_2$ on auscultation. LBBB occurs in sclerodegenerative disease of conduction tissue, cardiomyopathies, calcific aortic valve disease, and hypertensive or coronary heart disease. LV hypertrophy is commonly found in patients with LBBB. As opposed to RBBB, LBBB rarely occurs in patients without demonstrable heart disease, and the prognosis depends on the associated heart disease.

The ECG in LBBB demonstrates a broad monophasic R wave in leads I, $V_5$, and $V_6$, which is usually notched or slurred; deep S waves in $V_1$ and $V_2$; absence of the normal small septal Q waves in leads I, $V_5$, and $V_6$; and secondary T wave changes (Figure 35.15). LBBB is considered **complete** when the QRS width exceeds 0.12 sec and **incomplete** when it is 0.10 to 0.12 sec. By

A

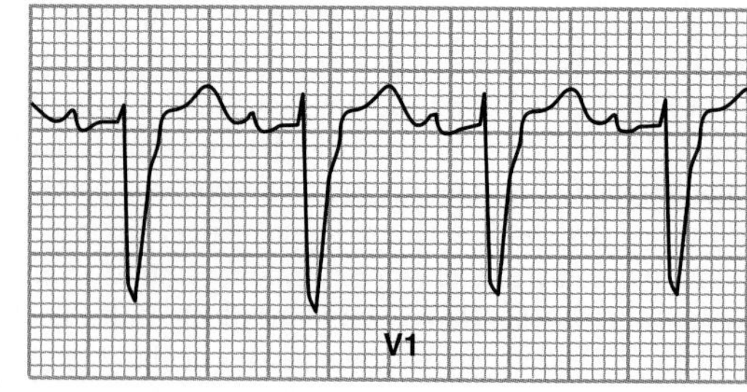


B

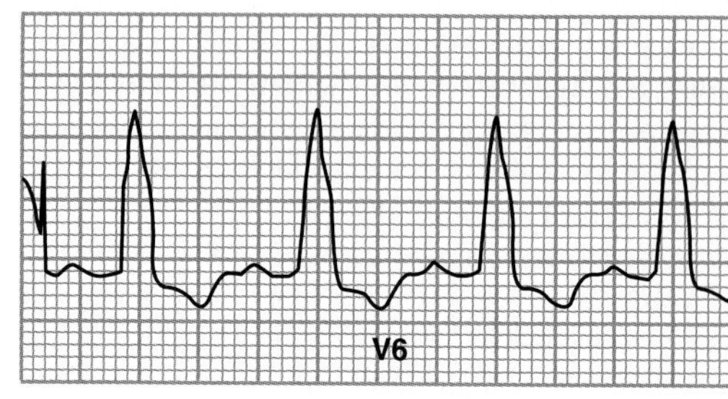


**FIGURE 35.15. Left Bundle Branch Block.** The rhythm is a sinus mechanism. Note the widened QRS complexes with a RsR pattern in V6. ST segment depression and T wave inversion are noted in V6.

affecting the initial portion of ventricular activation, LBBB interferes with the ECG diagnosis of myocardial infarction.

*Left anterior hemiblock*

Left anterior hemiblock (LAH) is the most common conduction abnormality. Impaired conduction in the anterior fascicle delays activation of the anterosuperior portion of the LV and produces the following ECG features: a left axis deviation beyond –30°; qR pattern in leads I and aVL; rS pattern in leads II, III, and aVF; and only negligible prolongation of the QRS. LAH may also cause persistence of S waves in leads $V_5$ and $V_6$ and the presence of a qrS pattern in leads $V_1$ and $V_2$, simulating anterior myocardial infarction.

*Left posterior hemiblock*

Impaired conduction in the posterior fascicle delays activation of the posteroinferior portion of the LV. ECG features consist of right axis deviation that exceeds +110°; presence of a qR pattern in leads I and aVL. Other conditions that cause right axis deviation, such as lateral infarction, RV hypertrophy, and vertical heart, must be excluded. Because it involves the broadest fascicle with a dual blood supply, isolated left posterior hemiblock is rare.

#### Bifascicular Blocks

Impairment of conduction can develop simultaneously in any two of the three fascicles; the impulse then propagates to the ventricles through the remaining fascicle. RBBB combined with LAH is the most common bifascicular block, and it features a mean QRS axis left of –30°; rSR′ in leads $V_1$ and $V_2$; and deep S waves in $V_5$ and $V_6$. Approximately 5% of patients with RBBB plus LAH develop second-degree or third-degree AV block. RBBB plus left posterior hemiblock feature ECG changes of RBBB and right axis deviation exceeding +110°. It progresses to advanced AV block in 5–10% of cases. Simultaneous block in the left anterior and posterior fascicles manifests as LBBB.

#### Trifascicular Block

Simultaneous block in all three fascicles manifests as complete AV block. Incomplete trifascicular block indicates bifascicular block plus a prolonged P-R interval, indicating slow conduction in the third fascicle. In most patients, a prolonged P-R interval results from a delayed impulse at the AV node rather than in the third fascicle. Patients with fascicular blocks can develop advanced AV block that may cause dizziness and syncope, at which time permanent pacemaker insertion is indicated. Asymptomatic patients need only periodic clinical follow-up.

### Sick Sinus Syndrome

Sick sinus syndrome implies sinus node disease leading to a variety of cardiac arrhythmias, including 1) sinus bradycardia unrelated to medications or excessive vagal tone, 2) sinus arrest or SA block, and 3) alternating episodes of tachyarrhythmia and bradycardia. Most patients also show some evidence of abnormal AV conduction.

The underlying cause of the syndrome is a degenerative process that destroys sinus nodal and surrounding atrial tissue. The AV node and His bundle may also be involved. A significant number of patients also have coronary artery disease, hypertension, or cardiomyopathy. Patients commonly report palpitations, dizziness, lightheadedness, and syncope. Ambulatory event recorders can often help in documenting the ECG manifestations of sinus node dysfunction.

Asymptomatic persons with sick sinus syndrome require no therapy. In patients with symptoms that are believed to arise from a conduction defect, permanent pacing is employed. In addition, antiarrhythmic drugs may be used to prevent or slow coexisting atrial tachyarrhythmias.

### Permanent Pacemakers

A permanent pacemaker consists of an electrode lead (or leads) and a pulse generator or battery. In the most common type, the electrode lead is inserted transvenously into the RV apex. The generator is inserted into a subcutaneous pocket below the clavicle. The power source is lithium cells with a life expectancy of 5–10 years.

A letter code designation is used to describe the complex function of pacemakers (Table 35.5). The first letter indicates the chamber paced; the second letter, the sensed chamber; the third, the mode of the pacemaker response to a spontaneous cardiac impulse; and the fourth letter indicates that the pacemaker has the property of rate modulation (i.e., the unit can increase its pacing rate in response to increased physiological need).

Most patients requiring a permanent pacemaker should be considered for dual-chamber pacing (Table 35.6). Pacer systems that include atrial pacing (as opposed to a simple VVI system, which paces and senses only the ventricle [Figure 35.16]) have the advantage of maintaining AV synchrony, reducing the incidence of congestive heart failure, the incidence of future atrial fibrillation (and thus the risk of embolization), and overall mortality. Contraindications for dual-chamber pacing include 1) fixed atrial fibrillation or flutter or any intractable supraventricular arrhythmia and 2) terminal disease or extreme debility where simple ventricular pacing would suffice. Simple VVI pacing may be adequate in those occasional patients with infrequent, symptomatic bradycardia.

Complications of permanent pacing include infection and erosion at the site of battery implantation, failure to capture (pace) the ventricular or atrial myocardium, and

**TABLE 35.5. North American Society of Pacing and Electrophysiology Pacemaker Code**

| Chamber Paced | Chamber Sensed | Response to Sensing | Rate Modulation |
|---|---|---|---|
| 0 = None | 0 = None | 0 = None | R = Rate modulation |
| A = Atrium | A = Atrium | T = Trigger pacing | |
| V = Ventricle | V = Ventricle | I = Inhibits pacing | |
| D = Dual (A+V) | D = Dual (A+V) | D = Triggers and inhibits pacing | |

**TABLE 35.6. Indications For Permanent Pacing**

| | |
|---|---|
| Acquired AV block | Complete AV block permanent or intermittent, symptomatic or asymptomatic<br>Mobitz type II AV block, symptomatic or asymptomatic<br>Type I (Wenckebach) AV block, symptomatic<br>Atrial fibrillation with complete AV block or advanced AV block and symptomatic bradycardia |
| Acquired AV block associated with myocardial infarction | Newly acquired bundle-branch block and transient advanced AV block<br>Type II second-degree AV block<br>Complete AV block |
| Chronic bifascicular and trifascicular block | Bifascicular block with intermittent symptomatic complete heart block<br>Bifascicular or trifascicular block with type II second-degree AV block, symptomatic or asymptomatic<br>Bifascicular or trifascicular block with syncope when other causes are not identifiable |
| Sinus node dysfunction | Sinus node dysfunction with documented symptomatic bradycardia (the bradycardia may be spontaneous or due to concomitant drug therapy)<br>Sinus bradycardia with bradycardia-dependent ventricular or supraventricular arrhythmias |
| Hypersensitive carotid sinus | Recurrent syncope or dizziness in a patient with easily-induced asystole (>3 sec) upon light carotid stimulation in the absence of drugs, which depress SA or AV node; symptoms should be clearly related to carotid stimulation |

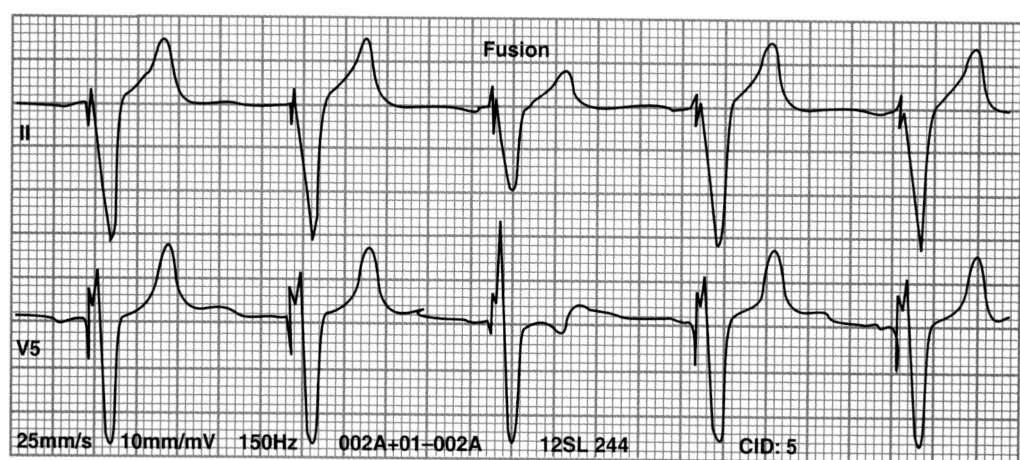


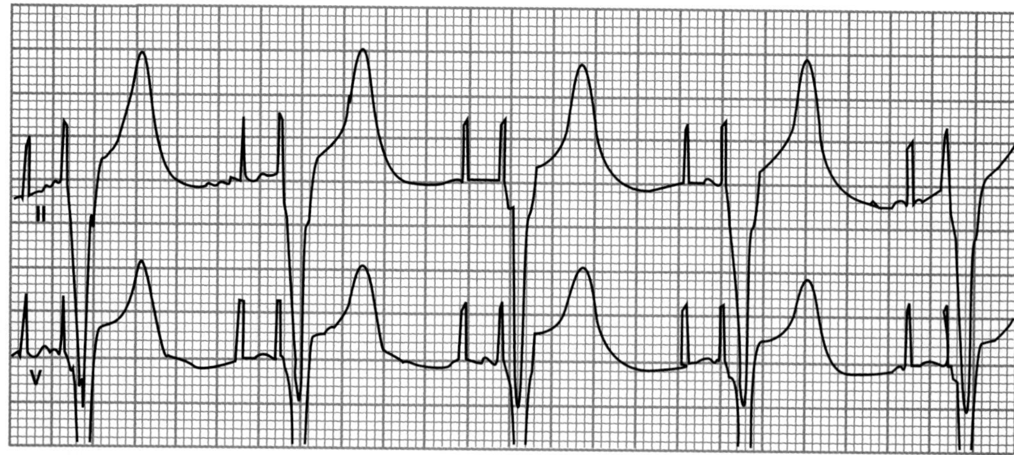


**FIGURE 35.16.** Artificially paced rhythms. **A. Ventricular pacing.** This strip demonstrates an electronic ventricular pacemaker maintaining a rate of 60 beats/min. Note the pacemaker "spike" preceding each QRS complex. The third complex in each lead represents a fusion beat, which occurs when the ventricles are excited simultaneously from both supraventricular and ventricular foci. The resultant complex appears to be a mixture of a supraventricular and ventricular complex. **B. AV sequential pacemaker.** With leads in both the atrium and ventricle, the first spike causes the atria to depolarize. The 200-msec delay that follows represents the programmed P-R interval. Ventricular depolarization then follows as the next spike.

failure to appropriately sense (owing to undersensing or oversensing).

Patients with permanent pacemakers should be monitored regularly to check the function and troubleshoot these complicated devices. The need for battery replacement is often heralded by a spontaneous, automatic slowing of the pacing rate—a property built into the pacemaker to alert the physician to the need for battery replacement.

# CHAPTER 36 SYNCOPE

Syncope is a sudden, and usually self-limited, transient loss of consciousness associated with a loss of postural tone, and a spontaneous recovery. Episodes are recurrent in about one-third of patients.

## Etiology

Syncope is a symptom, and not a disease. All forms of syncope involve a transient, global decrease in cerebral perfusion. Causes are legion, ranging from benign to life-threatening. In the 1990s, three groups—cardiac, non-cardiac and idiopathic, with their respective proportions being 33%, 26%, and 41% respectively—accounted for all cases of syncope. Widespread application of tilt-table testing and the recognition of neurally mediated mechanisms and psychiatric causes have redefined these proportions (Table 36.1). In elderly patients, cardiac causes predominate, whereas among younger patients, noncardiac diagnoses such as vasodepressor syncope, orthostatic hypotension, or emotional conditions are more likely causes.

### Cardiac causes

Although less frequent than other entities, cardiac cause for syncope needs primary consideration because it has been shown to be the most important predictor of the risk of death. Syncope may be caused by structural heart disease, cardiac arrhythmias, or both. **Structural heart disease** causing syncope commonly involves LV or RV outflow obstruction, such as aortic stenosis or some variants of hypertrophic cardiomyopathy. Syncope in aortic stenosis is exertional, since stroke volume fails to keep up with exercise-induced peripheral vasodilatation. Peripheral vasodilatation may also be reflexly induced in response to stimulation of LV mechanoreceptors by marked increase in LV systolic pressure during exercise. In mitral stenosis, syncope follows rapid tachycardias or atrial fibrillation. Patients with syncope and structural heart disease or an abnormal ECG have a high rate of death within the first year following the syncopal event and most arrhythmias that cause syncope occur in this subgroup. Effort syncope and chest pain also occur in pulmonary hypertension.

Cardiac arrhythmias are often responsible for syncope, especially in the elderly. The arrhythmias may be rapid or slow and supraventricular or ventricular. **Bradyarrhythmias** may follow sick sinus syndrome or administration of digitalis, β-blockers, and $Ca^{++}$ channel blockers with negative chronotropic effects. In high-degree AV block, the site of the block and the adequacy of ventricular escape rhythm determine the onset of syncope, with a more distal block and slow escape rhythm often evoking syncope.

A **supraventricular tachycardia** may cause syncope even with normal ventricular and valvular function. Not uncommonly, a paroxysmal supraventricular tachycardia causes the elderly to develop hypotension, cerebral hypoperfusion, and a feeling of faintness. Supraventricular arrhythmias complicating an accessory pathway that facilitates accelerated conduction are particularly liable to cause syncope.

**Ventricular tachycardia,** owing to structural heart disease, or **antiarrhythmic drugs**, especially class IA agents, may cause hypotension and syncope (e.g., torsades de pointes, see Figure 35.10). Syncope in **pacemaker** patients may be due to pacemaker malfunction (loss of capture or under-sensing).

**TABLE 36.1. Relative Frequency of the Causes of Syncope**

| Cause | Frequency (%) | |
|---|---|---|
| Neurally mediated* | 41–46% | |
| Heart disease | 18% | |
| Structural (organic) heart disease | | 4% |
| Arrhythmias | | 14% |
| Neurologic illness | 11–12% | |
| Psychiatric disorders | 6–10% | |
| Orthostatic hypotension | 8% | |
| Medication induced | 4–5% | |
| Unknown cause | 7–10% | |

*Defined as reflex mechanisms associated with inappropriate vasodilation, bradycardia, or both.

(Adapted from Kapoor, WN. Syncope. N Engl J Med 2000; 343:1856–1862.)

### Noncardiac causes

The noncardiac causes of syncope can be recalled with the mnemonic "SVNCOPE"—*s*ituational, *v*asodepressor, *n*eurologic, *c*arotid sinus hypersensitivity, *o*rthostatic hypotension, *p*sychiatric/emotional, and *e*xtra.

#### *Situational syncope*

Situational syncope may be mechanical (decreased venous return that occurs on a Valsalva maneuver) or neurally mediated (vagal stimulation or vasodepressor responses that cause sinus bradycardia, sinus arrest, or high-degree AV block). Examples include cough syncope (high intrathoracic pressure with low venous return), postmicturition syncope (rapid decrease in peripheral vascular resistance owing to drainage of distended urinary bladder), and defecation syncope (prolonged Valsalva maneuver). Elderly persons with hypertension—especially those receiving vasodilators—may suffer postprandial hypotension causing dizziness, syncope, and falls.

#### *Vasodepressor syncope*

The Bezold-Jarisch reflex is critical to the pathogenesis of vasodepressor syncope (Figure 36.1). Upright posture, vasodilation, and increased venous pooling decrease ventricular filling. This decrease in "preload" and systolic blood pressure causes catecholamine release, which causes vigorous contraction of the (small) ventricle. The Bezold-Jarisch reflex is activated via intracardiac vagal mechanoreceptors. Increased neural input to the brainstem via synapses with vagal efferents causes both bradycardia and hypotension; syncope ensues. Hypotension results from peripheral vasodilation. β-blockers, by short-circuiting the Bezold-Jarisch reflex, prevent bradycardia, hypotension, and syncope.

This type of syncope is a common sequel to emotional stress, threat of physical injury, sudden pain or discomfort, or the sight of blood or needles. Fatigue, hunger, fever, heat, and prolonged standing or recumbency are predisposing factors in susceptible persons. Patients often report a prodrome of a "queasy" feeling, nausea, sweating, lightheadedness, weakness, blurred vision, and tinnitus.

#### *Neurologic diseases*

A minority of syncope cases may be caused by seizures, which may be difficult to diagnose without a bystander account and without the patient's recollection of the events preceding the event. Syncope occasionally causes brief spells of tonic-clonic activity or irregular muscle twitching that are falsely interpreted as seizures. Patients with transient ischemic attacks, strokes, or cerebral emboli present with focal neurologic deficits rather than syncope; nonetheless, vertebrobasilar insufficiency may cause syncope.

#### *Carotid sinus hypersensitivity*

The normal response to carotid sinus massage includes brief slowing of the sinus rate and slowing of AV nodal conduction. Carotid sinus hypersensitivity may be suggested by syncope that follows turning of the head, shaving, or wearing a tight collar. The immediate responses may be cardioinhibitory (bradycardia), vasodepressor (a drop in systolic BP of

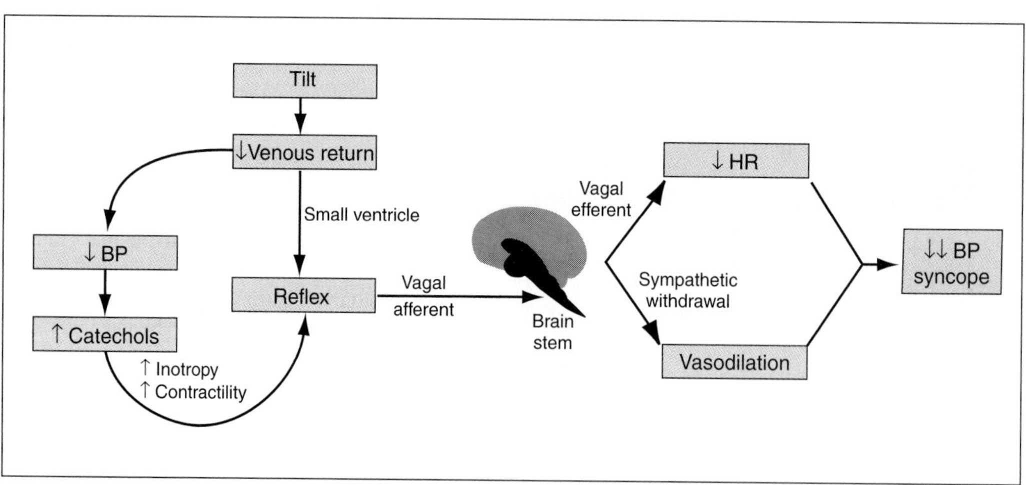


**FIGURE 36.1. Bezold-Jarisch reflex. The Bezold-Jarisch reflex is critical to the pathogenesis of vasodepressor syncope. The reflex is activated via intracardiac vagal mechanoreceptors. Increased neural input to the brainstem via synapses with vagal efferents causes both bradycardia and hypotension, with syncope ensuing. BP = blood pressure; HR = heart rate.**
(Redrawn from: Abi-Samra F, et al. PACE 1988;11:1201–1214 and Linzer M. Am J Med 1991;90:1–5. Used with permission.)

≥50 mm Hg), or a mixed-type with elements of both responses.

*Orthostatic hypotension*

When a person assumes an upright posture, normal homeostatic mechanisms (arteriolar and venous constriction, enhanced heart rate, and lower-extremity muscle tone) prevent a significant decrease in systolic blood pressure. Patients with orthostatic hypotension may have inadequate responses or impaired reflexes that cause postural symptoms. Symptomatic orthostatic hypotension may be related to inadequate volume, autonomic impairment (either primary or secondary, such as diabetes), or medications. Diuretics, vasodilators, tricyclic antidepressants, antihypertensives, phenothiazines, and long-acting nitrates commonly cause postural changes in blood pressure, particularly in the elderly.

*Psychogenic/emotional causes*

Emotional abnormalities are an important cause of syncope and should be suspected in young patients with recurrent syncope and no cardiac disease. Patients with generalized anxiety disorders, panic attacks, and somatization disorders may present with syncope.

## Diagnosis

The approach to evaluating syncope, as outlined in Figure 36.2, focuses on determining the presence of underlying heart disease because syncope of cardiac origin is more lethal than that of noncardiac or unknown cause. A detailed and accurate history, preferably corroborated by a bystander account, is critical (Table 36.2 and Table 36.3) and may help establish the diagnosis in over 45% of instances. Syncope must be distinguished from vague symptoms and syndromes not associated with loss of consciousness, such as vertigo, dizziness, faintness, drop attacks, and dysequilibrium (a sensation of imbalance). Medications should be thoroughly reviewed, including prescription, over-the-counter, and illicit drugs (Table 36.4).

Supine and upright heart rate and blood pressure should be checked. The pulse rate normally increases by at least 10 beats/min with an orthostatic systolic blood pressure drop of >10 mm Hg and a diastolic drop of >5 mm Hg. Failure of the pulse to rise may indicate autonomic impairment or medication effects. The neck should be inspected for jugular venous distention, and the carotid pulse wave and its amplitude. Cardiac auscultation can detect aortic stenosis, mitral stenosis, pulmonic stenosis, and hypertrophic cardiomyopathy with obstruction. If no carotid bruits exist and carotid sinus hypersensitivity is a diagnostic possibility, then carotid sinus massage should be performed while the patient's heart rate and BP are being monitored.

### Ancillary studies

The yield of various ancillary studies in establishing a cause for syncope is listed in Table 36.5. **ECG** may detect ischemic heart disease, prior myocardial infarction, chamber hypertrophy, conduction delays, a short P-R interval (accessory pathway), or a long Q-T interval. **Transthoracic and Doppler echocardiography** may confirm valvular heart lesions and quantify LV function; transesophageal echocardiography provides little additional information. Electroencephalograms (EEG) and computed tomography of the head are not indicated unless the history strongly suggests seizures or the physical examination shows a focal neurologic deficit.

**Ambulatory (Holter) monitoring** may uncover significant tachyarrhythmias or bradyarrhythmias or intermittent high-degree AV block. For those with infrequent symptoms or spells, cardiobeepers and memory loop recorders (transtelephonic continuous loops) may provide useful diagnostic information. Extended Holter monitoring (e.g., 72 hours) yields little additional information. Implantable continuous loop recorders can perform ECG monitoring for up to 18 months. Although this might benefit a few patients, its precise role is not yet defined.

**Signal-averaged ECG** (SAECG) amplifies and filters high-frequency late potentials in the terminal part of the QRS and is most useful when underlying ischemic heart disease is causing ventricular tachycardia. A normal SAECG excludes lethal ventricular arrhythmias as the cause of syncope, but such a test has a low positive predictive value when used in unselected patients.

### Electrophysiologic testing and tilt-table testing

The yield of electrophysiologic testing (EPT or EPS) depends on the presence of structural heart disease or an abnormal ECG which, when present, might serve as its surrogate. The major indication for EPT is the inability to confirm noninvasively an arrhythmia as the cause of syncope in patients with underlying heart disease. When positive, EPT will show ventricular tachycardia in 46%, bradycardia from SA or AV nodal disease in 30%, and supraventricular tachycardias in 23% of patients. Predictors of positive EPT are conduction system disease (left bundle branch block), LV dysfunction (ejection fraction <40%), and effort syncope. Predictors of a negative EPT are recurrent syncope, lack of injury during episodes, no underlying heart disease, normal baseline ECG, and normal Holter monitoring. A nondiagnostic EPT in syncope confers a low risk of sudden death (about 2%). Bradyarrhythmias induced on EPT are neither sensitive nor specific.

Indications for tilt-table testing are summarized in Table 36.6. Vasodepressor syncope may be unmasked with tilt-table testing. A positive study is the induction of

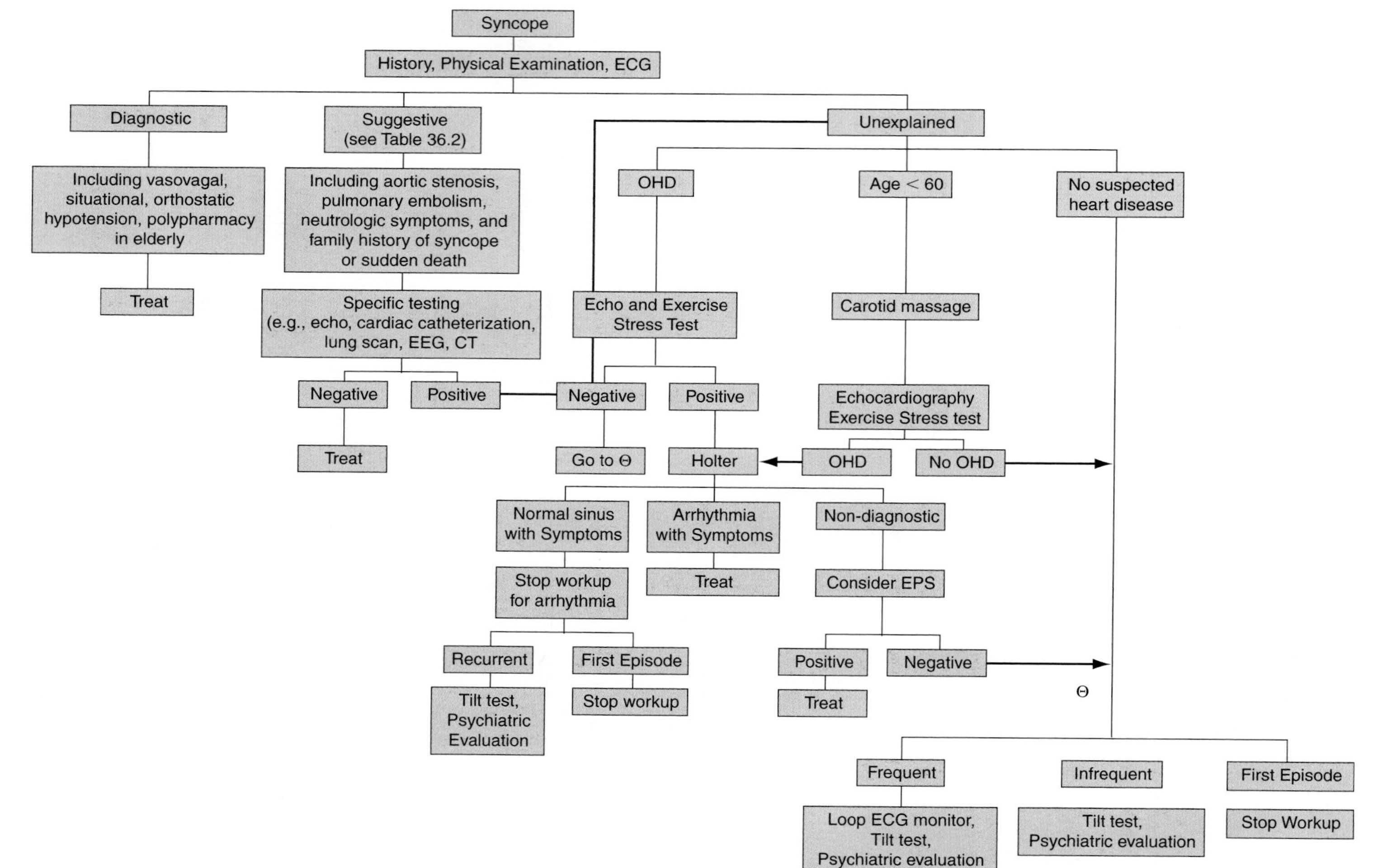


**FIGURE 36.2.** **Approach to the evaluation of syncope. EEG, electroencephalogram; CT, computed tomography; (Adapted from: Linzer M, Yang E, Estes MNA, et al.: Ann Intern Med 1997; 126:989–996. Used with permission.)**

**TABLE 36.2. Historical/Other Features That Suggest a Cause for Syncope**

| Syncope follows (F)/ Accompanies (A) syncope | Feature | Consider |
|---|---|---|
| F | Sudden pain, fear/sound/smell | Vasovagal |
| F | Prolonged standing | Vasovagal |
| F | Exertion in well-trained athlete, no heart disease | Vasovagal |
| F | Urination/cough/swallowing/defecation | Situational |
| F | Head rotation/pressure on neck* | Carotid sinus |
| F | Standing | Orthostatic hypotension |
| A | Headache | Migraine/seizure |
| A | Vertigo/dysarthria/diplopia | TIA, SS**, basilar migraine |
| A | Arm exercise | SS |
| Followed by | Confusion | Seizure |
| F/A | Exertion | AS, PH, MS, HCM, CAD |
| F | No prodrome (sudden and brief), + heart disease | Arrhythmia |
| F | Unexplained dyspnea, chest pain, risk factors for VTE | Pulmonary embolism |
| A | No heart disease, but (+) somatic symptoms | Psychiatric illness |
| — | (+) Family history | Long QT syndrome |

* = Shaving, tight collar, etc.; ** = may have difference between upper limbs in BP and pulse; AS = aortic stenosis; CAD = coronary artery disease; HCM = hypertrophic cardiomyopathy; MS = mitral stenosis; PH = pulmonary hypertension; SS = subclavian steal syndrome; TIA = transient ischemic syndromes of vertebrobasilar system; VTE = venous thromboembolism.

**TABLE 36.3. Important Elements of History in a Patient with Syncope**

- Activity immediately before blacking out
- Any apparent precipitating event(s)
- Any prodrome
- Time course of events
- If there were other symptoms, note their onset and progression
- Any injury related to the syncopal episode
- Any bowel or bladder incontinence
- The patient's recollection about "coming to"
- Duration of being "out"
- Any persistent symptoms
- Current medication(s)
- Any observer/witness
- Previous similar episode(s)

**TABLE 36.4. Common Drugs Causing Syncope**

| Diuretics | Vasodilators |
|---|---|
| Beta-blockers | Calcium channel blockers |
| Digitalis | Nitrates |
| Antiarrhythmics | Antidepressants |
| Phenothiazines | Hypoglycemics (including Insulin) |
| CNS depressants | Alcohol |
| | Cocaine |

(From Kapoor WN. Am J Med 1991; 90:91–106; with permission.)

**TABLE 36.5. Yield of Various Tests in Evaluating Syncope**

| Test | Yield (approximate %) |
|---|---|
| History/physical examination | 45 |
| Tilt-table with provocation tests* | 66 |
| Echocardiogram** | 5–10 |
| Continuous loop ECG recording | |
| Arrhythmia and syncope coincide | 8–20 |
| Symptoms, but no arrhythmia recorded | 12–27 |
| Holter monitoring† | |
| Arrhythmia and syncope together | 4 |
| Symptoms, but no arrhythmia | 17 |
| Electrophysiologic study†† | |
| With associated heart disease | 21 |
| With no associated heart disease | 1 |
| Electrocardiogram (ECG) alone | <5 |
| Head CT# | <4 |
| Basic laboratory tests## | 2–3 |
| Electroencephalogram (EEG) | <2 |
| Transcranial Doppler/carotid ultrasound | Not recommended |

*Among unexplained cases; provocation using isoprenaline or nitroglycerine.
**Yield shown is in situations where no heart disease is clinically suspected, but abnormal findings do not always indicate a relationship to the syncope.
†Overall yield <5–10%.
††Using inducible ventricular tachycardia as criterion; inducible bradycardia is not sensitive or specific.
#Usually with history consistent with seizures.
##Electrolytes, complete blood count, renal function tests, etc.

**TABLE 36.6. Indications for Tilt-Table Testing**

- Syncope with a profile of neurally mediated syncope
- Recurrent idiopathic syncope with or without prodrome
- To differentiate convulsive syncope from seizure disorder
- Evaluate recurrent dizziness/vertigo if associated with syncope or presyncope
- Diagnosis of psychogenic syncope

(From: Grubb BP et al. Am J Med 1991; 90:6–10.)

syncope or near-syncope associated with bradycardia, hypotension, or both.

## Management

### Cardiac syncope

A precise diagnosis is crucial to the rational management of cardiac syncope. Valvular disease that obstructs ventricular inflow or outflow may require surgery. With symptomatic bradyarrhythmias, offending drugs (e.g., β-blockers, digoxin) should be discontinued, if possible, before placement of a permanent pacemaker. Patients with documented sick sinus syndrome may need a permanent pacemaker. Paroxysmal supraventricular tachycardia owing to AV nodal reentry or an accessory pathway may be treated with drugs or catheter ablation.

Arrhythmias accompanied by hemodynamic compromise should be managed acutely. With symptomatic ventricular arrhythmias, precipitating factors (such as ischemia, hypoxia, or drugs) should be corrected. If ischemia is documented, antianginal regimens and possibly revascularization are appropriate treatments. Electrophysiologic testing should guide drug selection or placement of an automatic implantable cardioverter-defibrillator in those presumed to be symptomatic from ventricular arrhythmias; empiric antiarrhythmic drug therapy has no proven benefit.

### Noncardiac syncope

Patients with situational syncope should be educated about appropriate strategies to avoid recurrences. Treatment of recurrent vasodepressor syncope includes β-blockers or disopyramide (both negative inotropes), transdermal scopolamine (anticholinergic), or hydrofluorocortisone (a mineralocorticoid to promote salt retention and volume expansion).

Patients with autonomic insufficiency should be distinguished from those with volume-mediated or drug-induced orthostasis. In addition to maintaining an optimal circulating volume, avoiding excessive diuretic use, and discontinuing or adjusting doses of potentially offending drugs, patients may use mechanical measures, such as compression hose or body stockings. Beneficial drugs are ephedrine, hydrofluorocortisone, or prostaglandin synthesis inhibitors (indomethacin).

Patients with carotid sinus hypersensitivity may benefit from placement of a permanent pacemaker if a cardioinhibitory response is documented with carotid sinus massage. Patients with vasodepressor or mixed responses may benefit from denervation and/or local irradiation.

# CHAPTER 37 CONGESTIVE HEART FAILURE

Congestive heart failure (CHF) is defined clinically as a constellation of symptoms and signs denoting congestion of the systemic and/or pulmonary venous beds and low cardiac output due to the inability of the cardiac chambers to adequately discharge their contents. In this condition, despite adequate ventricular filling, cardiac output fails to meet the metabolic demands of the body. The impaired ventricular function is associated with diminished exercise capacity, a high incidence of ventricular arrhythmias, and reduced life expectancy. Several terms are used relative to CHF, as defined in Table 37.1.

Congestive heart failure is a common syndrome, afflicting approximately 1% of the U.S. population (about 3 million people) and contributing to almost 270,000 deaths annually.

## Pathophysiology

### Normal circulation

The pump function of the heart is dependent on the load placed on the heart during systole and diastole, myocardial contractility, and heart rate.

#### *Preload*

Ventricular end-diastolic volume represents preload. The relationship between preload and stroke volume is defined by **Starling's law,** which states that up to a limit, the stroke volume (or stroke work) is directly proportional to the end-diastolic volume of the ventricle (Figure 37.1). Factors such as total intravascular volume, venous return, and atrial function influence the end-diastolic volume. Normal left ventricular (LV) end-diastolic volume is attained at an end-diastolic pressure of up to 14

**TABLE 37.1. Various Forms of Congestive Heart Failure**

| | | |
|---|---|---|
| Left heart failure | — | Pulmonary venous congestion |
| Right heart failure | — | Systemic venous congestion |
| Acute heart failure | — | Typified by acute pulmonary edema |
| Chronic heart failure | — | Typified by congestive cardiomyopathy |
| High-output failure | — | Higher than normal cardiac output that is still inadequate to meet vastly increased metabolic demands, (e.g., thyrotoxic heart disease) |
| Low-output failure | — | Heart failure with lower-than-normal cardiac output |

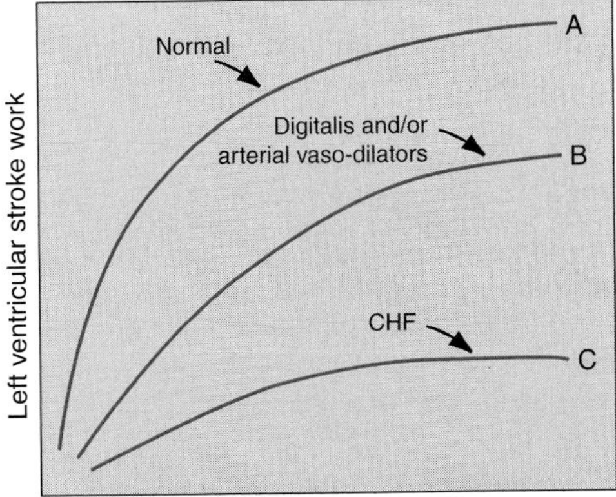


**FIGURE 37.1.** Ventricular function (Starling's) curves: In the normal individual (line A), a slight increase in left ventricular (LV) filling pressure should result in a large increase in LV stroke work. With the markedly depressed ventricular function of CHF (line C), even a large increase in LV filling pressure results in only a small increase of LV stroke work. Treatment with digitalis enhances contractility and treatment with arterial vasodilators decreases afterload in patients with CHF, shifting the ventricular function curve from C to B.

mm Hg. However, if the LV becomes more rigid (less compliant), as in LV hypertrophy, a higher end-diastolic pressure is required to distend the ventricle to a normal end-diastolic volume (Figure 37.2). Because measurement of LV volume is difficult in vivo, **LV filling pressure** (pulmonary capillary wedge-, pulmonary artery diastolic or LV end-diastolic pressure) is used as an indicator of preload.

*Afterload*

Afterload is the stress acting on contractile fibers in the ventricular wall after the onset of shortening. According to **Laplace's law,** afterload (wall stress) is directly proportional to ventricular pressure and ventricular radius and indirectly proportional to wall thickness. Aortic input impedance, systemic vascular resistance (SVR), and mean aortic pressure are indirect surrogates of afterload. SVR (in wood units) can be calculated as follows:

$$\frac{SVR = MAP - Mean\ RAP}{CO}$$

where MAP is mean aortic pressure, RAP is right atrial pressure (both in mm Hg) and CO is cardiac output (L/min).

For a given preload and contractility, LV stroke volume and afterload show an indirect relationship. Although a normal ventricle can adjust to changing afterload and deliver a normal stroke volume by using an intrinsic homeometric mechanism, a diseased ventricle loses this ability, and its systolic performance becomes profoundly afterload-dependent (see Figure 37.1).

*Myocardial Contractility*

Myocardial contractility (inotropic state) indicates the intrinsic capacity of myocardial fibers to shorten independent of their preload and afterload. The maximum velocity of contraction ($V_{max}$) is an index of contractility. Sympathomimetic amines, digitalis, glucagon, and tachycardias enhance myocardial contractility, while β-adrenergic-blocking agents reduce it. As shown in Figure 37.1, at a given preload and afterload, an upward and leftward shift of the ventricular function curve

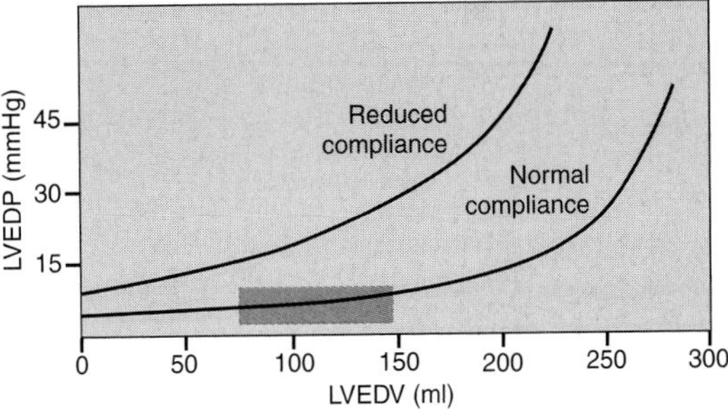


**FIGURE 37.2.** Diastolic pressure-volume (compliance) curves. The initial portion of the normal curve is fairly flat; consequently, a significant increase in left ventricular end-diastolic volume (LVEDV) results in only a small increase in left ventricular end-diastolic pressure (LVEDP). With increasing LVEDV beyond a certain limit, small increases in LVEDV cause rapid increases of LVEDP. With reduced compliance, the curve is shifted upward and to the left, indicating that even normal LVEDV is associated with high LVEDP. The shaded area indicates the normal range for LVEDV and LVEDP.

indicates increased contractility; a downward and rightward shift indicates decreased contractility.

*Systemic circulation*

Cardiac output is distributed to various organs according to their metabolic needs. Blood pressure is the product of cardiac output and systemic vascular resistance. Autonomically mediated vasomotor tone is pivotal in matching the perfusion of a particular organ to its demands.

*Circulatory reserve*

Increased oxygen demands during exercise are met by two mechanisms: augmented cardiac output and increased oxygen extraction by the tissues. Increased sympathetic activity on exercise augments both heart rate and myocardial contractility, thus raising cardiac output. Starling's law also becomes operational at high levels of exercise.

### Compensatory mechanisms in heart failure

Although either systolic or diastolic dysfunction can cause CHF, in approximately two-thirds of patients, the primary hemodynamic abnormality is systolic dysfunction (i.e., impaired myocardial contractility). With progressive impairment of myocardial contractility as the cardiac output declines, several compensatory factors evolve in order to restore normal cardiac output (Figure 37.3). However, as these mechanisms are expended to maintain the resting cardiac output, the cardiac reserve becomes eroded. Moreover, several deleterious effects are associated with these compensatory mechanisms (Table 37.2).

*Ventricular hypertrophy and dilatation*

Impaired contractility and pressure overload stimulate myocardial **hypertrophy.** The hypertrophied ventricle can generate greater force to overcome the increased afterload. In contrast, conditions associated with volume overloading, such as aortic regurgitation, cause ventricular **dilatation** to compensate for increased volume. An enlarged chamber can generate a greater stroke volume. However, as the ventricle enlarges, wall stress also increases, raising the myocardial oxygen demand. In both ventricular hypertrophy and dilatation, beyond a certain stage, myocardial $O_2$ demand outstrips the supply, resulting in diffuse myocardial fibrosis and further impairment of the contractile function.

After a large anterior wall infarction, the LV may

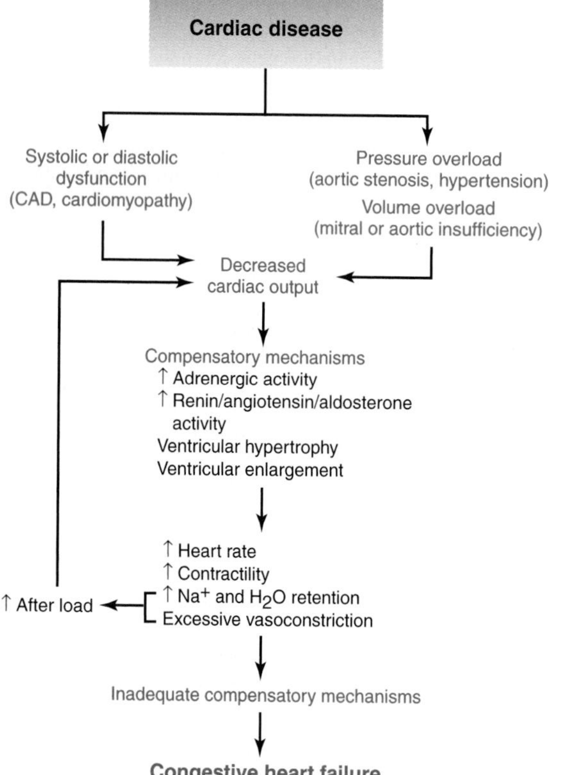


**FIGURE 37.3. Pathogenesis of congestive heart failure and the influence of various compensatory factors that become active in an attempt to maintain normal pump function. (CAD, coronary artery disease.)**

**TABLE 37.2. Compensatory Mechanisms in Congestive Heart Failure**

| Mechanism | Salutary Effects | Deleterious Effects |
|---|---|---|
| Ventricular hypertrophy | ↑ Force of contraction | ↑ $O_2$ demand, ↓$O_2$ supply<br>↓ Diastolic compliance<br>↑ Wall stress |
| Ventricular dilatation (increased preload, Starling's law) | ↑ Stroke volume | ↑ $O_2$ demand, ↑ wall stress, ↑ pulmonary congestion, ↑ systemic congestion |
| ↑ Sympathetic activity | ↑ Contractility, ↑ heart rate, ↑ Venous tone (preload) | ↑ $O_2$ demand, ↑ systemic arterial tone (afterload) causing ↓ stroke volume |
| ↑ Renin-angiotensin-aldosterone system | ↑ Salt and water retention; ↑ venous return and preload | ↑ Pulmonary congestion, ↑ systemic congestion, ↑ vasoconstriction (↑ afterload) |
| ↑ $O_2$ extraction | ↑ $O_2$ delivery | — |

enlarge and assume a spherical configuration (**ventricular remodeling**). Although this adaptive change maintains stroke volume, the remodeling process has deleterious long-term effects on global LV function and prognosis.

*Starling's law*

The ventricular function curve becomes progressively depressed (downward shift) with increasing severity of heart failure as large changes in preload result in only small changes in stroke volume (see Figure 37.1). In CHF, renal blood flow is markedly reduced, which activates the renin-angiotensin-aldosterone system, causing retention of sodium and water and expansion of the intravascular volume. Expanded central blood volume, by increasing the preload, activates the Starling's mechanism and increases the stroke volume. However, the deleterious effects of this mechanism include increased myocardial oxygen demands and pulmonary and/or systemic venous congestion manifested by dyspnea, edema, and hepatomegaly.

*Neurohormonal activity*

CHF is associated with increased levels of several neurohormones: norepinephrine, renin-angiotensin-aldosterone, antidiuretic hormone, endothelin, atrial natriuretic neuropeptide, and prostaglandins. In addition, cytokine levels (e.g., tumor necrosis factor) rise in CHF. Neurohormonal activation and the resultant apoptosis (programmed cell death) as well as ventricular remodeling (dilatation, hypertrophy, and fibrosis causing further ventricular dysfunction) play a key role in the progression of CHF.

Increased sympathetic discharge is beneficial in maintaining the normal circulatory status in heart failure through several different mechanisms, e.g., tachycardia, stimulation of contractility, arteriolar constriction, and venoconstriction. Despite the increased blood catecholamine level, the norepinephrine content of the failing myocardium decreases.

Increased activity of the systemic and tissue renin-angiotensin system in CHF has been well documented. A decrease in renal blood flow and reduced concentration of renal tubular $Na^+$ and $Cl^-$ ions as well as activation of atrial mechanoreceptors stimulate the renin-angiotensin system. A potent vasoconstrictor and stimulator of sympathetic nervous system, angiotensin II also contributes to cell growth and cardiac remodeling. It also stimulates secretion of aldosterone and vasopressin, which in turn promote sodium and water retention and loss of potassium and magnesium.

Plasma levels of arginine vasopressin (antidiuretic hormone) may be elevated in CHF. This hormone is also a potent vasoconstrictor, and its release is stimulated by angiotensin II. Levels of atrial natriuretic peptide are also increased in CHF. This compound, generated in the atrial tissue, promotes diuresis, natriuresis, and vasodilation. It inhibits the renin-angiotensin-aldosterone system as well as vasopressin.

The primary disadvantage of generalized arteriolar constriction is that it augments afterload, with increased resistance to LV ejection and a reduced stroke volume. This establishes a vicious cycle of reduced cardiac output, increased sympathetic activity, increased arteriolar constriction, and further reduction of cardiac output. A high level of circulating catecholamines indicates a poor long-term prognosis.

*Increased oxygen extraction*

Normally, peripheral tissues extract 3.5–5.0 ml of $O_2$ from each 100 ml of arterial blood. In low-output states, tissues extract greater amounts of oxygen, causing widening of the arteriovenous $O_2$ difference.

## Etiology

Several disease states affecting predominantly the left and/or right side of the heart account for CHF (Table 37.3). Despite some overlaps, heart failure is caused by predominantly systolic or predominantly diastolic dysfunction.

### Predominantly systolic dysfunction (depressed emptying)

*Abnormal loading conditions*

A **pressure overload,** or increased afterload, is imposed on the LV by conditions such as aortic stenosis, coarctation of the aorta, and systemic hypertension. Pulmonary stenosis and pulmonary hypertension place a pressure overload on the RV. Ventricular hypertrophy subsequently develops to overcome the increased outflow resistance. A hypertrophied ventricular wall is stiffer, causing end-diastolic pressure to rise. Progressive contractile failure follows several years of ventricular hypertrophy, culminating in ventricular dilatation and failure.

A **volume overload** is placed on the LV by conditions such as aortic or mitral regurgitation, patent ductus arteriosus, and ventricular septal defect. Tricuspid regurgitation, pulmonary regurgitation, and atrial septal defect impose a volume overload on the RV. To accommodate the increased volume, the ventricle dilates relatively early, and over several years, undergoes hypertrophy. The heart tolerates volume overload better than pressure overload.

*Myocardial contractile failure*

In myocardial infarction, maintenance of cardiac output depends on the infarct size: whereas in small infarcts, the residual normal muscle can compensate and maintain normal output, large infarcts lead to heart failure and/or cardiogenic shock. In cardiomyopathies, myocardial contractility is reduced diffusely, resulting in global ventricular dysfunction and heart failure (intrinsic myocardial failure).

### Predominantly diastolic dysfunction

Diastolic dysfunction implies impaired ventricular filling; however, the systolic function is preserved. LV hypertrophy—as in hypertrophic cardiomyopathy, aortic stenosis, or hypertension (especially in combination with diabetes mellitus)—reduces LV compliance. Filling such a stiff ventricle requires a powerful left atrial contraction. Left atrial pressure rises, causing pulmonary congestion and dyspnea (see Figure 37.2). If atrial fibrillation develops in this setting, the resulting loss of "atrial kick" and the reduced diastolic time for ventricular filling by tachycardia further aggravate the CHF. Intense myocardial ischemia can also reduce LV compliance and cause pulmonary edema.

Mitral stenosis and left atrial myxoma cause CHF by mechanically obstructing the mitral orifice, restricting LV filling, impeding left atrial emptying, and in turn, causing pulmonary vascular congestion. Similarly, systemic venous congestion develops in tricuspid stenosis, tricuspid atresia, and right atrial myxoma. In these conditions, ventricular filling is impeded by the mechanical obstruction, but the ventricle itself is normal.

## Clinical Features

The manifestations of heart failure are attributable to three main hemodynamic changes: 1) decreased cardiac output causing inadequate perfusion of various organ systems, 2) pulmonary venous congestion, and 3) systemic venous congestion. Depending on the

**TABLE 37.3. Etiology of Congestive Heart Failure**

| Predominantly Systolic Dysfunction | Predominantly Diastolic Dysfunction |
|---|---|
| **Conditions causing pressure overload:** | Marked left ventricular hypertrophy |
| Hypertension | Hypertrophic cardiomyopathy |
| Aortic stenosis | Hypertension |
| Coarctation of aorta | Severe myocardial ischemia |
| Pulmonary hypertension | Mitral stenosis |
| Pulmonary thromboembolic disease | Left atrial myxoma |
| **Conditions causing volume overload:** | Infiltrative cardiomyopathies (amyloidosis, hemochromatosis) |
| Aortic incompetence | Pericardial constriction |
| Mitral incompetence | Cardiac tamponade |
| Ventricular septal defect | |
| Atrial septal defect | |
| **Myocardial contractile failure:** | |
| Myocardial infarction | |
| Dilated cardiomyopathies | |

**TABLE 37.4. Clinical Manifestations of Congestive Heart Failure**

| Left Heart Failure | Right Heart Failure |
|---|---|
| **Symptoms** | |
| Dyspnea | Edema |
| Orthopnea | Dyspnea |
| Paroxysmal nocturnal dyspnea | Abdominal distension and discomfort |
| Acute pulmonary edema | Anorexia, nausea |
| Hemoptysis | Weight loss |
| Nocturia | Weakness |
| Fatigue | Anxiety |
| **Signs** | |
| Cardiomegaly | Positive hepatojugular reflux |
| Left ventricular $S_3$ | Jugular venous distension |
| Loud $P_2$ | Liver enlargement |
| Functional mitral incompetence | Spleen enlargement |
| Pulsus alternans | Dependent edema |
| Pulmonary rales | Ascites |
| Cheyne-Stokes breathing | Cyanosis |
| Pleural effusion | Cardiomegaly |
| | Right ventricular $S_3$ |
| | Functional tricuspid incompetence |
| | Cardiac cachexia |

**TABLE 37.5. New York Heart Association Functional Classification of Congestive Heart Failure**

| Class | Description |
|---|---|
| I | No symptoms on ordinary activity |
| II | Symptoms* occur on ordinary activity |
| III | Symptoms occur on less than ordinary activity |
| IV | Symptoms present at rest |

*Symptoms include dyspnea or fatigue

underlying mechanism, these features may occur in varying combinations (Table 37.4).

Signs and symptoms increase as CHF worsens, causing a progressive loss of functional capacity. The New York Heart Association (NYHA) Functional Classification is a widely used measure of disability in heart failure and provides important prognostic information (Table 37.5).

## Left Heart Failure

### Symptoms

**Dyspnea,** the cardinal symptom of left heart failure, implies awareness of breathing or shortness of breath. It is usually attributed to decreased compliance of the lungs due to pulmonary venous congestion and edema. With mild heart failure, dyspnea occurs only on exertion, but as CHF progresses, the activity threshold declines.

**Orthopnea** indicates dyspnea during recumbence, with relief on sitting up. Relief in an upright posture presumably follows an increase of intrathoracic space and reduction of pulmonary venous congestion, as the blood pools in the lower extremities.

In **paroxysmal nocturnal dyspnea** (PND), the patient typically sleeps 1–4 hours and then awakens acutely short of breath, feeling suffocated. The patient may sit upright and gasp for breath, walk for a few minutes, or open a window to obtain some fresh air. Associated signs may be sweating, pallor, cyanosis, cold extremities, and cough. The episode subsides in approximately 10–30 minutes, and the patient sleeps comfortably for the rest of the night. Wheezing may be present during PND ("cardiac asthma").

Acute **pulmonary edema** is a consequence of sudden, severe decompensation of the LV or severe mitral stenosis. The patient notes abrupt, agonizing dyspnea and persistent cough productive of white or pink, frothy sputum. Extreme anxiety and accentuated use of accessory muscles of respiration are its accompaniments. The skin is cold, pale, and gray with profuse sweating. The attack subsides spontaneously or with treatment, usually after a few minutes to a few hours. However, severe pulmonary edema can be lethal.

**Cheyne-Stokes breathing** is defined as periods of apnea alternating with hyperpnea (rapid breathing). It usually occurs in the elderly with left heart failure and concomitant central nervous system disease. It is ascribed to a disturbance of feedback control of the respiratory center secondary to prolonged circulation time, cerebrovascular disease, or sedation.

Expectoration of blood, or **hemoptysis,** may occur in severe left heart failure or pulmonary edema, varying from rusty-colored or pink, frothy sputum to frank blood. Hemoptysis also may arise from pulmonary thromboembolism, to which patients with heart failure are predisposed.

Patients frequently note **fatigue** on mild exertion. Low cardiac output causing decreased $O_2$ delivery to skeletal muscle, electrolyte depletion (hypokalemia), and physical deconditioning are possible causes.

Many patients report **dizziness,** weakness, and lack of balance. Most of these episodes are brief and occur when the patient is in an upright posture. Dizziness in patients with cardiac disease is due to low cardiac output resulting in poor perfusion to the brain. **Angina decubitus,** or nocturnal angina, may be another manifestation of left heart failure.

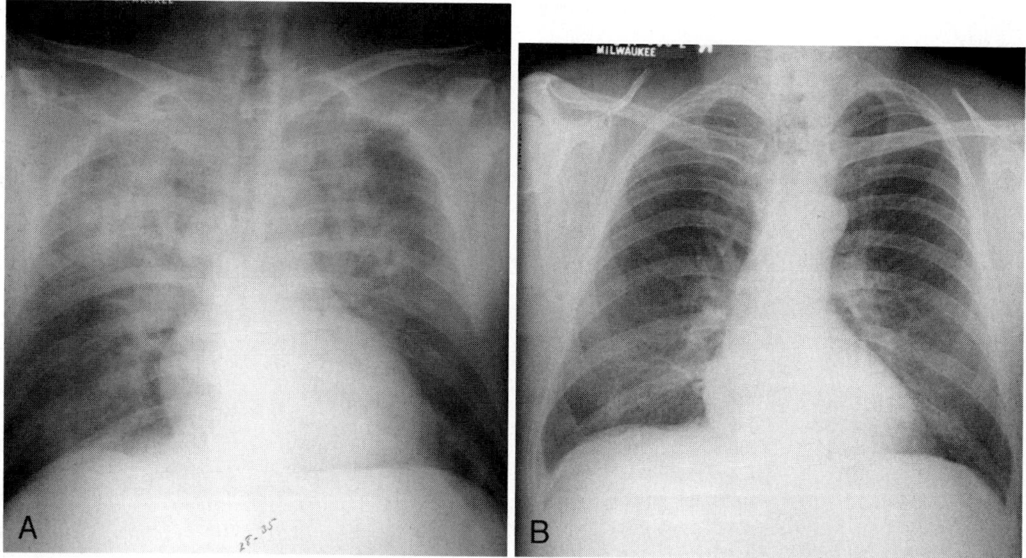


**FIGURE 37.4.** Chest radiograph in acute cardiogenic pulmonary edema showing bilateral confluent opacities ("bat wing"). (B) Follow-up x-ray a few days later, showing significant clearing, although some mild congestive changes remain. (Courtesy of the Radiology Museum, St. Joseph's Regional Medical Center, Milwaukee, Wisconsin.)

### Physical signs

A small-volume pulse is caused by low stroke volume. **Pulsus alternans** refers to a strong pulse alternating with a weak one, despite equal duration of the cardiac cycles. It implies severe myocardial failure. Tachycardia, pallor, cyanosis, and cold and clammy extremities indicate a hyperadrenergic state.

**Tachypnea,** or rapid, shallow breathing, is attributed to pulmonary venous congestion and decreased lung compliance. An audible **ventricular gallop** ($S_3$) over the cardiac apex is an early sign of left heart failure and indicates an enlarged and poorly contracting LV.

**Functional** ("secondary") **mitral regurgitation** may develop with LV enlargement and improper coaptation of the mitral valve leaflets. As the LV shrinks in response to therapy, this type of mitral insufficiency may disappear (see chapter 41).

Pulmonary findings in left heart failure arise from transudation of fluid into the alveoli and bronchiolar narrowing, and consist of **basilar crackles (rales)** bilaterally, and occasionally, bilateral rhonchi. Breath sounds may be diminished over the bases from pleural effusions, also caused by excessive transudation.

### Ancillary studies

**Chest radiography** is a valuable tool for detecting and assessing severity of left heart failure. Lung fields show vascular redistribution and Kerley B lines (see Figure 33.1). In frank pulmonary edema, confluent opacities appear in the central lung fields bilaterally near the hila, producing a "bat's wing" appearance (Figure 37.4). In persistent left heart failure, pleural effusion(s) may develop either on the right side or bilaterally. Pleural effusions, however, are more common in biventricular failure and usually occur when pulmonary capillary wedge pressure is significantly elevated. Cardiothoracic ratio is increased.

In early left heart failure, pulmonary function tests show premature closure of peripheral airways at low lung volumes, causing maldistribution of intrapulmonary air. Lung compliance is decreased.

**Echocardiography** and **radionuclide ventriculography** demonstrate enlarged LV end-diastolic and end-systolic volumes and depressed LV ejection fraction (usually $< 40\%$). **Cardiac catheterization** shows high pulmonary capillary wedge and LV end-diastolic pressures, and abnormally wide arteriovenous oxygen differences. However, severity of symptoms correlates poorly with the LV ejection fraction especially in chronic CHF.

Arrhythmias such as atrial flutter, atrial fibrillation, premature ventricular complexes, and bouts of nonsustained ventricular tachycardia are common in chronic CHF and indicate a poor prognosis. Ventricular tachycardia and ventricular fibrillation are frequent terminal events.

## Right Heart Failure

Two primary factors—systemic venous congestion and right ventricular (RV) dilatation—cause the symptoms and signs of right heart failure. Systemic venous pressure increases as a result of an increased blood volume secondary to inadequate RV emptying during systole and generalized venoconstriction in response to sympathetic overactivity. In the vast majority of patients, LV failure or mitral valve disease is the principal cause of right heart failure. Other causes include pulmonary emboli, chronic obstructive pulmonary disease, and pulmonary hypertension.

With left heart failure and/or pulmonary venous hypertension, passive pulmonary arterial hypertension develops to maintain forward flow. Once the pulmonary arterial pressure attains a certain level, pulmonary arterioles actively constrict by a reflex mechanism that worsens the pulmonary hypertension. This places a pressure overload on the RV, which subsequently fails as the compensatory mechanisms become ineffective in maintaining the forward output.

With progressive decrease of RV stroke volume, the signs and symptoms of pulmonary venous congestion (e.g., pulmonary vascular redistribution and dyspnea) become less marked. It is not uncommon for a patient with severe mitral stenosis to be free of orthopnea despite advanced right heart failure.

### Symptoms

Initially, patients usually note **edema** of the ankles and feet, which later spreads to the legs and abdomen. The edema is bilateral and pitting. In bedridden patients, edema may first develop over the sacrum. In its advanced stage, edema becomes widespread (anasarca), with ascites and edema of the external genitalia.

Right-upper-quadrant **abdominal pain** is caused by liver enlargement. Congestion of the gastrointestinal tract evokes **anorexia** and **nausea**. Nutrient absorption is impaired, and in persistent systemic venous congestion as seen in patients with constrictive pericarditis, significant protein loss may result (protein-losing enteropathy). All these factors cause gradual **weight loss** and, ultimately, **cardiac cachexia.** Other symptoms include fatigue, daytime oliguria, and nocturia.

### Physical signs

**Jugular venous distention** and jugular venous pressure (JVP) exceeding 3 cm above the sternal angle are indicative of right heart failure. The neck veins fill from below. A **positive hepatojugular reflux**—i.e., persistent elevation of the JVP during sustained pressure in the right upper abdomen—is an early sign of right heart failure. On close examination of the venous pulse, a sharp *y* descent is frequently found. RV gallop ($S_3$) is audible over the left lower sternal border and indicates increased RV end-diastolic volume.

**Hepatomegaly** and, occasionally, **splenomegaly** occur in right heart failure. The enlarged liver is tender to light pressure. After prolonged or recurrent episodes of right heart failure, widespread patchy necrosis, which is followed by fibrosis, develops in the liver owing to ischemic injury of the liver cells. Ultimately, cardiac cirrhosis follows.

**Functional tricuspid incompetence,** manifested by a pansystolic murmur over the left lower sternal border, prominent *v* -waves in the neck veins, and a pulsatile liver, develops as the RV dilates. Because the tricuspid valve no longer protects the systemic veins from RV systolic pressure, systemic venous congestion worsens. As the tissues extract more oxygen due to poor tissue perfusion and the capillary deoxyhemoglobin exceeds 5 g/dl, **peripheral cyanosis** becomes evident.

### Ancillary studies

The chest radiograph shows dilatation of the superior and inferior venae cava, right atrium, RV, and main pulmonary trunks. Associated pleural effusion indicates coexistent left heart failure. The **echocardiogram** may reveal dilatation of the RV and paradoxical septal motion indicating RV volume overload, especially when functional tricuspid incompetence develops. **Cardiac catheterization** reveals high central venous, right atrial, and RV end-diastolic pressures and pulmonary arterial hypertension. The pulmonary capillary wedge pressure is elevated when right-sided failure is associated with LV failure or mitral stenosis; however, it is normal when right heart failure arises from obstructive lung disease or pulmonary emboli.

Liver function tests become abnormal in advanced cases. Urinalysis commonly shows slight proteinuria and high specific gravity. Blood urea nitrogen may rise owing to poor renal perfusion (prerenal failure).

Recent studies suggest that brain natriuretic peptide (BNP) concentration in plasma is very helpful in diagnosing CHF, assessing its severity and evaluating response to therapy. This is very helpful in older patients in whom the diagnosis of CHF is particularly challenging. The levels increase in both systolic and diastolic heart failure.

### Prognosis

The overall 1-year survival in CHF varies from 10–60%. Milder degrees and initial episodes of CHF are easily controllable and have a better prognosis than chronic, severe CHF. Correctable causes, such as valvular lesions, hypertension, and some congenital abnormalities, when treated early, have a much better prognosis than uncorrectable abnormalities. Poor prognostic factors include LV dysfunction, poor exercise tolerance, presence of coronary artery disease, $S_3$ gallop, ventricular arrhythmias, atrial flutter or fibrillation, and increased neurohormonal factors.

## Management

The aims of management are to alleviate symptoms and improve quality of life, treat the primary cardiac disease to prevent recurrence of CHF, and improve survival.

### General measures

Depending on the severity of heart failure, complete bed rest or frequent rest periods should be advised to reduce the cardiac workload and promote diuresis. Supplemental $O_2$ is helpful in severe CHF. The head of the patient's bed should be elevated to decrease ventricular preload by pooling the blood in the legs. Use of elastic stockings, passive leg exercises, and low-dose heparin therapy are useful to prevent thromboembolic complications. Moderate exercise training should be encouraged to prevent or reverse physical deconditioning.

Caloric intake should be restricted in overweight patients. Influenza and pneumococcal vaccines may reduce the risk of respiratory infections. Factors that precipitate episodes of CHF should be identified and treated (Table 37.6).

## Pharmacologic Therapy

### Preventing cardiac remodeling

Long-term use of the following agents can improve clinical status, prevent disease progression, and reduce risk of major cardiac events. Although they may not immediately improve symptoms, their long-term benefits mandate their use in almost all patients with CHF unless contraindicated.

The beneficial effects of **angiotensin-converting enzyme (ACE) inhibitors** (Table 37.7) appear to be due to their vasodilatory effects, as well as the blockade of tissue ACE activity and breakdown of bradykinin. They have a proven benefit not only in all mild, moderate, and severe CHF but also in patients with asymptomatic LV dysfunction. ACE inhibitors reduce morbidity, improve symptoms and exercise capacity and prolong survival. ACE inhibitors minimize the loss of serum $K^+$ and blunt the stimulation of the renin-angiotensin system by diuretics. Captopril and enalapril are the representative agents. Hypotension, renal insufficiency, hyperkalemia, persistent cough, and angioedema are their important side effects.

Because angiotensin II can be formed through alternative pathways as well as through the converting-enzyme route, **selective blockers of type I angiotensin receptors** (ARBs) would block the angiotensin II, regardless of how it is generated. Since the clinical benefit of ARBs is not established, they should be used only in patients intolerant of ACE inhibitors.

An enhanced adrenergic drive occurs as a compensatory factor in CHF. While helpful over the short term for maintaining cardiac performance by increasing myocardial contractility and heart rate, long-term, continuous increase in adrenergic drive causes significant myocardial injury. Several recent studies have shown that long-term use of **beta-blockers** (Table 38.7) not only improves symptoms, increases exercise capacity, and decreases hospital admissions but also prolongs survival. Regression of myocardial mass, normalization of ventricular shape (reverse remodeling) and increase of left ventricular ejection fraction follow their use. Specifically, metoprolol, bisoprolol, and carvedilol have proven very beneficial. These agents are well tolerated by most patients with mild to moderate CHF. The mechanism underlying these beneficial effects is not entirely clear, although anti-ischemic and anti-arrhythmic effects are probably most important. Hypotension, fluid retention, worsening heart failure, and bradyarrhythmias are important side effects.

Marked hyperaldosteronemia occurs in patients with CHF. Aldosterone causes $Na^+$ retention, $K^+$ and magnesium depletion, sympathetic and parasympathetic inhibition, myocardial and vascular fibrosis, and baroreceptor dysfunction. ACE inhibitors are ineffective in blocking aldosterone activity on a long-term basis. Recently, **spironolactone** was shown to improve symptoms, reduce hospitalizations, and prolong survival.

Some other neurohormonal inhibitors such as endothelin receptor blockers are on the horizon for treatment of CHF.

**TABLE 37.6. Factors Contributing to Decompensation in CHF**

| |
|---|
| Cardiac |
| Recurrent myocardial ischemia |
| Acute myocardial infarction |
| Tachyarrhythmias |
| Infective endocarditis |
| Noncardiac |
| Systemic infections |
| Heavy alcohol consumption |
| Thyrotoxicosis |
| Excessive salt intake |
| Excessive fluid ingestion |
| Pulmonary embolism |
| Increased physical or emotional stress |
| Drugs |
| Poor compliance with medications |
| Use of negative inotropic agents (β-blockers) |
| Use of prostaglandin inhibitors (NSAIDs) causing fluid retention |

TABLE 37.7. Commonly Used Diuretics

| Drug | Dose | Route | Onset of Action (min) | Peak Effect (h) | Duration of Effect (h) | Class Site of Action | Class Adverse Effects |
|---|---|---|---|---|---|---|---|
| A. Thiazides | | | | | | | |
| Chlorthalidone | 25–50 mg qd | PO | 120 | 2–6 | 24–72 | Distal convoluted tubule | Hypokalemia<br>Hyponatremia |
| Hydrochlorothiazide | 25–50 mg qd | PO | 120 | 4–6 | 6–12 | (Metolazone acts in proximal convoluted tubule also) | Hypochloremic alkalosis<br>Glucose intolerance<br>Increased cholesterol |
| Indapamide | 2.5–5 mg qd | PO | 60–120 | 2 | 36 | | Nausea<br>Skin rash |
| Metolazone | 2.5–10 mg qd | PO | 60 | 2 | 12–24 | | |
| B. Loop Diuretics | | | | | | | |
| Furosemide | 20–200 mg | IV | 5 | 0.5 | 2 | Ascending limb of loop of Henle | Hypokalemia<br>Hypomagnesemia |
| | 20–240 mg qd or bid | PO | 30 | 1–2 | 6–8 | | Hypocalcemia<br>Hyponatremia<br>Hypochloremic alkalosis |
| Bumetanide | 0.5–1 mg (max 10 mg) | PO | 5 | 0.5–0.75 | 2 | | Increased cholesterol<br>Hearing loss |
| | 0.5–2 mg (max 10 mg) | IV | 30–60 | 1–2 | 4–6 | | |
| C. Potassium-Sparing | | | | | | | |
| Spironolactone | 25–200 mg qd | PO | 60–120 | (3 days) | 48–72 | Late distal convoluted tubule | Hyperkalemia<br>Hyponatremia<br>Hyperchloremic acidosis, gynecomastia and hirsutism |
| Triamterene | 50–100 mg qd or bid | PO | 120–240 | (2–4 days) | 7–9 | Collecting ducts | Hyperkalemia<br>Hyponatremia |
| Amiloride | 5–10 mg qd (max 40 mg) | PO | 120 | 3–4 | 24 | | |

### Lowering ventricular preload

Expanded intravascular volume due to abnormal salt and water retention by the kidneys as well as elevated ventricular filling pressure are responsible for the pulmonary vascular congestion that leads to dyspnea, orthopnea, and paroxysmal nocturnal dyspnea and for the systemic vascular congestion causing edema, hepatomegaly, distended neck veins, and ascites. One way to reduce this expanded intravascular volume is to limit salt intake to <3 g/day. A sitting or semi-sitting posture also reduces the ventricular preload by pooling blood in the periphery.

Judicious use of **diuretics** is the most effective way to reduce fluid retention (Table 37.8). Diuretics reduce renal tubular $Na^+$ reabsorption, causing natriuresis and diuresis. With the relief of pulmonary congestion, oxygenation of blood and exercise tolerance improve. Because the ventricles are operating at the flat portion of Starling's curve, cardiac output is only slightly changed, despite a reduction of the preload (see Figure 37.1).

The aim of diuretic therapy is to relieve symptoms of pulmonary and systemic venous congestion without compromising the cardiac output. The optimal dose of diuretics can be determined by performing serial clinical examinations, measuring body weight, measuring blood pressure for orthostatic changes, and assessing renal function. Persistent hydrothorax and ascites, by encroaching on the chest cavity, worsen dyspnea, and may necessitate thoracentesis and paracentesis, respectively, if refractory to diuretic therapy. Overzealous diuretic use should be avoided since it causes excessive contraction of intravascular volume, reducing cardiac output and also promoting thromboembolic complications. Hypokalemia, hypomagnesemia, hypotension, azotemia, and neurohormonal activation are side effects.

**Venodilators** such as nitrates also decrease the ventricular preload. By pooling blood in the periphery, they decrease venous return, reducing the filling pressures of both ventricles.

### Reducing left ventricular afterload

In CHF, aortic input impedance and ventricular afterload are inappropriately elevated, which tends to lower the stroke volume and increase myocardial $O_2$ demand. Arteriolar **vasodilators** break this cycle; they reduce aortic impedance, which facilitates systolic emptying of the LV, thus increasing cardiac output and decreasing myocardial $O_2$ demand (see Table 37.7). Vasodilators such as nitroprusside and ACE inhibitors are particularly useful in treating patients with left heart failure caused by acute mitral or aortic regurgitation because these drugs promote forward ejection into the aorta and reduce regurgitation into the left atrium and LV, respectively. On the other hand, in heart failure due to valvular stenosis, vasodilators may evoke hypotension because the stenotic valves do not allow increase in cardiac output to compensate for arterial dilatation.

Patients with heart failure frequently have venoconstriction that augments pulmonary blood volume and contributes to pulmonary congestion. Venodilators (e.g., **nitrates**) reduce pulmonary blood volume, preload, and pulmonary congestion, and thus relieve dyspnea and enhance exercise tolerance.

Because of its potency and rapid onset of action, IV **sodium nitroprusside** is an ideal agent for short-term use in patients with severe and refractory CHF. Pulmonary

**TABLE 37.8. Commonly Used Vasodilators**

| Drug | Mechanism of Action | Venodilation | Arteriolar Dilation | Dose | Route | Duration | Adverse Effects |
|---|---|---|---|---|---|---|---|
| NITRATES | | | | | | | |
| Nitroprusside | Direct | Major | Major | 5–150 μg/min | IV | Min | Hypotension, thiocyanate toxicity |
| Nitroglycerin | Direct | Major | Minimal | 10–100 μg/min | IV | Min | Hypotension, dizziness, syncope, headache, nausea |
| | | | | 0.3–0.6 mg | SL | Min | |
| | | | | 0.5–2 in. q 4–6 h | Topical | Hours | |
| | | | | 0.2–0.6 mg/h | Topical | Hours | |
| Isosorbide dinitrate | Direct | Major | Minimal | 2.5–10 mg q2–3h; | SL | Hours | |
| | | | | 10–40 mg q 6h | PO | Hours | |
| HYDRALAZINE | Direct | None | Major | 10–75 mg q 6 h | PO | Hours | Tachycardia, headache, nausea, drug-induced lupus |
| ACE INHIBITORS | | | | | | | |
| Captopril | ACEI | Major | Moderate | 6.25–25 mg TID | PO | Hours | Hypotension, hyperkalemia, cough, proteinuria, azotemia, angioedema, agranulocytosis |
| Enalapril | ACEI | Major | Moderate | 2.5–10 mg BID | PO | Hours | |
| Lisinopril | ACEI | Major | Moderate | 5–20 mg BID | PO | Hours | |

ACEI = angiotensin converting enzyme inhibition; PO = oral; SL = sublingual.

wedge pressure (left heart filling pressure), peripheral blood pressure, cardiac output, heart rate, and urine output should be monitored during sodium nitroprusside therapy. **ACE inhibitors** have a balanced vasodilatory effect on the arterial and venous beds. A combination of hydralazine and nitrates is an alternative in ACE inhibitors-intolerant patients.

#### Increasing myocardial contractility

Because depressed myocardial contractility is the underlying cause in most cases of heart failure, enhancing it would be expected to improve cardiac performance. Among the various positive inotropic agents, digitalis preparations are the most clinically useful. They improve myocardial contractility by promoting the availability of $Ca^{++}$ to actin and myosin. **Digoxin**, the most commonly used digitalis preparation, improves ventricular ejection fraction and exercise tolerance, but does not enhance survival.

Although digitalis is a direct vasoconstrictor, as the CHF improves and adrenergic tone is withdrawn, the net effect is vasodilation. In contrast to catecholamines, digitalis increases the myocardial contractility without concomitant tachycardia or systemic arterial constriction. It is particularly useful in patients with cardiomegaly, severe symptoms, reduced ejection fraction, and ventricular gallop.

Digoxin is available as 0.125-mg, 0.25-mg, and 0.5-mg tablets as well as for IV use. Slightly more than three-fourths of the oral dose is absorbed. Effects begin within 1–2 hours and reach a peak level 2–3 hours after ingestion. Its half-life is 1.6 days. It is excreted unchanged, predominantly by the kidneys. Therapy is usually begun with 0.75 mg of digoxin in divided doses during the first 24 hours, and then maintained at 0.125–0.5 mg daily. In patients with renal insufficiency, the dose should be reduced to 0.125 mg daily or administered on alternate days. The therapeutic serum level of digoxin is usually 1–2 ng/ml, with digitalis toxicity usually developing at serum levels exceeding 2 ng/ml. However, the diagnosis of digitalis toxicity is made by clinical and ECG findings because a wide range of digitalis levels can result in toxicity.

Digitalis in therapeutic doses produces ST-segment depression and Q-T interval shortening. Toxic amounts may initiate a variety of arrhythmias, such as multifocal premature ventricular contractions; bigeminy; atrial tachycardia with block; nonparoxysmal junctional tachycardia; atrioventricular dissociation; and first-, second-, or third degree AV blocks. Nausea, anorexia, vomiting, and altered vision (as if seeing through a green or yellow filter) may also occur. Hypokalemia, hypomagnesemia, hypoxia, and hypercalcemia may precipitate digitalis toxicity. Patients with acute myocardial infarction, myocarditis, and cor pulmonale are more sensitive to digitalis.

Treatment of digitalis toxicity consists of discontinuing the drug and administering a potassium supplement (if hypokalemia is present). In more severe toxicity, antiarrhythmic agents, such as lidocaine, procainamide, propranolol, or phenytoin, are necessary to control the tachyarrhythmias. A temporary pacemaker may be required when complete AV block develops with slow ventricular rate resistant to atropine. For severe digoxin toxicity causing life-threatening arrhythmias, digoxin immune Fab (free digoxin binding antibody fragments) is the treatment of choice.

**Dopamine** and **dobutamine** are sympathetic agonists with potent positive inotropic effects and without significant chronotropic effect. In addition, dobutamine lowers systemic vascular resistance. Neither dopamine in small doses nor dobutamine affects blood pressure significantly. These agents are available only for intravenous use. They are useful on a short-term basis, in patients with acute or refractory CHF.

Recently, a new class of positive inotropic agents with vasodilating properties, the bipyridine compounds, (e.g., **amrinone** and **milrinone**), have become available. They reduce systemic vascular resistance and preload, augment cardiac output, and improve symptoms. Their mode of action at the cellular level differs from that of digitalis and catecholamines: they inhibit cellular phosphodiesterase, resulting in an increase in the cyclic AMP level. Both agents are available in intravenous form for short-term use in patients with refractory heart failure. Although these agents improve hemodynamics and symptoms acutely, they have been associated with decreased survival.

### Treatment of CHF Due to Diastolic Dysfunction

Treatment is based on interventions that lower LV diastolic pressure and, at the same time, augment diastolic filling. Restriction of salt intake and careful use of diuretics as well as nitrates decrease LV end-diastolic volume and pressure, reduce pulmonary congestion, and relieve dyspnea. Control of tachycardia improves ventricular filling by increasing the diastolic filling period. Because a forceful atrial contraction can account for 35–40% of ventricular filling when a ventricle is hypertrophied, restoration of normal sinus rhythm in atrial fibrillation will greatly enhance ventricular filling. Calcium channel-blockers may favorably influence the compliance characteristics of the ventricular myocardium (lusitropic function). Because the systolic function is mostly normal in these patients, positive inotropic agents (digitalis) and arterial vasodilators (hydralazine, ACE inhibitors) may not be useful.

### Treatment of acute pulmonary edema

Pulmonary edema develops when the influx of fluid into the interstitial space or the alveoli from the intravascular space exceeds its efflux via the pulmonary lymphatics (see chapter 232). It may be cardiogenic (high-pressure form), when pulmonary capillary wedge pressure exceeds the plasma colloid osmotic pressure, or noncardiogenic (low-pressure form), when the pulmonary vascular permeability increases. Chest radiographs, while very helpful in diagnosis of pulmonary edema, cannot differentiate between high-pressure and low-pressure forms.

Acute pulmonary edema is a medical emergency and can be fatal unless promptly treated. Treatment goals are to maintain systemic arterial oxygenation and rapidly relieve pulmonary congestion (Table 37.9).

### Treatment of arrhythmias

Frequent premature ventricular complexes and bouts of nonsustained ventricular tachycardia are common in CHF. Structural myocardial changes, myocardial ischemia, electrolyte disturbances, and neurohormonal factors contribute to these arrhythmias. These arrhythmias increase the risk for sudden death. Conventional antiarrhythmic agents do not reduce this risk and may actually increase it.

Current recommendations for managing ventricular arrhythmias include optimizing therapy for CHF (especially with ACE inhibitors and β-blockers), maintaining serum potassium and magnesium levels in the high-normal range, and correcting ongoing myocardial ischemia. Ventricular arrhythmias associated with significant symptoms, such as presyncope and syncope, require evaluation with electrophysiologic studies and aggressive management with antiarrhythmic agents (e.g., amiodarone) and automatic implantable cardioverter-defibrillator.

### Refractory CHF

Patients with CHF refractory to standard therapy should be hospitalized, and evaluated and treated for any precipitating factors (see Table 37.6). They should be considered for individualized therapy under invasive monitoring with a pulmonary artery catheter. After the baseline hemodynamic status is evaluated, therapy with diuretics, vasodilators (IV sodium nitroprusside), and/or sympathomimetic amines (dopamine or dobutamine) is initiated. The goal is to achieve the optimal hemodynamic values (mean pulmonary capillary wedge pressure <15 mm Hg, systemic vascular resistance <1200 dynes/sec/cm$^5$, mean right atrial pressure <8 mm Hg, and mean systemic blood pressure >80 mm Hg). Patients are subsequently switched to oral medications and counseled regarding salt restriction, exercise, and flexible diuretic regimen. In patients refractory to intensive medical treatment, LV assist devices may be considered as a temporary bridge to heart transplantation. Nesiritide, a synthetic b-type natriuretic peptide with balanced arterial and venous dilation has become available for in-hospital use to treat severe decompensated CHF.

### Permanent pacing

Dyssynergy between the two contracting ventricles has been found to be an integral feature of chronic heart failure. Restoration of the synergy by mechanical pacing of both ventricles simultaneously through specially designed biventricular pacemakers has been found to be effective in treatment of chronic heart failure. Although such devices do not correct the abnormal contractility inherent in chronic CHF, they can improve the prognosis in chronic heart failure.

### Heart transplantation

Heart transplantation is reserved for patients with intractable functional Class III-IV CHF who have little likelihood of survival during the next 6–12 months. The ideal patients are relatively young (<60 years) and without multi-organ disease. In such patients, the chances of improved quality of life and return to employment are high. Significant pulmonary hypertension (pulmonary vascular resistance >6 Wood units), collagen vascular disease, positive HIV status, and severe, complicated diabetes mellitus are the major contraindications.

These patients are prone to acute and chronic rejection of the allograft. However, with the long-term use of immunosuppressant agents, 1- and 5-year survivals are 90% and 70%, respectively. The complications of heart transplantation include episodes of rejection, nephrotoxicity, bone marrow suppression, opportunistic infections, accelerated coronary atherosclerosis, and neoplasia.

## Prevention of Heart Failure

Controlling various risk factors for atherosclerosis and treating hypertension go a long way in preventing the initial LV dysfunction that eventually results in CHF. Once LV dysfunction begins, stimulation of neurohormones, vasoconstriction, LV remodeling, and salt retention, all interrelated processes, worsen LV dysfunction and convert asymptomatic LV dysfunction into symptomatic CHF. It is now well established that early use of ACE inhibitors and β-blockers at the stage of asymptomatic LV dysfunction can slow the progression of symptomatic CHF and enhance survival.

**TABLE 37.9. Treatment of Acute Cardiogenic Pulmonary Edema**

| Drug/Maneuver | Dose | Comments |
|---|---|---|
| Upright or Semi-upright Posture | — | Decreases venous return (preload); Increases lung volumes; decreases work of breathing. |
| Oxygen Therapy | 100%, 6–8 L/min by nasal prongs or mask; if ineffective, proceed to endotracheal intubation | Optimal oxygenation dilates pulmonary vasculature. |
| Continuous positive pressure breathing | | Improves gas exchange, reduces respiratory work and reduces preload. |
| Morphine sulfate | IV 2–5 mg, repeat every 20 min (total <15 mg) | Relieves anxiety, reduces preload by venodilation. |
| Loop Diuretics | | Reduce preload by vasodilation and rapid diuresis. |
| Furosemide | 20–120 mg IV | |
| Bumetanide | 1 mg IV | |
| Vasodilators | | |
| Nitroglycerin | 0.4 mg SL, | |
| or | 5–200 μg/min IV (inf) | Reduces preload and afterload. |
| Sodium nitroprusside | 5–10 μg/min (inf) | |
| Digoxin | 0.25–0.5 mg IV | Reduces ventricular rate if patient has atrial fibrillation, and also enhances contractility. |
| Bronchodilator | | |
| Aminophylline | 5 mg/kg IV over 15 min, then 0.5-0.9 mg/kg/hr (inf) | Relieves bronchospasm, vasodilator and positive inotropic agent. |
| Rotating tourniquets | Apply BP cuffs to three limbs, raise pressure up to 10 mmHg below diastolic BP, release pressure every 15 min and rotate to different limbs | Reduces preload. |
| Correct | Tachy-or brady-arrhythmias and AV asynchrony | |
| Dopamine or dobutamine | 2–5 μg/kg/min | Positive inotropic agents, useful especially if hypotension present. |
| Intra-aortic balloon counterpulsation | | Reduces afterload and improves myocardial blood flow, useful if hypotension is present. |
| Determine etiology | | Establish and correct the cause as rapidly as possible. |
| Diastolic dysfunction | | If etiology is predominantly diastolic dysfunction and systolic function is normal, use diuretics and nitrates cautiously; avoid digoxin and direct acting vasodilators; β-blockers and calcium channel-blockers may be required to control hypertension and/or ischemia, heart rate. |
| Ultrafiltration | | Removes excess water. |

Abbreviations: inf = infusion; SL = sublingual.

# CHAPTER 38 CORONARY ARTERY DISEASE

The clinical manifestations of coronary artery disease (CAD)—angina, myocardial infarction, sudden death, arrhythmias, and ischemic cardiomyopathy—arise from impairment of coronary blood flow that results from narrowing of the coronary arterial lumen by atheromatous plaques.

## Atherosclerosis

### Pathogenesis

Atherosclerosis, the process of hardening and thickening of medium and large arteries, begins in childhood and adolescence, and slowly progresses over decades to become clinically manifest during mid and late adulthood. The earliest lesions ("fatty streaks") are eccentric, yellowish, flat intimal lesions. These consist of foam cells (macrophages and smooth muscle cells filled with cholesterol esters) and T–lymphocytes, and they may progress to fibrous plaques during the second decade of life. Covered by pearly-gray, dense connective tissue matrix, fibrous plaques can protrude into the vessel lumen and restrict blood flow. They become complicated when the fibrous cap fissures or cracks, allowing platelet and fibrin mural clots to form. Calcification and bleeding also occur within these lesions.

The atheromatous plaques are mostly located in the epicardial segments of the coronary arteries, especially at branch points (bifurcations) and usually spare intramural segments. Smaller vessels may also be involved in smokers and diabetics.

While the precise mechanism of atherosclerosis is elusive, it is usually believed to follow endothelial injury brought about by shear forces, risk factors (oxidized low-density lipoprotein particles), and viral or immunologic factors, thus rendering the endothelium more permeable and thrombogenic. The release of several vasoactive, chemotactic, and growth factors leads to proliferative lesions.

### Risk Factors

Being water-insoluble, lipids are transported in blood as lipoprotein particles, of which there are five types: **chylomicrons**, **very–low-density** (VLDL), **intermediate-density** (IDL), **low-density** (LDL), and **high-density** (HDL) lipoproteins. LDL and IDL are the most atherogenic. HDL participates in reverse transportation of cholesterol from tissues to the liver and thus exerts a strong protective role from CAD.

Excess dietary saturated fat and cholesterol, obesity, hypothyroidism, nephrotic syndrome, and inherited conditions (e.g., primary hypercholesterolemia) lead to high levels of total cholesterol and LDL-cholesterol. Feminine gender, physical activity, and moderate alcohol intake correlate with high HDL levels; obesity, diabetes, smoking, and physical inactivity correlate with low HDL levels.

The prevalence of CAD increases with advancing age. In women, its prevalence is low before menopause but rapidly increases thereafter. Three primary risk factors (Table 38.1) are associated with most of the risk for CAD: hypercholesterolemia, smoking, and hypertension. Increasing one's **total cholesterol level** from 200 to 240 mg/dl increases the risk of CAD fivefold. **Smoking** one pack of cigarettes per day increases the risk of CAD three-to fivefold. The risk increases with heavier and prolonged smoking but declines by 50% within a few years of smoking cessation and to the level of nonsmokers in 5 years. Nicotine, an adrenergic agonist and a coronary vasoconstrictor, adversely affects clotting factors and serum lipids. Even a moderate degree of **hypertension** increases the incidence of CAD fivefold. Strong epidemiologic evidence (e.g., the Framingham study) shows that the coexistence of multiple risk factors amplifies the adverse impact. Thus, the risk of CAD increases tenfold in patients with all three risk factors when compared to subjects without any of these risk factors (14.6/1000 vs 1.6/1000).

### Clinical Syndromes

#### *Chronic Stable Angina Pectoris*

Classic angina pectoris (Heberden's angina) has three features: substernal location of discomfort, precipitating

**TABLE 38.1. Risk Factors for Coronary Atherosclerosis**

| Modifiable | Nonmodifiable |
|---|---|
| Hypercholesterolemia | Age (men, ≥45 yrs; women, ≥55 yrs) |
| Cigarette smoking | Family history (men, <55 yrs; women, <65 yrs) |
| Hypertension | |
| Physical inactivity | |
| Low HDL-cholesterol (<35 mg/dl) | |
| Diabetes mellitus | |
| Truncal obesity | |

factor (exercise or emotion), and relieving factor (rest or nitroglycerin). **Stable angina** implies that the pattern of angina—i.e., the activity threshold of developing angina and its intensity, duration, and relief with rest and/or nitroglycerin—is unchanged for months and years and is fairly predictable. The angina is termed **typical** when all three aforementioned features are present. When only two of three features are present, the episodes are described as **atypical** angina. With only one feature present, the episodes are termed non-anginal in nature.

Coronary arteriography shows significant CAD in approximately 90% of patients with typical angina and 50% of patients with atypical angina. CAD is demonstrable in fewer than 10% of cases with only one or none of the features of angina (nonanginal chest pain).

### Etiology

Atherosclerotic obstruction of one or more coronary arteries (>50% reduction in diameter) is the major cause of angina pectoris in about 90% of patients. Transient spasm of normal or atherosclerotic coronary arteries causes angina in some. A few patients have typical angina pectoris despite entirely normal coronary arteries (syndrome X); ischemia in these is attributed to small-vessel disease (microvascular angina). Aortic valve disease, especially aortic stenosis, marked RV hypertrophy, systemic lupus erythematosus, and polyarteritis nodosa are rare causes of angina.

### Pathophysiology

Angina results from an inadequate oxygen supply relative to the myocardial $O_2$ demand (Figure 38.1). Increased heart rate, contractility, LV chamber size, and/or systolic blood pressure increase the myocardial $O_2$ needs. Even under basal conditions, the myocardium extracts oxygen nearly maximally from coronary arterial blood, leading to a wide coronary arteriovenous $O_2$ difference. Thus, the only means of increasing the myocardial $O_2$ supply is to increase the coronary blood flow, which in turn is dependent on coronary vascular resistance and perfusion pressure (aortic diastolic pressure − LV end-diastolic pressure).

Coronary arteriolar dilatation is the primary means of enhancing coronary blood flow. With mild to moderately severe (50–90%) stenosis, arterioles distal to the obstruction dilate and tend to maintain normal blood flow at rest (but not during exercise). In severe (>90%) coronary stenosis, even maximal arteriolar dilatation is insufficient to maintain normal resting coronary blood flow, resulting in ischemia at rest. Enlargement of dormant collateral vessels is another compensatory mechanism to maintain coronary blood flow. Although it is inadequate to meet the myocardial $O_2$ demands, particularly during stress, collateral flow may prevent or limit the size of a

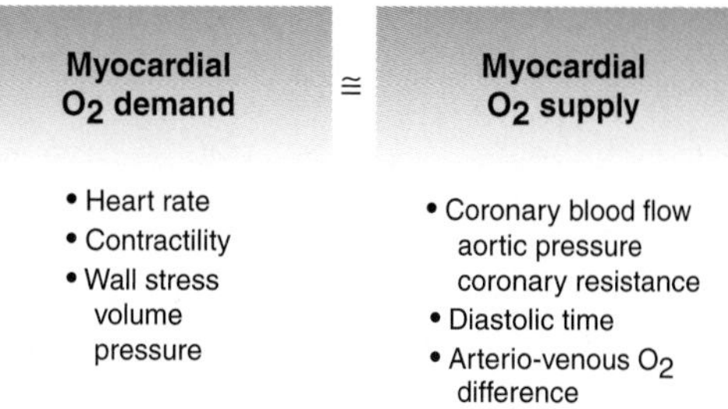


**FIGURE 38.1.** Factors determining myocardial oxygen demand and supply. Myocardial $O_2$ demand depends on heart rate, contractility, and left ventricular wall stress. Wall stress depends on the left ventricular diameter and systolic pressure. Normally, under physiological stress such as exercise, the myocardial $O_2$ supply can increase with the increase in demand. In coronary artery stenosis, the supply is inadequate relative to the demand, leading to myocardial ischemia.

myocardial infarction in the distribution of a slowly occluding coronary artery.

Minor atherosclerotic plaques may also inhibit the production of endogenous vasodilator and platelet inhibitors (e.g., nitric oxide and prostacyclin), thereby permitting platelet clumping with release of the vasoconstrictor thromboxane $A_2$, causing coronary vasospasm. Increased vasomotor tone mediated by an imbalance of autonomic nervous system and activation of serotonin receptors may also evoke vasospasm.

Thus, the spectrum of angina seen in patients consists of **exertional angina** (due to a fixed obstruction), **rest angina** (due to vasospasm or a very severe, fixed obstruction), and **mixed angina,** which has a varying activity threshold (owing to obstruction and vasospasm). As ischemia develops, the earliest change consists of diastolic dysfunction followed by systolic dysfunction, ECG changes, and angina (Figure 38.2).

### Clinical Features

Angina pectoris is episodic chest discomfort, precipitated by physical activity or emotional stress. Angina is a deep, aching, visceral pain, poorly localized and usually described as a tightness, heaviness, or burning or choking sensation in the chest. Occasionally, it is described as indigestion. The discomfort frequently rises to a crescendo, forcing the patient to rest. Less often, it builds up to a tolerable intensity, enduring until activity is discontinued. Rarely, angina abates itself during continued activity, enabling the patient to exercise even more vigorously without interruption ("walk-through" or "second-wind" angina). Acute anxiety, nausea, sweating, and dyspnea may accompany angina. The pain is most commonly felt beneath the sternum or across the anterior chest (occasionally in the precordial area) and may

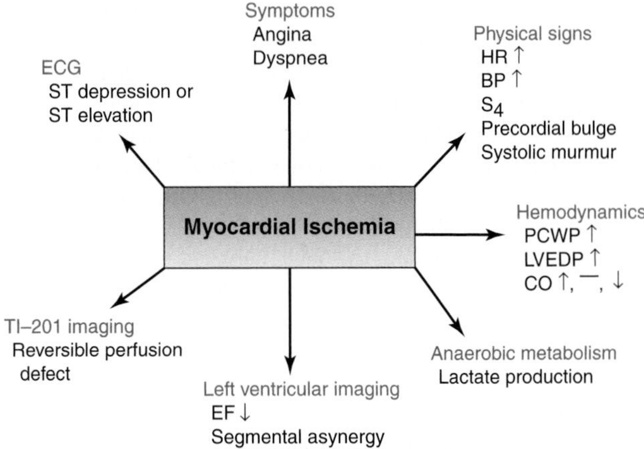


**FIGURE 38.2.** Manifestations of myocardial ischemia. HR = heart rate; BP = blood pressure; $S_4$ = fourth heart sound; PCWP = pulmonary capillary wedge pressure; LVEDP = left ventricular end-diastolic pressure; CO = cardiac output; EF = ejection fraction.

radiate to the inner aspect of the left arm, right arm, shoulders, neck, jaw, upper abdomen, and interscapular area. Pain in the region of the cardiac apex is not typical. The pain intensity may vary. Most episodes last 3–5 minutes, but severe attacks may last up to 30 minutes. Angina is usually more common during the morning hours. The Canadian Functional Classification of stable angina is shown in Table 30.3.

Physical examination during an episode of angina may reveal tachycardia, hypertension, abnormal precordial pulsation, and an atrial gallop ($S_4$) or mitral insufficiency murmur secondary to papillary muscle dysfunction. These cardiovascular findings are usually absent between episodes.

### Ancillary studies

*Electrocardiography*

In one-half to two-thirds of patients with stable angina, a standard 12-lead ECG is normal. In the remaining, evidence of old myocardial infarction or repolarization changes (ST-T abnormalities) may be seen. During spontaneous angina, most patients show an abnormal ST-segment depression (horizontal or down-sloping ST depression of >0.1 mV), indicating subendocardial ischemia.

*Exercise Stress Test*

Exercise stress tests help in evaluating patients with suspected CAD because most patients with stable angina have a normal resting ECG (Table 38.2). A focused history and clinical examination and a baseline 12-lead ECG are essential before the stress test to exclude the possibility of unstable angina or recent myocardial infarction (Table 38.3). The patient should be fasting for about 4–6 hours, and digitalis, diuretics, β-blockers, and nitrates should be withheld before the test. Exercise is performed on a treadmill or upright bicycle and the ECG is monitored continuously while the following variables are observed: the maximum extent of ST-segment depression or elevation, the level of activity causing > 1 mm of ST-segment depression, the duration of ST-segment depression during recovery, any arrhythmias, change in R-wave amplitude, and blood pressure.

A positive stress ECG is indicated by a horizontal or down-sloping ST-segment depression greater than 1 mm for 60–80 msec, using the P-R segment as the reference (Figure 38.3). ST depression indicates subendocardial myocardial ischemia. Elevated ST segment in leads with Q waves usually indicates underlying LV aneurysm, and

**TABLE 38.2. Indications for Exercise Stress Testing**

**CAD**
A. Diagnosis
  Men with atypical angina
  Women with typical or atypical angina
  Asymptomatic men:
  – in special occupations (e.g., pilots, firemen, bus drivers, railroad engineers)
  – 2 or more risk factors for atherosclerosis
  – before entering exercise training programs
B. Prognosis (risk stratification) with established CAD diagnosis
  Stable angina
  Post-myocardial infarction
C. Assessing treatment efficacy
  Medical
  Revascularization procedures (angioplasty, surgery)

**Non-CAD**
A. Evaluation and treatment efficacy of exercise-induced arrhythmias
B. Functional evaluation of valvular heart disease
C. Functional evaluation in heart failure

**TABLE 38.3. Contraindications to Exercise Stress Testing**

A. CARDIOVASCULAR
- Acute myocardial infarction
- Recent change in resting ECG
- Unstable angina
- Arrhythmias/conduction defects
  - Uncontrolled life-threatening arrhythmias
  - Second- or third-degree AV block
  - Fixed-rate pacemaker
- Decompensated heart failure
- Critical aortic stenosis
- Severe obstructive hypertrophic cardiomyopathy
- Acute myocarditis, pericarditis, or endocarditis
- Uncontrolled hypertension (BP > 200/105 mm Hg)

B. NON-CARDIAC
- Severe pulmonary hypertension
- Acute pulmonary embolism or infarction
- Any acute, systemic illness

in leads without Q waves, transmural ischemia. T-wave abnormalities, conduction defects, and arrhythmias are not specific signs of myocardial ischemia. A significant fall of systolic blood pressure (>10 mm Hg from baseline) indicates LV dysfunction.

The overall sensitivity and specificity of stress test for detecting CAD are 60% and 70% respectively. False-positive tests occur significantly more often in women.

The predictive value of exercise ECG test is highly dependent on the **pretest likelihood** of disease. For example, in a middle-aged man with several risk factors and typical angina (very high pretest likelihood of CAD), a positive exercise ECG does not add much to the diagnosis of CAD and a negative test is probably false negative. Similarly, in a young, premenopausal woman with atypical angina (low pretest probability of CAD), a positive exercise ECG is probably false positive and a negative test does not add much diagnostic information. Stress test provides the highest diagnostic yield in patients with intermediate pre-test likelihood of CAD. Conditions that frequently interfere with the interpretation of exercise ECG tests include left bundle branch block, LV hypertrophy, atrial flutter or fibrillation, and ST-T changes and/or Q waves in most leads on baseline ECG. Exercise testing with adjunctive myocardial imaging studies such echocardiography and nuclear perfusion imaging using thallium-201 or technetium-99m sestamibi are preferable in patients with an uninterpretable baseline ECG. Pharmacological stress agents such as dobutamine, adenosine, and dipyridamole can be employed in patients who are unable to perform exercise stress.

*Coronary arteriography*

Using selective **coronary arteriography,** one can visualize the coronary vessels, estimate the site and

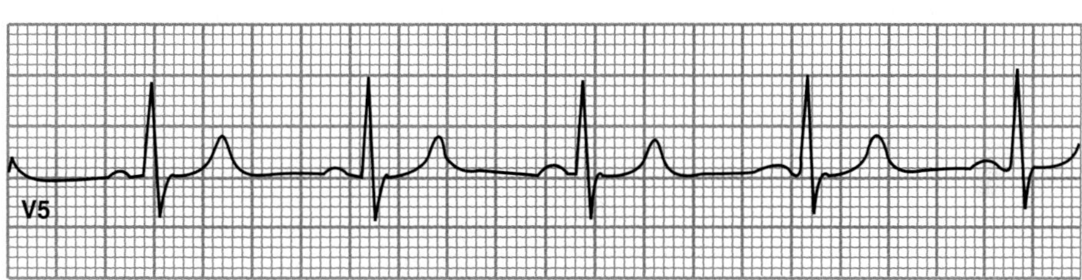


Baseline ECG Lead $V_5$
HR = 70 bpm, BP = 156/94 mmHg, ST ↓ = 0

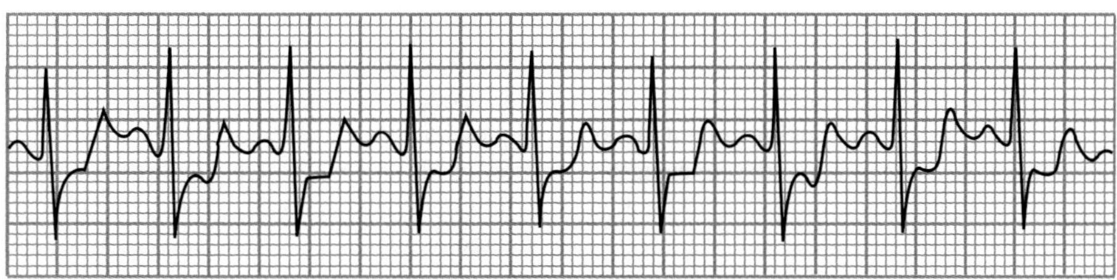

Peak exercise ECG Lead $V_5$
HR = 130 bpm, BP = 162/82 mmHg, ST ↓ = 2.5 mm

**FIGURE 38.3. ECG changes in angina.** A. Baseline ECG, with lead $V_5$ showing an isoelectric ST segment. B. During peak exercise, lead $V_5$ shows 2.5-mm horizontal ST-segment depression, indicating marked myocardial ischemia. HR = heart rate; BP = blood pressure.

**TABLE 38.4. Indications for Coronary Arteriography**

| Indication | Purpose |
|---|---|
| Disabling angina pectoris despite adequate medical therapy | To delineate coronary anatomy for potential revascularization |
| Angina and a strongly positive low level (<5 METS or heart rate <120 beats/min) exercise stress test | To assess the severity of CAD |
| Chest pain of unclear origin | As a diagnostic measure |
| Redevelopment of disabling angina after coronary artery bypass grafting | To differentiate graft occlusion from native CAD |

severity of narrowing, assess the status of the vessel distal to the lesion, determine the status of collaterals to the obstructed artery, and determine the number of diseased coronary arteries (Table 38.4). Coronary arteriography, however, yields little information about coronary blood flow. This procedure carries a 0.1% risk of death. Rarely, myocardial infarction, coronary artery dissection, embolic stroke, hypotension, arrhythmias, or thromboembolism occur, usually in patients with left main CAD or severe LV dysfunction.

**Left ventriculography** is routinely done in conjunction with coronary arteriography to assess global and regional LV function and to determine the existence of mitral insufficiency. During on-going ischemia, segmental asynergy and low ejection fraction are usually noted if a large area of myocardium is ischemic.

### Natural history

Patients with stable angina may progress to unstable angina, an acute myocardial infarction, sudden cardiac death, or multiple myocardial infarctions leading to ischemic cardiomyopathy.

Such clinical factors as advanced age, masculine gender, typical angina, diabetes mellitus, insulin use, prior myocardial infarction, heart failure, peripheral vascular disease and ST-T changes on the resting ECG portend severe CAD and indicate poor prognosis. The following ECG criteria from a symptom-limited stress test indicate a poor prognosis: reduced exercise capacity, marked down-sloping ST depression (>2 mm) at low levels of stress (stage 1 of Bruce's protocol or heart rate <120 beats/min), persistent ST depression for greater than 5 minutes after cessation of exercise, or systolic hypotension during exercise and ventricular ectopy along with ST depression. Left ventricular ejection fraction below 35%, large perfusion defect or perfusion defects in more than one vascular territory on perfusion imaging, left ventricular dilatation with increased lung uptake on thallium-201 imaging also indicate high-risk CAD. The number of obstructed coronary vessels and the status of LV function are the key long-term prognostic indicators. **Long-term prognosis** is excellent in patients with angina and normal coronary arteries. Single-, double-, and triple-vessel disease carry a yearly mortality of 2%, 6%, and 10%, respectively. Left anterior descending coronary artery stenosis has a yearly mortality of 4%. Left main coronary artery disease carries the worst prognosis; one-half of these patients die by the fifth year and 80% by the 10th year. Severe LV dysfunction with CAD has a mortality of 50% at 1 year and 85% at 5 years.

### Differential diagnosis

Several common conditions must be distinguished from angina (see Table 30.2). The pain of pulmonary hypertension is spontaneous, substernal, often prolonged, and accompanied by dyspnea. Diffuse esophageal spasm may be induced by cold liquids. Peptic ulcer pain is epigastric, related to food intake rather than exertion, relieved by antacids, and accompanied by epigastric tenderness. Pain from gallstones or biliary disease is spontaneous or postprandial, waxes and wanes, is epigastric or in the right upper quadrant, and remits on its own in a few hours or following spasmolytics and analgesics. Local tenderness and relationship to movement of the trunk are the main features of musculoskeletal pain. Cervical radiculopathy causes neck and upper chest pain, radiating into the arms.

### Management

Management strategies in chronic stable angina incorporate the following goals: 1) relieve acute episodes, 2) prevent future episodes, 3) prevent cardiac related death and myocardial infarction and the progression of atherosclerosis.

#### *Antianginal and anti-ischemic drug therapy*

Angina follows an imbalance of myocardial $O_2$ demand and supply, and drugs that improve this imbalance are useful in treating angina (Table 38.5).

##### Nitrates

Nitrates are well established for both the acute relief and prophylaxis of angina. They interact with guanylate cyclase in vascular smooth muscle cells, oxidize sulfhydryl groups, and are converted into S—nitrosothiols, which augment cyclic GMP, which in turn causes smooth muscle cell relaxation.

Glyceryl trinitrate **(nitroglycerin),** the drug of choice for immediate relief of angina, reverses myocardial ischemia by several mechanisms:

- It dilates the venous bed causing decreased venous return to the heart, thus reducing LV preload. As a result, the LV chamber becomes smaller, thus lowering the myocardial $O_2$ demand.
- By reducing the LV end-diastolic pressure, it increases the blood supply to the subendocardial region.
- By dilating the collateral coronary vessels, it enhances perfusion to ischemic myocardium.
- It also dilates stenotic segments of coronary arteries, thereby enhancing blood flow.

Nitrates are also spasmolytics, relieving any spasm of the major coronary arteries. Sub-lingual nitroglycerin may also be used prophylactically before performing activities likely to cause angina. Patients should avoid using nitroglycerin while standing up. If three tablets of nitroglycerin taken at 5-minute intervals do not relieve angina, the patient should be advised to go to the nearest hospital. The long-acting nitrates are indicated for angina prophylaxis. Commonly used nitrate preparations are listed in Table 38.6.

Nitrates may cause throbbing headache, hypotension, dizziness, and lightheadedness. Continuous use of nitrates over a 24-hour period induces tolerance, presumably from depletion of sulfhydryl groups; thus the necessity for a 12-hour nitrate-free interval during each 24-hour period to maintain responsiveness.

**TABLE 38.5. Effects of Antianginal Agents on the Determinants of Myocardial $O_2$ Demand and Supply**

| | Nitrates | β-Blockers | $Ca^{++}$ Blockers[‡] |
|---|---|---|---|
| *Demand:* | | | |
| LV wall stress | ↓↓ | ↑ | ↓ |
| Volume | ↓↓ | ↑ | ↓ |
| Pressure | ↓ | ↓ | ↓ |
| Contractility | ↑ | ↓↓ | ↓ |
| Heart rate | ↑ | ↓↓ | ↓ |
| Net change | ↓ | ↓ | ↓ |
| *Supply:* | | | |
| Perfusion pressure* | ↑ | ↓ | ↓ |
| Coronary resistance | ↓ | ↑ | ↓↓ |
| Diastolic period | 0, ↓ | ↑↑ | ↑ |
| Collateral flow | ↑ | 0 | 0, ↑ |
| Net change | ↑ | ↑ | ↑ |

Abbreviations: ↑ = increase; ↓ = decrease; 0 = no change; ↑↑ = significant increase; ↓↓ = significant decrease.
*Perfusion pressure = (aortic diastolic pressure) − (LV diastolic pressure).
[‡]Changes associated with verapamil and diltiazem; nifedipine causes reflex increase in heart rate and contractility.

BETA-ADRENERGIC BLOCKING AGENTS

These agents exert their antianginal effect primarily by lowering myocardial $O_2$ demand. Effective doses vary widely among patients and are determined by the abolition of angina, resting heart rate of about 50 beats/min, or the development of serious side effects (Tables 38.7 and 38.8). Beta-Blockers are often combined with nitrates for preventing angina. They offset nitrate-induced tachycardia and increased contractility, and nitrates prevent α-blocker-induced LV enlargement. Abrupt termination of beta-blockers may precipitate unstable angina or myocardial infarction.

CALCIUM ANTAGONISTS

Clinically available calcium channel blockers are verapamil, diltiazem, nifedipine, amlodipine, and felodipine; they are all potent vasodilators. Nifedipine and amlodipine are the most potent vasodilators, and verapamil and diltiazem also have negative inotropic effects. Diltiazem and verapamil have a depressant effect on the SA and AV nodes, whereas nifedipine, amlodipine, and felodipine lack any effect on the conduction system. Because of their negative inotropic effects, verapamil and β-blockers should not be combined in patients with LV

**TABLE 38.6. Commonly Used Nitrate Preparations**

| Preparation | Route | Dose | Onset (min) | Duration (hr) |
|---|---|---|---|---|
| Nitroglycerin | Spray | 0.4 mg | 2–5 | <0.5 |
| Nitroglycerin | SL | 0.3–0.6 mg | 2–5 | <0.5 |
| Isosorbide dinitrate | SL | 2.5–10 mg | 3–5 | 1–2 |
| Nitroglycerin | PO | 2.5–9 mg | 30–45 | 2–8 |
| Isosorbide dinitrate | PO | 5–30 mg | 15–30 | 3–6 |
| Isosorbide dinitrate (SR) | PO | 40 mg | 30–60 | 6–10 |
| Isosorbide mononitrate | PO | 20–40 mg | 30 | 6–8 |
| Nitroglycerin paste (2%) | Topical | 0.5–2 in | 20–60 | 3–8 |
| Nitroglycerin patches | Topical | 0.2–0.6 mg/hr | 30–60 | 8–14 |
| Nitroglycerin | IV | 10–200 μg/min | Immediate | Minutes |

Abbreviations: IV = intravenous; PO = oral; SL = sub-lingual; SR = sustained release.

**TABLE 38.7. Commonly Used Beta-Blockers**

| Drug | Route | Dose | Half-Life (hrs) | Cardioselective* | ISA |
|---|---|---|---|---|---|
| Propranolol | Oral | 10–120 mg QID | 4–6 | — | — |
| Propranolol LA | Oral | 40–160 mg BID | 4–0 | — | — |
| Metoprolol | Oral | 50–100 mg BID | 3–4 | + | — |
| Nadolol | Oral | 40–160 mg QD | 14–25 | — | — |
| Atenolol | Oral | 50–100 mg QD | 6–9 | + | — |
| Betaxolol | Oral | 15–20 mg QD | | + | — |
| Timolol | Oral | 10–20 mg BID | 3–4 | — | — |
| Pindolol | Oral | 10–30 mg BID | 3–4 | — | + |
| Acebutolol | Oral | 200–800 mg QD | 3–4 | + | + |
| Labetalol | Oral | 100–400 mg BID | 6 (α & β blocker) | | — |
| Propranolol | IV | 1 mg at 3–5 min intervals (max 0.1–0.15 mg/kg) | — | | — |
| Esmolol | IV | Loading, 500 μg/kg/min x 1 min<br>Maintenance, 50–200 μg/kg/min | — | | — |
| Metoprolol | IV | 5 mg at 5 min x 3 | — | | — |

*Noncardioselective agents block β-1 receptors in the heart and β-2 receptors in the bronchial tree and peripheral circulation.
+ = present; — = absent; ISA = intrinsic sympathomimetic activity; BID = twice daily; QD = once daily.

**TABLE 38.8. Adverse Effects of Beta-Blockers**

| Due to β-blockade | Unrelated to β-blockade |
|---|---|
| Bradycardia | Lethargy |
| Hypotension | Depression |
| Heart failure | Confusion |
| Cold extremities | Hallucinations |
| Bronchospasm | Nausea |
| Inhibition of metabolic and circulatory adjustments to hypoglycemia | Constipation |
| | Impotence |

dysfunction, as frank congestive heart failure may result. However, nifedipine instead may be safely combined with β-blockers.

*Medications to prevent myocardial infarction and cardiac death*

Use of **aspirin** (80–325mg/day) in chronic stable angina reduces the incidence of acute myocardial infarction and cardiac death. **Clopidogrel** can be used when there is intolerance to aspirin. **Lowering LDL-cholesterol** and **increasing HDL-cholesterol** have been shown to cause regression of atherosclerosis and marked reduction of adverse cardiovascular events. Modification of other risk factors such as smoking, hypertension, left ventricular hypertrophy, and C-reactive proteins is also beneficial in preventing adverse cardiovascular events.

### Myocardial revascularization procedures

*Percutaneous coronary interventions (PCI)*

Approximately 40% of patients with CAD and angina have discrete single-vessel or multivessel disease, making them amenable to treatment with PCI encompassing techniques such as balloon angioplasty, ablative atherectomy, and stent placement.

Balloon angioplasty consists of advancing a balloon catheter into the stenotic artery, positioning the balloon across the lesion, and inflating the balloon for a short period. A larger-diameter lumen results due to compression and disruption of atherosclerotic plaque and disruption of internal elastic lamina and, sometimes, the media of the artery. Balloon angioplasty is successful in dilating the stenosis and relieving angina in 85–90% of suitable patients. It is associated with a 1% mortality rate. The target vessel may abruptly occlude from dissection or clotting in approximately 4–5% of patients, resulting in severe ischemia and necessitating emergency bypass surgery. Following successful angioplasty, approximately 40% of arteries restenose within 6 months. Abrupt closure and restenosis rate are particularly high with angioplasty of vessels with severe, eccentric, long, and calcified lesions as well as lesions at branch points. Rotational atherectomy is more suitable for such lesions. While aspirin and heparin prevent early reocclusion of the treated vessel, no agent has so far been successful in reducing the long-term restenosis rate.

Availability of stainless steel stents has greatly helped in the treatment of abrupt or threatened closure after balloon angioplasty. At present, the majority of patients routinely receive stents in conjunction with balloon angioplasty or ablative atherectomy. Routine use of stents in the native coronary vessels has reduced the 6 month-restenosis rate to about 20%. Stenting of vein grafts is still associated with a significantly higher restenosis rate. Drug-coated stents are on the horizon and are expected to further reduce the restenosis rate.

Percutaneous procedures are less invasive and initially less expensive than bypass surgery and should be strongly considered in patients with disabling angina and/or objective signs of ischemia and suitable coronary anatomy.

*Coronary artery bypass surgery*

Coronary artery bypass grafting (CABG) consists of making aortocoronary bypasses using either segments of the saphenous vein or arterial conduits such as internal mammary or radial artery. The revascularization increases the amount of blood flow to the ischemic myocardium, thereby totally relieving angina in almost 60% of cases and markedly reducing it in another 20%. Approximately 85% of the vein bypasses are patent and functional at 1 year after surgery. While only 50% of the vein grafts are patent 10 years after surgery, 90% of mammary artery grafts remain patent.

The effectiveness of and indications for surgical therapy are outlined in Table 38.9. Important considerations in choosing CABG over medical therapy or PCI include the extent and severity of CAD, LV function, severity of angina and its response to medical therapy, results of the exercise stress test, and age, occupation, and general condition of the patient. The procedure has a hospital mortality of 1–2%, and a perioperative myocardial infarction rate of 5–10%.

Management strategies in chronic stable angina are defined in Figure 38.4.

## Prinzmetal's Angina

Some episodes of angina occur at rest and are accompanied by ST-segment elevation and ventricular ectopy or heart block. These episodes may be spontaneous, or precipitated by cocaine or tobacco smoking. The

**TABLE 38.9. Coronary Artery Bypass Surgery**

| |
|---|
| Effectiveness: |
| More effectively prevents unstable angina than medical therapy |
| Improves left ventricular function, especially during exercise |
| Improves the long-term survival in the following high-risk subsets: |
| Left main coronary artery stenosis |
| 3-vessel CAD with LV dysfunction |
| 2-vessel CAD when one of the vessels is LAD, with LV dysfunction |
| Proximal LAD and LV dysfunction |
| No advantage over medical therapy in one-vessel CAD |
| Indications: |
| Disabling angina, poorly controlled |
| Poorly tolerated medical therapy and unsuitable anatomy for PTCA |
| High-risk CAD (see above) |

Abbreviations: LAD = left anterior descending; LV = left ventricular; PTCA = percutaneous transluminal coronary angioplasty.

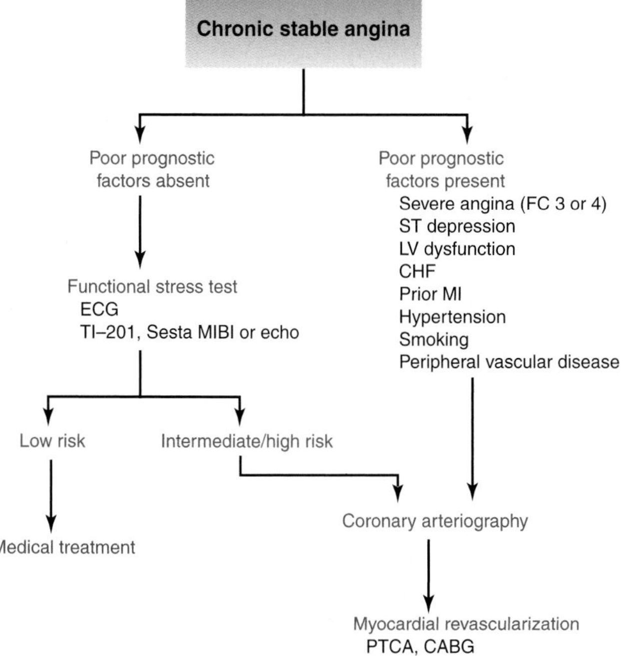


**FIGURE 38.4.** Management strategies for patients with chronic, stable angina.

attacks tend to occur at similar times of the day usually during the early morning hours. Angina and ST-segment elevation rapidly resolve following sublingual nitroglycerin. ST-segment elevation indicates transmural rather than subendocardial ischemia. Also called variant angina, they may be associated with history of migraine headaches or Raynaud's phenomenon.

Vasospasm, either in atherosclerotic or normal coronary arteries, is the causative mechanism, although in about two-thirds of patients with Prinzmetal's angina, coronary angiography shows severe, fixed, atherosclerotic lesions in the proximal region of one or more major coronary arteries. Coronary vasospasm can be shown angiographically during a spontaneous attack of variant angina or after induction with IV ergonovine maleate. About 18% of patients develop myocardial infarction or die suddenly within 3 months of diagnosis of variant angina. The active phase of disease lasts 3–6 months, following which some patients go into a long remission when coronary vasospasm cannot be induced, even with ergonovine.

Because therapy depends on the presence or absence of fixed coronary stenosis, coronary angiography should be the first step in the management. In patients with underlying severe atherosclerotic stenosis, myocardial revascularization using percutaneous interventions or CABG surgery is generally very effective in relieving angina. Drug therapy with aspirin, calcium channel blockers, and nitrates also should be implemented. In patients with absent or mild atherosclerotic disease, calcium antagonists and nitrates are the mainstay of treatment.

### Ischemic Cardiomyopathy

In some patients, atherosclerotic CAD causes multiple LV infarcts leading to dilated cardiomyopathy. Angina may or may not be reported. This entity is differentiated from the nonischemic congestive cardiomyopathy by coronary arteriography. The prognosis is poor. Besides controlling heart failure, treatment may include coronary revascularization and heart transplantation as appropriate. In some patients with preserved systolic function, diastolic dysfunction from severe myocardial ischemia may cause acute left heart failure and pulmonary edema. Angina may be absent; the ECG may show ischemic ST-T changes. Because revascularization may benefit most of these patients, coronary angiography should be performed.

## Silent (Painless) Ischemia

Most patients with CAD experience both painful and painless episodes of myocardial ischemia. However, some patients with CAD have only asymptomatic (silent) ischemic episodes. Despite being silent, these episodes adversely impact the prognosis. There is no agreement regarding the strategies to detect or treat such entirely asymptomatic patients. When a severe ischemic response is detected, coronary arteriography should be considered to define the severity of CAD.

# CHAPTER 39 ACUTE CORONARY SYNDROMES

The term **acute coronary syndromes** includes acute myocardial infarction (associated with and without ST-segment elevation) and unstable angina. Serial ECGs and serum cardiac markers are essential for clinical differentiation among the specific entities.

## Myocardial Infarction

Defined as necrosis of the myocardium, acute myocardial infarction (AMI) is characterized by severe and prolonged chest pain, progressive ECG changes, and a transient rise of cardiac enzymes. Of the nearly 1.5 million cases of AMI that occur yearly in the United States, roughly 30% are lethal; more than half of these deaths occur before arrival to the hospital.

### Etiology

Acute myocardial infarction typically follows the sudden formation of an occlusive thrombus at the site of a disrupted atheromatous plaque in a major coronary artery. A slowly evolving stenosis fosters the development of collaterals, which can limit or prevent infarction. Patients with multiple risk factors, unstable angina, and variant angina are more prone to develop AMI. Hypercoagulability, collagen vascular disease, and cocaine abuse are other risk factors for AMI.

Generally, occlusion of the left anterior descending artery can be demonstrated in an anterior wall MI. Occlusion of the right or circumflex artery occurs in an inferior, inferolateral or posterior MI. Rarely, MI occurs with normal coronary arteries, where coronary embolism or vasospasm has been incriminated.

## Pathology and Pathophysiology

The pathologic changes of AMI consist of coagulation necrosis followed by fibrosis. The earliest histologically recognizable changes begin 6–12 hours after the onset of AMI and include an eosinophilic appearance of myocardial fibers, with fuzzy and indistinct-appearing cross striations. Neutrophilic infiltration begins in 18–24 hours. By 48 hours, the infarct zone appears pale, with interspersed hemorrhagic and healthy areas. Fibrosis starts after the third week, and scar formation is complete in 6–8 weeks. Interruption of coronary blood flow causing hypoxia and accumulation of injurious metabolites, such as potassium, calcium, lipids, and oxygen-free radicals, impair LV function, leading to ventricular arrhythmias.

## Clinical Features

Although acute MI can occur at anytime of the day, it most commonly occurs within a few hours of awakening. Prior to the AMI, most patients report either new-onset angina or a change in the pattern of angina. **Substernal pain** radiating along one or both arms and the neck, lasting from 30 minutes to several hours (usually <24 hours) is the predominant symptom. It is usually associated with nausea, vomiting, sweating, weakness, and anxiety. The pain is refractory to nitroglycerin. The elderly and some diabetic patients may report no pain, presenting instead as arrhythmia, new or worsening heart failure, cerebrovascular accident, confusion, or severe weakness. In some, AMI is totally asymptomatic and is detected on a routine ECG.

During the initial few hours of AMI, the patient is in pain, with acute anxiety, pallor, and cold and clammy skin. Bradycardia and hypotension, signs of parasympathetic overactivity, are frequent, especially in inferior wall MI. Tachycardia and hypertension (signs of sympathetic overactivity) may be noted with anterior wall MI. As the pain is relieved, the blood pressure usually returns to the preinfarction level. In anteroapical MI, an abnormal precordial systolic bulge, representing the dyskinetic anteroapical segment of the left ventricle, may be visible and palpable. A soft $S_1$ due to reduced myocardial contractility and an apical atrial gallop ($S_4$) are common. A pericardial friction rub indicating pericarditis may arise on the second or third day and last for 1–2 days. Slight fever may also occur early in the first week.

Killip has suggested the following clinical classification of AMI:

- Class I—uncomplicated
- Class II—mild LV failure ($S_3$, pulmonary rales)
- Class III—acute pulmonary edema
- Class IV—cardiogenic shock

## Ancillary Studies

### Electrocardiography

In the evolution of AMI, the sequential ECG changes may include hyperacute (tall and spiked) **T waves, ST-segment elevation, T-wave inversion and Q-waves.** Hyperacute T-waves occur very early and briefly. ST-segment elevation occurs in the leads facing the infarct and the reciprocal ST-segment depression occurs in the leads away from it. The ST-segment elevation is attributed to an electrical gradient developing between the injured and the adjoining subepicardium. ST elevation, the only ECG sign of acute myocardial injury, is evanescent, becoming isoelectric by 2 weeks at most. In the vast majority of AMIs presenting with ST-segment elevation, Q-waves develop in the leads facing the infarct. Since the infarct segment is electrically inert, the initial electrical vector is directed away from it and is recorded as a negative wave (Q-wave). Q-wave develops early during the course of AMI but can persist indefinitely, an ECG indicator of an old scar. A symmetrically inverted T-wave appears as the elevated ST-segment regresses, reflecting transmural ischemia; this also may persist for months (see Figure 32.4).

Very early in AMI, an ECG may be unchanged; thus the need to get sequential ECG recordings. The standard 12-lead ECG can be helpful to localize the site of MI (see Figure 32.4): Q waves in leads $V_1$ and $V_2$, anteroseptal; $V_3$ and $V_4$, midanterior; I and aVL, anterolateral; $V_1$–$V_6$, extensive anterior, and Q in II, III, and aVF, inferior (diaphragmatic). In true posterior MI, $V_1$ and $V_2$ show tall and broad R-waves and upright T-waves, given the separation of these leads from the infarct by the healthy anterior wall.

The ECG has several limitations in diagnosing AMI. Associated conduction defects (left bundle branch block), Wolff-Parkinson-White syndrome, multiple prior infarcts, infarction of the LV apex or high lateral wall, or a small myocardial infarct anywhere may not show the typical ECG changes.

Patients with ST-segment elevation have a high likelihood of a coronary thrombus occluding the infarct-related artery. Therefore, an early ECG is vital in categorizing AMI into **ST-segment elevation** and **non ST-elevation** infarcts: This distinction is crucial in devising immediate treatment and assigning prognosis.

### Laboratory tests and imaging studies

Slight leukocytosis with a left shift usually occurs on the second day after AMI and lasts for 3–7 days. The erythrocyte sedimentation rate also rises during the second or third day and may persist for 1–2 weeks.

With myocardial cell death, several intracellular macromolecules **creatine kinase** (CK), cardiac specific

**troponins** (cTnT and cTnI), **myoglobin** and **lactate dehydrogenase** (LDH) leak into the circulation. These are collectively referred to as serum cardiac markers and their measurement provides important diagnostic and prognostic information. The serum CK level rises within 8 hours, peaks in 24 hours, and becomes normal within 72 hours. Troponin starts rising approximately 6 hours after onset of AMI and may remain high up to 7–14 days. Myoglobin may be detectable as early as 2 hours after onset of AMI. Serum LDH concentration rises in 24–48 hours, peaks at 48–72 hours, and becomes normal in 7–10 days. With the exception of troponins, which are cardiac specific, elevations of other macromolecules, however, is not specific for AMI. CK, being present in skeletal muscle and brain, rises after intramuscular injections and surgery, in skeletal myopathies, hypothyroidism, and electrical cardioversion, trauma, convulsions and central nervous system diseases. LDH, being present in the RBC, liver, kidneys, and lungs, rises in hemolysis, leukemia, liver disease, cancer and lung or renal infarction.

Isoenzymes of CK and LDH are somewhat more specific for detecting AMI. **CK-MB** usually peaks at 24 hours after the onset of AMI, and so, it should be measured on admission and sequentially thereafter until AMI is excluded. With successful restoration of flow in the infarct-related artery, CK-MB peaks at 12 hours. The fast-moving fraction of LDH, **LDH1,** rises in AMI and several other diseases, but an elevated LDH1/ LDH2 ratio exceeding 1 is highly suggestive of AMI. As mentioned earlier, troponins are the most specific markers for AMI and subforms of CK-MB and myoglobin are the first ones to rise.

**Serial Chest Radiographs** in AMI can help detect left heart failure, although bedside films do not reliably reflect cardiac size.

**Echocardiography and Radionuclide Angiography** can reliably estimate the LV ejection fraction (global function) as well as segmental wall motion abnormalities (regional function). Akinetic or dyskinetic segments correspond to old and new infarcts, and the ejection fraction helps determine the long-term prognosis following MI. Echocardiography can also identify intraventricular mural blood clots, pericardial effusion, mitral regurgitation due to a ruptured papillary muscle, ventricular septal rupture and right ventricular (RV) infarction.

### Hemodynamic monitoring

Because physical signs do not always reflect the underlying hemodynamic changes, and clinical and radiographic changes of heart failure lag behind intracardiac pressure changes, hemodynamic variables sometimes need to be measured directly (Table 39.1). The right atrial pressure does not reliably reflect the status of the LV following infarction, but the pulmonary capillary wedge pressure (PCWP) accurately mirrors the LV filling pressure.

A balloon-tipped, flow-directed (Swan-Ganz) catheter is used to measure right atrial and pulmonary artery pressures as well as cardiac output and PCWP and thereby stratify patients with AMI (Table 39.2). Using serial measurements of PCWP, cardiac output, systemic vascular resistance, and blood pressure, one can rationally manage heart failure and cardiogenic shock; also, by comparing the $O_2$ content of blood samples from various right heart chambers, a ventricular septal rupture can be differentiated from acute mitral regurgitation due to papillary muscle rupture.

Indications for **coronary angiography** include severe heart failure/cardiogenic shock, post-MI angina, or ischemia unresponsive to aggressive medical therapy as well as in association with primary coronary intervention (PCI) to restore flow in the infarct-related vessel (Figure 39.1).

**TABLE 39.1. Indications for Hemodynamic Monitoring**

Significant hypotension and hypoperfusion not easily corrected by fluids
Moderate to severe heart failure
Suspected mechanical complications, such as:
- Mitral insufficiency due to papillary muscle dysfunction/rupture
- Ventricular septal rupture with left-to-right shunt

Persistent ischemic pain
Refractory arrhythmias
Persistent sinus tachycardia, hypoxia, or acidosis

**TABLE 39.2. Hemodynamic Subsets of Patients With Acute MI**

| Subset | Systemic BP (mm Hg) | PCWP (mm Hg) | CI (L/min/m²) |
|---|---|---|---|
| Normal | N | ≤12 | 2.7 ± 0.5 |
| Hyperdynamic state | ↑ | <12 | >3.0 |
| Heart failure | N or ↓ | >18 | ≤2.5 |
| Hypotension | | | |
| Hypovolemia | ↓ | <9 | <2.2 |
| Cardiogenic shock | ↓ | >18 | <1.8 |
| RV infarction | ↓ | ≤18 | <1.8 |

BP = blood pressure; CI = cardiac index; N = normal; PCWP = pulmonary capillary wedge pressure; RV = right ventricular.
(Modified from Forrester JS, et al. N Engl J Med 295:1404, 1976.)

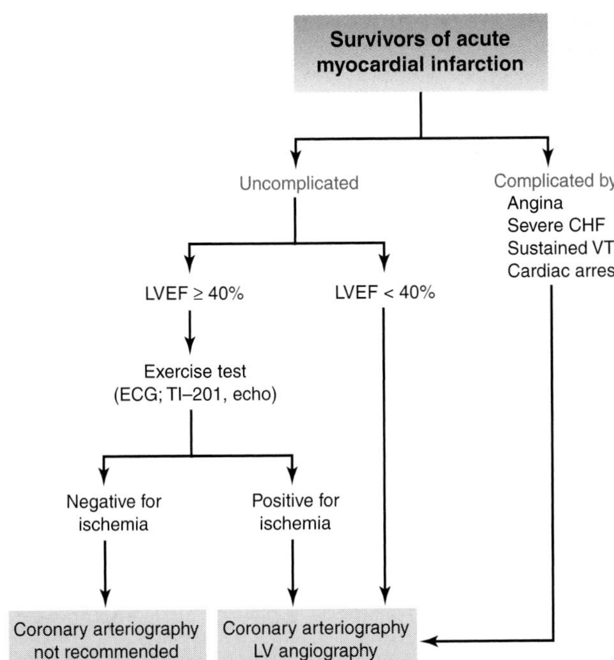


**FIGURE 39.1.** Indications for cardiac catheterization and arteriography in survivors of acute myocardial infarction. CHF = congestive heart failure; LVEF = left ventricular ejection fraction; VT = ventricular tachycardia.

## Differential Diagnosis

The initial presentation of AMI may be confused with several conditions, including acute pulmonary embolism, aortic dissection, acute pericarditis, acute pancreatitis, biliary colic, and ruptured peptic ulcer. When characteristic evolutionary ECG changes and rising serum cardiac markers are seen, the diagnosis of AMI is obvious.

## Natural History and Prognosis

Most deaths from AMI occur during the first 24 hours, and two-thirds of these occur during the first hour. Over 50% of all AMI deaths occur before the patients reach a hospital, with ventricular fibrillation causing most fatalities. For patients admitted to a coronary care unit, the hospital mortality is 8–10%, mostly during the first 48 hours. The in-hospital mortality declines progressively, and subsequent mortality depends on patient age, severity of LV dysfunction and coexisting diseases. Poor prognostic indicators are listed in Table 39.3.

## Management

The major management goals are: a) to relieve the symptoms, b) to reduce mortality by promptly detecting, treating and, where possible, preventing ventricular fibrillation and limiting infarct size, c) to rehabilitate patients for return to a normal life and d) to prevent progression of underlying atherosclerosis.

**TABLE 39.3. Indicators of Adverse Outcome in Acute MI**

| |
|---|
| Age >70 years |
| Heart failure ($S_3$ gallop, sinus tachycardia, rales, cardiomegaly, radiographic evidence of pulmonary congestion) |
| History of prior angina |
| Hypotension |
| History of prior MI |
| High enzyme rise |
| LV ejection fraction <40% |
| Persistent occlusion or reocclusion of infarct-related artery |
| Silent ischemia |
| Recurrent angina |
| ECG signs |
| Anterior location of infarct |
| Complex ventricular arrhythmias |
| Bundle branch block |
| Second- or third-degree AV block |
| Number of leads with ST elevation |
| Abnormal signal-averaged ECG |
| Associated diseases |
| Diabetes mellitus |
| Hypertension |
| Pulmonary disease |

Resuscitation promptly undertaken by trained bystanders or rescue personnel can reduce the prehospital mortality from AMI. Trained paramedics can also administer morphine for pain, atropine for bradyarrhyth-

**TABLE 39.4. Initial Management of Suspected Acute MI in the Emergency Department***

1. Establish the diagnosis
   Concise history and examination
   12-lead ECG and enzymes
2. Assess hemodynamic status (BP, rhythm, organ perfusion)
3. If ST elevation is present, administer 0.4 mg nitroglycerin sublingually, x 3 doses 5 min apart; repeat 12-lead ECG (avoid nitroglycerin if there is hypotension)
4. Obtain IV access
5. Start continuous ECG monitoring
6. Administer soluble aspirin, 325 mg po[†]
7. Start supplemental $O_2$, 4–6 L/min by nasal cannula
8. Initiate reperfusion strategy: IV thrombolytic treatment as soon as acute MI is diagnosed (ST elevation and no contraindications) or direct coronary angioplasty
9. Administer morphine sulfate for pain relief
10. Administer metoprolol if there is no contraindication
11. Admit to Coronary Care Unit
12. Emergency cardiology consult for possible direct coronary angioplasty/intra-aortic balloon counter pulsation (if hemodynamically unstable, severe heart failure, cardiogenic shock)

*These steps should be undertaken promptly and nearly simultaneously.
[†]Aspirin alone reduces early mortality by 21%.

**TABLE 39.5. Comparison of Various Fibrinolytic Agents**

| | SK | r-PA | rt-PA |
|---|---|---|---|
| Dose (IV) | 1.5 MU in 1 hr | 10 U given 30-min apart | 15–mg bolus; 0.75 mg/kg over next 30 min; then 0.5 mg/kg over next 60 min. |
| Recanalization | 50% | 75% | 75% |
| Hypotension | 5% | None | None |
| Half-life | 18 min | 14 min | 4 min |
| Allergic reaction(s) | Yes | No | No |
| Fibrinogen depletion | Severe | Mild | Moderate |
| Intracranial bleeding | 0.4% | 0.5% | 0.5% |
| Cost per dose | $100 | $2,200 | $2,200 |

SK = streptokinase, r-PA = reteplase, rt-PA = recombinant tissue plasminogen activator

mias, and lidocaine—and perform defibrillation—for ventricular arrhythmias. The initial management of suspected AMI after patients arrive at the emergency department is outlined in Table 39.4. Caring for patients in the coronary care unit (CCU) with continuous ECG monitoring helps identify and promptly treat arrhythmias, thus reducing arrhythmia-related hospital deaths.

Ischemia induced LV dysfunction is the major cause of in-hospital morbidity and mortality. Irreversible ischemic myocardial damage is nearly complete in 6 hours after the onset of AMI. However, in the early hours, a sizable amount of myocardium within the threatened area is still viable, with the potential for either recovery or necrosis, depending on the myocardial $O_2$ supply/demand balance. Pharmacologic agents (nitrates, β-blockers) can lower $O_2$ demands but their ability to salvage myocardium is limited. Because coronary thrombosis is the immediate cause of most AMIs, recent therapeutic interventions have aimed at restoring blood flow in the infarct-related artery. The degree of myocardial salvage correlates directly with the rapidity of flow resumption: ***So early reperfusion has become the mainstay of treatment for AMI.***

### Reperfusion therapy

*Fibrinolytic agents*

With successful reperfusion, chest pain and ST-segment elevation resolve and the CK and CK-MB levels peak earlier (about 12 hours). Large-scale trials of fibrinolytic agents have shown improvement in early and late mortality as well as preservation of LV function (Table 39.5). Also, patients with sustained patency of an infarct-related artery show less ventricular remodeling, infarct expansion, aneurysm formation, and late-potentials on signal-averaged ECG.

The indications and contraindications to fibrinolytic therapy are listed in Tables 39.6 and 39.7. Aspirin (160–325 mg/d), given concurrently, enhances the benefits of all fibrinolytic agents. Also, heparin, given in conjunction with tissue plasminogen activator (tPA) for 3–5 days, reduces the rate of reocclusion of infarct-related artery. Fibrinolytic agents may cause hypotension, bleeding, and intracranial hemorrhage. The incidence of hemorrhagic stroke with tPA is approximately 0.4–0.5%. The elderly and patients with hypertension (BP > 180/110) are more susceptible to hemorrhagic stroke.

Patients should be followed closely, with a 12-lead ECG about 90 minutes after starting fibrinolytic therapy. Rescue percutaneous intervention should be considered in patients who do not respond to fibrinolytic agents (continuing chest pain and/or persistent ST-segment elevation). Others should undergo cardiac catheterization only if angina or other evidence of myocardial ischemia recurs.

*Percutaneous coronary intervention (PCI)*

Direct (primary) PCI consisting of angioplasty and/or stenting is highly successful in opening infarct-related artery, restoring myocardial flow, relieving symptoms, preserving LV function, and reducing mortality. The indications for PCI are shown in Table 39.8.

**TABLE 39.6. Indications for Use of Fibrinolytic Agents**

- Typical chest pain lasting > 30 min, suggestive of acute MI
- 2 mm ST segment elevation in at least 2 contiguous precordial ECG leads (>1 mm in standard leads) and within 12 hrs of onset of chest pain

**TABLE 39.7. Contraindications to Fibrinolytic Therapy**

| Absolute | Relative |
|---|---|
| Active internal bleeding | Peptic ulcer disease |
| History of major GI or GU bleeding | Significant liver disease |
| Recent stroke (<8 wks) | Remote stroke >8 weeks |
| Major bleeding diathesis | Chronic renal failure |
| History of cerebral hemorrhage | Uncontrolled hypertension (>180/110 mmHg) |
| Intracranial tumor | Recent (<2 wks) biopsy, lumbar puncture, thoracentesis, paracentesis |
| Major surgery, trauma, head injury within 8 wks | Major arterial puncture, dental extraction |
| Prolonged or traumatic CPR within 2 weeks | Left heart thrombus |
| Diabetic or other hemorrhagic retinopathy | Oral anticoagulants |
| Acute pericarditis | Infective endocarditis |

**Routine care of patients in cardiac care units**

Most cases of uncomplicated AMI require 1–3 days of care in the cardiac care unit (CCU) and 6–7 days in the hospital. The general care of these patients in the CCU is summarized in Table 39.9.

*Drug therapy in the CCU*

Drug therapy consists mainly of analgesics, antithrombotic agents, β-blockers, nitrates, and angiotensin-converting enzyme (ACE) inhibitors.

Unless contraindicated, **aspirin,** 160–325 mg/day, is highly recommended at first patient contact and should be continued indefinitely. Given early in AMI, aspirin reduces hospital mortality by 21%. Even when given later, it reduces the long-term risk of AMI recurrence and cardiac death. **Clopidogrel** may be substituted when aspirin is contraindicated.

For pain relief, **morphine sulfate** is given 2–4mg IV every 5 minutes until pain is fully relieved or a total of 20 mg is given. Morphine, being vagotonic and sympatholytic, in excessive doses may cause hypotension, bradycardia, respiratory depression, nausea, and vomiting. Because persistent pain may denote ongoing myocardial ischemia, nitroglycerin (sublingually followed by

**TABLE 39.8. Indications for Direct PCI**

1. Thrombolytic agents contraindicated
2. Patients with acute MI in high-risk subsets:
   - Cardiogenic shock
   - Heart failure
   - Large anterior wall MI
3. Inferior wall MI complicated by:
   - Posterior extension
   - Right ventricular infarction
   - Third-degree AV block

Abbreviations: AV = atrioventricular; MI = myocardial infarction; PCI = percutaneous coronary intervention.

TABLE 39.9. Routine Care of Patients in Cardiac Care Units

| | |
|---|---|
| Complete bed rest (advisable) | First 24 h |
| Sit at bedside with or without assistance | Next 24 h, if improving |
| Bathroom privileges: | |
| Bedside commode | Unless contraindicated |
| Bladder catheterization | Avoid unless voiding is difficult |
| Supplemental oxygen by nasal prongs or mask | 2–4 L/min |
| IV fluids: | |
| Start IV access; keep open with 5% dextrose in 0.45% saline | Slow |
| Diet: | |
| Liquid (1000 calories) | First 24–48 h |
| Soft, easily digestible diet | After 24–48 h |
| Daily $Na^{++}$ | <4 g |
| Calorie restriction | If overweight |
| Stool softener: | |
| Bisacodyl (dioctyl calcium sulfosuccinate) (or milk of magnesia) | 200 mg |
| Patient education/behavior modification: | |
| Risk factor modification | Begin in CCU |
| Smoking | Forbidden |
| Alcohol | Forbidden |
| Prevention of venous thromboembolism: | Many measures |
| Full or prophylactic anticoagulation | |
| Thromboembolism stockings | |
| Pneumatic compression devices | |

IV) and β-blockers may also be given to relieve pain; however, hypotension *must* be avoided.

Bedrest predisposes to venous thromboembolism, and systemic embolism can follow the formation of a LV mural thrombus. Passive leg movements, early ambulation, and anticoagulation can prevent these complications. Full-dose intravenous **heparin** is given for 2–5 days, maintaining an activated partial thromboplastin time (aPTT) at 1.5–2.0 times control, especially in high-risk patients with prior thromboembolism, large anterior or apical MIs, heart failure, shock, atrial fibrillation, cardiomegaly, obesity, LV mural thrombi or when prolonged bed-rest is anticipated. Low molecular weight heparin (e.g., enoxaparin) is being increasingly used in place of unfractionated heparin. Heparin is followed by warfarin for at least 3 months, maintaining an INR level at 2.0–3.0. Long-term oral anticoagulation remains controversial especially in patients without atrial fibrillation. However, it should definitely be considered in patients with atrial fibrillation and others at high risk of thromboembolism.

**β-blockers** improve the myocardial $O_2$ supply/demand ratio, relieve ischemic pain, prevent arrhythmias, limit infarct size and reduce early as well as long-term incidence of non-fatal MI and mortality—with or without the use of fibrinolytic therapy. During the early hours of AMI, IV metoprolol is started at 5 mg every 5 minutes for 3 doses, followed by 50–100 mg orally twice daily. β-blockers without intrinsic sympathomimetic activity reduce sudden cardiac death and reinfarction rates (Table 31.7). Therefore, unless contraindicated, long-term β-blockers are strongly advocated in all AMI survivors, especially high-risk cases with tachyarrhythmias, recurrent angina, and impaired LV function.

**Nitroglycerin** is advisable when AMI is associated with hypertension, persistent or recurrent ischemia and/or heart failure. Early nitrate therapy also reduces the degree of LV remodeling. The infusion may be initiated at 5 mcg/min and gradually increased to reduce systolic blood pressure by approximately 10% from the baseline. The infusion should be given for 24–48 hours followed by oral or topical nitrates in patients with large MI and heart failure.

**ACE inhibitors** prevent LV remodeling, heart failure and reinfarction in patients with a LV ejection fraction less than 40%. Unless there is hypotension, captopril is started at 6.25 mg three times daily and increased up to 50 mg three times daily.

## Complications

### Postinfarction angina and infarct extension

Recurrent ischemic pain after relief of initial MI pain really represents unstable angina. It may be either ischemia in a vascular territory distant from the infarct ("ischemia-at-a-distance") or peri-infarction ischemia (in the same vascular territory as the infarct). ST-T changes during angina in leads without Q waves suggest ischemia-at-a-distance, indicating high risk. Urgent coronary angiography and suitable myocardial revascularization are indicated in all patients with recurrent post-MI angina, because such patients are at high risk for reinfarction and sudden death.

Infarct extension indicates occurrence of another MI within 3 weeks of the preceding one. Generally, ECG changes occur in the same leads, as the previous MI. Extension should be treated as a new AMI.

#### Cardiac arrhythmias

Atrial arrhythmias can result from sinus node ischemia, increased vagal tone, or due to LV failure.

**Sinus bradycardia** is common in early acute inferior-wall MI. When associated with hypotension, premature ventricular contractions or accelerated junctional or idioventricular rhythm, atropine (0.4–1.0 mg IV, repeated in 2 hours if necessary) is given, and if there is no response, a temporary pacemaker is placed. **Sinus tachycardia** is often due to heart failure, pulmonary embolism, pericarditis, or anemia.

**Atrial tachycardia, atrial flutter,** and **atrial fibrillation** are due to LV failure or atrial ischemia. These arrhythmias cause very rapid ventricular rates and hemodynamic impairment or angina and should be treated by electric countershock. The ventricular rate may be controlled in asymptomatic or mildly symptomatic patients by β-blockers, digoxin, or calcium channel blockers.

**Premature ventricular complexes** (PVCs) and other ventricular arrhythmias occur in almost 90% of patients with acute MI, but only symptomatic or sustained arrhythmias are treated. In these patients, serum potassium and magnesium levels should be maintained in the high-normal range. β-blockers also may help reduce the frequency of ventricular arrhythmias. Ventricular fibrillation occurs in 15–20% of patients with acute MI.

Primary **ventricular tachycardia** and **ventricular fibrillation** (due to acute ischemia) occur within the first 48 hours of MI and usually do not recur. Secondary ventricular tachycardia and fibrillation, which occur in the presence of predisposing factors (e.g., heart failure, shock, bundle branch block, or LV aneurysm) occur later than 48 h after MI, tend to be recurrent, carry poor prognosis, and require electrophysiologic testing for definitive therapy. Either situation requires immediate treatment.

When ventricular tachycardia develops, IV lidocaine is the drug of choice; if it fails, IV amiodarone or IV procainamide is generally effective. Ventricular tachycardia with stable hemodynamics should be treated with drugs first, and if refractory to drug therapy or associated with hemodynamic impairment, it should be treated by electric countershock (100 W-sec). Prophylactic lidocaine, although controversial, may be considered in patients below 70 years of age who are admitted during the first 6 hours of MI, because ventricular tachycardia or ventricular fibrillation is more frequent in early MI.

#### Conduction disturbances

Nodal and infranodal atrioventricular (AV) blocks may complicate acute MI. Because the right coronary artery supplies the inferior LV wall, AV node, and His bundle, these structures usually sustain ischemia in **acute inferior-wall MI,** leading to **first-degree-, second-degree-,** or **third-degree AV block.** The block is located in the AV node, and therefore with third-degree (complete) AV block, an escape rhythm usually arises from the His bundle, with a stable rate of 50–60 beats/min. These blocks are generally transient, lasting 2–3 days. Atropine or a temporary pacemaker is advisable if the escape rate is unusually slow and accompanied by hypotension or ventricular arrhythmias. Acute inferior-wall MI with third-degree AV block carries a mortality of 25–40%.

Occlusion of the left anterior descending artery leads to **anterior-wall MI,** which affects the right bundle and left anterior fascicle of the left bundle. These bundle-branch blocks (usually bifascicular, with left axis deviation and right bundle branch block) may progress to Mobitz type II and third-degree AV blocks. Complete heart block in acute anterior-wall MI invokes a slow and unstable escape rhythm from the distal bundle branches or Purkinje fibers, which often degenerates into ventricular fibrillation. Given the much greater myocardial damage in anterior MI, complete heart block in this setting is lethal in 70% of patients. A temporary pacemaker, while advisable when complete heart block or right bundle branch block (with or without left hemiblock) complicates the early course of anterior MI, does not reduce the high mortality because this conduction abnormality is merely symptomatic of necrosis of a relatively large amount of myocardium. Complete heart block in acute MI may last up to 2 weeks, but bundle-branch blocks may persist for longer periods of time, indicating a higher risk of recurrent complete heart block and sudden death during the ensuing year. Permanent pacemakers may be of benefit, particularly in patients with anterior wall MI who had transient high-grade atrioventricular block and continue to show bifascicular bundle branch block.

#### Heart failure

High LV filling pressures, due to either decreased compliance or heart failure, usually accompany acute MI. Large MIs (myocardial loss >28%) evoke a process of initial infarct expansion and later enlargement of normal myocardial regions, termed **ventricular remodeling,**

TABLE 39.10. Differential Diagnosis of a Systolic Murmur Developing During the Course of a Myocardial Infarction

| Ruptured Ventricular Septum | Mitral Regurgitation (MR) |
|---|---|
| More common after anterior wall MI | More common after inferior wall MI |
| Presents with severe congestive heart failure and shock | Involves papillary muscle (dysfunction or rupture) |
| Systolic murmur/thrill | Murmur generally audible in dysfunction, but may not be heard at all in rupture; rupture causes acute left heart failure, pulmonary edema, and hypotension |
| Doppler echo may be very useful | Echo shows MR |
| Prominent *v* **wave in LA pressure tracings** | ↑ LA pressure and *v* **wave in pressure tracings** |
| Step up in $SaO_2$ on moving catheter from RA into RV | No step-up in $SaO_2$ from RA into RV |

Abbreviations: Echo = echocardiography; LA = left atrium; RA = right atrium; RV = right ventricle; $SaO_2$ = $O_2$ saturation.

which causes heart failure. The degree of remodeling and severity of heart failure correlate with the amount of myocardium lost.

Oral or IV furosemide usually adequately controls symptoms of mild heart failure. In severe cases or pulmonary edema, furosemide or bumetanide is given IV, and if the blood pressure is normal, nitroglycerin or IV sodium nitroprusside may also be considered. Blood pressure, heart rhythm, urine flow, hemodynamics, blood urea nitrogen, creatinine, electrolytes, and serial chest radiographs are monitored. Unless there are atrial arrhythmias, digitalis is not very useful. Coexisting severe heart failure and cardiogenic shock call for dopamine or dobutamine (inotropic support). Ventricular septal or papillary muscle rupture should be detected early (see Mechanical Complications below).

### Right ventricular infarction

Approximately 35% of patients with inferior or posterior LV infarction also sustain a RV infarction. In patients with inferior-wall MI, an ST elevation in right-sided lead $V_4$ is highly suggestive of this entity. Its distinct hemodynamic pattern includes hypotension, markedly elevated right atrial and systemic venous pressures (jugular venous distention), equalization of diastolic pressures, and low cardiac output. Pulmonary capillary wedge pressure may be normal or moderately high. In most cases, hypotension improves on volume expansion; inotropic agents and AV sequential pacemaker may rarely be needed.

### Mechanical complications

**Ventricular septal rupture** occurs in 3% of cases of acute MI, usually in the first week after infarction. This catastrophe leads to a sudden, loud pansystolic murmur over the left lower parasternal area and severe congestive heart failure and/or cardiogenic shock. The differential diagnosis is from acute mitral regurgitation (MR) due to a ruptured papillary muscle (Table 39.10). Complete rupture of the body of the papillary muscle causes shock and rapid death. When the tip of one of the heads of the papillary muscle ruptures, acute MR follows with heart failure and/or cardiogenic shock; death may occur several days or weeks later.

In MR and septal rupture, the circulation should be rapidly stabilized with IV nitroprusside and intra-aortic balloon counterpulsation, followed by urgent coronary arteriography and left ventriculography, and then urgent surgical repair of the septal defect or valve. Coronary bypass surgery is also often required.

Rupture of the **LV free wall** causes 10% of all deaths in acute MI. More common in elderly, hypertensive women, it sometimes follows severe cough or straining at stool. Most patients die suddenly, and others, perhaps only with a slow oozing of blood, may survive for a few hours or days. Most patients report ongoing or recurrent chest pain from myocardial ischemia or pericarditis. A pericardial friction rub may be heard. The peripheral pulses may be thready, and neck veins grossly distended from cardiac tamponade. Electromechanical dissociation is common (see below). Hemopericardium evokes intense vagotonia with sinus bradycardia and AV junctional rhythm. When suspected, immediate pericardiocentesis, saline, and isoproterenol infusion, followed by emergency repair of the rupture, could be life-saving.

### Cardiogenic shock

A detailed discussion of cardiogenic shock follows in chapter 47.

### Electromechanical dissociation

In electromechanical dissociation (pulseless electrical activity), the force of ventricular contraction is severely impaired, despite regular electrical activity. This usually fatal condition occurs in acute mitral regurgitation due to ruptured body of the papillary muscle, massive pulmonary embolism, massive hemopericardium due to LV free wall rupture, after prolonged cardiopulmonary bypass, and in severe three-vessel coronary disease.

**Pericarditis**

Pericarditis often complicates acute MI, usually within the first 4 days, and is characterized by dull, achy precordial pain, which is worsened by stooping, bending, or breathing (pericardial-type chest pain), and atrial arrhythmias. The pericardial friction rub is usually evanescent. ECG may show diffuse ST-T changes. Salicylates, indomethacin, or a short course of corticosteroids promptly resolve various features of pericarditis. Anticoagulants are contraindicated.

**Thromboembolic complications**

A mural thrombus may form at the site of endocardial injury due to infarction and is seen much more often in anterior-wall MI (33%) than inferior-wall MI (2%). Systemic embolism may follow in a few days to weeks in high-risk cases (large anterior MI, congestive heart failure, or shock). While high-risk cases require full-dose heparin followed by short-term oral anticoagulation, all patients with acute MI should receive prophylaxis against venous thromboembolism from the legs and pelvis.

**Dressler's syndrome (postmyocardial infarction syndrome)**

Presumed to be an immunologic reaction to necrotic myocardium, Dressler's syndrome complicates about 3% of all cases of acute MI. Beginning most often 2 weeks to several months after an MI, it features recurrent fever, pericardial-type chest pain, pericardial friction rub, atrial arrhythmias, leukocytosis, and bloody pericardial and/or pleural fluid. Despite the recurrences, constrictive pericarditis is unlikely. Acute attacks are treated with aspirin, indomethacin, or steroids.

**True and false aneurysms of the left ventricle**

Left ventricular true aneurysm following Q-wave MI usually involves the anterolateral or apical segments and, when large, can cause congestive heart failure, systemic emboli from a mural thrombus, and/or ventricular arrhythmias. Large aneurysms produce abnormal chest wall pulsations. Chest radiographs may show a bulge on the left heart border and, occasionally, calcification in the aneurysm wall or mural thrombus. On ECG, persistent ST-segment elevation may be seen in leads showing Q waves. LV aneurysms carry an unfavorable long-term prognosis. Resection of aneurysm is indicated in cases of intractable heart failure and ventricular tachycardia despite medical therapy, or in recurrent systemic emboli despite anticoagulation; however, it is possible only if the remaining LV shows normal wall motion.

Rarely, the LV free wall ruptures, but the blood leakage into the pericardium is slow and contained by pericardial-epicardial adhesions. Such **pseudo-aneurysms,** whose walls have only pericardium, enlarge over time and may rupture fatally. Therefore, they should be corrected surgically.

## Non–ST Segment Elevation Myocardial Infarction

Traditionally, MIs were classified as **transmural,** if the ECG showed ST segment elevation and Q-waves, or **nontransmural** (subendocardial), if the ECG showed only ST segment depression and/or T-wave inversion. Because it is difficult to predict from the ECG whether a given MI is transmural (full ventricular wall thickness) or only subendocardial, MIs are presently categorized simply as **ST-segment Elevation MI** or **Non–ST-segment Elevation MI,** each having different pathoanatomy, prognosis and modes of treatment (Table 39.11). In non-ST segment elevation MI, the early mortality is lower, and myocardial damage relatively smaller with preservation of LV function. The infarct-related artery is usually open, albeit severely stenosed; if it is totally occluded, collateral flow is usually present. Given the relatively large amount of viable but threatened myocardium, these patients may suffer recurrent episodes of angina and reinfarction. These patients are usually grouped together with patients with unstable angina. Management in both conditions is similar.

### Predischarge Evaluation

The average 1-year mortality after hospital discharge is 10–15%. The risk for recurrent angina and reinfarction varies widely in post-MI patients, but most patients likely to develop these complications do so within the first 3 months after hospital discharge.

Before discharge, patients without clinical heart failure, LV dysfunction, or post-MI angina and arrhythmias should undergo a low-level exercise stress test, which is safe and helps to classify patients based on risk. Patients with a positive test (ST depression >1 mm,

**TABLE 39.11. Important Differences Between Non ST Elevation MI and ST Elevation MI**

| | Non-ST Elevation MI | ST Elevation MI |
|---|---|---|
| Patency of infarct-related artery | High | Low |
| Amount of myocardial damage | Small | Large |
| Incidence of recurrent angina and reinfarction | High | Low |
| In-hospital mortality | 2–5% | 5–10% |
| One-year mortality | 29% | 10–20% |

angina, systolic hypotension) should have coronary arteriography, and those with a clearly negative test can be safely managed on medical therapy.

### Posthospitalization Period

The goal in the posthospitalization period is to rehabilitate the patient physically and emotionally to return to work. Most patients with uncomplicated MI can safely return to work in 1–2 weeks. Minor chores are allowed, but not isometric exercise. The level of activity achieved later during the hospitalization should be maintained, and the pace and duration of exercise slowly increased. The development of angina, dyspnea, or undue fatigue generally implies that the exercise level should be reduced.

A symptom-limited exercise stress test 3–6 weeks after discharge can establish safe limits of activity and determine the level of exercise for body-conditioning programs. Achieving cardiovascular training requires 30 minutes of dynamic exercise (preferably involving both arms and legs, including warm-up and cool-down periods) 3 times weekly on alternate days, which attains 70% of a safely attained maximal heart rate during a symptom-limited stress test. Besides enabling extended work with a smaller rise in pulse and blood pressure, these long-term training programs enhance the patient's sense of well-being. Uncontrolled hypertension, heart failure, arrhythmias, and disabling angina are contraindications to exercise training and should be controlled before a high-intensity training program is begun.

### Secondary Prevention

Long-term use of β-blockers clearly reduces reinfarction and sudden death rates significantly (26–34%) in post-MI patients. Most cardiologists now recommend prophylactic β-blockers (unless contraindicated) for all intermediate-risk and high-risk patients following MI. Aspirin and oral anticoagulants provide long-term cardioprotection. Risk/benefit considerations, however, will dictate continuing aspirin indefinitely. ACE inhibitors can prevent heart failure and recurrent MI in patients with reduced LV function. Patients who continue cigarette smoking following MI increase their mortality by 25–50%. Besides modifying diet to achieve ideal body weight and reduce serum cholesterol levels, drug therapy should be undertaken to control hypertension and hyperlipidemia.

## Unstable Angina

In essence, worsening of previously stable angina, new-onset angina or angina occurring at rest represent unstable angina (Table 39.12). It is a very common syndrome, falling between chronic stable angina on one hand and the intense and prolonged pain of AMI on the other. Unstable angina portends a higher risk of AMI and sudden cardiac death—an important distinction from chronic stable angina.

**TABLE 39.12. Patterns of Unstable Angina**

1. New onset of severe angina (Class III or IV) within the previous 2 months
2. Worsening of previous stable angina to Class III or IV angina within the previous 2 months
3. Rest angina (usually prolonged ≥ 20 min) within the past 1 week
4. Post-myocardial infarction angina (>24 hours)
5. Variant angina

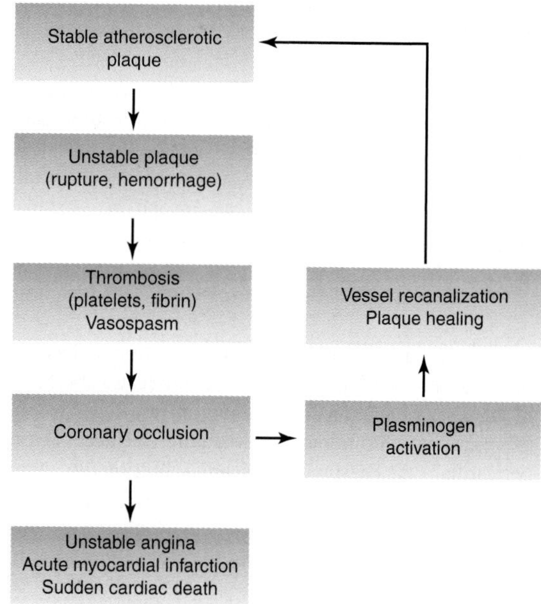


**FIGURE 39.2.** Pathogenesis of unstable angina.

### Pathogenesis

When extracardiac factors, such as anemia, tachyarrhythmias, hypertension, increased physical or emotional stress, and hyperthyroidism are excluded as contributory causes, unstable angina implies reduced coronary blood flow, most commonly due to formation of a nonocclusive, platelet-rich thrombus over a disrupted atherosclerotic plaque (Figure 39.2). Atherosclerotic plaques vulnerable to rupture are typically eccentric, rich in extracellular lipids within a large lipid pool and have a thin fibrous cap. Various metalloproteinases such as collagenases and elastases degrade the fibrous cap followed by its rupture and exposure of highly thrombogenic lipid pool to flowing blood. Inflammation is considered a prominent component of the unstable plaque. Plaque rupture stimulates activation, adhesion and aggregation of platelets as well as release of tissue factor, which in turn initiates coagulation cascade leading to the formation of platelet-rich thrombus. Vasospasm, severe stenosis or arteritis of coronary vessels less commonly cause unstable angina.

#### Diagnosis

The history is crucial to the diagnosis of unstable angina (Table 39.12). An atrial gallop and apical systolic murmur of mitral insufficiency may be audible during an episode of acute ischemia. The ECG may show ST-segment and T-wave changes. Generally, the ST-T changes accompany the episodes of chest pain and may normalize with relief of pain. Serum cardiac markers, especially total CK and CK-MB, are within normal range. However, cardiac specific troponin-T and troponin-I (cTnT and cTnI, respectively) may be slightly elevated.

Coronary angiography generally reveals multivessel CAD, with left main stenosis being found in 10% of patients. The angiographic appearances commonly suggest ruptured coronary plaques with associated thrombi. Coronary arteries are normal in 5–20% of cases, and in a significant number of these, vasospasm may be responsible for acute myocardial ischemia.

Left ventricular ejection fraction and segmental wall motion may be entirely normal in the absence of active ischemia. However, segmental wall motion abnormalities are usually present if critical stenoses compromise resting coronary flow (hibernating myocardium). Nitroglycerin administration by abolishing ischemia may improve left ventricular abnormalities.

#### Natural History

Adverse prognostic factors with an enhanced risk of myocardial infarction and mortality are summarized in Table 39.13. The overall mortality and AMI during hospitalization is 1–2% and 5–15%, respectively. Over a 30-month follow-up, a mortality rate of 10% and MI rate of 19% are noted. The acute phase of unstable angina usually lasts 3–4 months.

#### Management

In patients with unstable angina, treatment with anti-thrombotic and anti-ischemic agents is the first-line therapy to prevent thrombus extension, eliminate vasospasm and decrease myocardial oxygen demand. Symptom severity, hemodynamic status, history of prior revascularization procedures and drug therapy, coexistent medical conditions and above all the prognostic category impact the choice, timing, and aggressiveness of management (Figure 39.3).

Low risk patients indicated by normal or unchanged ECG; the absence of severe, prolonged (>20 min), or rest angina within the preceding 2 weeks; absence of heart failure or significant arrythmias, absence of elevated serum cardiac biomarkers such as cTnI can be medically managed (antiplatelet and anti-ischemic agents) on an ambulatory basis and further evaluated within 72 hours with a noninvasive stress test.

Patients with intermediate and high risk should be admitted to an intensive care unit and promptly started on the following therapy:

1. Antiplatelet agents. **Acetylsalicylic acid (ASA)** should be initiated immediately (160–325 mg/day). It prevents the formation of thromboxane A2 by irreversibly inhibiting cyclooxygenase-1 within platelets, thereby diminishing platelet aggregation. ASA reduces death or MI by 50–70% in unstable angina. **Thienopyridine drugs (ticlopidine, clopidogrel)** can be used in patients intolerant to ASA. They inhibit ADP receptors and prevent transformation of GP 2b/3a receptors into the high affinity stage. The antiplatelet efficacy of these agents is similar to that of ASA. Ticlopidine is associated with serious adverse effects such as neutropenia (2.4% patients)

**TABLE 39.13. Adverse Prognostic Factors in Unstable Angina***

| | |
|---|---|
| History | Age >65 years<br>Recurrent prolonged (>20 min) rest angina<br>Previous myocardial infarction |
| Physical examination | Hypotension<br>Cardiomegaly<br>New mitral regurgitation murmur<br>Heart failure (pulmonary edema, $S_3$, crackles) |
| Ancillary studies | ST-T changes in ECG<br>Complex ventricular arrhythmias<br>Elevated cTnI or cTnT<br>Low left ventricular ejection fraction<br>Large perfusion defect<br>Perfusion defects in > 1 vascular territories |
| Cardiac catheterization | Critical multivessel or left main disease<br>Abnormal LVEDP<br>↓ cardiac output<br>↓ left ventricular ejection fraction |

*Short-term risk of death or non-fatal myocardial infarction.
LVEDP = left ventricular end-diastolic pressure

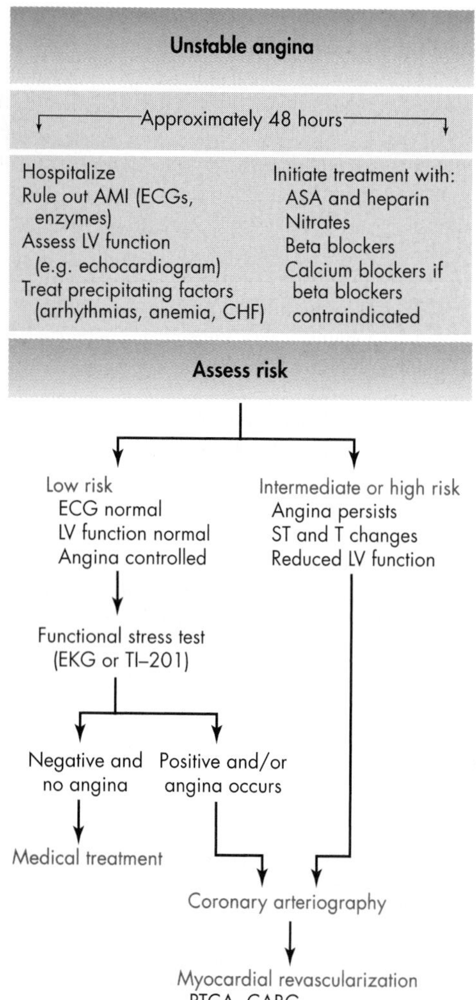


**FIGURE 39.3. Management strategies in unstable angina. AMI = acute myocardial infarction; ASA = aspirin; CHF = congestive heart failure.**

and thrombotic thrombocytopenic purpura (TTP). When compared to ticlopidine, clopidogrel has a more rapid onset of action and longer half-life with a much safer side effect profile. **Glycoprotein 2b/3a receptor antagonists (abciximab, eptifibatide, tirofiban)** by occupying the GP 2b/3a receptor sites on the platelets prevent fibrinogen binding and, thereby, platelet aggregation. These agents have been shown to significantly reduce death or MI in high-risk patients especially when PCI is performed.

2. Anticoagulants. In combination with ASA, **unfractionated heparin (UFH)** given for 2 to 5 days in patients with unstable angina has been shown to reduce the relative risk of death and MI by 56% and 33% respectively. The usually recommended dose is 60–80 U/kg as a bolus followed by 12–18 U/kg/h infusion rate to maintain the aPTT in the range of 1.5 to 2.0 times control. **Low molecular weight haparins (LMWH)** have been shown to be more beneficial, safer as well as easier to administer than UFH.

3. Anti-ischemic agents. **Nitroglycerin infusion** (10–200 mcg/min, goal is relief of chest pain or reduction of systolic BP by 10% from baseline) and adequate doses of **β-blockers** (target heart rate of 50–60 beats/min) should be initiated. Patients with an intermediate risk can be given medications orally. Rate-limiting calcium channel entry blockers (diltiazem, verapamil) can be used in patients with contraindications to beta-blockers.

Serial ECGs and serum cardiac markers should be monitored to detect AMI and LV function assessed by echocardiography. In most patients, ischemic symptoms are controlled with intensive medical treatment. If they remain symptom-free and hemodynamically stable during the 24 hours, they can be moved from the intensive care unit. Patients with prior revascularization procedures, LV ejection fraction below 0.5, heart failure, hypotension, malignant ventricular arrhythmias or severe AV block, recurrent angina or ST-T changes, and new mitral regurgitation murmur, should undergo coronary arteriography. The remaining patients can undergo a stress test for further triage. Coronary angiography should be performed in patients with ischemic response on functional testing or those with inconclusive results.

Other entities such as aortic dissection and pulmonary embolism should be ruled out if the initial chest pain does not respond to treatment within 30 minutes. If intractable myocardial ischemia is still the most likely possibility, the patient should undergo an emergent coronary angiography, preferably in conjunction with intraaortic balloon counterpulsation. Coronary artery bypass surgery or percutaneous coronary intervention should be performed in patients with suitable anatomy.

## Sudden Death

Sudden death is defined as unexpected death occurring instantly or within 1 hour after the onset of symptoms. It is more common in men and most frequently (about 80%) caused by atherosclerotic CAD. Nearly 50–60% of all deaths due to CAD are sudden.

The risk for sudden death is higher with heavy cigarette smoking, hypertension, LV hypertrophy or intraventricular block on ECG, complex ventricular arrhythmias, cardiomegaly, excessive obesity, and stressful lifestyle. About 25% of sudden death patients experience angina, palpitations, undue fatigue, or dyspnea on the day of death.

Ventricular fibrillation is often the immediate mechanism and is often associated with several underlying conditions (Table 39.14). About one-third of the survivors reveal an acute MI. Pathologically, the coronary arteries show severe multivessel disease in most patients and fresh thrombosis over old plaques in about one-third.

Cardiopulmonary resuscitation (CPR) instituted within 3–4 minutes of the onset of ventricular fibrillation can save some lives. Following CPR, patients should be admitted to a CCU for further observation, given the very high recurrence rate of ventricular fibrillation. Coronary angiography is indicated, followed by myocardial revascularization or aggressive anti-ischemic medical therapy. Implantation of cardioverter-defibrillator is the most effective treatment for preventing recurrent cardiac arrest.

**TABLE 39.14. Conditions Associated With Sudden Cardiac Death**

| |
|---|
| Coronary artery disease |
| Atherosclerosis |
| Acute myocardial ischemia |
| Previous MI |
| Congenital anomalies |
| Miscellaneous: spasm, embolism, trauma, dissection, arteritis |
| Myocardial diseases |
| Hypertrophic or dilated cardiomyopathies |
| Infiltrative cardiomyopathies, e.g., sarcoid, tumor, infection, dysplasia |
| Arrhythmogenic right ventricular dysplasia |
| Congenital heart diseases, e.g., tetralogy of Fallot |
| Valvular heart diseases, e.g., aortic stenosis, mitral valve prolapse |
| Electrophysiologic disorders |
| Long QT syndromes |
| Pre-excitation syndromes |
| Conduction system disorders |
| Miscellaneous |
| Acute, massive pulmonary embolism |
| Primary pulmonary hypertension |
| Aortic dissection |
| Severe cardiac tamponade |

# CHAPTER 40 CONGENITAL HEART DISEASES

Congenital heart disease occurs in 0.5 to 1.0% of all live births and, overall, shows a masculine predisposition. Maternal viral illnesses (e.g., rubella) and use of drugs (e.g., thalidomide) in early pregnancy are recognized causes, as well as certain chromosomal anomalies and single gene mutations. Children of affected parents also show a 2-fold to 4-fold rise in prevalence. A classification of these disorders is shown in Table 40.1. The clinical features, natural history, and complications of the more common congenital heart diseases are listed in Table 40.2; various diagnostic studies and therapy of these conditions are summarized in Table 40.3.

## Atrial Septal Defect

Atrial septal defects (ASD), which constitute almost one-third of all congenital heart disease in adults, are classified into several types by their location in the atrial septum (Table 40.4). However, the underlying theme in all ASDs is a shunting of blood from one atrium to the other. The normal fetal shunt is right-to-left through the foramen ovale. Soon after birth, pulmonary arterioles rapidly involute and the RV becomes more compliant. With the change in the inflow resistances of the two ventricles, left-sided filling pressure rises and right-sided filling pressure abates, and the foramen ovale closes functionally. A persistent, abnormal interatrial opening initiates a left-to-right shunt, owing to the gradually decreasing RV inflow resistance (compared to the LV). The size of the defect, the relative resistance in the two circulations, and the relative RV and LV compliance determine the shunt severity. Whereas large defects equalize the atrial pressures, hypertension and coronary disease lower LV compliance and increase the shunt. As age increases, rising pulmonary vascular resistance evokes pulmonary hypertension and RV hypertrophy, which raise the RV inflow resistance and reverse the shunt **(Eisenmenger's syndrome).**

Endocardial cushion defects have many derangements: left-to-right shunt through the ostium primum defect, left-to-right shunt via a ventricular septal defect, shunt from the LV to right atrium, and mitral or tricuspid incompetence through cleft mitral or tricuspid valves.

**TABLE 40.1. Classification of Congenital Heart Diseases**

| |
|---|
| **Abnormal pulmonic-systemic communications** |
| **Left-to-right shunt (acyanotic)** |
| Atrial septal defect |
| Ventricular septal defect |
| Patent ductus arteriosus |
| **Right-to-left shunt (cyanotic)** |
| Decreased pulmonary vascularity |
| Cyanotic type of tetralogy of Fallot |
| Complete transposition of great vessels with severe pulmonic stenosis |
| Increased pulmonary vascularity |
| Complete transposition of great vessels |
| Truncus arteriosus |
| **Vascular and valvular abnormalities** |
| Coarctation of the aorta |
| Aortic stenosis |
| Mitral valve incompetence |
| Pulmonic stenosis |
| Cor triatriatum |
| Ebstein's anomaly |
| **Cardiac malpositions (e.g., dextrocardia)** |

*Not a complete list of all congenital heart diseases.

The relative resistances in the pulmonary and systemic circuits determine the direction of the shunt. Both ventricles face an increased volume work that leads to biventricular failure.

Excess RV stroke volume prolongs RV ejection time, delaying pulmonic valve closure, while a smaller LV stroke volume shortens the LV ejection time, hastening aortic valve closure. The ensuing widely split $S_2$ from the early $A_2$ and late $P_2$ varies little with respiration (fixed split), because venous return to the atria during phases of respiration is equalized across the ASD.

## Ventricular Septal Defect

In adults, ventricular septal defects (VSD) constitute 10% of all congenital abnormalities, being equally frequent in men and women. Nearly 80% of the defects occur in the outflow area of the ventricular septum, between the pulmonary valve and septal tricuspid valve leaflet. The remainder occupy the inflow region (muscular portion) of the septum.

The extent and direction of the shunt depend on the size of the VSD and the relative resistances in the systemic and pulmonary circulations. A large VSD (cross-sectional area equal to that of the aortic valve) causes similar increase of systolic pressures in the LV, aorta, RV, and pulmonary artery and permits free blood flow from the LV to the RV. Thus, in a large VSD, pulmonary hypertension is severe. With the pulmonary vascular resistance well below the systemic levels, a large left-to-right shunt evolves. Volume overload causes the LV to distend and fail. A medium-sized VSD, being more restrictive, raises the RV and pulmonary artery systolic pressures only moderately, whereas in a small VSD, these remain normal. Over the years, large left-to-right shunts and pulmonary hypertension foster obliterative pulmonary vascular disease, raise pulmonary vascular resistance, and ultimately reverse the left-to-right shunt (Eisenmenger's syndrome).

## Patent Ductus Arteriosus

Patent ductus arteriosus (PDA) is the third most common congenital heart disease in adults, and is 2–3 times more common in women. Maternal rubella (German measles) during intrauterine life of the fetus is an etiologic factor. The pulmonary orifice of the ductus is located immediately distal to the bifurcation of the main pulmonary trunk, and the aortic orifice of the ductus lies distal to the origin of the left subclavian artery. In addition to pulmonic stenosis, PDA may occur with aortic coarctation and VSD.

During fetal life, oxygenated maternal blood bypasses the lungs and reaches the aorta via the ductus arteriosus, which closes functionally within several hours to 1 week and anatomically within a few days to several weeks after birth. The functional closure follows an increase in $PaO_2$ and changes in prostaglandins. However, a ductus remaining patent after birth shunts blood from the aorta to the pulmonary artery during both systole and diastole, causing LV volume overload. The caliber of the ductus and level of pulmonary vascular resistance determine the magnitude of the left-to-right shunt.

Other conditions causing a continuous precordial murmur include aortopulmonary septal defect, ruptured aneurysm of the sinus of Valsalva into the right heart chambers, combined aortic regurgitation and VSD, coronary or pulmonary arteriovenous fistula, and cervical venous hum.

## Eisenmenger's Syndrome

Eisenmenger's syndrome represents a reversed or bidirectional shunt through systemic-pulmonary communications, such as VSD, ASD, and PDA, which originally allowed a large left-to-right shunt. In these large left-to-right shunts, pulmonary vascular resistance gradually rises relative to the systemic resistance, thus effacing the left-to-right shunt. When resistances in the two vascular beds equalize, the shunt disappears or becomes bidirectional. If the pulmonary vascular resistance surpasses the systemic, a right-to-left shunt evolves. Pulmonary arterial pressure approaching systemic level imposes a pressure overload on the RV. The pulmonary blood flow decreases and is lower than the systemic, which remains normal.

## Tetralogy of Fallot

In adults, Fallot's tetralogy, or the combination of VSD with pulmonary stenosis, is the most common cyanotic congenital heart disease. It has a wide clinical and physiologic spectrum. At one extreme, pulmonary stenosis is mild to moderate, permitting a left-to-right shunt through the VSD (acyanotic type of tetralogy of Fallot). At the other extreme there is pulmonary atresia leading to right-to-left shunt, and the bronchial collaterals supply the pulmonary circuit. Most cases constitute a cyanotic type of tetralogy of Fallot, with severe pulmonary stenosis causing a right-to-left shunt. In addition to VSD and pulmonary stenosis, RV hypertrophy and a variable degree of overriding of the aorta complete the original tetrad. Pulmonary stenosis is often infundibular and occasionally valvular. Since pulmonary stenosis is progressive, acyanotic tetralogy of Fallot may progress to a cyanotic type.

The degrees of pulmonary valvular obstruction and systemic vascular resistance determine the hemodynamics. As the RV communicates with both the aorta (via its overriding origin) and LV (via VSD), its systolic pressure is always at a systemic level. When the resistance from pulmonary stenosis is low relative to systemic vascular resistance, the shunt is predominantly left to right. As resistance to ejection into the pulmonary artery increases due to progressive pulmonic stenosis, the left-to-right shunt decreases; when the pulmonary resistance exceeds the systemic resistance, the shunt is entirely right to left.

## Transposition of the Great Arteries

In transposition of the great arteries, the septum dividing the aorta from the pulmonary artery develops abnormally, and thus, the aorta arises from the RV, and the pulmonary artery arises from the LV. The aorta is anterior and parallel to a posteriorly located pulmonary artery.

Transposition in its pure form is incompatible with life; survival depends on mixing of blood between the right and left circulations through ASD, VSD, or PDA. Also, because the pulmonary and systemic circulations operate in parallel, rather than in series, the shunt has to be bidirectional. In **corrected transposition of the great arteries,** another congenital heart disease, inversion of the ventricles along with transposition of the great arteries results in physiologic correction of circulation. Systemic venous blood flows into the right atrium, across the mitral valve (bicuspid), into a ventricle having the anatomic characteristics of the LV (fine trabeculation and no infundibulum), and is ejected into the pulmonary artery. Oxygenated blood from pulmonary veins flows into the left atrium, across the tricuspid valve into a ventricle with RV characteristics (coarse trabeculation and an infundibulum), and is ejected into the aorta.

## Coarctation of the Aorta

Coarctation of the aorta occurs in 1 of every 2000 persons and is more common in men. Anatomically, there is a curtain-like infolding of the media that obstructs the blood flow. In the more common adult-type, the obstruction occurs just distal to the origins of the left subclavian artery and ligamentum arteriosum. Coarctation may coexist with bicuspid aortic valve, VSD, mitral regurgitation, endocardial fibroelastosis, cerebral aneurysms, and Turner's syndrome (in 20% of cases). Hypertension, the main feature of coarctation, is due to as-yet unknown mechanisms, but a lack of pulsatile renal blood flow, stimulating the renin-angiotensin system, seems to play a major role. Pseudocoarctation of the aorta (kinking and tortuosity without obstruction) and saddle embolism in the descending aorta should be considered in the differential diagnosis of coarctation of the aorta.

## Pulmonary Stenosis

A valvular type of pulmonary stenosis is the most common type of obstructive disease in the RV outflow tract; supravalvular and subvalvular obstruction is less common. RV hypertrophy follows the RV pressure overload.

## Ebstein's Anomaly

In Ebstein's anomaly, the tricuspid valve tissue is redundant and dysplastic, and the septal and posterior valve leaflets are attached lower than normal. Thus, the upper RV becomes a portion of the right atrium. The tricuspid valve is frequently incompetent, the RV is hypoplastic, and the foramen ovale is patent with a right-to-left shunt.

## Malpositions of the Heart

Normally, the cardiac apex is located on the left side of the midline and is described as levocardia. When the cardiac apex lies on the right side of the midline, it is termed **dextrocardia,** and when it is located in the midline, it is termed **mesocardia.** Generally, no serious abnormality of the heart exists when dextrocardia is a part of **situs inversus** (i.e., mirror-image reversal of all body organs). However, serious congenital heart malformations occur in patients with isolated dextrocardia or in levocardia with situs inversus.

**TABLE 40.2. Clinical Features, Natural History and Complications of Congenital Heart Diseases**

| Lesion | Clinical Features | Natural History | Complications |
|---|---|---|---|
| Atrial septal defect (ASD), ostium secundum type | No symptoms in most; fatigue and dyspnea. Atrial arrhythmias and heart failure after age 40.<br>Thin and frail, usually a child or adolescent; Pulse N or ↓ volume; equal *a* and *v* waves; HDN LPA; $S_1$ N; $S_2$ wide, fixed split; SEM from flow into pulmonary artery; MDM from flow across tricuspid; $S_3$. | Eisenmenger's syndrome in 20%, mostly with advancing age; PH lowers longevity; 1st, 4th and 6th decade mortality of 0.6%, 4.5% and 7.5% respectively. | Eisenmenger's syndrome, PH, Heart failure, atrial arrhythmias. Very low risk of infective endocarditis. |
| Atrial septal defect (ASD), ostium primum type | Heart failure, failure to thrive, and respiratory infections begin in late childhood or adolescence. Atrial fibrillation or flutter initiates heart failure. Symptoms develop during infancy in complete a-v canal defects; Down's syndrome in almost 50%.<br>Cyanosis, poor physical development; JVD if right heart failure; large *a* wave (PH) and *v* wave (from MR or TR or both); precordial bulge and Harrison's groove; holosystolic MR murmur and findings of MR; VSD and MR murmur superimposed. | Primum-type defect and mild MR: same as ostium secundum ASD.<br>If MR more severe, early heart failure. Complete a-v canal defects: heart failure during infancy and early death. | Eisenmenger's syndrome; associated mitral regurgitation enhances the risk of infective endocarditis. |
| Ventricular septal defect (VSD) | No symptoms with small VSD. Dyspnea, fatigue, effort intolerance respiratory infections, failure to thrive.<br>Arterial pulse N or brisk. No JVD; precordial bulge and Harrison's groove (±) HDN apical impulse with large shunts. $S_1$ usually covered by the holosystolic murmur, $S_2$ widely split, $S_3$ with ≥2:1 shunt; brief mid-diastolic murmur; holosystolic murmur in LP area most important sign, murmur only early systolic in very small VSD. | Defect commonly decreases in size and may disappear. Eisenmenger's syndrome rare in children but most frequent in young adults. | Eisenmenger's syndrome, Infective endocarditis, paradoxical embolism. |
| Patent ductus arteriosus (PDA) | No symptoms with small PDA. Heart failure during the third and fourth decades with large L-R shunts. Infective arteritis. Poor development and CHF.<br>Harrison's groove, pigeon chest, and wide pulse pressure with large PDA. Continuous thrill with systolic accentuation in the 1st and 2nd left intercostal spaces; typical rough, continuous (systole-diastole) murmur over the left upper sternal border. $S_3$ and mid-diastolic flow apical murmur from excess diastolic blood flow across the mitral valve. These suggest at least 2:1 L-R shunt. | Small PDA does not affect the cardiovascular system nor shortens longevity. Potential site for infective arteritis. | Eisenmenger's syndrome, PDA aneurysm; infective endarteritis, CHF, frequent respiratory infections and retarded growth. |
| Eisenmenger's syndrome | Symptoms more frequent in large VSD and PDA; onset often during infancy or childhood; in most ASD cases, onset in adulthood; fatigue, exertional dyspnea, angina, syncope, hemoptysis, and right heart failure; squatting (knee/chest position) uncommon. Patients with PDA tolerate it better since the head and neck blood flow maintained; with worsening disease, hemoptysis, predisposition to brain abscess, and strokes.<br>Central cyanosis; in PDA, toenails cyanotic, with pink fingernails (differential cyanosis); clubbing, low volume or normal pulse, "*a*" wave in neck veins and *v* wave with TR; RV heave, right-sided $S_4$, pulmonary ejection click, upper left parasternal SEM; pulmonary valvular incompetence from severe PH (early diastolic [Graham-Steell] murmur); loud $P_2$; $S_2$ narrowly split or absent; signs of right heart failure; tricuspid incompetence; arterial hypoxia, polycythemia, hyperuricemia. | Average survival into the mid thirties; death most commonly from hemoptysis, cardiovascular collapse, and heart failure; pregnancy carries a very high risk of maternal and infant mortality. | Cerebral thrombosis, cerebral abscess, paradoxical embolism and infective endocarditis. |

| | | | |
|---|---|---|---|
| Tetralogy of Fallot | Cyanosis early after birth; dyspnea relieved by squatting; syncope, physical underdevelopment.<br>Clubbing (fingers and toes), arterial and jugular venous pulses, N. $S_1$, N; soft and delayed or totally absent $P_2$, loud $A_2$; aortic ejection click due to a dilated aorta; SEM over the mid-left sternal border (pulmonary stenosis); murmur intensity inversely related to the stenosis severity; continuous murmur of bronchial collaterals over chest wall in severe Fallot's. | Prognosis depends on the magnitude of the R-to-L shunt. Survival into adulthood possible, and survival into the sixties not rare. | Infective endocarditis of pulmonary valve, paradoxical embolism, cerebral abscess and cerebral thrombosis. |
| Transposition of great arteries | More common among men and offspring of diabetic mothers; dyspnea, cyanosis, heart failure, and growth retardation.<br>Anteriorly located aorta causes very loud $A_2$. Associated VSD, PDA, or PS determine type of murmur. | Untreated, nearly 75% die by 6 months of age, and the rest rarely survive adolescence; patients with large ASD or VSD and significant PS may survive infancy. | |
| Corrected transposition | Symptoms depend on the nature of associated anomalies (such as tricuspid [left-sided] incompetence, VSD, pulmonary stenosis, and complete heart block). Anteriorly located aortic valve causes a very loud $A_2$. | | |
| Coarctation of aorta | No symptoms in many; headaches, nosebleeds, cold feet, chest pain and claudication.<br>Modest hypertension in the arms; absent, ↓, or delayed leg pulses; right arm to leg systolic pressure gradient >30 mm Hg; hypertensive retinopathy unusual; thrills and continuous murmurs over the scapular areas and ribs from enlarged collateral (intercostal) arteries; LV heave and $S_4$ due to LVH. $S_1$ N; loud $A_2$; aortic ejection click from dilated ascending aorta; SEM over right upper sternal edge; EDM due to aortic insufficiency; continuous murmur over left interscapular area from the coarcted segment. | Survival into adulthood in 25%; the remaining die from complications. Only 10% live beyond 6th decade. | Infective endocarditis, aortic rupture, heart failure, stroke due to rupture of cerebral aneurysm, mycotic aneurysm of the poststenotic dilated segment of aorta, myelopathy due to thrombosis of anterior spinal arteries, or CAD. |
| Pulmonic stenosis (PS) | Mild or moderate PS may be asymptomatic; fatigue, dyspnea, right heart failure and syncope with severe stenosis.<br>Prominent "a" wave in neck veins; palpable RV heave; $S_1$ N; soft and delayed or absent $P_2$; pulmonic ejection click; right-sided $S_4$; murmur length correlates with severity of PS; functional tricuspid incompetence and R-to-L shunt via a patent foramen ovale with onset of right heart failure. | | |
| Ebstein's anomaly | Symptoms most often develop in neonatal life or infancy and occasionally in adulthood with exertional dyspnea, fatigue, paroxysmal arrhythmias.<br>Cyanosis, atrial arrhythmias, tall "v" waves, pulsatile liver, systolic murmur with inspiratory accentuation, with or without Wolff-Parkinson-White syndrome; widely split $S_1$ and $S_2$; $S_3$ and $S_4$ frequent. | Many patients survive only into the third or fourth decade. | Infective endocarditis. |

CAD = Coronary artery disease; EDM = early diastolic murmur; HDN = hyperdynamic; LPA = Left parasternal area; LV = Left ventricle; LVH = Left ventricular hypertrophy; MDM = mid-diastolic murmur; MR = mitral regurgitation; N = normal; PH = Pulmonary hypertension; RV = Right ventricle; SEM = systolic ejection murmur; TR = tricuspid regurgitation; ± = may be present.

**TABLE 40.3. Diagnostic Studies in and Therapy of Congenital Heart Diseases**

| Lesion | ECG and Chest X-ray (CXR) | Echocardiography | Cardiac Catheterization | Therapy |
|---|---|---|---|---|
| Atrial septal defect (ASD), ostium secundum type | ECG: NSR in young, AF in old; Axis N or rightward; rSR′ or RSR′ in right chest leads. CXR: Heart N or increased size; RA and RV enlarged; PA enlarged, may be aneurysmal. | RV volume overload; ASD directly seen in subcostal, parasternal or apical views; Color-flow Doppler or contrast study can show the shunt. | Locates the ASD, excludes associated anomalies, measures PA pressures; can diagnose any associated CAD. | Surgical closure if shunt is $^{3}$1.5: 1.0, ideally between 3–6 years of age, closure in adolescents and adults if shunt is still left to right. No surgery if Eisenmenger's syndrome present. (Percutaneous catheter-based closure available.) |
| Atrial septal defect (ASD), ostium primum type | ECG: Left axis, p mitrale, p pulmonale, 1 st° or higher a-v blocks, atrial arrhythmias; rSR′ in right chest leads. LVH (MR) RVH (PH). CXR: same as secundum ASD; chamber enlargement variable; pulmonary plethora. | RV volume overload; anterior mitral leaflet lies in close proximity to the ventricular septum in systole *and* diastole; cleft in the anterior mitral leaflet on 2-D echo. | Step-up of $SaO_2$ at the right atrial level; left ventriculogram: gooseneck deformity of the LV outflow tract (sine qua non), MR and a LV-right atrial shunt. | Prevent infective endocarditis, treat heart failure and pulmonary infections. Surgical correction between 5–6 yrs or earlier. Marked MR: replace valve, operate at a later age. Total correction of complete a-v canal before 2 yrs of age may prevent Eisenmenger's syndrome. |
| Ventricular septal defect (VSD) | ECG: LVH, and/or RVH, left atrial hypertrophy, qRS pattern in left chest leads indicates LV volume overload. CXR: cardiomegaly, LV, RV, LA enlargement; enlarged PA and branches; pulmonary plethora. | 2-D and Doppler echo locate and quantitate VSD, assess the size of L-R shunt, and estimate RV and PA pressure. | Determines the extent of shunt, locates site of VSD, and detects any additional malformations. PA pressure depends on the size of the VSD. | Infective endocarditis prophylaxis and treatment of heart failure. Surgical closure before the child enters school for medium-sized VSDs with left-to-right shunt (>1.5:1). |
| Patent ductus arteriosus (PDA) | ECG: LVH with medium-sized or large PDA. CXR: cardiomegaly, enlarged LV, LA, Aorta and its arch and pulmonary artery and its branches; pulmonary plethora, ductus calcification in older persons. | PDA only occasionally seen directly on 2-D echo. LA, LV enlargement. Color-flow Doppler echo detects L-R shunt and extent of pulmonary hypertension. | Confirms diagnosis and identifies other anomalies. Step-up in the $SaO_2$ in the main PA above the RV. PA pressure either normal or high. Aortography precisely locates the PDA and measures its size. | Infective endarteritis prophylaxis. Surgical division of the ductus. Medical therapy for CHF in inoperable patients; Eisenmenger's syndrome contraindicates surgery. Risk of surgery exceeds the risk for infective endarteritis in asymptomatic middle-aged and elderly with a small ductus. |
| Eisenmenger's syndrome | ECG: Right axis deviation, RVH with strain and right atrial hypertrophy. CXR: marked enlargement of PA and major branches, marked attenuation of distal pulmonary arteries peripherally. Central pulmonary arteries enlarge most in Eisenmenger's due to ASD; enlarged RV and right atrium. | 2-D echo shows the intracardiac anatomy and RA, RV and PA enlargement. Doppler echo detects valvular regurgitation and estimates PA pressure. | PA and RV systolic pressures = systemic levels. Elevated right atrial pressure; large *"a"* wave; PA wedge pressure = N. Markedly high pulmonary vascular resistance (>10 Wood units). Moderate to marked arterial desaturation. Shunts may be right-to-left, bidirectional, or absent. Selective angiocardiography can locate the shunt. Can assess pulmonary vascular reactivity at baseline and after inhalation of 100% $O_2$ or administration of vasoactive agents. | Management of heart failure and various hematologic abnormalities; long-term anticoagulants for thromboembolic complications; nifedipine, prostacyclin and alpha-adrenergic blockade may be helpful. Single lung transplantation with repair of intra-cardiac defects promising. |

| | | | | |
|---|---|---|---|---|
| Tetralogy of Fallot | ECG: Moderate right axis deviation, moderate RVH, tall monophasic R in $V_1$, and rS in $V_2$-$V_6$; biventricular hypertrophy in the acyanotic type CXR: absent pulmonary artery segment and enlarged aorta; aortic arch right-sided (25%); normal/slightly increased heart size, boot-shaped heart shadow ("coer en sabot"); oligemic lung fields in cyanotic type and prominent or increased lung vessels in acyanotic type | VSD in the membranous septum and biventricular origin of dilated aorta; preserved continuity between posterior aortic wall and anterior mitral leaflet; narrowed subpulmonic RV outflow tract in the short-axis view. | Required to estimate the site and size of VSD, degree of pulmonary stenosis, and to detect other anomalies; selective angiocardiography for delineating RV outflow tract anatomy | Infective endocarditis prophylaxis, treatment of anemia and excessive erythrocytosis; propranolol to prevent anoxic spells. Total correction indicated whenever possible. Surgical mortality 2.5–3.0%; ventricular arrhythmias, complete heart block, right bundle branch block, RV aneurysm and aortic regurgitation postoperatively. Blalock-Taussig operation or a Waterson operation are temporary procedures |
| Transposition of great arteries | ECG: Right atrial enlargement, right axis deviation and RVH; LVH with PS CXR: Cardiomegaly and narrow mediastinum ("egg-shaped heart"); pulmonary plethora | 2-D echo: aorta located anteriorly; runs parallel to the pulmonary artery | $SaO_2$ much lower in aorta than in the PA. Sequential sampling can locate level of shunt. Angiocardiography can establish the diagnosis and define the precise anatomy | Treat heart failure; palliative procedures (atrial septostomy, PA banding, or systemic-pulmonary anastomosis may be needed in infants. Mustard's operation (rearranging the venous in-flow) and Rastelli's operation (correcting the ventricular outflow) may be successful |
| Corrected transposition | ECG: Absent septal forces (q waves) in the left chest leads. CXR: concave pulmonary segment and a smooth convexity of the high left border of the heart caused by a displaced ascending aorta | | Diagnosis established by angiocardiography | Surgical correction of associated abnormalities |
| Coarctation of aorta | ECG: LVH with strain. CXR: Heart size N or ↑; enlarged ascending aorta and aortic knuckle; enlarged left subclavian artery, concave coarcted region and poststenotic dilatation cause a figure-3 configuration of the left margin of the aorta at the coarcted area ("3" sign); notching of lower rib margins from enlarged intercostal vessels (Figure 33.1, Dock's sign). | 2-D echo, along with Doppler can identify the site and length of coarctation and assess pressure gradient across it. | Can measure pressure gradient across coarctation and detect associated anomalies (coronary artery disease in adults and bicuspid aortic valve). Aortography extremely important to define the degree and extent of coarctation. | Corrective surgery when systolic pressure gradient is ≥50 mm Hg, ideally between 8–16 years; surgical mortality <5%. In most cases, BP normalizes within several weeks after surgery; balloon angioplasty is an alternative; infective endarteritis prophylaxis and treatment of heart failure and high BP. β-blockers and ACE-inhibitors ideal for BP control. |
| Pulmonic stenosis (PS) | ECG: Right atrial enlargement, right axis deviation, and RVH with strain; height of R in $V_1$ correlates with the degree of PS. CXR: prominent poststenotic dilatation; pulmonary oligemia; right atrial and RV enlargement | 2-D echo and Doppler visualizes the valve morphology and determines pressure gradient. | Can localize the obstruction and estimate its severity (mold = systolic gradient across the pulmonic valve, <50 mm Hg; moderate, 50 to 80 mm Hg; severe, >80 mm Hg) and exclude associated abnormalities | Direct surgical relief of PS with low risk; percutaneous balloon valvuloplasty quite effective for severe or moderately severe PS. |
| Ebstein's anomaly | ECG: P pulmonale, right bundle-branch block, and prolonged P-R CXR: marked right atrial enlargement, small RV, and normal or oligemic lungs. | Tricuspid valve closure delayed; downward displacement of its septal leaflet. | On careful pullback of the electrode catheter from the RV apex a chamber is observed (between the right atrium above and RV below) with pressure curve characteristic of right atrium but electrogram characteristic of RV. | Control of heart failure and, in a few, surgical replacement of the tricuspid valve. Radiofrequency ablation of the bypass tracts to abolish atrial arrhythmias |

2-D = 2-dimensional; AF = Atrial fibrillation; CAD = Coronary artery disease; CXR = Chest x-ray; LV = left ventricle; LVH = Left ventricular hypertrophy; N = normal; NSR = normal sinus rhythm; PA = Pulmonary artery; PH = Pulmonary hypertension; RA = right atrium; RV = right ventricle; RVH = Right ventricular hypertrophy; $SaO_2$ = Arterial hemoglobin saturation.

**TABLE 40.4. Types of Atrial Septal Defects**

| Type | Location | Comment |
|---|---|---|
| Ostium secundum defect | Fossa ovalis region of the atrial septum | 2–3 times more common in women; may be familial, 1–3 cm in size; 75% of all ASD; associated mitral valve prolapse |
| Sinus venosus defect | Upper defect, superior vena caval opening area | Accounts for 10% of all ASD; associated anomalous drainage of pulmonary veins |
| Septum primum* | Low defect; often involves mitral valve | 2–3 times more common in women. Upper margin crescentic; lower margin is the mitral and tricuspid valve tissue; cleft anterior mitral valve leaflet and abnormal chordal attachments frequent; they cause mitral regurgitation; 15% of all ASD |
| AV canal defect* | Low defect; often involves mitral and tricuspid valves or upper ventricular septum | A complete defect has no gender predilection; associated high VSD and cleft mitral and tricuspid valves |

*Together called endocardial cushion defects.
ASD = atrial septal defect; VSD = ventricular septal defect.

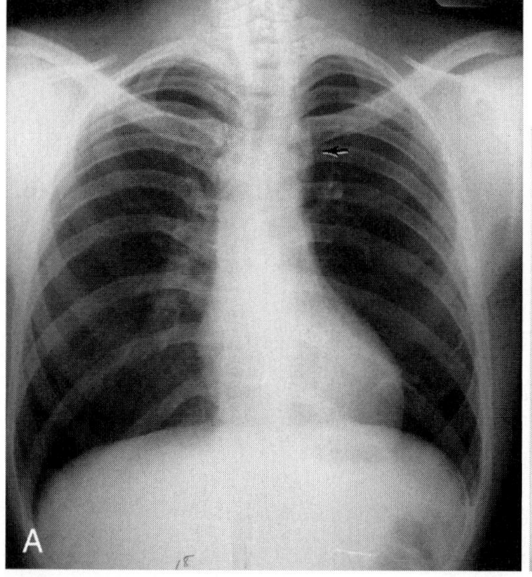

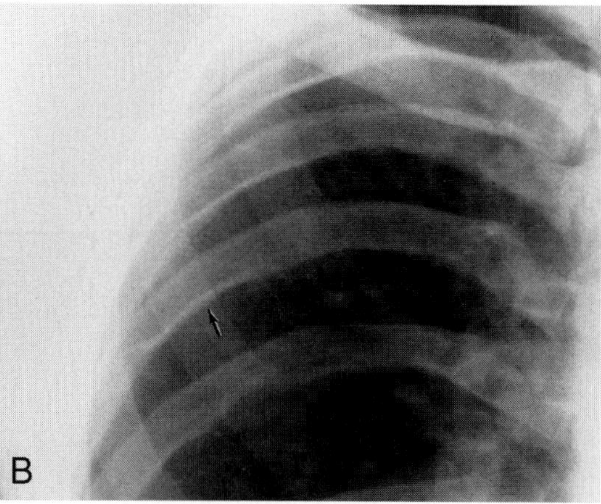

**FIGURE 40.1. A.** Chest x-ray of a patient with coarctation of the aorta. Note the bulge above and lateral to the aortic arch, probably due to an enlarged subclavian artery (arrow). **B.** Magnified view of the ribs showing notching in their lower borders ("Dock's sign").
(Courtesy of the Radiology Museum, St. Joseph's Regional Medical Center, Milwaukee, Wisconsin.)

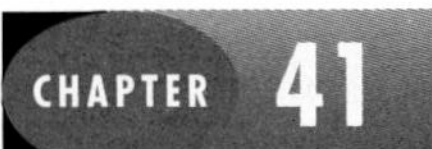

# VALVULAR HEART DISEASE

## Mitral Regurgitation

Mitral regurgitation (MR) is the abnormal ejection of a portion of LV stroke volume from the high-pressure LV to the low-pressure left atrium during all or part of systole. It is caused by abnormalities or dysfunction in any of the supporting structures of the mitral valve (anterior and posterior mitral leaflets, mitral annulus, chordae tendineae, papillary muscles, or regional LV segments).

### Pathophysiology

The pathophysiology of MR depends on its acuteness and severity and the extent of compensatory mechanisms to the regurgitant volume (Table 41.1). Because the left atrium cannot accommodate the sudden volume excess, **acute MR** is poorly tolerated; thus the left atrial, pulmonary venous, and pulmonary capillary wedge pressures rise severely, and pulmonary congestion follows. The contractility of the volume-primed LV increases via the Starling mechanism, evoking a supernormal ejection fraction.

In **chronic MR**, left atrial hypertrophy, dilation, and distensibility determine the left atrial and pulmonary venous pressures. An enlarging left atrium dampens the rise in these pressures. LV chamber hypertrophy and initial enlargement confer normal contractility. As the LV unloads a portion of its stroke volume into the LA, wall stress is lowered, thus sustaining normal or supernormal LV ejection fraction in mild to moderate MR. However, when the LV dilates and its end-diastolic volume (EDV) rises, symptoms evolve and functional status worsens.

### Etiology

The relative frequency of different diseases causing MR is shown in Figure 41.1. In myxomatous degeneration with mitral valve prolapse, the most common cause of **primary MR,** an abnormality of collagen tissue leads to loss of fiber orientation, thinning, and fragmentation of the normal fibrosa of the valve and its appendages. The affected valvular leaflet is stretched, redundant chordae elongate, and the mitral valve leaflet(s) prolapses into the left atrium. The ensuing MR is mild and mostly benign, but it may cause severe valvular leak and thus, congestive heart failure in some elderly patients.

A new systolic murmur and sudden onset of congestive heart failure immediately following a myocardial infarction (MI) (especially after an inferior-wall MI) may signify acute MR due to papillary muscle dysfunction and/or chordal rupture.

Ischemic papillary muscle dysfunction may also cause chronic MR.

**"Secondary" MR** results from LV dilatation and malalignment of the chordae tendineae-papillary muscle apparatus. Here, the normal mitral valve leaflets are unable to coapt normally owing to the dilated ring. The degree of MR varies with the severity of LV dysfunction.

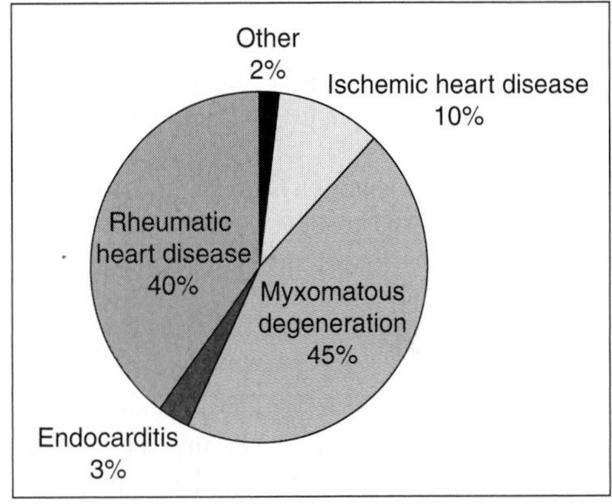


**FIGURE 41.1. Causes of mitral regurgitation.** (Redrawn from: Fenster MS et al. Curr Probl Cardiol 1995; 20:211, Figure 13. Used with permission.)

**TABLE 41.1. Longitudinal Changes in LV Mechanics in Mitral Regurgitation**

| Type of MR | Preload | Afterload | Contractility | EDV | ESV | EF | SV | LAP |
|---|---|---|---|---|---|---|---|---|
| Acute | ↑↑↑ | ↓ | Normal | ↑ | ↓ | ↑↑ | ↓↓ | ↑↑↑ |
| Chronic compensated | ↑↑↑ | N | Normal | ↑↑ | N | ↑ | N | ↑ |
| Chronic decompensated | ↑↑↑ | ↑ | ↓↓ | ↑↑↑ | ↑ | N | ↓ | ↑↑ |

EDV = end-diastolic volume; EF = ejection fraction; ESV = end-systolic volume; LAP = left atrial pressure; MR = mitral regurgitation; SV = forward stroke volume; ↑, ↑↑, ↑↑↑ = degrees of increase from normal; ↓, ↓↓ = degrees of decrease from normal; N = normal.
(From: Carabello BA. Curr Probl Cardiol 1993;18:423–478. Reprinted with permission.)

**TABLE 41.2. Clinical, ECG and Radiographic Features of Mitral Regurgitation**

| | Primary MR | Chronic MR |
|---|---|---|
| History | Previous rheumatic fever, MI, angina, endocarditis, or murmur helpful<br>In acute MR, dyspnea is acute, and pulmonary edema is usual. | The murmur usually precedes CHF by years (primary MR); palpitations (from atrial fibrillation) *and* fatigue (low cardiac output) frequent; some never report dyspnea, despite severely impaired LV function. |
| Physical examination | Acute MR with heart failure: tachypnea, late-inspiratory crackles, and bilateral or unilateral right-sided pleural effusions; tachycardia; rhythm generally regular, with atrial ($S_4$) gallop, and a loud, usually blowing apical systolic murmur. Murmur may be absent with severe MR. | Hyperdynamic precordium; LV lift; apical impulse laterally displaced; diffuse parasternal lift from systolic "ballooning" of the left atrium (all from ventricular and atrial dilatation); irregular rhythm with atrial fibrillation; soft $S_1$; widely split $S_2$ due to early $A_2$; $S_3$ gallop often but not always due to LV systolic dysfunction; typical MR murmur; brief middiastolic mitral murmur from excess flow. |
| ECG | Signs of myocardial infarction (MI) or ischemia with MI-related MR | No unique ECG findings except atrial fibrillation, left atrial enlargement (P mitrale), LV hypertrophy, and nonspecific ST-T changes |
| Chest X-ray | Usually no cardiomegaly; severe pulmonary vascular congestion and acute pulmonary edema | Cardiomegaly, pulmonary vascular congestion, and a double density at right heart border (enlarged left atrium); mitral valvular or annular calcification may be better seen on fluoroscopy |

## Clinical Features

An accurate history is critical in distinguishing whether MR is the cause or effect of LV dysfunction. The clinical, ECG and radiographic features of MR are listed in Table 41.2

The typical MR murmur is apical and holosystolic (see Figure 31.7), and it radiates to the left axilla, its intensity not always indicating the degree of MR. A midsystolic click and a late systolic murmur may occur in mitral valve prolapse, duly augmented by standing or a Valsalva maneuver, measures that lower ventricular volume. With heart failure, the click may vanish; with severe MR or ruptured chordae, the murmur turns holosystolic. Systolic murmurs may radiate to the spine in MR due to a flail anterior leaflet or to the base of the heart with a ruptured or perforated posterior leaflet.

## Ancillary Studies

Transthoracic Doppler echocardiography (Figure 41.2) may also provide important prognostic data regarding LV function, besides defining the etiology (flail leaflet, endocarditis, prolapse) and estimating the severity of MR. In early MR, the LV is hyperdynamic with normal end-systolic volume and supernormal ejection fraction. As disease worsens, end-systolic diameter (LVESD) increases greatly; an LVESD >55 mm denotes significant LV deterioration, and valve repair or replacement should be considered. Potential surgical candidates should undergo right and left heart catheterization to confirm the cause and severity of MR, identify other valvular disorders, assess LV function, and detect coexistent coronary artery disease.

## Management

Both the altered pathophysiology and the primary disorder need to be addressed. In acute MR, treatment goals are to reduce pulmonary venous pressures, decrease the regurgitant fraction, and increase forward cardiac output, which can usually be attained with a vasodilator-diuretic combination. Sodium nitroprusside, given its ability to lower afterload and to dilate venous capacitance vessels, is especially useful. Surgery should be considered in symptomatic patients with acute MR and normal LV function before the LV dilates greatly or its systolic function declines. In severe, acute MR, especially the post-MI type, temporary stabilization may be needed with an intra-aortic balloon pump. Surgical repair should be performed as soon as possible after stabilization.

The usual cardiotonic regimen (diuretics and preload and afterload reducers) is given to patients with more long-standing MR and congestive heart failure. Digoxin is given to treat systolic dysfunction and to control ventricular response in patients with rapid atrial fibrillation. Endocarditis prophylaxis is warranted in all patients with documented MR. Long-term oral anticoagulation may be required when atrial fibrillation complicates MR.

Asymptomatic patients with significant MR should be followed regularly to detect heart failure or progressive ventricular deterioration early. Early LV dilatation can be detected by echocardiography. Mitral valve surgery is appropriate when end-systolic diameter exceeds 50 mm or the ejection fraction is below 50%. The decision regarding mitral valve surgery in chronic MR depends on both the symptoms and LV function. Optimally, surgery should precede severe, chronic irreversible heart failure.

In general, mitral valve repair or reconstruction should be attempted whenever possible. Potential candidates for valve repair include those with MR of nonrheumatic, noninfective, and nonischemic causes. Uncomplicated mitral valve repair is durable, has a low operative mortality, and because the chordae and supporting apparatus are preserved, it better preserves LV function. Since no prosthesis is used, infections, thrombosis, and hemorrhage seem to be less.

## Mitral Valve Prolapse

Mitral valve prolapse (MVP) is a common abnormality affecting about 2–3% of men and 4–6% of women. The exact prevalence depends on the population under study and the diagnostic test used to establish its presence; however, MVP affects both genders and all age groups.

### Etiology

Often inherited as an autosomal dominant trait, MVP may also occur sporadically in normal persons or as part of a connective tissue anomaly (e.g., Marfan's or Ehlers-Danlos syndromes). MVP may also coexist with other clinical entities, including atrial septal defect, autonomic dysfunction, Graves' disease, Wolff-Parkinson-White syndrome, and ischemic heart disease. Ascribing a cause and effect relationship to these associations is difficult.

### Pathophysiology

MVP is a myxomatous degeneration of the valve and its supporting structures histologically, causing stretching of the affected leaflets, elongation of the chordae tendineae (which are often already redundant), and mid- to late-systolic prolapse of one or both mitral valve leaflets into the left atrium. Myxomatous degeneration is the most common cause of acquired MR in the adult. Despite the mild MR and benign clinical course in most cases, MVP can predispose to cerebral thromboembo-

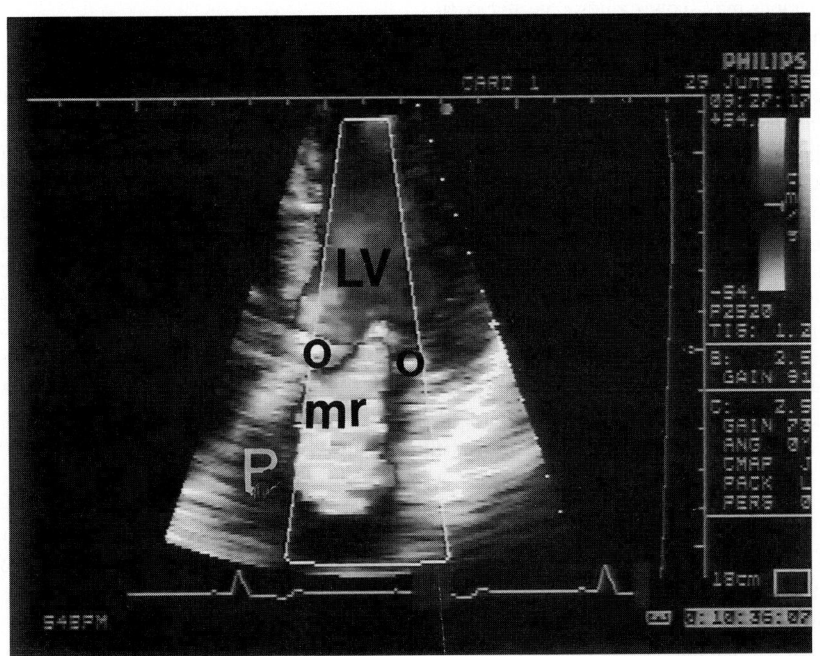


**FIGURE 41.2. Mitral regurgitation.** Doppler study showing turbulent, high-velocity flow across thickened mitral valve leaflets, indicating severe mitral regurgitation (mr). P = left atrium; o = mitral valve.

(Courtesy of Thomas Palmer, MD, and the Echocardiography Laboratory, St. Joseph's Regional Medical Center, Milwaukee, Wisconsin.)

lism, congestive heart failure, and infective endocarditis in some patients.

### Clinical Features

The actual prevalence of symptoms attributable to MVP is controversial. Almost 80% of patients report a panoply of nonspecific symptoms, including chest pain, dyspnea, fatigue, palpitations, dizziness, hyperventilation, and syncope. Anxiety, panic disorders, and other psychological disturbances also occur. The chest pain, being often nonexertional and prolonged, is usually unlike typical angina.

Physical examination may detect orthostatic hypotension or thoracic deformities (pectus excavatum, narrow anteroposterior diameter, loss of dorsal kyphosis and hypomastia) and classically, a mid- to late-systolic click, murmur, or both. The click is loudest at the left sternal border and apex and is usually followed by a mid- to late-systolic murmur (click-murmur syndrome). Valsalva maneuver or standing, by decreasing venous return, decreases the LV cavity size and hastens or worsens the prolapse of the mitral leaflets; thus, these move the click closer to $S_1$, prolonging the murmur and increasing its intensity. Squatting and handgrip have the opposite effect.

### Ancillary Studies

Chest radiographs may show scoliosis, pectus excavatum or -carinatum, or straight-back syndrome (loss of normal thoracic kyphosis), which, by distorting the cardiac silhouette, may feign cardiomegaly. The ECG may mimic myocardial ischemia in the inferior limb and lateral precordial leads, or it may exhibit paroxysms of supraventricular tachycardia and frequent premature atrial or ventricular beats at rest or exercise. The risk of sudden cardiac death is quite low, unless the valves are markedly thickened or LV function is abnormal.

Transthoracic echocardiography typically shows superior displacement of one or both mitral valve leaflets (more commonly, the posterior leaflet) into the left atrium. Usually, the diagnosis is confirmed by this test (Figure 41.3). Doppler echocardiography can determine the extent and severity of MR and establish MVP as the cause of MR. Cardiac catheterization is usually not indicated.

### Management

MVP mostly runs a benign course although complications may arise, especially in the elderly or those with marked thickening or redundancy of the valve leaflets with or without moderate to severe MR. Complications include endocarditis, chordal rupture, progressive MR, transient ischemic attacks, systemic emboli, and cardiac arrhythmias. Endocarditis prophylaxis is now recommended for all MVP patients with an MR murmur or those with great redundancy of mitral leaflets on echocardiography. β-blockers may relieve chest pain and/or palpitations. For those with transient ischemic attacks or other cerebral ischemic events, aspirin, 325 mg/day, is appropriate. Warfarin therapy (to produce an INR of 2–3) is reserved for those with recurrent emboli or associated atrial fibrillation. Patients with symptoms of congestive heart failure and severe MR due to MVP are candidates for mitral valve repair or replacement. Asymptomatic patients require reassurance.

## Mitral Stenosis

The normal cross-sectional area of the mitral valve orifice is 4–6 $cm^2$. Mitral stenosis is a narrowing or constriction of this orifice. Nearly all cases in the United States are presumably rheumatic, despite a past history of rheumatic fever being obtainable in only about half the cases. In rheumatic valvulitis, the valve leaflets scar and contract, the commissures fuse, and the chordae tendineae shorten. Mitral valve involvement is the hallmark of rheumatic heart disease. Mitral stenosis may less commonly follow severe mitral annular calcification and infective endocarditis. Left atrial myxoma or large left atrial thrombi may cause LV inflow obstruction that mimics mitral stenosis.

### Pathophysiology

Mitral stenosis leads to obstructed LV inflow and left atrial hypertension and hypertrophy, which ultimately cause atrial fibrillation. A rising left atrial pressure also raises pulmonary venous and capillary wedge pressures; pulmonary congestion and dyspnea follow. In long-standing cases, the high pulmonary vascular resistance (PVR) finally leads to pulmonary arterial hypertension. When the PVR rises to about 5 times normal, signs of RV failure (venous and hepatic congestion) appear.

The impaired LV filling may so reduce preload as to compromise cardiac output. Because the early (passive) LV filling is relatively more impaired than late (active) filling, a forceful atrial contraction is crucial to push blood across the stenotic valve. Factors that prolong diastole (β-blockers, bradycardia) augment filling, while those that shorten it (fever, tachycardia) may compromise filling. Thus, "flash" pulmonary edema and low output states may follow tachycardias, especially atrial fibrillation.

### Clinical Features

Mitral stenosis is 3–4 times more common in women than men. Nearly 50% of patients report slowly progressive symptoms, typically beginning in the fourth decade. Exertional dyspnea is the earliest and commonest

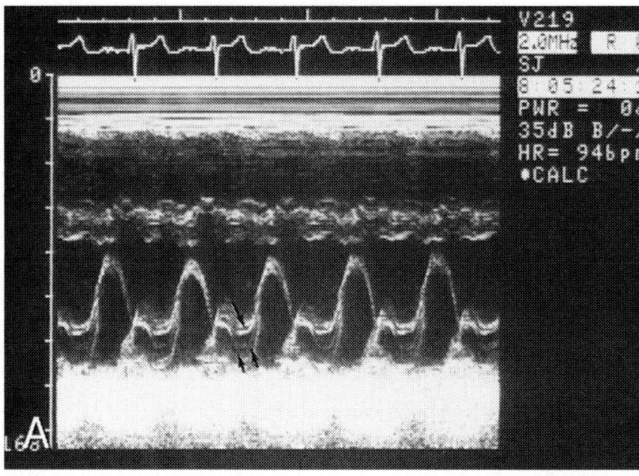


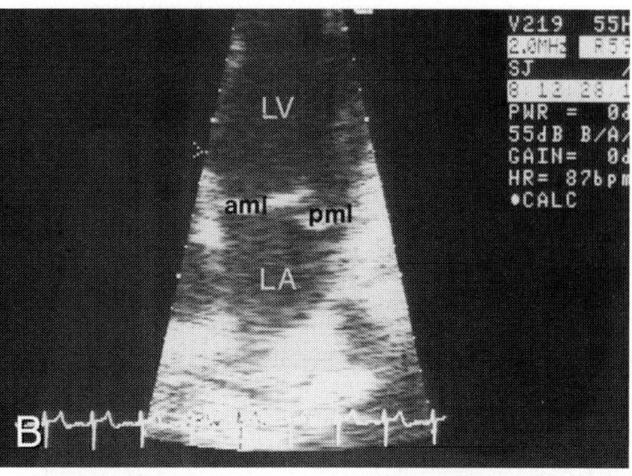


**FIGURE 41.3. Mitral valve prolapse. A.** M-mode echocardiogram showing systolic separation of the anterior and posterior mitral leaflets (arrows). **B.** Transthoracic echocardiogram (apical view) showing prolapse of the posterior mitral valve leaflet (pml). LA = Left atrium; aml = anterior mitral leaflet.

(Courtesy of Thomas Palmer, MD, and the Echocardiography Laboratory, St. Joseph's Regional Medical Center, Milwaukee, Wisconsin.)

symptom, with others including orthopnea, paroxysmal nocturnal dyspnea, fatigue (low output), palpitations, and edema. Bloody sputum occurs in about 50%, ranging from pink and frothy to frank hemoptysis. Chest pain occurs in about 10–15% of cases, often attributed to RV ischemia from pulmonary hypertension. Systemic emboli, sometimes the harbinger of mitral stenosis, occur in 15%, especially those with atrial fibrillation. In some, **tachyarrhythmias,** especially atrial fibrillation may cause an abrupt onset. Pulmonary edema may follow exertion, excitement, fever, anemia, tachycardia, coitus, and pregnancy.

With atrial fibrillation, peripheral pulses may be weak and/or irregular. On auscultation (see Figure 31.9), an accentuated $S_1$ and an opening snap (OS) are heard, followed by a diastolic rumble of variable duration. $S_1$ may be soft if the mitral valve is heavily calcified or if there is coexistent mitral regurgitation, aortic insufficiency, heart failure, or atrial fibrillation. The closer the $A_2$–OS interval or longer the murmur, the worse is the stenosis. The murmur is confined to the apex, and if it is not heard with the stethoscope bell in the left lateral position, mild exercise may unmask it. When normal sinus rhythm prevails, the forceful left atrial contraction produces a presystolic accentuation. As pulmonary hypertension evolves, neck vein distension, an RV lift, loud $P_2$, murmurs of tricuspid leak and/or pulmonic insufficiency, and pedal edema appear.

## Ancillary Studies

Chest radiograph shows a normal-sized LV. With significantly high left atrial pressures, signs of pulmonary vascular congestion emerge, and the distended interlobular septa cause Kerley's B lines (see Figure 33.2). The left atrial enlargement causes a "double density" (see Mitral Regurgitation), and the distended pulmonary arteries denote pulmonary hypertension. The small aortic knob, a bulging aortopulmonary window from a large central pulmonary artery, and a bulge below it from a large left auricle along with a small left ventricle together cause a straight left heart border (**mitralization,** Figure 41.4).

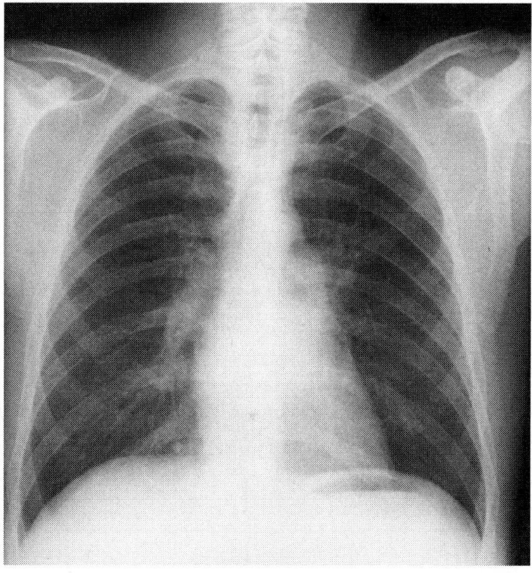

**FIGURE 41.4. Mitral stenosis.** "Mitralization" is evident on the left heart border—an enlarged left atrium is faintly seen as a double shadow.

(Courtesy of the Radiology Museum, St. Joseph's Regional Medical Center, Milwaukee, Wisconsin.)

The ECG shows left atrial enlargement and with pulmonary hypertension, right axis deviation, and RV

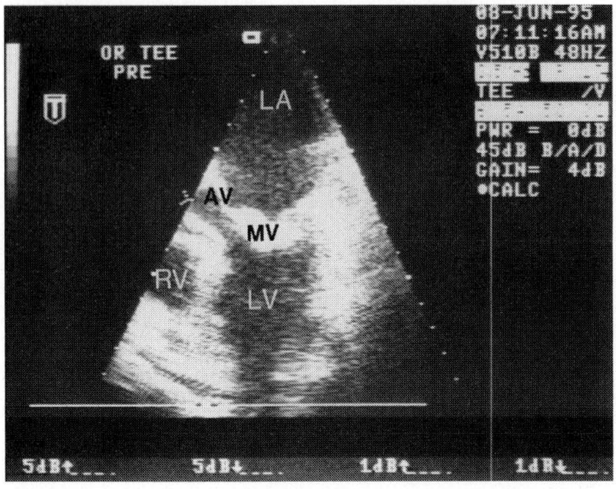


**FIGURE 41.5. Mitral stenosis. Transesophageal echocardiogram showing an enlarged left atrium (LA), a small under-filled LV, and markedly thickened and fused mitral valve leaflets (MV). RV = right ventricle; AV = aortic valve.** (Courtesy of Thomas Palmer, MD, and the Echocardiography Laboratory and Cardiac Diagnostic Unit, St. Joseph's Regional Medical Center, Milwaukee, Wisconsin.)

hypertrophy. Atrial fibrillation may be present. Transthoracic echocardiography is diagnostic.

Other associated valvular lesions may also be noted, as is common in rheumatic heart disease. Tricuspid regurgitation may be organic or functional due to dilated tricuspid annulus. The transvalvular gradient, the valve surface area, and pulmonary artery pressures can be estimated by Doppler echocardiography (Figure 41.5). When the valve orifice is 1 cm$^2$ or less, mitral stenosis is critical. Cardiac catheterization can confirm the severity of stenosis, diagnose other coexisting valve disease, and/or coronary artery disease, and quantitate the pulmonary hypertension.

### Management

Correct diagnosis and therapy for streptococcal pharyngitis and acute rheumatic fever (Table 41.3), penicillin V (250 mg b.i.d) or erythromycin (250 mg b.i.d) to prevent rheumatic fever in known rheumatic heart disease until age 35, and lifelong endocarditis prophylaxis form the essentials of preventive care. Long-term oral anticoagulation with warfarin, maintaining an INR of 2–3, is indicated in atrial fibrillation to prevent systemic emboli. Although elective cardioversion may restore sinus rhythm, it prevails in less than one-half of cases after 1 year. In atrial fibrillation with a rapid ventricular rate, digoxin, β-blockers, verapamil, and diltiazem are quite useful.

Usually, only moderate to severe mitral stenosis and pulmonary venous hypertension with symptoms require intervention, either mitral commissurotomy, valvuloplasty, or mitral valve replacement. Atrial fibrillation or single systemic embolic event alone rarely suffice as indications.

## Aortic Stenosis

Aortic stenosis (AS) is a narrowing of the aortic valve orifice from its normal 3–4 cm$^2$, causing obstruction to LV outflow. Most cases follow aortic valve disease due to a congenital bicuspid valve, calcific degeneration, or rheumatic valvulitis. Most congenital bicuspid aortic valves are not initially stenotic but narrow over several decades. Rheumatic AS almost always occurs with mitral valve disease, and so lone valvular AS is most likely nonrheumatic. Degenerative calcific AS, caused by wear and tear of normal valves, is common in the elderly, affecting men four times more often than women.

The etiology of AS varies with age (Figure 41.6). In persons under age 70, bicuspid valve disease is much more common; among those older than 70, calcific degenerative disease is more frequent. Dynamic LV outflow tract obstruction may occur in hypertrophic cardiomyopathy (chapter 44).

### Pathophysiology

Progressive LV outflow tract obstruction results from a series of events, including accelerated fibrosis and degenerative changes in the valve due to mechanical stress and turbulent blood flow across the valve, rigidity of valve leaflets, and immobility of the cusps from

**TABLE 41.3. Guidelines for the Diagnosis of an Initial Attack of Rheumatic Fever (Jones Criteria, 1992 Update)***

| Major Criteria | Minor Criteria |
|---|---|
| Carditis | Clinical findings |
| Polyarthritis | Arthralgia |
| Chorea | Fever |
| Erythema marginatum | Laboratory findings |
| Subcutaneous nodules | ↑ Acute phase reactants |
| | ↑ Erythrocyte sedimentation rate |
| | ↑ C-reactive protein |
| | Prolonged PR interval |
| **Supporting evidence of preceding group A streptococcal infection** | |
| Positive throat culture or rapid streptococcal antigen test | |
| Elevated or rising streptococcal antibody titer | |

*If a preceding group A streptococcal infection is proven, 2 major criteria or 1 major and 2 minor criteria denote a high probability of acute rheumatic fever.
(Adapted from: JAMA 1992; 268:2070. Used with permission.)

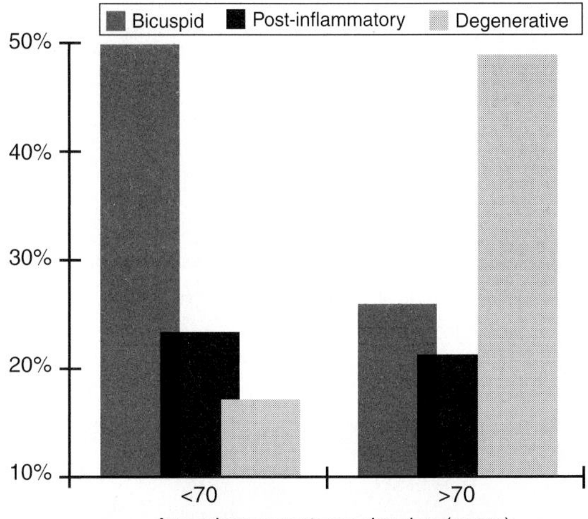


**FIGURE 41.6. Influence of age on the etiology of aortic stenosis. Bicuspid aortic valves predominate in those younger than 70 years old when symptoms develop. Degenerative valve disease predominates in those whose age at onset of symptoms is 70. Postinflammatory conditions causing aortic stenosis are believed to be predominantly rheumatic. Congenital abnormalities become a major consideration if age at onset of symptoms is less than 30.**

(Data from: Passik CS et al. Mayo Clin Proc 1987, 62:119. Used with permission.)

calcification. This obstruction leads to increased LV wall stress and filling pressures, LV hypertrophy, and finally, chronic LV pressure overload. These, along with the impaired epicardial-to-endocardial blood flow, increased myocardial $O_2$ demands, and abnormal relaxation response of a stiff, hypertrophied ventricle (diastolic dysfunction) explain many of the manifestations of AS. LV dilatation, systolic or diastolic dysfunction, and clinical deterioration eventually supervene.

## Clinical Features

AS is a slowly progressive disease. Angina, syncope, and dyspnea develop late in its course, as the valve area narrows to 1–1.5 $cm^2$. Nearly one-third of patients present with dyspnea and angina, and 15% with syncope. Dyspnea is primarily from pulmonary venous hypertension caused by diastolic dysfunction. Angina may be due to LV hypertrophy or associated coronary artery disease. Syncope is usually exertional and follows global cerebral hypoperfusion, due to low cardiac output or arrhythmia. Atrial fibrillation, which afflicts nearly 10% of patients, is poorly tolerated and may evoke both pulmonary congestion and low cardiac output. In late, severe AS, congestive heart failure may be due to LV dilatation and systolic dysfunction.

The arterial pulse is typically low volume and slow rising *(pulsus parvus et tardus)*. Best appreciated in larger arteries, it may be absent in the elderly. A narrow pulse pressure is characteristic, with a blood pressure of 100/60 mm Hg being typical. However, given the very high LV intracavitary pressures, a systolic blood pressure of 160–170 mm Hg does not rule out critical AS.

The apical impulse may be sustained, forceful, and heaving, reflecting the LV pressure overload; a laterally displaced impulse signifies LV dilatation. A thrill is often felt in the aortic area. $S_1$ is generally normal and may be followed by an ejection click, which suggests mobile valve cusps; it is not specific for AS. The aortic valve closure (**$A_2$**) may be soft, absent, late, or reverse-split. The $A_2$ is key in helping to distinguish AS from aortic valve sclerosis (in which $A_2$ retains its normal intensity and timing). Because LV hypertrophy is common in AS, an $S_4$ is often heard with prevailing normal sinus rhythm. $S_3$ gallops are sporadic and usually indicate systolic dysfunction.

The usual murmur of AS (see Figure 31.6) is a harsh, diamond-shaped, systolic murmur that is often best heard at the aortic area and may radiate to the neck. The later it peaks, the more severe the stenosis. A faint early diastolic murmur, signifying mild aortic regurgitation, may also be heard. In the elderly with degenerative calcific AS, an apical holosystolic murmur may coexist, due to mitral annular calcification. Clinically diagnosing the cause of a systolic murmur is often difficult; helpful hemodynamic maneuvers are listed in Table 41.4.

## Ancillary Studies

The ECG usually shows normal sinus rhythm, left atrial enlargement, and LV hypertrophy with associated ST-T wave changes. Conduction defects are common and left bundle branch block may be present. The chest radiograph often shows normal heart size, but cardiomegaly and poststenotic dilatation of aortic root may be present. Because the valve overlies the dorsal spine, aortic valve calcification may not be seen on posteroanterior projections, and lateral chest films and fluoroscopy may be more helpful in this regard.

Transthoracic echocardiography shows LV hypertrophy, thickened, calcific aortic valve cusps with decreased mobility, and the number of valve cusps (trileaflet or bicuspid). It also identifies any associated valvular disorders and assesses LV function (Figure 41.7). With Doppler echocardiography, the peak transvalvular (aortic valve [AV]-LV) gradient and valve surface area may be estimated. A peak AV-LV gradient of 50–75 mm Hg or a valve area of 0.5–0.8 $cm^2/m^2$ indicates moderate stenosis. Cardiac catheterization confirms these findings and is indicated in symptomatic patients over age 40 to exclude coronary artery disease.

**TABLE 41.4. Response of Systolic Murmur to Hemodynamic Maneuvers**

| Maneuver | AS | HCM | MVP | MR |
|---|---|---|---|---|
| Standing upright | ↓ | ↑ | ↑ | ± |
| Squatting | ± | ↓ | ↓ | ↑ |
| Valsalva | ↓ | ↑ | ↓↑ | ↓ |
| Isometric hand grip | ↓ | ↓ | ↓↑ | ↑ |
| Post-premature beat | ↑ | ↑ | ↓ | ± |

↑ = Increased; ↓ = Decreased; ↓↑ = Variable; ± = No change; AS = Aortic stenosis; HCM = Hypertrophic obstructive cardiomyopathy; MVP = Mitral valve prolapse; MR = Mitral regurgitation.
(From: Duthie EH et al. J Am Geriatr Soc 1981; 29:500. Used with permission.)

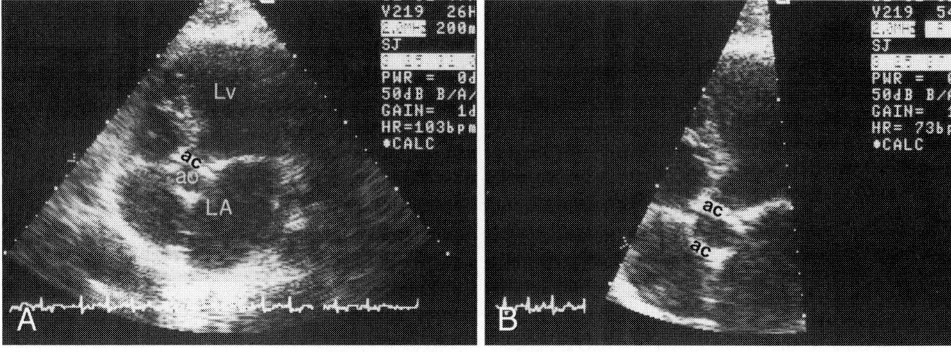


**FIGURE 41.7. Aortic stenosis. A. Transthoracic echocardiogram showing thickened aortic valve cusps (ac) and stenosis of the valvular area (ao). B. Magnified view. LA = Left atrium.** (Courtesy of Thomas Palmer, MD, and the Echocardiography Laboratory and Heart Care Center, St. Joseph's Regional Medical Center, Milwaukee, Wisconsin.)

## Management

The presence of any of the classic symptoms of AS dictates a thorough work-up so as to facilitate aortic valve replacement if high-grade obstruction is found. Patients with symptoms of heart failure should avoid vigorous exercise. Vasodilators are risky in AS, since the systemic vasodilation in the face of fixed cardiac output lowers blood pressure so severely as to imperil cerebral perfusion. Endocarditis prophylaxis is required in all cases.

Aortic valve replacement is necessary in all symptomatic patients with an AV-LV gradient above 75 mm Hg and/or valve orifice below 0.5 cm$^2$, and it should be considered in symptomatic patients with AV-LV gradient above 50 mm Hg or valve orifice of 0.5–0.8 cm$^2$. The procedure carries a mortality of about 5%. The choice of a mechanical valve over bioprosthesis partly depends on the feasibility of long-term anticoagulation. Mechanical valves require warfarin in doses sufficient to keep the INR between 2.5–3.5. Aortic balloon valvuloplasty is palliative in nonoperable, high-risk patients with advanced symptoms, but restenosis and poor long-term survivals are valid concerns.

Angina, syncope, or heart failure each portends a very poor prognosis. With angina or syncope, the average survival declines to about 3–5 years, and heart failure reduces survival to 18 months. Independent preoperative predictors of mortality include patient age, emergency status, presence of significant LV dysfunction, and lack of sinus rhythm.

## Aortic Regurgitation (Aortic Insufficiency)

Aortic regurgitation (AR) is the abnormal diastolic flow of blood from the aorta to the LV across an incompetent aortic valve. Most cases arise from two mechanisms: abnormalities of the aortic valve or the aortic root and its supporting structures. The former abnormalities, comprising cusp deformities (perforated or scarred cusps) and leaflet rupture or prolapse, include infective endocarditis, rheumatic valvulitis, myxomatous degeneration, and bicuspid aortic valve. Aortic root disorders include cystic medial necrosis, proximal aortic dissection, hypertension, aortoannular ectasia, and connective tissue diseases (ankylosing spondylitis, Reiter's syndrome, systemic lupus erythematosus, and rheumatoid arthritis). Ascending aortitis, another cause, was commonly caused by syphilis in the past.

### Pathogenesis and Pathophysiology

Patients with AR are generally hypervolemic, but the presence or absence of compensatory mechanisms largely determines the pathophysiology in any given patient. In acute AR, the LV end-diastolic volume and thus the LV end-diastolic pressure increase acutely, followed by an abrupt and marked rise in left atrial, pulmonary venous, and pulmonary capillary wedge pressures. Thus, acute AR is poorly tolerated. In chronic cases, LV dilation and hypertrophy initially increase the stroke volume, but after a long asymptomatic period, contractility may worsen, ushering in symptoms of overt heart failure.

### Clinical Features

AR has a clear predilection for men over women. Its clinical features largely depend on the underlying cause (e.g., endocarditis, dissection) and the presence of compensation for the hypervolemia. Symptoms of low cardiac output and pulmonary vascular congestion characterize acute AR, whereas a prolonged asymptomatic phase, often lasting decades, precedes the clinical presentation of most patients with chronic AR, even those with fairly severe AR. Symptoms, when they appear, often include palpitations, exertional dyspnea, and angina. Syncope is rare, but sudden death occurs in about 10%.

In acute AR, cardiac enlargement is minimal, and the apical impulse is only mildly displaced. Tachycardia is common, but the pulse pressure is normal. $S_1$ may be diminished in intensity or absent if the mitral valve closes prematurely. An early, high-pitched, diastolic murmur immediately follows $S_2$ and is heard best at the base and mid-left sternal border. When heard best to the right of the sternum, it may suggest aortic root disease. The murmur may be so faint as to be inaudible unless proper technique is used. A basilar systolic ejection murmur may also be present, due to excess forward flow across the aortic valve.

With long-standing AR, a wide pulse pressure, bounding peripheral pulses, and a bisferiens or "water hammer" pulse (see Figure 31.1) may be noted. Precordial palpation reveals a vigorously contracting and dilated LV. Heart sounds are generally normal. The typical murmur of AR is present. An $S_3$ gallop, a loud basilar systolic murmur, and occasionally, a mid-diastolic, low-pitched apical (Austin-Flint) murmur caused by vibrations from the regurgitant jet of blood on the anterior leaflets of the mitral valve may be noted.

### Ancillary Studies

The ECG may show evidence of LV hypertrophy. The chest radiograph often shows cardiomegaly and a dilated aortic root. Marked aortic root dilatation should arouse suspicion of a primary aortic root abnormality (e.g., Marfan's syndrome or aortic dissection). Transthoracic echocardiography usually shows left atrial hypertrophy, LV enlargement, and fluttering of the mitral valve leaflets. Doppler echocardiography can detect and quantify the degree of AR as well as assess LV size and function. In suspected infective endocarditis, transesophageal echocardiography may be better to detect vegetations.

Cardiac catheterization is indicated if valve replacement is contemplated. It can assess LV function, identify other valvular abnormalities, and detect and assess the severity of any associated coronary artery disease.

### Management

Long-term vasodilator therapy is recommended in AR, because it decreases the regurgitant volume and delays LV dilatation. Asymptomatic patients with severe AR and normal LV function may benefit from nifedipine, which may reduce or delay the need for aortic valve replacement.

Enalapril has also been shown to decrease mean wall stress, LV mass, LV end-diastolic pressure, and the end-systolic volume. If heart failure develops, digitalis, diuretics, and vasodilators should be initiated. With onset of heart failure, rapid deterioration is the norm, with an average survival of about 2 years. Prompt evaluation for aortic valve replacement should follow. In asymptomatic patients, periodic transthoracic echocardiography is useful to evaluate the end-systolic diameter; when it exceeds 50 mm or signs of LV dysfunction appear, aortic valve replacement should be considered, even with only mild symptoms.

## Tricuspid Regurgitation

Tricuspid regurgitation (TR) represents the abnormal systolic blood flow from the RV into the right atrium across an incompetent tricuspid valve. Clinically significant primary TR is uncommon. It may exist with or without underlying pulmonary hypertension. When pulmonary hypertension is present, secondary TR develops as a result of RV failure and dilatation, which stretch the tricuspid annulus. This type of "functional" TR commonly follows LV failure, mitral stenosis, and cor pulmonale due to chronic obstructive pulmonary disease. In the absence of pulmonary hypertension, acquired TR follows infective endocarditis (IV drug abuse), carcinoid syndrome, and RV dysfunction due to RV infarction. Tricuspid valve prolapse, Ebstein's anomaly, and atrial septal defect (ostium primum) are congenital lesions associated with TR.

The pathophysiologic consequences of TR include elevation of right atrial pressures, RV volume overload, and the development of signs and symptoms of systemic venous congestion. Symptoms of TR are primarily those of right heart failure and the underlying disease process responsible for TR. Physical examination shows jugular venous distension, prominent *v* wave with a rapid *y* descent and hyperdynamic parasternal impulse (RV lift), a holosystolic murmur along the lower left sternal border that waxes and wanes with respiration, an enlarged pulsatile liver, and peripheral edema.

The ECG may show right atrial enlargement and right ventricular hypertrophy. Atrial fibrillation and right bundle branch block are common. Transthoracic echocardiography may define the etiology of TR (prolapse, ruptured chordae, or vegetations). Doppler echocardiography, by measuring RV systolic and peak pulmonary artery pressures, can help assess its severity.

Except for endocarditis prophylaxis and the possible need for diuretics to manage peripheral edema, no specific treatment is indicated for mild to moderate TR. Tricuspid valve repair or annuloplasty may be performed in conjunction with mitral valve repair for severe TR due to mitral valve disease. In tricuspid valve endocarditis, excision of the tricuspid valve may be called for, especially for native valve infection due to *Staphylococcus aureus* or a fungal organism.

### Tricuspid Stenosis

Tricuspid stenosis (TS) is a narrowing or constriction of the tricuspid valve orifice that leads to obstruction to RV inflow. Pathophysiologic sequelae of this obstruction include the development of right atrial hypertension and hypertrophy and decreased cardiac output due to decreased ventricular filling.

TS is rarely an isolated valvular lesion. In adults, it is almost always due to rheumatic valvulitis, for which the pathology is similar to mitral stenosis. Other causes of TS include carcinoid syndrome, congenital heart disease, and fibroelastosis. Right atrial myxoma occasionally mimics TS.

Because rheumatic heart disease causes most cases, most patients with TS are women. Patients may report easy fatigability, which may be due to the associated mitral stenosis. Physical findings are a large *a* wave in the jugular venous pulse with a slow *y* descent, a loud $S_1$, and a low-pitched diastolic rumble along the left sternal border. This murmur typically increases with inspiration and often has a presystolic accentuation. Hepatomegaly, jaundice, presystolic liver pulsation, ascites, and pedal edema may also occur.

ECG and chest radiographs show evidence of right atrial enlargement. Chest films may also show a distended superior vena cava. Transthoracic echocardiography confirms the diagnosis and may identify other associated valvular lesions. Valve repair or replacement is required for symptomatic patients with TS.

# CHAPTER 42 PERICARDIAL DISEASES

### Pericarditis

Pericarditis, with its diverse causes, refers to the acute or chronic inflammation of the visceral and parietal pericardium (Table 42.1). Pericardial inflammation leads to fibrin deposition in the pericardium. The associated fluid exudation causes a pericardial effusion, which, depending on the underlying disease process, may be serous, bloody, or purulent. Large or rapidly evolving effusions may evoke serious hemodynamic consequences that impair ventricular filling and compromise cardiac output. An epicardial extension of pericarditis may sometimes produce an associated myocarditis.

#### Clinical Features

The onset of pericarditis may be insidious or abrupt. Typical symptoms are fever and chest pain. The pain varies in quality, location, and radiation, and may be associated with dyspnea. Some report an intense, steady, crushing, substernal discomfort that radiates to the shoulder, neck, or nape of the neck and may mimic an acute myocardial infarction. Typically worsened by a supine posture, coughing, or deep breathing, the pain is often relieved by sitting up and leaning forward—such posturing may presumably reduce local pressure on inflamed pericardial surfaces.

**TABLE 42.1. Frequent Causes of Pericarditis**

| Cause | Comment |
|---|---|
| **Idiopathic** | No unique features but resembles viral pericarditis. |
| **Infectious** | |
| Viral | Most cases are viral. Commonly due to Coxsackie B virus in young adults. Pneumonitis and pleuritis usually associated. |
| Bacterial | |
| Tuberculosis | Uncommon cause, but important in immunocompromised hosts. Pleural and/or systemic disease commonly associated. Eventually constrictive pericarditis may follow. |
| Purulent pericarditis | Follows pericardial "seeding" during bacteremia; extension of or contiguous infection; or penetrating chest wounds and esophageal perforation (Boerhaave's syndrome). |
| Rheumatic fever* | Pericarditis associated with valvulitis or myocarditis. |
| **Non-infectious** | |
| Uremia | Chronic end-stage renal disease generally present. Exuberant fibrinous pericardial reaction, often with hemorrhagic fluid. Reversible with dialysis. |
| Connective tissue diseases | Pericarditis part of panserositis in SLE, RA and PSS. Pericarditis and/or effusion develop sometime in the course of SLE and 30% of RA. May precede pancarditis in SLE. |
| Trauma | May follow significant closed chest trauma. Myocardial contusions and transient myopericarditis associated. |
| Post-MI | "Early" form commonly follows 10–15% of transmural MI in first few days, due to pericardial extension of epicardial inflammation directly from the injured myocardium. May be confused with recurrent ischemic pain and/or reinfarction.<br>"Late" form (Dressler's syndrome) follows MI by 2 wks to 2 yrs; may be recurrent. Autoimmune basis. Associated hemorrhagic pleural effusion, high fever. |
| Postpericardiotomy syndrome | Follows open-heart surgery or procedures involving opening the pericardium. Features similar to Dressler's syndrome. |
| Post-irradiation | May follow radiation to the chest for lung cancer, lymphoma, or breast cancer |

MI = myocardial infarction; PSS = progressive systemic sclerosis; RA = rheumatoid arthritis; SLE = systemic lupus erythematosus.
*Not actual infection of pericardium.

**Fever**, **tachycardia**, and **pericardial friction rub** are classic findings. The rub is best heard with the diaphragm of the stethoscope pressed firmly on the chest wall and with the patient sitting up and leaning forward. Intermittent, fleeting, positional, and of variable intensity, it may have a coarse, scratchy ("leather on leather") quality. The classic 3-component rub conforming to ventricular systole, early diastole, and late diastole (atrial contraction) is less common. With only 1 or 2 components, the rub may easily simulate a murmur.

## Ancillary Studies

Leukocytosis, elevated erythrocyte sedimentation rate, and high creatinine kinase (CK) levels are common. The CK-MB fraction rises when myocarditis is present. The chest radiograph shows cardiomegaly when a sizable pericardial effusion is present. Pleural effusions are common and are often left-sided.

ECG changes occur in about 90% of cases. Nearly one-half of these changes evolve through 3 phases. In phase I, the PR segment is depressed, the ST is diffusely elevated with an upward concavity, and the T waves are upright (Figure 42.1). The PR depression is an insensitive but specific ECG sign. Seen in two-thirds of all cases, it may be the sole ECG change in some patients. In several days, phase II follows, with isoelectric ST segments and flattened T waves. In phase III, T waves are inverted widely, often with low-voltage QRS complexes. Although atrial extrasystoles and atrial fibrillation may occur, ventricular arrhythmias are uncommon. The ECG distinction from acute myocardial infarction is listed in Table 42.2.

Further diagnostic testing depends on the clinical picture (e.g., tuberculin skin test for suspected tuberculosis and antinuclear antibody and double-stranded DNA if systemic lupus erythematosus is suspected). Echocardiography has no role in uncomplicated cases, although it can detect even small amounts of pericardial fluid. Characterizing pericardial fluid as either transudative or exudative is not helpful diagnostically. Thus, pericardiocentesis for strictly diagnostic purposes should be avoided. Large-sized pericardial effusions in patients with incipient tamponade or shock may need to be drained to improve hemodynamics.

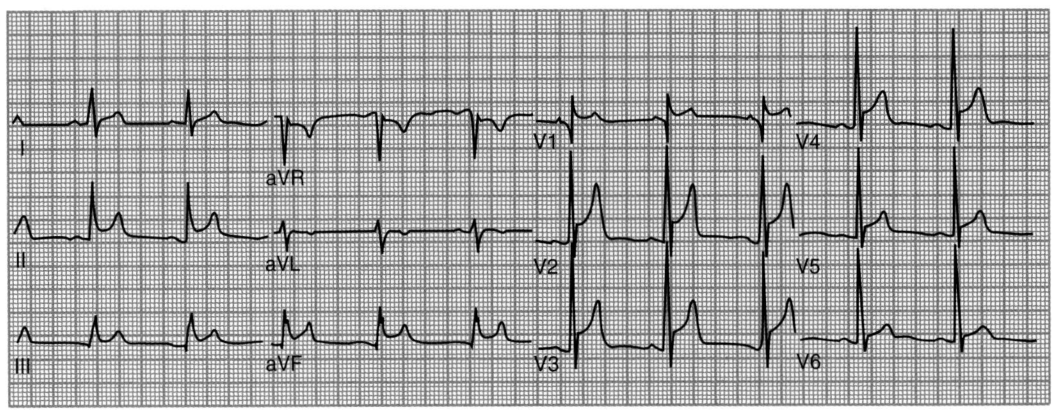


FIGURE 42.1. ECG changes in acute pericarditis. Note the elevated ST segments with upward concavity in all the leads except aVR and aVL. There is no reciprocal ST depression.

TABLE 42.2. ECG Differentiation of Acute Pericarditis and Acute Myocardial Infarction (MI)

| | Pericarditis | Acute MI |
|---|---|---|
| ECG leads involved | Usually diffuse; spares aVR, $V_1$ | Regional changes that correspond to distribution of coronary blood flow; may see reciprocal changes in other leads |
| PR segment | Usually depressed early | Normal |
| ST segments | Concave upwards | Convex upwards |
| Persistence of ST-segment changes | Days | Hours to days |
| Time course of T-wave changes | T waves invert after ST returns to baseline | T waves invert within hours while ST segment is still elevated |
| Q waves | Absent | Present unless non-Q wave infarct pattern |
| R-wave amplitude | Never lost | May be lost |

### Management

The specific medical management of pericarditis has 2 goals: to provide symptom relief and to treat the etiologic process, if needed. Symptomatic patients are usually given bedrest and aspirin (or nonsteroidal anti-inflammatory agents). Although pericarditis has a self-limited course in most cases, nearly one-fourth, especially those with immunologically mediated processes, may have prolonged pain or recurrent symptoms. Colchicine and tapering doses of prednisone may benefit these patients.

## Pericardial Effusion and Tamponade

The normal pericardium, an inelastic sac, contains less than 50 ml of fluid. Acutely, the pericardium can adjust to an accumulation of only about 100–200 ml of fluid without an abnormal rise in intrapericardial pressure (normally 0–3 mm Hg). With larger amounts, pericardial pressure rises sharply and intracardiac and pulmonary diastolic pressures rise. Chamber pressures equalize, and ventricular filling, and eventually cardiac output, decline. Ultimately, systemic blood pressure falls and shock supervenes. This condition is known as **cardiac tamponade**. With slower accumulations of fluid, the stretching pericardium blunts the rise in pericardial pressure. Thus, subacutely or chronically, relatively large amounts of pericardial fluid (>1 L) can accumulate before pericardial pressure rises sufficiently to impair cardiac filling.

### Etiology

Although pericardial effusions and pericarditis share similar causes (Table 42.1), the relative frequency of diseases causing each is different. For example, malignancy, the commonest cause of pericardial tamponade, causes pericarditis only infrequently. Hemopericardium (blood in the pericardium) may follow blood dyscrasias, anticoagulation, chest trauma, cardiac perforation during procedures (e.g., catheterization, pacemaker insertion), cardiac rupture, or dissecting aortic aneurysm. Causes of cardiac tamponade are listed in Table 42.3.

## Clinical Features

The clinical picture of pericardial effusion depends on the underlying disease as well as the compression and hemodynamic embarrassment due to the effusion. Hemodynamically trivial effusions are asymptomatic or evoke only vague, dull chest pain or dyspnea. Compression of adjacent organs, such as the major bronchi, recurrent laryngeal nerve, or esophagus, may evoke cough, hoarseness, or dysphagia, respectively. Only about one-third of patients with evidence of a pericardial effusion have a **pericardial friction rub**.

Patients with rapid accumulation of fluid may show classic signs of cardiac tamponade (Table 42.4). **Pulsus paradoxus** (a fall in systolic BP on inspiration by ≥12mm Hg) is seen in almost 75% of these cases. Inspiration normally augments venous return to the RV and its end-diastolic volume. RV filling displaces the interventricular septum toward the LV, thereby decreasing LV end-diastolic volume. In pulsus paradoxus, the inspiratory RV expansion is exaggerated and RV filling occurs at the expense of LV filling. Although pulsus paradoxus is an important bedside clue, it is neither sensitive nor specific. Many of the findings may be absent or attenuated in patients with hypovolemia who experience "low-pressure tamponade."

## Ancillary Studies

Workup of patients with pericardial effusion should include measurement of serum albumin, blood urea nitrogen, creatinine, thyroid-stimulating hormone (TSH), antinuclear antibody, urine protein, and tuberculin skin tests. Other diagnostic tests should depend on the clinical presentation.

At least 250 mL of fluid must accumulate in the pericardial sac before the chest x-ray shows cardiac enlargement. With more substantial accumulations, a symmetrically enlarged heart shadow may mimic a globular "water bottle". With large effusions, the ECG shows low-voltage QRS complexes and flattened T waves. *Electrical alternans*, a regular alteration of the amplitude of the QRS during sinus rhythm, seems to correlate specifically with hemodynamically important effusions.

**Transthoracic echocardiography** is the most sensitive and specific test in suspected, significant pericardial effusion. Small effusions (<300 mL) may appear on the subxiphoid view as an echo-free space between the posterior cardiac wall and parietal pericardium. Larger effusions may be seen both anteriorly and posteriorly. Right atrial compression and RV diastolic collapse are sensitive and specific echocardiographic signs of early tamponade (Figure 42.2). Because they appear before systemic hypotension and pulsus paradoxus and when the cardiac output is only modestly decreased, they foretell impending clinical cardiac tamponade with hemodynamic collapse.

Right-heart catheterization may detect coexistent conditions, such as LV failure or effusive-constrictive disease, and document hemodynamic improvement after pericardial drainage. Typically, the right atrial pressure is high with a preserved *x* descent and a decreased or absent *y* descent. Right-sided systolic pressures and the pulmonary capillary wedge pressure are moderately high. In tamponade, right atrial, RV, and LV end-diastolic pressures are all equal ("equalization of chamber pressures").

**TABLE 42.3. Common Causes of Pericardial Effusion: Mnemonic "VINDICATE"**

- **V**ascular (acute MI, hemopericardium) (6%)
- **I**nfectious (viral: Coxsackie B; bacterial: tuberculosis, *Staphylococcus aureus, Streptococcus pneumoniae*, Group A streptococcus, Enterobacteriaceae) (5%)
- **N**eoplastic (metastatic, [most common primary sites: lung, breast, leukemia/lymphoma]) (54%)
- **D**rugs (procainamide, hydralazine) (2%)
- **I**diopathic (14%)
- **C**onnective tissue disease (systemic lupus erythematosus, rheumatoid arthritis) (2%)
- **A**uto-immune (Dressler's and post-pericardiotomy) (2%)
- **T**rauma (aortic dissection with tamponade, penetrating chest wound) (<1%)
- **E**ndocrine/metabolic (chronic renal failure, myxedema) (14%)

Figures in parentheses indicate approximate frequency of each category.

**TABLE 42.4. Classic Signs of Cardiac Tamponade**

Dyspnea
Anxiety ("sense of impending doom")
Tachypnea
Signs of low cardiac output
  Fatigue, weakness, and confusion
  Tachycardia
  Hypotension (systolic BP often <100 mm Hg)
  Narrow pulse pressure
Marked neck vein distension (prominent *x* and absent *y* descents)
Pulsus paradoxus
Muffled heart sounds
Signs of compression of adjacent organs (see text)

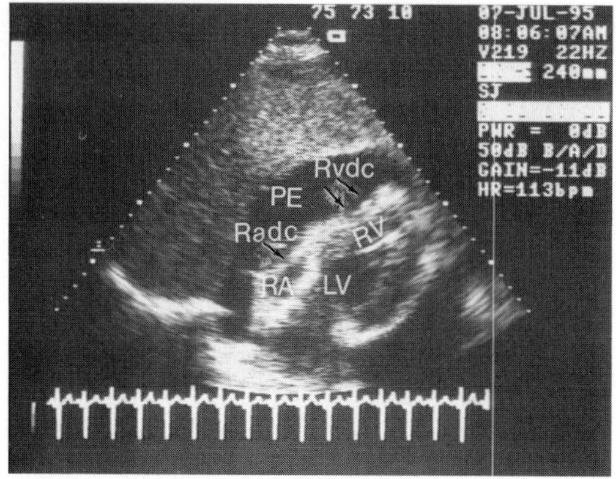


**FIGURE 42.2. Cardiac tamponade.** Two-dimensional echocardiogram (subcostal view) showing a large pericardial effusion (PE) and early-diastolic, concave indentation of right atrium (right atrial diastolic collapse, Radc) and right ventricle (right ventricular diastolic collapse, Rvdc), indicative of cardiac tamponade. LV = left ventricle. RA = right atrium. (Courtesy of Thomas Palmer, MD, and Echocardiography Laboratory of St. Joseph's Regional Medical Center, Milwaukee, Wisconsin.)

### Management

Pericardiocentesis, usually performed at the bedside using local anesthesia and echocardiographic localization and following a subxiphoid approach, rapidly lowers right atrial pressures and pulsus paradoxus, increases cardiac output, and allows measurement of intrapericardial pressure. Its major risks are pneumothorax and cardiac laceration.

Patients presenting with hypotension and suspected tamponade should be given IV fluids to expand the intravascular volume. This may delay the echocardiographic appearance of RV diastolic collapse or the clinical onset of hemodynamic compromise. A single pericardiocentesis rapidly relieves tamponade in many patients, as evidenced by improvement in hemodynamics thereafter. For recurrent, large effusions, additional options include the local instillation of nonresorbable steroids or creating a pleural-pericardial window. Persistently high right atrial pressure after effective pericardial drainage suggests combined effusive-constrictive disease, which may require more complete surgical pericardiectomies. Such effusive-constrictive features are most commonly seen with neoplastic pericardial involvement. **Hemopericardium** calls for urgent surgical drainage to prevent cardiac tamponade.

## Constrictive Pericarditis

In constrictive pericarditis, the pericardial space is partially or completely obliterated by fibrous adhesions formed during a previous bout(s) of acute pericarditis. Its diagnosis requires evidence of systemic venous congestion without myocardial dysfunction or other causes of congestion. Pericardium is calcified in one-half of these patients, especially when the initial effusion is hemorrhagic or the etiology is tuberculosis.

Common causes of constrictive pericarditis are neoplasms, irradiation, post-cardiac surgery, idiopathic processes, infections, chronic renal failure, connective tissue diseases, and asbestos exposure. Radiation-induced changes may not appear for many years following thoracic irradiation. Constrictive pericarditis may follow open heart surgery, even though the pericardium is not closed primarily.

### Pathophysiology

In constrictive pericarditis, because the heart is encased in a rigid shell, diastolic expansion is restricted and ventricular filling impaired. When the noncompliant pericardium is maximally stretched, systemic venous pressures rise and cardiac output eventually declines.

### Clinical Features

The onset is usually insidious, and symptoms progress gradually over months to years. Typical early features include fatigue, weight gain, hepatomegaly, and peripheral edema. However, cardiac output and systemic blood pressure are usually maintained.

Rising pulmonary venous pressures lead to symptoms of pulmonary congestion. Tachycardia and neck vein distension are noted on examination. The jugular venous pulse has a prominent and steep *y* descent along with a variable *x* descent (Figure 31.3), which contrasts with pericardial tamponade (where the *y* descent is absent or blunted, and the *x* descent is prominent). **Kussmaul's sign**, a paradoxical inspiratory rise in jugular venous pressure, may occur with constriction but not with tamponade. Difficult to appreciate when venous pressures are high, it is also nonspecific, being seen in restrictive cardiomyopathy and chronic RV failure. Pulsus paradoxus may occur but less commonly than in pericardial tamponade.

The apical impulse is not palpable. A pericardial knock is frequently heard at the apex. This sharp, high-frequency diastolic sound occurs earlier than an $S_3$ and corresponds to the sudden cessation of ventricular filling. Clear lung fields, ascites, and liver enzyme abnormalities are also common. Careful scrutiny of the neck veins is essential in differentiating constrictive pericarditis from chronic liver disease and nephrotic syndrome. Separating constriction from severe right heart failure is also a difficult feat.

### Ancillary Studies

Chest radiographs may show extensive pericardial calcification in about one-half of cases, but alone, calcification is not pathognomonic of constriction. The

ECG may show low-voltage QRS complexes and nonspecific ST–T changes. In severe cases, electrical alternans may occur. Atrial arrhythmias are common, and atrial fibrillation occurs in about 50% of patients.

Other than establishing normal LV function and ruling out cardiac tamponade and other causes of right heart failure, echocardiography has no diagnostic value. Cardiac catheterization may sometimes be necessary to assess hemodynamics. Computed tomography or magnetic resonance scans of the chest can document pericardial thickening and thus distinguish constrictive pericarditis from restrictive cardiomyopathy.

### Management

Once symptoms develop, the patient's functional status declines slowly and inexorably. In symptomatic patients, surgical pericardiectomy provides relief. It carries an operative mortality of 10% and a 5-year survival of nearly 80%. Symptoms slowly improve after surgery; persistent symptoms may be due to comorbid cardiac conditions or an incomplete resection, a common sequel in those with heavy pericardial calcification.

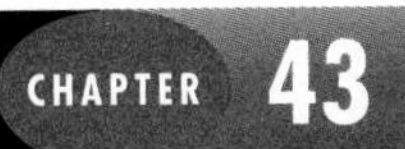


# INFECTIVE ENDOCARDITIS

## Definition and Epidemiology

Endocarditis, an inflammation of the endocardium, may be infective or nonbacterial. **Infective endocarditis** (IE) is caused by bacterial or fungal infections of the endocardium, whereas infection is absent in **nonbacterial endocarditis** (syn. verrucous or nonbacterial thrombotic endocarditis [NBTE]). Irregular excrescences (vegetations) form on the surface of the heart valves in most cases of endocarditis. Vegetations can also form on the endocardial surfaces of cardiac chambers/vessels, e.g., right ventricle in ventricular septal defect and pulmonary artery in patent ductus arteriosus; left ventricular outflow tract in hypertrophic cardiomyopathy. In IE, these consist of aggregates of platelets, fibrin, bacteria, and, rarely, neutrophils. Clots or shreds of fibrin form on an ulcerated valve surface in NBTE.

## Pathogenesis and Pathophysiology

The evolution of IE requires the interaction of two processes: an abnormal valve surface and transient bacteremia (Figure 43.1). High-velocity flow across an abnormal valve alters its surface, allowing deposition of platelet and fibrin aggregates on the valve's low-pressure side. During brief bacteremias, this sterile "vegetation" becomes a nidus where bacteria adhere. With bacterial colonization and further deposition of platelets and fibrin that follow, a bacterial "safe haven" evolves, where the microbes gain sanctuary from the body's cellular and humoral defenses. Valvular infection damages the valve architecture; progressive destructive changes cause or worsen valvular insufficiency. When infection extends into the valve annulus, abscesses and conduction disturbances result. Vegetations may detach and embolize systemically, involving the skin, brain, kidneys, and other organs. Emboli to the vasa vasorum of the brain may cause mycotic aneurysms; such extracardiac aneurysms are prone to rupture. In right-sided endocarditis, septic pulmonary emboli may cause multiple cavitating pulmonary infiltrates.

The intense interaction between the host and microbe generates abundant circulating antibodies and immune complexes, commonly exemplified by IgM antibody against IgG (rheumatoid factor), seen in almost half the cases of endocarditis that have lasted over 6 weeks.

## Etiology

Traditionally, IE is classified as acute or subacute; however, the etiology of IE is better viewed in the context of the two major pathogenetic processes responsible for its development: characteristics of the infecting organism and host factors.

### Characteristics of the microorganisms

Bacterial adherence to valve surfaces seems related to the microbe's ability to produce dextran, a complex extracellular polysaccharide. *Staphylococcus aureus, S. epidermidis*, viridans streptococci, and enterococci are common causes of IE, because of both the relatively high rate at which they cause transient bacteremia and their avid adherence to normal and abnormal valve surfaces. Over half of the cases of culture-proven native-valve endocarditis are due to streptococci, typically the viridans streptococci, which are normal inhabitants of the gingival crevices. Minor trauma from dental manipulations can evoke fleeting bacteremia and endocarditis. Enterococcal endocarditis often has a subacute course in older (>60) men, with genitourinary disorders or manipulations being frequent precipitating events. Enterococci pose special problems, given the recent emergence of drug-resistant strains. *Streptococcus bovis* bacteremia notably occurs with colonic polyps or colon cancer.

*S. aureus* causes up to 25% of all cases of culture-proven IE. Fungal IE should be considered in IV

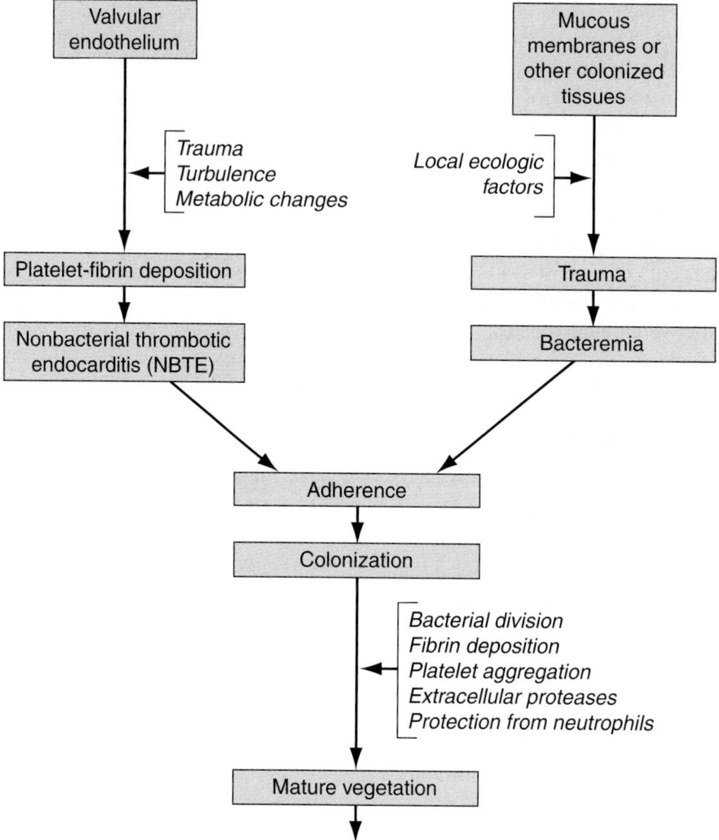


**FIGURE 43.1. Pathogenesis of Infective Endocarditis.** (Adapted from: Bayer AS, Scheld WM. Endocarditis and Intravascular Infections. In Mandell GL, Benett JE, Dolin R (eds.) Mandell, Douglas and Bennett's Principles and Practice of Infectious Diseases. Philadelphia: Churchill & Livingstone, 2000, Chapter 65, p. 859. Used with permission.)

drug abusers and those with recent cardiovascular surgery or prolonged IV antibiotic therapy. Recent antibiotic use and infections with slow-growing (HACEK group—***H****aemophilus parainfluenzae*, ***A****ctinobacillus actinomycetemcomitans*, ***C****ardiobacterium hominis*, ***E****ikenella* species, and ***K****ingella* species) or fastidious (nutritionally deficient streptococci, fungi, brucellae, chlamydiae, psittacosis, and Q fever) microbes may render cultures negative in nearly 5% of cases of IE.

### Host factors

Several host factors, including underlying illnesses and immune competence, largely determine the clinical presentation of endocarditis and its microbiology. Thus, IE may be classified into native-valve or prosthetic-valve IE (bioprosthesis or mechanical) or that related to IV drug abuse (IVDA), each with its unique list of causative organisms.

**Native-valve endocarditis** is most common in men aged over 50, especially elderly diabetic men. Predisposing valvular lesions are mitral valve prolapse (30–50%), rheumatic heart disease (30%), and congenital heart disease (10–20%) with a bicuspid aortic valve, pulmonic stenosis, ventricular septal defect, aortic stenosis, IHSS or patent ductus arteriosus. Degenerative disease of the aortic and mitral valves is responsible in some elderly patients. No predisposing valve lesion is found in a few cases.

**Prosthetic valve endocarditis** is discussed separately. **IE in IV drug abusers** generally affects younger men and has a predilection for right-sided valves. Staphylococcus is the most common causative organism.

## Clinical Features

IE affects persons of all age groups but mostly older men. Men are affected preferentially over women by a 2:1 ratio. The clinical features of IE may be constitutional, cardiac, embolic, and immunologic (Table 43.1).

**Constitutional symptoms**, being nonspecific, may

delay diagnosis of IE. The most common cardiac symptom of IE is **dyspnea**, which is usually related to congestive heart failure. Major **emboli** complicate one-third of cases, causing protean manifestations with involvement of different organs (skin, abdominal viscera, brain). Thus, sudden neurologic events in young patients should arouse suspicion of IE.

The virulence of the organism and its ability to adhere to the valve also influence the clinical picture. Thus, ***Staphylococcus aureus* endocarditis** presents as an acute, fulminant illness with high, hectic fever, predominant cardiovascular signs, and scant peripheral stigmata of endocarditis. Rapid valve destruction, hemodynamic instability, and extracardiac metastatic abscesses are its other features. Continuous, community-acquired *S. aureus* bacteremia should always be treated as endocarditis, especially if a primary nidus is not apparent. **Endocarditis due to the viridans streptococci** has an insidious onset with a low-grade fever and frequent extracardiac manifestations. A tendency for systemic emboli, ostensibly from large bulky vegetations, is typical of fungal endocarditis.

Fever and heart murmur are characteristic but not invariable. Fever may be absent in the elderly and in renal failure (urea has antipyretic properties), heart failure, and malnutrition. In many patients, particularly the elderly, the cardiac auscultatory findings of endocarditis are often inseparable from signs of prior valvular disease and high output (fever, anemia).

## Ancillary Studies

A normochromic, normocytic anemia is very common. In subacute cases, the WBC count may be normal or modestly high. The erythrocyte sedimentation rate (ESR) is almost always high, but a normal ESR does not exclude IE. Rheumatoid factor may be present. Proteinuria, occasionally in the nephrotic range, and microscopic hematuria are generally noted; gross hematuria may follow renal emboli or infarcts. RBC and WBC casts, when present, reflect an immune-complex-mediated glomerulonephritis.

**Blood cultures** are the key diagnostic test for IE, being positive in over 95% of cases. No more than 3 sets of cultures are routinely necessary in the first 24 hours unless antibiotics have been given in the preceding 2 weeks. The laboratory should be notified of the clinical suspicion of IE, so as to enable prolonged incubation and subculture techniques. The bacteremia is continuous, and therefore, in most patients, all sets of blood cultures will be positive. Persistent bacteremia without an identifiable source (e.g., an infected IV line) should arouse the suspicion of IE. Minimum inhibitory concentration (MIC) and minimum bactericidal concentration (MBC) should be measured in most cases to guide the choice and dose of antimicrobials. These provide critical data in patients who fail to respond to treatment or who harbor an unusual organism.

The chest x-ray may show heart failure. Septic pulmonary emboli (i.e, bilateral, multiple, small patchy infiltrates that may cavitate) are typical of right-sided endocarditis. In suspected prosthetic valve endocarditis, fluoroscopy typically shows abnormal valve motion or "rocking" by a loose prosthesis. With coronary artery emboli and myocarditis, the ECG may show signs of myocardial infarction and ST-T changes, respectively. Also, new conduction defects, the harbinger of a ring abscess, should be looked for.

Echocardiography has a critical role in the diagnosis and management of IE (Figure 43.2). Findings highly predictive of IE include characteristic vegetations, ab-

**TABLE 43.1. Clinical Features of Infective Endocarditis**

| Type | Common | Less Common |
|---|---|---|
| Constitutional | Fever (80%), chills, weakness (40%), sweats, anorexia, weight loss, malaise (each 25%) | Nausea, vomiting, abdominal pain, myalgias/arthralgias, back pain, headache |
| Cardiac | Dyspnea, which may be acute or insidious (40%); cardiac murmur (>85%) | Chest pain in 15%; myocardial infarctions due to emboli to coronary arteries from valvular vegetations; a new murmur/changing murmur very infrequent |
| Embolic | Major emboli (>35%) to different organs (e.g., abdominal pain due to splenic or mesenteric infarction; focal neurologic symptoms) | Janeway lesions (non-tender, hemorrhagic, macules on the palmar and plantar surfaces) seen in about 10% |
| Immunologic | Splenomegaly, clubbing, and skin manifestations (each in up to 50% of cases) | Conjunctival, oral mucosal, and lower-extremity petechiae; splinter hemorrhages in about 15% (very nonspecific); Osler nodes (multiple, 2–5 mm, tender, nodular lesions on the fingers or toes, seen in 15% (nonspecific) |

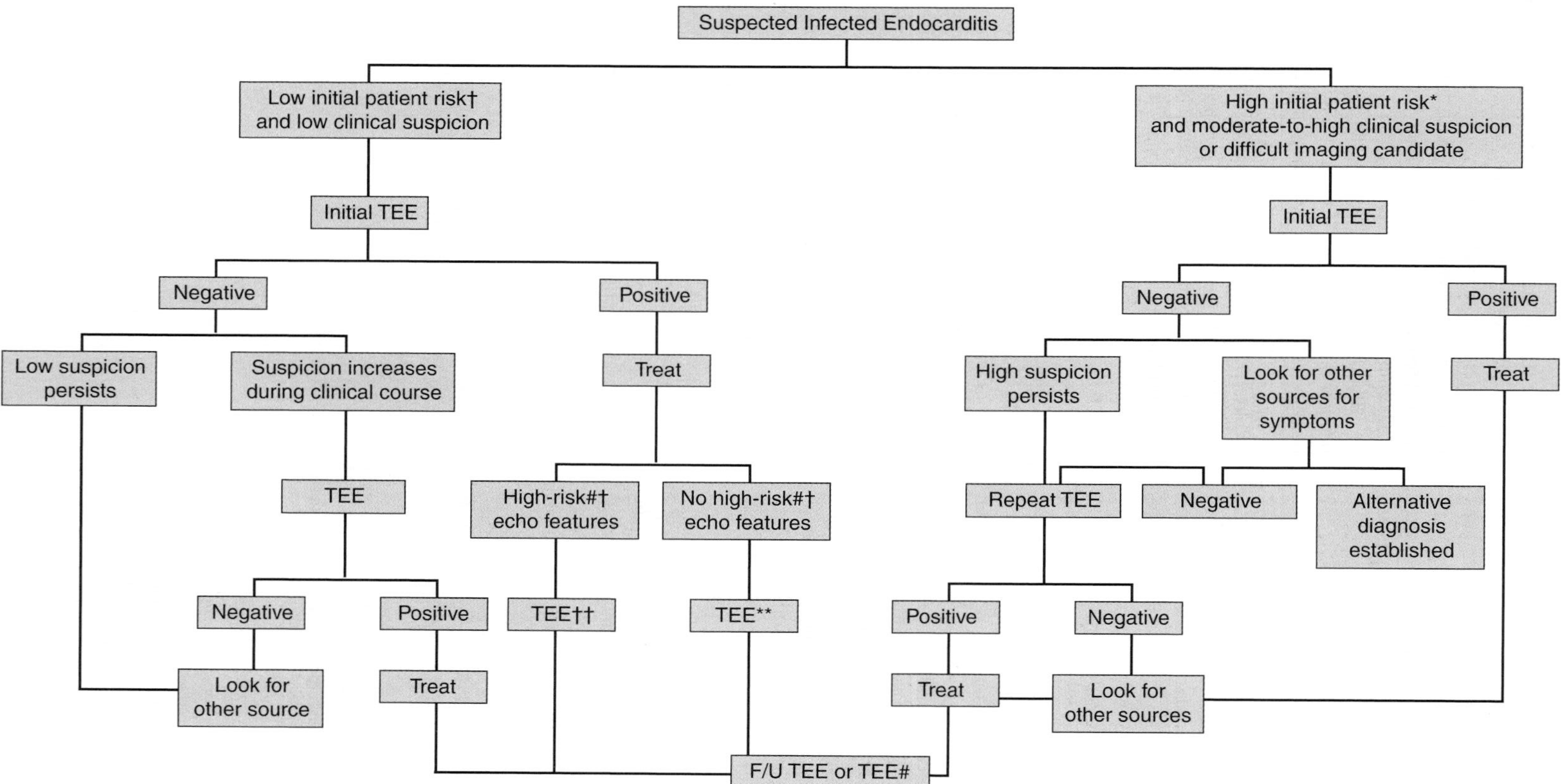


FIGURE **43.2. An Approach to the Patient with Suspected Infective Endocarditis.** # = TTE or TEE as follow-up to reassess vegetations, complications or treatment response as clinically indicated; #† = High-risk echo features include large and/or mobile vegetations, valvular insufficiency, suggestion of perivalvular extension, or secondary ventricular dysfunction; * = High patient risks include prosthetic valve, many congenital heart diseases, prior endocarditis, new murmur, heart failure, or other stigmata of endocarditis; ** = TEE only if clinical status deteriorates; † = Low suspicion for IE (e.g., patient with fever and a known heart murmur, but no other features of IE; †† = TEE to detect complications; TEE, = Transesophageal echocardiogram; Treat = Antibiotic treatment of IE; TTE, = Transthoracic echocardiogram.
Adapted from: Bayer AS et al. Circulation, 1998; 98:2938. Used with permission.

scesses, new prosthetic valve dehiscence, or new valvular regurgitation. Although echocardiography should be performed in all cases of suspected IE, it is not an appropriate screen for IE in clinical situations where fever or bacteremia is unlikely to represent IE. **Transthoracic echocardiography (TTE)**, with a sensitivity of about 70% for large (>5 mm) vegetations and very few false-positives, can assess the severity of valvular incompetence and detect vegetations and local complications (e.g., perforated leaflet, chordal rupture, myocardial ring abscesses). Nearly 80% of infected, native, left-sided valve vegetations may be detected. However, because small vegetations may be missed, a normal study does not exclude IE. Further, satisfactory imaging may not be achieved in patients with obesity, chronic obstructive lung disease, and chest wall abnormalities. **Transesophageal echocardiography (TEE)**, with a sensitivity of over 90% for detecting vegetations, can detect smaller vegetations and identify periannular abscesses, mycotic aneurysms, and pulmonic valve vegetations. It is the method of choice in patients who are difficult to image, those with suspected prosthetic valve IE, and those at high risk for complications as well as those with a high or intermediate clinical suspicion of IE.

## Management

Newly proposed criteria for diagnosing IE incorporate pathologic and clinical aspects, which includes both major and minor criteria (Table 43.2). The approach to the patient with suspected IE is outined in Figure 43.2.

General principles of treating infective endocarditis include:

1. Using bactericidal and not bacteriostatic antibiotics (failure to sterilize the vegetations increases the risk of relapse)

**TABLE 43.2. Proposed New Criteria for the Diagnosis of Infective Endocarditis**

***Definite IE***

**Pathologic criteria**
- Microorganisms demonstrated by culture or histology in a vegetation or in a vegetation that has embolized or in an intracardiac abscess or pathologic lesions
- Vegetation or intracardiac abscess present, histologically confirmed as active endocarditis

**Clinical criteria**
Using specific definitions as listed below
- 2 major criteria, or
- 1 major and 3 minor criteria, or
- 5 minor criteria

***Major criteria***

❑ ***Positive blood culture for IE***
- Typical organisms (*S. viridans, S. bovis,* HACEK group, or community-acquired *S. aureus* or enterococci without a primary focus from 2 separate blood cultures, or
- Persistently positive blood cultures for any microorganism (i.e., blood cultures drawn more than 12 hours apart, or all 3 or majority of ≥4 separate blood cultures, with the first and last drawn at least 1 hour apart)

❑ ***Evidence of endocardial involvement (echocardiographic)***
- Oscillating intracardiac mass on valve or supporting structure, or in the path of regurgitant jets, or on iatrogenic devices, with no alternative anatomic explanation, or
- Abscess, or
- New partial dehiscence of prosthetic valve or new valvular regurgitation

***Minor criteria***
- *Predisposition*: predisposing heart condition or IVDA
- *Fever* > 38°C
- *Vascular phenomenon*: arterial embolism, septic pulmonary infarcts, mycotic aneurysms, intracranial hemorrhage, Janeway lesions
- *Immunologic phenomenon*: Osler's nodes, Roth spots, glomerulonephritis
- *Echocardiogram*: consistent with IE but not meeting the major criteria noted above
- *Microbiologic evidence*: (+) blood culture but not meeting major criterion above, or serologic evidence of active infection with an organism consistent with IE

***Possible IE***: Findings consistent with IE that fall short of **Definite** but **not Rejected**
***Rejected***: Firm alternate diagnosis explaining evidence of IE, or resolution of endocarditis syndrome with ≤4 days of antibiotics, or no pathologic evidence of IE at surgery or autopsy, after antibiotics for ≤4 days

IE = infective endocarditis; IVDA = intravenous drug abuse; (+) = positive; HACEK = see text.
(Adapted from Bayer AS, Ward JI, Ginzton LE, Shapiro SM. Evaluation of new clinical criteria for the diagnosis of infective endocarditis. Am J Med 1994; 96:211–219. Used with permisson.)

2. Using IV therapy, which is almost always necessary
3. Ensuring high antibiotic concentrations for prolonged periods to eradicate slowly replicating organisms

### Antibiotic treatment

After appropriate cultures are obtained, empiric antibiotics may be given to patients with suspected IE, especially those who are acutely toxic or in heart failure. Ampicillin (3.0 g IV every 4 hrs) with nafcillin or oxacillin (2.0 g IV every 4 hrs) and gentamicin (1 mg/kg IV every 8 hrs with normal renal function) is appropriate. Given the high rate of methicillin-resistant *Staphylococcus aureus* (MRSA), vancomycin (15 mg/kg IV every 12 hrs) may be used instead of ampicillin and nafcillin. Once blood culture results are available, this regimen should be tailored to the specific organism and its in vitro sensitivities (Table 43.3).

Because the MIC for viridans streptococci is low (usually <0.1 μg/ml) and the cure rate is high (95–99%), there are several successful treatment options. Ceftriaxone is promising as a once-daily therapy. Aminoglycoside resistance, seen in 5–30% of enterococci, creates serious treatment difficulties.

Patients with isolated *S. aureus* bacteremia, an identifiable focus or source of infection, and normal heart valves should be treated for 2 weeks with IV therapy. The vast majority of patients with disseminated *S. aureus* infections should be treated for 4–6 weeks with this regimen. Rifampin (600 mg/day orally) can be added if metastatic abscesses are suspected.

### Endocarditis complicating intravenous drug abuse

Endocarditis may be responsible for 5–10% of hospital admissions for febrile intravenous drug abusers (IVDA). Despite the high rate of right-sided endocarditis among IVDAs (primarily the tricuspid valve), predicting IE among these patients is difficult. Thus, patients with fever and IVDA should be observed closely (usually in the hospital) until blood cultures are reported sterile.

IE in IVDA often presents with pleuritic chest pain and cough. In over half the cases, the responsible microorganism is *Staphylococcus aureus* (50%), followed by streptococci in 20%, gram-negative bacilli (esp. *Pseudomonas aeruginosa*) in 20%, and fungi (esp. *Candida* sp.) in 10% of cases. The geographical location (eastern vs western U.S.) may affect the microbial etiology. A murmur is common, but the classical triad of tricuspid regurgitation, a pulsatile liver, and the waxing-waning systolic murmur occurs in one-third of cases. Chest x-rays may show septic pulmonary emboli and/or pneumonia in about 50% of patients. Besides the tricuspid valve, mitral and aortic valves also may be involved.

Positive blood cultures are the cornerstone of diagnosis of IVDA-related IE. The cure rate in appropriately treated, right-sided *S. aureus* endocarditis exceeds 90%. The mortality in right-sided endocarditis averages 8–10%. Valve excision or debridement are usually reserved for those with persistent uncontrolled

**TABLE 43.3. Treatment of Infective Endocarditis Caused by Common Organisms**

**Viridans Streptococci and *S. bovis***

*Penicillin-susceptible* (MIC = 0.1 μg/ml)

1. Aqueous Penicillin G 12–18 MU/d in divided doses for 4 wks; OR
2. Penicillin G 10–20 MU/d in divided doses + Gentamycin 1 mg/kg IV q 8 h, both for 2 wks; OR
3. Vancomycin 15 mg/kg IV q 12 h for 4 wks.

*Relatively penicillin-resistant* (MIC >0.1-≤0.5μg/ml)

1. Penicillin G 18 MU/d in divided doses q 4 h or continuously + Gentamycin 1 mg/kg IV q 8 h, both for 4 wks, then continue penicillin G for 2 more wks; OR
2. Vancomycin 15 mg/kg IV q 12 h for 4 wks.

**Enterococci and viridans Streptococci**

(MIC >0.5μg/ml)

1. Penicillin G 18–30 MU IV in divided doses q 4 h or continuously for 4 wks; OR
2. Ampicillin 12 g/d in divided doses 4 h or continuously + Gentamycin 1 mg/kg IV q 8 h both for 4–6 wks; OR
3. Vancomycin 15 mg/kg IV q 12 h + Gentamycin 1 mg/kg IV q 8 h for 4–6 wks.

**Staphylococci**

Native valve

*Methicillin-sensitive* (*S. epidermidis* and *S. aureus*)

Nafcillin or oxacillin 2 g IV q 4 h for 4–6 wks. ± Gentamycin 1 mg/kg IV q 8 h for first 3–5 d.

*Methicillin-resistant*

Vancomycin 15 mg/kg q 12 h for 4–6 wks.

Prosthetic valve

*Methicillin-susceptible*

Vancomycin 15 mg/kg q 12 h for 6–8 wks. + Gentamycin 1 mg/kg q 8 h for first 2 wks.

*Methicillin-resistant*

Vancomycin 15 mg/kg q 12 h for 6–8 wks. + Gentamycin 1 mg/kg q 8 h for first 2 wks. If *S. epidermidis*, add Rifampin 300 mg q 8 h orally for 4–6 wks.

**Culture-Negative**

Ampicillin 3 g IV q 4 h + Gentamycin 1 mg/kg q 8 h.

d = days; h = hours; MIC = minimum inhibitory concentration; MU = million units; q = every; wks = weeks. In penicillin-allergic patients, one may give vancomycin or consider penicillin desensitization (Chapter 12). Gentamycin may be given IV or IM

(Adapted from Bartlett JG. In Pocket Book of Infectious Disease Therapy. Baltimore: Williams & Wilkins. 1996, pp. 274–276.)

bacteremia. Persistent fever and septic emboli are not indications for surgical intervention.

**Prosthetic valve endocarditis**

Because of differences in pathogenesis and pathogens, prosthetic valve endocarditis (PVE) may be classified as early (within 60 days of valve surgery) or late (>60 days after surgery). *Staphylococcus epidermidis* is the most frequent organism in early PVE, suggesting an important role for intraoperative contamination. Causative organisms in late disease resemble those of native-valve endocarditis. Suggested treatment of early PVE due to *S. epidermidis* (Table 43.3) takes into account the resistance patterns of this organism. Both early and late PVE often need reoperation for valve replacement.

**Role of surgery**

Valve surgery is required in about 25% of cases of IE. Common indications are congestive heart failure (>70% of cases), hemodynamic compromise, persistent infection or recurrent systemic emboli. Specific echocardiographic findings might also suggest the need for surgical intervention (Table 43.4). Ideally, patients are given antibiotics long enough to "sterilize" the vegetations before surgery, but hemodynamic issues often dictate the specific timing for surgery.

**TABLE 43.4. Echocardiographic Features That Suggest Potential Need for Surgery**

Vegetation
- Persistent vegetation after systemic embolization; systemic embolization during or following therapy

Valvular dysfunction
- Acute aortic/mitral insufficiency with left ventricular failure
- Heart failure refractory to medical therapy
- Valve perforation/rupture

Perivalvular extension
- Valvular dehiscence, rupture, or fistula
- New heart block
- Large abscess, or extension of abscess despite adequate therapy

(Adapted from: Bayer et al. Circulation 1998; 98:2936–2948. Used with permission.)

## Prognosis and Course

The patient's age, comorbid conditions, the valve affected, virulence of the organism, and complications of treatment all influence the prognosis. With optimal treatment, most patients (>90%) with native-valve endocarditis attain a microbiologic cure. Recurrent fever may reflect local complications (e.g., myocardial or valve ring abscess, metastatic abscesses) or drug fever. Recurrences and relapses mostly occur within a few weeks to a month of cessation of treatment. Relapses should be distinguished from reinfection, which is more common with IVDA and those with periodontal disease. Patients at high risk of complications are those with special issues determined by *clinical factors* (those with prolonged symptoms or poor response to therapy), *predisposition* (IE superimposed on prosthetic cardiac valves, cyanotic heart disease, previous endocarditis or systemic shunts), *site of lesion* (left sided IE), or *causative organisms* (staphylococci and fungi).

## Prevention

The use of **endocarditis prophylaxis** is rooted in medical practice, despite its empiric nature, increasing recognition of predisposition (underlying cardiac disease), and documented failures. However, it is recommended for all high-risk patients undergoing procedures likely to cause transient bacteremia (Table 43.5). The selection of antibiotic depends on the nature of the procedure, the ability for oral intake, and the presence or absence of penicillin allergy (Tables 43.6 and 43.7).

**TABLE 43.5. Indications for Endocarditis Prophylaxis**

| Prophylaxis Recommended | Prophylaxis Not Recommended |
|---|---|
| **High-risk category**<br>All prosthetic (including bioprosthetic and homograft) cardiac valves<br>Previous bacterial endocarditis<br>Complex cyanotic congenital heart disease<br>Surgically constructed systemic pulmonary shunts or conduits<br>**Moderate risk category**<br>Most other congenital cardiac malformations (other than above or below)<br>Acquired valvular dysfunction<br>Hypertrophic cardiomyopathy<br>Mitral valve prolapse with valvular regurgitation and/or thickened leaflets<br>**Surgical procedures**<br>Tonsillectomy and adenoidectomy; procedures in the oral mucosa; rigid bronchoscopy; sclerotherapy for varices*; esophageal stricture dilation*; ERCP with biliary obstruction*; bilary tract surgery*; procedures involving intestinal mucosa*; prostate surgery, cystoscopy; urethral dilation | **Negligible risk category**<br>Isolated secundum ASD<br>Surgical repair of ASD, VSD, or PDA without residua beyond 6 months<br>Previous coronary artery bypass graft surgery<br>Mitral valve prolapse without valvular regurgitation**<br>Physiologic, functional, or innocent heart murmurs<br>Previous Kawasaki disease without valvular dysfunction<br>Previous rheumatic fever without valvular dysfunction<br>Cardiac pacemakers and implanted defibrillators<br>**Surgical procedures**<br>Endotracheal intubation; fiberoptic bronchoscopy†; tympanostomy tube insertion; transesophageal echocardiography; vaginal hysterectomy; vaginal delivery; Cesarean section; urethral catheterization, uterine dilatation and curettage, sterilization procedures, insertion or removal or IUDs, and therapeutic abortion (all in uninfected tissue); cardiac catheterization; implanted pacemakers and defibrillators; circumcision; and incision or biopsy of surgically scrubbed skin |

ASD = atrial septal defect; ERCP= endoscopic retrograde cholangiopancreatography; IUD = Intrauterine devices; PDA = patent ductus arteriosus; VSD = ventricular septal defect.
(Adapted from: Dajani AS, et al: JAMA 1997; 277:1795.)
*Prophylaxis recommended in high-risk patients.
†Prophylaxis optional in high-risk patients.
**Individuals with prolapsing and/or myxomatous mitral valves that show regurgitation (audible on auscultation or shown on echocardiography) are at increased risk for bacterial endocarditis.

**TABLE 43.6. Endocarditis Prophylaxis for Dental, Oral, Respiratory Tract or Esophageal Procedures**

| Penicillin Allergy | Oral Intake | Agent | Dose, Route and Timing |
|---|---|---|---|
| None | Possible | Amoxicillin | 2.0 g p.o. within 1 h before |
| None | Not Possible | Ampicillin | 2.0 g IM or IV within 30 min before |
| Present | Possible | Clindamycin | 600 mg p.o. within 1 h before, OR |
| | | Cephalexin/Cefadroxil† | 2.0 g p.o. within 1 h before, OR |
| | | Azithromycin/Clarithromycin | 500 mg p.o. within 1 h before |
| Present | Not Possible | Clindamycin | 600 mg IV within 30 min before, OR |
| | | Cefazolin† | 1.0 g IV within 1 h before |

†Avoid if there is history of immediate hypersensitivity (urticaria, angioedema, or anaphylaxis) to penicillin.
(Adapted from: Dajani AS et al. JAMA 1997; 277:1798.)

**TABLE 43.7. Regimens for Endocarditis Prophylaxis for Procedures in Genitourinary/Gastrointestinal Tract (Excluding Esophagus)**

| Risk Category | Penicillin Allergy | Agents and Dosage | Comments |
|---|---|---|---|
| High | None | Ampicillin 2.0 g plus Gentamicin 1.5 mg/kg (not to exceed 120 mg) | First dose within 30 min; Ampicillin 1.0 g IV/IM or Amoxicillin 1.0 g p.o. 6 h later |
| High | Present | Vancomycin 1.0 g IV plus Gentamycin 1.5 mg/kg (not to exceed 120 mg) | Infuse vancomycin in 1–2 h; complete injection/infusion within 30 min before |
| Moderate | None | Amoxicillin 2.0 g p.o. OR Ampicillin, 2.0 g IM/IV | Amoxicillin 1 h before; Ampicillin within 30 min before |
| Moderate | Present | Vancomycin 1.0 g IV | Infuse vancomycin in 1–2 h; complete infusion within 30 min before |

(Adapted from: Dajani AS et al. JAMA 1997; 277:1799.)

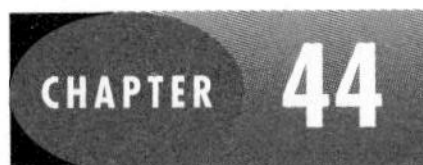

# DISEASES OF THE MYOCARDIUM

## Cardiomyopathies

The cardiomyopathies are primary myocardial diseases affecting the structure and function of heart muscle, but excluding ventricular dysfunction due to pericardial, valvular, hypertensive, or ischemic disease. They are generally divided into three clinical subgroups:dilated (congestive), hypertrophic, and restrictive (Figure 44.1). Dilated cardiomyopathies usually exhibit ventricular systolic dysfunction, whereas hypertrophic and restrictive types feature mostly diastolic dysfunction.

### *Idiopathic Dilated (Congestive) Cardiomyopathy*

Idiopathic dilated cardiomyopathy (IDC) is a primary myocardial disease of unknown cause, with ventricular dilatation and impaired myocardial contractility.

#### Etiology, Pathology, and Pathogenesis

Dec and Fuster postulate four basic but not mutually exclusive mechanisms for IDC: 1) familial and genetic factors, 2) viral and other cytotoxic insults, 3) immune abnormalities, and 4) metabolic, energetic, and contractile abnormalities. IDC is believed to have a genetic predisposition, with the affected locus being involved with immunoregulation. Antibodies against coxsackie B virus, while common in IDC, do not prove this agent as the etiology; however, the virus may alter the MHC-antigen expression or activate T cells or specific HLA antigens. The metabolic, energetic, and contractile derangements mark the disease progression, rather than initiate the disease.

IDC lacks any anatomic or histologic characteristics that set it apart from other causes of dilated cardiomyopathy (Table 44.1). The coronary arteries are normal. The chief microscopic features are myocyte hypertrophy and degeneration, with varying degrees of interstitial

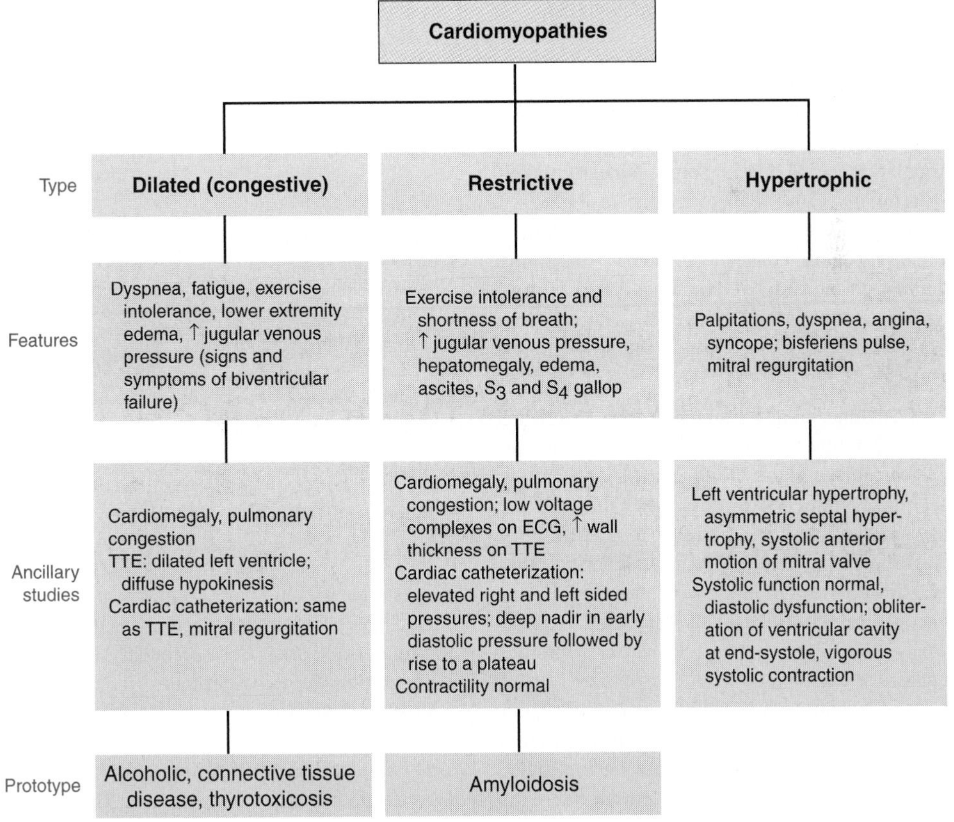


**FIGURE 44.1.** Classification and characteristics of cardiomyopathies. TTE = Transthoracic echocardiography.

**TABLE 44.1. Known Causes of Dilated Cardiomyopathy**

| | |
|---|---|
| *Toxins* | *Inflammatory or Infectious causes* |
| Ethanol* | Infectious |
| Chemotherapeutic agents: doxorubicin, bleomycin | Viral: |
| Cobalt* | Coxsackie virus, cytomegalovirus*, human immunodeficiency virus |
| Antiretroviral agents: zidovudine*, didanosine*, zalcitabine* | Rickettsial |
| Phenothiazines* | Bacterial: diphtheria |
| Carbon monoxide* | Mycobacterial |
| Lead*, Mercury* | Fungal |
| Cocaine* | Parasitic |
| | Toxoplasmosis* |
| *Metabolic abnormalities* | Trichinosis, Chagas' disease |
| Nutritional deficiencies | Noninfectious |
| Thiamine*, selenium*, carnitine* | Collagen vascular disorders |
| Endocrinologic disorders | Systemic lupus erythematosus, progressive systemic sclerosis, dermatomyositis |
| Diabetes mellitus, hypothyroidism*, thyrotoxicosis*, Cushing's disease, acromegaly*, pheochromocytoma* | Hypersensitivity myocarditis* |
| | Sarcoidosis*, peripartum dysfunction* |
| Electrolyte disturbances: | |
| Hypocalcemia*, hypophosphatemia* | *Neuromuscular causes* |
| *Familial cardiomyopathies* | Duchenne's muscular dystrophy, facioscapulohumeral muscular dystrophy, Erb's limb girdle dystrophy, myotonic dystrophy, Fredreich's ataxia |

*Potentially reversible either spontaneously or with treatment.
(Dec GW and Fuster V. N Engl J Med 1994; 331:1564–1575.)

fibrosis and inflammation. Inflammation is evident immunohistochemically in many cases, but this does not prove myocarditis.

Ventricular dilatation and impaired myocardial contractility eventually cause symptoms due to decreased ejection fraction, increased LV end-diastolic volumes, and pulmonary venous congestion. Excess circulating catecholamines chronically overstimulate cardiac receptors and damage an already depressed myocardium.

## Clinical Features

IDC has a distinct predilection for African Americans and men (by 2.5 times) compared to Caucasians and women. Signs and symptoms of advanced LV failure are the presenting features in most cases (Table 44.2). Despite normal coronary arteries, up to one-third of patients report angina-like chest pain. A minority experience atrial fibrillation or high-grade ventricular arrhythmias. Syncope strongly predicts sudden death. Pulmonary and/or systemic emboli may follow mural thrombi in the appropriate chambers.

Features of biventricular heart failure are typical, but signs of left heart failure usually predominate initially. Often, the blood pressure is low, with a narrow pulse pressure. Tachycardia is common and pulsus alternans may occur. The apical impulse is diffuse and laterally displaced. Atrial ($S_4$) and ventricular ($S_3$) gallops as well as systolic murmurs are common, particularly during periods of symptomatic decompensation. The systolic murmurs often arise from secondary mitral or tricuspid regurgitation due to ventricular dilatation and chordal geometric distortion.

Bilateral end-inspiratory crackles and pleural effusions signify left heart failure. Cool, pale extremities indicate poor peripheral perfusion. The neck veins are often distended; a prominent *v* wave follows tricuspid regurgitation. Ascites, tender hepatomegaly, and other

**TABLE 44.2. Presenting Symptoms of Idiopathic Dilated Cardiomyopathy**

| | |
|---|---|
| Dyspnea on exertion | 86% |
| Heart Failure | 75–85%* |
| Peripheral edema | 29% |
| Palpitations | 30% |
| Exertional chest pain | 8–20%† |
| Asymptomatic cardiomegaly | 4–13%‡ |
| Systemic/pulmonary emboli | 1.5–4% |
| Syncope | Rare |

*90% in NYHA Class III or IV.
†Chest pain eventually occurs in 35% of all patients.
‡Atrial fibrillation may be present in less than 25% of these.
(From: Dec GW and Fuster V. N Engl J Med 1994; 331:1564–1575.)

signs of right heart failure occur in less than one-half of patients. Atrial fibrillation is tolerated poorly.

### Ancillary Studies

The ECG typically shows tachycardia and nonspecific ST-T changes. Conduction delays occur in over three-fourths of all patients with IDC, their presence correlating with duration of symptoms and the extent of myocardial fibrosis. Sinus rhythm is mostly maintained, but in others, atrial fibrillation may prevail. The chest radiograph typically shows cardiomegaly and pulmonary vascular congestion. Pleural effusions, often bilateral, are common. Unilateral effusions are often right-sided.

Transthoracic echocardiogram shows ventricular dilatation (often involving all 4 chambers), normal wall thickness, and a decreased ejection fraction. While global hypokinesis is common, segmental wall motion may be abnormal in over one-half of the cases, owing to altered regional wall stress.

Cardiac catheterization should be reserved for patients with strong risk profiles for, or symptoms of, ischemia (typical angina, suspected ischemic LV dysfunction). Endomyocardial biopsy is done only when a treatable underlying disorder, such as sarcoidosis or hypereosinophilic syndrome, is suspected.

### Management

Nonpharmacologic therapy for IDC includes activity guidelines, salt restriction (2.0 g $Na^+$ diet), smoking cessation, and weight reduction. Vasodilators (either an ACE inhibitor or combined hydralazine-isosorbide dinitrate) improve symptoms and prolong survival in congestive heart failure. Digitalis not only controls resting heart rate in atrial fibrillation, but it also improves maximum exercise capacity and reduces symptoms of heart failure, even in those with prevailing sinus rhythm.

Patients with atrial fibrillation, mural thrombus on echocardiography, or prior thromboembolism should receive adjusted-dose warfarin to keep the INR between 2–3. Antiarrhythmic agents are reserved for survivors of sudden death and symptomatic patients with proven, sustained ventricular arrhythmias, usually after electrophysiologic testing. These patients may also benefit from an automatic implantable cardioverter-defibrillator (AICD).

### Natural History

The overall prognosis in symptomatic IDC is poor, with 5-year mortality rates averaging 20–50%. Many deaths occur within the first year after symptoms appear. Although LV function may spontaneously improve in some patients, symptoms typically progress and LV failure worsens over time in most. Not surprisingly, IDC remains a common indication for heart transplantation.

## *Hypertrophic Cardiomyopathy*

### Definition and Etiology

**Hypertrophic cardiomyopathy** (HCM) is a common genetic malformation whose central theme is a markedly hypertrophic, nondilated LV without systemic hypertension, aortic stenosis, or any other process capable of producing similar degrees of LV hypertrophy (LVH). Associated LV outflow tract obstruction may or may not be present.

Previously known as **idiopathic hypertrophic subaortic stenosis** (IHSS), HCM affects nearly 1 in 500 persons through an autosomal dominant inheritance. HCM is caused by one of the many mutations in the genes that encode the following cardiac sarcomere proteins: β-myosin heavy chain, cardiac troponin T, myosin-binding protein C, α-tropomysin, and β-myosin light chains. With over 50 mutations, the resulting phenotypic picture is highly variable.

### Pathology and Pathogenesis

The gross pathology of HCM consists of localized or diffuse ventricular hypertrophy. In 95% of endocardial biopsies, the histology shows myocardial cell disarray. The LVH and myocyte degeneration together cause abnormal LV relaxation, excessive LV stiffness, and impaired LV filling. Consequently, the filling pressures rise, leading to pulmonary venous hypertension and dyspnea. Excessive myocardial $O_2$ demands or impaired perfusion of hypertrophied muscle may provoke myocardial ischemia. Associated coronary disease may also cause ischemia through small-vessel disease from intimal thickening and medial fibrosis of the intramural coronary arteries. Nevertheless, the pathophysiology of the chest pain in HCM is poorly understood.

The majority of patients with HCM lack significant LV outflow obstruction. The obstruction, when present, is dynamic, and due to the hypertrophied ventricular septum. Sudden death in HCM patients appears to be due to tachyarrhythmias. Because HCM is the most common cause of sudden death in young athletes, its distinction from the ventricular hypertrophy that is common in well-trained athletes is crucial.

Decreased compliance and altered ventricular pressure/volume relationships also can jeopardize the cardiac output if the LV is "under-filled." For example, when effective atrial transport is lost (as in atrial fibrillation), the stiff and noncompliant LV fills inadequately, thus compromising the preload.

### Clinical Features

Clinical features of HCM vary widely, ranging from no symptoms to progressive heart failure. Symptoms, when present, usually appear in the third or fourth decade. Predominant symptoms are exertional dyspnea, fatigue, and chest pain that may or may not resemble classic angina, palpitations, dizziness, and exertional syncope. Many of these symptoms are exacerbated by tachycardias and/or atrial arrhythmias.

**Sudden death,** which affects 2–3% of adults with HCM, may be the sole initial manifestation of HCM, and most often caused by tachyarrhythmias. Such lethal arrhythmias may be precipitated either by an innate proclivity for them or through a vicious circle of myocardial ischemia, diastolic dysfunction, systolic dysfunction, lowered stroke volume, and decreased coronary perfusion. Major risk factors for sudden death include: previous history of sudden death, sustained ventricular tachycardia on Holter monitoring, a significant family history of sudden death or high risk mutation (e.g., Arg403Gln), prolonged or non-sustained ventricular tachycardia, onset of symptoms in childhood and significant ventricular hypertrophy.

Typical findings in HCM include a fast-rising arterial pulse, left atrial and LV hypertrophy, and a harsh, diamond-shaped systolic murmur heard typically at the base, and augmented by maneuvers that decrease LV cavity size (Valsalva, standing). A brisk carotid upstroke and bisferiens pulse, while not specific for HCM, can help distinguish HCM from valvular aortic stenosis. Other cardiac findings are an $S_4$ gallop and an apical murmur of mitral regurgitation. When there is no LV outflow obstruction, the murmur is usually absent, and the only auscultatory finding is an apical $S_4$.

## Ancillary Studies

The chest radiograph is normal (50% of cases) or may show left atrial enlargement and cardiomegaly. In over 90% of cases, ECG shows left atrial enlargement or LVH, or T-wave inversion (none being specific). Prominent, abnormal Q waves and diminished or absent R waves in lateral chest leads ("pseudoinfarct") often muddle the recognition of myocardial ischemia or infarction. Giant T-wave inversion may be with asymmetric apical involvement. Holter monitoring may show nonsustained ventricular tachycardia.

Echocardiography typically shows a nondilated, hypertrophied LV with a normal to supernormal ejection fraction and near-cavity obliteration at end-systole. Highly specific findings are asymmetrical septal hypertrophy (septal thickness >1.5 times that of the posterior wall or an interventricular septal thickness >15 mm). The anterior mitral valve leaflet comes in contact with the ventricular septum during systole—systolic anterior motion (SAM) of the mitral valve—producing dynamic outflow obstruction. SAM, which is seen in about one-half of cases, is quite specific for LV outflow tract obstruction. Doppler echocardiography may show mitral regurgitation and signs of impaired LV filling.

Cardiac catheterization measures chamber pressures, quantitates the LV outflow tract gradient, and assesses the presence and severity of associated coronary artery disease. Left ventriculography in HCM often shows massive septal and free wall hypertrophy, large papillary muscles, and an almost obliterated LV cavity at end-systole.

## Management

Because most patients with HCM lack significant left ventricular outflow obstruction, therapy aims to enhance ventricular diastolic filling and to reduce myocardial ischemia. The risk of sudden death mandates that patients with HCM not participate in high-intensity, competitive athletic activities. Dehydration and hypovolemia should be avoided.

Most agree that only symptomatic patients should be treated (Figure 44.2). Primary therapy is medical, using β-blockers as primary, and verapamil and disopyramide as secondary agents. One should avoid digoxin and vasodilators, and when there is significant outflow obstruction, or left heart failure, verapamil as well. Diuretics should be used with care, since they can lower ventricular filling pressures and thus, left ventricular output. Nitroglycerine should not be given for chest pain.

Atrial fibrillation worsens the clinical status in HCM. Amiodarone is the most effective agent for preventing recurrence of atrial fibrillation. Chronic or recurrent atrial fibrillation requires anticoagulant therapy. Those with significant outflow obstruction or with refractory symptoms should be considered for invasive, interventional strategies (e.g., percutaneous septal ablation by intracoronary alcohol injection, dual chamber pacing, treating atrial fibrillation with a-v nodal ablation and pacemaker). Dynamic outflow obstruction or mitral regurgitation mandate endocarditis prophylaxis.

Surgery (septal myotomy-myectomy) is reserved only for severe, refractory symptoms or an LV outflow tract gradient exceeding 50 mm Hg. Cardiac transplantation may be needed in some cases.

# *Restrictive Cardiomyopathy*

## Definition, Etiology, and Pathophysiology

Restrictive cardiomyopathy (RCM) is a heart muscle disease that causes impaired ventricular filling with normal or decreased diastolic volume of either or both ventricles. Systolic function is often normal, but there is diastolic dysfunction (i.e., impaired LV relaxation and filling and high pulmonary venous and right-sided pressures).

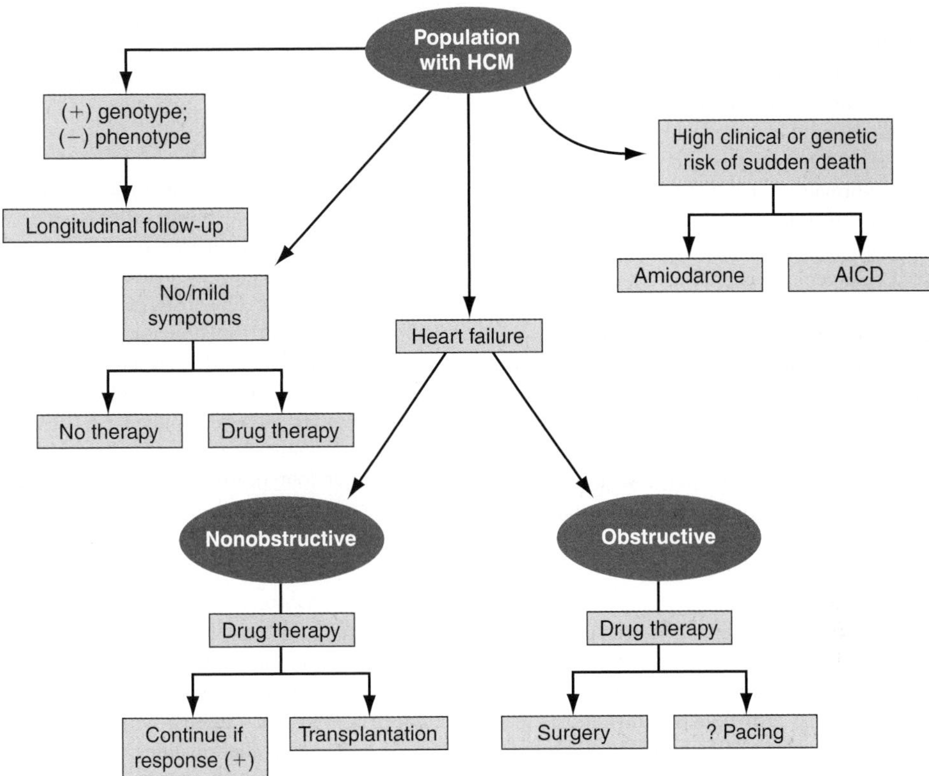


**FIGURE 44.2. Management of Hypertrophic cardiomyopathy (HCM). The size of the arrows indicate the approximate proportion of patients within each subgroup. The question mark indicates the uncertainty of the usefulness of pacing. The dotted lines indicate the current uncertainty of the size of this subgroup. AICD = automatic implantable cardioverter-defibrillator.**
Adapted from: Spirito P. et al. N Engl J Med 1997;336: p 377. Used with permission.

Among the major causes of RCM shown in Table 44.3, systemic **amyloidosis** (distinguished from senile cardiac amyloidosis) is one of the more common. **Hemochromatosis**, more often seen as a congestive cardiomyopathy, and **hypereosinophilic syndrome** (Loeffler's endocarditis) may present with RCM.

## Clinical Features

Although rare, the causes of RCM are potentially reversible or treatable (sarcoidosis, hemochromatosis). In general, RCM should be suspected when there is heart failure without cardiomegaly or systolic dysfunction. Features of biventricular failure are often the initial manifestation, and edema and ascites may sometimes become dominant. RCM may mimic constrictive pericarditis with neck vein distension and prominent $x$ and $y$ descents. Hepatomegaly, lung crackles, and a systolic murmur of tricuspid regurgitation are other common findings.

**TABLE 44.3. Causes of Restrictive Cardiomyopathy**

| Myocardial | Endomyocardial |
|---|---|
| Non-infiltrative | Endomyocardial fibrosis* |
| Idiopathic* | Hypereosinophilic syndrome |
| Familial | Carcinoid heart disease |
| Diabetic | Metastatic cancers |
| Infiltrative | Radiation* |
| Amyloidosis* | Anthracycline toxicity* |
| Sarcoidosis* | Drug-related fibrous endocarditis |
| Fatty infiltration | Serotonin |
| Gaucher's disease | Methysergide |
| Storage diseases | Ergotamine |
| Hemochromatosis | Mercurial agents |
| Fabry's disease | Busulfan |
| Glycogen storage disease | |

*More frequent than the others in clinical practice.
(Adapted from: Kushwaha SS, Fallon JT, Fuster V: Restrictive Cardiomyopathy. N Engl J Med 1997; 336: 267–276 used with permission.)

### Ancillary Studies

Sinus tachycardia, low voltage in the limb leads, nonspecific ST-T changes, left bundle branch block, and arrhythmias are common ECG findings. Chest radiography often shows mild cardiomegaly and pulmonary venous congestion. On transthoracic echocardiography, the valves are normal; the LV has thickened walls and normal systolic function, and it is not dilated. Two-dimensional images, particularly in amyloidosis, may show biatrial enlargement, interatrial septal thickening, and a peculiar "speckled" pattern. Computed tomographic scans show no pericardial thickening, an important differentiating point from constrictive pericarditis.

Cardiac catheterization may be needed to distinguish RCM from constrictive pericarditis, but the findings may be inconclusive. Endomyocardial biopsy should be performed in patients with a high index of suspicion for potentially treatable causes of RCM (hemochromatosis, sarcoidosis).

### Management

Diuretics and vasodilators should be used judiciously in RCM so that the LV preload is not compromised. Because systolic function is normal, digitalis is usually used only to treat atrial arrhythmias. Amyloidosis may predispose to digitalis toxicity. Calcium channel blockers and β-blockers may improve resting hemodynamics by promoting ventricular relaxation and prolonging filling time. Amyloid heart disease has the worst prognosis.

## Myocarditis

Myocarditis is often clinically diagnosed when heart failure complicates a febrile illness and when LV dysfunction (LV ejection fraction <45%) occurs in the absence of coronary artery disease or another specific etiology. Histologic diagnosis of myocarditis requires demonstration of an "inflammatory infiltrate with necrosis and/or degeneration of adjacent myocytes not typical of the ischemic change seen in coronary artery disease" (Dallas criteria). However, only 10% patients with the clinical definition of myocarditis show confirmatory results on endomyocardial biopsy. This dichotomy between the clinical and histologic criteria makes an accurate definition of myocarditis difficult.

### Etiology, Pathology, and Pathophysiology

The causes of myocarditis are listed in Table 44.4. Coxsackie virus infections occur commonly in young adults, usually in association with pleurisy or pericarditis. Lyme carditis often presents with a predominance of cardiac conduction abnormalities.

**TABLE 44.4. Causes of Myocarditis**

| Causes of Myocarditis |
|---|
| Infectious |
| Bacterial |
| Diphtheria (toxin), infective endocarditis, Lyme disease (*Borrelia burgdorferi*) |
| Fungal |
| Aspergillus |
| Mycoplasma |
| Parasitic |
| Toxoplasmosis, trypanosomiasis (Chaga's disease), trichinosis |
| Rickettsial |
| Rocky Mountain spotted fever |
| Viral |
| Adenovirus, Coxsackie groups A and B, cytomegalovirus (CMV), ECHO viruses, hepatitis B, HIV (may be opportunistic infections or drug effects also), influenza, poliomyelitis, rubella, rubeola |
| Inflammatory |
| Idiopathic giant cell myocarditis, rheumatic fever, sarcoidosis |
| Connective tissue diseases |
| Systemic lupus erythematosus, rheumatoid arthritis |
| Vasculitis |
| Polyarteritis nodosa, Churg-Strauss vasculitis |
| Hypereosinophilic syndrome |
| Toxic |
| Drugs |
| Aerosol propellants, daunorubicin, emetine, phenothiazines, tricyclic antidepressants |
| Physical agents |
| Radiation |

Cytomegalovirus infection, usually a self-limited illness, may be a more serious process in immunocompromised patients. Up to 40% of AIDS patients exhibit focal myocarditis due to multiple factors, including HIV, opportunistic infections, or drug effects. While 20% show LV dilatation and dysfunction (decreased ejection fraction, global hypokinesis), clinically apparent heart failure develops in only a minority of AIDS patients.

### Clinical Features

Myocarditis shows highly variable clinical features. Some patients are symptomatic during the early inflammatory phase and present acutely with fever, fatigue, palpitations, dyspnea, and chest pain. The chest pain may or may not simulate angina and, in some cases, results from associated pericarditis. Tachycardia is out of proportion to the fever. Signs of heart failure may be present.

The myocarditis may resolve uneventfully in some patients, but in others, it may evolve into a dilated cardiomyopathy. Thus, some patients may present initially with advanced heart failure and other complications of cardiomyopathy. An irregular rhythm, $S_3$ gallop, and signs of heart failure may be present.

### Ancillary Studies

The WBC count and erythrocyte sedimentation rate may rise, but both are nonspecific findings. CK-MB rises in less than 15% of cases. Acute and convalescent viral antibody titers may help define a specific etiology.

The ECG often shows tachycardia, low voltage, nonspecific ST-T changes, and a long QT interval. Atrial and ventricular extrasystoles, intraventricular conduction delays, and fleeting, high-degree AV block are also common. The chest radiograph may be normal or show signs of heart failure. Cardiomegaly may be due to LV dilatation or pericardial effusion. Echocardiography shows depressed LV systolic function and possibly a pericardial effusion. The LV cavity size may be normal or increased with some segmental wall motion abnormalities. About 15% of cases may harbor LV mural thrombi. Coronary angiography shows normal findings. Biopsy evidence of definite myocardial damage and T-lymphocyte infiltration is seen in only a minority of cases.

### Management

The usual treatment of myocarditis is supportive care. Because of concerns that exercise may enhance viral replication, physical activities should be limited in patients with suspected viral etiology. Congestive heart failure is treated with the usual measures.

Myocarditis does not appear to warrant immunosuppressive drug therapy. Therefore, routine gallium scanning and endomyocardial biopsy are not indicated.

# CHAPTER 45 DISEASES OF THE AORTA

The normal aorta is a conduit vessel with 3 major segments: the ascending aorta, aortic arch, and descending aorta. The aortic arch gives rise to brachiocephalic, left carotid, and left subclavian arteries. The thoracic and abdominal components of descending aorta are defined by their location above or below the diaphragm. The normal adult aorta is 3 cm wide at its origin and 1.8–2.0 cm wide at a level just below the renal arteries.

## Aortic Aneurysms

An aortic aneurysm is a permanent localized widening of the aorta with a diameter that is at least 50% greater than normal. Most follow vessel wall degeneration (caused by deficiencies in collagen and elastin, and abnormal proteolysis and serum elastolytic activity), which is closely related to risk factors for atherosclerosis. Thus, hyperlipidemia, hypertension, smoking, diabetes, and family history of aortic aneurysm enhance the risk for forming an aneurysm, which is further influenced by age-related changes (aortic elongation, tortuousity, inelasticity, and ectasia).

Cystic medial necrosis (CMN), the key pathologic finding, features fragmentation and loss of elastic tissue in the aortic media. In Marfan's syndrome, where CMN may occur prematurely, defective fibrillin (a glycoprotein) synthesis in the medial layer of the aorta leads to fewer microfibrils in the media, thus making the vessel prone to aneursymal dilatation. Whereas most ascending aortic aneurysms are due to CMN, atherosclerosis causes most descending aortic aneurysms.

### *Abdominal Aortic Aneurysms*

#### Clinical Features

Most (75–90%) aortic aneurysms are abdominal, commonly occupying the infrarenal segment between the renal arteries and aortic bifurcation. Abdominal aortic

**TABLE 45.1. Clinical Features of Ruptured Abdominal Aortic Aneurysms**

| Frequency | Clinical feature |
|---|---|
| Common (>60%) | Abdominal pain |
| | Abdominal tenderness |
| | Back or flank pain |
| | Leukocytosis (>11,000/$mm^3$) |
| Less Common (40–59%) | Pulsatile mass |
| | Systolic BP <110 mm Hg or orthostatic drop >10 mm Hg |
| Infrequent (<40%) | Vomiting |
| | Anemia (hemoglobin <11 g/dl) |

aneurysms (AAA) are often clinically silent and detected incidentally during a routine physical examination or imaging. However, some patients may report a steady thoracic or lumbar spinal pain that is caused by local pressure or expansion of the aneurysm. Unexplained back pain in an older person must arouse the suspicion of AAA. A pulsatile abdominal mass may be present but not invariably so (Table 45.1).

Rupture of an AAA, an ominous event, often causes abrupt hypogastric or back pain. Lethal hypovolemic shock quickly sets in unless there is urgent surgical intervention. Hypotension, a pulsatile abdominal mass, and back pain, the classic triad of signs, are seen in only about one-half of patients with ruptured AAAs. In patients with a suspected or confirmed aneurysm, peripheral vasculature must be thoroughly examined. An associated femoral artery bruit may signify coexistent occlusive disease in that segment.

## Ancillary Studies

Imaging—the procedure of choice for which is the abdominal ultrasound—most accurately confirms the AAA and quantitates its size; physical examination has significant limitations in this regard. Computed tomography offers results similar to ultrasound, but radiation, contrast use, and higher cost are drawbacks. Abdominal aortography—which not only determines the extent of the aneurysm, but also detects an associated renal artery stenosis in hypertensive patients—is usually limited to potential surgical candidates. Plain abdominal radiographs may often show a calcified aneurysmal wall (Figure 45.1).

**Aneurysm size** (measured in diameter) has important prognostic and therapeutic implications. Aneurysms below 4.0 cm rupture at an annual rate of 0–2%; comparable rate for those above 5.0 cm is 22%. Hypertension and smoking are other risk factors for rupture. Aneurysms expand by nearly 0.2–0.5 cm/yr, although the larger the aneurysm, the faster it dilates. Because aneurysms continue to enlarge with time, mortality also increases with time. Comparative mortality data for untreated thoracic-, thoracoabdominal-, and abdominal aortic aneurysms are shown in Figure 45.2.

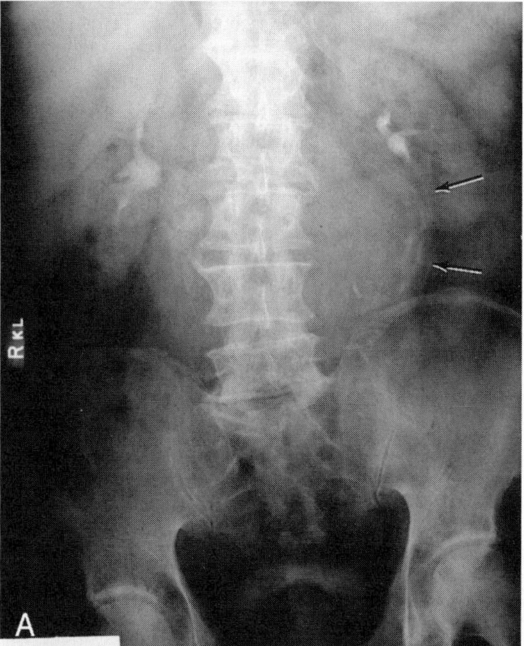


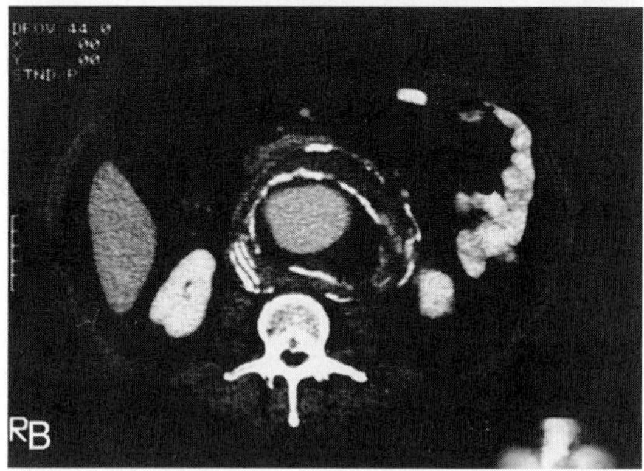


**FIGURE 45.1. Abdominal aortic aneurysm. A, A plain abdominal film shows the heavily calcified walls of a very large aneurysm (arrows). Aneurysms of this size, however, are quite uncommon. B, Computed tomographic scan confirms a large aneurysm with heavily calcified walls.** (Courtesy of the Radiology Museum, St. Joseph's Regional Medical Center, Milwaukee, Wisconsin.)

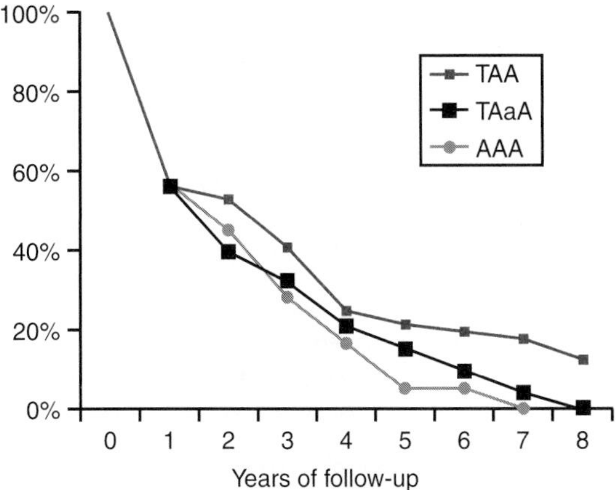


**FIGURE 45.2. Aortic Aneurysms: Survival data for patients that were not treated surgically. AAA = abdominal aortic aneurysm; TAA = Thoracic aortic aneurysm; TAaA = Thoracoabdominal aortic aneurysm.**
(Data from Perko MJ, Norgaard M, Herzog TM, et al.: Ann Thor Surg 1995; 59:1204–1209. Used with permission.)

## Management

The average surgical mortality for repair of nonruptured AAAs is near 4%, compared to 49% for repair of ruptured AAAs. Thus, the emphasis is on elective surgery and avoidance of rupture. All rapidly expanding AAAs or AAAs ≥6 cm should be electively repaired unless strong reasons prevail against surgery. Aneurysms below 4 cm can be followed with annual ultrasound monitoring. For those between 4–6cm, both early surgery and ultrasound monitoring provide similar survival results; however, in a 5-year period, the majority of these patients would require elective repair, thus underscoring the importance of regular, methodical follow-up. Elective AAA repair is contraindicated with recent myocardial infarction (past 6 months), unstable angina, refractory heart failure, severe lung disease (1 sec forced expiratory volume <50%), severe renal failure (serum creatinine >3 mg/dl), marked deficits from stroke, or life expectancy below 2 years. The recent availability of percutaneously introduced endovascular stents—experience with which is limited to centers with special expertise in that area—to repair aortic aneurysms has improved the outlook for these high-risk patients.

Successful aneurysm repair is followed by late complications (infection, aortoenteric fistula, false aneurysm, graft occlusion, and rupture) in about 10% of cases. Patients with graft infections may present with fever. Aortoenteric fistulae usually present with massive gastrointestinal (GI) hemorrhage. An aortoenteric fistula should generally be suspected in any patient with GI bleeding and (even a remote) past history of AAA repair or aortoperipheral vascular bypass graft. False aneurysms are contained ruptures, presenting as expanding abdominal, back, or groin masses.

# *Thoracic Aortic Aneurysms*

Nearly 25% of all aortic aneurysms involve the thoracic aorta, with the most common sites being the arch and descending aorta.

## Clinical Features

Thoracic aortic aneurysms (TAAs) are easily diagnosed because they are readily apparent on chest radiographs. Also, a TAA may compress adjacent structures and evoke symptoms before it expands to a critical size (e.g., hoarseness from compression of the recurrent laryngeal nerve). Others may manifest deep, diffuse chest pain, shoulder pain, dysphagia, hemoptysis, stridor, airflow obstruction, or cough. In ascending aortic aneurysms the aortic annulus may dilate, causing aortic insufficiency; with severe valvular insufficiency, heart failure may occur. Also, severe atherosclerosis of the thoracic aorta causes cerebral emboli leading to transient ischemic attacks and stroke. Nearly 42–70% of TAAs may rupture spontaneously; the 5-year survival rates vary from 13–39% (Figure 45.2).

## Ancillary Studies

Chest radiographs can be diagnostic of a TAA in the majority of patients, although they may be unrevealing in about 17%. Other imaging studies (CT, MRI, or transesophageal echocardiography) can confirm a TAA, quantitate its dimensions, and clarify its relationship to adjacent structures, aortography and coronary angiography are generally necessary before elective TAA repair, given the high risk of associated coronary artery disease. Aortic arch aneurysms generally enlarge at a rate of about 0.56 cm/year; other TAAs enlarge at about 0.42 cm/yr.

## Management

The most important predictor of rupture of a TAA is its size at initial presentation. Those ≥5–6 cm have the highest proclivity for enlargement and rupture. Those exceeding 6 cm are five times more likely to rupture and therefore, require elective repair. TAAs in Marfan's syndrome or with CMN should be repaired when they are larger than 5.0–5.5 cm, or even earlier if significant aortic valve disease is present. Associated coronary artery disease must be excluded or evaluated before surgery. Proximal TAA may require a composite graft with re-implantation of the coronary arteries.

Patients with a dilated aortic root are liable to develop aortic valvular insufficiency, dissection, or rupture. β-blockers, by reducing heart rate and the rate of change of pressure in the aortic root, may decrease the rate of enlargement and prevent or delay the onset of complications.

TAA surgery involves a 10% mortality and other major complications, including hemorrhage and paraplegia. Paraplegia occurs in about 5% of cases and is related to inadvertent interruption of the blood supply of the spinal cord. Early postoperative complications are related to advanced age, aneurysm size, coexisting diabetes mellitus, and technical factors (e.g., need for emergency surgery, prolonged aortic cross-clamp time and surgery of aortic arch). Early postoperative mortality is due to myocardial infarction, congestive heart failure, renal failure, respiratory failure, hemorrhage, and sepsis. Both early and late mortality are higher in surgery for aneurysms of the aortic arch.

## Aortic Dissection

### Definition and Etiology

Aortic dissection develops from an aortic intimal tear that allows blood to dissect into the vessel wall. Although all dissections may be potentially lethal, classifying them into either proximal or distal sites has important therapeutic and prognostic implications. **Proximal dissections** (type A) involve the ascending aorta, with or without the descending aorta. **Distal dissections** (type B) involve only the descending aorta, usually beyond the left subclavian artery. Proximal dissections are twice as common as distal ones.

Distal dissections and proximal dissections of the ascending aorta just above the aortic valve together constitute over 95% of all aortic dissections. Because proximal dissections frequently involve the vicinity of the aortic valve, they often cause aortic insufficiency, hemopericardium, cardiac tamponade, and disrupted arch vessels. Hypertension and cystic medial necrosis cause proximal dissections more often; atherosclerosis and hypertension more often cause distal dissections. Penetrating atherosclerotic ulcer and intramural aortic hematoma without an intimal tear have recently been found to render aortas prone to rupture and probably to dissection.

### Pathogenesis

Damage to the aortic media is a necessary prerequisite for aortic dissection. This damage, caused by cystic medial necrosis (CMN, see discussion on aortic aneurysm previously), is determined by chronic aortic wall stress and accelerated by long-standing hypertension. With a sudden intimal tear, blood under systemic pressure further disrupts the media and "dissects" the intima from adventitium.

### Clinical Features

Dissection affects men twice as frequently as it does women, except during pregnancy. Predisposing factors for aortic dissection are summarized in Table 45.2. The typical patient is a 50- to 60-year-old man with long-standing hypertension who develops severe chest or back pain. The pain may be tearing, ripping, stabbing, or sharp and is unrelated to respiration or position. It is severe and maximal from the very beginning, which contrasts with the pain of angina or myocardial infarction, which typically is progressive. Proximal dissections tend to cause anterior chest pain, and almost all distal dissections involve back or interscapular pain. The migration of pain may signify extension of dissection.

**TABLE 45.2. Predisposing Factors for Aortic Dissection**

| |
|---|
| Acquired Conditions |
| Risk factors for atherosclerosis |
| Penetrating atherosclerotic ulcer |
| Long-standing hypertension (50% of cases) |
| Intramural aortic hematoma |
| Hereditary connective tissue defects with premature cystic medial necrosis (Marfan's syndrome, Ehlers-Danlos syndrome) |
| Pregnancy (third trimester) |
| Aortic stenosis (abnormally high aortic wall stress) |
| Trauma |
| Blunt chest wall |
| Iatrogenic (arteriography, cannulation, or intra-aortic balloon pump insertion, or other operative manipulation) |
| Inflammatory conditions (e.g., syphilis, giant cell arteritis) |
| Congenital Conditions |
| Coarctation of the aorta, with or without associated bicuspid aortic valve |
| Bicuspid aortic valve |

Systemic blood pressure is often high despite apparent shock. Rapid, weak, and asymmetric peripheral pulses are typical. In one-half to two-thirds of patients with proximal dissection, aortic insufficiency may be present, manifest by syncope, cardiac tamponade (hemopericardium), or congestive heart failure. Focal neurologic deficits or hemiplegia are also common in proximal dissections, owing to involvement of the brachiocephalic vessels. In distal dissections, the left brachial and femoral pulses may be diminished or absent.

### Ancillary Studies

The ECG frequently shows LV hypertrophy due to the long-standing underlying hypertension. Chest radiographs show:

- A widened mediastinum, aortic shadow, or dilated aortic root;
- Separation of intimal calcification from the adventitial border by 1-cm or greater in older persons

with prior calcifications in the vessel wall (calcium sign); and

- Left-sided pleural effusions (due to either rupture of the dissection into the pleural space or by an inflammatory reaction).

In patients with chest trauma, these findings or a blurred aortic knob, left apical capping, mediastinal emphysema, or fracture of the first or second ribs should suggest traumatic aortic dissection.

Imaging studies (CT, MRI, transesophageal echocardiography, or aortography) can all visualize the intimal flap, delineate areas involved in the dissection, and identify the connections between true and false lumen (Figure 45.3, Table 45.3). Even in unstable patients with presumed traumatic dissections, transesophageal echocardiography can accurately, rapidly, and less invasively diagnose dissection (Figure 45.4). However, a later aortogram may be necessary to define the full extent of the dissection and to assess involvement of branch vessels, coronary arteries, and the aortic valve.

## Management

All patients with dissection need emergent medical therapy (Table 45.4). The patients should be managed in the intensive care unit with the goal of reducing the systolic blood pressure to 100–120 mm Hg and keeping the heart rate below 90 beats/min. Lowering the blood pressure and heart rate, attained by IV infusions of small incremental IV doses of β-blockers and sodium nitroprusside respectively, decreases the shear force on the aortic wall by lowering the velocity of LV ejection. Direct-acting vasodilators (hydralazine) should be avoided because they reflexly stimulate cardiac output, increase heart rate, and thus worsen the dissection.

Proximal dissections require immediate surgery, and those with aortic insufficiency may need placement of a composite graft with prosthetic valve and reimplantation of the coronary arteries. Stable, uncomplicated distal dissections can be medically treated initially and repaired electively later. A subset of patients with chronic dissections (i.e., stable dissections of >2 weeks) or those with only distal descending aortic dissections may be given chronic medical therapy alone. Intramural aortic

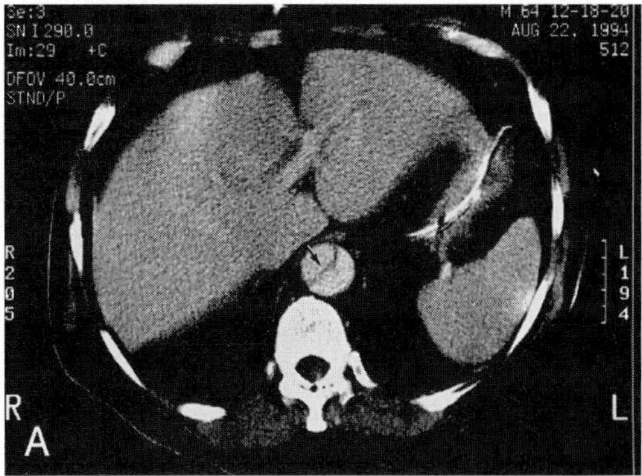


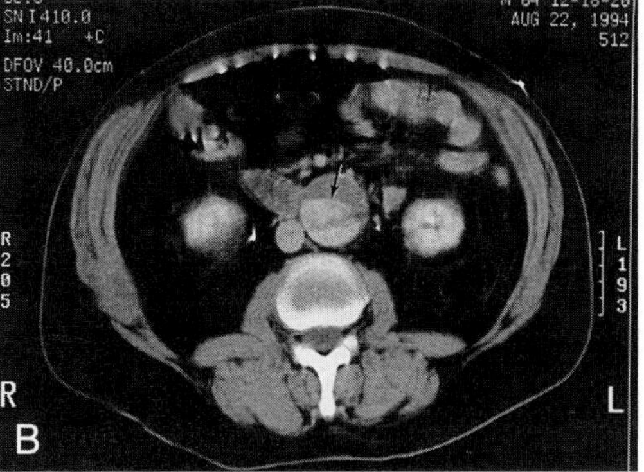


**FIGURE 45.3. Aortic dissection.** Computed tomographic scans showing a raised intimal flap (panel A) and false lumen (panel B).
(Courtesy of the Radiology Museum, St. Joseph's Regional Medical Center, Milwaukee, Wisconsin.)

**TABLE 45.3. Usefulness of Various Diagnostic Tests in Evaluating Suspected Aortic Dissection**

| Variable | Aortography | CT | MRI | TEE |
|---|---|---|---|---|
| Sensitivity | ++ | ++ | +++ | +++ |
| Specificity | +++ | +++ | +++ | ++/+++ |
| Site of intimal tear | ++ | + | +++ | ++ |
| Presence of thrombus | +++ | ++ | +++ | + |
| Presence of AR | +++ | – | + | +++ |
| Pericardial effusion | – | ++ | +++ | +++ |
| Branch vessel involvement | +++ | + | ++ | + |
| Coronary artery involvement | ++ | – | – | ++ |

Abbreviations: AR = aortic regurgitation (aortic valvular insufficiency); CT = computed tomography; MRI = magnetic resonance imaging; TEE = transesophageal echocardiography; +++ = excellent results; ++ = good results; + = fair results; – = not detected.
(From: Cigarroa JE, et al. N Engl J Med 1993; 328:35–43; with permission.)

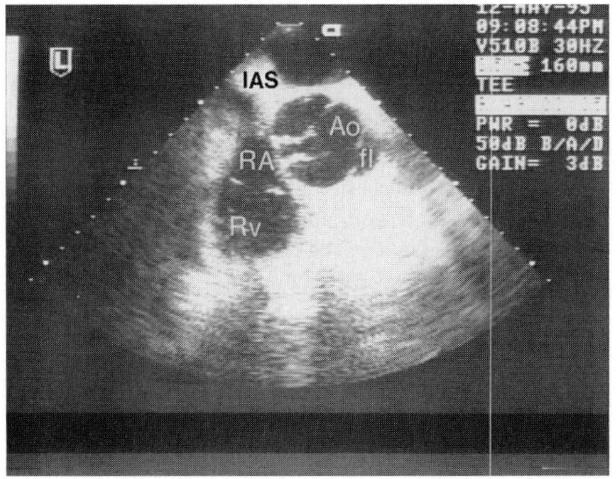


**FIGURE 45.4. Aortic dissection.** Transesophageal echocardiogram (TEE) obtained at the level of the aortic (Ao) root, showing a false lumen (fl) of the ascending aorta (Ao) posterior to the true lumen, indicative of an ascending aortic dissection. (IAS: Interatrial septum; RA: right atrium; RV: right ventricle.)
(Courtesy of Thomas Palmer, MD, and the Echocardiography Laboratory, St. Joseph's Regional Medical Center, Milwaukee, Wisconsin.)

**TABLE 45.4. Parenteral Drugs for Treatment of Acute Aortic Dissection***

| Drug | Dose | Onset of Action | Duration of Action | Adverse Effects |
|---|---|---|---|---|
| *Vasodilators* | | | | |
| Nitroprusside | 0.25–10 μg/kg/min | inst | 1–2 min | Nausea, vomiting sweating, muscle twitching, thiocyanate and cyanide intoxication |
| *Adrenergic inhibitors* | | | | |
| Trimethaphan | 0.5–5 mg/min | 1–5 min | 10 min | Orthostatic hypotension, paresis of bowel and bladder, blurred vision, dry mouth |
| Esmolol | 200–500 μg/kg/min for first 4 min; then 50–300 μg/kg/min | 1–2 min | 10–20 min | Hypotension, nausea |
| Labetalol | 20–80 mg IV bolus over 10 min; then 2 mg/ min | 5–10 min | 3–6 hrs | Nausea, vomiting, postural hypotension, dizziness, burning in throat, scalp tingling |

*All are given as IV infusion.
Abbreviations: inst = instantaneous.
(From: Kaplan, NM (ed). Clinical Hypertension (6th ed). Baltimore: Williams and Wilkins, 1994.)

hematomas are managed in a manner similar to that of dissection involving the corresponding part of the aorta.

## Prognosis

Untreated, aortic dissection has a 1-year mortality of 90%. Half of these deaths occur in the first week after presentation. Most of these early deaths in all types of dissection follow rupture of the aorta into the pericardial or pleural cavities. Untreated dissections involving ascending aorta carry a 3-month mortality of 90%. Almost 46% of patients with untreated intramural hematoma of the aorta die within 30 days. With prompt, appropriate therapy, survival in aortic dissection rises to 80%.

# CHAPTER 46 PERIPHERAL VASCULAR DISEASE

Occlusive arterial disease of the lower extremities is an extremely common disorder that increases in prevalence with advancing age. In persons over age 50, 2–3% of men and 1% of women report symptoms of vascular occlusion. Each year in the United States, over 400,000 hospitalizations are for peripheral vascular disease (PVD), with an estimated 110,000 bypass operations, 50,000 angioplasties, and 69,000 foot or lower-limb amputations.

Although many patients with PVD have a chronic, stable course, almost one-third develop progressive symptoms. Over 5–10 years of follow-up, intermittent claudication may worsen in 15–30% of patients. Incidence rates of vascular surgery for necrosis or rest pain average 2.5–5% per year.

## Etiology

Despite a component of impaired vascular reactivity, most patients with PVD have fixed atherosclerotic obstruction. Major risk factors for development of PVD are smoking, diabetes, hyperlipidemia, and hypertension.

**Thromboangiitis obliterans** (Buerger's disease) is a condition characterized by an inflammatory reaction that affects the small arteries and veins, typically in young smoking men, who display extensive, premature vascular disease. This inflammatory reaction leads to superficial thrombosis and arterial obstruction in the small, medium, and large-sized arteries of both the upper and lower extremities.

## Clinical Features

Patients with PVD present a wide spectrum, from asymptomatic to limb-threatening ischemia. Most patients with PVD report **claudication,** defined as muscle fatigue, pain, or cramping, provoked by exercise and relieved by rest. Quantitating the walking distance of patients with claudication is helpful to track the progression of their symptoms. With progressive vascular occlusion and inadequate collateral circulation, symptoms occur on minimal exertion or even rest. **Rest pain,** a burning discomfort in the affected extremity, is disabling and entails a high risk of gangrene and limb loss. Claudication should be distinguished from nocturnal leg cramps, which are not of vascular origin.

The site of claudication pain may help localize the site of obstruction. For example, stenosis of the proximal iliac vessels (Leriche syndrome) evokes exertional discomfort in the buttocks and thighs. Loss of morning erections and impotence in men are early clues to pelvic vascular disease. Patients with femoral-popliteal system disease often report exertional calf pain.

Given the systemic nature of atherosclerosis, one should search for its signs elsewhere when PVD is suspected. PVD is associated with high-grade (>75%) carotid artery stenosis and severe coronary artery disease in up to one-half of patients.

Although PVD may be discovered in asymptomatic patients during a routine physical examination, normal pulses do not exclude PVD. Other clues to PVD include a decreased capillary refill time (normally <1 sec), decreased hair distribution, dependent rubor, and chronic atrophic skin changes. With advanced PVD, extremities become cool and mottled, nonhealing ulcers develop, and acrocyanosis and digital gangrene may evolve.

Vasospastic conditions can also compromise blood flow. **Raynaud's phenomenon** (or Raynaud's disease) is a triphasic response to cold exposure: blanching followed by cyanosis, and then redness. Raynaud's phenomenon is usually benign, but underlying disease should be excluded, especially in those who present with unilateral signs and symptoms.

## Ancillary Studies

Ankle-brachial index (ABI) is a simple, noninvasive, office-based procedure that can be used as a screening tool in suspected PVD. In it, the systolic blood pressure is measured with a Doppler probe from both brachial arteries and the dorsalis pedis or posterior tibial arteries. The ABI is then calculated by dividing the lower-extremity systolic blood pressure by the upper-extremity reading. Because normal ankle blood pressure exceeds the brachial by 10–15 mm Hg, the normal ABI exceeds 1. An abnormal ABI may be defined as mildly (0.8–0.9), moderately (0.5–0.8), or severely diminished (<0.5).

Besides confirming the clinical diagnosis, ABI can also help to localize the site of obstruction (proximal versus distal) and track progression in patients with established disease. The ABI also provides prognostic information and helps to predict limb survival. Values below 0.5 indicate limb-threatening ischemia; ischemic rest pain is common, and ulceration and gangrene are likely with values below 0.4. Stiff, calcified, and noncompressible arteries render the ABI inaccurate, and in these cases, other diagnostic tests, such as measurement of toe blood pressures, might be useful.

Limb radiographs may show osteomyelitis with nonhealing ulcers. Arterial calcification is common, particularly in diabetics. In selected patients, Doppler ultrasound before and after exercise, duplex scanning, and transcutaneous oximetry may add important diagnostic information. Contrast angiography is generally reserved for patients in whom surgical reconstruction or balloon angioplasty is being considered. Neurologic and/or musculoskeletal conditions (radiculopathies, neuropathies, and "pseudoclaudication" due to spinal stenosis) can occasionally cause sufficient diagnostic confusion to warrant additional testing.

### Management

Patients with PVD should be advised to "stop smoking and keep walking." Profound deconditioning is common with severe PVD, and so exercise should be encouraged to the point of claudication. With a steady exercise training program, pain-free walking time is increased substantially.

Besides exercise, a vigorous risk-factor-modification program should be adopted. Smoking cessation is paramount. Good foot care is important in everyone, but especially in diabetic patients with sensory neuropathy. Patients should wear well-fitting, protective shoes, avoid injury, and inspect their feet daily for signs of skin breakdown or early ulceration.

Significant coronary artery disease is present in 75% of patients with PVD; thus, aspirin (325 mg/day) should be given to lower the risk of stroke, myocardial infarction, and vascular death. Presently, **pentoxifylline** (400 mg three times daily for at least 3 months) is the only approved drug for alleviating claudication. Pentoxifylline may act by decreasing blood viscosity and reducing the rigidity of red blood cells.

Chronic vasodilators and long-term anticoagulation appear to confer only minimal benefits. Concerns of potential harm from β-blockers in claudication have not been validated. Although Raynaud's phenomenon may improve with calcium channel blockers, avoiding cold exposure is very important.

Tissue necrosis (nonhealing foot ulcers, digital gangrene), rest pain, or disabling claudication with an ABI below 0.35 or toe pressure below 30 mm Hg warrants interventional therapy. **Angioplasty** may be the preferred initial step when limb claudication is due to a femoropopliteal stenosis. With proximal (below-the-knee) angioplasty, the long-term results are good, but the restenosis rate is generally high. Long-term patency with **surgical revascularization** depends on several factors, including the indication (intermittent claudication, limb-threatening ischemia), type of graft, site (axillary-femoral, femoral-femoral, femoral-popliteal, or more distal), and vessel characteristics (inflow, runoff distal to graft).

## ■ Acute Arterial Occlusion

Acute arterial occlusion, due to either thrombosis or embolism, is a surgical emergency. Such patients often present with the sudden onset of features of acute ischemic limb (i.e., the "5 Ps": pain, pallor, paresthesia, paralysis, and pulselessness). The pulseless, involved extremity is cold, pale, mottled, and occasionally "cadaveric" in appearance. Ischemic neuropathy is commonly present, with paralysis, decreased or absent reflexes, and loss of sensations. Untreated, myonecrosis quickly follows.

Acute **embolectomy** using a Fogarty catheter or infusion of **urokinase** results in 80–90 % limb salvage rates. Re-embolization occurs in about 25%. All patients should receive full heparinization sufficient to prolong the activated partial thromboplastin time to 1.5–2.0 times control. However, the role of long-term anticoagulation in such patients is less certain. Surgical revascularization should be considered when the anatomy is suitable and the stenosis is high-grade. Localized narrowing may be amenable to percutaneous transluminal angioplasty (PTA).

## ■ Atheroembolism

In patients with PVD, both large-vessel thrombosis and smaller atheromatous emboli may cause arteriolar occlusions and distal vessel infarctions. The resultant **"blue-toe syndrome"** is commonly due to atheroembolism, cardiac emboli, hyperviscosity states, systemic vasculitis, and hypercoagulable states. The atheroemboli are often composed of fibrin-platelet aggregates or cholesterol crystals. Disrupted atherosclerotic plaques in the more proximal vessels, especially the abdominal aorta, are frequently the source. Atheroemboli may follow catheterization or vascular surgery, and anticoagulation may sometimes be a cause by promoting hemorrhage into atherosclerotic plaques, which leads to their disruption.

Patients with lower-extremity atheroemboli may report bilateral limb pain and display a clinical picture resembling systemic vasculitis. Microinfarctions of the pancreas, kidneys, or bowel may result in pancreatitis, renal failure, or gastrointestinal bleeding. Physical findings include **livedo reticularis,** muscle tenderness, purpuric and ecchymotic skin lesions, acrocyanosis (blue toes), and occasionally digital gangrene. Laboratory findings are anemia, elevated sedimentation rate, leukocytosis, eosinophilia, and hyperamylasemia (all nonspecific findings). Wright's stain of the urine may reveal excess eosinophils.

A strong independent association exists between atherosclerosis of the ascending aorta or aortic arch and the risk of ischemic stroke. Ultrasonically detected atherosclerotic plaques exceeding 4 mm in thickness are risk factors for ischemic brain infarct and a possible source of cerebral embolism.

The management of atheroembolic disease and the response to therapy depend on the nature and severity of the underlying disease. Patients with operable and hemodynamically significant disease should undergo surgery. Antiplatelet agents or anticoagulants may be given on a long-term basis to patients with less severe or nonoperable disease (although anticoagulants may sometimes precipitate cholesterol embolism).

# CHAPTER 47 CARDIOGENIC SHOCK

## Definition and Etiology

Cardiogenic shock is a major abnormality of cardiac function that leads to systemic hypotension and severe, peripheral hypoperfusion. Its hemodynamic correlates are:

- Systemic hypotension (defined as a sustained [>30 min] and spontaneous drop in systolic blood pressure to below 90 mm Hg),
- Elevated intracardiac filling pressures (pulmonary capillary wedge pressure >18 mm Hg),
- Low cardiac output (cardiac index <2.2 L/min/$m^2$), and
- Low urinary output (<20 ml/hr).

With a patient in circulatory shock, it is critical to distinguish **hypovolemic shock** (preload failure) and **vasogenic shock** (afterload failure) from **cardiogenic shock** (pump failure) (Table 47.1). Frequent causes of hypovolemic shock are hemorrhage and excessive fluid losses from diarrhea, vomiting, and polyuria. Vasogenic shock may be due to a systemic inflammatory response syndrome (SIRS, previously called septic shock), neurogenic injury (spinal cord injury), anaphylactoid reactions, and vasodilator excess.

Although hypotension and hypoperfusion usually develop in patients with irreversible damage to over 40% of their myocardial mass, other conditions that decrease preload, increase afterload, or cause abnormal heart rate and rhythm can also cause cardiogenic shock. The etiology of cardiogenic shock is commonly subdivided into 3 categories: impaired contractility, decreased preload, and increased afterload (Table 47.2).

## Pathophysiology

Unless the hemodynamic status is rapidly restored to normal, the low cardiac output in cardiogenic shock quickly leads to multiple organ system dysfunction. In patients with acute myocardial infarction, decreased myocardial compliance causes both LV end-diastolic volume and pressure to rise. Accordingly, the pulmonary capillary wedge pressure increases, leading to pulmonary edema when the pressure exceeds 18 mm Hg.

Compensatory mechanisms, such as increased sympathetic tone and decreased parasympathetic tone, enhance myocardial contractility, heart rate, and central blood volume and produce peripheral arteriolar and venous constriction. Although some of these effects are clearly advantageous, others are not, if they lead to an imbalance between myocardial $O_2$ supply and demand. Counter-regulatory mechanisms—including acidemia, circulating myocardial depressant factors, and decreased coronary artery perfusion—also lead to decreased myocardial performance in the setting of cardiogenic shock.

## Clinical Features

The clinical evolution of circulatory shock is summarized in Table 47.3. Sustained systemic hypotension and peripheral hypoperfusion characterize cardiogenic shock. Systemic hypotension is also present when

**TABLE 47.1. Hemodynamic Profile in Circulatory Shock**

| | Hypovolemic (preload failure) | Cardiogenic (pump failure) | Vasogenic (afterload failure) |
|---|---|---|---|
| Central venous pressure | ↓ | ↑ | N or ↓ |
| Pulmonary capillary wedge pressure | ↓ | ↑ | N or ↓ |
| Cardiac index | ↓ | ↓ | N or ↑ |
| LV stroke work index | ↓ | ↓ | ↓ |
| Systemic vascular resistance | ↑ | ↑ | ↓ |
| Total $O_2$ consumption index | ↓ | ↓ | ↓ |

(Adapted from: Teba L et al. Postgrad Med 1992;91:123. Used with permission.)

**TABLE 47.2. Causes of Cardiogenic Shock**

**Impaired contractility/excessive preload**
- Acute myocardial infarction with markedly reduced LV function*
- Mechanical complications of acute myocardial infarction
  - Acute mitral regurgitation due to papillary muscle dysfunction/rupture, ventricular septal rupture
- Dilated cardiomyopathy (end–stage)
- Mitral insufficiency (subacute, chronic)
- Aortic insufficiency (subacute, chronic)
- Tachyarrhythmias
- Bradyarrhythmia including heart block
- Myocardial contusion
- Myocarditis, severe
- Myocardial dysfunction in septic shock
- Sequelae of cardiopulmonary bypass

**Decreased preload**
- RV infarction with RV pump failure
- Pericardial tamponade
  - Ventricular free wall rupture
  - Proximal aortic dissection (type 1)
- Pulmonary embolism, massive
- Pulmonary hypertension, severe
- Tension pneumothorax
- LV inflow tract obstruction
  - Mitral stenosis
  - Atrial myxoma

**Excessive afterload**
- LV outflow tract obstruction
  - Aortic stenosis
  - Hypertrophic cardiomyopathy (preload may also be reduced)
- Malignant hypertension
- Coarctation of the aorta

*Due to a massive infarction, preexisting LV dysfunction, associated dysrhythmias, and/or associated ischemic dysfunction.
(Data from: Grella RD, Becker RC. Current Probl Cardiol 1994; 19:693–742. Califf RM, Bengtson JR. N Engl J Med 1994; 330:175.)

**systolic blood pressure** is maintained at or above 90 mm Hg by vasopressors or inotropes. Some patients can present with a picture of clinical shock with a "normal" blood pressure, especially if prior hypertension has been present. Conversely, a systolic blood pressure below 90 mm Hg is not necessarily shock, as end-organ hypoperfusion also should be present, manifested by general fatigue and weakness and features of hypoperfusion of the kidneys, central nervous system, and skin.

Coronary hypoperfusion further worsens cardiac ischemia, predisposing to infarct extension and perpetuation of shock. Urine output below 20 ml/hr or less than 500 ml/24 hrs represents **oliguria,** which indicates renal hypoperfusion. Dyspnea, another common finding in cardiogenic shock, arises from the high pulmonary capillary wedge pressure, reflecting the severe LV dysfunction.

Physical examination discloses tachypnea and tachycardia, often with weak and thready peripheral pulses. Asymmetric peripheral pulses (aortic dissection) and pulsus paradoxus (cardiac tamponade) may provide important clues for specific causes. In hypovolemic shock, the neck veins are flat, but in cardiogenic shock, they may be distended. In inferoposterior wall myocardial infarction, distended neck veins, systemic hypotension, and clear lung fields together strongly suggest RV infarction. Atrial ($S_4$) and ventricular ($S_3$) gallops, as well as crackles, are heard. A new, holosystolic murmur in a post-infarct patient suggests a ventricular septal rupture or mitral regurgitation (due to papillary muscle rupture). An early diastolic murmur of aortic insufficiency is a key finding in suspected proximal aortic dissection.

## Ancillary Studies

Arterial blood gas analysis typically shows hypoxemia, hypocapnia, and metabolic acidemia from lactic acidosis. Leukocytosis, attributable to a stress response, is frequent. The ECG may show low-voltage complexes (tamponade), acute infarction, right heart strain (pulmonary embolism), conduction disturbances, or arrhyth-

**TABLE 47.3. Clinical Stages of Circulatory Shock**

| | Stage I (preshock) | Stage II (organ hypoperfusion) | Stage III (end-organ failure) |
|---|---|---|---|
| Mental State | Clear but distress present | Confusion, restlessness | Apathy, agitation or coma |
| Skin | Pale and cool | Cool and clammy | Cool, cyanotic, and mottled |
| Peripheral vasoconstriction | Mild | Marked | Intense |
| BP | Normal or slightly low | Hypotension | Undetectable by cuff |
| Urine output | Oliguria | Oliguria | Anuria |
| Heart Rate | Tachycardia | Tachycardia | Tachycardia |
| Other | Tachypnea, respiratory alkalosis | Respiratory failure; lactic acidosis; possible angina | Severe metabolic acidosis; multiple organ failure |

(From: Teba L et al. Postgrad Med 1992;91:124. Used with permission.)

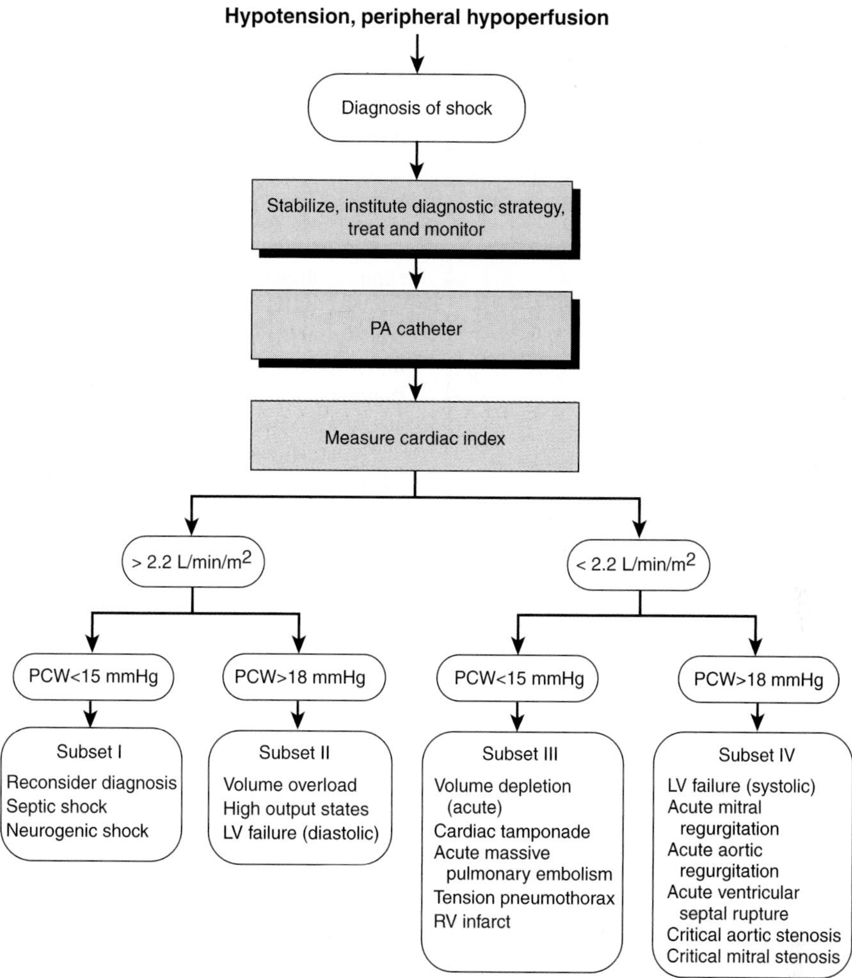


**FIGURE 47.1. Determination of hemodynamic subgroups in cardiogenic shock. Patients with a clinical diagnosis of shock can be characterized using the pulmonary artery catheter to provide hemodynamic information. (PA Catheter = pulmonary artery catheter; PCW = pulmonary capillary wedge pressure.)**
(Adapted from: Grella RD, Becker RC. Curr Probl Cardiol 1994; 19:693–742. Used with permission.)

mias. Right-sided precordial leads may help confirm RV infarction.

The chest radiograph may show pulmonary vascular congestion or pulmonary edema. Pneumothorax with tracheal shift (tension pneumothorax), or widening of the mediastinal and aortic silhouette with a positive calcium sign (aortic dissection) are examples of important radiographic clues to the etiology of shock. Bedside echocardiography may detect pericardial tamponade, acute valvular insufficiency, or RV hypokinesis.

## Management

The general approach to diagnosing an etiology for circulatory shock is outlined in Figure 47.1, and the therapeutic approach to cardiogenic shock is shown in Table 47.4. The first priority in managing cardiogenic shock is to stabilize the hemodynamic status and restore perfusion. With a recent myocardial infarction and acute heart failure, aggressive restoration of coronary blood flow and limiting of infarct size are attained by thrombolysis, angioplasty, and bypass surgery (chapter 39). Successful opening of the infarct-related coronary vessel can reduce the mortality from cardiogenic shock significantly.

Systemic hypotension should be aggressively treated with IV fluids and, if necessary, inotropes. Hypoxemia, electrolyte abnormalities, and acid-base imbalances must be quickly recognized and corrected. Through cardiac monitoring, one may detect arrhythmias that require medications, temporary pacemaker support, or electrical cardioversion. Placement of a pulmonary artery (Swan-Ganz) catheter can stratify patients into one of the

**TABLE 47.4. Therapeutic Approach to Cardiogenic Shock**

1. **General resuscitation**
   Monitor rhythm and blood pressure.
   Correct hypoxia, electrolytes abnormalities, and acid-base imbalance.
   Manage intravascular volume
2. **Improve systolic function**
   Administer catecholamines
   Intra-aortic balloon pumping
   Restore coronary blood flow
   - Angioplasty (PTCA)
   - Thrombolysis
   - Surgery
3. **Maximize preload and afterload**
   Administer saline or produce diuresis
   Vasodilation
4. **Diagnose and manage mechanical dysfunction of an intracardiac structure**
   Mitral valve
   Ventricular septum (rupture)
   Free wall (rupture, RV infarct)

PTCA = percutaneous transluminal angioplasty.
(Adapted from: Califf RM, Bengtson JR. N Engl J Med 1994; 330:1725. Used with permission.)

hemodynamic subsets (Table 47.5) and initiate the diagnostic algorithm of shock (Figure 47.1). Patients with RV infarcts may require large volumes of fluid to raise their central venous pressure, so as to provide adequate preload to the LV.

Afterload reduction is usually accomplished by continuously infusing **sodium nitroprusside** (0.25–10 µg/kg/min). Adverse effects include nausea, vomiting, sweating, muscle twitching, and, with long-term administration, thiocyanate and cyanide toxicity. Nitroprusside has balanced arteriolar and venous effects. IV nitroglycerin, primarily a venodilator, may be substituted for nitroprusside in some patients who have signs or symptoms of ongoing cardiac ischemia. Inotropic therapy in this setting specifically aims to improve myocardial contractility, increase cardiac output, and provide adequate systemic perfusion without increasing myocardial $O_2$ demands (Table 47.6).

**Dopamine** affects all adrenoreceptor sites in a markedly dose-dependent fashion. At low doses of 2–5 µg/kg/min (renal dose), it stimulates the DA1 receptors and increases the glomerular filtration rate and renal tubular sodium excretion. Slightly higher doses (5–10 µg/kg/min) stimulate α-1 and DA2 receptors, producing cardiac inotropic and chronotropic effects. At 10–20 µg/kg/min, peripheral vasoconstriction follows stimulation of α-1 receptors.

**Dobutamine,** a synthetic inotrope, lacks α-1-adrenergic-mediated vasoconstriction. Because it has no

**TABLE 47.5. Clinical and Hemodynamic Subsets of Patients With Acute Myocardial Infarction and Their Respective Mortality Rates**

| Hemodynamic | Clinical Subset | | Mortality (%) | |
|---|---|---|---|---|
| Subset | Pulmonary Congestion | Peripheral Hypoperfusion | Clinical | Hemodynamic |
| I. | – | – | 1 | 3 |
| II. | + | – | 11 | 9 |
| III. | – | + | 18 | 23 |
| IV. | + | + | 60 | 51 |

Subsets: I = no pulmonary congestion or peripheral hypoperfusion; II = pulmonary congestion without hypoperfusion; III = peripheral hypoperfusion without pulmonary congestion; IV = both peripheral hypoperfusion and pulmonary congestion.
(Adapted from Forrester JS, et al. N Engl J Med 1976;295:1356–1362.)

**TABLE 47.6. Adrenoreceptor Sites and Actions of Commonly Used Inotropic Agents**

| | Adrenoceptor Sites | | | | |
|---|---|---|---|---|---|
| Agent | α-1 | β-1 | β-2 | DA1 | DA2 |
| Norepinephrine | ++++ | ++++ | 0 | 0 | 0 |
| Dopamine | ++++ | ++++ | ++ | ++++ | ++++ |
| Dobutamine | + | ++++ | ++ | 0 | 0 |

Actions of various adrenoceptor sites: α-1 = vasoconstriction causing increased systemic arterial resistance; β-1 = increased cardiac index, contractility, and rate; β-2 = vasodilation of the systemic arterial resistance vessels; = DA1 = increase renal blood flow, decrease renal tubular resorption of sodium and water; DA2 = presynaptically regulate norepinephrine release from sympathetic nerve terminals.
(From: DiBona GF. Semin Nephrol 1994;14:34. Used with permission.)

activity at the dopaminergic receptor sites, it also lacks any DA1 or DA2 effects. By stimulating cardiac α-1 and peripheral α-2 receptors, it increases myocardial contractility and evokes peripheral vasodilation. The latter, along with the lack of significant vasoconstriction leads to net vasodilatation. Initial dose is 2–5 μg/kg/min.

**Norepinephrine** is a powerful vasopressor that has a limited role in the treatment of most patients with cardiogenic shock. Its main clinical indication is severe hypotension (<70 mm Hg) with normal or reduced systemic vascular resistance. Usually started at 1–4 μg/kg/min, its dose is further titrated according to the initial clinical and hemodynamic response.

In cardiogenic shock, dobutamine is often the "inotrope of choice" since it increases cardiac output with a smaller increase in heart rate and myocardial $O_2$ demands, and lowers systemic vascular resistance and pulmonary capillary wedge pressures. Because it is not a vasopressor, dobutamine should not be used as the sole inotrope in a severely hypotensive patient. Such patients require higher-dose dopamine or norepinephrine. Because it raises systemic blood pressure without incurring arrhythmias (unlike higher-dose dopamine), norepinephrine may be preferable.

All inotropic agents should be started at low doses and titrated upward to achieve the desired clinical response. Adverse effects include tachycardia, arrhythmias, provocation of myocardial ischemia, and local tissue necrosis (especially with extravasation into subcutaneous tissues). Dopamine and norepinephrine also have the potential to induce excessive vasoconstriction. Vomiting tends to be a more common side effect with dopamine because of stimulation of central dopaminergic receptors.

Cardiogenic shock not responding to appropriate pharmacologic therapy with IV vasodilators and inotropic agents requires placement of an **intra-aortic balloon pump** to temporarily stabilize the clinical status. Patients with mechanical complications of myocardial infarction (rupture of papillary muscle or ventricular septum) often need prompt referral for urgent surgery.

Despite aggressive and appropriate therapy, the in-hospital mortality of cardiogenic shock remains high, averaging about 70% in most large series. Successful PTCA has reduced the mortality of cardiogenic shock to about 40% in patients with acute myocardial infarction.

# CHAPTER 48 ASSESSMENT OF CARDIAC RISK FOR NONCARDIAC SURGERY

Cardiac complications, especially those related to coronary artery disease (CAD), are the leading cause of death following anesthesia and surgery. Patients with known or suspected cardiac disease commonly undergo risk assessment by internists or cardiologists before undergoing noncardiac surgical procedures. Through a detailed history and physical examination, combined with the use of selective testing procedures, the physician can identify individuals at low- and high-risk (risk stratification) for perioperative cardiac morbidity (PCM) (Table 48.1).

## Risk Stratification

Risk stratification serves important goals:

1. Avoids the risk and expense of specialized cardiac testing procedures in patients who are found to be at low-risk for PCM after a simple history, physical examination, and routine laboratory tests.
2. Defines a subset of patients at high risk for PCM. These patients have acute but correctable medical problems and may benefit from further medical or surgical treatment prior to the planned noncardiac surgical procedure.
3. In some patients at high-risk for PCM, modification of the proposed noncardiac surgical procedure to one that entails a lower risk or cancellation of the procedure may be appropriate.

## Noncardiac Predictors of Risk

### Age

Older patients are more likely to have associated CAD, comorbid medical problems, and depressed cardiac responses to catecholamine stress. Many studies have demonstrated a greater surgical mortality among the elderly when age is the only variable studied. However, functional status (i.e., physiological status or physiological age) is probably a significant factor to be considered besides chronological age.

### Type of anesthesia

Regional anesthesia offers no consistent advantage over general anesthesia in terms of improved surgical outcome. The one possible exception occurs in patients with a history of congestive heart failure, in whom regional anesthesia may be associated with a lesser incidence of postoperative pulmonary congestion.

**TABLE 48.1. Preoperative Cardiovascular Evaluation**

- Begin with complete history, physical examination, ECG and chest radiograph.
- Specific questions to address:
  1. Is angina pectoris or an anginal equivalent present?
  2. What is the functional capacity?
  3. Is there historical/ECG evidence of MI? If so, when did MI occur?
  4. Is there prior or current CHF? Is it systolic or diastolic? Define functional capacity.
  5. Is valvular disease or prosthetic valve present?
  6. Is antibiotic prophylaxis required?
  7. Is a temporary/permanent pacemaker present?
  8. Is there chronic obstructive pulmonary disease? If so, is the $FEV_{1.0}$ less than 1 liter?
  9. What is the general medical condition of the patient?
  10. What operation is planned? Assess risk:benefit.
  11. Is the current medical regimen appropriate/optimal?
  12. If surgery is risky, what are the alternatives?
  13. Is surgery necessary?

CHF = congestive heart failure; $FEV_{1.0}$ = 1-second forced expiratory volume.

**Site and type of surgery**

Emergency surgery is associated with a 2- to 5-fold increased risk of perioperative cardiac complications, including postoperative myocardial infarction (MI) or cardiac death. In addition, intrathoracic, intraperitoneal, orthopedic, aortic, and peripheral vascular procedures (particularly involving aortic cross-clamping) all also entail a higher risk of postoperative cardiac complications.

## Cardiac Predictors of Risk

**Ischemic heart disease**

In general, the presence of CAD increases the mortality of noncardiac surgery by 3- to 5-fold. In patients with CAD, important considerations include the presence of symptoms of myocardial ischemia and the workload that provokes them, the overall anginal pattern and its stability over time, the patient's overall functional capacity, a past history of MI (and if so, when it occurred), and the presence of any symptoms or signs of heart failure. However, the absence of angina and the presence of a normal resting ECG do not exclude significant CAD.

*Noninvasive testing for CAD in the preoperative patient*

Younger patients (<70 years of age) with no angina, prior MI, or heart failure and whose functional status is class I or II by the Canadian Cardiovascular Society angina scale are at **low-risk** for most surgical procedures and need no further specialized testing for myocardial ischemia (Figure 48.1).

Similarly, a **high-risk** subset of patients can also be defined by history, physical findings, and ECG characteristics who do not need further specialized noninvasive testing. This high-risk subset includes patients who have had refractory or poorly controlled congestive heart failure, unstable angina, or a recent non–ST-elevation MI with evidence for a large amount of jeopardized myocardium, or a recent MI complicated by heart failure or followed by angina. The majority of these patients can proceed directly to coronary angiography, assuming that they are candidates for potential revascularization.

The remaining large group of patients, who cannot be classified initially as low- or high-risk, form an **intermediate-risk** subset in which exercise stress testing or vasodilator perfusion imaging is helpful for risk stratification. This group consists of patients with known or suspected CAD but whose symptoms are currently stable, patients with a remote MI, patients with currently well-compensated congestive heart failure, or patients with diabetes mellitus. If these patients can exercise adequately, then **exercise stress testing** is generally performed. Exercise stress tests are most helpful when they provide clear evidence of myocardial ischemia at a low workload (<5 mets), indicating the patient is at high risk for PCM, or alternatively, when they demonstrate no ischemia at a high workload (>7 mets), indicating the patient is at low risk for PCM.

Unfortunately, many exercise test results do not fall into either category, and such patients carry an indeterminate risk of PCM. In these patients, as well as those whose history clearly precludes adequate exercise, **vasodilator perfusion imaging** may be used to test for the presence of significant CAD. Vasodilator perfusion imaging is most commonly performed with dipyridamole infusion, followed by either thallium-201 or technetium-99m sestamibi.

Numerous studies have demonstrated that the absence of reversible defects on vasodilator perfusion imaging is associated with a >95% negative predictive value for the occurrence of PCM (i.e., <5% of patients with no reversible defects will experience perioperative cardiac complications). The positive predictive value of reversible defects for PCM is only 20–30% (i.e., 70–80% of patients with reversible perfusion defects will not experience perioperative cardiac complications, but 20–30% will). It is up to the physician to decide which patients with reversible defects merit further investigation with, for instance, coronary angiography.

**History of previous myocardial infarction**

A history of previous MI is a risk factor for recurrent, perioperative MI, but the risk is decreasing. Recent data suggest that the risk of perioperative MI ranges from 1.5% in patients whose MI occurred over 6 months before the current planned surgery to 5.7% in patients whose MI occurred less than 3 months previously. The incidence of perioperative MIs tends to peak on the third postoperative day and entails a 40–70% mortality rate. Elective noncardiac surgery should be postponed for a minimum of 3 months following an MI.

### Congestive heart failure

Congestive heart failure (CHF) is a major risk factor for PCM. The risk of postoperative pulmonary edema is negligible (<2%) when a prior history of CHF is absent, modest (6%) when clinical findings suggest well-compensated CHF, and moderate (16%) when active heart failure is present preoperatively. Thus, it is important to resolve heart failure fully prior to surgery, as well as avoid hypokalemia and volume depletion from over-diuresis. Additionally, one must determine whether CHF is due to diastolic or systolic dysfunction, since management of these conditions differs greatly.

### Valvular disease

The risk of perioperative complications depends on the specific valve lesion, its degree of dysfunction, the state of LV systolic and diastolic function, and the patient's functional class. In general, significant aortic stenosis carries the highest mortality risk (10–15%) in patients undergoing noncardiac surgery.

Alterations in perioperative hemodynamics affect specific valvular/subvalvular lesions. For example, in patients with hypertrophic obstructive cardiomyopathy, careful fluid management (avoiding volume depletion) and avoidance of β-adrenergic agonists are both important, since these would increase the outflow obstruction. A relative tachycardia, by reducing regurgitant fraction, might benefit significant aortic regurgitation but could precipitate pulmonary edema in mitral stenosis. Periop-

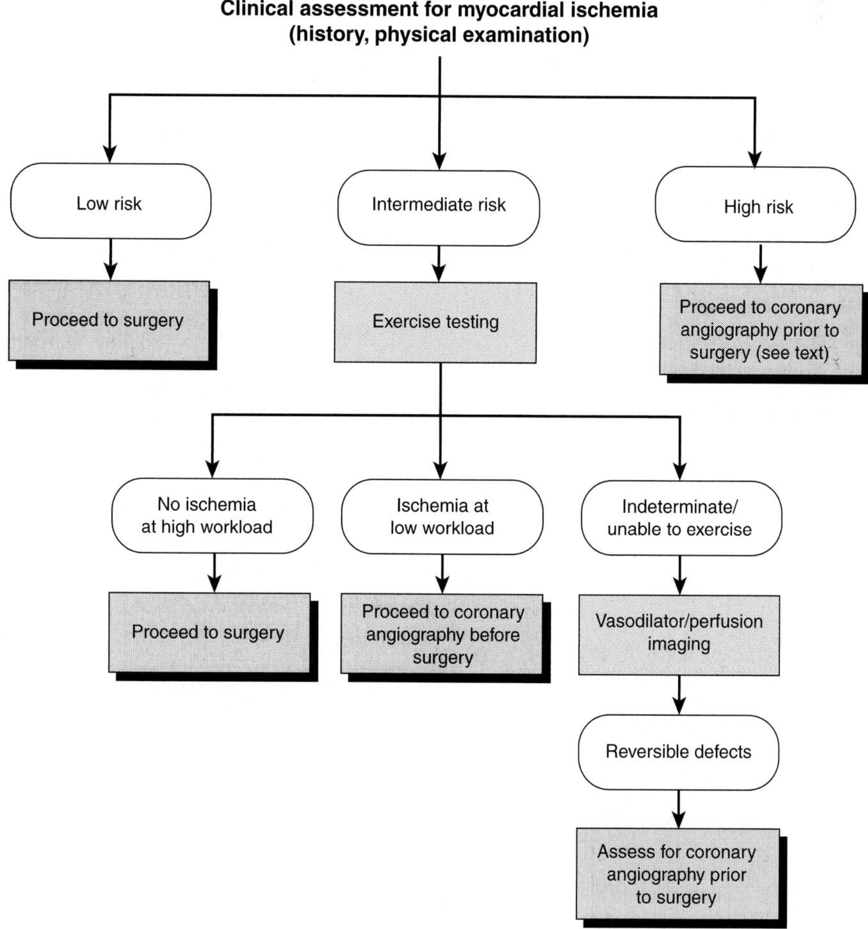


**FIGURE 48.1.** Evaluation of the preoperative patient for coronary artery disease.

erative hemodynamic monitoring with a pulmonary artery catheter is often helpful in patients with valvular disease.

### Hypertension

In patients with mild to moderate, well-controlled hypertension and no evidence of serious end-organ damage, general anesthesia is well tolerated. Medications should not be discontinued at the time of surgery, but rather, they should be continued up until surgery. There is no benefit in postponing surgery to gain better blood pressure control as long as the diastolic blood pressure is at or below 100 mm Hg.

### Arrhythmias

Ventricular and supraventricular arrhythmias commonly complicate the perioperative period. In general, the risk that arrhythmias pose to the patient is more closely related to the underlying heart disease. Ventricular arrhythmias discovered preoperatively should prompt a search for electrolyte abnormalities, ventricular or valvular dysfunction, pulmonary congestion, or myocardial ischemia. Medications such as digitalis, β-agonists, or theophylline may cause ventricular (or supraventricular) arrhythmias, and occasionally, an indwelling pulmonary artery catheter may cause mechanical irritation and hence ectopy.

If no reversible factor is evident, there are no data to support the prophylactic suppression of asymptomatic ventricular ectopy in the perioperative period. However, increased or new-onset ventricular ectopy in the postoperative patient with known or suspected CAD may reflect myocardial infarction or ischemia.

### Other issues

*Coronary revascularization*

The choice between coronary artery bypass graft (CABG) surgery or percutaneous transluminal coronary angioplasty (PTCA) prior to a proposed noncardiac surgical procedure must be made carefully. Besides exposing the patient to a higher risk of morbidity and mortality, **CABG** entails the additional risk of delaying the noncardiac surgical procedure. Additionally, some groups of patients, notably prospective vascular surgical patients, have a higher-than-usual mortality risk from CABG. Patients who survive CABG, however, tolerate the subsequent noncardiac surgery well. Often, however, the mortality risk of the prophylactic CABG offsets the survival advantage it confers on the patient during the subsequent noncardiac surgery. Thus, although CABG in the preoperative patient may not confer a short-term survival advantage, it likely does confer a long-term survival benefit.

In general, the decision for CABG should rest on standard guidelines for CABG, rather than on a perceived need for it to meet the needs of the proposed noncardiac surgery. The severity of ischemic symptoms, amount of jeopardized tissue, degree of functional limitation, state of LV function, patient age, and comorbid conditions all affect subsequent management decisions, including the need for myocardial revascularization.

**PTCA** is an additional option, although there is no definitive proof that performing PTCA prior to noncardiac surgery improves surgical outcome.

## Questions

**Instructions:** For each question below, select only **one** lettered answer that is the **best** for that question.

1. A 50-year old man complains of epigastric discomfort along with dyspnea during exercise and relief after several minutes of rest. Which ONE of the following diagnoses best represents his condition?
   A. Hiatus hernia
   B. Angina pectoris
   C. Aneurysm of the descending thoracic aorta
   D. Gastric ulcer
   E. Intestinal ischemia due to mesenteric arterial stenosis

2. All of the following factors enhance the myocardial $O_2$ demand, with the exception of:
   A. Enlarged LV chamber
   B. Slow heart rate
   C. Increased contractility
   D. Hypertension

3. A known hypertensive is admitted to the CCU with an acute anterior-wall myocardial infarction. He is diaphoretic and tachypneic. Pulse is 156 beats/min and BP is 98/50 mm Hg. The ECG reveals atrial flutter with 2:1 AV block. Which of the following is indicated now?
   A. Patient is in cardiogenic shock; start IV dopamine.
   B. Rapid heart rate is probably a major contributor for cardiogenic shock; immediate electrical cardioversion should follow.
   C. Ventricular rate is rapid; give IV propranolol.
   D. Start oral digoxin to improve contractility and slow the ventricular rate.

4. A 45-year-old man is hospitalized for acute inferior-wall myocardial infarction. His BP is 80/50 mm Hg, and the ECG rhythm strip shows sinus bradycardia (40 beats/min.). Which of the following is indicated now?
   A. Fluid challenge
   B. IV isoproterenol
   C. IV dopamine

D. IV atropine
E. Temporary pacemaker

5. His clinical status improves markedly after appropriate treatment. On the next day, the BP is 110/70 mm Hg and the ECG rhythm strip shows 5:4 Wenckebach type of second degree AV block. Which of the following is indicated now?
A. Temporary pacemaker
B. IV isoproterenol
C. IV atropine
D. Oral ephedrine
E. Observation

6. Sinus rhythm resumes on the fourth hospital day. On the same afternoon, sudden diaphoresis develops with dyspnea and rales at lung bases. His BP is 70/40 mm Hg. A faint, grade 2/6 systolic murmur is heard over the left lower sternal border. Which of the following conditions should be considered in the differential diagnosis?
A. Rupture of chordae tendineae
B. Rupture of ventricular septum or papillary muscle
C. Rupture of LV free wall
D. All of the above
E. None of the above

7. Which of the following will you do to diagnose and manage the above condition?
A. Pulmonary artery catheter; multiple blood samples for oximetry.
B. LV and coronary angiograms
C. Administer IV dopamine
D. Intra-aortic balloon counterpulsation
E. Surgical repair
F. All of the above

8. A 72-year-old man presents to the emergency department after 2 hours of anterior chest pain, profuse sweating, and confusion. The systolic BP is 80 mm Hg, and the chest reveals bilateral crackles. The 12-lead ECG shows sinus tachycardia at 118 beats/min and 2 mm ST-segment elevation in leads $V_1$ through $V_4$. Which of the following steps are appropriate for this patient's management?
A. Give IV esmolol to reduce the rapid heart rate.
B. Give soluble aspirin, 325 mg PO, and consult the cardiologist for emergent coronary angioplasty.
C. IV tissue plasminogen activator for a total dose of 100 mg in the next 3 hours.
D. Admit to the CCU and give IV fluids to treat hypotension.

9. A 55-year-old man is recovering from an inferior-wall MI in the CCU. On the third hospital day, he reports pleuritic-type chest pain, unrelieved by nitroglycerin. A house officer heard a pericardial friction rub about 3 hours before, but it is not audible now. Which of the following medications may be contraindicated?
A. Aspirin
B. Beta-blockers
C. Anticoagulants
D. Nonsteroidal anti-inflammatory agents

10. All of the following physical signs indicate the presence of a large intracardiac left-to-right shunt, except:
A. Loud $S_3$
B. Loud $S_4$
C. Mid-diastolic rumble across atrioventricular valves
D. Hyperkinetic precordium

11. A 19-year old man has a heart murmur. His BP is 110/60 mm Hg, jugular venous pulse is normal, and pulse is regular. The apical impulse is displaced downward and leftward. There is a systolic thrill over the left midsternal area. A grade 4/6 pansystolic murmur is audible over the left midsternal area. $S_1$ is covered by the murmur. $S_2$ is widely split with considerable respiratory variation. An $S_3$ followed by a mid-diastolic rumble is heard over the apex. ECG shows biventricular hypertrophy, and the chest radiograph shows increased pulmonary vascularity. Which of the following conditions can develop in the natural history of a ventricular septal defect?
A. Aortic regurgitation
B. Congestive heart failure
C. Infective endocarditis
D. Progressive decrease in the size of the defect
E. Eisenmenger's syndrome
F. Infundibular stenosis
G. All of the above

12. A 14-year-old girl is found to have a moderate left-to-right shunt through a patent ductus arteriosus (PDA). She is quite active in several sports and is entirely asymptomatic. What would you recommend?
A. Antibiotic prophylaxis against infective endocarditis until surgical division of PDA
B. Long-term antirheumatic prophylaxis
C. Curtailment of physical activity
D. Regular observation until the development of cardiac symptoms, and then recommend surgical treatment

13. All of the following are true except:
A. Atrial gallop indicates a large and poorly contractile ventricle.

B. Ventricular gallop may indicate a large and poorly contractile ventricle.
C. Atrial gallop implies decreased ventricular compliance.
D. Ventricular gallop may indicate hyperdynamic circulation.
E. Ventricular gallop may indicate a large left to right shunt.

14. Left axis deviation of QRS complex can occur in all of the following except:
A. Left anterior fascicular block
B. Inferior wall myocardial infarction
C. Ostium primum type of atrial septal defect
D. Left ventricular hypertrophy
E. Ostium secundum type of atrial septal defect

15. A 45-year-old man gives history of exertional substernal pain. Further evaluation reveals hypertension and moderate hypercholesterolemia. Which of the following findings on myocardial perfusion imaging with thallium-201 indicate high-risk coronary artery disease?
A. Fixed perfusion defect in inferior wall
B. Fixed perfusion defect in lateral wall
C. Reversible perfusion defect in inferior wall
D. Perfusion defects in two or more segments of left ventricle, left ventricular enlargement on stress images and increased lung-uptake of thallium-201

16. Echocardiography is useful for diagnosing all of the following except:
A. Cardiac tamponade
B. Pericardial effusion
C. Valvular vegetations
D. Ventricular aneurysm
E. Left ventricular systolic function
F. Pericarditis

17. A 45-year-old man is seen in the emergency department with palpitations. The ED physician performs carotid massage. All the following effects could be expected from the carotid sinus massage except:
A. Slowing of the ventricular response in atrial flutter
B. Termination of atrioventricular nodal reentrant tachycardia
C. Transient slowing of sinus tachycardia rate
D. Termination of non-paroxysmal junctional tachycardia

18. A 78-year-old man is admitted to the hospital with atrial fibrillation. All of the following might immediately follow new-onset atrial fibrillation except?
A. Systemic thromboembolism
B. Decreased cardiac output
C. Deep vein thrombosis
D. Increased angina

19. Which of the following statement(s) regarding ventricular tachycardia is false?
A. Ventricular tachycardia may result in syncope.
B. Digitalis toxicity may result in ventricular tachycardia.
C. In patients with left ventricular systolic dysfunction, non-sustained ventricular tachycardia increases the risk of sudden cardiac death.
D. Automatic implantable cardioverter defibrillator is associated with decreased risk of sudden cardiac death in patients with sustained ventricular tachycardia.
E. Sustained ventricular tachycardia commonly occurs without underlying structural heart disease.
F. Amiodarone is useful in the treatment of ventricular tachycardia.

20. A 75-year-old man, a retired minister, is brought to the emergency department, after having had an attack of shortness of breath that "descended on him like a bolt from the blue." He has had 2 previous myocardial infarctions. He is a non-smoker. Examination shows a blood pressure of 170/80 mm Hg, irregular pulse of 130/min, respirations of 40/min with air-hunger, diffuse crackles and wheezing all over his chest and moderate lower extremity edema. All of the following steps are useful for treating him, except:
A. Intravenous loop diuretics
B. Sitting posture
C. Intravenous morphine sulfate
D. Elevation of lower extremities
E. Supplemental oxygen

21. The ECG in the above patient shows atrial fibrillation, the most appropriate therapy for which in this patient would be:
A. Intravenous esmolol
B. Digoxin 0.5 mg orally immediately, followed by 0.25 mg every 6 hours; and quinidine 200 mg every 6 hours after the second dose of digoxin
C. Rapid anticoagulation with heparin to achieve an activated partial thromboplastin time (aPTT) of 2.5 times control, followed by warfarin; cardioversion in 4–5 weeks
D. Synchronized DC cardioversion immediately, followed by full heparinization and daily warfarin use to keep the INR in a range of 3x control

22. Heart failure may be due to hypertensive heart disease, coronary artery disease, and/or aortic and mitral valvular disease. Which of the following statement(s) regarding heart failure is true?
    A. In patients with mitral stenosis and atrial fibrillation with rapid ventricular rate, slowing ventricular rate improves symptoms of heart failure.
    B. Normal left ventricular ejection fraction precludes the diagnosis of congestive heart failure.
    C. In patients with valvular aortic stenosis and heart failure, markedly reduced left ventricular ejection fraction is a contraindication for aortic valve replacement.
    D. Normal cardiothoracic ratio on a chest X-ray rules out the diagnosis of heart failure.
    E. All of the above
    F. None of the above

23. With reference to treating patients with heart failure, which of the following medications is likely to increase survival?
    A. Digoxin
    B. Long-acting nitrates
    C. Angiotensin-converting enzyme inhibitors
    D. Diltiazem
    E. Diuretics

24. In patients with chronic severe aortic regurgitation, all of the following constitute indications for aortic valve replacement except:
    A. New York Heart Association functional (NYHA) class III or IV symptoms of heart failure and left ventricular ejection fraction (LVEF) > 50%
    B. NYHA functional class II symptoms of heart failure and LVEF > 50% but with progressive LV dilatation or declining EF at rest on serial studies or declining exercise capacity on exercise testing
    C. Significant angina with or without associated coronary artery disease
    D. LVEF of 25% to 49%
    E. Echocardiographic LV end-diastolic diameter > 75 mm or end-systolic diameter > 55 mm
    F. Asymptomatic patients with LVEF > 50% and mild to moderate LV dilatation

25. Which of the following is a false statement(s) regarding the valvular aortic stenosis and hypertrophic cardiomyopathy?
    A. Syncope may occur in both conditions.
    B. Bisferiens pulse is suggestive of hypertrophic cardiomyopathy, and anacrotic pulse is suggestive of valvular aortic stenosis.
    C. An apical holosystolic murmur signifying mitral regurgitation is often present in valvular aortic stenosis.
    D. Murmur of hypertrophic cardiomyopathy seldom radiates into carotid arteries.
    E. Murmur of valvular aortic stenosis often radiates into carotid arteries.

## Answers

| | | | | |
|---|---|---|---|---|
| 1. B | 2. B | 3. B | 4. D | 5. E |
| 6. B | 7. F | 8. B | 9. C | 10. B |
| 11. G | 12. A | 13. A | 14. E | 15. D |
| 16. F | 17. D | 18. C | 19. E | 20. D |
| 21. D | 22. A | 23. C | 24. F | 25. C |

## SUGGESTED READING

### *Textbooks and Monographs*

Agency for Health Care Policy and Research. Unstable Angina: Diagnosis and Management. Clinical Practice Guidelines. Rockville, MD: U.S. Department of Health and Human Services; 1994.

Alpert JS, Becker RC. Pathophysiology, diagnosis and management of cardiogenic shock. In: Schlant RC, Alexander RW, O'Rourke RA, Roberts R, Sonnenblick EH (eds.). The Heart, Arteries and Veins. 8th ed. New York: McGraw-Hill, 1994:907–925.

Bayer AS, Scheld WM. Endocarditis and Intravascular Infections. In Mandell GL, Benett JE, Dolin R (eds.) Mandell, Douglas and Bennett's Principles and Practice of Infectious Diseases. Philadelphia: Churchill & Livingstone, 2000. Chapter 65, pp. 857–902.

Braunwald E. Heart Disease: A Textbook of Cardiovascular Medicine. 6th ed. Philadelphia: W.B Saunders, 2000.

Chou TC. Electrocardiography in Clinical Practice. 3rd ed. Philadelphia: W.B. Saunders, 1991.

Constant J. Bedside Cardiology. 4th ed. Boston: Little, Brown & Company, 1993.

The Criteria Committee of the New York Heart Association. Nomenclature and Criteria for Diagnosis of Diseases of the Heart and Great Vessels. 9th ed. Boston: Little Brown & Company; 1994.

Nugent EW, Plantar WH, Edwards JE, et al. The pathology, abnormal physiology, clinical recognition, and medical and surgical treatment of congenital heart disease. In: Hurst JW, Schlant RC, Rackley CE, et al (eds.). The Heart. 7th ed. New York: McGraw-Hill, 1990.

Perloff JK. Physical Examination of the Heart and Circulation. 2nd ed. Philadelphia: W. B. Saunders Company; 1990.

Scheld WM, Sande MA. Endocarditis and intravascular infections. In: Mandell GL, Bennett JE, Dolin R (eds.). Principles and Practice of Infectious Disease. 4th ed. New York: Churchill Livingstone, 1995:740–783.

Tresch DD, Aronow WS. Cardiovascular Disease in the Elderly Patient. New York: Marcel Dekker, Inc., 1994.

Wagner GS. Marriott's Practical Electrocardiography. 9th ed. Baltimore: Williams & Wilkins, 1994.

Willms JL, Schneiderman H, Algranati PS. Physical Diagnosis: Bedside Evaluation of Diagnosis and Function. Baltimore: Williams & Wilkins, 1994.

### *Articles*

*Common presentations of heart disease in adults*

Manning HL, Schwartzstein RM. Mechanisms of disease: pathophysiology of dyspnea. N Engl J Med 1995; 333:1547–1553.

*Cardiovascular examination*

Duthie EH, Gambert SR, Tresch D. Evaluation of the systolic murmur in the elderly. J Am Geriatr Soc 1981; 29:498–502.

Lembro NJ, Dell'Italia L, Crawford MH, et al. Bedside diagnosis of systolic murmurs. N Engl J Med 1988; 318:1572.

Reddy PS, Salerni R, Shaver JA. Normal and abnormal heart sounds in cardiac diagnosis. Part II. Diastolic sounds. Curr Probl Cardiol 1985; 10(4):1–55.

Shaver JA, Salerni R, Reddy PS. Normal and abnormal heart sounds in cardiac diagnosis. Part I. Systolic sounds. Curr Probl Cardiol 1985; 10(3):1–68.

Swartz MH. Jugular venous pressure pulse: Its value in cardiac diagnosis. Prim Cardiol 1982; 8:197.

*Other noninvasive techniques of cardiac diagnosis*

Conversano A, Walsh JF, Geltmann EM, et al. Delineation of myocardial stunning and hibernation by positron emission tomography in advanced coronary artery disease. Am Heart J 1996; 131:440–450.

Popp RL. Echocardiography (pts 1 and 2). N Engl J Med 1990; 323:101,165.

Sansoy V, Glover DK, Watson DD et al. Comparison of thallium-$^{201}$ resting redistribution with technetium $^{99m}$sestamibi uptake and functional response to dobutamine for assessment of myocardial viability. Circulation 1995; 92:994–1004.

Schiller NB. Doppler echocardiography. Cardiol Clin 1990; 8:173–389.

Schiller NB. Transesophageal echocardiography. Cardiol Clin 1993; 11:355–537.

Verani MS. Pharmacologic stress myocardial perfusion imaging. Curr Probl Cardiol 1993; 18:481–528.

*Disorders of cardiac rhythm and conduction*

Akhtar M, Shenasa M, Jazayeri M, et al. Wide QRS tachycardia: reappraisal of a common clinical problem. Ann Intern Med 1988; 109:905–912.

Binah O, Rosen MR. Mechanisms of ventricular arrhythmias. Circulation 1992; 85:25–35.

Dreifus LS, ACC/AHA Task Force. Guidelines for implantation of cardiac pacemakers and antiarrhythmia devices. J Am Coll Cardiol 1991; 8:1.

Josephson ME, Wellens HJJ. Differential diagnosis of supraventricular tachycardia. Cardiol Clin 1990; 8:411–441.

Kudenchuk PJ. Atrial fibrillation: pearls and perils of management. West J Med 1996; 164:425–434.

Prystowsky EN, Benson DW Jr., Fuster V, et al. Management of patients with atrial fibrillation. Circulation 1996; 93:1262–1277.

Reiffel JA, Estes NAM, Waldo AL, et al. A consensus report on antiarrhythmic drug use. Clin Cardiol 1994; 17: 103–116.

Schweitzer P, Teichholz LE. Carotid sinus massage: its diagnostic and therapeutic value in arrhythmias. Am J Med 1985; 78:645–654.

Zipes DP, Akhtar M, Denes P, et al. Guidelines for clinical intracardiac electrophysiologic studies. J Am Coll Cardiol 1989; 14:1827–1842.

*Syncope*

Kapoor WN. Syncope. N Engl J Med 2000; 34:1856–1862.

Linzer M, Yang EH, Estes MNA, Wang P, Vorperian V, Kapoor, WN. Clinical Guideline: Diagnosing Syncope: Part I: Value of History, Physical Examination, and Electrocardiography. Ann Intern Med 1997; 126:989–996.

Linzer M, Yang EH, Estes MNA, Wang P, Vorperian V, Kapoor, WN. Clinical Guideline: Diagnosing Syncope: Part II: Unexplained Syncope. Ann Intern Med 1997; 127: 76–86.

Meissner MD, Akhtar M, Lehmann MD. Nonischemic sudden tachyarrhythmic death in atherosclerotic disease. Circulation 1991; 84:905–912.

*Congestive heart failure*

Bristow MR. α-Adrenergic Receptor Blockade in Chronic Heart Failure. Circulation. 2000; 101:558–569.

Cohn JN. Structural basis for heart failure: ventricular remodeling and its pharmacological inhibition. Circulation 1995; 91:2504–2507.

Costanzo MR, Augustine S, Bourge R, et al. Selection and treatment of candidates for heart transplantation. Circulation 1995; 92:3693–3612.

Garg R, Yusuf S. Overview of randomized trials of angiotensin-converting enzyme inhibitors on mortality and morbidity in patients with heart failure. Collaborative Group on ACE Inhibitor trials. JAMA 1995; 273:1450–1456.

Georghiade M, Bonow RO. Chronic heart failure in the United States: a manifestation of coronary artery disease. Circulation 1998; 97:282–289.

Intravenous nesiritide versus nitroglycerin for treatment of decompensated congestive heart failure: a randomized controlled trial. JAMA 2002; 287:1531–1540.

Lenihan DJ, Gerson MC, Hoit BD, et al. Mechanisms, diagnosis, and treatment of diastolic heart failure. Am Heart J 1995; 130:153–166.

Membership of the advisory council to improve outcomes nationwide in heart failure. Consensus recommendations for the management of chronic heart failure. Am J Cardiol 1999; 83:1A–38A.

Morrison LK, Harrison A, Krishnaswamy P. et al: Utility of a rapid β-natriuretic peptide assay in differentiating congestive heart failure from lung disease. J Am Coll Cardiol 2002; 39:202–209.

Pitt B, Zannad F, Remme WJ, et al. The effect of spironolactone on morbidity and mortality in patients with severe heart failure. Randomized Aldactone Evaluation Study Investigators. N Engl J Med 1999; 341: 709–717.

Williams JF Jr., Bristow MR, Fowler MB, et al. Guidelines for the evaluation and management of heart failure. J Am Coll Cardiol 1995; 26:1376.

Yusuf S, Sleight P, Pogue J, et al. Effects of an angiotensin-converting-enzyme inhibitor, ramipril, on cardiovascular events in high-risk patients. The Heart Outcomes Prevention Evaluation Study Investigators. N Engl J Med 2000; 342: 145–153.

*Coronary artery disease*

ACC/AHA/ACP-ASIM Guidelines for the management of patients with chronic stable angina. J Am Coll Cardiol 1999; 33:2092–2190.

ACC/AHA Guidelines for coronary artery bypass graft surgery. J Am Coll Cardiol 1999; 34:1262–1342.

ACC/AHA Task Force: Guidelines for clinical use of cardiac radionuclide imaging. J Am Coll Cardiol 1995; 25:521.

Glasser SP, Selwyn AF, Ganz P. Atherosclerosis: Risk factors and the vascular endothelium. Am Heart J 1996; 131: 379–384.

Gotto AM Jr.: Cholesterol management in theory and practice. Circulation 1997; 96:4424–4430.

Executive summary of the third report of the National Cholesterol Education Program (NCEP) expert panel on detection, evaluation, and treatment of high blood cholesterol in adults (Adult Treatment Panel III). JAMA 2001; 285:2486–97.

Opie LH. Calcium channel antagonists in the treatment of

coronary artery disease: fundamental pharmacological properties relevant to clinical use. Prog Cardiovasc Dis 1996; 38:273–290.

Pattillo RW, Fuchs S, Johnson J, et al. Predictors of prognosis by quantitative assessment of coronary angiography, single photon emission computed tomography, thallium imaging and treadmill exercise testing. Am Heart J 1996; 131:582–590.

Ross R: The pathogenesis of atherosclerosis: A perspective for the 1990s. Nature 1993; 362:801.

*Acute coronary syndromes*

ACC/AHA Guidelines for the management of patients with acute myocardial infarction. J Am Coll Cardiol 1996; 28:1328–1428.

Antman EM, Cohen M, Radley D, et al. Assessment of the treatment effect of enoxaparin for unstable angina/non-Q-wave myocardial infarction: TIMI 11B-ESSENCE meta-analysis. Circulation 1999; 100:1602–1608.

Braunwald E. Unstable angina. A classification. Circulation 1989; 80:410–414.

Braunwald E, Antman EM, Beasley JW et al: ACC/AHA guidelines for the management of patients with unstable angina and non–ST-segment elevation myocardial infarction:

Cairns JA, Hirsh J, Lewis HD, et al. Antithrombotic agents in coronary artery disease. Chest (suppl) 1995; 108:380S–400S.

CAPRIE Steering Committee. A randomized, blinded, trial of clopidogrel versus aspirin in patients at risk of ischemic events. Lancet 1996; 348:1329–1339.

DeServi S, Arbustini E, Marsico F, et al. Correlation between clinical and morphologic findings in unstable angina. Am J Cardiol 1996; 77:128–132.

Fletcher GF. Current status of cardiac rehabilitation. Curr Probl Cardiol 1992; 17:143–198.

Hamm CW, Katus HA. New biochemical markers for myocardial injury. Curr Opin Cardiol 1995; 10:355.

Libby P: The molecular bases of the acute coronary syndromes. Circulation 1995; 91:2844.

Maynard SJ, Menown IB, Adgey AA. Troponin T or troponin I as cardiac markers in ischemic heart disease. Heart 2000; 83:371–373.

Oler A, Whooley MA, Oler J, Grady D. Adding heparin to aspirin reduces the incidence of myocardial infarction and death in patients with unstable angina. A meta-analysis. JAMA 1996; 276:811–815.

Parker AB III, Waller BF, Gering LE. Usefulness of the 12-lead electrocardiogram in detection of myocardial infarction: electrocardiographic-anatomic correlations. Part I. Clin Cardiol 1996; 19:55–61.

Pitt B. Evaluation of the postinfarct patient. Circulation 1995; 91:1855.

Reeder GS. Identification and treatment of complications of myocardial infarction. Curr Prob Cardiol 1996; 21:585–667.

Savonitto S, Ardissino D, Granger CB, et al. Prognostic value of the admission electrocardiogram in acute coronary syndromes. JAMA 1999; 281:707–713.

Topol EJ. Toward a new frontier in myocardial reperfusion therapy. Circulation 1998; 97:211–218.

Topol EJ, Byzova TV, Plow EF. Platelet GPIIb-IIIa blockers. Lancet 1999; 353:227–231.

Yeghiazarians Y, Braunstein JB, Askari, A Stone PH. Unstable angina pectoris. N Engl J Med 2000; 342:10114.

1999 Update: ACC/AHA Guidelines for the management of patients with acute myocardial infarction. J Am Coll Cardiol 1999; 34:890–911. Part 7: The Era of Reperfusion. Circulation 2000; 102(Suppl I):I–172 to I–203.

executive summary and recommendations. Circulation 2000; 102:1193–1209. (2002 update available on acc.org).

*Congenital heart disease and valvular heart disease*

Brickner ME, Hillis LD, Lange RA: Congenital Heart Disease in Adults. N Engl J Med 2000; 342:256–263 and 334–342.

Duncan AK, Vittone J, Fleming KC, et al. Cardiovascular disease in elderly patients. Mayo Clin Proc 1996; 71:184–96.

Feldman T. Rheumatic heart disease. Curr Opin Cardiol 1996;11(2):126–30.

Fenster MS, Feldman MD. Mitral regurgitation: an overview. Curr Probl Cardiol 1995; 20:193–280.

Katz NM. Current surgical treatment of valvular heart disease. Am Fam Phys 1995; 52(2):559–68.

Passik CS, Ackermann DM, Pluth JR, et al. Temporal changes in the causes of aortic stenosis: a surgical pathologic study of 646 cases. Mayo Clin Proc 1987; 62:119–123.

Scognamiglio R, Rahimotoola SH, Fasolii G, et al. Nifedipine in asymptomatic patients with severe aortic regurgitation and normal left ventricular function. N Engl J Med 1994; 331:689– 694.

*Infective endocarditis*

Bayer AS, Bolger AF, Taubert KA, Wilson W, et al. Diagnosis and Management of Infective Endocarditis and Its Complications. Circulation 1998; 98:2936–2948.

Durack DT. Prevention of infective endocarditis. N Engl J Med 1995; 332:38–44.

*Diseases of the pericardium and myocardium*

Dec GW, Fuster V. Idiopathic dilated cardiomyopathy. N Engl J Med 1994; 331:1564–1575.

Fowler NO. Pulsus paradoxus. Heart Disease and Stroke 1994; 3:68–69.

Maisch B. Pericardial diseases, with a focus on etiology, pathogenesis, pathophysiology, new diagnostic imaging methods, and treatment. Curr Opin Cardiol 1994; 9: 379–388.

Sagristà-Sauleda J, Angel J, Permanyer-Miralda G, Soler-Soler J. Long-Term Follow-Up of Idiopathic Chronic Pericardial Effusion. N Engl J Med 1999; 341:2054–2059.

*Diseases of the aorta*

Amarenco P, Cohen A, Tzourio C. Atherosclerotic disease of the aortic arch and the risk of ischemic stroke. N Engl J Med 1994; 331:1474–1479.

Cigarroa JE, Isselbacher EM, DeSanctis RW, et al. Diagnostic imaging in the evaluation of suspected aortic dissection: Old standards and new directions. N Engl J Med 1993; 328:35–43.

Hallet JW. A Concise Review for Cinicians: Management of Abdominal Aortic Aneurysms. Mayo Clin Proc 2000; 75(4): 395–399.

Kouchoukos NT, Dougenis D. Medical Progress: Surgery of the Thoracic Aorta. N Engl J Med 1997; 336:1876–1889.

Lederle FA, Parenti CM, Chute EP. Ruptured abdominal aortic aneurysm: the internist as diagnostician. Am J Med 1994; 96:163–167.

Parodi JC. Endovascular Stent Graft Repair of Aortic Aneurysms. Curr Opin Cardiol 1997; 12:396–405.

*Peripheral vascular disease*

Hertzer NR. The natural history of peripheral vascular disease: Implications for its management. Circulation. 1991; 83: I12–I19.

Newman AB, Sutton-Tyrel K, Vogt MT, et al. Morbidity and mortality in hypertensive adults with a low ankle/arm blood pressure index. JAMA 1993; 270:487–489.

O'Keeffe ST, Woods BOB, Breslin DJ, et al. Blue-toe syndrome:causes and management. Arch Intern Med 1992; 152:2197–2202.

### *Cardiogenic shock*

Califf RM, Bengtson JR. Cardiogenic shock. N Engl J Med 1994; 330:1724–1730.

Teba L, Banks DE, Balaan MR. Understanding circulatory shock. Is it hypovolemic, cardiogenic, or vasogenic? Postgrad Med 1992; 91:121–129.

### *Assessment of Cardiac Risk for Noncardiac Surgery*

Guidelines for perioperative cardiovascular evaluation for non-cardiac surgery: report of the American College of Cardiology/American Heart Association Task Force on Practice Guidelines. J Am Coll Cardiol 1996; 27:910–948.

PART V

Melinda McCord
Janet A. Fairley

# DERMATOLOGIC DISORDERS

# CHAPTER 49 GENERAL APPROACH TO DERMATOLOGIC DISORDERS

Whereas 4–5% of outpatient visits are specifically for skin disorders, up to 20% of patients have some symptom related to the skin.

## History

The history should focus on specific aspects of the current skin problem and the relevant general characteristics of the patient (Table 49.1). Also important is the history of the lesions, their chronicity, and previous therapy. The latter may alter the appearance of some skin disorders or affect the findings of clinical tests. For example, use of over-the-counter antifungals not only alters the morphology of tinea infections, but also renders a negative potassium hydroxide (KOH) preparation result. General information about age, gender, and race also can be helpful because some disorders show predilections related to those factors.

## Physical Examination

Examination of the skin can be divided into the following three phases: (1) an overview of the patient, (2) a general inspection of the skin, and (3) a careful study of the morphology of the individual lesion(s). The purpose of the general overview is to look for signs of systemic illness, which may suggest that the skin lesion is a manifestation of a systemic disorder. A general inspection of the skin involves examining it for overall color, texture, and hydration (dry versus well-hydrated). A significant skin lesion such as a melanoma could be detected incidentally during such a general inspection. Morphologic diagnosis of skin disorders depends on identifying (1) the primary lesion;(2) secondary changes; (3) the configuration, extent, and distribution of the lesion; (4) the color of the lesion; and (5) changes in the rest of the skin or skin appendages, or both, including the nails, scalp, and oral mucosa.

A primary lesion arises from the disease process without alteration by the environment or by patient intervention (e.g., scratching), and its characteristics are the most important in determining a correct diagnosis; Table 49.2 lists common morphologic terms. The morphology of the primary lesion forms the basis for classifying skin disorders into broad groups, a process that helps determine a correct diagnosis. These broad groups are (1) papulosquamous, (2) vesicobullous, (3) tumor-nodule, (4) vascular reaction, and (5) dermatitis–eczema. Not all disorders are amenable to this classification; such groups help narrow the differential diagnosis. Secondary changes (Table 49.3) evolve from environmental or patient factors and often reflect the history of the lesion (e.g., lichenification, erosions from scratching, or crusting from secondary infection).

Configuration describes the shape of the lesions, which sometimes might be characteristic (e.g., target lesions of erythema multiforme). Discoid usually refers to discoid lupus erythematosus, whereas nummular usually implies a type of eczema. Likewise, guttate refers to the guttate form of psoriasis. The distribution of a lesion is generally less helpful for diagnosis than its morphology; however, in some instances, the distribution is so striking that it might suggest the cause—for example, the characteristic dermatomal distribution of herpes zoster. The color within skin lesions is generally attributable to melanin, oxyhemoglobin, reduced hemoglobin, carotene, and cellular infiltration. Other causes may be foreign substances such as deposition of a drug or tattoo. Palpation of the skin can help the clinician notice the subtle depression of an atrophic skin lesion, identify an infiltrated lesion, or better evaluate the texture and hydration of the skin.

**TABLE 49.1. Pertinent Aspects of Dermatologic History**

| |
|---|
| *Questions specific to the skin problem* |
| Acute or chronic? |
| What was the initial site of involvement and the pattern of spread? |
| Have any individual lesions changed from their initial appearance? |
| Does anything seem to cause or irritate the lesions, in the patient's opinion? |
| Are the lesions symptomatic—itching or pain? |
| Has the patient had any prior therapy (physician or over-the-counter preparations)? |
| *General information needed about the patient* |
| Age |
| Gender |
| Ethnic/racial background |
| Geographic origin and travel |
| Occupation and hobbies |
| Family history—do any other family members have skin problems? |
| *General medical history* |
| Allergies, asthma, diabetes, or other metabolic or chronic diseases |
| *Medications, including over-the-counter ones* |

TABLE 49.2. Morphologic Terms in Dermatology

| |
|---|
| *Primary lesions* |
| Macule—flat, circumscribed area of color change |
| Papule—an elevated, palpable lesion <5 mm in diameter |
| Nodule—an elevated lesion >5 mm in diameter |
| Tumor—large nodule, usually >2 cm in diameter; may be either benign or malignant |
| Plaque—a broad-based, elevated lesion in which the diameter of the lesion is greater than its height |
| Wheal—transient swelling caused by edema of skin |
| Vesicle—palpable, fluid-filled lesion <1 cm in diameter |
| Bulla—a fluid-filled lesion >1 cm in diameter |
| Cyst—circumscribed tumor containing semi-solid or liquid material |
| Pustule—an elevated lesion containing a focal accumulation of inflammatory cells and serum (pus) |
| Purpura—leakage of blood into the skin |
| Burrow—linear lesion caused by parasites in the skin |
| *Secondary changes* |
| Scale—accumulation of squamous debris from the epidermis |
| Crust—collection of dried serum, cellular, or bacterial debris overlying damaged epidermis |
| Fissure—cleft in epidermis extending into the dermis |
| Excoriation—loss of epidermis induced by scratching |
| Lichenification—exaggeration of skin markings associated with epidermal thickening and usually caused by scratching |
| Erosion—loss of epidermis; heals without scarring |
| Ulcer—loss of epidermis and at least part of the dermis; heals with scarring |
| Atrophy—loss of substance of skin; can be either superficial (epidermal) or deeper (dermal or subcutaneous) |
| Scar—new formation of connective tissue that replaces lost dermis or subcutaneous tissue |

## Diagnostic Procedures and Techniques

Once a differential diagnosis has been generated, specific diagnostic methods can follow. In general, nondermatologists tend to overdiagnose infectious disorders and underdiagnose inflammatory diseases. A few basic diagnostic techniques can help the physician avoid this pitfall.

### Potassium hydroxide preparation

A potassium hydroxide (KOH) preparation identifies fungal elements present on the skin. Scrapings are obtained from the skin, nails, or scalp and placed on a glass slide. A drop of 10–20% KOH is added, a coverslip is placed over the KOH, and the slide is gently warmed by passing it through the flame of an alcohol lamp. The KOH should not boil. If allowed to stand for 5–10 minutes, KOH dissolves much of the keratin from the skin scrapings, thus enabling the clinician to see more clearly fungal hyphae, spores, or both. Care should be taken to avoid getting KOH on the microscope because it will etch the lens. In dermatophyte infections, branched, segmented hyphae are present (see Color Plate 1, located in the color plate section at the end of the book); in tinea versicolor (a superficial fungal infection caused by *Pityrosporum*), shorter hyphae and spores cause a "spaghetti and meatballs" appearance.

Tinea capitis is more difficult to confirm with the KOH preparation. Even in experienced hands, a KOH test has an accuracy of only 60%; therefore, a culture of the scalp should supplement a KOH test to diagnose tinea capitis. Both scales and hairs plucked from an involved site should be examined. The spores in endothrix infections are found inside the distorted hair shaft, whereas in ectothrix infections, the spores and hyphae are outside of the hair shaft.

### Wood's lamp examination

A Wood's lamp emits light at a wavelength of 365 nm; it enhances the presence of hypopigmented and hyperpigmented epidermal lesions and causes fluorescence of certain superficial bacteria, fungi, and chemicals. A Wood's lamp is used to determine the depth of

TABLE 49.3. Descriptive Terms for the Configuration and Distribution of Skin Lesions

| |
|---|
| *Configuration* |
| Circinate—circular lesions |
| Discoid—disk-shaped |
| Nummular—coin-shaped |
| Annular—ring-shaped with clearing in the center |
| Polycyclic—annular but not forming complete rings |
| Guttate—multiple, small teardrop-shaped lesions |
| Serpiginous—snake-like |
| Iris or target—shaped like a bull's-eye with concentric rings |
| Herpetiform—grouped vesicles, papules, or erosions; similar to herpes |
| Zosteriform—a dermatomal distribution |
| Reticulated—interlacing, net-like |
| *Distribution* |
| Symmetry |
| Extensor versus flexural surfaces |
| Contact areas—confined to areas of contact with an exogenous agent |
| Seborrheic distribution—face, upper chest, and back |
| Photo distribution—in areas exposed to sunlight; spares the area under the chin and in the deep creases of the eyelid; also often shows some sparing in the shaded area below the nose |
| Koebnerization—formation of lesions in an area that has been traumatized. |

pigmentary disorders because it enhances epidermal pigmentary changes and diminishes dermal pigmentary changes. Vitiligo is enhanced, and the ash leaf macules of tuberous sclerosis are rendered visible. Another classic use of the Wood's lamp is for determining tinea capitis. Ectothrix infections caused by *Microsporum audouinii* or *Microsporum canis* fluoresce green. However, over 90% of tinea scalp infections in the United States are caused by *Trichophyton tonsurans,* an endothrix infection that fails to fluoresce—this greatly diminishes the role of Wood's lamp in identifying tinea capitis.

Other infections that can be detected with a Wood's lamp include erythrasma and tinea versicolor. Erythrasma, a superficial, cutaneous bacterial infection caused by the corynebacterium species, mimics tinea cruris. On examination with a Wood's lamp, erythrasma fluoresces a coral red because of the presence of porphyrins in the corynebacterium; tinea versicolor fluoresces yellow-green. In porphyria cutanea tarda, the urine, feces, and blister fluid may fluoresce a pinkish-orange. Because spot-testing of the urine does not always elicit fluorescence, it does not supplant quantitative measurement of the porphyrins.

#### Cytologic (Tzanck) smear

The Tzanck smear can confirm herpes infections rapidly. Despite being positive in herpes simplex types I and II and in varicella zoster infections, the smear cannot differentiate between these organisms. The test is performed by removing the top of an intact blister and scraping its base with a scalpel blade. The scraping is smeared onto a glass slide, air-dried, and stained, usually with methylene blue, Giemsa, or Wright stains. A coverslip is applied, and the smear is examined under the microscope. A positive result requires finding multinucleated giant cells (Color Plate 2), a task that is observer-dependent.

The Tzanck test requires an intact vesicle for accurate diagnosis. With intact vesicles, it is positive in over 70% of the cases, but the yield is much lower with crusted lesions. The Tzanck preparation correlates well with viral cultures in experienced hands; its other advantages are rapid results and almost universal availability. As an alternative to the Tzanck smear, many laboratories now offer rapid screening tests that rely on immunologic techniques and are usually available within 4–5 hours. Viral isolation, perhaps the most definitive test, is not 100% sensitive, and the results take several days.

#### Scabies preparations

Scabies, caused by the mite *Sarcoptes scabiei,* is a common infestation, and skin scrapings are extremely helpful in its diagnosis. Mites are most successfully detected from a site that has not been excessively scratched. For help with identifying a burrow, the clinician can apply washable ink to the affected areas, wash off the excess, and then look for burrows that retain the ink. Using a number 15 scalpel blade on which a drop of mineral oil has been placed, the clinician scrapes open an intact burrow and smears the contents on a slide. A common error is not scraping deeply enough because the scraping must be deeper than is required for fungal preparations. A coverslip is placed over the smear, and the preparation is examined with a microscope under low power. Identification of a mite, egg case, or feces is diagnostic (Color Plate 3). Some prefer the use of KOH in identifying scabies because it helps dissolve the keratotic debris and thus improves the visibility of the mite; however, KOH will destroy any feces present.

#### Diascopy

Diascopy is a simple procedure that can provide information regarding the cause of a color change within a lesion. A clear glass or plastic slide is used to apply firm pressure to the surface of a skin lesion. Blanching of lesions implies that any erythema is caused by vasodilation. Conversely, hemorrhage into the skin will not blanch. Exclusion of blood from the lesion also can reveal unusual color changes, such as a brownish-yellow hue in granulomatous disorders.

#### Skin Biopsy

Taking a skin biopsy is one of the most definitive ways to establish the diagnosis of skin disorders. The selection of the site, the technique used, and the interpretation of the report in light of the clinical examination are crucial to the success of such a biopsy procedure. In most disorders, a sample from a well-developed, representative lesion is most helpful. In bullous disorders, a biopsy specimen from the margin of a lesion is usually more helpful in determining the level of separation; secondarily infected or excoriated lesions should not be selected. Discoid lupus erythematosus and vasculitis are often identified by routine histology in slightly older lesions, but biopsy specimens for immunofluorescence testing for vasculitis should be obtained from recent lesions.

An incisional biopsy samples only a portion of the lesion, and an excisional biopsy removes it entirely. The most commonly used technique is the punch biopsy, which involves using a 3- to 4-mm punch (trephine). After local asepsis and local anesthesia, the punch is rotated while pressure is applied to drill it through the skin. The specimen is gently lifted and snipped from the underlying subcutaneous fat. The specimen should be handled gently, because damage from forceps can cause artifacts that can make histologic interpretation difficult. The site is closed with a suture, treated with a hemostatic agent such as 30% aluminum chloride, or packed with Gelfoam to stop the bleeding.

Sometimes a larger piece of tissue is required, such as that obtained in a wedge biopsy. A narrow, elliptical sample of skin and the subcutaneous fat are removed, and the wound is closed with a suture, leaving a linear scar. Biopsy specimens for routine histologic examination should be fixed immediately in 10% neutral-buffered formalin. However, immunofluorescence testing, electron microscopy, and many immunohistochemical techniques require special fixatives. Therefore, the reference laboratory should be consulted regarding the appropriate handling of the tissue before the biopsy.

# CHAPTER 50 PRINCIPLES OF TOPICAL TREATMENT

Dermatologic therapy emphasizes topical treatment, the advantage of which is that the affected site receives direct treatment, generally without systemic side effects. However, to the nondermatologist, the many topical agents and vehicles can make the choice of an appropriate medication a daunting task.

Although the skin is a barrier, the epidermis does permit selective transport of some molecules through it. Drugs are absorbed into the skin by passive diffusion, and the major barrier to absorption is the stratum corneum. Percutaneous absorption of medications is affected by many factors. Absorption of a medication is proportional to the concentration of the molecule applied up to a point, beyond which it plateaus. However, the percutaneous absorption of many compounds cannot be predicted on the basis of simple diffusion. Lipids and polar solvents—for example, acetone, alcohol, and dimethyl sulfoxide—enhance percutaneous absorption by alteration of the stratum corneum. Increased skin temperature results in increased absorption. Occlusion of medications will increase the surface temperature and enhance percutaneous absorption. Finally, maximum hydration increases percutaneous absorption fivefold. Ironically, by damaging the barrier, excessive dryness also might enhance percutaneous absorption.

Percutaneous absorption also varies with the body site and with age. For example, palmar and plantar skin absorbs much less than the skin of the trunk. The stratum corneum of a premature infant is only two to three cell layers thick, whereas that of a full-term infant is four to six cell layers thick. Within 2–3 weeks after delivery, the premature infant's stratum corneum matures to that of a full-term infant. However, infants and children may exhibit increased toxicity to some topically applied compounds because of their increased surface-to-volume ratio compared with adults. On the other hand, old age does not seem to impose any demonstrable changes on percutaneous absorption.

**TABLE 50.1. Amounts of Creams to be Used for a Two-Week Course of Therapy**

| Area of Application | Lotions | Creams, Ointments |
|---|---|---|
| Localized application | >1 oz | 15–30 g |
| Hands or feet | >2 oz | >60 g |
| Trunk | 4–8 oz | >120 g |
| Whole body | >6 oz | >480 g |

Note: Estimates based on twice-daily application.

Effective topical therapy depends on four major factors: the active ingredient, the vehicle, the condition being treated, and the patient (other medical problems, medications, compliance). The choice of the active ingredient and its vehicle—the two variables in the topical preparation—are most amenable to physician control. The choice of the correct active ingredient is dictated by the disorder being treated. A guide for the appropriate amount of topical preparations to prescribe is provided in Table 50.1.

The adage "If it is wet, dry it; if it is dry, wet it" has some general merit in that the selection of the vehicle has a significant impact on the response to therapy (Table 50.2). An eruption might be either wet (weeping, crusted, maceration, vesiculation) or dry (scale, lichenification, fissuring, and cracking). Vehicles can be divided into three groups: those that promote drying (wet dressings, powders, lotions, and sprays), those that moisturize (ointments and oils), and those with an intermediate effect (creams and gels). Table 50.3 lists the relative potency of topical steroids.

TABLE 50.2. Summary of Vehicles in Dermatologic Therapy

| Treatment | Principle | Ingredients | Advantages | Disadvantages |
|---|---|---|---|---|
| Open wet dressings | Moisturize areas by loosely wrapping many layers of moistened soft gauze or sheeting around them, leave in place for 1/2 to 2 hours, remove and remoisten | Normal saline, aluminum acetate (Burrow solution), aluminum diacetate (Domeboro), $KMnO_4$, or 5% acetic acid in *Pseudomonas* infections | Dries and cools by evaporation, decreases local blood flow in inflammation by vasoconstriction, cleanses the area, and removes crust and debris; increases skin hydration to foster cutaneous drug absorption | Simultaneously compressing large amounts of the body may lead to excessive evaporative heat loss; can apply compresses to only about one third of the body at a time |
| Closed wet dressings | Dressings covered by an impermeable wrap; otherwise same as above | Same as above | Same as above | May cause maceration and bacterial overgrowth; lacks the cooling effect of open dressings |
| Soaks | Useful for immersing extremities | Aluminum acetate, aluminum diacetate, and colloidal oatmeal (Aveeno) | Useful in treating widespread skin lesions; oatmeal soothes and is antipruritic; its oilated forms provide extra moisture | Useful in extremities only |
| Baths | Useful in immersing almost the entire body | Same as soaks Cornstarch (1/2 box in 6 inches of tub water) is inexpensive, soothing, and antipruritic | Same as soaks; oil may be added to the bath, which coats, lubricates, and moisturizes dry skin conditions | Oil could coat the bath tub and make it slippery |
| Lotions | A suspension or solution; liquid base cools by evaporation | Inert or active agents; liquid base of water, alcohol, or propylene glycol | Ideal in hair-bearing or intertriginous areas because it is easy to apply and does not cause occlusion folliculitis | Not helpful as lubricants for dry skin conditions because of high water and/or alcohol content |
| Ointments | Moisturize using a *small amount,* which is rubbed in | Emulsion of water droplets in oil; many agents | Gray or clear; have a greasy feel; very dry skin conditions can benefit from these | Patient acceptance is lower |
| Creams | Same as above | Emulsion of oil droplets in water; many agents | Patient acceptance is better; usually, a lighter and oilier base than ointment | Not as good at moisturizing as ointments because of volatile solvent or a high water content |
| Gels | Evaporate on contact and cause drying | Semisolid emulsions of agents in water, alcohol, or glycols | Useful in hair-bearing areas because they are not greasy or occlusive | Newer gels may lack the drying component seen in older types |

| | | | | |
|---|---|---|---|---|
| Pastes | Often used to protect a localized area—e.g., $ZnO_2$ paste in diaper area | A powder in an ointment base; many agents | High powder content provides more drying than ointment | Useful in localized lesions only |
| Powders | Promote drying and minimize friction between opposing folds of skin | May be inert—e.g., talc, cornstarch, and $ZnO_2$ powder; or active—e.g., nystatin | Best used in intertriginous areas that are normally moist and may potentially macerate | Foreign body reactions from insoluble powders near open wounds; a sticky mess may result if residual powder is not removed before reapplying |
| Topical steroids | Anti-inflammatory, antiproliferative and immunosuppressive; suppress the mitotic activity of both keratinocytes and fibroblasts | Many agents (see Table 50.3); potency relates to the vehicle and concentration of active ingredient; ointments more potent than creams or lotions | Class VII steroids are generally preferred for use in areas such as the face and groin (least likely to cause atrophy) | May cause steroid acne, purpura, and easy bruising (Color Plate 4), acneiform eruptions, perioral dermatitis or skin atrophy; may delay wound healing; fluorinated steroids are highly atrophogenic; use near eye can cause glaucoma, ocular hypertension, or cataracts if agents get in the eye |

**TABLE 50.3. Relative Potency of Selected Topical Steroids**

| | |
|---|---|
| *Class I* | *Class IV* |
| Betamethasone dipropionate | Desoximetasone |
| Clobetasol propionate† | Fluocinolone acetonide—ointment |
| Diflorasone diacetate | Flurandrenolide |
| Halobetasol propionate | Mometasone furoate |
| *Class II* | Triamcinolone acetonide 0.1% |
| Amcinonide—ointment | *Class V* |
| Betamethasone dipropionate—ointment | Betamethasone valerate—cream |
| Desoximetasone | Desonide |
| Diflorasone diacetate | Flurandrenolide |
| Fluocinonide—cream | Fluocinolone acetonide—ointment |
| Halcinonide | Hydrocortisone butyrate |
| Mometasone furoate | Hydrocortisone valerate |
| *Class III* | Triamcinolone acetonide 0.05% |
| Amcinonide—cream | *Class VI* |
| Betamethasone dipropionate—cream | Alclometasone dipropionate |
| Betamethasone valerate | Desonide |
| Diflorasone diacetate | Flumethasone pivolate |
| Triamcinolone acetonide | Fluocinolone acetonide cream—.01% |
| | Hydrocortisone butyrate |
| | Triamcinolone acetonide 0.025% |
| | *Class VII* |
| | Hydrocortisone acetate 1–2.5% |

*Suppression of hypothalamic-pituitary axis (HPA) is most common with use of higher potency (class I, II, or III) steroids under occlusion or in small children. Class I agents can cause HPA suppression, even without occlusion.

†Maximum dose: 60 g/week for a total of 2 weeks for clobetasol dipropionate to avoid HPA suppression. Occlusion should be avoided with these agents for the same reason.

(Adapted from: Stoughton RB. Vasoconstrictor Assay-Specific Applications. In: Maibach HI, Surber C (eds). Topical Corticosteroids. Basel, Switzerland: Karger AG, 1992, pp 42–53.

# CHAPTER 51 PAPULOSQUAMOUS DISORDERS

Papulosquamous disorders are characterized by primary lesions consisting of papules or plaques that are generally multiple and usually have sharp margins with secondary scaling. Among the papulosquamous disorders shown in Table 51.1, the more common ones are psoriasis, pityriasis rosea (PR), and lichen planus; others are secondary syphilis, dermatophytosis, pityriasis rubra pilaris, and parapsoriasis.

**TABLE 51.1. Papulosquamous Disorders**

| |
|---|
| Psoriasis |
| Pityriasis rosea |
| Lichen planus |
| Secondary syphilis |
| Dermatophytosis |
| Pityriasis rubra pilaris |
| Parapsoriasis |

## Psoriasis

### Definition

Psoriasis is a common, chronic inflammatory skin disorder that causes red papules and plaques covered by thick, silvery-white scales. The integral features of psoriasis are increased keratinocyte proliferation, altered keratinocyte maturation, and inflammation.

### Epidemiology, Etiology, and Pathogenesis

Psoriasis affects 1–2% of the United States population, without any gender predilection. The age of onset, although it is younger in women, has a bimodal distribution, with a larger peak between 15 and 25 years old, and the other in the fifth decade and beyond. The primary defect is unknown, but multiple factors seem to play a role, including local T cell activation, induction of keratinocyte receptors, and altered cytokine production in a genetically susceptible host.

Although psoriasis appears to be a heritable disorder, its exact mode of transmission remains elusive. It shows an association with the genes of the HLA loci HLA-Cw6 and HLA-DR7. An autosomal-dominant pattern, with reduced penetrance, is recognized in several large kindreds. However, the preponderance of data suggests that psoriasis is multigenic, and proposed susceptibility genes have been identified on chromosomes 1, 2, 4, 6, 8, 16, 17, and 20.

Psoriasis can be triggered or exacerbated by stress, excess solar irradiation, irritating topical therapy, infections (most commonly streptococcal), pregnancy, human immunodeficiency virus (HIV) infection, or drugs—the common medications in this context being β-blockers, antimalarial drugs, lithium, and perhaps nonsteroidal anti-inflammatory drugs (NSAIDs). Because systemic steroids can precipitate pustular psoriasis when their use is withdrawn, they should be used with extreme caution.

### Clinical Features

The hallmarks of psoriasis are the red, sharply demarcated papules and plaques covered by thick, silvery-white scales.Individual lesions can number anywhere from one to hundreds, and they vary in size and shape from small guttate papules to large circinate plaques (Color Plate 5). Symmetrically distributed, the lesions show a predilection for the scalp, genitals, nails, and extensor aspects of the arms and legs. Secondary excoriations or lichenification may develop with pruritic eruptions. The nails may develop pitting (Color Plate 6), onycholysis (lifting of the nail plate from the nail bed), brown "oil spots," subungual hyperkeratosis, grooving, and crumbling. The Koebner phenomenon, in which typical lesions form at the site of minor trauma, is characteristic (see Color Plate 5).

Psoriasis has numerous clinical variants, including eruptive or guttate, inverse, pustular, and erythrodermic types. Guttate psoriasis is characterized by 0.5- to 1.5-cm red papules and plaques that may be provoked by infections, particularly streptococcal ones. Inverse psoriasis is localized to the axilla, groin, and skin folds rather than the classic sites. Pustular psoriasis can be localized or generalized. The generalized form has an acute onset with crops of pustules and associated fever and leukocytosis. Erythroderma of any cause, including psoriasis, disrupts thermoregulation and fluid balance and thus signals a potential emergency. Erythrodermic psoriasis has many of the constitutional features of generalized pustular psoriasis. An inflammatory arthropathy, which is described in Chapter 264, occurs in 5–7% of patients with psoriasis.

### Differential Diagnosis

Chronic plaque-type psoriasis can resemble nummular eczema, mycosis fungoides, or tinea corporis. Guttate psoriasis should be distinguished from PR, secondary syphilis, and superficial tinea infections. Erythroderma may follow contact or atopic dermatitis, Sézary syndrome, drug eruptions, pityriasis rubra pilaris, or seborrheic dermatitis. Inverse psoriasis may resemble contact dermatitis, candidiasis, or Darier disease.

### Management

Psoriasis is a chronic disease with remissions and exacerbations. For limited disease, topical therapy may suffice. Commonly used preparations are topical steroids, tar preparations, anthralin, and the vitamin D analog, calcipotriene. Natural sunlight can sometimes be helpful, and ultraviolet light (UV), either UVB or UVA, combined with psoralen (PUVA) may be used in patients whose condition does not respond to topical compounds. UV should be administered in a supervised setting by personnel experienced with the treatment of psoriasis.

Systemic therapy is reserved for extensive disease, disease in sites that may affect one's ability to work (palms and soles), or psoriasis with severe associated arthritis. Low-dose methotrexate (2.5–35 mg) is given orally once per week. Given the risk for bone marrow or liver toxicity, patients who receive methotrexate must be carefully monitored. Acitretin is especially useful in pustular psoriasis, usually stopping pustule formation within a few days. Because acitretin is highly teratogenic and its metabolites can remain in the bloodstream for several years, women must use reliable birth control while taking acitretin and for 3 years after cessation of therapy. Other systemic agents, such as cyclosporin, hydroxyurea, and sulfasalazine, also may improve psoriasis.

## ■ Pityriasis Rosea

### Definition, Epidemiology, and Etiology

PR, which affects nearly 0.14% of the population, is a common, self-limited eruption occurring most frequently in children and young adults. Commonly seen during the spring in the United States, PR has neither a gender nor a racial predilection. Its etiology is unknown, but its seasonal occurrence, its tendency to cluster in close social groups, and the rare reports of particles resembling picornavirus on electron microscopy all suggest an infectious cause. However, it has not yet been definitively linked with a specific viral infection.

### Clinical Features

The initial lesion, a "herald patch," is a 2- to 5-cm oval, pink plaque or patch with fine peripheral scales. This precedes the remainder of the eruption and commonly occurs on the trunk but may involve the extremities also. Within hours or days, crops of oval, pink macules and papules with fine white peripheral scales arise symmetrically on the trunk, neck, and proximal extremities. The lesions form along the lines of cleavage on the trunk and usually spare the sun-exposed sites, eliciting a "Christmas tree" pattern (Color Plate 7). The herald patch is not always evident. Other than mild pruritus, symptoms or prodrome are usually absent.

### Differential Diagnosis and Management

Whereas the herald patch may be confused with tinea corporis, nummular eczema, psoriasis, or contact dermatitis, the most important disease in the differential diagnosis of the generalized eruption is secondary syphilis. Syphilis should be excluded by appropriate tests whenever PR is suspected. Other conditions include viral exanthem, nummular eczema, guttate psoriasis, seborrheic dermatitis, and dermatophyte infections. Many drugs—including bismuth, barbiturates, captopril, ketotifen, metronidazole, *d*-penicillamine, gold, mercury, isotretinoin, and arsenicals—may cause a similar eruption.

For most patients, the eruption requires only reassurance that it will eventually clear. Antihistamines or topical steroids may relieve mild pruritus, but more severe pruritus of generalized PR may require UVB treatment.

## Lichen Planus

### Definition and Epidemiology

Lichen planus is a common papulosquamous disease involving the skin, mucous membranes, and the nails and affects fewer than 1% of adults worldwide, most frequently those between 30 and 60 years old.

### Etiology

The etiology of lichen planus is unknown. It has been suggested that an unknown antigen (perhaps viral- or drug-induced) stimulates the migration and activation of lymphocytes in the skin. Lichen planus is more frequently associated with certain HLA types, especially HLA-DR1 and HLAB7 in familial cases. A certain complement of genes might predispose an individual to a lichenoid reaction to a given antigen. Recently, an association with hepatitis C in up to 20% of patients has been reported. Although hepatitis B surface antigen may be associated, lichen planus is not considered a direct result of hepatitis B infection.

### Clinical Features

The skin eruption consists of flat-topped, polygonal, purple papules arranged in a symmetric distribution on the extremities, commonly on the flexor surface of the wrists (Color Plate 8). Fine, lacy lines on the surface of the papules are called Wickham stria. Despite the associated severe pruritus, excoriations are rare. Mucous membrane lesions occur in 50% of patients and may occur without cutaneous disease. These consist of whitish, reticulated plaques that are most common on the buccal mucosa (Color Plate 9) but may involve other sites such as the mouth, vagina, or penis. Ulceration may occur with more severe mucosal involvement. In almost 25% of men with lichen planus, the genitals are affected. Nail dystrophy occurs in 1–10% of patients, consisting of thinning, splitting, longitudinal ridging, or pitting of the nail plate. Onycholysis and distal subungual hyperkeratosis also may occur. Pterygium formation (adhesion of the nail fold to the nail bed) may cause permanent scarring and nail dystrophy. These changes are not diagnostic; definitive diagnosis requires a nail biopsy.

Lichen planus has several morphologic variants: hypertrophic or verrucous (wartlike) plaques, follicular papules, vesicular or bullous lesions seen in conjunction with typical papules, actinic lichen planus involving sun-exposed sites, atrophy, and erosive mucosal lesions. In lichen planus of the scalp (lichen planopilaris), hyperkeratotic follicular papules progress to atrophy, scarring, and alopecia.

The role of liver dysfunction in lichen planus remains controversial; however, the recent reports of an association with hepatitis C suggest that laboratory screening of these patients may be warranted. A number of cases of lichen planus have been reported in conjunction with other autoimmune diseases, such as vitiligo, inflammatory bowel disease, and alopecia areata. These reports may imply autoimmunity or a viral etiology for lichen planus, suggest a genetic susceptibility to infection with hepatotoxic viruses, or both.

### Differential Diagnosis

The distribution and morphology of the eruption often suggest the diagnosis. Many drugs (gold, penicillamine, antimalarial drugs, arsenicals, hypoglycemic agents, tetracycline, thiazide diuretics, and angiotensin-converting enzyme inhibitors) and other agents (e.g., color film developers) may produce a lichenoid eruption. The other papulosquamous diseases should be considered in the differential diagnosis of the skin eruption. When lesions involve the palms and soles, syphilis should be excluded. The nail dystrophy may resemble psoriasis, onychomycosis, or alopecia areata. The mucous membrane lesions mimic lupus, leukoplakia, candidiasis, and syphilis.

### Management

In about half of the cases, the disease remits on its own in 6–18 months; in the remainder, it remains active for a prolonged period. Mild pruritus may be treated with antihistamines and topical steroids. With severe symptoms and extensive involvement, oral corticosteroids may be effective in a tapering dose over 2–6 weeks; however, activity often recurs when steroids are discontinued. They are best avoided in patients with chronic disease. PUVA therapy and systemic retinoids also have been reported to be effective. For oral lesions, a potent topical steroid may be given in gel form or mixed in an adherent vehicle such as Orabase. Topical retinoids (Retin-A) also have been used for oral lesions.

Newer approaches to psoriasis currently under development include a class of agents known as biologic response modifiers. These include inhibitors of TNFα as well as agents that inhibit components of the immune response in psoriasis. Humanized monoclonal antibodies, recombinant peptides that bind to the surface of T-cells and toxin-linked compounds are being used in research protocols. Some of the targets include CD11a (efalizumab), CD4 and CD2 (alefacept). Because of potential side effects, all of these agents are currently being studied in patients with more severe forms of the disease.

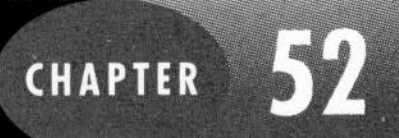

# CHAPTER 52 VESICOBULLOUS DISORDERS

## Pemphigus

### Definition and Epidemiology

Pemphigus refers to a group of autoimmune blistering diseases of the skin. In all forms of pemphigus, blisters arise because of the loss of cell-to-cell adhesion (acantholysis) within the epidermis. The onset of pemphigus vulgaris (PV) typically is in the fourth to sixth decades of life. Although no ethnic group is exempt, it is more common among Ashkenazi Jews and is associated with the HLA-DR4 or DRW6 haplotypes. The Brazilian endemic form of pemphigus foliaceus (PF), fogo selvagem, occurs in the forested regions of Brazil and is associated with the HLA-DR1-Dw20 haplotype. An environmental factor is strongly suspected in its pathogenesis. Pemphigus foliaceus (PF) is sporadic in the United States and shows no predilection for any specific group.

### Etiology and Pathogenesis

Both forms of pemphigus (PV and PF) are characterized by the presence of immunoglobulin-G (IgG) directed against the cell surface of keratinocytes. The stimulus for the development of these autoantibodies is unknown. They may be detected bound to the skin or in the circulation by immunofluorescence techniques. These autoantibodies are pathogenic by passive transfer into neonatal mice. Some cases of pemphigus appear to be drug-induced; the more common offenders are penicillamine, captopril, rifampin, phenobarbital, and piroxicam.

The histologic and clinical features of different forms of pemphigus are related to the level at which the keratinocytes detach (Table 52.1). For example, in PV, acantholysis occurs at the suprabasilar level of the epidermis, but in PF and fogo selvagen, acantholytic lesions are more superficial at the subcorneal level. Using molecular biologic methods, researchers have found the targets of the autoantibodies in PV and PF to be the cadherin type of cell adhesion molecules that are localized to the desmosomes of the epidermis. PF autoantibodies are directed against the desmosomal cadherin, desmoglein 1, and PV autoantibodies are directed against a closely related protein, desmoglein 3. Desmoglein 3 is strongly expressed in the basal layer of the epidermis, whereas desmoglein 1 is strongly expressed in the upper layers of the epidermis, which may explain these differences in the level of acantholysis and blister formation in PV and PF.

### Clinical Features

PV is characterized by the formation of flaccid bullae that arise on noninflamed skin. Pressure applied to the edge of the blister or the adjacent normal skin will cause these bullae to spread, termed Nikolsky sign. The blisters rupture, leaving erosions and large areas of denuded skin. The mouth is usually the first affected site. The scalp is another common site of early involvement. Although PV can remain localized for prolonged periods, it becomes widespread if untreated. Before the development of immunosuppressants, PV was frequently fatal because of extensive loss of the epidermal barrier.

In contrast, in PF the blisters are more superficial, and they easily rupture, leaving erosions. Erythema and

TABLE 52.1. Characteristics of the Major Vesicobullous Disorders

| Disease | Epidemiology | Clinical Features | Immunopathology and Histopathology | Therapy |
|---|---|---|---|---|
| Pemphigus vulgaris | Onset in fourth to sixth decade | Flaccid bullae arising on noninflamed skin; oral involvement common | IgG, C3 deposited on the cell surface of keratinocytes; suprabasilar acantholysis | Prednisone, 60–100 mg/day to suppress the blistering; add azathioprine (50–150 mg/day) or cyclophosphamide (50– 200 mg/day) if necessary |
| Pemphigus foliaceus | Onset in fourth to sixth decade | Flaccid bullae, crusting, and erosions mainly on the head, neck, and upper trunk; oral mucosa spared | IgG, C3 deposited on the cell surface of keratinocytes; acantholysis at the upper layers of the epidermis | Same as above |
| Bullous pemphigoid | Onset >60 years | Tense bullae (Figure 52.1) on an erythematous base; often worse in the intertriginous areas | IgG, C3 deposited at the basement membrane zone; subepidermal blisters | Compresses of Burrow solution, plus a high-potency topical steroid for localized disease; prednisone (0.6–1.2 mg/kg/day, initially; taper and use every-other-day dosing when disease is under control), with or without immunosuppressive agents (same as pemphigus vulgaris); tetracycline (500 mg four times daily) nicotinamide (500 mg three times daily) combination may be useful in selected cases |
| Dermatitis herpetiformis | Onset in second to fourth decade | Grouped vesicles on extensor surfaces; extreme pruritus | IgA in the dermal papillae; separation between tips of dermal papillae and the epidermis | Dapsone |

crusting often are prominent. Unlike PV, PF lesions are most frequent on the head and neck, and spare the oral mucosa; despite its chronic course, PF has a better prognosis.

### Diagnosis and Differential Diagnosis

PV and PF may be differentiated from each other clinically and histologically. At times, they can resemble pemphigoid, dermatitis herpetiformis, and erythema multiforme (EM). The oral lesions of PV may be mistaken for EM, erosive lichen planus, herpes, and cicatricial pemphigoid. In both PV and PF, circulating antibodies directed against the keratinocyte cell surface can be detected by indirect immunofluorescence (IF). In addition, lesional epidermis exhibits autoantibodies bound to the keratinocyte surface by direct IF. The titers of serum autoantibodies roughly correlate with disease activity; however, differentiating PV from PF by this method is difficult because the IF staining patterns are similar for both diseases.

### Management

The goal of therapy for all forms of pemphigus is to lower the autoantibody production, primarily through the use of high-dose corticosteroids, which are often combined with a steroid-sparing agent. Treatment is generally initiated with prednisone (see Table 52.1). If steroids alone do not produce an adequate response, or if their dose cannot be adequately tapered, azathioprine, cyclophosphamide, or methotrexate is added. Plasmapheresis may reduce the levels of circulating autoantibodies; however, unless antibody formation is suppressed, their titers may rebound when plasmapheresis is stopped.

Whereas untreated PV is highly lethal (50% within the first year), therapy lowers the mortality significantly to almost 10% over 5 years. Morbidity and mortality in the treated patient are usually caused by complications of therapy. Disease control and monitoring for these side effects are best achieved through close follow-up.

## Bullous Pemphigoid

### Definition and Epidemiology

Bullous pemphigoid (BP), the most common of the autoimmune bullous disorders, is generally a disease of the elderly, with no racial or gender predilections. Herpes gestationis, a related disorder that shares the histologic and immunologic features of BP, occurs during the second and third trimesters of pregnancy and generally resolves soon after birth. A proposed link between BP and cancer has not been proven. Other autoimmune diseases (pernicious anemia, diabetes, and rheumatoid arthritis) often are associated with BP.

### Etiology, Pathogenesis, and Pathology

The autoantibodies in BP patients are directed against two epidermal antigens of 230 kD and 180 kD (BP230 and BP180), both components of the hemidesmosome, an organelle of epithelial cells that functions in cell-substrate adhesion. Recent studies using a mouse model suggest that BP180 may be the more important pathogenic target of autoantibodies in human BP. The initial trigger for autoantibody formation is unknown. Histologically, these blisters show separation of the epidermis from the dermis through the basement membrane zone of the dermoepidermal junction. Binding of IgG and C3 also is demonstrable at the basement membrane zone by direct immunofluorescence.

### Clinical Features

An urticarial phase may precede the vesicobullous eruption of BP, in which patients develop plaques of erythema that mimic true urticaria but persist longer than 24 hours. Generalized pruritus also may precede the eruption. Although the lesions may be widespread, they most commonly affect the intertriginous areas, the flexor surface of the arms and legs, and the lower abdomen (Color Plate 10). Mucous membranes may be affected in up to 40% of patients, but this is rarely severe or a major feature. BP often has a chronic course, usually 2–6 years.

### Diagnosis and Management

Although the clinical features of BP are distinctive, biopsies for routine histology and direct immunofluorescence are used to confirm the diagnosis. Nearly 80% of patients will have detectable circulating autoantibodies against the basement membrane zone of the epidermis. BP may be confused with pemphigus, epidermolysis bullosa acquisita, EM, or dermatitis herpetiformis. In the urticarial phase, it may resemble true urticaria. Untreated, BP can become widespread, causing the patient considerable discomfort and increasing the risk of infection. The majority of BP patients will require systemic steroids (see Table 52.1) and perhaps other immunosuppressive agents.

## Dermatitis Herpetiformis

### Definition and Epidemiology

Dermatitis herpetiformis (DH) is a chronic, autoimmune, blistering disease, preferentially affecting men in their second to fourth decades. Its frequency varies among Caucasian populations, but is much less common among African-Americans or Asians. Initial studies revealed that 58% of patients with DH expressed HLA-B8 compared with 20–30% of normal controls; however, in patients with histologically confirmed DH, the frequency of HLA-B8 expression was 80–90%.

Recent studies show an even stronger association with HLA class II antigens: 90–95% of patients with DH express HLA-DR3 and DQw2 antigens. Most patients with DH have an associated gluten-sensitive enteropathy, although it is often asymptomatic.

### Etiology and Pathogenesis

In skin biopsy sections of patients with DH, the dermal papillae contain granular deposits of IgA; it is polyclonal and predominantly IgA1. However, the origin of the immunoglobulin and the antigenic site to which it is bound remain elusive. The association of the cutaneous eruption of DH with gluten-sensitive enteropathy suggests a role for the mucosal immune response in immunoglobulin production. Circulating immune complexes and an increased frequency of antireticulin, antiendomysial, antinuclear, and thyroid microsomal antibodies exist in the sera of patients with DH, but circulating antibodies against basement membrane (anti–basement membrane antibodies) are absent. Tissue transglutaminase has been identified as the target of the antiendomysial antibodies in DH. Antibodies to tissue translglutaminase are markers for the presence of bowel disease and correlate with adherence to a gluten-free diet, but their role, if any, in the pathogenesis of the skin lesions remains unknown.

### Clinical Features

The most notable feature of DH is the severe pruritus, which burns or stings and often precedes the primary lesion (a tense subepidermal blister) by 8–10 hours. However, examination rarely discloses blisters because the trauma of scratching causes excoriations, erosions, and crusting. Pruritus may be relieved as the blisters rupture. The lesions are symmetric with herpetiform clustering, and most often affect the extensor surfaces, including the knees, elbows, buttocks, sacrum, back, shoulders, and nuchal region. Mucosal surfaces are rarely affected. The course is one of remissions and exacerbations. Although spontaneous resolution does occur, remissions may be long-lasting.

Small bowel biopsy might show histologic changes of gluten-sensitive enteropathy; however, this enteropathy is often clinically silent, and laboratory evidence of malabsorption occurs in only 20–30% of patients. Intestinal lymphoma and, less commonly, an extraintestinal lymphoma, can complicate DH.

### Differential Diagnosis

A definitive diagnosis of DH depends on the correlation of the clinical features with histologic and immunologic data. Clinically, DH may mimic scabies, neurotic excoriations, EM, linear IgA disease, transient acantholytic dermatosis, bullous pemphigoid, and herpes gestationis. Characteristically, direct immunofluorescent examination of biopsy sections reveals granular IgA deposition in the dermal papillae.

### Management

Medical management and adherence to a gluten-free diet are two approaches to therapy of DH. Often, the skin manifestations alone respond to dapsone (100–200 mg/day). Symptoms often improve within hours of therapy, which confirms the diagnosis. Patients who do not tolerate dapsone may be given sulfapyridine (1–1.5 g/day). A gluten-free diet allows most patients to discontinue or reduce dapsone and clearly improves both the skin and bowel pathology, but patients are often intolerant of such a restrictive diet.

# CHAPTER 53 HYPERSENSITIVITY DISORDERS

This group of disorders consists of urticaria, angioedema, EM, vasculitis, and erythema nodosum. Urticaria is characterized by raised, usually pruritic lesions of variable size. Angioedema, occurring as indurated areas of swelling, most commonly affects areas of loose tissue (e.g., lips and eyelids). Urticaria and angioedema are discussed in Chapter 20.

## ■ Erythema Multiforme

### Definition, Epidemiology, and Etiology

EM, an acute hypersensitivity reaction with variable severity and manifestations, involves the skin and mucous membranes. Most common in persons in their second to fourth decades, EM increases during the spring and fall, paralleling the flux of infectious organisms. No age or race is exempt, and women are affected slightly more often than men. Patients infected with HIV are particularly susceptible to the development of EM.

Subclassified as EM major or minor, EM is triggered by infections, drugs, collagen vascular diseases, neoplasms, endocrinopathies, and environmental factors. EM minor is most commonly caused by the herpes simplex virus (HSV), with even subclinical herpes infections suspected in some cases. Other causes are pregnancy and, rarely, contact sensitization. EM major most frequently follows *Mycoplasma pneumoniae* infections and the use of drugs, which commonly include sulfa compounds, anticonvulsants (e.g., phenytoin), and NSAIDs (e.g., oxicam derivatives, butazones, and salicylates). Toxic epidermal necrolysis (TEN), considered by some in the spectrum of EM, is triggered by allopurinol, ethambutol, phenolphthalein, and pentazocine, in addition to the drugs previously listed. The interval between the exposure to the imputed drug and the onset of EM is variable and may be as long as 6 weeks.

## Clinical Features

Clinical features of EM minor and major and TEN are compared in Table 53.1. EM major (Stevens-Johnson syndrome) is the severe variant of EM minor. During its initial prodrome, many patients are given antibiotics or other drugs that may obscure the identification of a trigger. The loss of the cutaneous barrier produces abnormalities of fluid regulation and creates a risk of infection. TEN, a severe, progressive hypersensitivity reaction, is considered by some to be a variant of EM. The initial management problems involve fluid and protein losses, electrolyte imbalance, thermoregulatory failure, and infection.

## Diagnosis and Differential Diagnosis

EM major and minor are usually identified by the typical, symmetric target lesions on acral sites (Color Plate 11). EM major (Stevens-Johnson syndrome) is separated from EM minor by the involvement of two or more mucous membranes. Bullous lesions also are more likely to be present in EM major. An early eruption or an unusual presentation might make EM major difficult to distinguish from urticaria, urticarial vasculitis, BP, viral exanthems, staphylococcal scalded-skin syndrome, or toxic erythemas caused by drugs or

**TABLE 53.1. Features of Erythema Multiforme and Toxic Epidermal Necrolysis**

| | EM Minor | EM Major | Toxic Epidermal Necrolysis |
|---|---|---|---|
| Prodrome | Absent/mild; fever, malaise, cough | Acute prodrome in 50%, fever, malaise, rhinorrhea, cough, diarrhea, vomiting, myalgia and arthralgia, lasts 1–14 days | Similar to EM major |
| Lesions | Asymptomatic; symmetric, dull red macules and urticarial plaques that rapidly enlarge and develop central vesicles or papules; target/iris lesions; interior of each ring becomes violaceous or purpuric (Figure 53.1); there may be prominent hemorrhagic bullae | Initial lesions resemble EM minor but rapidly enlarge and become extensive; blistering and necrosis of skin and mucous membranes | Occur within 2 days of onset of initial symptoms; discrete, violaceous papules and macules; target lesions; lesions rapidly coalesce; minimal friction or pressure causes epidermis to slough (Nikolsky sign); tender erythema evolves into bullae |
| Location of lesions | Extensor surfaces of extremities and the dorsa of hands and feet, sites of trauma or sun exposure; trunk, face and neck less involved; one or multiple crops of lesions | Similar to EM minor; conjunctiva and perianal areas; conjunctivitis, keratitis, corneal ulcers, uveitis, two mucosal sites must be involved to diagnose EM major | Extensive, but predominantly face and trunk; rapid epidermal necrosis and exfoliation |
| Mucosal lesions | Oral lesions in 25%; only in the buccal mucosa, tongue, and lips; dehydration may develop | Most common mucosal site is oral cavity; thick crusts cover bleeding oral lesions | Large portions of mucosa may be affected |
| Other organ involvement | None; lymphadenopathy may occur | Pneumonitis, myositis, pericarditis, hepatitis, changes in mentation | Pneumonia, gastrointestinal bleed, hepatitis, shock, renal failure, sepsis |
| Course | 2–3 weeks; multiple crops of lesions develop; individual lesions last 1–2 weeks | 2–4 weeks | 4–6 weeks |
| Mortality | None | 5–20% | 15–20% |

infections. The distinction between EM major and TEN also may pose a diagnostic problem. TEN is more extensive and rapidly progressive, the skin is characteristically tender, and the initial eruption is morbilliform with early evidence of necrosis. TEN may be confused with burns, exposure to caustic substances, staphylococcus scalded-skin syndrome, and toxic shock syndrome. Cultures and histologic examination of a biopsy specimen or frozen section of denuded skin will establish the diagnosis.

### Management

The important management issues in EM are to identify and eradicate the causative agent. All drugs used before the onset of the eruption should be discontinued, and inciting herpetic, bacterial, and fungal infections should be treated. EM minor frequently responds to antihistamines and local care. Because oral lesions may make eating and drinking difficult, nutritional status should be monitored. With herpetic infections, recurrences of EM minor are not unusual.

The primary treatment for EM and TEN is supportive. Severe disease is best treated in a burn unit. Frequent assessment of the hematocrit, fluid, and electrolyte balance and pulmonary, renal, and hepatic function will allow early treatment of systemic complications. Cultures will indicate the need for antibiotic therapy. An ophthalmologic consultation should be obtained. Biologic dressings (e.g., Vigilon) will enhance healing, which occurs in 2–6 weeks with pigmentary changes but without scarring. Neutropenia, old age, renal failure, extensive skin involvement, and multiple medications are poor prognostic signs. The use of systemic corticosteroids is controversial. Whether early, high-dose corticosteroid therapy in EM will halt the progression of blistering is uncertain—given the paucity of controlled studies—and it may increase the risk of infection. A recent study suggests that intravenous immunoglobulin may be helpful for patients with TEN.

## Vasculitis

### Definition and Epidemiology

Hypersensitivity vasculitis includes a number of distinct clinical entities characterized histologically by inflammation and necrosis of small arterioles and postcapillary venules. This vascular destruction is neutrophil-mediated and the neutrophils' nuclear remnants are observed in a perivascular location. (The term leukocytoclasis describes the neutrophilic nuclear fragmentation.) Except for Schönlein-Henoch purpura, which is more frequent in children, neither an ethnic nor an age-group predilection has been noted.

### Etiology and Pathogenesis

Hypersensitivity vasculitis may result from many antigens, the sources of which include drugs (penicillin, sulfonamides, thiazide diuretics, and NSAIDs), bacteria (streptococci, staphylococci, mycobacteria), viruses (HIV and hepatitis B), and endogenous proteins (cryoglobulins). It is immune complex–mediated and may be idiopathic or associated with collagen-vascular diseases and neoplasms. In states of antigen excess, soluble antigen-antibody complexes are deposited in postcapillary venules, causing complement activation, release of chemotactic factors, mast cell degranulation, and neutrophil influx. Release of proteolytic enzymes and oxygen free radicals cause tissue destruction. Edema follows excess vascular permeability caused by vasoactive mast cell mediators.

### Clinical Features

Cutaneous symptoms are often mild and consist of burning or pruritus. Fever, malaise, arthralgias, and myalgias may occur. Palpable purpura (Color Plate 12), the hallmark of leukocytoclastic vasculitis, is caused by extravasation of red blood cells (RBCs) and plasma from pathologically permeable venules. Angioedema, urticaria, nodules, pustules, hemorrhagic vesicles or bullae, ulcers, gangrene, livedo reticularis, and subcutaneous edema are less common. The lesions usually arise in crops on the lower extremities or dependent sites, and heal in 1–4 weeks; residual hyperpigmentation or scarring may follow. With systemic disease, the gastrointestinal tract, kidneys, joints, muscles, heart, and nerves may be involved. Usually self-limited, the vasculitis may be recurrent or chronic.

### Diagnosis and Differential Diagnosis

In early cases, disorders causing nonpalpable purpura must be distinguished from those with palpable hemorrhage. Nonpalpable purpura may occur in thrombocytopenia, coagulopathies, thrombocythemia, systemic diseases (amyloidosis, diabetes, and uremia), trauma, stasis, and vascular fragility. The progressive pigmented purpuras (forms of capillaritis), distributed on the lower extremity, may cause confusion. A skin biopsy is diagnostic for hypersensitivity vasculitis; it reveals vascular wall disruption, fibrin deposition, neutrophils, and nuclear dust. Biopsy is most reliable when the specimen is acquired within 48 hours of onset of the eruption. Perivascular complement and immunoglobulin deposition shown by direct immunofluorescence studies can confirm an otherwise questionable diagnosis. Initial screening tests may include a complete blood count, sedimentation rate, urinalysis, and liver and renal function tests. Other studies [total complement (CH 50), antinuclear antibody, rheumatoid factor, hepatitis B antibody and antigen, and serum protein electrophoresis] may be used selectively.

### Management

The essentials of therapy are the removal of the suspected drug and the treatment of associated diseases. Vasculitis often resolves spontaneously in 1–4 months with supportive measures such as NSAIDs, rest, leg elevation, and antibiotics for infections. Dapsone and colchicine have both been used in patients with cutaneous disease. Patients with renal involvement or extensive necrosis respond to systemic corticosteroids or other immunosuppressive agents.

**TABLE 53.2. Common Causes of Erythema Nodosum (partial listing)**

| | |
|---|---|
| *Infections* | *Sarcoidosis* |
| Bacterial | *Inflammatory bowel disease* |
| β-hemolytic (upper respiratory) streptococcal infections | Ulcerative colitis |
| | Regional enteritis |
| | *Medications* |
| Primary tuberculosis | Penicillin |
| Fungal | Sulfonamides |
| Histoplasmosis | Some oral contraceptives |
| Coccidioidomycosis | Bromides |

## Erythema Nodosum

### Definition and Epidemiology

Erythema nodosum, a panniculitis, presents with tender, red subcutaneous nodules on the extensor surfaces of the lower extremities. The peak age of onset is between 20 and 30 years, and women are affected more often than men.

### Etiology and Pathogenesis

Erythema nodosum represents a reaction to a wide range of conditions (Table 53.2). An immune mechanism has been suspected, but not proven. β-Hemolytic streptococcal upper respiratory tract infections represent the most common and well-documented trigger, with erythema nodosum developing within 3 weeks after the infection. The most frequently implicated medications are oral contraceptives, sulfonamides, and bromides.

### Clinical Features

Before the onset of the cutaneous eruption, some patients experience a mild prodrome consisting of fever, chills, malaise, arthralgias, and myalgias, often reflecting the underlying disorder. Tender, red, single or grouped, 1- to 5-cm subcutaneous nodules are symmetrically distributed on the extensor surfaces of the lower extremities. They resolve after a few days or weeks, leaving brown-red to purple macules. Crops of nodules continue to occur for 3–6 weeks until they spontaneously resolve. In 20% of cases, the lesions are recurrent, and in a few, may be chronic.

## Differential Diagnosis and Management

Other entities that may pose a diagnostic problem are subcutaneous fat necrosis, erythema induratum, and other forms of panniculitis. Biopsy is frequently required to confirm the diagnosis. Erythema nodosum often responds rapidly to treatment of the primary disease. Bed rest and salicylates or NSAIDs can adequately mitigate symptoms and enhance resolution of this self-limited disease. Indomethacin and naproxen are especially effective. Corticosteroids, colchicine, potassium iodide, and support stockings may be useful in chronic or recalcitrant cases.

# CHAPTER 54 DERMATITIS–ECZEMA

Broadly defined, dermatitis is inflammation of the skin. The dermatitis group consists of many disorders (Table 54.1). In acute eczema, exemplified by rhus dermatitis (poison ivy, oak, or sumac), weeping vesicles and erythematous papules with secondary excoriations and crusting predominate, whereas chronic eczema typically has plaques with poor margins and papules with scaling and lichenification.

## Atopic Dermatitis

### Definition and Epidemiology

Atopic dermatitis is a relatively common chronic cutaneous disorder with a worldwide distribution affecting almost 7 in 1000 adults and 24 in 1000 children. Men are affected slightly more frequently than are women. The onset is rarely before 2 months of age.

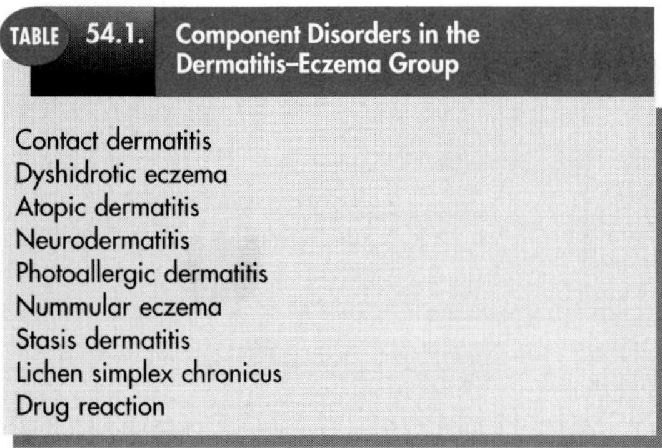

TABLE 54.1. Component Disorders in the Dermatitis–Eczema Group

| |
|---|
| Contact dermatitis |
| Dyshidrotic eczema |
| Atopic dermatitis |
| Neurodermatitis |
| Photoallergic dermatitis |
| Nummular eczema |
| Stasis dermatitis |
| Lichen simplex chronicus |
| Drug reaction |

### Etiology and Pathogenesis

The cause of atopic dermatitis is unknown. In genetically predisposed persons, environmental, immunologic, and physiologic factors contribute to the onset and perpetuation of the disease. Both cell-mediated and humoral factors are involved in its pathogenesis. Cell-mediated immunity is defective in almost three fourths of patients, with increased susceptibility to cutaneous viral and dermatophyte infections and decreased delayed hypersensitivity. T helper cells are increased relative to T suppressor cells. The predominant subset of T helper cells in atopic dermatitis secretes interleukin (IL)-4, IL-5, IL-6, and IL-10, and not $\gamma$-interferon. Serum IgE levels are high in 40–80% of patients, but its exact role in the pathogenesis of this disease is unknown.

The skin of atopic persons is heavily colonized with *Staphylococcus aureus*. In some studies, *Staphylococcus* has been isolated from lesional skin in more than 90% of patients, compared with less than 10% of normal controls.

### Clinical Features

Clinical features vary with the age of onset; thus, three patterns exist. Infantile eczema is characterized by acute dermatitis with an age of onset between 2 months and 2 years. Weeping, oozing, erythematous papules and plaques, which may become generalized, occur on the scalp, face, neck, and buttocks. Pruritus is severe with secondary excoriation, crusting, and infection. Exacerbations may follow immunizations, exposure to wool, and changes in the ambient humidity. In some cases, the severity of skin disease correlates with the consumption of certain foods. In most cases, the process is self-limited and resolves in 1–5 years.

Atopic childhood eczema is characterized by papular lesions in the antecubital and popliteal fossae, face, neck, and wrists. This dry eruption is very pruritic, and scratching leads to lichenification and secondary infection. Increased sensitivity to wool, animal hair, feathers, pollen, nickel, and neomycin may be noted. Adult (and adolescent) eczema is characterized by symmetric, erythematous, poorly demarcated plaques and patches preferentially localized to flexural sites. The plaques may consist of coalescent papules or vesicles and have scaling and lichenification. Hand dermatitis is more frequent among atopic individuals; rarely, the eruption may become generalized. Pruritus is intermittent and leads to excoriated, thickened, fissured skin. This symptom may improve with time if the cycle of itching and scratching is broken.

Patients with atopic dermatitis have frequent personal and family histories of allergic rhinitis and asthma. Anaphylactic reaction to penicillin is also more frequent. Other features include infraorbital folds, called Dennie-Morgan folds, allergic "shiners," facial pallor, follicular prominence or keratosis pilaris, hyperlinear palms and soles, ichthyosis vulgaris, and xerosis (dry skin). Cataracts occur in almost 20% of patients with severe disease. The excoriated, lichenified skin is more prone to disseminated viral (herpes simplex or vaccinia) infections. Other common secondary infections are verruca vulgaris, molluscum contagiosum, and dermatophytosis.

### Management

Daily bathing for 10–15 minutes, followed immediately by application of moisturizers, helps rehydrate the skin and prevent cutaneous evaporation. Petroleum jelly and viscous creams such as Eucerin® and Nivea® are more effective than lotions and should be applied frequently. A nonsoap cleanser or a gentle moisturizing soap is preferable to ordinary soaps. During the acute phase, compresses soaked in Domeboro solution are used to cool and dry oozing eczematous skin. Topical steroids are the most commonly used agents for atopic dermatitis; other topical agents are tar preparations. Topical tacrolimus may be particularly helpful for recalcitrant facial lesions. Antihistamines may help with pruritus. Secondary colonization may often develop with staphylococci; therefore, those with erosions and crusting should be considered for culture and antibiotics. Severe disease has been treated with light therapy and immunosuppressive agents (e.g., cyclosporin).

## ■ Stasis Dermatitis

### Definition, Epidemiology, and Etiology

Stasis dermatitis, an eczematous eruption occurring on the lower extremities of middle-aged and elderly adults with venous insufficiency, has a multifactorial etiology that is somewhat elusive. Patients with a history of deep venous thrombosis and venous varicosities are at risk. It is more common in women.

### Clinical Features

Erythematous patches develop above the medial and lateral malleoli, which become scaly and pruritic. There is often a background of persistent edema of the lower leg.

Frequently, excoriations cause erosions. Rarely, auto-eczematization produces a generalized eczematous or vesicular eruption due to cutaneous hyperirritability. Subacute and chronic inflammation evolve from xerotic, scaly, pruritic skin that is scratched. Hydrostatic pressure causes extravasation of RBCs from the vessels and the gradual deposition of hemosiderin, a brown pigment. Ulceration may occur and is usually found over the lower medial aspect of the leg. Patients with a history of deep leg vein thrombosis are more likely to develop ulceration.

### Management

The acute eczematous component of stasis dermatitis can be treated with soaks followed by the application of topical steroids. In the drier, more chronic dermatitic phase, topical steroids and bland emollients are used. Elevation of the legs when possible and use of compression stockings are vital to the long-term treatment of stasis dermatitis.

## ■ Seborrheic Dermatitis

### Definition and Epidemiology

Seborrheic dermatitis is a common inflammatory skin disorder characterized by red macules and irregular patches surmounted by yellow-white, fine, greasy scales.

### Etiology and Pathogenesis

The cause of seborrheic dermatitis remains elusive. Because of the abundant isolation of *Pityrosporum ovale*—a lipophilic, pleomorphic fungus from the scalp lesions—and because of the observed improvement with ketoconazole treatment, this fungus may have a role in the pathogenesis of this disease. Patients with HIV infection demonstrate severe seborrheic dermatitis, which supports a role for immune dysregulation and *Pityrosporum* overgrowth in these patients.

### Clinical Features

The most common presentation is fine, greasy scaling of the scalp. Other sites include nasolabial folds, eyelids, eyebrows, ears, chest, inframammary creases, axilla, and groin. Scaly red patches on the edges of the eyelids (marginal blepharitis) may be accompanied by conjunctivitis. In severe cases, an acute eczematous eruption develops on the trunk, and may evolve into erythroderma. The course is chronic, with exacerbations and remissions. The lesions often improve after exposure to sunlight during the summer, and the disease is aggravated by cold winter weather and stress.

### Differential Diagnosis and Management

The differential diagnosis includes atopic dermatitis, psoriasis, tinea capitis, nutritional deficiencies, and inborn errors of metabolism. A KOH examination will distinguish an atypical dermatophyte infection; with eyelid involvement, contact dermatitis should be considered.

Although usually well-controlled with intermittent treatment, seborrheic dermatitis frequently recurs. Scalp lesions respond to shampoos containing selenium sulfide, salicylic acid, zinc pyrithione, chloroxine, tar, or ketoconazole. Topical corticosteroid solutions may be applied once or twice daily in resistant cases. Facial and intertriginous lesions respond to low-potency topical corticosteroids (e.g., 1% hydrocortisone cream). The risk of atrophy of thin skin restricts the use of more potent steroids. Ketoconazole 2% cream may be used as a single agent or combined with topical corticosteroid creams.

## ■ Lichen Simplex Chronicus

### Definition and Epidemiology

Lichen simplex chronicus is a chronic, pruritic disorder featuring localized, red, lichenified, scaly patches or plaques. Women between 30 and 50 years old are more susceptible than others.

### Etiology

A cycle of itching and scratching is central to this disorder. The reason for the original pruritic sensation is rarely manifest. In some, the pruritus may be related to an atopic diathesis (asthma, hay fever, allergic rhinitis, and seasonal allergies) with inherent dry pruritic skin. Chronic mechanical trauma to the skin defines and perpetuates the cutaneous eruption. Chronic rubbing and scratching can induce neural hyperplasia, and this enhanced sensitivity sustains the cycle of itching and scratching.

### Clinical Features

Some lesions are papular or nodular and many are excoriated with overlying crusts. Common sites of involvement are the neck, extensor surfaces of the arms and legs, inner thighs, wrists, ankles, and anogenital region. Pruritus may be constant or paroxysmal. Patients report a pleasurable, comforting sensation when rubbing their skin; the cause of this reaction is unknown. In the nodular variant of lichen simplex chronicus, known as prurigo nodularis, the lesions are pruritic pink or brown nodules localized to the extremities. The severe pruritus is relieved only by vigorous scratching, which may produce bleeding and scarring.

### Differential Diagnosis

One helpful feature is the localization of lesions to sites within the patient's reach. Psoriasis, superficial dermatophytoses, and atopic eczema may cause diagnostic confusion. Psoriasis has characteristic white, coarse, silvery scales and pinpoint bleeding with their removal. Dermatophyte infections are evaluated with a KOH examination. Atopic dermatitis is seen in patients with an atopic diathesis and is localized to the flexor aspects of the extremities.

### Management

Management of the pruritus, which perpetuates the cycle of itching and scratching, is critical. Antihistamines with topical corticosteroids or intralesional corticosteroids are the most effective; mid-potency or high-potency topical steroids are used initially. In recalcitrant cases, they may be applied topically with occlusion. Lesions of prurigo nodularis may respond better to intralesional injection of the nodules with triamcinolone. Compresses with tepid water provide symptomatic relief and hasten healing. Doxepin, a tricyclic antidepressant and potent antihistamine, may also be useful in small doses. Oral or topical antibiotics are used for secondary infection.

## ■ Contact Dermatitis

### Definition and Epidemiology

Contact dermatitis is an eczematous dermatitis caused by exogenous agents. The dermatitis may be immunologically mediated (allergic contact) or may be a primary irritant response (irritant contact). The former requires a sensitization phase and is limited to persons who are genetically capable of being sensitized to that particular agent. Irritants, however, may elicit a reaction in any person who is exposed. Many more agents elicit irritant contact than allergic, and some may cause either type. Approximately 80% are irritant reactions, and the remainder are allergic. Contact dermatitis is common, affecting nearly 1% of the population and accounting for almost one fourth of all occupational disorders.

### Etiology and Pathogenesis

The pathogenesis of allergic contact dermatitis has been the focus of the majority of studies. It is a delayed (cell-mediated) type of hypersensitivity reaction. Sensitization to a compound involves three steps: formation of a protein-hapten conjugate, recognition of the conjugated antigen, and proliferation of sensitized lymphocytes on further exposure to the antigen. Memory and effector T lymphocytes then evoke an inflammatory cutaneous response. Because sensitization is involved, a period of 7–14 days may elapse between initial contact and a rash, thus often creating confusion regarding the cause. On re-exposure, the rash may manifest within 24–48 hours. Irritant dermatitis, in contrast, follows contact within 24 hours.

Myriad environmental agents can cause contact dermatitis. Irritant dermatitis is most frequently caused by acid or alkali compounds, detergents, and soaps. Poison ivy (rhus) dermatitis is the prototype of allergic contact dermatitis (Color Plate 13).

### Clinical Features

The acute phase of contact dermatitis consists of a pruritic, erythematous, weeping eruption, with occasional frank vesicles or bullae. The dermatitis is usually limited to areas of contact with the offending agent. With subacute or chronic dermatitis, the vesicles and weeping subside, and a scaly, lichenified appearance develops. Fissuring may be seen in chronic cases. Although irritants may elicit more burning and pain, and allergic reactions more pruritus, physical examination alone can rarely distinguish between the two.

### Diagnosis and Management

A good history and the pattern of localization give the most valuable clues to the correct diagnosis of contact dermatitis. Allergic contact dermatitis may be confirmed by patch testing. Dyshidrotic hand dermatitis, tinea pedis or manum, palmar-plantar psoriasis, or atopic dermatitis may cause diagnostic confusion.

In acute contact dermatitis, use of soaks or compresses combined with a potent topical steroid cream or lotion is the first step. An ointment-based steroid may be more appropriate as the vesiculation or weeping subsides and where scaling and lichenification are prominent features, as in more chronic cases. In some cases of widespread acute contact dermatitis, especially those involving the face, a short course of systemic steroids may be indicated. Oral antihistamines or topical anesthetic lotions (Sarna, pramoxine) will help with pruritus. Secondary staphylococcal infection is not uncommon and should be appropriately treated. Identification and elimination of the offending agent is key to successfully treating contact dermatitis.

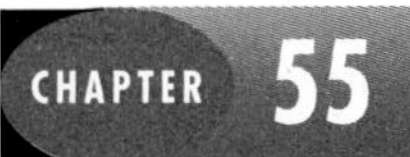

# BENIGN TUMORS OF THE SKIN

## Seborrheic Keratosis

### Definition, Etiology, and Pathogenesis

Seborrheic keratoses are benign cutaneous tumors usually involving the trunk and commonly affecting individuals in their fourth decade and beyond. Reports of patients with numerous lesions in familial clusters suggest but do not establish a genetic predisposition. Altered cytokeratin expression in seborrheic keratoses has been documented, but the significance is unknown.

### Clinical Features

Single or multiple lesions are most often observed on the trunk but also on the face, scalp, neck, and extremities. The palms, soles, and oral mucosa are spared. Initially, the lesions are well-demarcated brown macules. They evolve into papillated plaques with prominent follicular plugs. The "stuck-on" appearance and the greasy irregular surface are classic findings. When removed, the base is moist and pink. Usually, they are 2 mm to 3 cm and brown, but may appear black or flesh-colored. Some patients experience intermittent pruritus with these lesions and remove them by scratching.

The abrupt appearance of numerous pruritic seborrheic keratoses (the sign of Leser-Trélat) in adults may signal an internal malignancy. Slightly over half of the reported cancers are adenocarcinomas, the leading site being the stomach, followed by malignancies of the breast and lung, and leukemias. However, controlled studies have not proven such a relationship.

### Differential Diagnosis and Management

Although the clinical findings often suggest the diagnosis, some deeply pigmented lesions simulate malignant melanoma or a compound nevus. The sharp demarcation and the verrucous surface suggest seborrheic keratosis. Differentiation from verruca and solar keratoses is also needed. Seborrheic keratoses are effectively removed with liquid nitrogen or curettage. Atypical lesions and those resembling melanoma should be excised surgically.

## Actinic (Solar) Keratosis

### Definition and Epidemiology

Actinic keratoses are common premalignant lesions that develop on chronically sun-exposed areas. Related to cumulative sun exposure, they are the first clinical stage in the evolution of a squamous cell carcinoma. Risk factors for their development include fair skin type, failure to protect the skin with sunscreens, and exposure to high-intensity solar irradiation. Older adults with blue eyes, freckling, and a fair complexion and who live in sunny, warm regions are at greatest risk for developing actinic keratoses and skin cancer. In high-risk persons, these keratoses may occur even at the age of 20 or 30 years old.

### Clinical Features

Unless irritated or traumatized, the lesions usually cause no symptoms. The face, ears, dorsal hands, and forearms are the most commonly involved sites. The 1- to 10-mm flesh-colored, pink, or red macules or scaly papules are often more easily felt by palpation than identified visually. The surface is verrucous or hyperkeratotic with variable amounts of fine white scale. Hypertrophic actinic keratoses may form cutaneous horns; squamous cell cancer may develop later in the base. Other signs of excessive sun exposure may also be seen—for example, telangiectases, lentigines, and excessive wrinkling.

The rate of neoplastic transformation of actinic keratoses ranges from 5% to 15%. These squamous cell cancers are generally not aggressive, and their metastatic potential is limited. However, lesions in specific sites (e.g., the hands, ears, and lips) may be more aggressive, thus having a higher metastatic potential.

### Differential Diagnosis

The clinical findings usually suggest the diagnosis. Seborrheic keratoses, disseminated superficial actinic porokeratoses, Bowen disease, and squamous cell cancer may cause diagnostic confusion. Seborrheic keratosis has distinctive plugs on its surface and a "stuck on" appearance. In porokeratosis, the lesion has an elevated rim at the periphery. Bowen disease is more finely demarcated, and squamous cell cancers are more indurated. Erosion, ulceration, and progressive enlargement are more typical of squamous cell cancer.

### Management

Daily use of broad-spectrum sunscreens should be recommended to all patients with actinic keratoses. Lesions in limited numbers are often treatable with cryoablation with liquid nitrogen. Surgical excision, although rarely indicated as primary therapy, may sometimes be needed to establish the diagnosis. Topical 5-fluorouracil (5-FU), 1% or 5% cream, applied twice daily, is the most effective therapy for multiple lesions or large areas of involvement. 5-FU elicits an inflammatory reaction at the site of precancerous and cancerous lesions. Generally, the 5-FU creams are used for 2 to 3 weeks, or for 3 days after the most intense inflammation; topical steroids may be applied in conjunction with the 5-FU to reduce the severity of the reaction.

## Melanocytic Nevi

### Definition and Epidemiology

Melanocytic nevi are congenital or acquired benign neoplasms of melanocytes or nevus cells. Melanocytes are single, fusiform, or dendritic, and nevus cells are round or oval and grouped into nests; both are derived from the neural crest and may be distinguished by size and distribution.

Pigmented nevi are the most common tumors in adults and children. Benign melanocytic nevi are acquired from 6–12 months of age until around 40 years. The number of nevi is highest, averaging 40, at around age 25, after which they decline to almost zero by age 90. Caucasians and women acquire more nevi than persons of African descent and men, respectively. Nevi may be rapidly acquired during pregnancy, after intense sun exposure, or after therapy with corticosteroids, adrenocorticotropic hormone, or estrogen. True congenital nevi are present in only 1-2% of neonates.

### Etiology and Pathology

The exact origin of the nevus cell is uncertain. Based on their anatomic location, three primary variant nevi exist: junctional, compound, and intradermal types. Microscopically, junctional nevi show nests of nevus cells in the lower epidermis above the basement membrane zone. Compound nevi have both epidermal and dermal nests of nevus cells. In intradermal nevi, the cells are confined entirely to the dermis. Eventually, nevi regress with fibrous, fatty, or mucinous degeneration.

### Clinical Features

Benign, pigmented lesions are characterized by a smooth border, even color, and sharp circumscription. Any cutaneous or mucosal site may be affected, but lesions in the oral cavity are unusual. A nevus enlarges proportionate to body growth, with eventual regression. The junctional nevus, the most common type of nevus found on palms, soles, and scrotum, is a smooth, brown or tan, 1- to 10-mm macule without terminal hairs. Round or oval, it has a uniform pigment and sharp borders, and retains skin markings on its surface. A compound nevus is a brown, black, or flesh-colored papule with a smooth or gently papillated surface. It tends to be only slightly raised from the surrounding skin. Occasionally, its central portion is more darkly pigmented. Coarse, dark hair may be present. An intradermal nevus is either a dome-shaped or a soft pedunculated papule that may have hair. Although often flesh-colored, it may be brown or black. Usually smaller than 5 mm in diameter, intradermal nevi occur in adults.

### Differential Diagnosis and Management

Junctional melanocytic nevi may be difficult to distinguish from freckles, lentigines, or cafe au lait macules. Other entities in this differential diagnosis include a blue nevus, seborrheic keratosis, epidermal nevus, angiofibroma, Becker nevus, dermatofibroma, molluscum contagiosum, and early melanoma.

Most cases of benign melanocytic nevi require no treatment; the primary reason for removal is cosmetic. Symptomatic nevi from frequent trauma and features indicating possible malignancy may also warrant treatment. If a personal or family history of malignant melanoma is present, selected nevi may be excised if they are in a location that is difficult to follow. Giant congenital nevi (more than 10 cm in diameter) carry a small but significant risk for melanoma when compared with acquired nevi, and require staged excision, if possible.

## Acrochordon

Acrochordons (skin tags) are flesh-colored to brown papules located on the neck, eyelids, and axilla. Less frequently, these pedunculated or sessile lesions occur on the trunk and groin. They are soft and usually measure 1–3 mm. Giant acrochordons may be several centimeters long. Their appearance or their tendency to become traumatized by clothing or jewelry may cause patients to request their removal, which may be done by electrodesiccation or excision.

## Keloids

### Definition and Etiology

A keloid is an excessive overgrowth of fibrous tissue at the site of a previous wound; it presents as a firm, smooth, red to pink tumor. Persons of African and Hispanic descent tend to develop keloids more frequently, but the reasons are unclear.

### Clinical Features

Keloids have well-demarcated and angular borders with irregular extensions beyond the site of the original wound. The outline depends on the type of injury, the more common ones being burns and lacerations. Less often, they occur as sequelae of inflammatory acne. The sites of predilection are the sternum, neck, ear lobes, trunk, and extremities. Telangiectases may be evident through the thinned epidermis, and ulceration may occur. Patients often complain of tenderness or pruritus in early lesions.

### Differential Diagnosis and Management

The diagnosis of keloid is usually evident from the distinctive clinical features. The only entity that is likely to cause confusion is a hypertrophic scar, which spontaneously improves within the first 6 months of formation and lacks fibrous projections beyond the original site. Dermatofibroma, a rare fibrohistiocytic tumor, may occasionally resemble a keloid.

No treatment is uniformly effective. In many cases, intralesional injection of triamcinolone suspension produces flattening of the lesions and may be used every 6–8 weeks. Some keloids are amenable to surgical excision, but at a significant chance of recurrence, which may be lessened by instilling triamcinolone into the suture site at the time of surgery. Other less frequently used treatment options are x-ray therapy and methotrexate, which may be combined with surgery and Silastic gel sheeting.

## Epidermal Cyst

### Definition, Epidemiology, and Etiology

Epidermal cysts are known by various terms, including sebaceous cysts, keratin cysts, and epidermoid cysts. "Sebaceous cyst" is a misnomer because it involves differentiation toward keratin and not sebaceous gland lobules. These cysts are discrete, firm, elevated tumors located in the dermis or subcutis, and usually observed after puberty. Their etiology is uncertain. Although some lesions may be attributed to the traumatic inoculation of epidermal fragments into the dermis or embryonic entrapment of epidermal cells, most arise spontaneously from occlusion of pilosebaceous follicles. The cyst has an epidermal lining and is filled with keratin and lipid debris, which are white, malodorous, and rarely drain from the punctum. Enlargement occurs due to keratin production in a space that cannot drain to the surface.

### Clinical Features

The most common sites of involvement are the face, scalp, neck, back, and scrotum. With gradual enlargement, these cysts reach a final size of 0.5–5.0 cm. The epidermis above the lesion is normal or thinned from increasing pressure. The punctum in the skin represents the remnants of a ductal structure. Although adherent to the epidermis, the cyst is freely movable in the dermis. It is asymptomatic unless traumatized, infected, or ruptured, in which case intense inflammation and tenderness ensue.

### Differential Diagnosis and Management

The diagnosis, which is usually based on clinical information, may be made definitively with a biopsy. Lipomas, metastatic cancer, and occasionally neurofibromas may cause some confusion.

Both medical and surgical treatments are applicable. Inflamed cysts often diminish in size with the intralesional injection of corticosteroids. Ruptured and inflamed cysts may be incised and drained. At times, the cyst wall may be removed after the inflammation subsides. Surgical excision, the definitive treatment, is difficult if the lesion has been inflamed because fibrosis causes the cyst wall to adhere to the surrounding tissue. Unless the cyst wall is fully excised, the cyst will recur and inflammation will follow.

## Lipomas

### Definition and Clinical Features

Lipomas are benign subcutaneous tumors composed of fatty tissue, commonly seen on the trunk, forearms, posterior neck, buttocks, and thighs. These soft, rubbery, poorly demarcated, and freely movable nodules are generally less than 2 cm but can become large (10 cm). Single or multiple, the lesions are asymptomatic unless traumatized due to the location or size. The onset usually occurs between the ages of 30 and 40 years. Malignant change is rare, but may occur in large lesions. Midline lipomas may indicate spinal dysraphism and should be evaluated by magnetic resonance imaging of the spine before excision.

### Differential Diagnosis and Management

A lipoma may need to be distinguished from its variant forms (angiolipoma, hibernoma) or from an epidermoid cyst. An angiolipoma contains vascular elements and is tender to palpation. A hibernoma contains embryonic brown fat. Firm, well-demarcated borders are suggestive of a cyst. Lipoma is reliably diagnosed by examination of a tissue specimen. Unless cosmetic concerns or symptoms exist, treatment is not needed. Surgical excision with a primary closure is the treatment of choice.

# CHAPTER 56 MALIGNANT TUMORS OF THE SKIN

## Malignant Melanoma

### Definition and Epidemiology

Malignant melanoma, a cutaneous neoplasm with an increasing incidence in the United States and an increasing mortality rate, may develop in any tissue in which melanocytes are found, including the skin, mucous membranes, retina, and leptomeninges and within nevi. The common phenotype is a fair-skinned, sun-sensitive person with red or blond hair, blue eyes, abundant moles, and a tendency to freckle. Blistering sunburns in childhood indicate increased risk for melanoma. Intense sun exposure enhances the risk of melanoma for anyone.

Caucasians are more frequently affected than African-Americans or Hispanics. In Europe, melanoma afflicts Celtic or Nordic populations more often than Mediterranean populations, again because of skin type and patterns of sun exposure. African-Americans tend to develop melanoma in the palms, soles, nail beds, and mucosal surfaces.

The incidence of melanoma increases with decreasing latitude, as shown in the United States and Australia. Socioeconomic status indirectly influences the development of melanoma because the more affluent are more likely to develop a melanoma. It has been hypothesized that the affluent are more likely to receive intermittent, intense sun exposure through recreational activities, and this type of exposure may be more influential in the development of melanoma than chronic exposure.

### Etiology

Malignant melanoma is caused by multiple factors. Most investigators believe that tumor formation requires at least two separate genetic events. Oncogenes and antioncogenes are implicated in the cause of melanoma, with the antioncogenes that suppress neoplasia being the most important. Other genes that determine the susceptible phenotypes (e.g., those controlling pigmentation, DNA repair, and response to solar irradiation) probably also play a role. Although specific genes have been isolated, the involvement has been inconsistent. Genetic alterations may follow an environmental stimulus such as sun exposure and lead to lentigo maligna melanoma, but superficial spreading melanomas can arise in sun-protected sites. Thus, genetic factors are pivotal in the causation of melanoma as determinants of a phenotype with particular susceptibility, and as steps in tumor formation.

### Clinical Features

Features of a melanocytic lesion suggesting malignant melanoma are termed the "ABCDs": A = asymmetry; B = borders, irregular or notched borders; C = color, multiple shades of tan, brown, and black; and D = diameter, a diameter exceeding 6 mm. Among the four primary clinical subtypes with divergent histologic findings and clinical courses (Table 56.1), the outcome best correlates with the depth of tumor invasion (using the Breslow scale or Clark correlation measurement; see Differential Diagnosis and Management section) at diagnosis. Superficial spreading melanoma (Color Plate 14) may show signs of regression; because both favorable and adverse outcomes are related to regression, its relevance is controversial. Nodular melanoma often has a worse prognosis, probably because of the melanoma's greater depth at diagnosis. The acral lentiginous variant also has a poor outcome because its recognition is often delayed. Metastases in melanoma follow local extension and occur by lymphatic or hematogenous invasion.

### Differential Diagnosis and Management

All of the previously described characteristics of malignancy may not be present in an individual lesion. Entities that may cause confusion include seborrheic keratosis, solar lentigo, pyogenic granuloma, metastatic renal cell carcinoma, pigmented basal cell carcinoma, blue nevus, hemangioma, and pigmented Spitz nevus.

The rapid diagnosis of malignant melanoma is crucial to the survival of the patient because early detection and treatment lead to frequent cures. However, the rate of cure declines with the degree of vertical growth. Two classification systems were developed that provide predictive value for long-term outcome based on the vertical growth of the tumor. The Breslow depth relies on tumor thickness, and the Clark measurement relies on the anatomic level of invasion. A Clark level I lesion is an in-situ lesion (limited to the epidermis); level II is a tumor extending into the papillary dermis; level III is a tumor filling the papillary dermis and extending to the junction of the reticular dermis; level IV is tumor cells extending into the reticular dermis; and level V is tumor cells invading to the level of the subcutaneous tissue. Favorable prognostic features include a Breslow depth less than 0.76 mm, low mitotic rate, brisk infiltration of the tumor by lymphocytes, feminine gender, location on the extremities, and absence of regression or ulceration.

**TABLE 56.1. Clinical Subtypes of Malignant Melanoma and Their Characteristics**

| Subtype | Characteristics | Appearance of Lesions | Frequency | Comments |
|---|---|---|---|---|
| Superficial spreading melanoma (Color Plate 14) | Radial growth phase 1–5 years; predilection for the trunk in men and the lower extremities in women; median age at diagnosis is the fifth decade. | Flat papule or plaque, <3 cm in diameter, irregular borders, and patches of pink, brown, black, or white and areas of regression. | 70% of all cases | Dysplastic or congenital nevi are precursor lesions. Regression may also reflect depth inaccurately and underestimate the tumor growth. |
| Nodular melanoma | Brief or absent radial growth and rapid vertical extension; most develop in 6–18 months. Men more affected than women; the trunk, head, and neck are the favored sites; the mean age of onset is in the sixth decade. | Symmetric blue, gray, or black dome-shaped nodules or pedunculated papules, with average size of 1–2 cm. Pedunculated ones are particularly aggressive. A small fraction are amelanotic. | 15–30% | Aggressive lesions |
| Lentigo maligna melanoma | Slowly evolving. Present for 3–15 years at diagnosis. Most common in older women on the sun-exposed skin of the head and neck. Patients usually in the seventh decade of life. | Initially a tan macule, gradually enlarges to >3 cm. Exhibits asymmetry and varied color, and flecks of pigment may be noted within the brown or tan areas. After years of progression, the surface becomes irregularly elevated. | 5% of all cases | Low risk of metastasis. Some clinicians designate the flat lesion as lentigo maligna and the elevated lesion as lentigo maligna melanoma. |
| Acral lentiginous variant | Involves the palms, soles, mucosa, nail bed, and periungual regions. The sole is the most frequently described location. Affects older individuals of both genders. | Nail bed melanomas produce a visible, pigmented band. Pigmentation of the proximal nail fold (Hutchinson sign) is useful diagnostically. Diameter is often >3 cm. May initially resemble lentigo maligna type. Ulceration and hyperkeratosis observed in the nodular sections of the neoplasm. | 1–10% among Caucasians. Most common type in Asians, Hispanics, and American Indians. | Aggressive lesions. Often develop in 6 months. |

However, the tumor depth is clearly the strongest correlate with long-term survival.

Any suspicious pigmented lesion should be excised with adequate borders of normal skin (1–2 mm). If the lesion is too large or its location makes it difficult to remove entirely, then an incisional biopsy should be performed from the most unusual-appearing portion of the lesion. Photographs provide excellent documentation for subsequent examination. If the biopsy reveals a melanoma, then re-excision is necessary, with the borders determined by the depth of the tumor. Current recommendations for surgical margins are 0.5 cm for in-situ lesions, 1 cm margins for Breslow depth <1 mm, and 2 cm margins for Breslow depth >1mm. Resection should be to the fascia in depth. Elective regional lymph node dissection for mid-depth lesions (>1 mm but <4 mm) remains an area of controversy. Many centers currently biopsy the sentinel node, draining the area of the melanoma. The results of the sentinel node biopsy may then be used in decisions regarding node dissection or adjuvant therapy. Adjuvant therapy in advanced disease has been less than optimal. Interferon α-2B is approved for patients with a high risk for recurrent disease and may produce a moderate increase in survival in these patients. Other immune modulators and melanoma vaccines are currently under development and may provide promise in the future.

After treatment, patients with confirmed malignant melanoma should be monitored regularly, using the depth of the lesion as a guide for the interval between visits. At each visit, the skin, lymph nodes, liver, and spleen should be thoroughly examined. Liver function studies and annual chest radiographs are reserved for patients with thicker melanomas (>1.5 mm).

## ■ Dysplastic Nevus Syndrome

### Definition and Epidemiology

A dysplastic nevus is a large, irregular, melanocytic nevus with cytologic atypia and specific architectural features. The term "dysplastic nevus syndrome" continues to generate controversy because of incomplete agreement about the histologic definition of this lesion and its natural history. Most dermatopathologists use strict criteria to identify this entity but emphasize either architectural or cytologic features. A sporadic form and a familial variety are now recognized; the latter is inherited in an autosomal-dominant mode. Although patients with multiple dysplastic nevi are at increased risk for the development of melanoma, the degree of risk is still poorly quantitated.

A National Institutes of Health Consensus Conference in 1984 recommended categorizing those individuals with dysplastic nevi into four groups that correlated with risk of melanoma. The criteria considered in this classification were the following: personal history of melanoma and family history of multiple nevi and melanoma. Patients with the highest risk for the development of melanoma are those with a personal history of melanoma and two or more family members with a history of melanoma and multiple nevi. Those with the lowest risk have none of the pertinent criteria.

### Clinical Features

Dysplastic nevi measure 6–15 mm in diameter and are variegated with shades of pink, tan, and brown. The pink color is usually peripheral to the central tan and brown (creating a "fried egg" configuration). Often, the lesions are flat, but central papules or a cobblestone surface is not unusual. The border is irregular and poorly defined but lacks the scalloping of a malignant melanoma. Although commonly located on the back, they are also typically seen on the chest, abdomen, and extremities. Greater numbers of dysplastic nevi develop on sun-protected skin such as the buttocks, scalp, and breasts. They arise during puberty and continue to develop during adulthood. Many patients acquire more than 100 lesions.

### Differential Diagnosis and Management

The diagnosis of a dysplastic nevus and the dysplastic nevus syndrome is based on the characteristic clinical features, histologic criteria, and medical history. The differential diagnosis is mainly between a compound nevus and melanoma. The initial management for a patient with suspected dysplastic nevi includes a thorough family history and a full skin examination with attention to the scalp, feet, buttocks, and breasts. These are not only the sites where dysplastic nevi are found more commonly compared with regular nevi, but also the sites that are unlikely to be routinely examined. The measurements of all atypical nevi should be recorded. Most authorities advocate removing two representative lesions for histology. Biopsies should be taken from those nevi that have reportedly changed or are difficult to examine because of their location in hair-bearing areas. The patient should be told about the importance of sun protection and regular examination of the skin as well as the role of dysplastic nevi as potential markers for high risk of malignant melanoma. High-risk patients are examined every 3–6 months; low-risk patients are examined yearly.

## ■ Basal Cell Carcinoma

### Definition, Epidemiology, and Etiology

Basal cell carcinoma is the most common cancer and is strongly associated with excessive chronic sun exposure. This carcinoma usually affects older persons with fair skin. Its higher frequency among men may be explained by the fact that men have traditionally done outdoor work. This carcinoma is rare in African-Americans. The histologic features determine the natural history of an individual lesion. For poorly defined reasons, basal cell carcinomas are associated with scars and exposure to ultraviolet light, x-rays, and arsenic. Some recent studies implicate oncogenes and antioncogenes in the pathogenesis of this cancer.

### Clinical Features

Basal cell carcinoma has many clinical and histologic variants. The nodular basal cell carcinoma arises on the face or other sun-exposed (usually sun-damaged) site as a dome-shaped papule or nodule with a raised, pearly border and often with telangiectases (Color Plate 15). The surface is generally smooth and shiny but may be ulcerated, scaly, and crusted. The pigmented basal cell carcinoma, with a color ranging from shades of tan or brown to black, may mimic malignant melanoma. The sclerosing or morpheaform type is a scar-like plaque that is often lighter than the surrounding skin. It tends to have extension beyond the clinically visible margins of the lesion, which makes recurrence after treatment more common in this subtype. Superficial basal cell carcinomas are clinically subtle; these red, scaly plaques are often mistaken for solar keratoses, eczema, or psoriasis. Untreated, basal cell carcinoma may cause extensive local destruction, despite the rarity of metastases. Periorbitally located lesions may imperil vision by infiltrating the nerves and muscles. Nerve involvement and invasion of dermis by small discrete strands of cells signal a poor prognosis. Tumor size, location, and histologic features influence rates of recurrence. Spread to local nodes or viscera is rare, usually only occurring with very large, neglected tumors.

### Diagnosis and Management

Although the nodular basal cell carcinoma is easily identified, the recognition of the pigmented or scaly nodules and plaques is more difficult. Solar keratosis, psoriasis, melanoma, morphea, sebaceous hyperplasia, Bowen disease, and seborrheic keratosis frequently must be distinguished from a basal cell carcinoma. Definitive diagnosis requires a biopsy.

Treatment of a basal cell carcinoma varies with its size, site, and histology as well as its status as a primary tumor, local recurrence, or metastasis. The goal of any treatment is histologic cure with optimal cosmetic results. For the primary tumor, available methods are surgery, electrodesiccation and curettage, radiation, or cryotherapy. In Mohs micrographic surgery, the tumor mass is removed by serial tangential sections that are examined histologically for residual neoplastic cells at the time of surgery. This surgery is used for large, recurrent cancers; those that exhibit aggressive histologic patterns; or those that are present on sites with high recurrence rates. Selected patients may also benefit from retinoids, photodynamic therapy, and topical or systemic chemotherapy. The latter (with cisplatin and doxorubicin) is used for metastatic lesions. The role of education about protection from sun exposure cannot be overemphasized.

## Squamous Cell Carcinoma

### Definition and Epidemiology

Squamous cell carcinoma, an epithelial neoplasm, evolves from a clone of atypical keratinocytes. Some tumors are confined to the thickness of the epidermis and are called squamous cell carcinoma in situ or Bowen disease; others penetrate the basement membrane, extend into the dermis and subcuticular tissue, and have the potential to metastasize. Squamous cell carcinomas represent nearly 20% of all nonmelanoma skin cancers. They most commonly afflict older persons, persons with a fair complexion, and men. Many factors, particularly ultraviolet radiation, influence the incidence of squamous cell carcinoma. Patients receiving long-term immunosuppression, such as organ transplant patients, are also at high risk. Long-standing ulcers are another setting in which squamous cell carcinoma of the skin may arise.

### Etiology and Pathogenesis

#### Clinical Features

Squamous cell carcinomas frequently arise on sun-exposed sites as well-demarcated red plaques or nodules with a scaly, verrucous, or papillated surface. Compared with basal cell carcinomas, a predilection exists for the dorsal hands, scalp, and pinna. As the cancer cells invade the dermis and subcutis, the plaques become firm, indurated, and fixed to underlying structures. Ulceration and bleeding are common (Color Plate 16). These lesions often run an indolent course with many years of radial growth. Solar lentigines, actinic keratoses, and other signs of sun damage are usually seen on the surrounding skin.

The other common settings that harbor these cancers are scarred or chronically inflamed tissues. Lesions originating within burn scars, radiation ports, chronic ulcers, or sinuses behave aggressively, although they frequently are present for many months or years prior to diagnosis. The rate of metastasis is much greater in these patients. Invasive squamous cell carcinoma occurs in 5–15% of solar keratoses.

Many of the same factors that are predictive of recurrence and metastasis for basal cell carcinomas apply also to squamous cell carcinomas. Large, deep, and poorly differentiated lesions are more likely to be aggressive. The ear, lip, and inner canthus of the eye are sites with particularly high rates of recurrence and increased metastatic potential. Other poor prognostic factors are perineural spread, previous recurrence with adequate treatment, and formation within a scar. Patients treated with immunosuppressive drugs, especially for renal transplants, acquire greater numbers of tumors with an aggressive course. Widespread disease begins with lymph node involvement.

### Diagnosis and Differential Diagnosis

The diagnosis frequently requires a biopsy. Clinical suspicion is aroused by the appropriate setting and presentation, but squamous cell carcinomas may resemble superficial basal cell carcinomas, keratoacanthoma, verrucous lesions (warts and seborrheic keratoses), metastatic neoplasms, pyogenic granulomas, plaques of psoriasis or eczema, amelanotic or verrucous melanomas, and other papulosquamous disorders.

### Management

The treatment of squamous cell carcinoma is similar to that of basal cell carcinoma. Superficial lesions may be removed by excision, electrodesiccation and curettage, or cryosurgery using probes to assess the depth of tissue necrosis with freezing. Tumors that are large, deep, or localized to sites with a high risk of invasion are treated with Mohs micrographic surgery, which is also preferred for lesions with neurotropism or basosquamous histology.

# CHAPTER 57 ACNE

## Acne Vulgaris

### Definition and Epidemiology

Acne vulgaris, a very common skin disorder, is a self-limited inflammatory disorder of the pilosebaceous unit. Usually beginning at puberty and affecting mostly adolescents (85% of persons between 12 and 25 years old), acne predominantly appears in areas where the pilosebaceous follicles are the most dense—the face, neck, and upper trunk. In girls, it may precede menarche. The peak prevalence is age 14–17 years in girls and 16–19 years in boys, with a higher frequency and severity in boys. Most patients note significant improvement by age 20–23 years, but in 8–10% some activity continues into the fifth decade.

The inheritance pattern of acne vulgaris has not been established, but most experts invoke an autosomal-dominant trait with variable penetrance or a polygenic trait involving many genes. Because Caucasian Americans are affected more often than Japanese or African-Americans, genetics may play a role.

### Etiology and Pathogenesis

Acne develops from the interaction of multiple factors. Lipid is released into the follicular canal as part of a complex mixture called sebum that lubricates the skin. In acne, sebum is produced in excess, perhaps due to changes in androgen levels. The sebum composition is altered compared with those without acne, with a significantly lower level of linoleic acid. This abnormality may encourage the cohesion of cornified cells; their accumulation in sebaceous follicles results in comedones. These noninflammatory lesions are transformed into inflammatory lesions by *Propionibacterium acnes* in the follicular canal. *P. acnes* incites inflammation by generating free fatty acids and by recruiting lymphocytes and neutrophils, which release inflammatory mediators. The inflammatory products and sebum exert pressure on the epithelial wall, causing the follicle to rupture; inflammatory papules, pustules, and nodules follow.

### Clinical Features

Acne vulgaris has a number of clinical variants, with combinations of comedones, papules, pustules, nodules, and cysts. An open comedone is black because of the oxidation of accumulated material and the presence of melanin. A closed comedone is a flesh-colored papule with a minute ostium that inhibits the discharge of keratin debris. This is the primary lesion in the formation of inflammatory papules and pustules. In severe cases, nodules, cysts, and granulomatous lesions develop progressively. This intense inflammation finally leads to fibrosis, scars, and keloids. Individual papules and pustules resolve with transient erythema and postinflammatory hyperpigmentation, which can be particularly prominent in African-Americans and takes months to improve.

### Diagnosis and Differential Diagnosis

A complete history should be obtained to establish the cause, duration, localization, and severity. In susceptible individuals, the onset or exacerbation of acne is influenced by a family history of acne; menses; occupational exposure to oils, tars, greases, chlorinated hydrocarbons, and waxes; medications such as oral contraceptives, corticosteroids, iodides, isoniazid, lithium, phenytoin, and trimethadione; and cosmetics or hair preparations and androgen excess denoted by hirsutism or menstrual irregularities. Although typically distributed eruptions are diagnostic, acneiform lesions may occur in rosacea, perioral dermatitis, miliaria rubra, impetigo contagiosa, and folliculitis.

## Management

The treatment regimen is determined by the severity of the disease and the predominant type of lesion. Topical (Table 57.1) and systemic agents can reduce bacterial load, inhibit inflammation, decrease sebaceous gland activity, and impede corneocyte adhesion. Dietary restrictions have no role.

Inflammatory papules, pustules, and nodules are controlled with systemic antibiotics. They eliminate *P. acnes* from the skin, thus decreasing the free fatty acids in the sebaceous glands. Tetracycline, 1.0 g daily, tapered as clinical improvement occurs, is a safe, effective, and inexpensive initial choice. Significant response may take 4–6 weeks. Alternative agents are erythromycin, doxycycline, minocycline, and sulfonamides. Persons receiving tetracyclines should avoid sun exposure.

The only medication likely to produce a remission in patients with recalcitrant severe acne is isotretinoin, a vitamin A derivative. All forms of acne respond to it, but the side-effect profile restricts its use to only the most severe cases. Isotretinoin is given in a dose of 0.5–2 mg/kg/day; doses less than 1 mg/kg/day enhance the likelihood of recurrence. Its teratogenicity precludes its use in pregnancy or those not using adequate contraception. Other common complications are dry skin and mucous membranes, hyperlipidemia, mucositis, cheilitis, conjunctivitis, skin fragility, impaired night vision, transaminase elevations, desquamation of palms and soles, headache, and myalgia. An increased risk of pseudotumor cerebri exists, especially when tetracyclines are given simultaneously. Depression has been reported with a number of patients receiving isotretinoin therapy, but its relationship to the medication remains unclear.

Comedonal acne is best treated by one of the topical vitamin A derivatives, such as tretinoin, which normalize keratinization in the follicles and suppress bacterial proliferation. The formation of new follicular plugs is inhibited, and existing plugs are eliminated. Tretinoin is applied in a thin layer every night to dry skin. Early complications include burning, erythema, and peeling. The concentration of the preparation is increased according to response and tolerance. It is indicated for all types of acne because comedones are a common component.

The use of benzoyl peroxide as a topical bactericidal agent either alone or combined with tretinoin or antibiotics significantly reduces the density of *P. acnes* on the skin. Many different preparations contain benzoyl peroxide, with concentrations varying between 2.5 and 10%. Irritation is the most important side effect, related to the concentration of benzoyl peroxide and the vehicle. Another treatment option in mild to moderate acne vulgaris is topical antibiotics to decrease the population of *P. acnes*, the most effective ones being 1% clindamycin and 2% erythromycin. Bacterial resistance may follow topical and systemic antibiotic use. Selected patients may use oral corticosteroids, oral contraceptives, and dapsone. Other ingredients included in topical preparations are salicylic acid, resorcinol, sulfur, and metronidazole.

Acne surgery is the physical removal of the contents of comedones, pustules, and cysts to promote rapid

**TABLE 57.1. Commonly Used Topical Products for Acne**

| Agent | Formulation | Use | Action | Side Effects |
|---|---|---|---|---|
| Benzoyl peroxide | 5, 10% gel<br>2.5, 4% wash | 1–2 times daily | Keratolytic; some antibacterial action | Irritation; allergic contact dermatitis |
| Tretinoin (Retin A) | 0.025, 0.05, 0.1% cream<br>0.01, 0.025% gel<br>0.05% liquid | Once daily at bedtime | Comedolytic | Irritation; allergic contact dermatitis (rare); increased susceptibility to sunburn |
| Topical antibiotics | 1% clindamycin<br>2% erythromycin | 1–2 time(s) daily | Antibacterial | Irritation; allergic contact dermatitis (rare); gastrointestinal disturbances, including colitis (clindamycin, extremely rare) |
| Salicylic acid | 2% wash | 2–3 times daily | Keratolytic as a cleanser | Irritation |

improvement while the patient awaits the gradual effects of topical or systemic therapy. The intralesional injection of triamcinolone acetonide into large inflammatory cysts, pustules, and nodules leads to resolution of lesions with less scarring.

## Acne Rosacea

### Definition, Epidemiology, and Etiology

Rosacea, a chronic vascular and inflammatory disorder, occurs primarily on the central region of the face and has two primary components: (1) the vascular component consists of erythema and telangiectases; (2) the acneiform component consists of papules, pustules, and sebaceous gland hyperplasia. The inflammatory lesions exacerbate and remit and, when deep, may heal with scarring. Although associated with menopause and observed most commonly in women aged 30 to 50 years old, rosacea is more severe in men. It is rare in African-American patients.

The cause of rosacea is unknown. Vascular instability, with a consistent tendency to blush and flush easily, is an important element. Celtic origin and a fair complexion are also risk factors. Vasodilators (e.g., hot liquids, alcohol, spicy foods, and sun exposure) may exacerbate it. Although patients with increased numbers of *Demodex folliculorum* mites improve as the organism is eliminated by treatment, the association with *Demodex* is inconsistent. Sebaceous gland activity is stimulated, but not as the primary event. Unlike acne vulgaris, abnormal keratinization is absent.

### Clinical Features

The cheeks, chin, nose, forehead, eyes, and, less often, the seborrheic areas of the chest, scalp, and posterior ears are involved. The disease evolves from intermittent episodes of flushing and blushing to persistent erythema and telangiectasia on the nose and cheeks. This may occur as early as the second decade. Crops of papules and pustules develop, and the orifices of sebaceous glands become prominent. In severe cases, the nose becomes thickened and disfigured with the formation of rhinophyma. Rarely, inflammatory nodules are seen, which may be granulomatous or connected by sinus tracts, furuncles, and abscesses. The eyes are commonly involved, and blepharitis, conjunctivitis, iritis, keratitis, iridocyclitis, and hypopyon are common. Early eye involvement may be unnoticed by the treating physician.

### Differential Diagnosis

Acne vulgaris, seborrheic dermatitis, lupus erythematosus, and carcinoid syndrome simulate rosacea. Lack of comedones and distribution in the medial face help to distinguish it from acne vulgaris. The lesions of seborrheic dermatitis are red or pink macules covered with greasy yellow scales and localized to the eyebrows, nasolabial folds, scalp, chest, and ears. Lupus erythematosus and carcinoid syndrome can be established by measuring antinuclear antibodies and 5-hydroxyindoleacetic acid, respectively, especially in atypical cases.

### Management

Rosacea has a spectrum of severity, and its course is punctuated by exacerbations and remissions. However, even aggressive therapy rarely resolves all lesions completely. The use of a broad-spectrum sunscreen should always be encouraged. Mild disease needs no treatment except avoiding sun exposure and other vasodilatory agents. Moderate disease often responds well to oral tetracycline with or without topical metronidazole. Usually, tetracycline (1.0 g/day) for 4–6 weeks will suffice until the flare remits; it is then tapered to the smallest maintenance dose. Ocular involvement is considered an indication for systemic therapy. Alternative agents are erythromycin, minocycline, or oral metronidazole. Traditional acne therapy with benzoyl peroxide and topical erythromycin or clindamycin solutions may benefit some, but the benzoyl peroxide and the alcohol vehicle of these solutions may irritate sensitive, fair skin. Although topical steroids will initially help in cases of erythema, they should be used cautiously because their long-term use may worsen the telangiectases.

Rhinophyma and granulomatous lesions respond to isotretinoin, but relapses are frequent when the drug is discontinued. Additional options are pulsed dye laser or electrosurgery for telangiectases, laser or surgical therapy for rhinophyma, and antiparasitic drugs for exacerbations of rosacea due to *Demodex* infestation. Ketoconazole cream sometimes elicits good results because of its anti-inflammatory and antibiotic properties.

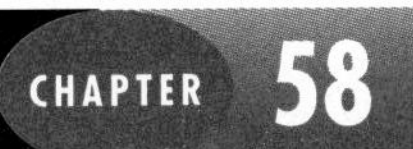

# FUNGAL INFECTIONS OF THE SKIN

## Dermatophyte Infections

### Definition and Epidemiology

Dermatophytosis (tinea or ringworm) is a superficial fungal infection of the skin, hair, or nails. The primary types of dermatophytoses are tinea capitis, tinea faciei, tinea barbae, tinea pedis, tinea manus, tinea corporis, tinea cruris, and onychomycosis. Some infections are inflammatory with fluctuant plaques and pustules, and others cause minimal scaling and erythema.

### Etiology and Pathogenesis

Dermatophytes live in the superficial, cornified epidermal cells. They are ubiquitous in the environment, and the source of an individual infection may be difficult to determine if there has not been family or animal contact. The host response to the infection in humans is influenced by the origin of the organism; species acquired from the soil or from animals induce a vigorous response, but those acquired from humans induce little inflammation.

Three genera of dermatophytes exist: *Microsporum, Trichophyton*, and *Epidermophyton*. The organisms causing a given type of infection vary with time and geographic location. Most cases of tinea capitis are caused by *Trichophyton tonsurans, Microsporum canis*, and *T. violaceum*, and most cases of tinea corporis arise from *T. rubrum, M. canis*, and *T. tonsurans*. Tinea pedis, tinea manum, and tinea cruris are caused by *T. rubrum, T. mentagrophytes*, and *Epidermophyton floccosum*. Tinea barbae is most commonly caused by *T. mentagrophytes* and *T. verrucosum. T. rubrum* and *T. mentagrophytes* are also present in onychomycosis.

### Clinical Features

Tinea pedis is the most prevalent adult dermatophytosis and has several distinct clinical presentations: the interdigital form; a sharply circumscribed "moccasin" distribution; and an acute inflammatory, vesiculobullous eruption on the soles of the feet. Tinea manum often coexists with bilateral tinea pedis or fingernail involvement and resembles the dry, scaly noninflammatory form of tinea pedis (Table 58.1 and Color Plates 17 and 18).

Dermatophytoses elicit two reaction patterns. The id reaction, representing hypersensitivity to fungal proteins, is the most common, with pruritic vesicles or papules on the trunk or extremities. Erythema annulare centrifugum, a chronic and recurrent disorder, consists of polycyclic, red plaques with central trailing scales localized to the trunk. Both eruptions respond to topical corticosteroid creams and ointments. Fungal elements are not present in the lesions of these reaction patterns.

### Diagnosis and Differential Diagnosis

Dermatophyte infections are diagnosed with a KOH preparation using scales from the surface of the lesion. When tinea capitis is suspected, hairs from the periphery of the patches are inspected for spores. However, the KOH examination is rarely helpful without alopecia (hair loss) or with intense inflammation. A fungal culture will confirm the diagnosis. When *M. audouinii* and *M. canis* commonly caused tinea in the past, the Wood's lamp examination rapidly diagnosed tinea by observing a blue fluorescence. Because these are less common etiologic agents in tinea currently, the Wood's lamp is now rarely used to diagnose tinea.

In addition to folliculitis, impetigo, seborrheic dermatitis, trichotillomania, psoriasis, and lupus erythematosus, may be mistaken for tinea capitis. Other entities to be differentiated from tinea corporis are seborrheic and contact dermatitis, nummular eczema, psoriasis, secondary syphilis, and PR. Tinea faciei is frequently mistaken for contact dermatitis, seborrheic dermatitis, or lupus erythematosus. Tinea barbae may be mistaken for bacterial and herpetic infections and contact dermatitis. Candidal intertrigo, erythrasma, seborrheic dermatitis, psoriasis, and irritant dermatitis resemble tinea cruris. Tinea pedis and tinea manum may mimic psoriasis, contact dermatitis, irritant dermatitis, dyshidrotic eczema, xerosis, or candidiasis. The differential diagnosis of tinea unguium includes trauma, lichen planus, psoriasis, damage from nail polish, and other primary nail dystrophies.

### Management

Tinea capitis, unguium, and barbae, and severe or recalcitrant infections of the palms, soles, groin, or glabrous skin require systemic antifungal therapy. Topical therapy usually suffices for tinea pedis, tinea manum, tinea corporis, and tinea cruris. Therapy of dermatophytoses and the role of local therapy such as soaks, solutions, and topical steroids are shown in Table 58.2.

## Tinea Versicolor

### Definition, Epidemiology, and Etiology

One of the most common dermatophytes causing superficial infections is *Malassezia furfur* (syn., *Pityrosporon orbiculare*), the agent causing tinea versicolor. Nearly 5% of people in the United States have had an

**TABLE 58.1. Characteristic Clinical Features of Dermatophytoses**

| Subtype | Characteristics | Comments | Causative Organism |
| --- | --- | --- | --- |
| Tinea pedis | The most prevalent dermatophyte infection in adults | May be complicated by lymphangitis and cellulitis | *Trichophyton rubrum* |
| Interdigital form | Maceration, scaling, and fissuring between the fourth and fifth toes; painful infection | Most common subtype; often extends to involve additional web spaces | *Trichophyton rubrum* |
| | Sharply circumscribed, red, scaly plaques with a hyperkeratotic surface on the soles and lateral aspects of the feet in a "moccasin" distribution | | *Trichophyton mentagrophytes* |
| Vesiculobullous type | Vesicles/bullae and eczematous changes in the soles of the feet | Acute inflammatory eruption; likely to be symptomatic with pruritus, burning, and tenderness | *Trichophyton mentagrophytes* |
| Tinea manum | Lesions most frequent on the palms and thumb web space in a unilateral distribution | Resembles the dry, scaly noninflammatory form of tinea pedis; often seen in conjunction with bilateral tinea pedis or fingernail involvement | *Trichophyton mentagrophytes* |
| Tinea cruris (jock itch) | Arcuate, red, generally symmetric, scaly patches with sharp margins, involving the inner thighs, inguinal folds, and rarely the perineum, buttocks, and scrotum; the enlarging rings are macerated, crusted, vesicular, or scaly | Heat and humidity perpetuate the infection; men affected more frequently than women; risk factors are obesity, tightly fitted clothing, and frequent, strenuous activity | *Epidermophyton floccosum* |
| Tinea capitis (Color Plate 17) | Initial lesions are erythematous, scaling patches of alopecia; variable inflammation; small patches of alopecia; hairs broken at the level of the skin, creating "black dots" (black-dot tinea); sharply circumscribed, boggy, highly inflammatory, tender mass (kerion); onset acute; papules and pustules often cover the surface | Superficial fungal infection of the scalp; occurs primarily in children<br>Less common in infants, adolescents, or adults; incidence greater in boys and African-American children; lymphadenopathy often present even with subtle cutaneous findings (important diagnostic clue for tinea capitis) | Most cases due to *Trichophyton tonsurans*, *Microsporum canis*, and *Trichophyton violaceum* |
| Tinea corporis | Single or multiple annular, erythematous plaques with fine white scale; vesicles or pustules may be present on the surface of some acute inflammatory plaques; sharply demarcated, raised borders; they enlarge progressively | Lesions are localized to glabrous (non–hair-bearing) skin (palms, soles, groin, and beard area excluded) | Most cases due to *Trichophyton rubrum*, *Microsporum canis*, and *Trichophyton tonsurans* |
| Tinea faciei | Erythematous lesions often have poorly defined borders; the scaling may be minimal | Unusual fungal infection to the cheeks and forehead | *Trichophyton rubrum* |
| Tinea barbae | Papules, pustules, nodules, and erythematous plaques in the beard area; with established infection, loosened and broken hairs form irregular patches of alopecia and crusting; fluctuant draining abscesses occur in some cases | Uncommon disorder, seen almost exclusively among male farm workers; spread by contaminated razors | *Trichophyton mentagrophytes*, *Trichophyton verrucosum* |
| Tinea unguium (Color Plate 18) | Gradual onset with a small patch of yellow, white, or brown discoloration forming at the edge of the nail; onycholysis develops as the nail plate lifts from the nail bed with the creation of crumbly subungual debris; with further infection, the nail becomes thickened and broken | Chronic dermatophyte infection of the fingernails or the toenails | *Trichophyton rubrum*, *Trichophyton mentagrophytes* |

**TABLE 58.2. Therapy of Dermatophytoses (partial listing)**

| Type | Comments | Therapy |
|---|---|---|
| Tinea capitis, Tenia unguium, Tinea barbae | Require systemic antifungal therapy; severe or recalcitrant infections of the palms, soles, groin, or glabrous skin are also treated with oral agents | Drug of choice: Griseofulvin, terbinafine or itraconazole. Duration: 6–8 week course of griseofulvin for tinea capitis and barbae; 4 weeks for oral terbinafine. Onychomycosis: 3 months for terbinafine, 5 months of pulse sporanox (treatment given for 1 week per month) or 12–18 months for griseofulvin. Response: more rapid in fingernails; duration of therapy usually approximately half of that for toenails. Alternative drugs: fluconazole |
| Tinea pedis, Tinea manum, Tinea corporis, Tinea cruris | Usually resolves with topical preparations of ketoconazole, miconazole, ciclopirox, clotrimazole, econazole, oxiconazole, or terbinafine | Improvement occurs in 2 weeks with topical agents but most cases require a full 4-week treatment; those with tinea corporis or tinea cruris who fail to improve in 4 weeks should be given an oral agent; patients with tinea pedis and tinea cruris should keep these sites cool and dry with powder containing miconazole or tolnaftate and nonocclusive clothing and shoes; compresses with Burrow's solution and short term use of a low-potency topical corticosteroid cream are useful in acute vesicular eruptions of tinea pedis. |

episode of tinea versicolor. Although no age is exempt, this infection is most common in adolescents and young adults (15–30 years old). *M. furfur* is found on normal skin in the yeast phase in small numbers. Clinical disease occurs when conditions enhance the growth of hyphal forms in large numbers. What stimulates this growth is uncertain, but such growth may be related to nutrition, immune competence, or genetic factors.

## Clinical Features

Tinea versicolor presents as multiple, oval, hypopigmented or hyperpigmented patches with fine scale distributed on the trunk, proximal arms, and face. Although mild pruritus may occur, tinea versicolor is asymptomatic in most cases. Many patients present during the summer months when they note the contrast between tanned and lesional skin. The race and complexion of the individual influence the color of the lesions. The inhibition of melanin production and transfer by azelaic acid produced by the fungus causes hypopigmentation, and the stimulation of melanogenesis by the inflammatory response causes hyperpigmentation.

## Differential Diagnosis

The diagnosis of tinea versicolor is usually evident by the characteristic cutaneous eruption. When the findings are subtle, the skin may be viewed in a darkened room with a Wood's lamp, which will enhance the differences in the lesional and uninvolved skin. The best confirmatory test is the KOH examination. Attempts to culture *M. furfur* are usually futile. Tinea versicolor should be distinguished from other papulosquamous diseases, seborrheic dermatitis, leprosy, pityriasis alba, and vitiligo. PR and secondary syphilis are the most likely papulosquamous diseases to cause confusion.

## Management

Tinea versicolor may be effectively treated with selenium sulfide 2.5% lotion or antifungal creams including miconazole, clotrimazole, ketoconazole, or econazole. Selenium sulfide lotion is applied to all involved areas and the bordering normal skin at night and scrubbed off in the morning. This may be repeated once a week for 4 weeks and then as needed to maintain complete clearing. Many different treatment schedules have been used with equal efficacy. Selenium sulfide should not be used in pregnancy. Patients with recalcitrant disease or poor compliance with a topical regimen are given oral ketoconazole. Ketoconazole, in a single 400-mg dose, is often curative, but some advocate a second dose after 1 week and further doses as needed. An alternative method is 200 mg per day for 2 weeks. An acidic environment is required for ketoconazole absorption; thus, it should be taken with orange juice or cola. Because this drug is excreted in the sweat, efficacy is enhanced by consuming it before exercising.

The response to therapy may be evaluated by re-examination of lesional scales dissolved in KOH. Relapses follow hot humid weather, immunosuppression, selective immunodeficiency, and pregnancy.

## Candidiasis

### Definition and Epidemiology

Candidiasis, or moniliasis, encompasses a variety of infections of the skin, mucous membranes, viscera, and nails. *Candida albicans* is the most common cause of these disorders, but other species may be identified, especially in immunocompromised patients. *Candida*, a normal inhabitant of the mouth, gastrointestinal tract, and vagina, will proliferate on other moist, warm, and macerated cutaneous sites such as the perianal region, intertriginous areas, digital web spaces, and nail folds. It acts as a pathogen when the cutaneous barrier is locally disrupted or the systemic immunologic defenses are altered.

### Clinical Features

Susceptibility to candidiasis is enhanced by obesity, endocrinopathies (diabetes mellitus and hypoparathyroidism), malignancies (leukemia and lymphoma), drugs (oral contraceptives, corticosteroids, antibiotics, and immunosuppressive agents), and inherited disorders (Down syndrome and chronic granulomatous disease of childhood). In addition, neonates are inherently predisposed to candidal infections and readily develop thrush, perlèche, or diaper dermatitis.

The most common cutaneous presentations of candidiasis are thrush, perlèche, diaper dermatitis, candidal vulvovaginitis, chronic paronychia, candidal intertrigo, and perianal candidiasis. Thrush, or oral candidiasis, is characterized by white adherent plaques on the tongue, gingiva, palate, buccal mucosa, and oropharynx. The base of the plaque is red and tender, and the organism is identified by examination of scrapings from the surface using a KOH solution. The most commonly affected are neonates (who acquire the fungus from the vagina at birth), the elderly, the malnourished, diabetics, persons receiving inhaled corticosteroid (asthmatics) or antibiotic therapy, and the HIV-infected.

Perlèche, or angular cheilitis, consists of superficial fissures, maceration, erythema, and pustules at the corners of the mouth. An inflammatory response in which moist, abraded skin is secondarily invaded by *C. albicans*, angular albicans is observed in children who drool because of braces, who lick their lips, or who suck their thumbs. Older adults are at risk for perlèche due to poorly fitting dentures and drooling from malocclusion. Perlèche is also present in patients with diabetes mellitus or HIV infection.

Several forms of cutaneous candidiasis are localized to intertriginous areas. In infants, moisture, maceration, and irritation from urine and stool in the diaper create an ideal habitat for candidal proliferation. The distinctive features of candidal diaper dermatitis are the formation of bright red patches with sharp borders, the involvement of the inguinal folds, and the presence of satellite macules or pustules peripheral to the initial lesion. The groin is tender and pruritic. A similar process leads to the development of smooth, red, pruritic patches with peripheral scale in skin folds of the axilla, groin, buttocks, umbilicus, and beneath the breasts. The pruritic patches are moist or dry with satellite pustules and fissuring. This form is called candidal intertrigo.

Although *C. albicans* is a component of the normal flora of the vagina and bowel, it often proliferates with pregnancy, diabetes mellitus, and therapy with oral contraceptives and systemic corticosteroids. Candidal vulvovaginitis is associated with edematous, red, pruritic labia; painful urination; and a gelatinous white discharge.

*C. albicans* is the most common pathogen in chronic paronychia. The proximal and lateral nail folds are red, swollen, painful, and raised from the nail plate. A purulent discharge may exude from the nail folds, and the nails become ridged and discolored in untreated infections. Workers at risk for this condition are food handlers, health care workers, launderers, and bartenders, whose hands are in water for many hours a day. Trauma sustained during nail care or other periungual disease creates a portal of entry for bacteria and fungi.

### Diagnosis and Differential Diagnosis

Candidal infections are diagnosed by microscopic examination of KOH preparations of scrapings from white plaques, scaly patches, pustules, or discharge. Pseudohyphae and spores are diagnostic of *Candida*. Fungal cultures are obtained to confirm the diagnosis if the clinician is uncertain.

Many of these disorders (chronic mucocutaneous candidiasis and candidal vulvovaginitis) have distinctive clinical presentations, but others require confirmation. Oral candidiasis should be distinguished from leukoplakia and lichen planus. Perlèche and riboflavin deficiency have similar clinical features. Diaper dermatitis must be distinguished from tinea cruris, irritant dermatitis, acrodermatitis enteropathica, seborrheic dermatitis, and histiocytosis. Candidal intertrigo may resemble an irritant dermatitis, superficial bacterial, or dermatophyte infection. Chronic paronychia may be confused with acute bacterial paronychia, onychomycosis, or psoriasis.

The diagnosis of systemic candidiasis requires the isolation of *Candida* from the blood or other body fluid. Multiple fungal cultures should be obtained in all immunocompromised or debilitated patients having intermittent fevers that are unresponsive to broad-spectrum antibiotics. The differential diagnosis includes systemic infections with bacteria or viruses.

### Management

To successfully treat candidal infections, the underlying risk factors should be adequately addressed. Although these infections will clear up when treated with antifungal agents, they will recur if chronic damage to the cutaneous barrier function exists. Thrush is treated with nystatin suspension or clotrimazole troches. Children and adults either swish nystatin liquid against their oral mucosa prior to swallowing or they slowly dissolve a clotrimazole troche in their mouths.

The treatment of perlèche depends on the cause. Macerated skin should be protected with petrolatum or zinc oxide. Fungi or bacteria should be treated with the appropriate topical antifungal or antibacterial agents. For intertrigo and diaper dermatitis, the principles of therapy are similar. The sites are kept cool and dry using powder, loose-fitting clothing, and compresses on the acutely inflamed areas. Use topical antifungals along with 1% or 2.5% hydrocortisone cream to relieve pruritus and inflammation, and use an antibiotic for suspected concomitant bacterial infection.

Topical antifungal agents, protective gloves, and avoidance of chronic moisture are pivotal to the successful treatment of paronychia. Occasionally, patients are treated with ketoconazole and oral antibiotics when evidence of superinfection is seen in recalcitrant cases. Vulvovaginitis is treated with intravaginal antifungal creams and suppositories of nystatin, clotrimazole, or miconazole. Most infections will resolve after 1 week of nightly therapy, but some require 2 weeks. In resistant cases, the candidal source is eliminated from the gastrointestinal tract with nystatin oral suspension, or the patient is given intravenous/intramuscular therapy for 2–4 weeks.

For chronic mucocutaneous candidiasis and candidemia, systemic treatment is also necessary. The drug of choice for systemic candidiasis is amphotericin B, which is often given along with 5-fluorocytosine for synergy. Although fluconazole is an effective, safer alternative, it may cause hepatotoxicity, which requires close monitoring with liver function testing. The nephrotoxicity caused by extended courses of amphotericin B limits its use in chronic mucocutaneous candidiasis, making oral ketoconazole the mainstay of therapy; oral itraconazole, clotrimazole, and intravenous miconazole are other options.

# CHAPTER 59 BACTERIAL INFECTIONS OF THE SKIN

## Impetigo

### Definition, Epidemiology, and Etiology

Impetigo, also called **impetigo contagiosa,** is a common superficial cutaneous infection with two basic subtypes: bullous and nonbullous. Both subtypes, exacerbated by hot, humid weather, are more frequent in children than in adults. Bullous impetigo, in which the blistered and denuded areas are a cutaneous response to the bacterial toxin, is caused by *Staphylococcus aureus* of phage group II and commonly with type 71. Nonbullous impetigo is due to group A β-hemolytic streptococci *(Streptococcus pyogenes),* often along with *S. aureus.*

### Clinical Features

Nonbullous impetigo is the most frequent skin infection in children, with lesions developing at sites of injury—for example, insect bites, abrasions, or other trauma. Poor hygiene, overcrowding, humidity, and warm environments favor its development. The highest incidence is during the summer, when a higher likelihood of injuries and factors that favor the development of lesions exist. Preferred sites of involvement are the face, extremities, and neck. The primary lesion, a red macule, evolves into a papule or vesicle and rapidly becomes crusted. Typical findings are multiple, thick, honey-colored crusts, ulcers, and erosions. Fever and lymphadenopathy are common. An uncommon but important late sequela is glomerulonephritis, which is caused by certain nephritogenic strains of streptococci. Superficial impetigo rarely causes scarlet fever.

Bullous impetigo is less common. Lesions develop on normal skin, most commonly in the axillae, groin, and hands. They consist of superficial, fragile, subcorneal bullae containing yellow-white opaque fluid. The bullae rupture rapidly, exposing erosions that are covered by thin, yellow-brown crusts.

### Diagnosis and Differential Diagnosis

Although the thick, honey-colored crusts of nonbullous impetigo are pathognomonic, the lesions of bullous impetigo, with their thinner amber crusts, are less distinctive. The Nikolsky sign (see Chapter 52) is negative, which distinguishes bullous impetigo from primary blistering diseases with secondary infection. Ecthyma may mimic impetigo, but on removal of the thick crust it reveals a deep ulcer with a halo of erythema. A culture of the blister fluid or base confirms the diagnosis.

### Management

Impetigo is effectively treated by suitable antibiotics and topical skin care. A semisynthetic penicillin (dicloxacillin for 14 days) is recommended, given the need to treat staphylococci and streptococci. Erythromycin is an alternative, but resistance to it is emerging. For superficial impetigo, topical mupirocin ointment is as effective as oral antibiotics. Extensive or deep lesions mandate oral agents. Gentle cleansing and warm compresses can remove crusts. To minimize autoinoculation and contagion, patients should practice good hygiene.

## Erysipelas

### Definition and Epidemiology

Erysipelas is a form of superficial cellulitis caused by group A β-hemolytic streptococci. Lymphatic involvement is a prominent feature. Erysipelas, in its most common form, occurs on the bridge of the nose and the cheeks. Chronic edema caused by venous or lymphatic insufficiency predisposes people to recurrent episodes of erysipelas. Other predisposing conditions are immunodeficiency syndromes, cachexia, malnutrition, diabetes mellitus, and poor general hygiene.

### Etiology and Pathogenesis

The most common pathogen is group A β-hemolytic streptococci. Other rarely isolated organisms are groups B, C, or G streptococci. The pathogen enters through an abrasion, surgical incision, puncture wound, ulcer, injury, or fissure in the nose, ears, or perineum. Any draining site may serve as a source of infection, but sometimes no portal of entry is apparent.

### Clinical Features

Fever, chills, headache, and malaise precede and accompany the onset of the skin eruption, and the patient appears toxic. Some report gastrointestinal symptoms, arthralgias, and changes in mental status. Typically, the lesions are sharply circumscribed, red, tender infiltrated plaques localized to the face and scalp (Color Plate 19); infrequently, they occur on the hands and genitalia. However, the infection is not limited to these areas. Leukocytosis is common, and often exceeds 20,000/mm$^3$. The lesions progress rapidly by peripheral extension of the raised indurated borders. In severe cases, the warm edematous plaques become blisters.

### Diagnosis and Differential Diagnosis

When erysipelas presents in its classic form (bright red, indurated facial plaque with distinct borders), little diagnostic difficulty results. Sometimes, the lesions may resemble allergic contact dermatitis, urticaria, scarlet fever, systemic lupus erythematosus, tuberculoid leprosy, or relapsing polychondritis. Culture of this closed infection is difficult to obtain and rarely of use in initial management.

### Management

Penicillin is the drug of choice for erysipelas. Improvement is rapid and dramatic. Penicillin-allergic patients are given erythromycin or clindamycin. A semisynthetic penicillin or cephalosporin is used when *S. aureus* is a potential second pathogen. Cool compresses provide symptom relief for tender, warm, blistered plaques, and swelling is controlled with immobilization and elevation. With chronic or recurrent infection, a bacterial reservoir and a possible portal of entry (e.g., macerated skin of tinea pedis) should be determined.

## Folliculitis

### Definition and Etiology

Bacterial folliculitis is an infection of the hair follicles, commonly caused by coagulase-positive staphylococci. Although *S. aureus* is the most frequent cause of superficial and deep folliculitis, superficial folliculitis is caused by streptococcus, proteus, pseudomonas, or other gram-negative organisms.

### Clinical Features

The clinical features depend on the age of the patient, the depth of infection, and the site of involvement. Superficial folliculitis (Bockhart impetigo) is a follicular pyoderma occurring most frequently on the scalps of children and on extremities and buttocks in adults. Small, dome-shaped pustules and red papules form in crops at the follicular ostia and resolve in 1–2 weeks. Hair growth continues, and lesions heal without scarring. Untreated infections may evolve into a deeper process with perifollicular extension of inflammation. Common variants of superficial folliculitis are *Pseudomonas aeruginosa* folliculitis, *Pityrosporum* folliculitis and gram-negative folliculitis. *Pseudomonas aeruginosa* is usually acquired in a hot tub or whirlpool and causes an eruption within days of exposure. Papules and pustules occur on the trunk, buttocks, arms, and legs. *Pityrosporum* folliculitis is a chronic pruritic infection of *Malassezia furfur* on the back, proximal arms, legs, face, and scalp. Gram-negative folliculitis occurs in patients with acne vulgaris after extensive courses of systemic antibiotics.

The prototype of deep folliculitis is sycosis barbae (folliculitis barbae). Follicular pustules and papules with central hairs form in the beard area. Men with dense facial hair are most predisposed. Without prompt therapy, the infection becomes chronic and recurrent. Crops of pustules recur at the same sites and rupture with shaving or cause excoriation. The trauma sustains and spreads the infection. Follicular papules coalesce into tender, red, crusted plaques.

### Diagnosis and Differential Diagnosis

The appearance of pustules in the appropriate distribution is usually characteristic. Lesions in recalcitrant disease should be cultured before initiating another course of antibiotics. Tinea barbae and pseudofolliculitis barbae may mimic sycosis barbae. Tinea barbae consists of erythematous nodules and plaques with distorted, damaged hairs, and rarely involves the upper lip. In pseudofolliculitis barbae, the curly facial hairs of black men curve back and pierce the skin.

## Furuncles and Carbuncles

### Definition and Etiology

Furuncles (boils) and carbuncles are inflammatory lesions of the hair follicles. A furuncle is a tender red nodule that often develops from a previous superficial folliculitis. A carbuncle forms when several furuncles coalesce into a larger, deeper abscess; *S. aureus* is the most common pathogen. Autoinoculation is an important mechanism in perpetuating the infection. Reservoirs of staphylococci for further infections derive from material draining from follicular openings, infected towels and linens, or nasal carriage of bacteria.

### Clinical Features

As the furuncle enlarges during the first 2–4 days, it is firm and red. Then it becomes fluctuant, and yellow-white material is visible through the thinned epidermis. As the nodule ruptures, pus and necrotic material are released onto the surrounding skin. The pressure and pain are reduced and healing follows, causing **fibrosis.** Furunculosis develops in areas with abundant hair follicles that are prone to friction and sweating—that is, the neck, face, axilla, and buttocks. Infestations and other pruritic disorders may be accompanied by impetiginization (the development of a contagious, superficial **pyoderma**) and furuncle formation. Malnutrition, diabetes mellitus, obesity, defective neutrophil function, alcoholism, immunosuppression, and hematologic disorders enhance susceptibility to the formation of furuncles and carbuncles, but these lesions usually occur in healthy patients.

Carbuncles are larger, deeper, and a source of greater morbidity than furuncles. Red, indurated plaques surmounted by multiple pustules evolve into very painful draining abscesses on the neck, back, and thighs. Fever, malaise, and leukocytosis may be present. After drainage, healing is slow and is accompanied by scarring. Complications, although rare, include bacteremia and cellulitis with either furuncles or carbuncles. Lesions on the lips or tip of the nose may cause bacteria to enter the cavernous sinus via the facial and angular veins, leading to its thrombosis.

### Diagnosis and Management

Both furuncles and carbuncles have deep, red, suppurative nodules. The lesions in folliculitis are more superficial; perifollicular induration and systemic symptoms are absent.

Aside from warm compresses, initial therapy consists of systemic antibiotics to cover *S. aureus*; its frequent penicillin resistance dictates use of a semisynthetic penicillin (e.g., dicloxacillin). Rifampin is added to potentiate the antimicrobial effect. Furuncles and carbuncles should not be incised and drained until lesions are fluctuant and the thinned epidermis reveals pus below. Mupirocin ointment and a sterile dressing are placed locally after drainage to prevent autoinoculation.

In recurrent or recalcitrant cases, a culture should be obtained to ensure that the organism is not methicillin-resistant *Staphylococcus* or some other form of bacteria that is not susceptible to the previous antibiotic regimen. The predisposing factors should be explored. Potential staphylococcal sources (e.g., the nasal carriage) are treated with mupirocin ointment and chlorhexidine or another antimicrobial soap for daily bathing. The patient's linen and clothing are laundered in hot water to eliminate the transmission of bacteria to other family members.

## Syphilis

### Definition and Epidemiology

Caused by *Treponema pallidum*, syphilis is an infectious disease with both cutaneous and visceral manifestations. It most commonly affects sexually active young adults and teenagers, but no age, race, or gender is exempt. Although sexual activity is the most common mode of transmission, any direct contact with its highly contagious lesions may cause infection. Congenital syphilis is transplacentally acquired. Other sexually transmitted diseases (STDs)—HIV, chlamydia, and gonorrhea—may coexist with syphilis; the diagnosis of any one of these should prompt a search for the others.

### Etiology

*Treponema pallidum*, the etiologic agent of syphilis, is a spirochete less than 20 μm in length. Identifiable with dark-field microscopy, it has a cell envelope, an axial filament, and a protoplast. These **treponemes** will not grow on culture media. Antibacterial drugs that impair cell wall synthesis are effective against *T. pallidum*. Spirochetes migrate through minute fissures in mucous membranes or skin in adults and can cross the placenta to infect a fetus.

## Clinical Features

The course is divided into early and late stages. Early syphilis is defined as the first 2 years of disease and encompasses primary syphilis, secondary syphilis, and early latent syphilis. Late syphilis includes late latent and tertiary syphilis.

The **chancre** is the hallmark of primary syphilis. Usually developing at the site of contact with the treponemes 3–4 weeks after exposure, a chancre is accompanied by bilateral, nontender regional adenopathy and resolves in 6 weeks, evolving from a red papule into an indurated, oval plaque with a superficial erosion and serous exudate.

Although usually solitary and localized to the genitals, chancres may be multiple and involve oral mucosa, rectum, face, axilla, breasts, or distal extremities. In women, a chancre may be overlooked because it may occur on the cervix. It can occur as a mixed infection with chancroid or become superinfected.

**Syphilids,** the skin signs of secondary syphilis, occur an average of 6 weeks after the onset of the chancre, which may not have resolved by then. The initial eruption may be transient, rapidly progressive red-brown macules, and the fully developed **exanthem** (skin eruption) is diffuse, symmetric, and polymorphous, consisting of macules, papules, and less often, nodules and pustules. Scaling is common, and lesions may follow the lines of cleavage in the skin. Although this suggests PR, involvement of the palms and soles suggests syphilis (Color Plate 20). The distribution of the lesions may be annular, follicular, or lichenoid. Other lesions observed at this stage are mucous patches, condyloma lata, syphilitic pharyngitis, and patchy "moth-eaten" alopecia. Characteristically, none of these lesions is pruritic. Mucous patches are white, eroded papules that arise on the tongue; tonsils; gingival, buccal, and labial mucosa; cervix; vagina; labia minora; glans; and corona of the penis. Condyloma lata are pink exophytic papules that are most infectious, affect moist intertriginous sites, and should be distinguished from condyloma acuminata. Fatigue, malaise, headache, nasal congestion, arthralgia, sore throat, and lymphadenopathy are usual symptoms. The gastrointestinal tract, kidneys, liver, central nervous system, prostate, lungs, and bones may be infected. Anemia, elevated sedimentation rate, leukocytosis, and increased alkaline phosphatase are notable. Resolution follows within 10 weeks, and lesions heal with pigmentary changes.

During the latent period, the disease manifestations are absent and the diagnosis is by reactive serologic tests. Tertiary syphilis, which usually follows after 3 or more years of latency, has three basic forms: benign, neurosyphilis, and cardiovascular syphilis. In benign disease, patients develop red coalescent nodules (gummas) that may ulcerate. These indolent asymptomatic lesions are distributed on the extensor arms, face, and back. Healing occurs with scarring and destruction of soft tissue.

## Diagnosis and Differential Diagnosis

Syphilis is diagnosed by correlation of the clinical findings and the results of serologic tests for syphilis. Observing treponemes by dark-field examination provides an immediate diagnosis of primary, secondary, and congenital syphilis. Serologic tests for syphilis are divided into nontreponemal or treponemal tests. The former detects reagins or phospholipids released from infected cells, the most common ones being the rapid plasma reagin and the venereal diseases reference laboratory tests. These nonspecific flocculation tests are used to screen patients with risk factors for syphilis. Quantitative antibody titers are used to follow up response to therapy. False-negative results may occur in patients with very high antibody titers **(prozone phenomena).** Treponemal tests use *T. pallidum* components as the antigen. The fluorescent treponemal antibody test and the microhemagglutination test are the most useful. In the fluorescent treponemal antibody test, a visible reaction results from the mixture of human serum with a fluorescein-labeled antihuman globulin on a slide to which *T. pallidum* has been adsorbed. The microhemagglutination test is less expensive and easier to perform.

*T. pallidum* induces a wide variety of different lesions, thus the vast differential diagnosis. The syphilitic chancre resembles the ulcers of chancroid or lymphogranuloma venereum, the eroded nodules of granuloma inguinale, and the blister base of HSV infection. Chancroid produces soft, painful ulcers with inflamed, undermined borders, a superficial membrane, and unilateral adenopathy. The friable granulation tissue of granuloma inguinale is characteristic. The lesions of lymphogranuloma venereum are painless, fleeting, and followed by lymphadenopathy. Pain or a burning sensation often precedes the grouped vesicles of herpes simplex infection. Secondary syphilis may be confused with other papulosquamous disorders such as PR, lichen planus, dermatophytosis, guttate psoriasis, and mycosis fungoides. Syphilids may be mimicked by drug eruptions, sarcoidosis, leprosy, urticaria pigmentosa, tinea versicolor, and streptococcal infections. Syphilitic cutaneous lesions are asymptomatic. Mucous patches may be confused with EM, candidiasis, leukoplakia, herpetic gingivostomatitis, erosive lichen planus, and aphthous stomatitis. Ulcerated oral gumma may mimic a squamous cell cancer.

### Management

Parenteral penicillin G is the most effective treatment for all forms of syphilis. The treatment for syphilis is shown in Table 157.4 (Chapter 157). Penicillin-allergic patients are given tetracycline hydrochloride 500 mg four times daily for 2 weeks or erythromycin (the same dose), but these alternate agents are less effective. Ceftriaxone may be useful in persons with neurosyphilis owing to its penetration of the central nervous system. The management of pregnant patients depends on the same criteria for antibiotic selection. Patients with concurrent HIV infection and syphilis may not be cured with the standard regimens. Many physicians treat these patients with higher doses or treatment of longer duration to prevent the potential neurologic involvement that results from inadequate therapy. Reevaluation of patients with early-stage syphilis is scheduled at 3, 6, and 9 months after treatment. HIV-positive individuals are reassessed more frequently.

For more information on syphilis, see chapter 157, Sexually Transmitted Diseases.

# CHAPTER 60 VIRAL INFECTIONS OF THE SKIN

## Verrucae

### Definition and Epidemiology

Warts, or verrucae, are common epidermal growths induced by a local infection with the human papilloma virus (HPV). Their characteristic appearance depends on the site of involvement and the viral type. Warts usually occur in children and adolescents, although no age is exempt. Patients with impaired cell-mediated immunity (e.g., immunosuppressive therapy) are particularly vulnerable and usually experience a protracted course. Patients with atopic dermatitis, AIDS, and lymphoma are also vulnerable. *Condyloma acuminata* (see Clinical Features section) occurs most frequently in sexually active adolescents and young adults, and its incidence has significantly risen since the 1970s.

### Etiology

HPV, a member of the papovavirus family, contains double-stranded DNA. These viral particles lack a lipoprotein envelope that confers greater resistance to freezing, chemicals, higher temperatures, and desiccation. They remain viable even without a human host, and therefore are transmissible by fomites. HPV is not pathogenic in other species.

Classified on the basis of the outer protein capsid antigens, more than 65 different types of HPV have been identified. Some these have been associated with malignant transformation in the involved lesion. DNA hybridization techniques, which are rarely clinically used unless concern exists regarding carcinogenic potential, allow identification of the viral type from a biopsy specimen. Current evidence suggests that HPV may inhibit the function of antioncogenes.

### Clinical Features

Verruca vulgaris (common warts) are flesh-colored papules with a rough, scaly gray or white surface; these warts are associated with HPV types 1, 2, 4, and 7. Single or multiple and of variable size (a few millimeters to several centimeters), they most frequently are found on the dorsa of the hands, but no epithelial site is exempt. Easily spread from the hands to the face or extremities, these warts may be inoculated into sites of trauma. Periungual and subungual warts are not uncommon and usually are difficult to eradicate. They can become irritated, fissured, and tender. Filiform or digitate warts occur on the head and neck. They have rough projections from the surface and are attached to the skin by a broad stalk.

Verruca plantaris (plantar warts) grow into the thick skin of the sole and appear as flat or slightly elevated papules or plaques. HPV types 1, 2, and 4 are usually isolated from these. Because these firm, coarse keratotic lesions localize to sites of pressure, walking is painful. Mosaic warts form when multiple single papules coalesce into a plaque. These may enlarge to several centimeters. On removal, superficial keratoses show a soft core with multiple bleeding points.

Verruca plana (flat warts) are 1- to 3-mm, pink or tan, flat-topped papules. The most common HPV types are 3, 10, 28, and 41. Variable numbers are distributed on the face, dorsal hands, wrists, and legs. Occurring in groups, they often coalesce into plaques, and they spread through autoinoculation. Shaving or other trauma induces new lesions in a linear distribution.

Condyloma acuminata arise in men on the penile shaft and in women on the vulva, perineum, or cervix; they also arise on the anal canal or the perianal skin. The soft, fleshy, clustered papules are tan, pink, or gray. Early lesions are minute, and diagnosed by applying dilute acetic acid compresses that whiten the altered epidermal surface. They may enlarge to form cauliflower-like masses. These larger lesions are frequently tender from recurrent trauma. HPV infection may be accompanied by a vaginal discharge, which may be malodorous because of secondary bacterial colonization. Pregnancy or immunodeficiency causes genital warts to become numerous. Transmission is via sexual contact or inoculation from a cutaneous site. Condylomata in children should prompt suspicion of sexual abuse and a workup for other STDs.

Genital warts have the following HPV types: 6, 11, 13, 16, 18, 30–33, 42–44, and 51–55. The isolation of HPV from penile, vulvar, and anal cancers, and the finding of HPV 6, 11, 16, 18, and other types in most cases of cervical cancer, attest to its malignant potential. In women who have condyloma of the vulva or sexual partners with condyloma, gynecological examination and Papanicolaou smears should be performed to detect internal condyloma or neoplasia.

### Diagnosis and Differential Diagnosis

Generally, the clinical appearance is diagnostic. Two important clues for the identification of skin warts are the presence of dilated, thrombosed capillaries that appear as brown or black dots and the disruption of the superficial skin lines. Lichen planus, lichen planus–like keratoses, molluscum contagiosum, and an epidermal nevus may be confused with verruca plana. Warts on the sole resemble corns or clavi. Paring the lesion will reveal a hard core of a clavus but a softer center with thrombosed vessels in a wart. Common warts occasionally need to be differentiated from seborrheic keratoses, nevi, acrochordons, and squamous cell cancer. Condyloma lata require differentiation from anogenital warts; syphilis serology is diagnostic. Condyloma acuminata may coexist with other STDs, which should be appropriately excluded.

### Management

Not all HPV infections require therapy because many types of warts will resolve on their own. Treatment depends on the age and the immune status of the patient; the extent, site, and duration of the lesions; presence of symptoms; and the patient's wishes. Because all modes of therapy are not equally effective in all persons, individualization is important. Most measures destroy the epidermal cells that harbor the virus. All methods carry high rates of recurrence because viral particles may be present even in skin that appears normal.

Cryotherapy is frequently used in treating all forms of HPV infection. Liquid nitrogen, which is effective without scarring, is sprayed on the lesion or applied with a swab for 2–15 seconds. Flat warts or condyloma require a shorter application, and verruca vulgaris requires a longer application; multiple applications may also be needed. Rarely, superficial digital nerves or vessels are damaged. Electrodesiccation and curettage rapidly reduces the size of the lesions but has a high rate of recurrence and scarring with healing. In contrast, the $CO_2$ laser can vaporize the infected keratinocytes without scarring. Both the operator and patient should be appropriately protected from the aerosolized viral particles in the laser plume. Cantharidin solution (Cantharone), a blistering agent, separates the infected cells of the epidermis from the dermis. The application is painless, and the site is simply washed to remove the infected cells.

Condylomata and warts without a highly keratinized surface are often treated with podophyllum resin (available in a 25% solution with tincture of benzoin or as a less-concentrated solution for home treatment). This irritating compound, which halts epidermal proliferation of virally infected cells, is carefully applied to individual lesions and removed in 4–6 hours. Other useful agents for verruca vulgaris or verruca plantaris include salicylic and lactic acid solutions and plasters, formalin, and 5-fluorouracil ointment. Resistant cases are treated with intralesional interferon or bleomycin, laser ablation, and, rarely, retinoids.

## Molluscum Contagiosum

### Definition, Epidemiology, and Etiology

Molluscum contagiosum is a common childhood viral disease, featuring single or multiple dome-shaped papules with central umbilication and a white core. The disorder is distributed worldwide and has a widely variable incidence. It is most commonly seen in children between the ages of 3 and 16 years and in sexually active adults. Persons with immunodeficiencies are especially susceptible, and men are more often affected. Patients with AIDS can develop generalized lesions that are very difficult to treat. The causative agent is molluscum contagiosum, a unique member of the poxvirus group. These are large, brick-shaped DNA viruses that measure 200–300 nm. There are two distinct pathogenic strains.

### Clinical Features

Initially, the papules are firm and flesh-colored or pink and, with time, become waxy and white or pearly gray. The lesions range from 2–5 mm in diameter but may exceed 1 cm. The most frequently involved sites are the face, trunk, and extremities in children and the anogenital region in adults. Mucous membrane involvement is not uncommon. In adults, transmission is associated with sexual activity. Generally, the eruption lacks symptoms, except perhaps mild pruritus. With rubbing, eczematous patches develop around some lesions. Eyelid lesions may incite conjunctivitis or keratitis.

## Diagnosis and Management

The shiny, dome-shape papules with central umbilication are characteristic. Sometimes they resemble milia, warts, varicella, papillomas, acne, epithelioma, and herpes virus infection. The diagnosis is confirmed by finding the viral inclusions (molluscum bodies or Henderson-Paterson bodies), which is accomplished by expressing the contents of a lesion onto a slide, flattening the material, and staining with Wright stain.

In immunocompetent persons, the disease is generally self-limited and resolves in 6–9 months. Not all cases require therapy; however, hundreds of lesions may form before spontaneous remission. Once the central keratin core is removed or destroyed, the lesions will heal. The disease is most reliably treated by curettage after topical anesthesia. Children tolerate this procedure poorly and are best treated with a brief application of liquid nitrogen or cantharidin. Light electrodesiccation, application of 50% trichloroacetic acid until whitening, or daily treatment with Duofilm are other options. Because new lesions may continually evolve from self-inoculation, all of these treatment regimens require multiple visits.

Molluscum contagiosum affecting immunocompromised persons is very difficult to treat. Trichloroacetic acid peels are useful in treating numerous facial, neck, and chest lesions in AIDS patients.

## Clinical Features

Transmission follows direct contact with lesional skin or secretions. The incubation period is 1–26 days, often 1 week. HSV infections may be primary or recurrent. Primary infections occur in persons without antibodies to HSV. In some, a prodrome of burning, tingling pruritus or neuralgia is followed by symptomatic localized or generalized eruptions or systemic involvement. The eruptions are superficial, clustered vesicles on an erythematous base. Most lesions resolve without scarring unless bacterial superinfection has prevailed. In others, the infection is subclinical, with a humoral response and without any cold sores. Serologic evidence of exposure to the virus is present in over 85% of some populations. After primary infection, the virus remains dormant in the sensory nerve ganglia until reactivation. Symptomatic primary infections are more severe than recurrent infections. Although herpes infection stimulates both humoral and cell-mediated immunity, the severity of the disease in the immunodeficient underscores the importance of cell-mediated immunity.

**Gingivostomatitis** is the most common clinical expression of primary HSV-1 infection in children, most of whom are 1–6 years old. Often, associated malaise, fever, salivation, irritability, fetid breath, and tender cervical lymph nodes exist. The gingival mucosa is red, edematous, and friable. Vesicles appear on the tongue, palate, buccal mucosa, and pharynx within 1 week of exposure to the virus. These evolve into gray ulcers with surrounding erythema. Oral pain inhibits eating and drinking, but the lesions resolve in 2–3 weeks. **Primary ocular herpes simplex infections** lead to a purulent conjunctivitis and superficial keratitis. Vesicles arise on edematous and erythematous eyelid margins. Pain, photophobia, lacrimation, discharge, and preauricular lymphadenopathy may be present. Generally, herpetic keratoconjunctivitis heals uneventfully in 2 weeks; scarring and blindness are rare.

In contrast, HSV-2 infection occurs most frequently in adolescents and young adults through sexual contact. **Genital herpes** evokes symptoms much more often than its oral counterpart. HSV-1 is isolated from 20–40% of genital lesions. Genital herpes in children is suggestive of sexual abuse.

Genital herpes infections are subdivided into herpes progenitalis and herpetic vulvovaginitis. Herpes simplex is the most common cause of genital ulceration in sexually active individuals. The most frequently involved site in men is the penis (glans, foreskin, and shaft) and, rarely, the scrotum or urethra. In women, the external genitalia and the mucosal surfaces of the vulva, cervix, and vagina are commonly involved. The vesicular eruption rapidly gives place to painful, superficial ulcers covered with gray exudate. Single or multiple 3-mm lesions develop on swollen, erythematous tissue and often coalesce into large, ulcerated plaques. Constitutional symptoms are severe in some patients, but resolution occurs in 3 weeks or less.

Several other forms of primary herpes virus infection exist. Inoculation of HSV directly into a skin fissure or abrasion induces vesicles, indurated papules, or bullae with regional adenopathy. Dentists may develop such herpetic whitlows on their fingers. In herpes gladiatorum, wrestlers and participants of contact sports may develop similar lesions on the face, scalp, and upper trunk through contact with the skin and mucous membranes of other players. Severe systemic symptoms often accompany the scattered, grouped vesicles and lymphadenopathy. Kaposi varicelliform eruption arises from the introduction of HSV into skin affected by atopic dermatitis or **Darier disease.** Neonates may develop a herpetic infection at the time of delivery from contact with lesions in the maternal genital tract (neonatal herpes).

Recurrent episodes of herpes virus infection have a shorter course and less severe symptoms than the primary infection. The vesicles are smaller and the distribution is more limited. A burning or tingling sensation often precedes the eruption, which resolves in 7–10 days without residual scarring. Common triggers include trauma, stress, menstruation, and ultraviolet radiation. In women, significant tenderness accompanies recurrent genital infections. Herpes may recur on the buttocks; regional lymphadenopathy and neurologic complaints may be associated. Eczema herpeticum, keratoconjuctivitis, and inoculation herpes are other primary infections that recur less often. Herpes infections may be complicated by EM with herpes labialis, cranial nerve or Bell palsy, neuralgia, disseminated disease, arthritis, and lymphedema with involvement of the extremities.

### Diagnosis and Differential Diagnosis

In most cases, the distinctive appearance of grouped vesicles on an erythematous base makes the diagnosis of herpes infection obvious. The most rapid method for confirming HSV is the Tzanck smear, which shows multinucleated giant cells among the keratinocytes scraped from the base of a vesicle. A viral culture is necessary to distinguish the viral type with certainty. Primary infections may be identified by the increase in antibody titer using the complement fixation test. Herpetic gingivostomatitis should be differentiated from hand-foot-and-mouth disease, aphthous stomatitis, EM, herpangina, diphtheria, and Behçet syndrome. Impetigo may be confused with herpes labialis, and the two may occur together. Herpes progenitalis resembles a syphilitic chancre or chancroid; however, the lesions of syphilis are painless.

### Management

Uncomplicated, localized herpetic infections do not require treatment. Acyclovir or famciclovir, orally or intravenously, shortens the duration of each episode and reduces recurrences. Both are effective in primary infections and recurrences, regardless of immune status. They have few significant adverse effects, but the dose should be reduced for patients with renal failure. Although acyclovir ointment may reduce viral shedding, it does not affect recurrence rate. Primary infections respond to oral acyclovir, 200 mg five times per day for 7–10 days. Acyclovir is given intravenously for neonatal herpes and severe infections. Recurrent disease is not suppressed unless the episodes are frequent or unless the cellular immunity is impaired. The most common regimen is acyclovir, 400 mg twice per day. Among the immunocompromised with HSV, acyclovir resistance is well known and is attributed to thymidine kinase–deficient viral clones. Foscarnet or vidarabine are useful in these cases.

Adjunctive treatment consists of compresses with Burrow solution to dry weeping lesions and therapy for superimposed bacterial infections. Factors that trigger recurrent episodes should be identified.

# CHAPTER 61 INFESTATIONS OF THE SKIN

Parasitic infestations are a common cause of pruritic eruptions. Primary lesions are often effaced by secondary changes, thereby obscuring diagnosis. The distribution of the lesions and a history of multiple affected persons within the same living group should arouse suspicion of these entities.

## Scabies

### Definition and Epidemiology

Scabies, an infestation of the skin with *Sarcoptes scabiei*, is contracted by close personal contact. Reported worldwide, scabies occurs in epidemics, with overcrowding and institutionalization perpetuating the disease. Scabies is rarely transmitted by fomites such as towels or linen because the organism cannot live for more than 5 days away from a warm human host. Thus, close human contact is essential for transmission. The two most common variants are nodular and crusted (Norwegian) scabies. Crusted scabies occurs most frequently among people with immune deficiencies and mental and physical disabilities (Down syndrome, neurologic disorders, and malnutrition).

### Etiology

*Sarcoptes scabiei* (var. hominis) is an arachnid that prefers a human host. Having an oval, gray, or translucent body, this arachnid measures 0.3–0.5 mm. After fertilization, the male mite dies; the female then enters the human stratum corneum, where she forms a tunnel and lays two to three eggs daily for 4–8 weeks. She dies after the egg laying is complete. The eggs hatch within 3–4 days of deposition, producing larvae, which develop into nymphs and then adults. An infested person who bathes frequently will have from 2–50 mites in the skin. Thousands of mites may exist on a person with Norwegian scabies.

### Clinical Features

The eruption consists of pruritic papules, vesicles, and burrows with pronounced secondary changes of crusting, infection, excoriation, and eczematization. Asymptomatic for the first 4–6 weeks, the parasite causes pruritus after the host is sensitized to its foreign proteins. The intense pruritus is often worse at night, and it may persist for weeks after treatment. Burrows are 0.2- to 1-cm, raised, linear lesions. The axilla, groin, and the web spaces of the hands and feet are commonly infected. In children and the elderly, lesions may exist above the neck on the forehead, cheeks, and hairline. Buttocks, nipples, flexor arms, and the waist should also be examined.

The nodular type of scabies consists of 3- to 5-mm red nodules that remain for months or years after treatment and classically occur on the scrotum and penis, among other sites. In the crusted type, the large, scaly, crusted plaques resemble psoriatic plaques and may be accompanied by nail dystrophy, subungual and periungual hyperkeratosis, and fissuring. The genitals, buttocks, scalp, hands, feet, and areas of pressure are the sites of predilection.

### Diagnosis and Differential Diagnosis

The differential diagnosis includes insect bite reaction, prurigo nodularis or neurodermatitis, atopic eczema, xerosis, or pruritus from systemic diseases with secondary excoriation. The history among multiple family members of a pruritic eruption that is present on the hands, wrists, axilla, and groin is suggestive of scabies. Although burrows are a reliable diagnostic clue, the frequency of secondary excoriations and crusting often makes them difficult to identify; applying black, washable ink to the skin and then wiping it off can outline these burrows and may help in their localization. Definitive diagnosis is through the recovery of a mite, eggs, or feces (see Chapter 49, Color Plate 3). Mites are most likely to be recovered from new lesions or burrows on the web spaces of the hands, subungual region of the digits, and wrists. Rarely, a biopsy is required to ascertain the diagnosis.

### Management

The two most frequently used therapeutic options are lindane (gamma benzene hexachloride) cream or lotion and Elimite cream (permethrin 5%). Lindane, the traditional treatment, is highly effective. However, because of its side-effect profile, its use has declined. Neurotoxicity may occur after its use in infants and children, owing to enhanced absorption. Inappropriate or frequent application may cause eczema, urticaria, and aplastic anemia. The cream or lotion is applied at night to all body surface areas below the neck in adults and older children, and washed off after 8 hours. Permethrin 5% cream is the treatment of choice in children and infants as young as 2 months of age; it is applied in the same manner but also on the face, neck, and hairline. All creases and folds should be carefully treated with all topical agents, and crusts should be removed with tepid soaks. On the evening of the first treatment, all linens are laundered in hot water and other bedding or clothing is dry-cleaned or placed in plastic bags for 5 days. Sulfur (5–10%) in petrolatum and 10% crotamiton (Eurax) are less effective alternatives. Other adjuncts include antihistamines and topical corticosteroid creams for relief of pruritus and antibiotics to treat bacterial superinfection. Family members and sexual contacts with or without pruritus should be treated to ensure eradication of the parasite.

## Pediculosis

### Definition and Epidemiology

Pediculosis is an infestation of the skin with lice that attack human hosts. Lice depend on their human hosts for blood. As they attach to the skin to obtain their meal, they inject noxious salivary secretions that are antigenic and may transmit some infectious diseases. Pediculosis affects both children and adults. Lice may be acquired by close human contact in a crowded environment and between individuals who share fomites such as combs, clothing, and upholstery. Poor hygiene contributes to the perpetuation of this disorder. Pediculosis capitis occurs most frequently in young girls and is rare in African-Americans. Patients with pediculosis pubis tend to be adolescents and young adults who acquire the disease through sexual activity.

### Etiology

The pediculi infecting humans are *Phthirus pubis* (the pubic or crab louse), *Pediculus humanus corporis* (the body louse), and *Pediculus humanus capitis* (the head louse). Each of these has a predilection for a defined site and rarely invades other areas. They have oval, gray, or translucent bodies with six legs and a proboscis for blood extraction. They range in size from 1–4 mm. The head louse is smaller than the body louse, but both have a slender abdomen and legs of equal size. The pubic louse resembles a crab with a rounded body, a pair of smaller legs near the mouth, and two sets of large legs. The ova or nits are oval, gray, or white concretions that adhere to hair and clothing and measure 0.3–0.8 mm. The eggs are deposited within 48 hours of fertilization and require approximately 2 weeks to mature.

### Clinical Features

Pediculosis capitis occurs in people of all ages but is most common in children. Severe pruritus leads to scratching with frequent secondary infections and adenopathy. The hair is dull, and ova or nits adhere to the hair shafts. In pediculosis corporis ("Vagabond's disease" or pediculosis vestimenti), the lice live in the seams of clothing in areas that are warmed by the body, such as the neck, waist, and groin; acral sites, however, are spared. The lice puncture the skin for nourishment, and their bites produce pruritic macules, papules, and urticarial wheals with prominent central puncta. These lesions are usually obliterated by secondary excoriations, lichenification, eczematization, crusting, and infection. Healing occurs with hyperpigmentation. Severe pruritus with parallel scratches in the interscapular region is characteristic.

Pubic lice induce pruritic red papules on the thighs, abdomen, and chest. Pediculi may also adhere to the hair of the beard area, axilla, eyebrows, and eyelashes. Eyebrows and lashes are most often infested in older children and may be accompanied by **blepharitis** (inflamed eyelids). With abundant parasites, maculae ceruleae are seen; they are 3- to 15-mm, blue, nonblanching, asymptomatic macules on the thighs, proximal arms, and ventral trunk. Transmission occurs via sexual intercourse or less often through infested bedding or other fomites. Other sexually transmitted diseases may also exist.

### Diagnosis and Differential Diagnosis

Pediculosis is usually diagnosed by the observation of nits and pediculi. Nits on scalp hair may resemble hair casts or scale, but nits adhere firmly to the hair shaft and fluoresce when a Wood's lamp is used. Examination of a hair with light microscopy should clarify the diagnosis of pediculosis capitis or pubis. At times, a superficial scalp infection is the only evidence of infestation. Pubic lice and their nits may be isolated near the skin surface in most cases. Body lice reside in the patient's clothes, not on the skin; an inspection of the clothing will reveal hundreds of eggs deposited in the seams.

### Management

Several shampoos are effective in treating pediculosis capitis. Lindane shampoo (Kwell, 1%) is the traditional treatment; it is applied to the scalp for 5 minutes and rinsed off, and is repeated in 1 week. However, concerns about toxicity now limit its use. Both permethrin 1% cream rinse (Nix) and pyrethrin with piperonyl butoxide 1% (Rid) are safe for children. After a 10-minute application, the agent is removed from the scalp and repeated in 1 week. A less convenient method is the use of crotamiton 10% cream or lotion for 24 hours. Nits are removed with a fine-toothed comb or tweezers after soaking the hair in a 5% solution of white vinegar. All items that come into contact with the scalp need to be cleaned or placed in plastic bags for 2 weeks.

Pediculosis pubis is treated with the same agents as above. Lindane is the treatment of choice and is applied to the affected area, adjacent normal skin, and perianal region. Sexual partners of infested individuals should be treated concurrently. Linen and clothing should be washed in hot water or dry-cleaned. If the eyelashes are infested, they should be treated with a thick coating of petrolatum 2 times a day for 1 week, followed by manual removal of the remaining lice. An alternative is physostigmine 0.25% ophthalmic ointment, 4 times per day for 3 days.

Body lice dwell in the clothing of the patient and remain on the skin only to feed. Frequent bathing and cleaning of clothing, bedding, carpets, upholstery, and mattresses should be sufficient to rid the host of this parasite.

# CHAPTER 62 PIGMENTARY DISORDERS OF THE SKIN

Pigmentary disorders are either (1) an acquired abnormality in melanin production and transfer or (2) a congenital absence of melanin or the constituents of its synthesis. The cosmetic consequences of these disorders can be psychologically devastating.

## Vitiligo

### Definition, Epidemiology, and Etiology

Vitiligo, which results from the loss of melanocytes, is a common disorder of patterned depigmentation affecting 1–2% of the population. It affects all races and both genders equally. The peak age of onset is between 10 and 30 years. Almost 30% of patients with vitiligo have another affected family member. In some families, the pattern of inheritance is autosomal dominant with incomplete penetrance. Further studies are likely to reveal a polygenic inheritance pattern.

Antibodies to melanocytes and melanoma cells have been observed in 80% of patients. It is proposed that an autoimmune process, by an antibody-mediated mechanism, causes melanocyte destruction. Melanocytes may be destroyed by a neurotransmitter released from nerve terminals or the accumulation of toxic intermediates in the synthesis of melanin. Another proposed factor in the pathogenesis of vitiligo is exposure to chemicals that produce depigmentation, such as thiols, phenol, derivatives of catechol, quinones, and mercaptoamines. Loss of pigment follows both inhibition of tyrosinase and direct injury to melanocytes.

### Clinical Features

The lesions are symmetrically distributed, ivory-white, depigmented, round, oval, or irregularly shaped macules, with sharp and sometimes hyperpigmented borders. The initial hypopigmentation progresses to depigmentation, and enlargement occurs with peripheral extension. Exposed sites such as the hands, distal arms, and periorificial regions of the face are often the first to be involved. Other typical locations include the axilla, groin, gluteal cleft, areolae, elbows, knees, knuckles, umbilicus, and shins. Some patients have extensive loss of pigment on the oral mucosa and in areas of minor trauma. In many patients—especially those with diffuse disease—a severe sunburn, chemical exposure, emotional stress, or physical illness is the triggering event.

Vitiligo is most commonly associated with premature graying and **halo nevi**—normal melanocytic nevi with a peripheral depigmented rim. Pigment loss may be noted in the retina. Vitiligo may also occur in patients with malignant melanoma at the primary tumor site and as a widespread progressive process. Several autoimmune disorders are also associated with vitiligo, including alopecia areata, Hashimoto thyroiditis, hyperthyroidism, hypothyroidism, parathyroid disease, myasthenia gravis, diabetes mellitus, pernicious anemia, and idiopathic adrenal insufficiency.

### Diagnosis and Differential Diagnosis

The diagnosis is based on history and skin examination. Important clues are the distribution, history of potential precipitating events, associated endocrinopathies, and family history of vitiligo or early graying of the hair. A Wood's lamp examination is important to enhance early subtle lesions and establish an accurate baseline. The physician should inquire about changes in vision. If signs or symptoms suggest an endocrinopathy or collagen vascular disease, a thyroid-stimulating hormone and antibody panel (antinuclear antibody, antiparietal cell, antithyroid antibodies) should be obtained. Other important entities in the differential diagnosis include tinea versicolor, lichen sclerosus et atrophicus, postinflammatory hypopigmentation, leprosy, lupus erythematosus, sarcoidosis, and mycosis fungoides.

### Management

Treatment is neither required nor consistently effective. Spontaneous repigmentation occurs in less than 25% of cases—more commonly in children and in lesions younger than 2 years old. Usually, extended periods of stability occur and then exacerbations are triggered by stress or illness.

The two primary forms of treatment are topical steroids and phototherapy. Topical corticosteroids are most effective in early-stage vitiligo and in localized disease. Treatment should be initiated with high-potency topical steroids in a test area. PUVA consists of psoralens plus UVA phototherapy. The psoralens enhance the effect of the ultraviolet light, and therapy may be complicated by severe phototoxic reactions. A protracted treatment course is often required to induce repigmentation. Eye protection must be worn for 24 hours after ingestion of psoralens because of its deposition in the lens of the eye. Because compliance with these restrictions may be difficult with children, PUVA should be used with great caution in this age group. Patients treated with topical PUVA soak the involved area in a psoralen solution and then expose the skin to ultraviolet light.

## Questions

**Questions 1–3:** For each of the patients described in questions 1–3, refer to items A through H below and select the procedure that is most appropriate. Each item in A–H may be selected once, more than once, or not at all.

A. Potassium hydroxide (KOH) preparation
B. Skin biopsy
C. Dark-field examination
D. Tzanck smear
E. Wood's lamp examination
F. Gram stain
G. Scabies preparation
H. Patch testing

1. A 16-year-old girl has had painful, tense vesicles on her groin for the past 2 days.

2. A 5-year-old African-American child has a 3-week history of a scaling, itchy scalp.

3. A 21-year-old man has an intensely itchy rash between his fingers and on the scrotum. The itching gets worse at night. Numerous excoriations and crusting are noted in the web spaces. The lesions on the scrotum are more nodular.

**Questions 4–5:** For questions 4 and 5, select the drug from A through H below that is most likely responsible for the condition described. Each item in A–H may be used once, more than once, or not at all.

A. Clonidine
B. Propranolol
C. Trimethoprim–sulfamethoxazole
D. Phenytoin
E. Methotrexate
F. Penicillamine

G. Dapsone
H. Furosemide

4. A 56-year-old man with a long history of mild psoriasis of the elbows and knees has sudden, widespread exacerbation of psoriasis.

5. A 62-year-old woman has a 3-week-old eruption involving the head and neck. Erosions and blisters are seen in a seborrheic distribution. The oral mucosa is clear.

**Questions 6–8:** For each patient described in questions 6–8, identify the organism from the items listed in A through H below that is most likely to be responsible. Each item in A–H may be used once, more than once, or not at all.

A. *Trichophyton tonsurans*
B. Group A β-hemolytic streptococci
C. *Phthirus pubis*
D. *Pediculosis hominis*
E. *Sarcoptes scabiei*
F. Herpes zoster
G. Herpes simplex
H. *Candida albicans*

6. A 43-year-old woman has a red face for 2 days. Well-demarcated, erythematous plaques are seen on the entire lower right side of the face, and she has a fever of 102°F.

7. A 7-year-old girl has sudden onset of guttate, papulosquamous lesions 2 weeks after an upper respiratory infection.

8. A 25-year-old man has intense pruritus localized to the groin. Excoriations in the groin and adherent, white lesions on the eyelashes are noted.

**Questions 9–12:** For each question below, select the **one** lettered answer that is **best** for that question.

9. An 82-year-old woman has had a blistering eruption for 2 months. Tense blisters are seen on an erythematous base, localized to the intertriginous areas, with sparing of mucous membranes. These clinical findings are most compatible with which of the following:
   A. Pemphigus vulgaris
   B. Pemphigus foliaceus
   C. Dermatitis herpetiformis
   D. Bullous pemphigoid
   E. Erythema multiforme

10. A 42-year-old man with lichen simplex chronicus is given a topical steroid for use. The major barrier to absorption of the medication into his skin will be which of the following:
   A. Lamina lucida
   B. Stratum basale
   C. Dermis
   D. Stratum corneum
   E. Stratum granulosum

11. A 36-year-old man has an atrophic nail with pterygium formation. The papulosquamous disorder most likely to cause these findings is which of the following:
   A. Psoriasis
   B. Lichen planus
   C. Pityriasis rosea
   D. Mycosis fungoides
   E. Discoid lupus

12. A 24-year-old man is placed on topical steroids for a rash in the periorbital region. You caution him not to get the medication into his eye because this can lead to which of the following:
   A. Pseudotumor cerebri
   B. Hypopyon
   C. Keratitis
   D. Iritis
   E. Glaucoma

## Answers

| | | | | |
|---|---|---|---|---|
| 1. D | 2. A | 3. G | 4. B | 5. F |
| 6. B | 7. B | 8. C | 9. D | 10. D |
| 11. B | 12. E | | | |

## SUGGESTED READING


***Textbooks and Monographs***

Champion RH, Burton JL, Ebling FJG (eds). Textbook of Dermatology. London: Blackwell Scientific, 1992.

Fitzpatrick TB, Eisen AZ, Wolff IC, et al. Dermatology in General Medicine. New York: McGraw-Hill, 1993.

***Articles***

*Therapy*

Thiers BH. Dermatology therapy update. Med Clin North Am 1998;82:1405–1414.

Lipper GM, Arndt KA, Dover JS. Recent therapeutic advances in dermatology. JAMA 2000;283:175–177.

Pierard GE, Pierard-Franchimont C, Ben Mosbah T, et al. Adverse effects of topical corticosteroids. Acta Derm Venereol 1989;69:26–30.

*Papulosquamous Disorders*

Boyd AS, Nelder KH. Lichen planus. J Am Acad Dermatol 1991;25:593–619.

Fox BJ, Odom RB. Papulosquamous diseases: a review. J Am Acad Dermatol 1985;12:597–624.

Stern RS. Psoriasis. Lancet 1997;350:349–353.

Simpson KR, Lowe NJ. Trends in topical psoriasis therapy. Int J Dermatol 1994; 33:333–336.

### *Vesiculobullous Disorders*

Nousari HC, Anhalt GJ. Pemphigus and bullous pemphigoid. Lancet 1999;354:667–672.

Scott JE, Ahmed AR. The blistering diseases. Med Clin North Am 1998;82:1239–1283.

### *Hypersensitivity Disorders*

Calabrese LH. Cutaneous vasculitis, hypersensitivity vasculitis, erythema nodosum, and pyoderma gangrenosum. Curr Opin Rheum 1991;3:23–27.

Weston WL, Badgett JT. Urticaria. Pediatr Rev 1998;19: 240–244.

Viard I, Wehrli P, Bullani R, et al. Inhibition of toxic epidermal necrolysis by blockade of CD95 with human intravenous immunoglobulin. Science 1998;282:490–493.

Roujeau JC. Treatment of severe drug eruptions. J Dermatol 1999;26:718–722.

Parsons JM. Toxic epidermal necrolysis. Int J Dermatol 1992;31:749–768.

### *Dermatitis—Eczema*

Sidbury R, Hanifin JM. Old, new, and emerging therapies for atopic dermatitis. Dermatol Clin 2000;18:1–11.

Hanifin JM, Tofte SJ. Update on therapy of atopic dermatitis. J Allergy Clin Immunol 1999;104:S123–125.

Leung DY. Pathogenesis of atopic dermatitis. J Allergy Clin Immunol 1999;104:S99–108.

Rietschel RL, Ray MC. Nonatopic eczemas. J Am Acad Dermatol 1988;18:569–573.

### *Benign Tumors of the Skin*

Gallagher RP, McLean DI, Yang CP, et al. Suntan, sunburn, and pigmentation factors and the frequency of acquired melanocytic nevi in children. Similarities to melanoma: the Vancouver mole study. Arch Dermatol 1990;126:770–776.

Lindelof B, Sigurgeirsson B, Melander S. Seborrheic keratoses and cancer. J Am Acad Dermatol 1992;26:947–950.

Murray JC. Keloids and hypertrophic scars. Clin Dermatol 1994;12:27–37.

### *Malignant Tumors of the Skin*

Bruce AJ, Brodland DG. Overview of skin cancer detection and prevention for the primary care physician. Mayo Clinic Proc 2000;75:491–500.

Skidmore RA Jr, Flowers FP. Nonmelanoma skin cancer. Med Clin North Am 1998;82:1309–1323.

Rigel DS, Carucci JA. Malignant melanoma: prevention, early detection, and treatment in the 21st century. CA Cancer J Clin 2000;50:215–240.

Jerant AF, Johnson JT, Sheridan CD, et al. Early detection and treatment of skin cancer. Am Fam Physician 2000;62:357–368, 375–376, 381–382.

Lange JR. The current status of sentinel node biopsy in the management of melanoma. Dermatol Surg 26:809–810, 2000.

### *Acne*

Healy E, Simpson N. Acne vulgaris. BMJ 1994;308:831–833.

Wilkin JK. Rosacea. Pathophysiology and treatment. Arch Dermatol 1994;130:359–362.

Thiboutot DM. Acne and rosacea. New and emerging therapies. Dermatol Clin 2000;18:63–71.

### *Fungal Infections of the Skin*

Brodell RT, Elewski B. Superficial fungal infections. Errors to avoid in diagnosis and treatment. Postgrad Med 1997;101: 279–287.

Lesher JL Jr. Oral therapy of common superficial fungal infections of the skin. J Am Acad Dermatol 1999;40: S31–34.

Gupta AK, Sauder DN, Shear NH. Antifungal agents: an overview (part 1). J Am Acad Dermatol 1994;30:677–700.

Gupta AK, Sauder DN, Shear NH. Antifungal agents: an overview (part 2). J Am Acad Dermatol 1994;30:911–933.

Mehregan DA, Mehregan DR, Rinker A. Onychomycosis. Cutis 1997;59:247–248.

### *Bacterial Infections of the Skin*

Dahl MV. Strategies for the management of recurrent furunculosis. South Med J 1987;80:352–356.

Elsner P. Treatment of bacterial sexually transmitted diseases. Semin Dermatol 1993;12:342–351.

Feingold DS. Staphylococcal and streptococcal pyodermas. Semin Dermatol 1993;12:296–300.

Grosshans EM. The red face: Erysipelas. Clin Dermatol 1993;11:307–313.

Johnson PC, Farnie MA. Testing for syphilis. Dermatol Clin 1994;12:9–12.

Kraus SJ. Diagnosis and management of acute genital ulcers in sexually active patients. Semin Dermatol 1990;9: 160–166.

Schachner L, Gonzalez A. Diagnosis and treatment of impetigo. J Am Acad Dermatol 1989;20:132.

### *Viral Infections of the Skin*

Cobb MW. Human papillomavirus infection. J Am Acad Dermatol 1990;22:547–566.

Corey L, Spear PG. Infections with herpes simplex viruses (I). N Engl J Med 1986;314:169–172.

Corey L, Spear PG. Infections with herpes simplex viruses (II). N Engl J Med 1986;314: 686–691.

Emmert DH. Treatment of common cutaneous herpes simplex virus infections. Am Fam Physician 2000;61:1697–706, 1708.

Green J. Therapy for genital warts. Dermatol Clin 1992;10: 253–267.

Williams LR, Webster G. Warts and molluscum contagiosum. Clin Dermatol 1991;9:87–93.

### *Infestations of the Skin*

Chosidow O. Scabies and pediculosis. Lancet 2000;355: 819–826.

Rasmussen JE. Scabies. Pediatr Rev 1994;15:110–114.

### *Pigmentary Disorders of the Skin*

Kovacs SO, Vitiligo. J Am Acad Dermatol 1998;38:647–666.

Halder RM, Young CM. New and emerging therapies for vitiligo. Dermatol Clin 2000;18:79–89.

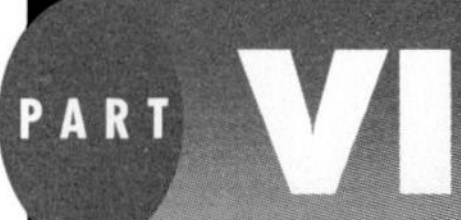

PART VI

Diana L. Maas
Albert L. Jochen
Irene M. O'Shaughnessy

# ENDOCRINE AND METABOLIC DISORDERS

# CHAPTER 63 DISEASES OF THE ANTERIOR PITUITARY GLAND

The pituitary gland has three lobes: the anterior (adenohypophysis), the posterior (neurohypophysis), and the intermediate. It is surrounded by important structures that can be affected by its enlargement, including the optic chiasm, cranial nerves, and the internal carotid artery; the latter two are contained within the cavernous sinuses. The infundibular stalk connects the pituitary gland with the hypothalamus and contains the portal plexus. The adenohypophyseal hormones are regulated by a neuroendocrine system of stimulatory and inhibitory peptides produced in the ventral hypothalamus and transported to the anterior lobe through the hypothalamic-hypophyseal portal system.

## Production and Function of Adenohypophyseal Hormones

Six major hormones are synthesized and released by the anterior pituitary: corticotropin (ACTH), thyroid-stimulating hormone (TSH), prolactin (PRL), follicle-stimulating hormone (FSH), luteinizing hormone (LH), and growth hormone (GH). Their major regulatory pathways and end-organ products are shown in Figure 63.1. All of the anterior pituitary hormones, except possibly prolactin, are feedback-controlled by their end-organ secretory products, at both the hypothalamic and pituitary levels. Prolactin is primarily regulated by an inhibitory factor, dopamine. Secretion of GH is pulsatile throughout the day, with the largest secretory peak in young, healthy adults occurring 60 to 120 minutes after the onset of stages 3 and 4 sleep. Secretion of ACTH and the levels of plasma cortisol that it evokes are widely pulsatile but strongly diurnal; both hormones peak at around 8 a.m., and the lowest levels are found between 6 p.m. and midnight. The normally pulsatile gonadotropin-releasing hormone (GnRH) secretion stimulates release of LH and FSH; when infused continuously, however, it inhibits LH and FSH release.

The major site of action of the hormone prolactin is the mammary gland, where it stimulates postpartum lactation. Prolactin inhibits GnRH release in the hypothalamus. Growth hormone exerts its effects directly and

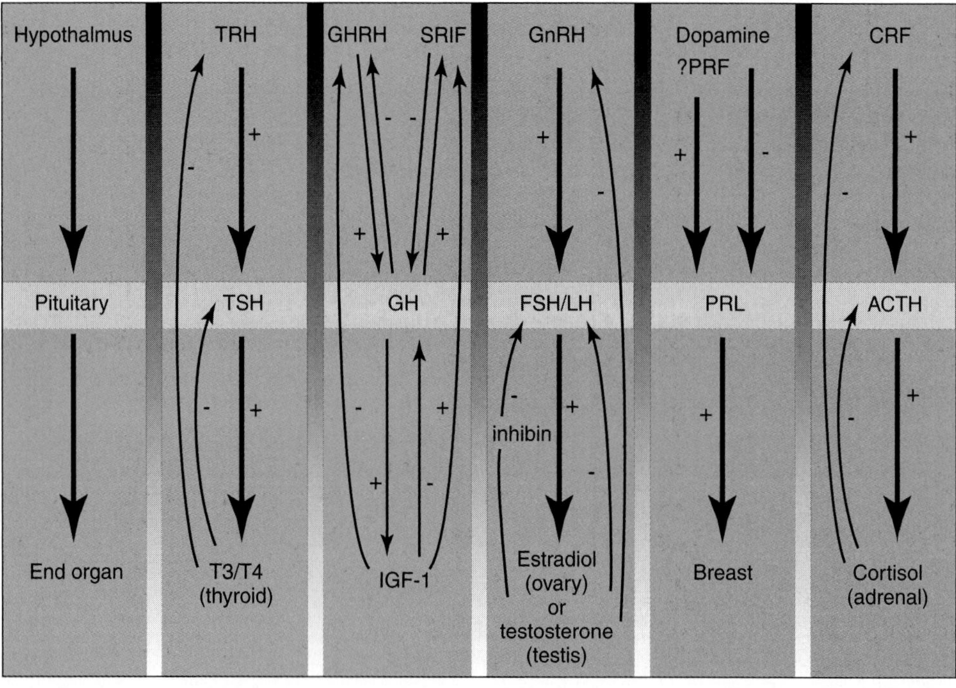


**FIGURE 63.1.** Regulatory pathways for the six major adenohypophyseal hormones. CRH = corticotropin releasing hormone; GHRH = growth hormone releasing hormone; GnRH = gonadotropin releasing hormone; IGF-I = insulin-like growth factor-I; PRF = prolactin releasing factor; SRIF = somatostatin.

indirectly through its synthesis of insulin-like growth factor I (IGF-I, somatomedin-C), mainly in the liver. Growth hormone also stimulates skeletal and soft tissue growth, lipolysis in adipose tissue, protein synthesis (especially) in muscle, and lactotropic activity by breast tissue; by antagonizing insulin, it inhibits cellular glucose uptake and stimulates hepatic gluconeogenesis and glycogenolysis. The effects on skeletal growth may be partially mediated through IGF-I. In both genders, the major functional roles of the gonadotropins LH and FSH include pubertal sexual development, fertility, and sexual activity; most of these functions are mediated through estrogen and progesterone in women and through testosterone in men. The major effect of ACTH is on the adrenal glands, where it stimulates synthesis and secretion of glucocorticoids and adrenal androgens. TSH stimulates all aspects of the synthesis and secretion of the thyroid hormones, thyroxine ($T_4$) and triiodothyronine ($T_3$).

## Pituitary Tumors

Pituitary tumors, which usually are benign, account for between 10% and 15% of intracranial tumors. A pituitary adenoma is the most common cause of pituitary insufficiency and pituitary masses in adults. Types of pituitary adenomas and their prevalence are listed in Table 63.1. These tumors are considered microadenomas if the vertical height on magnetic resonance imaging (MRI) or computed tomography (CT) is 10 mm or less, or as macroadenomas if vertical height exceeds 10 mm. Typically, a pituitary tumor presents with signs and symptoms related to mass effect or endocrine dysfunction.

Common clinical features of a pituitary mass include headache, visual field deficits, and cranial nerve palsies. The headache typically is retro-orbital or bitemporal. Its pathogenesis is unknown, but may be due to stretching of dura mater. The classic visual field abnormality, which is formally tested by Goldman perimetry, is bitemporal hemianopsia; it results from suprasellar tumor extension and compression of the optic chiasm. A pituitary tumor laterally invading into the cavernous sinuses may lead to dysfunction of cranial nerves III, IV, and VI, causing ophthalmoplegia, and of cranial nerves V1 and V2, causing facial pain.

The endocrine dysfunction may be due to hyposecretion or hypersecretion of a pituitary hormone by the tumor. Anterior pituitary hormone insufficiency is diagnosed biochemically (Table 63.2) and clinically (e.g., gonadal failure, hypothyroidism, and adrenal insufficiency). Hormonal insufficiency due to a pituitary

**TABLE 63.1. Incidence of Pituitary Adenomas**

| | |
|---|---|
| Prolactin-secreting | 27–29% |
| Nonsecretory or null cell | 25% |
| GH-secreting | 13–16% |
| ACTH-secreting | 10–14% |
| Plurihormonal | 8–12% |
| LH/FSH/alpha subunit-secreting | 2–9% |
| Silent adenomas (ACTH-staining) | 5% |
| TSH-secreting | 1% |

**TABLE 63.2. Evaluation for Pituitary Insufficiency**

| Pituitary Hormone | Laboratory Evaluation | Abnormal Results |
|---|---|---|
| ACTH | Insulin-induced hypoglycemia or CRF stimulation test | Cortisol level <18 μg/dl in response to symptomatic hypoglycemia (plasma glucose <40 mg/dl) or CRF injection |
| | Overnight metyrapone: Drug that inhibits the enzyme 11 β-hydroxylase which catalyzes the conversion of 11-deoxycortisol (compound S) into cortisol (compound F) | Cortisol level <5 μg/dl and 11-deoxycortisol <7 μg/dl |
| FSH, LH | Simultaneous assessment of basal FSH/LH/17 β-estradiol | Low 17 β-estradiol with low or inappropriately normal FSH and LH |
| | Simultaneous assessment of basal FSH/LH/testosterone | Low total testosterone with low or inappropriately normal FSH and LH |
| TSH | Simultaneous assessment of TSH/free $T_4$ | Low free $T_4$ with low or inappropriately normal TSH |
| GH | Insulin-induced hypoglycemia<br>Clonidine, 0.25 mg<br>Exercise for 20 minutes | GH level <7 ng/ml |

CRF = corticotropin-releasing factor; FSH = follicle-stimulating hormone; GH = growth hormone; LH = luteinizing hormone; TSH = thyroid-stimulating hormone.

tumor may involve any or all of the six major pituitary hormones; it usually results from compression of normal pituitary tissue by the tumor. The earliest and most common manifestation of pituitary hormonal deficiency is impotence in men and amenorrhea in women; in children, growth retardation and delayed puberty are common presenting signs. The tumor may compress the pituitary gonadotrophs, thus directly decreasing gonadotropin secretion. Alternatively, the elevated blood levels of prolactin **(hyperprolactinemia)** produced by a prolactin-secreting pituitary tumor inhibit the hypothalamic-derived GnRH, thus indirectly decreasing gonadotropin secretion. There are some variations, but pituitary hormones usually are lost in the following order: GH, FSH/LH, TSH, ACTH; prolactin deficiency is rare because pituitary macroadenomas usually produce mild hyperprolactinemia (PRL 20–100 ng/ml), which results from decreased dopamine inhibition due to infundibular stalk interruption.

Pituitary hormone replacement is discussed in Table 63.3. Although GH replacement is not routinely done in adults, some studies show positive effects on lean body mass and overall well-being.

A functional morphological classification of pituitary adenomas, which has gained wide acceptance, is useful in predicting the biologic behavior of the various tumor types and in planning appropriate treatment strategies. The initial laboratory work-up of a newly diagnosed pituitary tumor is shown in Table 63.4.

## Lactotroph Adenomas and Hyperprolactinemia

### Epidemiology

Hyperprolactinemia accounts for at least 20% of infertility in women and approximately 8% of sexual dysfunction in men, including infertility. The causes of pathologic hyperprolactinemia are diverse (Table 63.5), but a prolactin-secreting pituitary tumor is, by far, the most common cause. The pathogenesis of these tumors is unknown.

### Clinical features and diagnosis

The clinical presentation of prolactinomas varies with the patient's age and gender. Typically, young menstruating women report irregular menses (amenorrhea, oligomenorrhea, or delayed menarche), infertility, or galactorrhea. Galactorrhea occurs in 30% to 80% of affected women. Hyperprolactinemia directly suppresses hypothalamic GnRH secretion, resulting in amenorrhea. Because they cause early disturbance in the menstrual cycle, prolactinomas typically are microadenomas at the

**TABLE 63.3. Treatment of Panhypopituitarism**

| Pituitary Hormone | Hormone Replacement |
|---|---|
| ACTH | Cortisone acetate, 25 mg a.m., 12.5 mg p.m., or<br>Hydrocortisone 20 mg a.m., 10 mg p.m. |
| TSH | Thyroxine: dosage adjusted to keep free $T_4$ in the normal range |
| FSH/LH | Men: testosterone enanthate or cypionate, 200 mg IM q 2 weeks; testosterone patch or gel<br>Women: estrogen therapy, oral or transdermal, adjusted to relieve symptoms |
| GH | Synthetic GH subcutaneous injections:<br>In prepubertal children: 3-7× per week<br>In adults: 3× per week |

**TABLE 63.4. Laboratory Evaluation of Pituitary Tumors**

| Pituitary Tumor | Biochemical Features |
|---|---|
| Prolactinoma | Serum prolactin level usually >200 ng/ml |
| Acromegaly | Somatomedin C elevated above normal level for age. Nonsuppressible serum GH level >2 ng/ml 2 hours after 75-g oral glucose load |
| Cushing disease | Elevated 24-hour urinary free cortisol (always obtain simultaneous urine creatinine to ensure specimen is sufficient)<br>1-mg dexamethasone (given at 11 p.m. the night before) suppression test: abnormal if 8 a.m. fasting serum cortisol >5 μg/dl |
| TSH-secreting | Serum TSH inappropriately normal or elevated with elevated free $T_4$<br>Serum alpha subunit elevated, alpha subunit/TSH >1 |
| FSH/LH/alpha subunit–secreting | Elevated serum LH, FSH, or alpha-subunit |

TABLE 63.5. Causes of Hyperprolactinemia

| Category | Examples/Disorders |
|---|---|
| **Physiologic** | Pregnancy, nipple stimulation/suckling<br>Stress, exercise, sleep |
| **Pathologic** | |
| Pituitary adenoma | Prolactin-secreting pituitary tumor<br>Plurihormonal-secreting pituitary tumor (acromegaly) |
| Hypothalamic-pituitary disorders causing hyperprolactinemia in the absence of a prolactinoma | Tumor (e.g., craniopharyngioma, germinoma)<br>Histiocytosis X<br>Sarcoidosis<br>Pituitary stalk interruption<br>Surgery |
| Adrenal insufficiency | |
| Cirrhosis | |
| Primary hypothyroidism | |
| Renal failure | |
| Drug-induced | Estrogens/oral contraceptives<br>Psychotropic drugs (e.g. phenothiazines, tricyclic antidepressants)<br>Methyldopa<br>Metoclopramide<br>Opiates<br>Cimetidine<br>Cocaine |
| Neurogenic | Chest wall lesions/surgery<br>Spinal cord lesions |
| "Functional"/idiopathic | |

time of diagnosis. In contrast, men and postmenopausal women usually present with macroprolactinomas that produce tumor mass–related effects. Approximately 80% of affected men report decreased libido, and most are fully or partially impotent; galactorrhea occurs in 20% to 30%.

A serum PRL level higher than 200 ng/ml is diagnostic of a prolactinoma. Although a slightly elevated PRL level (20–200 ng/ml) may be the result of a microprolactinoma, mild PRL elevations also may result from one of several secondary causes (e.g., infundibular stalk compression, renal failure, primary hypothyroidism, or drugs).

### Management and prognosis

The dopamine agonists bromocriptine and cabergoline decrease serum prolactin levels consistently and rapidly and reduce tumor size in 80% of patients. Dopamine agonists are, therefore, the treatment of choice for all clinically significant microprolactinomas and macroprolactinomas. Many clinicians advocate initial treatment with a dopamine agonist for all patients, even those with visual abnormalities. Surgical resection is reserved for prolactinomas that do not respond to medical therapy or for patients who cannot tolerate the side effects of the dopamine agonists. External radiotherapy is reserved for the occasional patient who is refractory to or intolerant of these conventional therapies. The ultimate goal of therapy, whether medical or surgical, is decompression of the optic chiasm, correction of cranial nerve abnormalities, and resumption of normal pituitary hormone function.

## Somatotroph Adenoma or Acromegaly

### Definition and epidemiology

Acromegaly—abnormal enlargement of the extremities of the skeleton caused by hypersecretion of GH after maturity—has an estimated annual incidence of three to four cases per million, without any gender predilection. It can occur at any age, but is most commonly diagnosed in the fourth or fifth decade of life. Approximately 85% of cases result from a GH-secreting pituitary macroadenoma (Table 63.6). GH-producing pituitary tumors account for nearly 17% of all surgically resected pituitary tumors; about 30% of these tumors also secrete prolactin. Excessive GH secretion in a prepubertal child prior to the closure of the epiphyseal growth plates leads to gigantism; this condition is very rare.

### Clinical features and diagnosis

The manifestations of excessive GH secretion (Table 63.7 and Figure 63.2) usually develop gradually in older patients. Because these changes are insidious, they are

**TABLE 63.6. Causes of Acromegaly**

| Causes of Acromegaly |
|---|
| Pituitary adenoma |
| Pure growth hormone secreting |
| Mixed growth hormone/prolactin secreting |
| Ectopic pituitary tumor |
| Sphenoid sinus |
| Parapharyngeal sinus |
| Ectopic GHRH secreting tumor |
| Small cell carcinoma of the lung |
| Carcinoid |
| Pancreatic islet tumor |
| Adrenal adenoma |
| Pheochromocytoma |
| Ectopic GH secreting tumor (rare) |
| Pancreas |
| Lung |
| Ovary |
| Breast |

GH = growth hormone; GHRH = growth hormone releasing hormone.

**TABLE 63.7. Clinical Manifestations of Acromegaly**

| Clinical Manifestations of Acromegaly |
|---|
| Coarsening facial features/soft tissue swelling |
| Frontal bossing |
| Dental malocclusion with increased spacing between teeth |
| Headaches |
| Excessive sweating |
| Soft tissue swelling in hands/feet |
| Increased ring/glove size |
| Increased shoe size/width with thick heel pad |
| Skin tags |
| Colon polyps/cancer |
| Carpal tunnel syndrome |
| Hypertension |
| Diabetes mellitus |
| Deep, resonant voice/laryngeal thickening |
| Obstructive sleep apnea |
| Galactorrhea |
| Osteoarthritis—especially knees and hips |
| Visceromegaly |

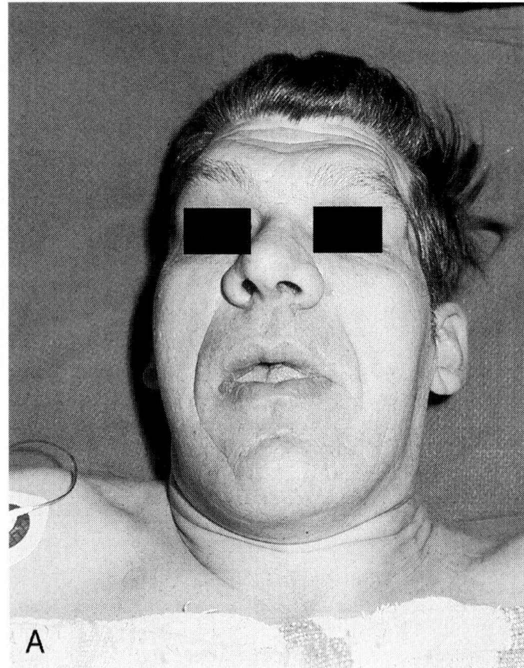


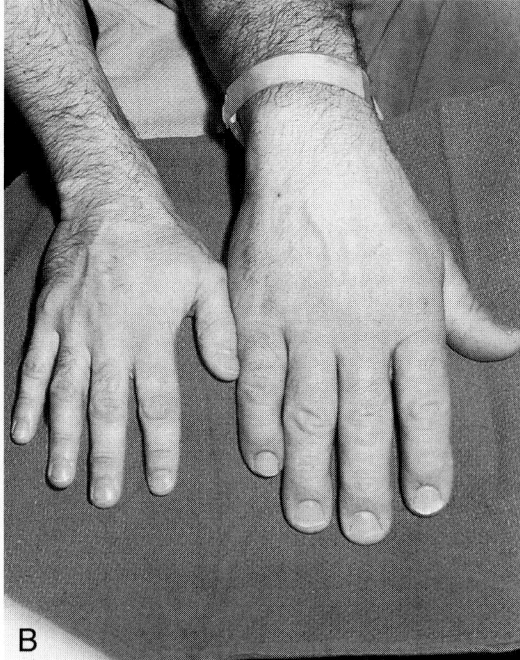


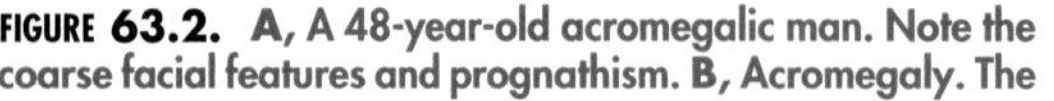

**FIGURE 63.2. A,** A 48-year-old acromegalic man. Note the coarse facial features and prognathism. **B,** Acromegaly. The hand on the left is that of a normal man; the one on the right is that of the man with acromegaly shown in part **A.**

often missed by the patient and, instead, are first noted by someone who has not seen the patient for a long time. In younger patients, these tumors are more aggressive; thus, the characteristic features evolve more rapidly. Besides the characteristic facial and acral soft tissue changes produced by excessive GH secretion, the sellar mass itself also may evoke symptoms from local effects. Nearly one half of patients with acromegaly harbor colonic polyps, and about 5% of all acromegalics develop colon cancer. Risk factors for neoplasia include age above 50, duration of acromegaly exceeding 10 years, and presence of three or more skin tags.

A serum somatomedin C level usually suffices as a screening test for acromegaly. Diagnostic biochemical criteria are elevated somatomedin C and nonsuppressible serum GH level above 2 ng/ml 2 hours after a 75-g oral glucose load.

### Management and prognosis

Acromegaly is difficult to cure. Treatment goals include lowering the serum GH level below 2 ng/ml 2 hours after a 75-g oral glucose administration; normalizing the somatomedin C level; and reversing associated medical problems, including diabetes mellitus, hypertension, soft tissue hyperplasia, and hyperhidrosis. Management options include surgery, radiotherapy, and medications; most patients require all three. Surgical removal or debulking of the tumor remains the first line of therapy. A surgical cure can be obtained in 80% of patients with microadenomas. Using the biochemical criteria listed earlier, surgery cures less than 30% of patients with macroadenomas. The somatostatin analogue octreotide, and the dopamine agonists bromocriptine and cabergoline, are used as medical therapy for acromegaly. Octreotide is useful as adjunctive therapy when cure is not achieved by surgery or radiation. It also can be used preoperatively to reduce the tumor size. Some patients respond to dopamine agonists; octreotide and a dopamine agonist also can be combined.

## Corticotroph Adenoma or Cushing Disease

### Definition and epidemiology

**Cushing syndrome** is a condition caused by excess amounts of cortisol in the bloodstream **(hypercortisolemia),** resulting from hypersecretion of the adrenal cortex or prolonged exposure to high therapeutic doses of glucocorticoids. It has widespread systemic effects (Table 63.8). **Cushing disease** refers to a subset of Cushing syndrome resulting from pituitary ACTH hypersecretion; it accounts for approximately 75% to 85% of adults with Cushing syndrome. The underlying pathology in about 90% of cases of Cushing disease is anterior pituitary microadenomas; pituitary hyperplasia underlies the remaining 10%. Cushing disease is six times more common in women than in men; the mean age at diagnosis is in the fourth decade.

| TABLE 63.8. Clinical Manifestations of Hypercortisolemia |
|---|
| Truncal obesity |
| Hypertension |
| Facial plethora (round face) |
| Hirsutism/vellus type hair growth |
| Gonadal dysfunction |
| Menstrual disorders |
| Impotence/decreased libido |
| Osteopenia/back pain |
| Supraclavicular/dorsocervical fat pads |
| Neuropsychiatric disorders/depression |
| Violaceous abdominal striae >1 cm wide |
| Proximal muscle weakness |
| Headache |
| Acne |
| Easy bruising |
| Superficial fungal infections |
| Poor wound healing |
| Hyperpigmentation |
| Glucose intolerance/diabetes mellitus |
| Nephrolithiasis |

### Etiology and pathogenesis

Iatrogenic (exogenous) causes are the most common, because of the widespread use of pharmacologic doses of glucocorticoids. Endogenous cases may be either ACTH-dependent (e.g., ACTH-secreting pituitary adenoma or ectopic ACTH-secreting neoplasm) or ACTH-independent (e.g., adrenal adenoma, adrenal carcinoma). Benign adrenal tumors causing Cushing syndrome predominantly produce glucocorticoids; adrenal cancers, however, often secrete high levels of adrenal **androgens** and **glucocorticoids.** Ectopic ACTH secretion occurs in a few neoplasms (e.g., small cell carcinoma of the lung, carcinoid tumors, pancreatic islet cell tumors), usually in men in the fifth decade and beyond.

### Clinical features

It is helpful to examine serial photographs of the patient (Figure 63.3), looking for evidence of progressive physical changes consistent with excessive cortisol exposure. The facial plethora (round face) may be subtle (see Figure 63.3) or quite obvious (Figure 63.4). Cushing syndrome also can be caused by ectopic production of ACTH by certain cancers, classically in small cell cancer of the lung. These patients more frequently present with severe proximal weakness, weight loss, and hypokalemia along with rapid development of the florid clinical manifestations of Cushing syndrome.

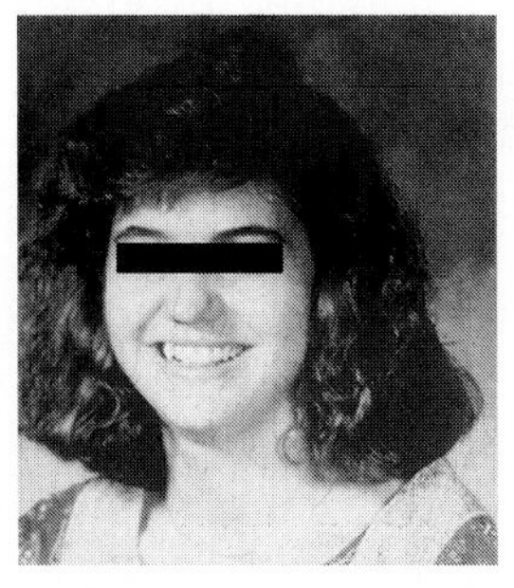
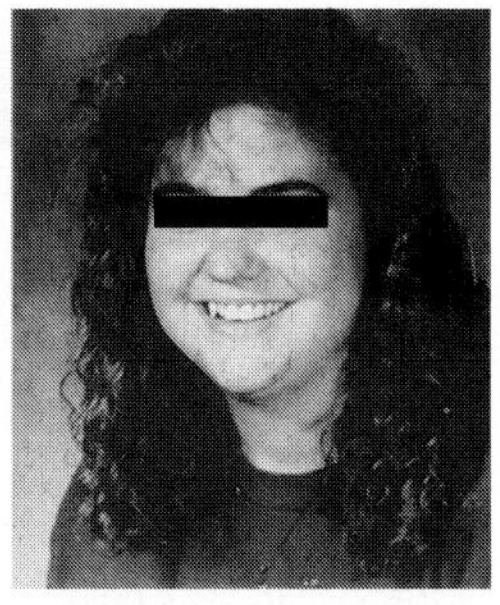

**FIGURE 63.3. These photographs of a young woman with Cushing syndrome show subtle changes in the facial outlines over a 3-year period.**
(Photographs courtesy of James Findling, MD, St. Luke's Hospital, Milwaukee, Wisconsin.)

## Diagnosis

The evaluation of a patient with suspected Cushing syndrome is outlined in Figure 63.5. Screening with the 24-hour urinary free cortisol results in very few false-positives; the 1-mg dexamethasone suppression test, however, may be false-positive from acute stress or illness, obesity, anticonvulsant agents, liver disease, high estrogen states, alcoholism, or affective disorders. Elevated salivary cortisol levels, obtained at 11 p.m., can also be used to confirm the presence of glucocorticoid excess. Once hypercortisolemia is established, the distinction between ACTH-dependence and ACTH-independence should follow, based on measurement of plasma ACTH; levels exceeding 20 pg/ml indicate ACTH-dependent hypercortisolism. Patients with primary adrenal neoplasms have a suppressed or low plasma ACTH (<10 pg/ml) and adrenal mass on CT scan. ACTH-dependent Cushing syndrome must be further separated into a pituitary tumor or an ectopic ACTH-secreting neoplasm. A normal CT or MRI of the sella cannot make this distinction, because only 50% to 60% of patients with Cushing disease have a sellar abnormality on MRI or CT.

### Management and prognosis

Transsphenoidal resection is the treatment of choice for the ACTH-secreting pituitary neoplasm; adrenalectomy is the preferred treatment in glucocorticoid-producing adrenal neoplasms. Remissions occur in approximately 80% to 90% of patients with Cushing disease who undergo transsphenoidal adenoma resection. Conventional external radiotherapy is not effective as a primary treatment, but it may be combined with pituitary surgery. Heavy charged-particle stereotactic radiosurgery (gamma knife) also is used as adjuvant initial therapy, but has a higher complication rate (e.g., cranial nerve palsies, visual field defects, and hypopituitarism). Ectopic ACTH production is managed by treating the primary tumor or by using adrenolytic agents such as mitotane, aminoglutethimide, or metyrapone. These agents also are useful in inoperable cases.

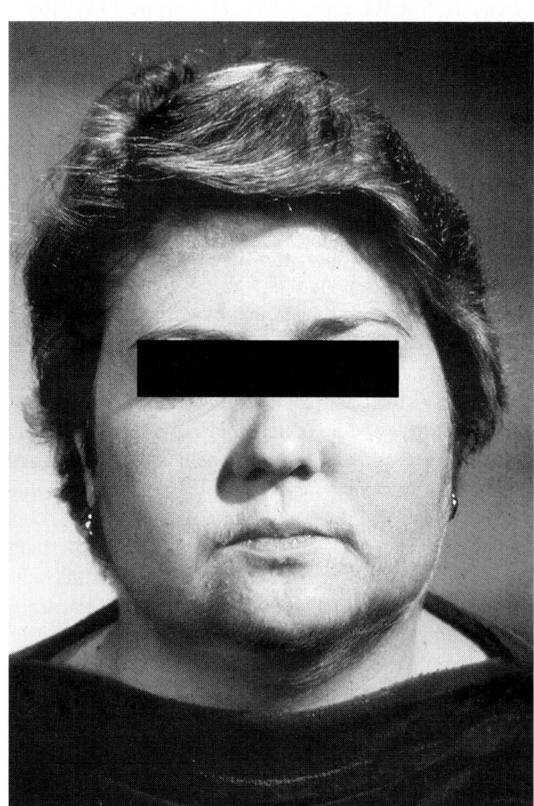

**FIGURE 63.4. This photograph of a middle-aged woman with Cushing syndrome demonstrates the characteristic plethoric facies.**
(Photograph courtesy of James Findling, MD, St. Luke's Hospital, Milwaukee, Wisconsin.)

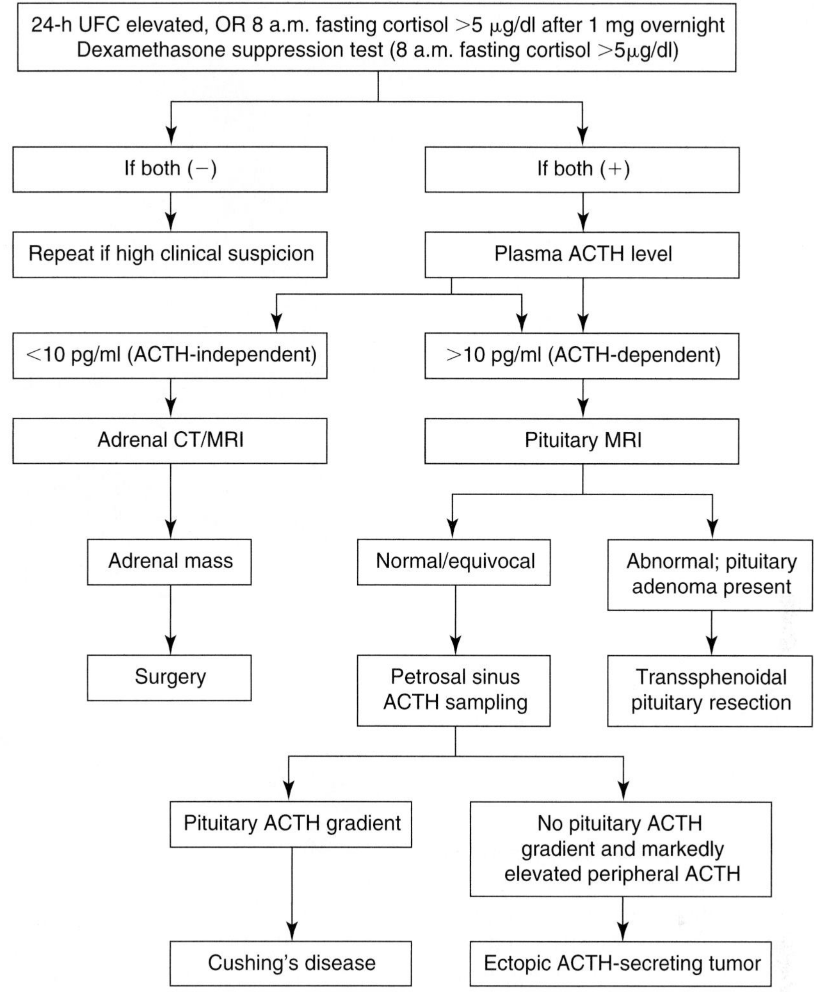


**FIGURE 63.5. Work-up for the diagnosis and further differentiation of Cushing syndrome. UFC = urinary free cortisol.**

# CHAPTER 64 DISORDERS OF THE POSTERIOR PITUITARY GLAND

The posterior lobe of the pituitary, which makes up only 20% of the total pituitary mass, is one of the three components of the neurohypophysis, the other two being the hypothalamic supraoptic and paraventricular neurons and the supraopticohypophyseal tract (Figure 64.1). The neurohypophyseal hormones are regulated by a direct neurosecretory pathway from the anterior hypothalamus.

The posterior pituitary secretes two major peptide hormones, **oxytocin** and **vasopressin** (which is known also as **antidiuretic hormone [ADH]**). Both of these hormones are synthesized in the hypothalamus, packaged into neurosecretory granules, transported along axons to the posterior pituitary gland, and stored until they are released into the blood stream (see Figure 64.1). Oxytocin stimulates uterine contraction, but its importance in normal parturition is unclear. Nipple stimulation by the suckling infant causes pituitary release of oxytocin, followed by milk ejection. Antidiuretic hormone is the major regulator of renal water excretion, and, therefore, of the total body water balance. Its deficiency causes diabetes insipidus (DI) with hypernatremia and

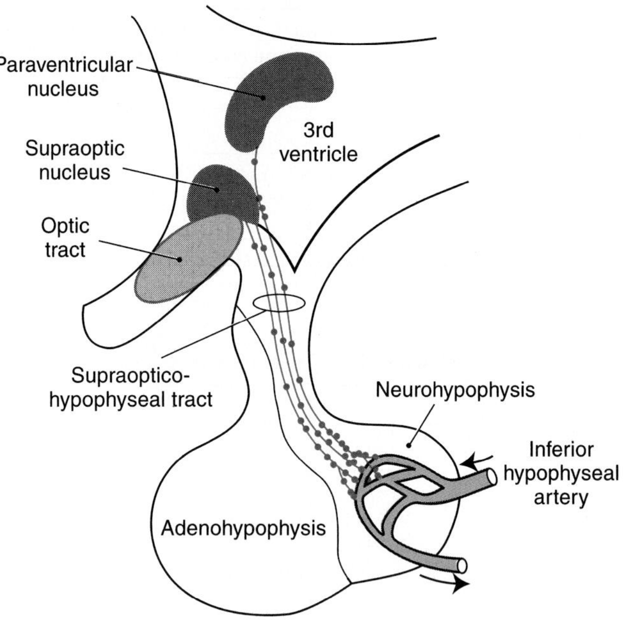


**FIGURE 64.1.** A schematic illustration of the neurohypophysis, including the hypothalamic paraventricular and supraoptic nuclei, supraopticohypophyseal tract, and posterior pituitary gland (neurohypophysis).

polyuria; excess ADH leads to syndrome of inappropriate ADH (SIADH) with hyponatremia and oliguria.

## Diabetes Insipidus

### Definition

**Diabetes insipidus** is characterized by **polyuria,** defined as the excretion of urine in excess of 2 to 3 L/24 hours. Large volumes of dilute urine are excreted, giving rise to severe **polydipsia** (excessive thirst) and a specific craving for ice water. Biochemical and clinical hallmarks of DI are listed in Table 64.1.

### Etiology, Pathogenesis, and Clinical Features

The three major types of DI are **hypothalamic** (central), **nephrogenic** or renal-resistant, and **dipsogenic primary polydipsia** (Table 64.2). There are two primary differences between hypothalamic and nephrogenic DI: (1) the plasma ADH concentration and (2) the response to vasopressin injection. Dipsogenic primary polydipsia results from overdrinking, with resultant polyuria and ADH suppression.

Hypothalamic DI is uncommon; it requires the destruction of at least 90% of ADH-synthesizing hypothalamic neurons. Diabetes insipidus caused by destruction of the posterior pituitary gland is not permanent, because the axons can regenerate new axon and capillary contacts to release ADH. Nearly two thirds of cases of traumatic and postsurgical DI are transient, but idiopathic DI is almost always permanent. Postoperative DI has a rapid onset, usually developing within 24 hours follow-

**TABLE 64.1. Biochemical and Clinical Hallmarks of Diabetes Insipidus**

| | |
|---|---|
| **Clinical** | |
| Polyuria | |
| Urine output | >200 ml/hr |
| Mild: | 2–4 L/day |
| Moderate: | 4–6 L/day |
| Severe: | >6 L/day |
| Polydipsia: | |
| Especially crave very cold fluids/ice water | |
| **Biochemical** | |
| Urine | |
| Specific gravity | ≤1.005 |
| $Osm_u$ | Inappropriately ↓ (for ↑ $Osm_{Pl}$) |
| Plasma | |
| *Hypernatremia | Serum $Na^+$ >145 mEq/L |
| *$Osm_{Pl}$ | >290 mOsm/L |
| ADH level | |
| Central DI | ↓ or inappropriately nl |
| Nephrogenic DI | ↑ |
| Water deprivation test | |
| Response to vasopressin | |
| Central DI | Partial or full |
| Nephrogenic DI | Partial or none |

OsmPL = plasma osmolality; $Osm_U$ = urine osmolality; ↓ = decreased; ↑ = increased; * = present if inadequate hypotonic fluid replacement or uncompensated.

**TABLE 64.2. Causes of Diabetes Insipidus**

**Central/Hypothalamic**
Idiopathic (30%)
Postcranial syndrome (20%)
Tumors (20%)
- Craniopharyngioma (most common)
- Pituitary macroadenoma
- Meningioma
- Dysgerminoma
- Metastatic carcinoma (lung, breast)

Head injury (16%)
- Vascular
- Sheehan syndrome
- Aneurysms
- Cerebral hypoperfusion

Granulomatous disease
- Sarcoidosis
- Histiocytosis

Infections
- Meningitis
- Encephalitis

Autoimmune

**Nephrogenic/Renal Resistant**
Idiopathic
Chronic renal disease
Hypokalemia
Hypercalcemia
Drug-induced
- Lithium
- Demeclocycline
- Methoxyflurane

Amyloidosis
Post–obstructive uropathy

**Dipsogenic Primary Polydipsia**
Idiopathic
Psychogenic
Drug-induced
- Tricyclic antidepressants
- Anticholinergic

ing surgery. Some patients with postoperative or traumatic DI may exhibit a "triphasic" response. The first phase is DI due to axon shock or lack of release of vasopressin, and lasts 5 to 10 days. The second phase, lasting for about a week, is characterized by antidiuresis due to the release of excessive amounts of vasopressin from the degenerating axon terminals. During this phase, the patient may require fluid restriction and cessation of desmopressin therapy. The third, or final, phase, which may be permanent or transient, is the return of DI after the pool of stored vasopressin is exhausted.

The key abnormality in nephrogenic DI is a refractoriness to vasopressin on the part of the renal collecting ducts, resulting in the output of inappropriately hypotonic urine compared with a hypertonic plasma. Renal resistant DI is further characterized by normal renal filtration rate and solute excretion, normal (if partial nephrogenic DI is present) or elevated plasma ADH level, and a failure of exogenous vasopressin to raise urine osmolality by 50% or to reduce urine volume. Lithium-induced nephrogenic DI may not be reversible, unlike nephrogenic DI due to hypokalemia, hypercalcemia, and prolonged polyuria.

**Primary or psychogenic polydipsia,** usually seen in psychotic patients, is an uncommon condition, featuring excessive water intake and polyuria; genuine thirst is absent. It requires the intake of gallons of water. This excessive drinking leads to plasma dilution, physiologic ADH suppression, and resultant polyuria. This disorder is diagnosed by demonstrating a normal osmoregulated ADH secretion and renal function during a standard water deprivation test. The treatment is fluid restriction; no therapy other than that of the underlying psychosis is required.

## Diagnosis

The diagnosis of DI and its etiology is established with a standard water deprivation test (Figure 64.2). The patient is deprived of all water intake until dehydration results, with a weight loss of at least 2% of body weight and a rise in plasma osmolality above 300 mOsm/kg. If polyuria remits, it practically excludes DI; if it persists, osmolality of two plasma and consecutive voided urine samples is measured. Aqueous vasopressin (5U) is given subcutaneously and urine and plasma osmolality measurements are repeated. Typical results in patients with central and nephrogenic DI as well as normal patients are shown in Table 64.3.

## Management and Prognosis

In acute postsurgical and traumatic hypothalamic DI, hypotonic oral or IV fluids are given to replace the losses and maintain hydration. Vasopressin, if needed, is given subcutaneously as a short-acting aqueous preparation. This procedure makes it possible to assess whether the DI is permanent while at the same time avoiding overtreatment, with resultant free water retention and hyponatremia. Chronic central DI is usually treated with the long-acting synthetic analogue 1-desamino-8-D-arginine-vasopressin (DDAVP, 10-20 μg, 1-2 intranasal insufflations daily or 0.1–0.2 mg, 1–2 oral tablets daily). Other than removing the underlying cause and ensuring adequate hydration, no specific treatment exists for nephrogenic DI. Reducing the solute load by medications and restricting the patient's salt intake help reduce polyuria and minimize nocturia; thiazides are the most effective agents in this context.

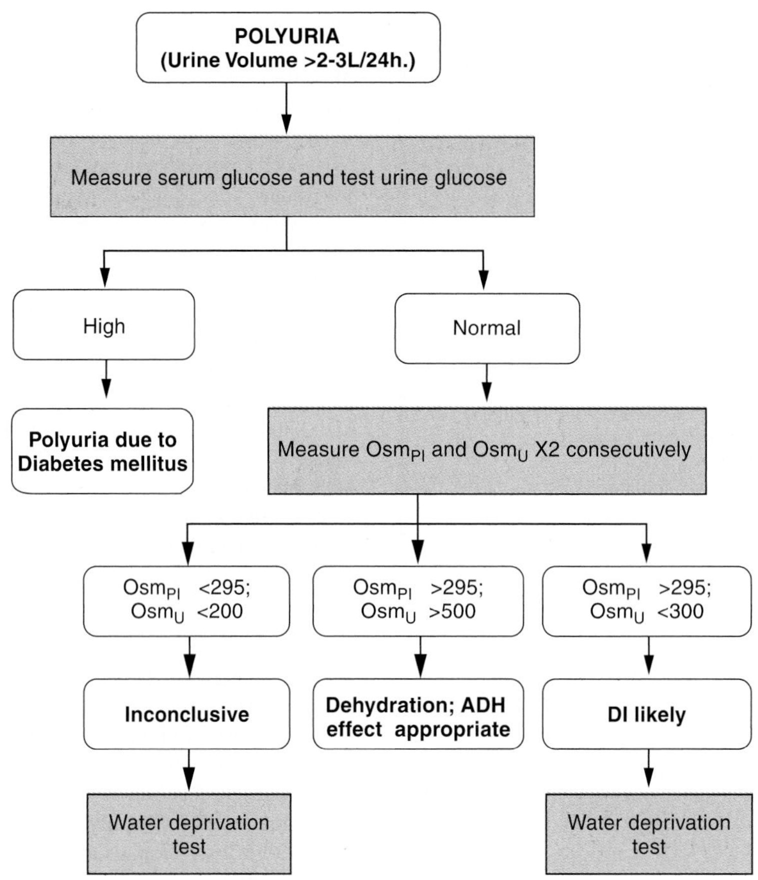


FIGURE 64.2. Work-up of polyuric states showing application of the water deprivation test.

TABLE 64.3. Interpretation of the Standard Water Deprivation Test

| | Ability to Concentrate Urine With Dehydration | |
|---|---|---|
| State | Before ADH | After ADH |
| Normal | +++ | ↑, <5% |
| Complete central DI | + | ↑, >50% |
| Partial central DI | + | ↑, >10% |
| Complete nephrogenic DI | ++ | No response |
| Partial nephrogenic DI | ++ | ↑, >10% |
| Primary polydipsia | +++ | ↑, <5% |

+++ = marked; ++ = moderate; + = minimal; ↑ = increased; DI = diabetes insipidus.

## Syndrome of Inappropriate Antidiuretic Hormone Secretion

### Definition and Epidemiology

SIADH is characterized by continual vasopressin release in the face of subnormal plasma osmolality or in the absence of either osmotic or nonosmotic stimuli. It accounts for more than 95% of hyponatremia in the hospital population.

### Etiology

Small cell lung cancer is the most common malignancy causing SIADH. Other underlying conditions are listed in Table 64.4.

### Clinical Features and Diagnosis

Clinical features usually are those of hyponatremia (lethargy, confusion, muscle cramps, coma, and seizures), those of the underlying cause, and, generally, diminished urine output. Significant thirst, edema, hypovolemia, orthostatic hypotension, diuretic use, and excessive water intake are absent. Biochemical criteria for the diagnosis of SIADH are serum $Na^+$ below 136 mmol/L; normal renal, adrenal, and thyroid function; normal triglycerides and glucose; urine osmolality exceeding that of serum; and excessive urinary $Na^+$ excretion (>20 mEq/L). Plasma ADH levels may be

**TABLE 64.4. Conditions Associated with SIADH**

| | |
|---|---|
| **Physiologic** | Nausea, pain |
| **Pathologic** | |
| Tumors | Carcinoma (lung, pancreas, urinary tract)<br>Thymoma<br>Lymphoma, leukemia<br>Mesothelioma |
| Pulmonary | Tuberculosis<br>Pneumonia, empyema, abscess<br>Chronic obstructive pulmonary disease |
| Intracranial conditions | Meningitis, encephalitis, abscess<br>Head injury<br>Brain tumor<br>Cerebral hemorrhage, subdural hematoma<br>Guillain-Barre syndrome<br>Seizures |
| Drug-induced | Vasopressin preparations<br>Carbamazepine, chlorpropamide, clofibrate, thiazides, vincristine, vinblastine, cisplatin, narcotics, phenothiazines |

clearly elevated or inappropriately normal in relation to the plasma osmolality.

## Management

The diagnostic evaluation and treatment of hyponatremia are outlined in Figure 64.3 and discussed further in Chapter 177. Determination of osmolality is critical; beyond osmolality, the diagnostic strategy to assess the cause of hypotonic hyponatremia is based on an initial evaluation of volume status.

Treatment of hyponatremia depends on the severity, the rate of evolution, and the underlying etiology of the hyponatremia as well as the presence or absence of symptoms. **Severe symptomatic hyponatremia** (serum $Na^+$ <120 mmol/L, with significant neurologic manifestations, i.e., confusion, seizures, coma) requires immediate therapy (see Chapter 177). Rapid or overcorrection of serum sodium can be very detrimental, resulting in **central pontine myelinolysis.** This condition is most likely to develop in patients undergoing rapid correction of **chronic asymptomatic hyponatremia** (duration of hyponatremia exceeds 48 hours). Central pontine myelinolysis, a demyelinating lesion of the pons with destruction of the myelin sheaths, features flaccid quadriplegia or paraplegia, facial weakness, dysphagia, dysarthria, and coma.

Mild to moderate, asymptomatic SIADH is treated by restricting fluid intake to less than the urine output, approximately 1000–1500 mL daily. If fluid restriction is unsuccessful, the antibiotic demeclocycline can be given. This agent inhibits the action of ADH at the level of the collecting duct. Persons with a light complexion should avoid direct sun exposure while receiving demeclocycline due to the photosensitivity caused by the medication.

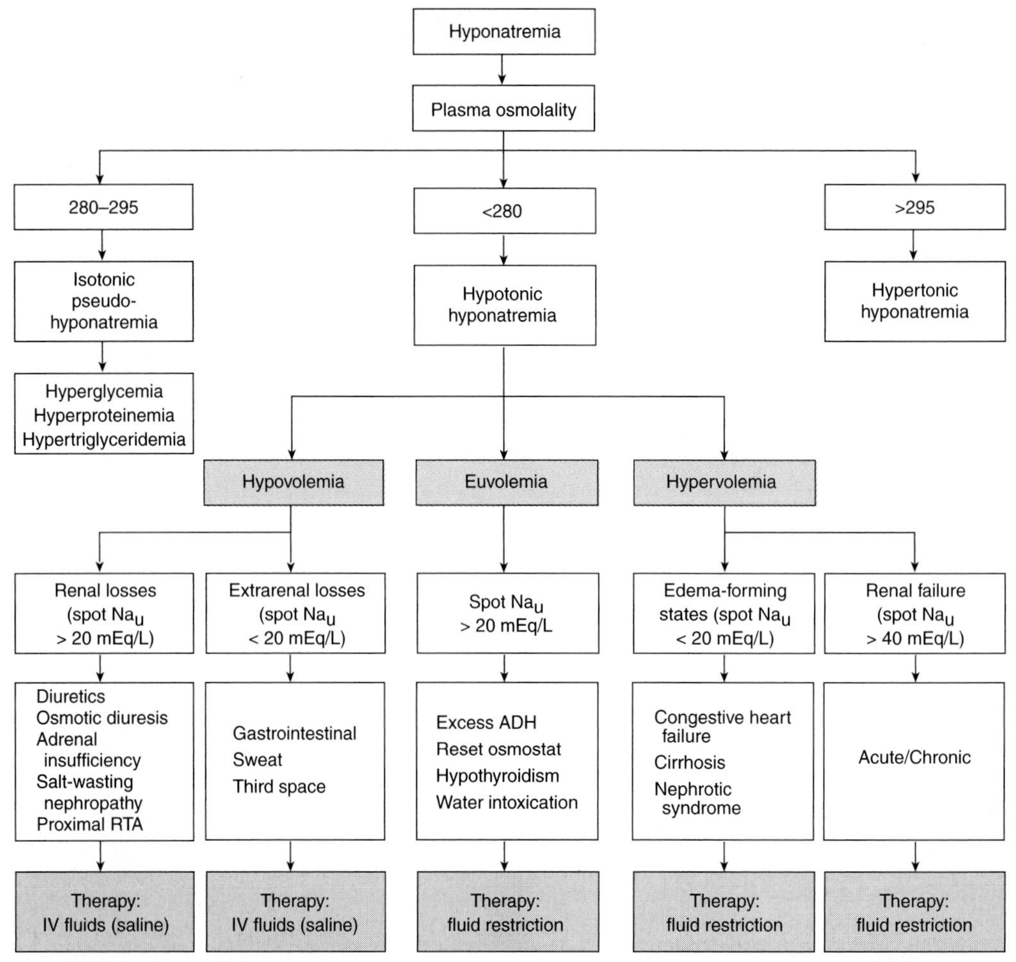


**FIGURE 64.3.** Diagnostic evaluation and therapy of hyponatremia.

# CHAPTER 65 THYROID DISEASES

## Thyroid Physiology and Thyroid Function

The thyroid gland, located anteriorly in the neck, weighs 15 to 20 g. It consists of a right and left lobe connected by an isthmus. A palpable pyramidal lobe extending upward from the isthmus occurs as a normal variant in many people. Accessory thyroid tissue is occasionally found along the course of the thyroglossal duct. Histologically, the structural unit of the thyroid is the follicle; the follicle consists of a single layer of cuboidal follicular cells enclosing a cavity filled with colloid, a gel-like material that serves as a reservoir of thyroid hormone. The thyroid gland also contains a small number of parafollicular cells **(C cells)** that secrete calcitonin and are unrelated to thyroid hormone metabolism. The gland receives its blood supply from superior and inferior thyroidal arteries.

Thyroid gland produces two thyroid hormones, **thyroxine** ($T_4$) and **triiodothyronine** ($T_3$), which are iodinated metabolites of tyrosine. The first step of their synthesis involves active transport and trapping of circulating iodides into the follicular cell (Figure 65.1). The iodine is oxidized and incorporated (by a process called organification) into the tyrosine residues of thyroglobulin (TG) by thyroid peroxidase, to form monoiodotyrosine (MIT) and diiodotyrosine (DIT). Most of the TG-bound MIT and DIT are later condensed to form $T_3$ and $T_4$ (coupling). The $T_4$ and $T_3$ are stored in the colloid of the thyroid gland, combined with TG. The final step involves resorption of colloid by the follicular cell and proteolysis of TG, releasing $T_4$ and $T_3$ into the circulation. The amount of $T_4$ released exceeds that of $T_3$ by nearly 10-fold. Each of these steps is physiologically regulated by TSH and can be inhibited by pharmacologic agents. Propylthiouracil and methimazole, drugs used to treat hyperthyroidism, block organification, and iodide in large doses inhibits thyroid peroxidase activity.

## Peripheral Circulation and Metabolism of Thyroid Hormones

$T_4$ and $T_3$ circulate in the bloodstream tightly bound to three serum proteins: thyroxine-binding globulin (TBG), albumin, and transthyretin (also called thyroxine-binding prealbumin). The quantitatively most important of the binding proteins is TBG, accounting for 70% of the total thyroid-binding capacity of the serum. More than 99% of both $T_4$ and $T_3$ are protein-bound. Although $T_4$ is more abundant than $T_3$ in the circulation, $T_3$ interacts with intranuclear receptors at a higher affinity and is more important in producing the biologic effects of thyroid hormone. $T_4$ is converted to $T_3$ intracellularly in its target cells by the action of 5′-deiodinase. $T_4$ also may be metabolized to metabolically inactive reverse $T_3$ by 5-deiodinase (Figure 65.2).

## Laboratory Testing of Thyroid Function

Serum free $T_4$ and TSH levels are the best tests of thyroid function. These tests, along with the traditional thyroid tests used in diagnosing hyperthyroidism, hypothyroidism, and thyroid hormone binding abnormalities, are summarized in Table 65.1. Assays to test for the autoimmune etiology of thyroid disease also are avail-

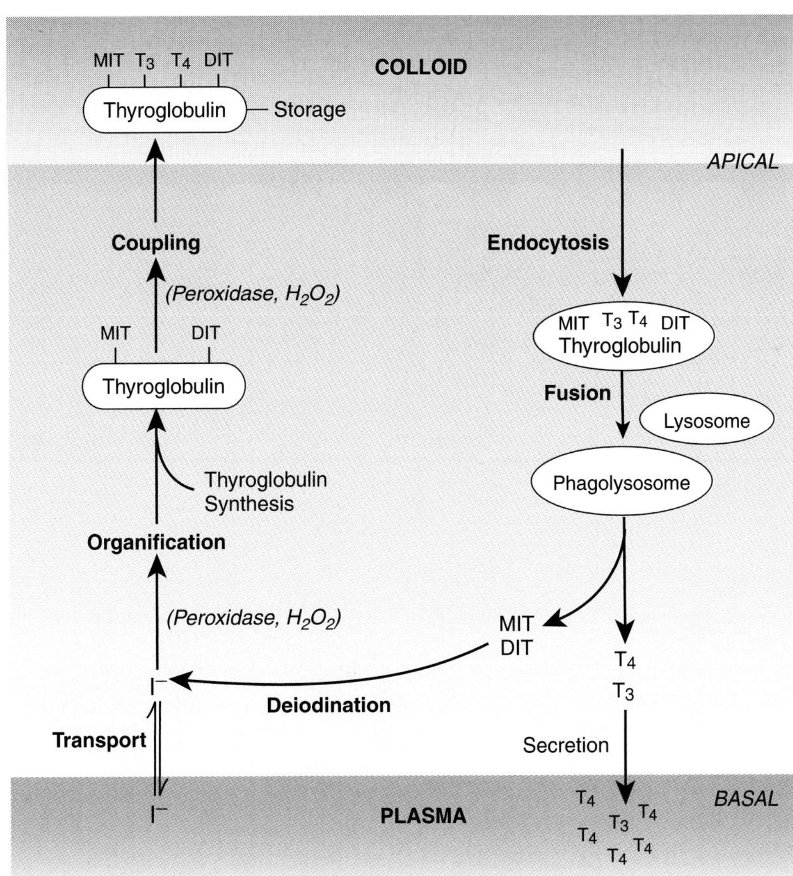


**FIGURE 65.1. Pathway of biosynthesis of thyroid hormones.**
(From: West JB (ed). Best and Taylor's Physiological Basis of Medical Practice. 12th ed. Baltimore: Williams & Wilkins, 1991, p. 813. Used with permission.)

able. Commonly used laboratory tests of thyroid function are described in the following text.

**Free $T_4$** is in reversible equilibrium with the bound hormone and represents the fraction of hormone that is biologically active. The changes in serum $T_4$-binding proteins (e.g., in pregnancy, oral contraceptive therapy, or nephrotic syndrome) that affect total $T_4$ concentration do not affect the concentration of free $T_4$. Therefore, the free $T_4$ concentration remains normal even in the presence of binding protein abnormalities. Free $T_4$ is measured by immunoextraction or enzyme immunoassay, or by equilibrium dialysis. **Serum TSH** is the best individual test of thyroid function. Except in secondary hypothyroidism due to pituitary insufficiency and the rare TSH-secreting pituitary adenomas, TSH is more sensitive than either total $T_4$ or free $T_4$ in diagnosing mild hypothyroidism or hyperthyroidism. **Total $T_3$ by radioimmunoassay ($T_3$RIA)** is used in the diagnosis of mild hyperthyroidism when the TSH is suppressed but the free $T_4$ is normal ("$T_3$ thyrotoxicosis"). Because many factors can affect the conversion of $T_4$ to $T_3$, measurement of $T_3$RIA is not useful in diagnosing hypothyroidism. Free $T_3$ can be measured in some laboratories.

The 24-hour **radioactive iodide uptake** (RAIU) test helps differentiate among the common causes of hyperthyroidism. The RAIU is an in vivo test involving the oral administration of a small dose of radioactive iodide, such as $^{123}I$ or $^{131}I$, with subsequent gamma counting over the thyroid bed to determine the percentage of administered counts concentrated in the thyroid after a specified period of time, generally 24 hours.

Many thyroid diseases are autoimmune. Thyroglobulin and thyroid microsomal proteins are common antigens involved in this process. Serum titers of **antithyroglobulin** and **antimicrosomal antibodies** can be quantitated and used to document the autoimmune etiology of primary hypothyroidism and goiters. Because thyroid peroxidase is the microsomal antigen

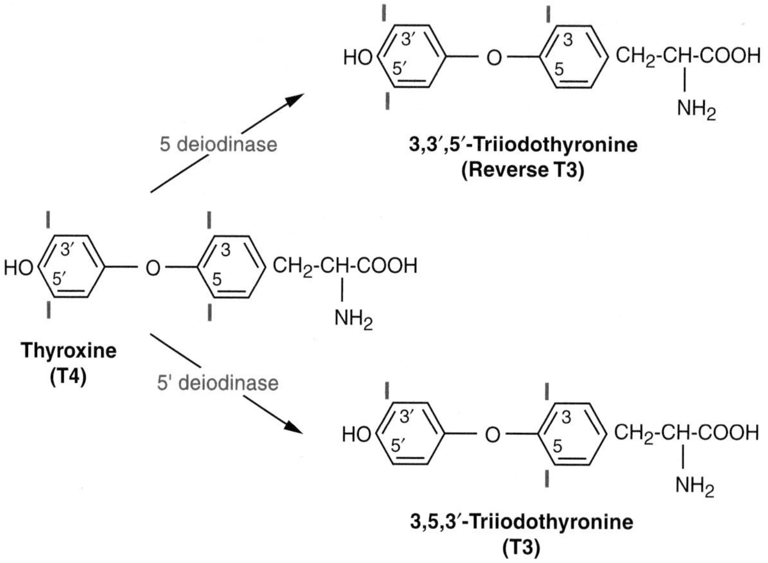

**FIGURE 65.2.** Structures of $T_4$, $T_3$, and reverse $T_3$.

**TABLE 65.1.** Laboratory Evaluation of Hyperthyroidism and Primary Hypothyroidism

| | Euthyroid, Normal TBG | Euthyroid, Low TBG | Euthyroid, High TBG | Hyperthyroid, Normal TBG | Hypothyroid, Normal TBG |
|---|---|---|---|---|---|
| Total $T_4$ (normal 5–12 μg/dl) | ↔ | ↓ | ↑ | ↑ | ↓ |
| $T_3$RU (normal 30-40%) | ↔ | ↑ | ↓ | ↑ | ↓ |
| FTI | ↔ | ↔ | ↔ | ↑ | ↓ |
| Free $T_4$ | ↔ | ↔ | ↔ | ↑ | ↓ |
| TSH | ↔ | ↔ | ↔ | ↓ | ↑ |

FTI = free thyroxine index; TBG = thyroid-binding globulin; TSH = thyroid-stimulating hormone.
↔ = normal; ↑ = increased; ↓ = decreased

**TABLE 65.2. Thyroid Imaging Studies**

| Test | Ability to Differentiate: Cold vs Hot | Solid vs Cystic | Benign vs Malignant | Resolution | Detecting Substernal Extension | Cost | Comments |
|---|---|---|---|---|---|---|---|
| Radionuclide scan | +++ | – | + | ++ | + | $300 | Most nodules are cold |
| Ultrasound | – | ++++ | – | ++++ | + | $200 | Supplements physical examination |
| CT | – | ++++ | – | ++++ | ++++ | $900 | Excellent for evaluating mass lesions |
| MRI | – | ++++ | – | ++++ | ++++ | $1500 | Same as CT |

**TABLE 65.3. Characteristics of Common Causes of Hyperthyroidism**

| | Demographics | Thyroid Gland | Ophthalmopathy | 24-h RAIU | Need for Definitive Therapy? |
|---|---|---|---|---|---|
| Graves' disease | Predominantly young to middle-aged women | Firm, diffusely enlarged with a bruit | Frequent | High | Yes |
| Toxic multinodular goiter | Middle-aged and elderly | Small to massive goiters with multiple nodules | Absent | High | Yes |
| Subacute thyroiditis | Young and middle-aged patients | Tender, modestly enlarged | Absent | Low | No |

RAIU = radioactive iodine uptake.

targeted by antimicrosomal enzymes, antimicrosomal antibodies also may be called antithyroid peroxidase antibodies.

Available thyroid imaging techniques include high-resolution ultrasound, radionuclide scan, computed tomography, and magnetic resonance imaging. Their relative merits, limitations, and indications are compared in Table 65.2. Imaging studies are rarely indicated in the hyperthyroid or hypothyroid patient. They are used more in evaluating thyroid nodules and masses in euthyroid patients.

## Hyperthyroidism

In **hyperthyroidism,** excessive activity of the thyroid hormones causes a hypermetabolic state. It arises from excess circulating quantities of free $T_4$ or free $T_3$. The causes of hyperthyroidism (Table 65.3) fall into three categories: conditions in which the thyroid gland is actively synthesizing and releasing excess thyroid hormone; conditions due to thyroid inflammation; and exogenous sources of thyroid hormone. (In the latter two categories, the thyroid itself is not synthesizing new $T_4$ or $T_3$ and takes up low amounts of iodide.) The first category is distinguished diagnostically by demonstration of an elevated 24-hour RAIU. Conditions with a "high uptake" include Graves' disease, toxic multinodular goiter, toxic adenoma, TSH-secreting pituitary tumor, and human chorionic gonadotropin (HCG) secreting tumor. Hyperthyroidism with a "low uptake" includes that caused by thyroid hormone use, the various forms of thyroiditis, and struma ovarii, or that following exposure to exogenous iodine, e.g., radiocontrast agents.

The three most common causes of hyperthyroidism—Graves' disease, toxic multinodular goiter (Plummer's disease), and thyroiditis—have distinctive clinical features (see Table 65.3).

### *Graves' Disease*

#### Pathogenesis

**Graves' disease** is the most common cause of hyperthyroidism. It is an autoimmune disease arising from the production of thyroid-stimulating immunoglobulins capable of interacting with the TSH receptors on thyroid follicular cells and mimicking the actions of TSH. Pathways of thyroid hormone synthesis and release are markedly increased despite the absence of TSH itself. Graves' disease is more common in women than in men, with an estimated incidence of 37 women and 8 men per 100,000 population. Histologically, the thyroid shows evidence of lymphocytic infiltration and a plethora of active, intact follicles.

## Clinical Features

The presentation of Graves' disease is influenced by the age of the patient, the severity of hyperthyroidism, and the presence of coexisting medical conditions (Table 65.4). Younger patients are apt to manifest heat intolerance, hyperhidrosis, anxiety, emotional lability, and tremors early in the course of their disease. In contrast, elderly patients often fail to manifest these symptoms, but, rather, tend to present only with atrial fibrillation, weight loss, or depression—a subtle and limited presentation, called **apathetic hyperthyroidism.** The thyroid is diffusely enlarged, firm, and nontender (Figure 65.3). In contrast to goiters from other causes, a bruit often is audible over the gland.

Patients with Graves' disease often have specific autoimmune diseases of selected nonthyroid tissues. **Ophthalmopathy** is especially common and results from inflammation of the tissues of the eye and the orbit. It includes conjunctival inflammation (chemosis), infiltration, and swelling of the eye muscles, producing ophthalmoplegia, corneal ulcerations, and proptosis (Figure 65.4). Retrobulbar swelling and edema cause the proptosis. Dermopathy and acropachy are much less common. **Dermopathy** results from mucopolysaccharide infiltration of the dermis and manifests localized myxedema, characterized by elevated, firm, thickened, erythematous patches, usually involving pretibial areas. Itching and pain may be present. **Acropachy** is clubbing and osteoarthropathy of the distal phalanges of the fingers, due to periosteal bone formation and associated soft tissue reaction.

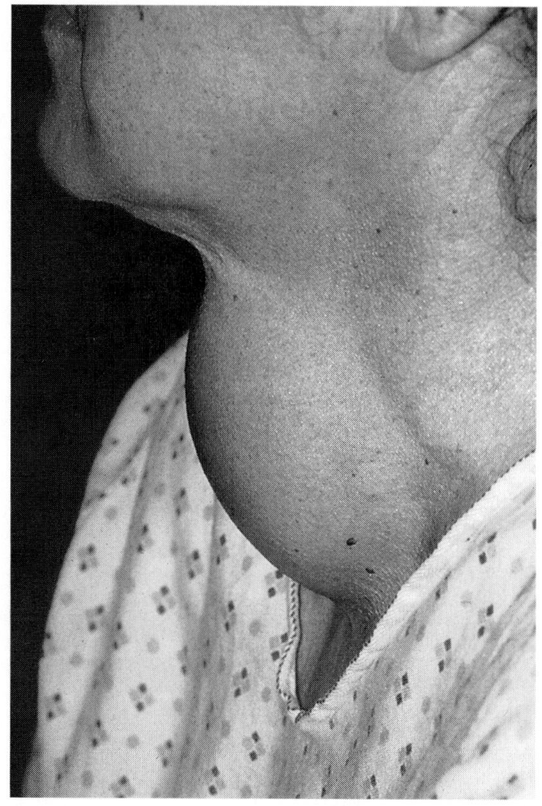

**FIGURE 65.3. A large, diffuse goiter as seen in Graves' disease.**
(Photograph courtesy of James M. Cerletty, MD, Department of Medicine, The Medical College of Wisconsin, Milwaukee, WI.)

**TABLE 65.4. Clinical Manifestations of Graves' Disease**

| Symptoms | Frequency (%) | Signs | Frequency (%) |
|---|---|---|---|
| Nervousness | 99 | Tachycardia | 100 |
| Increased sweating | 91 | Goiter | 100 |
| Heat intolerance | 89 | Skin changes | 97 |
| Palpitations | 89 | Bruit over thyroid | 77 |
| Fatigue | 88 | Eye signs | 71 |
| Weight loss | 85 | Atrial fibrillation | 10 |
| Tachycardia | 82 | Splenomegaly | 10 |
| Dyspnea | 75 | Gynecomastia | 10 |
| Weakness | 70 | | |
| Increased appetite | 65 | | |
| Eye complaints | 54 | | |
| Swelling of legs | 35 | | |
| Hyperdefecation (without diarrhea) | 33 | | |
| Diarrhea | 23 | | |
| Anorexia | 9 | | |
| Constipation | 4 | | |
| Weight gain | 3 | | |

(Adapted from Williams RH. J Clin Endocrinol 1946:6:1.)

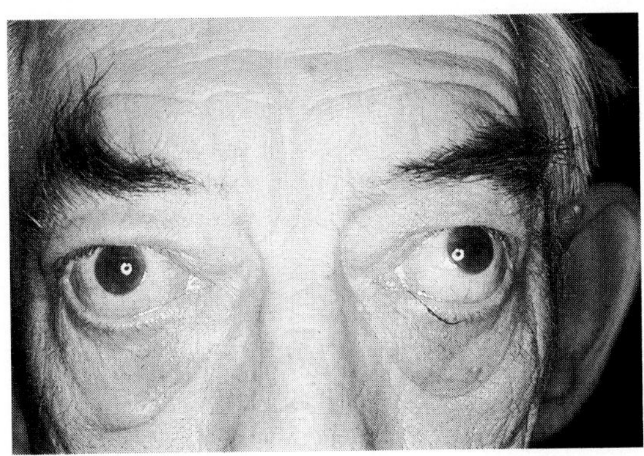

**FIGURE 65.4. Graves' ophthalmopathy.**
(Photograph courtesy of James M. Cerletty, MD, Department of Medicine, The Medical College of Wisconsin, Milwaukee, WI.)

## Diagnosis and Management

When thyrotoxicosis is suspected clinically, the diagnosis is confirmed by demonstrating a suppressed TSH level along with either increased "classical" thyroid function tests or an increased free $T_4$. The 24-hour RAIU is measured to confirm the presence of "high uptake" hyperthyroidism.

Spontaneous remission is unusual for the hyperthyroidism of Graves' disease. Thus, definitive treatment is indicated. Among the three available modes of therapy, thyroid ablation with radioactive iodine ($^{131}$I) is most commonly employed; prolonged therapy with antithyroid drugs and surgery are alternatives in selected subsets of patients. The patient should be apprised of the benefits and limitations of all three modes. Regardless of the mode elected, and unless contraindicated, all patients are given β-blockers (e.g., propranolol 20–40 mg q.i.d.) to reduce the adrenergic symptoms.

The treatment of choice for hyperthyroidism in adult men, and most adult women, is radioablation with $^{131}$I. The treatment sometimes produces euthyroidism, but more often results in permanent hypothyroidism, requiring life-long thyroxine replacement. Cumulative experience with use of $^{131}$I suggests no increase in the incidence of leukemias or other cancers. Its use is contraindicated in pregnancy; fears over potential, but unproven gonadal effects make its use in children and women of child-bearing age controversial. Destruction of the overactive thyroid gland with $^{131}$I causes rapid release of the stored thyroid hormone, and the hyperthyroidism worsens transiently but significantly (radiation thyroiditis). Therefore, depending upon the age and the general health of the patient and the severity of the thyrotoxicosis, treatment with antithyroid drugs for one or two months can be given before treatment with $^{131}$I, so as to deplete the gland of its stored thyroid hormone. In less severe hyperthyroidism, such pretreatment is not needed, but β-blockers are given.

**Subtotal thyroidectomy** is sometimes used for children and for those women of child-bearing age concerned about the effects of radioactive iodine on future pregnancies. Prior to surgery, the patient must be rendered clinically and biochemically euthyroid, using β-blockers, antithyroid drugs, and large amounts of nonradioactive iodine.

In mild hyperthyroidism with relatively small goiters, prolonged therapy with **antithyroid drugs** (propylthiouracil or methimazole) for 6 to 18 months sometimes induces a spontaneous remission in the hyperthyroidism. About one third of this select group maintain euthyroidism after the antithyroid drugs are discontinued, whereas the hyperthyroidism relapses in the remaining two thirds. Prolonged treatment with antithyroid drugs is also used to treat hyperthyroidism of all degrees in children.

## Course and Prognosis

Most patients become permanently hypothyroid as a result of therapy with $^{131}$I, generally over 3 to 5 months. Subtotal thyroidectomy also usually produces the same result, either immediately postoperatively or more gradually as the thyroid remnant is finally destroyed by the autoimmune process. Thus, most patients who have been treated for Graves' disease require lifelong thyroid hormone replacement. A small minority develop a euthyroid state without needing thyroid hormone replacement. Extrathyroidal autoimmune features of Graves' disease (e.g., ophthalmopathy) run a largely independent course; thus, ophthalmopathy may remain stable or even worsen upon treatment of the hyperthyroidism.

# *Toxic Multinodular Goiter*

Toxic multinodular goiter ("Plummer's disease), is where hyperthyroidism develops secondarily in a multinodular goiter of long standing.

## Pathogenesis and Pathology

Evidence of inflammation in toxic multinodular goiter is scant or absent. The nodular hyperplasia is of uncertain cause, but local growth-stimulating factors, growth-stimulating immunoglobulins, or neoplastic characteristics intrinsic to the cells themselves may be responsible. Iodine deficiency contributes in some geographical areas. Hyperthyroidism develops when the follicles become autonomous (i.e., when TSH is no longer required to stimulate thyroid hormone production). The overactivity of these nodules results in increased iodine trapping as well as the characteristic appearance on radionuclide scanning, showing "hot" nodules and areas of increased activity interspersed with "cold" zones; the latter arise from the low TSH levels, which suppress iodine uptake in the remaining normal tissue.

### Clinical Features

Hyperthyroidism typically develops slowly in patients with toxic multinodular goiters. In these patients, hyperthyroidism can be precipitated by iodine in iodide-containing IV radiologic contrast dyes or medications (e.g., amiodarone and saturated solutions of potassium iodide). Although most features are similar to those in hyperthyroidism of Graves' disease, the presentation of toxic multinodular goiter is more subtle, because of the more elderly population that it afflicts and the gradual onset of thyrotoxicosis. Unexplained weight loss, atrial fibrillation, and depression may thus dominate the clinical picture. The extrathyroidal autoimmune manifestations of Graves' disease are absent.

### Management and Prognosis

Toxic multinodular goiter is most commonly treated with $^{131}$I ablation of the gland. The 24-hour RAIU, although generally elevated, usually is not as high as that in Graves' disease. Thus, the usual $^{131}$I dose for toxic multinodular goiter generally exceeds that for Graves' disease. The hyperfunctioning follicles take up $^{131}$I much more avidly than the normal, suppressed follicles. The latter may regain normal function after $^{131}$I therapy, so that euthyroid state is more often restored in toxic multinodular goiter relative to Graves' disease. It is also prudent to administer β-blockers until hyperthyroidism is resolved and to give antithyroid drugs before $^{131}$I therapy. Subtotal thyroidectomy also is an option in selected cases.

## *Thyroiditis*

### Definition and Etiology

Thyroid inflammation, by disrupting normal follicular architecture and releasing the stored hormone, can cause **thyrotoxicosis** of limited severity and duration. Based on clinical features and thyroid histopathology, three types of thyroiditis can be recognized: subacute, postpartum, and silent. Subacute (also known as painful, de Quervain, or granulomatous thyroiditis) thyroiditis probably is viral, whereas postpartum thyroiditis is autoimmune. A subset of patients with silent thyroiditis manifest antithyroid antibodies, also implying an autoimmune etiology.

### Clinical Features

**Subacute thyroiditis** is a painful inflammation of the thyroid; acute onset of pain in the region of the thyroid sometimes is preceded by an upper respiratory infection. The pain may be severe and radiate to the jaw or ear. General malaise, muscle aches, fatigue, and fever may be associated. Nearly one half of patients with subacute thyroiditis develop symptoms of mild or moderate thyrotoxicosis. The thyroid may be moderately enlarged and tender to palpation. Cervical adenopathy usually is absent. The **erythrocyte sedimentation rate** (ESR) typically is high. The painful thyroid and the elevated ESR clinically differentiate subacute thyroiditis from silent thyroiditis. **Silent** (or painless) **thyroiditis,** less common than subacute thyroiditis, evokes mild, self-limited hyperthyroidism without neck pain. A normal ESR and the lack of neck pain and systemic symptoms differentiate it from subacute thyroiditis. Hyperthyroidism, which occurs with increased frequency postpartum, at times is due to a relapse of Graves' disease, but often it is due to postpartum thyroiditis, a form of painless thyroiditis. Often, thyroiditis has followed earlier pregnancies.

### Diagnosis and Management

Thyroiditis may be suspected when thyrotoxicosis is mild and occurs in a compatible clinical setting, as described earlier. The diagnosis is confirmed by obtaining a 24-hour RAIU showing low uptake.

Thyrotoxicosis in thyroiditis is treated symptomatically. Adrenergic symptoms (e.g., tachycardia) can be treated with propranolol. All other therapies previously cited for thyrotoxicosis are ineffective and contraindicated. The pain of subacute thyroiditis is treated with analgesics (aspirin and nonsteroidal anti-inflammatory drugs); high doses of glucocorticoids are required for severe pain.

### Course and Prognosis

The hyperthyroid stage of thyroiditis is self-limited (weeks). Hyperthyroid symptoms and TSH levels should be assessed monthly so that β-blockers can be discontinued when appropriate. The hyperthyroidism often leads to a hypothyroid phase, which occasionally is permanent and requires levothyroxine replacement. Therefore, patients should be closely monitored.

## Hypothyroidism

**Hypothyroidism** results from the functional inactivity of the thyroid gland. **Primary hypothyroidism** resulting from diseases intrinsic to the thyroid gland is much more frequent than hypothyroidism secondary to TSH deficiency. The causes of primary hypothyroidism are shown in Table 65.5.

### Pathogenesis

Primary hypothyroidism usually follows destruction of normal thyroid follicles by **chronic autoimmune**

**TABLE 65.5. Differential Diagnosis of Primary Hypothyroidism**

**Common Causes**
Autoimmune hypothyroidism
  Hashimoto's disease and atrophic variants
Iatrogenic
  Radioactive iodine
  Thyroidectomy
  External radiation therapy

**Less Common Causes**
Iodine deficiency
Inherited enzyme defects
Medications (e.g., lithium, amiodarone, anti-thyroid drugs)
Infiltrative diseases (e.g., cystinosis, hemochromatosis, scleroderma, amyloidosis)

**thyroiditis;** this form of thyroiditis has two forms: the **idiopathic** (atrophic) variant, with atrophy of the gland; or **Hashimoto's disease,** with a goiter. Both disorders have a high incidence of antibodies against thyroid antigens, specifically thyroglobulin and thyroid peroxidase; therapy for the two disorders is thyroid hormone replacement. Thus, it is not usually clinically useful to distinguish between these two variants.

The second most common cause of primary hypothyroidism is iatrogenic. It arises from a variety of causes: destruction of the thyroid gland by $^{131}I$ in treating Graves' disease; thyroidectomy for thyroid cancer or other reasons; and neck irradiation for lymphoma and other head and neck cancers.

### Clinical Features

Symptoms of primary hypothyroidism include fatigue, lethargy, increased sleeping, cold intolerance, coarsening of the hair, and dry skin. Weight gain, also typical, may be accompanied by nonpitting edema of the lower extremities and generalized puffiness of the face, particularly periorbitally. Also common are generalized cramps and aches in the lower back muscles. The thyroid may be enlarged, or may not be palpable. In Hashimoto's disease, the goiter is typically firm to rock-hard; its texture is multinodular or bosselated.

### Diagnosis and Management

Primary hypothyroidism is diagnosed definitively by a high TSH level in conjunction with a decreased free $T_4$. Thyroid antibodies are positive in 70% to 90% of cases, but it is not necessary to check them routinely. Treatment consists of oral administration of synthetic levothyroxine ($T_4$). The goal of $T_4$ therapy is to provide sufficient levels of thyroid hormone (starting dose of 75–100 μg/d in young people and 50 μg/d in the middle-aged; usual maintenance dose, 75–150 μg/d) to maintain a normal TSH level. Treatment markedly improves the symptoms, although it may take several weeks to months. $T_4$ replacement raises cardiac oxygen consumption; in a patient with significant coronary artery disease (CAD), it can precipitate crescendo angina or even a myocardial infarction. Thus, in older patients and in those with known CAD, $T_4$ is started in lower doses (25 μg/d); the biochemical and clinical euthyroid state is attained over a longer period of time and with close monitoring.

## *Secondary Hypothyroidism*

Destruction of the pituitary gland or the hypothalamus can cause TSH deficiency. Hypothyroidism follows, along with thyroid gland atrophy. Clinically, these patients differ from those with primary hypothyroidism because other pituitary hormones, most notably ACTH, also are deficient. Because treating hypothyroidism with $T_4$ in the setting of unrecognized **panhypopituitarism** (a state of inadequacy or absence of all anterior pituitary hormones) can precipitate an adrenal crisis, secondary hypothyroidism should be excluded.

# Thyroid Nodules and Thyroid Cancer

## *Thyroid Nodules*

Both benign and malignant conditions can produce thyroid nodules and goiters. Hyperthyroidism and hypothyroidism are routinely associated with benign goiters as a natural consequence of their pathogenesis; they are rarely associated with malignancies. Benign nodules are more common than malignant nodules, even in euthyroid patients (Table 65.6). Benign and malignant lesions can be differentiated by taking the patient's risk factors in conjunction with the cytology of thyroid cells obtained by fine needle aspiration. Consequently, it is impractical and unnecessary to surgically resect all thyroid nodules.

### Evaluation of Thyroid Nodules

Periodic palpation of the thyroid is all that is needed for evaluating a patient with a stable multinodular goiter and no worrisome risk factors such as history of neck irradiation. High-resolution ultrasound, by accurately quantitating the size and number of nodules, can supplement palpation. CT, by defining the relation of the goiter to the trachea and esophagus, is useful in assessing mass symptoms (e.g., dysphagia or hoarseness). An approach to thyroid nodules is shown in Figure 65.5.

**TABLE 65.6. Differential Diagnosis of Thyroid Nodules/Masses**

Colloid goiter (multinodular goiter)
Chronic autoimmune thyroiditis
  Hashimoto disease
  Euthyroid Graves' disease
Benign follicular adenoma
Simple cyst
Thyroid cancers
  Papillary
  Follicular
  Medullary
  Anaplastic
  Lymphoma

## Thyroid Cancer

### Epidemiology, Etiology, and Risk Factors

The incidence of thyroid cancer is 5 per 100,000 persons. Because the most frequent thyroid cancers are the low-grade papillary (60%) and follicular (25%) types, both of which have an excellent prognosis, overall mortality is low. Medullary cancer accounts for 10% of cases; anaplastic and lymphoma account for less than 5% each. Risk factors for thyroid cancer are listed in Table 65.7. Less than 15% of all solitary nodules are malignant.

### Specific Types of Thyroid Cancer and Their Management

Cancers that are histologically predominantly follicular but contain papillary elements behave biologically like papillary carcinomas—the least aggressive thyroid cancers. They tend either to remain localized in the thyroid gland or to metastasize to local lymph nodes. The

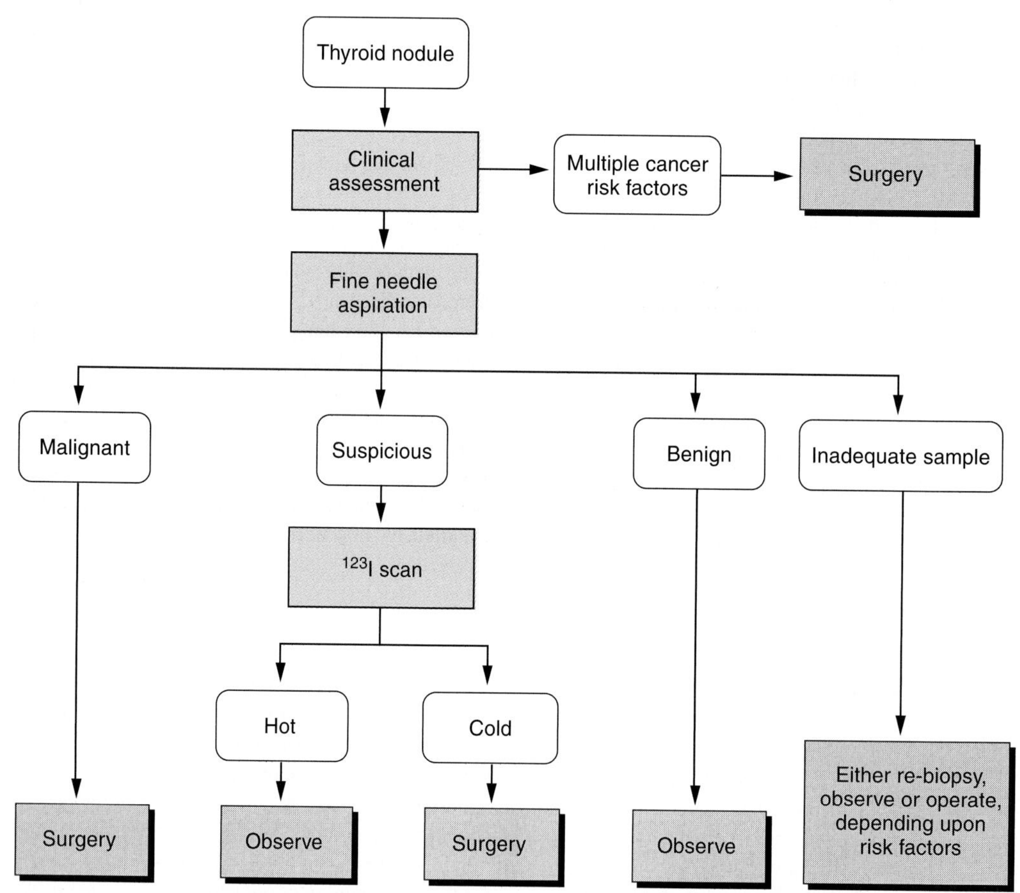


FIGURE 65.5. Algorithm for evaluation and therapy of thyroid nodules.

**TABLE 65.7. Features of Solitary Thyroid Nodules Associated With Increased Risk of Malignancy**

History
- Age < 20 or >60 years (~30% malignant)
- Gender: men affected more often than women
- Compression symptoms (dysphagia, hoarseness)
- History of neck irradiation (~30% malignant)
- Family history of medullary cancer

Physical examination
- Rapid growth of nodule
- Fixation
- Lymphadenopathy

Course
- Growth of nodule while on thyroid hormone suppression

Laboratory
- Euthyroid clinical status

Imaging
- Nodule cold on radionuclide scanning (10–15% malignant)

prognosis of papillary cancers is not materially affected by localized lymph node metastasis at diagnosis. The follicular type, while still indolent, is more aggressive than papillary cancer and tends to metastasize more readily to distant locations, including the bone and lung. Overall, about 3% of patients with these two types of cancer (usually those with larger tumors or extrathyroidal extension at initial presentation, or those in whom the thyroid cancer develops after age 70) eventually succumb to the malignancy.

Papillary and follicular carcinomas are treated by an individualized combination of surgery, $^{131}I$ therapy, and suppressive doses of $T_4$. The most appropriate regimen for a given patient remains controversial. Thus, lobectomy alone may suffice for small (<1.5 cm) papillary and follicular carcinomas, whereas total or near-total thyroidectomy typically is required for large tumors. Residual benign and malignant thyroid tissue can be ablated with large doses of $^{131}I$. Because papillary and follicular cancer cells possess TSH receptors, growth of residual tissue also can be slowed by $T_4$ given in sufficient doses to suppress the TSH to nonmeasurable levels. Recurrence of thyroid cancer can be detected by neck palpation, serum thyroglobulin levels, or radioactive iodine imaging (performed in the presence of a high TSH level produced from either holding levothyroxine therapy or injecting synthetic, recombinant TSH).

**Medullary carcinoma of the thyroid** (MCT) arises from the parafollicular cells of the thyroid gland. A sporadic form is well known, but MCT often is familial and inherited as part of the **multiple endocrine neoplasia-2 syndrome.** The characteristic feature of MCT is the production of calcitonin. Because MCT is not derived from thyroid epithelial follicular cells, it does not take up iodine, nor does it depend on TSH as a growth factor; thus, therapy with $^{131}I$ or with suppressive doses of $T_4$ is ineffective. Surgical resection is the treatment; if it is not curative, other modalities of therapy include medical therapy with octreotide, chemotherapy, and external irradiation, none of which are successful in completely stopping the usually slow growth of residual tumor tissue.

**Anaplastic carcinoma** accounts for less than 5% of all thyroid carcinomas. This highly aggressive lesion grows rapidly, invading surrounding structures, thereby causing compression symptoms in the neck, such as stridor, dysphagia, and hoarseness. Although surgery usually is attempted for diagnostic purposes and for initial tumor debulking, it rarely cures this aggressive cancer. As with MCT, $^{131}I$ and $T_4$ suppression are ineffective. External radiotherapy and chemotherapy have been used as palliative therapies for the compression symptoms. The overall prognosis is very poor. Survival exceeding 6 months after the diagnosis of anaplastic carcinoma is rare.

**Primary (non-Hodgkin) lymphomas** of the thyroid are being recognized with increasing frequency. The incidence of thyroid lymphoma is increased more than 50-fold in patients with Hashimoto's disease, suggesting that the lymphoma arises from the intrathyroidal lymphocytes present as a result of the chronic autoimmune process. Thyroid lymphoma should be suspected when a patient with known Hashimoto's disease develops a rapidly growing thyroid mass accompanied by symptoms of local compression. In this setting, needle aspiration can be helpful in identifying the lymphoma. In patients with localized disease or in those experiencing significant localized compression, surgical resection may be used. Subsequent therapy is similar to that used for other lymphomas and includes external radiation therapy and chemotherapy. Surgery is not the primary therapy in cases where subsequent staging with CT and bone marrow biopsy demonstrate extrathyroidal lymphoma.

## Miscellaneous Thyroid Disorders

**Thyroid crisis** (thyroid storm) is life-threatening hyperthyroidism. In most instances, it is ushered in by a precipitating event in previously untreated, severe hyperthyroidism. Precipitating events include infections, surgery, and trauma. Most patients have Graves' disease. The features include fever, which may be high, restlessness, confusion, and, possibly, frank psychosis. Cardiac arrhythmias are common, and cardiovascular collapse may supervene. Treatment includes propylthiouracil

(800–1200 mg) or methimazole (40 mg/day) given orally or by nasogastric tube. Iodide (10 drops of Lugol's iodine every 8 hours orally or as IV radiologic contrast, sodium ipodate 1 g/d) is given to block thyroid hormone synthesis and peripheral $T_4$ to $T_3$ conversion. Antithyroid drugs must precede the iodide, because iodide also is a substrate for thyroid hormone synthesis. β-blockers (propranolol 1–5 mg IV or 20–80 mg orally every 4 hours) are a critical component of the therapy. Glucocorticoids (hydrocortisone, 200–300 mg/day, or dexamethasone in equivalent doses) are administered to offset a relative adrenal insufficiency. Both propranolol and corticosteroids also lower the peripheral conversion of $T_4$ to $T_3$. A precipitating event should be searched for carefully and, if found, appropriately treated.

**Myxedema coma,** a medical emergency, is the end stage of advanced, untreated hypothyroidism. Its hallmarks are hypothermia, mental status changes, hypoventilation, and bradycardia. Paralytic ileus (generalized hypomotility of intestinal smooth muscle) and hyponatremia may occur. Precipitating events are exposure to cold weather, surgery, congestive heart failure, infection, and drugs, including anesthetics, tranquilizers, and narcotics. Diagnosis is based on classic signs and symptoms of severe hypothyroidism, hypothermia, and the features discussed earlier. In myxedema coma, a relative adrenal insufficiency may prevail due to the suppression of the pituitary-adrenal axis by advanced hypothyroidism. Therapy consists of aggressive $T_4$ replacement (200–500 μg initial IV bolus, followed by 50–100 μg daily, IV), glucocorticoids, (hydrocortisone IV, 100 mg every 8 hours for the first several days), and general measures. Precipitating factors should be sought and treated if present. IV preparations of triiodothyronine are available and may be used instead of $T_4$. Supportive measures are IV hydration, passive rewarming, and ventilatory support for hypoxemia and $CO_2$ retention. Rapid rewarming by external electric warming blankets ushers in vasodilatation and exacerbates hypotension.

In **euthyroid hyperthyroxinemia,** the serum total or free $T_4$ level is high, but without hyperthyroidism. It most commonly occurs with excess thyroid hormone binding proteins, in which case, measurement of free $T_4$ and serum TSH readily excludes hyperthyroidism. Iodine-containing medications (e.g., amiodarone) block peripheral $T_4$ to $T_3$ conversion, thus leading to high $T_4$. Free $T_4$ also is high in acute psychiatric illness and hyperemesis gravidarum.

Many medical and surgical illnesses affect thyroid function tests. In some patients, the serum $T_3$ level is low and is attributed to impaired conversion of $T_4$ to $T_3$, resulting in high reverse $T_3$. $T_4$ also is slightly reduced in most patients. This state is called **euthyroid sick syndrome.** Very low $T_4$ levels correlate with a high mortality. Serum TSH is typically normal, ruling out primary hypothyroidism.

# CHAPTER 66 DISEASES OF THE PARATHYROID GLANDS, VITAMIN D METABOLISM, AND CALCIUM HOMEOSTASIS

Calcium has two major physiologic functions: (1) calcium salts provide the rigidity and strength of the skeleton, and (2) ionized calcium plays critical roles in blood clotting, neuromuscular and membrane physiology, and signal transduction. Calcium kinetics are shown in Figure 66.1. Despite the high variability in dietary calcium intake, overall calcium balance is maintained principally by efficient regulation of intestinal calcium absorption. Circulating serum calcium takes three forms: free (ionized), albumin-bound, or complexed to citrate or phosphate. Only the ionized calcium is hormonally regulated and biologically active. Changes in serum albumin level affect the serum calcium level, but not the biological activity of calcium. When the albumin level is abnormal, it is possible to measure ionized calcium directly or to correct the total serum calcium by subtracting 0.8 mg/dl for each gram/dl the serum albumin level is below 4 g/dl.

The parathyroid gland secretes **parathyroid hormone** (PTH), an 84-amino acid polypeptide, in close and inverse relation to serum calcium level. Binding of extracellular calcium to the calcium-sensing receptor regulates PTH secretion. PTH maintains serum calcium levels in three ways: by stimulating (see Figure 66.1) osteoclast activity thereby causing bone resorption and effecting release of calcium into the circulation; increasing the distal tubular reabsorption of calcium in the kidney; and stimulating renal 1α-hydroxylase. PTH also increases urinary phosphate secretion.

The active form of vitamin D, 1,25-dihydroxyvitamin D, increases absorption of dietary calcium in the small intestine and maintains calcification of the bone matrix. Its two precursors are ergocalciferol (synthetically derived from vegetable sterols) and the naturally occurring 7-dehydrocholesterol, both of which are activated sequentially in the skin, liver, and kidneys (see

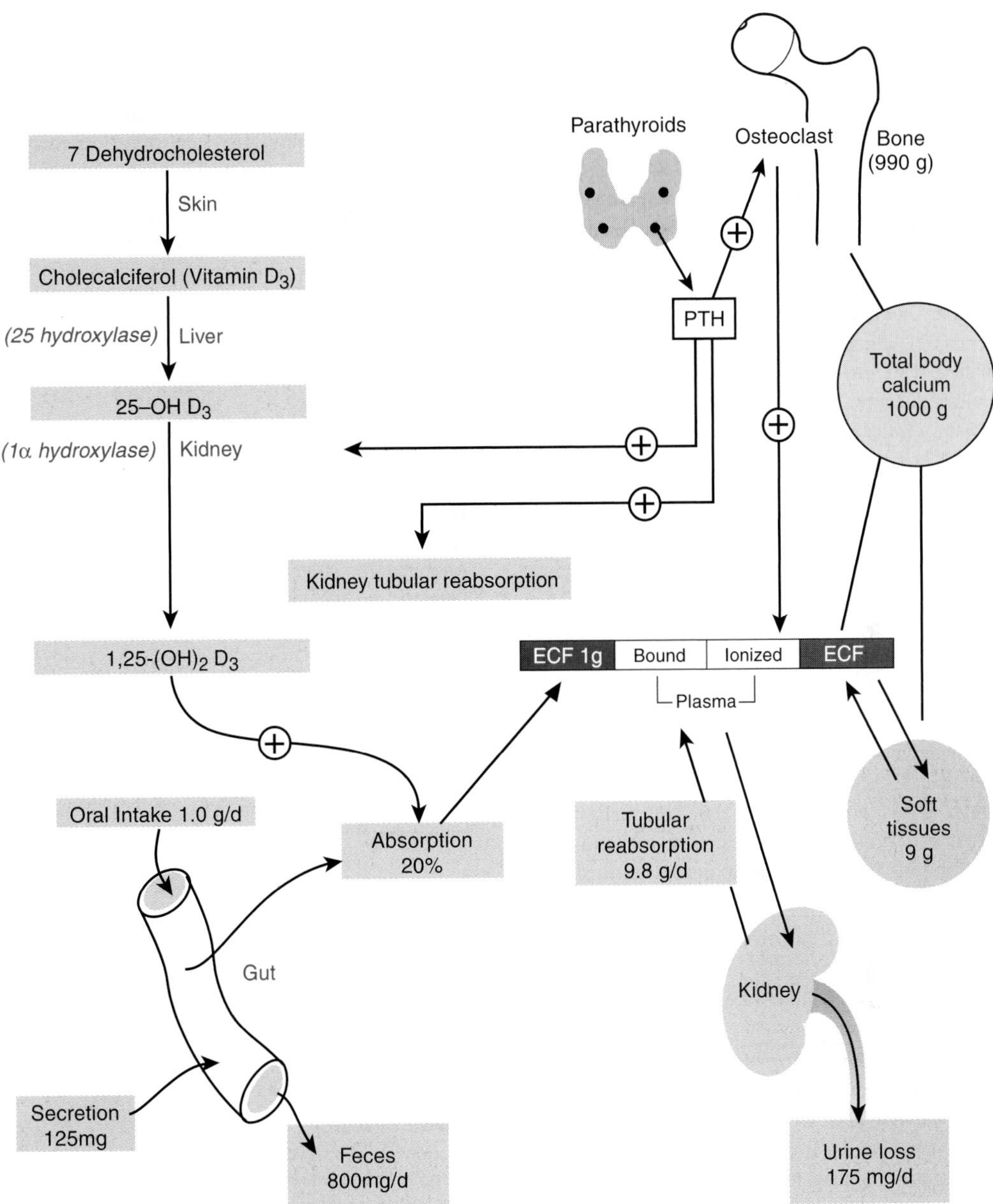


**FIGURE 66.1.** Calcium balance on an average diet. + = stimulatory pathways; PTH = parathyroid hormone.

Figure 66.1). The major storage form of vitamin D is 25-hydroxyvitamin D; its production is not homeostatically regulated. The conversion of 25-hydroxyvitamin D to 1,25-dihydroxyvitamin D is by a specific 1α-hydroxylase in the kidney, which is regulated primarily by PTH. 1,25-dihydroxyvitamin D acts by binding to high-affinity receptors in its target cells.

## Hypercalcemia

### Definition and Clinical Features

**Hypercalcemia** exists when the serum calcium level exceeds 10.4 mg/dl or when the ionized calcium exceeds 5.2 mg/dl. Hypercalcemia that is acute and severe (>14 mg/dl) can cause fatigue, anorexia, nausea, vomiting, and dehydration. When these symptoms are advanced or accompanied by confusion or coma, the diagnosis is **hypercalcemic crisis.** Hypercalcemia that is more chronic and mild evokes a variety of systemic signs (Table 66.1). The features of the underlying disease that cause the hypercalcemia also often influence the presentation.

## Diagnosis and Differential Diagnosis

Recognition of hypercalcemia has increased markedly in recent decades with the advent of routine, automated laboratory testing. The differential diagnosis of hypercalcemia is shown in Table 66.2. The underlying disorders often are **primary hyperparathyroidism** or malignancy, which together account for 90% to 95% of hypercalcemia cases. The two usually can be differentiated by the clinical presentations. Most patients with primary hyperparathyroidism have mild hypercalcemia (<13 mg/dl) and either are asymptomatic or manifest a complication of **chronic hypercalcemia,** such as **nephrolithiasis.** Patients with malignancy, however, usually present with advanced cancer and manifest more acute, severe hypercalcemia.

## Laboratory Evaluation of Hypercalcemia

The etiology of hypercalcemia usually is uncovered through the core tests listed in Table 66.3. Patients with primary hyperparathyroidism usually have a significantly elevated intact PTH level; it is low-normal or nondetectable in patients with hypercalcemia of malignancy. Measurement of urinary calcium excretion is useful (1) to exclude **familial hypocalciuric hypercalcemia** definitively when clinical and laboratory features suggest mild primary hyperparathyroidism, and (2) to determine the long-term risk for nephrolithiasis and **nephrocalcinosis** in patients with mild hyperparathyroidism.

# Primary Hyperparathyroidism

## Epidemiology and Pathogenesis

Primary hyperparathyroidism is the most common cause of hypercalcemia. It is seen more often in women than in men and its peak incidence is around the sixth decade. Primary hyperparathyroidism results from one of three pathologic conditions: a **single benign parathyroid adenoma** (85%) that produces excessive PTH; **diffuse hyperplasia** of all four glands, accounting for most of the remaining 15% and often occurring in the

**TABLE 66.1. Clinical Manifestations of Hypercalcemia**

| |
|---|
| **Renal** |
| Nephrolithiasis |
| Impaired concentrating ability (polyuria, polydipsia, and dehydration) |
| Renal tubular defects (natriuresis) |
| Interstitial nephritis |
| Nephrocalcinosis |
| Renal failure |
| **Gastrointestinal** |
| Constipation |
| Anorexia |
| Nausea |
| Peptic ulcer |
| Pancreatitis |
| **Neuromuscular** |
| Muscle weakness |
| Lethargy |
| Somnolence |
| Coma |
| Hyporeflexia |
| **Psychiatric** |
| Apathy |
| Depression |
| Psychosis |
| **Ectopic Calcification** |
| Pruritus (calcium deposition within the skin) |
| Band keratopathy (calcium deposition within the cornea) |
| **Cardiovascular** |
| Shortened QT interval on ECG (characteristic) |
| Increased sensitivity to digoxin |

**TABLE 66.2. Differential Diagnosis of Hypercalcemia**

| Common | Less Common | Factitious |
|---|---|---|
| Primary hyperparathyroidism | Medications (lithium, thiazides) | Acute hemoconcentration |
| Malignancy | Vitamin D intoxication | Increased calcium-binding proteins (e.g., hypergammaglobulinemia) |
| | Familial hypocalciuric hypercalcemia | |
| | Sarcoidosis (and other granulomatous diseases) | |
| | Acute immobilization | |
| | Renal failure | |
| | Hyperthyroidism | |
| | Milk-alkali syndrome | |

**TABLE 66.3. Laboratory Evaluation of Hypercalcemia**

| |
|---|
| **Core Work-Up** |
| Serum calcium, albumin, phosphate, and creatinine |
| Parathyroid hormone level |
| Urine calcium excretion (24-hour urine collection) |
| **Additional Tests Sometimes Useful** |
| Ionized calcium |
| SPEP, UPEP |
| Chest radiograph |
| CT, MRI of chest and abdomen |
| Parathyroid hormone-related protein |

CT = computed tomography; MRI = magnetic resonance imaging; SPEP = serum protein electrophoresis; UPEP = urine protein electrophoresis.

setting of the multiple endocrine neoplasia (MEN) syndromes; and **parathyroid carcinoma,** accounting for less than 1% of cases.

## Clinical Features

Patients with primary hyperparathyroidism can be completely asymptomatic or can manifest symptoms of either the hypercalcemia itself, or those of end organ damage. Serum calcium level typically ranges from 10.5 to 13 mg/dl; occasionally it is severely elevated. The bones and kidneys are typical targets for long-term complications. Nephrolithiasis is common and is the harbinger in many patients. **Hypercalciuria** can be severe and chronic so as to lead to nephrocalcinosis and renal failure. Increased bone resorption causes demineralization and osteopenia. Advanced, primary hyperparathyroidism classically leads to **osteitis fibrosa cystica** (Figure 66.2), with bone cysts, pathological fractures, and brown tumors.

## Management

Preoperative localization usually is not indicated. The definitive treatment of single adenomas is surgical removal. In cases of four-gland hyperplasia, three of the glands usually are removed. A portion of the remaining gland is either left in place or transplanted to the forearm to foster access, if hypercalcemia persists and reoperation is needed. Serum calcium falls postoperatively within several hours of successful surgery. Because the function of the remaining normal glands is suppressed by the adenoma, transient postoperative hypocalcemia may ensue. Because permanent hypoparathyroidism can follow if all four glands are removed surgically, observation for postoperative hypocalcemia is critical.

The treatment of asymptomatic hyperparathyroidism is not clearly defined. Some advocate deferring surgery in asymptomatic patients with mild hypercalcemia (<11 mg/dl), especially those who are elderly or frail and poorly suited for general anesthesia. If medical management without surgical intervention is selected, bone mass and renal function should be closely monitored.

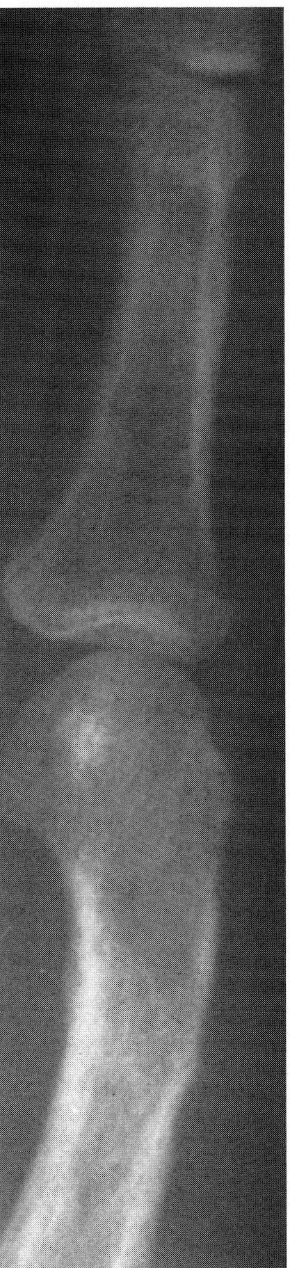

**FIGURE 66.2. Radiographs showing subperiosteal bone resorption in primary hyperparathyroidism. Excessive resorption of bone leads to an imperceptible blending of the cortex into the cancellous bone.**
(Courtesy of Radiology Museum, St. Joseph's Hospital, Milwaukee, Wisconsin.)

**TABLE 66.4. Medical Therapy of Hypercalcemic Crisis**

Step I: Intravenous normal saline to reverse dehydration and establish brisk urine output
Step II: Cautious use of furosemide (e.g., 20 mg b.i.d.) to promote further urine calcium excretion.
*Note:* Furosemide should be started only after adequate hydration has been established.
Step III:Individualized use of calcitonin or pamidronate.
Less commonly indicated are plicamycin, glucocorticoids, oral phosphate, indomethacin, dialysis, or gallium

## Hypercalcemia of Malignancy

### Pathogenesis

Malignancies are commonly associated with disorders of calcium metabolism, including hypercalciuria and hypercalcemia. Neoplasms may secrete **PTH-related protein (PTHrP),** which, although distinct from PTH, has amino-terminal homology with PTH and can mimic its effects on PTH receptors. PTHrP is produced most commonly by squamous cell cancers (head, neck, lung, and esophagus), renal cell carcinoma, and breast cancer. Metastases with extensive localized bone destruction constitute the second most common mechanism of tumor-related hypercalcemia. Hematologic neoplasms (e.g., multiple myeloma and lymphoma) cause hypercalcemia by releasing osteoclast-activating cytokines, and, occasionally (in lymphomas), 1,25-dihydroxyvitamin D.

### Clinical Features and Management

Most cancer-related hypercalcemia complicates an advanced malignancy, already diagnosed and associated with a poor prognosis. Rarely, the tumor is occult and requires an extensive work-up to unmask it (Table 66.3). The features of advanced cancer dominate the presentation, with weight loss, anorexia, fatigue, and pain from bone metastases. The hypercalcemia is more acute and severe **(hypercalcemic crisis)** than is typical for primary hyperparathyroidism and is more likely to cause nausea, vomiting, dehydration, and changes in mentation.

When possible, treatment is directed toward the primary tumor. Hypercalcemic crisis is treated medically (Table 66.4; see also Chapter 214). In many patients with terminal cancer one may elect not to treat the hypercalcemia, but to provide only palliative and supportive care.

## Hypocalcemia

### Definition and Etiology

**Hypocalcemia** is defined as a corrected serum calcium less than 8.2 mg/dl or ionized calcium less than 4.0 mg/dl. It can be due to a decrease in the albumin-bound or ionized (free) fraction of the serum calcium. Alterations in blood pH affect the ionized serum calcium without altering the total serum calcium. For example, acute acidosis increases ionized calcium by decreasing its binding to albumin, whereas acute alkalosis has the opposite effect. In true hypocalcemia, however, both the total and the ionized serum fractions are reduced.

Hypocalcemia usually is due to a deficiency in the production, secretion, or action of PTH or of 1,25-dihydroxyvitamin D. Measuring the serum phosphorus level is a key to its etiology. Since PTH decreases renal tubular phosphate reabsorption, hypocalcemia due to PTH deficiency is associated with hyperphosphatemia. In contrast, 1,25-dihydroxyvitamin D normally increases renal tubular phosphate reabsorption. Thus, vitamin D-related hypocalcemia is associated with hypophosphatemia.

### Clinical Features

Hypocalcemia often elicits no symptoms. Its clinical manifestations depend on the degree, rate of development, and duration of hypocalcemia. Among the many features listed in Table 66.5, two important ones are Chvostek's and Trousseau's signs. **Chvostek's sign** is elicited by tapping the facial nerve approximately 2 cm in front of the ear lobe and just below the zygomatic arch

**TABLE 66.5. Clinical Manifestations of Hypocalcemia**

**Cardiac**
Decreased myocardial contractility
Congestive heart failure
Prolonged QT interval (Figure 66.3)

**Dental**
Hypoplasia of teeth/enamel
Dental caries
Delayed eruption of teeth

**Neurologic**
Paresthesias (toes, fingers, and perioral regions)
Muscle cramps/fasciculations
Chvostek's sign (see Figure 66.4A)
Trousseau's sign (see Figure 66.4B)
Tetany
Seizures
Basal ganglia calcifications
Mental status changes

**Ophthalmologic**
Cataracts
Optic neuritis
Papilledema

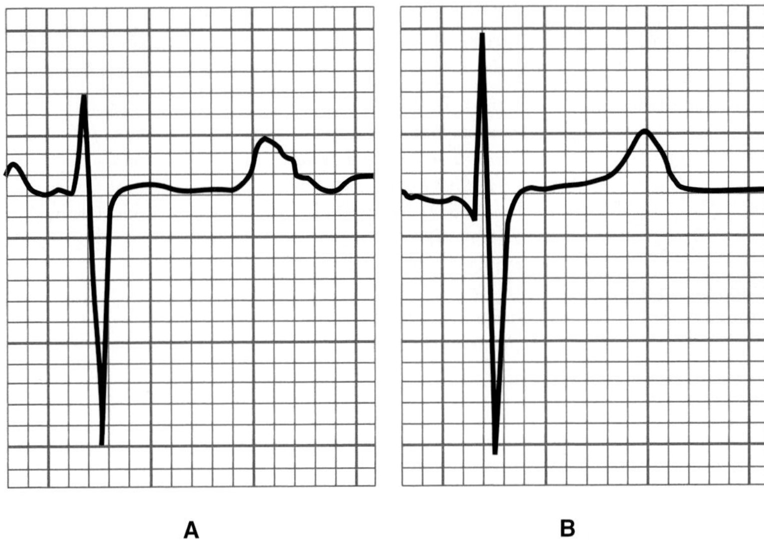


**FIGURE 66.3.** Prolonged QT interval in hypocalcemia. **A,** Baseline QT interval and the same corrected for rate (QTc) are 492 msec and 599 msec, respectively. **B,** After treatment, the QT and QTc are 432 and 442 msec, respectively.

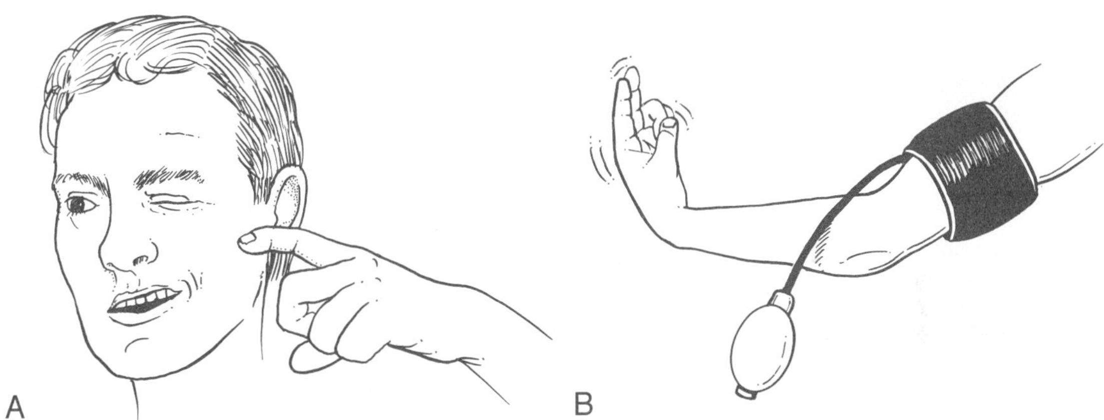


**FIGURE 66.4.** **A,** Positive Chvostek's sign. **B,** Positive Trousseau's sign.

(Figure 66.4A). A positive response is a twitching of the lip at the angle of the mouth. **Trousseau's sign** is tested by inflating a blood pressure cuff 10 to 20 mm Hg above the patient's systolic BP for 3 to 5 minutes, thus reducing the blood supply to the ulnar nerve. In hypocalcemia, this maneuver causes the classical **obstetrician's hand** (main d'accoucheur, Figure 66.4B). Whereas Chvostek's sign is positive in 10% to 20% of normal persons, Trousseau's sign is rarely present normally. The hallmark of severe hypocalcemia is tetany, caused by spontaneous sensory and motor discharges in peripheral nerves and featuring muscular twitching, spasms, or seizure. Acute respiratory distress may occur from laryngospasm and bronchospasm.

## Differential Diagnosis

The differential diagnosis of hypocalcemia based on the serum phosphate level is addressed in Table 66.6. Renal failure is the most common cause of endogenously produced **hyperphosphatemia** and subsequent hypocalcemia. As the glomerular filtration rate falls below 30 ml/min, PTH can no longer produce phosphaturia. Chronic **hypomagnesemia** can precipitate hypocalcemia by decreasing PTH secretion and by causing renal and

**TABLE 66.6. Causes of Hypocalcemia as Integrated With Serum Phosphate Level**

| Hyperphosphatemia | Hypophosphatemia | Variable Phosphate Levels |
|---|---|---|
| **Parathyroid Hormone–Related** | **Vitamin D–Related** | Osteoblastic metastasis |
| PTH deficiency | Deficient vitamin D | Acute pancreatitis |
| Congenital | Poor diet/no sun exposure | Hungry bone syndrome |
| Acquired | Malabsorption | Drugs |
| Post surgical | Impaired 25-hydroxylation of vitamin D | Critical illness/gram-negative sepsis |
| Autoimmune | Impaired 1-hydroxylation of 25-hydroxyvitamin D | Toxic shock syndrome |
| Infiltrative | Resistance to vitamin D | |
| Chronic hypomagnesemia (may cause PTH resistance also) | Vitamin D-dependent rickets, types 1 and 2 | |
| Idiopathic | | |
| PTH resistance | | |
| Pseudohypoparathyroidism | | |
| **Parathyroid Hormone–Unrelated** | | |
| Endogenous | | |
| Renal failure | | |
| Hemolysis | | |
| Rhabdomyolysis | | |
| Tumor lysis syndrome | | |
| Exogenous phosphate load | | |
| Laxatives and enemas | | |

**TABLE 66.7. Clinical Features of Albright Hereditary Osteodystrophy**

- Short stature
- Rounded facies
- Obesity
- Mental retardation
- Subcutaneous ossification
- Skeletal abnormalities
- Thickened calvarium
- Shortening and widening of the metacarpals, metatarsals, and phalanges of the hands and feet
- Short neck

skeletal resistance to the actions of PTH. In general, hypocalcemia does not develop until the serum magnesium falls below 1.0 mg/dl.

PTH resistance most commonly results from **pseudohypoparathyroidism** (PHP), a hereditary condition. In PHP, PTH administration does not raise serum calcium or evoke **phosphaturia.** Inheritance of PHP can be autosomal dominant or recessive and X-linked dominant. The classic biochemical and clinical features of PHP are hypocalcemia, hyperphosphatemia, elevated PTH, peripheral PTH resistance, parathyroid hyperplasia, and **Albright's hereditary osteodystrophy** (AHO; Table 66.7, Figure 66.5). The newer subtypes of PHP, however, present with different phenotypic appearances and different urinary biochemical responses to PTH infusion. In pseudopseudohypoparathyroidism, patients are normocalcemic but do harbor the physical features of AHO.

Hypocalcemia with hypophosphatemia usually implies a deficiency in or resistance to vitamin D. Vitamin D absorption depends on intact gastrointestinal function. Therefore, malabsorptive gastrointestinal disorders and some medications, including cholestyramine, can impair vitamin D absorption. Because the liver is the site of 25-hydroxylation, liver disease impairs this stage of vitamin D metabolism; similarly, formation of the biologically active metabolite 1,25-dihydroxyvitamin D is impaired in advanced renal disease. **Vitamin D–dependent rickets** (VDDR) types 1 and 2 are autosomal recessive syndromes of vitamin D resistance. Patients with type 1 VDDR have a selective resistance to vitamin D due to an isolated defect in 1-$\alpha$ hydroxylase activity, causing a deficiency in 1,25-dihydroxyvitamin D; patients with type 2 VDDR have a generalized vitamin D resistance owing to a mutation in the vitamin D receptor. Thus, in type 1 VDDR, the circulating 1,25-dihydroxyvitamin D level is low, whereas in type 2 VDDR, the level is high due to end organ resistance. High-dose calcium supplementation and 1,25-dihydroxyvitamin D are the primary therapy for type 2 and type 1 VDDR, respectively.

Pancreatic lipase, which is released in acute pancreatitis, liberates free fatty acids from the surrounding retroperitoneal and omental fat. These free fatty acids chelate calcium ions, resulting in hypocalcemia—a poor prognostic sign. The **hungry bone syndrome** occurs when calcium and phosphorus are acutely deposited into bones, causing hypocalcemia; it is typically seen within hours after a **parathyroidectomy** (excision of a parathyroid gland) for primary hyperparathyroidism. This condition may last for at least a month or until the remaining suppressed parathyroid glands resume functioning. Patients typically have a low serum phosphorus level, in contrast to patients with true PTH deficiency, who exhibit hyperphosphatemia. Several therapeutic agents also can cause hypocalcemia. Phenytoin, phenobarbital, and glutethimide impair 25-α hydroxylation of vitamin D; foscarnet may chelate circulating calcium; and cholestyramine may interfere with vitamin D absorption. Finally, cisplatin and pentamidine may produce urinary magnesium wasting.

## Diagnosis

Once hypocalcemia is detected, measuring the serum phosphorus guides the subsequent evaluation. A high level indicates either PTH deficiency or PTH resistance. A low level indicates a vitamin D–related disorder. When vitamin D deficiency is suspected, it usually is necessary to measure only the metabolite 25-hydroxyvitamin D, because it is consistently low in states of vitamin D deficiency. Circulating 1,25-dihydroxyvitamin D levels are less consistently depressed.

## Management

Acute hypocalcemia is treated by IV calcium gluconate or calcium chloride (Table 66.8). Vitamin D and calcium supplements are therapeutic mainstays of all

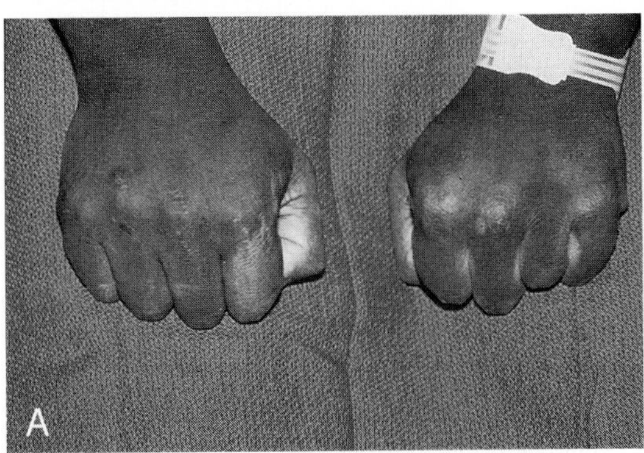


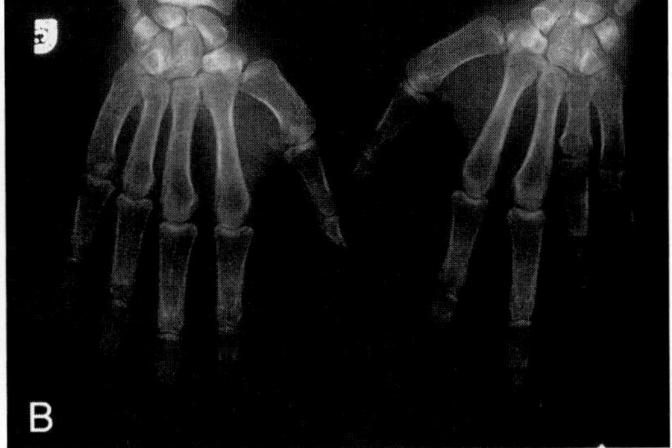


**FIGURE 66.5. Photograph (A) and radiograph (B) of the hands of a person with Albright's hereditary osteodystrophy.** (Courtesy of James M. Cerletty, MD, Department of Medicine, Medical College of Wisconsin, Milwaukee, Wisconsin.)

**TABLE 66.8. Therapy for Hypocalcemia**

**Acute Symptomatic Hypocalcemia (Tetany)**

1. 10% Calcium gluconate (90 mg of elemental $Ca^{2+}$/10 ml ampule)
   - Dilute 2 × 10-ml ampules of calcium gluconate in 50–100 ml of $D_5$ solution. Infuse 2 mg/kg body weight over 5–10 min.; or

   10% Calcium chloride (272 mg of elemental calcium/10 ml ampule)
   - Dilute 1 × 10-ml ampule in 50–100 ml of $D_5$ solution. Infuse 2 mg/kg over 5–10 minutes
2. Continue IV calcium until overt tetany is controlled

   This rapid infusion may ameliorate symptoms for 15 min to several hours
   - Follow rapid loading infusion by a slower infusion of 15 mg/kg of calcium gluconate mixed with $D_5$ infused over 6–12 hours

**Chronic Hypocalcemia**

1. Mild vitamin D deficiency
   Multivitamin containing 400 IU of vitamin D daily
   Oral calcium, 800–1200 mg daily
2. Hypoparathyroidism
   Oral elemental calcium 1-2 g in 3 divided doses
   Vitamin D replacement (approximate doses only)
   1,25-dihydroxyvitamin D: 0.25–2.0 μg/day
   Vitamin D: 25,000–100,000 IU/day

forms of parathyroid hormone and vitamin D deficiencies. If possible, the pharmacotherapy of vitamin D should allow for regulated production of 1,25-dihydroxyvitamin D. For example, if a hypocalcemic patient has normal renal function, a simple vegetable-derived vitamin D preparation should be used. Alternatively, 25-hydroxyvitamin D is used to treat patients with normal kidney function and liver disease, whereas 1,25-dihydroxyvitamin D is used for hypocalcemic subjects with advanced renal disease.

# CHAPTER 67 METABOLIC BONE DISEASE

Bone provides mechanical support for the body and is integrally involved in calcium homeostasis. There are two major forms of bone. The majority of skeletal mass is **cortical** or compact bone, found principally in the shafts of long bones. **Trabecular** or cancellous bone, found in vertebral bodies and at the ends of long bones, is less dense. Bone is composed of matrix, mineral, and cells. The **matrix** is the intercellular substance of bone tissue, consisting of collagen fibers, ground substance, and inorganic bone salts. The primary component of the matrix is type I collagen. Other glycoproteins, proteoglycans, and enzymes are present in the matrix, contributing to its mechanical strength and mediating its calcification. The rigidity of bone is derived from the calcium salts; hydroxyapatite $[Ca_{10}(PO_4]_6[OH)_2]$ is the most common calcium salt. Three specialized cells form and regulate the bone matrix and its calcification: the osteoblast, osteoclast, and osteocyte. The **osteoblast** synthesizes the enzymes involved in bone formation as well as most of the proteins of the bone matrix. **Osteocytes,** a matured form of osteoblasts, become embedded within the bone structure. **Osteoclasts,** giant multinucleated cells, are primarily responsible for bone resorption. The bone matrix and calcium salts are constantly remodeled and turned over by these cellular elements.

The three most prevalent metabolic bone diseases are osteoporosis, osteomalacia, and Paget's disease.

## Osteoporosis and Osteopenia

### Definition and Epidemiology

**Osteoporosis** is a common, age-related disorder characterized by reduced bone mass. Bone mineral and bone matrix are proportionally decreased. Decreased bone mass and decreased bone strength are correlated with fracture risk. **Osteopenia** is a more general term for radiographically decreased bone mass; in addition to osteoporosis, it also encompasses primary hyperparathyroidism, **osteomalacia** (vitamin D deficiency), and other metabolic bone diseases.

Osteoporosis may be a primary disorder, or it may follow a chronic disease. **Primary osteoporosis** sometimes is divided into **postmenopausal osteoporosis,** in which trabecular bone loss and vertebral fractures predominate, and **senile osteoporosis,** in which cortical and trabecular bone are lost equally and patients who fall are at increased risk for both vertebral and hip fractures. Multiple factors can cause primary osteoporosis (Table 67.1). Estrogen deficiency is an important factor in most women. For several years following menopause, the decline of bone mass accelerates. Therefore, early menopause is one of the strongest predictors for the development of osteoporosis. Because bone mass is higher in men than in women and in blacks than in whites, women, whites, and Asians are at greater risk of developing osteoporosis.

### Clinical Features

**Uncomplicated osteoporosis** is asymptomatic. Symptoms, when they occur, are related to fractures and their complications. Fractures most commonly involve the thoracic or lumbar vertebral bodies, the ribs, the proximal femur, and the distal radius; they result from minimal trauma and falls that ordinarily would not cause fractures. Fractures may cause local pain and loss of height, and they can lead to functional disabilities. Chronic pain from vertebral body collapse is especially common; it may be unremitting and disabling. Morbidity and mortality are high following hip fractures, particularly from venous thromboembolism.

**TABLE 67.1. Risk Factors for Postmenopausal Osteoporosis**

| |
|---|
| Early menopause |
| Caucasian or Asian race |
| Thin body habitus |
| Low calcium intake |
| Heavy alcohol use |
| Cigarette smoking |
| Physical inactivity |

**TABLE 67.2. Common Causes of Secondary Osteopenia and Osteoporosis**

| |
|---|
| Endocrine |
| Hyperthyroidism |
| Cushing's syndrome |
| Primary hyperparathyroidism |
| Hypogonadism |
| Diabetes mellitus |
| Gastrointestinal disease, malabsorption |
| Drugs |
| Anticonvulsants |
| Glucocorticoids |
| Levothyroxine (overreplacement) |
| Heparin |
| Neoplastic disease |
| Multiple myeloma |
| Diffuse metastatic disease |

## Differential Diagnosis

Several diseases can accelerate primary osteoporosis or can cause osteoporosis in patients otherwise at minimal risk (Table 67.2). In many of these conditions, an element of vitamin D deficiency is present, and patients may have a combination of osteoporosis and early osteomalacia (described in the following sections).

## Ancillary Studies

Because approximately one third of skeletal mass must be lost before it is appreciable on standard radiographs, radiographs are insensitive indicators of bone loss. Bone mass can be more accurately quantitated by specific bone densitometry techniques. **Single** and **dual photon absorptiometry** measure bone density in the radius, a largely cortical bone. **Dual energy x-ray absorptiometry** measures bone density in the spine and hip with minimal radiation exposure. Osteoporosis is defined by this technique as a bone density T-score (standard deviations below young adult peak bone mass) of less than or equal to −2.5. Bone densitometry is indicated in women with a history of early menopause, in patients with evidence of osteopenia on routine radiographs, and in most patients with diseases listed as secondary causes of osteoporosis (see Table 67.2). In general, patients with bone density exceeding 1.0 g/cm$^2$ have a low risk for fractures, whereas those with less than 0.6 g/cm$^2$ are at very high risk.

Secondary forms of bone loss should be excluded before primary osteoporosis is diagnosed. As part of the evaluation, vitamin D deficiency **(osteomalacia)** should be excluded. A careful review of systems can suggest the need for work-up for other conditions.

## Management

In established, advanced osteoporosis, therapy is more effective in preventing future bone loss than in restoring bone density to normal premenopausal levels. Thus, preventing bone loss in healthy women with normal bone density is a primary goal of therapy; the first step is to identify patients at risk (see Tables 67.1 and 67.2), including menopausal women. Treatment strategies include increasing physical activity, eliminating alcohol and smoking, and ensuring adequate dietary calcium. Unless there is history of nephrolithiasis, calcium supplementation of 1000 to 1500 mg/day is reasonable in most patients at risk. Supplementation with a daily multivitamin containing 200 to 400 units of vitamin D also is reasonable. Estrogen replacement can lower the rates of bone loss and fracture, particularly if it is begun within 3 years of menopause. The minimum effective dose for this purpose is 0.625 mg of conjugated equine estrogens. For women in whom a positive family history of breast cancer precludes use of estrogens, selective estrogen receptor modulators such as raloxifene can be used.

Treatment of **established osteoporosis** (low bone mass complicated by a history of nontraumatic fractures) also includes estrogen replacement, calcium supplementation, and addressing risk factors related to lifestyle (Table 67.3). In frail, elderly patients, it is critical to assess for risk of falls and to undertake any appropriate interventions. Newer bisphosphonates, such as alendronate and risedronate are proving to be effective, increasing bone density by approximately 5% per year. Calcitonin inhibits osteoclast activity and either improves bone mass or slows rates of bone loss in established osteoporosis. Calcitonin can be administered either as a nasal spray or as a subcutaneous injection.

## Osteoporosis in Men

Although osteoporosis is less common in men than in women, osteoporotic men are more likely than women to

**TABLE 67.3. Treatment of Primary Osteoporosis**

| |
|---|
| Core therapy |
| Estrogen replacement (or selective estrogen receptor modulator) |
| Reverse risk factors where possible |
| Oral calcium supplement (1000 mg/d) |
| Calcitonin |
| Bisphosphonates |
| Low-dose vitamin D |
| Occupational/physical therapy |

have one of the definable conditions (e.g., hypogonadism) listed in Table 67.2.

## Osteomalacia and Rickets

**Osteomalacia,** a disease characterized by a softening and bending of the bones, results when inadequate calcium is available for bone matrix calcification because of vitamin D deficiency. Therefore, in contrast to osteoporosis, where the decreases in bone mineral and matrix are proportional, osteomalacia is characterized histologically by decreased mineralization with increased bone matrix. It is caused by either vitamin D deficiency (inadequate diet, malabsorptive gastrointestinal disorders), or diseases or other factors that impair conversion of vitamin D to 1,25-dihydroxyvitamin D (liver or renal disease, or anticonvulsant therapy). The decreased intestinal absorption of calcium reduces its availability to mineralize bone matrix. A compensatory increase in parathyroid hormone levels leads to increased bone mineral resorption by osteoclasts.

Clinical features vary depending on the age at onset, the precipitating causes, and the presence or absence of concomitant hypocalcemia. **Rickets** is osteomalacia occurring in children prior to epiphyseal closure. Children with rickets have bowing of long bones, growth retardation, bone pain, and delayed dentition. Adults with osteomalacia present with bone pain and pathological fractures. Associated hypocalcemia leads to hypotonia, muscle weakness, and tetany.

Imaging studies show diffuse demineralization (osteopenia), increased trabecular markings, and pseudofractures (Figure 67.1). Serum calcium and phosphate often are low, and alkaline phosphatase is high. These two findings reflect secondary hyperparathyroidism. Therapy of osteomalacia includes administration of vitamin D or its active metabolite, 1,25-dihydroxyvitamin D, and, where possible, identification and treatment of the underlying disease or diseases.

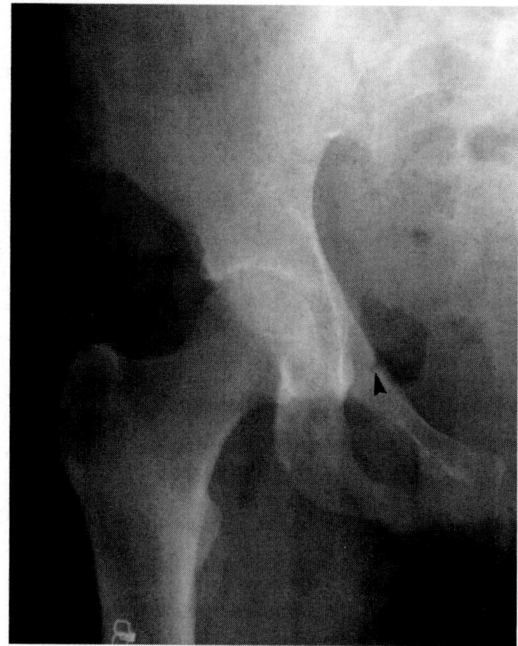

**FIGURE 67.1. Pelvic radiograph in osteomalacia showing pseudofracture (Looser zones). These fractures usually are best seen on the concave side of the affected bones.** (Courtesy of the Radiology Museum, St. Joseph's Hospital, Milwaukee, Wisconsin.)

## Paget's Disease of Bone

### Definition and Etiology

The hallmark of **Paget's disease** (osteitis deformans) is disordered bone remodeling with an increase in the rate of bone turnover. Although it usually is focal, Paget's disease may be widespread. The pelvic bones are most commonly involved, followed by skull, femur, lumbosacral spine, clavicles, ribs, and tibia. Excessive bone resorption results in areas of radiolucency on radiographs **(osteoporosis circumscripta).** The normal marrow is replaced by fibrovascular connective tissue. Excessive osteoblastic activity replaces resorbed bone, but new bone is organized haphazardly, with multiple, irregular cement lines; histologically, it has a characteristic mosaic pattern. Although the coarse, dense Pagetic bone appears abnormally dense on radiographs, its strength is not enhanced; the irregular structure makes it weaker than normal bone, thus causing fractures and deformities. The etiology of Paget's disease is unknown, but it may be caused by a slow virus infection.

### Clinical Features

Paget's disease is rare before middle age, but estimates suggest that it may be present in 3% of persons over age 40. Because most patients are asymptomatic, the disease usually is discovered incidentally on radiographs or by an isolated, otherwise unexplained rise in alkaline phosphatase. It also can present with swelling, deformity, or pain in a long bone. Skull enlargement may cause an increase in hat size over the years. Temporal bone involvement may cause hearing loss, and Pagetic bone growth and basal skull compression may evoke other neurologic symptoms. Vertebral and long-bone fractures may result from structural bone abnormalities; these fractures and deformities together may cause loss of height. With widespread disease, the high skeletal blood flow raises cardiac output, thus leading to heart failure. Osteogenic sarcoma occurs in less than 1% of cases.

## Laboratory and Radiologic Evaluation

Bone turnover in Paget's disease is focally increased. Therefore, markers of osteoblast activity (serum alkaline phosphatase) and of osteoclast activity (urine hydroxyproline) usually are high in active disease; observing changes in them can be helpful in monitoring response to therapy. Serum calcium and phosphate usually are normal. However, hypercalcemia can follow immobilization in patients with Paget's disease. Skeletal radiographs, especially of the pelvis, skull, femur and lower spine, are useful in diagnosis (Figure 67.2). Bone scans, which are more sensitive than radiographs, can define the extent of Paget's disease, but the findings are nonspecific and overlap with degenerative arthritis and metastatic cancer.

## Management

The major goals of drug therapy are to reduce pain, limit the development of further deformities, and prevent neurologic complications. Aspirin or nonsteroidal anti-

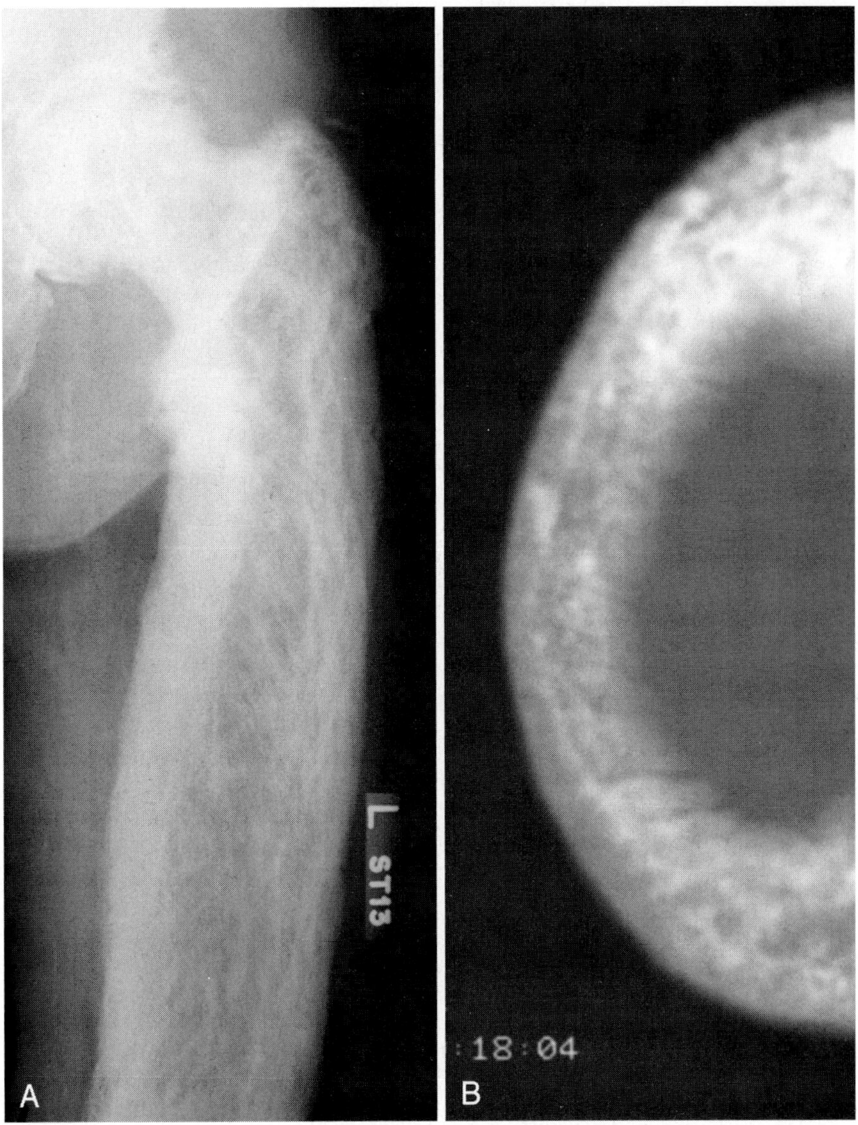


**FIGURE 67.2. A, Radiograph of the femur in a patient with advanced Paget's disease. B, CT scan of the skull of the same patient, showing coarse, dense, pagetic bone.** (Radiograph courtesy of Radiology Museum, St. Joseph's Hospital, Milwaukee, Wisconsin.)

inflammatory agents can help relieve pain. If symptoms are clearly attributable to Paget's disease, more specific therapy can be given, but it can be difficult to judge whether back pain in a patient with Paget's disease is due to Paget's disease or to coexisting degenerative disc disease. The use of calcitonin or bisphosphonate may suppress disease activity. Human or salmon calcitonin, 100 units daily, may be started subcutaneously. Following symptomatic improvement, the dose can be tapered to about 50 units 3 times per week; therapy can eventually be totally discontinued. The bisphosphonate etidronate is given orally cyclically (200–400 mg qd, 6 months on and 6 months off); alendendronate (40 mg qD, 6 months on and 6 months off) or risendronate (30 mg qD, 6 months on and 6 months off) may become the preferred alternatives; pamidronate is given in a series of IV infusions to produce a prolonged remission in symptoms. Mithramycin is less useful because of its hepatic, renal, and hematologic toxicity. Disease activity should be monitored during therapy.

# CHAPTER 68 DISEASES OF THE ADRENAL CORTEX

The adrenal glands, located at the superior pole of each kidney, consist of two concentric layers: the cortex and the medulla. The cortex is subdivided into three histological zones: the subcapsular **zona glomerulosa,** which secretes mineralocorticoids, and the **zona fasciculata** and **zona reticularis,** both of which secrete glucocorticoids and androgens.

The synthetic pathways for the steroid hormones produced in the adrenal cortex are shown in Figure 68.1. The major regulatory system for cortisol is through

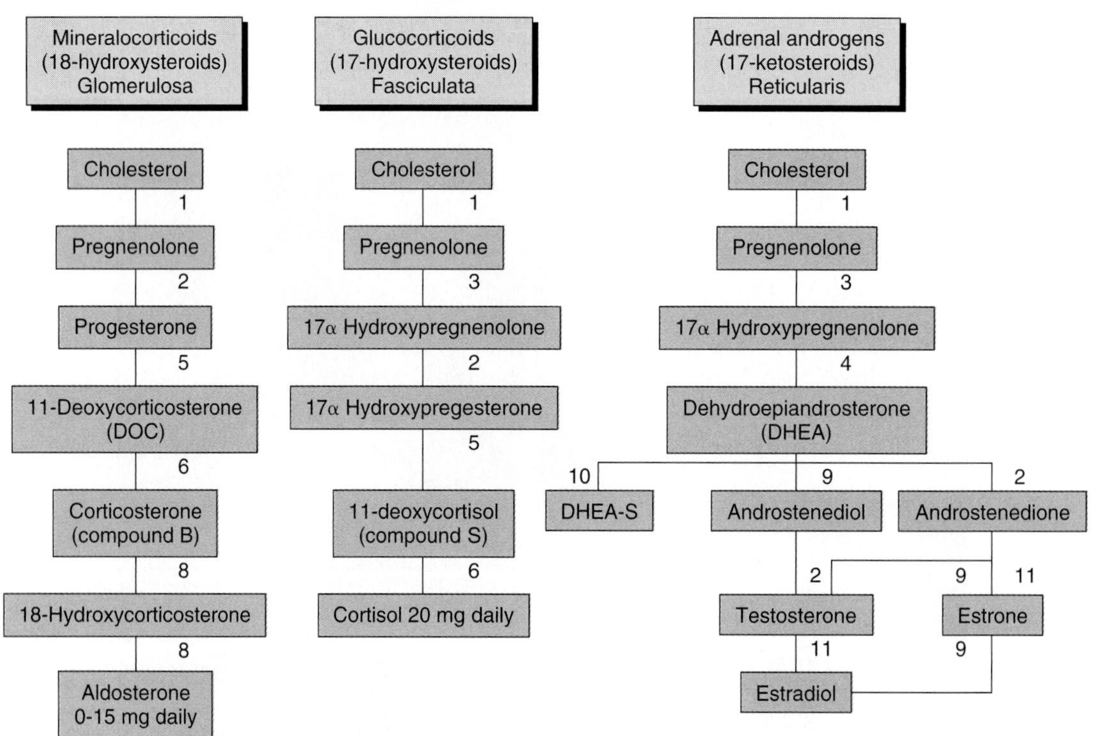


**FIGURE 68.1.** Synthetic pathways of adrenocortical steroids. Boxed numbers represent enzymes: 1 = 20,22 desmolase; 2 = 3β-hydroxysteroid dehydrogenase; 3 = 17-hydroxylase; 4 = 17,20-desmolase; 5 = 21-hydroxylase; 6 = 11β-hydroxylase; 7 = 18-hydroxylase; 8 = 18-aldehyde synthetase; 9 = 17-ketosteroid reductase; 10 = 3β-hydroxysteroid sulfotransferase; 11 = P-450 aromatase.

**hypothalamic corticotropin-releasing factor** (CRF) and **pituitary adrenocorticotropic hormone** (ACTH). Secretion of ACTH is pulsatile, creating a daily diurnal variation in cortisol secretion with maximal release in the morning. Cortisol circulates in plasma, bound to **corticosteroid-binding globulin** (CBG), a protein synthesized in the liver; only a small fraction occurs in the biologically active free form.

The renin-angiotensin system, hyperkalemia, and hyponatremia strongly stimulate aldosterone synthesis and release. Renin is produced by the juxtaglomerular cells of the kidney. It catalyzes the conversion of renin substrate to **angiotensin I** (A-I). The regulation of renin depends on intravascular volume. Upright posture, hemorrhage, diuretics, sodium restriction, and edematous states increase renin secretion by decreasing effective plasma volume. **Angiotensin-converting enzyme** (ACE) converts A-I to A-II, which up-regulates the enzyme that converts cholesterol to pregnenolone (the first step in adrenal steroid synthesis), and the conversion of corticosterone to aldosterone. Aldosterone promotes renal tubular $Na^+$ reabsorption as well as excretion of $K^+$ and $H^+$ ions.

**Dehydroepiandrosterone** (DHEA), **DHEA-sulfate** (DHEAS), and **androstenedione** are the major androgens synthesized in the adrenals. They exert their androgenic activity after peripheral conversion to the more potent androgens, **testosterone** and **dihydrotestosterone.** ACTH is the major stimulator of adrenal androgen secretion, but additional adrenocortical or other circulating regulators also may play a role in controlling their synthesis and release.

## Adrenal Insufficiency

### Definition

**Adrenocortical insufficiency** (Addison's disease), first described by Thomas Addison in 1885, has an estimated incidence of approximately 50 cases per million adults in Western countries. Development of the clinical manifestations of adrenocortical insufficiency requires loss or destruction of 90% or more of both adrenal cortices. Its treatment is simple, but if left undiagnosed and untreated, its consequences are devastating and often lethal.

### Etiology and Pathogenesis

Adrenocortical hormone insufficiency can result from primary destruction of adrenal cortices **(primary adrenal insufficiency),** insufficient pituitary ACTH **(secondary adrenal insufficiency),** or decreased hypothalamic CRF secretion **(tertiary adrenal insufficiency)**. **Acute adrenal insufficiency** most commonly occurs in a patient who is exposed to stress (e.g., sepsis, trauma or surgery) and who requires increased glucocorticoids that the underactive glands cannot provide. It also can follow acute bilateral destruction of the adrenal glands. The most common cause of adrenal insufficiency is **iatrogenic tertiary adrenal insufficiency;** this condition follows suppression of endogenous CRF/ACTH/cortisol owing to use of exogenous glucocorticoids in pharmacologic doses to treat unrelated diseases.

**TABLE 68.1. Disorders Associated With Autoimmune Addison Disease**

| |
|---|
| Thyroid disease |
| Hashimoto's hypothyroidism |
| Graves' hyperthyroidism |
| Diabetes mellitus (type 1) |
| Primary gonadal failure |
| Pernicious anemia |
| Myasthenia gravis |
| Hypoparathyroidism |
| Chronic mucocutaneous candidiasis |
| Alopecia |
| Vitiligo |
| Chronic active hepatitis |
| Malabsorption syndrome |

The **idiopathic** type is the most common primary adrenal insufficiency in the United States; it results from autoimmune destruction of all three layers of the cortex. Idiopathic primary adrenal insufficiency is more common in women; it may be familial, and it is usually diagnosed in the third to fifth decades of life. Nearly 60% of patients have circulating adrenal antibodies, and lymphocytic infiltration of the gland is noted early on. Addison disease shows a high association with autoimmune disorders of other endocrine glands (Table 68.1). The causes of primary adrenal insufficiency are listed in Table 68.2. Tuberculosis (TB) is the second most frequent cause in the United States and also is a common cause in developing countries. TB manifests with adrenal calcification on abdominal radiographs. The other entities listed in the table are rare.

### Clinical Features

Clinical features of adrenal insufficiency are presented in Table 68.3. Its evolution may be gradual or catastrophically sudden. The major physiologic derangements of adrenal insufficiency are fluid and sodium depletion. Mineralocorticoid and glucocorticoid loss reduces the ability to retain $Na^+$ and excrete $K^+$ and $H^+$ ions; cardiac output and renal perfusion are decreased. In acute adrenal insufficiency, intravascular volume, vascular tone, and cardiac output are all decreased; hypotension and, potentially, vascular collapse and shock fol-

**TABLE 68.2. Etiology of Adrenal Insufficiency**

| Primary Adrenal Gland Failure | Secondary and Tertiary Adrenal Insufficiency |
|---|---|
| Idiopathic/autoimmune | Long-term glucocorticoid steroid use |
| Tuberculosis | Congenital hormonal or releasing factor deficiencies |
| Adrenal hemorrhage | Neoplasms |
| Bilateral infarction | Inflammatory lesions |
| Fungal infection | Granulomatous disease |
| HIV/AIDS | Degenerative disease |
| Metastatic cancer | Trauma (infundibular stalk section) |
| Bilateral adrenalectomy | Radiation |
| Congenital adrenal hypoplasia | Necrosis (Sheehan syndrome) |
| Congenital adrenocortical hyporesponsiveness | |
| Congenital adrenal hyperplasia | |
| Adrenoleukodystrophy | |
| Drugs: mitotane, ketoconazole, metyrapone | |

**TABLE 68.3. Clinical Features of Adrenal Insufficiency**

| |
|---|
| Gastrointestinal |
| Anorexia |
| Nausea, vomiting |
| Diarrhea |
| Abdominal cramping |
| Cardiovascular |
| Hypotension |
| Tachycardia |
| Signs of dehydration |
| Fever |
| Muscle weakness |
| Restlessness |
| Hyperpigmentation of skin |

**TABLE 68.4. Typical Laboratory Abnormalities in Adrenal Insufficiency**

| |
|---|
| Hyponatremia |
| Hyperkalemia |
| Hypoglycemia |
| Metabolic acidosis |
| Azotemia |
| Na/K ratio usually < 20 |
| Eosinophilia |
| Lymphocytosis |
| Anemia |
| Hypercalcemia |

low. Characteristically, the skin pigmentation is absent when the adrenal failure is acute, secondary, or tertiary. Among the laboratory features summarized in Table 68.4, hyponatremia is due primarily to an impaired ability to excrete free water; thus, it is common to any type of adrenal insufficiency. However, hyperkalemia and metabolic acidosis are absent in secondary or tertiary adrenal failure, because aldosterone secretion is preserved.

## Diagnosis

In the case of **shock** with dehydration and intact adrenal function, a random plasma cortisol level should be at least 20 μg/dl; in most cases, the level exceeds 30 μg/dl. Adrenal insufficiency is best diagnosed by a rapid **cosyntropin stimulation test**. **Cosyntropin,** a synthetic fragment of ACTH, contains the first 24 amino acids of ACTH from the amino terminal end. The test is best done between 6 AM and 10 AM. Plasma samples are drawn for cortisol before and 60 minutes after administering 250 μg of cosyntropin IV. Normally, the plasma cortisol rises 7 μg/dl above the baseline, and it should exceed 20 μg/dl at 60 minutes. The plasma ACTH level separates primary from secondary adrenal failure; ACTH typically exceeds 250 pg/ml in the primary type, but it is low or inappropriately normal in other types.

## Management

The management of acute adrenal insufficiency is presented in Table 68.5. The most important point to remember in treating acute adrenal crisis is that if the diagnosis is considered, the patient should be treated immediately without waiting for confirmation. Once basal blood specimens have been obtained for diagnosis, fluid restoration and hormone substitution should follow promptly. IV glucocorticoids should be given in large quantities. If a cosyntropin stimulation test is performed, the patient initially receives an injection of dexamethasone, which does not affect plasma cortisol measurement. Hydrocortisone is the preferred glucocorticoid in the treatment of Addisonian crisis, because it inherently exhibits the greatest mineralocorticoid activity. Mineralocorticoid replacement is unnecessary if the total daily hydrocortisone dose exceeds 100 mg. With proper treatment, patients with adrenal insufficiency, even in Addisonian crisis, have a very good prognosis. Left untreated, acute adrenal crisis is lethal.

In managing chronic adrenal insufficiency (Table 68.6), it is important to educate the patient on three points: the need to take the glucocorticoid replacement regularly; the need to increase the dosage twofold to threefold for the few days of intercurrent illness or stress; and the need to revert to regular maintenance doses once the illness has resolved. It is not necessary to alter the mineralocorticoid dose. Cues for the patient to contact the physician include signs of dehydration, worsening of the intercurrent illness, or its persistence beyond 3 days.

## Cushing's Syndrome

Cushing's syndrome (see detailed discussion in Chapter 63) is a clinical disorder resulting from excessive cortisol production. The focus in this chapter is on Cushing's syndrome due to an adrenal neoplasm **(ACTH-independent hypercortisolemia)**. **Functioning benign adrenal adenomas** and **adrenocortical cancers** each give rise to less than 10% of cases of Cushing's syndrome. Usually, benign adenomas are small (<100 g at diagnosis) and synthesize cortisol very efficiently. In contrast, functioning adrenocortical cancers are very large at diagnosis and often produce adrenal steroids inefficiently. Because adrenal cancer is virulent, patients almost always present with a palpable abdominal mass and metastatic spread, but lack Cushingoid features.

Clinical features of hypercortisolemia are described in Table 63.8. In benign adrenocortical adenoma, the signs of cortisol excess usually begin gradually. Hyperpigmentation of the skin, hirsutism, and other virilizing signs often are absent. However, in functioning adrenocortical carcinomas, the course tends to be more acute and rapidly progressive, with hyperandrogenic effects predominating. Patients also report abdominal, back, and flank pain caused by the large tumor size. Hypercortisolemia with concomitant ACTH suppression (ACTH < 10 pg/ml) and an adrenal mass seen on CT or MRI are diagnostic.

Surgical removal of the benign adrenocortical adenoma through a **unilateral adrenalectomy** of the affected gland is curative. Glucocorticoid replacement is required to avoid acute adrenal crisis due to suppression and atrophy of the hypothalamus, pituitary, and contralateral adrenal. It may take as long as 1 to 2 years for these suppressed glands to resume functioning, so such replacement therapy must be tapered slowly. The prognosis for most adrenal carcinomas is dismal. These malignant tumors usually are treated with debulking surgery followed by chemotherapy with mitotane. Median survival after diagnosis in adults is 14 to 36 months; untreated, survival averages 3 months. Although mitotane lowers steroid production in 75% of patients and measurably reduces tumor size in 30%, there is no clear evidence that it actually prolongs life.

**TABLE 68.5. Managing Acute Adrenal Crisis**

1. IV fluid replacement
   Use normal saline (NS) or $D_5$ NS if hypoglycemia is present.
   Infuse rapidly initially to stabilize blood pressure.
   Monitor for signs and symptoms of fluid overload.
   Monitor serum $K^+$ carefully, because $K^+$ will drop precipitously. Replace as needed.
2. Glucocorticoid replacement
   Dexamethasone 4 mg IV for initial dose; *or*
   Hydrocortisone 100 mg IV immediately after cosyntropin stimulation test is completed and every 8 hours thereafter.
   Taper glucocorticoids rapidly to a maintenance dose, usually decreasing the dose by one half each day, if precipitating illness permits.
3. Treat the precipitating stress
   Search for and treat the illness that precipitated the adrenal crisis.

**TABLE 68.6. Management of Chronic Primary Adrenal Insufficiency**

1. Maintenance glucocorticoid replacement (any 1 of these regimens)
   Cortisone acetate, 25 mg in a.m. and 12.5 mg in p.m.
   Hydrocortisone, 20 mg in a.m. and 10 mg in p.m.
   Prednisone, 5 mg daily
   Monitor weight, clinical signs and symptoms of fluid retention, and Cushingoid features; adjust dosage accordingly.
2. Maintenance mineralocorticoid replacement
   Fludrocortisone, 0.05–0.2 mg daily
   Monitor standing and recumbent blood pressure and serum electrolytes.
3. Educate the patient about the disease, how to manage minor illnesses and major stresses.
4. Obtain a Medical Alert® bracelet or necklace and an emergency medical information card.

TABLE 68.7. Causes of Secondary Hyperaldosteronism

| Hypertensive | Normotensive |
|---|---|
| Renal artery stenosis | Cardiac failure |
| Renin-secreting tumors | Gastrointestinal disorders |
| Malignant hypertension | Renal tubular acidosis |
| Chronic renal disease | Renal tubulopathies (Bartter's syndrome) |
| | Hepatic cirrhosis |
| | Diuretic abuse |
| | Nephrotic syndrome |

## *Primary Hyperaldosteronism*

### Definition and Epidemiology

Mineralocorticoid excess causes hypertension by two patterns: aldosterone excess (primary hyperaldosteronism), and secondary hyperaldosteronism (Table 68.7). In 1955, Conn described primary hyperaldosteronism—a syndrome of hypertension and spontaneous hypokalemia due to aldosterone excess. Occurring in less than 1% of hypertensives, primary hyperaldosteronism is rare. It is seen most often in the third through fifth decades. In hypertensive patients with spontaneous hypokalemia ($K^+$ < 3.5 mEq/L), 40% have a variant of primary hyperaldosteronism.

### Etiology and Pathogenesis

Primary hyperaldosteronism most often results from **aldosterone-producing adenomas** (APA) and idiopathic hyperaldosteronism (IHA). Rarely, it may be due to **glucocorticoid-suppressible hyperaldosteronism** or an **aldosterone-secreting adrenal carcinoma.** APAs typically are solitary, unilateral, small (< 2 cm in diameter), and benign. In IHA, there is bilateral hyperplasia of the zona glomerulosa, possibly from hyperstimulation by an unidentified aldosterone-releasing factor. In primary hyperaldosteronism, the intravascular volume is typically high. Secondary hyperaldosteronism is hyperreninemic (elevated renin); patients may be normotensive or hypertensive. In normotensives with secondary hyperaldosteronism, the elevated circulating renin and aldosterone levels are due to decreased effective intravascular volume, whereas the hypertension in secondary hyperaldosteronism is more likely related to increased angiotensin II than to aldosterone.

### Clinical Features and Diagnosis

Key manifestations of primary hyperaldosteronism include hypertension, spontaneous hypokalemia, alkalosis, low plasma renin activity, and an elevated plasma aldosterone level. The hypertension usually is moderate and is due to the sodium-retaining effects of the mineralocorticoid. Rarely, the hypokalemia may evoke polyuria, easy fatigability, anorexia, muscle weakness, and cramps.

A screening for primary hyperaldosteronism is required for a hypertensive patient with spontaneous hypokalemia below 3.5 mEq/L, or a serum $K^+$ below 3.0 mEq/L while taking a diuretic. The first step is to confirm primary hyperaldosteronism, then to determine its etiology. Testing is optimal when the individual is salt loaded and when the hypokalemia is corrected. Before biochemical testing, the following medications should be discontinued: all antihypertensive agents except peripheral $\alpha$-1 antagonists and central $\alpha$-2 agonists, for at least 1 week; diuretics, for 4 weeks, and estrogen and spironolactone, for 6 weeks. The first phase of the work-up includes screening tests followed by multiple tests to confirm the diagnosis (Table 68.8). Approximately 80% of cases of primary hyperaldosteronism are due to either APA or IHA, so the second phase involves differentiating between these two causes. Imaging and bilateral adrenal vein catheterization are used to make the distinction. High-resolution CT is performed initially, because it localizes the APA in 70% to 80% of cases. Bilateral adrenal vein catheterization is the most effective means to distinguish between APA and IHA, but it is reserved for patients with equivocal CT scans and posture studies.

### Management and Prognosis

Patients with an APA who are at low surgical risk should undergo adrenalectomy. One year following a successful surgery, 80–90% of patients remain normotensive and normokalemic; after 5 years, however, 50% develop recurrence of the hypertension while remaining normokalemic. Because bilateral adrenalectomy usually is ineffective in controlling hypertension, medical management is chosen in all patients with IHA. Patients should follow a low sodium diet (<80 mEq/d), exercise regularly, and maintain an ideal body weight. Spironolactone, amiloride, and triamterene are the usual pharmaceutical agents for treating the hypokalemia of primary hyperaldosteronism. Spironolactone, the drug of choice, often is combined with nifedipine or an ACE inhibitor to adequately control blood pressure. If this therapy does not control the hypertension, the next step is empiric trials of other antihypertensive drugs, which usually are equally effective.

## *Congenital Adrenal Hyperplasia*

### Definition and Epidemiology

**Congenital adrenal hyperplasia** (CAH) is a family of autosomal recessive disorders resulting from defects in cortisol production. These disorders involve five enzymes: 21-hydroxylase, 11-hydroxylase, 3β-hydroxysteroid dehydrogenase, 17-hydroxylase, and 20,22-desmolase. Figure 68.1 shows the biosynthetic steps in the adrenal cortex that are catalyzed by these five enzymes. Deficient cortisol biosynthesis causes a compensatory rise in pituitary ACTH; therefore, adrenocortical hyperplasia and overproduction of the steroids that precede the enzymatic defect result. CAH can take two forms: a classic, congenital form with nearly total enzymatic deficiency; or, more often, a late-onset form with a partial enzymatic deficiency and onset after puberty.

## Clinical Features and Management

Clinical manifestations of each of the five enzymatic deficiencies depend on which steroids are deficient or in excess, as well as the absolute degree of deficiency or excess. The clinical and biochemical characteristics and diagnosis of the five forms of CAH are reviewed in Table 68.9. Classic 21-hydroxylase deficiency, the only HLA-linked type, accounts for more than 90% of cases of

**TABLE 68.8. Diagnostic Tests for Primary Hyperaldosteronism due to Aldosterone-Producing Adenoma or Idiopathic Hyperaldosteronism**

| Screening | | Confirmatory | | Localizing |
|---|---|---|---|---|
| 24-h (urinary) $K^+$ | >30 mEq | 4-h upright PAC/PRA | >20 | CT of the adrenals |
| PRA (ng/ml/h) | <2 | Captopril suppression test | | Adrenal vein catheterization |
| PAC (ng/dl) | >14 | PAC/PRA | >50 | |
| | | PAC (ng/dl) | >15 | |
| | | 4-h saline infusion test | | |
| | | PAC (ng/dl) | >10 | |

PAC = plasma aldosterone concentration; PRA = plasma renin activity.

**TABLE 68.9. Clinical and Biochemical Characteristics, and Diagnosis of the CAH Syndromes***

| Enzymatic Defect | Phenotypic Presentation** | Adrenal Hormone*** | Clinical/ Biochemical Features**** | Diagnosis |
|---|---|---|---|---|
| 21-hydroxylase | NM; VF to AG | AE, GD, MD | ±SW, ↑$K^+$A | ↑ Plasma 17-OH progesterone |
| 11-hydroxylase | NM; VF to AG | AE, GD, ME (↑DOC) | HBP, ↓$K^+$Alk | ↑ Plasma 11-deoxycortisol |
| 3β-hydroxysteroid dehydrogenase | UM to AG; VF to AG | AE, GD, MD | ±SW, ↑$K^+$A | ↑ Plasma pregnenolone<br>↑ Plasma 17-OH pregnenolone<br>↓ Plasma progesterone<br>↓ Plasma 17-OH progesterone<br>↑ DHEA<br>↓ Androstenedione |
| 17-hydroxylase | UM to AGF; lack of SSC | AD, GD, ME (↑DOC) | HBP, ↓$K^+$Alk | ↑ Plasma progesterone<br>↑ Plasma pregnenolone<br>↓ Plasma 17-OH progesterone<br>↓ Plasma 17-OH pregnenolone |
| 20,22 desmolase | UM to AG; NF | AD, GD, MD | ±SW, ↑$K^+$A, Massive adrenal enlargement | Deficiency of all adrenocortical steroids |

*Measurement of the plasma steroid precursor after exogenous ACTH stimulation may be necessary to diagnose mild or late-onset forms.
**NF = normal female; VF = virilized female; AGF = ambiguous genitalia female; NM = normal male; UM = undervirilized male; AG = ambiguous gentialia; SSC = secondary sexual characteristics.
***AD = androgen deficiency, AE = androgen excess, GD = glucocorticoid deficiency; MD = mineralocorticoid deficiency; ME = mineralocorticoid excess; DOC = 11-deoxycorticosterone.
****HBP = hypertension; SW =salt-wasting; ↑$K^+$A = hyperkalemic acidosis; ↓$K^+$Alk = hypokalemic alkalosis.

**TABLE 68.10. Differential Diagnosis of Adrenal Mass**

| |
|---|
| Benign nonfunctional adrenal cortical adenoma |
| Benign functional adrenal cortical adenoma |
| Cushing syndrome |
| Virilizing |
| Feminizing |
| Hyperaldosteronism |
| Primary adrenal cortical carcinoma |
| Nonfunctional |
| Functional |
| Tumors of the adrenal medulla |
| Pheochromocytoma |
| Ganglioneuromas/neuroblastoma |
| Benign adrenal cyst |
| Myelolipoma |
| Intra-adrenal hemorrhage |
| Metastases from other primary malignancies |
| Congenital adrenal hyperplasia |

CAH. The next most common, 11-hydroxylase deficiency, accounts for nearly 5% of all CAH cases.

The enzymatic defects that impair cortisol and mineralocorticoid synthesis are treated respectively with glucocorticoids and mineralocorticoids. The consequent reduction in release of pituitary ACTH results in suppression of the overproduced adrenocortical steroids.

## The Incidental Adrenal Mass

### Definition and Epidemiology

Since the advent of abdominal CT scanning, the unsuspected (incidental) adrenal mass **(adrenal incidentaloma)** has become a common diagnostic dilemma. The incidence of adrenal masses thus detected ranges from 0.5% to 10%. Because most of these masses have been found to be nonfunctional, and because primary adrenocortical cancer is exceedingly rare in adrenal masses smaller than 5 cm, a small, adrenal incidentaloma is usually considered to be benign and nonfunctional.

### Etiology and Pathogenesis

Common causes of an adrenal mass can be found in Table 68.10. Between 30% and 50% of primary adrenocortical carcinomas are nonfunctional; the rest are functional. Excessive cortisol is the most common secretory product for both benign and malignant adenomas. Primary malignancies that most commonly metastasize to the adrenals include those of the breast, lung, lymphoma, melanoma, and colon.

### Clinical Manifestations

The clinical characteristics of adrenal incidentalomas depend on their functional nature. A primary adrenal cortical carcinoma most commonly presents with abdominal pain and an easily palpable mass. The mean duration of symptoms prior to diagnosis is 6 to 9.5 months; most patients present in an advanced stage with a 5-year survival ranging between 15% and 25%, independent of the stage at diagnosis. Typical sites of metastases include lung, lymph nodes, liver, bone, and gastrointestinal tract.

### Diagnosis and Management

Initially, the CT or MRI appearance taken in context with a thorough history and physical examination may provide clues to the nature of the mass. **Myelolipomas** contain fat and are easily recognized on CT and MRI. Clinically, evidence is sought for Cushing's syndrome, **pheochromocytoma,** nonadrenal malignancies, virilization in a female, and feminization in a male. Cortical and medullary dysfunction should be determined using the screening tests shown in Table 68.11. Large masses should be removed. Needle aspiration is useful in cystic lesions and to help stage an extra-adrenal neoplasm (e.g., lung). For small lesions (less than 3–4 cm) associated with normal adrenal function, evaluation includes serial CT scans over a period of 12–18 months. If the lesion is stable in size, it is presumed to be a benign, nonfunctional, adrenal adenoma and no further follow-up is needed.

**TABLE 68.11. Screening Laboratory Assessment for Adrenal Incidentalomas**

| |
|---|
| Overnight 1-mg dexamethasone suppression test or 24-hour urinary free cortisol |
| Serum dehydroepiandrosterone sulfate |
| Serum potassium |
| Aldosterone: Plasma renin activity (if serum potasium < 3.5 mEq/L) |
| 24-hour urine metanephrines, VMA, and catecholamines |

VMA = vanillylmandelic acid.

# CHAPTER 69 DISEASES OF THE ADRENAL MEDULLA

The main secretion of the adrenal medulla is **epinephrine** rather than **norepinephrine**, owing to the presence of **phenylethanolamine-N-methyl transferase** (PNMT), which converts norepinephrine to epinephrine. **Epinephrine, norepinephrine,** and **dopamine,** collectively called **catecholamines,** are derived from tyrosine, the dietary amino acid; these structurally similar compounds are contained within the same biosynthetic pathway. All neurons and cells of the catecholaminergic lineage contain the enzyme **tyrosine hydroxylase.** Once tyrosine is hydroxylated to L-DOPA, the nature of the final hormonal product released by these cells is determined by their respective set of biosynthetic enzymes. Because most adrenomedullary chromaffin cells contain a full complement of all the enzymes outlined, epinephrine is the main secretion of these cells. Approximately 10% of the adrenal catecholamines are excreted directly into the urine as free epinephrine. All the remaining catecholamine derivatives are renally excreted (Figure 69.1).

The systemic effects of adrenomedullary catecholamine release are mediated through the activation of peripheral α- and β-adrenergic and dopaminergic receptors. The catecholamines are important mediators of central nervous system and autonomic nerve functions, and they are important regulators of the cardiovascular system. Because epinephrine has a slightly higher affinity for β-adrenergic receptors, the main hemodynamic effect

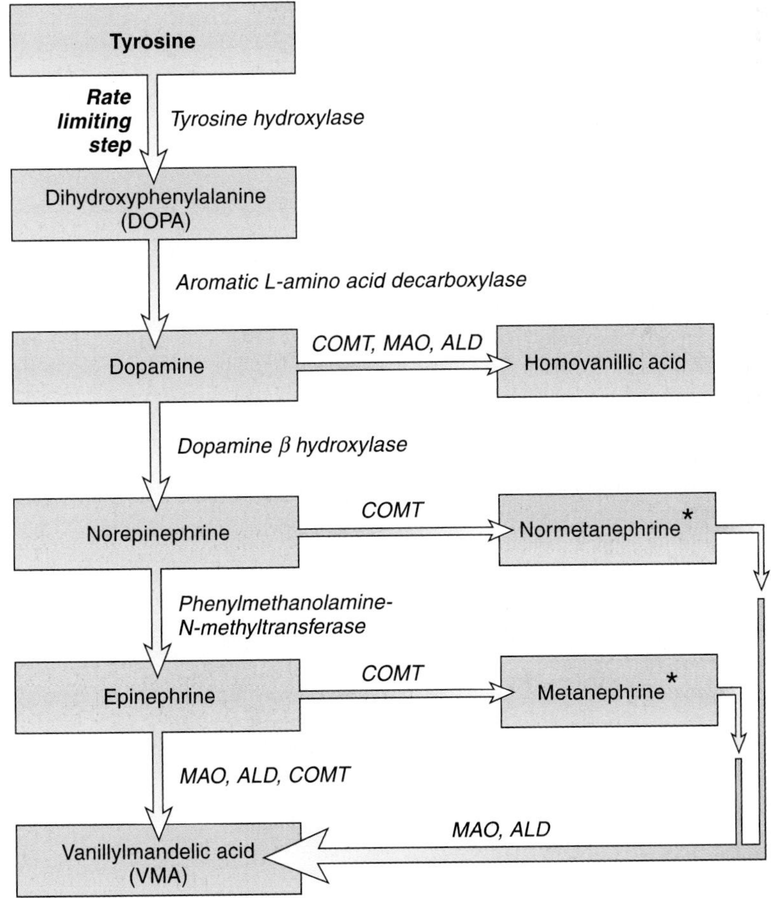


**FIGURE 69.1.** Biosynthetic and metabolic pathways for catecholamines. * = major urine metabolites; ALD = aldehyde dehydrogenase; COMT = catechol O-methyl transferase; MAO = monoamine oxidase.

of chromaffin cell secretion is cardiac, increasing both heart rate and contractility. Venous return, and, thus, preload to the heart, increase from $\alpha_1$-mediated vasoconstriction of capacitance vessels. Combined with an $\alpha_1$-mediated vasoconstriction of resistance vessels, these collective effects significantly raise the blood pressure. Catecholamines directly or indirectly affect all other endocrine systems. Circulating epinephrine levels alter fluid and electrolyte balance, because a $\beta$-mediated sympathetic mechanism controls the renin-angiotensin-aldosterone axis. Increased circulating epinephrine levels also enhance basal metabolism and facilitate the breakdown of stored fuels by directly stimulating lipolysis and enhancing glucagon-mediated glycogenolysis and gluconeogenesis.

Neoplasms are the most significant of all the adrenal medullary disorders. Their histology and functionality reflect the cell type of derivation. Tumors arise more often from the catecholamine-secreting cells of neural crest origin, presenting as pheochromocytomas in adults and as neuroblastomas in children (one of the common solid tumors of childhood).

## Pheochromocytoma

### Definition and Etiology

**Pheochromocytomas** are autonomously functioning, catecholamine-secreting, chromaffin-cell neoplasms. About 90% are benign solitary nodules found within the adrenal medulla itself. However, they can arise anywhere that neural crest tissue has migrated during the course of embryonic development; nearly 10% are located intra-abdominally in close proximity to the celiac or mesenteric sympathetic ganglia. Adrenal medullary pheochromocytomas are almost always (90%) unilateral. Bilateral lesions usually occur only as familial neoplasms, as in type IIa **(Sipple's syndrome)** or type IIb **multiple endocrine neoplasia syndrome** (MEN; Table 69.1). The MEN syndromes are transmitted as autosomal dominant diseases with incomplete penetrance and variable expression. Specific mutations of the RET proto-oncogene located on chromosome 10 cause familial predisposition to pheochromocytoma in MEN type II.

### Clinical Features

The hallmark of a pheochromocytoma is hypertension. The clinical triad of severe headache, palpitations, and excessive diaphoresis occurring with hypertension provides the best clinical clue for this tumor (Table 69.2). If this triad and hypertension are absent, the diagnosis of a pheochromocytoma can be set aside confidently. Although 80% or more of these patients are hypertensive on examination, nearly one half exhibit normotensive, symptom-free periods, interspersed with episodic and transient symptoms. Spectacular fluctuations in blood pressure are quite common. Excessive catecholamine

**TABLE 69.1. Classification of the Multiple Endocrine Neoplasia Syndromes**

| MEN Syndrome | Associated Disorders |
|---|---|
| MEN type I (Wermer's syndrome) | Hyperparathyroidism<br>Pituitary adenomas<br>Pancreatic islet cell tumor<br>Gastrinoma<br>VIPoma<br>Insulinoma<br>Glucagonoma |
| MEN type IIa (Sipple's syndrome) | Medullary carcinoma of thyroid<br>Pheochromocytoma<br>Hyperparathyroidism |
| MEN type IIb | Marfanoid habitus<br>Pheochromocytoma<br>Medullary carcinoma of thyroid<br>Mucosal and intestinal neuromas |

MEN = multiple endocrine neoplasia; VIP = vasoactive intestinal peptide.

**TABLE 69.2. Clinical Manifestations Associated With Pheochromocytomas**

| Symptoms | Incidence (%) | Signs | Incidence (%) |
|---|---|---|---|
| Headache | 75–100 | Hypertension | 75–100 |
| Palpitations | 50–75 | Tachycardia | 50–75 |
| Diaphoresis | 50–75 | Postural hypotension | 50–75 |
| Anxiety | 25–50 | Paroxysmal hypertension | 25–50 |
| Tremulousness | 25–50 | Weight loss | 25–50 |
| Chest pain | 25–50 | Tremor | 25–50 |
| Abdominal pain | 25–50 | Pallor | 25–50 |
| Nausea/emesis | 25–50 | | |
| Weakness/fatigue | 25–50 | | |

**TABLE 69.3. Normal Urine Levels of Catecholamines and Their Metabolites**

| Substance in Urine | Upper Limit of Normal |
|---|---|
| Total catecholamines | 100 μg/d |
| Norepinephrine | 75 μg/d |
| Epinephrine | 25 μg/d |
| Dopamine | 525 μg/d |
| Metanephrines | 1.1 mg/d |
| Vanillylmandelic acid | 7 mg/d |

secretion causing the constellation of these symptoms appears to be paroxysmal. During an attack, if BP and pulse rate both rise, the tumor is primarily releasing epinephrine. In contrast, if pulse rate declines as BP rises, the tumor is secreting mainly norepinephrine.

## Diagnosis

Pheochromocytomas are diagnosed biochemically. The most useful screening test is a 24-hour urine measurement of the levels of catecholamines (norepinephrine and epinephrine) and of their metabolites, metanephrine and vanillylmandelic acid (see Table 69.3 for normal values). The quantitation of total urinary metanephrines and catecholamines, especially norepinephrine, provides the most sensitive and specific proof of pheochromocytoma. Recently, the determination of free norepinephrine in a 24-hour urine sample was shown to be 100% sensitive and 98% specific for diagnosis. In most cases of pheochromocytoma, the **total urinary metanephrines and catecholamines** (norepinephrine + epinephrine) exceed 1000 μg/24 h and 150 μg/24 h, respectively. Because many medications influence the test results, all medications should be withheld for a minimum of 1–2 days, if possible, before collecting the urine sample. **Plasma norepinephrine,** another useful screening test in pheochromocytomas, typically exceeds 2000 pg/ml. However, because catecholamine secretion may be intermittent, single plasma catecholamine measurements may be less sensitive than urinary levels. Recently, measurement of plasma metanephrine levels showed higher sensitivity and specificity than the traditional biochemical tests for the diagnosis of both sporadic and familial pheochromocytoma. Specific pharmacologic stimulation/suppression tests often are used when the clinical features are equivocal and when urinary or plasma catecholamines are only slightly elevated. Provocative testing with intravenous glucagon bolus in these patients often elicits an exaggerated pressor response; agents that normally attenuate adrenomedullary catecholamine release (clonidine, $\alpha_2$-agonist) have no effect.

Once a pheochromocytoma is confirmed biochemically, localization with CT or MRI should follow. CT often is not the best initial imaging study when extra-adrenal or metastatic pheochromocytomas are suspected. Radionuclide tests with **$^{131}$I-meta-iodobenzylguanidine** (MIBG), a radioactive amine taken up and concentrated by adrenergic chromaffin cells, are quite useful in this setting.

## Management and Prognosis

Pheochromocytoma almost always is cured by surgical excision of the tumor. The recent development of laparoscopic surgical techniques has provided a safe alternative to open surgical techniques. Advantages of a laparoscopic approach include less postoperative pain, a shortened hospital stay and convalescent period, and a better cosmetic result. The 5-year postoperative survival rate exceeds 95%. An α-adrenergic blocking agent (phenoxybenzamine, 10 mg b.i.d., then increase by 10 mg every 2 days until blood pressure is controlled) is administered for at least 14 days prior to surgery in order to avoid an intraoperative hypertensive crisis. Unless **tachyarrhythmias** develop from complete α-blockade, preoperative β-blocking agents are not routinely given. **Phentolamine** (a reversible α-blocker) and **nitroprusside** (a direct-acting arterial vasodilator) usually are used to manage any hypertensive crises that arise during the induction of anesthesia or during surgery. Severe hypotension after tumor excision usually is avoided by perioperative plasma volume expansion with normal saline. **Metyrosine**, a tyrosine hydroxylase inhibitor that reduces tumor stores of catecholamines, also may be used for preoperative management of pheochromocytoma. Treatment with metyrosine lowers intraoperative fluid requirements, decreases the need for intraoperative medication to control blood pressure, and attenuates blood loss. Inoperable or malignant pheochromocytomas are medically managed, using both α- and β-adrenergic blockade. If these agents fail to produce adequate symptom relief, metyrosine may be added. In these rare patients, the 5-year survival rate is less than 50%.

Unrecognized pheochromocytomas are potentially lethal. Hypertensive crisis or lethal shock may be precipitated by drugs, anesthetic agents, surgery for unrelated conditions, or parturition. However, with early diagnosis, these patients enjoy an extremely high cure rate.

# CHAPTER 70 DISORDERS OF OVARIAN FUNCTION

## Ovarian Physiology

The ovary has two distinct regions: the **outer cortex,** with the **germinal epithelium** and **follicles,** and the **central medulla,** consisting of supportive stroma, blood vessels, nerves, and lymphatics. The **graafian follicle** contains both theca and granulosa cells. The interstitial and stromal ovarian cells arise from degenerating atretic follicles.

The ovaries have two major functions: cyclic **steroidogenesis** (the biosynthesis of steroids) and **ovulation** (oocyte maturation and release). **Estrogens, progestins,** and **androgens** are the major sex steroids synthesized by the three main functional components of the ovary: the **follicles,** corpus luteum, and **ovarian stroma** (Figure 70.1). Ovarian hormone production is controlled by the anterior pituitary gonadotropins, follicle-stimulating hormone (FSH) and luteinizing hormone (LH), which are necessary for follicle stimulation. Follicle stimulation results in estrogen production by the **theca interna** and **granulosa** cells found in the follicular wall. The main and most important estrogen produced by the germinal epithelium is **17β-estradiol**. The mid-cycle LH surge causes **ovulation** (discharge of the ovum from the graafian follicle), after which the corpus luteum secretes primarily progesterone. Androgens are produced mainly by the interstitial thecal cells and to a lesser degree by the ovarian stroma. The androgens include **dehydroepiandrosterone** (DHEA), **androstenedione,** and **testosterone**. Although the role of the ovarian androgens is not clear, the functions of the other ovarian hormones are shown in Table 70.1.

## Normal Menstrual Physiology

Menses is the monthly flow of blood from the female genital tract. **Menarche** (the onset of menses) occurs between 10 and 15 years of age. Menses cease **(menopause)** between 45 and 53 years of age. Normal menses occur every 28 days (range, 21–40 days) and last 2 to 7 days, with a blood loss of 30 to 100 ml during each cycle. The **menstrual cycle** is the interval between the first day of menses and the next onset of menses. It is the response of the uterus to the cyclic changes and interactions of hypothalamic GnRH, pituitary gonadotropins, and the secretion of ovarian estradiol and progesterone (Figure 70.2). The menstrual cycle is divided into the **follicular** (proliferative) and **luteal** (secretory) phases. The follicular phase marks the first half of the cycle; ovulation occurs at midcycle, and the luteal phase follows ovulation.

## Physiology of Androgen Secretion

The major circulating androgens in women are shown in Table 70.2. **Dihydrotestosterone,** formed from the conversion of testosterone by the enzyme 5α-reductase, appears to be the androgen responsible for androgen-dependent hair growth. Androstenedione, DHEA, and DHEA-sulfate possess little intrinsic direct androgenic activity before conversion to testosterone and dihydrotestosterone (see Table 70.2).

## Amenorrhea

### Definition and Etiology

**Amenorrhea** is defined as the absence of menses by age 16 in a nonpregnant woman **(primary)** or as no menses for over 3 months in a woman with previously regular cycles **(secondary)**. The differential diagnosis of amenorrhea is based on the anatomic structure primarily responsible for the problem (Table 70.3). **Oligomenorrhea** is infrequent menstruation. A defect at any level of the hypothalamic-pituitary-ovarian-genital tract axis may be responsible. Hypothalamic **hypogonadism** may result from tumors and infections; pituitary adenomas, craniopharyngiomas, germinomas, hamartomas, and teratomas are the most common underlying tumors. Infections that can have this effect include tuberculosis, syphilis, encephalitis, and meningitis. Almost 15% of cases of amenorrhea result from hyperprolactinemia, which inhibits hypothalamic GnRH release. Hyperprolactinemia is discussed in Chapter 63.

**Hypergonadotropic hypogonadism** is seen in patients with **gonadal dysgenesis** or Turner syndrome, a condition caused by a defect or absence of one of the two X chromosomes. **Turner syndrome,** the most common cause of primary amenorrhea, occurs in about 1 in 2000 female births. These girls typically have characteristic somatic abnormalities, including sexual infantilism, short stature, webbing of the neck, shieldlike chest, low-set ears with low posterior hairline, high arched palate, and **cubitus valgus** (increased carrying angle of the elbows). They also commonly manifest transient lymphedema of the hands and feet at birth (30%), cardiovascular anomalies (50%), renal defects (35%) and gonadal failure (95–100%). Other causes of hypergonadotropic hypogonadism include ovarian enzymatic deficiencies and premature ovarian failure. In addition to the conditions listed in Table 70.3, patients with polycystic ovary syndrome (Stein-Leventhal syndrome), adult-onset congenital adrenal hyperplasia, Cushing's syndrome, and

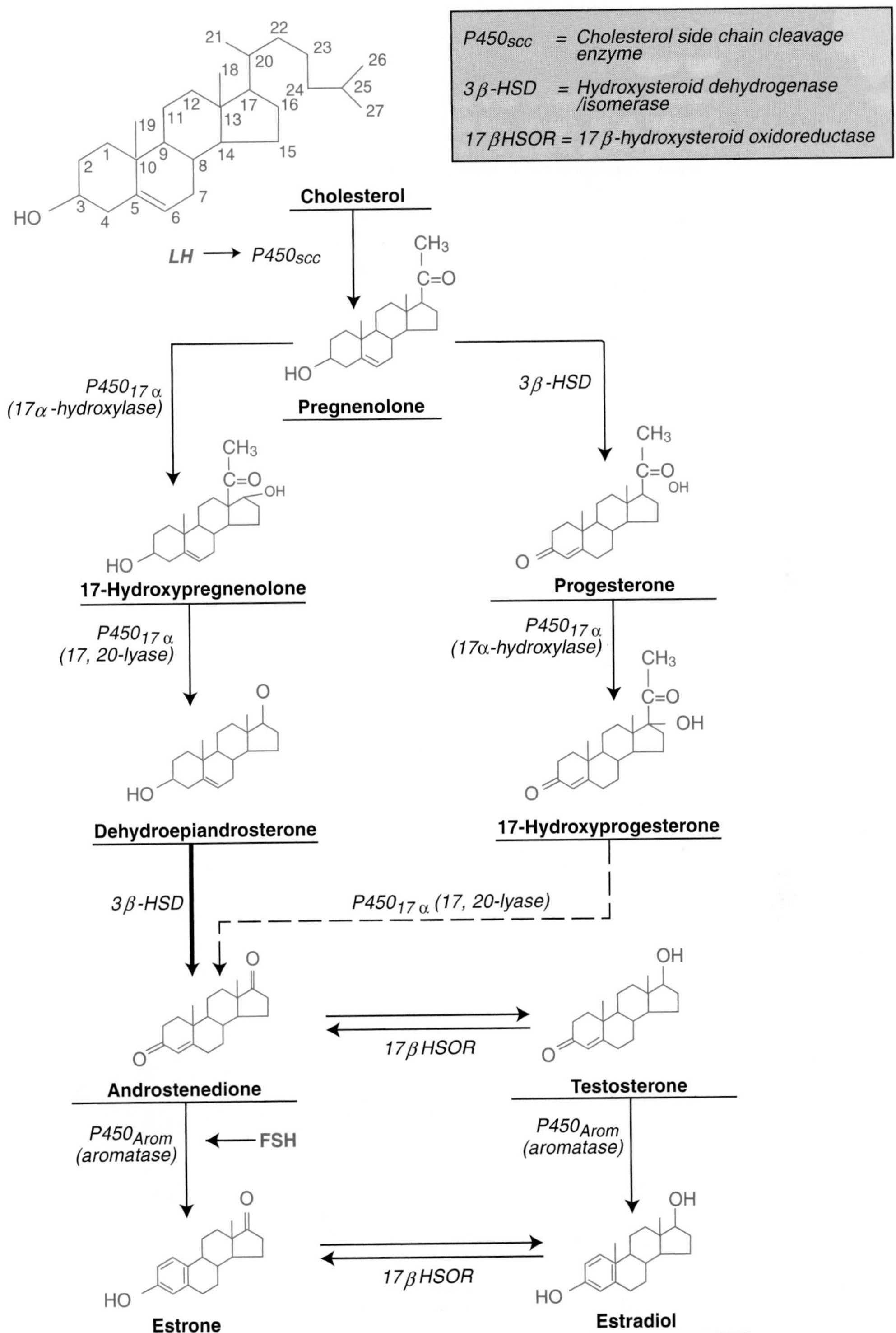


**FIGURE 70.1.** Principal pathways of ovarian steroid hormone biosynthesis. The major enzyme complements for the corpus luteum, theca, and granulosa cells are shown; these cells produce predominantly progesterone and 17-hydroxyprogesterone (corpus luteum); androgen (theca); and estrogen (granulosa). The horizontal arrows indicate the major sites of action of LH and FSH in mediating this pathway. The dotted line emphasizes the limited metabolism of 17-hydroxyprogesterone in the human ovary.
(Redrawn with permission from Carr BR, in Wilson JD, Foster DW (eds). Williams Textbook of Endocrinology. 8th ed. Philadelphia: WB Saunders, 1992, p. 745.)

**TABLE 70.1. Actions of the Ovarian Sex Steroids**

| Sex Steroid | Major Actions |
|---|---|
| Estrogen | Promotes development of secondary sexual characteristics in women<br>Promotes uterine, vaginal, and fallopian tube development and thickening of vaginal mucosa<br>Promotes thinning of cervical mucus<br>Promotes development of breast ductal system<br>Reduces bone resorption<br>Increases HDL cholesterol (oral estrogen only) |
| Progesterone | Induces secretory activity in the endometrium of the estrogen-primed uterus<br>Required for implantation of the fertilized ovum<br>Required for maintenance of pregnancy<br>Induces decidualization of the endometrium<br>Inhibits uterine contraction<br>Increases viscosity of cervical mucus<br>Promotes glandular development of breasts<br>Increases basal body temperature |

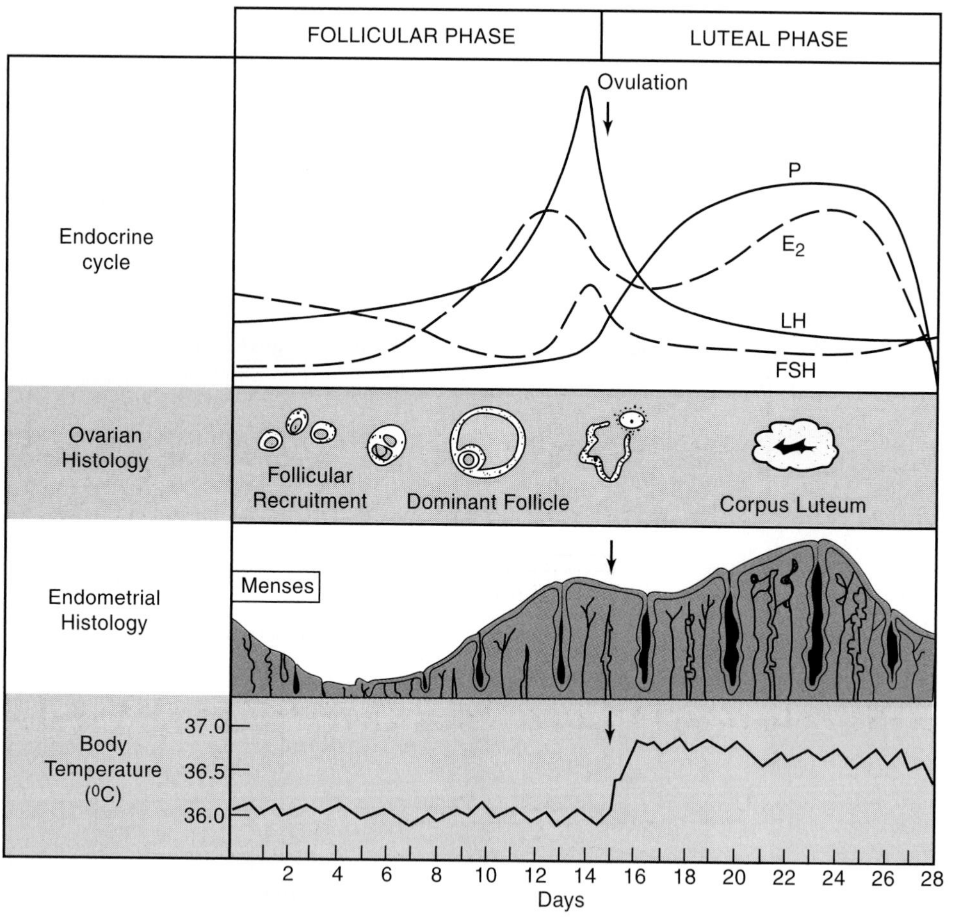


**FIGURE 70.2. Hormonal, ovarian, endometrial, and basal body temperature changes and relationship throughout the normal menstrual cycle.** (Redrawn with permission from Carr BR, Wilson JD. In: Isselbacher KJ, Braunwald E, Wilson JD, et al (eds). Harrison's Principles of Internal Medicine. 13th ed. New York: McGraw-Hill, 1994, p. 2022.)

TABLE 70.2. Major Androgens in Women

| Androgen | Sites of Formation[b] Ovary (%) | Adrenal (%) | Conversion (%) | Relative Androgen Activity[a] |
|---|---|---|---|---|
| Testosterone | 5–25 | 5–25 | 50–90 | 100 |
| Androstenedione | 45–50 | 30–45 | 5–25 | 10–20 |
| Dehydroepiandrosterone (DHEA) | 20 | 80 | – | 5 |
| DHEA-sulfate | <5 | >95 | – | minimal |
| Dihydrotestosterone | – | – | 100 | 250 |

[a]Relative to testosterone = 100.
[b]Percent of a particular androgen produced at each site.

TABLE 70.3. Causes of Amenorrhea

Pregnancy and/or breast-feeding
Hypogonadotrophic hypogonadism
- Hypothalamus
  - Tumors/infection
  - Hand-Schuller-Christian disease
  - Kallmann syndrome
  - Sarcoidosis
  - Idiopathic hypogonadotropic hypogonadism
  - Chronic debilitating disease
  - Anorexia, malnutrition, weight loss
  - Exercise-associated
  - Emotional trauma/stress
- Pituitary
  - Tumor compression
  - Hyperprolactinemia
  - Empty sella
  - Sheehan's syndrome
  - Sarcoidosis
  - Hemochromatosis
  - Post-surgical, irradiation, trauma

Hypergonadotropic hypogonadism
- Gonadal agenesis/dysgenesis
- Ovarian enzymatic deficiency
- Premature ovarian failure

Normal gonadotropins and estrogen
- Uterus/Vagina
  - Mullerian agenesis
  - Endometrial hypoplasia/aplasia
  - Labial fusion/imperforate hymen
  - Cervical stenosis/agenesis
  - Vaginal agenesis
  - Uterine scarring
  - Testicular feminization

TABLE 70.4. Clinical Evaluation of Amenorrhea

**History**
- General
  - Significant medical illness
  - Emotional stress
  - Weight loss
  - Exercise
  - Exposure to toxic chemicals/drugs/radiation
  - Past surgeries
  - Symptoms of estrogen deficiency (hot flashes)
  - Headaches
  - Visual field changes
  - Galactorrhea
  - Symptoms of hypothyroidism
- Developmental
  - Age and sequence of secondary sexual characteristics
  - Menarche
  - Menstrual history
  - Sexual history
- Family history
  - Reproductive problems
  - Age of mother's menarche and menopause

**Physical examination**
- Body habitus: muscle mass and fat distribution
- Skin: pigment, acne, hair distribution and type, striae
- Eye: visual fields
- Thyroid: size and consistency
- Breasts: Tanner stage, galactorrhea, atrophy
- Pubic hair: Tanner stage
- Pelvic: presence/absence/normalcy of internal and external genitalia, vaginal estrogenization, cervical mucus

hypothyroidism or hyperthyroidism often have amenorrhea with normal or near-normal estrogen levels.

## Evaluation

In assessing either primary or secondary amenorrhea, it is first necessary to exclude pregnancy. A thorough history and physical examination (Table 70.4) reveals the cause in most patients with amenorrhea. After assessing for the signs of Cushing's syndrome, hyperprolactinemia, and acromegaly, supportive laboratory tests should be scheduled. In addition to the mandatory pregnancy test, basal serum measurements of TSH, prolactin, 17-β estradiol, FSH, and LH are also generally required in all amenorrheic women, especially those with a normal physical examination. The work-up of amenorrhea is outlined in Figure 70.3. The progesterone withdrawal test or progestin challenge is a bioassay for estrogen production; it is performed by giving 5 to 10 mg of oral medroxyprogesterone acetate daily for 5 to 10 days or 100 to 200 mg of progesterone in oil intramuscularly as a single dose. Any vaginal bleeding within 7 to 10 days indicates adequate estradiol (estradiol level of at least 40 pg/ml) and confirms integrity of the uterine and vaginal tract. If withdrawal bleeding does not occur, cyclic estrogen followed by progesterone is given. Patients with normal or low FSH and LH who initially fail to bleed with progesterone alone, but who respond to sequential estrogen and progesterone, most likely have a hypothalamic or pituitary abnormality. Women who also fail to respond to the sequential estrogen and progesterone regimen usually have an outflow tract obstruction. High serum FSH levels (>40 mIU/ml) indicate ovarian failure. A karyotype should be analyzed in young women (<30 years old) with elevated FSH levels to look for Turner's syndrome.

### Management

The treatment of amenorrhea depends on the diagnosis and on patient goals. Influential factors include reversibility of the abnormality, adequacy of feminization, desire for fertility, need for contraception, problems due to estrogen deprivation, risk of endometrial hyperplasia and cancer with unopposed estrogen, and associated hirsutism and virilization.

If **functional hypothalamic amenorrhea** is induced by stress, weight loss, or excessive exercise, important treatment strategies include counseling and lifestyle changes. Women with a positive progesterone withdrawal test should be given **oral progesterone** (medroxyprogesterone acetate 5–10 mg daily) for 5 to 10 days every 1 to 3 months or an oral contraceptive pill to induce periodic bleeding, avoiding endometrial hyperplasia. Combined estrogen/progesterone therapy should be given when response to progesterone is absent, as in patients with ovarian failure and women with irreversible hypothalamic or pituitary disorders.

## Hirsutism and Virilization

### Definition

**Hirsutism** is defined as the presence in women of excessive body hair in areas associated with a masculine pattern of hair growth. There are two types of hair: vellus and terminal. **Vellus hair** is fine, soft, generally unpigmented hair that is not androgen-stimulated and is found diffusely over the body. **Terminal hair** is coarse, pigmented, androgen-dependent, and normally localized (in a masculine pattern) to the back, face, chest, abdomen, axilla, and pubic area. Hirsutism is generally more of a cosmetic problem capable of causing psychosocial difficulties than a pathological disorder. It is common, with 15% to 35% of normal women developing terminal hairs on the lower abdomen, upper lip, and chest. Terminal hair on the face, periareolar region, and lower abdomen is normal, but that on the upper back, shoulders, sternum, and upper abdomen suggests a more marked androgen effect. **Virilization** is defined as both decreased feminine secondary sexual characteristics (breast and vaginal mucosal atrophy) and increased masculine secondary sexual characteristics (hirsutism, temporal balding, voice deepening, clitoromegaly, and increased muscle mass). Virilization usually implies more significant hyperandrogenism.

### Etiology and Pathogenesis

Hirsutism in women results from increased androgen production or action, and its etiology may be androgen-dependent or androgen-independent. **Androgen-dependent hirsutism** has a male pattern of hair growth and typically is due to excessive adrenal or ovarian androgen production (Table 70.5) or increased follicle sensitivity to androgen. **Androgen-independent hirsutism** is characterized by increased growth of vellus-type hair. Most cases of hirsutism are idiopathic or due to polycystic ovarian syndrome.

Virilizing adrenal and ovarian tumors may be benign or malignant. Adrenal tumors produce primarily DHEA and DHEA-S; ovarian tumors produce primarily testosterone. Benign tumors usually produce androgens efficiently; therefore, they are small when diagnosed. In contrast, malignant tumors usually are inefficient in steroid hormone biosynthesis; they are large (>6 cm in diameter) and easily palpable at diagnosis.

### Clinical and Laboratory Evaluation

The primary goal in the diagnostic evaluation of a hirsute or virilized woman is to exclude a serious underlying cause. The first step consists of a thorough history and physical examination, with biochemical testing to pursue the clues thus obtained (Table 70.6). Abrupt, nonperipubertal onset, rapid advance of hirsutism, and additional signs and symptoms of virilization suggest serious disease. It is important to inquire about anabolic steroid use, especially in athletes. Constitutional symptoms (e.g., malaise, weight loss, and anorexia) suggest a malignancy. A thorough skin examination is essential, looking specifically for acne, **acanthosis nigricans** (diffuse, velvety, dark brown or black skin pigmentation chiefly on the back of the neck, axillae, and other body folds, thought to reflect the hyperinsulinemia

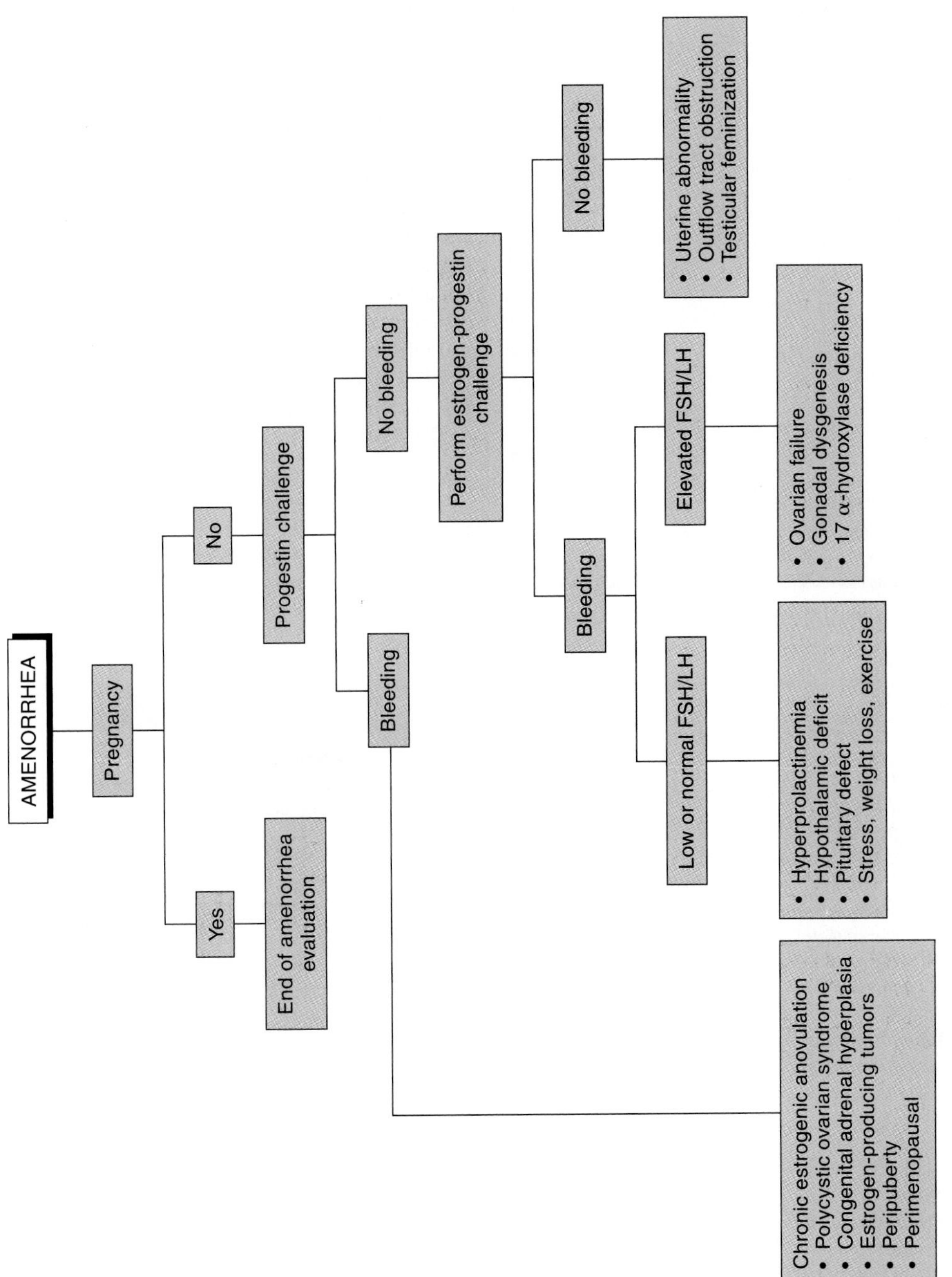


**FIGURE 70.3.** Assessment of amenorrhea.

**TABLE 70.5. Causes of Hirsutism and Virilization**

Androgen-dependent
- Adrenal causes
  - Virilizing adrenal neoplasms
  - Congenital adrenal hyperplasia
  - Cushing's syndrome
- Ovarian causes
  - Virilizing ovarian tumors
  - Severe insulin resistance
- Combined adrenal and ovarian causes
  - Polycystic ovary syndrome
  - Exogenous androgens

Androgen-independent
- Drugs
  - Phenytoin
  - Diazoxide
  - Minoxidil
  - Glucocorticoids
  - Cyclosporine
- Starvation/anorexia nervosa

Miscellaneous
- Idiopathic hirsutism
- Acromegaly
- Hyperprolactinemia
- Hyper- and hypothyroidism

accompanying polycystic ovary syndrome (PCOS), signs of Cushing's syndrome (wide violaceous abdominal striae, thin skin, facial plethora, and ecchymoses), and the quality and distribution of hair growth and virilization. Abdominal and pelvic masses should be noted.

A serum testosterone level above 200 ng/ ml usually suggests a virilizing ovarian tumor; an ultrasound should be obtained. If the DHEA-S level is more than twice normal, an abdominal CT should follow, to search for a virilizing adrenal tumor. A 17-hydroxyprogesterone level should be done 60 minutes after IV administration of Cosyntropin to exclude partial 21-hydroxylase deficiency; a poststimulation level above 1500 ng/dl diagnoses a homozygous deficiency. A mildly elevated prolactin is often seen in PCOS, but if the level is above 50 ng/ml, it is necessary to rule out a pituitary tumor. LH and FSH are used to evaluate for primary ovarian failure and PCOS. An LH:FSH above 2 or 3 is consistent with PCOS, although many experts dispute the usefulness of the LH/FSH ratio.

## Management and Prognosis

Therapy for hirsutism is primarily cosmetic, with medical therapy sometimes used as an adjunct to attenuate androgen production or responsiveness. Idio-

**TABLE 70.6. Clinical and Laboratory Evaluation of Hirsutism and Virilization**

**History**
- Time of onset
- Rate of progression
- Ethnic background
- Menstrual history
- Careful drug history
- Past medical history (hypertension and diabetes mellitus)
- Presence of constitutional symptoms
- History of weight gain

**Physical Examination**
- Deepening of the voice
- Amount and distribution of hair
- Temporal balding
- Skin changes
- Obesity (truncal)
- Galactorrhea
- Dorsocervical and supraclavicular fat pads
- Proximal muscle weakness
- Pectoral muscle development
- Abdominal mass
- Pelvic mass
- Clitoromegaly

**Laboratory Evaluation**

Ovulatory menses; mild to moderate hirsutism
- Routine hormonal evaluation not needed

Oligo- or amenorrhea; mild to severe hirsutism
- Total testosterone
- Dehydroepiandrosterone sulfate
- Prolactin
- LH, FSH
- Thyroid function tests
- 24-hour urinary free cortisol

  *or*
- 1-mg dexamethasone suppression test
- ACTH-stimulated 17-hydroxyprogesterone

ACTH = adrenocorticotropic hormone; FSH = follicle-stimulating hormone; LH = luteinizing hormone.

**TABLE 70.7. Therapeutic Approaches to Hirsutism**

| Mechanical | Drug Therapy |
|---|---|
| Shaving | Oral contraceptive agents |
| Bleaching | Spironolactone |
| Electrolysis | GnRH analogues |
| Laser hair removal | Cyproterone acetate |
| | Flutamide |

GnRH = gonadotropin-releasing hormone.

pathic hirsutism and hirsutism due to PCOS or attenuated congenital adrenal hyperplasia usually are treated with a combination of mechanical and drug therapy (Table 70.7). Oral contraceptive agents alone usually are ineffective for treating hirsutism; they are used in combination with spironolactone, which blocks the androgen receptor and is the drug of choice in the United States for treating hirsutism. However, drug therapy is not a cure, and it usually takes at least 6 months to evaluate the efficacy of any given agent. Lifelong therapy usually is required to prevent recurrence. Hirsutism does not resolve completely with combination therapy, but most patients report a satisfactory improvement.

## Polycstic Ovary Syndrome

### Definition and Etiology

**Polycystic ovary syndrome** (PCOS) is a heterogeneous disorder characterized by hyperandrogenism and chronic anovulation, with the exclusion of other causes of androgen excess. More than 90% of adult women presenting with clinical androgen excess have PCOS and some or all of the following: oligomenorrhea, obesity, hirsutism, and infertility. Virtually all circulating androgens (adrenal and ovarian) are mildly to moderately elevated in these women. Despite the name, enlarged, cystic ovaries are not essential for diagnosis, and, in fact, 25% of women with PCOS have normal-appearing ovaries. Although the cause of PCOS is unclear, many biochemical and physiological abnormalities of the ovaries, pituitary gonadotropins, and adrenal androgens have been described.

Insulin resistance and hyperinsulinemia are common metabolic abnormalities and important markers of cardiovascular risk in patients with PCOS. Among women with PCOS, 40% have impaired glucose tolerance (IGT), and 10% have frank type 2 diabetes. They often have lipid abnormalities. Women with PCOS have a higher risk of endometrial hyperplasia and cancer. The work-up for PCOS is presented in Table 70.8.

### Treatment

Traditionally, management of PCOS involved a symptom-oriented approach. If hirsutism or oligomenorrhea was the primary concern, suppression of the ovaries with oral contraceptives, with the possible addition of spironolactone, was the treatment of choice. If anovulation or infertility was the presenting complaint, stimulation of the ovaries with agents such as clomiphene citrate was attempted. More recently, treatment of PCOS has involved interventions to improve insulin sensitivity, which can result in lowered circulating androgens. These interventions include lifestyle modifications such as weight reduction, diet, exercise, and smoking cessation. Studies using insulin-sensitizing agents such as metformin and thiazolidinediones (primarily troglitazone) have been performed in PCOS patients.

## Menopause

### Definition and Etiology

**Menopause** is defined as the final episode of menstrual bleeding in a woman. Its median age of onset is 50 years. Menopause occurs when the ovaries are depleted of primordial follicles, resulting in decreasing estrogen secretion. Pituitary gonadotropins rise in response (FSH > 40 mIU/ml). Not all women experience an abrupt cessation of menses; many experience variable cycles with skipped periods and increasing intervals between cycles. Therefore, menopause usually cannot be diagnosed clinically unless menses have been absent for 6–12 months in women over 45 years of age.

**TABLE 70.8. Work-up of Polycystic Ovary Syndrome**

| |
|---|
| **History** |
| Menstrual history |
| Family history of DM and CVD |
| **Physical Examination** |
| Body mass index |
| Blood pressure |
| Skin (acne, hirsutism, acanthosis nigricans) |
| **Laboratory** |
| Total or free testosterone |
| Oral glucose tolerance test |
| Fasting lipids |
| Exclusionary labs (e.g. 17-hydroxyprogesterone, TSH, prolactin) |
| **Procedure (Not Usually Indicated)** |
| Transvaginal ultrasound |
| Endometrial biopsy |

CVD = cardiovascular disease; DM = diabetes mellitus.

## Clinical Features

Loss of estrogen leads to a number of signs and symptoms (Table 70.9). Although the prevalence decreases with time, nearly 50% of untreated women continue to experience flushing 5 years after menopause. The flushing may occur frequently throughout the day and night, leading to insomnia, irritability, and fatigue. The effects of estrogen deprivation on the skeletal system is of far greater medical significance. Bone mass begins to decrease after age 35 in both sexes, but this process accelerates rapidly at menopause. Although the beneficial effect of long-term estrogens in preventing bone demineralization and in reducing hip, wrist, and vertebral fracture rates is now well-documented, the potential risks of estrogen replacement therapy include uterine cancer, breast cancer, cholelithiasis, hypertension, and venous thrombosis.

**TABLE 70.9. Clinical Features of Postmenopausal Estrogen Deficiency**

| |
|---|
| Vasomotor instability |
| Hot flashes |
| Sweating |
| Decreased libido |
| Vaginal dryness |
| Urinary difficulties (e.g., incontinence) |
| Osteoporosis |
| Increased cardiovascular disease |
| Atrophy of urogenital epithelium and skin |
| Decreased size of reproductive organs and breasts |

## Management

Indications for **estrogen replacement therapy** (ERT) at the time of menopause include symptoms of estrogen deficiency and high risk for osteoporosis (see Chapter 8). ERT usually is contraindicated in women with estrogen-dependent tumors, undiagnosed genital bleeding, active liver disease, active thromboembolic disorders, porphyria, and pregnancy. For women with a uterus, an estrogen-progestin combination is used to prevent endometrial hyperplasia and cancer. Most clinicians use a cyclic or intermittent regimen: the estrogen is given for the first 25 days of the month and the progestin for the last 10 days of the ERT cycle (Table 70.10). In patients who receive combined continuous estrogen and progesterone therapy, endometrial atrophy with absence of bleeding eventually occurs. This state usually is reached in about 6 months. These women experience unpredictable intermittent bleeding, which may require endometrial biopsies. ERT and progestins commonly produce breast tenderness, bloating, weight gain, and depression.

**TABLE 70.10. Hormonal Replacement Regimens for Postmenopausal Women**

| Estrogen[a] | Dose (mg) | Progestin | Dose: Intermittent (mg)[b] | Dose: Continuous (mg)[c] |
|---|---|---|---|---|
| Conjugated estrogens | 0.3–1.25 | Medroxyprogesterone acetate | 5–10 | 2.5–5.0 |
| Micronized estradiol | 0.5–2.0 | Norethindrone | 1 | 0.35–1.0 |
| Transdermal estradiol | 0.0375–1.0 weekly to twice weekly | | | |

[a]Any of the estrogens could be paired with any of the progestins shown in the table.
[b]Intermittent = cyclic therapy.
[c]Continuous = daily, without cycling.

# CHAPTER 71 DISORDERS OF TESTICULAR FUNCTION

The **testicles** (the male gonads) are paired organs located in the scrotum, which acts as a temperature regulator and protects the gonads from physical injuries. The **testicular parenchyma** consists of the seminiferous tubules, which are embedded in a connective tissue matrix containing scattered Leydig cells, blood vessels, and lymphatics. The seminiferous tubules and the Leydig cells make up the two functional units of the testis. The **tubules** are a highly complex, convoluted network, responsible for spermatogenesis and transport of sperm to the excretory-ejaculatory ducts. The **Leydig cell,** the primary endocrine organ of the testes, produces testosterone. **Sertoli or nurse cells,** also located in the seminiferous epithelium, function as a supporting matrix for the germ cells; they also synthesize and secrete inhibin and clear damaged germ cells from the epithelium.

**Spermatogenesis** is the progressive maturation of the germ cell from **spermatogonia** (an undifferentiated male germ cell) to mature spermatozoa through the processes of mitosis, meiosis, and spermiogenesis; it takes approximately 70 days to complete and requires an intact hypothalamic-pituitary-gonadal axis (Figure 71.1). Transport of sperm through the epididymis to the ejaculatory duct takes between 12 and 21 days. The spermatozoa are initially released with fluid secreted by the Sertoli cells into the lumen of the seminiferous tubules. From here, they pass through the straight tubules to the Rete testis, then to the efferent ducts and into the ductus epididymis. During their transit through the epididymis, the spermatozoa undergo further maturation to become motile and attain fertilizing capacity. After passing through the epididymis, the sperm enter the **vas deferens,** which empties into the ejaculatory duct. There the semen is prepared for ejaculation through the urethra. The seminal vesicles and prostate add additional secretory factors to the semen before it is emptied into the ejaculatory duct.

Most testosterone is transported in the circulation protein-bound, with only 2% free (active). Almost 44% is bound to testosterone-binding globulin; another 54% binds to albumin and other proteins. Estradiol and dihydrotestosterone are the two major biologically active metabolites (Figure 71.2) of testosterone. Testosterone is secreted in a diurnal pattern, with peak levels in the morning and a nadir in the afternoon. **Estradiol** is synthesized by the aromatization of testosterone at extraglandular sites in peripheral tissues, catalyzed by aromatase. The conversion of testosterone to **dihydrotestosterone** is catalyzed by 5-$\alpha$ reductase. Dihydrotestosterone is localized to distinct tissues such as liver, skin, and accessory organs of reproduction (seminal vesicles and prostate); it leads to male sexual differentiation, including external virilization, and sexual maturation at puberty. The physiologic role of estradiol in men is unknown.

## Hypogonadism and Testicular Failure

### Definition

**Hypogonadism,** or testicular dysfunction, can be classified as **primary hypogonadism** (due to a defect of the testes), **secondary hypogonadism** (due to a hypothalamic-pituitary defect), or androgen resistance. Abnormal testicular function has different clinical presentations depending on the phase of sexual life in which it appears. This chapter focuses on adult abnormalities.

### Etiology and Pathogenesis

The hypo- and hypergonadotropic causes of hypogonadism are listed in Table 71.1. **Hypogonadotropic hypogonadism** can be due to a deficiency in hypothalamic gonadotropin-releasing hormone (GnRH) or the pituitary gonadotropins, follicle-stimulating hormone (FSH), and luteinizing hormone (LH). Permanent GnRH

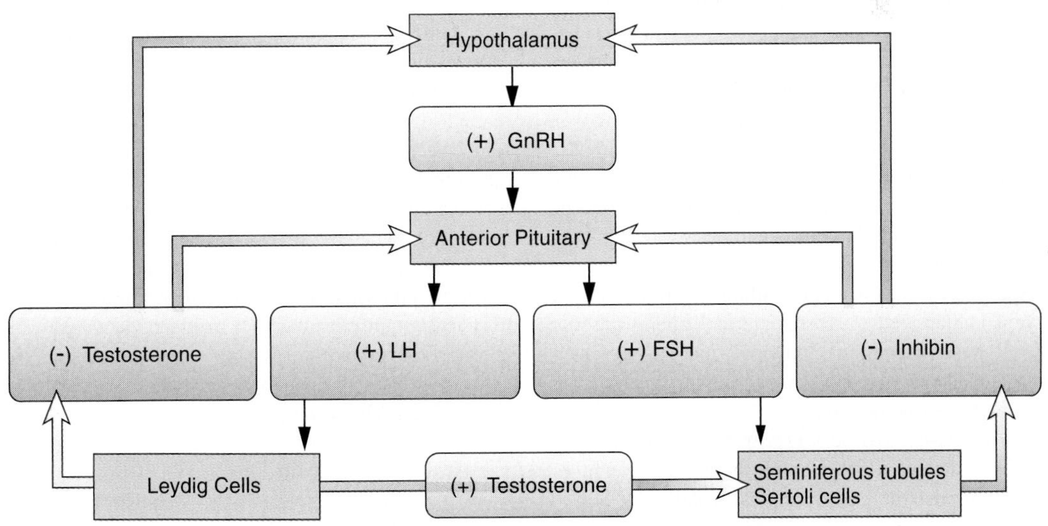


**FIGURE 71.1.** The hypothalamic-pituitary-gonadal axis. (−) = negative influence; (+) = positive influence.

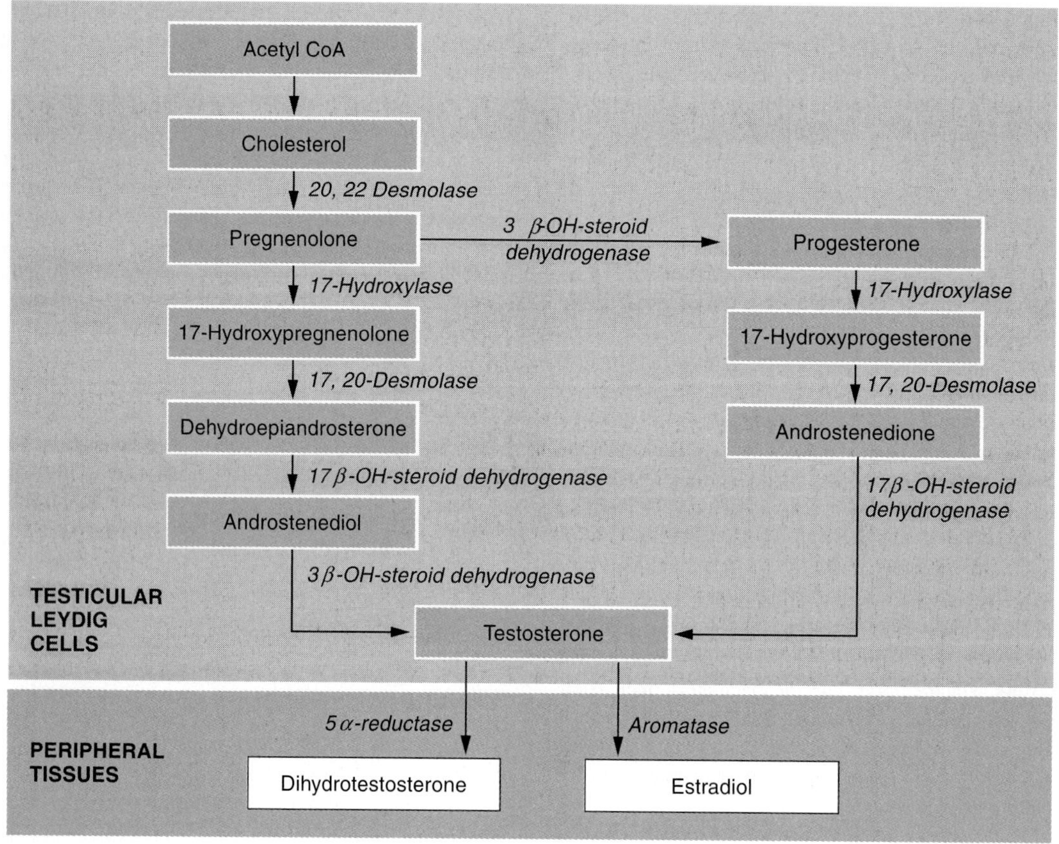


**FIGURE 71.2.** Biosynthesis and metabolism of testosterone. The first side-chain cleavage of cholesterol to pregnenolone is the rate-limiting reaction and is probably regulated by LH.

deficiency is seen with congenital disorders such as Kallmann's (male hypogonadism with anosmia) and Prader-Willi syndromes, external hypothalamic irradiation, and idiopathic acquired GnRH deficiency. **Primary or hypergonadotropic hypogonadism** can be congenital or acquired. **Klinefelter's syndrome,** affecting 1 in 500 male infants, is the most common cause of congenital testicular disease; it is caused by an early meiotic nondisjunction that leads to a 47 XXY karyotype. The syndrome is characterized by small testes, tall stature, increased arm span, long legs, gynecomastia, and azoospermia. Primary testicular failure may be associated with renal failure, liver disease, sickle cell anemia, febrile illness, paraplegia, and myotonic dystrophy. Spironolactone, ketoconazole, alcohol, and cyclophosphamide decrease androgen production.

Normal aging is associated with a gradual decline in testicular function, which may not be associated with a concomitant rise in gonadotropins. Total testosterone levels are commonly reduced in obese men, in part due to a decline in sex hormone–binding globulin (SHBG) concentrations. Free testosterone levels also may decline with massive obesity, however.

**Androgen resistance,** an uncommon cause of hypogonadism, can arise from either of two different mechanisms. The first involves an abnormality of the enzyme 5α-reductase, which converts testosterone to dihydrotestosterone; the second involves an intrinsic abnormality of the androgen receptor. This latter defect has variable severity; the mildest forms cause only infertility, whereas severe forms lead to ambiguous genitalia. Recent studies of patients with androgen receptor abnormalities or testicular feminization syndrome (a condition in which a genetic male, with 46 chromosomes and an XY karyotype, develops as a female) reveal that most patients have a single base substitution within the androgen receptor gene.

## Clinical Features and Diagnosis

Symptoms and signs of hypogonadism vary depending on whether the age of onset is before or after puberty. Adult men with androgen deficiency report decreased libido, infertility, impotence or erectile dysfunction, impaired masculinization, gynecomastia, and facial flushing. Physical examination should assess testicular size and consistency and look for signs of undervirilization, a palpable testicular mass, and gynecomastia. Laboratory tests should include serum testosterone, LH, FSH, thyroid-stimulating hormone (TSH), and prolactin, semen analysis if fertility is an issue, and a karyotype if Klinefelter syndrome is suspected.

### Management

Treatment of male androgen deficiency depends on whether the hypogonadism is primary or secondary and on whether the goal is only to normalize serum testosterone levels or also to stimulate spermatogenesis.

**TABLE 71.1. Causes of Hypogonadism**

| |
|---|
| **Primary Hypogonadism** |
| Autoimmune |
| Chemotherapy |
| Chromosomal abnormalities |
| Cryptorchidism |
| Drugs/alcohol |
| Radiotherapy |
| Systemic diseases |
| Trauma/castration |
| Viral orchitis (mumps) |
| **Secondary Hypogonadism** |
| Hyperprolactinemia |
| Pituitary tumors |
| Benign sellar tumors |
| Metastatic sellar tumors |
| Kallmann's syndrome |
| Infiltrative disorders |
| Idiopathic hypogonadotropic hypogonadism |
| Panhypopituitarism |
| Granulomatous disease |
| Autoimmune hypophysitis |
| Primary hyperthyroidism |
| **Androgen Resistance** |
| 5α-reductase deficiency |
| Androgen receptor defect |

Whether the problem is due to hypo- or hypergonadotropic hypogonadism, the serum testosterone can be increased by using transdermal or intramuscular (IM) testosterone (Table 71.2). However, spermatogenesis can be induced only in individuals with secondary hypogonadism. It requires IM injections of human chorionic gonadotropin or human menotropin or pulsatile GnRH injections.

## Impotence

### Definition and Epidemiology

Impotence is defined as the inability to obtain and sustain an erection satisfactory for sexual intercourse on more than 50% of coital attempts or the inability to sustain an erection, leading to a cessation of sexual intercourse. Erectile dysfunction of varying degrees of severity affects nearly 40% of men by age 40 and more than 75% by age 70.

### Etiology and Pathogenesis

Erection is a predominantly vascular event under strict neurologic control. Impotence may be related to three factors in aging men: decreased neurosensory activity, hypogonadism, and the effect of comorbid illness, including medications.

Evaluation of the male with erectile dysfunction should include a careful sexual history. Questions include whether the problem is primary or secondary, constant or intermittent, progressive or constant. A medical history and a detailed medication list should be obtained. Cardiovascular and psychiatric medications often are associated with erectile dysfunction. The physical examination should include an evaluation for the presence of peripheral neuropathy, testicular atrophy, and depression or other psychiatric disorder.

The general laboratory evaluation should include a screening for anemia, diabetes, renal insufficiency and liver disease, and a lipid profile to assess cardiovascular risk. Endocrine studies should include an ultrasensitive TSH test and serum testosterone level. A total testosterone may be drawn, but some experts advocate the

**TABLE 71.2. Testosterone Preparations**

| Preparation | Dose | Route |
|---|---|---|
| Testosterone enanthate or cypionate | 200–400 mg q 2–4 weeks | Intramuscular |
| Androderm | 2.5–5 mg patch/24 h | Transdermal (nonscrotal skin) |
| Testoderm | 4–6 mg patch/24 h | Transdermal (scrotal skin) |
| Testoderm-TTS | 5 mg patch/24 h | Transdermal (nonscrotal skin) |
| Testosterone gel (Androgel 1%) | 2.5–5.0 g daily | Transdermal (shoulders, upper arms, abdomen) |

measurement of non-SHBG-bound bioavailable testosterone as a more sensitive test.

### Management

Treatment of impotence is directed first at correction of any identifiable cause. Often this is not possible, however. Treatments are then directed specifically at improvement of erectile function. Sildenafil citrate (Viagra) was the first approved oral agent for erectile dysfunction. It inhibits phosphodiesterase type 5, which terminates the signal for erection, thus prolonging muscle relaxation and potentiating erectile function. Its use is contraindicated in patients on nitrates. Testosterone preparations may be indicated in patients with low serum testosterone and elevated gonadotropins. Other therapies include intracavernous injections of vasoactive agents such as papaverine, with or without phentolamine, and intraurethral injections of prostaglandin E1, vacuum therapy, and prosthetic surgery; vascular reconstruction may be indicated in some patients. Complications of self-injection therapy include prolonged erection, priapism, and, when papaverine is used, fibrosis of the erectile tissues. Potential complications of vacuum therapy include petechiae, ecchymosis, initial penile pain, and ejaculatory difficulty.

## Gynecomastia

### Definition and Epidemiology

In normal men, no breast tissue is palpable. Remnants of a duct system can be detected histologically, but the lining cells are atrophic. **Gynecomastia** is defined as the unilateral or bilateral enlargement of the male breast. It may be asymmetric, with one side larger than the other; the tissue may be a discrete subareolar plate or a diffuse mass of fibroadipose tissue. Gynecomastia is common, reportedly affecting 30% to 50% of normal men between the ages of 17 and 80 years and 70% of hospitalized men.

### Etiology and Pathogenesis

In general, any palpable breast tissue in men is abnormal except during three stages of life: (1) the transient gynecomastia of neonates; (2) the breast enlargement that occurs at puberty; and (3) the gynecomastia of senescence. In neonates, the breast enlargement is due to maternal estrogens and usually lasts a few weeks. Pubertal gynecomastia, which probably is due to testicular production of estradiol (which peaks initially before testosterone), affects 70% of pubertal boys and resolves within 2 to 3 years. In the seventh to eighth decade of life, the increased adipose tissue increases peripheral conversion of testosterone to estradiol (andropause); testosterone decreases slightly, and gynecomastia results.

Other than these three physiologic circumstances, any gynecomastia in an adult male is more likely to represent an underlying disease (Table 71.3). The growth, division, and elongation of the tubular duct system of the female breast is normally caused by estrogen and inhibited by androgens. Gynecomastia can, therefore, follow an alteration in the balance between these two opposing influences. Prolactin directly causes galactorrhea, but it does not directly stimulate breast enlargement; however, it may do so indirectly by inhibiting GnRH secretion. A history of recent sudden breast enlargement with pain and tenderness in a man usually implies an underlying disorder. Medications causing gynecomastia are listed in Table 71.4. Breast cancer is rare in men. However, gynecomastia in a patient with Klinefelter's syndrome is associated with a 10- to 20-fold increase in the incidence of breast cancer.

### Diagnosis

Mild asymptomatic breast enlargement is common in normal men. Generally, symptomatic and progressive cases warrant evaluation, with the primary goal of excluding breast cancer. For this purpose, it usually is sufficient to conduct a careful physical examination, observing for characteristics typically seen in women with breast malignancy, such as irregularity, hardness, fixation, eccentric location, ulceration, and axillary adenopathy. Mammography or ultrasonography can be helpful. Any suspicious finding on physical or radiologic examination should be biopsied.

Once breast cancer is ruled out, most causes of gynecomastia can be identified by careful clinical assessment and work-up. It is important to review medications carefully, note the age of onset and duration of gynecomastia, and check for the presence of impotence and subnormal virilization, galactorrhea and headaches, and symptoms of thyroid disease. Physical examination should stress breasts and testes (size, consistency, atrophy, and masses) and search for signs of liver disease and thyroid disease. Helpful laboratory studies (if dictated by clinical assessment) and their interpretations are shown in Table 71.5.

### Management and Prognosis

The initial emphasis is on correcting the underlying disorder (e.g., withdrawal of an offending medication). Unfortunately, long-standing gynecomastia may evoke significant fibrosis, which does not regress even after removing the cause. Regression may take many years; therefore, surgery is the mainstay of therapy and is often indicated for psychological and cosmetic reasons.

**TABLE 71.3. Causes of Gynecomastia**

| Mechanism | Causes |
|---|---|
| Exposure to exogenous estrogens | Vaginal creams<br>Occupational exposure<br>Anti-balding creams |
| Deficient production or action of testosterone | Anorchism (46,XY)<br>Klinefelter's syndrome (47,XXY)<br>Androgen resistance syndrome<br>Defects in testosterone synthesis<br>Gonadal toxins (drugs, radiation)<br>Viral orchitis (mumps)<br>Trauma<br>Castration<br>Renal failure |
| Increased endogenous estrogen production | True hermaphroditism<br>Testicular tumors<br>Germinal cell tumors (hCG-producing stimulate estrogen)<br>Stromal cell tumors (estradiol and testosterone-secreting)<br>Bronchogenic carcinoma and other hCG-producing tumors |
| Increased peripheral conversion of androgens to estrogen | Hyperthyroidism<br>Cirrhosis<br>Obesity<br>Senescence<br>Adrenal carcinoma<br>Refeeding/starvation |

hCG = human chorionic gonadotropin.

**TABLE 71.4. Medications Commonly Associated With Gynecomastia**

| Method of Action | Drug |
|---|---|
| Inhibits testosterone production | Chemotherapeutic agents (alkylating agents, vincristine, methotrexate)<br>Ketoconazole<br>Metronidazole |
| Androgen receptor antagonist | Spironolactone<br>Cimetidine<br>Marijuana<br>Digoxin |
| Increases peripheral conversion of testosterone to estrogen | Testosterone |
| Increases testicular estrogen production | hCG |
| Has estrogen-like actions | Estrogen<br>Diethylstilbestrol |
| Uncertain | Amiodarone<br>Calcium-channel blockers<br>Heroin<br>Phenothiazines<br>Methyldopa<br>Tricyclic antidepressants<br>Isoniazid<br>Theophylline<br>Diazepam |

TABLE 71.5. Biochemical Work-Up of Gynecomastia

| | |
|---|---|
| **Laboratory Studies** | |
| Liver function tests | |
| TSH | |
| Testosterone | |
| Estradiol | |
| LH, FSH | |
| hCG | |
| Androstenedione | |
| Prolactin | |
| Karyotype | |
| **Laboratory Interpretation** | |
| ↑LH with ↓ or normal testosterone | Suggests primary testicular insufficiency |
| ↓ LH with ↓ testosterone | Suggests estrogen-producing tumor or hypothalamic/pituitary deficiency |
| ↑ LH with ↑ testosterone | Suggests androgen resistance or pituitary gonadotropin-secreting tumor |

# CHAPTER 72 HYPOGLYCEMIA AND DIABETES MELLITUS

The plasma glucose concentration normally fluctuates between 70 and 120 mg/dl (3.9–6.7 mM). This normal blood level of glucose **(euglycemia)** is maintained by the interplay of three separate processes: dietary carbohydrate intake, endogenous glucose production, and peripheral glucose utilization. In the **postabsorptive "fasting" state** (5–6 hours after a meal), with dietary intake no longer a factor, the model is simply an equilibrium between glucose production and utilization. Under these conditions, most glucose utilization is by obligatory oxidative processes within tissues that function primarily on glycolysis; these include brain tissue and formed elements of the blood.

In the early post-absorptive state, **hepatic glycogenolysis** accounts for most of the endogenous glucose production. **Gluconeogenesis** is responsible for the balance; its importance increases as the fast continues. The quantity of hepatic glycogen available for mobilization as a potential source of circulating glucose is only about 70 g (an amount that is exhausted within 8 hours at the usual glucose utilization rate); consequently, gluconeogenesis becomes the only source of glucose with prolonged fasting. Because amino acids are the substrates for gluconeogenesis, muscle wasting eventually occurs. Fat tissue provides the largest source of stored calories as **triglycerides.** After about 48 hours, as the rates of lipolysis and ketogenesis increase, the brain adapts to ketone bodies as an alternative metabolic fuel. Because the brain utilizes most of the glucose at the cellular level, this adaptation allows lowering the rate of gluconeogenesis. After refeeding, glucose is absorbed across the intestinal mucosa at more than twice the rate of fasting endogenous glucose production. Glycogenolysis, gluconeogenesis, and lipolysis are then inhibited, and the many intracellular storage forms of metabolic fuel are repleted within the liver, muscle, and fat tissues.

Five hormones are key to maintaining euglycemia: insulin, glucagon, epinephrine, cortisol, and growth hormone. **Insulin** lowers blood glucose by stimulating its cellular uptake and utilization, and by curbing its endogenous production. Glucagon, epinephrine, cortisol and growth hormone all oppose insulin metabolically, and therefore are referred to as **counterregulatory hormones.**

**Insulin** is synthesized, stored and released by the β cells of the pancreatic islets. It is initially synthesized as a pre-prohormone, then converted to **proinsulin** as it is stored within the intracellular secretory granules. Before its release systemically, proinsulin is further modified proteolytically, producing the final form of insulin and a cleavage fragment called **C-peptide.** The insulin molecule has two disulfide linked subunits: a 21-amino-acid A chain and a 30-amino-acid B chain (Figure 72.1).

Pancreatic β cells secrete equimolar concentrations of C-peptide and insulin, at a basal rate of 0.5 units/h. Despite the islet innervation by both sympathetic and parasympathetic postganglionic fibers, β cells function largely independently, releasing insulin primarily in response to the local delivery of substrate; the most potent stimulus is the glucose level. Other substrates (arginine, free fatty acids, and ketone bodies) also stimulate insulin secretion. Following direct release into the portal circulation, insulin stimulates hepatic glycogen synthesis and inhibits hepatic glycogenolysis and gluconeogenesis. It also stimulates glucose uptake and utilization by other tissues (such as muscle and fat). Insulin possesses overall anticatabolic and anabolic effects. Collectively, these effects of insulin lower circulating blood glucose levels (Table 72.1).

All body tissues are capable of utilizing glucose. Glucose is transported across cell membranes by a facilitative diffusion mechanism, through several molecular subtypes of the **glucose transporter** (GLUT 1 through 5). Hepatocytes, pancreatic β-cells, and the absorptive epithelial cells of the intestinal mucosa all express GLUT 2, which facilitates free bidirectional movement of glucose across their plasma membranes; consequently, their intracellular glucose levels can be in continual equilibrium with ambient glucose levels. Tissues with a constant high level of metabolic activity (brain, kidney, smooth muscle, and red blood cells [RBC]) express GLUTs independently, regardless of insulin availability. Tissues whose activity levels fluctuate dramatically, most notably skeletal muscle and adipose tissue, require the presence of insulin to express their major GLUT on the cell surface.

**Glucagon,** a 29-amino acid polypeptide synthesized and secreted by the alpha cells of the pancreatic islets, is released into the portal circulation, with primarily hepatic effects. By increasing cAMP through G-protein activation of adenylate cyclase, glucagon strongly stimulates hepatic glycogenolysis and gluconeogenesis, effects directly opposed by insulin. Glucagon is the primary counterregulatory hormone. It is released from the α cells in response to decreases in circulating glucose level; the resultant increase in hepatic glucose output occurs within minutes. The main stimulant for glucagon release appears to be alterations in the local delivery of substrate to the islets, as is the case with insulin secretion.

**Epinephrine,** like glucagon, is an acute-acting counterregulatory hormone. Its secretion is neurally controlled in response to circulating glucose levels. By inducing $\beta_2$-adrenergic receptor-mediated increase in hepatocyte cAMP levels, epinephrine increases hepatic

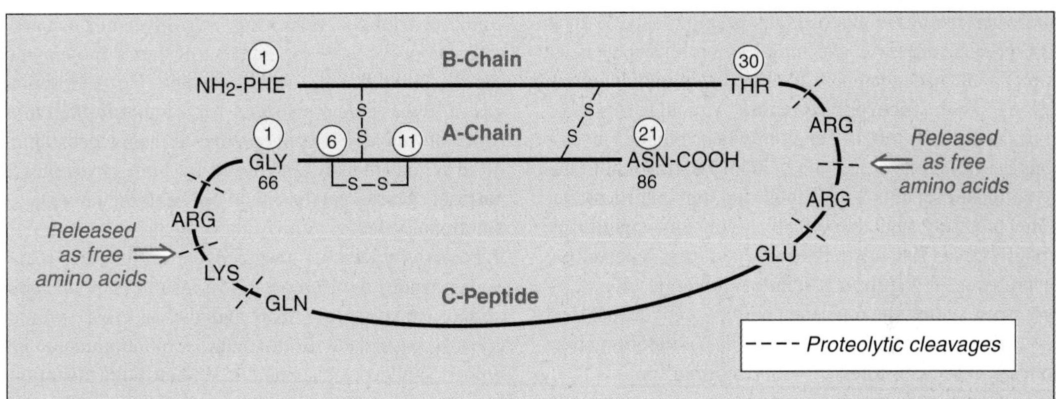


**FIGURE 72.1. Structure of proinsulin and insulin. Proinsulin is an 86-amino-acid protein that is cleaved at two sites to yield insulin, which is composed of A and B chains. An equal quantity of biologically inert C-peptide is produced as a byproduct.**

(Reprinted with permission from West JB (ed.). Best and Taylor's Physiological Basis of Medical Practice. 12th ed. Baltimore: Williams & Wilkins, 1991, p. 820.)

**TABLE 72.1. Metabolic Effects of Insulin**

| | Liver | Adipose Tissue | Muscle |
|---|---|---|---|
| Anticatabolic | ↓ glycogenolysis<br>↓ gluconeogenesis<br>↓ ketogenesis | ↓ lipolysis | ↓ protein catabolism<br>↓ amino acid output |
| Anabolic | ↑ glycogen synthesis<br>↑ fatty acid synthesis | ↑ glucose uptake<br>↑ glycerol synthesis<br>↑ fatty acid synthesis | ↑ glucose and amino acid uptake<br>↑ protein synthesis<br>↑ glycogen synthesis |

↑ = increased; ↓ = decreased.

glycogenolysis and gluconeogenesis. Epinephrine also indirectly affects the hepatic manipulation of glucose storage by inhibiting insulin secretion ($\alpha_2$-receptors on pancreatic $\beta$ cells). Besides, the activation of $\beta_1$-receptors on adipocytes stimulates lipolysis and generates free fatty acids, which can be used by the liver for ketogenesis. Glycogenolysis within skeletal muscle is also stimulated.

**Cortisol** and **growth hormone** also are counterregulatory hormones, but neither appears to have a primary role in correcting hypoglycemia. Mobilization of glucose does not occur until several hours following a rise in their circulating levels. Growth hormone initially has a paradoxical insulin-like effect, causing a transient lowering of blood glucose. Despite their delayed hyperglycemic effect, both these hormones appear to serve an integral role in glucose homeostasis.

**TABLE 72.3. Differential Diagnosis of Hypoglycemia**

| Fasting | Postprandial |
|---|---|
| Insulin | Alimentary |
| Oral sulfonylurea agents | Idiopathic |
| Ethanol | Early type 2 diabetes mellitus |
| Medications: | |
| Pentamidine | |
| Salicylates | |
| Propranolol | |
| Sulfamethoxazole | |
| Disopyramide | |
| Tumor hypoglycemia | |
| Insulinomas | |
| Adrenal insufficiency | |
| Prolonged starvation | |
| Liver failure | |
| Uremia | |

## Hypoglycemia

**Hypoglycemia,** a deficiency of glucose concentration in the blood, manifests clinically by symptoms of catecholamine release and/or neuroglycopenia (Table 72.2). Catecholamine release-related symptoms predominate when the blood glucose falls precipitously. With a more gradual decrease, the initial symptoms may be a reflection of inadequate substrate delivery to the central nervous system **(neuroglycopenia)**. Although hypoglycemic symptoms often develop when blood glucose drops below 45 mg/dl (2.5 mM), many healthy adults are asymptomatic at this level, thus making it difficult to define precisely and numerically, clinically significant hypoglycemia. Rather, definitive diagnosis depends on the presence of **Whipple's triad:** adrenergic or neuroglycopenic symptoms consistent with hypoglycemia, low blood glucose level, and relief of the symptoms when blood glucose is restored to within normal limits.

Hypoglycemia has diverse and numerous causes. It can be classified as one of two types, based on the temporal relationship between ingestion of a meal and the onset of clinically relevant symptoms (Table 72.3). **Postprandial** *(reactive)* hypoglycemia often occurs within the first few hours after food intake. On the other hand, **postabsorptive** *(fasting)* hypoglycemia is not seen until several hours later, after the meal has been fully digested and absorbed.

**TABLE 72.2. Symptoms of Hypoglycemia**

| Adrenergic | Neuroglycopenic |
|---|---|
| Sweating | Headache |
| Tremors | Irritability |
| Palpitations | Confusion |
| Pallor | Seizure |
| Hunger | Coma |

The best documented form of postprandial hypoglycemia in adults is ***alimentary hypoglycemia,*** caused by surgical procedures leading to the rapid movement of ingested food into the small intestine (e.g., pyloroplasty, gastric bypass, gastrectomy). An ***idiopathic*** *(functional)* form of reactive hypoglycemia remains debatable; it often is erroneously diagnosed by both physicians and patients. These persons tend to be thin, anxious, and emotionally labile, with somatic features of autonomic hyperactivity such as gastric hypermotility and irritable bowel syndrome. In most cases, insulin responds appropriately to a glucose load and the onset of symptoms correlates poorly with the nadir in blood glucose. Early type II diabetes occasionally is seen with postprandial hypoglycemia.

Fasting hypoglycemia is far more prevalent than the postprandial type, and most cases are **drug-induced.** Insulin and the sulfonylureas cause most episodes. **Iatrogenic hypoglycemia** is seen often in patients with type I diabetes attempting to maintain tight control with insulin. It also is seen, albeit less frequently, in patients with type II diabetes taking oral hypoglycemic agents. Ethanol potentiates the hypoglycemic effects of both of these agents, and also can induce hypoglycemia by itself, by directly inhibiting gluconeogenesis. Salicylates and $\beta$-blockers inhibit the mobilization of endogenous glucose stores. Quinine, pentamidine, sulfamethoxazole, and disopyramide promote release of excessive amounts of endogenous insulin.

**Insulinomas** (pancreatic $\beta$-cell tumors), are a rare but important cause of fasting hypoglycemia. Most of these tumors are benign and extremely small; they usually cause neuroglycopenic symptoms following a missed meal or exercise. Diagnosis of the insulinomas often is delayed because patients learn to avoid symptoms by eating frequently. As a result, many patients with insulinomas are obese. The evidence for insulinoma is an inappropriately high fasting level of insulin. During symptomatic episodes, blood glucose level tends to be below 45 mg/dl (2.5 mM), and the plasma insulin level is above 10 μU/ml (72 pmol/L). Some nonpancreatic neoplasms, which tend to be large, retroperitoneal, and mesenchymal, also can cause fasting hypoglycemia. Most of these tumors probably cause hypoglycemia due to the production of aberrant IGF-II, which has poor affinity for IGF-II binding protein 3 and, therefore, circulates disproportionately in the free form, with resultant hypoglycemia. The poor nutrition and inanition that often are associated are additional factors.

**Factitious hypoglycemia** also has been observed in nondiabetic psychiatric patients who have access to syringes and insulin. The presence of insulin antibodies, an inappropriately low C-peptide level, and high levels of circulating insulin often is diagnostic. Prescription errors can lead to inadvertent use of oral sulfonylureas, a possibility easily excluded by a negative urine screen for sulfonylurea metabolites.

The treatment of hypoglycemia depends on the cause. In adults, reactive hypoglycemia can be managed with small, frequent meals and reassurance. Anticholinergic drugs, by slowing GI transit, may be useful in managing alimentary hypoglycemia. If an insulinoma is diagnosed biochemically, CT, pre- and intraoperative ultrasound, and selective arteriography may help in anatomic localization. In most cases, surgical excision is curative. Diazoxide can help control hypoglycemia in multiple or metastatic insulinomas; it blocks insulin release from pancreatic β-cells by opening the same $K^+$ATP channels known to be blocked by sulfonylureas. In drug-induced hypoglycemia, therapy is directed toward the offending agent. Hypoglycemia from sulfonylureas, notably chlorpropamide, can be insidious and protracted. Because the brain is vulnerable to prolonged hypoglycemia, patients who develop severe hypoglycemia due to these drugs should be hospitalized and given IV glucose until stable.

## Diabetes Mellitus

**Diabetes mellitus** is a syndrome of altered carbohydrate, fat, and protein metabolism resulting from an absolute or relative deficiency of insulin. The most common biochemical abnormality is hyperglycemia. Long-standing diabetes is commonly associated with chronic complications of retinopathy, nephropathy, neuropathy, and accelerated atherosclerosis.

### Epidemiology and Classification

Diabetes mellitus affects approximately 3% to 4% of the U.S. population. It is a heterogeneous disorder with two subtypes. Type 1, or **insulin-dependent diabetes mellitus** (IDDM), caused by autoimmune destruction of the islet cells, accounts for approximately 10% of cases. It is characterized by a sudden onset of symptoms, insulin insufficiency, ketoacidosis, and dependence on insulin. Because it typically occurs in young subjects, IDDM formerly was called juvenile diabetes. Type 2 **diabetes mellitus** is the most common type; it is characterized by a more gradual and insidious onset of hyperglycemia and lack of susceptibility to ketoacidosis. Although insulin may be needed for optimal control of hyperglycemia, patients are not dependent on it to maintain life. Endogenous insulin levels may be high, low, or normal in these patients. Peripheral tissues, such as muscle, fat, and liver, are abnormally resistant to the effects of insulin; the result is decreased glucose uptake and inappropriate hepatic gluconeogenesis, despite insulin levels that may be normal. Because type 2 diabetes often debuts after the age of 40, it was formerly called mature (adult) onset diabetes. In other types of diabetes, entities such as pancreatic insufficiency (e.g., chronic pancreatitis, hemochromatosis, pancreatectomy), Cushing's syndrome, and acromegaly are the underlying cause. Drugs, including glucocorticoids and nicotinic acid, can produce hyperglycemia in patients predisposed to type 2 diabetes.

### Clinical Features and Diagnosis

The classic triad of polyuria, polydipsia, and polyphagia (excessive eating) arises from hyperglycemia, which leads to glycosuria upon exceeding the renal threshold. Glucose acts as an osmotic diuretic, leading to polyuria and, hence, polydipsia. Loss of calories evokes a sensation of excess hunger and polyphagia. Weight loss occurs frequently, despite excess food intake. These symptoms arise classically in patients with IDDM. Diabetic ketoacidosis also may be the initial manifestation of type 1 diabetes. Skin infections, vulvovaginitis (inflammation of the vulva and the vagina), and balanitis (inflammation of the glans penis) may cause the patient to seek medical care. Type 2 diabetes often is detected by screening examinations or because of fatigue accompanied by polyuria and polydipsia, albeit less severe than in type 1 diabetes. Peripheral neuropathy (pathological changes to the peripheral nervous system), often present when type 2 diabetes is diagnosed, may be the presenting feature in some cases. Less commonly, type 2 diabetes presents with vascular complications, such as myocardial infarction, peripheral vascular disease, or chronic renal failure.

Table 72.4 shows the accepted criteria for the diagnosis of diabetes in the nonpregnant adult as

**TABLE 72.4. Diagnosis of Diabetes Mellitus in Non-Pregnant Adults**

Random glucose > 200 mg/dl with symptoms of hyperglycemia;

or

Fasting venous plasma glucose (FBS) ≥126 mg/dl on two or more occasions

or

Oral glucose (75 g) tolerance test (GTT) showing a 2-hr glucose level of ≥200 mg/dl

developed by the National Diabetes Data Group. Commonly, type 1 diabetic patients are diagnosed by the first criterion; type 2 diabetes patients are diagnosed by the second. Oral glucose tolerance testing (OGTT) is reserved for individuals with potential symptoms of diabetes or its complications as well as FBS below 125 mg/dl.

## Management

### Goals of therapy

The aims of treatment are twofold: first, to relieve the symptoms of hyperglycemia, and second, to prevent or delay the onset of chronic complications. These goals should be accomplished while avoiding severe, recurrent hypoglycemia. Symptoms of hyperglycemia (e.g., thirst, polyuria, fatigue, blurred vision) are alleviated when the glucose level is generally maintained below the renal threshold for glucose of 180 to 200 mg/dl. Because glucose values in this range are associated with a high rate of long-term microvascular complications, the second goal of therapy is to lower the glucose further to achieve near-euglycemia. For optimal control, guidelines of the American Diabetes Association include fasting and pre-meal glucose levels of 70 to 120 mg/dl with postprandial excursions to less than 180 mg/dl. Glycated hemoglobin levels should be maintained below 7%.

### Diet

Dietary therapy is a key part of the treatment, regardless of the type of diabetes and whether or not oral hypoglycemic agents or insulin is administered. The principle of dietary therapy is to provide an adequate number of calories to meet energy needs. Depending on physical activity, nonobese adults require 25 to 40 calories/kg for weight maintenance. Patients with type 2 diabetes usually are obese and should be encouraged to lose weight by prescribing lower-calorie diets. Once the total caloric requirement has been determined, the distribution of calories should be decided, taking into account food preferences, work schedule, and other personal factors. Carbohydrates should provide 50% to 60% of total calories, protein should account for 15% to 20%, and fat should make up the remainder. The daily caloric intake usually is prescribed as three major meals with two or three snacks during a 24-hour period.

### Insulin therapy

Before 1982, insulin preparations were mixtures of beef and pork insulin. In 1982, human insulin, produced by recombinant molecular technology, became available and has replaced animal source insulins. Human, pork, and beef insulin have similar biopotencies and pharmacokinetics. The regular unmodified insulin acts rapidly. Two newer insulins, lispro and aspart, contains amino acid substitutions that accelerate insulin absorption and action relative to regular insulin. The other insulin preparations have been modified to prolong the insulin action (Table 72.5). NPH and Lente insulin may be mixed with regular insulin, if required, but the activity of regular insulin is better preserved when mixed with NPH insulin alone.

Insulin is given in such a way that it roughly approximates the idealized profile of insulin secretion in a nondiabetic person (Figure 72.2). This profile arises from **basal insulin secretion** (occurring in the absence of eating) and nutrient-stimulated insulin secretion with meals. Short-acting insulin (regular, lispro or aspart) is given before two or more meals to mimic nutrient-stimulated insulin secretion and to promote metabolism of the ingested calories. Intermediate- or long-acting insulin is given once or twice daily to mimic basal insulin secretion. Most diabetics require intermediate- or long-acting insulin in the evening in order to suppress the nocturnal hepatic gluconeogenesis that will otherwise occur in both types of diabetics; when unrestrained, it leads to pre-breakfast hyperglycemia (Table 72.6). The standard **split-mixed regimen** is a mixture of NPH (or lente) and regular insulin before breakfast and before the evening meal. In many patients, the pre-supper NPH peaks between 2 a.m. and 4 a.m., causing overnight reactions. These reactions can be avoided by giving the

**TABLE 72.5. Insulin Preparations**

| | Action Profile (hr) | | |
|---|---|---|---|
| **Type of Insulin** | **Onset** | **Peak** | **Duration** |
| **Rapid** | | | |
| Regular | 0.5–1 | 2–4 | 6–8 |
| Lispro | 0.25–0.5 | 0.5–1.5 | 3–5 |
| Aspart | 0.2–0.3 | 1–3 | 3–5 |
| **Intermediate** | | | |
| Lente | 3–4 | 6–12 | 16–20+ |
| NPH | 2–4 | 6–10 | 14–18+ |
| **Long-acting** | | | |
| Ultralente | 4–6 | 10–16 | 24–36 |
| Insulin Glargine | 1–2 | Flat | 24 |

NPH = neutral protamine Hagedorn.

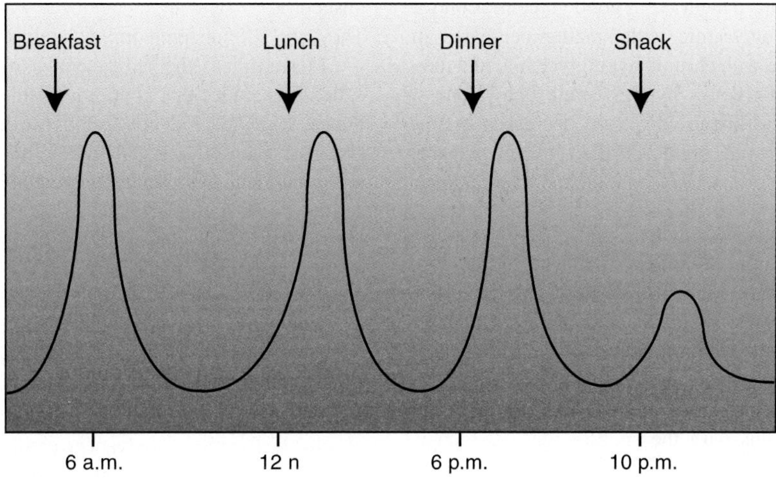


**FIGURE 72.2.** Idealized profile of a 24-hour insulin secretion pattern in a nondiabetic individual.

**TABLE 72.6. Common Insulin Regimens**

| Pre-Breakfast | Pre-Lunch | Pre-Supper (p.m.) | Bedtime (h.s.) |
|---|---|---|---|
| NPH/Reg | – | NPH/Reg | – |
| NPH/Reg (or lispro or aspart) | – | Reg (or lispro or aspart) | NPH |
| Reg (or lispro or aspart) | Reg (or lispro or aspart) | Reg (or lispro or aspart) | NPH |
| lispro or aspart | lispro or aspart | lispro or aspart | insulin glargine |

NPH = Neutral Protamine Hagedorn; Reg = regular insulin.

NPH (or lente) at bedtime. By also adding a dose of regular insulin pre-lunch, the morning NPH (lente) can be eliminated in many patients.

Premixed insulin preparations are available that consist of fixed ratios of two different insulins. These preparations can be used to simplify insulin administration in some patients. Insulin can be given subcutaneously by syringe or pen, or via an external insulin pump.

The most appropriate insulin dose for a given patient cannot be predicted. Rather, insulin adjustments are made prospectively based on the patient's glucose levels. Therefore, most diabetics should be encouraged to self-monitor capillary blood glucose (e.g., fingersticks or alternate site testing); the frequency of testing is individualized, based on the stability of the patient's glucose level and the goals of insulin therapy. In nonuremic patients, the pre-breakfast and pre-supper levels predominantly reflect the adequacy of the p.m. (or bedtime [h.s.]) and a.m. intermediate-acting insulin doses, respectively.

**TABLE 72.7. Side Effects of Insulin**

| |
|---|
| Hypoglycemia |
| Insulin atrophy |
| Lipoatrophy |
| Lipohypertrophy |
| Insulin edema |
| Weight gain |

The pre-lunch level can help adjust the a.m. regular insulin or lispro dose, just as the h.s. level can help adjust the p.m. regular or lispro insulin dose. **Glycosylated hemoglobin** (HbA1c) is covalent modification of hemoglobin by glucose; its assay rests on the premise that its amount is proportional to the mean glucose level. HbA1c is high in patients with sustained, prolonged hyperglycemia; thus, measurements help assess glycemic control during the two previous months. Measurements every 4 to 6 months can supplement self-monitoring and document glycemic control objectively.

Table 72.7 shows the complications of insulin therapy. The most common complication is hypoglycemia. Unfortunately, many insulin-dependent diabetics with long-standing diabetes cannot secrete adrenomedullary catecholamines following insulin-induced hypoglycemia. These catecholamines provide the adrenergic "warning" symptoms that prompt the diabetic to ingest carbohydrates immediately. Without this warning, the patient has ***hypoglycemic unawareness***; as a result, the first symptom of hypoglycemia may be cognitive impairment, seizures, or syncope. Catecholamine secretion depends on the extent and the rapidity with which hypoglycemia develops as well as the absolute level of hypoglycemia; thus, patients with good glycemic control can become hypoglycemic with smaller decreases in glucose than those with chronic hyperglycemia, and they are at heightened risk for hypoglycemic unawareness. Insulin allergy and lipoatrophy have decreased in frequency with improved, highly purified insulin preparations.

#### Oral hypoglycemic agents

The sulfonylureas stimulate insulin secretion from the pancreatic β cells. They can be used only in type 2 diabetes in whom blood sugar is not controlled by combined diet and exercise; they are contraindicated in type 1 diabetes and in pregnancy. (See Table 72.8 for dosages and duration of action.) Therapy with the sulfonylureas begins with the smallest dose, which is gradually increased until optimal control or maximum dose has been reached. If adequate glucose control is not achieved with the maximum dose, the drug should be discontinued and insulin therapy initiated. Side effects include anorexia, nausea, and diarrhea. Jaundice, skin rashes, and hematologic toxicity also have been reported. The sulfonylureas may cause severe and prolonged hypoglycemia, especially when there is impaired kidney function or no oral intake. Therefore, sulfonylureas should not be given under these conditions. Because they have far fewer side effects, the second-generation sulfonylureas now dominate the oral sulfonylurea market.

Like the sulfonylureas, two newer insulin secretagogues, repaglinide and nateglinide, stimulate the release of insulin from pancreatic islet cells. They have a rapid onset of action and are metabolized within several hours. They are administered immediately before each meal.

Metformin is the only member of a class of drugs called biguanides that is approved for use in the United States. Biguanides decrease glucose levels by multiple potential mechanisms, including anorexia, decreased intestinal glucose absorption, and potentiation of insulin action in its target tissues (principally inhibition of hepatic gluconeogenesis). Metformin is used in combination with either insulin or sulfonylureas in type 2 diabetes. It is contraindicated in type 1 diabetes and pregnancy. The side effects of metformin are primarily gastrointestinal. Lactic acidosis, sometimes fatal, has been reported. Metformin-associated lactic acidosis occurs primarily, if not solely, in patients with renal failure, hepatic dysfunction, or advanced cardiac disease. For this reason, use of the drug is contraindicated in these patients. Metformin should be withheld before patients undergo radiographic contrast studies.

Troglitazone was the first approved compound of the thiazolidinedione class of insulin-sensitizing agents. The thiazolidinediones bind to the nuclear receptor peroxisome proliferator-activated receptor-gamma (PPAR-gamma), which regulates the transcription of a number of insulin-responsive genes, resulting in improved insulin sensitivity and glucose transport. In response to a number of cases of troglitazone-induced hepatic necrosis, troglitazone was taken off the market in March of 1998. Two newer thiazolidinediones, rosiglitazone and pioglitazone, are currently available. The thiazolidinediones have been associated with weight gain and increases in plasma volume. They are contraindicated in patients with New York Heart Association (NYHA) class III or class IV heart failure. Liver transaminases should be monitored every 2 months for the first year of therapy and periodically thereafter.

Acarbose and miglitol are alpha-glucosidase inhibitors, which delay the absorption of carbohydrates from the gastrointestinal tract, significantly reducing postprandial hyperglycemia.

Oral agents are often combined with each other and some are combined with insulin to take advantage of their different mechanisms of action.

**TABLE 72.8. Oral Antidiabetic Agents**

| Agent | Starting Dose (mg/day) | Maximum Dose (mg/day) | Duration of Action (hr) |
|---|---|---|---|
| **Sulfonylurea Agents** | | | |
| Tolbutamide | 500 | 3000 | 6–10 |
| Chlorpropamide | 100–250 | 500 | 60 |
| Acetohexamide | 100–250 | 1500 | 12–18 |
| Tolazamide | 250 | 1000 | 16–24 |
| Glyburide | 1.25–5 | 20 | 24 |
| Glipizide | 2.5–5 | 40 | 15–24 |
| Glimepiride | 1–2 | 8 | 24 |
| **Other Antidiabetic Agents** | | | |
| Metformin | 1000 | 2500 | 8 |
| Pioglitazone | 15 | 45 | >24 |
| Rosiglitazone | 4 | 8 | >24 |
| Acarbose | 75 | 300 | 6 |
| Miglitol | 75 | 300 | 6 |
| Repaglinide | 1.5 | 16 | 3–4 |
| Nateglinide | 360 | 360 | 3–4 |

### Acute Complications of Diabetes: Diabetic Ketoacidosis and Hyperosmolar Coma

The term **diabetic coma** is loosely applied to diabetic ketoacidosis and hyperosmolar coma, but most patients are conscious and many have no alteration in mental status. The distinction between ketoacidosis and nonketotic diabetic coma is not absolute; mild ketonemia may be present in patients with a hyperosmolar state. Diabetic ketoacidosis is more common in type 1 diabetes, whereas nonketotic hyperosmolar coma occurs in type 2 diabetes.

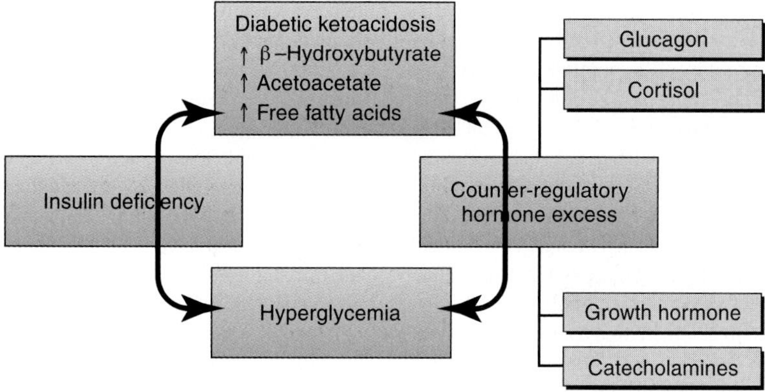


**FIGURE 72.3. The pathophysiology of diabetic ketoacidosis.** (Adapted from: Shade DS, Eaton RP. Diabetes 1977;26:597. Used with permission of American Diabetes Association, Alexandria, VA.)

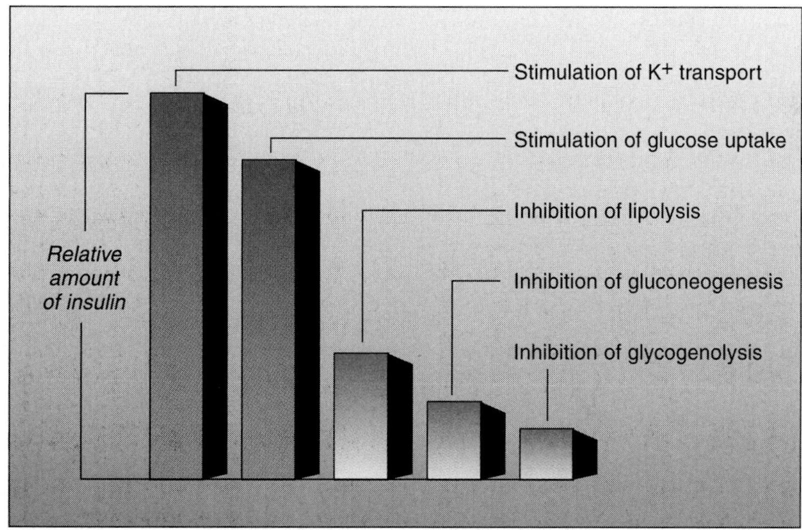


**FIGURE 72.4. Metabolic processes as dependent on relative levels of insulin. Gluconeogenesis is inhibited by minimal levels of insulin, whereas pharmacologic levels of insulin are needed to mobilize $K^+$ into the cells.** (Adapted from: Alberti KGMM, Nattras M. Med Clin North Am 1978;62:804. Used with permission of WB Saunders Co., Philadelphia, PA.)

The pathophysiology of diabetic ketoacidosis is summarized in Figures 72.3 and 72.4. The most important pathogenetic aspect is insufficient insulin action, further complicated by the unopposed action of anti-insulin hormones, namely, catecholamines, growth hormone, glucocorticoids, and glucagon. Hyperglycemia and ketoacidosis evolve as a consequence of insulin deficiency and counterregulatory hormone excess. Hyperglycemia leads to osmotic diuresis; dehydration and shock follow.

Insulin inhibits lipolysis by its effect on hormone sensitive lipase. This action of insulin is very sensitive, requiring less insulin than is needed to maintain euglycemia through increased cellular glucose uptake. Without insulin, increased lipolysis makes increased amounts of free fatty acids available to the liver; they are oxidized, and ketone bodies (acetoacetate and β-hydroxybutyrate) are formed as by-products. Ketone bodies can be utilized as a source of energy, but they accumulate in the blood if they are produced at a rate beyond which they can be excreted or oxidized. Ketone bodies are organic acids that readily dissociate and release hydrogen ions into the body fluids, causing the pH to fall, a metabolic state known as **ketoacidosis.**

### Diabetic ketoacidosis

The onset of diabetic ketoacidosis is characterized by an increase in symptoms of hyperglycemia, such as polyuria and polydipsia. Patients with previously undiagnosed diabetes may give a history of weight loss. Nausea, vomiting, and abdominal pain are common. Lethargy and some alteration of consciousness is generally present. Although most patients are not comatose at the time of admission, deep coma may result. On physical examination, signs of dehydration are evident (dry skin, a dry tongue, and hypotension). Increasing $H^+$ ion concentration leads to an increased rate and depth of respiration (**Kussmaul respiration**). Hypovolemia and shock or electrolyte abnormalities may be lethal. Precipitating events, such as infection, myocardial infarction, injury, or, often, noncompliance with insulin, may be present. Many patients either do not know of or ignore the need to continue insulin during a flu-like illness when they are eating poorly. In this setting, patients often discontinue insulin. Combined insulin deficiency and stress rapidly ushers in diabetic ketoacidosis.

#### *Diagnosis*

Ketoacidosis is diagnosed biochemically; its features are marked hyperglycemia, ketonemia, and acidosis. Blood glucose generally ranges between 400 and 800 mg/dl. The concentration of ketone bodies can be obtained semiquantitatively by using the Acetest tablet (**nitroprusside reaction**) with progressive dilutions of plasma. This reaction is sensitive to acetoacetate, but not to β-hydroxybutyrate. Measurement of electrolytes and pH reveals an **anion gap acidosis.** Normal anion gap ($[Na^+] - [Cl^- + HCO_3^-]$) is below 12 mEq/L; in general, the higher the level above 16 mEq/L, the greater the severity of ketoacidosis. (Some laboratories derive the anion gap by subtracting the total anions $[Cl^- + HCO_3]$ from the sum of cations $[Na^+$ and $K^+]$; the normal value then is below 16 mEq/L.)

#### *Management*

Diabetic ketoacidosis is a life-threatening situation, and management requires close observation and careful attention to details to achieve an optimal outcome. The essentials of treatment are insulin administration, replacement of fluid and electrolytes, and management of precipitating events. Only regular insulin is used in the treatment of patients with ketoacidosis. Low-dose insulin regimens, as opposed to high-dose regimens, evoke less frequent and less severe late hypoglycemia. Following an initial IV bolus of 10 to 20 units, insulin is administered preferentially as a continuous IV infusion, with an initial rate of 0.1 unit/kg/h. If no response to treatment is evident in 2 hours, the insulin infusion rate is doubled. In the presence of insulin resistance, larger insulin doses should be given. Plasma glucose should be monitored hourly; when it reaches approximately 250 mg/dl, the IV fluid is changed from normal saline to 5% glucose in half-normal saline. It is imperative to avoid hypoglycemia, because it may predispose to cerebral edema and brain damage.

The fluid losses in diabetic ketoacidosis range between 4 and 10 L. Although the fluid loss in ketoacidosis is hypotonic, fluid therapy is started with normal saline so as to achieve a prompt re-expansion of the circulating blood volume. In the first hour, 1 liter of normal saline is administered rapidly, followed by a liter of normal or half-normal saline in the next hour. The remainder of the fluids can be given more slowly until the patient's volume status is restored. Total body potassium is depleted, despite the deceptively normal or even high serum levels that appear initially. Hyperkalemia occurs when acidosis shifts potassium from the intracellular to the extracellular compartment. Insulin administration and correction of acidosis will reverse this shift; therefore, hypokalemia should be anticipated. Consequently, it is necessary to begin potassium administration at the rate of 20 to 30 mEq/L of fluid after adequate urinary output has been established. Potassium administration should be started at initiation of therapy if the initial serum $K^+$ is low or in the lower end of the normal range. Hypophosphatemia is common during therapy for ketoacidosis; because it reverses with refeeding, however, phosphate administration is not generally required. Most cases do not require administration of sodium bicarbonate, but it should be administered if the pH is below 7.0; some consider a pH below 7.1 as the indication.

A diligent search for precipitating causes should follow. If a bacterial infection is detected, appropriate antibiotics are required. It is necessary to rule out silent myocardial infarction by serial electrocardiography and appropriate blood tests. Gastric dilatation in the semiconscious patient requires nasogastric suction of the stomach contents.

### Nonketotic hyperosmolar coma

Hyperosmolar coma is much less common than diabetic ketoacidosis and usually occurs in older patients with type 2 diabetes. Conceptually, these patients have enough insulin to prevent ketosis and acidosis, but not enough to prevent hyperglycemia. (See Figures 72.4 and 72.5 for pathophysiology.) The evolution of the hyperglycemia, glycosuria, dehydration, and shock is similar to that in diabetic ketoacidosis. Patients usually present with a history of polyuria, polydipsia, and progressive fatigue of several days' or weeks' duration. The condition typically is precipitated by an associated illness, such as acute infection, myocardial infarction, cerebrovascular accident, heat stroke, hip fracture, or exacerbation of an underlying chronic illness. Decreased oral intake over a

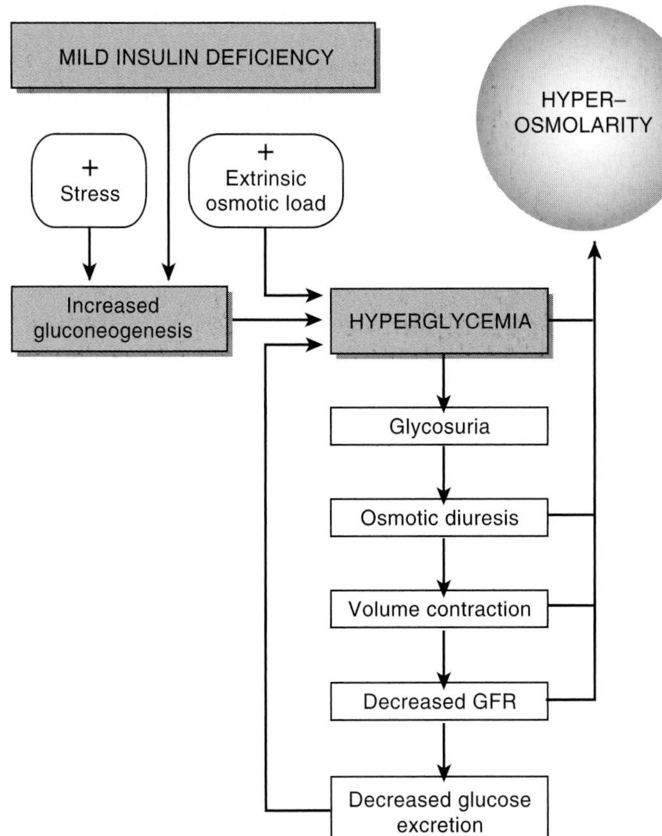


**FIGURE 72.5. Pathogenesis of hyperosmolar hyperglycemic non-ketotic state. GFR = glomerular filtration rate.**
(Adapted from: Greene DA. Top Emerg Med 1984; 5:49. Used with permission of Aspen Publishers, Inc., Gaithersburg, MD.)

period of time also is typical. Precipitating events occur at a higher frequency in nonketotic hyperosmolar coma than in diabetic ketoacidosis.

Physical examination reveals evidence of dehydration and impaired mentation. Focal neurologic signs, although often seen, usually resolve with treatment. Severe hyperglycemia is present; the blood glucose usually ranges from 800 to 1300 mg/dl. Plasma ketones usually are absent or, if present, occur in small amounts. The serum osmolarity is greatly increased, as measured directly or estimated by the following formula: serum osmolarity = 2(Na + K) + glucose/18 + BUN/2.8 (with serum osmolarity expressed in mOsm/L, sodium and potassium in mEq/L, glucose in mg/dL, and BUN in mg/dL). The principles of treatment are similar to those of diabetic ketoacidosis, although the dehydration usually is more profound than in diabetic ketoacidosis. It must be emphasized that the initial priority is to ensure adequate hydration.

## Chronic Complications of Diabetes

The availability of insulin has dramatically reduced the mortality from diabetic coma. The major morbidity and mortality due to diabetes now result from chronic complications, which consist of macrovascular disease (accelerated atherosclerosis) and microvascular disease (retinopathy, neuropathy, and nephropathy).

A major emphasis in the treatment of diabetes is prevention or delay of the onset of complications by modifications to the risk factors that increase the rate of complications. Tobacco use is forbidden, and hypertension is aggressively treated. Because hyperlipidemia is very prevalent in diabetes, cholesterol, HDL cholesterol, and triglycerides should be measured annually; hyperlipidemia, if present, should be treated. Obesity and inactivity portend risk of macrovascular disease. Suboptimal glucose control has a proven relationship with long-term complications, particularly of the microvasculature. Finally, most serious eye and foot problems can be avoided by proper preventive care by ophthalmologists and podiatrists.

### Macrovascular disease

#### *Coronary artery disease*

Atherosclerosis occurs more frequently, at an earlier age, and with greater severity in diabetic men and women than in nondiabetic persons. Even patients with impaired glucose tolerance are at a greater risk for the development of atherosclerosis. As in the general population, coronary artery disease is the leading cause of mortality in people with diabetes. Because of autonomic neuropathy, **myocardial infarction** in diabetes may be painless; it may present as diabetic ketoacidosis, and it is often diagnosed incidentally at a later date by a routine ECG.

*Peripheral Vascular Disease*

Involvement of large or medium-sized blood vessels in the lower limbs is a common complication of diabetes. Its prevalence is particularly high in older patients with type 2 diabetes. A diagnosis of arterial insufficiency is suggested by a history of **claudication**. Physical examination reveals absent or weak peripheral pulses. Noninvasive vascular testing involving measurement of arterial blood pressure and flow is used to confirm the diagnosis. Patients with peripheral vascular disease often cannot supply the increased blood flow needed to heal foot infections. The inability to heal these infections leads to **osteomyelitis, gangrene**, and **amputations**. Most foot infections are preceded by calluses. Therefore, routine foot care, including podiatric evaluation and proper footwear, is critical in preventing foot infections.

#### Microvascular disease

*Retinopathy*

**Diabetic retinopathy** is a leading cause of blindness in the United States. However, with yearly ophthalmologic examinations and preventive eye care, significant vision loss is prevented in all but a small fraction of patients. Some degree of diabetic retinopathy is detectable in more than 90% of patients who have had diabetes for 20 to 25 years. Diabetic retinopathy has two stages: **background retinopathy** and **proliferative retinopathy**. The earliest visible lesions of background retinopathy are exudates and microaneurysms. Capillary degeneration with fluid leakage and edema leads to exudates. Macular edema or a plaque of hard exudate may cause **visual loss**. In some patients, background retinopathy may progress to the proliferative stage; new vessels arise from the disc or from the retinal periphery. Traction on these new vessels may induce **vitreous hemorrhage** and visual impairment. Organization of these hemorrhages with fibrosis ultimately leads to **retinal detachment**. Careful follow-up is required in mild background retinopathy; if proliferative changes develop, appropriate treatment should follow promptly.

Proliferative diabetic retinopathy is treated by either xenon arc or laser beam photocoagulation to prevent vitreous hemorrhages and retinal detachments. The high-intensity light beam produces small spots of scarring. The rationale behind this treatment is based on the theory that new vessel growth is a response to areas of poor perfusion, releasing angiogenic growth factors. Controlled, scattered destruction of a portion of the retina prevents new blood vessels by eliminating their growth factor. In addition to retinopathy, **cataracts** and **glaucoma** are more prevalent in the diabetic population.

*Diabetic nephropathy*

**Diabetic nephropathy** often is present along with retinopathy, and occurs in approximately one third of patients. Nephropathy usually does not occur until 15 to 30 years after the initial diagnosis of diabetes. The specific lesion of diabetic nephropathy is nodular sclerosis (Kimmelstiel-Wilson lesion), visible on light microscopy as a rounded hyaline mass at the center of the glomerular lobules. More common, but less specific, is diffuse glomerulosclerosis with thickening of the glomerular basement membrane and an increased mesangial matrix. Nephropathy is first clinically evident by **proteinuria** (24-h urine protein > 500 mg). It is at first intermittent, but later becomes constant. **Microalbuminuria** (20–300 mg/24 h) heralds future development of gross proteinuria. Progressive nephropathy results in heavy proteinuria and the development of nephrotic syndrome, which typically progresses to renal failure within 5 years.

The treatment of diabetic nephropathy should be aimed at strict control of hypertension in addition to good glycemic control. Uncontrolled hypertension exacerbates worsening of renal function. A decrease in protein intake may slow the progression of nephropathy. Progression of proteinuria to overt renal failure also may be slowed by angiotensin-converting enzyme inhibitors. Insulin requirements fall as renal failure becomes manifest, and hypoglycemia may be frequent. Hemodialysis, peritoneal dialysis, and renal transplantation are used to manage end-stage renal disease.

*Diabetic neuropathy*

Diabetic neuropathy affects both the somatic and the autonomic nervous systems. Somatic neuropathy most commonly presents as symmetric peripheral neuropathy, with initial symptoms of numbness and tingling, usually in the feet and legs. Painful, burning, and aching variants occur and are especially bothersome at night. Tendon reflexes and response to sensory stimuli, particularly vibration, are decreased. Distal weakness may be noted. Peripheral neuropathy markedly worsens the risk of infection and amputation in patients with peripheral vascular disease and underscores the need for preventive foot care. Therapy of uncomfortable peripheral neuropathy involves the use of drugs with combined analgesic and sedative properties (e.g., gabapentin, tricyclic antidepressants, carbamazepine, phenytoin, and, in severe cases, narcotic analgesics). Topical agents (e.g., capsaicin) are effective at times. Neuropathy may less often involve a single peripheral nerve, causing motor or sensory deficit in the distribution of the affected nerve (mononeuropathy). Peripheral nerves may be affected either singly or in combination, producing a mononeuritis multiplex. Cranial nerves may be similarly affected, especially the third nerve.

Autonomic neuropathies can affect nearly all organs. The more notable examples include the skin (anhidrosis), the cardiovascular system (orthostatic hypotension and absence of reflex tachycardia), and the genitourinary system (neurogenic bladder dysfunction, impotence, and retrograde ejaculation). Impotence is seen in 75% of diabetic men 60 to 65 years old. Gastrointestinal autonomic neuropathy has varied features, including delayed emptying of the stomach (gastroparesis), symptoms of which are early satiety, nausea, and vomiting. Irregular gastric emptying complicates efforts at glycemic control. Therapy of gastroparesis with metoclopramide is partially effective in some patients. Constipation or frequent, profuse, nocturnal watery urgent bowel movements (nocturnal diabetic diarrhea) also may occur. In some instances, diabetic diarrhea may respond to a broad-spectrum antibiotic, but the treatment is mostly symptomatic. Evaluation for other causes of diarrhea is important.

# CHAPTER 73 NUTRITIONAL DISORDERS

## Estimating Energy Requirements

Understanding the body's basal energy requirements is a prerequisite to an effective nutritional assessment. Factors that contribute to the body's total energy requirements include the **basal metabolic rate** (BMR), the energy required for activity, and the thermic effect of food. The BMR, the energy expended by the body at rest and without food, is estimated by the **Harris-Benedict equation** (Table 73.1). The energy expended during various types of physical activity is **energy of activity;** it accounts for nearly one third of total energy expenditure, but varies with the type of activity. Sedentary activities (e.g., sleeping, reading) utilize 72 kcal/h, whereas strenuous activities such as running or construction work expend 600 kcal/h.

**Thermic energy** is the amount of energy required to carry out the digestion, absorption, and metabolism of food. The metabolism of all foods produces heat **(thermic effect of food);** the extent varies with different foods. These differences are expressed quantitatively as the **specific dynamic action** (SDA) or **calorigenic effect** of foods. Carbohydrate or fat increases heat production by approximately 5% of the meal's caloric content; protein has the highest thermogenic effect, approximately 30%. Inflammatory, febrile diseases increase BMR according to severity—mild illness by 10%, moderate illnesses by 25%, and severe illnesses by 50%.

Thus, the total daily energy requirement can be estimated by adding together the BMR, a compensation for the severity of illness, an allowance for physical activity, and the SDA. A less precise, but easier, method multiplies the estimated ideal body weight (see Table 73.1) by a factor that takes into account physical activity (sedentary = 30 kcal/kg; moderately active = 35–40 kcal/kg, and very active = 45 kcal/kg). Thus, a moderately active, healthy 70-kg man requires 2450–2800 kcal/d.

## Clinical Nutritional Assessment

An individual's nutritional status reflects the degree to which the physiologic need for nutrients is being met. Nutritional assessment consists of gathering data: (1) to identify persons who will require specialized nutritional care; (2) to ascertain the cause and degree of malnutrition, if present; and (3) to judge the potential risk for the development of malnutrition. A careful history, a physical

**TABLE 73.1. Estimation of BMR and Ideal Body Weight**

| | BMR[a] | Ideal Body Weight[b] |
|---|---|---|
| Women | 655 + (9.5 × W) + (1.8 × H) − (4.7 × A)[c] | 100 lb (45kg) for the first 5 ft (152cm) + 5 lb (2.2kg) for every inch (2.54cm) of H> 5 ft (152cm) |
| Men | 66 + (13.7 × W) + (5 × H) − (6.8 ×A) | 110 lb (2.2kg) for the first 5 ft (152cm) + 5 lb (2.2kg) for every 1 inch (2.54cm) of H >5 ft (152cm). |

BMR = basal metabolic rate; W = weight in kg; H = height in meters; A = age in years.
[a]Derived from the Harris-Benedict equation in Harris JA, Benedict FG. A Biometric Study of Basal Metabolism in Man. Washington DC: Carnegie Institute of Washington, Publ. No. 279, 1919.
[b]Adapted from Krause MV, Mahan K. Food, Nutrition and Diet Therapy. 7th ed. Philadelphia, WB Saunders, 1984.

examination, and appropriate laboratory data are essential. The different methods of assessing nutritional status have the same aims: to identify persons at nutritional risk and to intervene quickly with appropriate nutritional therapy.

**History and physical examination**

Historical data should include appetite, recent weight change, physical activity, dental and oral health, and food and drug allergies. Additional inquiries relate to gastrointestinal illness, chronic diseases, medications, eating disorders and nutritional problems, and a history of substance abuse. The patient's general appearance should be carefully noted. **Protein-energy status** is generally assessed by anthropometric and biochemical means. Height and weight are compared with standardized population tables (such as life insurance tables) (Table 73.2). The **body mass index** (BMI) is calculated by dividing weight (in kg) by height (in meters) squared, expressed as kg/m$^2$. The BMI correlates well with body fatness. A BMI of 24 to 27 for women or 24 to 25 for men indicates excess weight; a BMI above 30 indicates obesity.

**Ancillary studies**

Nutritional assessment also includes several biochemical measurements that primarily assess visceral (nonstructural) protein. Serum albumin often is included in these tests, but these levels may fluctuate for reasons other than nutritional depletion. Also, the relatively long half-life (about 14 days) limits its usefulness in evaluating malnutrition of short duration. Therefore, prealbumin (2-day half-life), is a better screening test for malnutrition. A total lymphocyte count below 1200 cells/mm$^3$ may indicate poor nutrition.

**TABLE 73.2. 1983 Metropolitan Life Height and Weight Tables**

| Height | | Weight (lb) | | |
|---|---|---|---|---|
| **Feet** | **Inches** | **Small Frame** | **Medium Frame** | **Large Frame** |
| **Men** | | | | |
| 5 | 2 | 128–131 | 131–141 | 138–150 |
| 5 | 3 | 130–136 | 131–113 | 138–153 |
| 5 | 4 | 132–138 | 135–145 | 142–156 |
| 5 | 5 | 134–140 | 137–146 | 144–160 |
| 5 | 6 | 136–142 | 139–151 | 146–164 |
| 5 | 7 | 138–145 | 142–154 | 149–168 |
| 5 | 8 | 140–148 | 145–157 | 152–172 |
| 5 | 9 | 142–151 | 148–160 | 155–176 |
| 5 | 10 | 144–154 | 151–163 | 158–180 |
| 5 | 11 | 146–157 | 154–166 | 161–184 |
| 6 | 0 | 149–160 | 157–170 | 164–188 |
| 6 | 1 | 152–164 | 160–174 | 168–192 |
| 6 | 2 | 155–168 | 164–178 | 172–197 |
| 6 | 3 | 158–172 | 167–182 | 176–202 |
| 6 | 4 | 167–176 | 171–187 | 181–207 |
| **Women** | | | | |
| 4 | 10 | 102–111 | 109–121 | 116–131 |
| 4 | 11 | 103–113 | 111–123 | 120–134 |
| 5 | 0 | 104–115 | 113–126 | 122–137 |
| 5 | 1 | 106–118 | 115–129 | 125–140 |
| 5 | 2 | 108–121 | 118–132 | 126–143 |
| 5 | 3 | 111–124 | 121–135 | 131–147 |
| 5 | 4 | 114–127 | 124–138 | 134–151 |
| 5 | 5 | 117–130 | 127–141 | 137–155 |
| 5 | 6 | 120–133 | 130–144 | 140–159 |
| 5 | 7 | 123–136 | 133–147 | 143–163 |
| 5 | 8 | 126–139 | 136–150 | 146–167 |
| 5 | 9 | 129–142 | 139–153 | 149–170 |
| 5 | 10 | 132–145 | 142–156 | 152–175 |
| 5 | 11 | 135–148 | 145–159 | 155–176 |
| 6 | 0 | 138–151 | 148–162 | 158–179 |

(Data from Society of Actuaries and Association of Life Insurance Medical Directors of America, 1979 Build Study, published 1980. Courtesy of Statistical Bulletin, Metropolitan Life Insurance Company. With permission.)

## Malnutrition

**Malnutrition** represents inadequate total calorie or protein intake to meet nutrient needs. Protein-energy malnutrition is common in as many as 50% of hospitalized patients. Worldwide, malnutrition most commonly affects infants and preschool children; however, no age group is exempt. Pathophysiologic changes that follow protein-energy malnutrition are listed in Table 73.3.

The treatment of protein-calorie malnutrition requires identification of patients at risk, often by hospital-based staff dietitians. Various grading systems categorize a patient's nutritional risk as mild, moderate, or severe, based on history, anthropometric indices, and laboratory testing; the patient's primary disease; anticipated duration of illness; and accessibility to nutrition (illnesses may limit patients' access to oral nutrition for protracted periods).

After careful nutritional assessment, a diet prescription must be created for each patient. Planning a diet begins with a review of the patient's usual food intake and a determination of its adequacy. Decisions regarding the route of feeding and the consistency of food are made based on the patient's ability to chew, swallow, and digest. No standard diet can meet every individual's needs, and modifications often must be made based on underlying conditions such as dysphagia, hypertension, diabetes, and hyperlipidemia (Table 73.4). For example, a diabetic patient should receive approximately 55% to 60% calories from complex carbohydrates, 20% from protein, and less than 30% from fat. The exchange list describing serving sizes of various foods in groups of similar nutrient value is a useful teaching tool for diabetics.

The American Heart Association and National Cholesterol Education Program have provided nutritional guidelines for patients with hyperlipidemia and coronary artery disease; they are used for both the primary prevention and the secondary treatment of established cardiovascular disease. The Phase 1 diet, a moderately low-fat, low-cholesterol diet for persons with normal lipids who wish to follow a preventive eating plan, is also useful in persons at moderate to high risk for the development of coronary heart disease. In general, the Phase 1 diet is continued for 2 to 4 months, at the end of which the serum cholesterol is reevaluated; if there has been insufficient response to the Phase 1 diet, the Phase 2 diet is initiated. It further reduces saturated fatty acid intake (to less than 7% of calories) and cholesterol (to less than 200 mg/day). If serum cholesterol levels still do not respond sufficiently, drug therapy is added.

In the malnourished patient or one at risk for malnutrition, the necessary nutrition can be effectively provided by two routes: enteral (by tube feeding through the **gastrointestinal** [GI] tract) and **parenteral** (by IV infusion, bypassing the GI tract). Decision-making regarding specialized nutrition support is illustrated in Figure 73.1.

Enteral feeding is preferred if the GI tract is functional. It is easier, less expensive, and safer, and it prevents intestinal atrophy and stress-induced gastritis. Many types of enteral feeding tubes are available (Table 73.5). Nasogastric and nasoduodenal or nasojejunal tubes may be placed nonsurgically. Introduced nasally, they can be left in place for several weeks. Ensuring accurate tube placement is essential before initiating feeding. This can be done by aspirating gastric contents and by radiographic evaluation for tubes with metallic weights at their tips. For long-term enteral feeding, surgically placed tubes are preferable. Gastrostomy and jejunostomy tubes can be placed via surgical, fluoroscopic, and endoscopic means.

A wide range of formulations is available for enteral feeding, with variable osmolality, caloric density, and composition. Disease-specific formulas also are available. When more specific nutritional support is required, a custom-made diet can be prescribed using commercially available components of carbohydrate, protein, and fat. Tube feeding usually is given full strength, but may need to be initiated in a diluted form, and increased

**TABLE 73.3. Pathophysiologic Response to Protein-Calorie Malnutrition**

Decrease in energy expenditure
Muscle wasting
Mobilization of body fat
Endocrine changes
  Euthyroid sick syndrome
  Decreased insulin and somatomedin
  Increased growth hormone, catecholamines, glucocorticoids, and aldosterone
Reduced red cell mass and oxygen transport
Decreased cardiac work and glomerular filtration rate
Reduced T-lymphocytes
Electrolyte abnormalities
Malabsorption of lipids
Decreased absorption of glucose
Diarrhea (due to bacterial overgrowth and abnormal intestinal motility)
Impaired central and peripheral nervous system(s)

**TABLE 73.4. Summary of Usual Hospital Diets**

| Diet | Purpose | Nutritional Value | Comments |
|---|---|---|---|
| General[a] | For adult patients who do not require diet modifications | Can be adequate in meeting all needs, based on menu selection | Can be modified according to personal taste in food |
| Soft | Provides food that requires little or no chewing | Can be adequate in meeting all needs, based on menu selection | Texture can be determined based on individual needs, from pureed to chopped. |
| Full liquid | Supplies fluid and nutrients for patients who are between clear liquid and solid foods | May be deficient in niacin, folic acid, and iron. Snacks may be necessary to increase caloric intake. | For postoperative or acutely ill patients; or those with gastrointestinal diseases and those unable to chew. Can serve as transitional diet. |
| Clear liquid | Short-term administration of fluid and 600–900 kcal/day | Falls short of providing adequate nutrition | Generally should not be continued more than 3–5 days |

[a]Contains 1600–2200 kcal, with 60–80 g protein, 80–100 g fat, and 180–300 g carbohydrate.

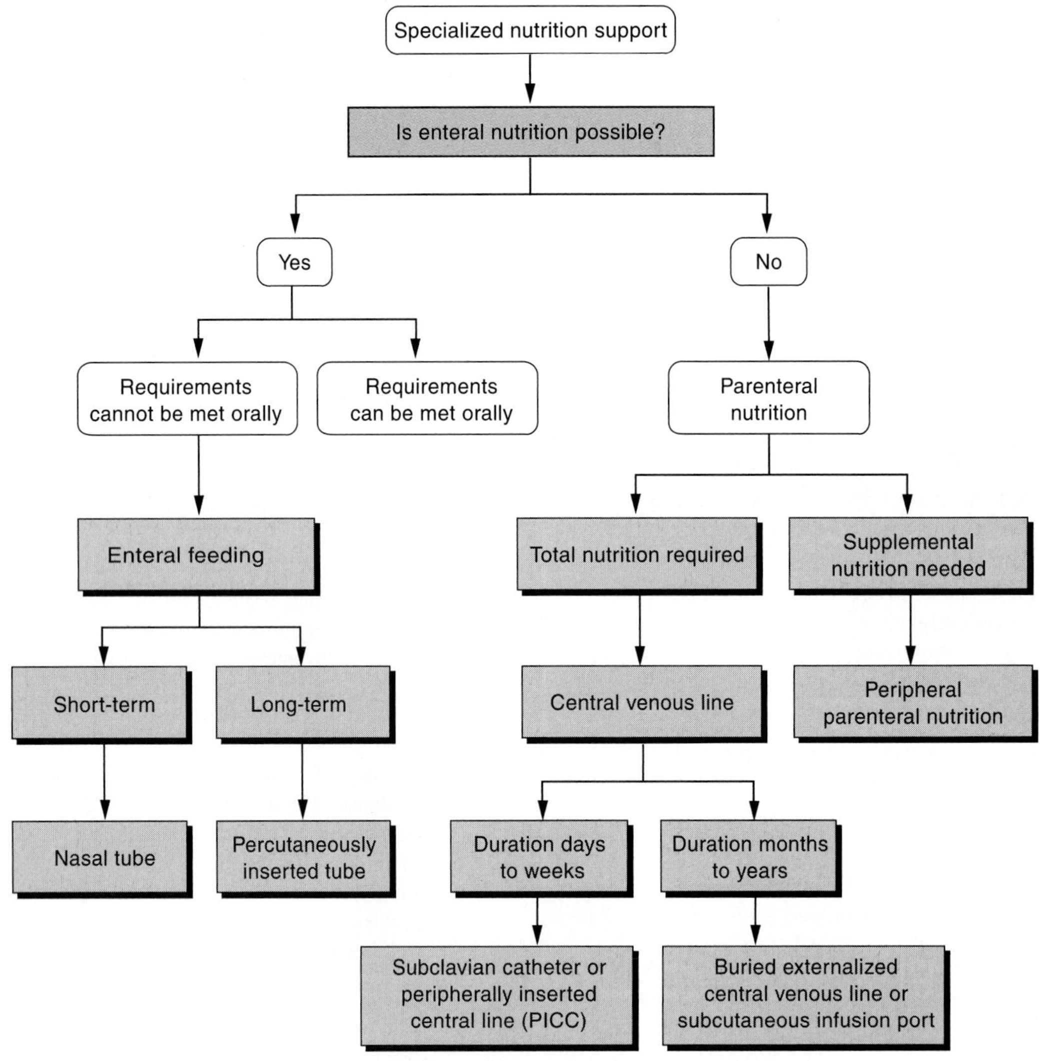


**FIGURE 73.1.** Algorithm for evaluation of specialized nutrition support.

**TABLE 73.5. Enteral Feeding Tubes**

| Type of Tube | Comments | Complications |
|---|---|---|
| **Nonsurgically Placed Tubes** | | |
| Nasogastric | For short-term use; easy to insert and reinsert | Tracheal intubation, aspiration, intestinal perforation, clogging |
| Nasoduodenal or nasojejunal | For short-term use; used when gastric emptying is impaired | Same as above |
| **Surgically Placed Tubes** | | |
| Gastrostomy tube | Long-term use; used when swallowing is impaired | Irritation at tube site; diarrhea |
| Jejunostomy tube | Long-term use; used when gastric emptying is impaired; usually need continuous feeding | Same as above |
| Combined gastrojejunostomy tubes | Allows for simultaneous gastric suction and jejunal feeding | Same as above |

incrementally to full strength. Feeding is administered continuously by pump or intermittently by gravity or pump over 30 to 60 minutes every 3 to 6 hours. Careful patient monitoring can help avoid the complications of enteral feeding (Table 73.6). Aspiration of gastric contents often is preventable (see Table 246.3).

Parenteral nutrition may supplement enteral feeding or may be the sole source of nutrients. It is given by two routes. **Peripheral parenteral nutrition** (PPN) (injected into arm veins) is limited to patients who require partial or short-term parenteral nutrition, with only low osmolar solutions (<600 mOsm/L). Most patients receiving parenteral nutrition require **central parenteral nutrition** (CPN), using external jugular, internal jugular, or subclavian veins. Subcutaneous tunneling of a central venous catheter is recommended when CPN is continued for more than 2 weeks. Components and complications of total parenteral nutrition (TPN) are shown in Tables 73.7 and 73.8, respectively. The presence of a terminal condition that precludes aggressive therapy and a functioning GI tract are relative contraindications to TPN.

**TABLE 73.6. Complications of enteral feeding**

| Mechanical | Gastrointestinal | Metabolic |
|---|---|---|
| Erosions | Nausea | Overhydration |
| Abscesses | Vomiting | Dehydration |
| Esophageal ulcerations | Diarrhea | Nutrient imbalances |
| Tube obstruction | Constipation | Hyperglycemia |
| | | Hypoglycemia |
| | | Electrolyte imbalance |

## Obesity

**Obesity,** an excess of **body fat** (adipose tissue), may be defined in terms of deviation from a presumed **ideal body weight** (IBW) for a given height (Table 73.9). It also can be defined by body mass index (BMI), or body weight in kilograms divided by the height in meters squared (kg/m$^2$). Obesity is a BMI greater than or equal to 30 kg/m$^2$. Morbid obesity is a BMI greater than or equal to 40 kg/m$^2$. Obesity is one of the most common health problems in the United States. An estimated 40 million Americans are obese, and the incidence is rising.

### Etiology

**Obesity** has multiple causes and pathophysiologic mechanisms. Genetic, behavioral, environmental, and

**TABLE 73.7. Components of Total Parenteral Nutrition**

| Component | Supplied As | Comments |
|---|---|---|
| Carbohydrate | 50% dextrose in water (D50W) | Monitor plasma glucose |
| Protein | 3–10% AA | Branched chain AA: in trauma and liver disease; essential AA: in renal failure |
| Fat | Weekly infusions of 0.5–1.0 L of 10% and 20% emulsions of soybean or safflower oil | Required for supplying essential free fatty acids and if TPN is continued for over 7–10 days |
| Vitamins and minerals | Added to the infusate | Based on RDA and patient's specific needs |
| Fluid | Generally 30–50 ml/kg for maintenance. | Replenish abnormal fluid losses; to avoid metabolic complications, check BUN and electrolytes daily for the first week; monitor intake, output, and daily weight |

AA = amino acids; RDA = recommended daily allowance; TPN = total parenteral nutrition.

**TABLE 73.8. Potential Complications of Parenteral Nutrition**

| Mechanical | Infectious | Metabolic |
|---|---|---|
| Pneumothorax (simple and tension) | Infection at catheter insertion site | Dehydration |
| Hemothorax | Seeding of catheter from distant infection | Hyperglycemia |
| Subclavian artery injury | Contamination of solution | Deficiencies of calcium, magnesium, or phosphorus |
| Central venous thrombosis | | Hyperphosphatemia |
| Air embolism | | Hyperchloremic metabolic acidosis |
| Cardiac perforation/tamponade | | Trace mineral deficiencies |

TABLE 73.9. Classification of Obesity Based on Ideal Body Weight

| | |
|---|---|
| Overweight | 0–20% above IBW<br>BMI 25–30 $kg/m^2$ |
| Obese | 20% or more above IBW<br>BMI > 30 $kg/m^2$ |
| Morbidly obese | 100% or more above IBW<br>BMI > 40 $kg/m^2$ |

BMI = body mass index; IBW = ideal body weight.

metabolic factors contribute to an energy imbalance. Specific genetic defects leading to obesity remain elusive in humans, but animal studies suggest that genetic factors influence energy balance and may increase susceptibility to obesity. The adipose tissue hormone leptin is felt to play an important role in maintaining body adiposity, and body weight. It's clinical implications are still unclear. Occasionally, obesity follows an underlying medical disorder.

**Overeating** (the ingestion of an amount of energy exceeding the body's needs) contributes to the development of obesity. Overeating is probably due to both biological and psychological factors. Obese individuals may harbor an aberration in one of many physiological signals that regulate feeding behavior, causing abnormal satiety; these signals may be metabolic (e.g., glucose, amino acids, and fatty acids), hormones (e.g., insulin), and GI events. A sedentary lifestyle may also cause obesity.

## Clinical Features and Complications

Obesity significantly increases morbidity and decreases life expectancy. Hypertension occurs three to five times more often in obese persons. Obesity, particularly abdominal obesity, often coexists with other risk factors for atherogenesis (hypertension and glucose intolerance); lipid abnormalities (including elevated total cholesterol, reduced **high-density lipoprotein** (HDL) cholesterol, and increased triglyceride levels), coronary heart disease (for which it also increases the risk for thromboembolic events); type 2 diabetes mellitus; and respiratory abnormalities, including hypoventilation and sleep apnea. In obesity, the risk of certain cancers (breast and endometrial) is enhanced; excess estrogens may be partly responsible. For unknown reasons, overweight men suffer a higher risk of fatal prostatic cancer; dietary factors (e.g., excess saturated fat in the diet) are suspected.

Liver abnormalities include abnormal liver tests and fatty liver. Cholelithiasis is strongly associated with obesity, with a prevalence of 30% among obese women. Many endocrine abnormalities complicate obesity, including adrenocortical hyperactivity. Cortisol production and cortisol turnover are high; however, 24-hour urine free cortisol levels are normal. In obese women, menstrual disorders (oligomenorrhea, amenorrhea, and dysfunctional uterine bleeding) and hirsutism are common. Obese men may have decreased libido and impotence; total testosterone levels are often low. The severity of these abnormalities parallels the degree of obesity and often, they can be reversed with weight loss. Obese patients commonly report joint pain, especially in the lumbosacral spine, hips, knees, and ankles. Excess weight contributes to the evolution of degenerative joint disease.

## Management

Because obesity has multiple causes, prevention and treatment are difficult. Obesity due to a medical cause (e.g., hypothyroidism, hypercortisolism, male hypogonadism, hypopituitarism, or hypothalamic abnormalities) should receive specific therapy.

If no underlying disorder is identified, treatment is then directed at weight reduction measures. Although short-term weight loss often is achieved, long-term weight reduction commonly fails: only 20% of obese persons maintain their weight loss 5 to 15 years after initial treatment. Thus, obesity should be considered a medical condition requiring lifelong therapy, the cornerstone of which is dietary therapy. In general, weight loss occurs when energy expenditure exceeds energy intake. Although many calorie-restricted diets exist, moderate calorie restriction using normal foods can be an effective and safe way to lose weight; the patient's age, medical condition, level of physical activity, and degree of obesity determine the degree of calorie restriction. Although a weekly weight loss of 2 pounds (1 kg) normally is a reasonable goal, underlying medical complications of severe obesity (heart failure, hypoventilation, or severe hyperglycemia), may require faster weight loss. Exercise (daily walking or swimming), initiated gradually, is also part of an effective weight reduction program. In severely obese persons, some weight loss may be necessary before exercise can be initiated. Long-term success in therapy also requires behavioral modifications, often involving attitudes toward eating, physical activity, socializing, and entertaining.

Currently, drug therapy plays a limited role in the treatment of obesity. Thyroid hormone and diuretics should be used only when medically indicated. Amphetamines should never be prescribed to treat obesity. Appetite-suppressing agents have been available for many years. A number of different brain receptors (including noradrenergic and serotoninergic receptors) can modulate appetite. Phenylpropanolamine (Dexatrim), formerly available over-the-counter, is no longer available due to safety concerns. The combination of fenfluramine and phentermine has been associated with valvular heart disease. Currently, only two prescription medications are approved for use for longer than 2 to 3 weeks. Sibutramine facilitates serotonin and norepinephrine release in neurons in the brain. Average weight loss after one year of treatment is 2.7% to 7.4%. Side effects include dry mouth, constipation, insomnia, anxiety, palpitations and increased heart rate, and increased blood pressure. Sibutramine should only be considered for individuals with a BMI >30, or if the BMI is 27 to 30 and the patient has one or more of the following: type 2 diabetes, dyslipidemia, or hypertension. Orlistat is a nonabsorbed inhibitor of gastric and pancreatic lipase that results in reduced absorption of fat and fat-soluble substances (i.e., cholesterol and certain vitamins). Orlistat is administered at each meal. Average weight loss is 5% at 1 year. Side effects are primarily gastrointestinal. A multivitamin is recommended at bedtime.

Occasionally, morbid obesity requires surgical treatment. It is considered in patients with a BMI greater than 40 kg/m$^2$. The most common procedures are gastroplasty and gastric bypass, and several centers are performing these procedures laparoscopically. Both procedures cause patients to limit food intake by delaying gastric emptying and causing the sensation of fullness after a small meal. Surgery should also be combined with behavior modification.

Anorexia nervosa and bulimia, are discussed in Chapter 27.

## Vitamins and Trace Elements

Vitamins are a group of unrelated organic compounds that share at least two common features: the body cannot synthesize them at all, or only to a very limited extent, and minute quantities are needed in the diet. Many vitamins act as coenzymes or as catalytic cofactors for biologic reactions. Single vitamin deficiencies now occur rarely; they appear more commonly with general malnutrition. Vitamin deficiencies occur in states of malabsorption, in individuals who follow radical diets or suffer from alcoholism, as a complication of total parenteral nutrition, and in inborn errors of metabolism. Vitamin excess states are now more common than vitamin deficiency because of increased public use of vitamin supplements.

Vitamins are generally divided in two groups: fat-soluble and water-soluble. The fat-soluble vitamins—A, D, E, and K—are found in foods in association with lipids. Conditions that interfere with fat absorption also interfere with the absorption of these vitamins. They can be stored in the body to some extent. The water-soluble vitamins include vitamin C and vitamins of the B complex. Water-soluble vitamins are not normally stored in the body in appreciable amounts, so a daily supply is desirable. Information regarding the various vitamins, their biologic functions, and symptoms of their deficiency and excess are shown in Table 73.10.

Trace elements are metals present in minute amounts in biologic fluids that are considered essential for optimal growth and development. They are constituents of, or interact with, larger molecules, such as enzymes or hormones. Many enzymes require a small amount of a trace metal for full activity. Metals can cause disease through deficiency, excess, or imbalance. Deficiency states can result from inadequate dietary intake, malabsorption states, and excessive loss through the urine, pancreatic juice or other exocrine losses. Deficiencies also may follow imbalances between metals. Trace element deficiencies also can occur in patients receiving total parenteral nutrition.

Metal toxicity, which can involve a number of metals including aluminum, copper, nickel, and zinc, can occur in several settings, including chronic renal dialysis. Early recognition can avoid significant neurologic, hematologic, and skeletal complications.

**TABLE 73.10. Vitamin Deficiency and Excess**

| Vitamin | Function | Signs of Deficiency | Signs of Excess |
|---|---|---|---|
| **Fat-Soluble Vitamins** | | | |
| Vitamin A | Vision<br>Growth<br>Reproduction, anti-cancer | Night blindness<br>Corneal ulcerations<br>Dryness and hyperkeratosis of skin | Fatigue, malaise, lethargy, bone pain and fragility, hepatomegaly, headaches, vomiting |
| Vitamin D | Calcium homeostasis<br>Bone mineralization | Rickets<br>Osteomalacia<br>Costochondral beading | Hypercalcemia, vomiting, anorexia, irritability, diarrhea, seizures |
| Vitamin E | Antioxidant<br>Absorption of Vitamin A | Hemolytic anemia in premature and newborn infants, red blood cell fragility | None known |
| Vitamin K | Production of prothrombin and clotting factors VIII, IX, and X | Hemorrhage | Warfarin resistance, jaundice in newborns |
| **Water-Soluble Vitamins** | | | |
| Vitamin C | Collagen cross-links<br>Wound healing<br>Antioxidant<br>Utilization of iron | Joint tenderness, scurvy (capillary hemorrhage), impaired wound healing, acute periodontal gingivitis, petechiae | Risk of renal oxalate stones |
| Thiamine (B1) | Metabolism of carbohydrates, fats and protein; nervous system function; coenzyme for carboxylation of 2-ketoacids | Beriberi, neuritis, edema, cardiac failure, anorexia, muscle weakness, confusion | None known |
| Riboflavin (B2) | Reactive portion of flavoproteins included in oxidation | Photophobia, cheilosis, glossitis, scrotal skin changes | None known |
| Niacin | Coenzyme in fat synthesis, tissue respiration and carbohydrate utilization, digestion | Pellagra (dementia, dermatitis, diarrhea), muscle weakness | Flushing, tingling of skin, head throbbing |
| Pyridoxine (B6) | Coenzyme in synthesis and breakdown of amino acids; synthesis of unsaturated fatty acids | Depression, nausea, vomiting, ataxia, convulsions, peripheral neuritis, hypochromic and macrocytic anemia | None known |
| Folic acid | Synthesis of nucleic acids; normal maturation of red blood cells; coenzyme | Megaloblastic anemia, Subacute combined degeneration of the cord | None known |
| Cyanocobalamin (B12) | Biosynthesis of nucleic acids and nucleoproteins; recycling of tetrahydrofolate | Megaloblastic anemia, Subacute combined degeneration of the cord | None known |
| Biotin | Synthesis and breakdown of fatty acids and amino acids | Anorexia, nausea, vomiting, glossitis, depression, skin and hair changes | None known |
| Pantothenic acid | Part of coenzyme A intermediate metabolism of carbohydrate, fat and protein | Infertility, abortion, depression, slowed growth | None known |

# CHAPTER 74 DISORDERS OF LIPID METABOLISM

The two major circulating lipids are triglycerides and cholesterol. Triglycerides, composed of three fatty acids esterified to glycerol, are stored in adipose tissue in the fed state and are mobilized during fasting; they provide the body's primary fuel reserves. Cholesterol serves several functions. It is a major structural component of the cell membrane and the synthetic precursor of steroid hormones and bile salts. Cholesterol and triglycerides must be efficiently transferred between their organs of origin (principally the liver and intestine) and their peripheral destinations. Because both lipids are highly hydrophobic and essentially insoluble in water, they are transported in spherical particles called lipoproteins; nonpolar triglycerides and cholesterol esters are concentrated in the central core of these lipoproteins. Phospholipids and apolipoproteins (apoproteins) make up a polar shell that allows the lipoprotein particle to remain suspended in the plasma. Apoproteins are specialized proteins that confer specific properties to the lipoprotein particles of which they are a part, permitting them to interact appropriately with their target tissues and with other lipoprotein particles. Six major lipoproteins are recognized, based on their functional roles, lipid composition, constituent apoproteins, electrophoretic mobilities, and particle density (Table 74.1).

Lipoprotein metabolism can be simplified into three interdependent pathways: the exogenous pathway, the endogenous pathway, and reverse cholesterol transport. These pathways interface with one another either at the hepatic level or via direct exchange of lipids and apoproteins between lipoproteins in the plasma. The exogenous pathway starts with the absorption of dietary fats from the small bowel; they are assembled into chylomicrons, stable droplets containing triglyceride fat, cholesterol, phospholipids, and protein (Figure 74.1). After entering the systemic circulation, the chylomicrons interact with lipoprotein lipase, an enzyme that lines the capillaries of adipose and muscle tissues. Lipoprotein lipase hydrolyzes chylomicron triglycerides into fatty acids and glycerol, which are then used by peripheral tissues. The triglyceride-depleted chylomicron remnants are removed from the circulation by the liver and catabolized.

In the endogenous pathway, hepatically derived triglycerides and cholesterol are secreted into the circulation in the form of very-low-density lipoproteins (VLDL; Figure 74.2). The lipid of VLDL is approximately 80% triglycerides and 20% cholesterol. VLDL also interacts with endothelial lipoprotein lipase, producing a triglyceride-depleted particle, the intermediate-density lipoprotein (IDL). Further catabolism and modification of IDL in the plasma largely yields low-density lipoprotein (LDL); LDL is taken up by the LDL receptor, a specific plasma membrane receptor in the liver. Extrahepatic tissues also possess LDL receptors. LDL thus provides cholesterol to the gonads and adrenal cortex for steroidogenesis. LDL can also be taken up by a less specific scavenger pathway by other cells, such as macrophages. In reverse cholesterol transport, the third basic lipoprotein pathway, the HDL takes up free cholesterol from peripheral tissues; it esterifies the free cholesterol with the enzyme lecithin-acyl cholesterol transferase (LCAT), then transfers the cholesterol ester to LDL in the plasma. Because HDL removes free cholesterol from tissue and plasma, high HDL levels tend to protect against atherosclerosis. The major morbidity of dyslipidemias results from the atherogenic nature of lipoproteins enriched with cholesterol-esters; elevated LDL is most strongly associated with atherosclerosis and coronary heart disease.

**TABLE 74.1. Properties of Lipoprotein Classes**

| Class | Density (g/L) | Diameter (nM) | Triglyceride: Cholesterol Ester | Characteristic Apoproteins |
|---|---|---|---|---|
| Chylomicrons | 0.93 | 75–1200 | 30:1 | B-48, C-II, E |
| VLDL | 0.93–1.006 | 30–80 | 4:1 | B-100, C-II, E |
| IDL | 1.006–1.019 | 25–35 | 1:1 | B-100, E |
| LDL | 1.019–1.063 | 18–25 | 1:7 | B-100, E |
| HDL | 1.063–1.210 | 5–12 | 1:4 | A, C, D, E |
| Lp(a) | 1.040–1.090 | 25–30 | 1:7 | B-100, apo[a] |

VLDL = very low-density lipoprotein
HDL = high-density lipoproteins; IDL = intermediate-density lipoproteins; LDL = low-density lipoproteins; Lp(a) = lipoprotein (a).

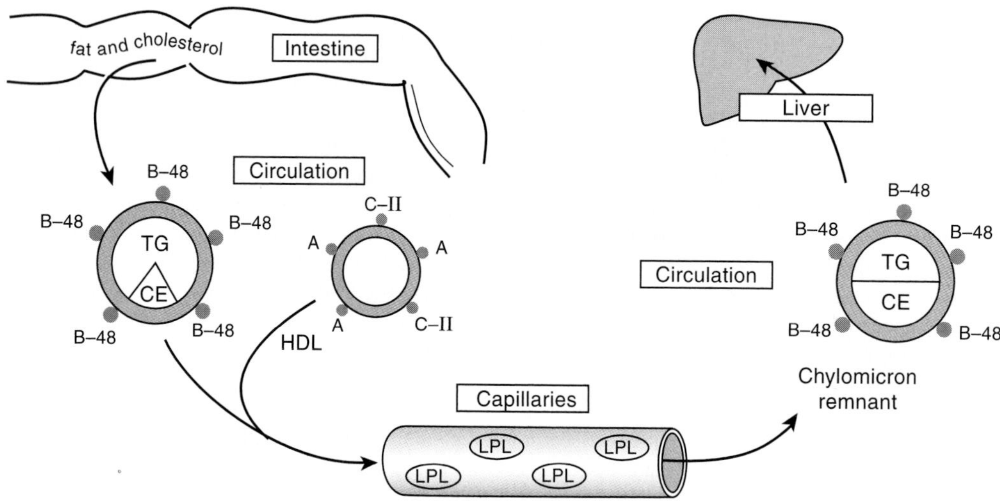


**FIGURE 74.1.** Absorption of dietary fat and its assembly into chylomicrons.

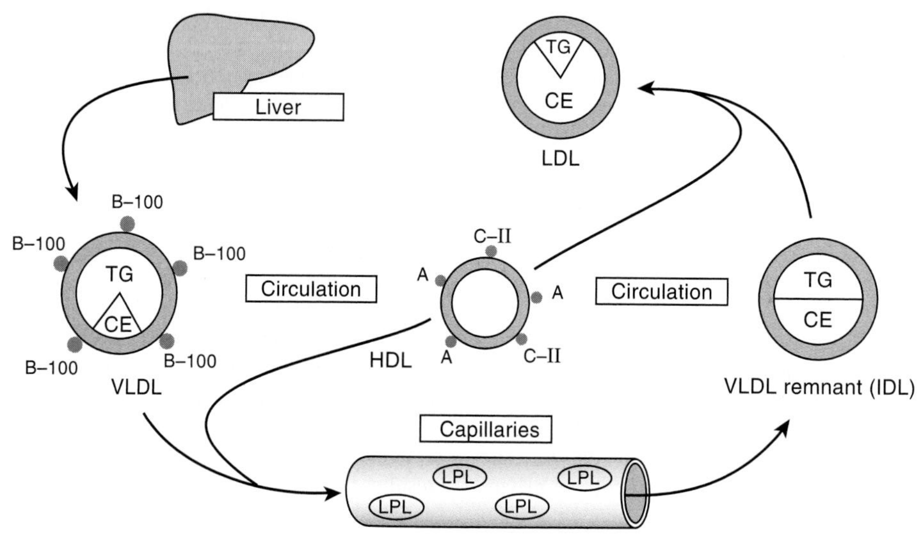


**FIGURE 74.2.** Formation of very-low-density lipoproteins (VLDL).

Hyperlipidemias originally were classified according to the profile of lipoprotein particles analyzed by electrophoresis or density ultracentrifugation. Thus, syndrome categories were based on which combination of chylomicrons, VLDL, LDL, and remnant particles (IDL) was present (Table 74.2). It is now recognized that each syndrome category includes multiple genetic syndromes and that a patient with a single defined genetic syndrome can be moved between categories by diet and other secondary factors. Therefore, it is more useful to consider hyperlipidemias according to their primary genetic disorder, as discussed below.

## Chylomicronemia Syndrome

The clearance of chylomicrons is defective in chylomicronemia syndrome, leading to a marked rise in fasting plasma triglycerides above 1000 mg/dl and sometimes as high as 10,000–20,000 mg/dl. Mild elevations usually cause no symptoms, but higher levels increase the chances of evoking one or more symptoms of the chylomicronemia syndrome (e.g., recurrent pancreatitis, eruptive xanthomas, lipemia retinalis, dyspnea, and changes in mentation). The xanthomas, which are nontender, yellowish papules, typically occur on the buttocks, elbows, and knees. They can resolve slowly as the triglyceride level is lowered. Accelerated atherosclerosis is absent.

Chylomicronemia is found either as a primary, full-blown, familial disorder or resulting from secondary factors superimposed on a milder, genetic predisposition to hypertriglyceridemia. The secondary disorders are more common (Table 74.3). Treatment of the disorder successfully lowers triglyceride levels in most patients, but some hypertriglyceridemia generally persists.

## Hypercholesterolemia

### Familial Hypercholesterolemia

Familial hypercholesterolemia results from defects in the gene coding for the plasma membrane receptor for LDL. Patients with one defective gene have heterozygous familial hypercholesterolemia and possess half the number of normal, functional LDL receptors. LDL is approximately twice normal, and total serum cholesterol varies from 300–600 mg/dl. Heterozygous familial hypercholesterolemia, which afflicts 1 in 500 persons, is associated with markedly accelerated atherosclerosis; most patients manifest clinically apparent coronary artery disease by age 40—many, by age 20. Tendon xanthomas, usually noted on the Achilles tendon and the extensor tendon of the hands and forearms, are virtually diagnostic. Tuberous xanthomas occur over extensor surfaces of elbows, knees, and hands. Premature arcus senilis (an opaque ring) is noted in the eyes at the corneal periphery. In homozygous familial hypercholesterolemia, LDL receptors are absent because both alleles encoding for the LDL receptor are defective; serum cholesterol is typically 600–1200 mg/dl. Aggressive atherosclerosis is apparent by early childhood. Response to medical therapy is poor, but extracorporeal LDL apheresis or plasma exchange may be partially effective. Portocaval anastomosis and liver transplantation are potential surgical approaches.

**TABLE 74.2. Classification of Lipoprotein Profiles in Hyperlipidemia**

| Type of Hyperlipidemia | Lipoprotein Elevated | Cholesterol Level | Triglyceride Level |
|---|---|---|---|
| Type 1 | Chylomicrons | ↑ | ↑↑↑ |
| Type 2a | LDL | ↑↑↑ | ↔ |
| Type 2b | LDL + VLDL | ↑↑ | ↔ or ↑ |
| Type 3 | Chylomicron + VLDL remnants | ↑↑ | ↑↑ |
| Type 4 | VLDL | ↔ or ↑ | ↑↑ |
| Type 5 | VLDL + chylomicrons | ↑ | ↑↑↑ |

↑ mild elevation
↑↑ moderate elevation
↑↑↑ marked elevation
↔ normal

**TABLE 74.3. Causes of Secondary Hypertriglyceridemia**

Diabetes mellitus
Obesity
Alcohol
Nephrotic syndrome
Uremia
Dysglobulinemia
Estrogens
Glucocorticoid excess
Systemic lupus erythematosus

### Polygenic Hypercholesterolemia

Patients with polygenic hypercholesterolemia have a mixture of genetic and environmental factors, leading to hypercholesterolemia of 200 to 350 mg/dl. Triglyceride levels generally are normal or modestly increased. Inheritance is not clearly autosomal dominant as in familial heterozygous hypercholesterolemia. Nonetheless, premature atherosclerosis often is present in first-degree relatives; significant hypercholesterolemia is noted in some first-degree relatives on screening.

### Treatment of Hypercholesterolemia

**Goals**

Goals for treating hypercholesterolemia are based on recommendations by the National Cholesterol Education Program Adult Treatment Panel (NCEP ATP III). The LDL cholesterol targets differ, depending on the presence of pre-existing coronary atherosclerosis, coronary heart disease risk equivalents and the number of other risk factors for it (Tables 74.4 and 74.5). The positive benefits of lowering cholesterol on reducing myocardial infarctions is well established. Secondary causes of hypercholesterolemia (hypothyroidism, nephrotic syndrome, acute intermittent porphyria, glucocorticoid excess, and dysglobulinemia) should be excluded in all patients with hypercholesterolemia. LDL cholesterol usually is not measured directly, but is calculated after quantitating triglycerides, total cholesterol, and HDL-cholesterol. The following formula is used to calculate LDL-cholesterol, provided fasting triglyceride levels are less than 400 mg/dl:

LDL cholesterol =
total cholesterol – (HDL cholesterol + triglycerides/5)

**TABLE 74.4. Target Levels for LDL Cholesterol**

| Risk Category | LDL Goal (mg/dL) | LDL Level at Which to Initiate Therapeutic Lifestyle Changes (mg/dL) | LDL Level at Which to Consider Drug Therapy (mg/dL) |
|---|---|---|---|
| CHD or CHD risk equivalents (10-year risk >20%) | <100 | ≥100 | ≥130 (100–129: drug optional)† |
| 2+ Risk factors (10-year risk ≤20%) | <130 | ≥130 | 10-year risk 10%–20%: ≥130<br>10-year risk <10%: ≥160 |
| 0–1 Risk factor‡ | <160 | ≥160 | ≥190 (160–189: LDL-lowering drug optional) |

*LDL indicates low-density lipoprotein: CHD, coronary heart disease.
†Some authorities recommend use of LDL-lowering drugs in this category if an LDL cholesterol level of <100 mg/dL cannot be achieved by therapeutic lifestyle changes. Others prefer use of drugs that primarily modify triglycerides and HDL, eg. nicotinic acid or fibrate. Clinical judgment also may call for deferring drug therapy in this subcategory.
‡Almost all people with 0–1 risk factor have a 10-year risk <10%; thus, 10-year risk assessment in people with 0–1 risk factor is not necessary.

**TABLE 74.5. Major Risk Factors for Coronary Heart Disease (CHD) That Modify LDL Goals**

Cigarette smoking
Hypertension (BP ≥ 140/90 mm Hg or on antihypertensive medication)
Low HDL cholesterol (<40 mg/dL)*
Familial history of premature CHD (CHD in male first degree relative ≤55 years; CHD in female first degree relative ≤65 years)
Age
Men ≥ 45 years
Women ≥ 55 years

*HDL cholesterol ≥ 60 mg/dl is considered a "negative" risk factor.
In NCEP ATP III, diabetes is regarded as a CHD risk equivalent.

**TABLE 74.6. Summary of Lipid-Lowering Drugs**

| | LDL-C | VLDL-TG | HDL-C | Side Effects |
|---|---|---|---|---|
| Bile acid resins | ↓ | ↑ | ↔ | Dyspepsia, constipation, proctitis |
| Fibric acids | ↑ or ↓ | ↓↓ | ↑ | Gallstones |
| HMG CoA-reductase Inhibitor | ↓↓ | ↓ or ↑ | ↑ | Myositis, abnormal LFTs |
| Nicotinic acid | ↓ | ↓ | ↑ | Glucose intolerance, abnormal LFTs, flushing, pruritus |
| Probucol | ↓ | ↔ | ↓ | Decreased HDL |

HDL-C = high-density lipoprotein–cholesterol; HMG CoA = 3-hydroxy-3-methylglutaryl coenzyme A; LDL-C = low-density lipoprotein–cholesterol; LFT = liver function tests; VLDL-TG = very-low-density lipoprotein–triglycerides.
↓ mild reduction
↓↓ moderate reduction
↔ no effect
↑ increase

### Diet

Many patients with mildly elevated LDL cholesterol are treated with diet therapy alone. The initial Step 1 NCEP diet contains less than 300 mg/day of cholesterol and 30% or less of total fat calories. Saturated fats are restricted to 10% of total daily calories, and most dietary triglycerides are polyunsaturated. The Step 2 NCEP diet is more restrictive; it contains less than 200 mg per day of cholesterol and 7% or less saturated fats. Because diet alone will usually reduce LDL cholesterol by no more than 25%, significant hypercholesterolemia requires drug therapy along with a continued Step 2 NCEP diet.

### Drug therapy

Table 74.6 shows the drugs used to treat cholesterol problems. The major drugs for lowering LDL cholesterol are bile acid resins, HMG CoA-reductase inhibitors, and nicotinic acid. Bile acid resins (cholestyramine and colestipol) bind bile acids in the intestine, preventing their reabsorption. Plasma LDL cholesterol is lowered as hepatic cholesterol is diverted to increased bile acid synthesis. Given in high doses (20 g/d), bile acid resins will reduce LDL cholesterol by approximately 20%. Long-term compliance is limited by gastrointestinal side effects. The HMG CoA-reductase inhibitors (lovastatin, pravastatin, simvastatin, atorvastatin, and fluvastatin) inhibit the rate-limiting enzyme for cholesterol synthesis in the liver. These agents usually are well tolerated and are the most potent LDL cholesterol–lowering agents, typically reducing LDL cholesterol by approximately one third. Nicotinic acid successfully lowers LDL cholesterol by approximately 25% in most patients. As with the bile acid resins, significant side effects impair long-term compliance. The most bothersome side effects—flushing and pruritus—can be partially blunted with aspirin and by starting with low doses (100 mg t.i.d.). Given in the short-acting crystalline form, in 2 to 3 divided doses, the total dose is gradually increased to 2 to 3 g/day. A controlled release preparation of nicotinic acid is also available and administered at bedtime.

Secondary drugs used to treat hypercholesterolemia are fibric acids and probucol. Fibric acid derivatives more effectively treat hypertriglyceridemia, but they will lower LDL cholesterol in a subset of patients. Probucol typically reduces LDL cholesterol by 10% to 20%, but it also lowers HDL levels.

## Lipid Disorders

### Familial Dysbetalipoproteinemia

Clearance of both chylomicron and VLDL remnants is defective in familial dysbetalipoproteinemia, causing remnant particles to accumulate. Cholesterol and triglycerides are symmetrically elevated to 300 to 450 mg/dl. Premature coronary artery disease occurs, and the clinical phenotype is characterized by plantar xanthomas.

### Familial Combined Hyperlipidemia

Familial combined hyperlipidemia is the most common disorder in patients with premature coronary artery disease. It is characterized by variable increases in both LDL and VLDL levels. Depending on diet, exercise, and the presence of secondary aggravating factors, patients may have elevated triglyceride levels, elevated cholesterol levels, or both. Decreased HDL levels are common. In this polygenic disorder, many genetic causes are likely.

### Treatment of Familial Combined Hyperlipidemia and Diabetic Dyslipidemia

#### Goals

Treatment goals in familial combined hyperlipidemia and diabetic dyslipidemia and diabetes include management of the patient's underlying diabetes or secondary causes of hyperlipidemia, diet and drug therapy. The typical lipid profile of such individuals is a low HDL cholesterol with elevated levels of LDL cholesterol and triglycerides.

#### Diet

Dietary recommendations are similar to those for patients with hypercholesterolemia and hypertriglyceridemia.

#### Drug therapy

An ideal drug for lowering LDL and triglycerides is niacin. This medication is relatively contraindicated in diabetic individuals. When triglyceride levels are only mildly elevated, HMG CoA-reductase inhibitors often are the treatment of choice. When concurrent moderate elevations of LDL cholesterol and triglycerides coexist, one can consider combination therapy with a fibric acid derivative and an HMG CoA reductase inhibitor. This combination must be used with caution because of the potential risk of severe muscle toxicity. If a combination is to be used, the least lipophilic HMG CoA reductase inhibitors (e.g., fluvastatin and pravastatin) should be combined with the least lipophilic fibric acid (fenofibrate). Fibric acids should be administered in the morning and the HMG CoA reductase inhibitor at night to separate the peak blood levels of the two drugs.

## Hypertriglyceridemia

### Primary Hypertriglyceridemia

Primary hypertriglyceridemia is characterized by elevated triglycerides in the range of 200–500 mg/dl. Plasma VLDL is elevated. The underlying genetic defects are heterogeneous and are related to either overproduction or defective clearance of VLDL. The presence of secondary factors (such as diabetes, obesity and alcohol) can markedly increase triglycerides in this disorder. In primary hypertriglyceridemia, plasma HDL levels are often low. In some families, premature atherosclerosis is present.

### Treatment of Hypertriglyceridemia

#### Goals

Treatment goals in hypertriglyceridemia are twofold, depending on the triglyceride level. In patients with the chylomicronemic syndrome and triglyceride levels above 1000 mg/dl, the goal is to reduce those levels below 1000 mg/dl in order to prevent immediate complications (such as recurrent pancreatitis and eruptive xanthomas). In patients with a more modest hypertriglyceridemia, there is an increased association with coronary heart disease (due largely to the relationship of hypertriglyceridemia with low HDL levels). In these patients, the goal is to lower triglyceride levels to as close to normal as possible, thus reciprocally raising HDL and reducing long-term risk for coronary heart disease.

#### Diet

Because the triglycerides within chylomicrons originate from dietary fat, diet is the only effective therapy for patients with the chylomicronemic syndrome. Dietary fat is restricted to 20% or less of total daily calories and, if need be, to 10%. It is essential to identify and correct causes of secondary hypertriglyceridemia (see Table 74.3). There are no drugs that effectively promote chylomicron metabolism. Milder hypertriglyceridemia resulting from VLDL is often associated with hypercholesterolemia as well. Dietary management follows the NCEP step 1 and 2 diets described above, duly modified as needed to lower the fat below 30%.

#### Drug therapy

The major drugs for reducing triglyceride levels are the fibric acids and nicotinic acid. The fibric acids gemfibrozil and clofibrate decrease the production of VLDL triglyceride and also enhance VLDL clearance by increasing lipoprotein lipase activity. Gemfibrozil is given at a dosage of 600 mg once or twice daily. Fenofibrate is given at 67 mg to 200 mg per day. Fibric acids are generally well tolerated, despite an increased incidence of gallstones. Nicotinic acid also reduces triglyceride levels. Its use in hypertriglyceridemia is somewhat limited due to its side effects and the high incidence of glucose intolerance and overt diabetes present in the hypertriglyceridemic population.

### Treatment of Low HDL Cholesterol

Low HDL cholesterol levels often are associated with elevated triglyceride levels, and treatment is similar to that for patients with familial hypertriglyceridemia. However, many patients have isolated low HDL cholesterol with relatively normal triglycerides. In these cases, treatment decisions are based on the other risk factors for heart disease and patient preference.

#### Nonpharmacologic approaches

Smoking cessation usually is associated with an increase in HDL. Weight loss can result in a significant increase in HDL cholesterol. Reduction in dietary fat, when associated with weight reduction, can raise HDL cholesterol but alone it may actually lower HDL. Exercise alone has a limited effect on HDL cholesterol, but when combined with weight reduction it can have a beneficial effect. Estrogen replacement, when given orally, can increase HDL cholesterol. Finally, although it raises HDL cholesterol levels, alcohol is not recommended as an HDL-raising tool.

#### Drug therapy

In patients with moderate hypertriglyceridemia and low HDL cholesterol, fibric acids are the treatment of choice. However, HDL cholesterol often remains low even after triglycerides are lowered.

In patients with relatively normal triglyceride levels, HMG Co-A reductase inhibitors, fibric acids, and niacin are considered. HMG CoA-reductase inhibitors raise HDL cholesterol moderately (5-10%). Fibric acids are not particularly effective if triglycerides levels are relatively normal. Niacin is the most effective HDL-raising medication available at this time (25-40% increases possible).

## Questions

**Questions 1–2:** You are asked to see a 64-year-old gentleman for an elevated TSH level of 12 μIU/ml. Clinically, the patient complains of recent onset of palpitations, heat intolerance, weight loss, and tremors. Significant findings on physical examination include a pulse of 112, his skin is slightly diaphoretic, his thyroid is mildly and diffusely enlarged, and he has a fine tremor of bilateral outstretched extremities.

1. What additional laboratory tests would you order on this gentleman?
   A. Free T4
   B. Prolactin
   C. Thyroid antibodies
   D. Testosterone
   E. None of the above

2. His free T4 comes back mildly elevated. His thyroid antibodies are negative and his alpha subunit is four times the upper end of normal. What is the cause of this patient's abnormal thyroid function tests?
   A. Transient thyroiditis
   B. Grave's hyperthyroidism
   C. Hashimoto's hypothyroidism
   D. Toxic multinodular goiter
   E. TSH-secreting pituitary adenoma

3. A 42-year-old diabetic woman has secondary amenorrhea. She takes insulin and metoclopramide. Her serum prolactin is 85 ng/ml (normal <20 ng/ml). If pregnancy is excluded, what is the most likely cause of her hyperprolactinemia?
   A. Prolactin-secreting pituitary tumor
   B. Metoclopramide
   C. Chronic renal failure
   D. Insulin

**Questions 4–5:** You are asked to see a 78-year-old gentleman with a history of small cell carcinoma of the lung and emphysema for mild hyponatremia. During one of his routine follow-up visits, a basic chemistry panel was obtained and his serum sodium was noted to be slightly low at 129 mEq/L (normal 135–145 mEq/L). He seems to be euvolemic clinically, his mental status is normal, and his urine sodium is mildly elevated.

4. What is the most likely cause of this patient's hyponatremia?
   A. Central diabetes insipidus
   B. Psychogenic polydipsia
   C. Nephrogenic diabetes insipidus
   D. Adrenal insufficiency
   E. Syndrome of inappropriate ADH

5. What is the most reasonable initial treatment for this patient's hyponatremia?
   A. Fluid restriction
   B. Hypertonic saline infusion
   C. Salt tablets
   D. DDAVP replacement
   E. High doses of glucocorticoids

**Questions 6–8:** A 37-year-old woman reports increased anxiety, tremulousness, diarrhea, palpitations, and heat intolerance over the last six months. Her appetite is reportedly "too good." She is on no medications. Her pulse is 120/min and BP, 122/76 mm Hg. She is thin and anxious, with warm and extremely moist skin; proptosis is noted; extraocular muscle movements are normal. The thyroid gland is firm and diffusely enlarged with a bruit; fine tremor of distal upper extremities and a shortened relaxation phase of her deep tendon reflexes are noted.

6. What is the most likely cause of this woman's signs and symptoms?
   A. Graves' hyperthyroidism
   B. Toxic solitary nodule
   C. Iodine-induced hyperthyroidism
   D. TSH-secreting pituitary adenoma

7. If you were to order a 24-hour radioactive iodine uptake (RAIU) in this patient, which of the following results would you expect?
   A. Normal
   B. Decreased
   C. Increased
   D. Nondetectable

8. The patient is placed on propranolol and propylthiouracil. One month later she develops a sore throat and fever of 103°F. What test should be obtained?
   A. Throat culture
   B. Chest x-ray
   C. TSH
   D. WBC count

9. Possible therapeutic agents used to treat thyroid storm include which of the following?
   A. Propranolol
   B. Propylthiouracil
   C. Dexamethasone
   D. All of the above

10. Production of PTH-related protein is most commonly associated with which of the following?
    A. Lymphoma
    B. Melanoma
    C. Colon cancer
    D. Squamous cell carcinoma of lung

11. Conditions that predispose patients to develop vitamin D deficiency include:
    A. Renal failure
    B. Malabsorption (steatorrhea)
    C. Being house-bound
    D. All of the above

12. Conditions associated with osteoporosis include which of the following?
    A. Cushing's syndrome
    B. Thyrotoxicosis
    C. Postmenopausal
    D. All of the above

13. A 63-year-old man presents with alcoholic cirrhosis and seizure disorder to the Emergency Department for evaluation after a fall on the ice. Examination shows severe mid-thoracic spinal pain and tenderness; thoracic spine x-rays confirm a T10 compression fracture and show generalized osteopenia. Labs show mild hypocalcemia and hypophosphatemia, with a normal albumin. The most likely cause of this patient's pathologic fracture is:
    A. Senile osteoporosis
    B. Metastatic prostate cancer
    C. Osteomalacia
    D. Hyperparathyroidism

14. During the past 6 months, a 47-year-old man has noted fatigue, 20-lb weight gain, proximal muscle weakness, and ankle swelling. His BP is mildly elevated. You note plethoric facies, truncal obesity, abdominal striae, and supraclavicular fullness. Which of the following tests would you now order?
    A. CT scan of the adrenals
    B. MRI of the pituitary gland
    C. Overnight 1-mg dexamethasone suppression test
    D. Random serum cortisol and ACTH levels2

15. A 65-year-old woman with a history of severe COPD presents to the Emergency Department with a one week history of nausea, vomiting, weakness, and an episode of syncope. She is found to have severe orthostatic hypotension and labs reveal serum sodium of 126 mEq/dl, potassium of 5.9 mEq/dl, and

a WBC count of 11,500 with 60% lymphs, 30% neutrophils, and 3% bands. Immediate evaluation and management should include:

A. Plasma osmolality and urine sodium; fluid restriction
B. Aldosterone and renin levels; fluid resuscitation
C. Cosyntropin stimulation test; fluid resuscitation and fludrocortisone
D. Cosyntropin stimulation test; fluid resuscitation and IV dexamethasone

16. In a patient with hypertension and paroxysms of diaphoresis, palpitations, and headache, which of the following is the best initial test to perform?
A. CT scan of the adrenal glands
B. Measurement of urinary catecholamines and metanephrine levels in 24-hour collection
C. Measurement of plasma renin activity and plasma aldosterone concentration
D. Measurement of plasma catecholamines

17. A 24-year-old female medical student presents with the chief complaints of hirsutism and irregular periods. Her menarche occurred at age 13, and her menstrual cycles have been irregular ever since. She has been going to an electrologist for facial hair removal on her chin and upper lip. She is otherwise healthy. Her ethnic background is English. On physical examination, she is 65 inches tall and weighs 145 pounds. She has evidence of acne on her face and coarse hairs on her chin and upper lip. The remainder of her examination, including a gynecologic examination, is normal. What is the most likely diagnosis in this young woman?
A. Ovarian androgen-secreting tumor
B. Polycystic ovary syndrome
C. Stress-induced amenorrhea
D. Late-onset congenital adrenal hyperplasia

18. A 29-year-old woman notes progressive acne, weight gain, and increasing hair growth on the face, chest, and shoulders for one year. A physical examination confirms these. The plasma testosterone level is 396 ng/dl. Which of the following is the most likely diagnosis?
A. Ovarian tumor
B. Adrenal tumor
C. 21-hydroxylase deficiency
D. Polycystic ovarian disease

19. A 46-year-old man presents to his doctor's office to discuss his impotence. He is in a stable relationship and has no significant stresses in his life. He has noted the gradual loss of interest in sex and attributed it to age and to a diagnosis of hypertension in the past two years with the initiation of beta-blocker therapy. He admits to periodic headaches and generally has noted a lack of energy. He needs to shave less frequently. On physical examination, his blood pressure is 125/70 and his pulse rate is 60/minute. His thyroid gland is normal and his testes are normal in size but slightly soft. What is your next step with this patient?
A. Change the patient's blood pressure medication and have him return to your office in 4 weeks.
B. Prescribe sildenafil (Viagra®).
C. Refer the patient for stress management.
D. Measure total testosterone, and if low, measure prolactin, FSH, and LH.

20. A 19-year-old man with a history of type 1 diabetes mellitus since age 12 presents to the Emergency Department with a 24-hour history of nausea, vomiting, and abdominal pain. Several members of his family have had the flu. Because he has not been able to eat or drink, he has not taken his scheduled insulin dose for the past 12 hours for fear of hypoglycemia. In the Emergency Department, he has a blood pressure of 85/50 and a pulse rate of 120 beats per minute. His oral mucosa is dry and his breath smells fruity. Laboratory studies reveal a blood sugar of 450 mg/dl, serum potassium of 5.0, and an anion gap of 25. An arterial blood gas shows a pH of 7.12. Which of the following statements is (are) true?
A. In spite of his high normal serum potassium level, this patient has total body potassium depletion, and will need supplemental potassium as treatment with fluids and insulin is initiated.
B. The preferred route of administration of insulin in DKA is by continuous infusion of regular insulin.
C. This patient may need as much as 6 to 10 liters of intravenous fluids to correct his fluid deficit.
D. All of the above.

21. A 25-year-old woman with type 1 diabetes mellitus since age 7 presents for a routine follow-up visit. She monitors her blood sugars 4 times per day and follows an insulin regimen that consists of NPH 15 units/lispro 5 units before breakfast and supper. She has noted several hypoglycemic reactions at 2AM, which have awakened her from sleep. She is 10 pounds overweight and would like to lose this weight in the next few months by diet and exercise. A hemoglobin A1c is 7.1%. What would you advise this patient to do?
A. Reduce her presupper NPH dose of insulin to 12 units.
B. Continue her lispro dose at supper and move her NPH dose to bedtime.
C. Have her double her current bedtime snack.
D. Decrease her morning NPH dose to 12 units.

22. A 45-year-old woman presents for evaluation. She is 66 inches tall and weighs 315 pounds. She has been obese since childhood, and multiple family members including her parents and siblings are overweight. Her family history is also positive for type 2 diabetes. She is becoming less and less active due to significant bilateral knee pain with ambulation. On physical examination, her blood pressure is 150/95. Her heart sounds are distant. She has dependent edema of the lower extremities. Which of the following statements is true regarding this patient's obesity?
    A. Due to her obesity, she is at higher risk for developing breast cancer and endometrial cancer.
    B. This patient is at risk for cholelithiasis.
    C. A lipid panel would likely reveal elevated levels of total cholesterol and triglycerides, and reduced HDL cholesterol.
    D. All of the above.

23. A 46-year-old woman presents for her first general physical examination since the birth of her last child 12 years ago. Her family history is positive for type 2 diabetes and hypertension. She had gestational diabetes with her last pregnancy. On physical examination, she is 66 inches tall and weighs 170 pounds. Her blood pressure is 158/90. She has central obesity. Her physical examination is otherwise unremarkable. Laboratory studies reveal a fasting plasma glucose level of 166 mg/dl, a hemoglobin A1c of 8.5%, and the following lipid profile:

| Total cholesterol | 223 |
|---|---|
| HDL cholesterol | 34 |
| LDL cholesterol | 128 |
| Triglycerides | 305 |

    Which of the following statements is correct?
    A. Based on NCEP ATP III (National Cholesterol Education Program Adult Treatment Panel) guidelines, diabetes is considered a coronary heart disease 'risk equivalent.'
    B. The approach to this patient should address her obesity, diabetes, hypertension, and hyperlipidemia, and should include dietary counseling, weight management, and increased physical activity.
    C. Based on NCEP ATP III guidelines, this patient's LDL cholesterol goal is less than 100 mg/dl.
    D. All of the above.

24. A 55-year-old woman presents to her gynecologist's office to discuss hormone replacement therapy. Her last menses was one year ago. She has minimal menopausal symptoms and no family history of osteoporosis. She was diagnosed with type 2 diabetes one year ago, which is well controlled on metformin. Which of the following statements regarding estrogen, lipids, and cardiovascular disease is true?
    A. Hormone replacement therapy (HRT) is indicated for both primary and secondary prevention of coronary heart disease (CHD) in women.
    B. Estrogen may increase this patient's mildly elevated triglyceride levels.
    C. HRT is typically associated with a decrease in HDL cholesterol levels.
    D. Based on NCEP ATP III guidelines, age >60 year in a woman is considered a major risk factor for CHD.

## Answers

| | | | | |
|---|---|---|---|---|
| 1. A | 2. E | 3. B | 4. E | 5. A |
| 6. A | 7. C | 8. D | 9. D | 10. D |
| 11. D | 12. D | 13. C | 14. C | 15. D |
| 16. B | 17. B | 18. A | 19. D | 20. D |
| 21. B | 22. D | 23. D | 24. B | |

## SUGGESTED READING


### *Textbooks and Monographs*

Becker KL (ed.) Principles and Practice of Endocrinology and Metabolism. 3rd ed. Philadelphia: Lippincott Williams & Wilkins, 2001.

Felig P, Frohman LA (eds). Endocrinology and Metabolism. 4th ed. New York: McGraw-Hill, 2001.

Wilson JD, Foster DW, Kronenberg HM, Larsen PR (eds.). Williams Textbook of Endocrinology. 9th ed. Philadelphia: WB Saunders Company, 1998.

### *Articles*

*Disorders of the Anterior Pituitary*

Klibanski A, Zervas NT. Diagnosis and management of hormone-secreting pituitary adenomas. N Engl J Med 1991; 324:822–831.

Melmed S. Acromegaly. N Engl J Med 1990;322:966–977.

Molitch ME. Gonadotroph-cell pituitary adenomas. N Engl J Med 1991;324:626–627.

Sarapura V, Schlaff WD. Recent advances in the understanding of the pathophysiology and treatment of hyperprolactinemia. Curr Sci 1993;5:360–367.

Snyder PJ. Clinically nonfunctioning pituitary adenomas. Endocrinol Metab Clin North Am 1993;22:163–175.

Vance ML. Hypopituitarism. N Engl J Med 1994;330:1651–1662.

*Disorders of the Posterior Pituitary*

DeFronzo RA, Thier SO. Pathophysiologic approach to hyponatremia. Arch Intern Med 1980;140:897–902.

Fraser CL, Arieff AI. Epidemiology, pathophysiology, and management of hyponatremic encephalopathy. Am J Med 1997;102:67–77.

Robertson GL. Physiology of ADH secretion. Kidney Int 1987;32:S20–S26.

Singer I, Oster JR, Fishman LM. The management of diabetes insipidus in adults. Arch Intern Med 1997;157:1293–1301.

Verbalis JG. Hyponatremia: endocrinologic causes and consequences of therapy. Topics in Endocrinology and Metabolism 1992;3:1–7.

*Thyroid Diseases*

Braverman LE, Utiger RD (eds). Werner & Ingbar's The Thyroid. 8th ed. Philadelphia: Lippincott Williams & Wilkins, 2000.

Cooper DS. Subclinical hypothyroidism. N Engl J Med 2001; 345:260–265.

Dayan CM, Daniels GH. Chronic autoimmune thyroiditis. N Engl J Med 1996; 335:99–106.

Magner JA. TSH-mediated hyperthyroidism. Endocrinologist 1993;3:289–296.

McDougal IR. Graves' disease: current concepts. Med Clin North Am 1991;75:79.

Ridgway EC. Clinician's evaluation of a solitary thyroid nodule. J Clin Endocrinol Metab 1992;74:231.

Weetman AR. Graves' disease. N Engl J Med 2000;343:1236–1248.

*Disorders of Parathyroid Glands, Vitamin D Metabolism, and Calcium Homeostasis*

Bilezikian JP. Management of acute hypercalcemia. N Engl J Med 1992;326:1196–1203.

Marx SJ. Hyperparathyroidism and hypoparathyroid disorders. N Engl J Med 2000;343:1863–1874.

Potts JT Jr. Management of asymptomatic hyperparathyroidism. J Clin Endocrinol Metab 1990;70:1489–1493.

Silverberg SJ, Bilezikian JP, Bone HG, et al. Therapeutic controversies in primary hyperparathyroidism. J Clin Endocrinol Metab 1999; 84:2275–2285.

*Metabolic Bone Disease*

Black DM, Thompson DE, Bauer DC, et al. Fracture risk reduction with alendronate in women with osteoporosis: the fracture intervention trial. J Clin Endocrinol Metab 2000; 85:4118–4124.

Eastell R. Treatment of postmenopausal osteoporosis. N Engl J Med 1998; 338:736–746.

Orwoll C. Assessing bone density in men. J Bone Miner Res 2000;15:1867–1870.

Proceedings of the third international symposium on Paget's Disease. J Bone Miner Res 1999; 14:S1–S104.

Riggs BL, Melton LJ III. The prevention and treatment of osteoporosis. N Engl J Med 1992;327:620–627.

*Diseases of the Adrenal Cortex*

Maas DL, Kochar MS. Primary aldosteronism. In Rakel RE (ed). Conn's Current Therapy. Philadelphia: WB Saunders, 1995.

Aron DC, Findling JW, Tyrrell JB. Cushing's disease. Endocrinol Metab Clin 1987;16:705–730.

Chodosh LA, Daniels GH. Addison's disease. Endocrinologist 1993;3:166–181.

Gill JR Jr. Primary hyperaldosteronism: strategies for diagnosis and treatment. Endocrinologist 1991;1:365–369.

Kloss RT, Gross MD, Francis JR. Incidentally discovered adrenal masses. Endocrinol Rev 1995;16:460–484.

*Diseases of the Adrenal Medulla*

Pacak K, Linehan WM, Eisenhofer G, et al. Recent advances in genetics, diagnosis localization, and treatment of pheochromocytoma. Ann Inter Med 2001;134:315–329.

Werbel SS, Ober KP. Pheochromocytoma. Update on diagnosis, localization, and management. Med Clin North Am 1995;79: 131–153.

*Disorders of Ovarian Function*

Azziz R, Carmina E, Sawaya ME. Idiopathic hirsutism. Endocrine Rev 2000;21:347–362.

Barnes R, Rosenfield RL. The polycystic ovary syndrome: pathogenesis and treatment. Ann Intern Med 1989;110: 386–399.

Franks S. Polycystic ovarian syndrome. N Engl J Med 1995; 333:853–861.

Grady D, Herrington D, Bittner V, et al. Cardiovascular disease outcomes during 6.8 years of hormone therapy: heart and estrogen/progestin replacement study follow-up (HERSII) JAMA 2002;288:49–57.

McDonough PG. Amenorrhea—an etiology approach to diagnosis. Fertil Steril 1978;30:1.

Rittmaster RS, Loriaux DL. Hirsutism. Ann Intern Med 1987;106:95–107.

*Disorders of Testicular Function*

Braunstein GD. Gynecomastia. N Engl J Med 1993;328: 490–495.

Krane RJ, Goldstein I, Saenz De Tejada. Impotence. N Engl J Med 1989;321:1648–1656.

*Hypoglycemia and Diabetes Mellitus*

Davidson MB. Clinical implications of insulin resistance syndromes. Am J Med 1995;99:420–426.

Gerich JE, Mokan M, Veneman T, et al. Hypoglycemia unawareness. Endocr Rev 1991;12:356–371.

Gearhart JG, Forbes RC. Initial management of the patient with newly diagnosed diabetes. Am Fam Phys 1995;51:1953–1962, 1966–1968.

Jaspan JB. Taking control of diabetes. Hosp Pract (Office Edition) 1995;30:55–62.

Konen JC, Shihabi ZK. Microalbuminuria and diabetes mellitus. Am Fam Phys 1993;48:1421–1428.

Laine C, Caro JF. Preventing complications in diabetes mellitus: the role of the primary care physician. Med Clin North Am 1996;80:457–474.

Raskin P, Arauz-Pacheco C. The treatment of diabetic retinopathy: a view for the internist. Ann Intern Med 1992;117: 226–233.

Service FJ. Hypoglycemic disorders. N Engl J Med 1995; 332:1144–1152.

Umpierrez GE, Khajavi M, Kitabchi AE. Review: diabetic ketoacidosis and hyperglycemic hyperosmolar nonketotic syndrome. Am J Med Sci 1996;311:225–233.

Valdovinos MA, Camilleri M, Zimmerman BR. Chronic diarrhea in diabetes mellitus: mechanisms and an approach to diagnosis and treatment. Mayo Clin Proc 1993;68:691–702.

*Nutritional Disorders*

Barrocas A, Belcher D, Champagne C, et al. Nutrition assessment: Practical approaches. Clin Geriatr Med 1995;11: 675–713.

Ham RJ. The signs and symptoms of poor nutritional status. Prim Care 1994;21:33–54.

Lipkin EW, Bell S. Assessment of nutritional status. The clinician's perspective. Clin Lab Med 1993;13:329–352.

Manning EM, Shenkin A. Nutritional assessment in the critically ill. Crit Care Clin 1995;11:603–634.

McMahon MM, Rizza RA. Nutrition support in hospitalized patients with diabetes mellitus. Mayo Clin Proc 1996;71: 587–594.

Reife CM. Involuntary weight loss. Med Clin North Am 1995;79:299–313.

*Disorders of Lipid Metabolism*

Jialal I. A practical approach to the laboratory diagnosis of dyslipidemia. Am J Clin Pathol 1996;106:128–138.

Knopp RH. Drug treatment of lipid disorders. N Engl J Med 1999; 341:498–511.

Rosenson RS, Frauenheim WA, Tangney CC. Dyslipidemias and the secondary prevention of coronary heart disease. Dis Mon 1994;40:369–464.

Executive Summary of the Third Report of the National Cholesterol Education Program (NCEP) Expert Panel on Detection, Evaluation and Treatment of High Blood Cholesterol in Adults (Adult Treatment Panel III). JAMA 2001;285: 2486–97.

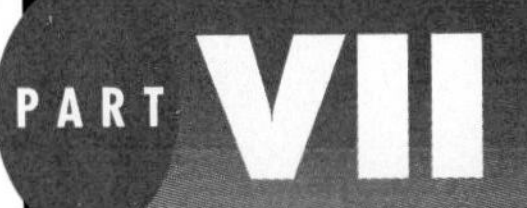
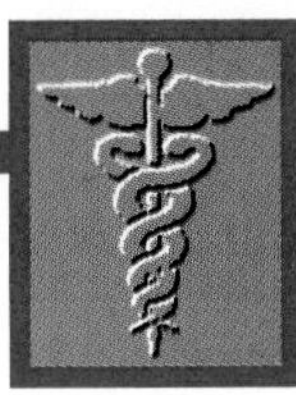

PART VII

Kulwinder S. Dua
David G. Binion
Kia Saiean

# GASTROENTEROLOGY AND DISEASES OF THE LIVER

Subpart A: Gastroenterology

CHAPTER 75

# GENERAL APPROACH TO THE PATIENT WITH GASTROINTESTINAL DISEASES

The gastrointestinal (GI) tract extends from the mouth to the anal canal. Associated structures include the pancreas and the hepatobiliary system.

Table 75.1 lists some typical GI symptoms in relation to the organ involved. Because GI disorders can be associated with other diseases or may be inherited, the importance of a thorough history cannot be overemphasized. The complete physical examination should include all the principal methods of examination, i.e., general examination and system specific inspection, palpation, percussion, and auscultation. It may be necessary to supplement the information thus gathered with general laboratory tests. In most instances, a reasonable diagnosis can then be made, thus allowing treatment to begin. In others, radiologic studies may be required as well. Patients with lesions requiring endoscopy, those whose symptoms persist despite therapy, and those whose conditions defy diagnosis are best referred to a gastroenterologist. Some patients may require additional specialized evaluation—for example, those being considered for a liver transplant, patients with inflammatory bowel disease, or those requiring endoscopic pancreaticobiliary intervention. These patients are best managed at specialized medical centers.

## Common Symptoms and Signs of Gastrointestinal Disease

### Dysphagia

Dysphagia is difficulty swallowing solids or liquids and results from conditions that impede orderly bolus transport from mouth to stomach (Table 75.2). In neuromuscular diseases, dysphagia results from dysfunction of the muscles of the mouth and pharynx involved in bolus formation and propulsion. This may lead to recurrent aspiration into the airway and nasal regurgita-

**TABLE 75.1. Symptoms of Gastrointestinal Disease**

| | |
|---|---|
| *General* | *Colon/Rectum* |
| Anorexia | Diarrhea |
| Malaise | Constipation |
| Symptoms of anemia | Abdominal pain/colic |
| Weight loss | Abdominal distention |
| *Pharyngeal* | Tenesmus |
| Difficulty initiating swallowing | Blood per rectum |
| Choking attack | *Hepatobiliary* |
| Nasal regurgitation | Anorexia |
| Pharyngeal residues after swallowing | Epigastric/right upper quadrant pain |
| *Esophageal* | Yellow discoloration of sclera |
| Heartburn | Dark urine |
| Regurgitation | Pale stools |
| Dysphagia: solids, liquids | Itching |
| Odynophagia | *Pancreatic* |
| Chest pain | Abdominal pain |
| *Gastroduodenal* | Weight loss |
| Upper abdominal pain | Anorexia |
| Postprandial fullness | Diarrhea |
| Vomiting | Symptoms of biliary obstruction |
| Hematemesis | |
| Melena | |
| *Small bowel* | |
| Diarrhea | |
| Abdominal pain/colic | |
| Abdominal distention | |
| Melena | |

TABLE 75.2. Selected Causes of Dysphagia

| Mechanism | Diseases |
|---|---|
| Neuromuscular | Brain stem neoplasms and vascular accidents |
| | Multiple sclerosis |
| | Poliomyelitis |
| | Muscular dystrophy |
| | Amyotrophic lateral sclerosis |
| | Myasthenia gravis |
| Abnormal peristalsis | Diffuse esophageal spasm |
| | Achalasia |
| | Cricopharyngeal dysfunction |
| Structural lesions of the esophagus | Stricture |
| | Web |
| | Ring |
| | Neoplasm |
| | Diverticulum |
| Extrinsic compression | Bronchogenic carcinoma |
| | Aberrant blood vessels |
| Psychogenic | |

tion of food. In cricopharyngeal muscle dysfunction, hypopharyngeal tumor, or Zenker's diverticulum, dysphagia resembles a neuromuscular disorder. Patients with dysphagia due to structural lesions or extrinsic compression of the esophagus feel as if the bolus is going "down the hatch" but then stops. The sensation produced by the arrested bolus may be felt substernally at the level of the obstruction, or may be referred, often up to the suprasternal notch. Patients with neuromuscular disorders usually report dysphagia for liquids and solids alike, whereas those with structural lesions have more difficulty with solids. A neoplasm is more likely when dysphagia is of recent onset. Dysphagia should be distinguished from *globus hystericus*, in which the patient feels a lump in the throat but has no actual difficulty swallowing.

## Heartburn

The most common esophageal symptom is *heartburn* or *pyrosis*, a burning discomfort in the subxiphoid or epigastric region, radiating substernally to the neck, and diminishing at the upper reaches. Occasionally, gastric contents may regurgitate into the mouth. Often relieved by swallowing saliva, water, or an antacid, heartburn is a common symptom of gastroesophageal (GE) reflux.

## Odynophagia

*Odynophagia* refers to pain upon swallowing. The symptom may occur in the oropharynx (e.g., acute pharyngitis). Esophageal odynophagia usually is perceived substernally. Infective esophagitis and corrosive injury commonly cause odynophagia. Odynophagia also may be caused by motor disorders of the esophagus (e.g., diffuse esophageal spasm), but it is rarely due to GE reflux disease.

## Dyspepsia

Dyspepsia is a sensation of discomfort in the upper abdomen—often perceived as "indigestion" by the patient—that is thought to reflect a disorder of the upper gastrointestinal tract. Usually linked to eating, dyspepsia may involve epigastric pain, fullness or bloating after meals, belching, nausea, and heartburn. Detailed inquiry may reveal a pattern suggestive of GE reflux, peptic ulcer disease, cholelithiasis, or chronic pancreatitis. Instances in which diagnostic studies exclude an organic basis for chronic dyspepsia are termed **"functional dyspepsia."** Despite significant overlap, symptoms of functional dyspepsia fall into three subgroups. In **ulcer-like dyspepsia,** symptoms mimic peptic ulcer disease, including relief with food, antacids, or $H_2$-receptor antagonists. In **dysmotility or stasis-type dyspepsia,** patients report symptoms of gastroparesis— early satiety, nausea, belching, and bloating after meals. In **flatulent or biliary-type dyspepsia,** the patients report postprandial fullness, epigastric discomfort, or flatulence. Despite the coexistence of dyspepsia and cholelithiasis, the two have no proven association.

The pathophysiology of functional dyspepsia has not yet been explained. Basal and peak acid outputs are normal in most affected patients, although gastric acid suppression benefits some of them. Delayed gastric emptying and reduced postprandial antral motility have been noted in some; in others, a reduced threshold has been found for discomfort after gastric distention, suggesting visceral sensory abnormality. Functional dyspepsia is largely a diagnosis of exclusion of other organic causes for dyspepsia. Management should include diet and lifestyle counseling (e.g., avoiding alcohol, tobacco, caffeinated drinks, and spicy, greasy foods). Patients with continuing symptoms can undergo empiric acid suppression with $H_2$-receptor antagonists/proton pump inhibitors (PPIs) or gastroduodenal motility enhancing by prokinetic agents.

## Abdominal Pain

Abdominal pain is one of the main symptoms of GI disorders for which patients seek medical help. Its expression and diagnostic evaluation are complex. The pain is best assessed using a sequence of dichotomous or similarly discrete descriptors. In this way, pain that is "terrible" and "all over" may be seen as acute or chronic, visceral or somatic, constant or intermittent, and centered in one area or another. Despite the frequent necessity for additional tests to make a diagnosis, in some instances abdominal pain is the only dependable means of diagnosis—for example, the right lower quadrant pain of acute appendicitis.

Abdominal pain can be visceral or parietal (Table 75.3). Pain originating from GI organs is *visceral*, carried by sympathetic nerve fibers. Because visceral organs have multisegmental innervation from both sides of the spinal cord, visceral pain usually is felt in the midline, and has indistinct borders with poor localization. Visceral pain is believed to result from stretching of a hollow GI viscus or the capsule of a solid organ, or from mediators released during inflammation or ischemia of GI structures. Sympathetic pain fibers in splanchnic nerves enter the posterior horn of the spinal cord, which may cause the pain sensation to spread retrogradely in the somatic sensory nerve of the corresponding dermatome. Thus, referred pain may be felt in areas remote from the source (e.g., right scapular pain from biliary tract disease). Pain may be *referred* to the abdomen from diseases outside the abdomen—for example, myocardial ischemia may present as upper abdominal pain alone or abdominal pain with chest pain. Diseases that extend to involve the peritoneum exhibit *parietal pain*, which is sharper and more severe, usually more accurately localized, and aggravated by movement or coughing. Occasionally, systemic diseases such as porphyria and diabetic ketoacidosis can present as abdominal pain.

The *location* of the pain, in terms of four quadrants, should be noted (Figure 75.1, Table 75.4); the nine-area section system also may be used. The *quality* of pain, as described by the patient, is also meaningful. Sharp and fairly localized parietal pain is secondary to peritoneal

**TABLE 75.3. Some Distinctions Between Visceral and Parietal Pain**

| Characteristic | Visceral | Parietal |
|---|---|---|
| Localization | Usually midline | More accurate |
| Nature | Dull, burning, cramping, gnawing, indistinct borders | Sharp, severe |
| Associated autonomic activity (e.g., sweating, nausea, vomiting) | May be present | Uncommon |
| Increase with movements, coughing, deep inspiration | | Present |
| Radiation to other areas | May be present | |

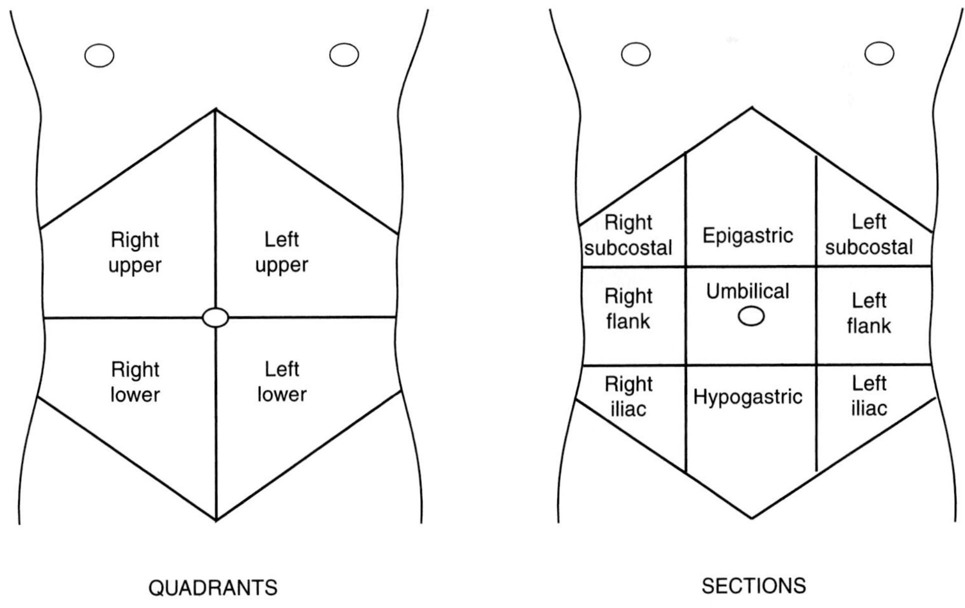


**FIGURE 75.1.** Two methods of designating abdominal area for describing findings: A. Four quadrantic divisions. B. Nine sections.

**TABLE 75.4. Frequent Causes of Abdominal Pain**

| Site | Acute | Chronic | Referred |
|---|---|---|---|
| Upper quadrants | Perforated gastric/duodenal ulcer<br>Cholecystitis<br>Biliary colic<br>Acute pancreatitis<br>Splenic rupture or infarction | Duodenal ulcer<br>Gastric ulcer<br>Non-ulcer dyspepsia<br>Chronic pancreatitis<br>Irritable bowel<br>Liver diseases | Cardiac<br>Pleuritic<br>Spinal root |
| Periumbilical | Appendicitis<br>Small bowel obstruction<br>Small bowel infarction<br>Dissecting aortic aneurysm | Inflammatory bowel disease<br>Intestinal ischemia<br>Irritable bowel | Spinal root |
| Lower quadrants | Appendicitis<br>Diverticulitis<br>Colon obstruction<br>Colon infarction | Inflammatory bowel disease<br>Colon ischemia<br>Irritable bowel | Spinal root<br>Pelvic diseases |

involvement by an inflamed GI viscus directly underlying the localized area. Generalized peritonitis due to perforation of a GI viscus could present as diffuse, severe abdominal pain. Visceral pain may be constant (e.g., right upper quadrant in acute hepatitis) or intermittent (e.g., colicky pain in small bowel obstruction).

The next consideration in the evaluation of abdominal pain is its *radiation*. Duodenal and pancreatic pain may radiate to the back, gallbladder pain to the right scapula, and pain from diaphragmatic irritation to the shoulder. The *timing* of abdominal pain and *factors aggravating or relieving* it also help in differential diagnosis. Nocturnal pain that interrupts sleep strongly indicates an organic cause for the pain. The effect of food, belching, passing flatus, defecation, and medications (e.g., antacids) on pain may help localize the pain to a specific viscus. *Change in pain* over time is particularly useful in the course of acute abdominal pain where sequential examinations will distinguish between acute illness requiring surgical or other intervention, and illness that is self-limited and often idiopathic. Finally, *other associated symptoms* should be noted. In the context of pain, vomiting may suggest bowel obstruction or gastric outlet obstruction; hematemesis or melena may suggest ulcer disease; and left lower quadrant pain with rectal bleeding could be due to colitis.

The combination of rebound tenderness and involuntary guarding on palpation implies localized or generalized peritonitis. Bowel sounds may be absent, because of peritonitis-related ileus. The patient tends to avoid movement and generally keeps the abdominal muscles tense (rigidity). By contrast, patients with visceral pain, as in acute pancreatitis, may be in severe distress but may have minimal abdominal signs on palpation. Visceral pain may evolve into parietal pain as the disease process extends to the peritoneum. Sequential physical examinations are useful in eliciting this change. Renal angles and hernial orifices should be examined systematically in patients with abdominal pain. In addition to detecting lower rectal lesions and abnormalities in the pouch of Douglas, a digital rectal examination can help assess the tone of the anal sphincter and the presence of frank or occult blood in the stool. The genitalia also should be examined. In women, a pelvic examination may be necessary.

Despite a thorough clinical assessment, the etiology of the abdominal pain may remain elusive. General laboratory tests (e.g., a complete blood count with differential, liver tests, and plain abdominal radiographs) may be required. Acute presentations may require urgent abdominal imaging with ultrasound or computed tomography (CT). Exploratory laparotomy may be urgently undertaken in some patients, whereas a more deliberate and selective approach may be pursued in others, especially those with long-standing abdominal pain. Laparoscopy is also being used in the diagnosis of abdominal pain and cancer and in the evaluation of abdominal trauma.

## Nausea and Vomiting

Nausea is the experience of revulsion to food and the anticipation of vomiting. Vomiting is a coordinated somatic and visceral motor activity, in which prolonged contractions of the abdominal muscles and the diaphragm raise the intra-abdominal pressure sufficiently to overcome the opposing hydrostatic and muscular forces of the gastric cardia, GE junction, and the esophagus. The proximal small bowel contents are thus moved into the stomach, and forcefully thereafter into the mouth and beyond. With retching, spontaneous contractions occur without fluid propulsion above the GE junction. Vomiting is controlled by the vomiting center in the medulla and triggered by afferent neural input to the medulla or stimulation of chemoreceptor trigger zone. Additional neural pathways also are involved. In contrast, GE reflux leading to oral regurgitation of gastric contents lacks the autonomic or somatic features (sweating and emotional distress) of vomiting.

Nausea and vomiting may be provoked by a myriad of disorders, some of which are not primarily gastrointestinal. Obstructive vomiting must be distinguished from the more common vomiting caused by sensory stimulation of the GI tract. In small bowel obstruction, patients vomit large volumes of bilious material, consisting of gastric and pancreatic secretions in addition to bile. Colicky periumbilical pain and a tympanitic, distended abdomen are associated. In pyloroduodenal stenosis and gastric outlet obstruction from peptic ulcer, patients usually vomit bile-free material, often containing food eaten many hours earlier. A succussion splash may be elicited. In colonic obstruction, vomiting follows constipation, abdominal pain, and distention. Nonobstructive GI causes of nausea and vomiting cover a full range of GI disorders with mucosal irritation or dysmotility—e.g., esophagitis, gastritis, peptic ulcer disease, and diabetic gastroparesis. Vomiting may be due to non-GI causes—toxic, metabolic, neurologic, or cardiac conditions (e.g., uremia, medications, pregnancy, ketoacidosis, raised intracranial pressure, or myocardial infarction). In some patients, the cause is elusive; emotional or psychiatric problems may be implicated.

Sustained, large-volume vomiting may cause dehydration and electrolyte imbalance. Loss of gastric acid results in metabolic alkalosis, often with hypokalemia. Nausea is a very potent stimulator of antidiuretic hormone (ADH) secretion; therefore, nausea and vomiting may lead to hyponatremia. Thus, treatment not only must address the cause and symptomatic control of nausea and vomiting but also must correct the fluid, electrolyte, and nutritional consequences. Antiemetics are not needed for controlling nausea and vomiting in patients with a treatable primary cause (e.g., gastric outlet obstruction), but for those who do require them, various drugs are available. These drugs may act centrally (antihistamines, anticholinergics, phenothiazines), peripherally (cisapride), or in both domains (dopaminergic antagonists).

### Diarrhea and Malabsorption

Diarrhea and malabsorption are discussed in Chapters 76 and 77, respectively.

## Radiographic Vs. Endoscopic Studies

Endoscopy is superior to radiography in several ways in the diagnosis and treatment of GI disease. It can demonstrate bleeding sites directly and detect flat or superficial mucosal lesions more readily. Endoscopically obtained biopsies can separate malignant from benign ulcers reliably. Whereas a cancer or retained food material, both can cause a filling defect in the esophagus on a barium swallow, the area can be inspected directly using esophagoscopy. Gastroesophageal reflux seen on barium studies cannot exclude associated Barrett's esophagus. The other facet of endoscopy, its ability for interventional therapy, clearly makes it the procedure of choice in patients in whom such intervention is planned. Dilating strictures, placing endoprostheses and feeding tubes, controlling GI bleeding, removing polyps, and decompressing the colon can all be done during endoscopy.

Nonetheless, there are some situations in which radiologic studies are superior to endoscopy. Plain abdominal films can reveal bowel gas patterns and intra-abdominal calcification that endoscopy cannot detect. Barium studies can assess GI motility, whereas endoscopy cannot. Subtle strictures are visualized better radiologically. In patients with suspected perforation, radiologic studies are more informative and safer. Despite the increasing availability of enteroscopy, i.e., endoscopic visualization of upper small bowel using a longer endoscope in some centers, large areas of the small bowel are inaccessible to endoscopy. Recently an electronic capsule has been introduced that can be swallowed and, while travelling down the GI tract, it transmits endoscopic images to a receiver. In situations in which full endoscopic facilities are not readily available, radiologic studies of the upper and the lower GI tracts are still excellent alternatives. Patients with dysphagia should have a barium swallow study first. Finally, radiologic studies are cheaper than endoscopy and carry a lower risk of complications.

In some situations, radiography and endoscopy are combined. For example, during endoscopic retrograde cholangiopancreatography (ERCP), biliary and pancreatic ducts are cannulated endoscopically and the cholangiopancreatogram is obtained radiologically. Transhepatic cholangiography may be required before the procedure to gain bile duct access in difficult or failed ERCP attempts.

Other imaging modalities play a major diagnostic and therapeutic role in GI diseases. Ultrasonography (US), computed tomography, and magnetic resonance imaging (MRI) can effectively image intra-abdominal structures not readily visualized otherwise (e.g., liver, gallbladder, pancreas, biliary system, kidneys, lymph nodes, masses, and fluid collections). The Doppler technique makes dynamic evaluation (using blood flow pattern) possible. Endoscopes with an attached ultrasound probe (endoscopic ultrasound [EUS]) can scan organs such as the pancreas, liver, and bowel wall in close proximity, and aspirate material for cytology with a targeted fine needle. Gastrointestinal bleeding site(s) that cannot be located endoscopically can be identified by angiography, and occluded by intra-arterial embolization or vasopressin injection. Available radionuclide imaging tests include $^{99m}$Tc-sulfur colloid (for liver parenchyma), $^{99m}$Tc-HIDA (for acute cholecystitis), $^{99m}$Tc-pertechnetate (for ectopic gastric tissue—e.g., Meckel's diverticulum), and $^{99m}$Tc-labeled red cells (for intermittent GI bleeding).

Diagnostic laparoscopy sometimes is indicated in the evaluation of patients with ascites in whom peritoneal disease is suspected. Sometimes it is used to biopsy hepatic surface lesions under direct visualization.

# CHAPTER 76 DIARRHEA

## Definition

Diarrhea is defined as stool weight exceeding 200 g/day in patients ingesting a typical Western diet (>300g/day on a high-fiber diet). The number or consistency of bowel movements per day does not define diarrhea. The stool water content is approximately 80%, and even higher in loose or watery stools. Therefore, diarrhea can be equated with increased fecal water loss. Symptoms of diarrheal illness may include increased stool frequency (>3/day), decreased stool consistency, abdominal pain, and fecal incontinence.

## Physiology and Pathophysiology

Of the 10 to 12 L of fluid that the intestines receive daily, oral intake is 2 L, and the rest comes from salivary, gastric, biliary, pancreatic, and small bowel secretions. The duodenum, jejunum, and ileum absorb about 9 L/day. The colon absorbs all but 0.1 L from the remaining 1.0 to 1.5 L. Water moves passively across the bowel mucosa to maintain isotonicity of its contents; the absorption and secretion of osmotically active solutes determine this flux. As shown in Figure 76.1, water transport is mainly *paracellular*, via the tight junction **(zonula occludens).** Solutes absorbed across the brush border exit into the lateral intercellular space (LIS), thus causing an osmotic gradient from LIS to the isotonic lumen contents. Water flows osmotically (hydraulic), so as to dispel this gradient; in the process, small solutes (MW <100) entrained in the water flow are absorbed by "solvent drag." This paracellular absorption of solutes depends on the permeability of the tight junction—jejunal tight junctions are "leaky," whereas those in the colon are much less permeable (see Figure 76.1). When solutes are not absorbed, excess water is needed in the lumen to maintain isotonicity, and diarrhea results. The normal colon is able to absorb up to 4 L/day, and can compensate partially for increased fluid delivery from the small intestine. Diarrhea occurs when the overall efficiency of intestinal water absorption falls below 99%. Flow rate and composition of bowel contents are presented in Table 76.1.

Inorganic ions and nutrients are absorbed through the mature cells on the villus tips in the small bowel and the surface epithelium in the colon. In both organs, the crypt cells secrete electrolytes and water. In the small bowel, $Na^+$ enters the enterocytes by two mechanisms: (1) by an $Na^+/H^+$ cation exchange and (2) in association with glucose, galactose, and most amino acids. The $Na^+/H^+$ exchanger is coupled to an anion transporter, which exchanges $Cl^-$ for $HCO_3^-$. This dual process (Figure 76.2), which occurs throughout the small bowel and colon, absorbs NaCl electroneutrally. Also, in the colonic brush border membrane, there are $Na^+$- selective channels that allow $Na^+$ to enter the cell by concentration gradients. Through the Na, K-ATPase ("sodium pump"),

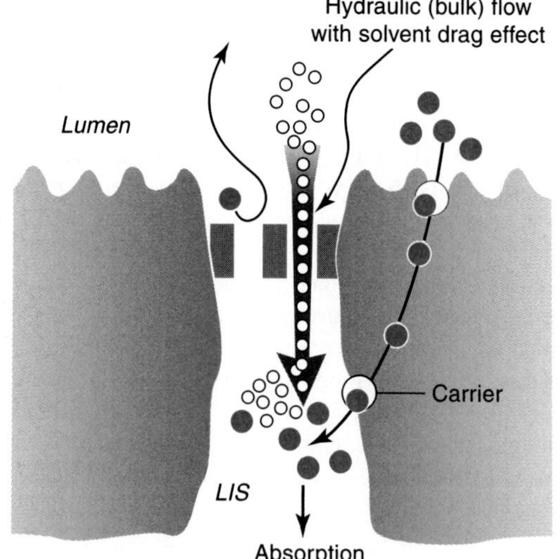


**FIGURE 76.1.** **Paracellular water absorption in response to active, carrier-mediated transport of a solute (large filled circles) from lumen to the lateral intercellular space (LIS). The water flow is driven by the osmotic gradient between lumen and the LIS, across the junction. The water flow carries with it a second, smaller solute (open circles)—i.e., solvent drag. The solute transported by carriers is too large to pass the tight junction; it is reflected from it.**

**TABLE 76.1. Intestinal Contents in the Postprandial State**

| | Flow Rate (L/d) | Na (mEq/L) | K (mEq/L) | Cl (mEq/L) | $HCO_3$ (mEq/L) |
|---|---|---|---|---|---|
| Proximal jejunum* | 10 | 60 | 15 | 60 | 15 |
| Mid-gut | 5 | 140 | 5 | 100 | 30 |
| Terminal ileum | 1.5 | 140 | 8 | 60 | 50 |
| Rectum/stool† | 0.1 | 15 | 85 | 15 | 30 |

*Varies with meals.
†Main anion: Short-chain fatty acids.

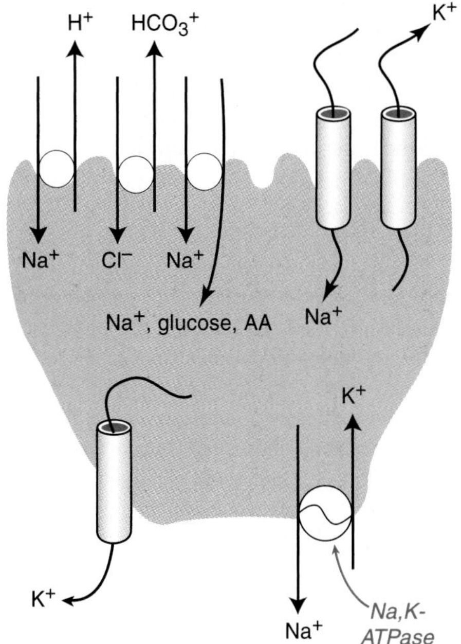


**FIGURE 76.2.** **Transporters of intestinal villus and/or colon surface epithelial cells. Left side: present in small bowel and colon. Middle: $Na^+$ uptake coupled to glucose, galactose or to amino acids; present in small bowel only. Right side: apical $K^+$- and $Na^+$-channels: colon only. Only the basolateral Na, K-ATPase provides energy.**

the $Na^+$ is ejected across the basolateral cell wall. This process leads to active $Na^+$ absorption and a low $Na^+$ in normal stool water. Potassium enters the colonic contents mainly by diffusion, and partly by active secretion. All active absorption in the entire bowel derives its energy from the sodium pump, which exchanges three $Na^+$ ions for two $K^+$ ions.

Multiple mechanisms regulate the intestinal absorption and secretion of electrolytes. These include mediators released from inflammatory and mast cells in the lamina propria (e.g., histamine, prostaglandins, leukotrienes, serotonin, interleukins); neurotransmitters, which act through receptors on the basolateral wall of enterocytes; hormones in circulating blood; neuropeptides released by specialized cells within the mucosa; and bacterial enterotoxins, such as cholera toxin and *Escherichia coli* enterotoxin. Most of these mechanisms decrease the absorption or increase the secretion of ions (some do both). Most mechanisms that produce gastrointestinal secretion inhibit the electroneutral absorption of NaCl by the villous cells, *and* open $Cl^-$ channels in the brush border membrane of crypt cells. Chloride ions enter the cell by basolaterally located $Na^+$ two $Cl^-$ $K^+$ uptake; the excess intracellular $K^+$ exits via basolateral $K^+$ channels and the $Na^+$ by the sodium pump (Figure 76.3). By contrast, $Na^+$ absorption coupled to sugars and amino acids is unaffected in secretory diarrhea; this is the basis for oral rehydration therapy.

## Classification

Diarrhea traditionally has been classified into osmotic, secretory, and miscellaneous types according to the underlying pathophysiologic mechanism. **Osmotic diarrhea** results when excessive, osmotically active solutes reach the rectum, accompanied by obligatory water to maintain isotonicity (Table 76.2). Carbohydrates are a common cause. Diarrhea results when intact sugars remain in the rectum and stool. Colonic bacteria anaerobically ferment carbohydrates to short-chain fatty acids (acetate, propionate, and n-butyrate) and $H_2$. The maximum fermentation capacity is 60 g/meal of carbohydrates, of which 15 g/meal is "physiologic" malabsorption. Carbohydrate-induced diarrhea occurs when the fermentation capacity of the colonic bacteria is surpassed—for example, during therapy with broad-spectrum antibiotics. The organic acids so produced are rapidly absorbed and play no role in the ensuing diarrhea.

**Secretory diarrhea** is due to reduced absorption or excess secretion of inorganic ions (Table 76.2). The 2-OH bile acids and some long-chain fatty acids impede colonic ion absorption, thus causing secretion. Diarrhea follows resection or extensive disease of the terminal ileum, where bile acids normally are actively absorbed, and may complicate cholecystectomy, which alters the physiology of bile secretion and absorption. Oleic acid, and its

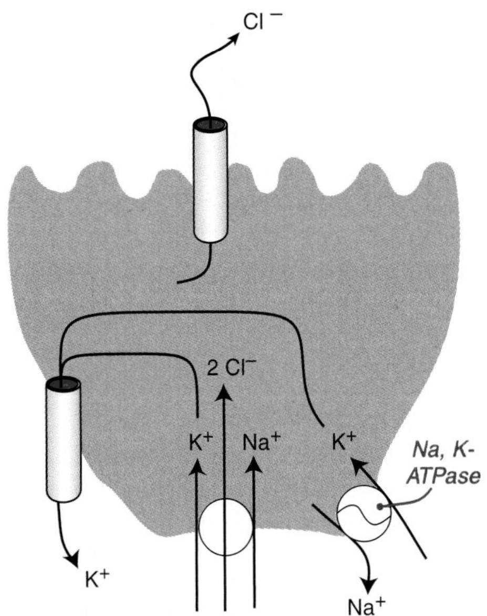


**FIGURE 76.3. Chloride secretion by intestinal and colonic crypt cells. The rate of secretion depends on the activation (opening) of the apical Cl⁻ channel. The energy is provided by the Na, K-ATPase.**

**TABLE 76.2. Causes of Osmotic and Secretory Diarrhea**

**I. Osmotic Diarrhea**
A. Carbohydrates escaping absorption and colonic fermentation
  1. Disaccharidase deficiencies
  2. Poorly absorbed dietary sugars: sorbitol, fructose, mannitol, lactulose
  3. Broad-spectrum antibiotic therapy
B. Poorly absorbed inorganic ions
  1. Magnesium: antacids, laxatives, food supplements
  2. Anions: Na-sulfate, -phosphate, -citrate
C. Miscellaneous: Polyethylene glycol 3250 (GoLYTELY)

**II. Secretory Diarrhea**
Bacterial enterotoxins
Stimulant laxatives
Diffuse small intestinal disease
Bile acid and fatty acid malabsorption
Microscopic/collagenous colitis
Hormonally mediated:
  1) Increased digestive secretions: gastrinoma
  2) Intestinal secretion: carcinoid syndrome, VIP-oma, medullary carcinoma of the thyroid
Congenital ion transport defects

bacterial hydroxylation product, 10-OH stearic acid, lead to excess stool water in steatorrhea. Stimulant laxatives (e.g., phenolphthalein, castor oil, bisacodyl, cascara) induce colonic secretion and stimulate colonic motility. One half of patients with gastrin-producing tumors have diarrhea, from excess gastric and pancreatic secretions that outstrip the absorptive ability of the entire gut. Serotonin, vasoactive intestinal polypeptide (VIP), and thyrocalcitonin bind to the enterocyte receptors, and incite secretory diarrhea.

Exudation from ulcerated ileal or colonic mucosa contributes to the diarrhea of **inflammatory bowel disease.** Increased luminal hydrostatic pressure proximal to a bowel obstruction lead to secretion, causing **"paradoxical diarrhea."** Rapid intestinal transit causes diarrhea after gastric surgery (dumping syndrome and postvagotomy diarrhea), and possibly in hyperthyroidism as well.

## Laboratory Tests

In theory, two simple tests distinguish between secretory and osmotic diarrhea. First, osmotic diarrhea from poorly absorbed solutes stops during 48 hours of fasting. While secretory diarrhea from malabsorption of bile or fatty acids does the same, continued diarrhea during fasting indicates a secretory cause. The second test is a stool water osmotic gap (stool water osmolality [290 mOsm/kg] − 2[measured stool $Na^+$ + $K^+$]). In secretory diarrhea, the gap is below 50 mOsm/kg. In osmotic diarrhea, the osmotic gap exceeds 50. However, these two tests have limited practical use since most diarrheas have more than one mechanism.

## Clinical Categories

Clinically, diarrhea is divided into acute and chronic (>3 weeks' duration). **Acute diarrhea** is usually caused by a pathogen, toxin, or food component ingested hours to one week before the onset of symptoms. Onset with watery stools, nausea, vomiting, and little or no fever reflects predominant small bowel involvement by a pathogen, without epithelial invasion. "Dysenteric syndrome"—that is, abdominal cramping, fever, and frequent small-volume bloody stools, suggest infection by an invasive organism, usually afflicting the colon. **Chronic diarrhea** frequently has a gradual onset and persists for over 3 weeks. All forms of confirmed chronic diarrhea should be considered pathologic, and warrant diagnostic evaluation.

## Diagnostic Evaluation

Acute diarrhea is marked by signs of dehydration, such as acute weight loss, orthostatic hypotension, poor capillary perfusion, and oliguria. Next, to determine a cause, inquiries should be directed to recent travel, similar illness among contacts, and food consumption. Stool tests for enteric pathogens, ova, and parasites are generally needed only in a dysenteric syndrome. Fecal leukocytes, when present, imply an invasive pathogen or inflammatory bowel disease. "False negatives" occur in enterohemorrhagic (O 157:H 7) E. coli, *C. difficile* and Yersinia infection, and amebic colitis. (See, also, chapter 86.)

A thorough medical history, the probability of specific causes (Figure 76.4), and the results of routine tests (complete blood count, serum electrolytes and albumin, sedimentation rate, stool testing for occult blood, ova, parasites, and enteric pathogens) are paramount in selecting tests for evaluating chronic diarrhea. **Functional diarrhea,** the most common cause, typically has a duration over 2 years, intermittent and daytime-only diarrhea, weight loss below 5 kg, normal routine tests, and a stool weight below 300g/day. A panoply of medications may cause diarrhea, including Mg citrate, phosphates, broad-spectrum antibiotics, antacids, colchicine, prostaglandins (Cytotec7), fluoxetine (Prozac7), olsalazine (Dipentum7), proton pump inhibitors, lactulose, and, occasionally, diuretics and nonsteroidal anti-inflammatory drugs (NSAIDs). **Surreptitious laxative and diuretic abuse** is frequently overlooked; the stool should be tested for phenolphthalein by adding 1N NaOH or KOH to observe the color change to a red-purple. When this is negative, urine can be analyzed for diuretics and for polyphenolic laxatives, including bisacodyl, and cascara. In some patients with acute, travel-related diarrhea, watery diarrhea continues, without a demonstrable pathogen. This post-infectious diarrhea abates within 6–24 months. Chronic watery diarrhea (Brainerd) syndrome is endemic in areas of the rural Midwest. The prognosis is good, although the pathogen remains elusive. Hormonally caused chronic diarrhea is rare—for example, carcinoid syndrome (elevated urine 5-HIAA), gastrinoma (Zollinger-Ellison and MEN-I syndrome), VIPoma, medullary thyroid carcinoma, adrenal insufficiency, and hyperthyroidism. These should not be sought routinely.

When initial evaluation does not yield a preliminary diagnosis, two studies are very helpful. The first is a 48- or 72-hour quantitative stool collection performed at home with the patient receiving a regular diet and no antidiarrheal medications. Stool weight less than 200g/d rules out diarrhea; 200–300g/d suggests a functional cause, and a weight above 800g/d indicates small bowel involvement. Stool fat should be measured in order to detect steatorrhea (>7g fat/d) as a sign of generalized malabsorption. The second test is a proctosigmoidoscopy with no (or only saline) preparatory enemas. Brown-black mucosal discoloration (melanosis coli) is diagnostic of long-term use of anthraquinone-type laxatives (e.g., cascara sagrada, senna, aloe). Biopsies should be done to exclude lymphocytic, microscopic, and collagenous colitis. A schematic approach to the diagnosis of chronic diarrhea is shown in Figure 76.5.

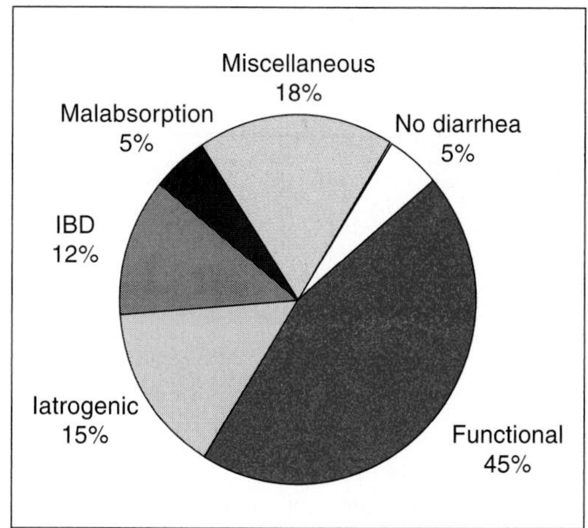


**FIGURE 76.4. Diagnosis in patients referred for evaluation of chronic diarrhea. IBD: inflammatory bowel disease. Miscellaneous: systemic diseases (e.g., diabetes, amyloid, immunosuppression), 5%; self-induced (laxative abuse, long-distance running), 5%; food/travel related (e.g., lactose deficiency, sorbitol, fructose, postinfectious diarrhea), 5%; hormonal causes, congenital transport defects, 3%.**

## Management

**Rehydration and acid–base balance**

Severe dehydration is defined as an estimated weight loss of over 4%—that is, an extracellular fluid deficit exceeding 2.5 L in a 60 kg patient. The deficit should be replaced in about 24 h with an IV solution of 0.45% NaCl (NaCl, 78 mEq/L) to which $NaHCO_3$, 50 mEq/L plus KCl, 10–20 mEq/L are added. For significant hypernatremia (>154 mEq/L), 1 L of 5% dextrose in water (D5W) is given for every 2 L of the above solution. Serum electrolytes, urine output, and BP should be monitored. Metabolic acidosis requires $HCO_3$ supplementation only with a serum $HCO_3$ below 15 mEq/L. Fluid should also be given for ongoing maintenance needs (about 2.5 L/d) as D5 0.45% NaCl, alternating with D5 0.25% NaCl; nearly 40 mEq of $K^+$ is added per 24 hours.

Oral rehydration solutions (ORS) are used to correct mild to moderate dehydration and for maintenance therapy of severe dehydration after initial rehydration (Table 76.3). In secretory diarrhea, glucose will stimulate $Na^+$ and water absorption; solvent drag will lead to absorption of $K^+$ and anions. ORS used for initial

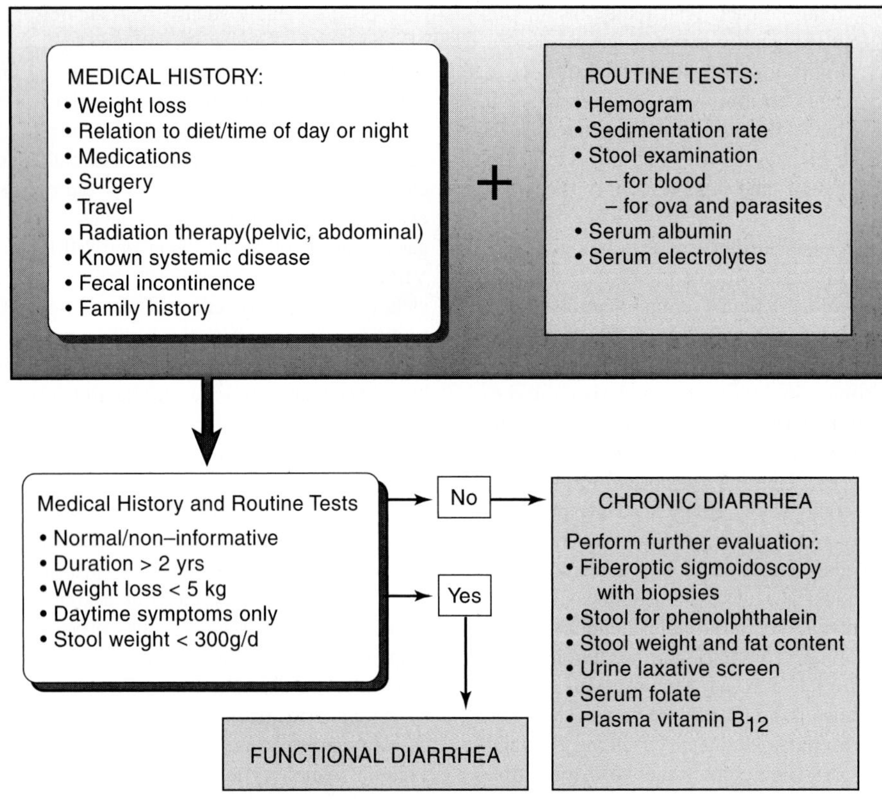


FIGURE 76.5. Evaluation of chronic diarrhea.

TABLE 76.3. Oral Rehydration Solutions

| | Source | Na | K | Cl | Base* | Glucose mmol/L |
|---|---|---|---|---|---|---|
| Rehydration solutions | | | | | | |
| WHO-UNICEF | — | 90 | 20 | 80 | 30 | 111 |
| Rehydralyte | Ross | 75 | 20 | 65 | 30 | 140 |
| Maintenance solutions | | | | | | |
| Pedialyte | Ross | 45 | 20 | 35 | 30 | 140 |
| Infalyte | Pennwalt | 50 | 20 | 40 | 30 | 111 |

*Bicarbonate or citrate.

rehydration has a higher $Na^+$ level than that used for maintenance hydration. Saccharides (e.g., sucrose, glucose polymers, or boiled rice flour) may be used in lieu of glucose. The volume administered equals the sum of the fluid deficit and the ongoing losses. Additional fluid and food intake are encouraged. Acute diarrhea frequently features transient acquired lactose deficiency; thus, dietary lactose should be low. Fructose, sorbitol, and caffeine should also be avoided.

### Anti–diarrheal medications

Anti–diarrheals are not indicated during acute, self-limited diarrhea, particularly when an invasive pathogen ("dysenteric syndrome") is suspected. Opiate-type agents are the mainstay of symptomatic therapy of chronic diarrhea. Loperamide (Imodium, 2 mg b.i.d.), diphenoxylate (Lomotil, 5 mg q 6–8h), and codeine (30 mg q 6–8h) are equally effective. They delay small bowel transit, and by interaction with the δ-type opiate receptor on enterocytes, may facilitate absorption. They may cause nausea and abdominal cramps. A long duration of action and the lack of central nervous system (CNS) effects make Loperamide the preferred agent; doses up to 10 mg b.i.d. may have to be given. Bulk-forming agents (e.g., bran, methylcellulose, and calcium polycarbophil) do not reduce stool losses of water and salts. At best, they increase stool consistency. Anti-spasmodics are not recommended.

## Special Situations

### Immunosuppressed patients

Most patients with AIDS develop diarrhea eventually, manifested either by large-volume diarrhea and weight loss or as the dysenteric syndrome. The latter indicates colitis caused by *C. difficile,* cytomegalovirus, or common bacterial pathogens. The former type is associated with infection by *Giardia lamblia*, cryptosporidia, microsporidia, *Mycobacterium avium-intracellulare*, or viruses. A cause may be elusive in nearly 50% of this group. Stool studies for bacteria, parasites, and viral pathogens are indicated. Colonoscopy and duodenoscopy with biopsies may be dictated by the clinical presentation. Management should be directed at the cause.

### Diabetic diarrhea

Rarely, chronic watery diarrhea complicates diabetes mellitus, usually with associated neuropathy and retinopathy. The autonomic neuropathy impairs intestinal motility and decreases $Na^+$ and $Cl^-$ absorption. The absorptive defect is due to reduced catecholamine content in the ileal mucosa, thus reducing activation of $\alpha$-2-adrenergic receptors on the enterocytes. Celiac sprue and intestinal bacterial overgrowth should be excluded, since both are more common in diabetics. Mild steatorrhea, found in nearly one-third of cases of diabetic diarrhea, is due to pancreatic atrophy. Treatment should be step-wise. "Sugar-free" diets with sorbitol or fructose are discontinued first. Opiate antidiarrheal drugs are given next; abdominal cramps may limit their use. Third, $\alpha$-adrenergic agonists (e.g., clonidine, 0.1 mg initially, with a maximum of 0.6 mg q 12h) may be tried, but their long-term efficacy is unknown. Pre-existing orthostatic hypotension may worsen. Oral antibiotics, pancreatic enzymes, and somatostatin should not be routinely used.

### Post-vagotomy diarrhea

Diarrhea follows truncal or selective vagotomy in up to 25% of patients; it is severe in 1–8%. The precise cause is unclear, but rapid gastric emptying of liquids ("dumping syndrome," chapter 83), rapid intestinal transit, and bacterial overgrowth may all be involved. The onset may be delayed by several years and the course is commonly episodic. Treatment is with small meals of low sugar content and, frequently, high doses of antidiarrheal opiates. Octreotide, a somatostatin analogue, may sometimes help.

### Antibiotic-associated diarrhea

Diarrhea occurs in up to 30% of patients receiving antibiotics, particularly penicillins, cephalosporins, and clindamycin. Colitis due to toxin-producing strains of *C. difficile* accounts for only 15–20% of cases; osmotic diarrhea due to decreased bacterial carbohydrate fermentation occurs in the remaining. Those with *C. difficile* toxin in the stool are given appropriate antibiotics (chapter 98). In those without, antibiotics should be stopped, if possible; poorly absorbed carbohydrates should be omitted from the diet.

### Tube-feeding diarrhea

Diarrhea may complicate liquid formula feedings through a nasogastric tube or a gastrostomy, with or without added fiber. Frequent causes include concurrent antibiotics or sorbitol-containing medications, a pre-existing intestinal disorder, or bolus feeding. Formula diets, including the elemental type, do not cause diarrhea when given by constant infusion into an otherwise normal intestinal tract.

Choleretic diarrhea, or bile acid induced diarrhea should be considered in patients who may have had pathology or surgery in the terminal ileum (i.e. Crohn's disease) which reduces the ability to efficiently absorb bile. A small minority of patients who have had cholecystectomy may also develop choleretic diarrhea (<10%), due to alterations in biliary secretion into the lumenal GI tract. Choleretic diarrhea may be characterized by severe cramping and visceral symptoms including sweating, urgency, and a rectal "burning" sensation with defecation. A diagnostic challenge of the bile acid binding resin cholestyramine (2–4 grams in the morning) may rapidly alleviate symptoms, and may be continued on a long term basis. It is important to note that cholestyramine will avidly bind medications, and patients should be cautioned not to take other medications for a minimum of two hours after a morning dose of the cholestyramine.

# CHAPTER 77 MALABSORPTION

Since the colon does not absorb nutrients, malabsorption can be characterized as the increased passage of single or multiple nutrients across the ileocecal valve, with or without diarrhea. Specific single nutrient malabsorption disorders may involve vitamin $B_{12}$, glucose-galactose malabsorption, amino acid transport defects, and disaccharidase deficiencies. Generalized malabsorption consists of defects of digestion and of nutrient malabsorption due to resection or extensive disease of the small bowel (Table 77.1).

## Physiology and Pathophysiology

Digestion and absorption are complex processes. The surface area available for absorption is limited to the top 10–20% of the intestinal villus surface. The pH of the fluid layer overlying the absorptive cells is 1–2 units below that of luminal contents; this fluid layer, about 40–100? thick, does not mix with intestinal bulk contents. Solutes need to cross this "unstirred layer" by diffusion, a process that limits the absorption rate of substances with a slow aqueous diffusion coefficient, such as the products of fat digestion. Digestion and absorption of carbohydrates is rapid and nearly complete in the jejunum; the ileum completes the fat and protein absorption. While the human digestive tract has considerable reserve capacity for digestion and absorption, it is limited in its capacity to absorb sorbitol and free fructose and to hydrolyze lactose to glucose and galactose.

### Digestion and absorption of fat

In the stomach, gastric lipase hydrolyzes fat to glycerol and fatty acids. The remainder of the fat is emulsified with proteins and the products of gastric lipase activity. The amphipathic conjugated bile acids stabilize the fat emulsion droplets. After pancreatic lipase binds to these droplets in the presence of colipase, fatty acids are released from positions 1 and 3 of the triglyceride, leaving intact 2-monoglycerides (2MG). The lipolytic products are then solubilized in bile salt micelles, which form when duodenal bile salts exceed a "critical micellar concentration" of approximately 2mM. The products of lipolysis diffuse out of the micelles, through the unstirred layer and across the apical cell wall into the cytoplasm of enterocytes. Further steps in fat absorption are shown in Figure 77.1. Chylomicrons and very low-density lipoproteins (VLDL), the final products of the absorptive process enter the intestinal lymphatics. Fat-soluble vitamins, cholesterol, and phospholipids are absorbed in tandem with the products of lipolysis. The highly efficient process of fat absorption is vulnerable at many steps, including duodenal acidification, which inactivates lipase and precipitates bile salts; duodenal bile salt concentrations below about 2mM, which precludes micelle formation; decreased lipase availability and a defective or reduced absorptive area. Further, lipase is the

**TABLE 77.1. Causes of Malabsorption**

*Impaired intraluminal digestion*
- *Pancreatic enzyme deficiency*
  - Deficient secretion in pancreatic disease; decreased cholecystokinin release
  - Enzyme inactivation: excess gastric acid secretion
  - Asynchrony: post-gastric surgery
- *Defective fat solubilization:* decreased bile salt concentration
  - Decreased synthesis: liver disease
  - Decreased bile flow: cholestasis
  - Excess bile salt inactivation: bacterial overgrowth, acid pH, binding (cholestyramine)
  - Bile salt loss: disease or resection of terminal ileum

*Impaired mucosal function*
- *Brush border enzyme deficiency*
  - Lactase, sucrase-isomaltase, trehalase deficiency: inherited or acquired
- *Impaired mucosal transport*
  - Global defect: diffuse intestinal disease, bypass or resection
  - Isolated defects: glucose-galactose malabsorption; Hartnup disease; cystinuria; congenital cobalamin deficiency
- *Drug effects*
  - Decreased crypt cell proliferation: colchicine, cytostatic drugs, neomycin
  - Decreased folate absorption: methotrexate, sulfasalazine, phenytoin

*Miscellaneous*
- *Disorders of mesenteric lymphatics*
  - Obstruction; primary ectasia
- *Intestinal ischemia*
- *Serum protein loss*
  - Menetrier disease
  - Lymphatic obstruction
  - Diffuse inflammation
- *Infiltrative disorders*
  - Amyloid
  - Lymphoma
  - Mastocytosis
- *Fibrosis*
  - Diffuse systemic sclerosis
  - Chronic radiation injury

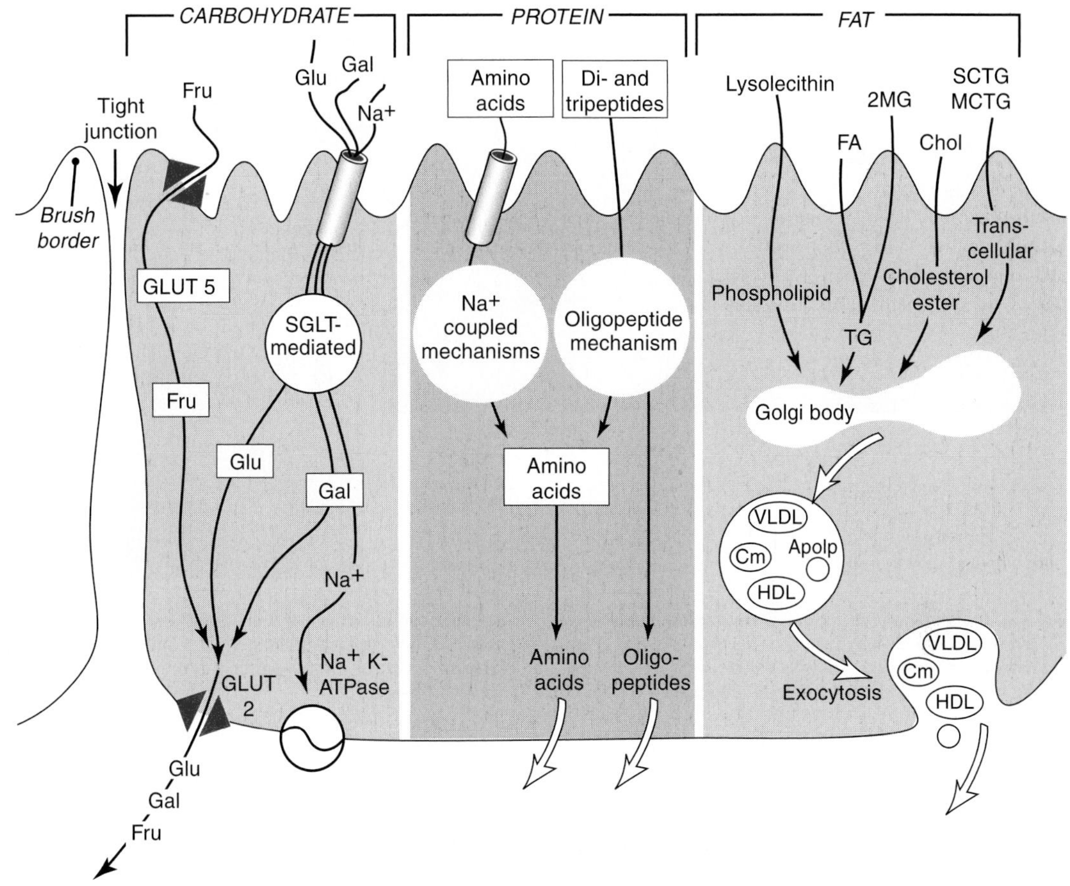


**FIGURE 77.1.** Schematic presentation of absorption of carbohydrate, protein and fat from the small bowel. Glucose transporters (GLUT), sodium-glucose transporters (SGLT) represent special transport mechanisms of absorption across the brush border. Components of absorbed lipid are reassembled in the Golgi body and transported across the cell using a process of exocytosis. 2MG = diglyceride; ApoLP = Apolipoprotein; Cm = chylomicron; FA = fatty acid; Fru = fructose; Gal = galactose; Glu = glucose; GLUT = glucose transporter; HDL = high-density lipoprotein; MCTG = medium-chain triglycerides; SCTG = short-chain triglycerides; SGLT = sodium-glucose co-transporter; TG = triglyceride; VLDL = very low-density lipoprotein.

pancreatic enzyme most vulnerable to tryptic digestion within the intestinal lumen.

### Digestion and absorption of proteins

The hydrolysis of proteins begins in the stomach, where pepsin digests collagen to OH-proline peptides. The action of pancreatic trypsin, chymotrypsin, and elastase produces oligopeptides, which are hydrolyzed at the brush border of the enterocytes to a mixture of tri- and dipeptides and amino acids. These small peptides are efficiently absorbed intact (see Figure 77.1). Carboxypeptidases A and B liberate free amino acids, which are absorbed by several distinct Na-coupled transport systems.

### Digestion and absorption of carbohydrates

Starch, the main dietary carbohydrate, consists of straight glucose chains connected by 1,6-glycosidic bonds. Salivary and pancreatic alpha-amylase splits starch, yielding maltose, maltotriose, and alpha-limit dextrins. Carbohydrate digestion, which involves several enzymes, is completed at the brush border membrane since only monosaccharides are absorbed. Glucose and galactose are actively absorbed by the Na-glucose co-transporter termed glucose transporter, termed SGLT 1. Fructose binds to a transporter termed glucose transporter (GLUT)5, and is taken up by facilitated diffusion. The exit of fructose, glucose, and galactose across the basolateral cell wall is mediated by GLUT2, a

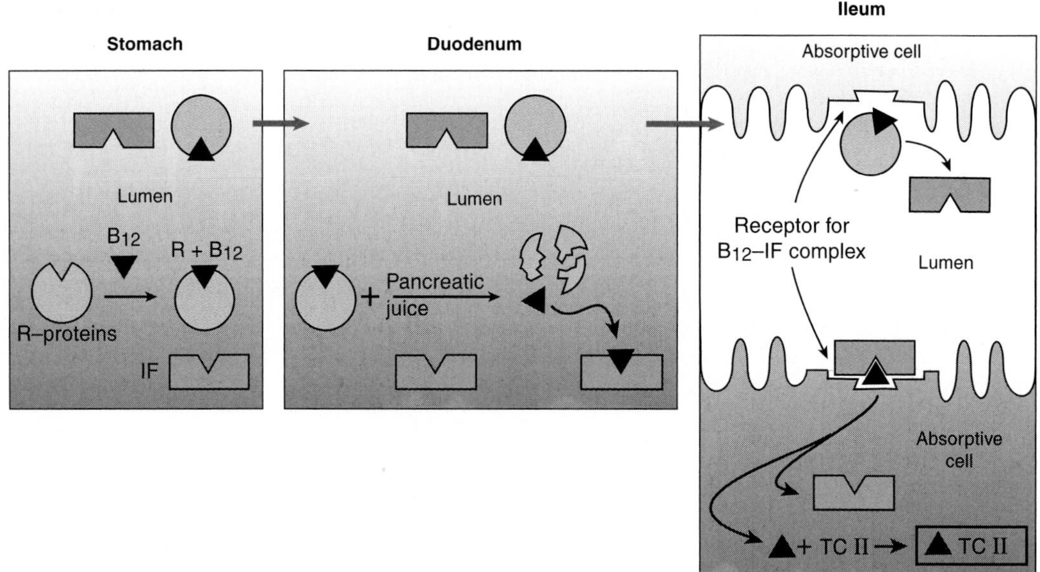


**FIGURE 77.2.** Schematic of vitamin $B_{12}$ (cobalamin) absorption. Lower halves of the three panels show the normal process of $B_{12}$ absorption. The top panels indicated by red lines represent $B_{12}$ malabsorption in pancreatic exocrine insufficiency, in which tryptic digestion of R-proteins is absent. TC II = transco balamin II; IF = intrinsic factor. Note that intrinsic factor binds vitamin $B_{12}$ only in the absence of intact R-proteins.

high capacity, rapidly inducible transport protein (see Figure 77.1).

### Regional absorption

The brush border enzyme, pteroyl polyglutamate hydrolase, acts on dietary folates to produce pteroyl monoglutamate, which is then absorbed. Both activities take place in the duodenum and proximal jejunum. Folate absorption is inhibited by sulfasalazine, phenytoin, and methotrexate. Similarly, the absorption of inorganic ferrous ions and active, vitamin D-dependent Ca2+ transport are limited to the proximal small intestine. By contrast, active reabsorption of bile salts and the uptake of the $B_{12}$-intrinsic factor complex (Figure 77.2) are located in the distal ileum.

## Etiology

The most common cause of impaired intraluminal digestion is deficient pancreatic enzyme secretion due to chronic pancreatitis, cystic fibrosis, or obstruction to the flow of pancreatic juice (see Table 77.1). The steatorrhea in high gastric acid secretory states **(Zollinger-Ellison syndrome)** results from acid inactivation of pancreatic enzymes. Rapid gastric emptying and the altered anatomy created by gastric operations may lead to poor mixing between pancreatic secretions and ingested food. The normal postprandial pancreatic enzyme output is 10 times what is required for food digestion; malabsorption occurs only when pancreatic enzyme output is below 10% of normal. Any process that reduces intraduodenal bile acid concentration may impair fat absorption.

Specific diseases causing malabsorption are discussed in chapter 80. **Disaccharidase deficiencies** are inherited, but may also be acquired with acute or chronic intestinal mucosal injury. Lactase is most vulnerable in this regard. **Diffuse small bowel disease** causes malabsorption of all nutrients, vitamins, and minerals. In contrast, **pancreatic enzyme deficiency** only affects the utilization of nutrients requiring digestion. **Bile salt deficiency,** in turn, impairs the absorption of fat as well as of fat-soluble vitamins (A, D, E, K).

## Diagnostic Evaluation

Clues to malabsorption include **anemia** without apparent blood loss, but with low serum iron, folate, or $B_{12}$; **koilonychia** (spoon nails) seen in iron deficiency; glossitis and cheilitis with folate deficiency, $B_{12}$, and iron deficiency; paresthesias and **tetany** due to $Ca^{2+}$ or $Mg^{2+}$ deficiency; **bleeding diathesis** from vitamin K deficiency; **bulky, malodorous stools** (visible fat droplets suggest pancreatic insufficiency); **spontaneous fractures** due to $Ca^{2+}$ and vitamin D deficiency; and **edema** from **hypoproteinemia.** Weight loss is nonspecific, and more often due to poor food intake than to malabsorption.

### Steatorrhea

*Identifying excess fat excretion is central to evaluating malabsorption.* Because long-chain triglycerides and fatty acids (FA) are not degraded in the colon, stool fat reliably and quantitatively indicates generalized malabsorption. Total FA is measured in a 2- or 3-day stool collection, while the patient receives a regular diet. A high-fat diet is generally neither needed nor feasible. Normal stool fat content is 6–7g/d, but may be as high as 15g/d during severe watery diarrhea. Thus, **steatorrhea** in patients with a stool weight over 600g/d is defined as a stool fat excretion exceeding 15g/d. Qualitative tests for fat malabsorption, while less onerous to perform, are also less accurate; they include Sudan III stain for fecal fat droplets, serum carotene, and breath tests for $^{14}CO_2$ after oral test doses of $^{14}C$-labeled fat compounds.

### Small intestinal biopsy

Mucosal biopsies can be obtained endoscopically or with special instruments from distal duodenum or proximal jejunum. When properly handled, biopsy is highly useful in the diagnostic evaluation of malabsorption (Table 77.2).

### Pancreatic exocrine function

In practice, pancreatic exocrine insufficiency is commonly inferred when pancreatic calcifications are noted on plain x-rays or atrophy on CT scans, or from abnormal pancreatic duct anatomy found during endoscopic retrograde pancreatography. The **secretin test,** the gold standard for assessing pancreatic exocrine function, involves aspiration and analysis of duodenal contents for volume and $HCO_3$ output following IV injection of secretin. It is expensive and requires specially trained personnel. In the **bentiromide (MBT-PABA) test,** pancreatic chymotrypsin hydrolyzes an orally administered peptide; the output of p-aminobenzoic acid thus liberated is measured in a 6-hour urine collection. In 80% of advanced pancreatic insufficiency and steatorrhea, less than 50% of the dose is excreted.

**TABLE 77.2. Uses of Proximal Small Bowel Mucosal Biopsy**

| |
|---|
| *Diagnostic* |
| Whipple disease |
| Amyloidosis |
| Giardiasis |
| Eosinophilic enteritis |
| Lymphangiectasia |
| Mastocytosis |
| Opportunistic pathogens (immunosuppressed patients) |
| Immunoglobulin A (IgA) deficiency |
| Lymphoma |
| *Suggestive* |
| Tropical sprue |
| Idiopathic intestinal pseudo-obstruction |
| Celiac sprue |
| Bacterial overgrowth (aspirated fluid) |
| Antroduodenal Crohn disease |

### Vitamin $B_{12}$ (cobalamin) absorption

**Schilling Test** (see Figure 135.4) is used to assess $B_{12}$ absorption. Essentially, the 24-hour urinary excretion of orally administered, radio-labeled $B_{12}$ is measured (Stage I). An abnormal Stage I establishes $B_{12}$ malabsorption. In Stage II, intrinsic factor (IF) is added to the oral test dose. Its results will be normal if the defect is absence of gastric IF (pernicious anemia). Four additional possibilities may explain abnormal Stage I and Stage II test results: (1) ileal disease or resection; (2) congenital absence of the ileal receptor for the $B_{12}$-IF complex; (3) $B_{12}$ uptake by bacterial overgrowth in the small intestine or by D. latum, the fish tapeworm; and (4) pancreatic insufficiency. Nonspecific salivary and gastric R-proteins successfully compete with IF for binding to $B_{12}$ at the acidic gastric pH. Pancreatic proteases destroy the R-proteins in the duodenum; the liberated $B_{12}$ then combines with IF, which resists digestion (see Figure 77.2). In pancreatic exocrine insufficiency, where proteolytic activity in the duodenum is low, the $B_{12}$-R-protein complex remains intact, but no ileal receptor exists for the absorption of this complex. Therefore, stages I and II of the test may be abnormal in patients with pancreatic insufficiency; it normalizes when the test is repeated with the administration of adequate doses of pancreatic enzyme supplements. It is important to note that clinical testing for serum vitamin $B_{12}$ levels may be falsely elevated during disease states, and other markers including plasma homocysteine and malonyl dialdehyde may better reflect the degree of vitamin $B_{12}$ deficiency.

### Breath tests

Malabsorption of test compounds can be surmised if their breakdown by colonic bacteria produces highly diffusible, measurable, exhaled gases. Incremental rises in breath $H_2$ concentration during colonic carbohydrate fermentation is widely used to detect carbohydrate malabsorption—for example, lactose and sucrose breath tests for diagnosing lactase and sucrase-isomaltase deficiency, respectively, and a glucose breath test to detect anaerobic bacterial overgrowth in the small bowel. The time of the rise in breath $H_2$ after an oral dose of a poorly absorbed sugar, such as lactulose, gives an indication of the orocecal transit time.

### Miscellaneous tests

While most serum proteins entering the GI tract are digested, reabsorbed, or degraded, serum $\alpha_1$-antitrypsin largely appears intact in the stool. Its GI clearance can be measured using serum level and its daily output in the stool. Other tests can suggest the malabsorption of specific nutrients—for example, low serum folate, $B_{12}$, iron, albumin, calcium, and magnesium; serum vitamin

D, urinary $Ca^{2+}$, and elevated alkaline phosphatase (bone fraction), and prothrombin time.

### Management

Treatment of malabsorption disorders is discussed in chapters 80 and 95. Dietary management is discussed here. Fat intake should be curtailed to 40–60 g daily because high stool fat causes diarrhea and abdominal discomfort. Carbohydrate restriction may be similarly needed in intestinal disease, but not in pancreatic insufficiency where little carbohydrate malabsorption occurs. Patients with infectious diarrhea and those with diffuse intestinal diseases frequently have transient lactase deficiency, and dairy products should be avoided. Medium chain triglycerides (MCT; fatty acids of $C_8$ and $C_{10}$ chain length) can be absorbed intact, without the need for digestion and solubilization, and have theoretical advantages in pancreatic insufficiency and bile salt deficiency states. However, MCT substitution for dietary fat leads to weight gain only in patients with cystic fibrosis and may actually cause osmotic diarrhea. Vitamin, calcium, and iron deficits should first be corrected by the oral route, but parenteral supplementation may have to be employed when the underlying malabsorption prevents a therapeutic response.

# CHAPTER 78 GASTROINTESTINAL HEMORRHAGE

### Definitions and Etiology

Blood loss from the gastrointestinal tract may be gross (obvious to the observer) or occult (not obvious). *Gross* bleeding is generally acute on presentation, with or without, generally without associated hypovolemia. GI bleeding may present as hematemesis, melena, hematochezia, or a combination of these. *Hematemesis* is vomiting blood that can be either red or acid-altered, appearing like "coffee grounds." It usually signifies bleeding proximal to the ligament of Treitz. *Melena* is black, tarry, foul-smelling stools, usually due to acute bleeding anywhere between the proximal GI tract and the right colon. *Hematochezia* is the passing of maroon or bright red stools originating from any site in the GI tract; when this site is the proximal GI tract, the bleeding is brisk enough to advance rapidly to the rectum. Chronic GI bleeding usually is occult. Patients with chronic GI bleeding present with symptoms of anemia—for example, dyspnea, fatigue, syncope, and angina. Others are identified by a positive fecal occult blood test, or on screening tests showing iron deficiency anemia.

**TABLE 78.1. Some Causes of Gastrointestinal Bleeding**

*Esophagus*
Esophagitis, varices, ulcer, neoplasm
*Stomach and duodenum*
Gastric erosions, Mallory-Weiss tear, ulcer, varices, neoplasm, vascular anomalies
*Small bowel*
Meckel's diverticulum, Crohn disease, infarction, vascular anomalies, aortoenteric fistula
*Colon*
Inflammatory bowel disease, infectious colitis, ischemia, neoplasm, vascular anomalies, diverticulosis
*Rectum/anus*
Proctitis, solitary ulcer, neoplasm, hemorrhoids
*Systemic conditions*
Thrombocytopenia, coagulopathies, chronic renal failure, swallowed blood

Among some of the causes of GI bleeding shown in Table 78.1, a few account for most of the bleeding episodes encountered clinically. More than 90% of upper-GI bleeds are secondary to peptic ulcer disease, gastric erosions, Mallory-Weiss tears, and esophageal varices (Figure 78.1). Common lesions causing lower-GI bleeding are hemorrhoids, diverticula, neoplasms, and colitis.

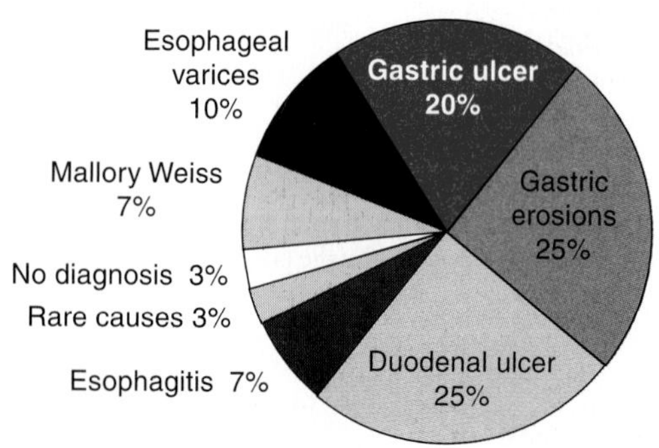


**FIGURE 78.1. Etiology of upper GI bleeding.**

### Management

The approach to a patient with acute GI bleeding begins with prompt assessment of hemodynamic stability. Patients with orthostatic hypotension or shock should first be stabilized with IV infusion of crystalloids; blood is sent for crossmatching, a complete count including platelets, coagulation profile, liver tests, electrolytes, blood urea nitrogen, and creatinine before embarking on diagnostic investigations. Upper GI tract bleeding is associated with a rise in blood urea nitrogen and, unlike renal failure, there is no parallel elevation of serum creatinine. Patients with acute GI bleeding are best managed in an intensive care unit with early surgical consultation. The amount of visible bleeding does not reliably indicate the degree of blood loss. For example, a little blood near the mouth or lower rectum might appear more impressive than bleeding that cannot be easily seen. In early, acute GI bleeding, hematocrit is unreliable, because it does not decrease until the extracellular fluid shifts into the intravascular compartment, which takes several hours. The need for blood transfusion is dictated by the presence of ongoing bleeding, hemodynamic instability arising from volume loss, and pre-existing medical conditions that lower the patient's tolerance to blood loss. An initially low hematocrit with relatively stable vital signs suggests chronic GI blood loss, particularly if the mean corpuscular volume (MCV) is low. Such cases do not require urgent resuscitation unless the anemia has exacerbated an associated condition such as heart failure or angina pectoris. Because there is no volume depletion, packed RBC should be transfused slowly, with a close watch for volume overload.

The timing of further diagnostic procedures depends on the rate of ongoing bleeding and the need for urgent therapeutic intervention. After resuscitation, patients with acute, significant GI bleeding require immediate diagnostic procedures, usually in the form of emergent endoscopic intervention. Patients with chronic GI blood loss usually can be investigated electively. A nasogastric tube may be passed first to examine the aspirate. A positive Gastroccult test on the gastric aspirate could be secondary to nasogastric tube-related trauma. However, an upper GI lesion is the likely source if the aspirate shows fresh or altered blood. Aspirate negative for visible blood, however, does not rule out an upper GI source, as seen, at times, with lesions distal to the pylorus. Endoscopy most accurately, rapidly, and safely identifies the bleeding site, with the additional advantage of allowing therapeutic interventions and obtaining tissue for histology. Upper GI endoscopy, anoscopy, proctosigmoidoscopy, and colonoscopy are some of the commonly performed endoscopic procedures. The small bowel can be evaluated by enteroscopy, single or double-contrast barium examination, or by capsule endoscopy.

In 5% to 10% of cases, endoscopy may not identify the site of bleeding, either because the lesion is beyond its reach or because brisk bleeding and large blood clots prevent adequate visualization. Angiography may be used in these patients, but it will not detect slow or intermittent bleeding. A radioisotope-labeled red cell scan, although more sensitive in this context, may not localize the bleeding site correctly.

Most patients with GI bleeding recover without active therapeutic intervention, especially those with esophagitis, gastritis, Mallory-Weiss tear, peptic ulcers, angiodysplasia, or diverticulosis. Those who continue to bleed or experience recurrent bleeding require urgent therapy. Significant comorbid conditions and visible active bleeding, a visible blood vessel, or a fresh blood clot in the ulcer base seen on endoscopy indicate a high risk of continued or recurrent bleeding. Many effective endoscopic therapies (e.g., thermocoagulation, electrocoagulation, argon plasma coagulation, laser photocoagulation, and submucosal injection of a sclerosant or epinephrine) can be applied in these patients. Bleeding esophageal and gastric varices may require either injection sclerotherapy or banding; other methods for controlling variceal bleeding include the insertion of an endoluminal compression device (Sengstaken-Blakemore or Minnesota tube) and IV vasopressin or somatostatin analog and transjugular intrahepatic portosystemic shunting (TIPS). Neoplastic lesions, such as polyps, can be removed endoscopically. Selective arterial embolization or vasopressin injection are options when endoscopy fails. Early surgery is indicated for persistent and life-threatening bleeding and in patients over 60 years of age, in whom the mortality risk rises with every episode of re-bleeding.

# CHAPTER 79 NONMALIGNANT DISEASES OF THE ESOPHAGUS

The esophagus is a hollow, muscular conduit that conveys swallowed material from the oropharynx to the stomach and prevents the reflux of gastric contents. Esophageal muscle, along with the cricopharyngeus, and the lower fibers of the inferior pharyngeal constrictor function as the upper esophageal sphincter (UES), which marks the proximal end of the esophagus. The esophageal body, about 25 cm long, terminates in the lower esophageal sphincter (LES), which has important functional properties but no distinctive anatomic features.

Swallowing is initiated voluntarily by pressing the tip of the tongue against the hard palate, after which the tongue rises against the hard palate, propelling the bolus back into the pharynx. The rest of the swallowing action is a reflex. The muscles of the soft palate and nasopharynx contract, shutting off the posterior nasal opening. The larynx is pulled upward and forward, away from the path of the food bolus and toward the base of the tongue, closing the airway, as the epiglottis retroverts to occlude the laryngeal orifice. Pharyngeal contractions move the bolus toward the esophageal introitus. Muscle relaxation, pull by the anteriorly and superiorly moving larynx, and bolus pressure, open the UES. Peristaltic esophageal contraction wave continues downward while the LES relaxes to allow the bolus to pass into the stomach.

The normal swallow wave, or *primary peristalsis*, comprises sequential contractions of the body of the esophagus starting at the upper end and propagating downward. It is associated with complete relaxation of the LES (Figure 79.1). Propagating motility patterns induced by esophageal distention are termed *secondary peristalsis*. Tertiary contractions occur simultaneously and are nonpropagating; they may be spontaneous or swallow-induced.

## Gastroesophageal Reflux Disease

Gastroesophageal reflux disease (GERD), one of the most common GI disorders, is characterized by clinical symptoms or histopathological changes produced by episodes of gastroesophageal reflux (GER).

### Etiology and Pathophysiology

Tonic contraction of the LES produces a pressure of 15 to 30 mm Hg above intragastric pressure. Normally, the LES tone helps prevent gastroesophageal reflux. During GER, gastric contents enter the esophagus through three major suggested mechanisms. During *transient lower esophageal sphincter relaxation* (tLESR), the LES relaxes without any antecedent swallow, and the relaxation persists longer than with swallow-induced relaxation. This may predispose to GER, especially during the postprandial period. *Hypotensive LES* (which is present in a few patients, including those with GERD due to scleroderma) allows free GER. Thirdly, sudden rises in *intra-abdominal pressure* may exceed the LES resting pressure and induce GER. When a hiatal hernia is present, the "pinchcock" effect of the crural diaphragm on the LES is absent, which facilitates GER with rises in intraluminal pressure. Refluxed material may become trapped in the hernia sac and becomes available for return to the esophagus. Nearly all the refluxate is cleared by esophageal peristalsis. The

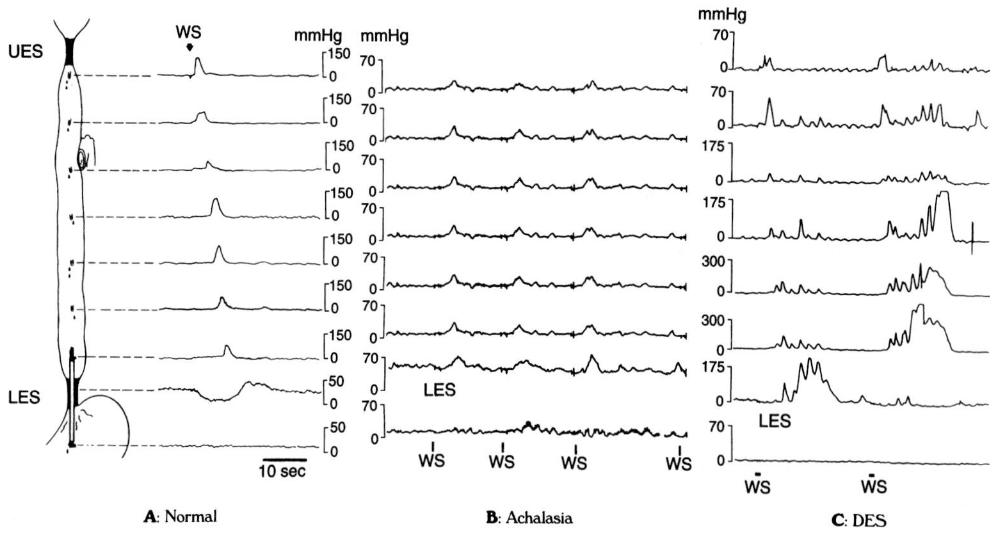


**FIGURE 79.1.** Esophageal manometry. A. Normal peristalsis showing propagating contractions in the body of the esophagus with complete LES relaxation. B. Patient with achalasia showing simultaneous low amplitude contractions in the body of the esophagus with incomplete LES relaxation. C. Patient with diffuse esophageal spasm (DES) showing peristaltic contractions followed by simultaneous high amplitude contractions. UES = upper esophageal sphincter; LES = lower esophageal sphincter; WS = water swallow.

minimal residual acidic material is eventually neutralized by swallowed saliva. The time that the esophagus remains acidified is called the *esophageal acid clearance time*.

Gastroesophageal reflux occurs regularly even in healthy people, usually secondary to tLESRs. GERD develops when there is a disturbed balance between the potency of the refluxate and the ability of the esophagus to withstand (mucosal resistance) and clear the refluxate. Although in most of the cases no predisposing condition is present, GERD also can occur in a variety of clinical settings. In scleroderma, the LES pressure is low and the amplitude of esophageal peristalsis decreased, predisposing to both GER *and* longer esophageal acid clearance time. Pregnancy-related reflux is secondary to raised intra-abdominal pressure and hormones lowering the LES pressure. Fatty meals, coffee, tea, alcohol, and smoking lower the LES pressure and delay gastric emptying. Certain drugs (calcium channel blockers and anticholinergics) also lower the LES pressure.

### Clinical Features

Most patients with GERD report frequent heartburn. However, heartburn may be absent in some patients with esophagitis or with complications such as esophageal stricture and Barrett's esophagus (in which the native esophageal squamous epithelium is replaced by specialized columnar epithelium). Sour and bitter fluid—occasionally even food—may regurgitate into the pharynx or mouth. Often, these symptoms are induced or worsened by bending forward or lifting. Dysphagia usually is due to peptic stricture, but it may also be secondary to esophagitis related dysmotility and decreased esophageal compliance. In some patients, esophageal acidification leads to hypersalivation (water brash), whereas others report chest pain. Gastroesophageal reflux with regurgitation/aspiration also can lead to chronic cough, pneumonia, pharyngitis, posterior laryngitis, worsening of asthma, chronic sinusitis, and dental caries (supraesophageal or extraesophageal complications of reflux disease)

### Diagnosis

In most cases, a careful history is sufficient to make a diagnosis. These patients can be started on acid suppression treatment. Endoscopy is indicated for symptoms refractory to medical therapy, dysphagia, odynophagia, chest pain, evaluation and dilatation of peptic strictures, weight loss, anemia, and GI bleeding, and to exclude Barrett's metaplasia. Patients with GERD may have normal-appearing esophageal mucosa also called as non-erosive reflux disease (N.E.R.D.). The differential diagnosis of GERD includes infections (e.g., candida, herpes, cytomegalovirus) or pill-induced esophagitis, dyspepsia secondary to peptic ulcer or biliary tract diseases, and chest pain due to coronary heart disease or esophageal motor disorders. Barium swallow may show GER, any associated motility disorder, and strictures. Two tests are useful in relating the symptoms of heartburn and chest pain to the reflux. One is the *Bernstein esophageal acid perfusion test*. Through a tube placed in the mid-esophagus, normal saline is infused and is switched to 0.1 N HCl without the patient's knowledge. If this reproduces the patient's usual symptoms, the HCl is replaced by normal saline, which should relieve the symptoms. The other test is *ambulatory esophageal pH monitoring* (usually for 24 hours) using an intraluminal pH probe placed transnasally. Evaluation of the tracings includes the percent of time the esophageal pH was acidic (pH $<4.0$), the number of reflux episodes, and the temporal relation between symptoms and the occurrence of reflux (symptom correlation index). Esophageal manometry is recommended prior to planned antireflux surgery.

### Management

Treatment of GERD ranges from simple measures (e.g., dietary control, sleeping with the head of the bed elevated, antacids as required, weight control) in uncomplicated cases to maximum acid suppression in patients with high-grade esophagitis (Figure 79.2). Acid suppression, using a proton pump inhibitor, is necessary in patients with persistent or severe symptoms and those with erosive esophagitis. I.V. PPI can be given to patients with erosive esophagitis who cannot take oral medication. Longer duration of treatment (2-3 months) may be required in those with supraesophageal symptoms. In these patients, maximum acid suppression also may be used as a therapeutic trial to determine if the supraesophageal symptoms are related to GERD. Prokinetic drugs (e.g., metoclopramide) raise LES pressure, and increase gastric emptying; they also can be used either alone or with acid suppression. Surgical management—that is, a fundoplication procedure—is reserved for those who have failed medical treatment, those who prefer not to be on long-term medications or are non-compliant (e.g., mentally retarded patients), or those with GERD-related complications (e.g., recurrent aspiration pneumonia). Endoscopic gastric plication using suturing devices and endoscopic application of radiofrequency to the LES are some of the newer techniques being used to treat GERD.

## ■ Complications of GERD

Benign esophageal stricture most commonly results from peptic esophagitis. Most patients present with slowly progressive dysphagia, although some may present acutely with food impaction. Distinction must be made from malignant strictures, motility disorders (acha-

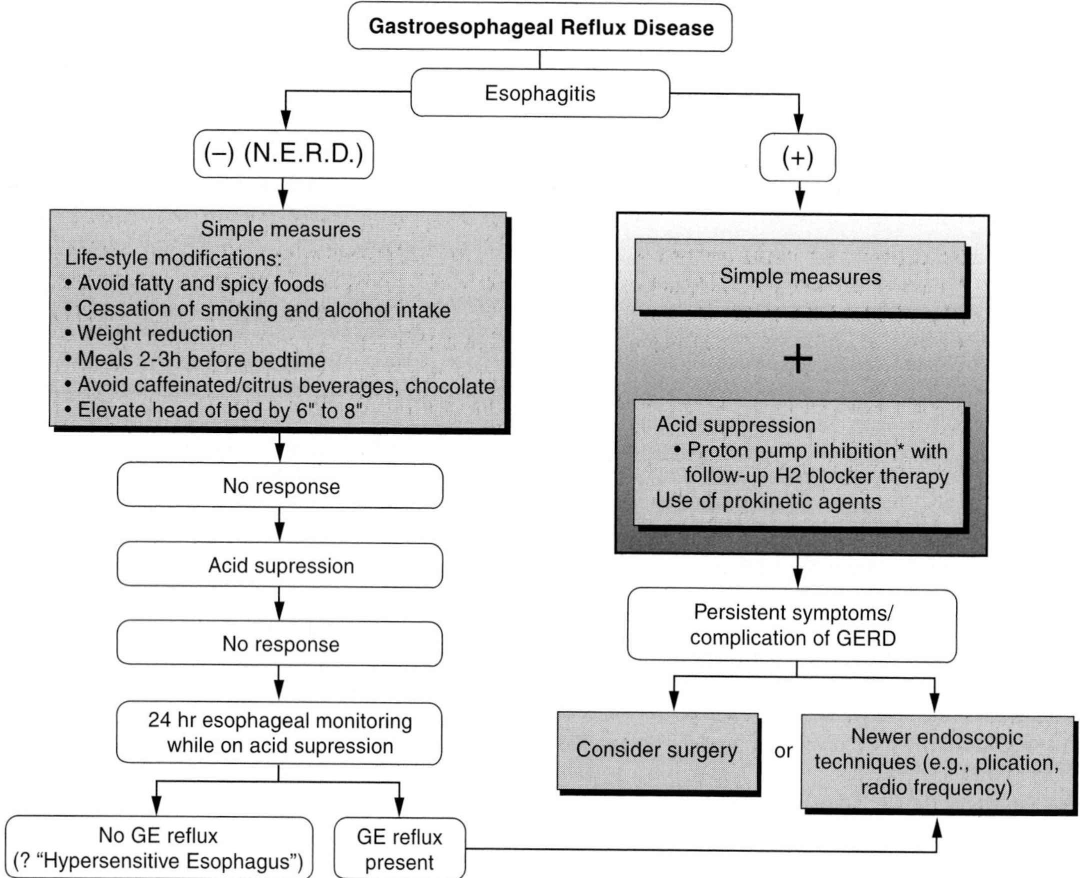


**FIGURE 79.2. Management of gastroesophageal reflux disease (GERD). * = In patients with erosive esophagitis whose symptoms recur while receiving $H_2$ blockers, proton pump inhibitors can be used on a long-term basis.**

lasia), strictures from other causes (infection, pill injury, lye ingestion), and esophageal webs, most commonly the Schatzki ring. Malignancy must be ruled out by biopsy, and dysphagia relieved by mechanical dilatation. Vigorous antireflux measures also are needed. Patients with *esophageal ulcer* may report retrosternal chest pain, odynophagia, or epigastric pain. Some may have acute bleeding as the first and only symptom. The differential diagnosis includes ulcers caused by infection, pill injury, or malignancy. Endoscopic evaluation and biopsy are a must. Bleeding in GERD usually is chronic and due to esophagitis. *Acute bleeding* in GERD usually is due to esophageal ulcer. Rigorous medical therapy, as outlined, is called for. Occasionally, chronic bleeding arises from an ulcer within a sliding hiatal hernia at the level of the diaphragmatic hiatus.

In *Barrett's esophagus,* the native esophageal squamous epithelium is replaced by specialized columnar epithelium, most commonly with goblet cells and a villous pattern, representing incomplete intestinal metaplasia and, less commonly, with cardia- or fundic-type mucosa. This change starts at the gastroesophageal junction and progresses upward during the course of GERD. Barrett's mucosa by itself evokes no symptoms. While more resistant to the effects of acid reflux, the new mucosa is prone to dysplasia and adenocarcinoma. The risk of such neoplasia being 30–50 times that of the general population, it calls for regular surveillance endoscopic biopsies. Esophagectomy is recommended for high-grade dysplasia. The underlying GER calls for vigorous therapy; however, the presence and extent of Barrett's mucosa are not alleviated by medical or surgical anti-reflux therapy. Although photodynamic therapy (PDT) has been used successfully for treating esophageal cancer, its role in ablating dysplasia associated with Barrett's esophagus requires further evaluation. In PDT, a photosensitizing agent (e.g., hematoporphyrin) is injected intravenously, which then preferentially concentrates within the dysplastic tissue or tumor. The cytotoxic effect is achieved by activating the compound endoscopically, using a laser of a specific wavelength.

## Motility Disorders of the Oropharynx and Esophagus

### Oropharyngeal Disorders

Oropharyngeal motility disorders causing dysphagia can be due to a variety of neuromuscular causes. Symptoms may arise gradually or abruptly, depending on the etiology. Patients may report difficulty initiating a swallow, pharyngeal food residue after swallowing, nasal regurgitation, food getting held up in the throat, and coughing while swallowing. Some may have recurrent pneumonia. Video fluoroscopy during barium swallow, direct endoscopic visualization of the pharynx during swallowing, and pharyngeal manometry can be used to assess oropharyngeal dysphagia. Treatment is directed at the primary cause. Many patients with cerebrovascular accidents recover with time. Others may require training in swallowing exercises best supervised by a speech therapist.

### Achalasia

Achalasia is a primary esophageal motility disorder featuring progressive dysphagia for liquids and solids, and delayed esophageal emptying, in the absence of an organic obstructing lesion. Postulated but unproven mechanisms include a viral etiology and defects in the esophageal neural pathways. Primarily, there is loss of ganglion cells in the esophageal myenteric plexus. Smooth muscle denervation leads to weak, nonprogressive, esophageal contractions, incomplete swallow-induced LES relaxation, and elevation of the basal LES pressure. An identical disorder occurs with chronic Chagas disease, where *Trypanosoma cruzi* destroys the intramural ganglia. Although achalasia may present at any age, the onset of symptoms is usually in the fifth to sixth decade. The yearly incidence is about 1 per 100,000 population.

The slowly progressive dysphagia may be associated with weight loss. Regurgitation of food while bending or recumbent is common, and may lead to pulmonary aspiration and pneumonia. Unlike gastroesophageal reflux, regurgitation in achalasia usually is not associated with heartburn. Some patients report chest pain (see the secion on "vigorous achalasia" later in this chapter). Esophageal cancer may be associated, especially in those who have had no (or unsatisfactory) treatment. Plain radiographs may reveal a widened mediastinum with an air-fluid level and no gastric air bubble. Esophagogram shows no peristalsis in the distal two thirds of the esophagus, and the lower esophagus tapers to a beak-like ending (Figure 79.3A). The esophagus may be of normal caliber or dilated and tortuous, and may contain retained food. Endoscopy should be done to rule out a cancer (of the gastric cardia or fundus) that mimics achalasia-like symptoms, the so called *pseudoachalasia.*

Characteristic findings on manometry (see Figure 79.1) include absent peristalsis, weak or repetitive contractions in the esophageal body, incomplete LES relaxation, raised LES, and intraesophageal pressures. The LES pressure may rise paradoxically after cholecystokinin octapeptide injection. A subset of patients have chest pain and high-amplitude, nonpropagating esophageal contractions *(vigorous achalasia).* Calcium channel-blocking agents (e.g., nifedipine) or nitrates may bring mild or modest symptomatic improvement and may be tried initially. However, patients eventually require pneumatic dilatation of the LES or surgery (Heller myotomy). Endoscopic injection of a muscle-weakening toxin (botulinum toxin) into the LES can be tried as a primary treatment, especially in those in whom surgery is contraindicated.

### Diffuse Esophageal Spasm

Diffuse esophageal spasm (DES) is a rare, idiopathic primary esophageal motility disorder in which high-amplitude tertiary contractions occur with normal peristalsis. The lower two thirds of the esophagus shows diffuse muscular thickening, but ganglion cells are preserved. Odynophagia, dysphagia, and substernal chest pain simulating angina, with radiation to the neck, jaw, shoulders, and back, and even relieved by nitroglycerin, are the main symptoms. The pain may be spontaneous or incited by emotional stress or drinking hot or cold liquids, but is not related to exercise or relieved by rest. The dysphagia varies in severity and may not accompany chest pain. Esophagogram shows tertiary contractions (Figure 79.3B); manometry shows more than 10% simultaneous contractions during water swallows and intermittent normal peristalsis (see Figure 79.1). Reducing stress, avoiding cold or hot foods, and therapy with long-acting nitrates and calcium channel blockers may help. Nitroglycerin may relieve acute attacks of pain. Pneumatic dilatation may help some patients while a long esophagomyotomy may benefit those with severe, intractable symptoms.

### Esophageal Webs and Rings

An *esophageal web* is structure 2 to 3 mm thick composed of mucosa and submucosa. A *ring* is a thicker structure containing mucosal and muscle tissue (except

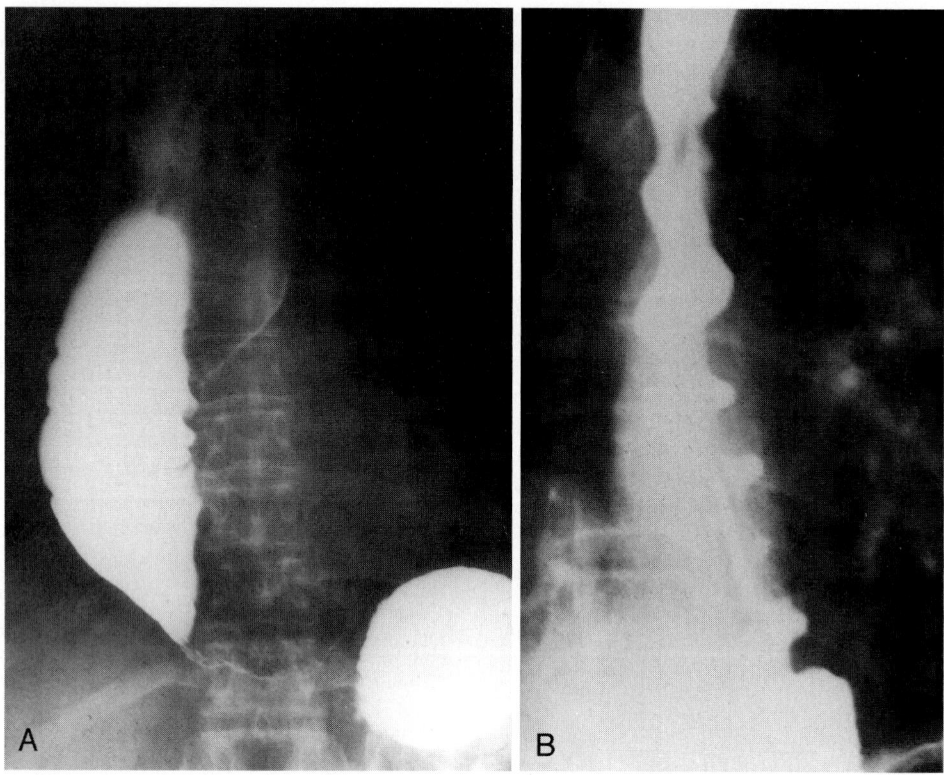


**FIGURE 79.3.** A. Achalasia. Barium swallow showing dilated esophagus, tapering to a beak-like narrowing at the lower end. B. Diffuse esophageal spasm with tertiary contractions.

Schatzki's ring, which is really a web). An anterior web at the upper end of the esophagus is seen in *Plummer Vinson syndrome (Patterson Kelly syndrome).* If dysphagia and iron deficiency anemia are associated, it is termed *sideropenic dysphagia.* Most patients are middle-aged or elderly women. A predisposition to develop postcricoid carcinoma is present. Esophagogram shows these webs best in the lateral projection. Circumferential cervical webs may require forceful dilatation.

The lower esophageal web (Schatzki's ring) is a persistent, annular, thin narrowing of the esophagus at the squamocolumnar junction, with squamous epithelium above and columnar mucosa below. Patients present with intermittent dysphagia. Typically, a bolus of meat gets impacted, and is then regurgitated; the patient then continues eating without further dysphagia. Occasionally, sudden, total dysphagia may occur, requiring endoscopic disimpaction. Schatzki's rings are best demonstrated by barium swallow. Dysphagia due to subtle webs and rings can be evaluated by barium marshmallow swallow study. Thicker rings probably represent short strictures due to reflux disease. Endoscopy is required to differentiate between lower esophageal ring and an annular stricture, which can be secondary to cancer. Those causing symptoms require dilatation.

## Other Conditions

### *Infectious Esophagitis*

*Candida albicans* is part of normal gut flora. Conditions that alter the normal gut ecology lead to colonization. Invasion of tissue by *Candida esophagitis* usually occurs with defects in body immunity (e.g., AIDS, leukemia, lymphoma, congenital immunodeficiency states, and chemo- or immunosuppressive therapy). It also can follow medical conditions such as diabetes mellitus, adrenal insufficiency, and malnutrition. Retention of food in the esophagus, such as occurs in esophageal stricture, diverticula, and achalasia, also can predispose to Candida esophagitis. The condition may be asymptomatic or may lead to retrosternal pain and odynophagia. Oral thrush is present in most cases. If untreated, mucosal sloughing and perforation may occur. Stricture may follow ulcerative esophagitis. Double-contrast barium esophagogram shows mucosal lesions—plaques, inflammation, shaggy outline, ulcers, or strictures. Endoscopy may show white plaques, confluent pseudomembranes, mucosal friability, ulceration, bleeding, and sloughing. Because the fungus is a normal commensal, brushing and cultures are not diagnostic. Only biopsies can diagnose tissue invasion accurately. Based on the severity of the esophagitis, one may use luminally active drugs (e.g., nystatin), systemically acting oral drugs (e.g., ketoconazole), or IV medications (e.g., amphotericin B). Oral drugs also are used prophylactically in immunosuppressed patients.

*Herpes simplex virus (HSV) esophagitis* can occur in normal or immunocompromised hosts. HSV invades the squamous epithelium, forming vesicles that slough. Discrete ulcers can coalesce, leading to widespread denudation of the esophageal mucosa. Patients usually report retrosternal pain, odynophagia, nausea, vomiting, and hematemesis. A presumptive diagnosis can be made if oral HSV infection is evident. Esophagogram shows multiple esophageal ulcers. Because HSV primarily invades the squamous epithelium, endoscopic biopsies are taken from the edge of an ulcer. HSV is identified by histology, immunohistology, or culture. Patients with intact immunity heal spontaneously, but immunodeficient patients require prophylaxis or treatment with acyclovir. Acyclovir-resistant strains may require foscarnet.

*Cytomegalovirus (CMV) esophagitis* is seen in immunosuppressed patients. It may be acquired (e.g., from blood product transfusion, organ transplant) or activated from a latent state. Unlike HSV, which infects squamous epithelium, CMV invades submucosal fibroblasts and endothelial cells, thus making endoscopic biopsies from the center and not the edge of an ulcer more relevant for its diagnosis. The lesions of CMV start as serpiginous ulcers that coalesce to form giant ulcers, usually in the mid- and lower esophagus. Patients report nausea, vomiting, odynophagia, or hematemesis, but unlike candida or HSV, acute severe retrosternal pain is unusual. Barium study may show a large esophageal ulcer. Endoscopic biopsies should be examined by routine histology, immunohistology, and culture. Ganciclovir is effective for prevention and treatment of CMV infection. Patients in whom it is refractory to ganciclovir can be given foscarnet.

## Esophageal Injuries

Accidental or suicidal ingestion of corrosive material (e.g., lye, drain cleaners, mineral acids such as HCl, $H_2SO_4$) can cause significant esophageal damage, leading to severe inflammation, bleeding, perforation, and long strictures. The presence or absence of oral burns correlates poorly with the degree of esophageal involvement. Urgent endoscopy is required to assess the extent of esophageal and upper GI tract injury. Treatment usually is supportive. Corticosteroids have been tried, with variable success, to reduce the degree of inflammation and subsequent fibrosis. Patients with lye injury of the esophagus are prone to develop esophageal cancer. *Pill injury* of the esophagus occurs when pills get held up in the esophagus, mostly at the level of the aortic arch, causing localized mucosal damage. Quinidine, iron salts, tetracycline, NSAIDs, and potassium are common offenders. The size, shape, and coating of the pill, and the habit of swallowing them without or with only minimum water, have all been implicated in the pathogenesis of pill injury. Most of these injuries occur in patients with a normal esophagus. Symptoms are chest pain, odynophagia, GI bleeding, perforation, or dysphagia secondary to a stricture. Most pill injuries resolve within 6 weeks. Esophageal injuries also follow radiotherapy, chemotherapy, and sclerotherapy or banding of esophageal varices.

## Mallory-Weiss Syndrome

Vomiting and retching generate high gastric pressures that can cause a longitudinal tear in the gastric mucosa just below the gastroesophageal junction that can extend into the lower esophagus. Patients often report vomiting gastric contents first, followed by bright red blood. Some patients lack a prior history of vomiting. Endoscopy is the best means of confirming the diagnosis, although the lesion can easily be missed. If an active bleeding site is identified, it can be treated endoscopically. Some patients may require surgical exploration. In most cases, the bleeding stops spontaneously.

### Perforation

Esophageal perforation can be either spontaneous or traumatic. Spontaneous perforation could follow vomiting (Boerhaave syndrome), esophageal ulcers, caustic injuries, pill injuries, infections, or neoplasms. Traumatic perforation may follow blunt or penetrating injuries or could be iatrogenic (instrumentation or surgery). The most common sites are the cervical and lower thoracic esophagus. Patients report chest pain. Fever and signs of mediastinitis, subcutaneous emphysema, or pleural effusion may be noted. Pleural effusions characteristically have a low pH, high amylase (salivary), abundant bacteria, and, sometimes, food particles. Lower esophageal perforation can mimic an acute upper abdominal crisis. Chest radiograph may reveal pleural effusion, pneumomediastinum, or subcutaneous air. Imaging with water-soluble contrast is invaluable in detecting intrathoracic perforation. Endoscopy is useless and unsafe, because it may extend an incomplete perforation during intubation or air insufflation. Contamination by saliva and food is avoided by not giving any food or fluids by mouth until follow-up water-soluble contrast study shows no leakage (usually around 2 weeks). Anticholinergics may be given to reduce salivary flow. Almost all patients require broad-spectrum antibiotics. Contaminated perforations and those that communicate with the pleural space or abdominal cavity require immediate surgery. However, in practice, most spontaneous perforations do require surgery, given their late recognition and significant contamination. An instrumentation-related perforation can be treated conservatively, provided it is recognized early. Perforation complicating esophageal cancer can be treated by placing an esophageal endoprosthesis.

# CHAPTER 80 CARCINOMA OF THE ESOPHAGUS

## Epidemiology

Delayed diagnosis and resultant incurability make esophageal cancer one of the most dismal of all cancer diagnoses. Several thousand people die with esophageal cancer annually. Despite advances in diagnosis and treatment, 5-year survival rates are less than 10%. Squamous cell carcinoma and adenocarcinoma are the main types of esophageal cancers. Although the *squamous cell type* is one of the most common cancers worldwide, it is relatively uncommon in North America. In the United States, it shows a distinct (3:1) preponderance among older (seventh decade) men. African-American men are at higher risk. Predisposing factors are alcohol consumption, smoking, corrosive esophageal injury, Plummer-Vinson syndrome with anemia, and achalasia. *Adenocarcinoma,* which arises from Barrett's mucosa or esophageal mucous glands, accounts for one third of esophageal cancers, and its incidence is rising among Caucasian men. Gastroesophageal reflux disease can predispose to the development of adenocarcinoma of the esophagus.

## Clinical Features and Management

Most patients present with recent dysphagia for solids that rapidly progresses to dysphagia for liquids. Odynophagia and bleeding also are common. More than half of patients note significant weight loss. Some experience pulmonary symptoms related to esophageal obstruction and aspiration or to tracheoesophageal fistula, or hoarseness due to paralysis of the recurrent laryngeal nerve. The chest radiograph may show metastases or complications such as pneumonia. The esophagogram may show a stricturing, polypoid, or ulcerated lesion (Figure 80.1). Endoscopy is essential for tissue diagnosis. Endoscopic ultrasound, CT scan, bronchoscopy, lymph node biopsy, and mediastinoscopy may all be required for staging, which is TNM-based.

Because the esophagus lacks serosa, most esophageal tumors have spread by the time of diagnosis. The survival rate for adenocarcinoma of the esophagus is similar to that for squamous cell carcinoma. Only about 50% of patients with esophageal cancer are considered operable, and less than half of these are resectable, leaving palliation as the only viable option for the majority of these patients at initial presentation. The major goal of palliation is to relieve dysphagia, which is

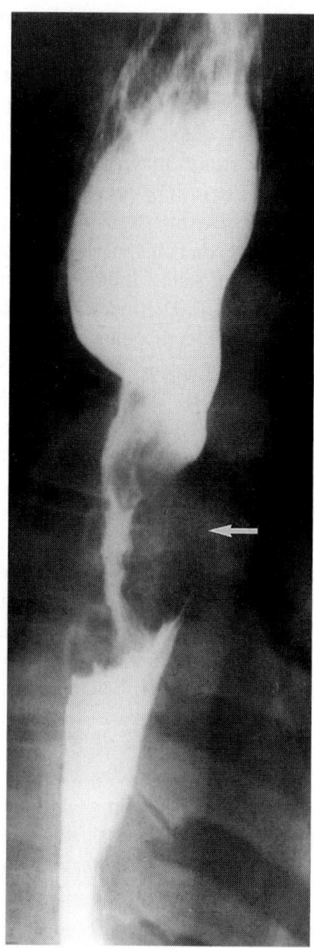

**FIGURE 80.1. Esophageal cancer. Barium swallow showing an irregular, ulcerated stricture (arrow) in the esophagus.**

achieved by *surgical removal* of the primary lesion with esophagogastric anastomosis or colonic interposition, or the *nonsurgical options* of radiotherapy, chemotherapy, dilatation, endoprosthesis placement (which also addresses esophagotracheal fistula), or tumor ablation with heat (BICAP), laser, (including photodynamic therapy [PDT]) or alcohol injection and irradiation. These can be combined as, for example, surgery with irradiation. Good nutritional support is essential, and in some cases, intensive therapy for pain may be required.

With screening programs for conditions such as Barrett's esophagus, an increasing number of esophageal cancers are now being diagnosed early. Esophagectomy in such patients has a 5-year survival rate greater than 90%. In some of these patients who pose a high surgical risk, PDT is being tried as an alternative therapy.

# CHAPTER 81 GASTRIC PHYSIOLOGY AND TESTS OF GASTRIC FUNCTION

The portion of the proximal stomach that is adjacent to the esophagogastric junction is the cardia, and the dome-shaped portion to the left of it and lying beneath the left hemidiaphragm is the fundus. Extending downward and to the right is the corpus, or body, the main portion of the stomach. The narrower distal stomach, or the antrum, ends in the pylorus, a narrow channel that connects with the first portion of the duodenum, known to radiologists as the "bulb."

Gastric motor functions include storage and volume adaptation, mixing of contents, trituration of solid food particles, and propulsion (emptying). The stomach has two distinct motor regions, each with a different functional role. The **proximal stomach** (the fundus and upper body) acts as a reservoir and is capable of receptive relaxation (increase in gastric volume without a corresponding increase in intragastric pressure). The proximal stomach exerts slow, sustained, or tonic contractions that, by steady pressure on its contents, gradually press them toward the distal stomach. This mechanism is largely responsible for emptying of liquids from stomach to duodenum. The **distal stomach (antrum),** which performs mixing and grinding, has a major regulatory role in the gastric emptying of solids; its motor activity is controlled by the gastric pacemaker, located in the smooth muscle cells in the midbody of the stomach.

## Gastric Acid Secretion

Gastric secretion is under neuroendocrine control, an integrated autoregulatory system with stimulatory and inhibitory influences acting to modulate and adjust gastric secretion to specific needs after food intake, as well as during the interdigestive period. The principal constituents of gastric juice are HCl, electrolytes ($Na^+$, $K^+$, $Cl^-$, $HCO_3$), mucus, digestive enzymes, and intrinsic factor. Gastrin, produced by G cells located mainly in the antrum, is the main hormone-stimulating gastric acid secretion under physiologic circumstances. The parietal cell secretes $H^+$-ions by an Mg-dependent $H^+$, $K^+$-ATPase (the proton pump), which is located exclusively in its luminal secretory membrane. The $H^+$ secretion is activated by histamine binding to H2-receptors and, to a lesser extent, by acetylcholine (ACh) binding to $M_3$-receptors, both located on the basolateral aspect of the parietal cell. Histamine is released from nearby enterochromaffin-like (ECL) and mast cells in response to the receptor binding of gastrin and ACh. The parietal cell secretion is down-regulated by paracrine release of somatostatin and prostaglandins. The histamine effect on the parietal cell is mediated by cyclic AMP-, and the ACh action by $Ca^{2+}$-dependent mechanisms (Figure 81.1).

Neural stimulation is triggered at different stages of eating a meal. Anticipation, sight, and smell constitute the **cephalic phase.** The tasting, chewing, and swallowing of food, and food in the stomach (probably via distention), all cause acid secretion through neural reflexes; distention also leads to gastrin release, which, in turn, stimulates parietal cells to produce HCl. Partially digested proteins, on contact with antral mucosa, a neutral pH in the antral lumen, antral distention, and vagal impulses, also evoke gastrin release. Calcium, in the lumen or blood, stimulates acid production, through gastrin release and direct parietal cell stimulation. Caffeine, roasting products in decaffeinated coffee, and fermented alcoholic drinks all stimulate acid production. Pure ethanol and distilled spirits have no effect on gastric secretion.

Inhibitory mechanisms for gastric secretion are located mainly beyond the pylorus. Secretin, cholecystokinin, and gastric inhibitory peptide (GIP) are released from duodenal or small bowel mucosa on stimulation variously by acid, fat, protein, and glucose in the lumen, and inhibit gastric acid secretion. Neural reflexes that originate in the duodenal bulb stimulated by acid inhibit acid secretion.

## Pepsin and Intrinsic Factor

Pepsinogen, especially the pepsinogen I fraction, originates in chief cells and correlates well with acid

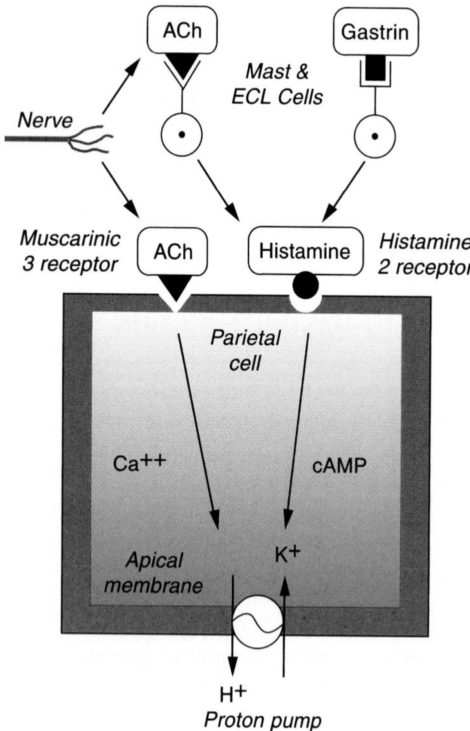


**FIGURE 81.1.** Parietal cell and acid secretion. See text for details. ACh = Acetylcholine; cAMP: = cyclic adenosine monophosphate; ECL = enterochromaffin-like cells.

secretory capacity. Stimuli that increase acid output also raise enzyme levels in the gastric juice. Pepsinogen, the proenzyme, is converted to pepsin by HCl and by pepsin. Intrinsic factor, a product of the parietal cell, depends only partially on stimuli for gastric acid secretion for its elaboration or secretion.

## Procedures for Investigating Gastric/ Duodenal Disease

### Measurement of gastric secretory capacity

Considerable inter- and intraindividual variation exists in measured acid secretory rates. Mean values are shown in Table 81.1. Secretory rates in patients with duodenal ulcer, as a group, exceed that of normals. Secretory rates for gastric ulcer patients, as a group, are about 60% of those for normals. Patients with gastrinomas (Zollinger-Ellison syndrome) show marked basal hypersecretion, with BAO over 15 mEq/h and the BAO:MAO exceeding 0.66.

Gastric secretory assessment has little value in the routine diagnosis of peptic ulcer. It should be measured in patients suspected of having Zollinger-Ellison syndrome, and in patients with abdominal pain or GI bleeding following partial gastric resection or vagotomy done for peptic ulcer disease. BAO or MAO values in the postoperative stomach exceeding 5 and 15 mEq/h, respectively, are highly predictive of recurrent ulcer. An intact response to modified sham feeding indicates persistent vagal innervation.

### Serum gastrin

The greatest value of determining serum gastrin is in identifying patients with ulcer disease due to hypergastrinemia, the hallmark of the Zollinger-Ellison syndrome. Hypergastrinemia also occurs in patients with achlorhydria (e.g., pernicious anemia, carcinoma of the stomach), renal insufficiency (mild to moderate hypergastrinemia), and may follow massive small bowel resection. The retention of antral mucosa in continuity with the duodenum following partial gastric resection and Billroth II anastomosis may lead to hypergastrinemia and stomal ulcer. Here, the antral gastrin cells are excluded from gastric acid or other inhibitory factors in the feedback regulation of antral gastrin release. Currently, the most common cause of hypergastrinemia is medication-induced hypo- or achlorhydria, particularly in patients treated with a "proton pump" inhibitor.

**TABLE 81.1. Mean Values of Gastric Acid Output (mEq/Hour)**

| | Men | Women |
|---|---|---|
| Basal acid output (BAO) | 4 | 2 |
| Maximum acid output (MAO) | 30 | 20 |
| Peak acid output (PAO) | 37 | 25 |
| BAO/MAO Ratio | <.6 | <.6 |

Modified sham feeding (MSF) test = 50% of PAO; lower limit = 10% of PAO.

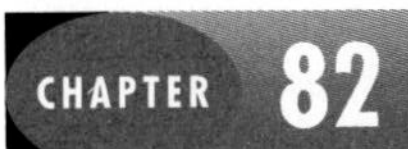

# GASTRITIS AND OTHER DISORDERS

## Gastritis

The term "gastritis" has suffered from a looseness of definition and application, because it can be defined according to clinical presentation, endoscopic appearances, or histopathology. Moreover, gastritis does not always imply inflammatory changes. Gastropathy is a condition where epithelial and vascular changes predominate with minimum inflammatory cell reaction.

## Erosive and Hemorrhagic Gastritis

An **erosion** is a break in the mucosa that does not penetrate the muscularis mucosae. Endoscopically, erosion appears as a whitish lesion with an erythematous halo. They are usually multiple. A black base implies recent bleeding. **Hemorrhagic gastritis** appears as petechiae, red streaks, or patches without any break in the mucosa. Patients with erosive or hemorrhagic gastritis may have no symptoms, or may report nausea, vomiting, GI bleeding, and upper abdominal pain. Endoscopy is the best means of diagnosis.

Aspirin and other NSAIDs cause gastritis, probably by topical mucosal effects and by suppressing endogenous prostaglandins. The fundic and corpus mucosa are more damaged than the antral mucosa. The onset is usually acute. Healing is rapid once the offending drug is withdrawn. Therapy with enteric coated NSAID preparations, or preventive therapy with synthetic prostaglandins (e.g., misoprostol) reduce NSAID-induced mucosal injuries. Gastritis may also follow alcohol intake, ingestion of corrosive agents, and drugs like potassium chloride. Severe stress, as in seriously ill patients, can compromise gastric mucosal defense and repair mechanisms, thus leading to lesions ranging from gastritis to complete ulcers. Gastritis may also follow radiation injury. Chronic erosive gastritis (diffuse varioliform gastritis), a disease of unclear etiology, has multiple erosions, seen endoscopically as small nodules with central umbilications. The condition may remit within months or persist for years.

## Chronic Active Gastritis

With or without mucosal atrophy, chronic active gastritis (CAG) can involve the fundic mucosa (type A gastritis), antral mucosa (type B gastritis), the whole stomach (pangastritis), or be multifocal. Antral nodularity or thin folds with prominent vessels may be seen endoscopically. Histology is required for evaluating the type of mucosal involvement (superficial, full-thickness, atrophic), the existence of metaplasia (e.g., intestinal metaplasia), and the etiology (e.g., *Helicobacter pylori*). When atrophic gastritis spares the antrum, the low acid output evokes hypergastrinemia.

*Helicobacter pylori (H. pylori)* is a gram-negative, comma-shaped rod with potent urease activity. Its relationship with peptic ulcer disease is discussed later. Superficial chronic active gastritis is the most common type of gastritis associated with *H. pylori*. The exact mode of transmission is unknown. Intrafamilial clustering suggests person-to-person spread. Higher prevalence rates are seen with increasing age, lower socioeconomic status, and among Latinos/Latinas and African Americans. On histology, the organism is seen in the mucous layer near the surface and pit epithelial cells. Though the antral mucosa is predominantly affected, lesser degrees of inflammation are seen in the fundic and corpus mucosa. The organism can also be found in the duodenum in areas with gastric metaplasia. Diagnosis and treatment of *H. pylori* are addressed in chapter 83.

Chronic active gastritis can be seen in patients having alkaline (bile) reflux, usually following gastric resection and pyloroplasty. Atrophic gastritis is seen in elderly patients or in autoimmune conditions like pernicious anemia. Adenocarcinoma of the gastric antrum and body can be associated with multifocal atrophic gastritis and intestinal metaplasia.

## Specific Gastritis

Cytomegalovirus, herpes virus, tuberculosis, and syphilis can cause gastritis. Gastritis can also occur in systemic conditions like sarcoidosis, Crohn's disease, chronic granulomatous disease, and graft-versus-host disease.

**Ménétrier's disease,** a rare disease seen mostly in men over the age of 50, features giant folds in the proximal stomach, with a greatly thickened mucosa showing foveolar hyperplasia (abnormal pit epithelium with lengthening of pit) and glandular atrophy. Abnormal mucosa and superficial ulcers cause gastric protein loss leading to hypoproteinemia. A true link to cancer has not been shown. Clinical features include epigastric pain, diarrhea, microcytic anemia from chronic blood loss, and peripheral edema. Barium x-ray shows large and tortuous gastric folds. Diagnosis requires full-thickness mucosal biopsies by laparotomy or open biopsy. Mild symptoms may require no therapy; severe symptoms may dictate total gastrectomy. Acid suppression, corticosteroids, anticholinergics, and tranexamic have been tried with variable success.

## Other Disorders of the Stomach

### Diaphragmatic Hernias

The diaphragm separates the "low-pressure" thorax from the "high-pressure" abdomen. Therefore, defects in the diaphragm may predispose to herniation of stomach or other abdominal contents into the thorax. The most common type of diaphragmatic hernia is the **sliding hiatal hernia,** in which the gastroesophageal (g-e) junction and a portion of the stomach slide through the diaphragmatic hiatus into the posterior mediastinum. Occasionally, reflux esophagitis may cause longitudinal shortening of the esophagus. Although hiatal hernia is not synonymous with g-e reflux, it may predispose to reflux disease. Patients with sliding hiatal hernias may be asymptomatic. Those with large hiatal hernias may report vague chest pain or present with chronic anemia due to either associated g-e reflux disease, or "kissing" erosions/ulcers on the crest of the mucosal folds as they pass through the hiatus.

In **paraesophageal hernia,** the g-e junction retains its normal anatomic position, but the stomach herniates alongside the g-e junction through the diaphragmatic hiatus. The entire stomach, oriented in an upside-down position, can herniate into the thorax. Stasis of food and secretions in the herniated stomach lead to erosions and ulcerations. Patients may, therefore, present with GI blood loss. A rare but serious complication of paraesophageal hernia is gastric volvulus. Delay in diagnosis and futile attempts at gastric decompression by a nasogastric tube may cause incarceration or strangulation of the herniated stomach. Inability to swallow, retching, and progressive severe pain suggest incarceration. **Congenital diaphragmatic hernias** result when structures involved in the development of the diaphragm fuse defectively. The posterolaterally located **foramina of Bochdalek** is the most common such congenital defect. The **foramina of Morgagni** are located anteriorly and 90% of the time the hernia is on the right side. Symptoms, when present, include obstruction, incarceration, strangulation, and respiratory distress. Post-traumatic diaphragmatic hernias result from injuries like stab wound, gunshot wound, or blunt trauma. The left diaphragm is more susceptible to injury as the liver protects the right diaphragm from blunt trauma, and as most assailants in stabbing incidents are right-handed. Rarely, the diaphragm may be injured during surgery or may rupture during coughing or severe straining.

Chest x-ray may show a mediastinal air fluid level. Barium x-rays, and not endoscopy, is the most useful means of diagnosis. Surgery is the treatment of choice for diaphragmatic hernias, except in the sliding type. When complications occur, surgery carries a higher risk; thus, it is advisable to consider it even in the asymptomatic patient. Management of GERD complicating sliding hiatal hernia is the same as that without hernia.

### Foreign Body Ingestion

All kinds of foreign bodies may be ingested, particularly by children (80% of the total), edentulous (denture-wearing) adults, prisoners, and the mentally ill. Immediate or delayed impaction with obstruction, perforation, and bleeding are potential complications. While plain x-rays of neck, chest, and abdomen are useful, some ingested foreign bodies (chicken bones, glass, plastic) will not be detected because they are radiolucent. All retained esophageal foreign bodies should be removed by endoscopy. Small, smooth objects (e.g., coins) in the stomach usually pass on their own, but sharp, pointed or larger (>5 cm long or >2 cm thick) objects must be removed by endoscopy or surgery.

**"Body packing"** refers to smuggling drugs (cocaine, heroin) in rubber or latex bags that are either swallowed or inserted into the rectum or vagina. These patients are admitted to an ICU until all packets are passed by GI tract lavage. For fear of rupturing a packet while it is still within the body, instrumentation is strictly forbidden.

# CHAPTER 83 PEPTIC ULCER DISEASE

Peptic ulcers are mucosal defects extending beyond the muscularis mucosae with implied pathogenic association with acid and pepsin ("no acid, no ulcer"). They can develop in the stomach, duodenum, lower esophagus, jejunum (after gastrojejunostomy), and in areas with ectopic gastric mucosa.

### Etiology and Pathophysiology

The mucus/bicarbonate layer is the first line of mucosal defense, followed by the epithelial cells. Adequate blood flow clears the back-diffused $H^+$ and supplies necessary nutrients to the cell. Prostaglandins enhance mucosal resistance to injury ("cytoprotection"). In simple terms, peptic ulcers follow when the balance between mucosal defense and acid-pepsin is disturbed. Duodenal ulcer is rare in persons with a maximal acid output less than 12–15 mEq/h. One-third of patients with duodenal ulcer also have increased basal acid output. However, gastric ulcer can occur even if acid secretion is low, although both gastric and duodenal ulcers heal with acid suppression. Acid with pepsin is more ulcerogenic than acid alone. A break in the mucosal defense by extraneous factors may be an additional, and possibly the primary, event in the pathogenesis of peptic ulcer. For example, NSAIDs cause peptic ulcers by their topical mucosal damaging effects or by their systemic effect of depleting mucosal prostaglandins.

An estimated 15% of persons with *H. pylori* will develop peptic ulcer. However, over 95% of patients with duodenal ulcer and around 75% of patients with gastric ulcer are infected with *H. pylori*. The exact mechanism by which *H. pylori* induces ulceration is unknown. The microbe itself or factors released by it may evoke inflammation that damages mucosal defense. *H. pylori* infection is also associated with elevated levels of gastrin and pepsinogen. As *H. pylori* is also found in a high percentage of people who never develop peptic ulcers, the exact pathogenesis of peptic ulcer is still unclear.

## Risk Factors

Peptic ulcer disease is slightly more prevalent in men than in women; the lifetime prevalence is about 10%. Duodenal ulcers are more frequent than gastric ulcers. Peptic ulcer incidence rises with age, reflecting a cohort phenomenon, possibly due to higher use of NSAIDs or increased prevalence of *H. pylori* in the elderly. Epidemiologic studies show higher incidence of gastric and duodenal ulcers in first-degree relatives of patients with similar types of ulcers. Patients with blood group O and nonsecretors of ABO antigens in body fluids are also at a higher risk of developing duodenal ulcer. Smoking increases the risk for both gastric and duodenal ulcers, besides impairing ulcer healing and promoting recurrence. Although tea and coffee stimulate acid production and alcohol may damage the mucosa, evidence is lacking to implicate them as risk factors. The role of psychological stress in the pathogenesis of ulcer remains unclear. Other diseases like cirrhosis, renal failure, chronic obstructive pulmonary disease, polycythemia vera, and hyperparathyroidism, for elusive reasons, are associated with an increased incidence of duodenal ulcer.

## Clinical Features

The most common symptom of duodenal ulcer is epigastric pain, which is usually burning, occurring 1–3 hours after meals, and relieved by food or antacids. Nocturnal pain may interrupt sleep. The pain may last for a few weeks followed by symptom-free intervals of weeks to months. Less typically, it may be a gnawing or crampy discomfort, or felt in the right or left upper quadrants, or may radiate to the back. While a sizable number of duodenal ulcer patients present initially with complications of ulcer, acute bleeding, or perforation, some report anorexia with nausea and vomiting, despite the lack of gastric outlet obstruction. Gastric ulcer patients are older and, more often than not, asymptomatic. They may present initially with GI bleeding or perforation. The typical pain-food-relief pattern may occur, but it is less distinct than with duodenal ulcer. In fact, food may worsen the pain. Vague or severe, diffuse upper abdominal pain may accompany nausea, anorexia, and weight loss. Nocturnal pain is less common. Except with complications or other associated diseases, physical examination is not generally very helpful for diagnosis. Epigastric tenderness may be noted.

Complications of peptic ulcer disease are shown in Table 83.1.

## Diagnosis

Peptic ulcer disease should be distinguished from non-ulcer dyspepsia, esophagitis, biliary diseases, pancreatitis, carcinoma, and infectious, granulomatous, or infiltrative diseases of the stomach and duodenum. History and physical examination lack sensitivity and specificity as diagnostic tools. Expertly done upper-GI barium radiology has a diagnostic accuracy of 80–90% for duodenal and 80% for gastric ulcer. Endoscopy detects a further 5–10% of ulcers and many consider it the procedure of choice. In some, peptic ulcer is discovered on urgent laparotomy for complications (e.g., perforation). Benign gastric ulcer has a regular, rounded edge and a smooth base. However, despite appearances, multiple biopsies to rule out malignancy are essential.

**TABLE 83.1. Complications of Peptic Ulcer Disease**

- Intractability
- Bleeding
- Perforation
- Penetration
- Gastric outlet obstruction
- Complications of therapy (H2 blockers antacids or proton pump inhibitors)
- Complications of surgery
  - Postgastrectomy syndrome
  - Dumping syndrome
  - Blind-loop syndrome
  - Anastomotic ulcer
  - Postvagotomy diarrhea

Several tests are available for diagnosing H. pylori infection. Bacterial urease activity can be tested by either the $^{13}$C-urea breath test (90–95% sensitivity) or rapid urease test (90–98% sensitivity). The latter is done by placing an endoscopically taken gastric biopsy specimen on a pellet containing urea and a pH color indicator. Urease produced by *H. pylori* converts urea to ammonia; the pH rises and color changes. The bacteria can also be found on histology or cultured (70–95% sensitivity). Serum antibodies, while highly sensitive (95%) cannot separate current from previous infection. Antral mucosal biopsy should be obtained on all endoscopically detected gastric or duodenal ulcers, to document H. pylori infection by rapid urease test. With eradication of H. pylori, antibody titers fall progressively. H. pylori antigen can be detected in the stools with >90% sensitivity. Serum gastrin and acid output studies have no role in the usual evaluation of peptic ulcer disease, unless hypersecretory states (e.g., Zollinger-Ellison syndrome) are suspected.

## Medical Management

The objectives of ulcer therapy are to promote ulcer healing and to prevent recurrences and complications. The strategy includes general measures, acid suppression, and promoting mucosal protection. Smoking and NSAID intake should be forbidden, as both of these are strong risk factors for ulcer nonhealing, recurrence, and complications. A causal relationship between alcohol abuse and ulcer disease is not proven; nonetheless, alcohol should be discouraged as it hampers the patient's compliance with the treatment. Specific dietary advice is not necessary but regular food intake should be encouraged. Stressful life situations reportedly delay ulcer healing.

Gastric acid can be reduced by either neutralization or inhibition of secretion. While antacids, which neutralize gastric acid, have been replaced by other anti-ulcer drugs, patients may still use them; one should be familiar with their role and side effects. Patient compliance is a problem and so is diarrhea due to magnesium-containing antacids. Ionized calcium in calcium-containing antacids stimulates gastrin secretion. Prolonged use of absorbable calcium-containing antacids with large amounts of milk leads to milk-alkali syndrome: hypercalcemia, alkalosis, nephrocalcinosis, and azotemia.

**H2-receptor antagonists** (cimetidine, ranitidine, famotidine, and nizatidine), which selectively block histamine H2-receptors on the parietal cells have been the most popular class of drugs used in treating peptic ulcer disease. Ulcer healing rates following therapy with these agents are 70–80% after 4 weeks and 90% after 8 weeks. Maintenance therapy with a single bedtime dose is also effective in reducing recurrence. Some of the side effects of these drugs are antiandrogenic effects, CNS symptoms, T-lymphocyte suppression, and pancytopenia. Through its effect on hepatic cytochrome protein pump inhibitors $P_{450}$, cimetidine and lansoprazole can inhibit the metabolism of many drugs like warfarin, phenytoin, and theophylline, leading to toxicity from these agents.

**Substituted benzimidazoles (protein pump inhibitors,** (PPI) e.g. omeprazole, lansoprazole rebeprazole, pentaprazole, esmaprazole) are the most potent inhibitors of acid secretion and will heal duodenal ulcers in 80–100% of cases at 4–8 weeks with very few side effects. Hypergastrinemia caused by sustained hypochlorhydria leads to enterochromaffin-cell hyperplasia in the gastric corpus and fundic mucosa, with progression to gastric carcinoid tumors in rats. No such complication has been reported in humans.

**Sucralfate,** a sulfated polysaccharide-aluminum complex, prevents mucosal injury and heals ulcers without altering gastric acid or pepsin secretion. Several mechanisms have been proposed for its anti-ulcer effect. It forms a viscous barrier over granulation tissue, thus preventing detrimental effects of acid and pepsin; it may also enhance healing by stimulating prostaglandin production, adsorbing pepsin, and reducing oxidant damage to epithelial cells. The usual dose is 1.0 g four times daily.

**Prostaglandins** (E and I groups) inhibit acid secretion and are also cytoprotective. Their acid inhibitory effect is mediated by suppressing histamine-related c-AMP generation in the parietal cell. Misoprostol is one such agent and is used mainly to prevent NSAID-induced ulcers. Side effects include crampy abdominal pain and diarrhea. Because misoprostol also has uterotropic effect, it can induce abortion.

### Approach to therapy

Nearly 30–40% of duodenal ulcers heal by 4–6 weeks spontaneously, and more than 75% heal with H2-receptor antagonists, and 80–100% with protein pump inhibitors. After initial healing, 70–80% of peptic ulcers recur within 6–12 months. Maintenance H2-blocker therapy greatly reduces recurrence, but the current emphasis is on eradicating *H. pylori.* As over 95% of duodenal ulcers are associated with *H. pylori,* and as eradication of *H. pylori* significantly lowers ulcer recurrence rate (to 0–21%), most of the newly diagnosed duodenal ulcers and *H. pylori*-positive gastric ulcer patients can also be treated against *H. pylori* initially. This approach, while more expensive than giving H2-receptor antagonist alone, is more cost-effective in the long run, given the significantly lowered recurrence rate. Several regimens are available. A bismuth drug (e.g., Pepto-Bismol) with two antibiotics (e.g., tetracycline and metronidazole; tetracycline and clarithromycin; or amoxicillin and clarithromycin) eradicates *H. pylori* by

90–96%; most instances call for an additional 4–6 weeks of follow-up treatment with ranitidine. However, PPIs are replacing H2-receptor antagonist and with clarithromycin *and* amoxicillin or metronidazole given for 2 weeks leads to excellent ulcer healing and eradication of *H. pylori.*

While it is unnecessary to document duodenal ulcer (they are rarely malignant) healing, endoscopy may be needed to obtain biopsies for *H. pylori* in patients with nonhealing ulcers. Ongoing *H. pylori* can also be determined using the breath test based on *H. pylori* urease activity or by testing stools for H. pylori antigen. Other causes of nonhealing ulcers like NSAID use and hypersecretory states like Zollinger-Ellison syndrome should be excluded. One should also consider infection with *H. pylori* strains that are metronidazole-resistant and/or clarithromycin-resistant. All gastric ulcers should be followed up until healed. Cancer should always be excluded by biopsy in unhealed gastric ulcers. Slowly healing gastric ulcers may require additional courses of treatment.

With modern medical management of peptic ulcer disease, total refractoriness to medical treatment is quite uncommon. Some may prefer surgery, but surgery is indicated mainly for complications. However, medical treatment does not eliminate the risks of ulcer recurrence, and for those who need maintenance therapy, or those with poor drug compliance, surgery is an excellent, drug-free alternative. A few patients will develop recurrent ulcers or experience chronic morbidity postoperatively.

The main objective of surgery is to reduce gastric acid secretion. **Subtotal gastrectomy** removes the bulk of the parietal cell mass and has an ulcer recurrence rate of 4–5%. Subtotal gastric resection is coupled with a gastroduodenostomy (*Billroth I*) or gastrojejunostomy (*Billroth II*) to restore continuity. Interrupting the neural path of acid secretion (vagotomy) and removing the main source of gastrin (antrectomy) can also accomplish acid reduction. Since truncal vagotomy will delay gastric emptying, a drainage procedure (e.g., pyloroplasty, gastrojejunostomy) must be added to this approach. In *proximal gastric vagotomy* (highly selective or superselective vagotomy), the vagal innervation to the fundus is interrupted and that to the antrum is preserved. As antral motility is intact, a drainage procedure is obviated. This operation has an ulcer recurrence rate of around 10%. Subtotal gastrectomy or antrectomy may be required for gastric ulcers. Vagotomy is not necessary as most patients with gastric ulcer have normal or low acid output.

## Complications

During their life-time, nearly one-third of patients with peptic ulcer will experience one or more complications. **Intractability** implies failure of the ulcer to heal despite 8–12 weeks of intensive therapy, ulcer recurrence, or development of complications despite maintenance therapy. Intractability may be due to hypersecretory states, penetrating or obstructing ulcers, smoking, and NSAID use. Eradication of *H. pylori* has significantly reduced the ulcer recurrence rate. When no remediable cause can be found, surgery is indicated.

**Bleeding** can complicate 15–20% of peptic ulcer cases, being more frequent in duodenal ulcers than gastric ulcers. It may be the first sign of peptic ulcer in 20–30% of patients. NSAID use accounts for the increasingly high incidence of ulcer bleeding in the elderly. Mortality from peptic ulcer bleeding has remained at 6–10%, the risk being higher in those over 60 years of age, or with concomitant diseases or continued bleeding or rebleeding. Deep ulcers in the posterior duodenal bulb and high lesser curve tend to erode large arteries and thus bleed briskly. Bleeding stops on its own in most patients with ulcer disease. Those found to have active bleeding on endoscopy or those at high risk for rebleeding (nonbleeding visible vessel, adherent fresh clot in the base of an ulcer) can be treated by endoscopic interventions. (See chapter 78 for general management of acute GI bleeding.) Surgery may be necessary when bleeding continues or recurs. Those unable to undergo surgery should be considered for angiographic embolization. Medical management of peptic ulcer should follow in all cases. Maintenance therapy after ulcer healing and eradication of *H. pylori* may reduce the rebleeding risk.

**Perforation** of an ulcer is less common than bleeding, but can be the first manifestation of peptic ulcer disease. It occurs in 5–10% of cases with duodenal ulcer and 2–5% of gastric ulcer cases. Perforation is more common with lesser curve gastric ulcers and anterior duodenal bulb ulcers. The use of NSAIDs has also increased the incidence of perforation in the elderly. Typical presentation is with the abrupt transition of vague, visceral pain of ulcer disease to the sharp, acute pain of peritonitis. Signs of acute peritonitis (muscle rigidity, rebound tenderness) are present with hypotension and tachycardia. Upright abdominal x-ray will show free intra-abdominal air. Endoscopy must be avoided as air insufflation can extend the perforation and further contaminate the peritoneal cavity. Spillage of duodenal contents may lead to hyperamylasemia. While the perforation seals without any intervention in a small minority, prompt surgery is indicated once perforation is diagnosed. While simple closure of the perforation is often enough, many surgeons carry out a more definite ulcer operation to avert further complications. **Penetration** is full thickness erosion of the gastric or duodenal wall into the pancreas, liver, biliary tree, or colon, but without free perforation. Penetration is identified in 20% of cases requiring surgery for peptic ulcer. Patients may note an alteration in their typical pain pattern—for example, the classical duodenal ulcer pain will begin radiating to the back once the duodenal ulcer penetrates the pancreas. Penetrating ulcers can respond well to medical therapy. Complicated penetrating ulcers (e.g., gastrocolic fistula) will require surgery.

Nearly 2% of patients with ulcer disease develop **gastric outlet obstruction,** arising from either inflammatory edema or cicatricial narrowing of the pylorus due to chronically recurring ulcer. Since obstruction is insidious and the stomach dilates as a result, the syndrome takes many weeks to develop. Vomiting is the most frequent symptom, which may cause severe esophagitis. Typically profuse, the vomit contains retained food, consumed many hours earlier. Abdominal pain, vague fullness after meals, anorexia, and weight loss may be reported. A succussion splash is a common and valuable sign besides dehydration. Hemoconcentration, prerenal azotemia, anemia, hyponatremia, low serum albumin, and in severe cases, hypokalemic alkalosis are typical laboratory findings. Barium study is diagnostic, but endoscopy is required to define the cause, especially to exclude malignancy. Nasogastric tube drainage of the stomach, IV rehydration, and restoration of electrolytes are immediate priorities. Acid suppression (H2-blockers, omeprazole) may relieve obstruction due to inflammatory edema. Gastric retention persisting beyond 5–7 days requires either endoscopic balloon dilatation of the pylorus or surgery.

## Zollinger-Ellison Syndrome

Zollinger-Ellison (ZE) syndrome is characterized by the autonomous production and release of gastrin by a tumor (gastrinoma) leading to severe ulcerative disease of the upper GI tract, diarrhea, hypergastrinemia, and hyperchlorhydria. Fewer than 1% of peptic ulcers are ZE syndrome-related. It mostly presents in patients between 30 and 50 years of age and is slightly more common in men.

Autonomous gastrin production by proliferating non-β islet cells leads to uncontrolled acid secretion by the parietal cells. Ninety percent of gastrinomas are found in the head of the pancreas and the wall of the duodenum. Slightly over one-half are multiple and a similar proportion are malignant. The tumor grows slowly and metastasizes mainly to regional lymph nodes and liver. About 30% of cases with gastrinomas have type I multiple endocrine neoplasia, and nearly all gastrinomas of this type are multiple.

The majority of patients have typical symptoms of peptic ulcer disease. Gastrinoma-related peptic ulcers tend to be persistent and poorly responsive to conventional therapy. Over one-third of patients report diarrhea, probably due to excess HCl in the small intestine that inactivates pancreatic digestive enzymes and thus reduces bile salt solubility. Some patients have diarrhea but no ulcer symptoms. In those with MEN-I syndrome, a family history—mainly of hyperparathyroidism with renal stones—is usually present. Most of the ulcers are located in the duodenal bulb or the stomach and may be multiple. However, ulcers may occur beyond the duodenal bulb (14%) and in the jejunum (11%). Recurrent ulcers may rapidly develop at or distal to the anastomotic site following conventional peptic ulcer surgery. Esophagitis and esophageal ulceration may also occur.

Severe, progressive, and recurrent peptic ulcer disease, peptic ulcers at unusual sites, and diarrhea should raise the suspicion of ZE syndrome. Besides demonstrating ulcers, barium study may show prominent gastric and duodenal folds, thickened and widened small intestinal folds, and excessive fluid in the small bowel lumen. Owing to the continuous stimulation of the parietal cells by gastrin, the ratio between basal and maximum pentagastrin-stimulated acid output is 0.66% or more. Both fasting serum gastrin levels and basal acid output are high. Gastrinomas thus confirmed are localized by CT, MR, ultrasound, or selective angiography with or without venous gastrin level sampling. Surgical resection is the ideal treatment for resectable tumors. If resection is not feasible, acid hypersecretion is suppressed by high doses of PPIs, or rarely, by total gastrectomy. Recently, I.V. pentaprozole has been approved for acid control in ZE syndrome. Chemotherapy (e.g., streptozotocin) reduces tumor size and serum gastrin in metastatic gastrinomas.

## Stress Ulcers

Severe physiological stress can result in gastroduodenal lesions ranging from mucosal erosions to life-threatening ulcers—for example, duodenal ulcers **(Curling's ulcers)** in severe burns, and gastroduodenal ulcers in CNS trauma or with other serious illnesses **(Cushing's ulcer).** The pathogenesis of stress ulcer is elusive. Physiological stress can compromise mucosal perfusion, and mucosal defense and repair. The usual presentation is acute GI bleeding in an ICU setting. Bleeding stress ulcers carry a high risk of rebleeding and mortality. Given the underlying serious illnesses, most of these patients respond inadequately to any form of therapy. Prevention is thus crucial. In clinical trials, keeping the gastric pH over 3.5–4 by antacid or sucralfate by nasogastric tube or by IV H2 blockers has lowered the rate of stress ulcer complications. I.V. pentaprozole may be used but need further trials.

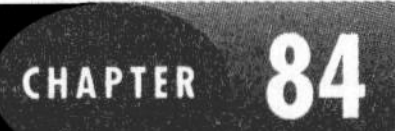

# NEOPLASMS OF THE STOMACH

## Gastric Cancer

### Epidemiology and Etiology

Gastric cancer, once common, has declined in incidence since the 1940s. Although it is most common in men older than 50 years, the gender difference is insignificant in cancers in younger persons. Gastric cancer has a striking geographic variation, with a higher incidence in Costa Rica, Japan, and China. Dietary factors (e.g., diets high in salt, pickled vegetables, smoked food, and salted fish) have been linked epidemiologically to its genesis. Patients with chronic atrophic gastritis with intestinal metaplasia, pernicious anemia, gastric polyps, hypertrophic gastropathy, and postgastrectomy gastric remnant also have a higher risk. Nitrite-forming bacteria that colonize the stomach in patients with hypo- or achlorhydria help convert dietary nitrates to nitrites. Nitroso compounds formed in this process are carcinogenic in animals. Antioxidants (e.g., vitamin C) inhibit this conversion. An epidemiological link has been noted between infection with *Helicobacter pylori* and later development of gastric adenocarcinoma. Chronic atrophic gastritis due to *H. pylori* infection may be the precursor. Both first-degree relatives of gastric cancer patients and persons with blood group A have a higher risk of gastric cancer, suggesting a genetic basis. Gastric cancer may present as an ulcer, but chronic benign gastric ulcer does not seem to be precancerous.

### Pathology

Over 90% of gastric cancers are adenocarcinomas. Cancers with intracellular mucus laterally displacing the nucleus (giving ring-like appearance) are termed **signet ring carcinomas. Colloid or mucinous carcinomas** are mucus-producing. Gastric carcinomas also may show glandular structures (papillary) or masses of cells (medullary). The cells can be highly, moderately, or poorly differentiated. Gastric carcinomas also are classified as *intestinal* or *diffuse* types. Intestinal carcinoma often arises from intestinal metaplasia. It is polypoidal or ulcerated, better circumscribed, and has a glandular structure resembling colon cancer. It is more common in older people. The diffuse type, more common in younger people, features rare glandular structures, indistinct margins, and frequent signet-ring cells. Early gastric cancer, which invades only the mucosa or submucosa, is diagnosed using a combination of endoscopy and histology.

### Clinical Features and Diagnosis

Patients with *early gastric carcinoma* usually are asymptomatic or may report vague, nonspecific epigastric symptoms. Such cancers usually are found by screening techniques being used in countries where gastric cancer is endemic (e.g., Japan). Symptoms of advanced gastric cancer are listed in Table 84.1.

Using the double-contrast x-ray technique, 90% to 95% of cases of gastric cancers can be diagnosed accurately. Malignancy is suggested by an ulcer within a mass, a polypoidal mass, interrupted or nodular folds approaching an ulcer, and rigidity with loss of peristalsis. However, appearances are deceptive; thus, all gastric ulcers, benign-appearing or otherwise, must be biopsied via endoscopy. Early gastric cancer may evoke only subtle changes; careful examination of the stomach is thus paramount. Computed tomography and endoscopic ultrasound can help define the depth of tumor invasion and presence or absence of metastases.

### Management

For patients with localized disease (early gastric cancer), surgery is the only hope of a cure. Patients with nonmetastatic but locally advanced disease also should be offered surgery to seek curative resection. If surgery is not possible, or if disease is disseminated, palliative surgery may be done to relieve symptoms (e.g., dysphagia, gastric outlet obstruction, bleeding); chemotherapy also should be considered. Using single agents such as 5-fluorouracil or mitomycin C, a response rate of 20% to

**TABLE 84.1. Manifestations of Gastric Cancer**

| Category | Symptoms |
|---|---|
| Constitutional/systemic | Anorexia, weight loss, thrombophlebitis, neuropathy |
| Local | Abdominal pain, gastrocolic fistula |
| Obstruction | Dysphagia (cardiac), vomiting (antral) |
| Bleeding | Hematemesis, melena, anemia |
| Metastasis | Pleural effusion, Virchow's nodes, periumbilical infiltration (Sister Joseph's nodule), ascites, ovarian metastasis (Krukenberg tumor) |

25% (i.e., ≥50% reduction in size) has been observed. This rate increases to 25% to 50% when combination chemotherapy with the FAM regimen (5-fluorouracil, Adriamycin, and mitomycin C) is used. Combining chemotherapy with radiotherapy confers no additional benefits. Because 10% to 50% of gastric cancers have estrogen receptors, giving tamoxifen with chemotherapy may have some advantage.

### Gastric Lymphoma

Gastric lymphomas are rare, accounting for less than 5% of gastric neoplasms. Most are extranodal non-Hodgkin lymphomas, arising from the submucosal lymphoid tissue, with a few arising from the mucosa-associated lymphoid tissue (MALT lymphoma). Epidemiological studies show a link between previous *Helicobacter pylori* infection and later development of MALT gastric lymphoma. Clinical features simulate those of peptic ulcer or gastric cancer. Systemic disease features lymphadenopathy and hepatosplenomegaly. Radiologic and endoscopic features rarely are able to differentiate lymphoma from adenocarcinoma. Thickened folds, duodenal extension, and multiple lesions with extensive ulcerations suggest lymphoma. Multiple biopsies are necessary for diagnosis. The Ann Arbor system is used for staging. Early disease is treated by surgery; when surgery is not feasible, radiotherapy can be used instead as the primary therapy. For later stages, chemotherapy and radiotherapy can be combined. A few cases of gastric MALT lymphoma have been cured by eradication of *H. pylori* infection.

# CHAPTER 85 ANATOMY AND PHYSIOLOGY OF THE SMALL INTESTINE

## Anatomy

The small intestine, approximately 600 cm long, extends from the pylorus to the ileocecal valve, and consists of the duodenum (the first 25–30 cm), the jejunum, and the ileum. The small bowel is supplied by the celiac and the superior mesenteric arteries; anastomotic channels exist between the superior and inferior mesenteric arteries, thus providing a collateral circulation. The vagus nerves that terminate in the myenteric and submucosal plexuses of the bowel wall provide the parasympathetic innervation; postganglionic fibers from the celiac and superior mesenteric ganglia provide the sympathetic efferents.

The mucosal surface of the intestinal folds is studded with slender villi with their bases encircled by pit-like crypts. The crypts and villi are lined by a continuous layer of columnar absorptive and mucoglycoprotein-producing goblet cells. Cell renewal begins from the undifferentiated crypt cells. In about 3 to 5 days, these newly formed cells migrate up the walls of the crypts and onto the villi, and mature into absorptive cells. When they reach the villus tips, the cells slough off into the lumen. The crypt epithelium also contains Paneth and enterochromaffin (enteroendocrine) cells. Endocrine cells present in the GI tract from the stomach to jejunum secrete gastrin, secretin, cholecystokinin, gastric inhibitory polypeptide, and motilin, whereas ileal and colonic cells produce peptide YY, enteroglucagon, and neurotensin. Somatostatin-producing cells are found throughout the GI tract.

The lamina propria, the loose cellular connective tissue beneath the epithelium, contains the capillaries, venules, and lymphatics serving the absorptive epithelium, as well as lymphocytes and plasma cells. The lymphocytes are seen between the columnar epithelial absorptive cells, in the lamina propria, and in focal aggregates called lymphoid follicles and Peyer's patches. Covering these aggregates are specialized epithelial cells (M-cells), which can endocytose antigens, and present them to the underlying T and B lymphocytes. It is thought that the antigen-sensitized B lymphocytes migrate to the lamina propria, and evolve into immunoglobulin-synthesizing plasma cells. Approximately 80% to 90% of these plasma cells synthesize and contain IgA, 12% to 16% contain IgM, and 2% to 4% contain IgG. The IgA, locally synthesized and secreted into the gut lumen, contains antibodies developed after exposure to antigens entering from the lumen. The secretory IgA has two IgA molecules joined by a J-protein to which a glycoprotein secretory component is added. The secretory component, synthesized by the epithelial cells and attached to the IgA before it enters the lumen, probably protects IgA from intraluminal enzymatic digestion. Secretory IgA is felt to exert a critical role in regulating gut bacterial flora, preventing and controlling tissue invasion by enteroviruses, and in preventing the absorption of undesirable antigenic material.

## Physiology

### Motor activity

An inherent, rhythmically fluctuating membrane potential occurs continuously and in synchrony in the adjacent cells of the longitudinal layer of small intestinal smooth muscle cells, known as the slow-wave activity (i.e., basic electrical rhythm, or electrical control activity). These slow waves occur as a distally migrating signal at 12 cycles/min in the duodenum to about 8 cycles/min in the terminal ileum. The spike potential is superimposed on the peaks of slow waves; the smooth muscles contract only in relation to them. The frequency of spike potentials and muscle contractions varies in time and in relationship to food intake, as well as in response to neural and hormonal stimuli. Meanwhile, slow wave activity runs constantly, unaffected by fasting, feeding, or hormonal or nervous stimuli.

The most common form of small intestinal motor activity is segmental contraction, a very brief, localized, ring-like contraction, usually 1 to 2 cm in length. These recur and disappear rhythmically, leading to movement of intestinal contents back and forth for mixing and better exposure to the mucosal surface.

While the patient is fasting, the small bowel demonstrates a motor pattern, the interdigestive myoelectric complex (migrating motor complex), that starts concurrently in the stomach and upper small intestine (Figure 85.1). At first, irregular segmental contractions occur (phase II), which slowly gather frequency and strength; then a slowly migrating contraction complex sweeps down to the ileum, with a velocity of 4 to 6 cm/min in the upper intestine, and 1 cm/min in the lower small intestine (phase III). A period of minimal, scattered contractions follows (phase I). As one complex reaches the ileum, another begins in the stomach or duodenum, thus repeating the cycle. After feeding, these complexes give place to frequent segmental contractions that are either stationary or migrate distally over short distances.

The act of vomiting also has a specific motor pattern. The medullary vomiting center receives signals from the chemoreceptor trigger zone. Receptors for serotonin (5-HT), dopamine, and histamine transmit the signals that trigger the act of vomiting via vagal fibers. Following a brief period of motor inhibition, a retrograde migrating contraction from the midgut empties bowel contents into the stomach. The abdominal wall muscles then suddenly contract, propelling gastric contents to the mouth.

### The epithelial cell and absorptive mechanisms

Digestion and absorption are discussed in Chapters 69 and 70. Carbohydrates consisting of starch (60–70%),

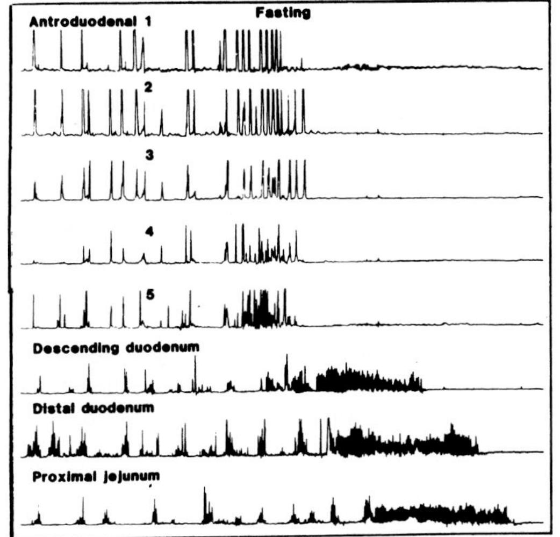


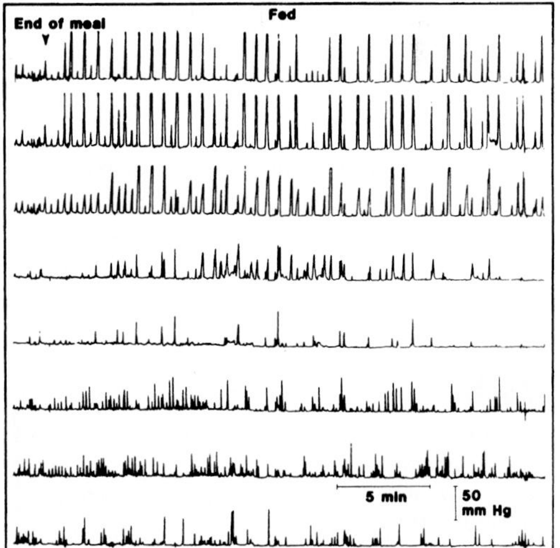


**FIGURE 85.1.** ***Left:*** **Normal interdigestive migrating motor complex in the fasting state.** ***Right:*** **Normal fed motor activity.** (Source: Malagelada JR, Camilleri M, Stanghellini V. Manometric Diagnosis of Gastrointestinal Motility Disorders. New York: Thieme Medical Publishers, 1986. Used with permission.)

sucrose (30%), and lactose (0–10%) make up 40% to 50% of total daily calories. Fat, nearly all of which is long-chain triglycerides, accounts for 30% to 40% of calories; the majority of fatty acids are palmitic, stearic, oleic, and linoleic. The remaining 5% of dietary fat consists of medium-chain triglycerides, phospholipids, fat-soluble vitamins, and cholesterol. Dietary protein averages 70 g/day. A nearly equal amount of endogenous protein, mostly secretions and desquamated mucosal cells and some plasma protein, enters the gut lumen.

## Congenital Abnormalities

Most congenital anomalies are discovered during infancy and childhood, and only occasionally are diagnosed for the first time in adulthood.

### Meckel's Diverticulum

Meckel's diverticulum, the most frequent congenital intestinal anomaly, affects almost 1.5% of the population. It arises from incomplete obliteration of the vitelline duct at the intestinal end, leaving a sac or diverticulum that arises from the antimesenteric border of the ileum, about 80 cm proximal to the ileocecal valve. These diverticula contain ectopic gastric, duodenal, colonic, and pancreatic mucosa, but gastric mucosa is the most common finding. Although the condition usually is asymptomatic, problems related to the diverticulum tend to arise most commonly during the first 2 years of life. Among the complications are bleeding, diverticulitis, perforation, and bowel obstruction; bleeding from ileal mucosal ulceration adjacent to ectopic gastric mucosa is the most common. Meckel's diverticulitis may mimic acute appendicitis.

Nonsurgical detection of the diverticulum is difficult, because it seldom fills with barium. Radioactive pertechnetate scanning may demonstrate those diverticula with gastric mucosa, but there are false negatives. Mesenteric angiography or tagged RBC scan may be helpful when there is significant bleeding.

### Other Abnormalities

Incomplete duodenal atresia may appear as an intraluminal diaphragm causing bilious vomiting. Anomalies of embryologic rotation and fixation may present as intestinal obstruction or a dilated cecum in the left upper abdominal quadrant in the adult.

# CHAPTER 86 INFECTIOUS ENTERITIS

### Definition and Epidemiology

Infectious enteritis (also known as acute gastroenteritis) is an acute illness with diarrhea and, depending on the causative agent, nausea, vomiting, abdominal cramps, fever, bloody stools, and headache. In the United States, the incidence of diarrheal illness is 1.5 to 1.9 per person per year, causing 10,000 to 20,000 deaths annually. Most of these enteritides occur in infants, particularly those living in areas with poor sanitation and a high incidence of malnutrition. Table 86.1 presents risk factors for acquiring infectious gastroenteritis. Additional information is given in Chapter 158. Special problems in immunocompromised patients are discussed in Chapters 164 and 165.

**TABLE 86.1. Risk Factors for Infectious Enteritis**

- Infants and preschoolers, especially in day care centers, kindergarten
- Travel to tropical and other areas with poor sanitation
- Contaminated food or drink
  - Poorly refrigerated food
  - Contaminated water supply
  - Raw or undercooked meat, fish, and shellfish
  - Nonpasteurized milk
- Low or suppressed gastric acid secretion

### Etiology

In the United States, bacteria and unicellular parasites account for 20% to 30% of episodes of infectious diarrhea, viruses for 30% to 40%, and undetermined agents (probably food toxins and viruses) for the remainder. The epidemiologic setting dictates the relative role of these agents in enteric infections, particularly in sporadic, large-scale epidemics. The major causes of traveler's diarrhea (*turista*) among travelers to Mexico and infectious enteritis are listed in Figure 86.1 and Table 86.2, respectively. The contribution of individual infectious agents according to the country visited.

### Pathogenesis

Gastric acidity provides an important initial defense by killing ingested organisms. Most pathogens need to attach to the epithelial brush border surface and to the specialized M-cells overlying Peyer's patches in order to proliferate, to produce toxins, and, for some pathogens, to invade the epithelium (Table 86.2).

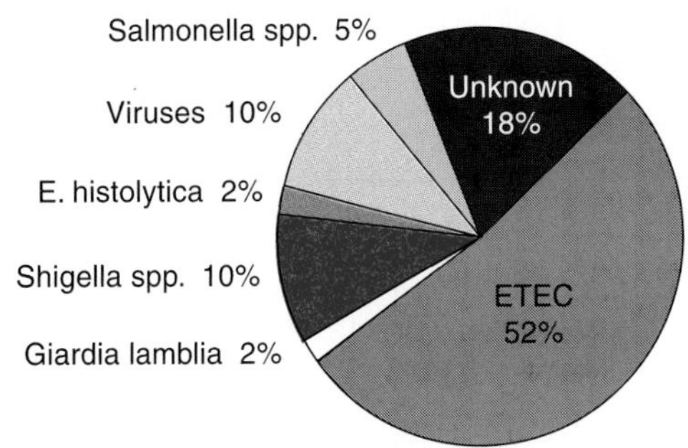


**FIGURE 86.1. Causes of traveler's diarrhea (turista) acquired in Central America. The incidence of Giardia varies from 0–50%, depending on the geographic location (see text). ETEC = enterotoxigenic E. coli.**

Specialized proteins in bacterial flagella and fimbriae interact with the epithelial cell membrane to effect attachment. Some pathogens invade the mucosa, causing inflammation, ulceration, bleeding, and, occasionally, bowel perforation. Others produce cytotoxins that destroy epithelial cells with or without ensuing tissue invasion (see Table 86.2). *Vibrio cholerae,* enteropathogenic *Escherichia coli,* and noninvasive *Salmonella* and *Shigella* species release enterotoxins that bind to cell surface receptors, initiating active $Cl^-$ ion secretion and reducing electroneutral NaCl absorption (see Chapters 76 and 77).

## Clinical Features

In broad terms, enteric infections cause either watery, secretory, **nonbloody diarrhea** with little abdominal pain and no fever, or the **dysenteric syndrome,** with cramps, bloody diarrhea, and fever. The incubation period ranges from hours (when the cause is ingested toxins) to 2 weeks. Physical findings may include signs of dehydration (see Chapter 76), diffuse abdominal tenderness without signs of peritoneal irritation (rigidity or rebound tenderness), and reduced, rather than absent, bowel sounds. Sensory and motor neuropathy may accompany enteritis acquired via seafood ingestion. The stool should be tested for blood. In the dysenteric syndrome, proctosigmoidoscopy is needed to obtain biopsy and aspirated exudate for microscopy (e.g., amebic trophozoites). In suspected infectious enteritis, expensive stool studies should be used efficiently (Figure 86.2). In secretory diarrhea, stool tests for pathogens may help define the source of the outbreak, but are not useful for guiding management.

## Management and Prognosis

Hospitalization and infection (enteric) precautions are indicated in patients with moderate or severe dehydration or the dysenteric syndrome. A stool sample should be sent to the laboratory before antibiotics, radiologic contrast material, or enemas are given. The management of dehydration and the use of antidiarrheal agents are discussed in Chapter 76. Antibiotic use in infectious diarrhea should be limited to specific situations (Table 86.3). Their empiric use is controversial and is not generally endorsed. Two factors limit the efficacy of antibiotics: (1) by the time the pathogen is identified, not only is the illness

**TABLE 86.2. Common Causes of Infectious Diarrhea**

| Causative Agent | Comment |
|---|---|
| **Bacteria** | |
| *Escherichia coli* | |
| Enterotoxigenic | Common |
| Enterohemorrhagic | Serious; from ingestion of undercooked beef, unpasteurized apple cider |
| Enteroadherent | Rare |
| Shigella | Foodborne |
| *Shigella dysenteriae*[†‡] | Low infectious dose |
| other spp. | Common |
| Salmonella | High infectious dose |
| *Salmonella typhi (paratyphi)*[†] | Rare |
| other spp. | Mild; obtained through handling of poultry, turtles |
| *Vibrio cholerae* | |
| –0.1; El Tor | Life-threatening diarrhea |
| Other spp. | Less severe. Fish, shellfish |
| *Campylobacter jejuni*[†‡] | |
| *Yersinia enterocolitica*[†] | Milk, pork |
| *C. difficile*[‡] | Antibiotic use; fecal-oral contamination |
| **Parasites** | |
| *Giardia lamblia* | Camping; Russia. May cause prolonged illness and mild malabsorption |
| Cryptosporidium spp | Low infectious dose, contaminated water supply |
| *Entameba histolytica*[†] | Rare |
| **Viruses** | |
| Rotavirus[‡] | Infants; in winter |
| Norwalk agent | Adults; water, food |
| Adenovirus spp. | All ages |
| **Food toxins** | Incubation period <12 hrs |
| *S. aureus* | Food |
| *C. perfringens*[†] | Food |
| Fish toxins (ciguatera, scromba) | Neurotoxins |

[†]Invasive
[‡]Produces cytotoxin

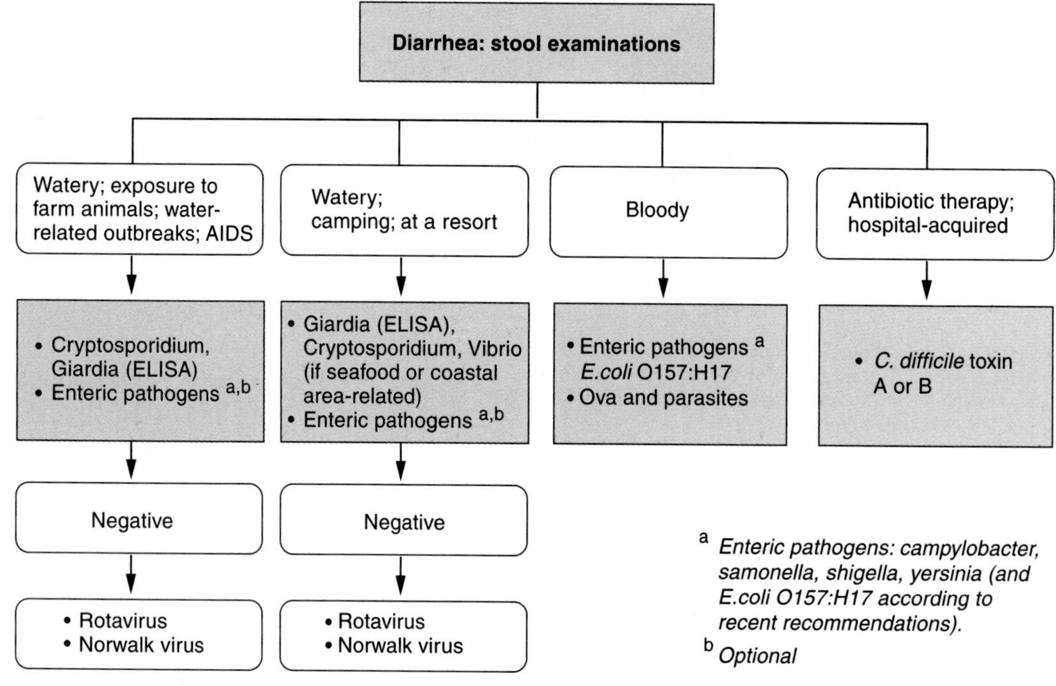


**FIGURE 86.2.** Recommended stool studies according to the clinical presentation of infectious diarrhea.

**TABLE 86.3. Guide to Antibiotic Therapy of Infectious Enteritis**

| Organism | Treatment |
|---|---|
| Shigella: dysenteric illness | TMP/SMX, 160/800 t.i.d. × 5 days<br>Ciprofloxacin, 500 mg b.i.d. × 5 days |
| Salmonella: dysenteric illness | Chloramphenicol, 0.5-1.0 g q.i.d., ×10–14 days<br>TMP/SMX, t.i.d. × 10–14 days<br>Ciprofloxacin, 500 mg b.i.d. × 10-14 days |
| *Campylobacter jejuni* | Erythromycin, 250–500 mg b.i.d. × 7 days<br>Ciprofloxacin, 500 mg b.i.d. × 7 days |
| *Yersinia enterocolitica* | Tetracycline, 500 mg q.i.d. (?) |
| *Giardia lamblia* | Quinacrine, 100 mg t.i.d. × 7 days<br>Metronidazole, 250 mg t.i.d. × 7 days |
| *Entameba histolytica* | Metronidazole, 250 mg t.i.d. plus diiodohydroxyquin, 650 mg t.i.d. × 20 days |
| Cryptosporidium | Paromomycin, 500 mg q.i.d. × 14 days<br>Clarithromycin, 250–500 mg b.i.d. × 14 days; efficacy not established |
| Acute infectious diarrhea with blood in stool; no pathogen identified or etiologic diagnosis | Ciprofloxacin, 500 mg b.i.d. × 3 days (?) |

TMP/SMX = trimethoprim-sulfamethoxazole.

subsiding, but the issue of specific therapy may be moot; and (2) enteric bacterial pathogens often alter their antibiotic susceptibility patterns. The prognosis is excellent in almost all patients. In the few in whom watery diarrhea lasts many months without a persistently identifiable pathogen, all that is needed besides antidiarrheals is reassurance that the diarrhea eventually will abate.

# CHAPTER 87 SELECTED SMALL BOWEL DISEASES CAUSING MALABSORPTION

General aspects of absorption, malabsorption, and the use of various laboratory studies in diagnosing malabsorption are discussed in Chapter 77. Among the many disorders that cause malabsorption, some specific small bowel diseases are considered in this chapter.

## Lactose Deficiency

Lactose, a disaccharide present only in milk, is composed of glucose and galactose. **Lactase** is required in the luminal surface of enterocytes to digest lactose to these readily absorbable sugars. Lactase deficiency, which occurs in the majority of the world's population (Figure 87.1), most commonly is an autosomal recessive disorder in which the enzyme disappears after the weaning period. Its symptoms are those of carbohydrate malabsorption—that is, abdominal distention, flatulence, and diarrhea. The relationship to ingestion of milk (cow's milk contains 5% lactose) and other dairy products—such as ice cream, pasteurized yogurt, and cheese—may be obvious. The diagnosis is established by a lactose—breath hydrogen test where breath $H_2$ rises above 20 ppm after a lactose test dose, or by a rise in plasma glucose not exceeding 20 mg/dl. Treatment is avoidance of nonfermented dairy products in the diet. Patients, particularly postmenopausal women, who need a constant source of calcium, phosphorus, and vitamin D, may consume milk with an added microbial lactase preparation (e.g., Lactonase, Lactrase). Nonpasteurized yogurt is well tolerated. Secondary lactase deficiency may follow any intestinal disease, causing widespread mucosal damage.

## Celiac Sprue

Celiac sprue, also known as **gluten-sensitive enteropathy,** is a prime clinical example of a mucosal absorptive defect causing malabsorption. There is a poorly understood sensitivity to (or inability to metabolize) gluten, a glutamine-rich protein component of wheat, rye, and barley. The higher prevalence of HLA-B6 and HLA-DR3 antigens suggests a genetic basis. The current notion is that gluten, or some peptide fraction derived from it, may induce immunologically mediated intestinal mucosal injury. The disease is more prevalent (normally 1/1000 to 1/2000) among diabetics. In untreated celiac disease, the mucosa reveals flattened surface with total loss of villi, elongated crypts, and flattened epithelial cells with some loss of brush-border microvilli. The lamina propria and the surface epithelium are infiltrated by lymphocytes and plasma cells. In symptomatic cases, serum folate levels are almost universally low. Circulating antibodies to gliadin, reticulin, and endomysium occur in most patients; the

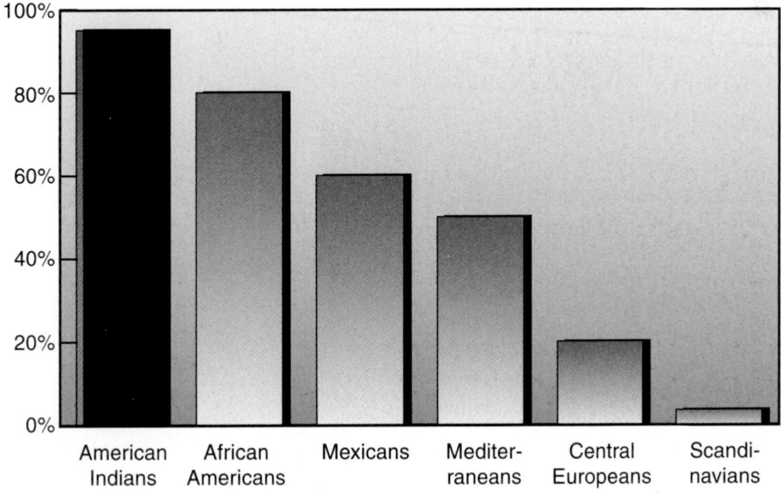


**FIGURE 87.1.** Prevalence of lactase deficiency in various populations of the world. Among Asians the prevalence ranges from 90 to 100%, among central Europeans from 15 to 25%, and among Scandinavians from 0 to 3%.

anti-endomysial antibody has the highest diagnostic accuracy.

### Clinical Features

Clinical manifestations vary widely, depending on the extent of the disease beyond the pylorus. The onset may be in infancy, shortly after weaning, or in childhood. It is not uncommon for it to remit in adolescence only to reappear later. In addition to steatorrhea, diarrhea, weight loss, cramps, abdominal distention, and malaise, nutritional deficiency states due to impaired absorption of iron, calcium, vitamin D, vitamin $B_{12}$, or vitamin K dominate the clinical picture. Physical examination may be normal or show signs of weight loss, decreased muscle mass, or signs of specific nutritional deficiencies, such as easy bruising, dependent edema, tetany, and glossitis. In severe cases, the abdomen is protuberant and has a doughy consistency.

### Diagnosis and Management

Laboratory findings may reflect any of the deficiencies just listed. The small bowel series shows a coarse fold pattern, irregular dilatation of gut loops, and, occasionally, transient intussusceptions. The diagnosis depends on mucosal biopsy followed by documentation of clinical, biochemical, and morphologic remission after excluding dietary gluten. A sprue-like small bowel mucosa on biopsy, IgA deposits in the dermis, mild malabsorption, and even remission of intestinal and skin lesions after a gluten-free diet occur in most cases of *dermatitis herpetiformis.*

Treatment is lifelong, with total gluten avoidance, best attained through careful patient education by an experienced dietitian, and by encouraging contact with the local chapter of a Celiac Disease or Sprue Society. Clinical and biochemical improvement follows within days or a few weeks of starting the diet, and bowel biopsies revert to normal within 3 to 12 months. Titers of circulating IgA antibodies to gliadin, endomysium, and reticulin also decline.

The prognosis is generally excellent on a gluten-free diet, but a favorable response is not universal in every patient with a biopsy suggestive of celiac sprue. This so-called **refractory sprue** usually responds to corticosteroids. **Ulcerative jejunitis,** a life-threatening complication, features worsening diarrhea and malabsorption, perforation, and occasional bleeding. In the **collagenous sprue** that develops in a few patients, jejunal biopsy shows a collagenous deposit beneath the epithelial basement membrane, extending into the lamina propria. The associated clinical worsening (i.e., weight loss, increasing malabsorption and diarrhea, anemia, and hypoproteinemia) does not respond to steroids and gluten withdrawal. Lifelong adherence to a gluten-free diet lessens the increased risk of malignancy that is a feature of this disease (generalized and intestinal lymphoma, squamous cancer of the oropharynx and esophagus, and adenocarcinoma of the small bowel).

## Tropical Sprue

Tropical sprue occurs in discrete tropical areas, including scattered islands in the Caribbean, the Indian subcontinent, and areas of southern Africa. The disease can be acquired during lengthy visits to endemic areas. Chronic contamination of the bowel by pathogenic bacteria is believed to be the cause. Progressive malabsorption, weight loss, and anemia commonly follow a bout of nonspecific, acute diarrhea. The small bowel biopsy shows varying degrees of villus shortening, crypt hypertrophy, and chronic inflammation of the lamina propria. Pharmacologic doses of folate along with tetracycline are highly effective.

## Intestinal Bacterial Overgrowth

Bacteria swallowed with saliva and food contaminate the normal small bowel only intermittently, because the gastric acid acts as an important bactericidal barrier. Bacterial overgrowth, usually resulting from coliforms and enteric anaerobes, occurs in several conditions (Table 87.1).

The gold standard of diagnosis, albeit expensive and not widely available because of the lack of laboratories with appropriate facilities, is quantitative aerobic and anaerobic culture of a fasting duodenal or proximal jejunal aspirate, showing in excess of $10^5$ viable bacteria/ml. Several screening tests are available, although none carry an accuracy over 80%. Two of these are as follows:

1. In the **glucose $H_2$ breath test:** a 50-g or 80-g glucose test dose should be totally absorbed. A rise

**TABLE 87.1. Conditions Associated with Bacterial Overgrowth in the Small Intestine**

| | |
|---|---|
| Reduced or absent gastric acid | Achlorhydria + pernicious anemia<br>Gastric operations, vagotomy, total gastrectomy |
| Intestinal stasis | Multiple duodenal and intestinal diverticula<br>Afferent loop of Billroth II gastrectomy<br>Proximal to intestinal strictures<br>Pseudo-obstruction syndromes |
| Contamination by colonic contents | Resection of ileocecal valve<br>Intestinal-colonic fistula |

in breath $H_2$ implies bacterial fermentation in the small bowel.

2. In the **$^{14}$C-D-xylose and $^{14}$C-cholylglycine tests,** bacterial D-xylose fermentation and bile acid deconjugation, respectively, cause $^{14}CO_2$ to appear in the breath, signaling overgrowth.

In bacterial overgrowth, bacteria consume both the free vitamin $B_{12}$ and the $B_{12}$-intrinsic factor complex, thus causing $B_{12}$ malabsorption. Bacteria also deconjugate bile acids, which are then absorbed by passive diffusion; the reduced intestinal bile acid concentration may then lead to steatorrhea. $H_2$ and $CO_2$ produced by bacterial carbohydrate fermentation cause abdominal distention and pain, which leads patients to reduce their nutrient intake. Empiric antibiotics are used; drugs and dosages may have to be altered over time as symptoms recur during therapy. Tetracycline or cephalexin (250 mg q.i.d.) elicits a response in 40% of patients. Amoxicillin/potassium clavulanate, 250–500 mg t.i.d. or ciprofloxacin, 500 mg b.i.d., plus metronidazole, 250–500 mg t.i.d., lead to better results. Once clinical success is achieved, antibiotics are given monthly, for 10 to 14 days on a recurring, long term basis.

## Whipple Disease

Whipple disease is a rare, progressive multisystem disease, seen mostly in middle-aged men. It is a bacterial infection that does respond to treatment with antibiotics. In untreated patients, even without diarrhea and malabsorption, jejunal biopsies show periodic acid-Schiff (PAS)-positive macrophages and intra- and extracellular rod-shaped organisms in the lamina propria of the jejunal villi. Many organs also contain PAS-positive macrophages. The organism appears to be a gram-positive actinomycete bacillus, *Tropherymya whippleii*, despite its lack of consistent isolation from cultures of affected tissues. A host defect is likely, because the phagocytized bacteria are not destroyed, and a strong inflammatory response is lacking, despite bacteria lying free in various organs.

Episodic arthralgias and nondeforming arthritis of large joints typically antedate GI symptoms by several years. Pneumonia, cough, and pleurisy occur, with occasional low-grade fever, anorexia, nausea, vomiting, diarrhea, edema, ascites, and lymphadenopathy. Hyperpigmentation occurs in the exposed skin in about 50% of patients. In 10–40% of cases, central nervous system (CNS) symptoms are manifest, including headache, dementia, myoclonus, ataxia, supranuclear ophthalmoplegia, and blindness.

Laboratory manifestations of malabsorption commonly occur. Small bowel radiographs usually show dilated loops with coarse, irregular folds. Diagnosis is made by duodenal or jejunal biopsy showing swollen and distorted intestinal villi; abundant PAS-positive macrophages and, often, dilated lacteal vessels are seen in the lamina propria. Electron microscopy shows rod-shaped bacilli. Penicillin, 1.2 million units/day, and streptomycin, 1 g/day for 14 days, are given initially, followed by oral trimethoprim-sulfamethoxazole (160/800 mg b.i.d.), or tetracycline, 1 g/d for 1 year, to ensure penetration of the antibiotic into the CNS. Complete remission regularly follows this regimen, but relapses occur in up to 35% of cases followed for at least 1 year. CNS involvement is very serious. Relapsed CNS disease is less amenable to retreatment.

## Protein-Losing Enteropathy

Protein-losing enteropathy is a pathophysiologic process in which excess plasma protein (>1.5 g/d) is lost by leakage into the gut. All plasma proteins participate in this process. Hypoproteinemia results when the proteins enter the distal GI tract, where they cannot be digested and absorbed, or when the liver's capacity for plasma protein synthesis from absorbed amino acids and oligopeptides is exceeded. Many clinical disorders exhibit this syndrome, including Ménétrier disease, enteritis (allergic, viral, and bacterial), and diseases with increased pressure in the intestinal lymphatic system, such as inferior vena caval obstruction, constrictive pericarditis, and congestive heart failure. Some patients present with dependent edema or anasarca; others basically exhibit features of the primary disorder. The diagnosis is made by IV infusion of Cr-labeled albumin and collection of stools for 96 hours to measure the level of radioactivity. Serum and stool α-1-antitrypsin is very useful for clearance tests, because it is not reabsorbed or digested after leakage from blood into bowel lumen.

## Short Bowel Syndrome

Short bowel syndrome describes the losses of fluids and electrolytes as well as malabsorption that are seen following extensive intestinal resection. Several factors determine the clinical consequences: (1) *the length of the remnant*, because loss of up to 50% of intestinal length is generally well tolerated; (2) *adaptation by the remnant*, because it increases absorptive capacity over the first 3–12 postoperative months; (3) *the site of resection*, because that determines malabsorption of specific nutrients; (4) *the presence of colonic capacity* for water and salt absorption and for the bacterial production of short-chain fatty acids and their absorption; and (5) *the integrity of the remnant.*

Resection of less than 100 cm of ileum from the ileocecal valve (e.g., for Crohn disease), reduces bile salt absorption, which is offset by increased hepatic bile salt synthesis. Excess delivery of bile salts into the colon disturbs colonic water and salt absorption. However, resection of more than 100 cm of terminal ileum leads to heavy losses of bile salts into the colon, which outstrips the hepatic synthesis. The lowered bile salt levels in bile and small intestinal contents lead to steatorrhea and a predilection for cholesterol gallstones. Dietary fat restriction can minimize the diarrhea, because colonic water and salt absorption is compromised by long-chain fatty acids. However, vitamin $B_{12}$ absorption is likely to suffer. Steatorrhea increases colonic absorption of dietary oxalate, resulting in urinary calcium oxalate stones.

Management of the short-bowel syndrome must address many issues. **Caloric losses** from the GI tract tend to decrease during the initial period of adaptation of the remaining intestine. Frequent, high-caloric feedings should be encouraged, but elemental diets are not indicated. Supplemental home parenteral nutrition may be needed in patients with very little intestine remaining. **Water and electrolyte deficits** are more likely with small bowel stomas than with an intact colon. Minor deficits are correctable by daily use of an oral rehydration solution, but electrolyte solutions may need to be infused overnight. Refractory patients may require the use of the parenteral somatostatin analog octreotide, which decreases vascular perfusion of the small bowel, and ultimately may decrease the volume of intestinal secretion and diarrhea. It is necessary to monitor for and treat any **nutrient deficits** from excessive losses of minerals, especially calcium, magnesium, potassium, and zinc, and of fat-soluble vitamins. **Vitamin $B_{12}$ malabsorption** is the rule after extensive ileal resections, necessitating $B_{12}$ replacement by monthly injections. **Diarrhea** due to excess bile salt delivery can be abolished by a bile salt-binding resin (e.g., cholestyramine). Because calcium ions precipitate oxalate and prevent its intestinal absorption, dietary calcium should be increased and oxalate intake restricted. **D-lactic acidosis** with confusion and ataxia is a rare but serious complication, which resolves with antibiotics and cessation of carbohydrate intake.

# CHAPTER 88 MESENTERIC VASCULAR DISEASE AND INSUFFICIENCY

Mesenteric arterial insufficiency is a formidable problem for the clinician, the surgeon, and the radiologist. The collateral interconnecting arteries between the celiac, superior mesenteric, and inferior mesenteric arteries endow the gut with a significant degree of protection from ischemia.

## Chronic Intestinal Ischemia

Chronic mesenteric ischemia (also known as abdominal angina) is the result of atheromatous stenosis or occlusion of two of the three major gut arteries, often at or near their aortic origins. Patients report steady and often severe mid-abdominal or generalized pain, occurring 20 to 30 minutes after meals. However, the relation between food intake and pain is not always constant. Fear of pain on eating leads to decreased food intake and weight loss. Physical examination usually is unrevealing, save for abdominal bruits. However, elderly patients often exhibit asymptomatic bruits. Angiography, the major diagnostic tool, also shows equivalent stenosis in asymptomatic persons. The more common causes of chronic abdominal pain must be excluded before diagnosing intestinal angina or embarking on surgical revascularization or balloon angioplasty.

## Acute Mesenteric Ischemia

Acute bowel infarction, a life-threatening intra-abdominal calamity, is due to sudden compromise of the intestinal blood supply. Serious cardiovascular, renal, or other systemic disease is often associated. At least one half of the cases represent nonocclusive intestinal ischemia and infarction, which particularly afflicts those above age 50, with chronic congestive heart failure, cardiac arrhythmias, recent myocardial infarction, hypotension, and hypovolemia. Splanchnic vasoconstriction is the central theme here. It may be brief but long enough to damage mucosa. Thromboembolic arterial occlusion leads to 35% of cases, with the clinical setting of emboli being arrhythmias (atrial fibrillation), recent myocardial infarction, or infective endocarditis. Aortic dissection, vasculitis, and venous thrombosis account for 15%.

Abdominal pain is the most common initial symptom, along with an urge to defecate. Early on, abdominal findings are sparse or absent. Bloody stools are common. With time, nausea, vomiting, and back pain appear, along with fever, peritoneal signs, leukocytosis, metabolic acidosis, hyperamylasemia, and blood-tinged peritoneal fluid that denotes progressive intestinal necrosis. The diagnosis of acute mesenteric ischemia must be considered in any older patient with persistent, acute abdominal pain without other abdominal findings or abnormalities on plain radiographs, especially because this often indicates that the process is at an early stage. The diagnosis is difficult, but delays are fatal. In this setting, rapid assessment of the cardiovascular status and prompt resuscitation should be carried out to alleviate or correct congestive heart failure, pulmonary edema, or arrhythmias.

Abdominal radiographs are obtained to exclude other acute abdominal events and to detect signs of ischemic bowel. A duplex ultrasound can detect blood flow and its direction in the three major visceral arteries. With angiography, the diagnostic "gold standard," the state of the splanchnic vessels can be assessed; if the findings justify it, a vasodilator such as papaverine can be given. The decision for surgery is extremely difficult. At surgery, it often is not possible to confidently assess the limits of viable bowel, and a "second-look" laparotomy 12 to 36 hours later may help identify and resect any additional nonviable bowel. Atherosclerotic or thrombotic obstruction of the celiac and superior mesenteric artery, near their origin, may be treated by percutaneous balloon angioplasty, but recurrent occlusion is common.

# CHAPTER 89 NEOPLASMS OF THE SMALL INTESTINE

Neoplasms of the small bowel are uncommon. The majority are benign, and are quiescent or detected incidentally. Polyposis syndromes involving the small bowel are discussed in Chapter 100.

## Adenocarcinoma

**Adenocarcinoma** is the most common small bowel cancer, occurring mainly in the duodenum and jejunum. It may, rarely, complicate the course of long-standing Crohn ileitis. Symptoms occur due to obstruction, ulceration, bleeding, and, occasionally, intussusception or perforation. Adenocarcinoma in the region of the papilla of Vater tends to develop from villous adenomas. It may produce ulcer-like symptoms but also frequently obstructs the common bile duct or ampulla, thus clinically simulating cancer of the head of the pancreas with jaundice. Most adenocarcinomas of the duodenum and small bowel are discovered too late for curative surgical resection. The prognosis is grim.

## Lymphoma

Most GI lymphomas arise from monoclonal proliferation of intestinal B lymphocytes. Primary lymphoma of the small intestine occurs most commonly in the ileum and has several forms. The multifocal, nodular form can produce a picture resembling regional enteritis by producing localized polypoid, infiltrative, and ulcerative lesions affecting several segments. Diffuse involvement of the small bowel by lymphoma may mimic celiac disease, including radiographic and biopsy features, with evidence of malabsorption. Fever, abdominal pain, and anorexia are more suggestive of diffuse lymphoma. In a subset, an abnormal, IgA-type immunoglobulin is produced, composed of heavy chains of the $\alpha$-1 subclass (**$\alpha$-heavy chain disease**). It occurs among adolescents and young adults of Middle Eastern countries, Asia, and South America. New symptoms (e.g., pain, weight loss) occurring in patients with established celiac disease or lack of response to a gluten-free diet could be an indication of lymphoma of the small intestine. Treatment and prognosis depend on the extent of bowel involvement and the presence or absence of extraintestinal lymphoma. Localized or small-segment disease is best treated by surgery, with or without postoperative radiotherapy or chemotherapy. Primary diffuse lymphoma of a long intestinal segment is less amenable to surgery; radiotherapy and chemotherapy are the mainstays.

### Kaposi Sarcoma

**Kaposi sarcoma** may involve any part of the GI tract. It presents as a submucosal infiltrative process and usually is clinically silent. The typical skin manifestations are present in nearly all patients, most of whom have AIDS. Metastases to the small intestine originate predominantly from malignant melanomas and lung cancer. Bleeding, obstruction, and perforation are the usual symptoms.

### Carcinoid Tumor

Carcinoid tumors are most common in the terminal ileum, the appendix, and the rectum. The great majority are small, asymptomatic, and found incidentally at surgery or autopsy. However, some are clinically malignant. Metastases, which seem to correlate best with size, occur in 20% to 30% of cases at diagnosis. These slow-growing neoplasms may cause partial bowel obstruction; liver metastases may produce the "carcinoid syndrome," with cramps and watery diarrhea, cutaneous flushing, bronchial constriction, telangiectasias, and right heart valvular lesions. Food and alcohol intake may precipitate flushing in patients with foregut tumors. Carcinoid tumor cells hydroxylate and decarboxylate tryptophan to serotonin, which is later metabolized to 5-hydroxyindoleacetic acid (5-HIAA) and excreted abundantly in the urine.

Widespread metastases are rare. Although liver metastases may be present, tumor resection should be considered to prevent intestinal obstruction and bleeding. Combined 5-fluorouracil and streptozotocin chemotherapy has shown a 35% to 50% temporary response rate. Hepatic artery ligation or embolization followed by chemotherapy is another option. Diarrhea may respond to diphenoxylate and loperamide. Infusion of octreotide, a somatostatin analogue, can help prevent "carcinoid crises" during anesthesia and surgery. Carcinoid tumors and their metastases grow quite slowly, with many patients surviving 5 to 10 years or more; almost 25% survive 5 years, even with liver metastases. Death usually is caused by hepatic or cardiac failure.

# CHAPTER 90 INTESTINAL OBSTRUCTION AND PARALYTIC ILEUS

## Etiology and Clinical Features

Mechanical obstruction or generalized hypomotility of intestinal smooth muscle (paralytic ileus) may cause intestinal and abdominal distension. Features of mechanical obstruction and paralytic ileus are compared in Table 90.1. In mechanical obstruction, rhythmic cramps reach a peak, causing the patient to writhe, and then recede. The cramps are accompanied by loud, often high-pitched, or hollow bowel sounds **(borborygmi)**. Abdominal distention is present unless obstruction is at a high level. Constipation depends on the level of the lesion; the lower the level and more complete the obstruction, the sooner obstipation (severe constipation) ensues. Repeated vomiting and sequestered fluid in the bowel lumen cause dehydration. If strangulation, infarction, or peritonitis develops, signs of shock and sepsis will follow, and surgery is urgently needed.

**TABLE 90.1. Features of Mechanical Obstruction and Paralytic Ileus**

| | Mechanical Obstruction | Paralytic Ileus |
|---|---|---|
| Etiology | Intraluminal blockage (tumors, foreign bodies, gallstones, worms) or extrinsic compression and obstruction (adhesions, tumors, herniations, volvulus) | Secondary to a primary derangement, e.g., trauma, peritonitis, uremia, sepsis, post-operative atony from manipulation of abdominal viscera; pelvic and spinal fractures, narcotics, anticholinergics, hypokalemia, hypocalcemia |
| Evolution | Rapid with high obstruction; less rapid for lower levels | Slow. Clinical picture dominated by the underlying illness |
| Abdominal pain | Colicky, appears in bouts that reach a peak, borborygmi heard during contraction | Usually painless; discomfort and dyspnea depend on extent of distention |
| Other symptoms | Nausea, vomiting, distention, and obstipation | Nausea, vomiting, distention, and obstipation |
| Abdominal examination | Soft and tympanitic, visible outlines of dilated intestinal loops, borborygmi (early); bowel sounds are absent in late disease complicated by peritonitis | Abdomen may be distended but is characteristically silent |
| Radiographs | Single or multiple loops of distended small bowel (Figure 83.1) with air-fluid levels | Multiple, distended, gas-filled small and large intestinal loops, with gas also in the lower colon and rectum. |
| Course and treatment | Progressive unless obstruction relieved; surgery must be considered early | Often self-limited. Responds to correction of the underlying illness through intestinal decompression and management of fluid/ electrolyte problems |

## Diagnosis

Hernial orifices should be carefully checked for incarcerated or strangulated hernias. Metabolic acidosis or alkalosis, leukocytosis, hyperamylasemia, and hemoconcentration are seen, but these are nonspecific. Plain supine, upright, and lateral abdominal radiographs should be obtained, and, if inconclusive, repeated in a few hours. Besides air-fluid levels (Figure 90.1), bowel gas patterns might suggest inguinal or other internal hernias, volvulus, or air in the biliary tree (a bilioenteric fistula with gallstone passage) or in the portal vein (bowel infarction). A cautiously performed barium enema often shows the level and nature of mechanical colon obstruction. Treatment consists of correcting fluid and electrolyte imbalance, relieving emesis, and decompressing the small bowel of its fluid and swallowed air. In suspected mechanical obstruction, early surgery should be considered before strangulation (creating a nonviable bowel segment) occurs.

Colonic obstruction most often is due to cancer (see Chapter 100). Its course is gradual, but obstipation occurs early. Plain abdominal radiographs show a gas-filled colon, up to a point distal to which no gas is seen. In *cecal volvulus*, a large, left-upper-quadrant, gas-filled viscus is seen with a paucity of gas distal to it. In *sigmoid volvulus*, a large, dilated colonic loop arises from the pelvis. On a barium enema, a normal rectum and distal sigmoid taper to a "bird's beak" at the site of the volvulus. Barium enema or sigmoidoscopy is successful in reducing most cases of sigmoid volvulus.

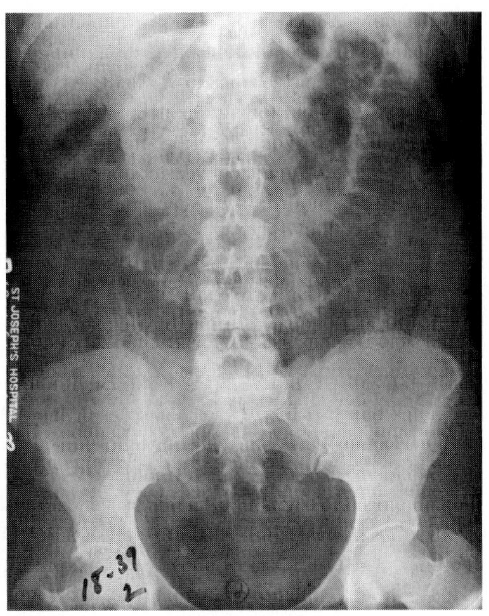


**FIGURE 90.1. Plain x-ray of abdomen showing small bowel obstruction.**

# CHAPTER 91 REGIONAL ENTERITIS

## Definition and Epidemiology

Regional enteritis, or **Crohn disease of the small intestine,** is a chronic inflammatory disorder of unknown cause, potentially involving the GI tract from mouth to anus with secondary involvement of regional lymph nodes, liver, skin, eyes, and joints. (Crohn colitis is discussed in Chapter 95.) The incidence of Crohn disease has risen substantially during the past few decades; in the past, it was particularly common among Jews of eastern European heritage and people residing in areas with a cold or temperate climate; more recent demographic studies suggest that all ethnic groups in westernized nations are at risk. No defined pattern of inheritance is apparent, but first-degree relatives of index cases have a 5% to 15% lifetime risk of acquiring this disease. Intriguingly, studies of monozygotic twins, with one affected member, suggest that the unaffected twin has only 50% to 60% risk of developing Crohn disease. The disease is diagnosed before 30 years of age in 75% of patients, and before 20 years of age in 30% of patients.

## Pathology

The cellular reaction in the intestine is lymphoplasmacytoid; mononuclear cells aggregate to form non-caseating granulomas with giant cells in one half of cases. This inflammation, along with edema and fibrosis, involves all layers of the gut wall. The initial lesion consists of micro-ulcers overlying mucosal lymph follicles (aphthae). Irregular ulcers and the formation of deep fissures typify evolving Crohn disease. The inflamed and swollen intervening mucosa gives it a "cobblestone" appearance. Crohn disease of the small bowel typically tends to form fistulae and single or multiple fibrotic strictures. The bowel wall is thick and stiff. Normal intervening "skip areas" may be present between grossly diseased segments of the GI tract.

The small bowel, mainly the distal ileum, is solely involved in 30% of cases; in 50% of cases, ileitis contiguously extends into the colon; 20% of cases involve only the colon. Duodenal and antral involvement occurs in 1% to 3% of cases. Perianal disease, with fistulae and abscesses, as well as deep anal and perineal ulcers, develops in 30% of patients at some time and is the initial presentation in 1% to 3% of patients.

## Clinical Features

The clinical picture is determined by the site of GI involvement. Given the distal ileal involvement in 80% to 90% of patients, nonbloody diarrhea is the rule; steatorrhea and vitamin $B_{12}$ malabsorption are related to the length of the affected ileum. Abdominal pain (usually in the right lower quadrant) is very common. A steady ache indicates serosal extension and possible perforation; a palpable, tender inflammatory mass may form and evolve into an intra-abdominal abscess. Such perforations lead to sinus tracts, or fistulae into another viscus (bowel, urinary bladder, or vagina), or to the abdominal wall. Colicky pain with distention and its relief after bowel movements suggest partial ileal obstruction, due to inflammatory ileal swelling or fibrotic strictures. Weight loss may follow anorexia, fear of pain after eating, or malabsorption. Rectal bleeding most often is occult. Gross bleeding occasionally occurs, especially in young persons during their first attack with extensive Crohn colitis.

Perineal disease may be severe, often with dusky, anal skin tags and perianal or ischiorectal abscess, draining perineal fistulas, and anorectal stricture. Antroduodenal involvement may cause ulcer-like pain and pyloric or duodenal obstruction. Low-grade fever is usual; with spiking fever, an abscess is suspect. Extra-intestinal complications are erythema nodosum, arthritis, uveitis, oral aphthous ulcers, and primary sclerosing cholangitis. Malabsorption caused by ileal disease or resection leads to metabolic bone disease, anemia, bleeding diathesis, gallstones, renal oxalate stones, and weight loss (see Chapter 87).

## Diagnosis

There is no single test that confirms the diagnosis of Crohn disease; rather, the diagnosis is made from a constellation of clinical, laboratory, histopathologic, endoscopic, and radiographic findings. Laboratory abnormalities reflect inflammation, malnutrition (including hypoalbuminemia), blood loss, and malabsorption. Anemia has multiple causes, including myelosuppression by chronic disease. Urinalysis may demonstrate oxalate crystals, suggestive of fat malabsorption and enteric hyperoxaluria, or gross fecal contamination suggestive of a enterovesicular fistula. Imaging of the ileum by a small bowel series or barium enema may show mucosal edema, aphthous ulceration, luminal narrowing ("string sign"), fistula formation, and inflammatory mass effect (Figure 91.1), but these findings are typical of patients with longstanding disease. Crohn disease of the small intestine must be distinguished from ileocecal tuberculosis, lymphoma, and ileal carcinoid. Endoscopic evaluation with biopsies of the terminal ileum and throughout the colon may identify crypt architectural distortion, which is a hallmark feature of chronic, destructive intestinal inflammation. Colon radiographs or colonoscopy can identify colon and terminal ileal involvement. "Skip areas" in the colon and absence of rectal disease negate the diagnosis of ulcerative colitis. Work-up for intestinal obstruction is necessary if symptoms suggest it. Abdominal/pelvic CT can detect inflammatory masses, abscesses, fistulae, and extrinsic ureteral obstruction.

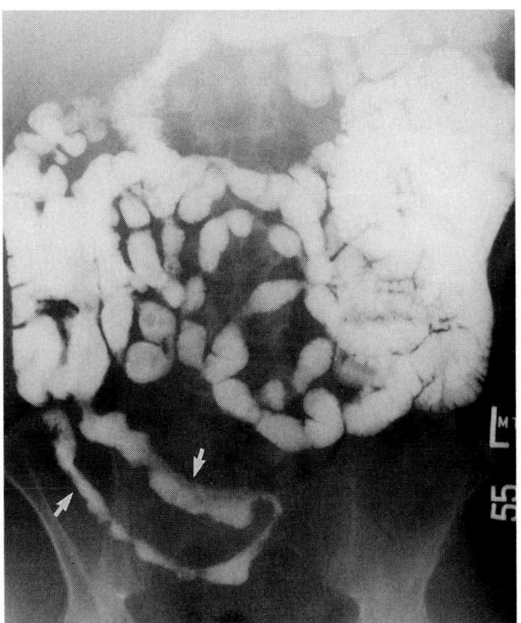


**FIGURE 91.1.** Crohn's disease of the small bowel. Small bowel barium x-ray shows the entire small bowel and the proximal and transverse colon; the transit time to the cecum was 55 min. Two separated loops (*solid arrows*) represent about 40 cm of terminal ileum with irregular narrowing and eccentric dilatation (pseudosacculations). The loops are separated by transmural inflammation and thickening of the mesentery. No abscess or intestinal fistula was found. The colon is spared.
(Courtesy of Edward Stewart, MD, Milwaukee, Wisconsin.)

## Management

The overriding goal of treatment is to achieve and maintain clinical remission, preserving the quality of life in patients with this chronic, recurrent disease, which has no specific treatment. Pain and diarrhea respond to codeine and antidiarrheal agents (e.g., loperamide). Nutritional support should correct vitamin and mineral deficiencies and ensure adequate caloric intake. Liquid formula diets are useful in some cases of severe and extensive disease. Patients with narrow strictures should avoid high-residue foods (e.g., corn, Chinese cabbage, pulp of citrus fruit, and enteric-coated tablets). Parenteral alimentation may be needed to prepare for surgery or as part of short-term therapy to induce a remission. The rare case of short bowel syndrome from extensive bowel resection requires home parenteral nutrition.

A few medications can help spur clinical remission but do not help in managing complications, such as abscesses and bowel strictures. In patients with mild disease, enteric-coated 5-ASA (mesalamine) products begin to release the active agent in the small bowel, while the release of 5-ASA from sulfasalazine and olsalazine (DIPENTUM) occurs entirely within the colon. In patients with moderate to severe disease, prednisone, 20–40 mg/day, is useful, but it does not prevent recurrences and its use should be limited to 2 to 4 months. Chronic steroid use is associated with multiple adverse reactions, including adrenal insufficiency, bone demineralization, and avascular necrosis of major joints. Patients who require steroids for the induction of remission should be considered for the use of immunomodulatory agents such as azathioprine, 6-mercaptopurine, and methotrexate, which can be steroid-sparing and maintain remission for several years. Their use must be weighed against their serious potential side effects (bone marrow suppression, pancreatitis, and predisposition to infections, allergies, and a higher risk of developing neoplasms). In patients with moderate to severe disease that has not responded to immunomodulator therapy, newer biologic agents such as the chimeric monoclonal antibody Infliximab, which targets the key cytokine TNF-α, have emerged as powerful forms of therapy for rapidly inducing remission. Long-term metronidazole may aid in closing fistulae. Maintenance therapy with therapeutic doses of mesalamine or immunomodulators (e.g., azathioprine, 6-MP) may lower the 1-year relapse rate from about 60% to about 25%. Surgery is indicated for complications that cannot be treated medically (e.g., abscesses, bowel obstruction, enterocutaneous fistulae, and incapacitating pain unresponsive to medical measures, and the rare case of adenocarcinoma of the ileum). The life-time risk of requiring surgery is about 70%; 30% to 50% of patients require further surgery. Disease recurrence following an ileocolonic resection regularly begins at the surgical anastomosis and extends proximally. The use of postoperative therapy to maintain surgically induced remission is currently under investigation.

# CHAPTER 92 PHYSIOLOGY OF THE COLON

## Colonic Motility

Unlike the small bowel, the colon has no uniform pattern of fasting and postprandial motor activity. Its primary motor activity is the nonpropulsive, ring-like segmental contraction, which produces mixing and to-and-fro movement of contents. Coordinated but irregular contractions propel intraluminal contents aborally over varying distances. The cecum and ascending colon delay the transit of solids until liquefied. Segmental contractions, more frequent in the distal colon, retard the flow into the rectum; the distention of the colon with feces causes a sensation of fullness that evokes an urge to defecate. A normally distensible rectum can accommodate rather large volumes of material. Giant migrating contractions frequently accompany colonic inflammation; they rapidly fill the rectal ampulla, prompting urgent defecation.

Cholecystokinin (CCK), gastrin, and motilin stimulate colonic smooth muscle, whereas secretin, glucagon, and vasoactive intestinal polypeptide (VIP) inhibit it. The final step in the motor inhibition of the colon and its sphincters is believed to be the local release of nitric oxide (NO). Prostaglandins of the E type diminish segmental activity and increase propulsion.

## Fluid and Electrolyte Transport in the Colon

Colonic epithelium differs functionally from that of the small bowel. The colonic mucosa is a tight membrane with lower effective pore size, lower osmotic permeability for water, higher electrical resistance and transmucosal potential difference, and higher ability to absorb $Na^+$ against electrochemical gradients. More than 95% of the large amount of short-chain fatty acids (SCFA) produced by carbohydrate fermentation is absorbed, most of it in exchange for bicarbonate. Absorption of these organic acids (acetate, propionate, n-butyrate) also stimulates the colonic absorption of $Na^+$ and water. SCFA, especially n-butyrate, is the major and essential substrate of colonocyte metabolism. Most of the n-butyrate entering colonocytes is metabolized by the cells and does not enter the portal system. Decreased SCFA production causes colonic absorptive dysfunction and, possibly, inflammation.

Ileal flow into the colon in a healthy person approximates 1500 ml/24 h, containing 200 mEq of $Na^+$. Stool output has 100 to 150 ml of water/24 h and 1 to 5 mEq of $Na^+$. The maximal, estimated absorptive capacity of the colon is 4 to5 L of water and 800 mEq $Na^+$ daily, provided the inflow from the terminal ileum is constant.

Thus, the colon can compensate for a two– to threefold rise in the volume normally delivered to it.

### Bacteriology of the Colon

Distal to the ileocecal valve there is an abundant, metabolically active bacterial population averaging $10^{10}$–$10^{12}$ bacteria/ml, composed mainly of strict anaerobes such as bacteroides and bifidobacteria. *Escherichia coli* is the most common facultative aerobic organism; anaerobic gram-positive cocci are also common. One-third of fecal weight consists of bacteria. Their activities alter bowel contents in many ways, such as the fermentation of both simple and complex (e.g., fiber) carbohydrate, deamination and decarboxylation of proteins and amino acids, ammonia formation from urea, hydroxylation of fatty acids, degradation of bilirubin to urobilins, deconjugation and dehydroxylation of bile acids, and the synthesis of vitamin K and folate. Bacteria also deconjugate glucuronide conjugates or convert inert compounds to pharmacologically active metabolites (e.g., splitting sulfasalazine into 5-ASA and sulfapyridine).

# CHAPTER 93 PROCEDURES IN THE DIAGNOSIS OF COLONIC DISORDERS

## Radiography

Plain films of the abdomen can detect "toxic" colonic dilatation (as in inflammatory bowel disease) and mechanical obstruction. Barium contrast enema is useful in detecting diverticulosis, inflammatory bowel disease, ischemic colitis, and motility disorders, such as Hirschsprung disease.

## Proctosigmoidoscopy

Proctosigmoidoscopy is indicated in patients with changes in bowel habit, rectal bleeding, anorectal pain, persistent constipation or diarrhea, weight loss, or anemia. Besides observing the mucosal appearance and the vascular pattern and looking for lesions such as polyps and tumors, it is possible to biopsy and to take specimens for parasitologic examination and bacterial culture. Biopsies should be obtained routinely in patients with chronic diarrhea. Rigid proctoscopy allows inspection of only the distal 25 cm of rectosigmoid. However, prior pelvic surgery, irradiation, and diverticulosis may cause sufficient fixation and angulation to limit full passage of the rigid scope. Flexible sigmoidoscopes not only surmount these problems, but extend inspection to 60 cm; they are routinely used to screen for cancer and polyps, but should not be considered to provide complete evaluation of the colon, even if no pathology is detected. Colonoscopy may be required to complete the evaluation of the lower GI tract, but it requires preparation using a colonic lavage solution as well as sedation in most patients.

## Stool Examination

Stool obtained by routine digital examination should be inspected and tested for occult blood. A variety of products, using a color indicator method, can detect fecal occult blood. In the presence of hydrogen peroxide, the peroxidase activity of heme hastens the oxidation of guaiac to a quinone; a blue color develops, indicating the presence of blood. False-positive results may follow ingestion of raw or undercooked red meat, turnips, or horseradish. The finding of RBCs and WBCs in the stool of patients with diarrhea points toward the possibility of acute or chronic inflammatory colonic disease. Proper collection and handling of fresh stool samples are necessary for successful bacteriologic and parasitologic examinations in evaluating diarrhea. Guidelines established by the clinical laboratory must be observed, and the stool collected before administering antibiotics and laxatives or barium radiographs.

## Colonoscopy

Fiberoptic colonoscopy is invaluable for confirmation and biopsy of findings on barium enema, in detecting and removing colon polyps, and in evaluating known or suspected inflammatory bowel disease. It is widely used for screening individuals at high risk for bowel cancer. In some situations, it complements barium radiograph examination, but several reports indicate a higher yield of significant pathology than barium enemas, albeit at a higher cost.

### Miscellaneous Tests

**Defecography**

Anorectal morphology and functional dynamics during defecation can be investigated by defecography. This radiology technique uses a stool-consistency barium paste and is useful for evaluation of rectal prolapse and fecal continence, and to assess the rectoanal angle and perineal descent during rest and straining.

**Colorectal transit time**

In the colorectal transit time technique, the subject ingests radiopaque markers (e.g., Sitzmarks) and progression of markers is monitored by abdominal radiographs until all of the markers have been expelled. Segmental transit times can be measured by counting markers in the right colon, left colon, and rectosigmoid areas.

**Anorectal manometry**

Rectal distention evokes rectoanal inhibitory reflex—that is, brief relaxation of the internal anal sphincter and contraction of the striated muscle external sphincter. Recording pressures from the anal canal and rectum, before and during rectal balloon distention, can diagnose Hirschsprung disease (absent rectoanal reflex), and detect the cause of fecal incontinence (by increased rectal sensation and reflex thresholds, decreased rectal compliance, or impaired internal or external sphincter function).

# CHAPTER 94 MOTILITY DISORDERS OF THE COLON

## Aganglionic Megacolon

Aganglionic megacolon is a congenital, familial motility disorder commonly known as **Hirschsprung disease,** that is thought to result from failure of the intramural ganglion cells to migrate into certain parts of the GI tract. Most commonly, a variable length of distal colon, involving the internal sphincter and adjacent rectum, is devoid of myenteric ganglion cells. Rarely, more extensive portions or even the entire colon are involved. The aganglionic segment is narrowed and unable to transport fecal contents, causing constipation and progressive dilatation of the normal proximal bowel, which leads eventually to abdominal distention. The clinical history is one of obstipation dating from birth. On digital rectal examination, the ampulla usually is empty. Radiographs show a narrowed distal colon and dilatation of the remainder of the bowel. Anorectal manometry reliably separates chronic idiopathic constipation from Hirschsprung disease by demonstrating in the latter the absence of the **rectoanal inhibitory reflex** (see Chapter 93). The confirmatory finding is the absence of myenteric ganglion cells on mucosal/submucosal suction or punch biopsy or deep surgical biopsy of the rectal wall of the narrowed segment. Treatment includes surgical resection of the aganglionic segment.

## Acquired Motility Disorders

### *Constipation*

Constipation, with or without colonic enlargement, is a common symptom; it is seen more often in women than in men, and its incidence rises with advancing age. A widely used definition is less than two bowel movements weekly, but the primary symptom may be hard, pellet-like stools or difficult emptying with excess straining at stool.

#### Etiology

Several medications impair bowel transit, including opiates, anticholinergics (including tricyclic antidepressants), calcium channel blockers, and ganglionic blockers. Endocrine-metabolic causes are hypothyroidism, hypercalcemia, and uremia. Neurogenic and myogenic constipation may follow heavy metal intoxication, spinal cord lesions, Hirschsprung disease, Parkinson disease, muscular dystrophy, multiple sclerosis, and autonomic neuropathy. Finally, any stenotic lesion of the colorectum and anus, including rectal prolapse, may cause constipation of recent onset. When no underlying cause is found, idiopathic constipation is diagnosed.

### *Idiopathic Constipation*

In adults, the etiology of idiopathic constipation is obscure, and treatment remains a challenge. Eventual success depends on step-wise treatment (Table 94.1), the aims of which are to evoke artificial bowel regularity, reduce symptoms, and prevent fecal impaction. The merits of increasing stool weight by a high-fiber diet are unclear. Bulk laxatives (e.g., methylcellulose, polycarbophil, psyllium) or stool softeners (e.g., docusate) are useful, as are hyperosmotic cathartics given periodically (orally or rectally,) including saline cathartics ($Mg^+$ salts) PEG-electrolyte solution (GoLYTELY), lactulose or sorbitol syrup, and hypertonic phosphate solutions (Fleets).Cisapride, a prokinetic drug, 10–20 mg t.i.d.,

**TABLE 94.1. Treatment of Idiopathic Constipation**

*Step 1:*
- Rule out metabolic and medication-related causes
  - Reassure and educate patient
  - Advise and encourage regular physical exercise
  - Instruct patient to attempt daily defecation
  - Recommend stool softeners
  - If small, hard stool: recommend bulk laxatives; add bran (20 g/d); mineral oil
  - Try cisapride, 10–20 mg q.i.d.

*Step 2:*
- Osmotic cathartics
  - Nonabsorbed sugars (sorbitol, lactulose)
  - PEG–electrolyte solution
  - Enemas: saline; hypertonic phosphate
  - Psychologic evaluation?

*Step 3*
- Stimulant laxatives

*Special situations:*
- Pelvic outlet obstruction: biofeedback therapy to coordinate pelvic floor relaxation with defecation act
- Normal transit constipation: reassurance/psychologic evaluation
- Delayed colonic transit (colonic inertia) with massive fecal retention: consider colectomy with ileoproctostomy.

may be used. Stimulant laxatives (phenolphthalein, danthron, bisacodyl, and cascara) should be used sparingly.

### Fecal Impaction

Symptoms and findings of bowel obstruction may be caused by the accumulation of firm, immovable fecal masses, 70% of which form in the rectum. This condition occurs mainly in chronically debilitated and immobile patients. Potential complications are dehydration, the formation of stercoral pressure ulcers, and colonic perforation. Treatment consists of hydration and careful disimpaction by digital means or by repeated retrograde irrigation and suction.

### Overuse of Laxatives

Known or surreptitious laxative use may cause the conditions discussed in this section. **Melanosis coli** is marked by a reticular, brown-black discoloration of the colonic mucosa. Lipofuscin-laden macrophages accumulate in the lamina propria. Although specific for long-term use of anthracene-type laxatives (e.g., senna, cascara, aloe, danthron), the condition has no functional significance. **Cathartic colon** is a featureless, moderately dilated colon occasionally found on barium enema examination. Mild, nonspecific abdominal symptoms may occur. Damage to the myenteric plexus of the colon reportedly follows chronic stimulant laxative use. **Factitious diarrhea** is an underdiagnosed cause of chronic watery diarrhea. By definition, the patient does not confess to using laxatives. The condition often is reflective of a complex psychiatric disorder, including the so-called Münchhausen syndrome (see Chapter 76).

## Colonic Pseudo-obstruction

Acute pseudo-obstruction of the entire colon **(Ogilvie syndrome)** is a transient motor abnormality associated with systemic illnesses, such as congestive heart failure, myocardial infarction, sepsis, and assisted ventilation. Stool output ceases and abdominal distention may develop; bowel sounds are reduced but not absent. The condition is diagnosed by plain abdominal radiographs after excluding mechanical obstruction by proctosigmoidoscopy or a limited barium enema. Opiates and anticholinergic agents must be stopped. Nasogastric suction, parenteral fluids, and colonoscopic decompression often are successful. Surgery is necessary for impending perforation.

## Irritable Bowel Syndrome

### Definition and Epidemiology

Irritable bowel syndrome (IBS) is defined as abdominal pain with changes in bowel habits, without detectable organic causes. Two or more of the following symptoms are present in most patients: (1) intermittent abdominal distention; (2) more frequent and loose bowel movements with the onset of pain; (3) pain relief after bowel movements; (4) difficult or painful defecation. Nearly 15% of adults have symptoms that qualify for this diagnosis, but only 20% of these consult a physician. The prevalence is twice as high in women as it is in men. Symptoms commonly begin in the second or third decade and rarely after the sixth. Irritable bowel syndrome is a major cause of time lost from work and is the most common diagnosis among patients with abdominal complaints. The terms "spastic colon" and "mucous colitis" are no longer used.

### Pathophysiology

Irritable bowel syndrome is a symptom complex likely to include several disorders and pathophysiologic mechanisms. Several abnormalities in colonic motor activity have been observed. Compared with control subjects, affected patients experience a delayed but increased colonic motor response after eating (gastrocolic reflex), possibly related to abnormal sensitivity to postprandial release of cholecystokinin. The patients have a lower pain threshold to balloon distention and gas insufflation throughout the GI tract, from esophagus to rectum, indicating increased visceral pain perception. Abnormal psychologic features are found in 70% to 90%

of patients, predominantly depression, anxiety, and somatization disorders. Such personality disorders are more common in patients with IBS symptoms who consult a physician than in those who do not. The prevalence of a history of sexual and physical abuse in IBS patients of either gender is quite high.

### Clinical Features

The symptoms are quite variable, but alternating constipation and diarrhea, often with lower abdominal pain, are the most common. Flatulence and a sense of abdominal distention are common. The pain rarely is localized to one specific site. A common bowel pattern is the passage of a formed stool, followed by two or three loose, watery stools with mucus, soon after waking. Symptoms tend to be worsened by environmental stresses, by depression, and by a variety of foods. Bowel movements are small in volume, and the daily stool weight is usually normal (<200 g), rarely exceeding 300 g/day. Features that should suggest a cause other than IBS include weight loss, nocturnal stools, soiling, progressive severity of symptoms, blood in the stool, and onset after the age of 50. The diagnosis is based on a careful medical history, physical examination, complete blood count, flexible sigmoidoscopy, stool test for occult blood, and, when indicated, a lactose tolerance test. Extensive and repeated diagnostic testing should be avoided. IBS does not predispose to diverticular disease, inflammatory bowel disease, or to cancer.

### Management

The patient should be reassured about the absence of organic disease and the good prognosis of the disorder. Counseling regarding changing from or adapting to a stressful environment may be needed, and, perhaps, formal psychological counseling. Biofeedback therapy and relaxation training may help. Foods that evoke symptoms should be avoided, especially gas-forming items (e.g., legumes, dark bread, and products high in sorbitol and fructose). Despite little evidence that a high-fiber diet is helpful in IBS, psyllium and polycarbophil may be tried. Antidiarrheal drugs (e.g., loperamide and diphenoxylate) are safe and should be taken before diarrhea tends to occur. Similarly, anticholinergics (dicyclomine, propantheline, hyoscyamine) may help with the painful colonic spasms if taken before their expected onset. Some patients may benefit from carefully monitored, low-dose antidepressants (e.g., amitriptyline).

# CHAPTER 95 INFLAMMATORY BOWEL DISEASE

The term *inflammatory bowel disease* (IBD) embraces primarily two diseases, chronic ulcerative colitis and Crohn's disease. In up to 10% of patients with IBD colitis, it is difficult to distinguish between Crohn's disease and ulcerative colitis; these patients often are characterized as having "indeterminate" colitis, even following colectomy and histologic evaluation. Crohn's disease of the small intestine is discussed in Chapter 91. Only Crohn's colitis and ulcerative colitis are reviewed in this chapter.

## Chronic Ulcerative Colitis

### Definition and Epidemiology

Chronic ulcerative colitis (CUC), an idiopathic inflammatory disease of the colonic mucosa, in the past was most prevalent among Caucasians, particularly Ashkenazi Jews. With an annual incidence in the U.S. of 5 to 10 per 100,000, its prevalence in the United States is 45 to 80 per 100,000 people. Two incidence peaks seem to occur, one at ages 20–30 and a second peak at around age 60. A minority of patients offer a family history of inflammatory bowel disease (IBD), but the concordance rate among identical twins is low (approximately 5%), and no genetic pattern of inheritance has yet emerged.

### Etiology

No evidence favoring an infectious, allergic, immunologic, genetic, or psychosomatic cause has held up to scrutiny. The incidence is higher in nonsmokers and ex-smokers and possibly in oral contraceptive users. Appendectomy seems to be protective. The number of $IgG_1$- and $IgG_2$-producing plasma cells in the lamina propria is increased, and the mucosal synthesis of the interleukin (IL)-1 receptor antagonist reportedly is lower than normal. Autoantibodies have been noted against a colonocyte-associated protein (also present in skin and bile ducts). The ability of the colonocytes to metabolize n-butyrate is markedly decreased. The role of these epidemiologic and laboratory observations in causing CUC remains uncertain.

### Pathology

The disease invariably begins at the anal verge with varying degrees of proximal extension. It involves only the rectosigmoid in 40% to 50% of patients, the left colon in 30% to 40% of patients, and proximal extension beyond the splenic flexure (pancolitis) in about 20% to 40% of patients. In 20% to 30% of patients with disease initially limited to the distal colon, there is proximal extension over time. The inflammation is confined to the colonic mucosa and submucosa, with mononuclear cell infiltration at the base of the lamina propria. In the acute stages, neutrophils and eosinophils invade the surface and crypt epithelium with crypt abscess formation. Changes in crypt architecture (crypt branching and atrophy) are a constant feature that separates IBD from acute infectious colitis. As the crypts are destroyed, the mucosa thins, but foci of regenerating mucosa often develop into inflammatory pseudopolyps. The chronic and recurrent inflammation often leads to shortening and stricturing of the colon ("lead-pipe" colon on barium studies). The rectum may contract. The ulceration and inflammation in severe, fulminant cases extends into the muscle layers with intramural plexus damage, causing dilatation, impaired motor function and, ultimately, perforation—the so-called **toxic megacolon.** Up to 10% of patients may present with fulminant colitis at the time of diagnosis.

## Clinical Features and Course

The symptoms of CUC vary from mild and frequent bloody rectal discharges with tenesmus (a painful spasm of the rectum with an urge to defecate, and passage of little fecal matter), to a fulminating form with severe systemic and abdominal symptoms. The onset of CUC usually is gradual, with small, bloody stools and tenesmus. Abdominal pain preceding urgent defecation is due to frequent, giant migrating colonic contractions. Fever, weight loss, anemia, and hypoproteinemia occur in more severe cases. Fecal losses of water, sodium, and potassium are not severe, given that bowel movements are small-volume and contain only blood and mucus. Eighty percent of patients have intermittent exacerbations with total remissions, but 10% to 15% remain continuously active without a remission. Historically, 5% of patients have gone into permanent remission after the initial episode of colitis; however, many of these patients are now felt to have been suffering from hemorrhagic bacterial dysentery, most probably *Escherichia coli* 0157:H7, and were misdiagnosed.

Extracolonic manifestations occur in about 10% of patients and occasionally may precede the bowel symptoms. Oral aphthous ulcers, episcleritis, uveitis, pyoderma gangrenosum, erythema nodosum, and an asymmetric nondeforming arthropathy of large joints tend to parallel the course of the colitis; sacroiliitis, **primary sclerosing cholangitis (PSC),** ankylosing spondylitis, and secondary amyloidosis, however, may progress even without active colitis and even after proctocolectomy. Most patients with PSC have associated CUC. Primary sclerosing cholangitis features chronic inflammation, fibrosis, and stricture formation of the intra- and extrahepatic bile ducts. Cholestatic jaundice, pruritus, and bouts of suppurative cholangitis follow in the ensuing years, causing secondary biliary cirrhosis and liver failure. A raised serum alkaline phosphatase is the earliest laboratory finding; endoscopic retrograde cholangiography or magnetic resonance cholangiopancreatography is required for diagnosis. Ursodeoxycholic acid can slow the worsening of liver tests, but the only effective treatment in patients with progressive disease is liver transplantation. Cholangiocarcinoma ultimately develops in 10% or more of patients with PSC.

## Diagnosis

The physical examination may be normal, but patients often look ill and pale and have a moderate fever. Abdominal examination commonly shows tenderness over the colon. Abdominal distention, tympany, and increased tenderness in acutely ill patients suggest fulminant colitis, and potentially toxic megacolon. A slightly granular texture is noted on digital rectal examination; bloody mucus often is seen on the glove (mucosal friability).

There are no diagnostic laboratory abnormalities. All patients with a dysenteric syndrome (tenesmus and frequent, bloody stools) should undergo fiberoptic sigmoidoscopy without patient preparation by enemas or laxatives. Beginning at the dentate line, the mucosa is uniformly friable, hyperemic, finely ulcerated, and granular. Edema obscures the usual fine tracery of blood vessels beneath the mucosa. With limited distal disease, these gross changes are demarcated proximally by normal mucosa within the viewing range of the sigmoidoscope.

A plain abdominal radiograph can assess the colonic diameter in suspected toxic megacolon (Figure 95.1), and an upright view can detect free intra-abdominal air. In extensive CUC, the gas-filled, dilated transverse colon shows a shaggy, thickened mucosal profile with few or no haustrations. Barium enema can determine the extent of the disease and better define its nature. It may be nearly normal in early or mild disease. In the acute stage, spasm and irritability are more prominent. Ulcerations, usually tiny and difficult to see, often appear as fuzzy serrations or fine spiculations (Figure 95.2). Large ulcerations resemble a collar button. In less active stages, the mucosal surface may be nodular and finely polypoid, reflecting inflammatory pseudopolyps. Air-contrast study makes these details clearer. In chronic disease, the colon is shortened and the lumen is tubular and narrowed with absent haustra (i.e., the "lead pipe" colon). When the entire colon is involved, "backwash ileitis" is not uncommon, with a dilated ileal segment showing a smooth mucosa. Full colonoscopy with inspection and biopsy of the terminal ileum can supplant barium enema, but neither should be done in acute, severe

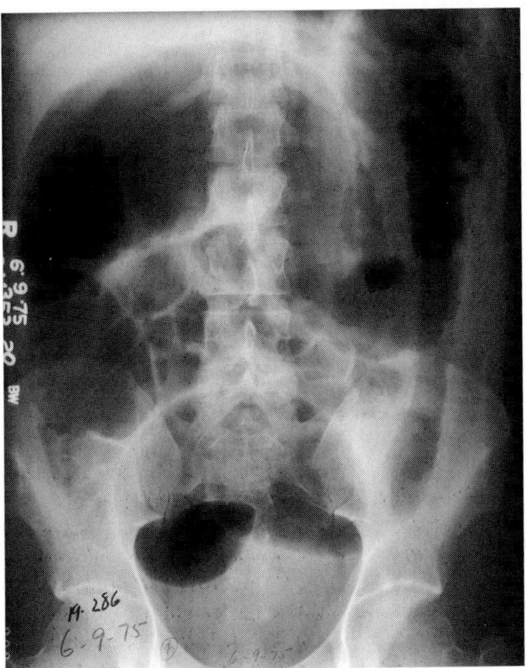

**FIGURE 95.1.** Toxic megacolon. Pronounced distension of the cecum and ascending colon are noted. Note the absence of haustrations in the air-filled descending colon.

colitis for risk of perforation or precipitating toxic megacolon.

The differential diagnosis includes infectious, Crohn's, indeterminate, ischemic, and radiation colitis. Acute infectious colitis due to *Entameba histolytica*, *Salmonella* species, *Shigella* species, *Yersinia* species, *Campylobacter* species, and enterohemorrhagic *E. coli* O157:H7 may mimic IBD at sigmoidoscopy, but their onset is more abrupt than CUC and Crohn's colitis. On endoscopy, the hallmark of CUC is the uniformity of inflammatory changes in the circumferential and longitudinal direction, beginning at the anal verge and ending with a clear demarcation to normal-appearing mucosa located within the colon or at the ileocecal valve.

## Medical Management

Medical management aims to control the acute attack, prevent recurrences, and correct nutritional, fluid, and electrolyte deficits. Although both corticosteroids and 5-aminosalicylate (5-ASA) compounds shorten acute attacks, corticosteroids act faster and are more effective than 5-ASA; however, corticosteroids do have cumulative side effects that are more serious. Patients whose CUC ends distal to the splenic flexure usually can be managed by self-administered hydrocortisone as enemas or rectal foam and 5-ASA as enemas or suppositories. Patients with mild to moderate, extensive colitis may be given sulfasalazine (4–6 g/d), or oral prednisone (30–60 mg/d) if the clinical severity requires it. A severe attack is one with more than six bloody stools daily with systemic signs (fever, tachycardia, anemia, or erythrocyte sedimentation rate [ESR] >30 mm/hr). Despite the lack of precision, this definition remains useful when applied with clinical common sense. Such patients are hospitalized and closely watched for abdominal distention, increasing tenderness, fever, tachycardia, and rectal bleeding; hydrocortisone (100 mg q6h) is given intravenously and by rectal drip. Most patients tolerate only clear liquids and require parenteral nutrition. Early surgical consultation is mandatory; emergency proctocolectomy is indicated in the 20% to 30% of patients who fail to improve within 1 week.

Because 5-ASA is absorbed in the small intestine, sulfasalazine functions by delivering 5-ASA to the colon. The sulfonamide is a mere carrier, with no therapeutic

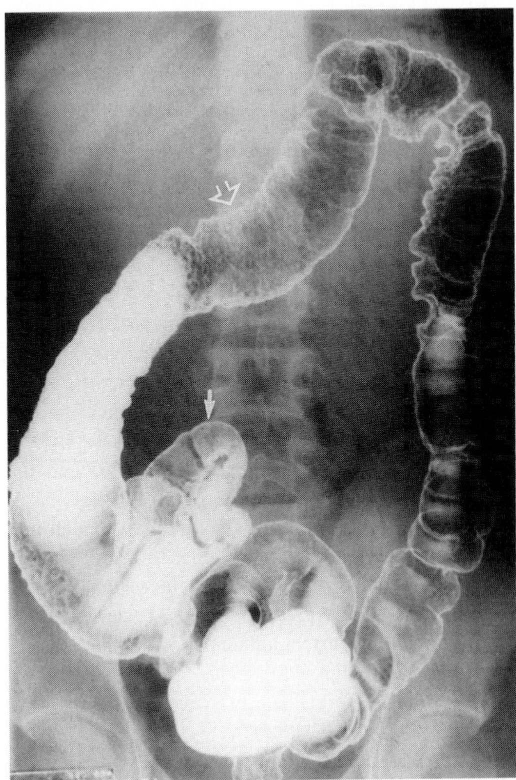

**FIGURE 95.2.** Acute ulcerative colitis. The colon and rectum are diffusely involved. Normal haustral pattern is lacking in the proximal and transverse colon segments. Note superficial ulcerations, causing the spiculated contours of the transverse colon (*open arrow*). The terminal ileum (*solid arrow*) is normal.
(Courtesy of Edward Stewart, MD, Milwaukee, Wisconsin.)

effect in CUC; colonic bacteria split the azo-bond that links 5-ASA and sulfapyridine. Side effects, which are common, usually are due to sulfapyridine. Dose-related effects are nausea, vomiting, headaches, and folate malabsorption. Other side effects are skin rash, fever, hemolytic anemia, alveolitis, hepatitis, and reversible male infertility because of non-viable sperm. Once remission occurs, patients are maintained indefinitely on a 5-ASA drug (e.g., sulfasalazine, 1 g b.i.d), to reduce the risk of clinical relapse. Patients who are intolerant of sulfasalazine and men who are concerned about fertility impairment may use one of the newer 5-ASA drugs, such as 5-ASA encapsulated in a pH-sensitive resin (Asacol7), or impregnated in a methylcellulose for gradual delivery (Pentasa) and olsalazine (Dipentum7), which has two 5-ASA molecules linked by an azo-bond. Olsalazine causes watery diarrhea in 10% to 15% of patients. Patients who are intolerant of the 5-ASA medications can be treated with immunomodulatory therapy in hopes of maintaining remission (e.g., azathioprine, 6-mercaptopurine). However, the use of immunomodulators includes the potential risk of infection, pancreatitis, allergy and neoplasia, and must be weighed against the potential benefit of a curative proctocolectomy.

### Surgical Management

Indications for surgery are a severe attack unresponsive to medications, toxic megacolon, chronic disease activity uncontrolled by medical therapy, or unacceptable side effects from drugs. Total proctocolectomy cures CUC. Less extensive surgical resections or temporary colon bypass are not appropriate. A standard, right lower quadrant end-ileostomy works well, but has cosmetic ramifications and requires self-care of the ileostomy. An increasingly chosen alternative is the creation of an ileal pouch that is anastomosed to the preserved anal sphincter. Fecal continence is attained in most cases when this two-step operation is done by experienced surgeons. In patients with indeterminate colitis, the ileal pouch anal anastomosis has a success rate similar to that of patients with CUC. Patients with Crohn's colitis should not be offered the restorative pouch operation, because complication rates with recurrent inflammation and fistulization are unacceptably high.

### Risk of Colorectal Cancer

Chronic ulcerative colitis carries an annual risk of 0.8–1% for developing colorectal cancer (CRC), beginning 10 years after initial presentation. Patients with pancolitis are at the highest risk, but the risk also is increased in patients with left-sided involvement. The diagnosis of cancer in CUC is difficult, because the symptoms mimic those of the underlying colitis, and radiography and endoscopy are less accurate than in the normal colon. Dysplastic changes of the colonic mucosa occur in many patients before CRC develops and are nearly universal when a cancer is diagnosed. Yearly surveillance colonoscopy with multiple biopsies obtained at 10-cm intervals, beginning 10 years after diagnosis, is currently recommended for all CUC patients, regardless of the amount of disease activity. Both high- and low-grade dysplasia, when identified by an experienced pathologist in patients without inflammatory disease activity, warrants evaluation for proctocolectomy. The identification of adenomatous changes in polypoid lesions in the colon suggests dysplasia; however, the development of multiple pseudopolyps in patients with longstanding disease may make endoscopic surveillance difficult, again making evaluation for proctocolectomy important. When adjusted for tumor stage at diagnosis, CRC complicating CUC has the same prognosis as CRC in general. The surveillance colonoscopy confers a survival advantage due to the early detection of CRC.

## ■ Crohn's Colitis

In 20% of patients, Crohn's colitis (Crohn's disease of the colon) involves only the colon, with pathological features similar to those of colitis of the small bowel. The rectum is affected in 60% of patients, pancolitis occurs in 30% of patients, and "skip areas" develop in 20% of patients. Fistulas with adjacent organs and colonic obstruction, as well as perforation with abscess formation (Figure 95.3), may follow. Mucosal biopsies contain granulomas in only 25% of cases.

### Clinical Features

Most patients have diarrhea, abdominal pain, and weight loss, often with an insidious onset. Painful defecation is a harbinger of anal and perianal disease. Whereas pneumaturia and fecal matter in the urinary sediment suggest an ileovesical or colovesical fistula, dyspareunia and a brownish, malodorous vaginal discharge are clues to a rectovaginal fistula. Physical examination may reveal a tender, inflammatory abdominal mass. The anal canal often is narrowed, with dusky skin tags representing inflamed anal papillae, and perianal openings of fistulous tracts. Digital rectal examination may cause exquisite pain, especially when there are anal canal ulcers and perianal abscesses. Such anal disease may precede the intestinal and colitis symptoms by months or years. The terminal ileum should be evaluated by imaging or by colonoscopy in patients presenting de novo with such lesions. Extraintestinal complications usually parallel those of CUC, but erythema nodosum is more common and PSC and pyoderma gangrenosum are less common in Crohn's colitis than in CUC.

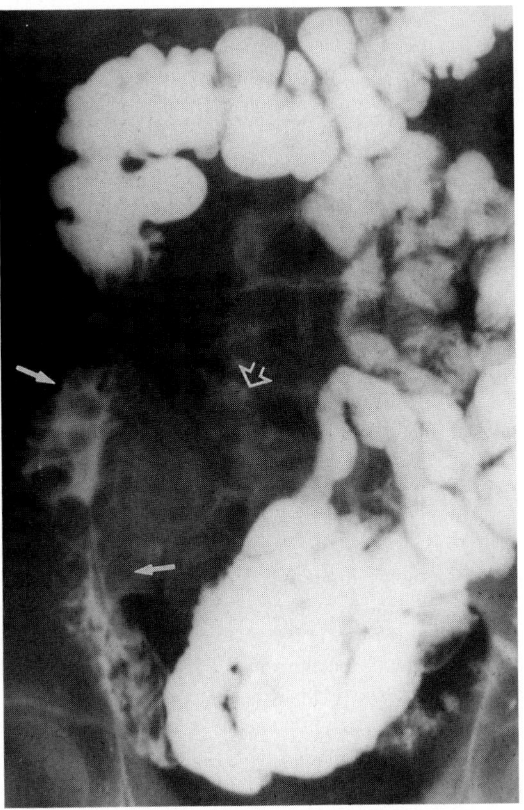

**FIGURE 95.3.** Crohn's ileocolitis. Small bowel x-ray shows ulcero-nodular Crohn's disease of terminal ileum and ascending colon (*solid arrows*). The x-ray distinction between terminal ileum and colon is no longer possible. Note the large area in the right hemiabdomen without bowel. The bowel is displaced by extramural inflammation. The open arrow shows the collection of contrast material in this area, which is an abscess communicating with the diseased bowel. A palpable, tender mass was noted clinically.
(Courtesy of Edward Stewart, MD, Milwaukee, Wisconsin.)

## Diagnosis and Management

When proctosigmoidoscopy shows mucosal inflammation, other types of colitis, including infectious, must be excluded, as for CUC. The distinction from CUC is important but challenging; helpful features for making that distinction are listed in Table 95.1. In 5% to 10% of patients with IBD, however, CUC cannot be separated from Crohn's colitis— the so-called "indeterminate colitis."

The management principles are much the same as for Crohn's disease of the small bowel. Drugs with established effectiveness are 5-ASA, corticosteroids, azathioprine/6MP, methotrexate and Infliximab. Bowel rest and total parenteral nutrition do not influence the disease, but may provide short-term rehabilitation. High-dose metronidazole, given for many months, may help temporary fistula closure, although the drug may induce a neuropathy, particularly in doses over 1 g per day. Patients with mild disease can be maintained in remission with mesalamine. In patients with moderate to severe disease, who require steroids for induction of remission, maintenance therapy with azathioprine/6-MP, with dosages adjusted for individual metabolism, can be used. However, azathioprine/6-MP may cause pancreatitis early in its use and bone marrow suppression at any time. Infliximab, the chimeric monoclonal antibody against the cytokine TNF-α, is effective in patients with refractory and fistulizing Crohn's disease. Concurrent therapy with immunomodulators is recommended, because the duration of response to Infliximab is short-lived, and may require retreatment at 2- to 3-month intervals.

Surgery by an experienced surgeon is reserved for treating intractable disease and local complications. The implications of proctocolectomy for Crohn's colitis differ from those for CUC. The disease may not be eradicated; 20% to 50% of patients later develop Crohn's disease in the remaining terminal ileum. An ileoanal pouch anastomosis is not indicated, given the risk of ileal recurrence. In contrast to CUC, an ileorectal anastomosis and segmental colectomy are options, depending on the location of severe involvement. Severe perirectal and anal disease require definitive surgery.

**TABLE 95.1. Differential Diagnosis of Ulcerative vs. Crohn's Colitis**

| | Chronic Ulcerative Colitis | Crohn's Colitis |
|---|---|---|
| *Distribution* | Continuous | Segmental |
| Ileal involvement | 0* | Diagnostic, if present |
| *Histology:* | | |
| Inflammation | Diffuse | Focal |
| Granulomas | 0 | ++ (~30%) |
| Transmural | 0 | 4+ |
| *Clinical:* | | |
| Perianal lesions | 1+ | 3+ |
| Fistulae | (+) | 2+ |
| Strictures | 1+ | 3+ |
| Hemorrhage | 2+ | (+) |
| *Endoscopy:* | | |
| Friability | 3+ | 1+ |
| Aphthoid lesions | 0 | 4+ |
| Granularity | 3+ | 1+ |
| Cobblestone | (+) | 3+ |
| Linear, deep ulcers | 1+ | 3+ |
| Involvement | Uniform | Non-uniform |

*The scale of 0–4+ indicates the frequency of a finding in each of the two diseases, with 0 being the least frequent/

### Risk of Colorectal Carcinoma

The risk of colorectal carcinoma in extensive Crohn's colitis approaches that in CUC. As in CUC, surveillance colonoscopy with multiple biopsies is widely practiced. A number of cases of adenocarcinoma of the ileum have been reported in patients with ileal Crohn's disease; however, no guidelines exist for regular surveillance of the small bowel for premalignant changes or early cancer.

# CHAPTER 96 DIVERTICULAR DISEASE OF THE COLON

True colonic diverticula, involving all bowel wall layers, are rare. Most are pseudodiverticula, with only mucosal herniations through the muscular layer of the colonic wall, commonly occurring at points of penetration of the circular muscle by intramural blood vessels, located between the mesenteric and the two anti-mesenteric taenia. Diverticula most commonly involve the sigmoid. Nearly unknown in developing countries, the high incidence of diverticulosis in the West is felt to be due to lifelong, low dietary fiber intake. High intraluminal pressure is a postulated mechanism. The incidence rises with age, and two thirds of individuals have diverticula by age 85. No association exists between irritable bowel syndrome and colonic diverticulosis. Complications, mainly diverticulitis and hemorrhage, arise in about 12% of patients.

## Uncomplicated Diverticulosis

Although readily apparent during colonoscopy, diverticula often are diagnosed incidentally on barium enema examination (Figure 96.1). In the early, prediverticular state, the radiographs suggest muscular thickening of the sigmoid with an irregular, sawtooth appearance of the mucosal outline. Most patients are asymptomatic, but a minority report episodic abdominal pain, often in the left lower quadrant, lasting several days and often temporarily relieved by bowel movements. On palpation, the area of reported pain may be tender. Anticholinergics, including hyoscyamine, rarely relieve this type of abdominal pain. Increased dietary intake of fiber, such as unprocessed wheat bran, often is helpful. An amount of up to 20 g of fiber per day is reached over several weeks, thus allowing the patient to adjust to the initial fullness and flatulence associated with high fiber intake. Methylcellulose or psyllium also are useful and are better tolerated, albeit more expensive.

## Diverticulitis

Diverticulitis occurs in as many as 10% of patients with diverticulosis, and follows perforation of one or more diverticula, causing extracolonic inflammation, which may be complicated by abscess, sinus tracts running parallel to the lumen, colovesical or colovaginal fistulae, and, rarely, by free perforation and peritonitis. Extraluminal compression by an inflammatory mass may cause obstruction and closely mimic an obstructing cancer. The features are severe pain; a tender and palpable mass, usually in the left lower quadrant; fever; and, rarely, rectal bleeding. Rebound tenderness and involuntary abdominal rigidity are unusual and indicate perforation of a diverticulum or a retroperitoneal abscess into the peritoneal cavity. The differential diagnosis includes colonic infarction, acute infectious colitis, an attack of ulcerative or Crohn colitis, and an obstructing or perforating colon cancer. The diagnosis is confirmed by abdominal CT or ultrasound (US). Colonoscopy and barium enema should be avoided during the active stage. Most episodes are mild and can be managed medically. Oral intake is restricted to clear liquids. Antibiotic treatment is empirical; metronidazole and a third-generation cephalosporin, or imipenem/cilastatin, often are used. Recurrent and complicated attacks mandate

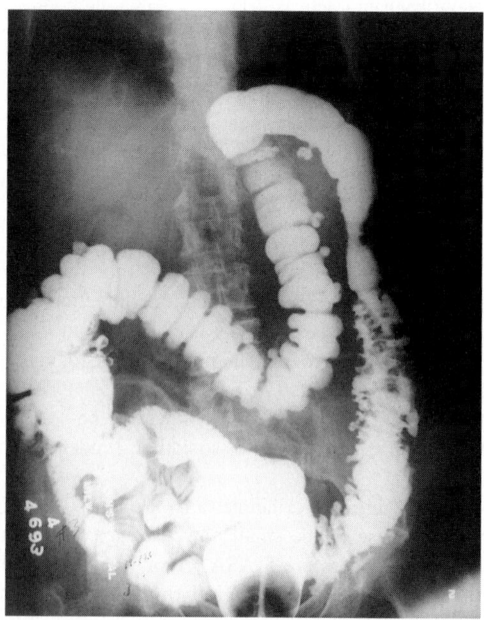


**FIGURE 96.1.** Barium enema showing diverticulosis of the colon.

resection of the involved segment, usually the sigmoid. Abscesses require drainage (surgically or under US or CT guidance), followed by bowel resection when the inflammation has subsided.

### Diverticular Bleeding

Almost 3% of patients, often elderly, develop sudden, potentially severe, but rarely fatal, painless rectal bleeding. Up to 70% of these episodes of bleeding arise from proximal colonic diverticula. Selective angiography, $^{99m}$Tc-labeled RBC scans, and colonoscopy are helpful diagnostic tests, but none of them is useful once active bleeding stops. The major differential diagnosis is bleeding from angiodysplasia, which also tends to occur in the proximal colon. Selective arterial infusion of vasopressin can control bleeding, but rebleeding is common. Repetitive, severe bleeding requires partial colectomy; its success depends on correct preoperative localization of the bleeding site.

# CHAPTER 97 APPENDICITIS

Appendicitis is the most common abdominal disease requiring surgical intervention. No age is exempt, but the incidence is highest in young adults. It is rare before the age of 2 years, and it is not uncommon in the elderly. The lifetime risk of acute appendicitis is nearly 10%, with a preponderance of men being affected.

Obstruction of the lumen by a fecalith, causing stasis, followed by ischemia, mucosal ulceration, infection, vascular thrombosis, infarction, and occasional perforation, is a commonly outlined sequence. In many cases, however, no obstruction, foreign body, or precipitating event is found. Some acute attacks reverse spontaneously, and the process subsides. Usually, the symptoms evolve over 24 hours; the appendix perforates in 15% to 20% of cases.

Classically, the patient reports periumbilical pain, followed by anorexia, nausea, and low-grade fever. Pain in the early stages is visceral and, thus, is felt in the midline. As the serosa and adjacent peritoneum are involved, the pain shifts and becomes somatic in the right lower quadrant. Localized, rebound tenderness and muscle spasm are apparent at McBurney's point, which is about halfway between the anterior superior iliac spine and the umbilicus. With a retrocecal inflamed appendix, abdominal signs may be absent but pain may be elicited by iliopsoas muscle stretching.

Many conditions mimic acute appendicitis, including mesenteric lymphadenitis, acute gastroenteritis, referred abdominal pain from pneumonia, pelvic inflammatory disease, acute Crohn disease, ureteric colic, ruptured ovarian follicle or tubal pregnancy, and right-sided diverticulitis. The diagnosis rests mainly on the history and physical findings, including a rectal and pelvic examination. Abdominal or transvaginal ultrasound may demonstrate an enlarged, thick-walled appendix in about 85% of cases and can effectively exclude other conditions such as ectopic pregnancy, ovarian cysts, and other adnexal diseases. Computed tomographic scanning may be required to diagnose periappendiceal abscess in those suspected of having appendiceal perforation. Diagnostic uncertainty should not delay surgical exploration. Surgery confirms the diagnosis in about 70% of patients; another diagnosis is found in 15% of patients, and no diagnosis is made in the remaining 15% of patients.

# CHAPTER 98 ACUTE INFECTIOUS COLITIS

Acute inflammatory diseases of the colon, such as shigellosis, amebic colitis, salmonellosis, pseudomembranous colitis, and *Campylobacter* and *Escherichia coli* O157:H7 infection, lead to cramps and tenesmus, watery or bloody stools, fever, and, at times, nausea and vomiting, which most often reflect tissue invasion.

Both stool examination for ova and parasites, and bacterial culture, should precede other GI diagnostic studies. Sigmoidoscopy can then follow to inspect the mucosa for hyperemia, edema, friability, exudate (pseudomembranes), and ulceration. Wet smears should be examined for amebae, and biopsies from ulcerated areas should be stained for amebic trophozoites. Serology (indirect hemagglutination) testing can also reliably diagnose amebiasis. *Campylobacter fetus spp jejuni,* an organism that exists widely in the animal kingdom and has been isolated in water, unpasteurized milk, and poultry, recently has emerged as an important pathogen causing a dysenteric syndrome. It often produces a prodrome of malaise followed by abdominal cramps, diarrhea (often grossly bloody), anorexia, fever, nausea, and vomiting. Proctoscopic findings may mimic pseudomembranous colitis or inflammatory bowel disease. Laboratory evaluation of all acute diarrheas should include tests to identify this organism. Erythromycin therapy is commonly used, but it may not alter the natural course of the disease if begun several days after the onset of illness.

Acute colitis sometimes occurs without apparent etiology—thus the term "acute self-limited colitis." The central dilemma is to differentiate this transient condition (2–4 weeks) from the first attack of idiopathic IBD—that is, ulcerative colitis or Crohn disease. Gross and histologic morphology can be useful.

## Pseudomembranous Colitis

Pseudomembranous colitis, caused by strains of *Clostridium difficile*, a sporulating anaerobe, may occur during or following a course of broad-spectrum antibiotics, most commonly penicillins, cephalosporins, and clindamycin. Watery diarrhea, abdominal cramps, and fever are extremely common; rebound tenderness, bloody diarrhea, and leukocytosis are less frequent. Erythema, edema, erosions, and cream-colored pseudomembranes usually are seen on sigmoidoscopy. Occasionally, only the proximal colon is involved. *C. difficile* produces two toxins concurrently: toxin A, an enterotoxin causing the mucosal damage, and toxin B, a cytotoxin. The diagnosis requires a combination of listed symptoms *and* finding toxin A or B in the stool. Very few healthy adults and 10% to 15% of hospitalized patients are carriers of *C. difficile*. Isolation of patients with this disease and enteric precautions are essential, given its transmissibility by the fecal-oral route. Only symptomatic cases with toxin-positive stools require therapy. Metronidazole, 250 mg q.i.d., and Vancomycin, 125 mg q.i.d., for 10 days are equally effective. Metronidazole is preferred, given its lower cost. Clinical response is prompt, but relapses occur in 25% of cases; these usually abate after a second course of therapy. Half of those re-treated may relapse again, requiring metronidazole or vancomycin for a further 4 to 6 weeks. Clostridial toxins may be bound by cholestyramine. Carriers need not be treated.

## *Enterohemorrhagic* E. coli *Infection*

Enterohemorrhagic *E. coli* (EHEC) infection is caused by verotoxin (Shigella toxin I and II)-producing *E. coli,* predominantly the O157:H7 strain. Transmitted via undercooked beef, unpasteurized milk, unpasteurized apple cider, drinking water, and possibly person-to-person, the infection leads to severe abdominal cramps, diarrhea (which may become bloody after 1–2 days), and, in 50% of cases, fever. Because the right colon is principally involved, sigmoidoscopy may be normal. The disease, which usually lasts 5–7 days, occurs as local outbreaks. The diagnosis requires bacteriologic confirmation. The hemolytic-uremic syndrome (acute renal failure, hemolytic anemia, and thrombocytopenia) develops in about 5% of those affected, particularly in the very young and the very old. Antibiotic therapy has not been effective, possibly because of delays in the diagnosis.

# CHAPTER 99 OTHER COLORECTAL DISORDERS

## Ischemia of the Colon

Colonic ischemia, most commonly seen in patients over 50 years of age with atherosclerotic disease elsewhere, may be part of the syndrome of mesenteric insufficiency (see Chapter 88). It is primarily seen as an isolated event, but it may follow acute interruption of the inferior mesenteric artery during intra-abdominal aneurysm or bowel surgery. Association with vasculitis, amyloidosis, or oral contraceptive use is rare.

The usual features are acute lower abdominal pain and cramps, rectal bleeding, and, perhaps, fever and vomiting. Tenderness, guarding, and leukocytosis are common and may mimic acute diverticulitis. Life-threatening infarction and perforation may follow, requiring urgent laparotomy. More often, the blood supply to that segment of the colon remains sufficient to ensure viability, but with tissue changes termed *ischemic colitis*. Characteristically segmental, these particularly affect the splenic flexure and the rectosigmoid, the "watershed" areas with respect to blood supply. Sometimes, patients are seen after the acute episode, or may give a history suggestive of prior ischemic events. Colonoscopy has been useful in early diagnosis. Barium enema (Figure 99.1) shows "thumbprinting"; it reflects intramural edema and bleeding, causing some segmental narrowing. There is no specific therapy; usually the process subsides, restoring a normal-appearing colon. The sporadic, residual stricture or ulceration that follows may mimic Crohn disease or even adenocarcinoma.

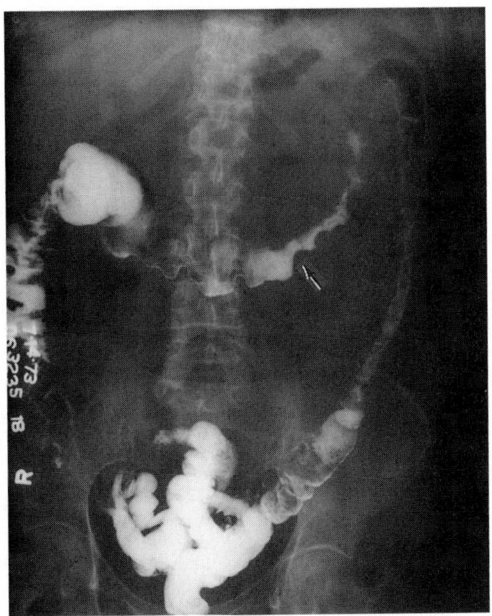

**FIGURE 99.1. Ischemia of the colon. Barium enema examination showing thumbprinting (arrow).**

## Radiation Proctocolitis

**Acute radiation colitis** often is seen in patients during or soon after radiotherapy for cervical, ovarian, uterine, rectal, or prostatic cancers. Usual symptoms are nausea, vomiting, cramping, tenesmus, diarrhea, and rectal bleeding. Sigmoidoscopy often shows a hyperemic, edematous mucosa with variable friability and, occasionally, ulcerations. **Chronic radiation colitis** may occur months or years after therapy, due to progressive occlusive changes in small mural arteries, leading to ischemic necrosis, **mucosal ulceration, and stricture formation.** Crampy abdominal pain, tenesmus, and stool with blood and mucus are the usual symptoms; obstruction may develop. Sigmoidoscopy usually shows a granular, friable membrane, variable-sized ulcers, and prominent telangiectases (neovascularization). Surgery rarely is necessary, and laser therapy may control bleeding if it is severe enough to require attention. The distal ileum may be involved as well due to its location within the pelvis. Consequently, malabsorption of vitamin $B_{12}$ and of bile salts may result. In the latter case, diarrhea will respond to cholestyramine therapy.

## Collagenous and Lymphocytic Colitis

Patients with collagenous and lymphocytic colitis present with chronic watery diarrhea; abdominal pain is minor or absent. Most are in their fifth or sixth decade, with a striking predominance of women. The colon is normal on endoscopic and radiologic examination, and there are no consistent laboratory abnormalities. The daily stool volume may be as high as 1.5 L, although dehydration and weight loss are rare. The diarrhea tends to wax and wane without any therapy. There is an unexplained association with autoimmune disorders, such as rheumatoid arthritis, scleroderma, and the sicca syndrome. The diagnosis is established by mucosal biopsies obtained proximal to the rectum. These show increased intraepithelial lymphocytes, accumulations of mononuclear cells in the lamina propria, and a disarray of the surface epithelium; the crypt architecture remains intact. Patients with marked thickening of the collagen plate beneath the surface epithelium are designated as having collagenous colitis; those without this thickening are said to have lymphocytic colitis. Both probably represent a single disease entity, sometimes termed microscopic colitis. The prognosis is excellent. Initial treatment consists of antidiarrheal drugs. Patients who do not respond receive a trial of sulfasalazine or one of the newer 5-ASA formulations. A few patients require short courses of systemic corticosteroids.

## Pneumatosis Cystoides Intestinalis

Pneumatosis cystoides intestinalis is a rare condition characterized by multiple gas-filled mural cysts with surrounding chronic inflammation in the small or large intestine (Figure 99.2), encountered incidentally on abdominal radiographs. In most cases, an underlying condition can be identified that allows gas to dissect into the intestinal wall. Treatment consists of a formula diet that is free of complex carbohydrates and provides high $O_2$ supplements, to promote the diffusion of $N_2$ and $H_2$ out of the gas-filled cysts.

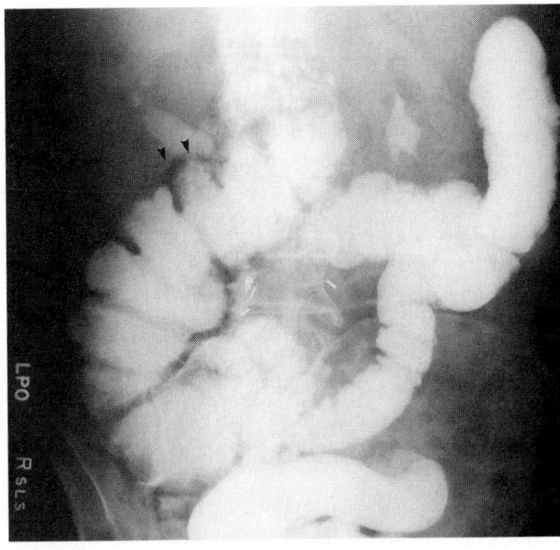


**FIGURE 99.2. Pneumatosis intestinalis. Barium enema examination showing accumulation of air (arrows) in the colonic walls.**

# CHAPTER 100 COLORECTAL NEOPLASMS

## Incidence

Adenomas and cancers arising from the colorectal epithelium form a sequential development from benign to malignant neoplasms. Their incidence, linked to dietary factors, has great geographic variation. Strong epidemiological data link colorectal neoplasia with heavy consumption of a high-fat, red meat, low-fiber diet. In the United States, the lifetime risk of colorectal cancer (CRC) is from 5% to 6%, with 160,000 new cases and 60,000 deaths yearly. The incidence of both adenoma and carcinoma rises with age. About 40% to 60% of persons over 60 years of age harbor one or more colon adenomas.

## Pathogenesis

### The adenoma-carcinoma sequence

Most, if not all, CRCs are thought to arise within benign adenomas; the probability of malignant transformation depends on the size, histology, and degree of epithelial dysplasia of an adenoma. The progression from normal epithelium through adenoma to cancer is determined by accumulated genetic alterations that manifest as hypomethylation of DNA and aneuploidy, signifying an abnormal DNA content. Specific genetic changes involve somatic mutations of proto-oncogenes and of tumor suppressor genes; the latter include adenomatous polyposis coli gene (APC) and mutated in colon cancer gene (MCC), both located on chromosome 5q; deleted in colon cancer gene (DCC) on 18q; and p53, located on 17p. Inactivation of one allele has no effect on cell proliferation. Abnormal growth occurs only when the second allele mutates or is deleted (loss of heterozygosity [LOH]). Proto-oncogenes, such as K-ras (12p) and C-myc, may be activated or amplified by a point mutation and then act as mitogenic signals. Mutation or allelic loss of APC and MCC results in a hyperproliferating epithelium; the progression to adenoma formation is associated with K-ras mutations and DCC inactivation and the appearance of carcinoma with the loss or mutation of the tumor suppressor gene, p53. More than 90% of CRC exhibit two or more of these gene alterations (Table 100.1).

## Neoplastic Polyps

Tubular adenomas are characterized by branching adenomatous glands and epithelial dysplasia. When the glands elongate to the center of the polyp, finger-like projections result; the polyp is termed **villous adenoma.** About 85% of all neoplastic colorectal polyps are tubular, and 5% are villous adenomas. The remaining 10% are of the mixed type. Polyps grow either pedunculated (on a stalk) or sessile (broad-based). Approximately 90% of neoplastic polyps are less than 1 cm in size. Among patients with one identified polyp, one half harbor multiple lesions. Approximately 70% of all polyps detected during colonoscopy occur distal to the splenic flexure—that is, within reach of a fiberoptic sigmoidoscope. In only 5% to 10% of patients are neoplastic polyps located solely in the proximal colon. The degree of epithelial dysplasia ranges from mild to moderate to severe or high-grade. In high-grade dysplasia (carcinoma in situ), the neoplastic cells do not extend beyond the basement membrane. Intramucosal carcinoma, the next step in the progression to overt malignancy, invades the lamina propria, but not the muscularis mucosae. Because lymphatics are absent above the muscularis mucosae, these malignancies are not invasive. Neoplastic polyps with foci of carcinoma in situ or intramucosal carcinoma are often called "malignant polyps." High-grade dysplasia and noninvasive carcinoma are more common in larger polyps, particularly the villous type. Diminutive polyps, less than 5 mm in size, do not pose an increased risk of developing cancer.

Colorectal polyps usually are asymptomatic and rarely bleed; fecal occult blood testing (FOBT) is positive in only 20% to 30% of affected patients. In general, only polyps larger than 2 cm in size tend to bleed intermittently. Patients with large rectosigmoid villous adenomas occasionally present with all the sequelae of secretory diarrhea, including dehydration and hypokalemia, owing to rectal discharge of copious amounts of mucoid fluid.

Colorectal polyps should be removed completely, usually by endoscopy. The entire polyp is studied histologically to establish its nature (neoplastic or not) and the degree of dysplasia. Polypectomy is efficient

**TABLE 100.1. DNA Alterations Commonly Present During the Evolution of Colorectal Carcinoma**

| Tumor Suppressor Gene: Deletion and/or Mutation | Oncogene: Activation | Result |
|---|---|---|
| APC, MCC* | – | Hyperproliferation |
| DCC | K ras | Adenoma |
| p53 | C-myc | Carcinoma |

*The sequence and numbers of genetic alterations are variable. Mutations and deletions of additional genes are likely to be discovered in the future.

TABLE 100.2. Screening and Surveillance for Colorectal Polyps and Carcinoma: Provisional Recommendations

| | Group | Start | Procedure |
|---|---|---|---|
| *Screening* | General population | Age 40 | Annual FOBT |
| | | Age 50 | FFS. When negative, repeat once after 5 years |
| *Surveillance* | ≥1 first-degree relative with CRC | Age 35 | C every 3–5 years |
| | Ulcerative colitis | 10 yrs after onset | Annual C with biopsies |
| | Extensive Crohns colitis | 10 yrs after onset | Annual C with biopsies |
| | Family history of FAP, Turcot syndrome | Age 12 | Annual FFS |
| | Family history of HNPCC | Age 25 | C every 2 years |
| | Patients with Peutz-Jeghers syndrome; juvenile polyposis | ? | C in kindreds with associated CRC; frequency ? |

C = colonoscopy; FAP = familial adenomatous polyposis; FFS = flexible fiberoptic sigmoidoscopy; FOBT = fecal occult blood test; HNPCC = hereditary nonpolyposis colorectal carcinoma.

therapy of malignant polyps when extension beyond the muscularis mucosa is absent. Diminutive polyps (<5 mm) may be simply fulgurated without biopsy in view of the very low risk of subsequent cancer associated with them. If neoplastic polyps are found during sigmoidoscopy, complete colonoscopy is required with removal of all lesions. Follow-up surveillance involves colonoscopy in 3 years and then every 5 years.

### Surveillance and Screening for Colorectal Neoplasia

*Surveillance* is aimed at individuals with increased risk (see Table 204.1) for colorectal carcinoma. Individuals with an affected first-degree relative have a four-fold increased risk for CRC at a relatively young age—that is, less than 60 years old. Surveillance colonoscopy is needed every 3 to 5 years, starting at age 35. Screening is discussed in Chapter 197, with suggestions in Table 100.2 and Figure 204.2.

## Familial Adenomatous Polyposis

Familial adenomatous polyposis (FAP) inherited in an autosomal dominant mode accounts for approximately 1% of all cases of CRC. An estimated 20% of affected patients represent new mutations. The genetic basis is a germline mutation in one allele of the APC gene on chromosome 5q21; cancer develops as additional mutations occur, including deletion or mutation of the second allele of the APC gene (see Table 100.1). Myriad small adenomatous polyps develop throughout the colon; 50% of patients develop this by age 25. Nearly all patients progress to CRC, on average by age 42. Retinal pigment epithelium hypertrophies and polyps develop in the upper GI tract. The incidence of duodenal and ampullary carcinoma is increased. Approximately 15% of families affected by FAP additionally develop mesodermal abnormalities, including osteomas, dental abnormalities, and desmoid tumors **(Gardner syndrome).** A rare association of FAP with malignant brain tumors is called **Turcot syndrome.**

Potentially affected family members should undergo annual surveillance sigmoidoscopy starting at age 12. Those with established FAP should also have upper endoscopy performed every 1 to 3 years. Proctocolectomy is mandatory when colonic polyps are detected. Ileoanal anastomosis with creation of an ileal pouch obviates the need for a permanent ileostomy in these young persons. If an ileorectal anastomosis is done, frequent follow-up for rectal cancer is required. Sulindac causes polyps to regress in this syndrome, but it is not a substitute for colectomy, nor for regular surveillance of a remaining rectum.

### Hereditary Nonpolyposis Colorectal Carcinoma

Hereditary nonpolyposis colorectal carcinoma (HNPCC), formerly called the Lynch syndrome, is an autosomal dominant disorder, characterized by 100 or fewer adenomas in the proximal colon and the development of predominantly right-sided CRC by approximately age 45. The rather stringent so-called **Amsterdam criteria** form the current basis for the diagnosis of HNPCC: (1) three or more blood relatives of the proband have CRC, one of whom is a first-degree relative of the other two; (2) the relatives with CRC belong to more than one generation; and (3) at least one relative with CRC was diagnosed prior to age 50. Type I HNPCC affects only the colon. Type II presents with additional non-colonic cancers of the endometrium, breast, ovary, stomach, and other organs. The genetic defect consists of germline mutations in several genes involved in DNA repair. Approximately 5% of all CRC patients are estimated to have HNPCC. Diagnostic molecular biology testing for the presence of the implicated germline mutations is expected to become available in the near future. Such testing probably will establish the diagnosis of HNPCC in many patients who do not meet the current, family history–based criteria. Patients at risk should undergo screening colonoscopy every 2 years, beginning at age 25.

## ■ Colorectal Carcinoma

Colorectal carcinoma (CRC) is the end-stage of the evolution from normal mucosa through adenoma, and severe dysplasia, to noninvasive and then to invasive adenocarcinoma. Inflammatory bowel disease and HNPCC are the only conditions in which adenoma formation is omitted from this sequence. The risk and the time interval for adenoma to evolve into carcinoma correlate with the size and histologic features of the adenoma; on average, this process takes nearly 10 to 12 years. A 50-year-old person has a 5% chance of developing CRC and a 2.5% risk of dying from it. Approximately 4% of patients have a second CRC at the time of diagnosis (synchronous), and 3% develop it subsequently (metachronous). Rectal carcinoma represents nearly one third of all cases of CRC.

### Clinical Features, Diagnosis, and Management

The clinical presentation depends on the site and size of the tumor. Right-sided lesions commonly present with anemia from chronic blood loss, palpable right lower quadrant mass, and enlarged liver with an irregular surface due to metastases; colonic obstruction, tenesmus, decreased stool caliber, pencil stools, and visible blood separate from the stool are more common with left-sided lesions. Rectal bleeding should not be ascribed to co-existing hemorrhoids without further evaluation.

Digital rectal examination may show blood in the stool or a tumor in the lower rectum. Barium enema may reveal a polypoid or annular filling defect (see Figure 204.1), or wall infiltration with mucosal destruction; this radiologic approach can miss rectal tumors. The diagnostic procedure of choice is full colonoscopy with biopsy. The entire colon must be inspected preoperatively to exclude a synchronous carcinoma and to remove adenomas beyond the area of planned resection. Carcinoembryonic antigen (CEA), a cell surface glycoconjugate, is elevated in one third of patients with early CRC and in three fourths of those with advanced CRC. Cancers of other organs, colitis, and smoking also may elevate CEA, which seriously limits its use as a diagnostic or screening tool for CRC. Serial postoperative CEA monitoring can help detect local and distant recurrences following surgical resection.

Management of colorectal cancers is discussed in Chapter 204. Briefly, surgical resection in the form of partial colectomy or low anterior resection of the rectum remains the standard treatment. Palliative resection often is needed for relief of symptoms (e.g., bleeding, obstruction) even when all tumor tissue cannot be removed. Prognosis and further management decisions depend on the operative tumor staging. (Table 100.3 shows a widely used system, and Table 204.3 shows the TNM staging.)

## *Nonneoplastic Colorectal Tumors*

**Hyperplastic colon polyps** are small and usually sessile. Their incidence approaches that of adenomatous polyps; most occur in the distal colon and rectum. These polyps are not premalignant, and their detection in the rectosigmoid does not call for colonoscopy or regular surveillance.

**Peutz-Jeghers syndrome** consists of autosomal, dominantly inherited hamartomatous polyps throughout the GI tract, especially the small bowel, and mucocutaneous pigmentation of the lips, oral mucosa, and fingers. The polyps may cause intussusception, obstruction, and bleeding. An increased incidence of colonic and upper gastrointestinal carcinomas has been noted in several affected families.

**TABLE 100.3. Staging of Colorectal Carcinoma Astler-Coller Modification of the Dukes Classification**

| Stage | Extent | Incidence at Time of Diagnosis | 5-Year Survival |
|---|---|---|---|
| A | Limited to mucosa | 14% | 90–100% |
| $B_1$ | Into muscularis propria | 38% | 65% |
| $B_2$ | Through muscularis propria (and serosa) | | 45% |
| $C_1$ | Same as $B_1$, plus regional node metastases | | 43% |
| $C_2$ | Same as $B_2$, plus regional node metastases | 25% | 15% |
| D | Distant metastases | 23% | 0–5% |

# CHAPTER 101 ANATOMY AND PHYSIOLOGY OF THE PANCREAS

## Anatomy

The pancreas is entirely retroperitoneal and lacks a capsule. It is 12 to 15 cm long and weighs 70 to 100 g. The head and the uncinate process lie within the curve of the duodenum; the body and tail extend obliquely to the splenic hilus. Its blood supply comes from branches of the celiac and superior mesenteric arteries; the splenic artery branches supply mainly the body and tail. The venous drainage is to the splenic and the portal vein. Nonunion of the dorsal (Santorini) and the ventral (Wirsung) ducts occurs in 7% of individuals *(pancreas divisum)*. It has both parasympathetic and sympathetic innervation.

The exocrine tissue is arranged as a tubuloacinar gland consisting of acini and intercalated intra- and interlobular ducts, which converge on the main pancreatic duct. Acinar cells synthesize and export proteins; ductal cells secrete bicarbonate in exchange for chloride.

## Physiology

The pancreatic acinar cells synthesize nearly 20 digestive enzymes, the pancreatic secretory trypsin inhibitor (PSTI), and colipase. Although some of the digestive enzymes are released in the active form (e.g., amylase, lipase, ribonuclease), the proteases (e.g., trypsin, chymotrypsin, carboxypeptidases, elastase) and phospholipase are released as proenzymes or zymogens. Enterokinase, released from the duodenal mucosa, converts trypsinogen to active trypsin, which activates all other proenzymes within the duodenal lumen. The PSTI protects against the digestive action of small amounts of trypsin that may be prematurely liberated from trypsinogen in acinar cells and the pancreatic duct system.

Enzyme synthesis and secretion (Figure 101.1) are stimulated by circulating cholecystokinin (CCK), by central vagal pathways, and by gastro- and enteropancreatic reflexes. CCK is released from the proximal small intestine by the products of protein and fat digestion; this release is inhibited by free intraduodenal trypsin (feedback inhibition). In patients with low duodenal protease activity due to pancreatic insufficiency, plasma CCK levels rise; feeding trypsin-containing pancreatic extracts lowers them. At the intracellular level, lysosomal enzymes are segregated from proteins destined for export into the acinar lumen, a process that is believed to be disturbed in the pathogenesis of acute pancreatitis.

The pancreatic ductal cells are stimulated by secretin to add a bicarbonate-rich fluid to the acinar proteinaceous secretion. The action of secretin is potentiated by CCK and acetylcholine. The cystic fibrosis transmembrane regulator (CFTR), which functions as an apical $Cl^-$ channel, and the $Cl^-/HCO_3^-$ anion exchanger participate in this process. Secretin is released from the duodenal mucosa when the luminal pH decreases to 4.5 or less. This mechanism, plus direct duodenal $HCO_3^-$ secretion, account for the continued neutralization of gastric acid leaving the stomach. Pancreatic secretions are supersaturated with $Ca^{2+}$ ions; their precipitation in the form of $CaCO_3$ is prevented by lithostathine, a protein produced and secreted by the acinar cells.

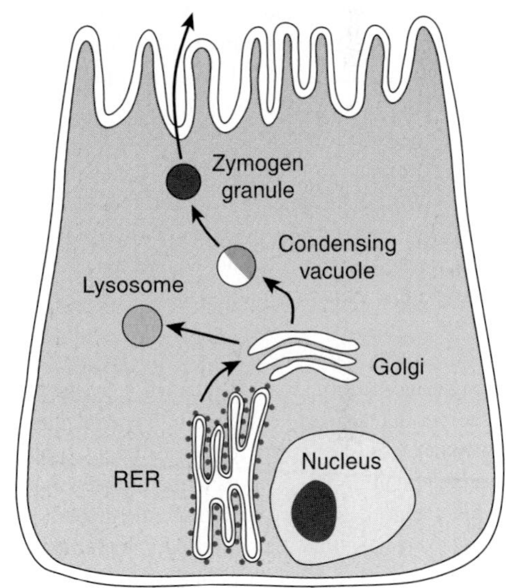


**FIGURE 101.1. Synthesis, sorting, and secretion of zymogens and hydrolytic enzymes in the pancreatic acinar cell. Posttranslational processing occurs in the Golgi apparatus. The subsequent sorting step separates lysosomes from condensing vacuoles. Without this separation, the acid pH and the hydrolases within lysosomes will activate trypsinogen to trypsin. The content of zymogen granules is discharged into the acinar lumen by exocytosis.**
(Reprinted from Soergel KH. Acute pancreatitis. In: Sleisenger MH, Fordtran JS (eds.). Gastrointestinal Disease. 5th ed. Philadelphia: W.B. Saunders Co., 1993: 1630. Used with permission.)

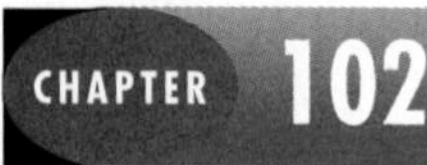

# PANCREATITIS

## Acute Pancreatitis

### Definition and Incidence

Acute pancreatitis is a process of autodigestion by prematurely activated zymogens and enzymes escaping from acinar cells and pancreatic ducts into periacinar and periductal connective tissue. The course is determined by the degree and extent of digestion and inflammation within the gland and by variable involvement of adjacent and remote organs. In contrast to chronic pancreatitis, the pancreas eventually regains normal structure and function. Unless the precipitating cause is removed, the risk of recurrence is nearly 50%. The annual incidence is close to 10 per 100,000 population.

### Etiology and Pathogenesis

In animal models, the rate of exocytosis of the content of zymogen granules is decreased, leading to accumulation of zymogens within the acinar cells. The isolation of zymogens from lysosomal enzymes fails, with the consequent activation and misdirected exit of active enzymes across the basolateral cell wall. The factor initiating this chain of events is unknown, but obstruction of the pancreatic duct at or near the ampulla of Vater may explain some—but not all—episodes of acute pancreatitis. Reflux of duodenal contents or bile into the pancreatic duct does not play a role. Certain causes of acute pancreatitis (e.g., hypercalcemia, ethanol, hypoperfusion) increase pancreatic duct permeability, allowing pancreatic enzymes and zymogens to escape into the periductal tissue. Circulating trypsin inhibitors partially inactivate pancreatic proteases released into the blood; the remaining active trypsin liberates several kinin peptides from their inactive blood precursors. These peptides exert harmful systemic effects, including vasodilatation, excessive vascular permeability, and lowered pain threshold.

Several conditions and drugs lead to acute pancreatitis in humans (Table 102.1). Gallstones cause acute pancreatitis when they impact in the ampulla of Vater; these stones rarely are larger than 5 mm in diameter because they must first pass through the cystic duct. Viruses and bacteria (e.g., mumps, and *Campylobacter jejuni*) are very rare causes.

### Pathology

Initially, there is periacinar and periductal fat necrosis, which progresses to inflammation involving the secretory cells in the acinar periphery, pancreatic ductules and duct, and local blood vessels. The process often spreads to peripancreatic tissue and adjacent organs. Fatty acids liberated from lipid containing cells combine with $Ca^{2+}$ to form calcium soaps. Local complications include (1) fluid collections, frequently multiple and lacking a defined wall; (2) patchy pancreatic necrosis, which may remain sterile or become infected by enteric bacteria transmigrating across the colonic wall; and, rarely, (3) pancreatic abscess, representing an area of liquefied pancreatic necrosis that is infected.

### Clinical Features

Steady midepigastric pain is the key feature. It peaks rapidly in intensity (15–60 min), often radiates straight to the back, and often is relieved by sitting and leaning forward. Nausea, vomiting, and low-grade fever are common. Hypotension occurs in about 30% of patients, owing to retroperitoneal fluid sequestration, generalized excessive vascular permeability, and low peripheral vascular resistance. The abdomen is tender, but without rigidity and rebound tenderness (i.e., no peritoneal irritation). Bowel sounds are sparse or absent (possible onset of paralytic ileus). Painless ecchymoses may develop later in the flanks (Grey-Turner sign) or

**TABLE 102.1. Conditions Frequently Associated with Acute Pancreatitis**

| | |
|---|---|
| *Obstruction* | *Trauma* |
| Choledocholithiasis* | Blunt abdominal trauma |
| Tumors | Abdominal operations |
| Sphincter of Oddi stenosis | ERCP procedure |
| *Metabolic* | *Vascular* |
| Hypertriglyceridemia | Shock |
| Acute hypercalcemia | Vasculitis |
| *Toxins* | *Drugs* |
| Ethanol* | Valproic acid |
| Methanol | Azathioprine (6-MP) |
| Scorpion venom | Metronidazole |
| Congenital | Sulfonamides |
| Pancreas Divisium | Most diuretics |
| | Pentamidine |
| | Tetracycline |
| | Mesalamine |
| | ACE inhibitors |
| | DDI (2′ 3′ dideoxyinosine) |
| | Cocaine abuse |

*Common cause.
ACE = angiotensin converting enzyme.

**TABLE 102.2. Prognostic Signs in Acute Pancreatitis (Ranson Criteria)**

| On Admission | | During Initial 48 Hours of Therapy | |
|---|---|---|---|
| Age | >55 yrs | Hematocrit | >10% decrease |
| WBC | >16,000/mm$^3$ | BUN | >5 mg/dl increase |
| Serum glucose | >200 mg/dl | Serum calcium | <8 mg/dl |
| Serum LDH | >350 IU/l | $PaO_2$ | <60 mm Hg |
| ALT | >250 SFU | Base deficit | >4 mEq/l |
| | | Fluid sequestration | >6 liters |

Fewer than three signs present: benign clinical course.
Three or more signs present: serious clinical illness/death in up to 67% of patients.
ALT = serum alanine-aminotransferase; BUN = blood urea nitrogen; LDH = lactate dehydrogenase; $PaO_2$ = arterial oxygen tension; SFU = sigma Frankel units.
(Modified from: Ranson JH, Rifkind KM, Turner JW. Surg Gyn Obstet 1976;143:210. Used with permission.)

periumbilical area (Cullen's sign). No complications arise in the 80% of cases with a mild course and brief hospitalization (<1 week); the 6% to 10% overall mortality occurs in the remaining 20%.

## Diagnosis

Acute pancreatitis is diagnosed by a combination of clinical, laboratory, and, in some cases, radiologic findings. Serum amylase activity, the most commonly used test, rises within 2 to 12 hours after the onset of pain and is normal within 3 to 5 days. The probability of acute pancreatitis rises with the degree of rise in serum amylase; it is nearly 100% with values more than five times the upper limit of normal. With lipemic serum, results may be falsely negative. Determining pancreatic (P) and salivary (S) isozymes of amylase, or measuring urine amylase, or estimating the amylase-creatinine clearance ratio serves no added benefit. Many other conditions may elevate serum amylase—for example, gastric, duodenal, or jejunal perforation, mesenteric infarction, chronic pancreatitis, salivary adenitis, ovarian neoplasms, renal failure, ethanol intoxication, upper GI endoscopy (including endoscopic retrograde cholangiopancreatography [ERCP]), and critical illness. Serum lipase has a similar diagnostic value; it tends to remain high longer than amylase. Together, these two tests are 95% sensitive and 90% specific for diagnosing pancreatitis.

Other laboratory features include leukocytosis (75%), mild hypocalcemia (30%) with normal ionized calcium (which explains the rarity of tetany), transient hyperglycemia that requires no therapy, and, regardless of the etiology of the attack, moderate increase in serum aspartate transaminase (AST). High serum C-reactive protein (>120 mg/L) can predict pancreatic necrosis reliably. Together, many tests obtained during the first 48 hours of illness may help predict prognosis. However, the Ranson and the Glasgow criteria and the APACHE II (Acute Physiology and Chronic Health Evaluation) score can reliably predict a mild versus a complicated course only in 70% to 80% of cases (Table 102.2).

### Imaging studies

Plain abdominal radiographs should always be obtained; they may show free air due to a perforated viscus, pancreatic calcifications of chronic pancreatitis, radiopaque gallstones, and paralytic ileus. Chest radiographs often show pleural effusions and basilar atelectasis due to the subphrenic inflammation. Abdominal ultrasound is the preferred method for detecting gallstones and bile duct dilatation. The latter findings combined with elevation of more than three laboratory tests (bilirubin, GGT, ALT, ALT/AST ratio >1.0, alkaline phosphatase) indicate gallstone-related pancreatitis. Abdominal CT (Figure 102.1), while abnormal in 90% of cases of acute pancreatitis, is not required routinely.

## Management

Mild pancreatitis (i.e., uncomplicated illness) requires only supportive care. The goals are prompt rehydration to achieve euvolemia, full pain relief with opiates, and resting the intestines by avoiding all oral intake. Nasogastric suction is employed for vomiting or evolving paralytic ileus. Routine antibiotic use is of no benefit. Small feedings of a diet low in fat and protein are started once the pain subsides and the bowel sounds resume. The patient must be watched closely for early signs of complications. Persistent shock, increasing abdominal tenderness, fever, and dyspnea require prompt evaluation.

## Complications

Systemic complications tend to occur during the first week of illness, whereas local complications and involvement of adjacent organs follow during the next two weeks

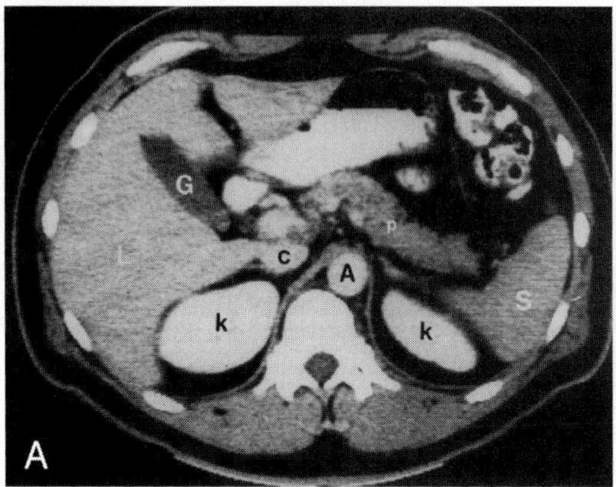


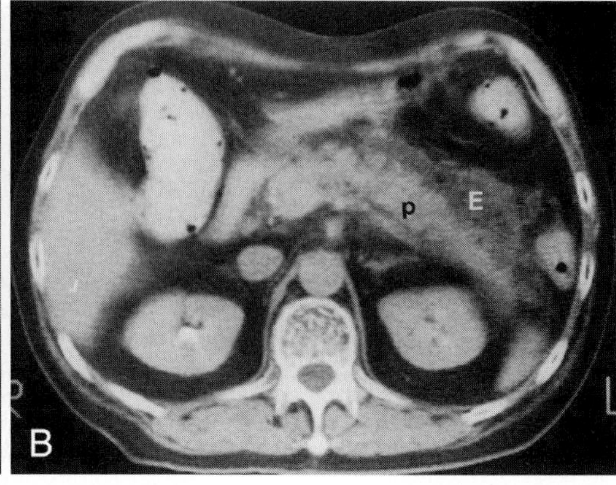


**FIGURE 102.1.** A. Normal pancreas. B. Mild acute pancreatitis with thickening of the pancreas and peripancreatic edema. CT scans at the head of the pancreatic body and tail after IV contrast administration. G = gallbladder; k = kidney; S = spleen; A = aorta; c = inferior vena cava; p = pancreas; E = peripancreatic edema. (Reprinted from Soergel KH. Acute pancreatitis. In Sleisenger MH, Fordtran JS (eds.). Gastrointestinal Disease. 5th ed. Philadelphia: W.B. Saunders Co., 1993: 1641, Fig. 80-6. Used with permission.)

**TABLE 102.3. Complications During Acute Pancreatitis**

| Systemic | Local | Adjacent Organs |
|---|---|---|
| Shock | Impacted common bile duct stone | Splenic vein occlusion |
| Acute renal failure | Pancreatic necrosis | Splenic infarct |
| ARDS* | Sterile | Bleeding |
| Sepsis | Infected | Colonic necrosis |
| Miscellaneous | Fluid collection | Pleural effusion |
| DIC** | Sterile | Pancreatic fistula |
| Hyperglycemia | Infected | |
| Hypocalcemia | Pancreatic abscess | |
| | Bleeding | |

*Adult respiratory distress syndrome.
**Disseminated intravascular coagulation.

(Table 102.3). About 20% of patients develop one or more complications.

Early *circulatory shock*, an ominous sign, often signals pancreatic necrosis; admission to ICU, aggressive hydration, and vasopressors are indicated. Shock later in the course may reflect gram negative sepsis. *Acute renal failure* due to acute tubular necrosis may arise from the combination of shock and high renovascular resistance. The *adult respiratory distress syndrome* (ARDS) often complicates severe, acute pancreatitis, and is ascribed to alveolar surfactant damage by phospholipases and circulating free fatty acids; hypoxemia unrelated to other causes is an early clue. Treatment consists of oxygen, and, in severe cases, ventilatory support with positive end-expiratory pressure (PEEP). *Sepsis* may follow ascending cholangitis and infected pancreatic necrosis. Hyperglycemia and hypocalcemia, while common, rarely need therapy. Distinguishing toxic psychosis from delirium tremens and opiate effects may be a challenge in diagnosis and therapy.

*Persistent impaction of a gallstone* in the ampulla of Vater delays the resolution of pancreatitis. Progressive jaundice and spiking fevers follow, reflecting ascending cholangitis. In addition to prompt endoscopic or surgical disimpaction of the stone, antibiotics also are indicated. *Pancreatic necrosis* (PN) occurs in 80% of patients with a clinically severe course during the second or third week of illness. Prognosis and management critically depend on whether the necrotic tissue is infected (see below). A dynamic CT with rapid IV contrast injection is performed, and necrotic areas, defined by the lack of contrast enhancement (Figure 102.2), are aspirated using a CT-guided fine needle. Gram stain of the aspirate diagnoses or excludes infection. Patients with sterile PN are treated conservatively. In infected PN, unless the affected tissue is promptly excised surgically, the mortality exceeds 60%. Combined excision and antibiotics (fluoroquinolones or imipenem/cilastatin, plus metronidazole) lowers the mortality to 10% to 20%. *Fluid collections* form in up to 50% of patients with severe pancreatitis. Most resolve spontaneously; persistent collections over 6 weeks old evolve into pseudocysts. For enlarging or infected collections (pancreatic abscess) percutaneous aspiration and drainage can be employed.

*Splenic vein thrombosis* may later result in gastric fundic varices. *Splenic infarcts and necrosis* result from thrombosis of the splenic artery or vein or from direct extension of the inflammation to the splenic hilum. Extension of the inflammatory process into the mesocolon may cause bleeding and *perforation of the transverse colon. Bleeding* may have several sources, including antral and duodenal erosions and erosion of splenic or pancreatic vessels, in which case blood may enter a disrupted pancreatic duct and empty into the duodenum. *Pleural effusions* are common and arise from a variety of mechanisms, and tend to resolve spontaneously.

#### Preventing recurrence

The care of the patient with acute pancreatitis mandates a thorough search for the cause (see Table 102.1). If abdominal US shows gallstones, cholecystectomy should follow, with surgical or endoscopic exploration of the common bile duct as soon as pancreatitis subsides. Hypertriglyceridemia and hypercalcemia should be ruled out. At this point, nearly 20% of patients would remain in whom a cause is elusive. These patients, after experiencing one severe or two mild attacks, should undergo magnetic resonance cholangiopancreaticography (MRCP) and, if required, an elective ERCP, which will reveal a variety of correctable causes. A systematic search, as shown in Figure 102.3 will identify only 5% to 10% of patients as having "idiopathic pancreatitis."

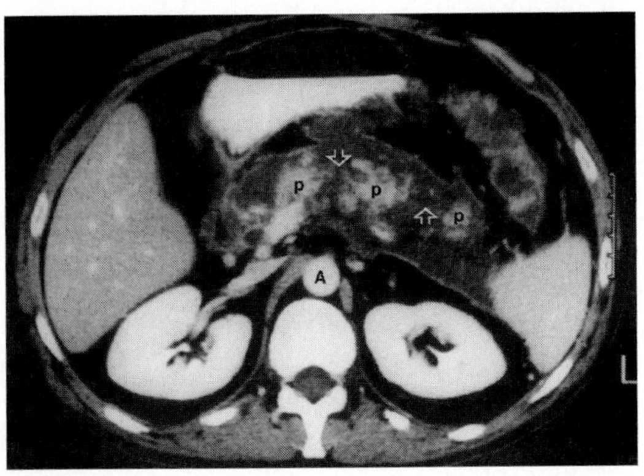


**FIGURE 102.2. Necrotizing pancreatitis. CT scan during rapid IV bolus injection of contrast material. P: normally perfused areas of the pancreas. Open arrows: nonperfused necrotic areas. A. Aorta. The pancreas is surrounded by fluid that extends into the small bowel mesentery.**

(Reprinted from Soergel KH. Acute pancreatitis. In Sleisenger MH, Fordtran JS (eds). Gastrointestinal Disease. 5th ed. Philadelphia: W.B. Saunders Co., 1993:1642, fig. 80-10. Used with permission.)

## Chronic Pancreatitis

### Definition and Pathogenesis

Chronic pancreatitis is marked by irreversible, usually progressive, fibrosis of the gland, along with decreased exocrine and endocrine function. Episodes clinically resembling acute pancreatitis may occur, especially during the early years of alcoholic pancreatitis. The 10-year mortality approaches 25%.

The disease occurs in two major categories, chronic calcifying pancreatitis and chronic obstructive pancreatitis; *chronic calcifying pancreatitis* the most common. The initial event in chronic calcifying pancreatitis is the precipitation of proteins in pancreatic duct radicles and, later, in the main duct. An abnormal lithostathine metabolism—that is, either its decreased acinar secretion or its proteolysis within the ducts, yielding a fibrillar, insoluble peptide—is said to be responsible. These protein plugs eventually calcify and cause irregularly distributed obstruction of the small and large ducts, leading to duct dilatation, acinar atrophy, chronic inflammation and fibrosis. The islets of Langerhans are progressively destroyed late in the disease. *Chronic obstructive pancreatitis* follows tumors or duct strictures, obstructing the flow of pancreatic juice. A special form is *pancreas divisum,* in which a narrow dorsal duct and small-caliber minor papilla may initiate chronic pancreatitis.

### Etiology

Most cases of chronic pancreatitis arise from alcohol abuse. Pancreatitis in an alcoholic is really chronic pancreatitis from the start. Subsequent alcohol abstinence does not alter the progression to pancreatic exocrine insufficiency, but may decrease pain and delay the onset of diabetes mellitus. The onset of symptoms is typically between the ages of 35 and 45. *Senile pancreatitis/atrophy,* seen in older (>60 years) nonalcoholics, occurs mainly as malabsorption along with pancreatic calcification; pain is either mild or absent. *Familial pancreatitis,* an autosomal dominant disorder, accounts for about 2% of patients. Gene defects in familial pancreatitis have been identified. Episodic abdominal pain begins between the ages of 10 and 14 years, with pancreatic calcifications visible on radiographs; pancreatic adenocarcinoma reportedly is common. Chronic pancreatitis seen with *primary hyperparathyroidism* and *hyperlipidemia,* and after *renal transplantation,* has an elusive mechanism and frequency. In *obstructive pancreatitis,* removing the obstructing lesion can halt the course of chronic pancreatitis. No cause is found in one fifth of cases; however, bouts of recurrent acute pancreatitis, regardless of cause, do not cause chronic pancreatitis. *Tropical pancreatitis,* presenting mainly with calcifications, pain and diabetes mellitus, is common in teenagers and young adults in southeast Asia and Central Africa.

## Clinical Features and Diagnosis

The leading symptom is intermittent or chronic epigastric pain that often radiates straight through to the back and may be aggravated after eating and on the morning after a drinking bout. The pain may be due to raised intrapancreatic tissue and duct pressure from ductal obstruction by fibrosis or stones, and perineural fibrosis. Weight loss, diabetes mellitus due to progressive destruction of islets of Langerhans, steatorrhea, and local complications tend to develop 5 to 15 years after onset of pain.

The diagnosis of chronic pancreatitis rests on symptoms, radiological studies, and, rarely, tests of exocrine pancreatic function. Blood tests add little to the diagnosis. Serum amylase and lipase may be normal, or may rise during episodes of pain. Plain abdominal radiographs may reveal intraductal pancreatic calcifications (Figure 102.4); this finding, along with a typical pain pattern, is diagnostic. Abdominal CT and ERCP (Figure 102.5) frequently show ductal dilatation; their main value lies in revealing potentially correctable lesions (tumors, stones, and pseudocysts). M.R.C.P. is now gradually replacing the need to do diagnostic ERCP.

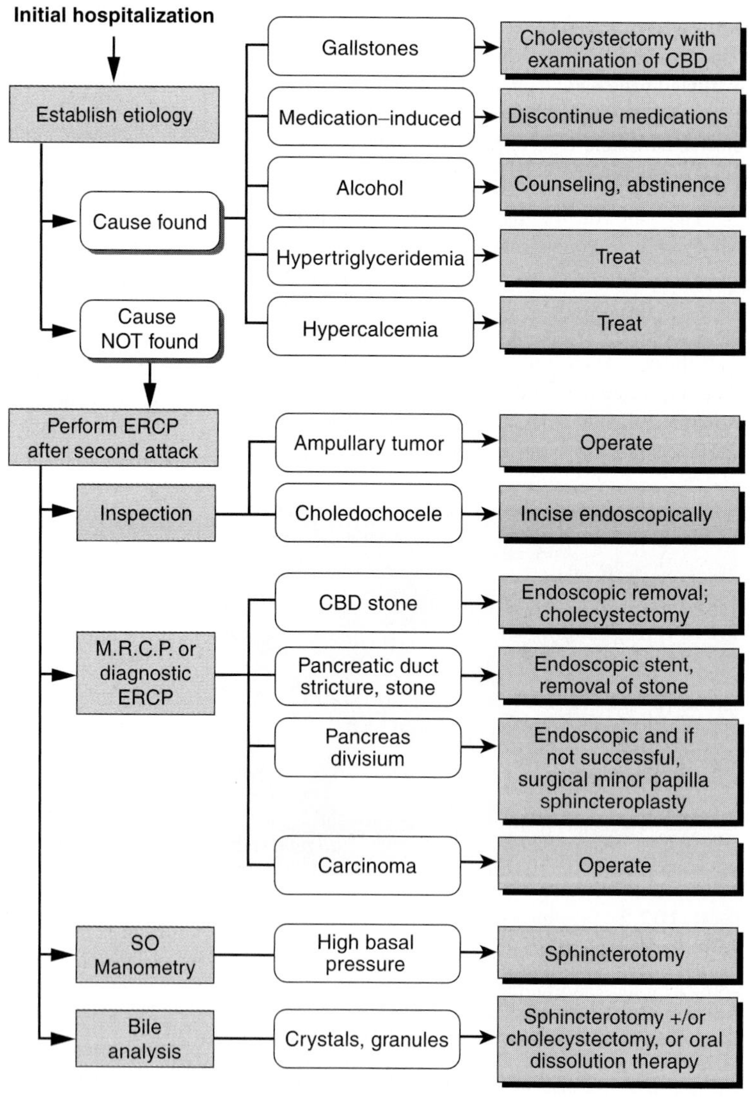


**FIGURE 102.3.** Suggested approach to identifying the cause of acute pancreatitis. CBD = common bile duct; Dissolution therapy = therapy with chenodeoxycholic acid or ursodeoxycholic acid; ERCP = endoscopic retrograde cholangiopancreatography; SO = sphincter of Oddi.

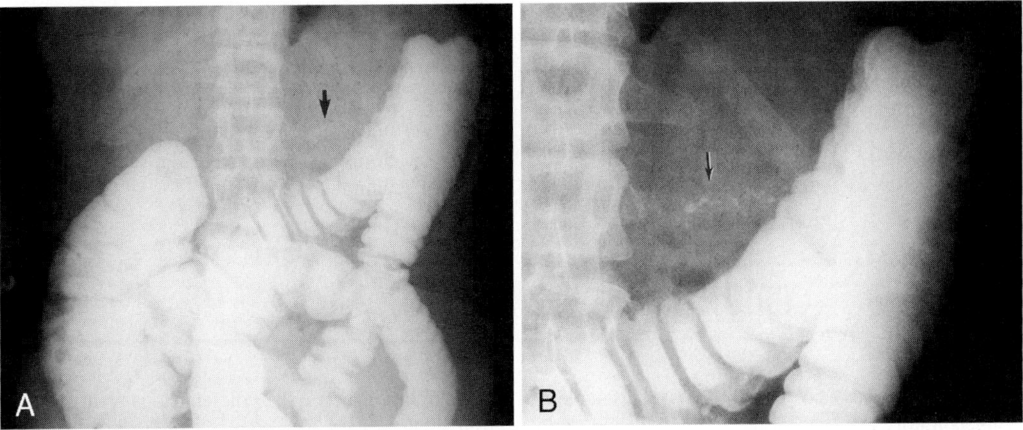

**FIGURE 102.4.** A. Pancreatic calcification. (A barium enema was being performed for other reasons.) B. Magnified view.

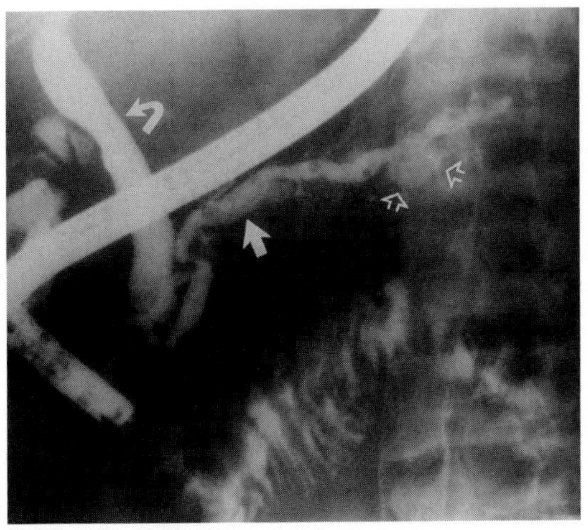

**FIGURE 102.5.** ERCP in chronic pancreatitis. The pancreatic duct (straight solid arrow) is irregularly dilated and contains several round filling defects (stones). Contrast material extravasates into a small pseudocyst (open arrows). The common bile duct (CBD), indicated by the curved arrow, is moderately dilated (11 mm diameter). The terminal portion of the CBD is narrowed by pancreatic fibrosis.

## Management and Complications

Chronic, often disabling, *upper abdominal pain* is the main therapeutic challenge. Acute exacerbation of the pain may warrant brief hospitalization, cessation of oral feeding, and parenteral analgesics. Opiate analgesics eventually are required in most patients; they should not be withheld or curtailed because of concomitant alcoholism or concerns about addiction. The pain resolves spontaneously in about 60% of patients after 5 to 10 years. Orally administered pancreatic extract (6 tablets/meal of Viokase, Cotazym, or Isozyme) reduces pancreatic secretion by feedback inhibition of CCK release; an $H_2$-receptor antagonist or PPI should be coadministered to prevent their inactivation at low gastric pH. This approach lessens pain in a minority of patients with idiopathic chronic pancreatitis. Percutaneous injection of the celiac ganglion with alcohol or phenol transiently relieves pain in about 50% of patients. Patients with intractable pain and a dilated main pancreatic duct should be considered for ERCP or surgical decompression. A longitudinal pancreaticojejunostomy relieves pain in almost 70% of patients, provided they abstain from alcohol.

*Malabsorption* occurs late in the course, when pancreatic enzyme secretion is reduced by 90% or more. Deficiencies of vitamins, including $B_{12}$, and of iron and calcium usually do not develop owing to intact intestinal absorptive function. Treatment is indicated only when weight loss continues despite attempts at increasing caloric intake. Pancreatic extracts, as described earlier, or enteric-coated preparations that dissolve only at the alkaline pH of the duodenum and upper jejunum, may be tried (e.g., Pancrease or Creon, 2–3 capsules/meal).

*Diabetes mellitus* eventually develops in about 70% of patients with pancreatitis, and one half of those require insulin. In contrast with the usual diabetic, the risk of iatrogenic hypoglycemia is even greater, given the combined deficiency of insulin and glucagon, erratic dietary habits, and alcohol-induced hypoglycemia. *Pancreatic pseudocysts* appear in about 60% of patients, representing a type of retention cyst from pancreatic duct destruction or disruption. Surrounded by a rim of chronic inflammation and fibrosis, and located within or adjacent to the pancreas, they may compress the distal common bile duct. Enlarging or nonresolving large (>5 cm in diameter) pseudocysts or those complicated by obstruction (pancreatic duct, bile duct or duodenum) should be considered for drainage (endoscopic vs guided, percutaneous or surgical).

*External compression* of the common bile duct by a pseudocyst or by pancreatic fibrosis with resulting jaundice calls for surgical correction to prevent secondary biliary cirrhosis. *Pancreatic ascites,* a form of chemical peritonitis caused by leakage of pancreatic juice from a disrupted ductal structure, is rare; the levels of amylase and lipase in the fluid are far greater than those in the serum. The treatment is surgical—that is, a partial pancreatectomy or drainage of the leaking duct into a loop of jejunum.

# CHAPTER 103 CYSTIC FIBROSIS

General aspects of cystic fibrosis (CF) and its respiratory manifestations are discussed in chapter 223. Malabsorption and intestinal obstruction from cystic fibrosis are discussed here. *Malabsorption*, with steatorrhea, occurs in about 85% of affected persons, starting in early childhood, and is caused by pancreatic exocrine insufficiency due to painless obstruction of the pancreatic duct system by proteinaceous, inspissated secretions. The resulting growth failure and malnutrition can be ameliorated by administering high doses of pancreatic extracts. Partial substitution of dietary fat by medium-chain triglyceride may produce additional weight gain.

Colicky abdominal pain and distention signaling acute or **chronic intestinal obstruction** occur frequently in these patients. This complication, due to accumulation of masses of tenacious, putty-like material in the ileum or proximal colon, is treated acutely by 20% N-acetylcysteine (30 ml in 120 ml of water) given orally or rectally as a retention enema. Chronic cases may be given less expensive agents, including diatrizoate (Gastrografin) or 1–2L of a polyethylene glycol-electrolyte solution (GoLYTELY) orally. The dosage of pancreatic extract should be increased and poorly digestible, stringy cellulose materials (e.g., the pulp of citrus fruit) should be avoided. Patients with CF cannot respond to bacterial enterotoxins with $Cl^-$ secretion given the absence of CFTR gene product from the apical cell membrane throughout the bowel. Thus they are protected against secretory diarrhea mediated by increases in intracellular cAMP or calcium concentration.

# CHAPTER 104 NEOPLASMS OF THE PANCREAS

Pancreatic neoplasms with endocrine manifestations originate in the islet cells. Examples of these rare neoplasms are insulinomas (see Chapter 72) and gastrinomas (see Chapter 83).

The great majority of nonendocrine pancreatic neoplasms are malignant. Their etiology remains unknown except for some rare types of familial tumors. Pancreatic cancer is the fifth most common carcinoma as a cause of death; it accounts for more than 20% of all gastrointestinal cancers. Its incidence has increased steadily during the past 40 years; it now causes almost 25,000 deaths annually in the United States.

## ■ Adenocarcinoma

About 90% of pancreatic tumors are mucinous adenocarcinoma of ductal origin, predominantly seen in men (2:1) and associated with cigarette smoking, beer drinking, certain industrial carcinogens, and, probably, chronic pancreatitis. It affects all age groups, but is most common in the seventh and eighth decades of life.

### Clinical Features

Pain and weight loss, lasting several months, occur in up to 75% of patients. The pain is upper abdominal, vague, dull, and constant; it implies retroperitoneal extension or perineural infiltration by tumor. Anorexia due to pain or liver metastases, pancreatic exocrine insufficiency, and onset of diabetes mellitus all lead to weight loss. Obstructive jaundice occurs in over 50% of cases, particularly with a tumor located in the pancreatic head and compressing the intrapancreatic common bile duct. Rarely, it presents with an episode of otherwise unexplained acute pancreatitis. Anorexia, loss of weight, and vague abdominal pain in the face of negative diagnostic studies may mimic depression. Duodenal or gastric wall invasion may cause vomiting, bleeding, or obstruction. The tumor usually is not palpable. The liver may be enlarged, firm, and irregular due to metastases. Jaundice along with a palpably enlarged gallbladder (Courvoisier's sign) signals common bile duct obstruction by a pancreatic or ampullary cancer. Most patients are surgically incurable by the time of diagnosis.

### Diagnosis

Early diagnosis of pancreatic cancer is a clinical challenge; no practical screening test for early pancreatic cancer is available. The emphasis should be on the detection of small tumors, less than 2 to 3 cm in diameter, that might be resectable for cure. Such small lesions, however, tend to be subclinical and often are beyond the limits of abdominal US and CT. Positive findings on current diagnostic testing imply a tumor that has less than a 2% chance for cure. Finally, the presenting complaints are shared by many other abdominal disorders; thus, the tests for this tumor must be highly specific. Clues for pancreatic cancer include upper abdominal or back pain suggesting a retroperitoneal origin, unexplained dyspepsia and weight loss with negative conventional work-up, recent onset of mild diabetes in the elderly without predisposing factors, and acute pancreatitis with no obvious cause in the sixth decade and beyond.

Routine blood tests have limited use. Mild anemia or hyperglycemia may be present. Serum amylase and lipase are moderately high in only 10% to 20% of patients. Hyperbilirubinemia and cholestatic liver tests are found with common bile duct encroachment and with extensive liver metastases. A raised plasma carcinoembryonic antigen level (CEA) occurs in one third of cases. The level of carbohydrate antigen CA 19-9, the sialylated blood group Lewis A, is high in 70% of patients, with the degree of elevation correlating with the tumor size. However, CA 19-9 levels are moderately high in 20–30% of patients with acute and chronic pancreatitis.

Several imaging tests can yield findings suggestive of, but not completely diagnostic of, pancreatic cancer. Transabdominal US may suggest the disease in 60% of cases, CT in 80% of cases, and ERCP in 93% of cases. MRI scan is a useful adjunct to CT and can also be used as an alternative to CT in those who cannot be given iodinated contrast. Although MRI has a greater contrast resolution, it is still a secondary imaging modality, with CT being the examination of choice. In experienced hands, endoscopic US can demonstrate lesions that are beyond the resolution of the other techniques. It can detect tumors less than 2 cm in size and also give information on resectability with high accuracy rates. EUS guided fine needle aspiration of suspected lesion can be performed. With evidence of unresectability, CT- or US-guided fine-needle aspiration for cytology can confirm the diagnosis with a high degree of accuracy. When a small, potentially resectable, tumor is found, its resectability can be confirmed preoperatively by endoscopic US, selective visceral arteriography and by diagnostic laparoscopy. Tumor invasion of stomach or duodenum can be demonstrated by upper GI series or by endoscopy.

### Management

The objectives are palliation or an attempt to cure. If the need for palliation is obvious, excessive testing should be avoided in favor of confirming the diagnosis at surgery. Gastric and duodenal obstruction can be bypassed by a gastrojejunostomy without any resection. Obstructive jaundice with pruritus, anorexia, or bacterial cholangitis is palliated by endoscopic insertion of plastic or expandable metal stents into the obstructed common bile duct. When this attempt fails, surgical or percutaneous decompression can be attempted.

Approximately 15% to 20% of patients with carcinoma of the head of the pancreas have an apparently resectable lesion at operation, with only a few cures. Essentially, all carcinomas of the body and tail have progressed beyond the curative resection stage. Choice of the operative procedure lies between resection of the duodenum and head of the pancreas *(Whipple operation)* and total pancreatectomy, both with regional node removal. The results of the Whipple operation for ampullary carcinoma are considerably better. Irradiation therapy by high-dose external beam techniques or by intraoperative radiation may provide limited palliation of symptoms and minor prolongation of survival. Debilitating abdominal and back pain in advanced pancreatic carcinoma may be relieved or significantly improved by percutaneous block and chemical neurolysis of the celiac and superior mesenteric sympathetic ganglia. This procedure should be more widely employed. Chemotherapy, so far, has been unable to provide measurable benefits to patients with this disease.

## Ampullary Carcinoma

Ampullary carcinomas, which tend to occur in middle-aged persons, arise from either the ampulla of Vater itself or adjacent structures such as the distal common bile duct, pancreatic head, or the duodenum that involve the ampulla. A common presenting feature is jaundice due to biliary obstruction, which may remit as the tumor erodes into the duodenum. Ulceration can lead to overt or occult GI bleeding. Cholangitis or pancreatitis are other presentations. Biochemical studies may show features of cholestatic jaundice. The ampulla can be directly visualized and biopsied using a side-viewing endoscope. Endoscopic ultrasonography can define the depth of the lesion. Surgery is the treatment of choice. Endoscopic resection for superficial lesions is also possible. Biliary obstruction can also be palliated endoscopically.

## Cystic Lesions of the Pancreas

Most common cystic lesions are pseudocysts, accounting for 70% to 90% of cystic lesions seen in the pancreas. About 10% to 15% of these lesions are primary neoplasms of the pancreas. *Serous cystadenoma* usually are seen in women in the sixth decade of life. Malignant transformation is rare and, therefore, many recommend observation unless patient has symptoms. *Mucinous cystic neoplasms,* on the other hand, can undergo malignant transformation; therefore, surgical removal is advisable. These tumors occur at around 50 years of age and are seen predominantly in women. Intraductal papillary mucinous tumors (IPMT) of the pancreas are characterized by ectasia of the pancreatic duct with mucinous filling defects seen on ERCP. These lesions also can undergo malignant transformation, and, therefore, surgery should be considered.

## Questions

**INSTRUCTIONS:** For each question below, select only **one** lettered answer that is the **best** for that question.

1. A 53-year-old man, who was diagnosed as having a gastric ulcer on upper GI radiographs, was given omeprazole (20 mg daily) for 12 weeks. On follow-up, his epigastric pain persists. The next step in his management should be to:
   A. Continue omeprazole for another 4 weeks.
   B. Increase the dose of omeprazole until the patient responds.
   C. Repeat barium upper GI examination.
   D. Evaluate the gastric ulcer endoscopically.
   E. Treat the patient for *Helicobacter pylori* infection.

2. A 58-year-old man has a 15-year history of recurrent duodenal ulcer disease. His ulcer heals promptly with $H_2$-receptor antagonists, but recurs within 2 to 6 months after stopping treatment. There is no history of NSAID use. Management of this patient should include which of the following?
   A. Long-term treatment with $H_2$-receptor antagonists
   B. Treatment with omeprazole instead of an $H_2$-receptor antagonist
   C. Consideration of treatment for *H. pylori* infection
   D. CT scan of abdomen to rule out gastrinoma
   E. Referral for duodenal ulcer surgery

3. A 72-year-old man has a 6-month history of dysphagia, mainly for solids, and a 15-lb. weight loss. He is a heavy smoker but claims to have stopped smoking 4 months ago. The most likely diagnosis is:
   A. Esophageal carcinoma
   B. Gastric carcinoma
   C. Achalasia
   D. Peptic esophageal stricture
   E. Pill injury of the esophagus

4. A 28-year-old woman has a 1-hour history of passing maroon stools. Her pulse is 120/min and blood pressure is 100/60 mm Hg. She feels dizzy on standing. Her hematocrit is 44%, hemoglobin is 13 g/dl, and mean corpuscular volume (MCV) is 88 fl. This patient has which of the following?
   A. Acute, significant blood loss
   B. Acute, minimal blood loss
   C. Acute and chronic blood loss
   D. Chronic blood loss
   E. None of the above

5. A 45-year-old patient has a history of recurrent vomiting. Upper GI examination shows evidence of gastric outlet obstruction. Which of the following could be expected?
   A. Projectile and bilious vomiting
   B. Gastric volvulus
   C. Paraesophageal hernia
   D. Hypokalemic acidosis
   E. Hypokalemic alkalosis

6. In Barrett's esophagus:
   A. Gastroesophageal reflux should be aggressively treated to make the metaplastic epithelium disappear.
   B. Periodic endoscopic evaluation should be done with biopsy.
   C. Anti-reflux surgery is the treatment of choice.
   D. Patients have a higher incidence of esophageal infection.
   E. Squamous epithelium extends below the gastroesophageal junction.

7. All of the following are true about *Helicobacter pylori*, EXCEPT:
   A. Over 90% of patients with duodenal ulcer are positive for *H. pylori.*
   B. Eradication of *H. pylori* lowers duodenal ulcer recurrence rate.
   C. Prior infection predisposes to gastric adenocarcinoma.
   D. Prior infection predisposes to gastric mucosa-associated lymphoid tissue (MALT) lymphoma.
   E. Infected patients have a higher incidence of achalasia.

8. A 42-year-old woman has had watery diarrhea and mild lower abdominal cramping distress for 4 months. She has lost 4 kg through attempts at weight reduction. Systemic symptoms, blood in the stool, and recent foreign travel are absent. All the following considerations are appropriate, EXCEPT:

A. Laxative abuse.
B. Idiopathic ulcerative colitis.
C. Consumption of sorbitol-containing diet foods.
D. Functional diarrhea.
E. Microscopic colitis.

9. Based on the information in question 8, which of the following approaches to the patient is NOT indicated?
   A. Proctosigmoidoscopy with biopsies
   B. Esophagogastroduodenoscopy (EGD) with duodenal biopsies
   C. Urine laxative screen
   D. Thorough dietary history
   E. Stool testing for occult blood

10. A 28-year-old married man with a 12-year history of ulcerative colitis suffers his eighth relapse, with tenesmus, frequent bloody stools, abdominal cramps, and a fever of 100.5°F. Each previous attack responded to a 2-month course of corticosteroids; he took no medications during remissions. His serum alkaline phosphatase is 2.5 times the upper limit of normal. Endoscopic retrograde cholangiopancreatography (ERCP) shows caliber irregularities of intra- and extrahepatic bile ducts. All of the following issues are relevant, EXCEPT:
    A. Proctocolectomy should be considered to prevent progression of primary sclerosing cholangitis.
    B. The patient should have received maintenance therapy with a 5-ASA–containing medication.
    C. The couple's plans to have children need to be considered in choosing the type of 5-ASA-containing medication.
    D. The patient needs surveillance colonoscopy with biopsies in the near future.
    E. The patient may have osteoporosis.

11. A 32-year-old nonalcoholic man has recovered from an initial episode of acute pancreatitis. Abdominal ultrasonography showed no gallstones, and serum triglyceride and calcium levels were normal. All of the following may help determine the etiology of pancreatitis, EXCEPT:
    A. ERCP
    B. Review of pre-illness medication intake
    C. Bile analysis for cholesterol crystals
    D. Inquiries about possible cocaine abuse
    E. Upper gastrointestinal series

12. The following conditions are associated with, or may be a consequence of, celiac sprue, EXCEPT:
    A. Diabetes mellitus
    B. Lymphoma of the small intestine
    C. Carcinoma of the colon
    D. Ulcerative jejunitis
    E. Squamous carcinoma of the oropharynx

13. A 1.2-cm tubular adenoma was removed from the sigmoid colon of a 65-year-old man. Colonoscopy shows no additional lesions. He has no symptoms, and his family history is unremarkable. A fecal occult blood test (FOBT) is negative. Which of the following statements is correct?
    A. He should undergo fiberoptic proctosigmoidoscopy in 6 months.
    B. Further follow-up depends on the results of serial FOBT.
    C. An abdominal CT scan should be ordered.
    D. He should undergo colonoscopy in 3 years.
    E. His risk of developing colorectal carcinoma remains high despite regular colonoscopic surveillance and removal of any new polyps.

14. A 45-year-old man with well-established alcoholic chronic pancreatitis has lost 5 kg during the past 4 months. Possible direct causes of this weight loss include all of the following, EXCEPT:
    A. Excessive consumption of ethanol
    B. Newly developed diabetes mellitus
    C. Malabsorption with diarrhea
    D. Decreased food intake due to constant pain
    E. Lack of funds to purchase food

15. If a 3-day stool collection obtained from the patient described in question 14 yielded a daily stool weight of 360 g and 38 g of fat/day, which of the following tests is expected to be abnormal?
    A. A serum iron level
    B. A glucose breath $H_2$ test
    C. The blood folate concentration
    D. A test of vitamin $B_{12}$ absorption
    E. The serum vitamin D concentration

## Answers

| | | | | |
|---|---|---|---|---|
| 1. D | 2. C | 3. A | 4. A | 5. E |
| 6. B | 7. E | 8. B | 9. B | 10. A |
| 11. E | 12. C | 13. D | 14. A | 15. D |

## SUGGESTED READING

### *Textbooks and Monographs*

Arias IM, Boyer JL, Fausto N, et al (eds). The Liver: Biology and Pathology. 3rd ed. New York: Raven Press, 1994.
Blaser MJ, Smith PD, Ravdin JI, et al (eds). Infections of the Gastrointestinal Tract. New York: Raven Press, 1995.
DeDombal FT. Diagnosis of Acute Abdominal Pain. 2nd ed. Edinburgh: Churchill Livingstone, 1991.
Feldman M, Friedman LS, Sleisenger MH (eds). Sleisenger & Fordtran's Gastrointestinal and Liver Disease. 7th ed. Philadelphia: WB Saunders, 2002.

Go VLW, DiMagno E, Gardner JD, et al (eds). The Pancreas: Biology, Pathobiology and Disease. 2nd ed. New York: Raven Press, 1993.

Gollan JL, Kalser SC, Pitt HA, et al (eds). Proceedings of the NIH Consensus Development Conference on gallstones and laparoscopic cholecystectomy. Am J Surg 1993;165:388–548.

Sherlock S, Dooley J (ed.). Diseases of the Liver and Biliary System. 10th ed. Boston: Blackwell Scientific Publications, 1997.

Targan SR, Shanahan F (eds). Inflammatory Bowel Disease. From Bench to Bedside. Baltimore: Williams & Wilkins, 1994.

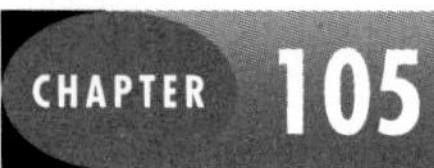


# ANATOMY AND PHYSIOLOGY OF THE LIVER AND LABORATORY EVALUATION OF LIVER FUNCTION

## Anatomy

The liver, which normally is located in the right upper abdomen, has a median weight of nearly 1800 g in men and 1400 g in women. Anatomists traditionally have used the falciform ligament to divide the liver into the right and left lobes. During deep inspiration, the liver usually descends below the right costal margin and becomes palpable on examination. Elongation of the right lobe, a variation called **Riedel's lobe**, may be mistaken for hepatomegaly. Under normal conditions, the **portal vein** supplies approximately 70% of the blood flow to its parenchyma; the hepatic artery, a branch of the celiac axis, supplies the remainder. The normal liver can withstand ligation of the hepatic artery, but the cirrhotic liver cannot because of compromised portal vein perfusion. The three main hepatic veins drain most of the liver; the caudate lobe, however, drains directly into the inferior vena cava. This separate drainage explains the compensatory hyperplasia of the caudate lobe during acute hepatic vein thrombosis.

The polyhedral **hepatocytes** (liver cells) are arranged in single-cell plates separated by blood-filled sinusoids. Endothelial cells and phagocytic **Kupffer cells** line the sinusoids and enclose the **space of Disse.** The space of Disse contains lipid-storing **stellate cells** (Ito cells), which function as the principal hepatic fibroblasts, as well as interstitial lymph fluid, which drains via the lymphatics through the porta hepatis. Bile canaliculi, the terminal radicles of the biliary system, are interspersed between nonsinusoidal surfaces of adjoining liver cells.

There are two different conceptual models that describe the organization of the hepatic parenchyma: the **classic lobule** and the **liver acinus**. The classic lobule is a two-dimensional structure with a central vein serving at its center and portal triads (portal vein, hepatic artery, and bile duct) surrounding it. The liver acinus is a more elegant model and provides structural and functional relevance. In the acinar model, oxygen- and nutrient-rich blood from the portal vein and hepatic artery flows toward terminal hepatic venules located at the apex of an acinus (Figure 105.1). The liver acinus consists of three distinct zones: hepatocytes in zone 1 (periportal) receive blood with the highest oxygen content; hepatocytes in zone 3 (pericentral) are the furthest away from oxygen and, thus, most vulnerable to ischemic injury. Zone 3 hepatocytes also are actively involved in the metabolism and disposition of drugs. Thus, hepatotoxic medications (e.g., acetaminophen) may induce zone 3 necrosis.

## Physiology

An in-depth discussion of the elegant cellular biology and function of the liver is beyond the scope of this text. However, understanding the pathophysiology of liver disease does require a basic understanding of the important role of the liver in bile formation, protein synthesis, and the metabolism of medications, carbohydrates, lipoproteins, and ammonia.

### Bile Formation and Metabolism

The normal liver excretes between 500 and 600 ml of bile daily. The excreted bile consists predominantly of water, bile acids, cholesterol, bile pigments, electrolytes, and phospholipids. Bile acids are either primary (synthesized from cholesterol in the liver, e.g., chenodeoxycholic acid) or secondary (produced by bacterial degradation in intestine, e.g., ursodeoxycholic acid or deoxycholic acid). The presence of hydrophilic or hydrophobic side chains determines the ability of these bile acids to assist in fat digestion and absorption. The beneficial effects of ursodeoxycholic acid (a hydrophilic bile acid) are believed to depend on its ability to replace hydrophobic bile acids, which are thought to play a role in bile duct and hepatocyte injury.

An end-product of heme degradation, **bilirubin,** a lipid-soluble linear tetrapyrrole, is produced via a complex process at a rate of 4 mg/kg in healthy adults. Jaundice results from accumulation of bilirubin due to disorders of bilirubin metabolism, hemolysis, hepatocyte injury, or obstruction of the bile ducts.

### Protein Synthesis

The major protein synthesized by the liver is albumin, which is pivotal in maintaining plasma oncotic pressure and in the transport of many compounds,

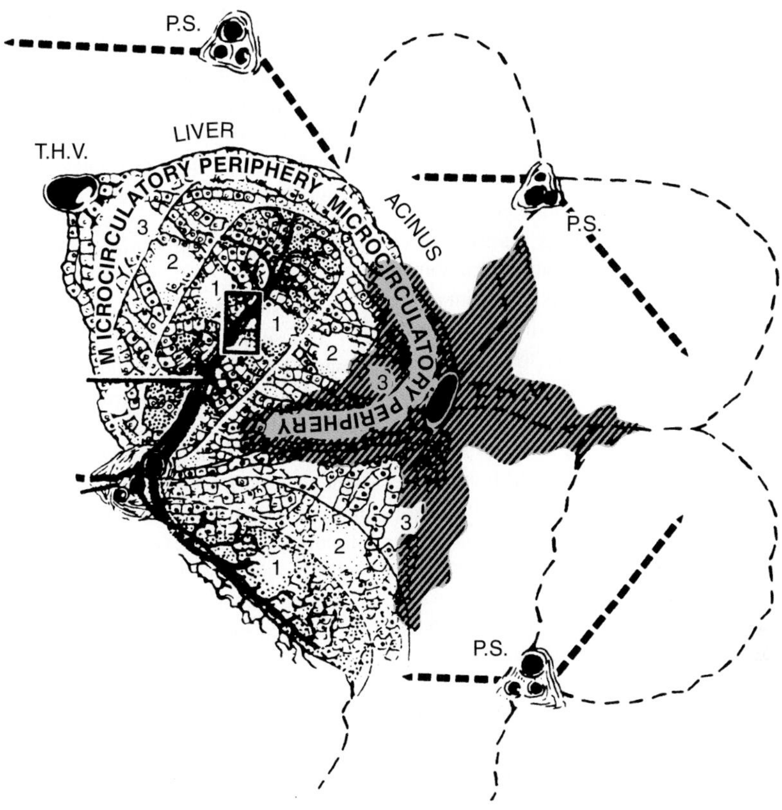


**FIGURE 105.1.** **Blood supply of the simple liver acinus, the zonal arrangement of cells, and the microcirculatory periphery.** (From Farber and Fisher (eds.). Toxic Injury of the Liver. (New York: Marcel Decker, Inc., 1979. Used with permission.)

including medications. Under normal conditions, albumin is synthesized and exported at a rate of almost 10 g per day. Nutritional needs, osmotic pressure, corticosteroids, and inflammation modulate the rate of production. The synthesis of a number of coagulation factor proenzymes (factors I, II, V, VII, IX, X) and plasma inhibitors of hemostasis antithrombin III, protein C, and protein S also takes place in the liver.

Through the process of urea synthesis, the liver disposes of ammonia, the toxic byproduct of nitrogen metabolism. The serum ammonia level may rise in acute as well as chronic liver disease. In the former, it rises as a result of severe hepatocellular necrosis, whereas in the latter, portosystemic shunting and loss of glutamine synthesis (a mechanism of intrahepatic ammonia scavenging) are responsible.

## Metabolism of Drugs, Carbohydrate, and Fat

The liver metabolizes certain drugs and biotransforms others for more efficient hepatic or urinary elimination. A number of enzyme families, the best studied of which is the cytochrome p450 system, usually are involved in the metabolism and detoxification of drugs. On occasion, they also produce toxic intermediates that may evoke liver injury. The biotransformation of drugs occurs via phase I or II reactions. Phase I reactions involve oxidation or reduction, leading to increased polarity, and, thus, water solubility of the compound. Phase II reactions also enhance the water solubility of the compound, but through sulfation or glucuronidation.

In the fasting state, the liver supplies glucose on demand from glycogen by **glycogenolysis** and converts amino acids, lactate, and glycerol to glucose via **gluconeogenesis.** In a fed state, glycogen is synthesized from glucose and glycolysis. In most patients with chronic liver disease, carbohydrate metabolism remains intact. However, in acute hepatic failure, hypoglycemia may follow depletion of glycogen stores.

Cholesterol and lipoprotein homeostasis is under hepatic control. Cholesterol accumulates in the liver from either de novo synthesis or uptake of lipoproteins. Synthesis of bile acids from cholesterol and biliary excretion of cholesterol both lower hepatic cholesterol stores. These processes are exquisitely controlled through feedback inhibition involving the enzyme 3-hydroxy-3-methylglutaryl-coenzyme A (HMG-CoA) reductase as well as bile acid synthesis. The liver utilizes large amounts of hepatic fatty acids as a major energy source or partially metabolizes them to ketones, thus providing an energy substitute for skeletal and cardiac muscle.

## Liver Function Blood Tests

A number of widely used blood tests are commonly called "liver function tests." This term is a misnomer, because only serum albumin, bilirubin, and prothrombin time truly assess liver function. Hepatocellular injury is signaled by elevated aminotransferases, whereas elevations of bilirubin, alkaline phosphatase, and gamma-glutamyl transpeptidase (GGT) reflect cholestatic injury.

### Serum Aminotransferases

Serum aminotransferases, formerly called transaminases, are catalytic enzymes, and their elevation usually reflects leakage from damaged cells in hepatocyte injury. **Alanine aminotransferase (ALT)** is more specific to the liver, whereas **aspartate aminotransferase (AST)** also is elevated in muscular, kidney, and brain injury, or even hemolysis. An elevated AST/ALT ratio greater than 2:1 is typical of alcoholic liver disease and may help identify this form of liver injury, although other forms of liver disease also may manifest a high ratio.

Up to an eight-fold elevation of aminotransferases is relatively nonspecific, but marked increases (> 1000 IU/L) should narrow the potential causes to acute viral hepatitis, ischemia or passive congestion, drug-induced injury (e.g. acetaminophen), or hepatotoxins (e.g., carbon tetrachloride). Most other forms of acute and chronic injury result in modest aminotransferase elevations, with the exception of acute choledocholithiasis. In the first 48 hours this may result in aminotransferases in the thousands, followed by a rapid decline.

### Serum Bilirubin

In healthy subjects, serum bilirubin ranges from 0.2 to 1.0 mg/dL and is almost completely in the unconjugated form. Unconjugated hyperbilirubinemia may result from increased production (e.g., hemolysis or ineffective erythropoiesis), or reduced clearance (e.g., neonatal jaundice, or drug-induced injury, or one of the genetic syndromes associated with bilirubin-uridinediphosphate glucuronyl transferase [bilirubin-UGT] deficiency). In adults, isolated, chronic unconjugated hyperbilirubinemia most commonly is due to **Gilbert syndrome,** a benign disorder associated with reduced bilirubin-UGT activity and total bilirubin below 6 mg/dL. Crigler-Najjar syndrome is an uncommon autosomal recessive disorder of unconjugated hyperbilirubinemia associated with absent (type I) or markedly reduced (type II) bilirubin-UGT function.

Conjugated hyperbilirubinemia may be the result of obstructive jaundice, intrahepatic cholestasis due to hepatocellular disease, or rare and benign defects of hepatic storage or excretion (e.g., **Dubin-Johnson syndrome** and **Rotor syndrome**). In conjugated hyperbilirubinemia, total bilirubin values greater than 30 mg/dL reflect hepatocellular injury rather than obstructive jaundice. Obstruction may lead to such values when there is concomitant renal failure or profound hemolysis.

### Serum Alkaline Phosphatase

The serum alkaline phosphatase level comprises a group of isoenzymes found mainly in the liver, bone, first-trimester placenta, intestine, and kidney. Electrophoretic isoenzyme fractionation reliably distinguishes its source, and heat sensitivity also may be used (a bone-derived fraction is heat-labile—"bone burns, liver lives"). Hepatic alkaline phosphatase is a marker of cholestasis; it is elevated fourfold or more in 75% of patients with prolonged cholestasis. It does not distinguish intrahepatic from extrahepatic cholestasis and may be elevated in infiltrative and malignant diseases of the liver.

### Gamma-Glutamyl Transpeptidase

Gamma-glutamyl transpeptidase (GGT) is a sensitive marker of liver dysfunction and particularly of biliary obstruction. Although it also is found in other tissues, GGT is essentially absent from bone and, thus, is very useful in confirming the hepatic origin of an elevated serum alkaline phosphatase. A number of drugs and other substances, especially alcohol, induce microsomal enzyme activity and elevate GGT.

### Prothrombin Time

Hepatocytes synthesize all of the major coagulation factors except factor VIII. The **prothrombin time (PT),** which measures the integrity of factors I, II, V, VII, and X (the so-called extrinsic pathway), serves as a useful marker of liver function. The factor V level also is used to assess hepatic synthetic function and prognosis in acute fulminant liver failure. Because a number of the clotting factors are vitamin K–dependent (II, VII, IX, and X), a prolonged PT—particularly in the cholestatic patient—may signify vitamin K malabsorption rather than liver disease. If exogenous vitamin K administration lowers the PT by more than 30% within 24 hours, cholestasis or malabsorption is indicated rather than hepatocellular dysfunction.

### Serum Albumin and Immunoglobulins

**Albumin** is synthesized exclusively by the liver and is commonly used as a marker of hepatic synthetic function. Extrahepatic factors such as volume and nutritional status, thyroid hormone, corticosteroids, ongoing inflammation, and acute alcohol ingestion all affect serum albumin levels. Because of its prolonged half-life (20 days), the serum albumin is not as useful a marker as the PT in assessing the severity of acute liver failure. Although serum immunoglobulins often are elevated in chronic liver disease, they do not reflect liver function. Rather, B-lymphocytes appear to overproduce immunoglobulins in response to impaired reticuloendothelial function in the hepatic sinusoids and shunting of portal venous blood.

## Imaging of the Liver

### Ultrasound

Because it is noninvasive, readily available, and relatively inexpensive, an abdominal ultrasound is often the initial radiological investigation of hepatobiliary disease, particularly in the jaundiced patient. Sensitivities of over 90% for gallbladder stones and solid and cystic liver lesions over 2 cm in size have been reported, but the yield is highly operator-dependent. Concurrent Doppler flow analysis makes it possible to perform noninvasive assessments of hepatic and portal vein flow and portosystemic shunt patency.

### Computed Tomography

Although more accurate than ultrasound (US), the expense and inconvenience of abdominal computed tomography (CT) renders it a second-line investigation. When used with intravenous contrast, CT accurately evaluates the size, shape, density, and mass of the liver. It reliably detects and characterizes solid and cystic lesions, abscesses, and hemangiomas. Although less accurate than US in detecting dilated bile ducts, CT better defines extrahepatic structures and lesions causing biliary obstruction.

### Magnetic Resonance Imaging

Modern magnetic resonance imaging (MRI) yields excellent anatomical information. However, its high cost relegates it to assessment of lesions that require better delineation after CT, or for patients with renal insufficiency, which precludes CT with intravenous contrast. It is particularly useful in detecting and confirming small liver hemangiomas. Magnetic resonance cholangiopancreatography (MRCP) provides noninvasive, three-dimensional images of the biliary tract, albeit without any therapeutic options.

### Radionuclide Scintiscanning

The advantages of ultrasound, CT scanning, or MRI scanning surpass technetium Tc 99m sulfur colloid scanning, so that it is now used only rarely. The Kupffer cells of the liver take up the technetium Tc 99m. On external imaging of the liver, primary liver cancer, metastases, cysts, hemangiomas, and abscesses appear as filling defects, because these lesions lack Kupffer cells. In cirrhosis, fatty liver, and hepatitis, the uptake usually is low and inhomogeneous.

## Invasive Tests

### Liver Biopsy

Liver biopsy may be done percutaneously, transvenously, or laparoscopically. Indications and contraindications for **percutaneous liver biopsy** are listed in Tables 105.1 and 105.2. The point of maximal liver dullness, usually between the sixth and ninth intercostal spaces, is prepared aseptically. One of these intercostal spaces is infiltrated with local anesthesia and is used for the needle biopsy. Evanescent pain commonly follows, at the needle site or in the right shoulder. In most cases, only outpatient observation is required following biopsy. Hemorrhage, bile leak, and hypotension are uncommon and, when encountered, usually occur within 3 hours of the procedure. CT- or US-guided fine-needle aspiration and biopsy often are safer and more accurate for space-occupying lesions. A **transvenous liver biopsy** is more appropriate for liver biopsy in patients with severe and uncorrectable coagulopathy or ascites. The interventional radiologist cannulates the internal jugular or femoral vein, and obtains liver tissue under fluoroscopic guidance, using a biopsy forceps or needle. Any associated bleeding recirculates within the venous circulation. Biopsy specimens are smaller than those obtained by the percutaneous route, and a risk for capsular puncture is present. **Laparoscopy**, when combined with directed biopsy, is particularly useful in assessing lesions on the surface of the liver or peritoneum, and when ascites precludes percutaneous biopsy. Although laparoscopic biopsy is better than percutaneous biopsy for diagnosing

**TABLE 105.1. Indications for Percutaneous Liver Biopsy**

Evaluate abnormal liver enzyme elevation, unexplained acute hepatitis, or hepatomegaly
Stage and grade chronic hepatitis
Diagnose and stage chronic cholestatic liver diseases, hemochromatosis, Wilson disease, nonalcoholic steatohepatitis, occasionally alcoholic liver disease, suspected drug-induced injury or infiltrative disease (e.g., sarcoidosis, amyloidosis)
Evaluate for allograft rejection/dysfunction after transplantation
Monitor drug toxicity (e.g., methotrexate)
Evaluate fever of unknown origin

**TABLE 105.2. Contraindications for Percutaneous Liver Biopsy**

| |
|---|
| INR > 1.5 |
| Platelet count < 60,000/$mm^3$ |
| Uncooperative patient |
| Ascites |
| Right-sided subdiaphragmatic or pleural infection |
| Suspected echinococcal cyst |
| Suspicion of vascular mass |

INR = international normalized ratio

cirrhosis, it is not routinely used for this purpose, given its higher costs and invasiveness.

### Endoscopic Retrograde Cholangiopancreatography

The use of a side-viewing endoscope allows for cannulation of the duodenal papilla with imaging of the biliary and pancreatic tree in endoscopic retrograde cholangiopancreatography (ERCP). ERCP allows many options, both diagnostic (e.g., brushings or biopsy of suspected malignancy) and therapeutic (e.g., endoscopic sphincterotomy, stone extraction, and stent placement). It is the gold standard for diagnosis of primary sclerosing cholangitis and the procedure of choice in managing post-cholecystectomy common bile duct stones. It is invasive and has a number of complications, including pancreatitis, bleeding, perforation, and infection.

# CHAPTER 106 CLINICAL PRESENTATIONS OF LIVER DISEASE

## Elevated Liver Enzymes

The approach to the patients with abnormal liver tests—many of whom are asymptomatic—consists of a directed history and physical examination as well as classification of the type of liver injury as hepatocellular, cholestatic, or mixed. Symptoms of liver disease often are nonspecific, and include fatigue, anorexia, weight loss, fever or chills, arthritis, pruritus, and change in urine or stool color. Specific inquiries should be made regarding transfusions, intravenous and other illicit drug use, tattoos, alcohol use, sexual history, travel, use of over-the-counter and prescribed medications or remedies, contacts with sick persons, associated disorders such as inflammatory bowel disease, and occupational exposures. Successful prior blood donations may indicate previously normal liver tests. Family history of liver disease is important. In addition to a thorough general physical examination, specific features to look for include signs of chronic liver disease, including icterus, muscle wasting, spider angiomata, palmar erythema, gynecomastia, hepatosplenomegaly, ascites, abdominal masses, and gallbladder enlargement; signs of hepatic encephalopathy, including asterixis; and evidence of other associated disorders such as congestive heart failure or hyperthyroidism.

The specific approach to further evaluation of patients with abnormal liver tests then should be based on whether there is a hepatocellular, cholestatic, or mixed pattern of injury, as outlined in Figures 106.1 through 106.3.

## Jaundice

Jaundice refers to a yellow appearance of skin and eyes resulting from retention and deposition of excessive bile pigment. Although hemolysis may cause jaundice, hepatobiliary disease is a more common cause. Both extrahepatic biliary obstruction and parenchymal liver disease leading to intrahepatic cholestasis may lead to jaundice. Once hemolysis has been excluded, an abdominal ultrasound should be done to assess whether there is biliary dilatation or nondilated bile ducts; further studies can then follow, as outlined in Figure 106.2.

When the ultrasound shows a dilated biliary tree, cholangiography, typically via ERCP (or percutaneous transhepatic cholangiography [PTC] when ERCP is not feasible/available), is the next step. In this setting, ERCP offers diagnostic (e.g., brushings of strictures) and therapeutic (e.g., gallstone extraction) options. If the biliary tree is nondilated, evaluation for parenchymal liver disease, including primary biliary cirrhosis and primary sclerosing cholangitis. should be pursued. A focal lesion requires further imaging with CT or MRI.

## Fulminant Hepatic Failure

Fulminant hepatic failure (FHF) formerly was defined as the onset of encephalopathy within 8 weeks of onset of illness. A more recent definition requires rapid onset of hepatocellular dysfunction exhibited by jaundice or coagulopathy, encephalopathy, and absence of previously established liver disease. Cerebral edema, hypoglycemia, metabolic acidosis, a high rate of infectious complications, and multi-organ failure may complicate management of these patients. Common causes of FHF include drug-induced injury (particularly acetaminophen), acute hepatitis A, acute hepatitis B (with or without concomitant hepatitis D), and "cryptogenic hepatitis." Hepatitis C rarely, if ever, leads to FHF. Less common causes include acute Wilson disease, Budd-Chiari syndrome, ischemia, fatty liver of pregnancy, Reye syndrome, and other viral infections. Prompt recognition of FHF, intensive medical care, and immediate referral to a liver transplant facility are imperative in the management of patients with FHF.

## Hepatomegaly

Hepatomegaly may be detected on physical examination or by liver imaging. It has many causes (Table 106.1), some of which can be diagnosed only by imaging. In North America, alcoholic hepatitis is an important and common cause of hepatomegaly. Often, a patient admits to alcohol abuse only after alcoholic liver disease is diagnosed. Primary biliary cirrhosis and autoimmune hepatitis may present with hepatomegaly. The presence of systemic disease elsewhere (e.g., sarcoidosis), metabolic tests (e.g., hemochromatosis), and liver biopsy results (e.g., amyloidosis) all may be involved in elucidating a cause.

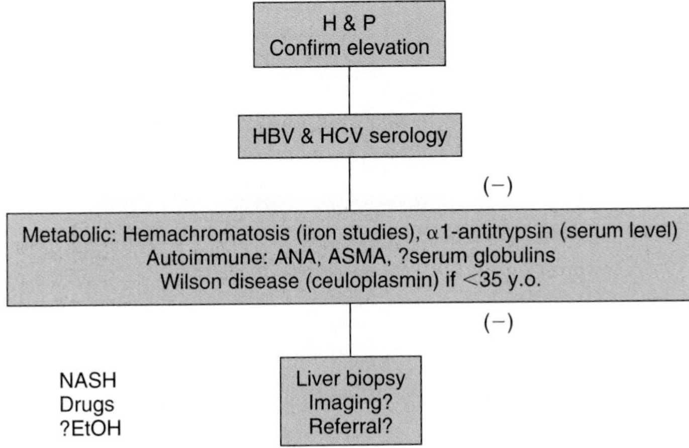


**FIGURE 106.1.** Evaluation of Elevated Aminotransferases.

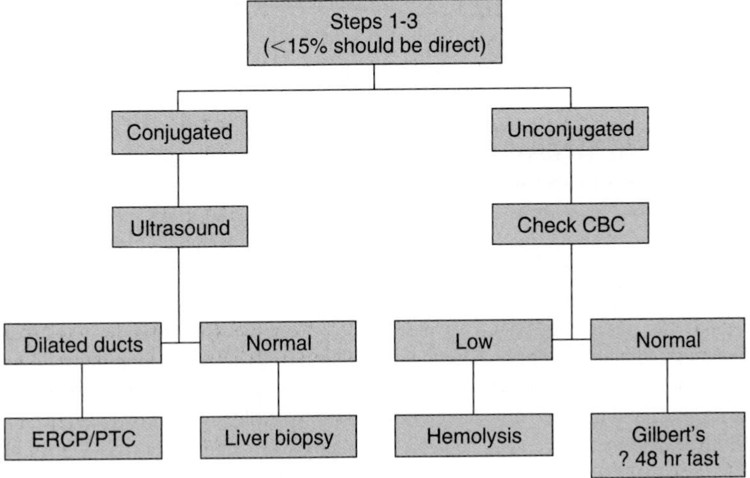


**FIGURE 106.2.** Evaluation of Elevated Bilirubin.

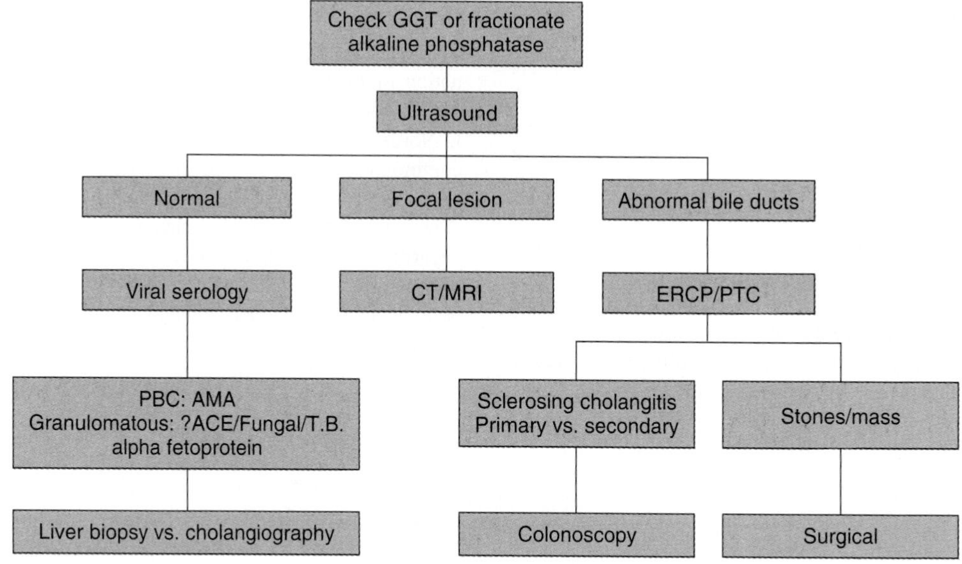


**FIGURE 106.3. Evaluation of Elevated Alkaline Phosphatase.**

**TABLE 106.1. Etiology of Hepatomegaly**

| | |
|---|---|
| Hepatic tumors | Infiltrative liver disease |
| Primary | Hemochromatosis |
| Benign | Amyloidosis |
| Malignant | Sarcoidosis |
| Secondary | Vascular |
| Hepatic cysts | Passive hepatic congestion |
| Benign | Hepatic vein thrombosis |
| Malignant | Inflammatory |
| Alcoholic hepatitis | Primary biliary cirrhosis |
| | Primary sclerosing cholangitis |
| | Autoimmune hepatitis |

# CHAPTER 107 VIRAL HEPATITIS

Besides the six identified hepatitis viruses classified as A, B, C, D, E and G, a number of other viruses, including the Epstein-Barr virus, herpes simplex virus, cytomegalovirus, parvovirus B19, TT virus, and adenovirus, also may cause acute hepatitis. Although found in patients with liver disease, some of these viruses, including hepatitis G and the TT virus, have not been shown to *cause* liver disease. Acute viral hepatitis typically presents with nonspecific systemic manifestations, including anorexia, nausea, vomiting, abdominal pain, and arthralgias. Jaundice is not necessarily present. In fact, infants and children often are anicteric following acute hepatitis, whereas as many as 70% of adults with acute hepatitis A develop jaundice.

**Chronic hepatitis** is a clinical syndrome, with chronic liver inflammation leading to necrosis and possibly progressing to fibrosis, cirrhosis, and liver failure. Prolonged enzyme elevation for at least 6 months along with compatible liver biopsy findings are essential for diagnosis and classification. Biopsy findings of chronic hepatitis include portal inflammation, with a new histologic classification system including grading (reflecting the amount of inflammation) and staging (degree of fibrosis). Chronic hepatitis develops in patients with hepatitis B and hepatitis C but is not seen with the other viral hepatitides.

## Hepatitis A

Hepatitis A virus (HAV) is an RNA virus transmitted via the oral-fecal route and is the most common identified cause of infectious hepatitis. Infection is followed by an incubation period of about 30 days. The virus is detectable in stool from 2 weeks before the onset of jaundice and up to 8 days thereafter. Transmission may occur by person-to-person contact or ingestion of contaminated food. Uncooked shellfish is a particularly frequent culprit. Certain parts of the world, including Eastern Europe, Russia, Africa, the Middle East, and parts of South America, are areas of high endemicity where immunity before the age of 10 is nearly universal.

### Clinical Features

Viral hepatitis has a wide range of presentation, from clinical infection to fulminant hepatic failure. Patients younger than 4 years of age often are anicteric, whereas 40% to 70% of those older than 15 years of age develop jaundice. About 85% of patients have nonspecific symptoms, as noted earlier. When jaundice develops, it resolves within 2 weeks in 85% of patients. Interestingly, cigarette smokers tend to lose interest in smoking. Examination in most persons reveal tender hepatomegaly, and a small percentage may have splenomegaly, rash, and lymphadenopathy. A minority (<10%) develop a relapsing course that may lead to cholestasis. Patients with sickle cell disease are more susceptible to this particular pattern. Extrahepatic manifestations include immune-complex–mediated glomerulonephritis, vasculitis, and other autoimmune phenomena. Mortality is rare among young patients, but rates as high as 1% to 2% have been reported in those over the age of 40 years. Concomitant liver disease and pregnancy appear to result in more severe disease. Aminotransferases are elevated, beginning in the prodromal phase, and normalize in most patients by 2 months, although 15% of patients have persistent elevations for approximately 6 months. Diagnosis is confirmed by detection of IgM anti-HAV antibody, which becomes undetectable in approximately 75% of patients at 6 months. Although rarely indicated, liver biopsy findings include spotty necrosis with portal and periportal inflammation.

### Management

Management consists of supportive measures with treatment of symptoms. Contrary to earlier belief, bed rest does not accelerate recovery, and early ambulation should be encouraged. The great majority of patients do not require hospitalization, with the exception of those with severe or persistent anorexia, mental status changes, or coagulopathy. Although no specific medications are indicated for treatment of acute hepatitis A, corticosteroid therapy is useful in accelerating resolution of the cholestatic phase. Prevention of infection is possible via passive immunization and vaccination. Passive immunization is the method of choice for postexposure prophylaxis because immunity develops within 3 to 5 days and lasts up to 3 months. The inactivated vaccine confers immunity for at least 5 to 10 years and consists of a sequence of two injections, although some clinicians advocate a third dose to lengthen the duration of protection.

## Hepatitis B

The hepatitis B virus (HBV), a double-stranded DNA virus, remains the leading cause of chronic hepatitis, with 350 million infected individuals worldwide and some 1.25 million infected individuals in the United States. In the United States, HBV is largely a disease of adulthood and is associated with parenteral and sexual exposures.

### Clinical Features

Once an adult is infected by HBV, the outcome is variable, with the majority (about 65-70%) developing a subclinical, transient hepatitis followed by development of lifelong immunity, indicated by the presence of hepatitis B surface antibody (HbsAb). Another 25% develop overt hepatitis but still develop lifelong immunity and HbsAb. Approximately 1% develop fulminant acute hepatitis B, which has a high mortality. In contrast to neonates, approximately 90% of whom develop hepatitis B infection, only about 5% of adults develop this complication. A positive hepatitis B core IgM antibody (HBcAb IgM) test indicates acute infection (Table 107.1). Among those with chronic infection, a subgroup (the so-called "healthy carriers") exhibits *only* hepatitis B surface antigen (HBsAg); others with more active viral replication exhibit hepatitis B e antigen (HBeAg) and/or hepatitis B viral DNA (those with chronic active infection). "Healthy carriers" also exhibit hepatitis B e antibody (HBeAb) which indicates less viral replication. The presence of hepatitis B surface antibody (HBsAb) indicates immunity. All patients with chronic infection, including the "healthy carriers," are at higher risk for development of hepatocellular carcinoma. In the United States, HBV currently accounts for 10% to 15% of hepatocellular carcinomas and 5% to 10% of cases of end-stage liver disease.

### Management

Therapy for chronic HBV infection consists of either (1) a 16-week course of alpha-interferon in doses of 5

**TABLE 107.1. Hepatitis B Virus Markers**

| | Anti-HBc Total | Anti-HBc IgM | HBs Ag | Anti-HBs | HBeAg | Anti-HBe | HBV DNA |
|---|---|---|---|---|---|---|---|
| Acute hepatitis B | (+) | (+) | (+) | (–) | (+) | (–) | (+) |
| Vaccinated for hepatitis B | (–) | (–) | (–) | (+) | (–) | (–) | (–) |
| Prior hepatitis B exposure—immune | (+) | (–) | (–) | (+) | (–) | (+) | (–) |
| Chronic hepatitis B "healthy carrier" | (+) | (–) | (+) | (–) | (–) | (+) | (+)/(–) |
| Chronic hepatitis B active replication | (+) | (+)/(–) | (+) | (–) | (+) | (–) | (+) |

million units daily or 10 million units three times weekly or (2) a 1- to 2-year course of lamivudine, 100 mg per day. Clearance of HBV DNA and loss of HBeAg are seen in only 25% to 35% of interferon-treated patients. Adverse effects of interferon include flulike symptoms, joint pains, thrombocytopenia, leukopenia, and irritability. Not only is treatment with interferon expensive and poorly tolerated by many, it also is contraindicated in decompensated liver disease. Lamivudine, a nucleoside analogue, is much better tolerated, and may be used in decompensated liver disease; it leads to clearance of HBV DNA and loss of HBeAg in about 25% of patients after a 2-year course. Unfortunately, viral resistance develops in 15% to 25% of patients after 1 year of treatment. Adefouir, a newly introduced nucleoside analogue, appears to be effective against these resistant strains. All sexual and household contacts of HBV-infected patients should be immunized with the very effective hepatitis B vaccine. Acute exposures should be treated with hepatitis B immune globulin and vaccination.

## Hepatitis C

Molecular cloning technology identified the hepatitis C virus (HCV) in 1989. Several geographically distributed genotypes of HCV have been identified, and the two most common genotypes in the United States are 1a and 1b. HCV, a single-stranded RNA virus, typically is transmitted parenterally, and accounts for approximately 20% of cases of acute viral hepatitis. The acute hepatitis rarely is fulminant, but does lead to chronic infection in 55–85% of patients. A staggering 60% to 70% of the cases of chronic hepatitis in the United States—some 2.7 million persons—are due to HCV. Although many people with chronic hepatitis C are asymptomatic, an estimated 25% develop cirrhosis over a span of 25 years. Factors that might promote progression to more aggressive disease include high viral load, viral genotype, 1a/1b, male gender, concomitant alcohol use, and viral co-infection. Each year, hepatocellular carcinoma develops in 1% to 3% of patients with cirrhosis due to hepatitis C. End-stage liver disease from HCV is now the top indication for liver transplantation in the United States.

### Clinical Features

The incubation period of hepatitis C is 7 to 8 weeks. Antibody to HCV (anti-HCV) may be detectable by the time of or up to 8 weeks after the onset of symptoms. Unfortunately, this antibody is not protective. Serologically, acute hepatitis C can be diagnosed by the presence of HCV RNA in the serum as early as 10 days after exposure, well before the onset of ALT elevation or symptoms. Acute hepatitis C leads to jaundice in about 21% of patients. Once chronic HCV infection is documented, a liver biopsy is the procedure of choice in assessing the severity of the disease and determining prognosis.

### Management

Routine specific treatment of acute hepatitis C is effective but waiting at least 3 months to determine whether chronicity develops is prudent. The best currently available therapy for chronic hepatitis C is combination therapy with alpha-interferon and the oral nucleoside analogue, ribavirin. Although ribavirin has little effect on HCV RNA levels by itself, the addition of ribavirin to alpha-interferon as the initial treatment for chronic hepatitis C for 48 weeks has yielded a sustained response (absence of HCV RNA) rate of 41%. The introduction of pegylated alpha-interferon use along with ribavirin has raised the response rate to 54%. Whereas treatment with alpha-interferons has many potential side effects, ribavirin is well tolerated, with its most common side effect being a mild hemolytic anemia. No vaccine is available for hepatitis C, and immune globulin is *not* protective. Hepatitis C universally recurs after liver transplantation.

## Hepatitis D

Hepatitis D virus (HDV) is a single-stranded RNA virus that requires the presence of HBV for complete virion assembly and secretion. Hepatitis D always occurs in association with either acute or chronic HBV infection. Interestingly, in chronic HDV infection, HBV activity is suppressed. Although reported worldwide, HDV appears most frequently in the Mediterranean basin. Diagnosis of acute HDV infection is signaled by the presence of IgM anti-HDV, although this may be transient and a positive IgG anti-HDV may be the only sign of recent infection. New polymerase chain reaction (PCR) assays for HDV RNA are available. Management of HDV infection is similar to that of the underlying HBV infection, with alpha-interferon as the only currently approved treatment choice. Preventive measures are directed at prevention and eradication of HBV.

## Hepatitis E

Hepatitis E, previously called epidemic non-A, non-B hepatitis, is an RNA virus that was first isolated in 1983 and cloned in 1990. Although most often seen in India, the Far East, the Middle East, and parts of Latin America, a worldwide distribution has been noted. The hepatitis E virus has been associated with the largest epidemics of infectious hepatitis in the world. Transmission, symptoms, and overall clinical presentation are quite similar to those of acute hepatitis A infection.

A positive IgM anti-HEV confirms the diagnosis and may be positive as early as 4 days after onset of symptoms. Liver histology is indistinguishable from hepatitis A virus infection. The overall fatality rate appears somewhat higher than hepatitis A and is particularly high in pregnant women in the second and third trimester. In addition, the cholestatic phase is more common than hepatitis A. A second pattern characterized by ascites and other signs of FHF without encephalopathy also has been reported. Once again, chronicity is not seen. Abnormal aminotransferases normalize over a 6-week period. As with hepatitis A infection, management consists of supportive measures.

# CHAPTER 108 AUTOIMMUNE HEPATITIS AND CHOLESTATIC LIVER DISEASE

Hepatocytes and biliary epithelium provide potential targets for autoimmune diseases that affect the liver. Three major diseases make up this category, including autoimmune hepatitis, which targets hepatocytes, and primary biliary cirrhosis (PBC) and primary sclerosing cholangitis (PSC), both of which appear to target the biliary epithelium.

## Autoimmune Hepatitis

Autoimmune hepatitis (AIH) is defined as a chronic periportal hepatitis associated with hypergammaglobulinemia, positive serum autoantibodies, and absence of viral hepatitis and other causes of chronic liver disease. There is a female predominance with AIH, and an association with HLA DR3 and DR4 alleles has been noted. Approximately 70% of patients are women, with the peak incidence between 16 and 30 years of age. Other autoimmune syndromes commonly associated with AIH include autoimmune thyroiditis, vitiligo, rheumatoid arthritis, diabetes mellitus, and ulcerative colitis. There is no single test that documents the presence of AIH, so the diagnosis may be difficult. Autoimmune hepatitis is categorized into three types based on the autoantibody profile. Positive antinuclear antibody (ANA) titers 1:160 or greater or anti-smooth muscle antibodies (ASMA) titers 1:80 or greater define type 1 AIH; anti–liver-kidney microsomal autoantibodies (anti-LKM) define type 2 AIH; and autoantibodies against soluble liver antigens (anti-SLA) define type 3. Autoimmune hepatitis is a rare disorder, with an incidence currently reported as 50 to 200 cases per 1 million persons in Caucasian populations. Although the precise mechanism of the pathogenesis of AIH is not clear, there is evidence for 1) a viral etiology with a subsequent overly aggressive immunologic reaction, 2) a disorder in cellular community and/or 3) a genetic predisposition.

### Clinical Presentation

About one half of patients with AIH have an acute clinical presentation of hepatitis and jaundice, but acute liver failure occasionally may be the initial manifestation. About 25% of patients present with already established cirrhosis at the time of diagnosis and suffer from its concomitant complications. In type 1 AIH, elevated IgG levels are seen in 97% of cases. Approximately one half of patients have other coexisting autoimmune disorders. Both AIH types 2 and 3 are quite rare in North America, whereas 20% of AIH cases in Western Europe are classified as type 2. The liver enzyme pattern of AIH is similar to that seen with acute viral hepatitis, and biopsy findings are similar except for the predominance of plasma cell infiltration with AIH. A number of syndromes overlapping with other autoimmune liver diseases, such as primary biliary cirrhosis and primary sclerosing cholangitis, also have been reported.

### Management

The level of inflammation initially present largely determines the natural history of AIH. Without treatment, the 10-year mortality of patients with a 10-fold elevation of aminotransferases and two-fold elevated IgG levels is 90%. Treatment usually is with corticosteroids alone or in combination with azathioprine. Relative indications for treatment include aminotransferase levels elevated over 1.5-fold, IgG levels elevated two-fold, or moderate periportal hepatitis on biopsy. Severe fatigue also may be an indication for treatment. Evidence of severe inflammation on biopsy or aminotransferase levels elevated more than 10-fold are absolute indications for treatment. Patients need to be treated for at least 12 months, with a slow taper over 4–6 weeks. About 65% of patients achieve remission after 24 months of treatment; these patients may require long-term azathioprine. A number of patients without maintenance therapy do relapse, however. Approximately 10% of patients do not respond to standard therapy. If liver transplantation is required, patients do extremely well, with a 5-year survival higher than 92%.

## Primary Biliary Cirrhosis

Primary biliary cirrhosis (PBC) is a destructive cholangiopathy that results in nonsuppurative inflammation and subsequent destruction of both small- and medium-sized bile ducts. In spite of its name, cirrhosis is not invariably present at diagnosis, and the rate of progression is quite variable. There is a strong female predominance (10:1), and the median age is approximately 50 years at the time diagnosis. The prevalence of PBC is between 20 and 240 cases per 1 million population and appears to the highest in northern Europe, although no clear racial predominance exists.

### Clinical Presentation

Patients often are diagnosed at the presymptomatic stage based on a finding of elevated liver enzymes. Typically, alkaline phosphatase is elevated three- or fourfold, with mild elevation of the aminotransferases. The bilirubin may be normal in early disease but is an extremely useful marker of disease progression. Approximately two thirds of patients with PBC complain of fatigue, whereas only 10% of patients are jaundiced at presentation. Pruritus also is a common complaint. Osteopenia, hypercholesterolemia, and xanthomas, as well as steatorrhea, also may be encountered. Portal hypertensive bleeding may occur in the absence of cirrhosis due to presinusoidal portal hypertension. This bleeding is believed to result from obliteration of portal venules by regenerative nodules. Positive serum antimitochondrial antibody (AMA) at a titer of 1:40 or higher is highly specific for PBC and has a sensitivity of about 95%. The AMA appears to be directed against the E2 antigen of the pyruvate dehydrogenase complex on the internal mitochondrial membrane. An elevated serum quantitative IgM level helps confirm the diagnosis. Histology reveals inflammatory cells infiltrating the interlobular and septal bile ducts. Granulomas, the classic florid duct lesion, and ductular proliferation may be seen.

### Management

If PBC is untreated, cirrhosis typically follows in 15 to 20 years. An elevated serum bilirubin level, advanced age, a low albumin, elevated prothrombin time, and edema have been associated with a worse prognosis. All are components of the well-validated Mayo Clinic model used to predict survival. Treatment with ursodeoxycholic acid, 13-15 mg/dL, has been shown to improve transplant-free survival in patients with moderate to severe PBC. The only long-term cure appears to be liver transplantation, which has excellent results.

## Primary Sclerosing Cholangitis

Primary sclerosing cholangitis (PSC) is a chronic inflammatory condition of the intrahepatic and extrahepatic biliary system associated with inflammatory bowel disease. Although genetic predisposition and immunologic factors are believed to play a role, the exact etiology of PSC is unknown. Approximately 60% to 70% of all patients with PSC have inflammatory bowel disease, but only 5% to 7.5% of inflammatory bowel disease patients develop PSC. The severity of one disease does not necessarily affect the development or progression of the other.

### Clinical Presentation

Patients often present in the third decade of life and are predominantly men. Secondary causes of sclerosing cholangitis include AIDS cholangiopathy, recurrent choledocholithiasis, ischemic injury, biliary malignancy, congenital abnormalities, and intra-arterial administration of fluoxuridine. Laboratory tests show cholestasis with a marked elevation of alkaline phosphatase. Hypergammaglobulinemia, positive p-ANCA, and mildly elevated aminotransferases may be seen. Impaired synthetic function is present with advanced disease. Diagnosis is made based on cholangiography (ERCP, MRCP, or PTC) revealing strictures with intervening areas of normal-appearing bile ducts and a beaded appearance. Dominant strictures are found in a minority of patients.

Liver biopsy findings range from portal inflammation to progressive fibrosis and eventual disappearance of bile ducts and cirrhosis. The classic "onion-skin" lesion is seen in approximately 40% of biopsies. Primary sclerosing cholangitis is a progressive disease, with a mean survival ranging from 11 to 17 years after diagnosis. In addition to typical cholestatic liver symptoms, PSC also has a number of unique complications, including cholelithiasis and choledocholithiasis, as well as cholangiocarcinoma, which is difficult to detect and even more difficult to treat.

### Management

Therapy for PSC involves symptomatic treatment and management of complications. Cholestyramine is the first-line agent for treatment of pruritus. Antihistamines, ursodeoxycholic acid, and rifampin are used for refractory patients. Replacement of fat-soluble vitamins and aggressive monitoring and treatment of bone disease are required. Endoscopic dilation of dominant strictures may be helpful in a minority of patients, but unnecessary biliary intervention should be avoided because of the high risk of cholangitis. Because of the diffuse nature of most strictures, biliary surgery is successful in the minority of patients with isolated extrahepatic disease. There are no satisfactory long-term medical, endoscopic, or non-transplant surgical options for most patients with PSC. Surveillance for cholangiocarcinoma is suboptimal, because biliary brushings and biopsies miss 30% to 50% of lesions, and other potential tools, such as serum CA 19-9, have not been found to be reliable. Surveillance for colonic dysplasia should not be neglected in patients with associated inflammatory bowel disease, regardless of the course of PSC. Liver transplantation provides the only means of long-term survival in patients with end-stage liver disease. Timing of the transplantation is controversial, mainly because of the specter of cholangiocarcinoma and the limited supply of donor organs. Patients who receive transplants do extremely well, with 5-year survival rates of 85%. Patients transplanted with incidental cholangiocarcinoma (unknown prior to transplantation but discovered incidentally in explanted liver) however do very poorly. Most PSC patients who undergo liver transplantation receive a choledochojejunostomy to avoid retaining any of their diseased bile duct.

# CHAPTER 109 ALCOHOLIC LIVER DISEASE

Alcohol remains the leading cause of cirrhosis in the Western world and causes a spectrum of disease ranging from fatty liver to alcoholic hepatitis and cirrhosis. One glass of wine, a half-pint of beer, or a shot glass of liquor contains approximately 7 g of alcohol. For the average person, consumption of approximately 40 g of alcohol per day is required for development of alcoholic cirrhosis. Lifelong alcoholics have a 20% to 30% risk of developing cirrhosis. Patients with underlying or concomitant liver disease are more susceptible to developing alcoholic liver disease, even with ingestion of smaller amounts of alcohol. Decreased fatty acid oxidation, increased triglyceride synthesis, and generation of acetaldehyde lead to a dose-related acute swelling of hepatocytes and development of a fatty liver. Stellate cells eventually are activated, resulting in pericellular fibrosis and development of cirrhosis.

### Clinical Presentation

Alcoholic liver disease should be suspected in patients with a history of heavy alcohol use, patients without other evident causes of liver disease, or patients with other complications of alcoholism. The clinical syndrome of acute alcoholic hepatitis has a high mortality of up to 60% in severe cases. There often is no obvious predisposing factor. Acute onset of jaundice, fever, and right upper quadrant discomfort, often with florid stigmata of chronic liver disease along with markedly elevated bilirubin levels, is encountered. An AST:ALT ratio greater than 2, especially one greater than 3 with the ALT less than 300 IU is highly suggestive. One exception is acute Wilson disease, which may present with AST/ALT ratio of 4 or greater. The reason for the elevated ratio in alcoholic liver disease is a relative lack of ALT synthesis due to a deficiency of pyridoxal 5′-phosphate in alcoholics. The cardinal histologic features of alcoholic hepatitis include ballooning degeneration, Mallory bodies, and neutrophil infiltration of the parenchyma. Histologic confirmation rarely is required.

### Management

Cirrhosis may already be present but is not universal in patients with alcoholic hepatitis. Continued alcohol intake has the strongest adverse impact on outcome. The presence of encephalopathy, impaired synthetic function, or variceal hemorrhage also predicts poor outcome. The severity of alcoholic hepatitis may be assessed by the discriminant function (DF), determined by:

*4.6 × elongation of prothrombin time (seconds) over baseline + bilirubin (mg/dl).*

Values of 32 or higher indicate very severe disease. The DF does not distinguish reversible (pure alcoholic hepatitis) from end-stage liver disease. In patients with an elevated discriminant function score over 32, pure alcoholic hepatitis, and no contraindications (e.g., active infection or GI hemorrhage), therapy with corticosteroids (prednisone, 40 mg/day) may be of some benefit. Pentoxyfilline (400 mg 3x/day) has also been shown to enhance survival. Alcohol abstinence is required, and management of other complications is similar to that for other forms of liver disease.

## Fatty Liver

Hepatic steatosis, commonly found on liver biopsies, is the result of accumulation of lipid within hepatocytes. The course of fatty liver often is benign, but when associated with a necroinflammatory process, as in nonalcoholic steatohepatitis (NASH), chronic alcohol ingestion, continued use of culprit medications, or uncorrected jejuno-ileal bypass progresses to fibrosis, and significant complications may follow. Fatty accumulation in the liver may be categorized based on histology as microvesicular or macrovesicular, based on size of the fat droplets. Although macrovesicular steatosis most often is due to excessive alcohol intake, it also may be associated with obesity, diabetes mellitus, hyperlipidemia, jejuno-ileal bypass, and medications such as estrogen or corticosteroids.

Microvesicular steatosis is encountered in Reye syndrome, medications such as amiodarone and tetracycline, acute fatty liver of pregnancy, and inborn errors of metabolism. Acute fatty liver of pregnancy is a potentially life-threatening entity that may lead to FHF and usually occurs in the third trimester of the woman's first pregnancy. An urgent liver biopsy is indicated to establish the diagnosis. Rapid induction of labor and a swift delivery should be performed. Rarely, liver transplantation has been required.

**TABLE 109.1. Causes of Nonalcoholic Steatohepatitis**

| |
|---|
| Obesity |
| Hypertriglyceridemia |
| Non-insulin dependent diabetes mellitus (NIDDM) |
| Rapid weight loss: gastric bypass, jejuno-ileal bypass |
| Short bowel syndrome |
| Bacterial overgrowth |
| Drug-related: corticosteroids, amiodarone, tamoxifen, estrogens, perhexiline maleate |
| Abetalipoproteinemia |
| Total parenteral nutrition |

## Non-alcoholic Steatohepatitis

Histologically identical to alcoholic hepatitis, nonalcoholic steatohepatitis (NASH) is fatty liver with inflammation. The diagnostic criteria for NASH include exclusion of significant alcohol use, exclusion of other known causes of liver disease, and consistent liver biopsy findings. Although the cause of NASH is unclear, it has been associated with obesity, diabetes mellitus, hyperlipidemia, and jejuno-ileal bypass (Table 109.1). Laboratory test findings are similar to but less pronounced than those for alcoholic hepatitis. Unlike alcoholic hepatitis, however, the ALT is typically greater than AST in NASH. Management of NASH is directed at treatment of associated disorders, and ursodeoxycholic acid has been shown to be of some benefit in a few small studies.

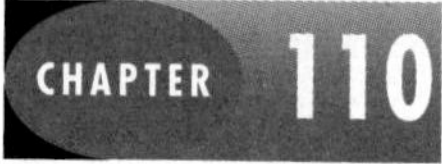

# CHAPTER 110 DRUG-INDUCED LIVER DISEASE

The liver is a major site for biotransformation and metabolism of drugs (see chapter 105). Drug-related hepatotoxicity arises from interaction of hepatotoxic medications and their metabolites within hepatocytes. This may be related to intrinsic hepatotoxins or may result from idiosyncratic reactions.

### Clinical Presentation

The clinical syndromes and histopathology produced by drug-induced liver injury are quite varied and may mimic all known types of hepatobiliary disease. In addition, a single medication may lead to several different histologic findings—for example, methyldopa may lead to hepatitis, cholestasis, or granuloma formation. Although drug-induced liver damage is rare, it does account for 2% to 5% of hospital admissions for jaundice in the United States. Drug-induced fulminant hepatic failure may account for up to 30% of cases of FHF.

Certain individuals appear to be at higher risk for development of toxicity. Reduced hepatic blood flow, decreased activity of cytochrome enzyme systems, and decreased renal clearance make elderly persons more susceptible to damage from NSAIDs and isoniazid. Obese patients are at increased risk because of prolonged exposure to fat-soluble drugs stored in adipose tissue. Depleted glutathione stores in patients with malnutrition and chronic alcohol use make them susceptible to acetaminophen toxicity (Figure 110.1). Because of the nonspecific nature of the findings of drug-induced injury, diagnosis may be difficult. A high index of suspicion is required. The onset of illness usually occurs sometime between 4 days and 8 weeks after initial exposure.

### Management

In most cases, improvement occurs after withdrawal of the offending medication. A drug rechallenge should be avoided. In progressive cases, however, liver transplantation may be necessary.

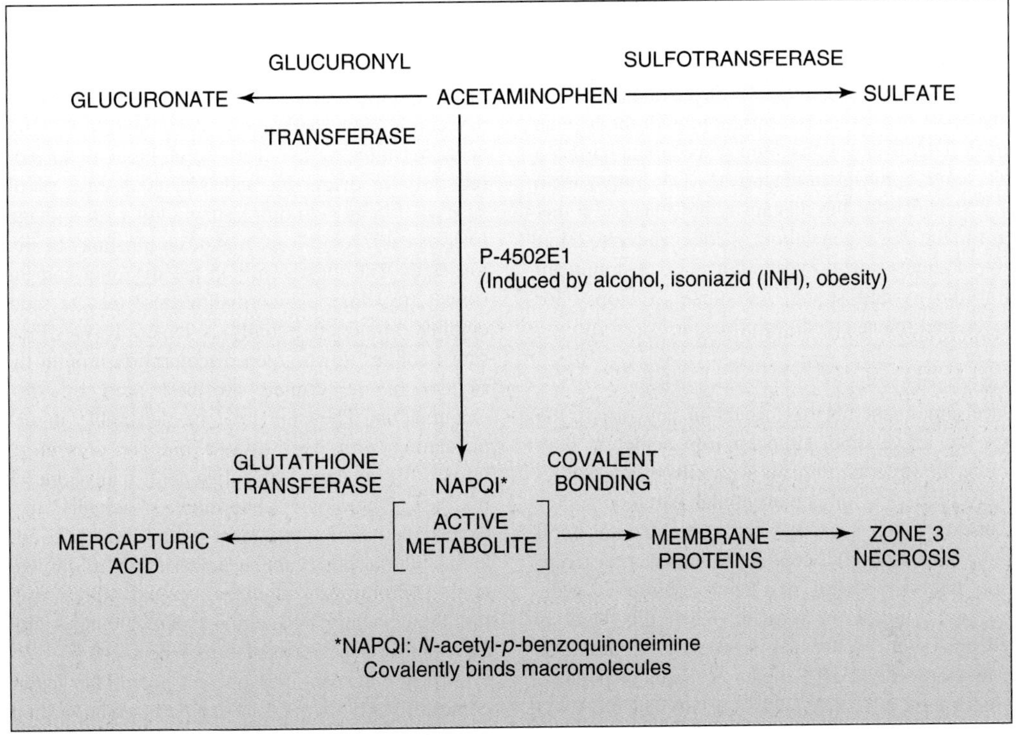


FIGURE 110.1. Acetaminophen metabolism and route of potential toxicity.

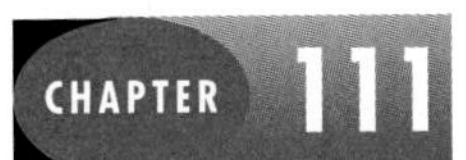

# CHAPTER 111 METABOLIC LIVER DISEASES

## Hemochromatosis

Hereditary or genetic hemochromatosis is an autosomal recessive syndrome of iron overload attributed to a defect in the *HFE* gene, which has been identified on the short arm of chromosome 6. Most cases are attributable to a single substitution of tyrosine for cysteine at position 282 (*C282Y*) of the *HFE* gene. A second single substitution of histidine for aspartate mutation at position 63 (*H63D*) does not result in iron overloading in the homozygous state, but is associated with disease in the mixed heterozygote state (*C282Y/H63D*). Hemochromatosis should be distinguished from hemosiderosis (sometimes referred to as secondary hemochromatosis), which refers to tissue deposition of iron and may be a consequence of iron loading from repeated transfusions.

The *HFE* gene encodes for a transmembrane protein known to bind $\beta_2$-microglobulin. The precise mechanism has not been elucidated, but the *HFE* gene defect apparently disrupts tightly regulated iron homeostasis by disrupting the elegant feedback mechanisms within the intestinal epithelial cell. Thus, there is persistent excessive iron absorption despite elevated iron stores. Excessive iron accumulation results in induction and propagation of free radicals, with subsequent damage to lipids, proteins, and DNA. Iron deposition and, eventually, fibrosis occur not only in hepatocytes and Kupffer cells but also in cardiac tissue, pancreatic acini, endocrine organs and the kidney.

### Clinical Presentation

The "classic" presentation of a middle-aged man with bronzed skin, diabetes, and hepatomegaly, with or without cirrhosis, is not often seen. Abnormal liver enzymes or elevated iron studies are more common presentations that allow detection in the preclinical phase. Hypogonadotropic hypogonadism due to pituitary iron deposition, chondrocalcinosis, and metcarpophalangeal arthritis (particularly of the 2nd and 3rd metacarpals) also are seen. Cardiomyopathy appears to be more common in those who drink alcohol on a regular basis. Women are less affected and typically present at a later age due to the protective effects of menstrual blood loss. If hemochromatosis is suspected, fasting transferrin saturation should be the first laboratory test, with a value greater than 55% necessitating further evaluation. The quantitation of liver iron concentration, with the hepatic iron index (HII) over 1.9 on a biopsy specimen, has been the gold standard means of diagnosis. Liver biopsy is no longer mandatory for the diagnosis, however, now that testing for the *HFE* gene (both *C282Y* and *H63D*) is available. Patients over 40 years of age are at significant risk for fibrosis and should still undergo biopsy for prognostic and management purposes.

### Management

Once significant fibrosis occurs in any organ, the changes are irreversible, although iron depletion may ameliorate the severity. Patients with cirrhosis are at an extremely high risk for hepatocellular carcinoma. Removal of excess iron stores by weekly phlebotomies (450 ml blood = 250 mg iron) is continued, with a target serum ferritin of less than 50µg/L or a hemoglobin of 12 g/dL in men or 11 mg/dL in women. When this level is reached, phlebotomy is used less frequently. Screening of family members for the HFE mutation should be pursued if the index case is C282Y/C282Y or H63D/C282Y.

## Wilson Disease

Wilson disease is a rare autosomal recessive disorder that results from a defect in copper transport. Within the liver, copper is avidly absorbed and eventually carried to the Golgi apparatus, where it binds to the Wilson disease protein (WDP). Copper bound to WDP is then transported and either inserted into apoceruloplasmin (forming ceruloplasmin) or carried to the bile membrane for excretion. In Wilson disease, a gene defect in chromosome 13 results in a lack of WDP, which then results in accumulation of cytotoxic copper within the liver, the basal ganglia (CNS symptoms), and the iris (Kayser-Fleischer rings), as well as low serum ceruloplasmin levels and enhanced urinary copper excretion.

### Clinical Presentation

Wilson disease has protean clinical manifestations. Approximately half of the patients present with the liver disease (usually between the ages of 3 and 12 years), whereas the other half present with neurologic or psychiatric symptoms (usually in adolescence and early adulthood). Onset of disease is before the age of 35. Liver disease may present with either acute liver failure associated with hemolysis, decompensated cirrhosis, acute hepatitis, or jaundice. A high index of suspicion is required for diagnosis, and Wilson disease should be suspected in any child or young adult with undiagnosed liver disease. Neurologic manifestations may be difficult to detect. The most common are dystonia and Parkinsonism; psychiatric abnormalities also may be seen, and cognitive function initially is intact. Kayser-Fleischer rings, subtle brown-green discoloration around the periphery of the cornea, are best seen by slit-lamp examination. They may not be detectable in patients presenting with liver disease but are present almost universally in those presenting with neurologic abnormalities. Neurologic abnormalities actually may be exacerbated when treatment is initiated. Glycosuria, aminaciduria, renal tubular acidosis, or full-blown Fanconi syndrome may manifest as renal tubular dysfunction. Acute hemolytic anemia, nephrocalcinosis, arthritis, and sunflower cataracts also may be seen.

Early diagnosis may prevent potentially lethal outcomes. Liver biopsy and slit-lamp examination should be obtained. Diagnosis requires at least two of the following features: low plasma ceruloplasmin, increased urinary copper concentration, and a hepatic copper concentration greater than 250µg/g dry weight. Molecular techniques for genetic diagnosis are not widely available.

### Management

The first-line treatment is oral penicillamine, which chelates copper, depletes body stores of copper, and enhances urinary copper excretion. Penicillamine may not be tolerated in cases with bone marrow suppression, an urticarial rash, drug-induced lupus, and proteinuria. Trientine is second-line therapy, and zinc also may help by decreasing copper absorption. Certain foods with a particularly high copper concentration, including chocolate, shellfish, and organ meats, should be avoided.

A number of other metabolic disorders, including alpha-1 antitrypsin deficiency, urea cycle defects, glycogen storage diseases, porphyrias, and cystic fibrosis also may lead to chronic liver disease.

# CHAPTER 112 VASCULAR LIVER DISEASE

Hypoperfusion, as in prolonged shock or acute heart failure, results in reduced hepatic arterial and portal venous blood flow. The resultant liver injury consists of zone 3 necrosis with extremely elevated aminotransferases, cholestasis, and coagulopathy. In right heart failure, raised venous pressures are transmitted to the liver, causing sinusoidal dilatation and congestion, perivenular hemorrhage, and centrilobular liver cell necrosis. Over time, collagen formation and fibrosis follow and produce cardiac cirrhosis. Jaundice, tender hepatomegaly, and ascites are typical findings of passive congestion. Liver test abnormalities are not typically distinctive, although markedly elevated LDH levels may provide a clue. Constrictive pericarditis with or without cirrhosis should always be considered in patients with portal hypertensive ascites and an elevated total protein.

## Budd-Chiari Syndrome

Budd-Chiari syndrome is caused by obstruction of the major hepatic veins and, thus, hepatic venous outflow, characterized by right upper quadrant pain, hepatomegaly, and high-protein-content ascites. Occlusion may be due to myeloproliferative disorders, malignancy, hypercoagulability, oral contraceptive use, pregnancy, and an inferior vena cava "web" or malformation.

### Clinical Presentation

Rapid onset of upper abdominal pain, hepatomegaly, and ascites occurs. The course is commonly progressive, with subsequent cirrhosis or liver failure. The caudate lobe often is markedly enlarged, because its separate drainage into the inferior vena cava provides the only venous outflow for a congested liver. Patients undergoing high-dose chemotherapy and bone marrow transplantation, particularly those with preexisting liver disease, are susceptible to a similar syndrome called veno-occlusive disease. Aminotransferases are elevated, and coagulopathy may denote progressive liver failure. Ultrasonography with Doppler flow imaging is diagnostic and is the first-line test. Hepatic venography documents extent of occlusion and also permits pressure measurements, which may be imperative in planning surgical intervention.

### Management

Urgent transplantation is required for fulminant hepatic failure (FHF) or if cirrhosis develops. Treatment of the acute syndrome with thrombolytic agents occasionally is successful within the first few weeks. Decompression of the venous system with portacaval, mesocaval, mesoatrial, and splenorenal shunts may be indicated in the absence of cirrhosis. The role of transjugular intrahepatic portosystemic shunting (TIPS) is unclear. Chronic and less progressive cases are treated with supportive measures.

# CHAPTER 113 CIRRHOSIS

### Definition and Classification

Cirrhosis is defined by the presence of fibrous bands that divide the liver into regenerative nodules. Cirrhosis is classified as **micronodular** when nodules are less than 3 mm in diameter and **macronodular** when nodules are 3 mm or more in diameter. The former type is associated with alcoholic liver disease, NASH, and hemochromatosis, whereas the latter is seen with chronic viral hepatitis. The liver architecture and the microvasculature are markedly distorted in cirrhosis. A large proportion of hepatic blood flow bypasses the parenchymal cells within the regenerative nodules and may lead to encephalopathy. Portal hypertension, impaired synthetic function, portosystemic shunting, and predisposition to malignant transformation may follow but are not universal.

### Clinical and Laboratory Features

Cirrhosis and liver failure share common clinical and biochemical features. Well-established cirrhosis may be asymptomatic, or patients may experience fatigue, weakness, confusion, upper GI hemorrhage, leg edema, or abdominal distention due to ascites. There may be abdominal wall venous collaterals, splenomegaly, reduced muscle mass, and Dupuytren's contractures. Abdominal and inguinal hernias may be worsened by ascites. Stigmata of cirrhosis include palmar erythema, spider angiomata, gynecomastia, and testicular atrophy. Patients with cirrhosis are predisposed to bacterial infections; spontaneous bacterial peritonitis portends a particularly poor prognosis.

**Anemia,** often macrocytic, is common. Splenic sequestration causes **leukopenia** and **thrombocytopenia.** A prolonged prothrombin time (PT) usually is refractory to vitamin K. **Hypoalbuminemia** is due to decreased albumin synthesis or hemodilution. Serum bilirubin and aminotransferases may be normal or slightly elevated. Renal failure with oliguria, azotemia, and avid $Na^+$ retention are ominous signs. Prognosis and surgical risk can be estimated by assessing Child's class (Table 113.1). Focal abnormalities on abdominal ultrasound or CT should raise suspicion for hepatocellular carcinoma (HCC). The serum α-fetoprotein (AFP) level is a useful marker for HCC but has a sensitivity of only 50% to 70%. Liver decompensation occurs when a patient with cirrhosis develops encephalopathy, variceal bleeding, or ascites.

**TABLE 113.1. Child-Pugh Score for Severity of Liver Disease**

| Criterion | 1 point | 2 points | 3 points |
|---|---|---|---|
| Prothrombin time (seconds ⇑) or | < 4 | 4–6 | > 6 |
| INR | < 1.7 | 1.7–2.3 | > 2.3 |
| Albumin (g/dl) | >3.5 | 2.8–3.5 | <2.8 |
| Ascites | None | Slight | Moderate |
| Encephalopathy (grade) | None | 1–2 | 3–4 |
| Bilirubin (mg/dl) | < 2 | 2–3 | > 3 |

Grade A: 5–6; Grade B: 7–9; Grade C: ≥10
INR = international normalized ratio

## Complications

### Portal hypertension

Gastrointestinal bleeding is a common life-threatening complication of portal hypertension. The site of obstruction (Figure 113.1) helps classify obstruction of portal venous flow resulting in portal hypertension. The most common cause is cirrhosis, which results in sinusoidal obstruction. Portal hypertension also may result from presinusoidal obstruction (portal vein thrombosis, primary biliary cirrhosis, sarcoidosis, schistosomiasis) or post-sinusoidal obstruction (Budd-Chiari syndrome, veno-occlusive disease, congestive heart failure [CHF], pericarditis). In the setting of portal hypertension, only 10% of normal blood flow reaches the hepatic veins; 90% is shunted to collaterals. Most dangerous are the gastroesophageal collaterals emanating from the left gastric and short gastric veins to the esophagus. Collaterals also develop from the inferior mesenteric vein to the hemorrhoidal veins and from the umbilical veins to those of the abdominal wall.

Normally, the pressure gradient across the liver from the portal vein to the hepatic vein is approximately 3 mm Hg. This is called the wedged hepatic venous pressure (WHVP) and is measured by a balloon catheter wedged in the inferior vena cava. Portal hypertensive bleeding may occur when the WHVP is elevated to 12 mm Hg or more.

*Clinical presentation*

Patients may present with prominent abdominal wall veins radiating from the umbilicus, ascites, and splenomegaly. The portal-systemic collaterals predispose to bleeding from esophageal varices, gastric varices, or hemorrhoids. Splenomegaly may result in left upper abdominal discomfort, leukopenia, and thrombocytopenia.

**FIGURE 113.1.** Classification of portal hypertension.

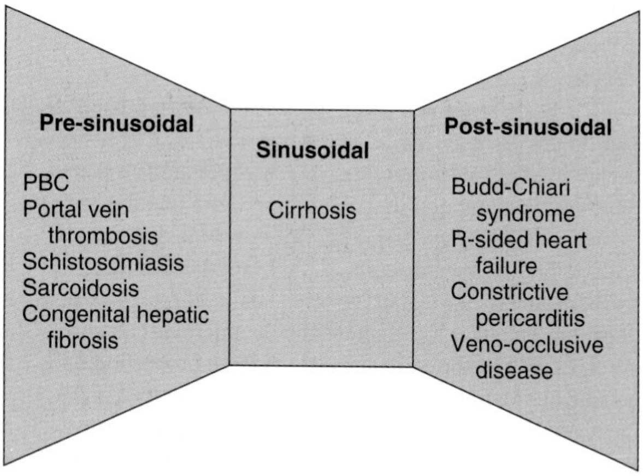

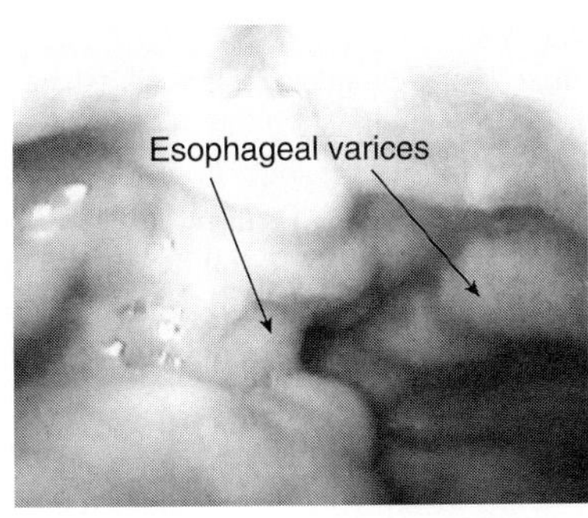


**FIGURE 113.2.** Esophageal varices noted on endoscopy.

Esophageal varices usually are identified by endoscopy (Figure 113.2). Patients with known portal hypertension should be screened for the presence of esophageal or gastric varices in order to implement appropriate prophylactic therapy. Nonselective β-blockers, such as **propranolol,** have been shown to lower portal hypertension and effectively prevent the first episode of variceal bleeding. The dosage is titrated to reduce the resting pulse rate by 25%. Isolated gastric varices should raise suspicion for splenic vein thrombosis. Ultrasound with Doppler and venous phase mesenteric arteriography may be required in those with suspected portal vein or hepatic vein thrombosis.

*Bleeding esophageal varices*

Hemorrhage from distended esophageal varices is the most common emergency in cirrhotics with portal hypertension and has a high mortality. It may not be possible to identify a specific precipitating factor, but a history of aspirin or nonsteroidal anti-inflammatory drug ingestion should be sought. Nonvariceal sources of bleeding account for up to half of the cases of upper GI bleeding in cirrhotics. Bleeding may be slow and gradual or abrupt and massive with hematemesis, melena, or both. Urgent upper GI endoscopy assesses the size of varices, identifies any high-risk stigmata, best estimates the varices' bleeding risk, excludes other sources of bleeding, and provides therapeutic options.

Patients with bleeding esophageal varices should be hospitalized promptly. Urgent resuscitation and correction of coagulopathy should be followed by urgent endoscopy. The primary treatments consist of **endoscopic band ligation** and **endoscopic injection sclerotherapy. Sclerotherapy** is direct injection of the varix with a sclerosant (e.g., sodium morrhuate). **Band ligation** is a newer endoscopic technique of suctioning and then deploying a small rubber band around the varix. Both techniques cause thrombosis, local ulceration, and, ultimately, fibrosis to prevent variceal recurrence and bleeding. Band ligation is as effective but has fewer adverse effects than sclerotherapy. Scheduled repeated treatments may be required to obliterate any remaining veins, with band ligation having been shown to require fewer sessions. Endoscopic therapy is successful in controlling acute bleeding 80% to 90% of patients, but is associated with complications such as esophageal ulcers, strictures, perforation, fever, and mediastinitis.

Acute and massive variceal hemorrhage not controlled by endoscopic therapy may require the use of vasoactive drugs. Octreotide, a synthetic analog of somatostatin, has been shown to be a safe and effective agent. It is administered intravenously with a 50-μg bolus followed by an infusion of 50 μg/hr. It is effective in stabilizing bleeding for up to 72 hours until more definitive treatment can be undertaken. Vasopressin is no longer used due to its adverse side-effect profile. Esophageal balloon tamponade (e.g., using a Sengataken-Blakemore tube) provides direct compression of varices and temporarily controls bleeding but is now very infrequently used.

Variceal bleeding refractory to endoscopic therapy requires decompression with a transjugular intrahepatic portosystemic shunting (TIPS) or surgical shunt. A TIP involves placement of an expandable intrahepatic stent to create an intrahepatic portacaval shunt under fluoroscopic guidance. It effectively controls acute and recurrent variceal bleeding and ascites by reducing portal hypertension. Placement of a TIPS does predispose to encephalopathy but less so than a surgical shunt, because less blood flow is diverted. Transjugular intrahepatic portosystemic shunt stenosis due to intimal hyperplasia or thrombosis is a common problem but can be managed by vigilant surveillance with Doppler ultrasound and subsequent dilation, as necessary. The surgical shunt decompresses the portal venous system, but it also decreases hepatic blood flow, thus potentially worsening liver function and predisposing to hepatic encephalopathy. This procedure usually is performed in persons with adequate liver function in whom liver transplantation would not be anticipated for several years. A distal splenorenal shunt appears to be effective in preventing rebleeding with less encephalopathy and mortality. Endoscopic therapy is not successful in long-term control of gastric variceal bleeding and usually requires TIPS or surgical intervention.

### Ascites

Ascites is the accumulation of intraperitoneal fluid. A combination of abnormalities in renal function resulting in sodium and fluid retention, hypoalbuminemia leading to decreased plasma oncotic pressure and expansion of extracellular volume, and increased lymph formation due to increased portal capillary pressure all contribute to ascites. Sodium retention is believed to be a consequence of arterial underfilling, which triggers homeostatic mechanisms that control sodium balance. Plasma renin activity, antidiuretic hormone, plasma norepinephrine levels, and aldosterone are all increased.

*Clinical presentation*

Ascites may develop insidiously or it may follow worsening liver function during an episode of hemorrhage, infection, toxic injury or surgery. Physical examination has a poor sensitivity except for large amounts of ascites. Shifting dullness, a fluid wave or bulging flanks may be noted. Pleural effusions may signal the presence of hepatic hydrothorax. Hepatic hydrothorax is seen in approximately 5% of cirrhotics and typically is right-sided. Tense ascites may cause respiratory distress. Ventral, inguinal, and umbilical hernias may be induced or worsened. Ascites is readily demonstrated by abdominal ultrasound.

All patients with new-onset ascites should undergo a diagnostic paracentesis, and the fluid should be sent for albumin, protein, total and differential cell count, and culture (collected in blood culture bottles at the bedside). An elevated serum ascites albumin gradient (SAAG) higher than 1.1 confirms that ascites is related to portal hypertension (Table 113.2). A low fluid protein (< 1.1) indicates susceptibility to developing bacterial peritonitis, whereas an elevated protein should raise suspicion for high-protein causes of ascites. More specific testing for glucose, LDH, amylase (pancreatitis), triglyceride (chylous ascites) and cytology should be done when warranted.

*Management*

The first step in management is strict sodium restriction, to no more than 2 g/day. This restriction may be difficult to maintain, but it is instrumental in management (Figure 113.3). Oral spironolactone (50-400 mg daily) and furosemide (20-160 mg/day) usually are required and should be used in a 5:2 ratio for best effect. Electrolyte disturbances, worsening of hepatic encephalopathy, renal dysfunction, gynecomastia, and muscle cramps may limit diuretic use. The goal of treatment should be a weight loss of 1 kg/day in patients with peripheral edema and 0.5 kg/day in those without.

For diuretic-resistant ascites, repeated large-volume paracentesis (up to 4–6 L) is safe and effective. Concomitant administration of intravenous albumin

**TABLE 113.2. Serum Ascites Albumin Gradient for Source of Ascites**

| |
|---|
| High (>1.1) |
| Cirrhosis |
| Hepatocellular carcinoma |
| Budd-Chiari syndrome |
| Right ventricular failure |
| Constrictive pericarditis |
| Low (<1.1) |
| Peritoneal carcinomatosis |
| Pancreatic ascites |
| Nephrotic syndrome |
| Peritoneal tuberculosis without cirrhosis |

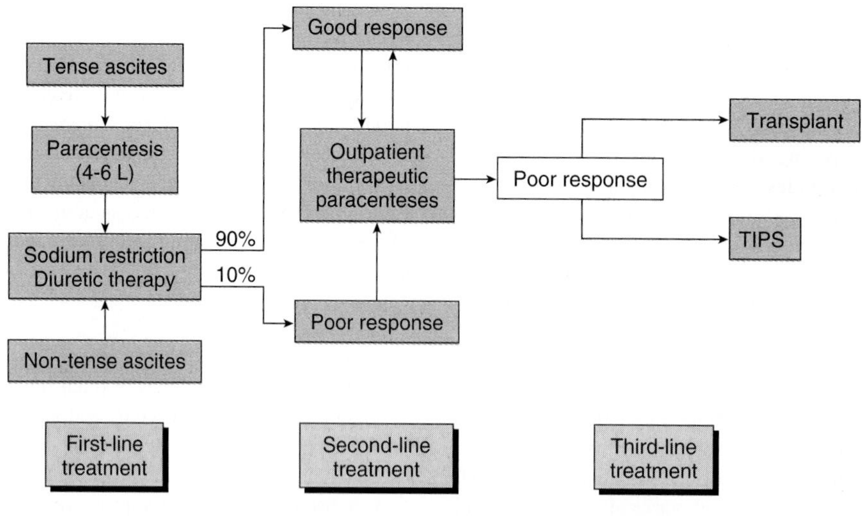


**FIGURE 113.3.** Treatment of Ascites.

(8–10 g/L of fluid expected to be removed) may be beneficial in patients with renal insufficiency and in those in whom more than 5 L is removed. Diuretic resistance portends poor prognosis and may necessitate listing for liver transplantation. Placement of a TIPS has been found to be effective in these patients and yields better outcomes than repeated paracentesis. Surgical peritoneal-venous shunts (the LeVeen shunt or Denver shunt) involve placement of a catheter between the peritoneum and the central veins. They may be useful in a minority of cirrhotics with good liver function but are now rarely used because of problems with side effects (e.g., vena cava thrombosis, shunt occlusion, peritoneal fibrosis) and the availability of alternative treatments.

### Spontaneous bacterial peritonitis

Bacterial translocation from the gut lumen in the setting of impaired reticuloendothelial system phagocytic function and ascitic fluid antimicrobial activity results in spontaneous bacterial peritonitis (SBP). Between 10% and 30% of hospitalized cirrhotic patients with ascites have SBP.

#### *Clinical presentation*

Classic signs of SBP such as abdominal pain, rebound tenderness, and fever often are absent. Diagnosis of SBP should be considered in any patient with cirrhosis who demonstrates clinical deterioration, particularly those with hepatic encephalopathy or shock. Renal failure accompanies approximately one third of cases and denotes a poor prognosis. Enteric gram-negatives are the most common pathogens, with streptococci and staphylococci also frequently encountered. Diagnostic paracentesis and ascitic fluid analysis with cell count and inoculation of culture bottles at the bedside for culture are required. Ascitic fluid absolute neutrophil count exceeding 250/mm$^3$, a positive Gram stain, or a positive culture are all diagnostic of SBP. A multibacterial Gram stain or culture, markedly elevated LDH or decreased glucose, or inability to achieve a decrease of at least 50% in the absolute neutrophil count on repeat paracentesis at 48 hours warrant investigation for secondary causes of bacterial peritonitis (e.g. gut perforation, diverticulitis, appendicitis, cholangitis).

#### *Management*

Intravenous administration of a second-generation cephalosporin is the treatment of choice. Aminoglycosides should be avoided due to prolonged renal toxicity. Treatment should continue for at least 5 days, and repeat paracentesis should be done to confirm resolution. Prophylaxis with norfloxacin (400 mg/day) or ciprofloxacin (500 mg 3x/week) in patients with prior history of SBP, or an ascitic fluid protein below 1 g/dL, has been shown to decrease the incidence of SBP. Cirrhotic ascites also predisposes to **peritoneal tuberculosis,** but AFB stains and cultures are insensitive. A diagnostic laparoscopy with biopsy of peritoneal lesions demonstrating granulomas may be required.

**TABLE 113.3. Staging of Hepatic Encephalopathy**

| Stage | Features |
|---|---|
| I | Mental slowing, confusion, or altered motor behavior. Psychometric defects are detectable. |
| II | Agitation, greater confusion, inappropriate behavior |
| III | Stupor, but arousable |
| IV | Coma, without response to pain; possible seizure activity |

### Hepatic encephalopathy

Hepatic encephalopathy, also called portosystemic encephalopathy (PSE), is a neuropsychiatric syndrome seen with both acute and chronic liver failure. It is believed that a "toxin," which would normally be metabolized with intact liver function, accumulates, reaches the brain, and results in PSE. Although many candidate agents—including ammonia, fatty acids, gamma aminobutyric acid, mercaptans, and other false neurotransmitters—have been implicated, the true etiologic "toxin" is not known. The current hypothesis is that PSE results from the combined effect of various cerebral toxins, the individual contributions of which in any one patient may differ. Urea cycle defects in children may precipitate PSE in the absence of cirrhosis.

#### *Clinical presentation*

The stages of PSE are shown in Table 113.3. On examination, **asterixis** should be tested with the patient's hands outstretched, wrists hyperextended, and fingers separated. Asterixis is the inability to maintain this flexed posture demonstrated by rapid flexion-extension movements of the hands. Asterixis is not specific to PSE and may be seen with other cause of metabolic encephalopathy (e.g., uremia, respiratory failure, or sedative overdose). Other neurological abnormalities also may be seen in advanced PSE, especially spasticity, hyperreflexia, and extensor plantar responses. **Fetor hepaticus** (a fishy, ammonia-like odor on the breath) also may be noted. Simple bedside tests of cerebral function (e.g., Reitan trail test) help diagnose early encephalopathy and monitor its response to therapy. Arterial and venous blood ammonia is elevated in the majority of patients, but it correlates poorly with the degree of coma, and sequential measurements are not typically required. Persistent

**FIGURE 113.4. Precipitants of encephalopathy.**

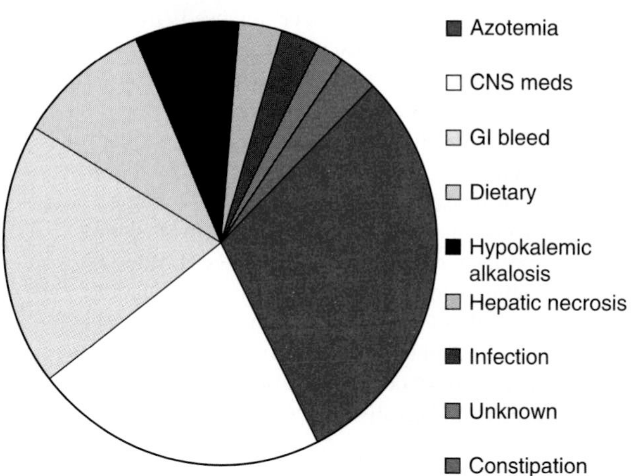


lateralizing signs are not typically seen with PSE and may indicate a secondary process.

*Management*

Initial measures should include evaluation for and appropriate treatment of precipitating factors such as gastrointestinal hemorrhage, infection, hypokalemia, hyponatremia, severe alkalosis, excessive sedative use, and renal dysfunction (Figure 113.4). Next, empiric measures are directed at decreasing ammonia levels. A diet should be high in fiber and moderate in protein (~ 100 g/day). Anorexia and malnutrition are common in liver failure, and, therefore, aggressive protein restriction below 100 g/day often is detrimental. Careful maintenance of electrolyte and volume status is critical, especially if diuretics are used. Sedation with medications should be avoided if at all possible. Constipation exacerbates PSE and should be treated aggressively.

Oral lactulose, a nonabsorbable disaccharide, is the mainstay of treatment for PSE. Its site of action is the colon, where it is metabolized to short-chain organic acids, which acidify the colonic contents and cause an osmotic diarrhea. Some postulate that the putative toxins are thus acidified and "trapped" within the colonic lumen. The dose of lactulose is titrated to cause at least three loose stools per day, but severe diarrhea must be avoided. In patients unable to take medications by mouth, lactulose enemas (300 ml lactulose/700 ml $H_2O$) may be administered. Oral antibiotics such as metronidazole and neomycin, which eradicate anaerobic colonic bacteria, are useful adjuncts when response to lactulose alone is inadequate. Many enteral and parenteral nutritional products enriched in branched-chain amino acids are advocated for use in PSE, but their efficacy is unproven. Recurrent PSE has a poor long-term prognosis, and early referral for transplantation should be considered.

**Hepatopulmonary syndrome**

Hepatopulmonary syndrome is characterized by the combination of liver disease, hypoxemia, and intrapulmonary vascular dilatation related to nitric oxide. The dilated intrapulmonary shunts are not oxygenated, and blood flow through them is accentuated with the patient standing. This accounts for the phenomena of platypnea (shortness of breath that is more pronounced when erect) and orthodeoxia (hypoxemia that is more pronounced when erect). The intrapulmonary shunts can be documented by contrast-enhanced ("bubble") echocardiography. Perfusion scan using technetium-labeled, macroaggregated albumin allows quantitation of the shunt. Hepatopulmonary syndrome is an indication for liver transplantation. Patients with partial oxygen tensions ($PaO_2$) below 60 mm Hg or inability to increase $PaO_2$ to more than 150 mm Hg on 100% oxygen do poorly after transplantation.

**Hepatorenal syndrome**

Hepatorenal syndrome is development of renal failure in severe liver disease (acute or chronic) in the absence of other identifiable causes of renal disease. Decreased renal blood flow and renal filtration are involved in the pathogenesis. Infection, hemorrhage, overaggressive diuresis or paracentesis, and nephrotoxic medications may mimic or precipitate the syndrome. Decompensation of liver disease also is commonly present. The diagnosis is made in the appropriate setting if there is oliguria (urine volume < 500 ml), a low urine sodium (< 10 mEq/ml), absence of proteinuria or hematuria (< 50 RBC per high-power field) and documentation of adequate intravascular volume. The prognosis is quite poor, with a mortality of 50% to 95%, depending on the underlying cause. If liver transplantation is an option or recovery of liver function is anticipated, hemodialysis may be useful.

# CHAPTER 114 BENIGN TUMORS OF THE LIVER

The incidental finding of a focal hepatic lesion on imaging studies in an asymptomatic patient is a common clinical scenario. The first steps in the evaluation should be to determine whether the lesion has arisen within normal or diseased parenchyma and whether there is an underlying condition (e.g., hepatitis B [HBV] or hepatitis C [HCV]) that carries a high risk of malignancy. If there is no underlying liver disease or high-risk condition, the patient is asymptomatic, and the radiologic characteristics are benign, conservative management is warranted.

## Hepatocellular Adenomas

**Hepatocellular adenomas** are rare tumors seen predominantly in women using long-term high-dose oral contraceptives, but also are seen androgenic anabolic steroid use. Current low-dose contraceptives do not appear to have a significant association. Most are solitary lesions, may measure up to 10 cm in size, and are highly vascular, predisposing to infarction and hemorrhage. Patients may be asymptomatic, have episodic pain, or present with acute right upper quadrant pain. The latter often is due to infarction or, more ominously, hemorrhage if accompanied by shock. Because these lesions are estrogen-sensitive, pregnancy and menstruation increase the risk of rupture. Malignant transformation to hepatocellular carcinoma may occur. Imaging studies are helpful in management but are not always diagnostic. Routine biopsy is not warranted, because of the risk of bleeding. Patients presenting with shock should undergo emergent angiographic embolization before definitive surgical resection is undertaken. In asymptomatic stable patients, all lesions larger than 10 cm (because of the risk of hemorrhage) should be electively resected. Other patients should have hormonal therapy withdrawn and serial imaging performed, and should undergo resection if symptoms develop.

**Focal nodular hyperplasia,** the second most common liver tumor, is a congenital malformation in which the connective tissue elements of the liver are contained within a stellate scar. It appears to reflect a hyperplastic response to abnormal blood flow from a pre-existing vascular malformation. Typically, there is a stellate scar near the center of the lesion from which fibrous septa radiate into the mass with histologically normal but disorganized hepatocytes. Oral contraceptive use is not implicated in its pathogenesis, but because it most often occurs in women during their reproductive years, making the distinction from a hepatocellular adenoma often is a clinical problem. MRI scanning is the best imaging modality, offering increasing enhancement of the central scar on delayed images. Asymptomatic patients with characteristic imaging features should be reassured without further investigation. Biopsy occasionally is required for atypical cases. Surgical excision is not indicated unless symptoms can truly be associated with the lesion.

## Hemangiomas

**Hemangiomas** are the most common benign liver tumor. They predominate in women and are composed of cavernous vascular spaces lined by a single layer of blood-filled epithelium. Often asymptomatic, they may be single or multiple and vary in diameter from less than 1 cm to more than 20 cm. The majority are solitary, smaller than 5 cm, in the right lobe, and asymptomatic. A minority of patients with lesions larger 4 cm in diameter are symptomatic, with mild to moderate abdominal fullness or discomfort. Hemangiomas that thrombose, involute, or calcify may become symptomatic. Spontaneous bleeding is extremely rare. Physical examination may reveal a soft bruit over the liver. Ultrasound (Doppler flow in 10-50%), CT (centripetal contrast enhancement), and MRI (marked hyperintensity on T2-weighted images) as well as labeled RBC radionuclide scanning are all diagnostic. Needle biopsy should be avoided. Surgical resection seldom is warranted except for clearly related symptoms or rare hemorrhage.

# CHAPTER 115 MALIGNANT TUMORS OF THE LIVER

## Hepatocellular Carcinoma

Hepatocellular carcinoma (HCC) is the sixth most common cancer worldwide and accounts for 75% to 85% of all primary liver tumors. Pre-existing liver disease, male gender, geography, and environment all affect the prevalence of HCC. Hepatocellular carcinoma is very common in Southeast Asia and Africa but relatively uncommon in Northern Europe and the United States. Most cases are associated with cirrhosis (Table 115.1), and patients actively infected with hepatitis B (relative risk of ~ 100) or hepatitis re at particularly high risk. In Taiwan, hepatitis B immunization has led to a reduction in the incidence of HCC.

### Clinical Presentation

The triad of right upper quadrant pain, weight loss, and hepatomegaly in a cirrhotic patient is a common presentation. Abrupt decompensation of liver function, marked change in liver size, and acute onset of pain and peritoneal signs (due to rupture and hemorrhage) should raise suspicion for HCC. A vascular bruit may be heard in up to 25% of cases, as can a liver rub. Paraneoplastic syndromes including erythrocytosis, gynecomastia, hypercalcemia, and hypoglycemia are recognized but rare.

Elevated cholesterol in a cirrhotic patient due to de novo HCC production occurs in up to 38% of cases and may be a clue. Alpha-fetoprotein (AFP), a normal fetal serum protein, also is produced by HCC cells and rises significantly in approximately 50% of patients with HCC in North America. A level higher than 400 ng/ml accompanying a focal liver lesion is considered diagnostic of HCC. Marked elevation also may be seen with other causes of hepatocyte injury, such as viral hepatitis. Patients at particularly high risk for HCC (e.g., HBV, HCV, or hemochromatosis) currently undergo serial 6-monthly to annual AFP tests and liver US. The cost-effectiveness of this protocol has not been demonstrated. Particularly in Western countries, CT provides a higher yield for HCC but is not routinely employed, due, in part, to its higher cost. Lesions accompanied by AFP levels above 400 ng/ml do not require biopsy. Biopsies should be performed on other lesions unless the patient has significant coagulopathy and hepatic decompensation.

**TABLE 115.1. Risk Factors for Hepatocellular Carcinoma**

| Risk Factors |
|---|
| Chronic hepatitis B |
| Chronic hepatitis C |
| Cirrhosis |
| Hemochromatosis |
| Alpha-1-antitrypsin deficiency |
| Anabolic steroid use |
| Hereditary tyrosinemia, glycogenosis |
| Dietary aflatoxins, alcohol, smoking (?) |
| Thorotrast exposure |
| Industrial carcinogens |

### Management

Surgery, including orthotopic liver transplantation, currently offers the only potential curative treatment. Unfortunately, only a minority of patients may undergo resection due to poor hepatic reserve or extent of tumor involvement. Liver transplantation leads to poor outcome unless a solitary lesion is small (< 5 cm) or multiple (≤ 3) lesions are extremely small (≤ 3 cm). Systemic chemo- and radiation therapies have no role. Radiological and surgical interventions, including percutaneous alcohol injection, chemoembolization, radiofrequency ablation, and cryotherapy, are effective for palliation and prolong survival but are not curative. Better means of early detection are needed to achieve better outcomes in the treatment of HCC. The fibrolamellar variant of hepatocellular carcinoma appears to have a more benign course.

## Metastatic Cancer of the Liver

After lymph nodes, the liver is the most frequent site of extrahepatic cancer metastases; they are noted in about 40% cases in autopsy studies. Primary neoplasms of the alimentary tract, pancreas, breast, and lung most commonly metastasize to the liver. Most metastases are hematogenous, and only about 10% are solitary. When present on the liver surface, metastases typically are white, umbilicated, and round.

### Clinical Presentation

Patients may present with progressive, right upper quadrant abdominal pain, anorexia, and hard hepatomegaly. With advanced disease, ascites and lower extremity edema may follow, particularly if the tumor is causing inferior vena cava compression. Elevation of serum alkaline phosphatase may be a clue but has a low sensitivity. Aminotransferases and the total bilirubin typically are mildly elevated. The diagnosis is made by abnormalities on imaging, and guided needle biopsy is diagnostic.

### Management

Treatment usually consists of the systemic chemotherapy indicated for that particular extrahepatic malignancy. Despite treatment, most liver metastases portend a poor prognosis, with less than 10% of patients alive at 1 year. Careful selection of a subgroup of patients with solitary lesions, particularly those with colorectal cancer without other evidence of residual disease, may yield better results, however. The 5-year survival rate after resection of metastatic cancer is nearly 25% in this group. In general, for patients with newly diagnosed extrahepatic malignancy, routine screening of the liver is neither cost-effective nor warranted and should be reserved for those with symptoms or abnormal liver blood tests.

## Cholangiocarcinoma

Cholangiocarcinoma is a primary malignancy of the biliary ductular epithelium. Tumors may develop anywhere along the length of the biliary tree. If the lesion is at the hilum (junction of the left and right main hepatic ducts), where it may expand into the liver and cause bilateral obstruction, it is called a Klatskin tumor. Because of the slow growth at this site, the clinical picture evolves slowly and mimics benign cholestatic disorders. Risk factors for cholangiocarcinoma include choledochal cysts, primary sclerosing cholangitis, Caroli disease, Oriental cholangiohepatitis due to *Clonorchis sinensis*, and exposure to thorium dioxide.

### Clinical Presentation

Patients may present with jaundice, pruritus, right upper quadrant pain, anorexia, weight loss, and fatigue. There usually is no significant pain, and secondary bacterial cholangitis is uncommon. A nontender, enlarged, palpable gallbladder is a useful sign of malignant biliary obstruction **(Courvoisier's sign)** but is not specific for cholangiocarcinoma. Liver test abnormalities reflect a cholestatic picture, and CA 19-9 levels usually are elevated but are not sufficiently specific to differentiate from benign disease. The diagnosis is made by cholangiography along with positive biliary cytology or biopsy. The cholangiogram may reveal a polypoid lesion or demonstrate a stricture suggestive of a benign disease or sclerosing cholangitis. The yield of brushings and biopsies is suboptimal, with reported yields of 50% to 75%.

### Management

The few patients with locally confined, resectable tumors may benefit from surgical resection. Results with transplantation are very poor. Standard chemo- and radiotherapeutic regimens are ineffective. Nonoperative management using endoscopically or percutaneously placed stents may provide relief from jaundice and pruritus. The benefits of brachytherapy with iridium implants placed via percutaneous stents are being investigated.

# CHAPTER 116 LIVER TRANSPLANTATION

Liver transplantation has become widely accepted as an effective treatment for patients with irreversible acute and chronic liver diseases for which there were no viable options previously available (Table 116.1). Advances in immunosuppression, organ preservation, and surgical techniques have improved overall 1-year survival to about 85% and 5-year survival to 75% or greater. Patients with certain indications, such as those with primary biliary cirrhosis, do particularly well, with 10-year survival rates of 80-90%. Excellent quality of life, return to work, and a productive lifestyle should be expected. The current shortage of donor organs fuels current controversies regarding the appropriateness of certain indications such as hepatocellular carcinoma and alcoholic liver disease. Recurrence of hepatitis C and hepatitis B is almost universal but can be managed in most patients.

**TABLE 116.1. Common Indications for Liver Transplantation**

| |
|---|
| Hepatitis C cirrhosis |
| Alcoholic cirrhosis |
| Hepatitis B cirrhosis |
| Primary biliary cirrhosis |
| Primary sclerosing cholangitis |
| Fulminant hepatic failure |
| Wilson disease |
| Budd-Chiari syndrome |
| Autoimmune hepatitis |
| Hepatocellular carcinoma |
| $\alpha_1$-antitrypsin deficiency |

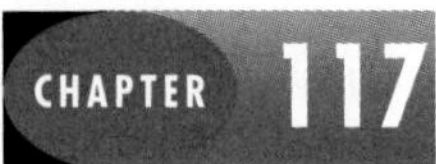

# CHAPTER 117 FIBROCYSTIC DISEASES OF THE LIVER AND BILIARY TREE

Fibrocystic diseases of the liver include autosomal dominant polycystic kidney disease (ADPKD), solitary hepatic cysts, biliary cystadenomas, congenital hepatic fibrosis, choledochal cysts, and Caroli disease. The latter four entities communicate with the biliary tree and are susceptible to cholangitis. Congenital hepatic fibrosis is a rare autosomal recessive disorder characterized by fibrotic enlargement of the portal tracts, portal hypertension, and association with autosomal recessive polycystic kidney disease, ADPKD, and Caroli disease. Caroli disease is a rare developmental malformation of the intrahepatic biliary tree with cystic dilatations separated by relatively normal intervening bile ducts. Recurrent cholangitis, portal hypertension, and cholangiocarcinoma may complicate Caroli disease.

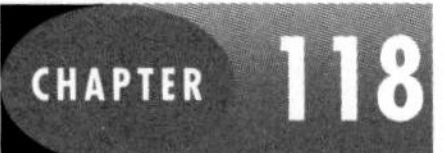

# CHAPTER 118 DISEASES OF THE GALLBLADDER AND BILIARY TRACT

## Cholestasis

Cholestasis is defined as impaired bile formation and flow. The anatomic location of the abnormality resulting in cholestasis varies, with anywhere from the interior of the liver cell to the duodenum being possible. Mechanical obstruction is a common cause of cholestasis; however, cholestasis does not necessarily mean mechanical obstruction. Isolated hyperbilirubinemia in the absence of liver dysfunction results from interference with the transport and metabolism of bilirubin within hepatocytes (Table 118.1).

Cholestasis classically has been divided into intra- and extrahepatic forms, based on the anatomic location of impairment of bile flow (Table 118.2). A more detailed conceptual scheme classifies cholestasis according to more specific sites, as follows:

1. **Intrahepatic cholestasis** at the hepatocellular level (e.g., cholestatic forms of alcoholic hepatitis and viral hepatitis, cholestasis caused by drugs such as chlorpromazine and sulfonamides)
2. **Cholestasis due to lesions at the bile canalicular membrane** (e.g., cholestasis caused by sex hormones, cholestasis occasionally seen with Hodgkin disease, the cholestatic jaundice of pregnancy in the third trimester, and the unusual syndrome known as benign recurrent intrahepatic cholestasis
3. **Cholestasis due to lesions of the interlobular bile ducts,** which includes that due to primary biliary cirrhosis, primary sclerosing cholangitis, sarcoidosis of the liver, allograft rejection, and graft-versus-host disease
4. **Cholestasis due to obstructing lesions of the extrahepatic bile ducts,** including that caused by choledocholithiasis, cholangiocarcinoma, benign strictures, primary sclerosing cholangitis, choledochal cysts, and stenosis of the distal common bile duct due to pancreatic tumor or inflammation.

## Histopathology of the Liver

Many histologic features in the liver are common to cholestasis, regardless of the cause. Bile stasis is most prominent in the centrilobular regions, with only minimal

**TABLE 118.1. Hyperbilirubinemic Syndromes**

| Characteristic | Gilbert's | Crigler-Najjar | Dubin-Johnson |
|---|---|---|---|
| Prevalence | 5% of population | Very rare | Rare |
| Bilirubin type | Unconjugated | Unconjugated | Conjugated |
| Age of onset | Young adult | Infant | Adult |
| Inheritance | Autosomal dominant | Autosomal recessive | Autosomal dominant |
| Mechanism | Uptake, conjugation | Conjugation | Canalicular secretion |
| Outcome | Harmless | Kernicterus/death<br>Liver transplant | Harmless |

cellular necrosis and foci of mononuclear cells. In prolonged cholestasis, portal fibrosis and round cell infiltration develop, with fibrous strands connecting adjacent portal tracts, plus ductal proliferation. With further prolonged cholestasis, portal fibrosis becomes more extensive, with septa developing between portal tracts and hepatic veins, followed by nodular regeneration and the picture of secondary biliary cirrhosis. Grossly, the liver is enlarged, green, and nodular.

## Clinical Features

Common symptoms of cholestasis are jaundice and pruritus, which may precede jaundice. Hyperlipidemia, xanthomas, and xanthelasmas may follow long-standing cholestasis. Other features of cholestasis include acholic stools, owing to the lack of bile reaching the duodenum; steatorrhea due to the absence of bile acids in the small bowel; dark urine due to bilirubinuria; osteomalacia and osteoporosis, probably due to several factors, such as impaired vitamin D and calcium absorption from the gut; easy bruising or hemorrhage due to vitamin K malabsorption in the liver; and excoriations from scratching.

**TABLE 118.2. Etiology of Cholestasis**

- Intrahepatic
  - Primary biliary cirrhosis
  - Primary sclerosing cholangitis
  - Drug-induced
  - Pregnancy
  - Sarcoidosis
  - Sepsis
- Extrahepatic
  - Common bile duct obstruction
    - Stone
    - Stricture
    - Carcinoma
    - Choledochal cyst
    - Primary sclerosing cholangitis
  - Pancreas
    - Pancreatitis
    - Pseudocyst
    - Carcinoma

## Laboratory Features

Some degree of conjugated hyperbilirubinemia is usually present in cholestasis (see Table 118.2). With complete bile duct obstruction, serum bilirubin rises to 15 to 20 mg/dl but then stabilizes due to extrahepatic bilirubin disposal mechanisms. Serum alkaline phosphatase usually rises more than threefold, due to increased synthesis in the obstructed liver. Often, a unique lipoprotein X, thought to be a low-density lipoprotein, appears in the serum. Serum bile acids are the most sensitive indicator of cholestasis, because their concentration rises in all forms of cholestasis even before jaundice appears.

## Diagnosis and Management

Important elements in the history include fever, chills, pain, and colic, suggesting mechanical obstruction and cholangitis; current and recent drug use (e.g., oral contraceptives, phenothiazines); weight loss; prior abdominal or biliary tract surgery; prior diseases clinically associated with cholestasis; and family history. The examination should include careful palpation of the liver and spleen, and a search for an enlarged, palpable gallbladder (Courvoisier's sign), lymph nodes, and xanthomas. The first imaging procedure in cholestasis usually is an ultrasound or CT, performed to answer the critical question, "*Is there dilation of the intra- or extrahepatic bile ducts?*" The advantages of these imaging methods are shown in Table 118.3. If the biliary tree appears dilated, then direct cholangiography is indicated, usually through endoscopic retrograde cholangiopancreatography (ERCP), because it offers expanded therapeutic options, such as the ability to do sphincterotomy (severing the muscle fibers of the sphincter of Oddi in order to enlarge the outlet of the biliary tree into the duodenum), extract gallstones, or dilate strictures or place stents over mechanically obstructing mass lesions. Magnetic resonance cholangio-pancreatico graph (MRCP) is now replacing the need to do diagnostic ERCP.

**TABLE 118.3. Diagnosis of Cholestasis: Computed Tomography vs. Ultrasound Examination**

| Procedure | Advantages | Disadvantages |
|---|---|---|
| Ultrasound | Better at detecting gallstones in the gallbladder | Only uncommonly detects gallstones in the common bile duct |
| | Accurately measures diameter of common bile duct | Less than optimal visualization of pancreatic tumor, cyst, etc. |
| Computed tomography | Better visualization of pancreas | Poor sensitivity for detecting gallstones within gallbladder or common bile duct |

If the initial imaging examinations fail to demonstrate bile duct dilation, a needle biopsy of the liver needs to be considered. Biopsy is indicated if the clinical picture strongly supports alcoholic hepatitis, drug-induced cholestasis, or autoimmune disease of the liver.

## Gallstones

Bile contains three lipid polar amphipaths: cholesterol, lecithin, and bile acids. Cholesterol, with only one hydroxyl group, is practically insoluble in water; lecithin can interact with water and forms liquid crystalline complexes; bile acids have a major hydrophilic side and thus have detergent properties and form micelles (Figure 118.1). Bile acids in water form micelles and incorporate lecithin, greatly increasing the capacity to incorporate cholesterol in the hydrophobic interior of the micelle.

Several methods have been devised for expressing the solubility relationships of the three biliary lipids. They illustrate that the solubility of cholesterol is finite and that bile with insufficient bile acids and lecithin to dissolve all the cholesterol in micellar solution is supersaturated with cholesterol. Such bile is termed *lithogenic*, in that it fosters cholesterol nucleation and crystal formation, leading to crystal growth and gallstone formation. Patients with cholesterol gallstones have been shown to have lithogenic bile. Either the biliary level of solubilizing lipids is decreased (diminished hepatic bile acid secretion, a smaller bile acid pool, excess loss of bile acids in stool due to terminal ileal disease, or use of bile acid binders) or there is increased secretion of cholesterol (from increased activity of HMGCoA reductase, or diminished activity of 7-hydroxylase).

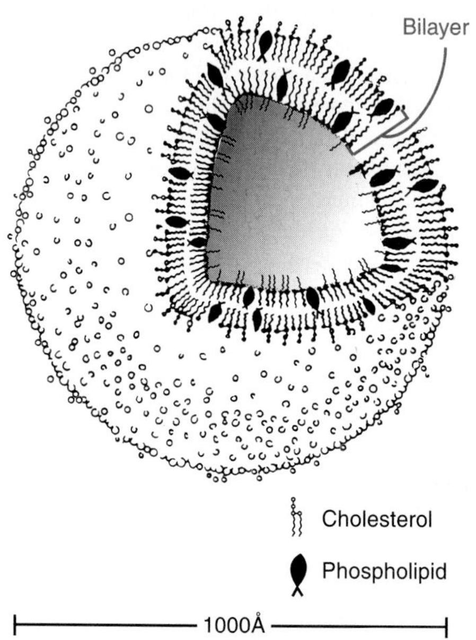


**FIGURE 118.1. Biliary unilamellar vesicle.**
(From: Sleisenger M, Fordtran J. Gastrointestinal Disease. Pathophysiology, Diagnosis, Management, 4th ed. Philadelphia: W.B. Saunders, 1989. Used with permission.)

**TABLE 118.4. Risk Factors for Gallstones**

| |
|---|
| Age |
| Feminine gender |
| Caucasian race |
| Obesity |
| Diabetes mellitus |
| Rapid weight loss |
| Chronic oral contraceptive or estrogen use |
| Terminal ileal disease (e.g., Crohn's disease) |
| Bile salt sequestrants (e.g., Cholestyramine) |

Gallstone disease afflicts 10% of Americans; its incidence increases with age, with nearly one third of elderly persons having gallstones. They are more prevalent in women (Table 118.4). In the United States and most Western countries, cholesterol gallstones predominate; bile pigment stones account for about 20% of all gallstones. Pigment stones contain less than 25% cholesterol, appear as dark or black calculi, are radiopaque, and are seen in chronic hemolytic states, cirrhosis, and chronically obstructed bile ducts, such as those due to benign strictures. Pigment stones predominate in the tropics and the Orient. The association of gallstones with pregnancy remains inconclusive.

### Natural History of Gallstones

Most gallstones are asymptomatic; most are detected incidentally during ultrasound examination of the abdomen. In patients with asymptomatic gallstones, the cumulative probability of symptoms developing is about 10% at 5 years and no greater than 20% at 15 to 20 years. In most patients, biliary symptoms precede the onset of complications. Thus, cholecystectomy is not indicated in the asymptomatic patient. Some gallstones become symptomatic, but the mechanisms are unclear (Figure 118.2). Abdominal pain usually follows impaction of a gallstone or gallstones at the cystic duct (acute cholecystitis and chronic cholecystitis) or their migration through the cystic duct and impaction within the common bile duct (choledocholithiasis). Common bile duct stones are particularly dangerous, because they may evoke gallstone pancreatitis and bacterial cholangitis. Symptoms from gallstones, albeit episodic, have a high rate of recurrence. Thus, once gallstones evoke symptoms, cholecystectomy is recommended, even though symptoms may be absent at the time of surgery. Finally, in a small group of patients, the gallstone disease is "complicated" by pancreatitis, fistula formation, gallstone ileus, cholangitis, or liver abscess. These patients clearly mandate therapy for ongoing active disease.

## Diagnosis

Only 10% of gallstones, mostly pigment stones, are radiopaque. Some are lucent but have calcium rings near the surface. Oral cholecystography (Figure 118.3) identifies most gallstones, but a successful study requires reliable ingestion and normal absorption of the contrast medium, a healthy liver, and a patent cystic duct. Ultrasound (Figure 118.4), a highly reliable and accurate imaging technique for identifying gallstones, has replaced oral cholecystography for this purpose. Common duct and gallbladder stones also may be identified by MRCP and ERCP.

## Management

The patient's age and concomitant health problems weigh heavily in the decision on appropriate therapy. Cholecystectomy remains the most effective treatment for cholelithiasis. The most significant advance in surgical techniques for gallstones in recent years has been the revolutionary development of the laparoscopic technique for cholecystectomy. This technique, which has become the preferred method for cholecystectomy worldwide, permits a cholecystectomy to be performed safely and effectively using instruments that are introduced into the abdomen through a few stab punctures. Consequently, a formal laparotomy is avoided and the recovery time is greatly curtailed.

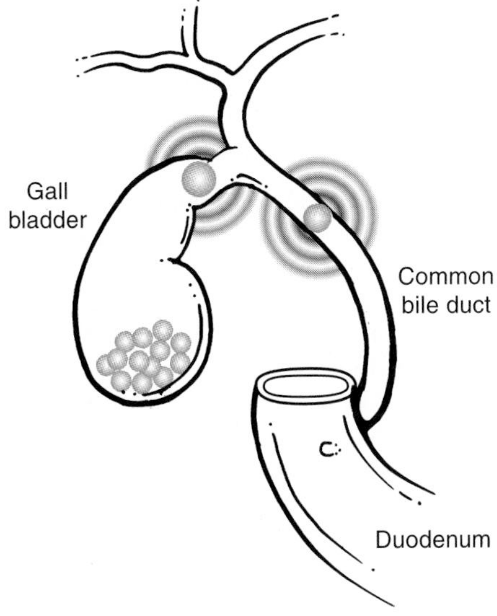


FIGURE 118.2. Symptomatic gallstone.

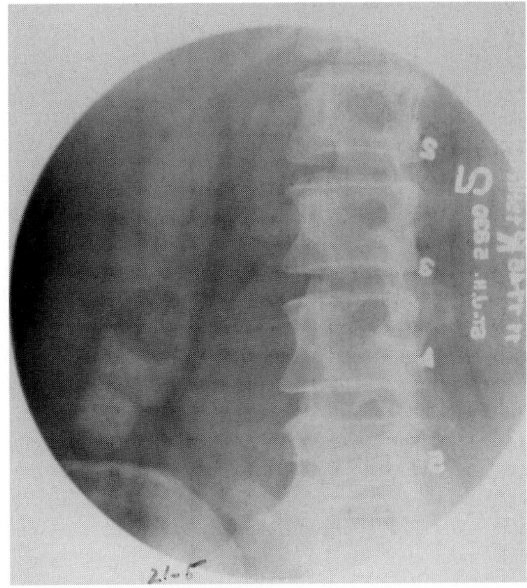

FIGURE 118.3. Oral cholecystogram showing opacification of the gallbladder, which contains gallstones.

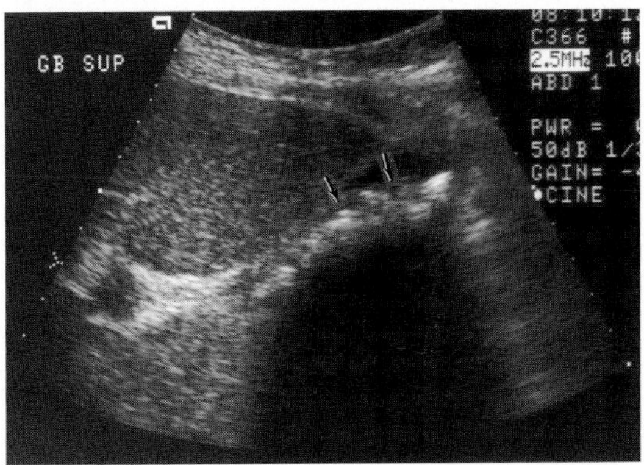


FIGURE 118.4. Ultrasonogram showing gallstones (arrow).

A great deal of research has gone into the use of oral medications to dissolve gallstones, based on the premise that patients with cholesterol gallstones who have a small bile acid pool could expand it with oral use of bile acids to produce unsaturated bile. Two agents, chenodeoxycholic acid and ursodeoxycholic acid, have been approved for this indication. A functioning gallbladder, radiolucent stones, and a patent biliary tract are prerequisites for their use. With optimum dosages, only 30% to 50% of this select group show complete stone dissolution, however; even after dissolution, there is significant recurrence.

## Acute Cholecystitis

Most instances of acute cholecystitis result from impaction of a gallstone in the cystic duct. The classical attack is discrete, comes on rather suddenly, often at night, and lasts hours to days. There may be history of similar episodes in the past. The patient usually reports epigastric pain, generally unrelated to movements or respiration, and, often, nausea and vomiting. Later, the pain commonly shifts and localizes in the right upper quadrant; it may radiate to the shoulder and the right scapular area. Tenderness to palpation (Murphy's sign) and signs of peritoneal irritation are noted. Fever and leukocytosis are common. There may be the impression of a tender mass in the right subcostal area.

The diagnosis depends largely on the history and physical findings. Cholecystitis may simulate perforation or penetration of peptic ulcer, myocardial infarction, acute pancreatitis, pneumonia, hepatitis and acute right-sided pyelonephritis. Ultrasonography accurately detects cholelithiasis and gallbladder wall edema. The hepatic dimethyl imino-diacetic acid (HIDA) scan, in which, following IV administration, the radiopharmaceutical is taken up by hepatocytes and excreted into the biliary tree, which may be imaged, also is useful in this setting. With an obstructed cystic duct, no radioactivity is noted in the gallbladder (i.e., positive HIDA scan).

Hospitalization is required for pain relief and IV fluids, and surgical consultation. Cholecystectomy usually is performed during the same admission. Cultures of the gallbladder and bile are positive in at least one half of patients with acute cholecystitis at surgery. The most common organisms are aerobic coliforms, streptococci, clostridia, and bacteroides. Therefore, fever or leukocytosis mandates antibiotics.

## Other Types of Cholecystitis

Some patients have recurrent attacks of mild to severe acute cholecystitis. Almost all have gallstones and require cholecystectomy. Many others with gallstones may experience vague symptoms without such attacks. Chronic cholecystitis could be present in such a setting, and cholecystectomy should be given careful consideration.

Acalculous cholecystitis occurs in the absence of gallstones. Gallbladder ischemia is believed to be responsible, causing inflammation and secondary infection. It is seen largely in older persons with recent trauma or recent surgery or with vasculitis on corticosteroid therapy. It has been reported in patients with AIDS and with *Cryptosporidium* spp infection of the biliary tract. The clinical presentation is the same as for acute cholecystitis. Ultrasound examination often shows an inflamed gallbladder wall with sludge but no stones. The HIDA scan is positive, and these patients require urgent surgery.

## Choledocholithiasis

In Asian and African countries, calcium bilirubinate stones predominate; these appear to arise, not only in the gallbladder, but also primarily in intra- and extrahepatic portions of the biliary tract. Bile duct stones produce biliary colic with nausea and vomiting. A common bile duct stone may acutely obstruct the common bile duct with jaundice and liver enzyme elevations or acute pancreatitis. However, 20% of patients with bile duct stones have no pain, and 25% to 30% of patients have no jaundice.

### Diagnosis and Management

Elevated serum alkaline phosphatase and mild hyperbilirubinemia are the most characteristic abnormalities. The former may occur without pain, jaundice, or other symptoms. Common bile duct stones with acute bacterial cholangitis cause spiking fever and a picture of sepsis. With acute pancreatitis, abdominal pain is more epigastric and radiates to the back. Leukocytosis is common; bacteremia due to enteric organisms may occur. Plain abdominal radiographs may show an ileus and, uncommonly, gallbladder stones. Ultrasonography usually shows biliary tract dilation, but this finding may be absent.

Symptomatic common duct stones should be treated with antibiotics, analgesics, and IV fluids. As soon as the patient has been stabilized, ERCP should follow, to establish a diagnosis and to extract the gallstones. Following recovery, the patient should also undergo a laparoscopic cholecystectomy. If the common bile duct stones cannot be removed by endoscopy, then open cholecystectomy and common bile duct exploration are required.

## Internal Biliary Fistulae

Biliary-enteric fistulae may form due to chronic inflammation from long-standing cholelithiasis, adhesions of the duodenum, or hepatic flexure at the gallbladder. This condition has no characteristic clinical picture, but patients may report symptoms of biliary colic or chronic cholecystitis and sometimes have associated cholangitis. A plain abdominal radiograph may reveal air in the biliary tree (pneumobilia). Gallstone ileus may follow erosion of a gallstone into the intestinal tract with mechanical obstruction, most commonly in the terminal ileum.

## Benign Stricture of the Bile Ducts

Benign strictures arise in the common bile duct from operative trauma at the time of biliary tract surgery, choledocholithiasis, or chronic pancreatitis. Jaundice insidiously develops a few weeks or months following surgery, often with abdominal pain, fever, chills, and pruritus. Bile pigment stones may form above the stricture in more chronic cases. Unrelieved obstruction leads to secondary biliary cirrhosis and bacteremia and hepatic abscess. Liver tests show variable but chronic cholestasis. Ultrasonography shows dilation of the bile ducts above the stricture, and ERCP accurately defines the biliary anatomy. Until recently, surgery to bypass the stricture was the only treatment available. Recent advances allow the passage of stents, and balloon dilation of strictures to relieve obstruction and cholestasis without surgery. Primary sclerosing cholangitis, ischemia (e.g., post–liver transplant), radiation, and cholangitis are other rare causes of strictures of the bile ducts.

# CHAPTER 119 NEOPLASMS OF THE BILIARY TREE

## Carcinoma of the Bile Ducts

Carcinoma arising from the intrahepatic ducts *(cholangiocarcinoma)* may mimic hepatocellular carcinoma. Chronic biliary tract disease resulting from primary sclerosing cholangitis, sclerosing cholangitis due to chronic *Clonorchis* spp infection, and Caroli disease are its predisposing factors. Cirrhosis itself may be a risk factor for cholangiocarcinoma, but this association is not as strong as that for hepatocellular carcinoma. The diagnosis and management are essentially the same as for hepatocellular carcinoma.

A common site for bile duct carcinoma is the junction of the right and left main hepatic ducts at the porta hepatis; it may extend locally into the liver, a condition named *Klatskin tumor.* Slow and insidious growth at this site produces a gradually evolving clinical picture of cholestasis that mimics a nonneoplastic cholestatic disorder. A collapsed gallbladder and dilation of the intrahepatic bile ducts as detected by ultrasonography and confirmed by cholangiography usually establish a diagnosis.

Primary common bile duct cancers may be polypoid but more commonly are scirrhous and produce a stricture that may simulate a benign stricture or sclerosing cholangitis. Jaundice and pruritus are the most common presenting features. There usually is no significant pain, and secondary bacterial cholangitis is uncommon. The liver usually is enlarged and rounded. A nontender, enlarged, palpable gallbladder is a useful sign of malignant biliary obstruction (Courvoisier's sign). Laboratory findings are those of cholestasis; diagnosis is best established by cholangiography.

Because these cancers rarely can be cured by surgery, the nonoperative management of bile duct cancer, using endoscopically placed stents over the obstructing lesions, has become increasingly important. Relief from jaundice and pruritus, and improved quality of life, follow endoscopic stenting techniques. No effective chemotherapy has evolved thus far for biliary tract cancer.

## Questions

**Instructions:** For questions 1 through 4 below, select only **one** lettered answer that is the **best** for that question.

1. A 45-year-old alcoholic man with known cirrhosis but no prior history of variceal bleeding is admitted because of hematemesis. His platelet count is 33,000, and the INR is 2.31. He appears malnourished and has an albumin of 1.9.

   All of the following are appropriate management measures for this patient except:

   A. Urgent upper endoscopy
   B. Intravenous octreotide
   C. Intravenous propranolol
   D. Subcutaneous vitamin K
   E. Administration of fresh frozen plasma

2. In a patient with new-onset ascites, fluid analysis should **routinely** be performed for all of the following except:

   A. Amylase
   B. Albumin
   C. Total protein
   D. Cell count
   E. Gram stain and culture

3. A 42-year-old woman with known hepatitis C and ascites is referred for evaluation and treatment. She has never experienced encephalopathy or variceal bleeding. Initial results of ascitic fluid analysis are as follows: WBC 890/mm$^3$; 7% PMN, 82% monos, 6% Lymphs; albumin 1.1 g/dl (serum albumin 2.9 g/dl); total protein 1.7; Gram stain negative; cytology negative; amylase 22.

   Which one of the following is appropriate?

   A. Intravenous cefotaxime
   B. Initiation of α-interferon and ribavirin therapy

C. Referral for liver transplantation
D. Upper endoscopy to evaluate for presence of esophageal varices
E. TIPS placement

4. All of the following conditions are at high risk for development of malignancy except:
   A. Wilson disease
   B. Hereditary hemochromatosis
   C. Primary sclerosing cholangitis
   D. Hepatitis B infection
   E. Hepatitis C infection

**Instructions:** For questions 5-9, match any of the following scenarios with the most appropriate diagnostic test:

A. Cholangiography
B. C282Y/H63D mutation
C. Serum p-ANCA
D. Serum anti-mitochondrial antibody (AMA)
E. Serum anti-nuclear antibody (ANA)
F. Ceruloplasmin
G. $\alpha_1$-antitrypsin level

5. A 19-year-old man presents with fulminant hepatic failure, anemia, and acidosis.

6. A 35-year-old man with a history of intermittent bloody diarrhea presents with fever, right upper quadrant pain, and elevated liver enzymes.

7. A 22-year-old woman with hypothyroidism presents with fatigue and markedly elevated aminotransferases.

8. A 40-year-old man presents with stigmata of chronic liver disease, a history of social alcohol use, and new-onset diabetes.

9. A 48-year-old woman presents with pruritus and fatigue and is found to have an elevated alkaline phosphatase.

## Answers

| | | | | |
|---|---|---|---|---|
| 1. C | 2. A | 3. D | 4. A | 5. F |
| 6. A | 7. E | 8. B | 9. D | |

## SUGGESTED READING


### *Textbooks*

O'Grady JG, Lake JR, Howdle PD (eds). Comprehensive Clinical Hepatology. London: Mosby, 2000.

Schiff ER, Sorrell MR, Maddrey WC (eds). Schiff's Diseases of the Liver. 8th ed. Philadelphia: Lippincott-Raven, 1999.

Zakim D, Boyer T. Hepatology: A Textbook of Liver Disease. 2nd ed. Philadelphia: WB Saunders, 1997.

### *Articles*

*Laboratory and Clinical Evaluation*

Cattau EL, et al. The accuracy of the physical examination in the diagnosis of suspected ascites. JAMA 1982;247:1146.

Desmet VJ, Gerbert M, Hoofnagle JH, Manns M, Scheuer PJ. Classification of chronic hepatitis: diagnosis, grading and staging. Hepatology 1994;19:1513-1520.

Friedman LS. Elevated aminotransferase levels as an incidental finding: Differential diagnosis. Gastrointestinal Diseases Today 1997;6:10-17.

Moseley RH. Evaluation of abnormal liver function tests. Med Clin North Am 1996;80:887-906.

Pratt DS, Kaplan MM. Evaluation of abnormal liver enzyme results in asymptomatic patients. N Engl J Med 2000;342: 1266-1271.

*Viral Hepatitis*

Fattovich G, Giustina G, Degos F, et al. Morbidity and mortality in compensated cirrhosis type C: a retrospective follow-up study of 384 patients. Gastroenterology 1997;112:463-472.

Lee WM. Hepatitis B virus infection. N Engl J Med 1997;337: 1733-1745.

Lemon SM, Thomas DL. Vaccines to prevent viral hepatitis. N Engl J Med 1997;336:196-204.

McHutchison JG, Gordon SC, Schiff ER, et al. Interferon alfa-2b alone or in combination with ribavirin as initial treatment for chronic hepatitis C. Hepatitis Interventional Therapy Group. N Engl J Med 1998;339:1485-1492.

Proceedings of the National Institute of Health Consensus Development Conference on the Management of Hepatitis C. Hepatology 1997;26[Supplement 1].

*Autoimmune Hepatitis and Cholestatic Liver Disease*

Franco J, Saeian K. Biliary tract inflammatory disorders: Primary sclerosing cholangitis and primary biliary cirrhosis. Current Gastroenterology Reports 1999;1:95-101.

Johnson PJ, McFarlane IG. Meeting report of the International Autoimmune Hepatitis Group. Hepatology 1993;18:998-1005.

Kaplan MM. Primary biliary cirrhosis. N Engl J Med 1996;335: 1570-1580.

*Alcoholic, Fulminant, and Drug-induced Liver Disease*

Diehl AM. Alcoholic liver disease: natural history. Liver Transpl Surg 1997;3:206-211.

Lee WM. Drug-induced hepatotoxicity. N Engl J Med 1995; 333:1118-1127.

Mas A, Rodes J. Seminar: fulminant hepatic failure. Lancet 1997;349:1081-1085.

Morgan MY. The treatment of alcoholic hepatitis. Alcohol 1996;311:117-134.

*Metabolic Liver Disease*

Bacon BR, Olynyk JK, Brunt EM, et al. HFE genotype in patients with hemochromatosis and other liver diseases. Ann Intern Med 1999;130:953-962.

Sheth SG, Gordon FD, Chopra S. Nonalcoholic steatohepatitis. Ann Intern Med 1997;126:137-145.

*Cirrhosis and Complications*

Arroyo V, Gines P, Gerbes A, et al. Definition and diagnostic criteria of refractory ascites and hepatorenal syndrome in cirrhosis. Hepatology 1996;23:164-176.

Cello JP, Ring EJ, Olcott EW, et al. Endoscopic sclerotherapy compared with percutaneous transjugular intrahepatic portosystemic shunt after initial sclerotherapy in patients with acute variceal hemorrhage: a randomized, controlled trial. Ann Intern Med 1997;126:858-865.

Cordoba J, Blei AT. Treatment of hepatic encephalopathy. Am J Gastroenterol 1997;92:1429-39.

D'Amico G, Pagliaro L, Bosch J. The treatment of portal hypertension: a meta-analytic review. Hepatology 1995;22: 332-354.

Garcia-Tsao G. Treatment of spontaneous bacterial peritonitis with oral ofloxacin: inpatient or outpatient therapy? Gastroenterology 1996;11:1147-1150.

Krowka MJ, Porayko MK, Plevak DJ, et al. Hepatopulmonary syndrome with progressive hypoxemia as an indication for liver transplantation: case reports and literature review. Mayo Clin Proc 1997;72:44-53.

Runyon BA, Montano AA, Akriviadis EA, et al. The serum-ascites albumin gradient is superior to the exudate-transudate concept in the differential diagnosis of ascites. Ann Intern Med 1992;117:215-220.

*Tumors of the Liver*

Bruix J. Treatment of hepatocellular carcinoma. Hepatology 1997;25:259-262.

Reddy KR, Schiff ER. Approach to a liver mass. Semin Liver Dis 1993;43:423-435.

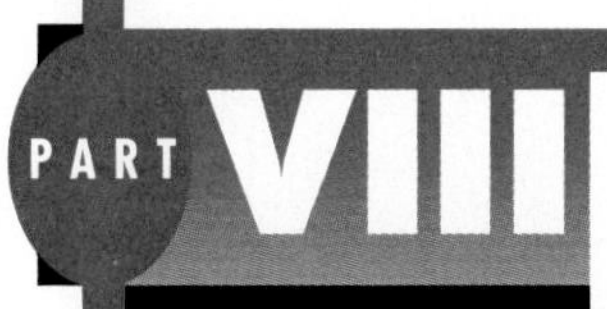
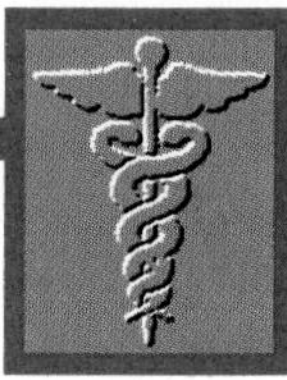

# PART VIII GERIATRIC MEDICINE

Mary E. Cohan
Edmund H. Duthie, Jr.

# CHAPTER 120 AGING PROCESS

Aging refers to the physiological changes that occur in living beings with the passing of time. The aging process, the subject of a number of theories based on empirical evidence, is not yet completely understood. Programmed cellular senescence, free radicals, and random gene mutation have all been proposed as causes of aging. The ability to recognize and distinguish normal aging processes from disease processes is important in the clinical treatment of older patients.

The U.S. population older than age 65 has increased dramatically since the beginning of the twentieth century. Life expectancy is the average number of years of expected life remaining from birth or a stated age. Since 1900, life expectancy at birth has dramatically increased in the United States for both men and women and for all races. During the same period—most remarkably since 1980—mortality rates have declined among older persons. Death rates from both cardiovascular disease and cerebrovascular disease—two of the foremost killers of the aged— also have been declining. As a result, the number of elderly people has increased dramatically, creating challenges in health care, the political arena, and the economy that have yet to be met.

A thorough knowledge of gerontology and geriatric medicine is essential for the physician of the future. Older persons currently occupy approximately one third of U.S. hospital beds and more than 90% of nursing home beds. (The latter now outnumber acute care hospital beds.) Although they constitute only 12% of the U.S. population, elderly persons account for one third to one half of an internist's encounter time with patients. Public expenditures for the elderly—Social Security, Medicare, and Medicaid—are rising, and major changes in reimbursement systems and practice styles have occurred as a consequence. Certainly, these costs will escalate as the number of older persons steadily increases through this century.

Age itself is less important than the influence of concomitant disease processes and physiologic parameters in predicting outcomes in older patients. Careful attention to physiologic organ reserve and the principles of functional assessment and multidisciplinary care enhance the treatment of older patients and optimize outcomes.

# CHAPTER 121 CLINICAL APPROACH TO THE ELDERLY PATIENT

## Bedside Techniques

The fundamental skills of history taking—with some modification—are basic to accurate diagnosis and promotion of well-being in the elderly. Traditional teaching requires assessment of the patient's reliability as a historian; this assessment is especially necessary with older patients because of the increased prevalence of delirium and dementia in this population. Thus, some type of mental status examination should be administered formally to elderly patients. Questionnaires and other aids help the practitioner perform a complete assessment within a reasonable period of time (e.g., the Short Portable Mental Status Questionnaire, shown in Table 121.1). Sensory deficits, pain, illiteracy, nonorganic mental illness, poor motivation, and aphasia may all interfere with the interpretation of such test results.

Multiplicity of problems is almost the rule in elderly persons. It is estimated that 85% of persons age 65 and older are afflicted with at least one chronic illness; among nursing home patients an average of five or six illnesses is quite common. The physician must consider these factors and expect multiple and complex problems, especially in the frail or dependent elderly person. The principle of economy of diagnosis (i.e., attempting to explain a patient's signs and symptoms with one unifying hypothesis) has less applicability in the aged. Identifying problems and addressing each with an appropriate treatment plan are challenging clinical activities. The clinician must give highest priority to acute conditions and those chronic conditions that most adversely affect the patient's functioning.

The elderly patient may have communication difficulties; the physician must allow more time to take a history and also develop strategies to deal with common communication problems. Patients with hearing and eyesight impairments should be urged to bring their hearing aids and eyeglasses to the visit. Patients with obvious hearing difficulties should be given an otoscopic

**TABLE 121.1.**

Short Portable Mental Status Questionnaire (SPMSQ)
Eric Pfeiffer, M.D.

Instructions: Ask questions 1–10 in this list and record all answers. Ask question 4A only if patient does not have a telephone. Record total number of errors based on ten questions.

| ↓/– | |
|---|---|
| | 1. What is the date today? ______ Month ______ Day ______ Year |
| | 2. What day of the week is it? ______ |
| | 3. What is the name of this place? ______ |
| | 4. What is your telephone number? ______ |
| | 4A. What is your street address? ______ (Ask only if patient does not have a telephone) |
| | 5. How old are you? ______ |
| | 6. When were you born? ______ |
| | 7. Who is the President of the U.S. now? ______ |
| | 8. Who was President just before him? ______ |
| | 9. What was your mother's maiden name? ______ |
| | 10. Subtract 3 from 20 and keep subtracting 3 from each new number, all the way down. |
| ______ | Total Number of Errors |

0–2 errors = intact
3–4 errors = mild intellectual impairment
5–7 errors = moderate intellectual impairment
8–10 errors = severe intellectual impairment

To Be Completed by Interviewer

Patient's Name: ______ Date: ______

Sex: 1. Male
2. Female

Race: 1. White
2. Black
3. Other

Years of Education: ______
1. Grade School
2. High School
3. Beyond High School

Interviewer's Name: ______

**TABLE 121.2. Geriatric System Review: Special Issues**

| | |
|---|---|
| Sensory function | Falls |
| Sexuality | Constipation |
| Incontinence | Nutrition |
| Dental health | Depression |

examination and cerumen disimpaction if needed. Hearing-impaired persons function much better in quiet surroundings. The physician should face the patient at eye level in a well-lit room and speak at a reasonable pace. Yelling into the patient's ear is ineffective and should be avoided. Hearing-impaired patients depend on visual cues; their eyeglasses must be put on before the interview begins and must be worn throughout the interview. When interviewing aphasic persons, it may be best to use questions that require a simple "yes" or "no" response.

Taking a history of the present illness proceeds as it might for any other patient. However, presentations of acute illnesses or exacerbations of chronic conditions differ in the elderly patient compared to the young. For example, myocardial infarction may be painless and present with signs or symptoms of heart failure; dyspnea caused by exertion may represent an anginal equivalent; a fall may presage a serious infection or represent a cardiac arrhythmia or stroke. Such lists of atypical presentations are almost endless, and texts of geriatric medicine are replete with them.

Obtaining a history of medication use in the aged person is critically important. Significant morbidity in this population results from drug side effects and interactions. Patients must be instructed to bring all their medications to the interview. Many elderly patients see more than one physician (e.g., internist, ophthalmologist, urologist, or dermatologist), with each prescribing a drug or two, and often not mindful of some of the other agents being prescribed. Elderly persons also commonly use over-the-counter preparations (e.g., vitamins, herbal supplements, antacids, laxatives, and aspirin), which may cause side effects that necessitate medical attention. Over-the-counter agents and herbal supplements may also complicate an established treatment plan.

The review of systems in an elderly patient should highlight a few areas, as listed in Table 121.2.

## Functional Assessment and the Team

Determining functional ability is a critical element in the assessment of the aged patient. In contrast to the younger patient, disability in the elderly patient may be multifactorial, owing to multiple illnesses. In the frail or dependent elderly person, the interplay of multiple and complex illnesses creates the need for teamwork. The goal of the geriatric health care team is to provide the elderly patient with the highest level of function in the least restrictive environment. For elderly patients, the emphasis often is on quality of life rather than on life prolongation. Dependent elderly persons are stressed not only biologically, but psychologically and socially as well. For optimal patient care, the physician must work closely with colleagues in nursing, social work, dietetics, dentistry, pharmacy, rehabilitation, psychology-psychiatry, podiatry, and chaplaincy. It is important for such interdisciplinary teams to be able to clearly identify groups of patients who will benefit maximally from a team approach so that resources are expended optimally. Discharge planning teams in many hospitals also involve the physician in optimizing the disposition and treatment plan.

The term *activities of daily living (ADL)* refers to those practical dimensions required for patients to function daily. In elderly persons, the decline and recovery of physical function in response to diseases occur in a sequential manner, regardless of their cause. Bathing, dressing, using the toilet, transferring, and feeding abilities are lost in that order during decline and regained in the reverse order during recovery. Many scales and instruments are available to help assess the ADL domains. One popular scale helps describe components by a simple mnemonic, "CADET" (Table 121.3). ADL also may be measured by many other tools; the Eastern Cooperative Oncology Group (ECOG) scale or the Karnofsky scale (Table 121.4), both widely used in oncology, can be applied to the elderly patient to assess the global disability caused by multiple, chronic illnesses.

Higher functioning levels have been described as the *instrumental* activities of daily living (IADLs). The IADLs include cooking, cleaning, doing laundry, shopping, using the telephone, handling finances, and managing transportation. Function is best assessed by directly observing the patient performing the tasks. Because direct observation is not always possible, obtaining the information from the patient or a caregiver often is necessary. The physician should assess these domains in each elderly patient evaluated. If screening reveals deficits, a physiatrist, occupational therapist, speech therapist, audiologist, or physical therapist can assist in defining the problem more accurately and instituting treatment.

**TABLE 121.3. The CADET Functional Assessment**

**C:** Communication
**A:** Ambulation
**D:** Dressing
**E:** Eating
**T:** Toileting

**TABLE 121.4. Performance Status Scale: Eastern Co-operative Oncology Group (ECOG) Compared to Karnofsky Scale**

| ECOG Scale | Karnofsky Scale |
|---|---|
| 0 Asymptomatic | 100 Asymptomatic |
| 1 Symptomatic, fully ambulatory | 90 Normal activity, minor signs or symptoms<br>80 Normal activity with effort |
| 2 Less than fully ambulatory, but in bed less than 50% of each day | 70 Cares for self, unable to carry on normal activity or work<br>60 Requires occasional assistance but self-care for most needs |
| 3 In bed more than 50% of each day | 50 Requires considerable assistance<br>40 Disabled, requires special care and assistance |
| 4 Bedridden | 30 Severely disabled, hospitalization indicated<br>20 Very sick, hospitalization needed<br>10 Moribund<br>0 Dead |

**TABLE 121.5. Clinical Pharmacology in the Elderly Patient**

| Variable | Mechanism | Clinical Example | Clinical Correlates |
|---|---|---|---|
| 1. Drug absorption | — | — | No important clinical effect |
| 2. Drug distribution | Total body water decreases | Water soluble drugs have a high initial concentration | Alcohol has a higher concentration for a given dose |
| | Total body fat increases | Lipid soluble drugs have prolonged half-life | Diazepam has a prolonged half-life in elderly |
| 3. Hepatic metabolism | Decreased rate of Phase I hepatic metabolism | Diazepam, quinidine have prolonged biotransformation | These medications needed in smaller doses; more opportunities arise for drug interaction; when possible, monitor drug levels |
| 4. Renal excretion | Decreased creatinine clearance | Renally excreted drugs will have a prolonged clearance | Adjust dose and timing of administration of aminoglycoside and other renally excreted drugs based on creatinine clearance*; measure serum levels whenever possible |
| 5. Pharmacodynamic changes | Change in target organ sensitivity to drugs | β-agonists have decreased cardiostimulatory effect; benzodiazepines cause more sedation | Drug dose may need to be adjusted depending on pharmacodynamic effect |

*Creatinine clearance (Cockcroft-Gault equation):

$$\text{CrCl} = \frac{(140 - \text{age}) \times \text{wt (kg)}}{72 \times \text{serum creatinine (mg/dl)}}$$

0.85 (CrCl) = CrCl for women

## Clinical Pharmacology

Adverse effects of drugs are common in elderly persons, some of which result from physicians' prescribing habits and lack of insight regarding geriatric physiology. The pharmacokinetic and pharmacodynamic factors altered by age are listed in Table 121.5.

The following practical suggestions should be kept in mind when prescribing for an elderly patient:

1. Establish whether drug therapy is really required. The need for constant and critical review of the older patient's drug regimens cannot be overemphasized.

2. Start low and go slowly.
3. Educate the patient about his or her drugs, their importance to well-being, and their possible side effects.
4. Simplify dosing schedules as much as possible.
5. Consider the cost of agents and, whenever possible, choose less expensive products that have equal efficacy.
6. Consider the type of container to be used. It should display the name of the drug and easy-to-read instructions; it should also be easy to open.

# CHAPTER 122 AGE-RELATED CHANGES IN ORGAN SYSTEMS

The physician must understand the changes that occur in the body as a result of age and be able to differentiate these changes from disease. This section delineates some of the age-related changes that occur in different organ systems (Table 122.1). At times, reference is made to common pathology. More detailed discussions of pathology can be found in other chapters.

## Cardiovascular System

Arteriosclerosis affects the media of blood vessels and causes them to become less distensible or more "stiff." This change, which appears to be a physiologic result of aging, contributes to a progressive rise in systolic blood pressure throughout life. Diastolic blood pressure, however, rises steadily into middle age, and then it plateaus; it may actually decline in late life. Hypertension has been defined as a systolic blood pressure greater than 140 mm Hg and diastolic greater than 90 mm Hg. Using these criteria, as many as 40% to 50% of elderly persons may be classified as hypertensive. Isolated systolic hypertension (systolic pressure >140 mm Hg and diastolic pressure < 90 mm Hg) is a condition found almost exclusively in the aged. Older adults have no change in cardiac output—either at rest or with exercise—when compared to younger adults. It is noteworthy, however, that the aged have a lower heart rate response to stress than the young. It appears, therefore, that cardiac output with stress is maintained in the aged by increased diastolic filling and reliance on the Frank-Starling mechanism.

Echocardiography of healthy elderly subjects reveals that left ventricular wall thickness increases with advancing age, possibly from increasing afterload. Ambulatory electrocardiographic monitoring in healthy aged subjects shows that 88% of subjects have supraventricular ectopic beats and 80% have ventricular ectopic beats. Holter monitor results in aged patients must be interpreted cautiously.

Systolic heart murmurs are not a normal consequence of aging, but they can be heard frequently (a prevalence as high as 50–60%) in aged patients.

## Neurologic, Sensory, and Psychologic Systems

Older people maintain intellectual performance as measured by tests of verbal abilities, such as vocabulary, information, and comprehension. However, their performance on timed tasks declines progressively throughout adult life. Experimental measurements reveal that learning does occur in late life, but that it takes longer than in youth or middle age. Immediate recall and long-term memory are preserved into late life, but short-term memory shows impairment when tested experimentally. The clinical significance of these findings is not obvious. In general, healthy elderly people should score well on the bedside mental status examinations used by most clinicians; thus, deficits in performance require an explanation.

Even the untrained observer recognizes differences in the gaits of the young and the old. When ambulating, elderly persons have a shorter stride; they flex more at their elbows, trunk, and knees and lift their heels and toes less. Tests of balance show that older persons are less able than younger persons to control sway when standing still. Even healthy older persons have problems balancing on one leg for more than a few seconds.

The pupils of the eye become smaller and less able to dilate maximally with advancing age. The lens undergoes degeneration, becoming less pliable; it develops a yellow hue and often becomes opacified. These age-related changes in the eye lead to several vision problems: difficulty seeing in low light or in areas with significant glare; problems with depth perception; decreased perception of blues and greens; and difficulty focusing on nearby objects (accommodation). This constellation of changes often is referred to as presbyopia.

Hearing decline, or presbycusis, also accompanies aging. Characterized by a loss of ability to hear consonants and some high-frequency sounds, presbycusis also is coupled with difficulty screening out background noise.

## Oral System

Tooth loss is not a normal part of the aging process. Until the latter part of the 20$^{th}$ century however, most

**TABLE 122.1. Clinically Relevant Age-Related Organ System Changes**

| System and Pattern of Change | Clinical Significance |
|---|---|
| *Cardiovascular* | |
| Decreased distensibility of blood vessels | Senile purpura, bounding arterial pulse |
| Increased peripheral vascular resistance | Systolic hypertension |
| Unchanged cardiac output | |
| Increased left ventricular wall thickness | Diastolic dysfunction |
| Impaired baroreceptor function | Orthostatic hypotension |
| Decreased heart-rate response to stress | Modification of maximum predicted heart rate with exercise stress testing |
| *Nervous System* | |
| Impaired temperature regulation | Hypothermia and hyperthermia |
| Impaired baroreceptor response | Orthostatic hypotension |
| Brain atrophy | Predisposition to delirium |
| Decreased neurotransmitter concentration | Predisposition to delirium |
| Altered gait and balance | Propensity for falls |
| Short-term memory loss | More time required to learn new material |
| *Special Senses* | |
| Presbyopia | Visual difficulties (see text) |
| Presbycusis | Hearing difficulties (see text) |
| Increased threshold for taste | Potential for altered dietary intake (e.g., sodium) |
| Arcus senilis | |
| Decreased pupil size | Difficulty seeing in dim light |
| Decreased color sensitivity | |
| *Pulmonary* | |
| Decreased lung elasticity | |
| Decreased vital capacity, increased residual volume | |
| Decreased $PaO_2$ | |
| Decreased mucus clearance | ? Higher incidence of bronchitis and pneumonia |
| *Renal/Genitourinary* | |
| Decreased creatinine clearance | Alterations in drug clearance |
| Decreased capacity to concentrate urine | Potential for dehydration |
| Prostatic hypertrophy | Nocturia, hesitancy, and hematuria |
| *Musculoskeletal* | |
| Degeneration of intervertebral discs | Loss of height |
| Decreased bone mass | Predisposition to osteoporosis |
| Articular cartilage degeneration | Propensity for osteoarthritis |
| Increased fat to lean body mass ratio | May reduce serum creatinine |
| *Endocrine* | |
| Menopause | Accelerated bone loss and arteriosclerosis; vaginal mucosal atrophy |
| Impaired glucose tolerance | Can cause misdiagnosis of diabetes mellitus |
| Selected impaired hormonal responses to stimulation | May affect endocrine function tests |
| *Hematologic/Immunologic* | |
| Mild elevation of sedimentation rate | |
| Impaired cell-mediated immunity | May enhance risk of reactivation of tuberculosis or varicella |
| *Skin* | |
| Gray hair | Change in appearance |
| Decreased dermal thickness | Makes assessment of skin turgor unreliable |
| Increased wrinkling | Change in appearance; scars may be difficult to detect |
| Atrophy of sweat glands | Decreased sweating and tendency for hyperthermia |

people older than 65 were edentulous (without teeth). Salivary flow is unchanged from youth. Xerostomia (dry mouth) is not attributable directly to old age. It is due most commonly to drugs (i.e., agents with anticholinergic side effects), connective tissue diseases, or radiotherapy. It can cause discomfort, diminished food intake, and impaired taste, and also can accelerate caries. Alterations in pain perception may keep older patients from promptly seeking the dental treatment they require.

Flavor perception, a product of both taste and olfaction, declines with advancing years. The thresholds for salty taste and bitter taste increase in older subjects; data for sweet and sour tastes are conflicting. Changes in taste may cause a decrease in eating pleasure and an increased reliance on salt and other spices to improve palatability of food.

## Pulmonary System

Changes in the connective tissue of the lung and chest wall reduce the elasticity of the lung and increase the stiffness of the chest wall in aged patients, and pulmonary function declines. Total lung capacity remains unchanged; however, vital capacity drops and residual volume rises. A decline in the forced expiratory volume in the first second ($FEV_1$) has been noted in numerous studies. Arterial blood gas measurements indicate that the $PaO_2$ declines with advancing years. The following formula is used to calculate the $PaO_2$ of patients at different ages: $104 - (0.27 \times \text{age})$.

## Gastrointestinal System

An increased frequency of atrophic changes of the gastric mucosa has been noted with advancing age. Gastric secretion diminishes, and frank achlorhydria is five to seven times more prevalent in the aged than in the young.

Nutrient absorption is not changed significantly, but a decrease in metabolism and absorption of sugars, calcium, and iron may occur. Colonic diverticula are common but by no means universal in old people. A low-residue diet throughout life has been implicated as one potential pathogenetic factor for this problem.

## Renal and Genitourinary Systems

Studies of renal function demonstrate a steady fall in creatinine clearance with advancing age. This change may not be readily apparent to the clinician, however, because older people do not demonstrate a dramatic rise in serum creatinine (because of reduced production of creatinine due to loss of lean muscle mass from aging). In a given elderly patient, creatinine clearance is difficult to predict. When the patient is undergoing drug therapy, attention to blood levels and close monitoring are required to predict the precise dose and interval for agents renally excreted.

Urine-concentrating ability declines with advancing age. This decrease, combined with an altered thirst mechanism, may easily predispose elderly patients to dehydration during periods of stress. Lower values for renin and aldosterone are found in either the basal or stimulated state in elderly persons.

In men, benign hyperplasia of the prostate represents a common aging phenomenon. Bladder physiology in the aged has not been completely elucidated. Nocturia is reported by large numbers (60–70%) of nonselected elderly persons. Incomplete bladder emptying may occur in subjects who have no urinary symptoms, and residual volumes of 75 to 100 ml of urine may be acceptable. Bacteriuria is relatively common in elderly men and women (10–30%). The prevalence rises in frail, institutionalized populations. Usually, treatment of asymptomatic bacteriuria is not warranted in older patients. The cause for the bacteriuria should be considered; the extent of evaluation varies with the individual clinical circumstance.

In elderly women, atrophic changes of the introitus and vagina follow estrogen loss. However, sexual activity remains possible into late life and should continue to be pleasurable—despite decreases in vaginal barrel elasticity, vaginal lubrication with sexual arousal, and the intensity and duration of orgasm. In older men, erections require more genital stimulation. In addition, seminal fluid volume is reduced, with less expulsive pressure and less need to ejaculate with orgasm. Orgasm shortens, and penile flaccidity may quickly follow. The time from orgasm to achievement of next erection (refractory period) lengthens with age and may last 12 to 24 hours. Impotence or symptoms of sexual dysfunction should be pursued and should never be attributed to age alone.

## Musculoskeletal System

From adolescence through middle age (30–50 years of age), body weight steadily increases and then plateaus. (Although weight loss may occur in the later years, it is not predictable.) Body composition changes simultaneously. As a percentage of body weight, the total body water decreases, as does lean body mass; total body fat, however, increases.

Although loss of bone mass is normal in men and women throughout adult life, it does not produce clinical sequelae in all people. Thus, osteoporosis is not part of normal aging. Population studies of nonselected elderly show up to 50% of people have radiographic or clinical evidence of degenerative joint disease.

## Endocrine System

### Sex hormones

Menopause is characterized by declining serum estrogen and rising gonadotropin levels. These changes affect estrogen-sensitive tissues: subcutaneous vulvar fat is lost, and the vaginal mucosa become atrophic, with loss of rugae. Estrogen loss also accelerates age-related bone loss. Total and free testosterone levels decline in elderly men. The Baltimore Longitudinal Study of Aging has reported a high frequency of age-related hypogonadism in healthy elderly men. The normal range for testosterone levels is wide; subnormal values in elderly men should prompt investigation of whether the hypogonadism is primary or central and whether a specific disease mechanism is causing the hypogonadism. Depressed testosterone levels should not be attributed to old age.

#### Thyroid hormone

The similarities between normal aging and hypothyroidism are so striking that the diagnosis of hypothyroidism may easily be missed in older patients. Serum levels of thyroid hormone and thyroid-stimulating hormone remain constant into later life. The elderly hypothyroid patient requires a lower dose of thyroid replacement than a young counterpart; changes in body weight and loss of metabolically active lean body mass in later life may be responsible.

#### Glucose metabolism

Glucose tolerance declines gradually in older persons as the result of age-related relative insulin resistance. Standard criteria for the diagnosis of diabetes incorporate this age-related change and should prevent misdiagnosis of diabetes mellitus. Nomograms are available to assist with the interpretation of glucose tolerance tests. Fasting blood sugar is not significantly influenced by age.

### Hematologic and Immunologic Systems

An apparent age-related decline in hemoglobin reported in some studies is mostly due to diseases or conditions that influence hemoglobin concentration. The adult norms for hemoglobin also apply to the elderly person.

The erythrocyte sedimentation rate (ESR) increases slightly in older subjects. The meaning of this increase remains unclear. However, marked elevations of ESR (such as those seen in polymyalgia rheumatica) should never be interpreted as related to old age. Leukocyte count and function remain stable into late life. The increased prevalence of bacterial infection in the aged may be explained by diseases that alter leukocyte function or by changes in organ systems that alter barrier function or impede leukocyte response to pathogens. Both the number and function of T and B lymphocytes decline. Impaired cell-mediated immunity may enhance the risk of reactivation of tuberculosis or varicella.

The prevalence of autoantibodies (e.g., rheumatoid factor and antinuclear antibodies) in low titer increases in elderly patients. Although the clinical significance of this increase is unclear, the clinician should correlate such results carefully with the clinical findings to avoid misdiagnosis of rheumatoid arthritis or systemic lupus erythematosus in the elderly patient.

### Skin

To the patient and physician alike, aging is most obvious on the skin and hair. Pigment production within hair follicles declines; thus, graying of the hair occurs. Hair loss occurs in both men and women. Scalp hair loss usually is androgen-dependent, and a male pattern of baldness in a woman should raise suspicion of androgen production, possibly as the result of a neoplasm.

The skin becomes dry, wrinkled, and lax with age. Loss of dermal thickness gives the skin a transparent quality. Skin turgor is a notoriously unreliable key to assessing hydration in an elderly person. Flat, pigmented lesions over sun-exposed areas are called lentigo senilis (liver spots or age spots); their incidence increases in elderly persons. Interestingly, the prevalence of melanocytic nevi (moles) decreases in older patients; they are rarely seen in those older than 80. Ecchymoses on the forearms and dorsum of the hands are frequent in older people; in the absence of any coagulopathy, they can be termed senile purpura. Changes in the connective tissues of the blood vessels and their surrounding skin may account for the leakage of blood into the skin with incidental trauma. Benign neoplastic proliferation of blood vessel components results in the frequently observed capillary hemangiomas (cherry red spots); these punctate, raised, bright red lesions are of no pathologic consequence.

Although not part of normal aging, a number of other dermatologic conditions are noted in elderly persons; these include seborrheic keratoses and seborrheic dermatitis. The physician should assess the skin of the older patient for actinic keratoses and malignant neoplasms (such as basal cell carcinoma or squamous cell carcinoma), because their prevalence increases with age. The clinical features of these conditions are fully outlined in Chapters 55 and 56.

Xerosis (dry skin) with or without pruritus is probably the most common dermatologic symptom among older patients. The physician should consider and exclude conditions known to cause pruritus (e.g., renal disease, liver disease, hypothyroidism, diabetes, malignancies, and myeloproliferative disorders). Symptomatic treatment should include avoidance of excessive hydration by reducing the frequency of bathing or showering; using soaps such as Basis, Dove, or Tone; and using topical emollients immediately after the skin has been wetted.

# CHAPTER 123 DELIRIUM AND DEMENTIA

Delirium and dementia are significant geriatric concerns. The physician should approach dementia and delirium as brain failure. Just as with any other major organ failure (cardiac, renal, or hepatic), the physician must determine whether the problem is acute or chronic and whether it is reversible—fully or partially.

## Delirium

Acute reversible brain failure, referred to as delirium, is present in about 30% of elderly patients admitted to general medical and surgical wards. The search for a cause can be painstaking in view of the many possibilities (Table 123.1). Drugs notorious for precipitating delirium are the sedative-hypnotics, minor tranquilizers, major tranquilizers, and tricyclic antidepressants. Other agents are listed in Table 123.2.

Patients with delirium are difficult to evaluate. History must be obtained from family, friends, or the nursing staff. The physical examination is hindered by patient uncooperativeness. The cardinal features of delirium are a decreased awareness of the environment and impaired attention span (clouding of consciousness), perceptual disturbance (e.g., visual hallucinations and illusions), incoherent speech, sleep-wake disturbance, increased or decreased psychomotor activity (e.g., tachycardia, diaphoresis, mydriatic pupils, and fever), disorientation and memory impairment, rapid onset with fluctuating course, and the presence of some underlying organic factors. The foremost consideration in differential diagnosis should be a drug-induced delirium.

**TABLE 123.1. Common Causes of Delirium**

Drug toxicity (see Table 123.2)
Infections
Fluid and electrolyte abnormalities
Acid–base disturbances
Hypoxemia/hypercarbia
Hypoglycemia or hyperglycemia
Hypotension
Intoxication (alcohol, other)
Hypothermia or hyperthermia
Sensory deprivation (ICU psychosis)
Fecal impaction
Urinary retention
Congestive heart failure
Primary CNS disturbance

CNS = central nervous system; ICU = intensive care unit.

**TABLE 123.2. Drugs Reported to Cause Delirium in the Aged**

Amantadine
Antiadrenergic agents (e.g., β-blockers and central alpha-blockers)
Anticholinergic agents
Cimetidine
Digoxin
Lithium
Nonsteroidal antiinflammatory agents
Psychotropics (e.g., hypnotics, major and minor tranquilizers, and antidepressants)
Corticosteroids
Theophylline

The prognosis of delirium depends on the underlying cause. Given a mortality risk as high as 25%, delirium is a true medical emergency, requiring skillful evaluation to define the underlying cause.

Therapy requires a gentle approach that optimizes sensory function, diminishes extraneous environmental stimuli, and incorporates familiar people, such as family members. Restraints should be used sparingly and caution exercised to avoid decubitus ulcers, peripheral nerve damage, and aspiration. Restraints are potentially injurious to agitated patients. Sedation should be used sparingly, especially in cases in which a drug is the suspected cause. Adding a second agent may only complicate matters further, because many of the same agents used to treat delirium may also produce it. However, in instances in which the patient is a danger to self or others and cannot be managed with nonmedical measures alone, drug therapy may be necessary. One approach in using drug therapy is to use a major tranquilizer to sedate the patient and then gradually wean him or her off the drug. Management of such patients is further complicated by the possibility that delirium may be superimposed on dementia, with the premorbid mental status abnormal as well (Table 123.3).

## Dementia

Dementia is the chronic form of brain failure, afflicting roughly 10% of the population older than 65 and almost half of those older than 85. The major causes of dementia are primary degenerative dementia (Alzheimer disease or senile dementia of the Alzheimer's type), vascular dementia, and a combination of these two. Together, these causes account for three fourths or

**TABLE 123.3. Clinical Features Differentiating Delirium From Dementia**

| Characteristic | Delirium | Dementia |
|---|---|---|
| Onset | Sudden | Insidious |
| Course over 24 hours | Fluctuating, with nocturnal exacerbation | Stable |
| Consciousness | Reduced | Clear |
| Attention | Globally disordered | Normal, except in severe cases |
| Cognition | Globally disordered | Globally impaired |
| Hallucinations | Usually visual, or visual and auditory | Often absent |
| Delusions | Fleeting, poorly systematized | Often absent |
| Orientation | Usually impaired, at least for a time | Often impaired |
| Psychomotor activity | Increased, reduced, or shifting unpredictably | Often normal |
| Speech | Often incoherent, slow or rapid | Difficulty finding words, perseveration |
| Involuntary movements | Often asterixis or coarse tremor | Often absent |
| Physical illness or drug toxicity | One or both are present | Often absent, especially in senile dementia of the Alzheimer's type |

Adapted from Lipowski ZJ. N Engl J Med 1989; 320:580.

**TABLE 123.4. Causes of Dementia**

Alzheimers disease
Vascular (cerebrovascular accident)
Drugs (alcohol, others)
Posttraumatic
Degenerative diseases of central nervous system (Creutzfeld-Jakob, Parkinson, Huntington, Pick)
Space-occupying lesion (tumor, infection)
Normal pressure hydrocephalus
Vitamin deficiencies (vitamin $B_{12}$, thiamine)
Metabolic disorders
Major organ dysfunction (cardiac, renal, hepatic)
Depression (pseudodementia)
Infectious (HIV, syphilis)
Vasculitis

more of all cases of dementia. Other causes are listed in Table 123.4.

Dementia has several main features: loss of intellectual abilities of sufficient severity to interfere with social or occupational functioning; memory impairment, impairment of abstract thinking (e.g., concrete proverb interpretation or the inability to find similarities and differences between related words); impaired judgment; disturbances of higher cortical function (e.g., aphasia, apraxia, agnosia, and an inability to copy three-dimensional figures); personality change; normal level of consciousness; and an organic factor judged to be causative. Isolated memory loss, especially short-term memory, differs from dementia and is termed mild cognitive impairment.

The distinction between dementia and pseudodementia (depression masquerading as dementia) is important, because depression is usually treatable. Depression is suggested when the patient is actively seeking medical attention; the onset is more rapid and is known with precision; the patient is aware of cognitive loss; depressed affect is present with vegetative signs; "don't know" answers are given to questions on the mental status examination; and behavior is observed that is not congruent with the severity of the cognitive loss. Neuropsychological testing, referral to a psychiatrist, or an empiric trial of antidepressant therapy may help differentiate depression from dementia in cases in which the diagnosis is in doubt.

The evaluation of dementia includes history, physical examination, and adjunct laboratory testing (Table 123.5). A history of hypertension, transient ischemic attack, stroke, abrupt onset, and stepwise deterioration indicates vascular dementia. Focal neurologic findings on physical examination suggest a localized central nervous system (CNS) pathology. Usually, a reversible or treatable condition is uncovered through evaluation in only a small number of cases. However, the human suffering that could be alleviated and cost savings achieved by reducing needless institutionalization through such an evaluation cannot be discounted. As with many areas of medicine, the evaluation should be tailored to the individual clinical circumstance.

As noted, Alzheimer disease (primary degenerative dementia) is the most common cause of dementia, but its cause remains obscure. Genetic factors may play a role, but no clear-cut pattern of genetic transmissibility has been identified. A few families have shown an autosomal dominant pattern of transmission. Evidence suggests that

**TABLE 123.5. Evaluation of Dementia**

History
- Symptoms (nature, onset, progression)
- Associated symptoms (e.g., urinary incontinence, behavioral abnormalities)
- Medications
- Alcohol use
- Past medical history (neurologic disorders, cardiovascular disorders, depression)
- Family history

Physical examination
- Blood pressure
- Pulse oximetry
- Mental status
- Sensory examination
- Neurologic examination

Psychological examination
- Depression screen

Laboratory
- CBC
- Glucose
- Electrolytes
- Renal function
- Hepatic function
- Thyroid function
- Vitamin $B_{12}$, folate
- Calcium, phosphate

Other*
- Neuroimaging (CT scan, MRI, PET, SPECT)
- HIV
- EEG
- Formal psychiatric evaluation
- Neuropsychological evaluation
- Speech/language evaluation
- Syphilis serology
- Lumbar puncture

CBC = complete blood count; CT = computed tomography; EEG = electroencephalogram; HIV = human immunodeficiency virus; MRI = magnetic resonance imaging; PET = positron emission tomography; SPECT = single photon emission computed tomography.
*Studies may be appropriate in certain clinical situations.
Adapted from Anonymous. JAMA 1987;258:3411–3416.

the gene for familial Alzheimer disease is located on chromosome 21. Data from twin studies indicate the importance of both genetic and nongenetic factors in the development of this illness. Putative nongenetic factors include slow-acting viral agents, environmental toxins and trace metals, chromosomal abnormalities, and deficiencies of neurotropic hormones. Neurotransmitter deficits in the CNS have been noted, especially concerning acetylcholine. However, attempts to modulate neurotransmitter levels have had limited success. Microscopic hallmarks of the illness include selective neuronal death, neurofibrillary tangles, and neuritic plaques.

In order to diagnose Alzheimer disease, the patient must first meet the clinical criteria for dementia. Next, other known causes of dementia should be considered, using history, physical examination, and laboratory tests (see Table 123.5).

Alzheimer disease progresses through mild, moderate, and severe stages. Patients with mild disease exhibit mild changes in memory and language. In the moderate stage, many behavioral domains are involved, and the classic syndrome is identifiable. Severe Alzheimer disease is characterized by marked impairment of all intellectual abilities. Motor dysfunction may emerge. Death may be caused by aspiration pneumonia, sepsis from decubitus ulcers or urinary tract infection, or concomitant medical illnesses.

No cure currently exists for Alzheimer disease. Physicians caring for these patients should help patients and their family try to cope with the illness. A comprehensive approach is needed in the management of patients with dementia, who often require the coordination of many resources. Some key management principles are outlined in Table 123.6.

**TABLE 123.6. Managing Patients with Dementia**

Optimize function
- Treat medical conditions and provide ongoing medical care
- Optimize sensory function—glasses, hearing aids
- Avoid medications with CNS side effects
- Encourage physical and social activity
- Educate about good nutrition
- Assess the environment and recommend adaptations, e.g., OT home safety evaluation

Identify and manage complications
- Psychosis
- Agitation and aggression
- Depression
- Wandering
- Incontinence

Educate patients and families
- Nature of the disease
- Prognosis
- Advance directives
- New treatments and research protocols

Provide social service and legal information
- Community resources
- Legal and financial counseling
- Respite or institutional care
- Ethical issues

CNS = central nervous system; OT = occupational therapy.
Adapted from Confusion. Pp. 125–153. Kane RL, Ouslander JG, Abrass IB. Essentials of Clinical Geriatrics. 4th ed. New York: McGraw-Hill, 1999.

Medications are being developed to ameliorate signs and symptoms of dementia. Vitamin E, an antioxidant, in pharmacologic doses has been beneficial in Alzheimer's disease. Acetylcholinesterase inhibitors such as Donepezil and Rivastigmine have also shown some effect. Their use has been recommended in patients with mild to moderate degenerative dementia.

# CHAPTER 124 URINARY INCONTINENCE

Involuntary voiding of urine is common in elderly persons and is underreported to physicians. An estimated 15% to 30% of elderly community dwellers and up to 50% of institutionalized geriatric patients suffer from this condition. Transient incontinence should be excluded before evaluating this problem in depth. The mnemonic DIAPPERS (Table 124.1) is helpful in recalling causes of transient incontinence. Correction of these conditions may rectify the incontinence, thus obviating any further exploration.

Chronic persistent incontinence can be evaluated in the ambulatory setting. Important elements of the history, physical examination, and initial investigation are outlined in Table 124.2. Measurement of the postvoid residual volume helps categorize the type of incontinence. Patients with large residual volumes (>150 ml) need evaluation for anatomic obstruction or detrusor dysfunction. Incontinence with a small residual volume can mean a normally functioning bladder (functional incontinence) or detrusor instability (involuntary detrusor muscle contractions). It also occurs in patients (primarily women) with stress incontinence. In most cases the type of incontinence can be identified after the initial office evaluation, but urologic consultation for cystoscopy and urodynamic testing may be required in some instances.

**TABLE 124.1. Common Causes of Transient Incontinence**

**D**elirium or confusional state
**I**nfection, urinary (symptomatic)
**A**trophic urethritis or vaginitis
**P**harmaceuticals
- Sedatives or hypnotics, especially long-acting agents
- Loop diuretics
- Anticholinergic agents (antipsychotic agents, antidepressants, antihistamines, anti-Parkinsonian agents, antiarrhythmics [disopyramide], antispasmodics, opiates, and antidiarrheal agents)
- Alpha-adrenoceptor agonists and antagonists
- Calcium-channel-entry blockers
- Vincristine

**P**sychological disorder, especially depression
**E**ndocrine disorder (hypercalcemia or hyperglycemia)
**R**estricted mobility
**S**tool impaction

Adapted from Resnick NM. Medical Grand Rounds 1984;3:284. Used with permission.

The main types of urinary incontinence are listed in Table 124.3. The most common types in older women are urge and mixed stress and urge incontinence. Treatments for incontinence fall into three main categories: behavioral interventions, drug therapy, and surgery. Therapy depends on the cause of the incontinence. Stress incontinence is managed by weight loss for obese patients, pelvic floor exercises, and systemically or topically administered estrogens in women. Failure of conservative measures and demonstration of improper urethral anatomy may warrant surgical correction of the anatomic problem. Pads and diapers are adjuncts for refractory nonoperative patients or patients with a poor surgical result.

Treatment of detrusor instability may include behavioral measures such as adequate fluid intake, scheduled voiding, and pelvic floor muscle exercises. Drug therapy using oxybutynin, tolterodine, and anticholinergic agents (imipramine), have been used with varying clinical results. Whenever possible, urinary catheterization with an indwelling Foley catheter should be avoided because of the high risk of infectious complications. However, such catheterization may be necessary in patients with anatomic obstruction who cannot be managed surgically or patients with an underactive detrusor who cannot be intermittently catheterized. Patients with indwelling catheters should receive antibiotics only for symptomatic urinary tract infections, because they may rapidly develop resistant organisms. The frequency of catheter change is empirical. Although monthly changes have been advocated, there are few data to support this practice. Catheterization can precipitate meatal damage, bladder stones, and urosepsis.

**TABLE 124.2. Clinical Evaluation of the Incontinent Patient**

History
- Type (urge, reflex, stress, overflow, or mixed)
- Frequency, severity, duration
- Pattern (diurnal, nocturnal, or both; temporal relationship to medication administration)
- Associated symptoms (straining to void, incomplete emptying, dysuria)
- Alteration in bowel habit/sexual function
- Other relevant factors (e.g., cancer, diabetes, acute illness, neurologic disease, pelvic or lower urinary tract surgery)
- Medications, including nonprescription agents (diuretics, anticholinergics, sedative-hypnotics, and adrenergic agents)
- Incontinence chart (frequency, timing, and amount of continent and incontinent voids)

Functional assessment (CADET)

Physical examination
- General medical examination
- Test for stress-induced leakage when bladder is full
- Observe or listen to voiding
- Palpate for bladder distention after voiding
- Pelvic examination (atrophic vaginitis/urethritis; pelvic muscle laxity; pelvic mass, cystocele, rectocele)
- Rectal examination (resulting tone and voluntary control of anal sphincter; prostate nodules; fecal impaction)
- Neurologic examination (mental status and screening examination, including sacral reflexes and perineal sensation)

Initial workup
- Metabolic survey (measurement of electrolytes, calcium, glucose, and urea nitrogen)
- Measurement of postvoid residual volume (straight catheterization or ultrasound)
- Urine analysis and culture

Adapted from Incontinence. Pp 181–230. Kane RL, Ouslander JG, Abrass IB. Essentials of Clinical Geriatrics. 4th ed. New York: McGraw-Hill, 1999.

**TABLE 124.3. Basic Types and Causes of Persistent Urinary Incontinence**

| Type | Definition | Common Causes |
|---|---|---|
| Stress | Involuntary loss of urine (usually small amounts) with increases in intraabdominal pressure (e.g., cough, laugh, or exercise) | Weakness and laxity of pelvic floor musculature, bladder outlet or urethral sphincter weakness |
| Urge | Leakage of urine (usually larger volumes) because of inability to delay voiding after perceiving sensation of bladder fullness | Detrusor motor or sensory instability, isolated or associated with one or more of the following: local genitourinary condition (cystitis, urethritis, tumors, stones, diverticula, and outflow obstruction); CNS disorders (stroke, dementia, Parkinsonism, suprasacral spinal cord injury or disease*) |
| Overflow | Leakage of urine (usually small amounts) resulting from mechanical forces on an overdistended bladder or from other effects of urinary retention on bladder and sphincter function | Anatomic obstruction by prostate, stricture, cystocele<br>Non-contractile bladder associated with diabetes mellitus or spinal cord injury<br>Neurogenic (detrusor-sphincter dyssynergy), associated with multiple sclerosis and other suprasacral spinal cord lesions |
| Functional | Urinary leakage associated with inability to toilet because of impairment of cognitive or physical functioning, psychological unwillingness, or environmental barriers | Severe dementia and other neurological disorders<br>Psychological factors such as depression, regression, anger, and hostility |

*When detrusor motor instability is associated with a neurological disorder, it is termed "detrusor hyperreflexia" by the International Continence Society.
Reprinted with permission from Incontinence. Pp 181-230. Kane RL, Ouslander JG, Abrass IB. Essentials of Clinical Geriatrics. 4th ed. New York: McGraw-Hill, 1999.

# CHAPTER 125 DISTURBANCES OF TEMPERATURE REGULATION

Despite the association of heat illness with athletes or military recruits who perform in high ambient temperatures, and of hypothermia with winter sports or alcohol debauch, the fact is that both conditions are most prevalent in elderly people.

The body maintains a constant temperature through a balance between heat generation and heat dissipation (see chapter 153, Temperature Homeostasis). Aging alters the body's ability both to generate and to dissipate heat. Older adults experience impaired temperature perception, sweating, vasoconstriction, vasodilatation, chemical thermogenesis, and shivering, all of which place them at an increased risk of developing hypo- or hyperthermia.

## Hyperthermia

Hyperthermia (heat illness) includes a spectrum of conditions marked by heat cramps, heat exhaustion, and heat stroke. Whenever the environmental temperature exceeds the body's ability to dissipate heat, the possibility of heat stroke arises. Body temperature of 105°F to 106°F in the setting of abnormal mental status, anhidrosis, and warm skin suggests the diagnosis. Some investigators have found that elderly persons show many differences from the young when exposed experimentally to a heat stress; older subjects may have a delayed return of core temperature to baseline levels, sweat less, and vasodilate less efficiently than the young. Factors other than age that are associated with heat illness include reduced activity; alcoholism; the use of major tranquilizers, anticholinergics, or diuretics; and the inability of persons to care for themselves.

Full-blown heat stroke is a serious medical condition, involving multiple organ systems. The manifestations of heat stroke include altered mental status, volume depletion, acid-base disorders (mixed picture of metabolic acidosis and respiratory alkalosis), renal dysfunction, disseminated intravascular coagulation, rhabdomyolysis, and hepatic dysfunction.

Physicians should identify susceptible patients in their practices, especially frail elderly persons who live in inner-city urban areas and use the previously listed drugs. During periods of prolonged high environmental heat, these patients should be advised to wear loose-fitting clothing, ingest adequate amounts of fluid and salt (diuretic therapy may have to be suspended for a few days), take cool tub or sponge baths, and spend some time in air-conditioned environments, if possible. Windows should be open with fans blowing the hot air out of the home during extreme heat, and shades should be closed to keep out the direct sunlight.

## Hypothermia

Hypothermia is defined as a core body temperature less than 95°F. Studies of elderly persons suggest problems with both heat production and heat conservation when subjects are exposed to a cold stress. Environmental temperatures need not be extreme to precipitate this condition; even temperatures in the 60s (°F) may be sufficient to overwhelm certain patients. As with heat illness, certain elderly persons are predisposed to this condition. Risk factors include living alone, low income that prevents adequate home heating, the use of phenothiazines or alcohol, hypothyroidism, central nervous system disease (e.g., stroke or Parkinson disease), overwhelming sepsis, and malnutrition.

Patients present with mental obtundation; cool skin (especially over the abdomen or low back) that may be edematous; bradycardia (sometimes irregular); and hypotension. Muscles may be rigid from shivering. Neurologic findings, such as miotic pupils and upgoing plantar responses, can be noted. The key to diagnosis is suspecting the condition and checking the core body temperature.

Laboratory evaluation can show evidence of volume depletion (e.g., high hemoglobin and elevated serum proteins), acid-base disorders (e.g., metabolic acidosis), disseminated intravascular coagulation, and hyperamylasemia. The electrocardiogram often shows atrial fibrillation with a slow ventricular response; the Osborne wave, or J-wave, may be seen in the terminal portion of the QRS complex.

As with heat illness, patients who are at risk for hypothermia should adopt preventive measures. Sick or frail elderly should not keep room temperatures too low. Although 65°F may be adequate for healthy elderly people, 70°F may be required for sick or frail elderly persons.

# CHAPTER 126 MISCELLANEOUS SYNDROMES WITH INCREASED PREVALENCE IN THE ELDERLY

## Accidents and Falls

Injuries rank as the fifth leading cause of death in aged persons. Elderly persons, who constitute 12% of the general population in the United States, sustain 75% of all fatal falls. Prevalence surveys indicate falls among one half of all elderly women and one third of elderly men.

In addition to death, sequelae to falls include fractures of the hip, spine, skull, or radius; disabling soft tissue injuries; subdural hematoma; and accidental hypothermia if the patient falls in a cool environment and is unable to get up. The loss of confidence and family anxiety that these episodes cause are more difficult to quantify, but they have significant impact. Falls are an indication of poor functional status and are a contributing reason for nursing home placement.

The differential diagnosis for falls is lengthy (Table 126.1). Most falls are caused by neurologic factors, not cardiac abnormalities. In addition, many falls are multifactorial.

Obtaining a careful history is essential. Observers of the event should be closely queried about whether loss of consciousness ensued or preceded the fall, and exactly how the fall occurred. Drug and alcohol history is important. The physical examination should be comprehensive and include a survey for serious injury. No standard laboratory evaluation is recommended for these patients. Instead, laboratory tests should be selective, based on the history and physical examination.

Most falls in elderly persons are multifactorial. Patients can compensate for a single disability, but a number of problems can cause decompensation with stress. Corrective action in multiple areas simultaneously may improve the situation. Therapy depends entirely on the cause identified. The temptation to immobilize or restrain the "faller" must be balanced against the patient's wishes and the risks from immobility. Patients may decide that the risk of a fall outweighs the isolation and depression that accompany impaired mobility.

## Osteoporosis

A significant proportion of elderly people are prone to fractures of the hip, wrist, and vertebrae, which result in a serious burden of morbidity and cause a major economic drain on medical resources. Based on observed fracture rates, osteoporosis afflicts about one third of elderly persons, primarily women. The approach to patients with fractures often emphasizes operative therapy and perioperative management; however, diagnostic studies to assess the etiology of the bone disease receive little emphasis. The usual radiographs employed to diagnose fractures cannot distinguish among the possible causes. (Osteoporosis is fully discussed in Chapter 67.) Assessing and treating older patients for risk factors for osteoporosis is important.

## Macular Degeneration

The leading cause of irreversible blindness in elderly patients is macular degeneration. It presents with a loss of central vision. Examination of the fundus may reveal drusen and retinal pigmented epithelial changes. Advanced cases can show disciform scars, neovasculariza-

**TABLE 126.1. Causes of Falls**

| Cause | Nursing Home* % (Range) | Community Living† % (Range) |
|---|---|---|
| Gait and balance disorder or weakness | 26 (20–39) | 13 (2–29) |
| Dizziness or vertigo | 25 (0–30) | 8 (0–19) |
| "Accident" or environment-related | 16 (6–27) | 41 (23–53) |
| Confusion | 10 (0–14) | 2 (0–7) |
| Visual disorder | 4 (0–5) | 0.8 (0–4) |
| Postural hypotension | 2 (0–16) | 1 (0–6) |
| Drop attack | 0.3 (0–3) | 13 (0–25) |
| Syncope | 0.2 (0–3) | 0.4 (0–3) |
| Other specified causes | 12 (10–34) | 17 (2–39) |
| Unknown | 4 (0–34) | 6 (0–16) |

*4 studies; 1076 falls
†7 studies; 2312 falls
Reprinted with permission from Rubenstein LZ, Josephson KR, Robbins AS. Ann Intern Med 1994;121:443.

**TABLE 126.2. Pressure Sores: Staging and Treatment**

| Stage | Description | Treatment |
|---|---|---|
| Stage I | Nonblanchable erythema of intact skin, the harbinger of skin ulceration | Pressure relief |
| Stage II | Partial thickness skin loss involving epidermis and/or dermis; superficial ulcer that presents clinically as an abrasion, blister, or shallow crater | Pressure relief and maintenance of a moist physiologic environment |
| Stage III | Full thickness skin loss involving damage or necrosis of subcutaneous tissue that may extend down to, but not through, underlying fascia. The ulcer presents clinically as a deep crater with or without undermining of adjacent tissue. | Pressure relief<br>Cleansing<br>Debridement |
| Stage IV | Full thickness skin loss with extensive destruction, tissue necrosis, or damage to muscle, bone, or supporting structures (for example, tendon or joint capsule). Note: Undermining and sinus tracts may also be associated with Stage IV pressure ulcers. | Pressure relief<br>Cleansing<br>Debridement<br>Skin grafts and myocutaneous flaps in special cases |

Reprinted from Clinical Practice Guideline, No 3. AHCPR Publication No. 92-0047. Rockville, MD: Agency for Health Care Policy and Research, Public Health Service, U.S. Dept. of Health and Human Services. May 1992.

tion, and retinal detachments. Therapy with laser photocoagulation has proved beneficial in selected cases; concurrent management with an experienced ophthalmologist is critical for success. Patients with irreversible poor visual acuity should be referred to a low-vision clinic. Local agencies are present in most large communities to help the visually impaired.

## Pressure Sores

Pressure sores are localized areas of tissue injury that occur after prolonged exposure to pressure. Four factors contribute to the development of tissue injury: pressure, shearing forces, friction, and moisture. The National Pressure Sore Advisory Panel has developed the staging system in Table 126.2.

Two thirds of pressure sores develop in the hospital setting, and more than one half of all persons with pressure sores are 70 years old or older. Pressure sores increase hospital costs, prolong length of hospital stay, and increase mortality. Risk factors for the development of pressure sores include immobility, poor nutrition, advanced age, urinary or fecal incontinence, and impaired level of consciousness.

The key element in pressure sore management is prevention, particularly in high-risk individuals. Preventive strategies relieve pressure and minimize the effects of risk factors (including immobility, incontinence, and poor nutrition). Pressure relief can be achieved with repositioning and the use of specialized cushions or mattresses.

The treatment of stage I pressure sores is pressure relief. Treatment of stage II sores involves both pressure relief and maintenance of a moist physiologic environment. Occlusive, vapor-permeable dressings (e.g., Op-site, Tegaderm) and hydrocolloid dressings (e.g., DuoDerm, IntraSite) often are used for stage II ulcers. Stage III and IV ulcers take months to heal and require pressure relief, cleansing, and debridement of necrotic tissue. Debridement can be accomplished surgically, with wet to wet saline gauze, with irrigation, or with enzymatic debriding agents. Patients with a compromised vascular supply who have ulcers on their feet and legs should be referred to a vascular surgeon for debridement. The use of topical antibiotics is controversial. Systemic antibiotics are indicated for cellulitis, sepsis, or osteomyelitis, but not for routine pressure sore treatment. Surgical treatments (such as skin grafts or myocutaneous flaps) are reserved for special circumstances such as non-healing stage III or IV pressure sores.

## Preventive Geriatric Health Care

The concept of prevention applies to the treatment of elderly as well as younger patients. Certain measures can stave off morbidity, and its attendant suffering and consequent loss of independence. For example, diet or lifestyle modifications that affect the risk for osteoporosis or falls can improve the patient's chances for a better quality of life. Immunization schedules, cancer screening, and treatment recommendations for hypertension are discussed in other sections of this text. Chapter 7 presents recommendations on immunizations and cancer screening. Treatment recommendations for hypertension are considered in Chapter 183.

### Nutrition

In general, the vast majority of community-dwelling elderly persons are adequately nourished. Obesity may be a more prevalent problem than malnutrition in the aged population in the United States. Studies vary in their findings of nutrients that tend to be deficient in the diets of the aged. Calcium, iron, and total caloric intake have been found deficient in the diets of some elderly subjects surveyed, and deficiencies of several vitamins and minerals are more common in older adults: calcium, vitamin D, vitamin $B_{12}$, folate, thiamine, and zinc. Reliable serum levels are readily available for detection of vitamin $B_{12}$ and folate levels, but screening for the others should be guided by the history and physical examination.

A clinical assessment should include a history of weight loss or gain, edema, anorexia, vomiting, diarrhea, or chronic illness. Other factors that contribute to poor nutrition include poor dentition, sensory loss, disability that impairs food preparation or shopping, loss of taste or smell, alcoholism, mental deterioration, certain drugs (especially those used to treat malignancies), low socioeconomic status, and living alone with few social contacts. The physician should evaluate the patient's height and weight and look for signs of cachexia (e.g., muscle wasting and loss of subcutaneous fat), cheilosis (B vitamins), glossitis (vitamin $B_{12}$, folate, iron), edema (protein), or jaundice.

These simple measures should suffice for a screening evaluation when coupled with laboratory tests (such as hemoglobin, white cell count with differential, red cell indices, and serum protein and albumin). If undernutrition is suspected, a more detailed dietary history, physical assessment, and, possibly, further laboratory evaluation are necessary; a dietitian may conduct these procedures. Forming a plan for treatment requires identifying the reasons for the poor nutrition. (Clinical nutritional assessment is discussed in Chapter 73.) A careful assessment of dietary calcium intake should be made for patients with osteoporosis. At present, the Recommended Daily Allowance (RDA) is similar for middle-aged and elderly adults, with the exception of caloric intake, which has been modified downward for the older patient.

### Physical activity

The value of physical activity in elderly persons cannot be overemphasized. Exercise has been demonstrated to yield a training effect in populations studied into their ninth decade. Thus, improved cardiovascular function can be achieved with a regular program of exercise, even in elderly people. Although there is as yet no proof, several other benefits are believed to accrue from physical activity in this population. Retaining muscle strength and joint flexibility may allow the elderly individual to maintain better agility and thereby lessen the propensity to fall. As mentioned earlier, bone mass appears to increase with activity. Finally, from a psychologic standpoint, a program of regular physical activity may contribute to the individual's sense of well-being and improve the overall quality of life.

## Questions

**Instructions:** For each question below, select only **one** lettered answer that is the **best** for that question.

1. You are called to see an 84-year-old woman who is one-day post op from a hip fracture repair. This evening she became confused and combative and the nurses are asking for physical restraints. Her temperature is 100.8 F, blood pressure 100/70, pulse 100. Lungs have bibasilar crackles. Her medications include morphine sulfate prn pain, diphenhydramine for sleep, enalapril, and docusate sodium. Possible causes of her delirium include:
   A. Narcotics
   B. Pneumonia
   C. Dehydration
   D. Sedative hypnotics
   E. Hypoxemia
   F. All of the above
   G. A and B only

2. The usual decline in function in the elderly follows a hierarchical pattern. Which one of the following is the correct order of the decline in functioning?
   A. Dressing, feeding, bathing, toileting, transferring
   B. Toileting, bathing, dressing, transferring, feeding
   C. Bathing, transferring, toileting, feeding, dressing
   D. Transferring, bathing, feeding, dressing, toileting
   E. Bathing, dressing, toileting, transferring, feeding
   F. None of the above

3. A 74-year-old woman has urinary incontinence. It was previously sporadic, but in the last two months it has worsened, much more so in the last week. At this point in her care, each of the following measures might have a potential role EXCEPT:
   A. The topical use of estrogen-containing creams in the vulvovaginal areas
   B. A 10-day course of trimethoprim-sulfamethoxazole if evaluation suggests a urinary tract infection
   C. A careful review of medication use
   D. The prescribed use of pads/diapers
   E. An inquiry about her loss of interest in her surroundings, disturbance in sleep patterns, and weight loss

4. A 70 year old man has fallen several times in the past month. He has no associated symptoms or dizziness. He takes digoxin 0.25 mg daily and warfarin 2.0 mg

daily for atrial fibrillation and nortriptyline 20 mg at bedtime for depression. Supine BP is 140/80 mm Hg, pulse 70/min, standing BP is 110/70 mm Hg, pulse 78/min. Initial management will include which of the following?
   A. Discontinue nortriptyline
   B. Discontinue warfarin
   C. Prescribe full length elastic stockings to promote venous return
   D. Prescribe fludrocortisone 0.1 mg qd

5. The most important factor when selecting a benzodiazepine for an older patient is which of the following?
   A. Antidepressant effect
   B. Half-life
   C. Potency
   D. Rate of absorption
   E. Sedative effect

6. Which of the following is true regarding dementia?
   A. Dementia is a normal part of aging.
   B. Patients have an alteration in their sensorium (i.e. there is clouding of consciousness).
   C. Most cases are reversible.
   D. Alzheimer's disease is the most frequent cause.

7. An 80 year old, 72 kg woman with a history of coronary artery disease presents with paroxysmal nocturnal dyspnea and orthopnea. Exam shows an irregularly irregular tachycardic pulse. EKG confirms atrial fibrillation with rapid ventricular response. Labs show a creatinine of 1.2 mg/dL. After initial loading, the estimated maintenance dose of digoxin is:
   A. 0.125 mg po qd [creatinine clearance <20 mg/min]
   B. 0.125 mg alternating with 0.25 mg po qod [creatinine clearance 20-50 mg/min]
   C. 0.25 mg po qd [creatinine clearance 50-90 mg/min]
   D. 0.375 mg po qd [creatinine clearance >90 mg/min]

## Answers

1. F 2. E 3. D 4. A 5. B
6. D 7. B

## SUGGESTED READING


### *Textbooks and monographs*

Duthie EH and Katz PR (eds). Practice of Geriatrics. 3rd ed. Philadelphia: WB Saunders, 1998.

Hazzard WR, Blass JP, Ettinger WH, Halter JB, Ouslander JG (eds). Principles of Geriatric Medicine and Gerontology. 4th ed. New York: McGraw-Hill, 1999.

Kane RL, Ouslander JG, Abrass IB (eds). Essentials of Clinical Geriatrics. 4th ed. New York: McGraw-Hill, 1999.

### *Articles*

*Clinical pharmacology*

Beers MH. Explicit criteria for determining potentially inappropriate medication use in the elderly. Arch Intern Med 1997;157:1531-1536.

*Delirium and dementia*

Inouye SK et al. A multicomponent intervention to prevent delirium in hospitalized older patients. N Engl J Med 1999;340:669–676.

Mayeux R, Sano M. Drug therapy: treatment of Alzheimer's disease. N Engl J Med 1999;341:1670–1679.

*Falls*

Jensen J, Lundin-Olsson L, Nyberg L, Gustafson Y. Fall and injury prevention in older people living in residential care facilities. Ann Inter Med 2002;136:733–741.

Lipsitz LA. An 85-year-old woman with a history of falls. JAMA 1996;276:59-66.

Rubenstein LZ, Josephson KR, Robbins AS. Falls in the nursing home. Ann Intern Med 1994;121:442–451.

Tinetti M, Williams C. Falls, injuries due to falls, and the risk of admission to a nursing home. N Engl J Med 1997; 337:1279–1284.

*Urinary incontinence*

Urinary Incontinence Guideline Panel. Urinary Incontinence in Adults: Clinical Practice Guidelines, 2 1996 Update. AHCPR Pub NP 96-0682. Rockville, MD: U.S. Dept. of Health and Human Services. March 1996.

*Senile macular degeneration*

Ferris FL. Senile macular degeneration: Review of epidemiologic features. Am J Epidemiol 1983;118:132–151.

Fine S, Berger J, Maguire M, Ho A. Age-related macular degeneration. N Engl J Med 2000;342:483–492.

*Pressure sores*

Panel for the Prediction and Prevention of Pressure Ulcers in Adults: Prediction and Prevention. Clinical Practice Guideline, No 3. AHCPR Publication No. 92-0047. Rockville, MD: Agency for Health Care Policy and Research, Public Health Service, U.S. Dept. of Health and Human Services. May 1992.

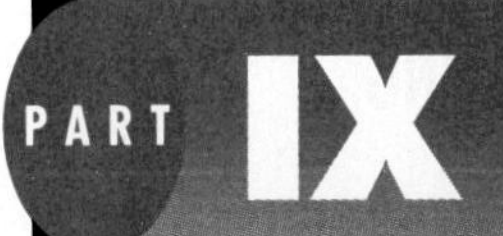

PART IX

Christopher R. Chitambar
Tom Anderson
Jerome L. Gottschall
Janet R. Hosenpud

# HEMATOLOGIC DISORDERS

# CHAPTER 127 PROLIFERATION AND DIFFERENTIATION OF CIRCULATING BLOOD CELLS

Peripheral blood cells originate from uncommitted **multipotential stem cells,** which are essential for self-renewal of bone marrow lines. These cells also give rise to the precursors of each of the committed cell lines morphologically recognizable in the bone marrow, and whose mature products appear in the peripheral blood as the normal elements—leukocytes (including neutrophils, eosinophils, basophils, and monocytes), erythrocytes, and platelets. Each of these committed cell lines proliferates under the influence of growth factors, which are now cloned and generally available in clinical practice for supportive care. Figure 127.1 demonstrates the conceptual development of these cell lines. Operationally referred to as colony-forming units (CFUs) because of their historical identification in the spleens of irradiated mice, these **committed** stem cells also are referred to as burst-forming units (BFUs); an accompanying suffix delineates lineage. Thus, CFU-G refers to CFU of granulocytic lineage, that is, giving rise to granulocytes; CFU-E refers to CFU of erythrocytic lineage, giving rise to red blood cells, and so forth. In the milieu of a healthy bone marrow, and under the appropriate hormonal stimulation (e.g., erythropoietin–erythrocyte stimulation; thrombopoietin–megakaryocyte proliferation; G-CSF–granulocyte colony forming factor), these colonies proceed to produce a large but limited number of mature progeny, resulting in a normal blood profile. These committed colonies, however, lack self-renewal capability. Therefore, the uncommitted stem cell replenishes these clones of cells as it responds to various feedback stimuli that still are being intensively studied.

The morphologic identification of each clone of committed cells in the bone marrow is critical to sophisticated hematologic diagnostic consultation. Each cell lineage is recognizable; aberrations of individual morphology, absolute number, and proportion in relation to other marrow elements allow the hematologist or pathologist to render a diagnosis. The earliest recognizable granulocytic precursor is the myeloblast; during subsequent divisions and morphologic maturation, succeeding generations of cells evolve into progranulocytes (with their unique primary granules), then sequentially into **metamyelocyte, myelocyte, band,** and, ultimately, **granulocyte** (neutrophil) forms. Unique variants of these intermediary stages of maturation also are recognizable for the eosinophilic, basophilic, and monocytic cell clones. During this process, the cells transform their appearance as their intracellular organelles shift from replication imperatives to those required for physiologic function (e.g., granulocytes and monocytes require critical recognition and phagocytic abilities for defense against infections).

A similar process occurs in erythrocytic proliferation and maturation. The earliest recognizable erythroid cell is the **pronormoblast,** which evolves into a **normoblast.** During this maturation process, the intracellular cytoplasm changes from supporting replication to the synthesis of hemoglobin; this latter function is under exquisite, precise control, aberrations of which lead to significant consequences (e.g., thalassemia syndromes). Morphologically the cell cytoplasm transforms from an RNA-rich appearance (basophilic) to a hemoglobin-rich appearance (eosinophilic). The nucleus of the maturing erythrocyte becomes progressively involuted and ultimately is extruded from the cell. Imprecise retention of nuclear remnants is morphologically recognizable in the peripheral circulation as **Howell-Jolly bodies** or **nucleated red cells.**

Megakaryocyte precursors are converted from a mononuclear precursor to clones of cells with 4, 8, and even 16 individual nuclei, which undergo secondary fusion. The resulting characteristic bone marrow element, the megakaryocyte, is volumetrically 10–50 times larger than most other marrow elements and contains characteristic azurophilic granules and the serpiginous cytoplasmic boundaries. Through a unique budding process, each megakaryocyte, during its finite life-span, gives rise to thousands of individual platelets. The unique appearance of the megakaryocyte allows the experienced morphologist to recognize otherwise subtle underlying bone marrow dysfunctional states, because many dysplastic conditions produce smaller cells lacking characteristic granules, paradoxically termed **micromegakaryocytes.**

During fetal development, hematopoiesis is widely distributed throughout the marrow cavity of most bones. Hematopoiesis in the fully matured adult occurs only in the medulla of the flat bones, the ribs, the vertebra, the sternum, and pelvis (the latter two sites allow marrow aspiration and biopsy). Proliferating cells in marrow normally constitute 30–50% of marrow volume in adults; the rest is fat. At times of need (e.g., blood loss or infection), the marrow cellular area expands to fill the fatty sites and even replaces the fat in the long bones. The presence of active marrow replication in the long bones of adults is always a manifestation of an underlying disease state.

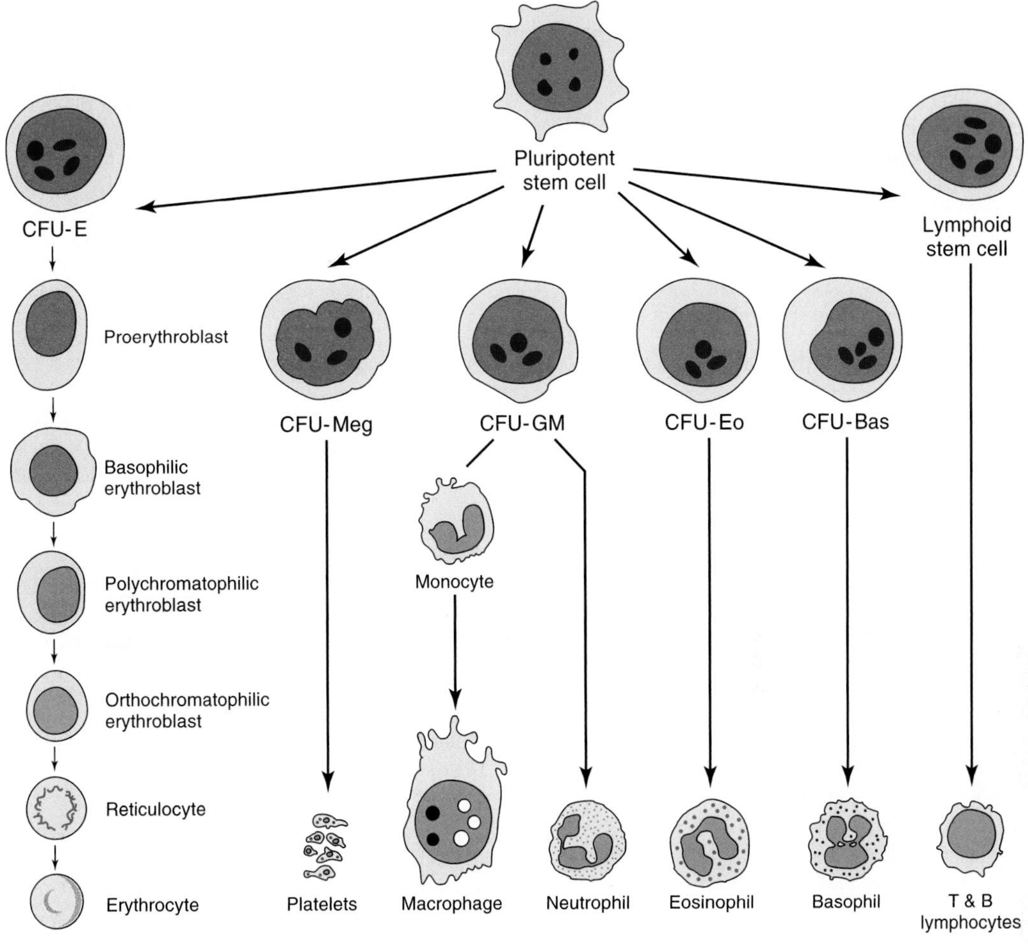


**FIGURE 127.1.** Schematic representation of the development of various cell lines.

# CHAPTER 128 GENERAL ASPECTS OF ANEMIA

In anemia, the hemoglobin and volume of packed RBCs **(hematocrit)** are reduced; with the exception of some thalassemias, the actual number of RBC also is reduced. Most anemias are secondary to other diseases or conditions; therefore it is imperative that the physician attempt to identify and correct the underlying etiology whenever possible. Symptomatic and supportive therapy of anemias is important, even critical in many circumstances, but one should avoid immediate intervention unless the patient is critically ill or a diagnostic evaluation has been initiated. Although most underlying causes ultimately can be identified, indiscriminate use of transfusions before simple straightforward tests have been obtained should be discouraged.

The pattern and severity of anemia, coupled with the patient's history, provide many clues; patients with profound degrees of anemia with minimal symptoms usually have conditions that produce anemia over prolonged periods of time so that the body is able to adapt to a lower oxygen-carrying capacity in the blood (e.g., pernicious anemia, slow chronic GI or menstrual blood loss). In contrast, sudden significant anemia in a previously healthy person causes significant symptoms (e.g., dyspnea on exertion, easy fatigability). The physician should inquire about diet, alcohol consumption, and blood loss. Because patients do take notice of and usually seek medical attention for bright red blood per rectum, such rectal bleeding often does not cause severe anemias;

**TABLE 128.1. Anemia: Some General Physical Findings and Their Significance**

| Finding(s) | Significance |
|---|---|
| Pallor + icterus + splenomegaly | Hemolytic anemia, pernicious anemia, liver disease |
| Neck, axillary, inguinal lymphadenopathy | Lymphoma, leukemia, infection |
| Hepatosplenomegaly | Myeloproliferative or lymphoproliferative disorders, chronic liver disease |
| Sternal tenderness | Acute leukemia |
| Absent vibration/position sense + a positive Romberg test | Subacute combined degeneration of the spinal cord in pernicious anemia |
| Transient, focal neurologic disturbances + obtundation/coma + hemolytic anemia and thrombocytopenic purpura | Thrombotic thrombocytopenic purpura (TTP) or hemolytic uremic syndrome (HUS) |
| Spooning of the fingernails (koilonychia, Figure 128.1), + dry coarse hair | Severe iron deficiency |
| Small (1 mm), well circumscribed red lesions on the lips or nasal mucosa | Hereditary hemorrhagic telangiectasia (HHT) causing severe iron deficiency. |

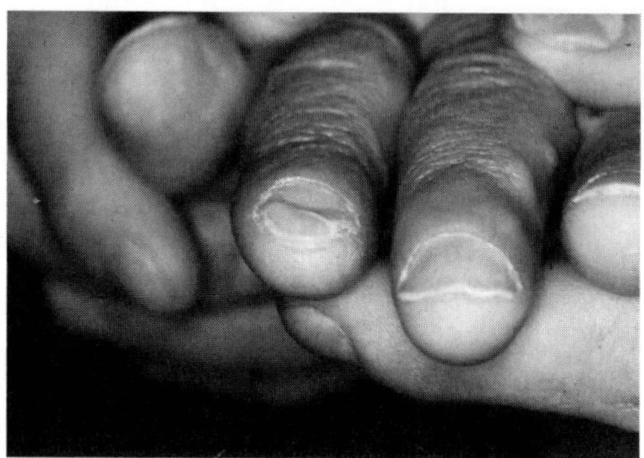

**FIGURE 128.1. Nails of a patient with severe iron deficiency anemia showing koilonychia.**

**TABLE 128.2. Required Basic Laboratory Studies in Anemia**

| | Normal Values | |
|---|---|---|
| **Test(s)** | **Men** | **Women** |
| Hemoglobin (g/dl) | 13–16 | 11–15.5 |
| Hematocrit (%) | 38–50 | 36–48 |
| RBC count (% $10^{12}$/L) | 4.5–6 | 4–5.6 |
| Mean cell hemoglobin (MCH [pg]) | 28–34 | 1 |
| Mean cell volume (MCV) (fl) | 80–95 | |
| WBC count ($10^{12}$/L) | | 4–11 |
| Platelet count ($10^{12}$/L) | 150–450 | |
| Reticulocyte count (%) | | 0.5–1.5 |

Calculation of red cell indices

$$\text{MCV} = \frac{\text{Hematocrit (L/L)}}{\text{Red cell count } (\times 10^{12}/\text{L})}$$

In Femtoliters (fl: $10^{15}$/L)

$$\text{MCH} = \frac{\text{Hemoglobin (g/L)}}{\text{RBC } (\times 10^{12}/\text{L})}$$

In picograms

$$\text{MCHC} = \frac{\text{Hemoglobin (g/dl)}}{\text{Hematocrit (L/L)}}$$

many patients, however, fail to notice chronic melenic stools, or the chronic GI bleeding may be inapparent, so that severe anemia develops insidiously. Many women underestimate the degree of their menstrual blood losses. In those with consistently excessive menses, the mere reproducibility of that excess may cause a false sense of "normalcy." The number of pregnancies gives a clue regarding prior stress on a women's baseline iron stores, which may severely compound other iron losses. Besides information about occupational or environmental exposure to potentially toxic chemicals, solvents, or medications, other useful data include a family history of anemia, icterus, splenectomy, or gallstones at an early age.

Physical examination may detect pallor. Although not always a reliable finding, pallor may give clues, especially when coupled with other findings of atrophic glossitis or neurologic abnormalities (e.g., pernicious anemia–vitamin $B_{12}$ deficiency) or cutaneous and retinal hemorrhages (e.g., iron deficiency secondary to a bleeding diathesis). Cardiovascular examination may disclose tachycardia, cardiac dilatation, or flow murmurs; high-output heart failure may be present with prolonged or severe anemia. Pelvic or rectal examination may show bleeding or its causative lesion (e.g., uterine fibroids with menometrorrhagia, hemorrhoids, cancer). Hypothyroidism is suggested by the facial appearance, slowly relaxing reflexes, and body alopecia. (Some other physical findings and their significance are shown in Table 128.1; categories of anemia are listed in Table 128.2; and laboratory studies required in anemia are presented in Figure 128.2.)

The RBC morphology in anemia has diagnostic significance. Because the normal erythrocyte population has characteristic features, deviations from the norm give clues as to the general categories of anemias, suggest possible causes, and, thus, guide the clinician regarding prioritization of diagnostic testing. Although examination of the peripheral smear by light microscopy is ideal, it is becoming a lost art among physicians; however, the clinician should at least be able to interpret the laboratory technician's report of the smear or the newer computerized values, including such modalities as nomograms, which calculate parameters with diagnostic implications. Variations from normal result from imbalances in nuclear or cytoplasmic development. Persistence of normal parameters in the face of significant anemia usually indicates that the anemia is secondary to multiple causes or syndromes, which also must be identified and assessed. Anemia occurs in three categories based on cell morphology and calculated red cell indices: hypochromic microcytic anemia, macrocytic anemia, and normocytic normochromic anemia (see Figure 128.2). Normocytic anemias have two subtypes: those with normal or low reticulocyte count (<2% or <0.085 $10^6/mm^3$) and those with elevated reticulocytes (>2% or >0.1 $10^6/mm^3$). Variations in the size of RBC are indicated by **red cell distribution width** (RDW), normally 11% to 15%.

**Normocytic, normochromic anemias** are those anemias in which the indices suggest that the RBC production has not been perturbed by serious disorders in nuclear or cytoplasmic maturation, but the production rate is simply inadequate, either because the marrow is suppressed or because there is an increased destruction rate or loss of cells. Most often this is due to a concomitant, clinically active disease that is readily apparent. Depending on the identification of such entities, these anemias are historically characterized as the anemia of

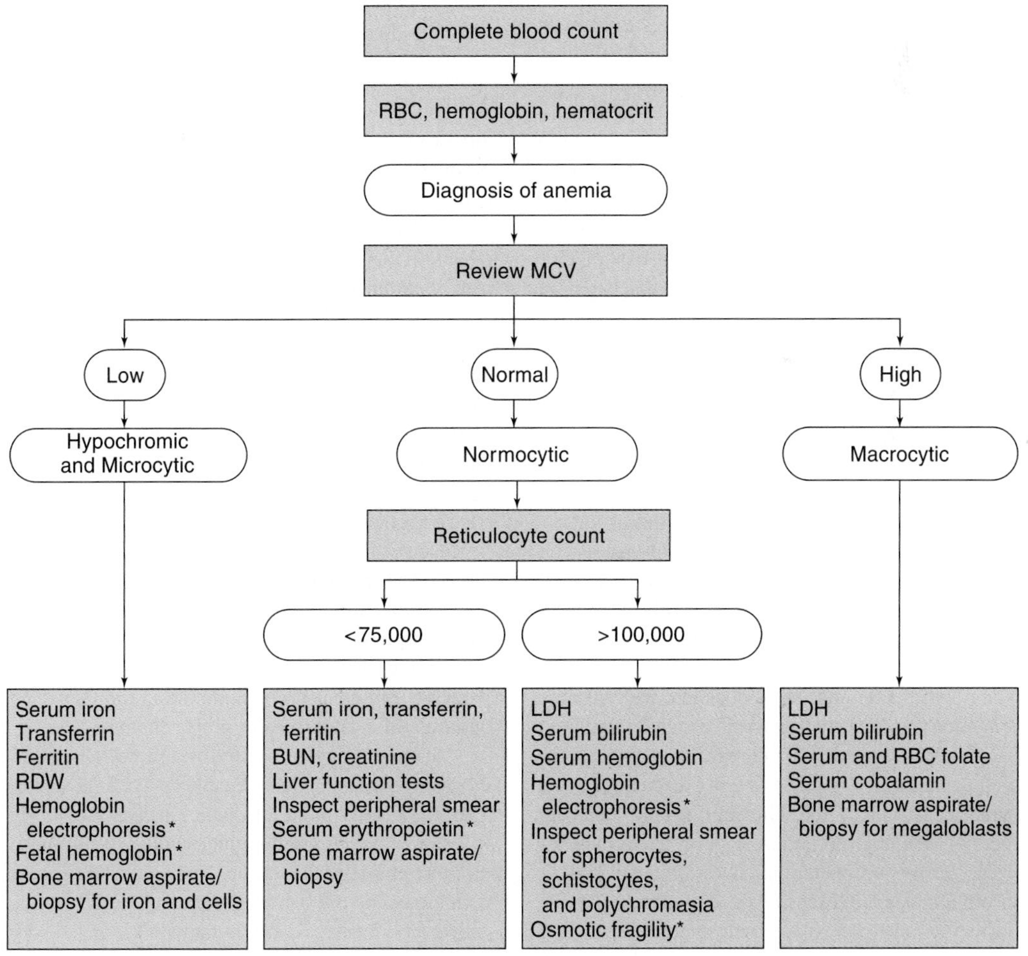


**FIGURE 128.2. Categories of anemia and suggested studies. * = not routinely required.**

**TABLE 128.3. Causes of Normochromic Normocytic Anemia with Normal or Low Reticulocyte Count**

| Abnormal Morphology | Normal Morphology |
|---|---|
| Aplastic anemia | Chronic Disease |
| Metastatic malignancy | Renal insufficiency |
| Leukemia/lymphoma | Endocrine Disorders |
| Myeloma/macroglobulinemia | HIV Infection |
| Myelodysplastic anemia | Hepatocellular disorders |

chronic renal failure, anemia of hepatic disease, anemia of inflammation, and so forth. In essence, if one identifies a clinically active co-morbid condition requiring intervention, and especially if there is clinical or laboratory evidence of other organ dysfunction, a mild anemia with relatively normal indices most likely is a secondary anemia and need not be aggressively evaluated unless its severity is out of proportion to the co-morbid condition, does not correlate with subsequent changes in the co-morbid condition, or is of such severity that treatment is required. In any of these situations one must test for other concomitant forms of anemia that also might be present, and for which treatment can be readily effected (Table 128.3). Normocytic anemias with low reticulocytes and a normal morphology occur in systemic disorders, whereas those with elevated reticulocyte counts accompany active hemorrhage, hemolytic anemia, or removal of a myelotoxic factor. The anemias mentioned are discussed in greater detail later in this chapter.

The clinician should be alert to the presence or absence of abnormal numbers or forms of other blood elements as additional clues. Immature leukocyte precursors such as metamyelocytes may suggest infections, whereas myeloblasts suggest underlying malignancies, including leukemias; if accompanied by abnormal platelet forms, this picture of **leukoerythroblastosis** suggests an underlying myelophthisic condition due to metastatic cancer to the bone marrow. RBC rouleaux suggests a circulating paraproteinemia consistent with an inflammatory state if polyclonal, and multiple myeloma if monoclonal.

**Macrocytic anemias** are associated with disease states in which nuclear maturation is delayed relative to the cytoplasmic production of hemoglobin. Although the list of specific causes is extensive (as discussed in the following paragraphs), the clinician should consider disorders of cobalamin (vitamin $B_{12}$) or folate metabolism (e.g., pernicious anemia [an autoimmune disorder], malabsorption states, GI diseases). Many drugs may be responsible for iatrogenic macrocytic anemias, including all the anticancer antimetabolites such as 5-fluorouracil and methotrexate (which is also used in many patients with rheumatoid arthritis), Imuran (used in systemic lupus erythematosus and solid organ transplant recipients), and alkylating agents for cancers. An interesting syndrome, common among members of the dental profession and teenagers, is nitrous oxide abuse, which interferes with vitamin $B_{12}$ metabolism, causing macrocytosis and, ultimately, anemia and other effects of vitamin $B_{12}$ deprivation.

**Microcytic anemias** are associated with disease states in which cytoplasmic production of hemoglobin is delayed relative to nuclear maturation. If the patient can be documented to have had a normal complete blood cell count (CBC) within the past few years, this implies a diagnosis of iron deficiency in adults, and testing must be done to confirm or refute this possibility. If documented, iron deficiency must prompt a diagnostic search for the cause of blood loss. If there is previous evidence of a microcytic anemia, especially dating back to childhood, an inherited congenital form of hemoglobin synthesis dysfunction—a hemoglobinopathy state such as thalassemia—should be suspected.

## Etiologic Factors for Anemia

Anemias can be conceptualized in many ways. One straightforward way is to realize that anemias are due to one or more of the following conditions: (1) inadequate production of RBCs; (2) excessive loss of RBCs; or (3) excessive destruction of RBCs.

**(1) Inadequate production.** Several substances are essential for the manufacture of hemoglobin or RBC: iron, vitamin $B_{12}$, folic acid, and certain hormones (such as thyroxine, testosterone, or hematopoietic growth factors, e.g. erythropoietin). Iron deficiency in adults almost invariably is the result of chronic blood loss caused by a localized lesion or lesions, or from an inability to absorb iron following certain surgical procedures. The list of causes of iron deficiency is extensive; however, one should think in terms of anatomic causes, e.g., diverticula or angiodysplasia (bowel), peptic ulcer (stomach), menstrual losses, excessive reproductive losses, and fibroids (uterus). Iron malabsorption may result from iatrogenic or other causes in the proximal small intestine (e.g., gastric bypass surgery), or disorders affecting gastric acidification (e.g., atrophic gastritis). Parasitic infections are uncommon in the United States, but are still a major health problem worldwide.

Vitamin $B_{12}$ requires **intrinsic factor** (IF), produced by gastric parietal cells to enable its systemic absorption from the gut. Without adequate intrinsic factor, vitamin $B_{12}$ cannot be absorbed in the terminal ileum, the site of its most efficient absorption. Thus, atrophic gastritis or pernicious anemia can cause inadequate IF production, and, consequently, cause vitamin $B_{12}$ malabsorption. Similarly, diseases that cause inflammation or injury to the mucosa of the terminal ileum (e.g., Crohn's disease) interfere with absorption; surgical resection for such conditions produces a permanent iatrogenic mechanism for vitamin $B_{12}$ malabsorption.

Anemia from folic acid deficiency may follow nutritional deprivation or enhanced demand (as in late pregnancy) in the face of prior nutritional deficiency. It is exacerbated in hematologic conditions that cause a constant excessive stress on folate metabolism (e.g., hemoglobinopathies, such as sickle cell disease, or immunologic states, such as autoimmune hemolytic anemia with markedly reduced RBC lifespan), requiring a more rapid production rate. In the United States, folate deficiency is only rarely an isolated problem unless the patient's lifestyle produces a constant behavior of nutritional deficiency (e.g., chronic alcoholism).

Important, potentially life-threatening conditions associated with inadequate production include bone marrow failure states such as aplastic anemia, myelodysplastic syndromes, myelofibrosis, or myelophthisic anemias (bone marrow infiltration by diseases, including cancer). Anemias of chronic infection, inflammation, or renal failure all represent dysfunctional inadequate production due to concomitant illnesses. These conditions should be identified and, if possible, corrected; failure or inability to do so will lead to a chronic condition that may expose the patient to otherwise unnecessary expense, discomfort, or blood replacement therapy.

**(2) Excessive blood loss.** Chronic blood loss is complicated by the resultant iron deficiency so that the patient's anemia is secondary to both excessive losses and compromised production. Blood loss should be relatively easily to identify by performing a careful history, physical examination, and selected diagnostic tests. Durations of signs and symptoms are important, as are inquiries regarding whether the patient is aware of previous medical encounters that can retrospectively document the presence or absence of anemia. (For example, has this mother of five children, still menstruating heavily at age 45, *had* a normal hemoglobin/hematocrit, mean cell volume (MCV), or iron studies? Has the patient ever been prescribed iron therapy? At the time of elective surgery in the recent past was the patient anemic? Has the patient used aspirin or other nonsteroidal medications for chronic arthritic problems? Does the patient [and family] have a history of easy bruisability, irregular menses, etc.? Is there a family history of anemias?) Laboratory tests can identify many sources of blood loss quickly, e.g., repetitive examination of stool or urine for blood. The CBC findings, especially the RBC numbers and the mean cell volume (MCV), give clues to the underlying mechanisms of anemia.

**(3) Excessive destruction of RBCs** usually results from immune challenges (e.g., autoimmune hemolytic anemia alone or as a manifestation of a more general immunologic disorder such as SLE), a pharmacologic stress (use of certain antibiotics in patients with underlying G6PD deficiency), or a congenital hereditary hemoglobinopathy such as sickle cell disease. Pernicious anemia exemplifies how physiologically complex anemias can be: although pernicious anemia follows nutritional vitamin $B_{12}$ deficiency leading to inadequate production, technically, the failure to produce erythrocytes is due to intramedullary destruction of defective RBC owing to the vitamin $B_{12}$ deficiency. The component of hemolysis in severe pernicious anemia exceeds all but the most severe and unusual immune hemolytic states.

# CHAPTER 129 HYPOCHROMIC, MICROCYTIC ANEMIAS

**Hypochromic microcytic anemias** result from a failure to synthesize normal amounts of hemoglobin. Iron deficiency anemia is the most common form of this type of anemia in adults; thalassemias are most common in children, and less common in adults, as are the sideroblastic anemias, a subcategory of myelodysplastic syndromes. Laboratory differentiation of these anemias is illustrated in Figure 129.1.

## Iron Deficiency Anemia

Most functioning iron is included as constituents of porphyrin compounds (hemoglobin and myoglobin) and as trace elements of respiratory enzymes (e.g., cytochrome C, catalase). The balance of the total body iron is nonporphyrin, set aside for transport and storage. Iron is a highly reactive substance with the potential to cause serious oxidative damage to cells, especially as a cofactor with other oxidative stresses. Hence it can be transported safely only when bound to specialized proteins such as **transferrin.** Normally, 100 ml plasma contains about 300 to 400 mg of transferrin, which binds 50 to 150 μg of iron. About one third of the plasma transferrin normally is saturated with iron. Iron is stored in the liver, spleen, and marrow as ferritin or hemosiderin. **Ferritin,** a composite of iron-containing micelles, is water-soluble, and is leached from cells during staining procedures; it is

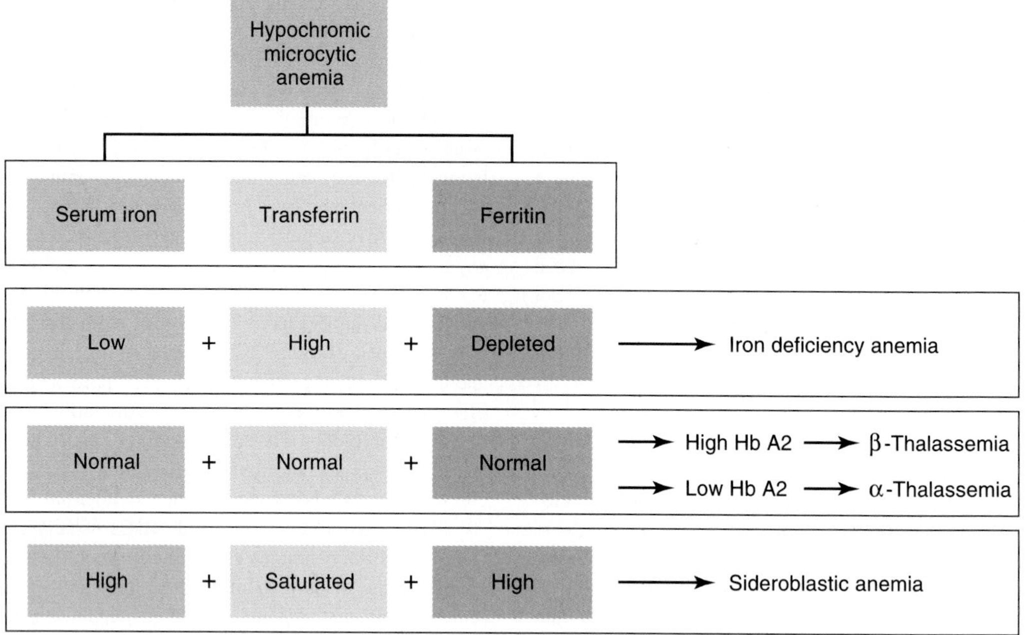


**FIGURE 129.1.** Hypochromic, microcytic anemias—an overview.

invisible in marrow on ordinary microscopy. **Hemosiderin,** an insoluble product made of multiple ferritin micelles (molecular aggregates) bound to insoluble proteins, is seen microscopically with the Prussian blue stain.

## The Iron Cycle

The iron cycle is depicted in Figure 129.2. About 10% of dietary ferrous iron is absorbed into the bloodstream from the duodenum. Bound to transferrin, it is taken to the liver and marrow for storage or use in erythropoiesis. In the normoblastic mitochondria, ferrous iron joins with protoporphyrin to assemble heme (Figure 129.3). Heme is transported to the ribosomes. It then combines with two alpha and two beta polypeptide chains to create the intact hemoglobin molecule. This molecule consists of four heme moieties integrated into the four discrete polypeptide chains, creating the intact hemoglobin structure with its intricate tertiary structure and intermolecular charges, which facilitate oxygen binding. Hemoglobin synthesis abates as the RBC matures, manifested by extrusion of the nucleus and cessation of ribosomal RNA-directed protein and heme synthesis. Once this occurs, the human RBC has a discrete lifespan, because there is no mechanism to further synthesize the proteins necessary to maintain the functional and structural components of the RBC. After a lifespan of 120 days, the enzymatically depleted RBC is phagocytosed by macrophages (see Figure 129.2). Some of the iron is recycled back to the marrow via transferrin for new hemoglobin synthesis. Unused iron is deposited in reticuloendothelial cells as ferritin and hemosiderin (Figure 129.4). Excess ferritin is released into plasma; it serves as an index of iron deficiency or overload because its serum level reflects tissue iron turnover.

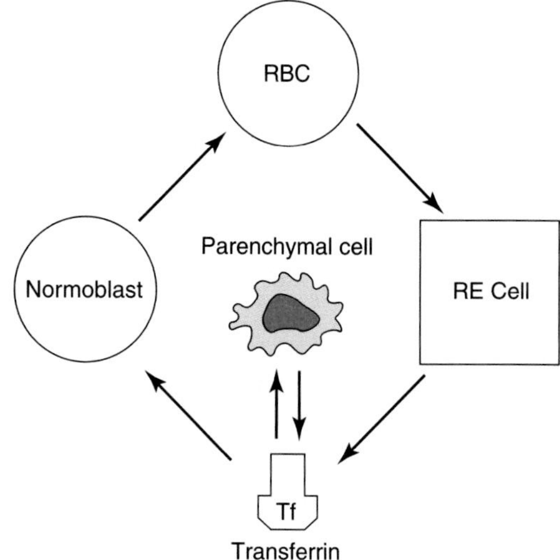


**FIGURE 129.2.** The iron cycle.

## Iron Absorption and Distribution

The infant starts life with an adequate supply of iron, acquired at the expense of its mother's own iron stores. During the early years of growth, the demand for iron is met through diet. By the time of puberty, body iron stores are established. Adult men lose about 1 mg of iron daily (through desquamation, minor bleeding, hair loss, etc.); this loss is readily offset by a normal diet that provides more than 10 mg of iron daily. Women, during their menstruating years, require about 2 mg of iron daily, depending on menstrual frequency, flow, and duration. Iron loss is further exacerbated during pregnancy; each pregnancy entails a net transfer to the infant, and loss to the mother, of 700 mg iron, even before the continued increased losses caused by lactation and resumption of menses. After the menopause, iron requirements in men and women equalize at 1 mg per day, but many women enter menopause iron-deficient, or at least iron-depleted.

Iron exchange is almost entirely endogenous. The body is physiologically designed to retain iron avidly, and lacks a mechanism to secrete or otherwise eliminate excess iron. Hence, any evidence of iron deficiency in an adult requires a careful search for the site of chronic bleeding. The major sources of bleeding are disorders of the gastrointestinal tract (e.g., peptic ulcers, reflux esophagitis, carcinoma, polyps, hemorrhoids), menstruation, and pregnancy. Less common sites of blood loss include the nasal cavity, oral cavity, and lungs (e.g., hemoptysis due to hereditary hemorrhagic telangiectasia or pulmonary hemosiderosis). Urinary blood loss, as hemosiderin, occurs in intravascular hemolysis from paroxysmal nocturnal hemoglobinuria (PNH).

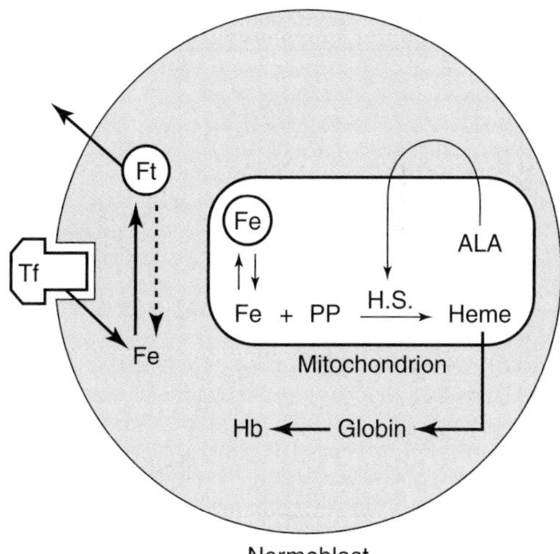


**FIGURE 129.3. Heme synthesis in the mitochondria of normoblast. ALA = aminolevulinic acid; Fe = iron; H.S. = heme synthetase; Hb = hemoglobin; PP = protoporphyrin; Ft = ferritin; Tf = transferrin.**

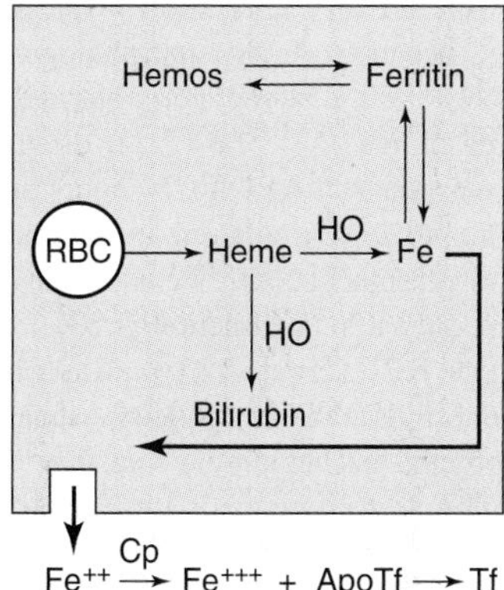


**FIGURE 129.4. Iron disposition in the reticuloendothelial cell. ApoTf = apotransferrin; Cp = ceruloplasmin; Hemos = hemosiderin; HO = heme oxygenase; Tf = transferrin.**

## Clinical Features

Both the degree of anemia and the rapidity with which it develops influence the clinical picture. Symptoms may be completely absent, or the patient may report variable weakness, light-headedness, and palpitations. Muscular weakness may occur, because iron is an integral component of myoglobin. Dyspnea may be caused by a diminished oxygen-carrying capacity, although a deficiency in respiratory enzymes also may be responsible. The hair may be coarse and lusterless and the fingernails brittle. In far advanced iron deficiency, fingernails show spooning (**koilonychia**). (See Fig. 128-1).

## Laboratory Features

Normal values for iron studies in the adult and their aberrations in iron deficiency are shown in Table 129.1. Iron deficiency anemia evolves through several stages. Early in the development of iron deficiency, storage iron is greatly diminished, as indicated by low ferritin values and depleted stainable marrow iron. The peripheral blood smear may be normal. As the disorder progresses, red cell distribution width (RDW) increases, followed by hypochromia and microcytosis (Color Plate 22), then by anemia. Simultaneously, serum iron gradually declines, with a corresponding increase in transferrin and a progressive drop in the percent saturation of transferrin. With the cessation of blood loss and initiation of iron therapy, these values gradually become normal, in reverse order. The ferritin level and the bone marrow storage iron are the last to be restored to normal.

## Management

The goal of management of iron deficiency is twofold: to give therapeutic iron and to locate and correct

TABLE 129.1. Laboratory Studies in Various Stages of Iron Deficiency

| Laboratory Test | Early | Advanced | Iron Deficiency Anemia |
|---|---|---|---|
| Peripheral smear | Normal | Slight hypochromia | Marked hypochromia and microcytosis |
| MCV (fl) | >80 | 75–85 | <80 |
| MCH (pg) | >32 | 28–32 | <27 |
| RDW | 14–18 | 14–18 | >18 |
| Serum iron (μg/dl) | >35 | <30 | <10 |
| Transferrin (μg/dl) | 250–350 | 300–450 | >450 |
| % Saturation | 35 | 15–30 | <10 |
| Ferritin (μg/mL) | 15–20 | 10–20 | <10 |
| Bone marrow iron | | | Completely depleted |

the site of blood loss. **Therapeutic iron** is administered in the form of simple iron salts, such as ferrous sulfate or gluconate; composite capsules are best avoided. Oral ferrous sulfate, 325 mg daily, provides 65 mg of elemental iron, far in excess of what the normal GI tract is capable of absorbing, even in the iron-depleted state in which the mucosal cell receptors are upregulated to increase iron absorption. Thus, the practice of increasing the daily iron dosage to 2 to 3 tablets should be discouraged unless there is a reason to assume underlying iron malabsorption. Higher iron doses cause GI side effects and tend to promote noncompliance. Many experienced physicians prefer to use only one tablet daily, thereby enhancing patient compliance for longer periods of time. Adequate replacement produces a recovery of hemoglobin of 1 g/dl/week (Figure 129.5). Oral iron should be continued for at least 6 months after the hemoglobin level reaches normal, assuming the cause of blood loss can be corrected; if it cannot be corrected, lifelong replacement may be necessary. If anemia is not corrected by an adequate trial of oral iron in a compliant patient, then an α or β thalassemia trait must be suspected, although malabsorption remains a possibility.

Transfusions are not necessary for most types of anemia for which effective medications are available. Furthermore, transfusions sometimes are hazardous, and they may lead to a false sense of security by ignoring the basic cause of the infirmity. Transfusions should be given for an exsanguinating hemorrhage or to prepare for impending major surgery, but most patients with iron deficiency respond adequately to oral iron. Parenteral iron, despite its perceived risks, normally is well tolerated and can very effectively reverse serious iron deficiency. However, it should be administered carefully under the supervision of a hematologist.

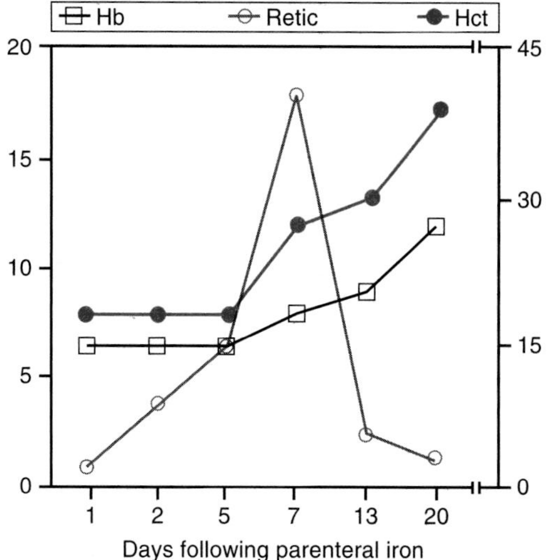


FIGURE 129.5. Response of blood elements to iron therapy.

## Anemia of Chronic Inflammation

### Pathogenesis and Pathophysiology

**Anemia of chronic inflammation** (also called anemia of chronic disease) is a common form of anemia. It is grouped with the iron deficiencies because it is associated with a major aberration in the way iron is handled, not because of any morphologic similarity. Normally, when $^{59}$Fe is administered intravenously, half of the plasma radioactive $^{59}$Fe (T1/2) disappears in 90 minutes; it reappears in RBC in 24 hours and peaks in 7 days with 80–90% accumulation. In contrast, in chronic inflammation, plasma T1/2 of $^{59}$Fe occurs in less than 30 minutes, and only a small fraction (<20%) of the dose reappears in the RBC (Figure 129.6). Most of the cleared iron is sequestered in the spleen, suggesting that reticuloendothelial tissues play a role in iron clearance during infection. Iron compounds are required to promote bacterial proliferation as well as hematopoiesis. Thus, iron sequestration may, in a manner of defense, help deprive invading bacteria of a required growth factor. Anemia of chronic inflammation appears to be mediated by negative regulatory cytokines, such as IL-1, tumor necrosis factor alpha (TNFα), and transforming growth factor beta (TGFβ), all of which inhibit erythropoietin production and produce hypoproliferative anemia with defective RBC lifespan.

## Clinical and Laboratory Features

Many chronic inflammatory disorders cause anemia—pyelonephritis, osteomyelitis, bacterial endocarditis, tuberculosis, HIV, pleuritis, and rheumatoid arthritis, to name a few. Each dominates the clinical picture; the anemia is incidental to or part of the clinical picture. A low serum iron (frequently <10 μg/dl) and a low transferrin (as low as 100 mg/dl) indicate aberrations in iron metabolism. In contrast to iron deficiency, because both the serum iron and transferrin levels are low, the transferrin saturation is normal. An elevated serum ferritin (Figure 129.7) and abundant iron deposition in bone marrow macrophages attest to increased iron storage. The iron, iron-binding capacity (transferrin), and serum ferritin levels in various clinical disorders are shown in Figure 129.8.

The anemias of chronic inflammation usually are normocytic and normochromic, although they may become hypochromic in later stages. The RBC or platelets lack a distinctive morphology, but an underlying infection may cause leukocytosis. Reticulocytes are less than 1.5% (75,000/cμm). The granulocytes and their precursors often display exaggerated ("toxic") granulation, which is an index of accelerated granulocytopoiesis. Dohle inclusion bodies in the WBCs are an important indicator of pyogenic infection. The bone marrow shows granulocytic hyperplasia. Prussian blue staining of marrow aspirates confirms excess stainable iron, much of which is contained in the cytoplasm of the macrophages. The anemia and abnormal iron values all normalize if the infection is overcome. Erythropoiesis may be accelerated by use of recombinant erythropoietin. Transfusions rarely are indicated, because the anemia is not severe, but they may be necessary to prepare for, or recover from, intercurrent surgery.

## Anemia of Chronic Renal Insufficiency

Anemia of chronic renal insufficiency is similar in morphology to that of chronic inflammation, but with some notable differences. Whereas $^{59}$Fe is cleared rapidly during inflammation (T1/2 = <30 min), its plasma T1/2 is prolonged (>120 min) in renal failure. The RBC lifespan is reduced by half when measured in the patient's body, but it is normalized if the same cell is introduced into a normal person. This diminished survival is attributed to

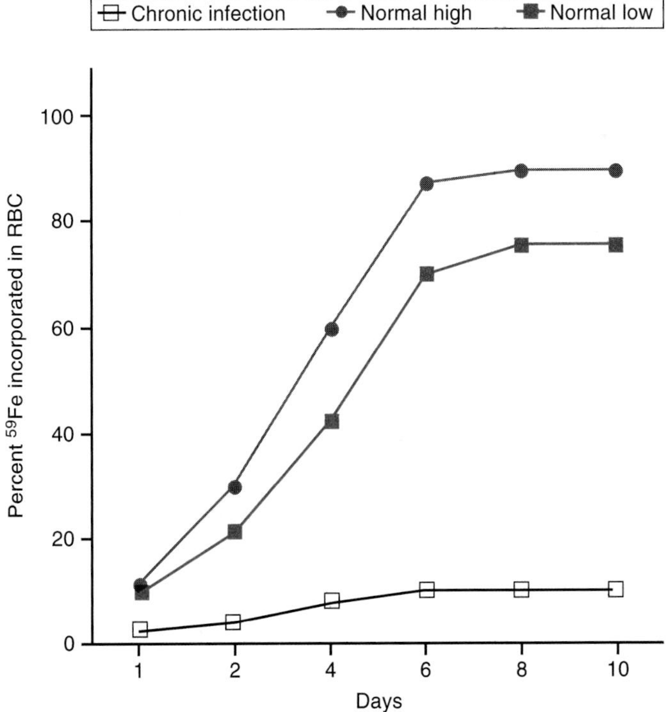


**FIGURE 129.6. Incorporation of radiolabeled iron in healthy individuals and those with anemia of chronic infection.**

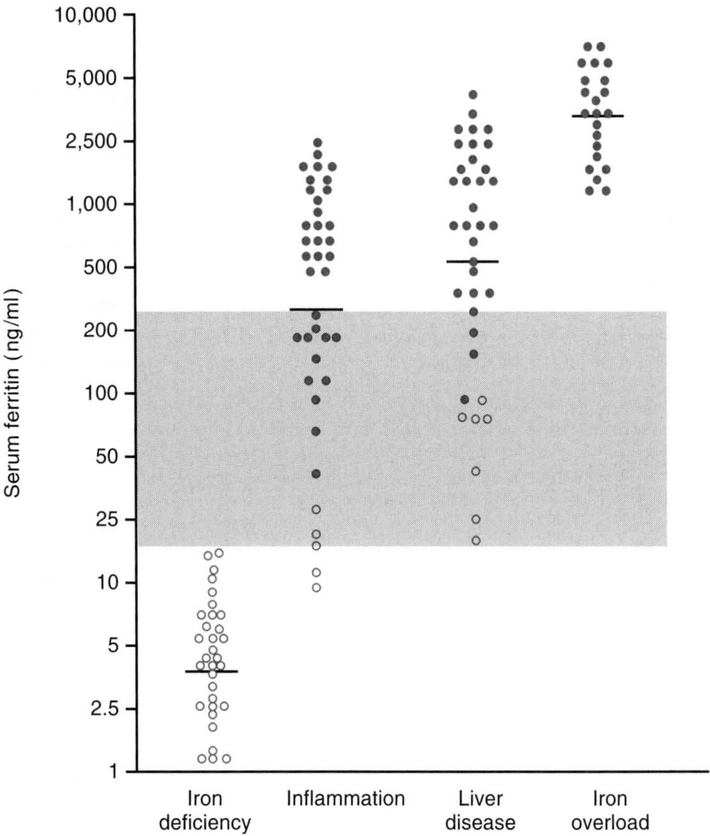


**FIGURE 129.7. Serum ferritin in various clinical disorders.** Horizontal lines indicate geometric means. Open circles show iron deficiency (total iron-binding capacity <400 mg/dl and transferrin saturation <16% and/or absent marrow iron). Shaded area shows the normal range.

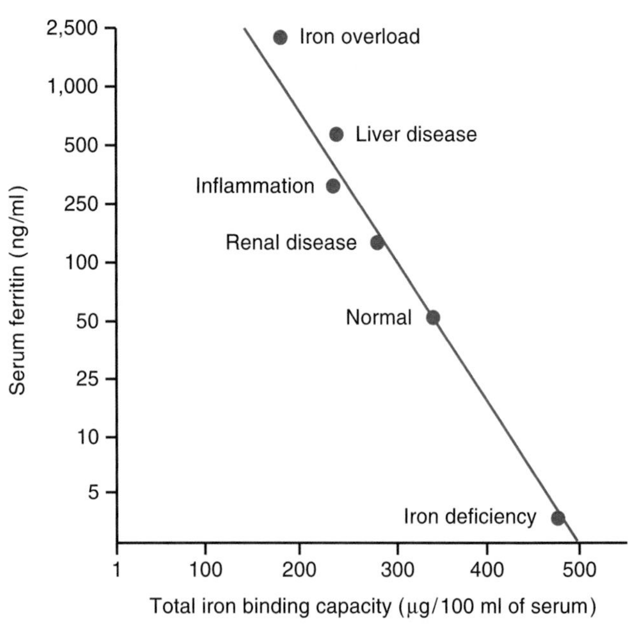


**FIGURE 129.8.** Serum ferritin and total iron-binding capacity in various clinical disorders. (Redrawn with permission from: Lipshitz DA et al. N Engl J Med 1974; 290: 1215.)

chemical damage from azotemia, oxidation by free radicals, and mechanical damage due to RBC fragmentation and membrane loss; this often is manifested morphologically in the peripheral smear by the presence of "burr cells." Erythropoiesis is somewhat suppressed by abnormal amounts of inactivated cytokines (IL-1, TNF-γ, and interferon-γ), but the major cause of anemia is inadequate production of **erythropoietin,** a glycoprotein hormone made in the kidney; patients with advanced renal failure have a defect in erythropoietin production. Because of this combination of a shortened RBC lifespan (~50 days), and inadequate production due to erythropoietin deprivation, RBC transfusions were common in the past, often leading to iatrogenic iron overload states. The development of synthetic erythropoietin to treat anemia of chronic renal insufficiency has somewhat ameliorated this problem.

## Sideroblastic Anemia

**Sideroblastic anemia** is caused by a defect of iron incorporation into the heme molecule. The iron is retained in the mitochondria, where it accumulates, leading to a functional blockade of iron incorporation in RBC, and deposition of excess iron in reticuloendothelial cells in the marrow and liver. As a result, iron rises in plasma and eventually saturates all of the transferrin. The peripheral RBCs display a biphasic distribution curve; some are large, but others are small with low hemoglobin content. Ringed sideroblasts, representing RBC precursors with excess iron retained in the perinuclear mitochondria are easily seen in marrow (Color Plate 23), and are diagnostic.

Several clinical types of sideroblastic anemia are known. One is a rare hereditary sex-linked disorder involving only men; it responds to a degree to pharmacologic doses of pyridoxine, which partly corrects an enzymatic defect in the first stage of heme synthesis. **Acquired sideroblastic anemia** may follow exposure to certain drugs or chemicals that interfere with various enzymes required in heme synthesis; possible environmental or medical causes include alcohol (inhibits heme synthetase), lead exposure (inhibits multiple enzyme steps), chloramphenicol (an antibiotic that inhibited mitochondrial protein synthesis, once the most frequent cause of sideroblastic anemia but rarely used anymore), and isoniazid (interferes with pyridoxine utilization, jeopardizing early stages of heme synthesis). Another type, without obvious cause **(idiopathic sideroblastic anemia),** occurs most often in elderly persons; it is included among myelodysplastic anemias. Currently, sideroblastic anemias are not curable unless an offending drug can be identified and removed.

# CHAPTER 130 THE MACROCYTIC ANEMIAS

In **macrocytosis,** erythrocytes appear large on visual evaluation, with an increase in both mean cell volume (MCV) and RDW. RBCs in normal newborns normally exhibit macrocytosis. In liver disease and alcohol ingestion, cholesterol may be adsorbed onto RBC membranes, producing increased distensibility with resulting unusual morphology. Plasma cholesterol often is decreased correspondingly in this type of macrocytosis. An unusually large proportion of reticulocytes may elevate the MCV, because reticulocytes are larger than mature RBC. Finally, RBCs may agglutinate when hyperglobulinemia or cold agglutinins are present, causing falsely high indices as the automated machine inadvertently counts clusters of cells. As a result, the MCV is falsely elevated.

Macrocytic anemias are disparate entities. In megaloblastic anemias, functional proliferation fails, because defective DNA synthesis leads to effective diminished mitosis; the result is large RBCs. Megaloblastic anemias are caused by a deficiency of vitamin $B_{12}$ or folic acid or the failure to incorporate folate because of iatrogenic factors such as antimetabolite drugs used in treating malignancy or autoimmune diseases. Occasionally, myelodysplastic syndromes such as idiopathic sideroblastic anemia may demonstrate macrocytosis associated with ineffective erythropoiesis.

## The Megaloblastic Anemias

### Definition and Pathophysiology

Megaloblastic anemias are characterized by accumulations of large cells with disordered maturation. In cobalamin (vitamin $B_{12}$) and folate deficiency, all dividing cells show a similar abnormality: large size, inadequate chromatin because of deficient DNA content, and profuse cytoplasm with excessive RNA. Vitamin $B_{12}$ is an important cofactor in converting homocysteine to methionine to produce methyl groups. Folic acid transports these methyl groups (as $N^{5,10}$-methylene tetrahydrofolate) to the site of cellular proliferation in order to convert uridylate (RNA base) to thymidylic acid (DNA base). Without vitamin $B_{12}$, methyl groups are not formed; without folic acid, they are not transported to sites of activity. However, with either deficiency, DNA synthesis becomes defective and cytoplasmic RNA accumulates. The marrow and blood pictures associated with vitamin $B_{12}$ and with folate deficiencies are indistinguishable from each other. However, serious, even irreversible, neurologic disturbances may follow cobalamin deficiency because of its unique role in providing fatty acids to protect the spinal cord. Although folic acid may correct the abnormal blood picture of vitamin $B_{12}$ deficiency, it offers no protection from neurologic disease. Thus, it is essential to distinguish between these two deficiencies and to correct a vitamin $B_{12}$ deficiency. Incorrect presumption of folate deficiency with repletion may precipitate an irreversible neurologic injury in patients with significant underlying vitamin $B_{12}$ deficiency.

## Etiology and Pathogenesis

Cobalamin is available only from diet. The adult daily requirement is 1.0–2.0 μg. In the gastrointestinal tract, cobalamin binds first to R-proteins and then to intrinsic factor (IF), a glycoprotein from gastric parietal cells (see Chapter 71 and Figure 71.2). Cobalamin is released from the cobalamin-IF complex in the ileum, where it is absorbed. Vitamin $B_{12}$ is transported by several transcobalamins. Dietary vitamin $B_{12}$ deprivation is exceedingly rare because of its ubiquitous distribution, its minuscule daily requirement, and its long biologic half-life; vegans (strict vegetarians), exceptions to this rule, sometimes manifest vitamin $B_{12}$ deficiency after many years of following this dietary lifestyle. However, the normally $B_{12}$ replete patient will not manifest megaloblastic anemia for many months, often years, after discontinuation of vitamin $B_{12}$ replacement or the development of malabsorption.

In **pernicious anemia** (PA), IF deficiency causes vitamin $B_{12}$ malabsorption. Autoantibodies are directed against gastric parietal cells, more specifically, the gastric $H^+/K^+$-ATPase. The gastritis that follows impairs IF secretion; ultimately, IF deficiency develops. Also, antibodies to IF that occur in the gastric juice bind to the vitamin $B_{12}$-binding sites in the IF, thus preventing formation of vitamin $B_{12}$-IF complex. Partial gastrectomy severely impairs vitamin $B_{12}$ absorption by removing parietal cells. Vitamin $B_{12}$ absorption may also be curtailed by ileal disease or resection; more unusually, this effect may result from competition for vitamin $B_{12}$ from bacterial overgrowth in blind intestinal loops or infestation with the fish tapeworm, *Diphyllobothrium latum*. Rarely, the cause may be exposure to nitrous oxide (either during anesthesia or by illicit use). Vitamin $B_{12}$ malabsorption ultimately causes vitamin $B_{12}$ depletion.

## Clinical Features

Anemia from cobalamin deficiency develops very slowly, thus allowing ample cardiovascular compensation. Patients whose cobalamin deficiency is the result of PA usually are elderly. Pernicious anemia, an autoimmune disorder, is unusual in younger patients. Patients with full-fledged cases exhibit severe anemia and pallor. An acquired intracorpuscular defect and ineffective erythropoiesis cause hemolysis, and, thus, mild icterus. Characteristic signs include papillary atrophy and an extremely pallid appearance of the tongue and buccal mucosa (resembling boiled veal). Angina, dyspnea, and, eventually, high-output heart failure follow. Palpitations, vertigo, and syncope are reported. Because of the unique role of cobalamin in myelin metabolism, a deficiency predisposes to several neurologic changes: subacute combined degeneration of the spinal cord (impaired vibration and position senses, hyporeflexia, and a positive Romberg test); bizarre behavior (paranoia); and "megaloblastic madness" (psychosis). Because pernicious anemia is an autoimmune disease, it often is associated with concomitant autoantibodies directed against other glands as well. Thus, all patients with PA should be evaluated for hypothyroidism and the presence of antithyroid antibodies. Gastric cancer develops in 8% of patients with pernicious anemia, a rate greater than expected in the general population.

## Diagnosis

In PA, there is complete achylia and achlorhydria (absence of gastric juice). The serum vitamin $B_{12}$ level usually is diminished. The diagnostic findings of PA are severe anemia, macrocytosis, leukopenia, and thrombocytopenia. The red cell distribution width (RDW) is increased, and the RBCs show great **anisocytosis** and **poikilocytosis** (i.e., vary in size and shape), often with large, oval-shaped RBC (macro-ovalocytosis). The neutrophils also are large, with increased nuclear lobulations (hypersegmented cells, Color Plate 24) and "giant" metamyelocytes. The bone marrow is megaloblastic, with large cells (large nuclei) due to disordered maturation (Color Plate 25). These changes quickly disappear when vitamin $B_{12}$, folate, or transfusions are given; thus, if a bone marrow biopsy is delayed even a few days the morphology may have reverted to normal, leading to a misdiagnosis. Patients should always have serum vitamin $B_{12}$ and folate levels drawn prior to replacement therapy. In emergent situations, a bone marrow aspiration should be performed to confirm the diagnosis.

The Schilling test (Figure 130.1) is definitive for PA even after the blood picture is completely reversed by treatment; it also distinguishes PA from other megaloblastic anemias (e.g., malabsorption or bacterial overgrowth, Table 130.1). Normally, more than 10% of the

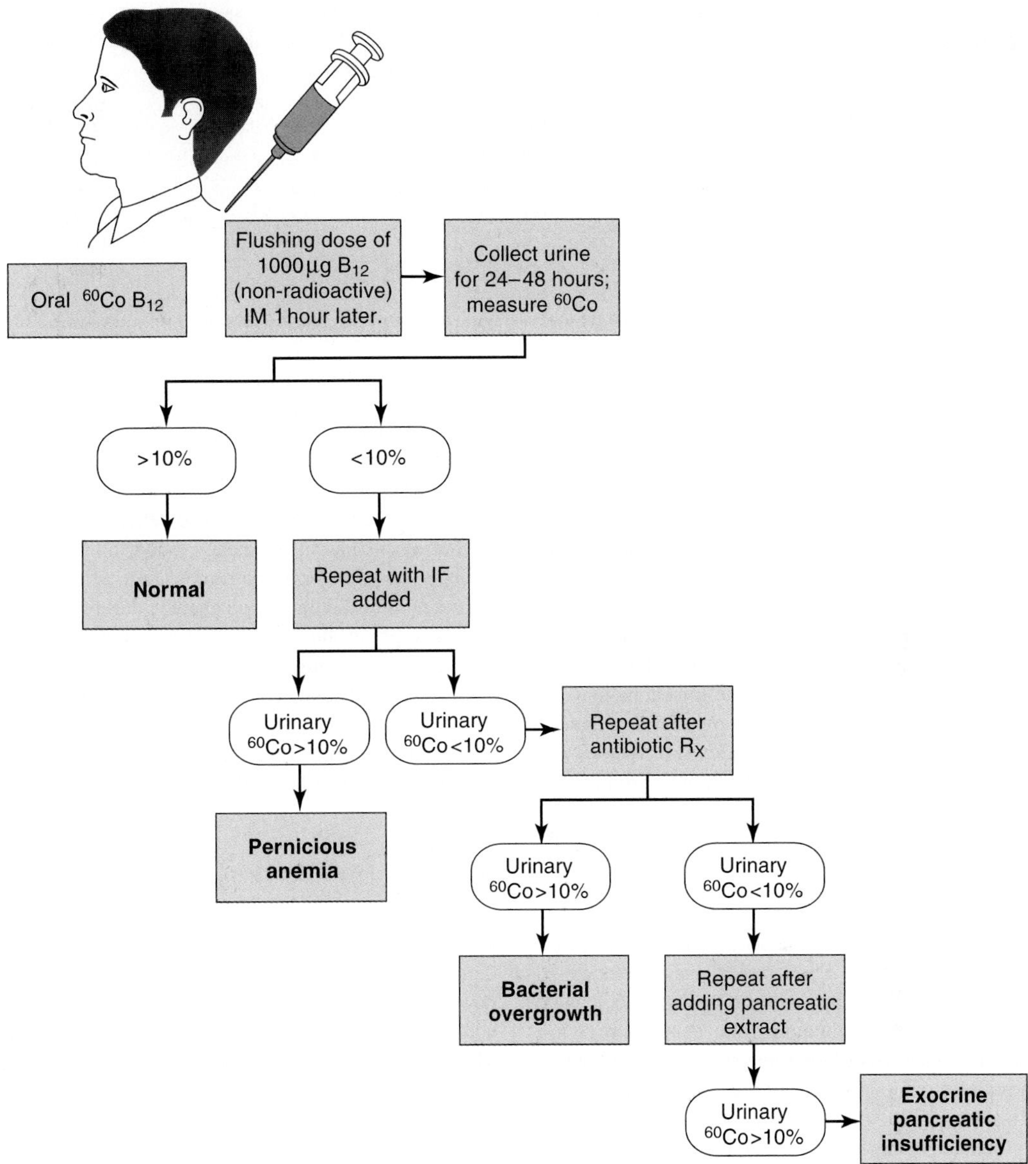


**FIGURE 130.1. The Schilling test.** The initial test is Stage 1; Stage I + IF is Stage II. Tests after antibiotics and pancreatic extracts are Stages III and IV.

oral $^{60}$Co-cobalamin appears in the urine. The diagnosis of PA is confirmed by the Schilling test and corroborated by a subsequent transient reticulocytosis (10–40%), which appears 5 to 10 days after the first injection. Antibodies to parietal cells occur in 90% of patients with PA and antibodies to IF occur in 60%; neither of these findings is specific or as definitive as the Schilling test. The serum or urine methylmalonic acid level, which is 10 times higher in vitamin $B_{12}$ deficiency than in folate deficiency or normal patients, can be used to confirm subtle, ambiguous cases in which the vitamin $B_{12}$ level is normal, but the bone marrow suggests pernicious anemia. If the bone marrow is not examined, then these tests should be done before an empirical trial of vitamin $B_{12}$ replacement. In subtle cases of pernicious anemia the serum vitamin $B_{12}$ test may be normal and the Schilling test equivocal. Measurement of serum methylmalonic acid and homocysteine levels, the substrates of the

TABLE 130.1. Radioactive Cobalamin Absorption (Schilling) Tests

| | Materials Given | | | |
|---|---|---|---|---|
| **Condition** | **Stage I: $B_{12}$** | **Stage II: $B_{12}$ + IF** | **Stage III: $B_{12}$ After Antibiotics** | **Stage IV: $B_{12}$ + Pancreatic Extract** |
| Normal | Normal | Normal | Normal | Normal |
| Pernicious anemia | Low | Normal | Low | Low |
| Blind loop syndrome | Low | Low | Normal | N.A. |
| Pancreatic insufficiency | Low | Low | Low | Normal |
| Malabsorption syndrome, bowel resection | Low | Low | Low | Low |

N.A. = Not applicable.

enzymatic processes noted above, may confirm a suspected diagnosis.

### Management

Pernicious anemia is treated by daily injection of vitamin $B_{12}$, 1000 µg for 1 week, with careful observation of the reticulocyte and RBC response. A lack of improvement means that a disorder other than vitamin $B_{12}$ deficiency is present, and the search for the etiology must be continued. After 1 week, the injections may be continued at weekly intervals for 1 month, then once a month for the rest of the patient's life. Transfusions are not necessary as long as the patient responds promptly to cobalamin.

## ■ Folic Acid Deficiency

### Pathogenesis

Folic acid, as it occurs in natural foodstuffs (e.g., fresh leafy vegetables), is a complex macromolecule—polyglutamic folic acid. Before it can be absorbed, it must be converted to monoglutamic folic acid (pteroylglutamic acid) by enzymes in the intestinal wall. Following absorption and bloodstream transport, folic acid passively diffuses into the cell, where it is restored to a polyglutamate storage form, which prevents counterdiffusion out of the cell. The average daily requirement is 50 µg/day; its biologic half-life is 3 weeks. Total folate body stores are small. After total dietary deprivation, serum folate levels decline rapidly. Sequential morphologic features of folic acid deficiency consist of hypersegmented polymorphonuclear leukocytes (PMN), macro-ovalocytosis, and megaloblastic changes in bone marrow. Four to five months of total dietary deprivation culminate in macrocytic anemia, in contrast to 4–5 years for vitamin $B_{12}$ deficiency.

The blood picture in folic acid deficiency is identical to that of cobalamin deficiency, but it often is seen in younger subjects. Truly nutritional folic acid deficiency occurs toward the end of pregnancy, during anticonvulsant therapy, in alcoholism, and in malabsorption syndrome (tropical sprue, gluten sensitivity, or ileal resection). Increased folate requirements in pregnancy (or in sickle cell and other hemolytic anemias) may hasten its depletion. Anticonvulsants are believed to inhibit the enzymes that convert polyglutamates, causing a failure to absorb folate.

### Management

Treatment of folic acid deficiency first requires recognition of the possible causes. In simple nutritional deficiencies or late-stage pregnancy, folic acid (1 mg/day) administration may be followed by reticulocytosis, and, later, by restoration of normal hematologic values. The treatment of folate and other nutritional deficiencies in alcoholism is complicated by the many psychosocial issues of alcoholism. However, the nutritionally deprived alcoholic usually shows a reticulocyte surge soon after folate replacement, either through diet or as folate tablets, assuming cessation of direct alcoholic toxicity to the marrow. Folate deficiency caused by anticonvulsant therapy may be treated by the concurrent use of folic acid. In malabsorption syndromes due to intestinal disease or inflammation, folate and other nutrients may require parenteral restoration.

# CHAPTER 131 APLASTIC ANEMIAS

**Aplastic anemias** result from bone marrow failure, which may be total or selective for RBCs, WBCs, or platelets. The hallmark of aplastic anemia is **pancytopenia:** anemia, leukopenia, thrombocytopenia, and reticulocytopenia; the precursors of these cells—normoblasts, granulocytes, or megakaryocytes—are absent in the bone marrow. Pancytopenia occurring with a hyperplastic marrow is not aplastic anemia; megaloblastic anemias, paroxysmal nocturnal hemoglobinuria (PNH), aleukemic leukemia, or related malignancies and myelodysplastic states warrant consideration. **Hypoplastic anemia** differs in degree, and usually there is some degree of persistence of neutrophil and megakaryocytic proliferation.

## Etiology

Ionizing radiation (accidental, therapeutic, or military) damages proliferating cells or stem cells. Some anticancer drugs produce dose-dependent marrow depression, damaging committed stem cells or hematological cell lines in sufficient dosage. Cis-platinum toxicity also includes renal failure with its concomitant erythropoietin deficiency. Unless uncontrolled hemorrhage or infection proves lethal, the cytopenia is often self-limited: the unharmed, committed stem cells will repopulate the marrow when the drug is stopped. A few drugs (chloramphenicol, phenylbutazone, mephenytoin, etc.) produce marrow suppression only in rare, susceptible individuals. Benzene and its derivatives, which cause aplastic anemia or leukemia, are classic examples of chemicals or solvents that can enter the body by ingestion, inhalation, or through the skin.

Almost half of the cases of aplastic anemia are idiopathic (i.e., they have no discernible etiology). An immunologic attack on uncommitted stem cells has been postulated in some cases, because studies have shown that lymphocytes from some patients with aplastic anemia can suppress granulocytopoiesis (CFU-GM) or erythropoiesis (CFU-E) in normal marrows in culture. Adding antithymocyte globulin to cultures of aplastic marrows may help annul such suppression. Similar cell-bound antibodies are noted in the lymphocytes or serum of congenital hypoplastic anemia of the Blackfan-Diamond variety. In some cases immunosuppressive therapy (using antithymocyte globulin, cyclosporin, or doses of chemotherapy drugs in preparation for a subsequently aborted bone marrow transplantation) has led to restoration of marrow function. Marrow aplasia may be due to a defect in the marrow microenvironment. Bone marrow transplantation, either by ablating the endogenous immune system or by replacing a pool of stem cells, is an effective strategy to treat aplastic anemia regardless of whether the aplastic anemia follows immunosuppression of stem cells, injured stem cells, or damaged microenvironment.

Pancytopenia with an empty bone marrow has been found to occur before or after paroxysmal nocturnal hemoglobinuria. In fact, if reticulocytosis suddenly develops during the course of treating a patient for aplastic anemia, it is worthwhile to do an acid hemolysis test to help distinguish between PNH and recovery from aplasia.

## Management

Effective treatment of aplastic anemia is difficult, calling for interaction with a well-trained hematologist. It is extremely important to confirm the diagnosis of aplastic anemia, and to identify its etiology if possible, as the therapy is extremely expensive and potentially toxic, even lethal. Aplastic anemia should be distinguished from acute leukemia, myelodysplastic syndromes, PNH, and acute or chronic granulomatous infection. Potentially toxic substances must be removed from the patient's environment. This step is not curative, but continuing exposure to the toxic agent could otherwise protract the course of the anemia, and might prove lethal. The patient and all siblings should be typed for human leukocyte antigen (HLA) compatibility.

Once the diagnosis is established, a comprehensive program of blood component support, and concomitant therapy should follow. Transfusions are life-supporting, but may cause subsequent bone marrow transplantation (BMT) failure. Thus the physician must provide support, but also must begin an evaluation for possible BMT as soon as supportive care and immunosuppression have begun. Initial therapy is designed to stimulate any residual clones of marrow precursors using androgens, and to oppose the offending immunosuppression by using antithymocyte globulin and cyclosporin. A limited number of patients respond to this therapy, but rarely is complete hematopoietic restoration achieved. Unless the patient responds to therapy in the first few weeks, a search for a BMT donor must follow via family or national registry programs. Although BMT is inherently dangerous, it also is highly effective, and for practical purposes, is the only cure for patients who fail to respond to initial therapy within weeks. If an HLA-matched sibling is available as a donor, and the patient not subjected to excessive blood component therapy, BMT is curative in 85% of cases.

If a suitable donor is not available, packed RBC should be transfused, as for any severe anemia. All blood products should be screened for cytomegalovirus (CMV) infection, and should be filtered or irradiated to reduce the likelihood of inadvertent transfusion of viable lymphocytes, which may induce transfusion-mediated graft-versus-host disease if the patient is immunosuppressed or may immunize the patient, compromising future transfusions and possible transplantation. Platelets are transfused only as an emergency stopgap measure in limited circumstances: if the platelet count is below 10,000, if active hemorrhage is present, or if surgery is planned. A platelet count should be done 1 hour after the platelet transfusion to detect an acceptable rise in the count. If there is no such rise, anti-platelet antibodies are suspect; HLA-matched platelets are then the only possible way to provide platelets for emergencies. Infections should be promptly treated. CMV, *Candida* spp, and *Aspergillus* spp often are the causative agents. Broad-spectrum antibiotics are required if specific microbes are not found.

Testosterone, with or without prednisone, although no longer recommended as initial therapy, may be used to augment the therapy with cyclosporin and antithymocyte globulin. Thymectomy is beneficial in the rare thymoma-associated pure red cell aplasia, but is not effective in true aplastic anemia.

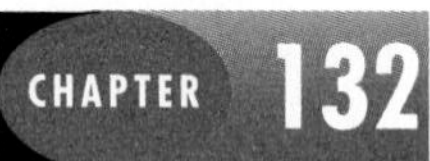

# CHAPTER 132 GENERAL ASPECTS OF HEMOLYTIC ANEMIAS

## Definition

**Hemolytic anemia** is characterized by a diminished red cell survival time, which is followed by anemia unless compensated by increased marrow production. An RBC survival time between 20 and 100 days may be offset by increased bone marrow activity. Anemia, if any, is mild, demonstrating that the normal marrow can sustain an increased RBC production of 2- to 5-fold. However, the limit of compensatory bone marrow activity is reached when the red cell survival time is less than 20 days. Any intercurrent illness that partially suppresses marrow production, even transiently, will exacerbate a previous borderline, compensated anemia. Successful management of hemolytic anemia requires careful confirmation of the diagnosis and then identification of the specific cause.

## Diagnosis and Differential Diagnosis

General features of hemolytic anemias are summarized in Table 132.1. Several general clues suggest hemolytic anemia: an unexplained, abrupt drop in hemoglobin or hematocrit; sustained reticulocytosis; and elevated serum lactate dehydrogenase (LDH). If the marrow is otherwise healthy, it often compensates for the anemia by developing hyperplasia of the myeloid precursors and megakaryocytes, along with hyperplasia of the erythroid precursors (normoblasts). Leukocytosis often occurs, as does thrombocytosis. More specific signs include elevated serum hemoglobin if hemolysis is acute and of significant magnitude, and a predictable decline in unbound haptoglobin (see caveats in Table 132.1), and the appearance of blood pigments in the urine. Table 132.2 shows the classification of hemolytic anemias. Other conditions in which anemia develops rapidly may mimic hemolytic anemia, but careful clinical correlations can avoid this confusion (Table 132.3). Note the unfortunate nomenclature: "haptoglobin" levels refer, in reality, to unbound haptoglobin levels. Thus, with hemolysis the free hemoglobin binds to haptoglobin; hence, the subsequent assay for unbound sites results in a low level, even though this acute-phase protein increases rapidly to a variety of physiologic stresses.

## Pigment Metabolism in Hemolytic Anemia

Red blood cell senescence occurs when the RBCs' supply of energy-related enzymes is depleted with resultant adenosine triphosphate (ATP) depletion. Once this occurs, the RBC can no longer actively pump sodium and water back out of the cell, leading to engorgement and relative membrane rigidity and fragility; such cells get trapped in the splenic macrophages and undergo hemolysis. Their components are then recycled or excreted. Iron is returned to the iron pool for hemoglobin synthesis, and amino acids are reused for protein synthesis. Heme is recycled but may be converted to bilirubin faster than it can be conjugated or excreted by the normal mechanisms demonstrated in Figure 105.3, leading to jaundice. In the intestine, bilirubin is converted to the fecal pigments known as **stercobilin,** and to **urobilinogen,** a soluble, colorless product.

Part of the hemoglobin discharged to the plasma during intravascular hemolysis is oxidized to **methemoglobin,** which binds to plasma albumin to form **methemalbumin,** an elevated level which indicates intravascular hemolysis. The remaining (90%) hemoglobin from hemolyzed RBC is conjugated by haptoglobin

**TABLE 132.1. General Features of Hemolytic Anemias Feature**

| Feature | Finding/Observation | Comment |
|---|---|---|
| Degree of anemia | Highly variable | Hb ranges from 11–12 g when well compensated to <2 g when severe |
| Pattern of anemia | Normocytic and normochromic | May be macrocytic with reticulocytosis |
| Morphologic abnormalities | Not specific; none<br>Spherocytes | In PNH, hereditary spherocytosis/ certain immune hemolytic anemias |
| | Peculiar RBC structures (sickle cells, target cells, or RBC inclusion bodies) | The hemoglobinopathies |
| | Schistocytes | Microangiopathy |
| Serum lactate dehydrogenase (LDH) | Increased from release of contents of hemolyzed cells into plasma | Non-specific for hemolytic anemia |
| Serum hemoglobin | Rises in intravascular hemolytic anemias | Must be drawn and interpreted with care (normal RBC may disintegrate on venipuncture) |
| Serum haptoglobin | Disappears | Haptoglobin depleted in severe liver disease; interpret test carefully if there is decompensated liver disease. |
| Urinary hemoglobin, hemosiderin, methemalbumin | Present in and confirms intravascular hemolysis | Hemoglobin not bound by haptoglobin spills into the urine |
| Splenomegaly | Frequent in hemolysis primarily by phagocytosis in reticuloendothelial sinusoids | |
| Sustained reticulocytosis | Often indirectly identifies hemolytic anemia | Highly sensitive, but not specific |
| Normoblasts in peripheral blood | Present with brisk hemolysis | Nonspecific |

**TABLE 132.2. Classification of Hemolytic Anemias**

A. According to duration or length of course
  1. Acute
  2. Chronic
B. According to RBC abnormality
  1. Intracorpuscular defects
    a. Hereditary
      i) Spherocytosis
      ii) Non-spherocytic
        a. Abnormalities in Embden-Meyerhof pathway
        b. Deficiency of G6PD
      iii) The hemoglobinopathies
        a. Sickle cell anemia
        b. Hemoglobin-C disease
        c. Unstable hemoglobin—the Heinz body anemias
    b. Non-hereditary
      i) Paroxysmal nocturnal hemoglobinuria
  2. Extracorpuscular—all acquired
    a. Immune
    b. Nonimmune
    c. Drug-induced
    d. Mechanical fragmentation

**TABLE 132.3. Disorders That May Be Confused With Hemolytic Anemias**

| Disorder/Condition | Cause for Confusion |
|---|---|
| Rapid hydration in severe dehydration | Sudden drop in hemoglobin and hematocrit |
| Anemia with severe hemorrhage | Reticulocytosis |
| Folate, iron, or $B_{12}$ replacement in anemias due to their deficiencies | Reticulocytosis |
| Nutrition and alcohol cessation in alcohol-related marrow failure | Reticulocytosis |
| Anemia + jaundice, but no bilirubinuria | Unconjugated hyperbilirubinemia |
| Myoglobinuria (traumatic/ exertional) | Positive test for urine hemoglobin |
| Bleeding into muscle or a body cavity (e.g., ruptured ectopic gestation) | Anemia, icterus and reticulocytosis |

and recycled to the bone marrow and other iron storage sites. Although haptoglobin is an acute-phase reactant, its production can increase. When hemolysis shortens RBC survival below 30 days, free haptoglobin disappears from the plasma, and serum free hemoglobin begins to rise. Serum free hemoglobin above 100 mg/ml is freely filtered by the kidney and enters the urine as methemoglobin and hemosiderin. The presence of any or all of these pigments in urine is prima facie evidence for significant intravascular hemolysis.

# CHAPTER 133 HEMOLYTIC ANEMIAS DUE TO INTRACORPUSCULAR DEFECTS

The RBC membrane is a complex structure that provides important structural integrity to the cell; even more importantly, it provides the matrix for a complex series of enzymatic and metabolic activities that are pivotal for cell integrity. The cell membrane keeps critical intracellular elements from leaking out of the cell and depleting it prematurely of metabolic support. It functions to anchor critical intracellular processes to the submembrane region of the cell, maintaining cation and water transport. Besides being a barrier to exogenous and often dangerous compounds, it maintains the basic structure of RBC as a biconcave disc. It must maintain its normal plasticity and distensibility to allow RBCs to traverse the extensive capillary structures in all organs. Protein makes up 50% of the RBC membrane; it consists of spectrin, actin, ankyrin, and protein 4.1. About 10% of the RBC membrane is carbohydrate, organized as glycophorin and sialic acid; it produces a negative charge, enabling RBC to repel each other to remain in discrete suspension. Thus aberrations of RBC membrane structure and function lead to a complex and diverse spectrum of hemolytic anemias referred to as (inherent) intracorpuscular defects.

## Hereditary Spherocytosis

**Hereditary spherocytosis** (HS) is an autosomal dominant disorder with mild hemolytic anemia in which RBCs maintain a normal mean volume but a smaller surface area. The RBCs are small, with a dense, globular appearance, and lack central pallor.

### Pathophysiology

The RBC membrane is very permeable to sodium and water, which require active ejection by an energy-consuming adenosine triphosphate (ATP) pump. Hereditary spherocytosis is characterized by a deficiency of spectrin, ankyrin band 3, or protein 4.2 in the RBC membrane; this abnormal protein structure results in dysfunctional changes in membrane distensibility, which, in turn, confer a spherical appearance and peculiar thickness to the RBC. These cells also are poorly deformable and thus undergo retention and stasis in the narrow splenic sinusoids. The erythrocyte suffers a relative depletion of plasma and glucose, compromising the ATP pump function; the entrapped, now rigid, spherocytes are then phagocytized by splenic macrophages. Transfused normal RBC survive normally in the HS patient, and the HS RBC survive normally when transfused into a splenectomized individual (normal T1/2 using $^{51}$Cr tagged RBC, 25–35 days). However, the HS RBC survival is considerably shortened in HS patients with an intact spleen (T1/2 <10 days).

### Clinical Features

Patients with HS adapt so well to their mild anemia, which has been present since birth, that they often are asymptomatic. The medical interview may elicit a history of gallstones at an early age in the patient, a sibling, or a parent; often there is a family history of "yellow eyes" and splenectomy. The icterus is mild and often is overlooked. Obvious splenomegaly is always present, unless there has been prior splenectomy; intractable leg ulcers sometimes are seen over bony prominences.

Severe crises may occur, frequently preceded by brief fever, myalgia, and malaise ("viral syndrome"); these are caused by a parvovirus B-19 infection, which inhibits cellular proliferation. Cluster cases of aplastic crisis may affect multiple members of the same family, if in close proximity. The crises display a life-threatening, precipitous drop in RBC because of inhibition of RBC production and a persistently shortened RBC lifespan. The previous compensatory reticulocytosis is aborted. Consistent with the theory of an intercurrent viral infection, mild leukopenia and thrombocytopenia also are noted. Chronic hemolysis creates an increased demand for folate, and unless a higher folate intake is maintained, such patients can develop a concomitant megaloblastic anemia; such a superimposed ineffective erythropoiesis may greatly intensify anemia in the setting of chronic increased hemolysis.

### Laboratory Features

The characteristic blood picture consists of well-compensated anemia and a double erythrocyte population (also indicated by a high red cell distribution width [RDW]), consisting of spherocytes (small diameter, a globular shape, and a dense appearance with no central pallor) and reticulocytes (bluish-gray, polychromatophilic cells). Reticulocytosis is a constant, invariable compensatory phenomenon, unless there is aplastic crisis or splenectomy, or both. Spherocytosis is determined indirectly by **increased osmotic fragility** wherein these cells demonstrate increased hemolysis to hypotonic solution because of the aforementioned membrane deficiency. Thus the RBCs of the HS patient begin to undergo lysis at saline concentrations of 0.64% and are virtually completely hemolyzed in saline concentrations as low as 0.5%, the level at which normal RBCs just begin to hemolyze. Unless there is a viral infection or marked folate depletion, the bone marrow shows pronounced normoblastic hyperplasia. In an aplastic crisis, no RBC precursors are present.

### Management

With an established diagnosis of HS, the only treatment is splenectomy. Splenectomy produces a normal RBC life span, restores the erythrocyte count to normal, dispels the risk of future aplastic crises, and removes the risk of further bilirubin gallstone formation. However, the spherocytic defect and the increased osmotic fragility remain and can be confirmed by laboratory testing. Because of the risks of overwhelming sepsis from encapsulated bacteria, all afflicted teenagers should receive pneumococcal vaccination and have splenectomy delayed until adulthood if possible.

## Other Hereditary Intracorpuscular Defects

The mature erythrocyte consumes glucose as its chief source of energy; each step is controlled by a different enzyme. The glycolytic process consists of two major components: the anaerobic (Embden-Meyerhof) pathway and the aerobic hexose monophosphate shunt (Figure 133.1). Hereditary defects at certain stages of each component can lead to nonspherocytic hemolytic anemia.

### The Anaerobic Pathway

In the RBC, 90% of glucose undergoes anaerobic glycolysis; this process generates ATP in order to maintain active transport. The key enzymes involved are phosphoglycerate kinase (which produces 2 moles of ATP per mole of glucose) and pyruvate kinase (which produces 2 more moles of ATP later in the sequence). The end product of the Embden-Meyerhof pathway is lactate (see Figure 133.1), but there is also a net gain of 4 moles of ATP. Without ATP generation at each of these loci, less ATP is produced and active transport is lost. Notably, the resulting hemolysis from accumulation of cations and

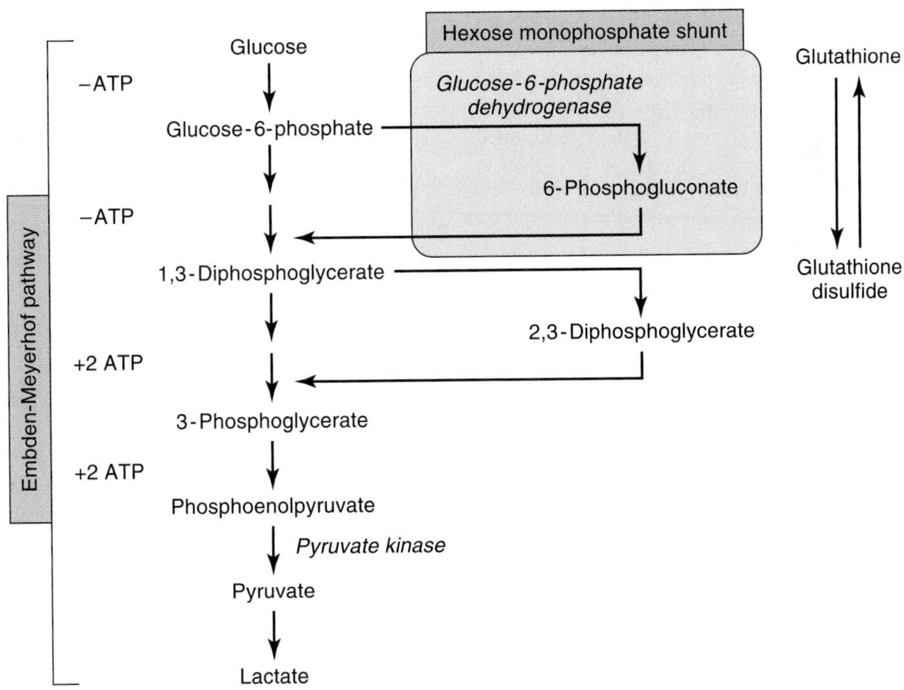


**FIGURE 133.1.** Embden-Meyerhof pathway and the hexose monophosphate shunt.

**TABLE 133.1. Drugs That Cause G6PD Deficiency-Related Hemolysis**

| Analgesics | Antimalarials | Nitrofurans | Sulfonamides | Sulfones |
|---|---|---|---|---|
| Acetanilid | Chloroquine | Nitrofurantoin | Sulfamethoxazole | Dapsone |
| Acetylsalicylic acid (in large doses) | Primaquine | | Sulfapyridine | Thiazolsulfone |
| Phenacetin | | | Sulfacetamide | |

**TABLE 133.2. Some Hemoglobinopathies**

| Example | Amino Acid Substitution | Clinical Abnormality | Functional Abnormality |
|---|---|---|---|
| Hb.G Philadelphia | α 68 (E17) ASN Lys | None | None |
| Sickle cell anemia | β 6 (A3) Glu Val | Hemolytic anemia, Painful crises | Reduced solubility with $O_2$ tension |
| Hb. Koln | β 98 (FGS) Val Met | Heinz body hemolytic anemia | Unstable |
| Hb. Chesapeake | α 92 (FG4) Arg Len | Erythrocytosis | Increased $O_2$ affinity |
| Hb. M-Milwaukee | β 67 (E11) Val gln | Cyanosis | Decreased $O_2$ affinity; methemoglobinemia |
| α-Thalassemia trait Hb. Bart's disease Hb. H disease | α Chain gene deleted | Hypochromic anemia | Rate of α chain synthesis diminished or absent |
| β Thalassemia | β Chain gene deleted | Hypochromic anemia | β chain synthesis suppressed or deleted |

water in the RBC primarily affects the older cells, which have diminished concentrations of ATP and enzymes.

Laboratory tests to confirm red cell enzymopathies and intracorpuscular hemolytic anemias require direct assays for pyruvate kinase or other key enzymes. These assays are expensive, tedious, and not generally available. Indirect evidence for glycolytic defects is provided by an estimate of increased autohemolysis that is corrected entirely by ATP, or by glucose and ATP.

### The Hexose Monophosphate Shunt

When malaria prophylaxis was instituted in the U.S. military, almost 10% of African American men who received primaquine suffered severe intravascular hemolysis; the outcome was attributed to an inherent defect in their RBC that remained subclinical until exposed to an oxidant drug (e.g., primaquine). It was accompanied by an accumulation of **Heinz-Ehrlich bodies** and unstable glutathione of RBC subjected to oxidants. Later, disordered glycolysis within the hexose monophosphate shunt (HMS) was identified as the cause.

**Glucose-6 phosphate dehydrogenase** (G6PD) is a vital component of the HMS; it keeps triphosphopyridine nucleotide (TPN) in a functional or reduced state (TPNH). This system continually provides hydrogen ions, which maintain glutathione in the reduced state (GSH) to maintain methemoglobin reductase and eventually to protect hemoglobin from oxidation. Diminished HMS activities generate $H_2O_2$. This oxidant denatures hemoglobin to produce Heinz bodies and compromises the RBC membrane integrity. The lifespan of the RBCs is believed to be limited by G6PD activity. A mutant enzyme with a lifespan less than that of normal RBC correspondingly diminishes the RBC survival. G6PD deficiency is an X-linked recessive trait. Hemolysis from exposure to various oxidant drugs (Table 133.1), vegetables (fava beans, henna, senna), diabetic ketoacidosis, and infections affects only RBC. Platelets and WBCs, however, turn over more rapidly than the T1/2 of G6PD and never grow old enough to undergo lysis due to G6PD deficiency.

## The Hemoglobinopathies

Hemoglobinopathies are summarized in Table 133.2. Many of these mutations have been found in single individuals or families. The most common hemoglobinopathies are more widely dispersed, and are described further in the following paragraphs.

### *Sickle Cell Anemia*

**Sickle cell anemia** is a hereditary disorder of hemoglobin structure produced by a mutant replacement of valine for glutamic acid in position 6 of the β polypeptide chain

(Table 133.2). The hemoglobin polymerizes to an elongated fibrocrystalline structure, especially during hypoxia, dehydration, or infection. These rigid crystals force the RBC membrane to elongate; the intertwined, affected RBCs occlude small blood vessels. Areas supplied by the occluded blood vessels undergo necrosis. Hemolytic anemia is a constant feature, arising from shortened RBC lifespan due to these relatively rigid cells, and is confirmed by evidence of anemia, with accompanying reticulocytosis, decreased haptoglobin, elevated LDH, and sickle cells (Color Plate 26).

## Clinical Features

Symptoms of sickle cell anemia develop around 4 to 6 months of age, concomitant with the physiologic change from fetal to adult hemoglobin synthesis. Recurrent vascular occlusion can occur in almost any organ. Repeated, painful bone infarcts with malformation and avascular necrosis are common. Pulmonary fibrosis and progressive pulmonary hypertension also evolve from repeated infarcts. Myocardial infarcts cause ventricular dysfunction. Cerebral infarcts produce strokelike syndromes. Recurrent renal infarctions lead to an inability to concentrate urine (isosthenuria), which further exacerbates sickle crisis during periods of pyrexia. Functional asplenism resulting from splenic infarcts leads to encapsulated bacterial sepsis. The presence of a palpable spleen is a priori evidence that an adult patient does not have SS (homozygous sickle cell) disease, but rather has sickle trait combined with another hemoglobinopathy. Persistent mucosal infarcts in the gastrointestinal tract can lead to achlorhydria. The chronic hemolysis in this disorder produces bilirubin gallstones in virtually all affected adults.

These organ injuries are compounded by the risk of **thromboembolism.** A particularly life-threatening and painful condition is known as the **acute chest syndrome,** wherein the patient suffers a major infarct of the lung with severe pain, and a potentially vicious cycle of severe hypoxia and intravascular sickling throughout the circulation. In men, sickle crisis in penile veins produces protracted painful priapism, often requiring surgical intervention. Because of the severe obligatory hemolysis in SS disease, the cells of these patients often have a lifespan of only 10–15 days; hence, these patients are anemic in spite of a dramatic compensatory reticulocytosis. They also are susceptible to aplastic crises produced by intercurrent viral infections or folate depletion. Frequent acute illness leads to days lost at school and work; repeated tissue injury threatens normal organ function throughout the life of affected patients. Prompt symptomatic therapy and intervention are highly desirable.

## Diagnosis

The diagnosis of sickle cell anemia requires that the heterozygous sickle cell trait be differentiated from homozygous sickle cell anemia. The patient with sickle cell *trait*, who usually has a normal or borderline hemoglobin level, is rarely anemic except during an intercurrent disease, and does not exhibit a significant baseline reticulocytosis. Because these cells "sickle" only with profound hypoxic stresses (e.g., reduced oxygen tension, as in military exposures), the lifespan of these heterozygous RBCs is relatively normal. Sickling can be induced in vitro by exposure to extreme hypoxic states during laboratory testing, thus providing a simple way to screen for sickle cell trait. As shown in Figure 133.2, only one of the two sets of hemoglobin molecules has the mutant valine amino acid substitution, whereas the other is normal unless another aberrant mutation occurs from another hemoglobinopathy, such as thalassemia. In contrast, the homozygous patient manifests anemia, reticulocytosis, icterus, and virtually absent haptoglobin. The diagnosis is suspected by the appearance of sickle cells on the routine peripheral smear, and confirmed by hemoglobin electrophoresis. Identification of sickle cell *disease* versus sickle cell trait is important, as is the presence of additional concomitant hemoglobinopathies such as hemoglobin C, thalassemias, and others whose presence modulates disease behavior, thus altering prognosis.

## Management

The goal of management is to maintain an adequate proportion of normal hemoglobin and, conversely, a relatively low proportion of hemoglobin S. Because spontaneous sickling crises are rare unless the concentration of hemoglobin S exceeds 50–60% of total circulating hemoglobin, systematic transfusion may be sufficient to maintain this proportion and a total hemoglobin of about 10 g/dl. Such an aggressive transfusion approach includes limited exchange (e.g., 5 units packed RBC transfused with concomitant phlebotomy of 4 units of whole blood sufficient to maintain S Hg below 30%). Sickle cell crises are exquisitely painful. Affected people usually are started on narcotic analgesics for painful crises at an early age; consequently, there is a risk of developing addiction, especially if the patient is noncompliant or has inadequate access to supportive care and early intervention. Simple analgesics (e.g., salicylates, ibuprofen) are adequate for pain control of minor infarcts, but narcotics often are required for more severe episodes. Need for narcotic analgesia can be minimized by strict attention to supportive care, such as hydration, oxygen administration during crises, and the judicious use of transfusions.

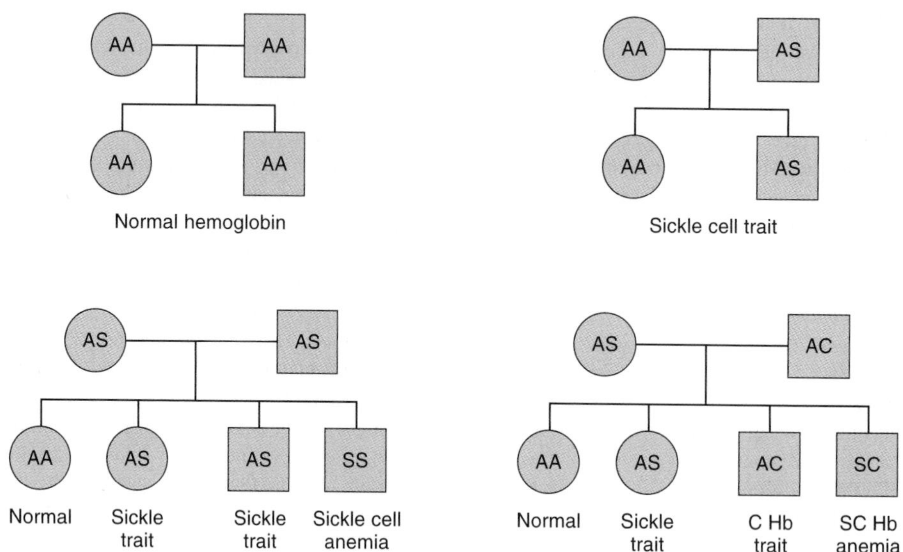


**FIGURE 133.2. Inheritance of the sickle cell trait.**

Because infants with high levels of fetal hemoglobin (Hgb F) do not have sickling phenomena, and occasional adults with sickle cell disease who have endogenously elevated Hgb F production have fewer crises, pharmacologic approaches have been made to increase Hgb F production. Judicious doses of hydroxyurea, usually 500–1500 mg/day, may paradoxically induce Hgb F production; HgF levels above 5% often significantly decrease the frequency, duration, and severity of sickle crises. The benefit from hydroxyurea may also be related to its suppressive effect on white blood cells and inflammation. In higher doses, hydroxyurea suppresses bone marrow production of all cell lines. Its use must be monitored carefully and frequently by an experienced hematologist. The importance of careful compliance and the potential need for repetitive dose modification by the treating physician must be emphasized to the patient.

### Complications

Iron overload (nonhereditary hemochromatosis, or hemosiderosis) may develop in sickle cell patients as a result of ongoing hemolysis and repeated blood transfusions. Its hallmarks are a high serum ferritin, high serum iron, and a high transferrin saturation—even as high as 100%. Stainable iron is abundant in the bone marrow; it is deposited in the macrophages or in the interstitium. Excess iron is deposited in the liver, causing liver dysfunction, hepatomegaly and, ultimately, cirrhosis; the myocardium, leading to cardiomegaly, cardiac dysfunction, and congestive heart failure; the pancreas, causing diabetes mellitus; and the testicles, producing testicular atrophy, gynecomastia, and feminization. This type of iron overload, which closely mimics hereditary hemochromatosis, is treated by chelation with desferrioxamine.

## Hemoglobin C Disease

Hemoglobin C disease results when leucine is substituted for glutamic acid in the 6th position of the β chain. The resulting mutant hemoglobin precipitates to form crystals within the RBC, producing RBCs with relatively rigid cell membranes, which cause the cells to be trapped and phagocytized by the reticuloendothelial cells. Clinical features include splenomegaly, mild anemia, reticulocytosis, and the presence of many target cells in the peripheral blood (Color Plate 27). The diagnosis is established by hemoglobin electrophoresis. The characteristic crystals may be noted on a Wright-stained smear.

Hemoglobin C disease is moderately severe, but the association of hemoglobin C with S hemoglobin **(SC disease)** causes even more problems, because of the added risk of intravascular sickling events. Pregnancy poses a significant physiologic challenge to patients with SC disease. Besides the risk to the fetus because of injury to the placenta, such patients are at extremely high risk of thromboembolism or aseptic necrosis.

## The Unstable Hemoglobins

Amino acid substitutions in the vicinity of the heme pocket may make the hemoglobin molecule unstable, which causes the hemoglobin to precipitate and form **Heinz-Ehrlich bodies**—the harbinger of unstable hemoglobins (Color Plate 28). Red blood cells with Heinz bodies are trapped in the spleen or destroyed as they circulate. **Heme fragments** (dipyrrholes), which are diagnostic, escape into the urine as a mahogany brown pigment.

Affected patients develop hemolytic anemia and splenomegaly. Viral infections or therapy with sulfonamides or oxidants may worsen the hemolysis. Paradoxically, some of the mutant hemoglobins have a higher oxygen affinity, causing slight erythrocytosis rather than anemia. Hemoglobin electrophoresis is not helpful in these cases because the location of these mutations fails to significantly alter the conformational shape or molecular charge of the hemoglobin molecules. A reliable diagnosis is made only by determining the amino acid sequence of the hemoglobin molecule or by finding Heinz-Ehrlich bodies. (Unstable hemoglobins are "heat labile" because the hemoglobin comes out of solution if hemolysates are heated to 50° C for 1–2 h.)

## The Thalassemias

The thalassemias are characterized by absent or diminished production of alpha chains (α-thalassemia) or beta chains (β-thalassemia). Varying degrees of hemolysis occur because of the intracellular deposition of excessive amounts of the opposite form of hemoglobin chains, leading to shortened RBC lifespan. However, the major defect is the diminished hemoglobin production, causing a hypochromic microcytic anemia, which often is confused with iron deficiency. The ensuing individual molecules of hemoglobin are normal, but the disrupted regulation of intact hemoglobin chains causes an imbalance in hemoglobin production. The functional result is a lowered hemoglobin concentration within the cell.

### Alpha-Thalassemia

Alpha chain synthesis is controlled by four separate genetic loci on chromosome 16. The position of the affected alleles determines the resulting abnormality. A deletion of one or two genes, typical of patients with an African heritage, leads to the α-thalassemia trait, a mild form of anemia with hypochromic, microcytic erythrocytosis, mimicking iron deficiency. A three-gene deletion, as in some patients of Asian heritage, causes a chronic, severe, debilitating homozygous hemolytic anemia, which is associated with intracellular inclusions (hemoglobin H disease). With deletion of all four genes, the fetus has no α chains, becomes severely anemic, and dies at birth of **hydrops fetalis** (Figure 133.3).

Affected persons display a hypochromic, microcytic anemia; it usually is mild and may even feature a high RBC count **(hypochromic erythrocytosis),** an important, essentially pathognomonic clue, because the RBC count invariably is low in iron deficiency. Unless this is recognized, because the mean cell volume (MCV) and MCH are low, such patients often are mistakenly treated

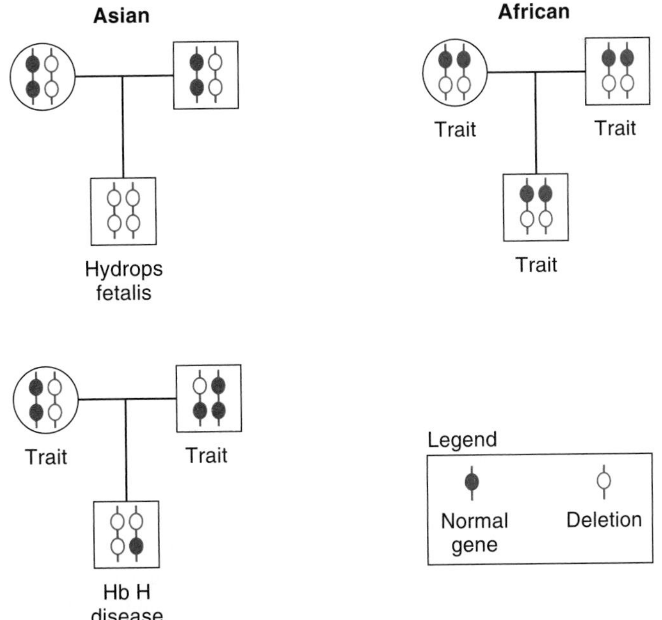


**FIGURE 133.3. Hereditary patterns of alpha-thalassemia.**

with iron for years without improvement. Serum iron, transferrin, and ferritin are normal, and also are clues that this is an underlying hemoglobinopathy rather than iron deficiency. The bone marrow shows normal stainable iron. The hemoglobin electrophoresis pattern is normal, because these mutations rarely alter the electrophoretic charge on the hemoglobin molecule. Often, this is a diagnosis of exclusion by ruling out iron deficiency and other hemoglobinopathies; evaluation of other family members often is helpful.

### Beta-Thalassemia

#### Background

Beta-thalassemia is more common in people of Mediterranean origin. However, the mutant gene has been introduced into the non-Mediterranean population through migrations, military incursions into northern Europe, and intermarriages.

Beta polypeptide chains are controlled by two genes located on chromosome 11. Deletion of one gene with a normal second gene results in the β-thalassemia trait, which is characterized by mild anemia with low MCV and MCH. Hemoglobin electrophoresis shows a compensatory elevation of minor component $A_2$ or increased hemoglobin F. If both β genes are deleted, the offspring have a markedly diminished β chain production rate, leading to imbalanced production of α and β chains. The excess α chains then precipitate, leading to hemolysis.

Clinically, homozygous β-thalassemia features severe hypochromic microcytic anemia, with increased serum bilirubin and hemoglobin F and a hyperplastic bone marrow with marked erythroid hyperplasia; physical examination reveals splenomegaly, resorption of bone as a result of expansion of the medullary compartment within, and characteristic facies. Pathologic fractures are common. Peripheral blood smear shows many misshapen target cells.

Through analysis of DNA isolated from circulating peripheral nucleated cells (a common finding in these patients), it is possible to identify specific mutations using restriction fragment length polymorphism analysis. These and similar tests can be used to identify the specific genetic defect and assess its otherwise occult presence in family members. With the potential of gene insertion technologies, such biologic probes will gain practical importance.

#### Management

Beta-thalassemia trait requires no treatment, but it is important to distinguish it from iron deficiency to avoid needless iron therapy. Homozygous β-thalassemia should be regularly and frequently treated with packed RBC transfusions to keep hemoglobin values at about 10 g/dl in order to minimize bone resorption and skeletal deformities. Frequent transfusions in these patients combined with their inability to use iron in hemoglobin synthesis lead to severe iron overload. As a result, these individuals assume a peculiar grayish-brown pallor with deposition of iron into the skin and parenchymal organs. Because many patients require frequent, lifelong transfusions, serial ferritin determinations should be performed. Chelation therapy with desferrioxamine should be begun early in life, and administered comprehensively to reduce the intracellular iron stores and resulting parenchymal damage. Splenectomy may be helpful in controlling severe hemolytic anemia. Bone marrow transplantation currently is the only curative procedure.

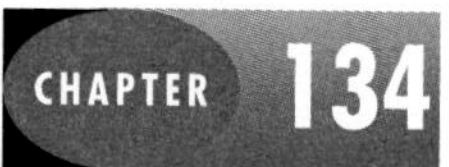


# HEMOLYTIC ANEMIAS DUE TO EXTRACORPUSCULAR DEFECTS

## Autoimmune Hemolytic Anemia

First described in 1907, autoimmune hemolytic anemia (AIHA) is characterized by a hemolytic antibody capable of causing both intravascular and in vitro hemolysis of the individual's own RBCs. The breakthrough that led to the discovery of thousands more cases of AIHA was the demonstration of an antibody—through the Coombs test, named after its discoverer—that adheres directly to the surface of RBCs, inducing hemolysis by fixing complement and damaging the cell membrane. Antibodies that can cause hemolysis are themselves immunogenic and antigenic; thus, antibodies known as Coombs sera (or antiglobulins) can be developed against either broad-spectrum classes of naturally occurring antibodies (e.g., IgG classes), or specifically identified antibodies.

The immune hemolytic anemias vary widely in their clinical presentation and treatment. Warm antibodies, produced in limited amounts, usually do not occur free in serum, but may be demonstrated by the Coombs' reaction, using a murine antihuman monoclonal antibody directed against human autoantibodies adherent to RBC surface antigens. It is possible to elute this autoantibody from the RBC surface in order to study its characteristics in the laboratory at physiologic temperatures, hence the historical term "warm antibody." The specificity of the antibody, and its agglutination or hemolytic capabilities, can be defined through transfer to various RBCs in blood banks. Warm antibodies usually are polyclonal, and contain both IgG and IgM components, commonly directed against typical RBC antigens. Hemolysis varies depending on the classes and subclasses of the antibody present; for example, IgG1 fixes complement poorly, whereas IgG3 fixes complement avidly; hence, patients with a high IgG3 autoantibody titer would be more prone to severe hemolysis than those with IgG1 autoantibodies.

Warm hemolytic anemia is mediated by reticuloendothelial macrophages that have membrane receptors for IgG; they phagocytize any particulate matter to which IgG adheres. As the RBC with its adherent antibody, with or without complement, is exposed to macrophages, that component of the cell membrane is phagocytized by excising the cell membrane (antigen)-antibody complex. This occurs repeatedly, such that the original morphology of the cell is gradually transformed, from a cell with maximal surface area per unit volume (biconcave disc) to a cell with the minimal surface area per unit volume (a spherocyte). As this process evolves, the spherocyte becomes progressively smaller, until it ultimately meets its demise in the spleen. Immune-mediated hemolytic anemias produce spherocytes (Color Plate 29), unlike mechanical hemolysis, which confers blatant microangiopathic changes on the RBC, and yields schistocytes (typical of disseminated intravascular coagulation [DIC], endocarditis, and other such disorders).

Warm hemolytic anemias have diverse causes. Approximately one half of all cases are idiopathic; the remaining patients have an underlying spontaneous or iatrogenic autoimmune disease, or a lymphoproliferative disorder. The diagnosis of AIHA mandates a workup to exclude one or more of the associated conditions noted in Table 134.1; conversely, hematologic parameters should be monitored in patients with a previous diagnosis of these conditions to identify the development of an associated autoimmune hemolysis.

Table 134.2 presents the classification of Coombs reactivity according to immunologic criteria. In some circumstances autoantibodies also are directed against other blood elements, e.g., platelets, and can be associated with autoimmune insults against solid organs such as those seen in systemic lupus erythematosus (SLE).

Autoimmune hemolytic anemia is treated initially by immunosuppression, with prednisone, 1–2 mg/kg body weight. Side effects include glucose intolerance, hyperkalemia, gastritis, and insomnia; patients must be monitored closely for the first few weeks to manage possible side effects as well as to assess response. Signs of a favorable response include a rising hemoglobin/hematocrit and RBC numbers, as well as a decreasing reticulocyte count and antibody titer. Steroids should be used aggressively initially, and once a response is documented, tapered weekly over a period of months. In many cases, successful discontinuation of steroids may not be possible; in such cases, the physician must evaluate the benefit of long-term use of steroids against the complications, such as immunosuppression, cataracts, and osteoporosis, or consider other alternatives (e.g., splenectomy or alternative immunosuppressive, such as cyclophosphamide or Imuran). Packed cell transfusion is limited to severe or critical situations, because the transfused cells share the same target membrane antigens recognized by the autoantibody and thus will be rapidly destroyed.

## Cold Agglutinin-Associated Hemolytic Anemia

The presentation and treatment of cold agglutinin-associated hemolytic anemias differ entirely from those of the warm agglutinins. Patients often are more symptomatic, although the degree of anemia may not be as severe as that seen in the warm antibody type. The cold agglutinin syndrome is dominated by the clinical features not only of hemolysis, but of compromised microcircu-

**TABLE 134.1. Disorders Associated With Warm Autoimmune Hemolytic Anemia**

| | |
|---|---|
| **1. Lymphoproliferative disease** | **3. Other immunologic disorders** |
| Chronic lymphocytic leukemia | Hypogammaglobulinemia |
| Non-Hodgkin lymphoma | Dysglobulinemia |
| Hodgkin disease | **4. Gastrointestinal disease** |
| Thymoma | Ulcerative colitis |
| Myeloma | **5. Ovarian tumors** |
| **2. Collagen disease** | Dermoid cysts |
| Systemic lupus erythematosus (SLE) | |
| Scleroderma | |
| Rheumatoid arthritis | |

TABLE 134.2. Antiglobulin Sensitization Patterns

| Adhering Immunoglobulin | Characteristics | Serologic Specificity |
|---|---|---|
| IgG alone | Reacts at 37°C<br>Non-agglutinating except with Coombs serum<br>Non-hemolyzing | Rh antigen |
| IgG + C′ | Same but may hemolyze | Same |
| IgM + C′ | Cold agglutinins (3°C) | Anti-I |
| | Mycoplasma (polyclonal) | Anti-i |
| | Infectious mononucleosis | Anti-i |
| | Lymphoma (monoclonal) | |
| C′ alone | Donath-Landsteiner | Anti-P |
| C′ alone | SLE | Polyclonal |

SLE = systemic lupus erythematosus.

lation, especially in anatomic areas exposed to ambient temperatures significantly below physiologic temperatures. Thus, patients invariably have features similar to Raynaud's phenomenon or characteristic acrocyanosis, with recurrent capillary thrombosis in the malar areas of the face and ears. An early avascular pale appearance results, with later progression to a livedo reticularis syndrome of violaceous and ultimately permanent disfigurement.

In contrast to warm hemolytic anemias, cold-agglutinin disease produces a monoclonal autoantibody, which almost always targets the "I"-antigen system. (This system has an adult type "I" antigen which develops after birth, and a downregulated but present fetal type "i" antigen; clinicians refer to "anti-big I" or "anti-little I," respectively.) The idiopathic form of the disease, which usually occurs in elderly patients, as well as those associated with underlying autoimmune or lymphoproliferative diseases, feature an anti-I antibody. In contrast, infections such as ***Mycoplasma pneumoniae***, which usually occur in younger persons, produce an anti-i antibody.

The natural history of this condition relates to the possible underlying etiology. If determined to be anti-i, and especially if temporally associated with a known or suspected infectious episode, the syndrome probably will be self-limiting. Conversely, anti-I usually is chronic and necessitates protracted therapy analogous to that used in warm antibody syndromes. Similarly, diagnosis of an anti-I syndrome mandates a workup for the same spectrum of associated conditions. Careful analysis of the complement-fixing capability of the antibody, and its thermal amplitude, can be helpful. Besides educating the patient regarding the need to avoid exposure to cold, the physician should recognize that transfusions, especially of blood not warmed to the physiologic temperature, may provoke a clinical crisis by aggregating in the microcirculation, and that immunosuppression and splenectomy, although fortunately not often needed, also are less effective.

# CHAPTER 135 DISORDERS OF PHAGOCYTIC CELLS

The sequential proliferation, maturation, and differentiation of WBCs are discussed in Chapter 120. Table 135.1 presents normal total and differential WBC counts; the distribution of WBC appears in Tables 135.2 and 135.3.

## Morphology

The granulocytes are characterized functionally and morphologically by cytoplasmic granules. Early granulocyte precursors (i.e., progranulocytes) bear only primary granules (primary granules consist of lysosomal membranes that encase hydrolytic enzymes, myeloperoxidase, and cationic proteins, all of which have bactericidal properties). As maturation proceeds, primary granules are replaced by secondary granules; secondary granules have specific staining features that identify them as neutrophils, eosinophils, and basophils (e.g., neutrophils: diffusely dispersed, fine lavender–staining cytoplasmic granules; eosinophils: bright red, acidic [eosin] staining, large and round granules that are fewer per cell than neutrophilic granules; basophils: large, irregular granules that are even fewer and attract basic [black] dyes).

Mature polymorphonuclear leukocyte (PMN) granules consist of lactoferrin and proteolytic enzymes. Quantitative fluctuations of alkaline phosphatase play a diagnostic role in certain myeloproliferative disorders. Granulocyte precursors derive energy through mitochondrial respiration. As the PMN mature, mitochondria disappear; energy is then derived from glycolysis.

**TABLE 135.1. Numbers of White Blood Cells in Normal Blood**

| | |
|---|---|
| A. Total white blood cells: | 4.5–11.0 × $10^{12}$/L |
| B. Types and proportion of WBC: | % |
| Band form—neutrophils | <3 |
| Segmented—neutrophilic PMNs | 40–70 |
| Lymphocytes | 25–45 |
| Eosinophilic PMNs | 3 |
| Basophils | 0.5 |
| Monocytes | 4 |

PMN = polymorphonuclear leukocyte.

**TABLE 135.2. Distribution of Phagocytes**

| Total Number of WBC × $10^{12}$/L — 4.5–11.0 | |
|---|---|
| **Type of Phagocyte** | **Predominant Location** |
| Polymorphonuclear leukocyte | Blood, tissues |
| Monocyte | Blood, tissues |
| Tissue macrophage | Spleen lymph nodes, bone marrow |
| Kupffer cells | Liver sinusoids |
| Alveolar macrophages | Lungs |

## Phagocytic Properties

The major function of polymorphonuclear cells is phagocytosis. The particle (e.g., bacteria) is identified by appropriate immunoglobulin markers so as to be recognizable to membrane receptors. The external membranes of both PMN and macrophages contain receptors for both complement and immunoglobulins, which is necessary for their physiologic phagocytic function. PMN motility, also critical to phagocytosis, is directed by chemotaxis to a specific target so that PMNs are attracted to the site of the bacterial invasion. Complement components 3a and 5a and fibrinopeptide B are important chemotactic stimuli. Products of tissue damage (such as denatured proteins) and arachidonic acid metabolites share in this function. Energy for phagocytosis is driven by glycolysis; lactate and $CO_2$ are released as final products.

Once a bacterial particle is engulfed, the leukocyte granules deploy around the phagosome; the lysosomal and vacuolar membranes eventually fuse. As the lysosomal contents are discharged into the vacuole, the granules disappear. For cell protection, the proteolytic contents of lysosomes cannot come in contact with PMN interior structures. With the appropriate enzymes, bacteria may be killed or digested. Bacterial killing is mediated by membrane oxidase enzymes that obtain electrons from reduced pyridine nucleotides (NADPH). These enzymes convert oxygen ($O_2$) to superoxide anion ($O_2^-$) and hydrogen peroxide ($H_2O_2$), which, together with myeloperoxidase, are highly bactericidal. $H_2O_2$ is detoxified by glutathione derived from the hexose monophosphate shunt (Figure 133.1). The entire process of phagocytosis is accompanied by a short respiratory burst resulting in

**TABLE 135.3. Distribution of Granulocyte Compartments**

| | | |
|---|---|---|
| 1. Proliferative pool—capable of mitosis, 10-20 × circulating pool | | |
| *Stage* | *Characteristic* | *Frequency (%)* |
| a) Myeloblast | No granules, 1-3 nucleoli | 0.2–1.5 |
| b) Promyelocyte | Primary granules, 0-1 nucleoli | 2–4 |
| c) Myelocyte | Secondary granules, oval nucleus | 8–16 |
| 2. Nonproliferative (reserve) pool | | |
| a) Metamyelocyte | Progressively indented nucleus | 10–25 |
| b) Band cell | Elongated nucleus | 10–15 |
| c) PMN | Segmented nucleus | 6–12 |
| Mature polymorphonuclear leukocytes (PMN) are deformable because of lobed nucleus. May change shape to penetrate between endothelial cells and enter circulation or tissues. | | |
| 3. Peripheral blood pool | | |
| a) Circulating pool | | |
| b) Marginating pool | | |

$CO_2$ release (see Neutrophil Kinetics and Function in Chapter 148).

## Reactive Leukocytosis

Leukocytosis may arise from infectious or noninfectious causes. It is caused physiologically during parturition, exercise, and stress, probably mediated by the effect of endogenous epinephrine on marginated PMN. Neutrophilia (high neutrophil count) is primarily due to infection. Absolute neutrophilia, a normal response to infection, consists of a "left shift" in myeloid elements, a term meaning the increased number of mature and immature neutrophils and precursors thereof that have been released from the marginated pool of cells in the circulation, as well as from the marrow cavity as a stress response. The presence of myelocytes, metamyelocytes, and even promyelocytes or myeloblasts can be observed transiently if the infectious stress is severe and the patient's marrow is capable of responding. Absolute or relative lymphocytopenia often is present in severe infection; the former results from acute lysis or apoptosis of circulating lymphocytes by the endogenous corticosteroids secreted physiologically, whereas the latter is the artifact of the laboratory reporting system. Clinicians are encouraged to assess the lymphocyte count critically in such laboratory reports. An absence of lymphopenia is unexpected and raises the possibility of concurrent viral infections or lymphoproliferative diseases.

Polymorphonuclear cells in mild infections show "toxic" granules (i.e., azurophilic granules from accelerated granulocytopoiesis). In more severe infections, neutrophils (polymorphonuclear cells) contain Dohle bodies (grayish-blue membrane-attached inclusions). Leukocyte alkaline phosphatase (LAP) content rises. Fever follows pyrogen release from damaged leukocytes. These changes dissipate as the infection resolves. Noninfectious factors also cause leukocytosis (e.g., uremia, gout, acidosis, burns, eclampsia, severe dehydration and hemoconcentration, acute hemorrhage, or hemolysis). Tissue necrosis in major surgery, myocardial infarction, and malignancies are other causes.

Neutrophilia may be due to certain physiologic substances and medications. Corticosteroids and epinephrine enhance delivery of neutrophils from reserve marrow pools. Lithium promotes granulocytopoiesis. Overwhelming infection by invading microorganisms or infections in "closed" serosal cavities may engender overwhelming leukocytosis ($>100\ 10^9/L$). This leukemoid reaction may seemingly resemble chronic myelocytic leukemia (CML). Leukemoid reactions occur only in acutely ill patients with a serious infection. In recently diagnosed CML, patients are asymptomatic and fully ambulatory. LAP score is high in infectious leukocytosis; it is depleted in CML.

## Leukopenia

Leukopenia occasionally follows overwhelming infections, including bacterial infections, when the bone marrow fails to provide neutrophils in sufficient numbers. In leukopenia, total WBCs decline, the ratio of neutrophils and bands to lymphocytes increases, and small numbers of metamyelocytes and myelocytes appear. The polymorphonuclear cells display heavy toxic granulation or degranulation, Dohle bodies, and cytoplasmic vacuolization. The usual setting is an immunocompromised host, an alcoholic, or a patient with metastatic malignancy. Leukopenia in these settings suggests a limited leukocyte response to infection. Thus, it is a poor prognostic sign.

Leukopenia also accompanies other disparate clinical states besides infection (Table 135.4). In pseudoleukopenia, an enhanced leukocyte response to epinephrine is characteristic. Leukopenia is regularly noted in systemic lupus erythematosus and autoimmune leukopenia. Increased peripheral destruction or sequestration in large spleens gives rise to leukopenia (3,000–4,000) and thrombocytopenia (60,000–90,000). Leukoerythroblastosis (normoblasts appear together with immature granu-

**TABLE 135.4. Causes of Leukopenia**

Physiologic
- Otherwise normal blacks and people of Middle Eastern heritage

Pseudoneutropenia—increase in marginating pool
Chronic benign neutropenia
Systemic lupus erythematosus
Aplastic anemia
- Drugs and chemicals—e.g., chloramphenicol
- Viral disease
- Congenital—Fanconi's syndrome
- Idiopathic acquired

Infections
- Gram-negative bacteria—e.g., typhoid, *Brucella* spp virus, and rickettsial disease
- Protozoa—malaria, kala-azar
- Overwhelming infection—e.g., septicemia, miliary tuberculosis

Splenomegaly (hypersplenism): e.g., cirrhosis, Felty's syndrome, Gaucher's disease, sarcoidosis
Aleukemic and preleukemic leukemia, metastatic carcinoma, myelofibrosis
Megaloblastic anemia–e.g., folate and vitamin $B_{12}$ deficiency
Paroxysmal nocturnal hemoglobinuria
Congenital neutropenia—Kostmann syndrome
Drug-induced agranulocytosis
- Immune-mediated, e.g., aminopyrine
- Toxic suppression, e.g., chlorpromazine

locytes in periphery) accompanies leukopenia due to malignancies. In "aleukemic" leukemia, replacement of granulocyte precursors in the marrow leads to leukopenia. Because blasts are not always present peripherally, the diagnosis is confirmed by bone marrow biopsy.

## Drug-Induced Leukopenia and Agranulocytosis

Some drugs (e.g., antineoplastic agents) given in a sufficiently high dosage regularly and universally suppress hematopoiesis. Agranulocytosis is a rare complication of drug therapy in which affected individuals develop precipitous leukopenia in response to doses of the drug that ordinarily are not toxic to the population at large. Usually a latent period of 30–50 days of therapy with the offending drug precedes the sudden drop in neutrophils. These events occur selectively in persons with specific characteristics.

### Basic Mechanisms of Agranulocytosis

Although the clinical and hematologic expression of drug sensitivity is remarkably similar for most offending drugs, the mechanisms differ profoundly for different medications. The basic abnormality exists in the host rather than the drug. Despite overlap and specific differences, two basic mechanisms are proposed:

1. **Nonimmunologic**
   a. Direct chemical suppression in a host with a pre-existing proliferative defect
   b. Accumulation of toxic metabolic end-products in a host who is constitutionally unable to detoxify or excrete them
2. **Immunologic**
   a. Immune destruction by drug-related antibodies (or their precursors) that destroy peripheral polymorphonuclear cells.

Causes of drug-induced agranulocytosis are listed in Table 135.5. **Immunologically related agranulocytosis** is ushered in by abrupt symptoms, such as chills, fever, and collapse. The symptoms are explained by the peripheral lysis of WBC with the release of toxic pyrogens. Rapidly escalating sepsis is almost inevitable when patients suddenly are deprived of the protection afforded by polymorphonuclear cells. The usual incubation period (time from drug exposure to the development of symptoms) is 40 days.

**Nonimmune toxic marrow suppression** is dose-dependent, and develops concomitantly with treatment. Hence the clinical history is important because the interval between drug exposure and development of neutropenia usually is shorter than that seen in immunologically mediated types, usually is precipitous, but fortunately is rapidly reversible if the offending agent is withdrawn promptly. If not recognized, this syndrome may progress to involve other cell lines, producing an aplastic anemia, which may or may not be reversible.

**TABLE 135.5. Drug-Induced Agranulocytosis**

I. Immune
   A. Mediated by WBC antibodies
      Aminopyrine
      Thiouracil
      Methimazole
      Chlorpropamide
      Sulfanilamides
      Levamisole
      Clozapine
   B. Immune lupus reaction
      Procainamide
      Hydralazine
   C. Antibiotics
      Penicillin-nafcillin
      Cephalosporins
      Stibophen
II. Toxic chemical depression
   Chlorpromazine
   Depression by accumulation of toxic metabolites
   Carbamazepine
   Phenytoin

### Etiology

Although it is no longer used, the immunogenic drug aminopyrine is the prototype of all drug-induced neutropenia or agranulocytosis syndromes, and the first drug identified that causes immunologic suppression of granulocytes. Consistent with known attributes of immunologic reactions, the initial aberrant response is the development of an IgM class immunoglobulin that can attach to the neutrophil, binding complement, and inducing cell lysis. A secondary IgG response follows; although this may fix complement less avidly, it can recognize granulocyte precursors and inhibit committed stem cells once they acquire typical granulocytic membrane antigens. This can be documented by assessing in vitro growth of precursor clones of cells known as CFU-Gs. Addition of patients' sera will inhibit the growth of CFU-G clones obtained from normal volunteers; adsorption of these antibodies from patients' sera before exposure to normal marrow cells abrogates its inhibitory effects. Presence of the antibody is self-limiting unless the patient is rechallenged with the offending agent. In the case of phenothiazine derivatives, the neutropenia may be self-limiting and relatively mild, and unless monitored for, not recognized. However, any intercurrent challenge to granulocytopoiesis may be catastrophic.

**TABLE 135.6. Conditions Associated With Monocytosis**

| |
|---|
| Infections |
| Brucellosis |
| Fever of unknown origin |
| Infective endocarditis |
| Recovery phase from infection (transient) |
| Syphilis |
| Tuberculosis |
| Inflammatory conditions |
| Autoimmune diseases |
| Polyarteritis |
| Rheumatoid arthritis |
| Systemic lupus erythematosus |
| Granulomatous diseases |
| Crohn disease |
| Sarcoidosis |
| Ulcerative colitis |
| Neoplastic disorders |
| Acute myeloid leukemia |
| Hodgkin disease |
| Monocytic leukemia |
| Myelomonocytic leukemia |
| Preleukemia |
| Solid tumors (malignant) |
| Others |
| Histiocytoses |
| Postsplenectomy |
| Recovery phase of agranulocytosis (transient) |

### Management

Identification and discontinuation of the offending drug are critical to the successful treatment of drug-induced agranulocytosis. The serious risk of infection dictates the use of reverse isolation and broad-spectrum antibiotics (see Chapter 164). Recovery from agranulocytosis may be hastened by the prompt injection of GM-CSF or G-CSF for the duration of the leukopenia. Once the offending drug is identified, it must never be administered again.

## ■ Monocytosis, Eosinophilia, and Basophilia

### *Monocytosis*

Monocytosis is present if the number of monocytes exceeds 900/µl (9–10%). Monocytes divide and transform into other phagocytic cells, release cytokines (CSF and IL-1), and process and present antigen to lymphocytes. Thus, they modulate immune and lymphocyte function.

Clinically, monocytes rise transiently during **recovery from infection** or from agranulocytosis, where they play a role in clearing debris from the inflammatory sites (Table 135.6). With **chronic infection** (bacterial endocarditis, tuberculosis, syphilis, and brucellosis), they persist longer in the peripheral blood. Monocytes are harbingers of **chronic granulomatous disorders** (e.g., sarcoidosis, systemic lupus erythematosus [SLE], rheumatoid arthritis). In **hematologic malignancies**—notably monocytic leukemia, myelomonocytic leukemia, and Hodgkin disease, persistent monocytosis often exceeds $25 \times 10^9$/L.

### *Eosinophilia and Basophilia*

**Eosinophilia** is present when the absolute or the proportional count of eosinophils exceed 700/µl or 10%, respectively. It occurs in conditions shown in Table 135.7, most of which represent **allergic or atopic diseases** or inflammatory skin diseases. Eosinophilia is an important finding in **parasitic infestations** associated with tissue invasion (e.g., trichinosis, schistosomiasis, hookworm, echinococcosis, or filariasis). **Hypereosinophilic syndrome,** defined as eosinophilia exceeding 1500/µl, is a progressive disorder with tissue necrosis and multiple organ damage. It can be controlled with corticosteroids or hydroxyurea. **Eosinophilia-myalgia syndrome,** which followed the use of contaminated L-tryptophan, is characterized by skin rashes, dyspnea, peripheral neuropathy, eosinophilia, and myositis. Characterized now as **eosinophilic fasciitis,** this syndrome may occur episodically without an apparent inciting event, presumably due to some unrecognized environmental insult. Specific inquiry regarding drug or chemical exposures is important, because it may progress to irreversible bone marrow aplasia.

Basophils are the least numerous of the granulocytes and rarely exceed 150/µl. Whereas transient increases may occur in allergic or inflammatory states, chronic progressive basophilia is related to chronic myelocytic leukemia. Late-stage basophilia is a harbinger of impending blast transformation.

**TABLE 135.7. Causes of Eosinophilia**

1. Allergy (asthma, hayfever, atopy)
2. Dermatitis
3. Parasitic infestations
4. Malignant disease, e.g. Hodgkin disease
5. Pulmonary infiltrates with eosinophilia
6. Irradiation
7. Hypereosinophilic syndrome
8. Eosinophilic leukemia
9. Miscellaneous disorders (polyarteritis, eosinophilia-myalgia syndrome)

## Infectious Mononucleosis

**Infectious mononucleosis** is an acute viral disorder caused by **Epstein-Barr** virus (EBV), affecting young adults and characterized by fever, pharyngitis, lymphadenopathy, splenomegaly, and absolute lymphocytosis with many atypical cells (Color Plate 30). Palatal exanthem in the form of red petechiae at the junction of the hard and soft palates, although not diagnostic, is quite characteristic. Patients treated with ampicillin experience an increased incidence of macular skin rash. Development of transient heterophil antibodies (HA) and persistent EBV antibodies are characteristic. With a typical clinical and hematologic picture, a high HA titer is diagnostic. HA are antibodies to sheep RBC that can be absorbed by beef RBC, but not by guinea pig kidney cells.

Heterophil antibiodies have been replaced by a highly sensitive and specific commercial Monospot test, which depends on the rapid development of an IgM antibody, but only 85–95% cases are positive in the first week of the illness. If infectious mononucleosis is strongly suspected but the test results are negative in the first week, retesting in the second or third week of illness is useful. Detection of antibodies against specific components of EBV is useful, making the diagnosis in the rare situation where the Monospot test is negative, or when the presence of chronic infections is of concern. IgM antibodies to the viral capsid antigen (VCA) are diagnostic of a primary EBV infection. IgG anti-VCA antibodies occur almost universally in all cases at first presentation and persist for life, but they cannot reliably diagnose primary infection. Abnormal liver tests are not uncommon. Cold agglutinins are frequently elevated; clinical hemolysis is rare. Because the clinical syndrome of "mononucleosis" occasionally is due to cytomegalovirus (CMV) rather than EBV, when Monospot test is negative, CMV titers should be performed.

Treatment is symptomatic in uncomplicated cases. Recovery is almost universal. Complications are extremely rare; Coombs-positive hemolytic anemia has been reported. Splenic rupture, severe hepatitis, and toxic encephalopathy may be lethal in a few cases. Corticosteroids are indicated for hemolytic anemia, thrombocytopenia, neurologic complications, and respiratory problems.

## Myeloproliferative Disorders

The myeloproliferative disorders represent a diverse group of clinical disorders caused by the uncontrolled clonal proliferation and expansion of an identifiable marrow cell line. Interestingly, although each of these entities has a predominant clonal expansion, the other marrow and blood elements often also are increased, indicating that the mutation occurred prior to the discrete differentiation into a selected cell line. Thus although **polycythemia vera** (P. vera) is an entity dominated by marked erythrocytosis, most patients have at least mild elevation of neutrophils or platelets, or both. **Chronic myelogenous leukemia** (CML) often shows thrombocytosis at presentation, and, in fact, the platelet count in CML has some prognostic significance. In **essential thrombocythemia,** abnormalities of other elements may rarely be noted. Thus the differential diagnosis of these conditions often is difficult and requires careful clinical and laboratory evaluation. Because the mutational event precedes true selective differentiation, one form of disease can later evolve into another (e.g., from P. vera into essential thrombocythemia, or myeloid metaplasia, etc.); therefore, diagnosis of any of these conditions calls for careful follow-up and monitoring. Such morphologic and pathological transformations also alter disease behavior mandating changes in treatment, and alter prognosis. The clinical and laboratory features of the myeloproliferative disorders and their therapy are reviewed in Chapters 134 through 138.

# CHAPTER 136 EVALUATION OF THE PATIENT WITH A BLEEDING DISORDER

The approach to the patient with a suspected bleeding or thrombotic disorder begins with a complete history, a physical examination, and basic screening tests of the hemostatic system. Thorough, careful questioning in patients with hereditary bleeding disorders often yields a history of excessive bleeding. Although the family history can be very helpful in diagnosis in younger patients, mild congenital coagulation factor deficiencies may not surface until adulthood, when excessive bleeding follows a surgical procedure or trauma.

The clinical profile of the bleeding may offer diagnostic clues. Although localized, excessive, postoperative bleeding may require only local therapy, such bleeding from multiple sites calls for consideration and confirmation of a more generalized hemostatic defect. Delayed bleeding after surgery or trauma may follow certain factor deficiencies, drugs, or blood vessel factors.

Prolonged bleeding after superficial trauma often indicates platelet function defects, whereas hemarthrosis and deep hematomas often suggest a coagulation disorder.

## Coagulation Cascade

The normal hemostatic system often is described as a "cascade" of chemical reactions occurring after the system is activated, and continuing until an irreversible hemostatic plug is formed (Figure 136.1). The system consists of three intertwined and interdependent parts, designed to produce effective hemostasis yet prevent excessive thrombosis. The first of these is the coagulation system, consisting of coagulation factor proenzymes (factors VII, IX, X, XI, and XII, prothrombin) and nonenzymatic cofactors (factors V or VIII). When activated, these generate thrombin from prothrombin. The platelets that form a reversible platelet plug are the second part of the system. They also provide the phospholipid surface necessary for coagulation factor activation. The fibrinolytic and antithrombin systems complete the picture, limiting the cascade, and thus preventing unwanted and excessive thrombus generation.

The central event in the coagulation system is the generation of activated factor Xa, the only known enzyme that can activate prothrombin. This event follows either the exposure of inactive factor VII to tissue factor on fibroblasts or an altered endothelial surface or exposed subendothelial proteins. The commonly used terminology reflects the underlying concept that when exposed to negatively charged protein surfaces, the coagulation factors become activated, and the cascade proceeds. As hemostasis proceeds, this activation of X to Xa is inhibited, and the direct VIIa–tissue factor effect on X must be supplemented by the IXa-phospholipid-VIIIa complex. Once factor Xa is generated, it can link up with Va, phospholipid, and prothrombin to produce thrombin.

Thrombin is the linchpin of coagulation. It breaks down fibrinogen to form fibrin monomers and it activates factor XIII, promoting the cross-linking of fibrin polymers into an insoluble fibrin meshwork. It can activate

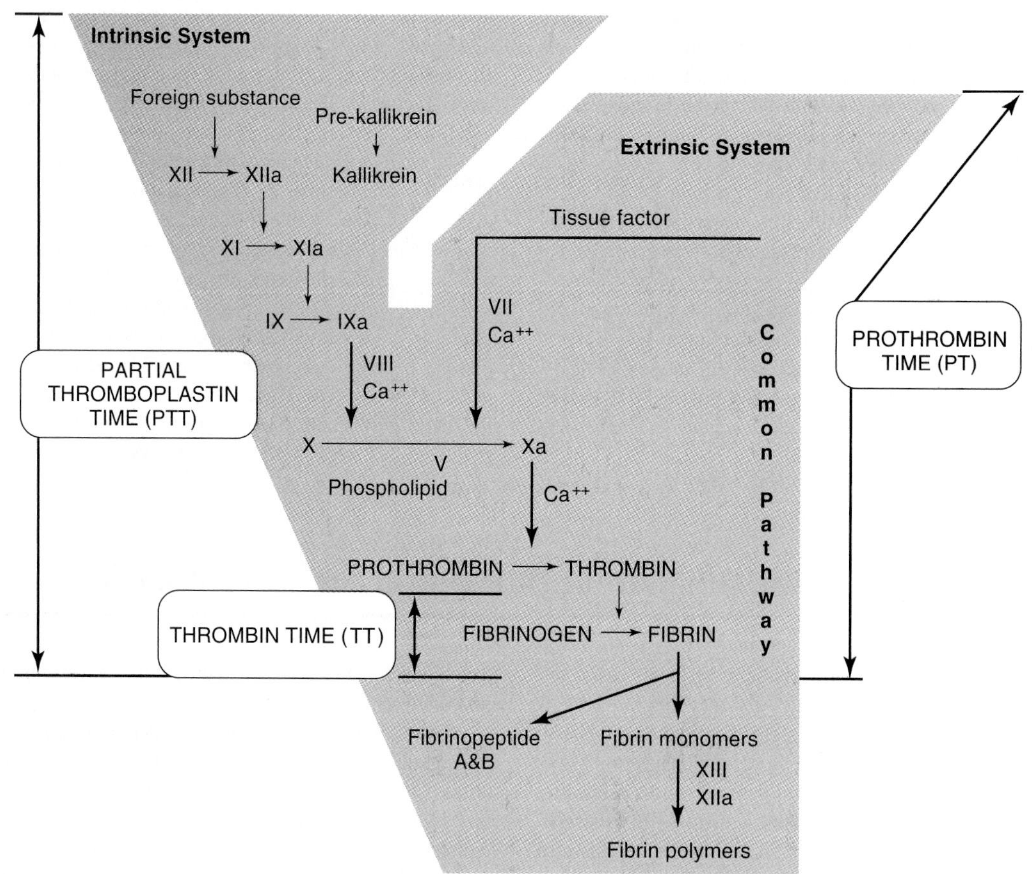


**FIGURE 136.1.** Simplified schema of blood coagulation.

factors V and VIII to promote its own formation, and it can activate platelets and induce the platelet release and aggregation reactions. Fibrin monomers ultimately congeal into fibrin polymers, which create a stable, hemostatic thrombus. The entire coagulation system is a sequence of amplified reactions. Interestingly, the concentrations of coagulation factors in the early portion of the cascade are markedly less (often by a factor of several hundred) compared to fibrinogen, or even prothrombin. Thus most bleeding disorders are due to deficiencies of these factors. Only some nutritional deficiencies, liver disease, or consumption of coagulation factors affects factors I and II. Hemophiliacs can survive on just fractions of normal plasma factor levels (about 5%, or only 10–20 μg/dl), compared to 4,000 μg/dl for fibrinogen. However, depletion of factor VIII below a critical threshold is catastrophic.

## The Fibrinolytic and Antithrombin Systems

The coagulation cascade is inhibited both by "natural" anticoagulants and by the fibrinolytic system. The most important natural anticoagulant is antithrombin (AT) III. ATIII inhibits thrombin and several other activated proteins (VIIa, Xa, IXa, XIa, kallikrein, and plasmin) by forming stable bonds to these factors. Heparin accelerates the reaction. Thrombomodulin, a component of the endothelial cell membrane, is another important anticoagulant. When bound to thrombin, thrombomodulin can activate protein C. Activated protein C can join with protein S and phospholipid to break down factors Va and VIIIa.

The fibrinolytic system is a series of proteins that, when activated, can degrade cross-linked fibrin. Plasminogen requires activators to convert into plasmin, the enzyme able to degrade fibrin. Some natural plasminogen activators are factor XII and prekallikrein. Several drugs are capable of plasminogen activation (streptokinase, urokinase, and recombinant tissue plasminogen activator, tPA). Like all parts of the coagulation system, this system also has inhibitors.

## Platelets

Endothelial injury also results in the activation of platelets. In response to such injury, platelets adhere to one another and release their granules into the microenvironment of the injury. This release reaction generates the formation of a reversible platelet plug, capable of combining with the fibrin polymers to create a stable, irreversible platelet thrombus. The platelet release reaction is affected by many drugs, of which aspirin is the most studied and potentially therapeutic. Aspirin decreases cyclooxygenase and thus prevents thromboxane A2 synthesis, thereby inhibiting the release reaction (Figure 136.2).

## Laboratory Evaluation

Although there is no substitute for a complete clinical history in the diagnosis of bleeding disorders, laboratory screening tests are the key to their diagnosis. (See Table 136.1.)

### Prothrombin time

The prothrombin time (PT) measures the function of the proteins of the "extrinsic" and the common (fibrinogen, II, V, X) pathways. The vitamin K–dependent proteins (II, VII, IX, X) are measured by the PT, and levels are affected by warfarin. The PT is most sensitive to deficiencies of factors V, VII, and X, or prothrombin, but it also may be prolonged when the fibrinogen is low, or when heparin or fibrin split products are present. An elevated hematocrit prolongs the PT, because it affects the relative amount of anticoagulant and plasma in the test. Because responsiveness of the test varies with thromboplastins of varying sensitivity, the test results have been standardized, and the results are reported as the **international normalized ratio (INR).**

### Partial thromboplastin time

The partial thromboplastin time (PTT) measures the "intrinsic" (factors XII, XI, IX, VIII, prekallikrein) and the common (fibrinogen, II, V, X) pathway factors and detects circulating anticoagulants. Heparin inhibits many of the same factors in its role as an antithrombin III cofactor. Thus, the PTT also is used to monitor heparin dose. Because the PTT is more sensitive to deficiencies of the early intrinsic pathway factors and less sensitive to deficiencies of the later common pathway factors, occasionally fibrinogen deficiency prolongs only the PT and not the PTT. In general, the PTT is prolonged when factors V, VIII, IX, X, XI, or XII, or prothrombin is low, or in the presence of an inhibitor to any of these factors, a high fibrinogen level, fibrin split products, heparin, or disseminated intravascular coagulation (DIC).

The PT and PTT are the basic screening tests of the coagulation system. If one of them is abnormal, a mixing study is the next step. Normal plasma and the patient's plasma are mixed in a 1 : 1 ratio. Normal plasma has such a surplus of factors that the test should become normal if a factor is simply deficient. If the test is abnormal because of the presence of an inhibitor, the test remains abnormal, and further studies are necessary to locate the specific inhibitor. In rare coagulation disorders with a strong history of bleeding (e.g., factor XIII deficiency), PT and PTT may be normal, necessitating additional tests.

### Thrombin time

The thrombin time indicates the time needed for plasma to clot when thrombin is added to the mixture. It can screen for decreases in fibrinogen, abnormal fibrino-

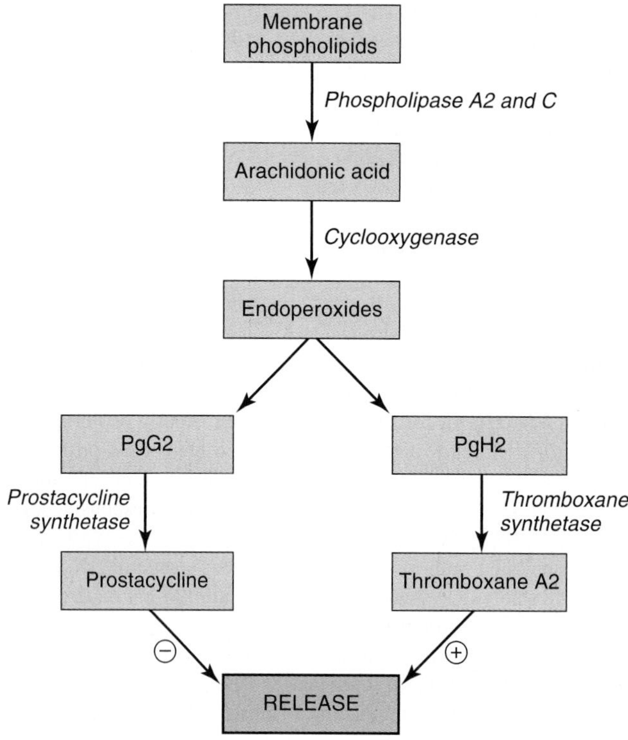


**FIGURE 136.2.** Steps in platelet release reaction. ⊕ = stimulation; ⊖ = inhibition.

**TABLE 136.1. Laboratory Evaluation of Bleeding Disorders: Causes of Abnormal Screening Tests**

| Condition/Cause | ↑PTT | ↑PT | ↑TT |
|---|---|---|---|
| Deficiency of: | | | |
| HMW kininogen | + | | |
| Prekallikrein | + | | |
| XII | + | | |
| XI | + | | |
| IX | + | | |
| VIII | + | | |
| VII | | + | |
| V | + | + | |
| X | + | + | |
| Dysfibrinogenemia | | + | + |
| Afibrinogenemia | + | + | + |
| Hypofibrinogenemia | | + | + |
| Lupus anticoagulant | + | + | |
| Oral anticoagulant | + | + | |
| Liver disease | + | + | |
| Polycythemia | + | + | |
| Heparin | + | | + |

gens, the presence of fibrin split products, or the presence of heparin.

### Fibrin or fibrinogen degradation products

The **fibrin or fibrinogen degradation products** (FDP) test detects breakdown products of fibrin or fibrinogen and can confirm the diagnosis of **DIC**. These tests determine the highest dilution of plasma at which the specimen agglutinates; they usually are reported semiquantitatively. The d-dimer test uses monoclonal antibody that is very specific for cross-linked FDP only. Both tests are positive in DIC, often in acute venous or arterial thrombosis, in late pregnancy, and, often, immediately postoperatively.

### Euglobulin clot lysis time

The euglobulin clot lysis time test evaluates the presence of systemic fibrinolysis. The plasma fraction used is free of the lytic system inhibitor. If the fibrinogen is normal, the clot formed should be rapidly dissolved. If the test clot dissolves more rapidly than the control clot, it is evidence of activation of the fibrinolytic system.

### Reptilase time

The reptilase time test is used to evaluate fibrinogen. It measures fibrin formation after the snake venom cleaves fibrinopeptide A from the fibrinogen molecule.

### Platelet studies

The peripheral smear should be examined to exclude thrombocytopenia as a cause of bleeding. Abnormal platelet morphology may suggest abnormal platelet function in thrombotic disorders, in the storage pool diseases, or in the myelodysplastic or myeloproliferative diseases. If the count is normal and the history suggests a bleeding disorder due to abnormal platelet function, a qualitative abnormality may be suspected. The bleeding time (BT) is the basic test of the ability of the platelets to form a hemostatic plug. A small cut is made in the skin, and the time until bleeding stops is measured. A prolonged BT may indicate either abnormal platelet function or abnormal skin and blood vessel fragility. It is a difficult test to standardize and perform, and its unreliability limits its usefulness. Because of the difficulties in interpretation and the lack of predictive value, it is used as a screening test for the evaluation of bleeding disorders but not as a preoperative screening test. A normal test does not exclude a significant platelet function abnormality.

Platelet aggregation tests can be performed to further define the functional characteristics of platelets. Platelet-rich plasma is added to various known aggregating agents (ADP, epinephrine, ristocetin, thrombin), and the solution is placed in an aggregometer. If the platelets aggregate, increasing amounts of light are able to pass through the specimen. The patterns of aggregation after each agent often may suggest whether the platelet function abnormalities are congenital or due to drugs.

### Factor assays

Specific functional assays have been developed for all of the factors listed in Table 136.2. Generally, levels of 50–150% are considered normal. For many of the factors, antigenic assays also are available. An abnormal functional assay coupled with a normal antigenic assay suggests a structurally abnormal protein. More recently, using the polymerase chain reaction (PCR), amino acid substitutions causing functionally abnormal factors have been identified. An example is the guanine-to-adenine substitution at nucleotide position 1691 of the factor V gene, leading to the substitution of arginine (R) by glutamine (Q) at position 506 of the polypeptide chain of factor V (factor V Leiden). The resulting inability of activated protein C to inactivate factor V—**activated protein C (APC) resistance**—leads to a thrombotic tendency. The most common manifestations are deep vein thrombosis and superficial thrombophlebitis. This allele (factor V:$Q^{506}$) is highly prevalent among Caucasians, with a frequency of 2–15%. Conversely, in patients with venous thrombosis, studies show a prevalence of 10–40% for factor V:$Q^{506}$ allele. Retrospective studies show a very high prevalence of factor V:$Q^{506}$ in pregnancy-associated deep vein thrombosis and deep vein thrombosis associated with oral contraceptive use. It is not uncommon for it to coexist with other genetic thrombotic disorders, which may alter the severity, pattern, and frequency of thrombotic events.

**TABLE 136.2. Coagulation Factors and Their Kinetics**

| Factor Number | Coagulation Factor | Biologic Half-Life (h) |
|---|---|---|
| I | Fibrinogen | 90 |
| II | Prothrombin | 72 |
| III | Tissue thromboplastin | – |
| IV | Calcium | – |
| V | Labile factor | 16 |
| VII | Stable | 5 |
| VIII | Antihemophilic A (AHF) | 12 |
| IX | Antihemophilic B (AHB) (Christmas factor) | 24 |
| X | Stuart-Prower factor | 48 |
| XI | Plasma thromboplastin antecedent (PTA) | 60 |
| XII | Hageman factor | 60 |
| XIII | Fibrin stabilizing factor | 120 |
| | Prekallikrein (Fletcher factor)* | |
| | High-molecular-weight kininogen (Fitzgerald, Williams, or Flaujeac factor)* | |
| | von Willebrand factor* | |
| | Protein C* | |
| | Protein S* | |

*Not usually referred to by a Roman numeral, or has not been assigned a number.

Factor VIII, the protein involved in the coagulation cascade, is attached to the much larger von Willebrand carrier protein, which also is responsible for platelet aggregation and adhesion to the endothelium. Functional assays of factor VIII protein are designated VIII:C; antigenic assays are designated VIII:Ag. The **von Willebrand factor** (vWF) is a large, multimeric protein composed of vWF monomers joined by polymerization to form the large multimers of plasma vWF. Functional assays for vWF are the ristocetin cofactor assay, and the antigenic assay is the vWF:Ag. These multimers can be measured in the plasma, and results are important to define the various types of von Willebrand disease.

# CHAPTER 137 BLEEDING DISORDERS DUE TO FACTOR DEFICIENCIES

The diagnostic approach to a bleeding disorder varies depending on the clinical circumstance, as well as on the results of a careful drug, family, and overall medical history. Most severe congenital bleeding disorders become apparent very early in childhood, but the less severe factor deficiencies may escape detection until adulthood or until the system is unable to cope with the stress of either surgery or trauma.

## Hereditary Bleeding Disorders

### *Hemophilia A*

**Hemophilia A** is an X-linked bleeding disorder (incidence, 1:10,000 men) caused by a deficiency of factor VIII. Because spontaneous mutations may cause up to 30% of cases, the family history may be negative. Chromosome changes consist of frame shift, deletions, inversions, and point mutations within the factor VIII gene. A true deficiency of the protein occurs in up to 90% of severe cases. The severity of the bleeding usually correlates with factor VIII levels. Severe hemophilia (factor VIII <1%) presents in childhood with spontaneous hemarthroses and internal hematomas. The risk of long-term complications (e.g., joint fibrosis and intracranial hemorrhage) has been decreased dramatically by prophylactic infusions of factor VIII concentrates. Although the risk for spontaneous bleeding is proportionately less in moderate (factor VIII = 2–5%) and mild (factor VIII = 5–30%) hemophilia, the risk for bleeding after even minor surgical procedures or trauma persists (Table 137.1).

The PTT is variably prolonged, depending on the severity of the factor deficiency. The VIII:C is decreased, but the PT, bleeding time, and vWF:Ag are normal. Women who are carriers have low VIII:C levels (20–50%) and normal vWF:Ag levels, and usually present with a mild bleeding disorder.

**TABLE 137.1. Clinical Bleeding in Relation to Coagulant Factor Levels in Hemophilia**

| Severity | Coagulant Factor Activity (%) | Type of Bleeding |
|---|---|---|
| Severe | <1 | Spontaneous bleeding |
| Moderate | 1–5 | Severe bleeding after minor injury, occasional spontaneous bleeding |
| Mild | 5–20 | Severe bleeding after major hemostatic stress, no spontaneous bleeding |

#### Management

Mild deficiency often requires prophylaxis before dental or surgical procedures, but prophylactic factor VIII concentrate infusions usually are not needed. **Intravenous desmopressin** (DDAVP) induces the release of stored factor VIII and vWF from endothelial cells. Whereas mild or moderate cases often respond to desmopressin, severe cases do not, because they have no stored factor VIII. These individuals require both prophylactic and therapeutic infusions of factor VIII concentrates.

One unit of factor VIII/kg raises the factor VIII level by 2%. The dose of concentrate required to achieve a desired factor VIII level is calculated by the following formula: Units factor VIII = desired level (%) × weight (kg) × 0.5. The type of bleeding to be stopped determines which dose is required—15–20% to control spontaneous joint or muscle bleeding, 30–40% for more severe bleeding, 50–100% for major surgery, and 30–50% for prophylaxis 10–14 days postoperatively. Factor VIII has a half-life of nearly 12 hours. Thus, it should be infused every 12 hours, or as indicated by the factor VIII level, to achieve the levels mentioned. Patients with mild hemophilia A who are undergoing dental procedures also may be adequately treated with oral epsilon-aminocaproic acid or tranexamic acid, inhibitors of fibrinolysis.

The management of hemophilia A has been complicated by the transmission of contaminating viruses in the blood supply. Since 1985, all factor VIII concentrates in the United States have undergone some type of viral inactivation procedure, so that the risk of transmitting hepatitis, HIV, and other viruses has declined substantially. Unfortunately, though, more than 70% of hemophiliacs exposed to concentrates have acquired HIV, and immune suppression in HIV-negative hemophiliacs with hepatitis is a continuing problem as a result of prior exposure to contaminated concentrates.

Inhibitor-related resistance to factor concentrates occurs in nearly 15% of severe hemophiliacs on replacement therapy; it is usually apparent when the infusions no longer raise the factor level in a previously responsive patient, or when the PTT fails to normalize in a 1:1 mix of the patient's and pooled plasma.

**TABLE 137.2. Laboratory Abnormalities in von Willebrand Disease by Type**

| | Type I | Type IIA | Type IIB | Pseudo | Type III |
|---|---|---|---|---|---|
| PT | N | N | N | N | N |
| PTT | Mild ↑ | Mild ↑ | ↑ | ↑ | ↑ |
| BT | ↑ | ↑ | ↑ | ↑ | ↑↑ |
| Platelet count | N | N | N or ↓ | N or ↓ | N |
| VIII: C | Sl ↓ | N or Sl ↓ | N or ↓ | N or ↓ | ↓↓ |
| VWR: Ag | Sl ↓ | ↓ | ↓ or N | N or ↓ | ↓↓ <5 |
| Multimer | N distribution ↓ numbers | ↓ large & intermediate; ↑ small | No large multimers | ↓ large | None |
| RCvWFA | ↓ | ↓ | ↓ or N | ↓ or N | ↓↓ <1 |
| Comments | Most common | 10–15% of cases | Autosomal dominant | Really a platelet disorder | Often homozygous |

RCvWFA = ristocetin cofactor vWF; Activity: ↓ = decreased; ↑ = increased; N = normal; For others, see text.

Inhibitors, measured in **Bethesda units** (BU), are IgG antibodies. An inhibitor below 5 BU (low responder) may be overcome by high doses of factor VIII concentrate. Most inhibitors are species-specific, so that inhibitors to human factor VIII may be evaded by infusing porcine factor VIII, thus still attaining an increase in factor VIII level. Cross-reactivity of the inhibitor to the porcine factor VIII should be excluded. With higher inhibitor activity (>10 BU; high responder), anamnestic response is likely on factor infusion. Options are porcine factor VIII, factor IX complex concentrates, or recombinant factor VIIIa concentrates. Immunosuppression of the inhibitor output is not always successful. Inhibitors cause management problems and a 20% mortality rate.

## Hemophilia B

Hemophilia B (also known as factor IX deficiency or Christmas disease) also is an X-linked recessive trait (1:50,000 male births). Its clinical features and correlation of bleeding to factor levels resemble hemophilia A. The PTT is prolonged; the PT, BT, and platelet count are normal. The liver produces factor IX; thus, severe liver disease may lower factor IX level. Required factor IX levels for treatment or prophylaxis are similar to those for hemophilia A. However, factor IX diffuses extravascularly, so that to attain factor levels similar to those in hemophilia A, it takes twice as much factor infusion (units factor IX = desired level (%) × weight (kg) × 1.0).

The half-life of factor IX exceeds 24 hours, so that once-daily (twice on the day of surgical procedures) infusions usually suffice. Factor IX complex concentrates contain varying amounts of factors II, VII, and X, and may cause thrombotic complications (**disseminated intravascular coagulation** [DIC], deep venous thrombosis, and pulmonary embolism). These patients also develop inhibitors, with outcomes and management similar to hemophilia A.

## Von Willebrand disease

Von Willebrand disease (vWD), an autosomal dominant and variably expressed illness, is the most common (1 per 125 persons) heritable coagulation disorder. The **vW protein** (vWF), a very large, multimeric protein produced by endothelial cells and megakaryocytes, is stored in the platelet α granules and the Weibel-Palade bodies of the endothelial cells. A carrier of factor VIII, it helps the platelets aggregate among themselves and adhere to the endothelium, leading to a platelet plug. Thus, loss of vWF resembles decreased platelet function (easy bruising, menorrhagia, and mucosal and gastrointestinal bleeding). Severe vWF deficiency occasionally may cause a bleeding pattern resembling a coagulation factor deficiency (e.g., bleeding after surgery or trauma, spontaneous hemarthrosis). The diagnosis of mild vWD can be difficult in stressed patients, because the stored vWF in the endothelial cells is released as an acute phase reactant, and vWF levels may become normal.

Using the multimeric pattern on plasma electrophoresis (Table 137.2), several subtypes of vWD may be identified. Type I is the most common. In type IIB, the vW molecule has an abnormal affinity for the platelet surface. The large multimers are intravascularly bound, and vWF levels are low. Platelet aggregates form and are removed, causing thrombocytopenia. Use of desmopressin in these patents may worsen the thrombocytopenia by increasing the release of abnormal vWF; it is thus contraindicated. **Pseudo-von Willebrand disease** (or "platelet type" von Willebrand disease) mimics type IIB. The vWF is normal, but the platelet receptor has an abnormally high affinity for the large vW multimers, causing platelet aggregation as the protein is released. Circulating large multimers are low. Cryoprecipitate induces spontaneous platelet aggregation in the pseudo-vW type, thus differentiating it from type IIB. In type III, the vWF and VIII:C decline severely, and all multimers are completely absent; the severe bleeding here resembles severe hemophilia A or B (hemarthrosis and soft tissue bleeding). Screening studies may be normal in a significant number of patients, thus making the diagnosis difficult.

### Management

Treatment of von Willebrand disease depends on the type (Table 137.2). At the time of diagnosis, desmopressin often is infused to document response and to help anticipate therapy if a bleeding emergency arises. Thirty minutes after infusion, the platelet count, factor VIII, and vWF/ristocetin cofactor levels are drawn. Desmopressin often suffices in less severe deficiencies or for minor surgery (e.g., tooth extractions). It usually is quite effective in type I, but responses are variable in type IIA. Because it only releases stored vWF and VIII:C, desmopressin is not useful in severe deficiencies or in those not producing these factors, nor should it be given in type IIB and platelet-type vWD. Either cryoprecipitate or vWF concentrate is used in severe deficiency and type IIB. Oral antifibrinolytic agents often are used in mild or moderate deficiency to prevent bleeding after dental surgery or for arduous mucosal bleeding (e.g., epistaxis) or menorrhagia.

# CHAPTER 138 BLEEDING ASSOCIATED WITH PLATELET DISORDERS

Platelets, fragments of the megakaryocyte cytoplasm, have a normal life span of 10 days in the circulation. Their surfaces provide the phospholipid base for many of the coagulation factors to function, and their storage granules provide procoagulant and vasoactive proteins that are key to the ability to form a hemostatic plug. Young platelets appear to be more hemostatically active. Disorders in platelet numbers or function, therefore, often cause bleeding disorders, whether hereditary or acquired. The normal blood has 140,000 to 400,000 circulating platelets per $mm^3$. Roughly one third of the circulating platelets are pooled in the spleen.

## Thrombocytopenia

### Definition and Etiology

Thrombocytopenia is a decrease in the number of circulating platelets in the blood. Due to poor platelet plug formation, a bleeding diathesis results, the severity of which correlates with the degree of thrombocytopenia. No significant hemostatic abnormalities follow thrombocytopenia when the platelet count exceeds 100,000/$mm^3$. In uncomplicated thrombocytopenia, spontaneous bleeding is unusual when platelet count exceeds 40,000/$mm^3$. An inverse linear correlation is noted between bleeding time and a platelet count below 100,000/$mm^3$.

Thrombocytopenia may result from **decreased production, increased destruction,** or **increased pooling** of platelets (Table 138.1). Decreased production of megakaryocytes and platelets follows damage to the marrow or occurs as a part of aplastic anemia. Megaloblastic anemias, myeloproliferative disorders, and certain hereditary disorders (e.g., Wiskott-Aldrich syndrome, May-Hegglin anomaly) often are associated with ineffective thrombopoiesis. Accelerated platelet destruction, caused by an autoantibody, often causes thrombocytopenia, or the platelets may be consumed by intravascular thrombosis (e.g., disseminated intravascular coagulation and microangiopathic processes). The bone marrow in these instances usually shows an increase in megakaryocytes. It is important to obtain a history of drug ingestion in any patient with thrombocytopenia, because drugs may directly suppress the bone marrow or they may act as antigens and stimulate antibody formation.

## Immune Thrombocytopenic Purpura

### Clinical Features and Diagnosis

Immune thrombocytopenia may be either primary (idiopathic) or secondary (Table 138.2). Acute **idiopathic immune thrombocytopenia** most commonly affects children from 2 to 6 years of age, and the chronic form most often affects young women. Autoantibody-coated platelets are rapidly sequestered in the spleen, causing thrombocytopenia.

Patients usually report petechiae or mucosal bleeding. Blood-filled blisters may be seen in the oral cavity. Neither lymphadenopathy nor splenomegaly occurs in **idiopathic thrombocytopenic purpura** (ITP). Clinical features of the associated disease are seen in secondary types. The platelet count is low, and the bleeding time is

**TABLE 138.1. Pathogenesis and Frequent Causes of Thrombocytopenia**

| | |
|---|---|
| Decreased production | Aplastic anemia<br>Radiation, cytotoxic drug therapy<br>Pancytopenia<br>Marrow infiltration<br>Myelofibrosis, cancer<br>Ineffective megakaryopoiesis<br>Vitamin $B_{12}$ or folate deficiency<br>Drug-induced<br>Ethanol, gold, sulfonamides, trimethoprim-sulfamethoxazole, quinine ("cocktail purpura") |
| Increased destruction | Immune destruction<br>Immune thrombocytopenic purpura (ITP), lymphomas, SLE<br>ITP with Coombs positive hemolytic anemia (Evan's syndrome)<br>Drug-induced (some involving anti-platelet antibody)<br>Thiazides, acetaminophen, phenytoin, heparin, quinidine, quinine<br>Nonimmune destruction<br>Infections<br>Infectious mononucleosis, septicemia<br>Disseminated intravascular coagulation (DIC), microangiopathic hemolytic anemia, thrombotic thrombocytopenic purpura (TTP), hemolytic uremic syndrome (HUS) |
| Normal production | Peripheral pooling<br>Splenic sequestration |

**TABLE 138.2. Principal Causes of Immune Thrombocytopenia**

Idiopathic
- Acute
- Chronic

Secondary
- Lymphoproliferative disorders
- Systemic lupus erythematosus

Drug-related

prolonged; the blood smear shows a reduced number of platelets, some of which may be large. Bone marrow examination reveals an increased or normal number of megakaryocytes. The platelet antibody test is positive in most but not all patients.

Idiopathic thrombocytopenic purpura is a diagnosis of exclusion. In some patients with ITP, especially if associated with autoimmune hemolytic anemia (Evans syndrome), systemic lupus erythematosus (SLE) or lymphoma eventually develops. Any history of drug ingestion should be noted. In a thrombocytopenic patient, all but the very essential drugs should be stopped. Drug-related immune thrombocytopenia usually resolves rapidly after the offending drug has been stopped. In children, ITP may exhibit spontaneous remissions.

### Management

Adults with ITP or children without spontaneous remission are treated with corticosteroids. In some patients with ITP, platelet counts may rise transiently following a transfusion, but most cases do not exhibit this feature. High-dose prednisone is initiated (1–2 mg/kg/d). If thrombocytopenia resolves, prednisone is slowly tapered and eventually stopped. Patients who do not respond to prednisone or require large maintenance doses (>10 mg/d) require splenectomy, which can induce a remission in about 70% of patients. All patients with ITP should receive a Pneumovax vaccination in anticipation of possible future splenectomy. Patients with a prior response to prednisone are more likely to respond to splenectomy. If splenectomy fails, immunosuppression is begun with cyclophosphamide, vincristine, or azathioprine (Imuran). The following agents may be useful in resistant cases: high-dose intravenous (IV) IgG, plasmapheresis, and danazol, an androgen with reduced virilizing ability. Intravenous IgG, which transiently increases platelet count, has been more effective in children than in adults with ITP; it is useful in certain situations (e.g., before splenectomy or other surgical procedures, or in suspected CNS bleed). Danazol traditionally has been used for the long-term management of refractory ITP.

Patients with secondary thrombocytopenia are treated in the same manner; additional treatment for the primary disorder may be needed.

## Acquired Platelet Function Defects

Acquired platelet function defects, the most common cause of bleeding (Table 138.3), most commonly are caused by drugs, but underlying diseases also may be responsible. Although the cause of the defect in uremia is unclear, uremic platelets appear to bind the von Willebrand factor defectively, interfering with aggregation and with the subendothelial adhesion of platelets. Dialysis sometimes corrects the abnormality partially, and life-threatening bleeding may be treated with platelet concentrates. Lesser bleeding episodes often respond to either cryoprecipitate, desmospressin (DDAVP), or estrogen.

**TABLE 138.3. Acquired Platelet Function Defects**

| |
|---|
| Uremia |
| Myeloproliferative diseases |
| Myelodysplastic syndromes |
| Paraproteinemia |
| Autoimmune |
| Collagen vascular disease |
| Antiplatelet antibodies |
| Immune thrombocytopenia |
| Liver disease |
| Cardiac surgery |
| Drugs |
| Alcohol |
| Ampicillin |
| Aspirin |
| Cephalothin |
| Chlorpromazine |
| Clofibrate |
| Cocaine |
| Cyclosporin A |
| Dipyridamole |
| Vincristine, vinblastine |
| Nitrofurantoin |
| NSAIDs |
| Penicillins |
| Phenylbutazone |
| Sulfinpyrazone |
| Tricyclic antidepressants |

In myeloproliferative and myelodysplastic syndromes, the platelets commonly are abnormal; however, the pattern of aggregation and adhesion abnormalities usually is not characteristic or diagnostic. Most commonly, aggregation and release to epinephrine, ADP, or collagen are abnormal. The bleeding time, although often abnormal, does not reliably gauge the risk of bleeding. Paraproteinemias often cause platelet defects, apparently by abnormal protein coating of the platelet surface. The abnormality is independent of the type of paraprotein, and it usually improves with either treatment of the underlying disorder or plasmapheresis.

A variety of drugs adversely affect platelet function, a feature with therapeutic merit in some drugs (e.g., aspirin) and adverse sequelae in others (Table 138.4). A significant bleeding diathesis may arise during cardiopulmonary bypass (CPB), partly due to platelet dysfunction; platelets seem to degranulate while circulating in the CPB and often appear as "ghosts" in the peripheral smear. Although therapeutic doses of antiplatelet drugs before CPB may enhance the bleeding risk, platelet transfusions usually correct the defect promptly.

## Hereditary Platelet Disorders

### *Bernard-Soulier Syndrome*

In Bernard-Soulier syndrome, an autosomal dominant disorder, the platelets lack the membrane glycoproteins necessary for binding vWF to the platelet surface. Clinical features include easy and sometimes spontaneous bruising, epistaxis, menorrhagia, petechiae, and purpura. The peripheral blood smear shows giant platelets. The bleeding time and ristocetin aggregation tests are abnormal, but the VIII:C and VIII:RAg are normal, differentiating this disorder from von Willebrand disease. Severe, life-threatening hemorrhage requires transfusion of normal donor platelets. Heterozygotes often are asymptomatic.

### *Glanzmann's Thrombasthenia*

In Glanzmann's thrombasthenia, an autosomal recessive disorder, the lack of glycoprotein IIb/IIIa complex on the platelet surfaces renders the platelets unable to bind fibrinogen to their surface. Mucosal bleeding, spontaneous bruising, petechiae, and, rarely, hemarthrosis are the features. Platelet-to-platelet interaction is abnormal, and the bleeding time is prolonged. The disorder tends to become less severe with age. Severe hemorrhage requires platelet concentrates, but because antibodies may develop to glycoprotein IIb/IIIa, platelets should be transfused only in severe bleeding episodes. Epsilon-aminocaproic acid may be used for relatively minor mucosal bleeding.

### *Hereditary Storage Pool Diseases*

These secondary aggregation disorders are more common than primary aggregation defects. Other con-

**TABLE 138.4. Drugs Affecting Platelet Function**

| |
|---|
| Antihistamine |
| Aspirin |
| β-blockers |
| Cephalosporin antibiotics |
| Dextran |
| Diltiazem |
| Nifedipine |
| Nitroglycerin |
| Nitroprusside |
| NSAIDs |
| Penicillin |
| Prostacyclin |
| Quinidine |
| Tricyclic antidepressants |
| Verapamil |

genital abnormalities, such as Wiskott-Aldrich syndrome, thrombocytopenia with absent radii (TAR) syndrome, or Chédiak-Higashi syndrome occasionally may be associated, but inheritance is variable, and most patients are otherwise normal. Mucosal bleeding, epistaxis, easy bruising, and hematuria are reported. The bleeding time is prolonged, and platelet adhesion and aggregation are abnormal in the presence of collagen. Severe hemorrhage requires platelet concentrates.

# CHAPTER 139 ACQUIRED BLEEDING DISORDERS

## Etiology

Acquired coagulation disorders may be caused by a panoply of medical conditions. As a cause of bleeding diathesis, they are much more common than hereditary coagulation or platelet disorders. Some major clinical issues include acquired bleeding problems due to liver disease, disseminated intravascular coagulation (DIC), drugs, malignancies, massive transfusions, thrombotic thrombocytopenic purpura, and hemolytic-uremic syndrome.

### Liver Disease

Liver disease, through multiple mechanisms (Table 139.1), probably is the most common cause of coagulation abnormalities in a general hospital population. Deficiencies of coagulation factors synthesized in the liver may lead to life-threatening bleeding, and profound thrombocytopenia may arise from cirrhosis and splenic sequestration. The spectrum of abnormalities is wide, from a normal coagulation profile in a patient with mild liver disease to life-threatening severe hemorrhage with disseminated intravascular coagulation (DIC) or fibrinolysis.

**TABLE 139.1. Hemostatic Abnormalities in Liver Disease**

| Mechanism | Result |
|---|---|
| Decreased synthesis of vitamin K–dependent factors | Elevated PT |
| Splenic sequestration | Thrombocytopenia |
| Circulating platelet inhibitors | Platelet dysfunction |
| Synthesis of abnormal coagulation factors | Dysfibrinogenemia |
| Increased factor consumption | Primary fibrinolysis<br>DIC |
| Decreased clearance of factors | DIC<br>Fibrinolysis |
| Decreased AT-III and protein C Production | DIC |

AT-III = antithrombin III; DIC = disseminated intravascular coagulation.

### Disseminated Intravascular Coagulation

Disseminated intravascular coagulation is a pathologic process that activates the coagulation, fibrinolytic, and platelet systems. Many underlying disorders seem to cause the expression of tissue factor to initiate the process. Coagulation factors and platelets are consumed as the coagulation cascade is continuously activated; although the initial event is thrombin generation, excessive bleeding usually dominates the clinical picture. Thrombin converts fibrinogen to fibrin, elevates the fibrin degradation products, activates platelets, and initiates fibrinolysis (Figure 139.1). Disseminated intravascular coagulation may occur as a fulminant bleeding event with end-organ ischemia related to intravascular microthrombi, or as a chronic complication of malignancy featuring recurrent thrombosis and compensated factor consumption. Table 139.2 presents a partial list of causes of DIC.

Diagnosis of acute, fulminant DIC usually is easy in an actively bleeding patient. However, the diagnosis of chronic DIC may be difficult, especially if the underlying disease remains elusive. Laboratory results indicate coagulation factor consumption, evidence of fibrin and fibrinogen degradation, fibrinolytic activity, and evidence of microangiopathy on a peripheral smear (schistocytes and erythrocyte fragments). In severe DIC, virtually all coagulation tests are abnormal. Fibrinogen degradation products (FDP) rise in 80% to 100% of patients with DIC, and the protamine sulfate or ethanol gel tests (indicating circulating soluble fibrin monomers) usually are positive. The d-dimer assay is specific for FDP, and it is the most reliable test for diagnosing DIC. Some other tests for diagnosing DIC are listed in Table 139.3.

Treatment of DIC is primarily of the underlying cause, thus removing the stimulus for the coagulation activation. In addition, replacement of factors, individualized to fit the pace of the patient's consumption and guided by repeated laboratory monitoring, usually is necessary to prevent fulminant hemorrhage. Low-dose heparin (5–10 U/kg/h) occasionally is used if the cause of the DIC is ongoing. It also is used to try to lower the rate of factor consumption so that replacement therapy

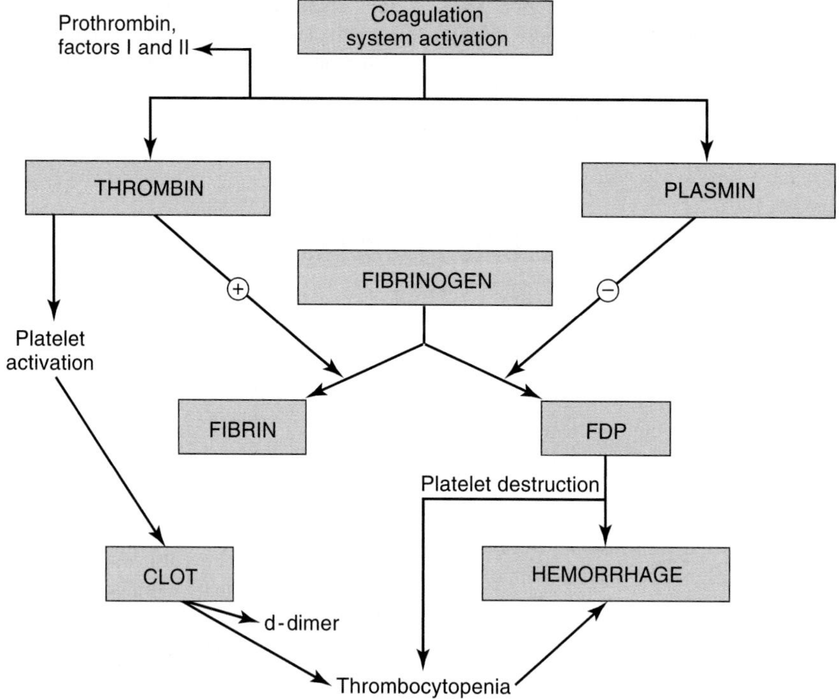


**FIGURE 139.1.** The evolution of disseminated intravascular coagulation (DIC).

**TABLE 139.2. Causes of Disseminated Intravascular Coagulation**

*Infection*
Gram-negative and gram-positive bacteremia, viruses (herpes, Lassa, dengue), Rocky Mountain spotted fever, fungi (*Candida* spp, *Aspergillus* spp) and others (clostridia, toxic shock syndrome, malaria)
*Trauma*
Crush injuries, brain injuries, thermal injuries
*Vascular injuries*
Giant hemangioma, aortic aneurysm, vasculitis, aortic balloon pump, acute myocardial infarction, pulmonary embolism, malignant hypertension
*Obstetric complications*
Abruptio placentae, eclampsia, amniotic fluid embolism, hydatidiform mole, uterine rupture, retained dead fetus/missed abortion
*Malignancies*
Adenocarcinomas, tumor lysis syndrome, acute leukemia
*Other*
Adult respiratory distress syndrome (ARDS), amyloidosis, inflammatory bowel disease, cirrhosis, fulminant hepatic necrosis, pancreatitis, snake bites, Reyes syndrome, hypovolemic/hemorrhagic shock

**TABLE 139.3. Laboratory Abnormalities in Disseminated Intravascular Coagulation**

| Test | Reliability (% abnormal) |
|---|---|
| d-dimer | 93 |
| Antithrombin III | 89 |
| Fibrinopeptide A | 88 |
| FDP titer | 75 |

FDP = fibrinogen degradation products.

can keep up with the demand. Heparin resistance occasionally develops because of low antithrombin III levels; ATIII concentrates may be helpful. Cryoprecipitate is used for severe hypofibrinogenemia and as a source of VIII:C, and platelets are transfused to maintain counts of 20,000/μL.

## Thrombotic Thrombocytopenic Purpura

Thrombotic thrombocytopenic purpura (TTP) and the closely related hemolytic-uremic syndrome (HUS) are of uncertain etiology, and, until recently, were uniformly fatal. These disorders are compared in Table 139.4. They accompany pregnancy, malignancies, rheumatoid arthritis, HIV infection, certain chemotherapy agents (e.g., mitomycin C), and, ironically, the platelet inhibitory drug ticlopidine. A high-molecular-weight form of von Willebrand protein and a platelet-aggregating protein have been noted in TTP plasma, either or both of which may play a pathogenetic role. It appears that an acquired antibody inhibits the enzymatic degradation of these larger forms; thus plasma transfusions or exchange functions to replace or remove the enzyme and its inhibitor. Most often, the blood vessel lumen throughout the body show a PAS-positive hyaline material deposition. Besides general supportive measures, the management of TTP usually includes emergent, daily plasmapheresis along with relatively large doses of corticosteroids. If plasmapheresis cannot be started rapidly, fresh frozen plasma may be infused in large volumes as a temporary measure. Rarely, splenectomy may be effective in TTP unresponsive to these measures. With aggressive plasmapheresis, 80% to 90% of patients with TTP recover.

## Drugs

Drugs are a major cause of bleeding disorders. Bleeding may occur as a result of drug therapy for thrombosis or sometimes as an unwanted secondary effect of drugs on the function of platelets (see Table 138.4). Aspirin and the nonsteroidal anti-inflammatory agents inhibit platelet cyclooxygenase and thereby decrease platelet aggregation. Unless the hemostatic system is otherwise compromised, few drugs with antiplatelet effects cause clinically significant bleeding. Heparin is widely used in the treatment of thrombotic disorders. Serious bleeding during carefully monitored heparin therapy is unusual; however, the risk is higher in older patients, after recent surgery, in hypertensive patients, or in patients with other bleeding diatheses.

A modest thrombocytopenia develops in nearly 5% of patients undergoing heparin therapy; it is noted within 4 days of beginning heparin and usually requires no intervention (type I). However, a more severe, progressive form, with autoantibodies against heparin-platelet factor 4 complexes may occur, generally within 4 to 6 days of beginning heparin. The antibody leads to extensive platelet aggregation in the presence of heparin (type II). The thrombocytopenia is associated with thromboembolism. The antibodies also may react with the heparin bound to the endothelial cells, thereby causing an immune-mediated endothelial cell injury. This, in conjunction with the platelet aggregation, may predispose to arterial or venous thrombosis.

**Heparin-induced thrombocytopenia** (HIT) may be managed by changing the type of heparin (e.g., from bovine to porcine). If this does not suffice, heparin is discontinued. Diagnostic studies include heparin-induced platelet aggregation, platelet factor-4 immunoglobulin (PF4-Ig) by ELISA, and serotonin release assay. Low-molecular-weight heparin, warfarin, platelet transfusions, and inferior vena caval filters should be avoided, but antithrombotic therapy should be continued, using alternative agents such as danaparoid or Lepirudin. Plasma exchange may be beneficial in selected cases. In most cases, the risk for developing HIT may be decreased by beginning warfarin and heparin simulta-

**TABLE 139.4. Comparative Features of Thrombotic Thrombocytopenic Purpura (TTP) and Hemolytic-Uremic Syndrome (HUS)**

| | TTP | HUS |
|---|---|---|
| Age group | Mostly adults | Mostly children |
| Etiology | Unknown | Illness often follows gastroenteritis by *Escherichia coli* O157:H7 |
| Prodrome | Less common | Bloody diarrheal illness |
| Clinical features | Hemolytic anemia, thrombocytopenia, renal failure, fever, and neurologic symptoms | Hemolytic anemia, thrombocytopenia, and acute renal failure; either hemoglobinuria or anuria in most |
| Renal involvement | Occurs, but renal failure is usually less severe | Integral part of illness, very severe |
| Central nervous system (CNS) involvement | Profound; headache, blurred vision, seizures, coma | Unlikely |
| Recurrences | Common (up to 20%) | Rare |
| Coombs test | Negative | Negative |
| Therapy | Steroids, plasmapheresis, splenectomy | Dialysis, transfusions |
| Peripheral smear | Schistocytes | Schistocytes |
| Lactate dehydrogenase (LDH) | High | High |

neously, and discontinuing heparin as soon as thrombocytopenia develops. By 4 to 6 days of such combined therapy, warfarin usually would have attained a therapeutic level, thus ensuring adequate anticoagulation despite withdrawal of heparin. Patients who develop HIT should not be given heparin subsequently.

Warfarin is the most widely used long-term oral anticoagulant. It blocks the regeneration of vitamin K, thereby blocking synthesis of factors II, VII, IX, and X, protein C, and protein S. The risk of bleeding in patients on warfarin is directly proportional to the intensity of anticoagulation, as determined by the **international normalized ratio** (INR). Various drugs profoundly affect warfarin clearance and, therefore, the risk of bleeding (Table 139.5). In unselected patients, the risk of bleeding while on warfarin varies from 0.1% to 3% per year. Warfarin overdose is treated with oral or intravenous vitamin K, or infusions of fresh frozen plasma; the choice depends on the severity of the anticoagulation and whether or not there is active bleeding. Because of the prolonged half-life of warfarin, a bleeding patient may require repeated plasma infusions.

Massive transfusions, usually following trauma, cause bleeding from multiple mechanisms; these include dilution of clotting factors from replacement fluids lacking factors, consumption of available factors in a bleeding patient, DIC due to hypovolemia, acidosis, or sepsis, dilutional thrombocytopenia, and acquired platelet dysfunction, possibly due to degranulation by traumatized platelets. Patients are treated with infusions of fresh frozen plasma, platelets, red blood cells, and cryoprecipitate, with repeated laboratory monitoring.

**TABLE 139.5. Drugs That Influence Warfarin Effect***

| Intensify Warfarin Effect | Decrease Warfarin Effect |
|---|---|
| Phenylbutazone | Barbiturates |
| Metronidazole | Penicillin |
| Sulfinpyrazone | Rifampin |
| Trimethoprim-sulfamethoxazole | Cholestyramine |
| Amiodarone | Quinidine |
| Tamoxifen | |
| Isoniazid | |
| Ketoconazole | |
| Thyroxine | |
| Cimetidine | |
| Erythromycin | |
| Phenytoin (Dilantin) | |

*not a complete list

# CHAPTER 140 THROMBOTIC DISORDERS

Disturbances in the balance of the coagulation system may lead to a hypercoagulable state as a result of a congenital lack of one of the natural anticoagulants, congenital defects in the fibrinolytic system, or a variety of acquired defects in the coagulation system. The term "hypercoagulable state" in general refers to an abnormality in the coagulation system predisposing to recurrent thrombotic events.

## Factor V Leiden [V506Q] Syndrome

Ironically, the most recently recognized form of congenital hypercoagulable states is the most common. Factor V Leiden syndrome (named for the recognition of a high frequency of this mutation in Germany) is an inheritable form of factor V that is enzymatically relatively resistant to degradation by activated protein C—hence its original designation, activated protein C resistance (APC resistance). Estimates of its frequency range from 6% of the Caucasian American population to >40% in some discrete European communities. It is now diagnosed by genetic testing for the mutation. This test can be accurately performed even after a patient has been started on emergent anticoagulation, or after a functional assay of APC resistance has been obtained. As one would expect, the factor V Leiden mutation places the patient at increased risk of thrombosis, especially when stressed by injury, e.g., catheter placement, pregnancy, hormone replacement therapy, or treatment with selective estrogen receptor modulators (SERMs) such as tamoxifen, or raloxifene used to treat breast cancer. Such patients have a 7-fold increased risk of spontaneous thrombosis. When exposed to oral contraceptives, heterozygotic patients should be treated like any other thrombotic patients; the first episode can be treated with standard short-course anticoagulation. Homozygous patients, or "double heterozygotes," i.e., patients with another congenital hypercoagulable condition, should be anticoagulated for life because of their lifelong risk of thromboses. For instance, homozygous factor V Leiden patients have an 80-fold increased risk, i.e., ~1% annual risk for life.

## Prothrombin G20210A Syndrome

Another recently diagnosed congenital thrombophilic state is a mutation of the prothrombin gene in which the amino acid glutamic acid is substituted for arginine; thus, it also can be tested after anticoagulation initiation. This disorder results in an increased prothrombin level, leading to relative resistance to the normal effects of antithrombin III, which normally binds thrombin 1:1. This genetic abnormality, now detectable by mutational analysis, produces a propensity to thrombosis similar to that of factor V Leiden, although it is much less common, at ~0.5% (but still more common than the traditionally recognized thrombophilic states discussed subsequently). It produces a 2.8-fold increase in the risk of spontaneous thrombosis, and often is encountered in combination with the factor V Leiden mutation; patients with this syndrome require lifelong anticoagulation.

## Hyperhomocysteinemia

Hyperhomocysteinemia is an inheritable form of a hypercoagulable state that occurs because of a mutation in the enzyme required to metabolize this compound, **methylene tetrahydrofolate reductase.** Thus, patients with poor dietary intact of folic acid may have elevated levels of homocysteine, as may individuals with the aberrant MTHR enzyme. This abnormality should be considered in any patient with unusual or recurrent thromboses or when arterial thromboses occur. Like the acquired anticardiolipin antibody syndrome, this is a thrombophilic state that causes arterial as well as venous thromboses. Furthermore, it is relatively treatable in that pharmacologic doses of folic acid usually can correct the deficiency, so diagnosis facilitates prophylaxis against future events with a virtually nontoxic vitamin. Research underway suggests a linear relationship between serum homocysteine levels and risks of coronary artery disease, with profound implications.

## Antithrombin III Deficiency

Antithrombin III (AT-III), a glycoprotein, inactivates factors XIa, Xa, IXa, and thrombin by forming a 1:1 insoluble complex with each of these activated factors. AT-III is produced by the liver, and its deficiency is inherited in an autosomal dominant mode, with an incidence of 1 per 2500 to 5000 persons. The homozygous state is felt to be incompatible with life. Heterozygotes may have either low levels (50–70%) of functionally normal protein (type I), or normal levels of abnormal protein (type II). Acquired deficiency may occur in nephrotic syndrome. Typical initial thrombotic events, which usually occur by age 35, are pulmonary emboli, Budd-Chiari syndrome, or thrombosis of deep veins, renal veins, or mesenteric or iliofemoral vessels. Other factors (e.g., surgery, pregnancy, oral contraceptive use, or trauma) may precipitate these events.

Other tests of the coagulation system typically are normal. Because AT-III levels normally decrease with acute thrombosis or after heparin therapy, the diagnosis of AT-III deficiency should be confirmed by checking levels when the patient is off anticoagulation (except warfarin) and not experiencing an acute thrombotic event. Prophylactic heparin treatment is given during pregnancy, and AT-III concentrates may be given to all others at risk (surgery, childbirth, or trauma). Replacement is given to maintain AT-III levels above 80%. Because congenital deficiency states produce not only thrombophilia, but also relative heparin resistance (AT-III is the required cofactor for unfractionated heparin efficacy), this rare diagnosis is important to consider whenever relative heparin resistance is encountered in treating a thromboembolic event.

## Protein C Deficiency

Protein C, a vitamin K–dependent protein, is produced in the liver. It exerts its anticoagulant effect by inactivating factors Va and VIIIa. Its deficiency is inherited as autosomal dominant, albeit with incomplete penetrance. Before the advent of concentrates, the homozygous state was fatal. A heterozygous protein C deficiency state (30–50% of normal) causing thrombosis occurs in fewer than 1 in 1000 persons. A deficiency leads to recurrent thromboembolism, often in early life, and usually is precipitated by some other event. Protein C concentrates or antithrombotic therapy with warfarin is an appropriate treatment. Initiation of warfarin in affected persons causes the already low protein C levels to decline even further and faster than the procoagulant factors, because of the shorter half-life of circulating protein C. The initial result is a net prothrombotic state. Thrombosis of the dermal vessels and skin necrosis follow. Full heparinization concurrent with initial warfarin doses prevents this complication. Activated protein C resistance is discussed in chapter 136.

## Protein S Deficiency

Protein S, a vitamin K-dependent factor produced by the liver, circulates both free and protein-bound. Free protein S is a cofactor of protein C in its inhibition of factors Va and VIIIa (Figure 140.1). Its deficiency is inherited as an autosomal dominant trait. Its clinical features are similar to protein C deficiency. Acquired deficiency occurs in nephrotic syndrome. Warfarin decreases protein S levels, and should be stopped for at least 1 week before testing protein S levels. Heparin does not lower protein S level, but acute thrombosis does. The treatment is long-term warfarin to prevent spontaneous thrombosis.

## Fibrinolytic Defects

The fibrinolytic system is illustrated in Figure 140.2. Nearly 30% of patients with thrombosis may have abnormalities of their fibrinolytic systems. **Tissue plasminogen activator** (tPA) is made by endothelial cells; its deficiency, an autosomal dominant trait, manifests with venous or arterial thrombosis, or both. Acquired tPA deficiency may contribute to cancer-related hypercoagulability. Plasminogen abnormalities and dysfibrinogenemias (both inherited and rare) lead to thrombosis. Homocystinuria, an autosomal recessive disease, also is rare and manifests with vascular abnormalities and thrombosis.

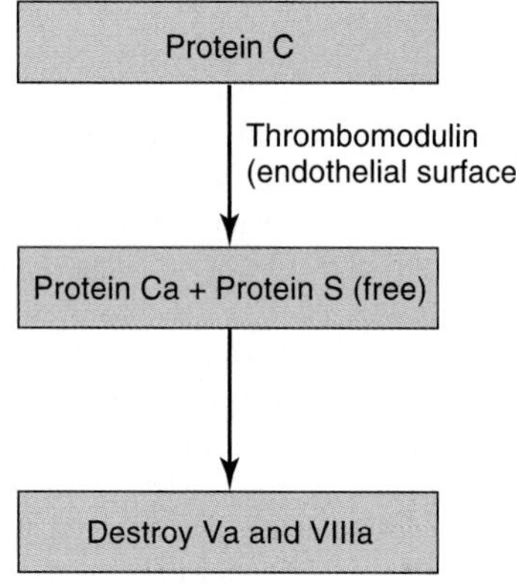


**FIGURE 140.1.** Protein C and Protein S system.

## Acquired Thrombotic Defects

The **lupus anticoagulant** (LA), which often is implicated in recurrent thromboses, is a heterogeneous group of antiphospholipid immunoglobulins that interfere with prothrombin activation and exert procoagulant activity by increasing platelet adhesiveness and activation, interfering with protein C activation and causing abnormal AT-III activity. Lupus anticoagulants occur in infections, systemic lupus erythematosus, and lymphoproliferative disorders. Venous thrombosis and pulmonary embolism are the major features; however, other major arterial or venous thromboses occur as well. An autoimmune thrombocytopenia coexists in some patients because of the autoimmune basis of LA; however, the usual clinical features are thrombotic. Lupus anticoagulant usually is recognized when thrombosis is evaluated in young patients or when a prolonged PTT is seen in asymptomatic persons. The type of phospholipid reagents used and the antiphospholipid antibody interference prolong the PTT, but the clinical picture is clotting, not bleeding.

Patients without lupus or other autoimmune diseases may have **anticardiolipin antibodies,** an antiphospholipid antibody syndrome that also causes venous and arterial thrombosis. These antibodies have been implicated in coronary artery disease, recurrent coronary bypass graft occlusion, retinal artery occlusion, and stroke. Drugs associated with this syndrome include

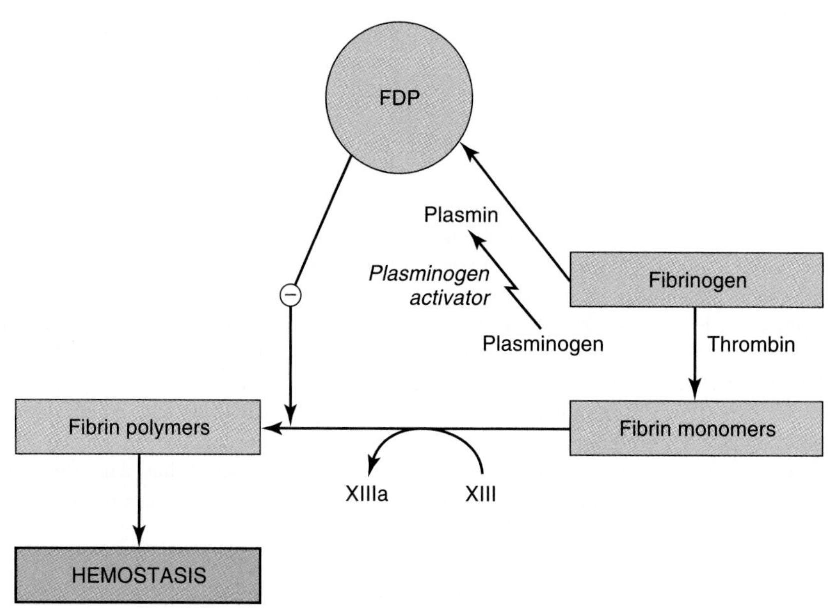


**FIGURE 140.2.** The fibrinolytic system.

phenytoin, quinine, phenothiazines, alpha-interferon, cocaine, and hydralazine. Assays are available to detect IgG, IgM, idiotype, and IgA anticardiolipin antibodies. Treatment is with long-term oral anticoagulation to prevent recurrent thrombosis. Treatment of refractory cases is controversial, and includes possible attempts to immunosupress the patient, or even concurrently inhibit platelet aggregation, which can be difficult and dangerous.

## Other Diseases Associated With Hypercoagulability

The myeloproliferative disorders have all been associated with both bleeding and thrombosis, but most of these disorders tend to exhibit only one or the other. **Polycythemia vera** leads to thrombosis, whereas patients with myeloid metaplasia tend to bleed. Patients with essential thrombocytosis may thrombose, but also paradoxically bleed. Hyperviscosity, platelet dysfunction, and hyperaggregability, or acquired storage pool disease may cause excessive clotting. All types of thrombosis are seen. The usual types include pulmonary embolism, deep venous thrombosis, and coronary or cerebrovascular occlusions; unusual types include Budd-Chiari syndrome and microvascular thrombosis. **Paroxysmal nocturnal hemoglobinuria** may present with thrombosis as the first symptom. Here, the hypercoagulability results from increased sensitivity and aggregation of platelets to the complement, accompanied by an increased sensitivity to thrombin.

**Malignancy,** by unclear mechanisms, also leads to a hypercoagulable state. Solid tumors may activate factor VII by the tissue factor pathway, whereas mucin-secreting tumors may activate factor X directly. Some anticancer agents (e.g., cyclophosphamide, methotrexate, fluorouracil) confer an increased risk of thrombosis. Migratory thrombophlebitis in malignancies (Trousseau syndrome) usually occurs with adenocarcinomas of the stomach, pancreas, or prostate. The apparent intrinsic hypercoagulable state in any cancer may be augmented by the immobility, advanced age, and increased tissue trauma also common to these patients. Tumor impingement on vessels increases the turbulence of flow and predisposes to local hypercoagulable conditions (e.g., superior vena cava syndrome or pelvic thrombosis).

Laboratory evaluation in these patients may show high fibrinogen, thrombocytosis, a short PTT, and, occasionally, d-dimers. The risk of thrombosis may be lessened by treating the primary condition. Acute thrombotic events are treated in the usual way with heparin. Many of these may be refractory to oral anticoagulation, requiring heparin therapy on an ambulatory basis.

# CHAPTER 141 ERYTHROCYTOSIS

**Erythrocytosis** represents a significantly elevated RBC count, hemoglobin (Hgb), and hematocrit (Hct). Its classification is shown in Table 141.1. In dehydration, burns and shock, erythrocytosis is considered *relative*, because the plasma volume is diminished and the total red cell volume is normal. Chronic hypoxia increases erythropoietin (EPO) secretion, leading to erythrocytosis. Carbon monoxide from heavy cigarette smoking stimulates RBC production. Smoking also may cause airflow obstruction; the resulting hypoxemia leads to excessive EPO secretion. A similar hypoxia-mediated mechanism operates in erythrocytosis of high altitude and other cardiopulmonary diseases, because any condition that effectively lowers $O_2$ saturation elicits release of EPO as a normal physiologic response. In high-affinity hemoglobinopathies, mutant hemoglobins yield oxygen less readily to the tissues, thus stimulating RBC production. A hormonally mediated mechanism occurs in Cushing syndrome and with androgen-secreting tumors.

**TABLE 141.1. Causes of Erythrocytosis**

A. Primary erythremia—polycythemia vera
B. Secondary
  1. Relative (reduced plasma volume and normal RBC volume)
    Burns
    Dehydration
    Shock
  2. With elevated erythropoiesis
    Cigarette smoking ↑ CO
    Hypoxia—cardiopulmonary, high-altitude living
    Renal cysts or masses
    Infratentorial tumors
    Cushing syndrome
    Androgens
      (i) Therapeutic
      (ii) Androgen-secreting tumors
    High $O_2$ affinity hemoglobinopathy

## Polycythemia Vera

Primary erythremia, or **polycythemia vera** (P. vera), derives from increased or hyperproliferative stem cells that proliferate independently of EPO. The resulting peripheral picture is one of erythrocytosis, and to a lesser extent leukocytosis, and thrombocythemia.

### Pathophysiology

Among the physiopathologic alterations in P. vera (Table 141.2), the risk of hemorrhage is an important issue, attributed to stasis, vascular distention, and increased blood viscosity. The platelets also function abnormally; these, in conjunction with a relatively low plasma volume and limited total fibrinogen, cause **frequent, fragile blood clots,** followed by **hemorrhage.** The chief morbidity of leukocytosis is histamine release from the polymorphonuclear leukocytes (PMN), which causes **pruritus** and peptic ulcer. Excessive hematopoiesis leads to overproduction of purine substrates for nucleic acid synthesis; **hyperuricemia** and **gout** follow. Megakaryocytes and platelets stimulate fibroblastic proliferation via platelet-derived growth factor; myelofibrosis and myeloid metaplasia of the spleen eventually result. The cellular proliferation in P. vera is monoclonal. The stem cells of P. vera are capable of independent growth and do not require the addition of EPO to ensure in vitro proliferation of CFU-E.

### Clinical Features

Polycythemia vera is relatively rare and usually affects older persons, with a slight preponderance in men. Because of its insidious onset, years go by before patients realize that anything is wrong with them. Symptoms, if present, are caused by the large RBC mass, and may include **headache, tinnitus, vertigo, visual disturbances, paresthesias,** and **erythromelalgia.** Severe pruritus, especially after a hot bath, is caused by histamine release from the neutrophils. The excess blood viscosity causes thrombosis, and, paradoxically, hemorrhage. **Venous thromboembolism** and intermittent claudication are very common. Other sites of thrombosis are the myocardium, spleen, brain, mesentery, and gastrointestinal tract. The **peptic ulcers** that develop in about 10% of patients are attributed to increased histamine release. The patient with fully expressed P. vera is plethoric, with marked conjunctival injection and **splenomegaly.** Central cyanosis is absent, a helpful distinction from hypoxic disorders that cause erythrocytosis.

### Laboratory Features

Differentiation among the various causes of erythrocytosis depends on three major findings (Table 141.3).

**TABLE 141.2. Pathophysiology of Polycythemia Vera**

| Predominating Marrow Cell | Pathophysiology | Complication |
|---|---|---|
| Erythroblast | Blood viscosity | Vascular stasis, hemorrhage, thrombosis, impaired cerebral blood flow |
| Megakaryocytes | Platelets | Hemorrhage |
| | Hypercoagulable | Thrombosis |
| | Ineffective platelets | |
| Granulocytes | Cobalamin-binding | Pruritus |
| | Histamine | Peptic ulcer |
| | | Gout |
| Fibroblasts | Platelets | Leukoerythroblastosis |
| | Myelofibrosis | Massive spleen |
| | Myeloid metaplasia | Anemia |
| Primary mechanism | Proliferation of a single clone, which grows independently of EPO | |

EPO = erythropoietin.

**TABLE 141.3. Differentiating Among Causes of Erythrocytosis**

| Condition | Arterial $O_2$ Saturation | Total RBC Volume | Splenomegaly | EPO Value |
|---|---|---|---|---|
| Cigarette smoking | ↑ CO | Slightly ↑ | 0 | N |
| Hypoxia | ↑ | Normal | 0 | ↑ |
| Renal disease | Normal | ↑ | 0 | ↑ |
| Polycythemia vera | Normal | ↑ | ↑ | ↓ |

CO = carbon monoxide; EPO = erythropoietin.

The first and most important is an elevated total RBC volume, as shown by $^{51}$Cr-RBC with normal plasma volume (normal RBC volume is 32–34 ml/kg in men and 30–32 ml/kg in women). In P. vera, the figure is significantly higher, unless there has been recent major hemorrhage or repeated phlebotomies. Secondly, the arterial oxygen saturation ($SaO_2$) must exceed 92% in P. vera, in contrast to hypoxia-mediated erythrocytosis, where $SaO_2$ is below 87%. Blood samples removed for $SaO_2$ also should be examined for CO content (normally <2%) and for P50 (normal value is 27 mm Hg; value is lower [left-shifted] in high-affinity hemoglobins). When these findings are present, splenomegaly confirms P. vera. If not, two of the three may be considered diagnostic when one minor criterion also is present. Minor criteria include leukocytosis (>20,000/$10^{12}$/L) or thrombocytosis (>800,000/$10^{12}$/L) in the presence of greatly increased marrow cellularity (>80–90%). With early myelofibrosis, reticulin fiber deposition may be increased.

In P. vera, as well as other members of the myeloproliferative group, the leukocyte alkaline phosphatase (LAP) score exceeds 190 (the normal score is 80–100). In contrast, it is depleted in chronic myelocytic leukemia (CML). Leukocytes play a role in vitamin $B_{12}$ transport through their transcobalamin II content. With high WBC turnover, excess transcobalamin II is released into the plasma. Cobalamin binding capacity is thus enhanced in P. vera. Frequently, serum iron is diminished, transferrin is increased, and ferritin is very low, a pattern suggesting iron deficiency from repeated phlebotomies. Besides, most available iron is used preferentially for erythropoiesis, leading to diminished iron stores. With increased RBC, endogenous EPO synthesis should cease, and serum EPO levels are low. In contrast, in secondary polycythemia from hypoxia, the serum EPO level increases.

### Management

Once the diagnosis of P. vera is established, the RBC volume should be reduced rapidly through weekly phlebotomy. As the hematocrit declines to 45% to 48%, the choice must be made of phlebotomy alone, myelosuppressive agents (hydroxyurea [HU]), or $^{32}$P. Phlebotomy rapidly regulates hematocrit, but it does not control the splenomegaly, pruritus, or thrombosis. Myelosuppressives should be limited to patients over 50 years of age. (With HU, the dose is adjusted to maintain WBC at $10 \times 10^9$/L, and platelets at $500 \times 10^9$/L). However, phlebotomies must still be done for hematocrit above 45% to 48%. Probably the most convenient treatment is $^{32}$P. The initial dose often is effective for more than 1 year, but aggressive disease may recur sooner. If the platelet count increases to more than $800 \times 10^9$/L, $^{32}$P is readministered. Even with $^{32}$P, or HU, phlebotomy should be employed when the hematocrit exceeds 45%.

Within 10 years following $^{32}$P therapy, about 10% of patients develop burned-out P. vera, myelofibrosis, or leukemic transformation. The oncogenic properties of HU remain a hazard, but its leukemogenic potential remains unknown. Surgery in patients with P. vera must be undertaken with the utmost caution because of the severe risk of immediate postoperative hemorrhage and thrombosis in these patients; each patient about to undergo surgery should be warned of the profound hazards. Surgery should be done only if the platelet count and hematocrit are sufficiently regulated.

### Course and Prognosis

Polycythemia vera eventually stabilizes, because RBCs no longer increase. During this spent phase, therapy is no longer required. Hematopoiesis shifts from a bone marrow that becomes fibrotic to myeloid metaplasia of the liver and spleen. These organs enlarge massively within 10 years of onset. Paradoxically, erythrocytosis transforms to anemia; transfusion, and not phlebotomy, may now become necessary. The most limiting prognostic factor is the transformation to acute leukemia, which is terminal and rapidly fatal.

# CHAPTER 142 CHRONIC MYELOCYTIC LEUKEMIA AND MYELOFIBROSIS

## Chronic Myelocytic Leukemia

### Definition

**Chronic myelocytic leukemia** (CML) results from massive clonal expansion of granulocyte marrow precursors. The resulting extreme and progressive peripheral leukocytosis manifests all of the various morphologic stages of developing granulocytes. The characteristic marker is the Philadelphia chromosome (Ph), found in all the bone marrow-derived cells; it establishes CML as a clonal disorder derived from a disordered proliferation of uncommitted stem cells. Ph appears as a minute structure derived from chromosome 22, in which part of the long (p) arm is broken off and adheres to the short (q) arm of chromosome 9 in a rearrangement known as (t 9:22)(q 34:11). Genetic material (C-abl) is thus transposed from chromosome 22 to chromosome 9, creating a new fusion gene between 5′-bcr and C-abl. Uncontrolled cellular proliferation follows the production of a new hybrid messenger RNA and a new product—tyrosine kinase. The abnormal RNA transcript can be noted on a Northern blot. Using polymerase chain reaction (PCR), the bcr-abl fusion RNA may be amplified by 100,000-fold, thus allowing detection of the genetic abnormality, even when the disease is in remission. Ph is found in 90% of cases of CML. The 10% of CML patients who lack Ph are more refractory to treatment. However, even in these cases, the bcr-abl fusion RNA can be detected by amplification using PCR.

### Clinical Features

The onset of typical Ph-positive CML is asymptomatic. CML often is found incidentally during an examination for unrelated reasons. Weight loss may develop later in the course, despite a good appetite; hyperthyroidism may be suspected. Slowly developing mild anemia leads to fatigue, loss of vigor, and exercise intolerance. Early satiation, a feeling of abdominal fullness, and left upper quadrant or left shoulder pain are related to splenomegaly. As in P. vera, serum histamine levels may rise with leukocytosis and cause pruritus. With high granulocyte turnover, urate production increases, leading to gout. Splenomegaly, often massive, is the outstanding clinical sign. Hepatomegaly and bony pain and tenderness (from increased intramedullary pressure causing pressure on nerve-rich endosteum) may be noted. Pallor, fever, and lymphadenopathy are late manifestations. Splenic infarction occurs as the spleen enlarges and outstrips its blood supply.

Late in the course of disease, the number or function of the platelets may be compromised. Bleeding into the skin or from the mucous membranes may then follow. Infection rarely is a problem because the polymorphonuclear leukocytes (PMN) retain their normal phagocytic function. However, if PMN eventually are replaced by nonfunctioning blast cells, uncontrolled infection may result.

### Laboratory Features

The total WBC count almost invariably exceeds 50 $\times$ $10^9$/L. The WBCs are distributed in the peripheral smear in all developmental stages in descending proportions (segmented PMN [60–70%], band forms, metamyelocytes, myelocytes, promyelocytes, and blasts). The total aggregate of granulocyte precursors often exceeds 20% to 25%. Notably, the basophils increase to 3% to 4% or more during remission. Monocytosis, while variable, may be 20% or higher in Ph-negative CML or CMML. The RBCs usually are normal or slightly elevated early in the course of the disease, but decline later. Similarly, the platelet count is elevated at first but may diminish preterminally.

A major objective manifestation of CML is the low or suppressed leukocyte alkaline phosphatase (LAP) score, which distinguishes CML from other myeloproliferative disorders (P. vera, myelofibrosis, or essential thrombocythemia) in which it is high. A low LAP score occurs in very few conditions other than CML; exceptions are paroxysmal nocturnal hemoglobinuria, gout, or chronic liver disease, conditions readily separable from CML clinically or by laboratory means. Serum uric acid is elevated, and there may be evidence of urate deposition. Increased vitamin $B_{12}$–binding capacity results from increased granulocyte turnover. A bone marrow biopsy, although rarely needed for diagnosis, may differentiate CML from myelofibrosis, or help detect the Ph chromosome, especially if nonproliferating cells are present in the peripheral blood.

## *Philadelphia Chromosome-Negative CML*

About 10% of patients with CML are Philadelphia chromosome–negative. Their WBC count is elevated, but not to the same level as in the Ph-positive type. The monocyte count is elevated more characteristically, leading to the designation **chronic myelomonocytic leukemia** (CMML). Serum and urine muramidase (lysozyme) values are elevated. More important, this group fails to respond to conventional chemotherapy, thus indicating a worse prognosis.

### Course

The clinical course of CML is determined by the presence or absence of the Ph chromosome. The initial phase of Ph(+) CML is asymptomatic, indolent, and fully responsive to chemotherapy. In the accelerated phase that develops eventually, mature and immature granulocytes as well as basophils increase in number, and previously effective chemotherapeutic agents become ineffective. Abnormal forms of PMN also emerge, with two nuclear lobes **(Pelger-Huet cells).** The bone marrow may become difficult to aspirate. The spleen enlarges massively; anemia and thrombocytopenia worsen. In the blast phase that follows, nucleated blast cells replace the peripheral PMNs. Some blasts harbor a pathologic enzyme, **terminal deoxyribonucleotide transferase** (TDT), which normally is manifested by thymus-derived cells. Despite an occasional, transitory response to vincristine and prednisone, the ensuing course inexorably deteriorates and is rapidly lethal.

### Management

Truly effective therapy for CML is the elimination of the Ph chromosome and the restoration of normal hematopoiesis, which currently are possible only through bone marrow transplantation. The recipient must be young enough to withstand the rigors of transplantation, and the donor must be exactly matched to his or her HLA type. The recipient's marrow is completely ablated with total body irradiation and high-dose chemotherapy, a process that would be fatal unless the donor's marrow cells completely engraft. If there is no suitable sibling donor, a nonrelated donor may suffice if a suitable match can be found through a marrow registry. Another alternative is autotransplantation of the patient's own marrow, harvested previously during periods of remission.

Chemotherapy must be employed if conditions for successful marrow transplant cannot be achieved. Historically, hydroxyurea has been the most widely used drug for treating CML. Successful treatment restores the spleen size and WBC to normal. However, the Ph chromosome remains, as does a slowly increasing LAP score. Most physicians prefer to maintain the patient on a small dose of hydroxyurea, but a few prefer intermittent use. Recombinant human α-interferon, an alternative agent, also is effective. Given alone or in combination with chemotherapy drugs, it can produce prolonged remissions with disappearance of Ph(+) cells from the bone marrow. Blast transformation must be aggressively treated with daunorubicin and cytosine arabinoside. Patients with TDT-positive blasts may respond temporarily to vincristine plus prednisone.

The most significant recent advance in the treatment of CML has been the development of Imatinib (Gleevec), a drug that inhibits BCR-ABL tyrosine kinase and induces major remissions in patients in chronic phase.

## Myelofibrosis

**Myelofibrosis** is the conversion of the aspiratable, semi-fluid bone marrow to a nonaspiratable, solid collection of fibrous tissue. The spleen enlarges, sometimes massively, because it engages in hematopoiesis to compensate for the loss of marrow. The disease arises from a single clone of pluripotent stem cells. Because megakaryocytes and platelets persist in marrow, the fibrosis appears to be stimulated by platelet-derived growth factor.

### Clinical Features

Characteristically, myelofibrosis affects older individuals and is more frequent in men. Often, it develops late or preterminally in polycythemia vera or CML. Its clinical hallmark is splenomegaly and, often, gout. Its symptoms include those of anemia, as well as an enlarging fullness in the left upper abdominal quadrant (LUQ) and early satiation. Splenic infarction, a distressing complication, manifests with pain in the LUQ and left shoulder. Ascites and pleural effusions are apt to occur if the extramedullary hematopoiesis involves pleural and peritoneal sites. Weight loss, progressive splenomegaly, and increasing anemia are prominent events with preterminal infections, hemorrhage, or leukemic transformation.

### Laboratory Features

Anemia may be moderate or severe, with variable WBC and platelet counts. The RBC resemble teardrops, with a small projection at one end. The peripheral smear is leukoerythroblastic (i.e., immature WBC and normoblasts seen simultaneously). A simple distinction from CML is that the total of WBC precursors rarely exceeds 20%. Many large platelets are present peripherally; some of them are megakaryocytic fragments. Bone marrow usually is not aspiratable **(dry tap).** Diagnosis requires biopsy with a Jamshidi-type needle, which shows bundles of fibrous tissue and many residual megakaryocytes. The Ph chromosome is absent unless the myelofibrosis has evolved from CML.

### Management

Myelofibrosis has no treatment; its course is indolent, and the disease smolders for 5 years or longer. Related anemia may require occasional blood transfusions. Hydroxyurea sometimes is given to control the size of the spleen, with its dosage carefully regulated by titration of WBC and platelets. Oxymetholone (a form of testosterone) may be helpful, but it requires careful monitoring for the development of icterus or edema. Splenectomy, while not recommended, may be necessary to relieve pain, or occasionally, to allay severe cytopenias arising from sequestration and hemolysis.

# CHAPTER 143 ESSENTIAL THROMBOCYTHEMIA

### Etiology

The platelet count may rise in a variety of clinical situations (e.g., specific stimulatory disorders, postsplenectomy, chronic blood loss, hemolytic anemia, and iron deficiency). If all of these causes are excluded, what remains is **essential thrombocythemia** (ET). Essential thrombocythemia is comparable to polycythemia vera, because it represents an uncontrolled clonal proliferation of stem cells that produces too many platelets.

### Clinical Features

Essential thrombocytopenia occurs predominantly in persons over the age of 50. It usually is asymptomatic. When symptoms do develop, they usually are of a thromboembolic nature. However, ET also causes hemorrhage, because the platelets, although abundant, are abnormal and nonfunctional. The thrombosis may occur at various sites, including the cerebrum, myocardium, mesentery, and peripheral veins or arteries. Splenomegaly is the only outstanding physical sign. Patients with exceptionally large spleens may develop painful splenic infarctions. Eventual transformation to acute leukemia is rare.

### Laboratory Features

Serial platelet counts are very high (they must exceed 800,000/mm$^3$). Hematocrit and RBC usually are normal in ET (but if Hct >48% or RBC >6.0 $10^{12}$/L, confirmation is required by a $^{51}$Cr RBC red cell volume; red cell volume is >34 ml/kg in P. vera, but <30 ml/kg in ET). The bone marrow is hypercellular in ET, with clumps of megakaryocytes. Marrow iron stores are normal. Absent stainable iron suggests iron deficiency as the cause of thrombocytosis; iron should then be given continuously for 1 month and hematologic tests redone thereafter. Bone marrow biopsy readily shows myelofibrosis and excess reticulin. The Ph chromosome is present in chronic myelocytic leukemia (CML), but absent in ET. The **leukocyte alkaline phosphatase** (LAP) score is very high, as opposed to CML, in which it is low or absent.

### Management

No consensus exists as to whether all patients with ET, especially young women, should be given myelosuppressives. In young women, especially if the menses are heavy, a month's trial of oral iron may help lower the platelet count. However, older persons with persistent thrombocytosis and splenomegaly are better treated with myelosuppression. Elderly patients (age >70) who are unable to visit their physician frequently are best treated with $^{32}$P, which may be required only about once a year; it does, however, carry a risk of leukemic transformation.

Most physicians prefer to treat ET with hydroxyurea. Other agents include busulfan, chlorambucil, and 6-thioguanine, but their leukemogenicity or toxicity makes HU preferable. Recently, anagrelide has been approved by the FDA.

# CHAPTER 144 THE MYELODYSPLASTIC SYNDROMES

The myelodysplastic syndromes (MDS) are examples of irreversible, disordered proliferation of clonal growth that feature profoundly atypical hematopoiesis (usually with cytopenias), increased bone marrow cellularity, malfunctioning peripheral blood cells, and eventual conversion to leukemia.

### Classification and Subtypes

The MDS represent a collection of dissimilar cytopenias grouped by predominant features. **Refractory anemia** (RA) consists of normocytic to macrocytic anemia, accompanied by leukopenia and a small number of blasts (<5%) in the bone marrow (the term is a misnomer, because it was used to describe an anemia unresponsive to common hematinic drugs—vitamin $B_{12}$, folic acid, and iron). The marrow often is hypercellular, with increased iron content.

## ■ Refractory Anemia With Ringed Sideroblasts

Refractory anemia with ringed sideroblasts (RARS) shows increased numbers of dysplastic erythroblasts, many of which resemble megaloblasts. The key finding is an increased number of ringed sideroblasts where stainable iron is present in mitochondria disposed around the nucleus (Color Plate 23). Ringed sideroblasts may occur in younger persons as a sex-linked hereditary abnormality or after toxicity (e.g., by alcohol or isoniazid. The **myelodysplastic syndrome with ringed sideroblasts** (MDS-RS) is most common in older patients (>60 years) and is characterized by macrocytic anemia and varying degrees of leukopenia and thrombocytopenia. Although the marrow is megaloblastic, RARS fails to respond to vitamin $B_{12}$, folic acid, pyridoxine, and other hematinics. About 15% of patients succumb to total marrow failure or leukemia.

## ■ Refractory Anemia With Excess of Blasts

Refractory anemia with excess of blasts (RAEB) features anemia and leukopenia, sometimes with peripheral (usually <5%) blasts. Bone marrow is inappropriately hyperplastic; the presence of less than 20% blasts provides arbitrary distinction from leukemia. Commonly, megakaryocytes are represented by micromegakaryocytes and giant platelets with bizarre granulation. The peripheral PMN are hypogranular and show bilobed structures **(Pelger-Huet cells)** or a peculiar ropy nucleus with clumped chromatin.

### Chronic Myelomonocytic Leukemia

Chronic myelomonocytic leukemia (CMML) has a number of features atypical for MDS. Some argue that this entity does not even belong to this group. Such patients present with chronic anemia, leukocytosis, and thrombocytopenia. The leukocytosis suggests chronic myelocytic leukemia, but the Ph chromosome is absent and the peripheral blood shows monocytosis and monoblasts. The monocytes contain excess muramidase (lysozyme), which is detected in the serum and urine. The LAP score may or may not be low.

### Refractory Anemia With Excess of Blasts-in-Transition

Sooner or later, refractory anemia with excess of blasts-in-transition (RAEB-t) progresses to the point that blasts exceed 25%. Although many blasts contain Auer rods, they do not fulfill the criteria for acute leukemia. Certain cytogenetic abnormalities may be seen in MDS, especially deletions of all or part of chromosome 5, that do not necessarily correlate with the morphologic subtype.

#### Management

Therapy usually is discouraging, but, fortunately, most of the MDS disorders are indolent. Transfusions of RBC and platelets often are required. Hematopoietic growth factors (G-CSF and EPO) may improve peripheral blood counts temporarily. Small doses of cytosine arabinoside, 13 cis-retinoic acid, and 5-azacitidine may produce a therapeutic response. If a suitable HLA-matched donor is found, allogeneic bone marrow transplantation may be "curative," especially in recipients younger than 40 years of age.

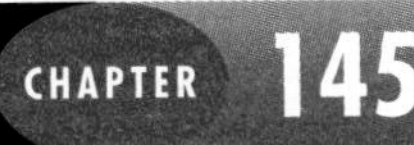

# CHAPTER 145 CHRONIC LYMPHOCYTIC LEUKEMIA (CLL)

#### Definition

**Chronic lymphocytic leukemia** (CLL) is a clonal expansion of mature-appearing, nonfunctioning, and exceptionally long-lived lymphocytes. Unlike chronic myelocytic leukemia (CML), there is no single cytogenetic abnormality; rather, a variety of mutations, often involving chromosome 11 or 13, have been discovered. Monoclonality may be shown by a uniform surface immunoglobulin expression. As in low-grade lymphomas, the basic pathophysiology is the loss of apoptosis (programmed cell death) such that progenitor cells retain their replicative rate, but the defective malignant cells accumulate in the circulation and sites of lymphoid tissue, e.g. lymph nodes, bone marrow, spleen, and liver.

#### Clinical Features

At its onset, CLL is insidious and is found incidentally during routine laboratory testing or during the course of other disorders. In many patients, the initial finding in CLL is an absolute lymphocytosis exceeding 10,000/μl. The Rai system of classification (Table 145.1) effectively stages clinical and prognostic indices. Only rarely do new patients present with lymphadenopathy or hepatosplenomegaly. With progressive disease, the lymphocytosis increases slowly. A doubling time of less than 1 year carries the most serious prognosis. Lymphadenopathy or hepatosplenomegaly during observation has prognostic and therapeutic significance.

Because lymphocytes synthesize and transport immunoglobulins, the effect of CLL on the immune system has clinical implications. The failure of nonfunctional lymphocytes to secrete immunoglobulins leads to a slow decline in serum IgG, IgM, and IgA levels, and, consequently, to an increased susceptibility to infection, especially pneumonia and viruses. In addition, an increased sensitivity to insect antigens causes an exaggerated response (huge welts) to mosquito and other insect bites. Patients with CLL often lose their ability to distinguish between native and foreign cells. As a result, autoimmune diseases evolve, e.g., autoimmune hemo-

**TABLE 145.1. The Rai Staging System**

| Stage | Characteristic Feature | Median Survival (Yrs) |
|---|---|---|
| 0 | Lymphocytosis | >12.5 |
| 1 | Lymphocytosis + lymphadenopathy | 8–10 |
| 2 | Lymphocytosis + splenomegaly | 6 |
| 3 | Lymphocytosis + anemia | 2–4 |
| 4 | Lymphocytosis + thrombocytopenia | 2–4 |

lytic anemia or immune thrombocytopenia. Immune neutropenia and pure red cell aplasia also occur, although they are more difficult to prove because of the preponderance of lymphocytes in the marrow.

## Management

Most patients with Rai stage 0-1 CLL require only periodic clinical, hematologic, and immunologic documentation. Treatment may be started if the lymphocytes double in less than 1 year (or if they exceed 150,000/μL). Most patients in stages 3 or 4 need treatment. Anemia or thrombocytopenia requires therapy once the cause is established. Recurrent infections, progressive weight loss, or immunologic abnormalities also call for treatment. CLL predisposes to other neoplasias, so a regular and diligent search for malignancies is needed. Treatment, when indicated, usually is begun with an alkylating agent (e.g., chlorambucil or cyclophosphamide) alone or in combination with prednisone. Lymphadenopathy and splenomegaly plus systemic symptoms require aggressive treatment. Treatment may be with traditional multidrug regimens developed for lymphoma; more recently, though, fludarabine-based regimens have been shown to produce higher remission rates of longer duration, but at the risk of increased infections. There is no evidence yet that such treatments used initially will change the ultimate outcome of this disease, but they demonstrate the first important treatment advance for this disease in more than 30 years. The use of monoclonal antibodies, e.g., CAMPATH-1, directed against the CD-59 antigen as with low-grade lymphomas, has been shown to be effective. Many patients with advanced-stage CLL develop hypogammaglobulinemia, and thus are at risk for recurrent viral or encapsulated bacterial infection; such patients may require maintenance therapy with intravenous human IgG. Conversely, the aberrant clone of lymphocytes can produce autoimmune hemolytic anemia or immune thrombocytopenia requiring immunosuppressive therapy in this same concomitantly immunosuppressed patient. As with idiosyncratic idiopathic thrombocytopenic purpura (ITP) or autoimmune hemolytic anemia (AIHA), one may use steroids, and must consider splenectomy, if the patient is refractory to medical management of the CLL or pharmacologic immunosuppression.

# CHAPTER 146 ACUTE LEUKEMIA

## Definition

**Acute leukemia** is a clonal malignancy of immature hematopoietic cells in which the malignant clone proliferates, but fails to mature. The immature cells accumulate in the bone marrow and suppress normal hematopoiesis. Diagnosis requires at least 30% immature cells or blasts in the bone marrow.

## Classification

Acute leukemias usually are classified by both the histologic and the immunologic appearance of the malignant cells. The **French-American-British** (FAB) classification, the standard nomenclature used to subtype the leukemias, relies on morphology and the results of cytochemical stains to differentiate the various leukemias (Tables 146.1 and 146.2). However, some leukemic blasts lack morphologic features to indicate whether their lineage is myeloid or lymphoid. For these, a variety of specialized stains are used to clarify the lineage. For instance, peroxidase-positive granules indicate myeloid lineage, whereas PAS **(periodic acid-Schiff)**-positive cytoplasm indicates erythroid or, occasionally, lymphoid differentiation.

Unfortunately, leukemic blasts do not always follow

**TABLE 146.1. FAB Classification of Adult Acute Lymphoblastic Leukemia**

| Subtype | Morphology | Cytochemistry | Immunophenotype | CR (%) | 3-Yr Remission (%) |
|---|---|---|---|---|---|
| L1 (Childhood) | Small uniform blasts<br>Small nucleoli | Myeloperoxidase<br>PAS (++) | CD 10+<br>(CALLA+) | 85 | 40 |
| L2 (Adult) | Larger blasts, irregular nucleoli | Myeloperoxidase<br>PAS (+) | Same as L1 | 35 | |
| L3 (Burkitt-like) | Large blasts, basophilic cytoplasm, vacuolated large nucleoli | Myeloperoxidase<br>PAS (–) | CD 10–<br>CD 19, 20+ | 10 | |

CR = complete remission.

TABLE 146.2. Subtypes of Acute Myeloid Leukemia

| FAB | | Monoclonals | Cytogenetics |
|---|---|---|---|
| M0 | Undifferentiated | CD13+<br>CD14+<br>CD33+<br>CD34+ | |
| M1 | AML with minimal differentiation | CD13+<br>CD14+<br>CD33+<br>CD34+ | Various, includes +8, del7 |
| M2 | AML with differentiation (granules, Auer rods) | | t(8;21) |
| M3 | Acute promyelocytic leukemia | | t(15;17) |
| M4 | Acute myelomonocytic<br>M4EO—with eosinophils | | 11q<br>inv(16)<br>t(16;16) |
| M5 | Acute monocytic leukemia | | t(9;11) |
| M6 | Erythroleukemia | | del(7a)<br>del(5a) |
| M7 | Megakaryocytic leukemia | Antiplatelet<br>GP11b/111a | |

TABLE 146.3. Cytochemical Stains Used to Identify Leukemic Cells

| Stain | Significance |
|---|---|
| Myeloperoxidase (MPO) | Myeloid cells containing peroxidase |
| Nonspecific esterase (NSE) | Monocytes and precursors<br>Some ALL weakly +<br>Some APL |
| Periodic acid-Schiff (PAS) | + when glycogen present, especially erythroid precursors, occasional myeloid or lymphoid |
| Terminal deoxyribonucleotide transferase (TdT) | Nuclear enzyme present in immature lymphoid neoplasms |

ALL = acute lymphocytic leukemia; APL = acute promyelocytic leukemia.

rules. Blasts may be negative or equivocal on stains, making it necessary to focus on the results of leukemic blast reactivity with monoclonal antibodies, rather than on histochemistry. The monoclonal antibodies react to antigens found on cells only at specific times in their maturation; they are specific for leukemic blasts that have undergone maturation arrest. Classification schemes are available based on the surface antigenic "appearance" and the cytogenetic make-up of leukemia cells (Table 146.3).

In approximately 70% of patients with acute leukemia, nonrandom, specific genetic rearrangements can be observed, many of which not only are diagnostic of a myeloid or lymphoid lineage, but also have prognostic significance. These rearrangements or translocations appear only in the neoplastic clone, and not in the patient's normal hematopoietic cells; in many cases they not only supplement the histologic and immunologic testing of myeloblasts, but have become the foundation for diagnosis. For instance, **acute myelomonocytic leukemia with an inverted chromosome 16** and eosinophilia (M4Eo) in the bone marrow is a specific AML subtype (see Table 146.1). It carries a high rate of complete remission (>90%) and a 40% to 50% chance of remaining in complete remission after treatment. Similarly, **acute promyelocytic leukemia** is associated with the translocation of genetic material between chromosomes fifteen and seventeen, **t(15:17).** This unique leukemia invariably presents with disseminated intravascular coagulation (DIC), and is best treated with the differentiating agent all-trans retinoic acid—tretenoin (Vesanoid)—before using cytotoxic therapy. The best prognosis for response to therapy and remission duration is in inv(16), t(8;21), and t(15;17). A poorer prognosis is associated with 11q, +8, 20q-, and -5q, and -7q, and 9;22. Leukemias with normal karyotypes have an intermediate prognosis.

### Clinical Features

The clinical features of acute leukemia are related to the depression of normal blood counts. Fatigue, weakness, mucosal bleeding, and recurrent infection are all common presenting symptoms; despite the term "acute," they may have been present for weeks or months beforehand. Occasionally, more acute symptoms will prompt a diagnostic evaluation (e.g., serious bleeding due to **disseminated intravascular coagulation**, sepsis, pyoderma gangrenosum, or neurologic symptoms due to leukemic central nervous system involvement or leukocytosis). Some leukemias (e.g., the monocytic variants) tend to infiltrate tissues, and may present with respiratory compromise.

Acute leukemia usually is a problem not of diagnosis, but, rather, of management. **Hyperleukocytosis** (blood blast counts of 100,000/mm$^3$ or more) predisposes to **leukostasis syndrome,** in which aggregates of blast cells occlude small arteries in multiple organs. The features of this rapidly fatal syndrome include coma, obtundation, confusion, intracranial hemorrhage, massive hemoptysis, respiratory failure, and myocardial infarction. Emergent leukopheresis and initiation of antileukemic therapy are required. Disseminated intravascular coagulation requires emergent coagulation replacement therapy. When caused by acute promyelocytic leukemia (APL; M3 leukemia), treatment with all-trans-retinoic acid (ATRA) minimizes the transient exacerbation of DIC normally produced when chemotherapy induces rapid cell lysis. Extramedullary presentations of acute leukemias occasionally occur, more commonly in acute myelogenous leukemia (AML) than in acute lymphoblastic leukemia (ALL). Although these chloromas usually occur concurrently with the bone marrow leukemia, they also arise independently thereof.

## ■ Acute Myelogenous Leukemia

Acute myelogenous leukemia (AML; also known as acute nonlymphocytic leukemia, acute myeloblastic leukemia, acute myelocytic leukemia, and granulomatous leukemia) is a disease of advancing age, with a slightly higher incidence in men. More than 50% of all cases occur in patients over 60 years of age. The etiology of AML is unknown, but heredity, radiation exposure, and exposure to certain chemicals and drugs exposure are implicated. Patients with Down syndrome are 20 times more prone to acute leukemia (ALL and AML) than normal. Increased risk prevails in other diseases as well (e.g., Wiskott-Aldrich, Bloom syndrome, ataxia-telangiectasia). Despite the implication of viruses in animal leukemias, conclusive evidence of a viral etiology in human leukemia is lacking.

Following treatment with almost every antineoplastic agent, whether for cancer or autoimmune disease, there is a small but finite risk of developing myelodysplastic syndrome or AML. The alkylating agents, nitrosoureas, and etoposide are particularly known for this fatal complication. The use of radiation concurrently with chemotherapy appears to confer an additive risk in this context. These secondary leukemias tend to be resistant to standard treatment and often involve cytogenetic abnormalities of chromosomes 5, 7, and 8.

In the standard FAB classification system, AML has seven subtypes. Monoclonal antibody phenotyping and cytogenetics are listed in Table 146.2. This subclassification is increasingly important, because treatment and prognosis vary depending on the FAB type and the cytogenetic findings.

### *Acute Leukemias (M0 through M2)*

In **acute undifferentiated leukemia** (M0), the abnormal blasts do not resemble either myeloblasts or lymphoblasts, and there are no Auer rods. The blasts are not lineage-specific. The group probably includes true AML, some mixed-lineage leukemias, and some stem cell malignancies. In **acute myeloblastic** (M1) leukemia (Color Plate 31), the blasts are mainly undifferentiated, but some have Auer rods. The cells usually show clear myeloid differentiation on monoclonal antibody staining. In **acute myeloid leukemia with differentiation** (M2), leukemic cells show a more clearly myeloid lineage. They typically are positive for myeloperoxidase staining and have Auer rods; the 8:21 translocation has been associated with this phenotype, and it has a relatively good prognosis, even without transplantation therapy.

### *Acute Promyelocytic Leukemia (M3)*

These leukemias show dramatic granularity and multiple Auer rods. As noted, the 15:17 translocation is invariably present. The coagulation system is virtually always activated, with DIC either at diagnosis or with the initiation of treatment; patients require aggressive blood and platelet support in addition to consumed factor replacement. Overall, patients are younger, and survival is greater than 70% with current therapy. Recognition of this subtype is important before the initiation of induction therapy, so that the coagulopathy is treated early and serious bleeding prevented. Treatment with the differentiating agent **all-trans-retinoic acid** (ATRA) induces a hematologic and bone marrow morphologic response, while avoiding exacerbation of DIC, allowing the physician to treat subsequently with conventional cytotoxics with a relative margin of safety.

## Acute Leukemias (M4 through M7)

M4 leukemic cells, while still mainly myeloid, show some monocytic features. A variant is the M4Eo subtype with the inverted chromosome 16, as described previously. **Acute monocytic leukemia** (M5) is "pure" monocytic leukemia, in which the leukemic cells are either **monoblasts** (M5a) or **promonoblasts** (M5b). Tissue infiltration is common, with hypertrophy of the gums (Figure 146.1) or pulmonary or CNS infiltrates due to leukemic blasts. This tissue-invasive form of acute leukemias mandates special therapeutic intervention to treat or give prophylaxis against leptomeningeal involvement. In **acute erythroleukemia** (M6), the blasts show clear erythroid features with dysplastic, megaloblastic erythroid maturation. Typical cytogenetic abnormalities include -7 and -5. The malignant cells are of erythroid lineage, and the criteria require that at least 30% of the cells be proerythroblasts. Finally, in **acute megakaryocytic leukemia** (M7), the blasts are relatively undifferentiated; small "microblasts" often are seen in the blood. The bone marrow may show extensive fibrosis. The blasts must have surface glycoprotein IIb/IIIa or von Willebrand protein in the cytoplasm, or stain positive for factor VIII to confirm megakaryocytic lineage. Acute megakaryocytic leukemia is the most common leukemia in Down syndrome (trisomy 21).

### Management

Therapy of AML, with the exception of M3, initially involves induction therapy and some postinduction "consolidation." Induction attains a complete remission—i.e., normal bone marrow with fewer than 5% blasts, plus adequate bone marrow function to attain normal peripheral blood counts. Usually, profound bone marrow hypoplasia is produced by treatment with an anthracycline (e.g., idarubicin, or daunorubicin) plus a 7-day infusion of cytosine arabinoside; the hypoplasia usually lasts 3 to 6 weeks, until the patient's normal bone marrow can recover hematopoiesis.

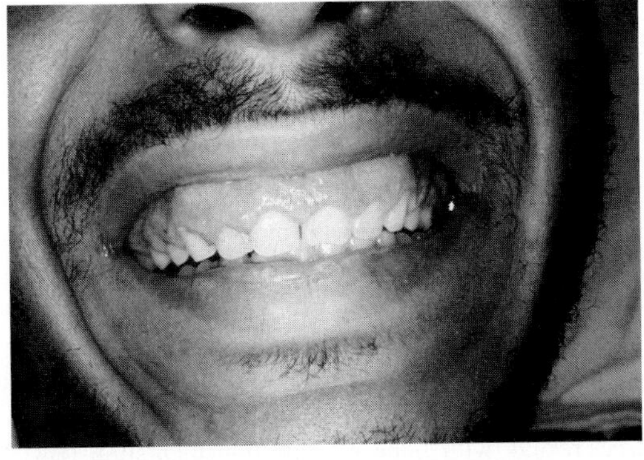

**FIGURE 146.1.** Gum hypertrophy in M5: the patient had swollen, bleeding gums and febrile episodes.

Blood products are transfused in the interim to maintain hemostasis, and antibiotics are given for fevers and infections. By 21 to 36 days after the initiation of therapy, the marrow produces sufficient normal cells, thus lessening the need for transfusions and antibiotics. Complete remission occurs when the marrow turns normal (<5% blasts and normal morphology) and the peripheral counts have recovered. The incidence of mortality during induction—usually as a result of infection or uncontrolled bleeding—is nearly 10%, although it may be 60% to 80% in older (>65) persons. A reduction in the dosage of chemotherapy in elderly patients to lessen toxicity also lowers the antileukemic effect. It is more promising to attenuate the duration of cytopenias in these patients by using G-CSF or GM-CSF. Many patients require a second, usually lesser, dose of therapy during induction to attain a remission. About 10% of patients are primarily resistant to chemotherapy; they usually have secondary leukemias; prior myelodysplastic abnormalities of chromosomes 5, 7, 8, and 13; and blasts positive for CD34.

Some postinduction treatment is necessary. Without it, the leukemia invariably recurs within 4 to 18 months. Consolidation therapy improves both the duration of remission and overall survival. It is usually chemotherapy, given soon after recovery from induction, in doses that produce less bone marrow hypoplasia than the induction schedule. It may be given 2 to 4 times as the marrow recovers from each cycle of therapy. A popular form of consolidation is the use of high-dose cytosine arabinoside; this treatment can obviate relative pharmacologic resistance, and can penetrate the leptomeninges, thus providing prophylaxis to high-risk leukemias, e.g., M4 and M5 subtypes. Although some form of postinduction therapy is needed, the duration and intensity after a documented remission are not yet clearly standardized. The median survival is 18 to 24 months. Approximately 15% to 20% of all AML patients appear to achieve long-term remission and, possibly, cure. Patients with M2 t(8:21), M3 t(15:17), and M4E (inv 16) have much better prognoses.

**Bone marrow transplant** (BMT) is conceptually a late intensification therapy. High-dose chemotherapy and, usually, radiation are given to destroy native leukemic bone marrow completely, in the process also destroying normal bone marrow; it is followed by transplantation of donor marrow to restore the hematopoietic abilities. It is now clear that this technique is in essence a form of "adoptive immunotherapy" wherein a new immune system is transplanted into the recipient, which is crucial in controlling or eradicating residual clones of leukemic cells refractory to the ablative chemotherapy with or without radiotherapy. Bone marrow transplant appears to be most effective in the first remission, with approximately 50% of patients surviving at 10 years. For BMT done during either the first relapse or second remission, survival drops to 15% to 20%. Leukemia relapse is the major cause of failure in these patients. The same transplanted immune system, depending on the degree of histocompatibility, can produce highly morbid, even lethal, graft-versus-host disease involving the liver, skin, gut, and lung. During transient immunosuppressive periods, infection—especially interstitial pneumonia and respiratory failure—is life-threatening, as is veno-occlusive disease of the liver, a vascular injury to the venules of the liver. The risk for developing veno-occlusive liver disease depends on both prior and ablative treatment characteristics. The rigors of BMT make it an option only in relatively young, otherwise healthy patients with an excellent histocompatible match. Because there is only about a 30% chance that an American patient, usually from a family with a limited number of siblings, will have a good related match, a worldwide matched unrelated donor (MUD) program has been developed to find compatible donors. This program has dramatically increased the number of feasible transplants worldwide. Unfortunately, members of ethnic or racial minorities rarely can be matched successfully, even with this technique. Transplantation with cord blood, rich in bone marrow stem cells, or poor in preconditioned lymphocytes, currently is being tested.

## Acute Lymphoblastic Leukemia

Acute lymphoblastic leukemia (ALL) is most common in children, with a peak incidence between 2 and 6 years. The term "adult ALL" usually refers to patients older than 15 to 18 years, and it is biologically different from childhood ALL. Acute lymphoblastic leukemia has a second peak incidence in adults over the age of 60. The diagnosis of ALL is based on the morphology of the malignant blasts, plus their immunophenotypic and cytochemical characteristics. Three subtypes of ALL are recognized by the FAB (see Table 146.1).

### Clinical Features and Diagnosis

In general, the diagnosis of acute leukemia is not difficult, with the signs and symptoms of bone marrow failure, including fatigue, bleeding, or fever, depending on the degree of cytopenias at the time of the diagnosis. As a result of tissue infiltration by malignant lymphoblasts, ALL manifests testicular enlargement, skin nodules, lymphadenopathy, splenomegaly, and cranial nerve palsies. The peripheral blood may show dramatically high WBC with circulating lymphoblasts, or it may show neutropenia and few abnormal cells. The bone marrow usually is hypercellular because of the lymphoblastic infiltration, and normal marrow elements may appear to be completely absent. Although the morphology of the blasts distinguishes ALL from AML, in very undifferentiated cells the diagnosis occasionally must rely on the results of either special stains or monoclonal immunocytochemistry stains.

The lineage of 75% of all adult ALL is B-cell, including leukemic cells with a more mature B-cell phenotype (expressing surface immunoglobulin) and others with a "pre–B-cell" phenotype (a rearrangement of the immunoglobulin genes only, with no surface immunoglobulin). The remaining adult ALL are of T-cell lineage, with either mature T cells or pre–T cells. Cytogenetic findings occasionally are needed to pinpoint the exact lineage of the malignant cells. Up to 20% of adult ALL have some myeloid antigens. Rarely, the leukemic cells—otherwise typical blasts—show similar expression of both myeloid and lymphoid antigens on their surface. Some of these cells appear to be best classified as M0-AML, and may best be treated using an AML regimen. Others are truly ALL with myeloid antigens, and it is controversial whether or not this confers a poor prognosis.

### Management

Conventional treatment of ALL in general involves a sequence of induction; consolidation and intensification (given several times in sequence); and maintenance chemotherapy (for 1–2 years). Induction usually involves some combination of vincristine and prednisone, plus an anthracycline. The complete remission rate is 65% to 85%, with a mortality of 3% to 20%. The value of consolidation and intensification treatments in adult ALL is controversial; however, the more intensive, multiple-drug programs seem to confer longer remissions and survival. Likewise, the benefit and necessary duration of maintenance therapy in adult ALL is unknown. Most maintenance therapies include methotrexate, 6-mercaptopurine, and, possibly, vincristine, L-asparaginase, or prednisone. All therapy regimens in ALL include some type of prophylactic treatment of the central nervous system (CNS). Leukemia recurs in the CNS in 30% of untreated cases, and 5% of adults present initially with CNS disease. CNS prophylaxis, historically done with craniospinal radiation, more recently has been accomplished by intrathecal drugs or high-dose methotrexate or cytosine arabinoside administered systemically.

Twenty-five percent of adults with ALL are cured with conventional chemotherapy. Efforts to improve these results with bone marrow transplantation (BMT) have been made. Allogeneic BMT currently is reserved for patients following their first relapse, after they have attained a second remission. It also may be used in the first remission in patients in a poor-risk group, patients presenting with high WBC, patients with unfavorable translocations [e.g. t(4;11), t(1;19)], or L3 patients. Autologous BMT may be used in older patients, in patients with a poor prognosis as a intensification maneuver, or in patients without tissue-matched donors. Current treatment programs in adult ALL lead to remission rates of 70% to 80% and cure rates of 20% to 30%.

# CHAPTER 147 CLINICAL USES OF BLOOD AND BLOOD COMPONENTS

## Blood Donation, Processing, and Storage

Blood transfusion practices have steadily improved as greater physician awareness of risks vs. benefits and advances in the safety of the blood product have helped achieve this progress. Despite this improvement, the need to continue to improve on transfusion practices and to provide an adequate and safe blood supply is greater than its ever been.

Blood and blood products are a limited resource. An individual may donate 450 to 500 ml of whole blood as often as every eight weeks. Donors are asked a series of health questions and questions about behaviors that put them at risk for transfusion-transmitted infections. Following collection, the donor blood is routinely tested for the ABO and RhD antigen and then tested for the presence of infectious disease markers associated with hepatitis B, hepatitis C, HIV-1/2, HTLV-I/II, and syphilis. Recently, a new research test, nucleic acid testing (NAT), is now being tested on all blood donations with the intended value of shortening the window between infectivity and positivity to the standard serological tests for hepatitis C and HIV. Units with positivity for infectious disease markers are discarded and the donors are deferred from future blood donation. Units are drawn in an anticoagulant preservative solution that permit the easy separation of blood into its components, which then allows the use of specific component therapy. Red blood cells can be stored up to 42 days following donation. Platelets are stored for five days, and fresh frozen plasma and cryoprecipitate are stored at −18°C or colder for one year.

## Transfusion Orders

After carefully assessing the patient's transfusion needs, the physician orders the appropriate blood product. The transfusion order should include the type of blood component to be transfused, its amount (in ml or units), the urgency of the need for the product (i.e., routine, STAT, specific date, etc.), time to administer the product, and the duration of the transfusion. In addition, any special needs (i.e., irradiation, leukocyte reduction, CMV antibody negative) should be clearly specified.

## Compatibility Testing

Upon physician's order, the patient's blood sample is obtained and correctly labeled. The need to meticulously follow hospital policy concerning the collection and labeling of the blood sample cannot be overemphasized. The patient's blood is typed for ABO and RhD (RBC transfusions must be ABO, Rh compatible) and screened for alloantibodies (from prior transfusion or pregnancy) that are directed against an RBC antigen on the donor red cells. The crossmatch between the patient and the donor unit done either serologically or electronically helps ensure compatibility. Finally, at the bedside, the unit to be transfused is carefully identified and matched with the appropriate patient before transfusion is begun. It is to be noted that crossmatching is done for whole blood and red blood cell transfusions, but not for FFP, cryoprecipitate, or routine platelet transfusions. Should an antibody to a red cell antigen be identified, then blood is selected that lacks the antigen to which the antibody is directed. In a STAT situation, a fully crossmatched unit of blood can be ready for transfusion in approximately 45 minutes from the time the work begins in the blood bank.

The **maximum surgical blood ordering schedule** (MSBOS) is a list devised to compare transfusion needs with specific surgical procedures. It ensures the proper preoperative blood order (i.e., order for type and crossmatch, or type and screen). One option, called the type and screen (T & S), is utilized when there is only a small chance (<10%) that a patient undergoing a particular procedure or need will require a blood transfusion. No blood will be crossmatched and set aside for the patient's surgery unless an unexpected need for transfusion develops during surgery. Blood can be made readily available since the patient has been typed and screened. The MSBOS and type and screen effectively employ blood resources without increasing risk to the patient.

If blood is needed in an emergency situation prior to the completion of a type and crossmatch, type O red blood cells (RBCs), usually RhD negative, may be transfused. The physician ordering emergency blood must consider the possible benefit of transfusion against the risk of infusion of potentially incompatible blood. During emergency situations attention to proper identification of the recipient and the blood obtained for compatibility testing is essential.

## Blood Product Therapy

### Guidelines for Issuing and Transfusion of Blood

Careful identification of the recipient with the identification information on the blood container is essential to ensure safety for the patient. Most major hemolytic transfusion reactions occur because of a clerical error involving identification of a patient, patient sample, or unit assigned to the patient. Proper equipment for transfusion of the product should be available including the fact that all blood must pass through a blood filter prior to entering the patient's blood stream. In general, drugs or medications should not be added to a blood product. However, normal saline may be added. The rate of infusion of the blood product will depend on the clinical situation. In non-emergent situations a unit of red cells should be transfused over two to four hours. Blood should be infused slowly at the start unless an emergency situation exists. This allows time to identify possible major incompatibilities without large quantities of blood product being transfused. When large quantities of blood (massive transfusion) are required, the use of an approved blood warmer is essential to prevent hypothermia and the associated risks.

### Whole Blood

Whole blood transfusions must be ABO identical to the patient. They are indicated for patients who require both oxygen carrying capacity and volume expansion (usually an actively bleeding patient). Whole blood contains red blood cells, plasma proteins, and a satisfactory amount of all clotting factors, except for reduced Factor V and Factor VIII. Platelets in whole blood are not viable. Whole blood is expected to reduce the symptoms associated with decreased intravascular volume and anemia.

### Red Blood Cells

The vast majority of red blood cell transfusions are given as packed red blood cells (PRBCs). They are indicated for patients who require an increase in oxygen carrying capacity for symptomatic anemia or to prevent the symptoms of anemia in patients at risk. PRBCs are not good intravascular volume expanders. Patients requiring a red cell transfusion may have signs and symptoms of tachycardia, shortness of breath, pallor, fatigue, syncope, posteral hypotension, angina, or cerebral hypoxia in association with their low hemoglobin-hematocrit level. There is no specific hemoglobin or hematocrit "trigger" at which patients should be transfused. This approach has been replaced by an emphasis on transfusion avoidance in the absence of signs or symptoms attributable to anemia. Transfusion is deferred until compensatory mechanisms become insufficient to alleviate the signs and symptoms of anemia. If the anemia can be corrected by iron, vitamin $B_{12}$, folate, or in selected cases erythropoietin, then these medications should be used prior to transfusion unless the patient's condition is unstable. Many patients can tolerate a hemoglobin level of 7–9 g/dL without the need for transfusion. Comorbid conditions, such as cardiovascular disease, pulmonary disease, states of excessive oxygen consumption, or cerebral vascular disease, may require that a patient's hemoglobin be kept at a higher level than noted above. This is because symptoms and signs of anemia may develop at higher hemoglobin levels in such patients. One unit of PRBC generally raises the hematocrit by about 3% and the hemoglobin by about 1 g/dL.

### Leukocyte-Reduced RBCs

Filtration is the most effective method for removing leukocytes from red blood cells. The use of "third generation" leukocyte reduction filters remove at least 99.9% of the leukocytes contained in a red blood cell product. The indications for leukocyte-reduced red blood cells include the following: 1) the prevention of non-hemolytic febrile transfusion reactions; 2) the reduction in occurrence of alloimmunization against HLA antigens in patients receiving multiple transfusions such as those with acute leukemia or aplastic anemia; and 3) the prevention of post-transfusion cytomegalovirus infection. The use of leukocyte-reduced blood products is a growing trend in the United States.

### Fresh Frozen Plasma

Fresh frozen plasma (FFP) is the plasma separated from whole blood and frozen at -18°C or below within 8 hours of blood collection. It contains all of the coagulation factors and anticoagulant proteins (i.e., protein C, protein S, antithrombin-III) at normal levels. FFP does not contain viable platelets.

Fresh frozen plasma is indicated in the following: 1) acquired or congenital deficiency of coagulation factors for which a specific, safe clotting factor concentrate is not available, 2) massively transfused patients who have developed a dilutional coagulopathy and microvascular bleeding, 3) serious bleeding or emergency surgery requiring rapid reversal of warfarin, 4) acquired coagulopathy in an actively bleeding patient or one who is about to undergo an invasive procedure, and 5) thrombotic thrombocytopenic purpura (TTP). FFP is transfused as ABO compatible, does not require a crossmatch, and a reasonable dose is 10–15 ml/kg body weight (2–4 units of FFP followed by laboratory evaluation to determine the response and to assess the interval between doses). FFP must be transfused within 24 hours of thawing if used for coagulation factor replacement. It should not be used routinely as a volume expander.

## Platelet Transfusions

Platelets—random donor platelets (RDPs) are prepared by separating platelets from a single unit of whole blood, containing a minimum of $5.5 \times 10^{10}$ platelets, and can be stored for up to five days at room temperature. Plateletpheresis—pheresis platelets or single donor platelets (SDPs) are collected by apheresis technique from a single donor using a blood cell separator and contain a minimum of $3.0 \times 10^{11}$ platelets suspended in approximately 200–400 ml of plasma. HLA matched platelet concentrates are an apheresis platelet concentrate selected for matching of the donor's HLA type with the recipient's HLA type for patients who have become alloimmunized to HLA antigens. A pheresis platelet is the equivalent of approximately six RDPs.

Platelet transfusions are indicated to control active bleeding or prevent hemorrhage associated with a deficiency in platelet number or function. Platelets are most commonly used prophylactically to prevent bleeding when the platelet count is <10,000–20,000/μl in patients with temporary myelosuppression from hematologic malignancy or those receiving chemotherapy. For patients undergoing minor surgical procedures such as a line placement, the platelet count may need to be greater than 50,000/μl. For surgical procedures in thrombocytopenic patients, it may be necessary for the platelet count to be >75,000/μl, and patients having neurosurgical or eye procedures may require platelet counts >100,000/μl prior to the procedure. Platelets are also used in some patients who develop a platelet function abnormality following cardiopulmonary bypass for open heart surgery. The average platelet concentration dose is one unit of RDPs per 10 kg of body weight. It is common in a number of hospitals to define a standard "dose" of platelet concentrates with a standard dose ranging from 4 to 6 platelet concentrates per institution. An apheresis platelet is commonly considered a therapeutic dose of platelets. Platelet transfusions should result in prevention or resolution of bleeding caused by thrombocytopenia or abnormal platelet function. A standard dose of platelets should raise the platelet count 30,000-50,000/μl.

The platelet count may fail to rise as expected in patients with fever, sepsis, splenomegaly, or disseminated intravascular coagulation, or in patients with antibodies to HLA or platelet-specific antigens. Refractoriness to platelet transfusion, that is, failure to obtain a rise in platelet count shortly after platelet transfusion, is most commonly, but not always, due to the development of antibodies against Class I HLA antigens on transfused platelets. HLA-matched or platelet crossmatched transfusions have been used to provide adequate platelet increments in this situation.

Patients with idiopathic thrombocytopenic purpura, drug-induced immune thrombocytopenia, thrombotic thrombocytopenic purpura, and post-transfusion purpura, in general, should not receive platelet transfusions unless there is major or life-threatening hemorrhage. This is because the recovery and survival of infused platelets is diminished in these conditions. If at all possible, ABO compatible platelets should be transfused since ABO incompatibility may decrease the survival of transfused platelets. Platelet transfusions in thrombotic thrombocytopenic purpura should be avoided since it may exacerbate intravascular thrombosis.

## Granulocyte Transfusions

Granulocyte transfusions are obtained by apheresis technique and should contain a minimum of $1 \times 10^{10}$ granulocytes. Recent use of corticosteroids and granulocyte colony stimulating factor (G-CSF) to stimulate the donor's white count prior to apheresis has resulted in the ability to collect three to five times as many granulocytes as previously. Granulocyte transfusions are used infrequently because antibiotic therapy has been effective in treating or preventing infectious complications in patients at risk. Granulocyte transfusions should be used in patients who have an absolute granulocyte count of <500/μl with documented sepsis or serious infection that has not responded to antibiotic therapy and for which the patient is expected to have a significant period of neutropenia.

## Cryoprecipitate

Cryoprecipitate is the cold precipitated protein fraction derived from fresh frozen plasma when it is thawed at 1–6°C. It contains ample fibrinogen, Factor

VIII, von Willebrand factor, and Factor XIII and fibronectin. Cryoprecipitate had been used in the past to treat hemophilia A and von Willebrand disease, but those diseases are now treated by safer commercial concentrates. Cryoprecipitate is specifically indicated for the treatment of hypofibrinogenemia and for use as a fibrin sealant (fibrin glue, a surgical adhesive). In an average size adult with significant hypofibrinogenemia, an appropriate dose is 8–12 units of cryoprecipitate.

### Special Blood Products

Some patients require the use of specialized blood products to meet their transfusion needs (e.g., cytomegalovirus (CMV) antibody negative, leukocyte-reduced and gamma irradiated blood products). CMV transmission is a known complication of blood transfusion since the 1960s, especially in immunosuppressed patients. Individuals at risk include fetuses receiving intrauterine transfusions, premature infants of less than 1,200 gram weight born to CMV-seronegative mothers, CMV-seronegative pregnant individuals receiving blood transfusions, and CMV-seronegative recipients of renal, heart, liver, lung, or bone marrow transplants. CMV infection can be reduced by providing blood from donors that are CMV-antibody negative or by leukocyte-reducing the blood product prior to transfusion.

Gamma irradiation of blood products is used to prevent post-transfusion graft vs. host disease. This is a disease that is mediated by lymphocytes in the blood product that recognize the transfusion recipient as foreign and mount an immune response. The disease is characterized by fever, skin rash, diarrhea, liver abnormalities, and pancytopenia due to bone marrow aplasia. Patients at risk for post-transfusion graft vs. host disease include, but are not limited to, bone marrow transplant patients, both allogenic and autologous, patients treated with high dose chemotherapy such as acute leukemias, other malignant states treated with chemotherapy, patients with Hodgkin's or non-Hodgkin's lymphoma, congenital immunodeficiency disorders, low birth weight neonates, and those receiving intrauterine transfusion. Because of the rare occurrence of post-transfusion graft vs. host disease when a blood relative donates a directed unit, such units are also irradiated. Gamma irradiation of blood products with 2,500 cGy will prevent post-transfusion graft vs. host disease.

Leukocyte-reduced blood products are used to prevent 1) febrile non-hemolytic transfusion reactions; 2) alloimmunization to HLA antigens in recipients of multiple transfusions, and 3) CMV infection in at risk patients. In addition, blood transfusions are thought to cause a down regulation in the immune system, and it is hypothesized that the white cell in the blood product may be responsible for this effect. Some physicians advocate leukocyte-reducing all blood products to prevent potential complications associated with down regulation of the immune system.

### Autologous Blood Transfusion

An autologous unit of blood (i.e., blood obtained from the patient for transfusion to the patient) is the safest blood product for the patient to receive. The use of autologous blood continues to be an important manner of increasing the safety of a blood transfusion. Autologous blood transfusion methods include preoperative autologous donation, preoperative hemodilution (collecting 1 to 2 units immediately preoperatively and replacing with saline, and then transfusing the units during the surgery), and intraoperative and postoperative blood cell salvage (recovery of shed blood and reinfusion into the patient). Physicians should ensure that all patients who may benefit from autologous blood transfusion are given the opportunity to do so.

## Complications of Blood Transfusion Therapy

Transfusion reactions can be classified as acute or delayed, immunologic or non-immunologic (Table 147.1). Tremendous strides have been made in reducing the infectious complications of blood transfusion, particularly those of HIV and hepatitis C. It is important to remember that there are other significant, serious, and sometimes fatal complications associated with blood

**TABLE 147.1. Classification of Transfusion Reactions**

| |
|---|
| Immediate—immunologic |
| Acute hemolytic transfusion reaction |
| Non-hemolytic febrile transfusion reaction |
| Allergic reaction, anaphylactic reaction |
| Transfusion-related acute lung injury (TRALI) |
| Immediate—Nonimmunologic |
| Hypervolemia |
| Complications of massive transfusion |
| Bacterially contaminated blood product |
| Delayed—Immunologic |
| Delayed hemolytic transfusion reaction |
| Post-transfusion graft vs. host disease |
| Post-transfuion purpura |
| Delayed—Nonimmunologic |
| Iron overload |
| Infections |
| Hepatitis B, Hepatitis C |
| HIV, HTLV-I |
| Cytomegalovirus |
| Malaria, Chagas' disease, Babesiosis |
| Syphilis |

transfusion. Prevention of such adverse events has not been as successful as those for many of the serious infectious consequences of blood transfusion. Thus, the use of blood only when clinically indicated is an extraordinarily important responsibility of the transfusing physician. Clinicians must be aware of the alternatives to allogenic transfusions such as the use of various forms of autologous blood transfusion, use of hematopoietic growth factors, and pharmacologic agents that foster hemostasis.

## Immediate Complications—Immunologic

### Acute Hemolytic Transfusion Reaction

The most severe, life-threatening, hemolytic transfusion reactions result from the inadvertent administration of ABO incompatible blood to a recipient who has an antibody directed against the A and/or B antigen of the transfused red cell. Acute hemolytic transfusion reactions, both ABO and non-ABO, occur with the frequency of approximately 1 in 6,000–1 to 25,000 components infused. Hemolysis may be intravascular or extravascular depending on the antibody involved and its ability to activate complement. Fever or fever accompanied by chills is the most common finding in a hemolytic transfusion reaction. Other signs and symptoms may include generalized flushing, nausea, dyspnea, chest pain, back pain, and hypotension. The most severe complications from a hemolytic transfusion reaction includes shock, acute renal failure, and disseminated intravascular coagulation. These are most commonly associated with ABO incompatible blood transfusion.

When a hemolytic transfusion reaction is suspected, the blood transfusion should be immediately stopped and the patient evaluated for this possible complication. Treatment should include keeping an intravenous line open with 0.9% normal saline and correcting hypotension and/or bleeding should that occur. A diuretic such as Lasix should be administered in a potential severe ABO hemolytic transfusion reaction. Mannitol (20 g in 100 ml infused over 5 minutes) has also been used. Urine output should be maintained at >100 ml per hour. The blood bank should be immediately notified of any suspected transfusion reaction.

### Non-Hemolytic Febrile Transfusion Reaction

Non-hemolytic febrile transfusion reaction is defined as a febrile response of at least 1°C shortly after a blood transfusion. Such reactions are associated with antibodies to white cell antigens present in the transfused product or from the production of various cytokines during storage, particularly with platelet products that are stored at room temperature. Prevention of febrile non-hemolytic transfusion reactions is accomplished by removing the white blood cells from the blood product. This is best done through pre-storage leukocyte reduction. Blood transfusion should be stopped when a non-hemolytic febrile reaction is suspected since fever is also a common finding of a hemolytic transfusion reaction.

### Allergic Reactions

Allergic reactions are some of the most common transfusion reactions but fortunately are usually mild. Symptoms usually include urticaria (hives) and itching. They usually result when the patient has an antibody to a plasma protein present in the transfused blood product. These reactions can be treated with antihistamines or even potentially prevented by premedication with antihistamines prior to the transfusion. Occasionally, life-threatening anaphylaxis occurs with blood transfusions. The classic occurrence is in patients who are IgA deficient and who have developed antibodies to the IgA molecule. These patients require transfusion with IgA deficient blood, washed red cells, frozen deglycerolized blood. These reactions are treated in a similar manner to other types of anaphylaxis.

### Transfusion-Related Acute Lung Injury (TRALI)

This condition is characterized by pulmonary infiltrates and the development of a non-cardiogenic pulmonary edema occurring shortly after a blood transfusion and is thought to be a result of passively transferred donor antibodies that react against recipient leukocyte antigens causing leukocyte activation resulting in damage to pulmonary endothelium. Patients present with fever, dyspnea, and hypoxia shortly after receiving a blood transfusion. The chest x-ray demonstrates pulmonary edema, yet left atrial and pulmonary wedge pressures are usually within normal limits and may even be low. Recovery usually occurs within 48 hours, although death has been reported. Patients may require respiratory support and may even require fluid replacement rather than fluid restriction.

## Immediate Complications—Non-Immunologic

### Volume Overload

One of the most under-reported complications of transfusion is the development of mild to moderate congestive heart failure after blood transfusion. Patients at risk for heart failure following a blood transfusion should be carefully monitored and may require diuretics. Red blood cell transfusions, not whole blood, should be used for patients with euvolemic anemia. Patients at risk for volume overload should have their blood infused slowly over a number of hours.

### Adverse Effects of Massive Blood Transfusion

Massive blood transfusion may be associated with a number of adverse effects. These include dilutional thrombocytopenia, dilutional coagulopathy, hypothermia (if massive amounts of whole blood are rapidly infused without a blood warmer), and citrate reaction (development of hypocalcemia). Physicians should be aware of these complications and carefully monitor the patient for these possibilities.

### Bacterial Contamination

Rarely, units of blood may contain bacteria that can cause a severe septic transfusion reaction. Bacterial contamination has been reported in red cell units but has been most associated with platelet concentrates since platelets are stored at room temperature. Clinical presentations are those of chills or rigors associated with nausea and vomiting, shortly after a blood transfusion. Fever and hypotension frequently develop and may progress to shock and disseminated intravascular coagulation. The Blood Bank should be immediately notified when a septic transfusion reaction is suspected. The transfusion should be stopped and the unit disconnected from the patient. The patient should be treated with broad-spectrum antibiotics until the organism is identified.

## Delayed Complications—Immunologic

### Delayed Hemolytic Transfusion Reaction

Delayed hemolytic transfusion reactions are usually manifested by a fall in the hemoglobin and hematocrit. The reaction occurs several days to weeks following a transfusion. Such clinical reactions occur with a frequency of approximately 1 per 1,500–8,000 units transfused and are usually mild and not life-threatening. Such reactions are caused by the development of an alloantibody to a red blood cell antigen either by primary immunization or by secondary anamnestic response. Signs and symptoms include unexplained anemia, fever, jaundice, and occasionally hemoglobinuria. Patients suspected of such reactions should have both a direct and indirect antiglobulin test evaluated. Future transfusions will require blood that lacks the antigen to which the antibody in the patient's plasma is directed.

### Post-Transfusion Graft vs. Host Disease

Post-transfusion graft vs. host disease has been explained under the subsection of special blood products.

### Iron Overload

Iron overload occurs in adults who receive large quantities of blood transfusion (60–210 units) for conditions that cause chronic anemia. The accumulation of iron that is present in these blood products may cause endocrine, cardiac, and liver dysfunction. Iron chelation therapy is effective in some patients.

### Post-Transfusion Purpura

This uncommon syndrome is manifested by profound thrombocytopenia that develops approximately 5–9 days after transfusion. The exact pathogenesis is not fully understood. Diagnosis is made by recognizing thrombocytopenia after a blood transfusion, although other causes of thrombocytopenia need to be excluded. Patients with this disorder develop an antibody against a platelet-specific antigen that is not present on their own platelets. The $Pl^{A1}$ antigen is the most common platelet-specific antigen associated with this disease. Treatment includes the use of intravenous gammaglobulin and/or therapeutic plasma exchange.

## Delayed Complications—Non-Immunologic

### Infectious Complications

Approximately 4 million individuals in the United States are affected with hepatitis C, with about 10% (400,000) having been infected due to a blood transfusion. Remarkable advances have been made since the discovery of the hepatitis C virus in the late 1980s. At the present time, the current estimated risk of hepatitis C is thought to be approximately 1 per million units transfused.

Hepatitis B can also be transmitted by blood. Its current estimated risk is between 1 in 63,000 to 1 in 230,000 components transfused.

Prior to the development of a test for HIV in 1985, over 8,000 individuals in the U.S. became infected with HIV from a blood transfusion. Since implementation of testing in 1985, there have been only 47 reported cases of HIV infection. This has been due to advances in the sensitivity and specificity of the test used to weed out the donors who are HIV positive. The current risk for acquiring HIV infection through transfusion is approximately 1 per 1.9 million units infused.

There are a number of other infectious complications associated with blood transfusion. These include the human T-cell leukemia virus type 1, cytomegalovirus, spirochete infections, parasitic infections such as Chagas' disease, malaria, and others. Currently, there is a great deal of active research going on in the United States and other parts of the world to develop methods that would essentially sterilize a blood product while maintaining the function of the product itself. It is possible that in the near future blood products may be treated in such a way rendering them free of being able to transmit either bacterial, viral, or other infectious organisms.

## References Articles


1. American Society of Anesthesiologists Task Force on Blood Component Therapy: Practice Guidelines for Blood Component Therapy. Anesthesiology 1996; 84:732–747.
2. Blajchman MA. Allogenic blood transfusion—immunomodulation and postoperative bacterial infection. Do we have the answers yet? Transfusion 1997; 37:121–125 (editorial).
3. Dzik D, Aubuchoun J, Jeffries L, et al. Leukocyte reduction of blood components, public policy and new technology. Transfusion Medicine Reviews 2000; 14:34–52.
4. Pisciotto PT, Vincent K. Prophylactic vs. therapeutic platelet transfusion practices in hematology and/or oncology patients. Transfusion 1995; 35:498–502.
5. Popopsky MA, Chaplin HC, Moore SB. Transfusion-related acute lung injury: a neglected serious complication of hemotherapy. Transfusion 1992; 32:589–592.


## Questions

**Instructions:** For each question below, select only **one** lettered answer that is the **best** for that question.

1. Pernicious anemia is characterized by which of the following?
   A. Abnormal serum transport of vitamin $B_{12}$
   B. Increased degradation of vitamin $B_{12}$
   C. Impaired DNA synthesis of all dividing cells
   D. Erythroid hypoplasia of bone marrow
   E. Development of antibodies against vitamin $B_{12}$

2. Which of the following is characterized by decreased serum iron concentration, increased serum transferrin, diminished serum ferritin, and hypochromic microcytic erythrocyte indices?
   A. Iron-deficiency anemia
   B. Sex-linked hereditary pyridoxine responsive anemia
   C. The third trimester of pregnancy
   D. Thalassemia minor
   E. Osteomyelitis

3. Which of the following is the most important safeguard against iron overload?
   A. Urinary excretion of iron if a serum concentration is exceeded
   B. Chronic blood loss from the gastrointestinal tract
   C. Selective absorption of dietary iron
   D. Retention of iron by phagocytic macrophages
   E. Oxidation of ferrous iron to nonabsorbable ferric iron

4. The anemia associated with total gastrectomy is caused by:
   A. Folic acid deficiency due to anorexia.
   B. Iron deficiency due to achlorhydria.
   C. Antiparietal cell antibodies.
   D. Malabsorption of vitamin $B_{12}$ due to diminished intrinsic factor.
   E. Failure to generate erythropoietin.

**Questions 5–9:** Match the items in column I with those in column II

| I Substance | II Function |
|---|---|
| 5. Transferrin | A. Tissue respiration |
| 6. Ferritin | B. Oxidation of iron |
| 7. Cytochrome | C. Oxygen transport |
| 8. Hemoglobin | D. Iron transport |
| 9. Ceruloplasmin | E. Iron storage |

**Questions 10–16.** Select only **one** lettered answer that is the **best** for that question.

10. Release of mature polymorphonuclear leukocytes from the bone marrow into the circulating blood depends, in part, on:
    A. Microtubular ultrastructure.
    B. Function of actin and myosin.
    C. Glycolysis.
    D. Replacement of primary granules by secondary granules.
    E. Cellular deformability.

11. The presence of toxic granulation in a mature polymorphonuclear leukocyte is indicative of which of the following?
    A. Accelerated granulocytopoiesis
    B. An abnormal serum factor that causes coagulation of leukocyte granules
    C. Residual ribosomal RNA that persists after cellular maturation
    D. The effect of endotoxin on lysosomal membranes
    E. Accelerated leukocyte destruction

12. Leukocytes that adhere to endothelial surfaces may be mobilized and identified by which of the following?
    A. Injection of endotoxin
    B. The skin window test
    C. Activation of $C'_3$ and $C'_5$ to $C'_{3A}$ and $C'_{5A}$
    D. Injection of epinephrine
    E. The phagocytic index

13. The chief function of folic acid is to:
    A. Transport vitamin $B_{12}$ to reactive site.
    B. Protect against oxidation of iron compounds.
    C. Enhance production of erythropoietin.

D. Provide methyl groups to convert uridylic to thymidylic acid.
E. Protect against proliferation of malignant (leukemic) cells.

14. A stimulus that is known to promote production of erythropoietin is:
A. Colony-stimulating factor.
B. Hypoxia.
C. Plethora.
D. Decompensated renal disease.
E. IL-3.

15. A 65-year-old man is admitted for severe epistaxis. History reveals a recent transient ischemic attack complicating atrial fibrillation; he receives daily warfarin. The patient states that his eyesight has been less than satisfactory lately. His vital signs are a pulse of 92/min; BP, 120/68 mm Hg; and respirations, 22/min. Physical examination is otherwise normal, except for continuing nasal bleeding. His hemoglobin is 13.1 g/dl and hematocrit, 36%. The INR is 6.5. Besides cessation of warfarin therapy, the management of this patient includes which one of the following?
A. Cryoprecipitate
B. Fresh frozen plasma
C. Type and cross-match for 2 units of PRBC; transfuse one unit as soon as available
D. Desmopressin (DDAVP) infusion
E. Aquamephyton, 10 mg IV now

16. A 74-year-old asymptomatic man is noted to have a normal physical examination, but his WBC count is 26,000/mm$^3$. The peripheral smear shows 23% PMNs, 62% lymphocytes, 8% monocytes, 5% basophils, and 2% eosinophils. The lymphocytes are mature-appearing. The hemoglobin and platelet counts are normal. The most appropriate management for this patient is which of the following?
A. Fludarabine with prednisone
B. Cyclophosphamide with prednisone
C. Chlorambucil with prednisone
D. Consider splenectomy
E. Observation with periodic documentation of clinical and hematologic data

## Answers

| | | | | |
|---|---|---|---|---|
| 1. C | 2. A | 3. C | 4. D | 5. D |
| 6. E | 7. A | 8. C | 9. B | 10. E |
| 11. A | 12. D | 13. D | 14. B | 15. B |
| 16. E | | | | |

## SUGGESTED READING

### *Books and Monographs*

Gross S, Roath S (eds). Hematology: A Problem-Oriented Approach. Baltimore, MD: Williams & Wilkins, 1996.

Lee GR, Foerster J, Lukens J, et al. (eds) Wintrobe's Clinical Hematology. 10th ed. Philadelphia, Lippincott Williams & Wilkins, 1999.

Petz L. Platelet Transfusions. In Pisciotto PT (ed). Blood Transfusion Therapy: A Physician's Handbook. 3rd ed. Arlington, VA: American Association of Blood Banks, 1996.

Rossi EC, Simon TL, Moss GS. Principles of Transfusion Medicine. 2nd ed. Baltimore, MD: Williams & Wilkins, 1995.

### *Articles*

*Proliferation and Differentiation of Circulating Blood Cells*

Armitage JO. Emerging applications of recombinant human granulocyte-macrophage colony-stimulating factor. Blood 1998; 92:4491–508.

Cazzola M, Mercuriali F, Brugnara C. Use of Recombinant Human Erythropoietin Outside the Setting of Uremia. Blood 1997; 89:4248–4267.

Metcalf D. Cellular hematopoiesis in the twentieth century. Seminars in Hematology 1999; 36:5–12.

*Microcytic and Macrocytic Anemias*

Goodnough LT, Skikne B, Brugnara C. Erythropoietin, iron, and erythropoiesis. Blood 2000; 96: 823–833.

Kis AM, Carnes M. Detecting iron deficiency in anemic patients with concomitant medical problems. J Gen Intern Med 1998; 13:455–61.

Means RT Jr. Advances in the anemia of chronic disease. Int J Hematol 1999; 70:7–12.

Stabler SP, Allen RH, Savage DG, Lindenbaum J. Clinical spectrum and diagnosis of cobalamin deficiency. Blood 1990; 76:871–881.

Stabler SP, Lindenbaum J, Allen RH. The use of homocysteine and other metabolites in the specific diagnosis of vitamin B-12 deficiency. Journal of Nutrition 1996; 126:1266S–72S.

Toh BH, van Driel IR, Gleeson PA. Pernicious anemia. N Engl J Med 1997; 337:1441–8.

*Aplastic Anemias*

Young NS, Maciejewski J. The pathophysiology of acquired aplastic anemia. N Engl J Med 1997; 336:1365–72.

*Hemolytic Anemias and Hemoglobinopathies*

Ballas SK. Management of sickle cell pain. Curr Opin Hematol 1997; 4:104–11.

Domen RE. An overview of immune hemolytic anemias. Cleveland Clinic Journal of Medicine 1998; 65:89–99.

McMullin MF. The molecular basis of disorders of the red cell membrane. Journal of Clinical Pathology 1999; 52:245–8, 1999.

McMullin MF. The molecular basis of disorders of red cell enzymes. Journal of Clinical Pathology 1999; 52:241–4.

Steensma DP, Hoyer JD, Fairbanks VF. Hereditary red blood cell disorders in middle eastern patients. Mayo Clinic Proceedings 2001; 76:285–93.

Steinberg MH. Management of sickle cell disease. N Engl J Med 1999; 340:1021–30.

Tabbara IA. Hemolytic anemias. Diagnosis and management. Med Clin North Am 1992; 76:649–668.

Weatherall DJ. Pathophysiology of thalassaemia. Baillieres Clinical Haematology 1998; 11:127–46.

Weatherall DJ. The thalassaemias. BMJ 1997; 314:1675–8.

*Bleeding Disorders*

Bajaj SO, Joist JH. New insights into how blood clots: implications for the use of APTT and PT as coagulation screening tests and in monitoring of anticoagulant therapy. Semin Thromb Hemost 1999; 25:407–18.

Furie B, Limentani SA, Rosenfield CG. A practical guide to the evaluation and treatment of hemophilia. Blood 1994; 84:3–9.

George JN. Platelets. Lancet 2000; 355(9214):1531–9.

George JN, Raskob GE, Shah SR, Rizvi MA, Hamilton SA, Osborne S, et al. Drug-induced thrombocytopenia: a systematic review of published case reports. Ann Intern Med 1998; 129:886–90.

Kitchens CS. Approach to the bleeding patient. Hematol Oncol Clin North Am 1992; 6:983–989.

Mann KG. Biochemistry and physiology of blood coagulation. Thromb Haemost 1999; 82:165–74.

Mannucci PM. Drug therapy: hemostatic drugs. N Engl J Med 1998; 339:245–52.

Mannucci PM. How I treat patients with von Willebrand disease. Blood 2001; 97:1915–9.

The American Society of Hematology ITP Practice Guideline Panel. Diagnosis and treatment of idiopathic thrombocytopenic purpura: recommendations of the American Society of Hematology. Ann Inter Med 1997; 126:319–26.

*Thrombotic Disorders*

Hooper WC, Evan BL. The role of activated protein C resistance in the pathogenesis of venous thrombosis. Am J Med Sci 1998; 316:120–8.

Huisman MV, Rosendaal F. Thrombophilia. Curr Opin Hematol 1999; 6:291–7.

Levi M, Cate H. Current Concepts: Disseminated Intravascular Coagulation. N Engl J Med 1999; 341:586–592.

Van Cott EM, Laposata M. Laboratory evaluation of hypercoagulable states. Hematol Oncol Clin North Am 1998; 12:1141–66.

Warkentin TE. Heparin-induced thrombocytopenia: a ten-year retrospective. Annual Review of Medicine 1999; 50:129–47.

*Myeloproliferative Disease*

Tefferi A. Myelofibrosis with myeloid metaplasia. N Engl J Med 2000; 342:1255–65.

Tefferi A, Solberg LA, Silverstein MN. A clinical update in polycythemia vera and essential thrombocythemia. Am J Med 2000; 109:141–9.

*The Myelodysplastic Syndromes*

Heaney ML, Golde DW. Medical Progress: Myelodysplasia. N Engl J Med 1999; 340:1649–1660.

*Leukemias*

Deininger MW, Goldman JM, Melo JV. The molecular biology of chronic myeloid leukemia. Blood 2000; 96:3343–56.

Kipps TJ. Chronic lymphocytic leukemia. Curr Opin Hematology 2000; 7:223–34.

Lowenberg B, Downing JR, Burnett A. Acute myeloid leukemia. N Engl J Med 1999; 341:1051–62.

Mauro MJ, Druker BJ. Chronic myelogenous leukemia. Curr Opin Oncol 2001; 13:3–7.

Pui CH, Evans WE. Acute lymphoblastic leukemia. N Engl J Med 1998; 339:605–15.

Thomas ED. Bone marrow transplantation: a review. Semin Hematol 1999; 36:95–103.

Willman CL. Molecular evaluation of acute myeloid leukemias. Semin Hematol 1999; 36:390–400.

*Clinical Uses of Blood and Blood Products*

Goodnough LT, Brecher ME, Kanter MH, AuBuchon JP. Medical Progress: Transfusion Medicine (First of Two Parts)—Blood Transfusion. N Engl J Med 1999; 340:438–447.

Goodnough LT, Brecher ME, Kanter MH, AuBuchon JP. Transfusion medicine. (Second of Two Parts)—Blood Conservation. N Engl J Med 1999; 340:525–33.

PART X

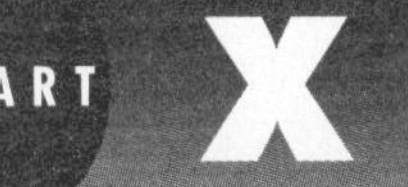

David K. Wagner

# INFECTIOUS DISEASES

# CHAPTER 148 HOST DEFENSES

An individual is protected against invading microorganisms in a variety of ways (Table 148.1). These protective mechanisms involve **nonspecific host defenses,** including the skin, mucosal membranes, and components of the immune system such as the complement system and granulocytic phagocytes. The cellular and humoral immune systems are categorized as **specific host defenses** because they respond to specific antigens and because there is a memory of a preceding encounter with that same organism in the immune response. In the following sections, the function of the normal host defenses is described, followed by clinical examples of infections that occur in immunocompetent individuals. Chapter 21, Immunodeficiency, in the Allergy and Immunology part, and Chapter 164, Infections in Immunocompromised Patients, later in this part, discuss the types of infections seen in immunocompromised persons.

## Nonspecific Host Defenses

### Intact skin and normal flora

Intact skin and mucous membranes form a physical barrier to external microbes. These surfaces, especially the mucous membranes, are normally colonized by bacterial species, which vary according to the site (Table 148.2). The resident microorganisms perform a protective function primarily by competing with nonresident flora for cutaneous or mucosal attachment sites. In addition, certain bacteria, such as the viridans streptococci, produce a high-molecular-weight antibiotic called bacteriocin that may inhibit pathogenic bacteria. Others may stimulate phagocytosis and production of natural antibodies at mucosal sites. Natural antibodies, found in previously healthy persons without a history of specific infection, are believed to be important in immunity to certain encapsulated organisms (e.g., *Haemophilus influenzae, Neisseria meningitidis*).

**TABLE 148.1. Host Defenses: An Overview**

| Nonspecific | Specific |
|---|---|
| Intact skin and normal flora | Cellular immune system |
| Local antimicrobial factors | T lymphocytes |
| Nutrition | Humoral immune system |
| Stress and exercise | B-lymphocytes |
| Hormonal factors | |
| Immune system | |
| Complement phagocytic cells | |

**TABLE 148.2. Common Bacteria Colonizing at Various Sites**

| Site | Organisms |
|---|---|
| Skin | Staphylococci (usually *S. epidermidis*)<br>Corynebacteria<br>Propionibacteria |
| Intestinal tract | Anaerobes and gram-negative bacilli |
| Oropharynx | Streptococci and anaerobes |
| Female genital tract | Anaerobes and gram-positive bacilli |

The barrier defense provided by normal skin or mucous membranes breaks down with traumatic injuries, surgical incisions, burns, vascular insufficiency, radiation injury, chemotherapy, and various inflammatory conditions. Such breakdown allows for the invasion of bacteria, leading to cutaneous or mucocutaneous infection. For instance, *Streptococcus pyogenes,* which usually dies on intact skin, requires a breakdown in the epidermis to cause cellulitis. In certain other cutaneous infections that occur in the presence of epidermal trauma, the microbiologic cause is suggested by the mechanism of injury (Table 148.3).

Breakdown of the normal microbial flora can result in colonization by potentially pathogenic and invasive bacteria. Chronic diseases (diabetes mellitus and alcoholism) as well as severe illness that leads to general debilitation favor the adherence of gram-negative bacilli to oropharyngeal mucosal cells, predisposing to pneumonia. However, antibiotic use is the biggest factor leading to altered microbial flora. The frequent use of broad-spectrum antibiotics can cause the depletion of normal flora and lead to colonization and infection by more pathogenic organisms.

### Local antimicrobial factors

Factors that locally inhibit invading microorganisms include excretory secretions, ciliary movement, local production of antimicrobial substances (e.g., lysozyme), and gastric or urinary acidity (Table 148.4).

### Complement system

The complement system contains a number of plasma proteins that are important mediators in host defense against a variety of organisms. These proteins cooperate in a series of interactions via either the **classical** or the **alternate pathway** (Figure 148.1).

Complement-deficient states may be acquired or inherited (Table 148.5). Acquired deficiencies include severe burns, in which the deficiency follows a loss of all serum proteins, or nephrotic syndrome, in which only some factors (B) are reduced, with the other complement components remaining normal. Some autoimmune diseases, such as systemic lupus erythematosus, may be associated with consumption of complement or with development of serum inhibitors to specific complement components. Inherited complement deficiencies are uncommon.

**TABLE 148.3. Relationship of Setting of Epidermal Trauma to the Type of Cutaneous Infection**

| Setting | Organism |
|---|---|
| Dog or cat bite | *Pasteurella multocida;* oral aerobes and anaerobes |
| Wound contamination by fresh water | *Aeromonas hydrophila* |
| Burn wounds | *Staphylococcus aureus* (commonly), Candida, *Pseudomonas aeruginosa, Klebsiella pneumoniae, Escherichia coli* |
| Lower extremity ulcers in diabetic people | Mixture of gram-positive, gram-negative and anaerobic organisms |
| Radiation and chemotherapy | Usual residents of intact skin or mucosa |
| Secondary infection complicating atopic dermatitis or eczema | Usual residents of intact skin |

**TABLE 148.4. Local Antimicrobial Factors**

| Site | Factor | Normal Mechanism | Mechanism Interfered By |
|---|---|---|---|
| Respiratory tract | Turbulent airflow | Deposition of large particles | Endotracheal intubation/tracheostomy<br>Clearance of aspirated material impeded by diminished cough during altered states of consciousness |
| | Lysozyme | Antibacterial activity | Phagocytic cell dysfunction |
| Gastrointestinal tract | Gastric pH | Mucosal barrier for ingested organisms | Decreased acidity fosters bacterial overgrowth—*Salmonella enteritis* more common in achlorhydric patients; use of antacids in critically ill patients leads to colonization of the upper GI tract with gram (−) bacilli |
| | Pancreatic enzymes, bile, and intestinal secretions | Antimicrobial action | Obstruction |
| | Peristaltic action | Propels and removes microbes | Antimotility agents |
| Genitourinary tract | Urinary flow | Stimulates a flushing mechanism | Obstruction to urinary flow predisposes to infection, which may ascend into the kidney |
| | Hypertonicity of renal medulla, urine pH, and urea | Inhibitory for bacteria | |
| | Acidic pH of vagina | Maintained by the commensal flora | Antibiotic use |
| Eyes | Tears | Exerts bathing action; expels bacteria mechanically | Obstruction or decreased production of tears |
| | Lysozyme | Antibacterial action | |

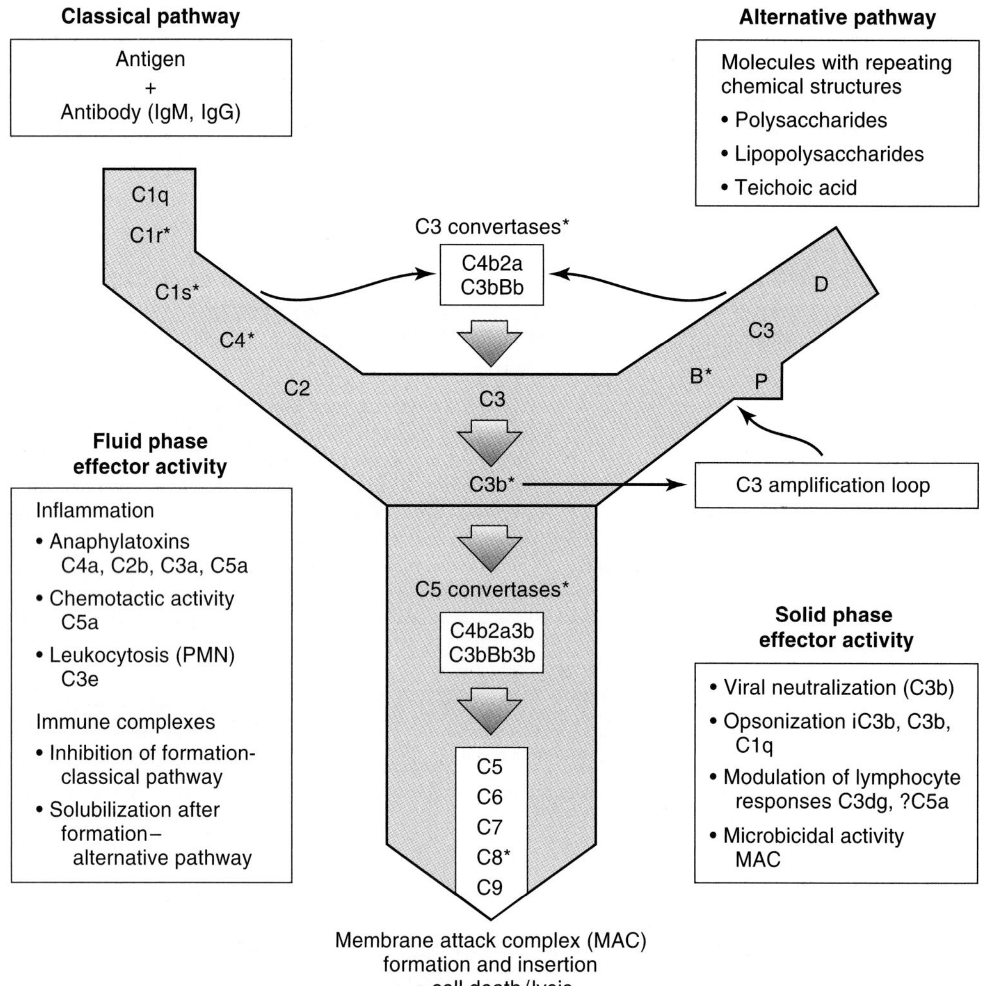


**FIGURE 148.1.** The **complement cascade**, showing both classical and alternate pathways, with the components arranged in order of their activation. Sites of downregulation of complement activity are indicated by asterisks. (Reprinted with permission from Densen P. Complement. In Mandell GL, Bennett JE, Dolin R (eds). Principles and Practice of Infectious Diseases. 4th ed. New York, NY: Churchill Livingstone, 1995, p 60, Figure 1.)

**TABLE 148.5. Major Complement Deficiencies**

| Acquired | Inherited |
|---|---|
| Severe burns | Classical pathway |
| Nephrotic syndrome | Alternative pathway |
| Sickle cell disease | Terminal complement components |
| Autoimmune diseases | |

### Phagocytic cells

*Neutrophil kinetics and function*

Neutrophil precursors are the major cell type in the bone marrow. It takes about 10 days for myeloblasts to develop into mature neutrophils, which then are released into the circulation. Circulating neutrophils normally survive 6–10 hours, but during severe infections, their survival may be reduced to even less than 1 hour.

The neutrophil's function involves migration to a site of infection, followed by killing the invading organism. The first step in activating neutrophils is through **chemoattractants** (e.g., complement C5a), which are produced at sites of inflammation. The neutrophil moves toward the chemoattractant and adheres to the vascular endothelial cells. It then enters the extravascular space and migrates toward the infection, where it engulfs the offending organisms in a process known as **phagocytosis.** Complement component C3b may aid in the phagocytosis process. The ingested microorganisms are killed by either oxidative ("respiratory burst," Figure 148.2) or oxygen-independent mechanisms.

*Quantitative and qualitative neutrophil defects*

Defects in neutrophil function may be due to inadequate cell numbers (quantitative) or to defective cell function (qualitative) (Table 148.6).

Peripheral neutrophil counts normally range from 1500–8000 cells/μl. The risk of infection increases as counts decrease below 1000/μl, and it increases dramatically at counts below 100/μl. The most common infecting organisms in patients with low neutrophil counts (neutropenia) include enteric gram-negative organisms *(Escherichia coli,* Enterobacter, *Pseudomonas), Staphylococcus aureus,* and fungi (e.g., *Candida albicans, Aspergillus).* The most common quantitative defect is due to bone marrow toxicity resulting from drugs or infection. Myelotoxicity is most frequently associated with cytotoxic chemotherapy but also may be due to other drugs, such as chloramphenicol, trimethoprim-sulfamethoxazole, and zidovudine.

Qualitative neutrophil defects are mostly hereditary and usually diagnosed in childhood. However, some disorders of neutrophil motility may be associated with autoimmune disorders, diabetes mellitus, alcoholism, or corticosteroid use. Alcohol also causes neutropenia, in addition to other negative effects, including depressed barrier defenses (depressed glottic reflex, aspiration) and decreased cell-mediated immunity. Corticosteroids, on the other hand, raise the neutrophil count (neutrophilia) due to demargination. They also can affect cell-mediated and humoral immunity (antibody formation).

## Specific Host Defenses

The specific host defenses consist of the cellular and humoral immune systems. These systems respond to specific antigens that are recalled through an immunologic memory of a preceding encounter with a specific organism.

### Cellular immunity

*T-lymphocyte development and function*

The cellular immune system is the linchpin of specific host responses. T-lymphocytes mature in the fetal thymus, where they develop distinct surface receptors, including those for antigens. The T-cell receptor is a heterodimeric protein that contains four parts (the variable, diversity, joining, and constant regions) and that recognizes a foreign antigen with its variable region structure. The variable region of the T cell, which is expressed in conjunction with the CD3 molecule, is capable of changes to match the multitude of antigens, although each T-lymphocyte will have only one variable region structure specific for only one antigen.

T-lymphocytes do not respond to foreign antigens by themselves, but do so in conjunction with **antigen-presenting cells** (Figure 148.3). Antigen-presenting cells are primarily macrophages or dendritic cells. After a foreign antigen (microbe) is engulfed by a macrophage, the antigen is processed and expressed on the surface of the macrophage in conjunction with **major histocompatibility complex (MHC) class II** molecules. The T-lymphocyte receptor recognizes the antigen–MHC complex with the help of the accessory molecules CD4 or CD8. After attachment of the receptor to the antigen–MHC complex, a **cytokine** signal (usually interleukin1

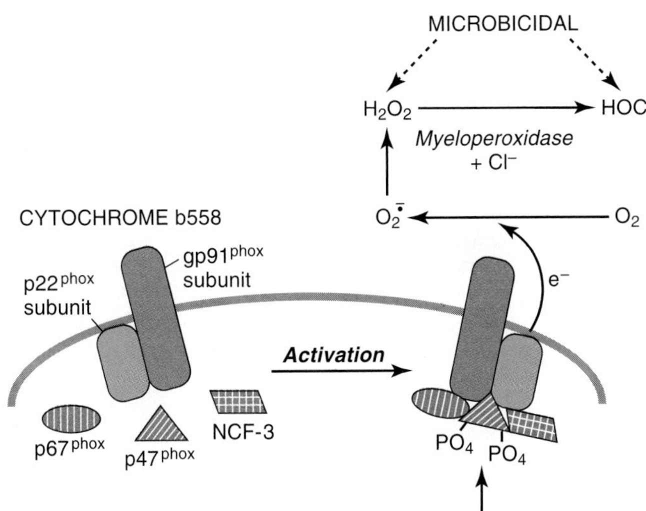


**FIGURE 148.2.** Components of the phagocytic cell respiratory burst. The cytochrome b558 is an integral membrane protein, and the p47phox, p67phox, and neutrophil cytosol factor 3 (NCF3) are cytoplasmic proteins. When activated, the p47phox is phosphorylated and translocates to the membrane together with the other cytoplasmic factors; NADPH oxidase is formed following interaction with the cytochrome. When electrons are transferred from NADPH to molecular oxygen, superoxide is formed, which breaks down into $H_2O_2$. Interaction with myeloperoxidase in the presence of chloride generates hypochlorous acid. The $H_2O_2$ and hypochlorous acid are extremely microbicidal.

(Reprinted with permission from: Gorbach SL, Bartlett JG, Blacklow NR (eds). Infectious Diseases. Philadelphia, PA: Saunders, 1992, p 49, Figure 7–3.)

**TABLE 148.6. Major Quantitative and Qualitative Neutrophil Defects**

| Quantitative Defects | Qualitative Defects |
|---|---|
| Marrow toxicity from drugs or infection | Chronic granulomatous disease |
| Autoimmune disorders | Chediak-Higashi syndrome |
| Acquired cyclic neutropenia | Myeloperoxidase deficiency |
| Inherited cyclic neutropenia | Specific granule deficiency |
| | Leukocyte adhesion deficiency |
| | Motility disorders |

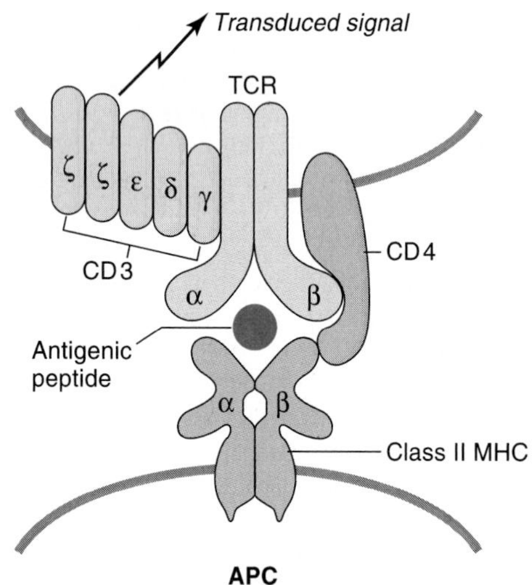


**FIGURE 148.3.** **Antigen recognition by and activation of T cells. Antigen is presented by an antigen-presenting cell (APC) in the form of peptide bound to MHC molecules on the APC surface, which in turn is recognized by the α/β-T-cell receptor (TCR). Most CD4 positive T cells recognize peptides bound to class II MHC, whereas most CD8 positive T cells recognize peptides bound to class I MHC. After recognition of antigen, the CD3 complex of proteins, which is associated with the α/β-TCR, produces an intracellular signal that causes T cell activation.**

(Reprinted with permission from: Lewis DB, Wilson CB. In Remington JS, Klein JO (eds). Infectious Diseases of the Fetus and Newborn Infant. 4th ed. Philadelphia, PA: Saunders, 1995, p 22.)

[IL1] produced by the macrophage) initiates a clonal expansion of the T-lymphocyte population.

T-lymphocytes respond usually by differentiating into one of three types:

- T-lymphocytes that express CD4 molecules are called **helper T cells.** These cells respond to foreign antigens by producing other cytokines, which regulate the immune response by other cells, including T-lymphocytes and B-lymphocytes.
- T-lymphocytes that express CD8 molecules are called **suppressor T cells.** These cells down-regulate the immune response once the offending organism is controlled. These CD8-expressing cells are also able to mature, through cytokine stimulation, into cytotoxic T-lymphocytes. Cytotoxic T-lymphocytes recognize antigen in conjunction with MHC class I antigens and are important in killing virus-infected cells.
- The third cell type, termed the **natural killer cells,** are lymphocytes with the ability to lyse target cells in a non–HLA-directed manner. They are important in resistance to tumors and viruses.

*Cellular immune defects*

Cellular immune defects may be either acquired or congenital (Table 148.7). The most widely recognized example of an acquired defect is infection with the human immunodeficiency virus (HIV). Other viruses (e.g., influenza, Epstein-Barr virus [infectious mononucleosis], and cytomegalovirus), fungi (e.g., coccidioidomycosis), tuberculosis, and parasites (e.g., *Toxoplasma*) also have been associated with depressed cellular immunity. Malignancies that suppress cellular immunity include Hodgkin disease and certain other lymphomas. Cellular immunity may also be depressed by pharmacologic agents (cytotoxic agents [e.g., cyclophosphamide and methotrexate], corticosteroids, and cyclosporin). Radiation therapy used for malignancies affects cellular immunity in a way similar to cytotoxic agents, by reducing lymphoid populations. Both nutrition and alcohol can inhibit cellular immune responses.

### Humoral immunity

*B-lymphocyte development and function*

**Antibodies** are antigen-specific immunoglobulins produced by B-lymphocytes and play several roles in

**TABLE 148.7. Defects in Cellular Immunity**

| Acquired Defects | Congenital Defects |
|---|---|
| Infections | DiGeorge syndrome |
| Malignancies | Severe combined immunodeficiency |
| Pharmacologic agents | |
| Radiation | |
| Nutrition | |
| Alcohol | |

protection against infection. At mucosal sites, in conjunction with nonspecific host defenses, local immunoglobulin (Ig) A antibody may inhibit attachment of pathogenic organisms. Systemically, antibody may interact with complement to enhance phagocytosis (opsonization) or to achieve complement-mediated cytolysis. Other cytolytic processes involving antibody include **antibody-dependent cellular cytotoxicity** (ADCC) and IgE mediated parasitic immunity. In these respective processes, lymphocytes or eosinophils, with the aid of antibodies, kill antigen-bearing target cells. Antibodies also act in neutralization processes, either with cell-free bacterial products (toxins) or cell-free viruses.

**TABLE 148.8. Immunoglobulin-Deficient States**

| Acquired Defects | Primary Deficiencies |
|---|---|
| Multiple myeloma | X-linked hypogammaglobulinemia |
| Chronic lymphocytic leukemia | Ataxia-telangiectasia |
| Severe burns | Wiskott-Aldrich syndrome |
| Nephrotic syndrome | Common variable hypogammaglobulinemia |
| Splenectomy | Selective IgA deficiency |
| HIV infection | |

*Immunoglobulin-deficient states*

Several major causes of immunoglobulin-deficient states are listed in Table 148.8. In some malignancies, such as multiple myeloma and chronic lymphocytic leukemia, expansion of malignant cells occurs at the expense of normal immunoglobulin production. Primary B-cell deficiencies usually have an X-linked inheritance pattern and are discovered in infancy or early childhood, although common variable hypogammaglobulinemia and selective IgA deficiency are more likely to be discovered or treated in adulthood.

# CHAPTER 149 MANIFESTATIONS OF INFECTION

Although some infectious diseases are classically localized to an organ system with a textbook list of symptoms, their severity can vary greatly, depending on the resistance pattern of the organism and the sensitivity of the host. For instance, herpes zoster presents classically in a dermatomal pattern (Figure 149.1), but it may present in a widely disseminated form in an immunosuppressed host.

Infections also may involve one or several organ systems. The clinician must therefore be aware of not only the range of symptoms that might suggest a particular organ system infection, but also the combination of symptoms and signs that are consistent with a multisystemic infectious disorder. Certain simple **historical features** may suggest an infection. For example, acute rhinorrhea and a sore throat in the winter months might be consistent with a rhinovirus-associated rhinitis. Dysuria and frequency in a non–sexually active woman would be consistent with *Escherichia coli*–associated cystitis. Abrupt onset of fever above 103°F with cough, purulent sputum, and pleuritic pain is characteristic of pneumococcal pneumonia.

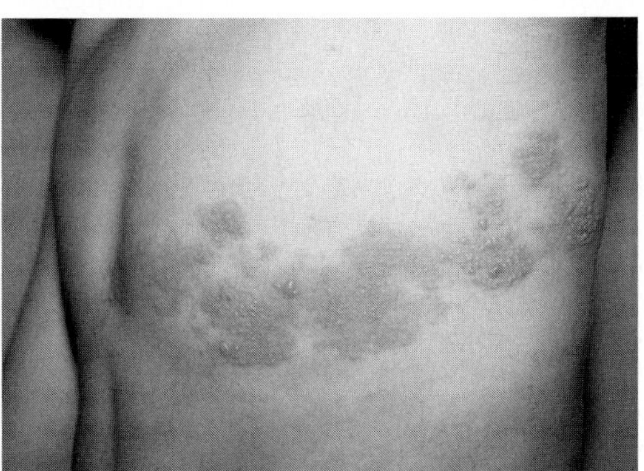

**FIGURE 149.1.** Herpes zoster (shingles) showing a dermatomal distribution.

On the other hand, many other infectious diseases are more difficult to diagnose, and the diagnosis rests on a compilation of historical factors, physical findings, and clues from the laboratory. In some cases, despite all the information, there still may be confusion as to whether the particular clinical presentation is consistent with an infectious disorder, a connective tissue disease, or a neoplasm.

## Patient History

In all diseases, the history is important in establishing a list of possible entities for the differential diagnosis; this is particularly true in infectious diseases. Important historical considerations include geographic factors, which determine the range of potential infectious exposure, and several host factors, which determine the susceptibility of an individual to a particular infection.

### Geographic and environmental factors

Geographic factors can be divided roughly into travel considerations and local geographic or environmental concerns. **Travel** is an ever increasing concern, given the ease and frequency of international travel and immigration. Many infectious disorders, especially parasitic infections, are endemic outside the United States. For example, a life-long resident of Wisconsin with new onset of seizures would not likely have neurocysticercosis as the cause. However, this etiology would be considered in a patient from, or with an appropriate travel history to, Mexico, Africa, or South America. Similarly, febrile episodes in a patient from Wisconsin would not warrant a consideration of malaria in the differential diagnosis, unless that person had recently returned from places endemic for malaria (e.g., Africa, South America, Southeast Asia).

One must next consider **local geographic or environmental factors,** which include place of residence, place of work, and other environmental factors, such as contact with a person having a transmissible infection. **Place of residence** includes both the geographic region and dwelling where the person resides. Local geography is an important consideration for certain infections. For example, a febrile pulmonary process in a patient in the southwestern United States could represent coccidioidomycosis, whereas the same in the Mississippi River Valley could be blastomycosis.

The other important consideration in place of residence is the type of dwelling in which a person resides or is housed at the time the infection occurs. In the etiology for a pneumonia, for example, the differential diagnosis differs for a community-acquired versus hospital-acquired or nursing home–acquired (nosocomial) pneumonia. In general, patients who are institutionalized have a greater risk for exposure to more resistant pathogens, and those pathogens may cause a more severe illness. Other examples involving the place of residence would include a building with a contaminated air-conditioning system, leading to legionellosis, or incarceration, predisposing to tuberculosis or penicillin-resistant pneumococcal infection.

The **place of employment** sometimes may hold important clues as to the nature of the infection. The differential diagnosis of a systemic febrile illness in abattoir workers (slaughterhouse workers), for example, includes brucellosis, a diagnosis that is unusual in most other occupations. A febrile illness with nausea and right-upper-quadrant tenderness might represent acute hepatitis or cholecystitis with cholangitis in a typical patient, but if the individual were a day-care worker, acute hepatitis A would be more likely, especially if other cases have recently occurred in such a facility. Attendance at a school or day-care center and **avocational activities** (hobbies) should also be considered.

Other **environmental concerns** might include sporadic exposures to infectious diseases that should be pursued in the history. Certain diseases, especially common respiratory illnesses, can spread easily among family members. Therefore, eliciting a history of illnesses, such as streptococcal pharyngitis or mycoplasmal pneumonia, in another family member is an important finding and underscores the importance of known contacts in evaluating many infectious disorders. Although many infectious diseases are sporadic, in others, contact tracing is important in the workup (e.g., sexually transmitted diseases, hepatitis, influenza, and tuberculosis).

### Host-specific factors

The type of host is of utmost importance in assessing the manifestations of infection, both in terms of the entities to be considered and the potential severity of the infection. **Age** (e.g., hepatitis A is generally seen in younger people), **coexisting disease** processes (e.g., cirrhosis is a major risk factor for tuberculous peritonitis), and **immune status** (e.g., HIV infection or immunosuppressive drug therapy) are key considerations.

Infections in immunocompromised patients are outlined in more detail in other chapters of this section. Suffice it to say that the **type of defect in host defense** affects the differential diagnosis, certain conditions being more likely depending on the defect. A patient with a pulmonary infiltrate will arouse certain considerations, such as *Streptococcus pneumoniae* or *Haemophilus influenzae* pneumonia, but if the same patient is receiving high-dose corticosteroids for some period of time, other pathogens may need to be considered, including *Aspergillus* or *Mycobacterium tuberculosis.*

Certain infections also may be much more fulminant in an immunocompromised host. For example, a pneumococcal pneumonia may assume a lobar configuration in many instances, but the splenectomy patient may manifest bacteremic pneumococcal disease with severe septic shock and disseminated intravascular coagulation.

## Physical Signs

Organisms encountered by the host from the environment either are killed, or colonize the skin or mucosal surfaces and become part of the normal flora, or are pathogenic. Pathogenic microorganisms either cause a local inflammatory response or invade the tissues. However, even bacteria that are part of the normal flora may, in the right circumstances, cause infection (e.g., cystitis or pyelonephritis due to *Escherichia coli*). It is the inflammatory response in the tissues that leads to the physical signs or manifestations of infection.

**Manifestations due to inflammatory responses**

Particular pathogenic microorganisms may be fairly organ-specific, having **tropism** to certain tissues, whereas other pathogens have a more varied effect. Some organisms, in fact, are named for their target organ. For example, the family of hepatitis viruses all have tropism for the liver. Hepatitis viruses, therefore, predictably cause an inflammatory reaction in the liver with the attendant physical signs of hepatic enlargement and tenderness.

Other organisms also may affect one organ system most commonly but, not uncommonly, will affect other organ systems, too. For example, *Streptococcus pneumoniae* most commonly causes pneumonia (with bronchial breath sounds, rales, or egophony; lobar consolidation may or may not be present) although it may also cause meningitis (with signs of meningeal irritation, such as nuchal rigidity) and infection of other organs.

Infectious disorders are not always simple to categorize in terms of etiology and may manifest with constellations of findings that do not immediately suggest the diagnosis. For instance, endocarditis, which may be due to a number of organisms, can manifest acutely with fever and a new murmur, or the physical manifestations may be more subacute, with fever, malaise, and weight loss. The acute presentation is most likely associated with *Staphylococcus aureus,* whereas the subacute process is often due to the viridans streptococci. The findings with the subacute presentation, however, may or may not immediately suggest endocarditis, and they might initially suggest a malignancy or a collagen vascular disorder.

Both the microbe and host influence the physical manifestations of an infection. Compared with the normal host, the immunocompromised patient not only tends to have more severe physical manifestations of infection in the involved organ system, but also suffers an enhanced risk of disseminated infection. A striking example mentioned earlier is pneumococcal sepsis and disseminated intravascular coagulation seen in the splenectomized patient. The clinician must be especially diligent, careful, and complete when examining these patients so that no clues are overlooked.

**General signs: fever**

Fever is one of the first physical clues to a potential infectious disease. Although some localized infections, such as rhinitis, urethritis, or vaginitis, are usually not accompanied by fever, most patients with a significant infection of an organ system will be febrile. Fever is by no means specific to infection, because patients with malignancy or connective tissue disorders can also be febrile. The clinician should also be aware that hypothermia can occasionally accompany a significant infection, such as gram-negative sepsis, and portends a poor prognosis (see Chapter 153).

### Laboratory Findings

A complete blood count is frequently obtained to support the possible diagnosis of infection. Bacterial infections commonly, but not invariably, manifest with an elevation of the total leukocyte count with an increase in immature forms (bands)—"a shift to the left." Similarly, a lymphocytosis may correlate with a viral infection (e.g., influenza), and eosinophilia may correlate with helminthic infections (e.g., strongyloidiasis). Anemia of chronic disease may be related to an underlying subacute or chronic infection. Numerous other laboratory tests are also used to support the diagnosis of infection, as described in more detail in subsequent chapters.

# CHAPTER 150 LABORATORY DIAGNOSIS OF INFECTIOUS DISEASES

Although knowledge of the patterns of infections in different clinical settings is essential in the diagnosis and differential diagnosis of specific infections, the laboratory is vital in helping make specific therapeutic decisions. The laboratory diagnosis of infectious diseases first involves proper collection and processing of specimens, so that the results can be interpreted appropriately. The importance of good communication with the microbiology laboratory cannot be overemphasized. Information about the suspected disease process helps the laboratory personnel to process the specimens properly.

Once in the laboratory, the specimen is subjected to various types of direct visualization (e.g., microscopy) and culture, as directed by the clinician. Some organisms are fastidious or grow poorly on culture, but they may elicit certain types of immunologic responses in the host that can be assayed. The clinician needs a clinical understanding of the possible tests in order to know which tests will give the best information in a particular clinical setting.

## Collection of Specimens

Before specimens are collected from a patient with a suspected infection, it is important to remember that the body has a normal microbial flora on all of its mucocutaneous surfaces. In sampling most normally sterile sites (e.g., blood, cerebrospinal fluid), one must traverse this normally nonsterile skin or mucosal surface to access the sites of collection. Avoiding contamination by normal flora requires that special attention be given to maintaining a sterile procedure.

When specimen collection is contemplated, there also should be a reason for obtaining a particular specimen. The practice of so-called "pan-culturing," or culturing all potentially available sites, is appropriate in some, but not all, settings. Especially with cultures of nonsterile sites, one must always anticipate what potential culture results the microbiology laboratory may return so that interpretation can be made in view of the clinical setting.

### Culture of blood and other normally sterile sites

1. A disinfectant is applied to the skin for at least 30 seconds before blood cultures are drawn.
2. The samples should be obtained percutaneously. Because skin contaminants may interfere with the results of blood cultures, at least two separate blood cultures should be obtained for adequate interpretation.
3. When preparing blood cultures, microbiology laboratories routinely use systems that allow for the detection of both aerobes and anaerobes. Thus, it is necessary to inoculate blood into two separate bottles or devices.
4. For suspected peritonitis, peritoneal fluid should be inoculated directly into blood culture bottles at the bedside.
5. In evaluating catheter-related sepsis, some routinely obtain one culture through the catheter and one percutaneously. However, catheters are often colonized, and these colonizing organisms will grow on the culture. When catheter-related sepsis is suspected, the catheter should be removed and its distal 2 inches aseptically clipped into a sterile container, which then should be sent to the laboratory for quantitative culture. In addition, blood cultures should be obtained.
6. After the samples have been obtained, they should be properly labeled and expeditiously transported to the laboratory. Repeating the test, especially from sterile sites (e.g., lumbar puncture), may not be easily accomplished.

### Culture of normally nonsterile sites

The practice of "pan-culturing" is especially problematic when obtaining cultures from nonsterile sites. The clinician must anticipate what potential culture results the microbiology laboratory may return and order tests as dictated by the clinical setting. For example, culturing of respiratory secretions frequently yields numerous organisms; deciphering the finding of organisms in the sputum (i.e., which ones are pathogenic versus simply colonizing) then rests with the clinician.

To make optimum use of culture results from nonsterile sites, the physician should exercise care in collecting specimens. Laboratories often screen samples from nonsterile sites, and samples that do not meet certain requirements for appropriate culture may be rejected.

1. Because the mouth cannot be sterilized to avoid contamination, the patient should be encouraged to expectorate after a deep cough. To be suitable for culturing, the sputum specimen should contain a predominance of neutrophils and, if at all, scant epithelial cells (see sputum examination, Chapter 216).
2. For urine samples obtained from women, the best sample is a midstream specimen procured after meatal cleaning. A urine specimen may need to be leukocyte esterase–positive before being processed for culture by the laboratory.
3. Sampling of open wounds, such as decubitus ulcers, is especially difficult due to the presence of numerous colonizing organisms. If a soft tissue abscess is present or suspected, the abscess material should be aspirated into a syringe through a sterile needle. The needle is then removed, the syringe is capped with a sterile cap, and the whole syringe then sent to the laboratory.
4. It is important to inform the laboratory of the suspected diagnosis.
5. Body sites that have an abundant endogenous microbial flora (e.g., oral cavity, vagina) should not be sampled for anaerobic pathogens. Sputum, because of passage through the oral cavity during expectoration, suffers from this limitation.
6. Use of appropriate transport media is important in delivery of samples to the microbiology laboratory. Pus or purulent material is best injected into

anaerobic transport vials; syringes used for aspiration are best avoided for transportation of specimens because of risk of needle-stick injury and diffusion of oxygen across the plastic syringe walls.

## Direct Examination of Specimens

### Microscopy

Pathogenic organisms can often be directly visualized through a **light microscope** in a variety of clinical specimens. A number of stains are used in the laboratory, the most common being the Gram stain.

*Gram staining*

Because using the Gram stain is a common procedure, the clinician should be familiar with its performance and interpretation (Table 150.1). The Gram stain is helpful in identifying organisms through their staining characteristics, and also through the morphology (see Figure 155.1).

Bacterial organisms are classified as either **gram-positive** or **gram-negative,** meaning they enhance with the stain or not. Organisms are further classified by their shape, either round **(cocci)** or rodlike **(bacilli).** Gram-positive cocci, for instance, indicate staphylococcal or streptococcal species. Gram-positive organisms may be further differentiated visually by their relationship to each other. Staphylococci tend to **cluster,** whereas streptococci tend to form **chains.** Similarly, gram-negative organisms can be differentiated somewhat by their morphology. For example, abundant, small, gram-negative coccobacilli might indicate *Haemophilus influenzae.*

### Other staining techniques

Because the Gram stain does not stain all types of organisms, other stains or visualization methods are helpful in selected circumstances.

**TABLE 150.1. Gram Stain Procedure**

1. Air dry and heat fix specimen on a glass slide.
2. Flood the slide with crystal violet and allow to sit for 10–15 sec.
3. Rinse the slide with water.
4. Flood the slide with Gram iodine and allow to sit for 10–15 sec.
5. Rinse the slide with water.
6. Decolorize with 95% ethyl alcohol until blue color just disappears from thin portions of the smear.
7. Rinse the slide immediately with water.
8. Flood the slide with safranin for 10–15 sec.
9. Rinse the slide with water.
10. Air dry and examine.

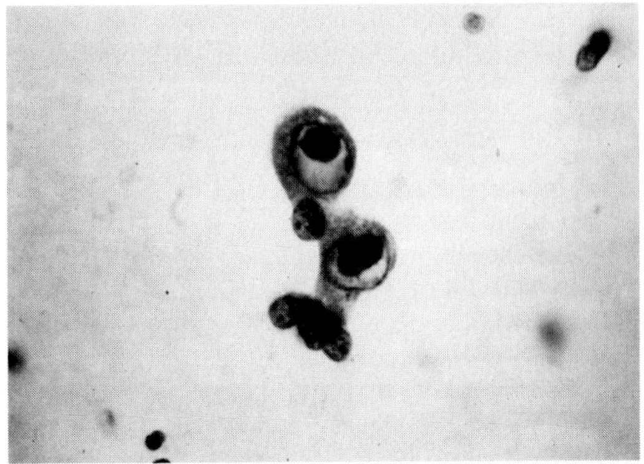

**FIGURE 150.1.** Intranuclear inclusion bodies of cytomegalovirus seen on hematoxylin-eosin staining.

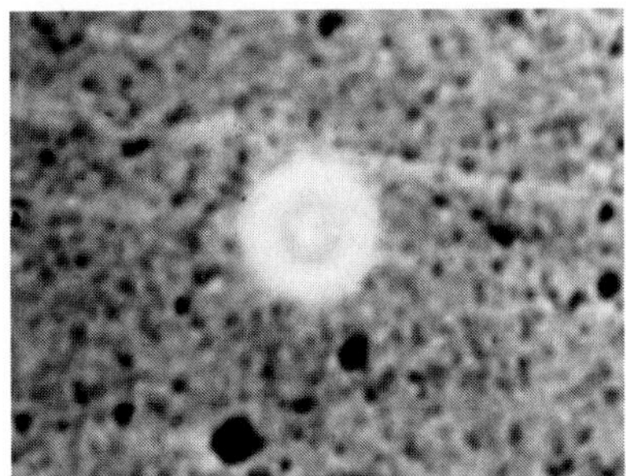

**FIGURE 150.2.** India ink preparation showing the capsule of *Cryptococcus neoformans.*

Mycobacteria are best seen with an **acid-fast stain,** on which they appear pink and beaded. These organisms may be difficult to detect, and an experienced technologist is needed to examine the specimen. Most bacteria, except for *Nocardia* and some *Legionella* species, do not retain the pink dye of the acid-fast stain.

Viral inclusion bodies (e.g., cytomegalovirus) may be seen by direct examination of smears stained with **hematoxylin and eosin** (Figure 150.1).

A **potassium hydroxide** (KOH) preparation helps to identify fungi in selected specimens (see Figure 223.1) A drop of KOH applied to a slide containing sputum, skin, or oral or vaginal scrapings destroys bacteria and mucus but allows the fungal elements to be visualized.

Other methods of staining fungi include the **india ink** preparation, which, for example, will stain the capsule of *Cryptococcus neoformans* (Figure 150.2). Fungal elements also can be seen in biopsied tissue samples with the use of other stains (Gomori or methenamine silver) and can indicate invasion of these tissues by the fungus.

Direct visualization using a variety of stains is also commonly used when examining for intestinal parasites.

TABLE 150.2. Examples of Antigenic Immunoassays

| Disease/Microbe | Sample/Specimen | Immunoassay |
|---|---|---|
| **Meningitis** | | |
| • *Streptococcus pneumoniae* | Cerebrospinal fluid | Latex agglutination |
| • *Haemophilus influenzae* | | |
| • *Neisseria meningitidis* | | |
| • *Cryptococcus neoformans* | | |
| **Respiratory tract/pneumonia** | | |
| • Respiratory syncytial virus | Respiratory secretion | DFA |
| • *Bordetella pertussis* | Respiratory secretion/urine | DFA/RIA |
| • *Legionella pneumophila* | | |
| **Hepatitis** | | |
| • Hepatitis B virus | Serum | RIA |
| **Sexually transmitted diseases** | | |
| • Herpes simplex virus | Vesicle fluid or exudate | ELISA |
| • *Chlamydia trachomatis* | Exudate | ELISA |
| • *Treponema pallidum* | Serum | Fluorescent assay (FTAABS) |
| **Diarrhea/colitis** | | |
| • *Clostridium difficile* | Stool | ELISA |

DFA = direct fluorescent antibody; ELISA = enzyme-linked immunosorbent assay; FTAABS = fluorescent treponemal antibody absorption; RIA = radio immunoassay.

Extensive experience is required in interpreting wet preparations of stool samples.

*Dark-field microscopy*

Another method of directly visualizing organisms, besides light microscopy, is with the use of a special dark-field microscope. Spirochetes are best seen by this method. Motile spirochetes, for example, can be seen in the exudate from lesions in primary syphilis. Because these spirochetes are infectious, gloves should be worn when obtaining samples for dark-field examination.

**Immunoassay techniques**

For rapid diagnosis of infections, various immunoassays have been developed that rely on antibody reactions to unique antigens of the suspected organisms (Table 150.2). The immunoassay is a standard method for diagnosing several diseases (e.g., syphilis, *Treponema pallidum*) or active carrier states (e.g., hepatitis B), because these organisms are not cultivable in clinical laboratories.

## Microbial Isolation and Identification (Culture)

Although it is helpful to visualize microorganisms directly, a definitive diagnosis of most bacterial infections resides with standard **culture** methods. Clinical specimens are cultured in appropriate media, and microbial identification is based on numerous factors, such as selective growth in media containing certain nutrients, the appearance of the colonies, presence of hemolytic properties, the odor produced, and the microscopic appearance. A number of biochemical tests are also used, especially with gram-negative bacteria.

Some microbes grow slowly or have selective culture requirements (fastidious), causing delays in diagnosis (e.g., *Mycobacterium tuberculosis*). Good communication with the laboratory is critical in obtaining optimal culture results. If the laboratory is aware that a particular pathogen is suspected (e.g., *Legionella* pneumonia), then appropriate selective plates will be used.

**Antibiotic susceptibility** of bacteria, testing the bacteria for antibiotic resistance, is pivotal in making or altering an antibiotic selection in particular clinical settings. Susceptibility is determined by disk diffusion testing on plates or by testing serial dilutions of an antibiotic against a known inoculum of organism. A **minimum bactericidal concentration** (MBC) and **minimum inhibitory concentration** (MIC) are thus determined. If the culture medium is a broth, subcultures are made to a medium free of antimicrobial agent and reincubated to determine the MBC, which is the smallest concentration of the antimicrobial agent that on subculture fails to show growth of the microbe. The MIC is the minimum amount of the test agent that will inhibit visible growth of the microorganism. Determining mycobacterial sensitivities is limited to specialized laboratories, and determining fungal or viral susceptibilities is limited to research facilities. Molecular techniques, such as **DNA probes** and **polymerase chain reaction (PCR)**, are sensitive and specific techniques for identifying pathogens. In PCR, the microbial DNA is amplified to make adequate nucleotide sequences. A specially labeled oligonucleotide ("gene probe") is then used to mark the results of the PCR, thus affording their detection. PCR/DNA probe is highly specific and extremely sensitive. Specific DNA probes and PCR assays are presently available for many infectious agents, most notably *Mycobacterium tuberculosis* and HIV. DNA probes are also quite useful in the investigation of outbreaks of infections, often enabling identification of the source.

# CHAPTER 151 MICROBES THAT CAUSE INFECTION

The field of infectious diseases is ever-changing. New organisms are discovered in association with established clinical syndromes (e.g., *Helicobacter pylori* in peptic ulcer disease), but also with relatively new syndromes (e.g., HIV and AIDS, hantavirus pulmonary syndrome). In addition, familiar organisms sometimes reemerge (e.g., tuberculosis) or develop new antimicrobial resistance, making treatment more difficult (e.g., multidrug-resistant tuberculosis and vancomycin-resistant enterococcus).

## Viruses

Viruses are composed of either RNA or DNA (which may be single-stranded or double-stranded). Although they usually have an outer protein coat (capsid), some viruses have an outer lipid envelope as well.

### Viral replication

Because viruses encode only a restricted number of proteins, they depend on the machinery of the host cell to accomplish their replication cycle. To initiate the replication cycle, viruses must first enter the host cell, via a process known as **endocytosis.** Some viruses use specific host receptors to accomplish this goal (e.g., CD4 receptors for HIV).

Inside the cell, a process of viral uncoating (a series of changes to the viral capsid) follows that allows replication of viral genetic material. **DNA viruses** enter the host nucleus, where they use host enzymes to produce mRNA. The mRNA encodes a DNA polymerase that is used for viral replication. **RNA viruses,** however, replicate through an RNA polymerase. (An exception to this pattern of RNA replication involves the retroviruses, which use a virally encoded reverse transcriptase to make a DNA copy of the viral RNA. This DNA integrates into the host DNA and becomes latent. After a period of time, host machinery is used to make viral proteins.) After sufficient viral components are synthesized, they are assembled and released to infect other cells.

### Pathogenic effects

Viruses may have several effects on the host cell. They may integrate into the host genome and remain dormant, or they can redirect the host genome into a malignant transformation. When activated in a replicative mode, the virus may be lytic to the host cell, or through transformed surface markers, the host cell may be damaged through self-directed immunologic mechanisms.

### Viral taxonomy

There are six families of **DNA viruses,** as listed in Table 151.1. Of this group, the herpesvirus family is probably the most ubiquitous and well-recognized clin-

**TABLE 151.1. Families of Human DNA Viruses**

| Family | Examples of Viruses | Examples of Clinical Manifestations |
|---|---|---|
| Herpesviridae | Herpes simplex virus | Mucocutaneous ulcers |
| | Varicella-zoster virus | Chicken pox |
| | Epstein-Barr virus | Infectious mononucleosis |
| | Cytomegalovirus | Disseminated infections in immunocompromised hosts |
| | Human herpesvirus 6 | Roseola |
| Adenoviridae | Adenovirus | Respiratory tract infection |
| Hepadnaviridae | Hepatitis B virus | Hepatitis |
| Parvoviridae | Parvovirus B19 | Erythema infectiosum, red cell aplasia |
| Papovaviridae | Papilloma virus | Warts, genital warts |
| | Polyoma virus | Progressive multifocal leukoencephalopathy |
| Poxviridae | Molluscum contagiosum | Molluscum contagiosum |

**TABLE 151.2. Families of Human RNA Viruses**

| Family | Examples of Viruses | Examples of Clinical Manifestations |
|---|---|---|
| Picornaviridae | Rhinovirus | Common cold |
| | Hepatitis A | Acute hepatitis |
| | Coxsackievirus | Aseptic meningitis |
| | ECHO virus | Aseptic meningitis |
| | Poliovirus | Poliomyelitis |
| Orthomyxoviridae | Influenza virus | Respiratory tract infection |
| Paramyxoviridae | Parainfluenza virus | Respiratory tract infection |
| | Respiratory syncytial virus | Respiratory tract infection |
| | Mumps virus | Parotitis |
| | Measles virus | Rubeola (measles) |
| Retroviridae | Human immunodeficiency virus | AIDS |
| Reoviridae | Rotavirus | Diarrhea |
| Togaviridae | Rubella virus | Rubella (German measles) |
| | Alphavirus | Eastern equine encephalitis |
| Flaviviridae | Dengue virus | Dengue fever |
| | Yellow fever virus | Yellow fever |
| | St. Louis encephalitis virus | Encephalitis |
| Bunyaviridae | California encephalitis virus | Encephalitis |
| | Hantavirus | Hantavirus pulmonary syndrome |
| Arenaviridae | Lassa fever virus | Hemorrhagic fever |
| Filoviridae | Ebola virus | Hemorrhagic fever |
| Coronaviridae | Coronavirus | Upper respiratory tract infection |
| Rhabdoviridae | Rabies virus | Rabies |

ically. These viruses can become latent after a primary infection and reappear at a later time (e.g., recurrent mucocutaneous ulcers from herpes simplex or herpes zoster manifesting years after chickenpox). These recrudescent infections may be especially severe in immunocompromised patients. Examples of **RNA viruses** pathogenic for humans are shown in Table 151.2.

## Bacteria

Bacteria are a diverse group of prokaryotic organisms, classified according to structural properties, production of enzymes or toxins, metabolic activities, and molecular homology. The Gram stain, which highlights differences in cell wall structure, is commonly used to separate large groups of bacteria (Table 151.3).

### Gram-positive bacteria

Pathogenic **gram-positive cocci** are from the genera *Staphylococcus*, *Streptococcus*, and Enterococcus. Morphology may help to distinguish among these organisms, as staphylococci tend to form clusters, whereas streptococci and enterococci tend to form chains.

Based on the coagulase test, staphylococci may be categorized as coagulase-positive or coagulase-negative. *Staphylococcus aureus* is pathogenic by tissue invasion (e.g., abscess) or by toxin production (e.g., toxic shock syndrome, food poisoning, scalded skin syndrome). Antibiotic sensitivity of *S. aureus* should be tested, because methicillin-resistant strains are becoming more common.

Streptococci, which typically appear in pairs or chains, are divided into several serogroups (A through H and K through V). Streptococcal infections in humans most often result from groups A, B, C, D, and G. Organisms in group D have been reclassified recently into enterococci, which cause genitourinary and wound infections as well as endocarditis. In recent years, the emergence of vancomycin-resistant enterococcus (VRE) has been of major concern. *Streptococcus pneumoniae,* an important member of the streptococcal group, causes pneumonia, meningitis, and bacteremia. Although most strains remain sensitive to penicillin, the incidence of resistance of *S. pneumoniae* to penicillin and other antibiotics has dramatically risen in recent times.

Of the **gram-positive bacilli,** the more common, clinically significant organisms are *Corynebacterium*, *Bacillus* species, and *Listeria monocytogenes.* Corynebacteria are club-shaped on Gram staining and have a "Chinese letter" configuration on microscopic examination.

### Gram-negative bacteria

Clinically significant disease due to **gram-negative cocci** most commonly involves two species of *Neisseria*,

*N. gonorrhoeae* and *N. meningitidis*. Both are fastidious in their growth requirements and are identified biochemically. Another organism, *Moraxella (Branhamella) catarrhalis,* has become an increasingly common cause of lower respiratory tract infections in the elderly and in patients with underlying chronic bronchitis and emphysema.

**The gram-negative bacilli** comprise a large group of pathogens, the largest group of which is the Enterobacteriaceae family (see Table 151.3). The lipopolysaccharide component of Enterobacteriaceae causes many of the major features of sepsis. *Helicobacter pylori* is an important cause of peptic ulcer disease.

### Anaerobic bacteria

Anaerobic bacteria are the predominant commensal organisms at many body sites, including the oral cavity, intestine, and female genital tract. Infection may be associated with a defect in host defenses (e.g., trauma, diabetes) or with invasion by exogenous organisms (e.g., tetanus). Some common anaerobic pathogens are listed in Table 151.4.

### Spirochetes

Spirochetes are spiral or coiled organisms that are best observed under a dark-field microscope. They are difficult to isolate on artificial media, and demonstration of the organism or serologic tests are usually required to

**TABLE 151.4. Important Pathogenic Anaerobic Bacteria**

**Gram-positive cocci**
*Peptostreptococcus* spp.
*Peptococcus* spp.
**Gram-positive bacilli**
*Clostridium* spp. (*perfringens, septicum, difficile, tetani, botulinum*)
*Lactobacillus* spp.
*Propionibacterium* spp.
**Gram-negative bacilli**
*Bacteroides fragilis*
Other *Bacteroides*
*Prevotella* spp.
*Fusobacterium* spp.

**TABLE 151.3. Important Pathogenic Aerobic Bacteria and Some Typical Diseases They Produce**

| Gram-Positive Bacteria | | Gram-Negative Bacteria | |
|---|---|---|---|
| **Cocci** | | **Cocci** | |
| *Staphylococcus epidermidis* | UTI, bacteremia, catheter related infections | *Neisseria gonorrhoeae* | Urethritis, cervicitis, PID |
| | | *Neisseria meningitidis* | Meningitis |
| *Staphylococcus aureus* | Abscess, cellulitis, TSS | *Moraxella catarrhalis* | Bronchitis, pneumonitis |
| *Streptococcus viridans* | Endocarditis | | |
| *Streptococcus pneumoniae* | Pneumonia, meningitis | **Bacilli** | |
| *Streptococcus pyogenes* | Pharyngitis, pyoderma | Enterobacteriaceae (*Escherichia, Enterobacter, Klebsiella, Proteus*) *Serratia, Shigella, Salmonella* | UTI, sepsis, respiratory infection, gastroenteritis |
| Enterococcus species | UTI, endocarditis | | |
| **Bacilli** | | | |
| *Corynebacteria* species | Diphtheria, pharyngitis, endocarditis | *Pseudomonas aeruginosa* | Pneumonia, bacteremia, UTI |
| *Bacillus* species | Meningitis, bacteremia | *Acinetobacter* species | UTI, bacteremia, respiratory infection |
| *Listeria monocytogenes* | Meningitis | *Haemophilus influenzae* | Respiratory infection |
| | | *Legionella pneumophila* | Pneumonia |
| | | *Helicobacter pylori* | Peptic ulcer disease |
| | | *Vibrio* species | Cholera, wound infections |
| | | *Campylobacter* species | Diarrhea |
| | | *Pasteurella multocida* | Infected dog/cat bites |
| | | *Bartonella* species | Cat scratch disease, bacteremia |
| | | *Brucella* species | Brucellosis |

PID = pelvic inflammatory disease; TSS = toxic shock syndrome; UTI = urinary tract infection.

confirm a diagnosis. Members of the genera *Treponema, Borrelia, Leptospira,* and *Spirillum* are known to cause human disease.

Treponema species pathogenic for humans include *T. pertenue, T. carateum,* and *T. pallidum. T. pallidum,* the agent of syphilis, is the most common treponeme encountered in this country. It should also be noted that treponemal species can be part of the normal oral flora. Two disease processes caused by species of *Borrelia* include Lyme disease, caused by *B. burgdorferi,* and relapsing fever. Louse-borne relapsing fever is caused by *B. recurrentis* and *B. hermsii,* and tick-borne relapsing fever is caused by *B. turicatae, B. parkeri,* and others.

Leptospirosis is due to two species of *Leptospira, L. interrogans* and *L. biflexa.* Humans are infected through accidental exposure to water or soil that is contaminated with urine of infected animals.

*Spirillum minor* causes rat bite fever.

### Mycobacteria

Clinically significant mycobacteria can be divided into tuberculous (infection caused by *Mycobacterium tuberculosis,* see Chapter 225) and nontuberculous mycobacteria (see Chapter 226). These mycobacteria share the property of acid-fast staining. Because of a high lipid content in the cell wall, acid-fast bacilli retain dye after acid-alcohol washing.

Leprosy due to *M. leprae* is a common worldwide infection but is uncommon in the United States. It is a chronic granulomatous disease primarily involving skin and peripheral nerves.

### Rickettsiae

The family Rickettsiae includes species from the genera *Rickettsia, Coxiella,* and *Ehrlichia.* All are obligate intracellular bacteria but with different replication cycles. The rickettsiae are engulfed by vascular endothelial cells (and sometimes smooth muscle cells), where they proliferate and damage the host cell. Rickettsial infections are transmitted by arthropods (tick, mite, body louse, or flea) from an animal host. The rickettsioses consist of a **spotted fever** group (e.g., Rocky Mountain spotted fever due to *R. rickettsii* and rickettsialpox due to *R. akari*) and a **typhus** group (e.g., *R. prowazekii* causing epidemic typhus and Brill-Zinsser disease and *R. typhi* causing murine typhus). Both groups have prominent fever and a rash that is mainly due to damage to small blood vessels.

*Coxiella burnetii* infects humans via aerosols of infected soil and dust; the clinical syndromes that result include Q fever and pneumonia.

Ehrlichiosis is a new syndrome similar to Rocky Mountain spotted fever. This febrile illness with transient leukopenia and thrombocytopenia is transmitted via a tick bite.

### Chlamydiae

Chlamydiae were originally thought to be viruses, but they contain both RNA and DNA and are able to divide. They depend on the host cell primarily for energy, because they do not generate their own adenosine triphosphate (ATP). The developmental cycle of chlamydia is fairly unique, with two morphologic forms. One form, the **elementary body,** is suited for extracellular life but does not divide. Once attached to and internalized by the host cell, the elementary body transforms into the metabolically active **reticulate body,** which is able to divide.

There are three chlamydial species that are pathogenic to humans, *C. pneumoniae, C. psittaci,* and *C. trachomatis. C. pneumoniae* is a cause of community-acquired pneumonia. *C. psittaci* produces a systemic disorder with prominent pulmonary findings, termed psittacosis (or ornithosis); exposure to parrots, parakeets, and several other types of birds is an important historical clue. *C. trachomatis* in adults causes primarily eye disease and genital tract disorders. Trachoma, a chronic follicular keratoconjunctivitis, is a common cause of blindness worldwide. Genital tract infection causes urethritis, epididymitis, pelvic inflammatory disease, proctitis, and lymphogranuloma venereum (LGV).

### Mycoplasmas

The mycoplasmas are small organisms like the chlamydiae and rickettsiae, yet they are able to replicate outside the host cell. Unlike bacteria, they lack a cell wall. Mycoplasmas are very difficult to culture.

The family Mycoplasmataceae contains several *Mycoplasma* species as well as *Ureaplasma urealyticum.* The ability of *Ureaplasma* to hydrolyze urea differentiates it from the *Mycoplasma.*

Most *Mycoplasma* species are not disease-producing and are found to colonize the upper respiratory or genital tracts. A few species are pathogenic: *M. pneumoniae, M. hominis, M. genitalium,* and *U. urealyticum.*

Mycoplasmas tend not to be invasive. They produce disease by local damage to mucosal cells or by sensitizing host membranes into autoimmune reactions. *M. pneumoniae* is an important cause of upper respiratory tract infections and, sometimes, pneumonia in young individuals. *M. hominis* is a cause of vaginitis and pelvic inflammatory disease and may cause disease outside of the genital tract. *U. urealyticum* is an important cause of nongonococcal urethritis. *M. genitalium,* although less common, has been implicated in both nongonococcal urethritis and pelvic inflammatory disease.

The structure of these organisms necessitate therapy with antibiotics active at sites other than the cell wall, such as macrolides or tetracyclines.

### Nocardia and *Actinomyces*

*Nocardia* and *Actinomyces* are higher bacteria in the order Actinomycetales. They are weakly gram-positive and resemble fungi with filamentous branching but lack cell walls characteristic of fungi. *Nocardia* species are aerobic and weakly acid-fast method), whereas *Actinomyces* species are anaerobic and not acid-fast.

*Nocardia* species are more commonly seen in patients with cellular immune defects, in whom they can produce a necrotizing pneumonia. Hematogenous dissemination to the brain is common. *Actinomyces* species, which are not usually opportunistic, are oral saprophytes that can penetrate intact tissues after local trauma or infection. Actinomycosis is usually a chronic infection that can extend to superficial tissues and form a soft tissue swelling that will subsequently drain. Drainage material contains characteristic "sulfur granules" visible on microscopy, which consist of clumps of organisms.

## Fungi

Fungi, unlike bacteria, have rigid cell walls composed of chitins and polysaccharides. Fungi are classified as yeasts or molds. **Yeasts** are round or oval and reproduce by a budding process, whereas **molds** are composed of tubular hyphal structures that grow by branching. Some fungi, called dimorphic fungi (e.g., *Histoplasma capsulatum, Blastomyces dermatitidis, Sporothrix schenckii, Coccidioides immitis*), grow in patients as yeasts but as molds in vitro at room temperatures.

Common pathogenic fungi and their clinical manifestations are listed in Table 151.5. However, many other presentations occur, particularly in immunosuppressed people. *Pneumocystis carinii, Candida albicans, H. capsulatum, Cryptococcus neoformans,* and *C. immitis* are prominent pathogens in AIDS.

**TABLE 151.5. Important Pathogenic Fungi**

| Fungi | Clinical Manifestations |
|---|---|
| *Candida albicans* | Esophagitis, bacteremia |
| *Pneumocystis carinii* | Pneumonia |
| *Histoplasma capsulatum* | Pneumonia, systemic dissemination (Chapter 221) |
| *Blastomyces dermatitidis* | Pneumonia, systemic dissemination (Chapter 223) |
| *Cryptococcus neoformans* | Pneumonia, meningitis |
| *Coccidioides immitis* | Pneumonia, meningitis (Chapter 222) |
| *Aspergillus* spp. | Pulmonary syndromes (Chapter 224) |
| *Sporothrix schenckii* | Cutaneous nodules |

## Parasites

Table 151.6 lists the important **protozoal parasites** and their major clinical manifestations. Most of these protozoa are recognized on microscopic examination of appropriate clinical specimens; however, *Microsporidium* requires electron microscopy for detection.

**TABLE 151.6. Important Protozoal Parasites**

| Examples of Protozoa | Clinical Manifestations |
|---|---|
| *Giardia lamblia* | Diarrhea |
| *Entamoeba histolytica* | Dysentery, hepatic abscess |
| *Toxoplasma gondii* | Brain and eye lesions (very important in AIDS) |
| *Trichomonas vaginalis* | Vaginitis |
| *Plasmodium* spp. | Malaria (consider in the returning traveler) |
| *Cryptosporidium parvum* | Diarrhea (very important in AIDS) |
| *Isospora belli* | Diarrhea (very important in AIDS) |
| *Enterocytozoon bieneusi (Microsporidium)* | Diarrhea |
| *Babesia microti* | Fever, hemolysis |
| *Trypanosoma* | Chagas disease, African sleeping sickness |

The **helminths** (worms), a greater problem in the developing parts of the world and not common in the United States, are divided into three categories: the **nematodes** (round worms), **trematodes** (flukes), and **cestodes** (tapeworms) (Table 151.7). Helminths commonly pass eggs in the intestinal tract, and the characteristic morphology of eggs on stool microscopy is helpful diagnostically. Eosinophilia, an immune response that is a helpful diagnostic sign, may be seen with helminths that have a tissue cycle.

**TABLE 151.7. Important Helminthic Parasites**

| Helminths | Clinical Manifestations |
|---|---|
| **Nematodes (roundworms)** | |
| *Trichuris trichiura* | Anemia, rectal prolapse (may be asymptomatic) |
| *Ascaris lumbricoides* | Intestinal obstruction |
| *Enterobius vermicularis* | Anal pruritus (pinworm) |
| *Strongyloides stercoralis* | Diarrhea, autoinfection (may be life-threatening in AIDS, lymphoma, or in the immunosuppressed) |
| *Trichinella spiralis* | Myositis (trichinosis) |
| **Trematodes (flukes)** | |
| *Schistosoma mansoni* | Hepatosplenomegaly |
| *Schistosoma haematobium* | Hematuria, hydronephrosis |
| *Clonorchis sinensis* | Biliary obstruction, cholangiocarcinoma |
| **Cestodes (tapeworms)** | |
| *Echinococcus granulosus* | Hepatic (hydatid) cysts |
| *Taenia saginata* | Abdominal cramps, bowel obstruction |
| *Taenia solium* | Seizure (neurocysticercosis) |
| *Diphyllobothrium latum* (fish tapeworm) | Megaloblastic anemia |

# CHAPTER 152 ANTIMICROBIAL THERAPY AND GENERAL PRINCIPLES OF ANTIBIOTIC USE

The past decade has witnessed the development of a plethora of antimicrobial agents. Although particularly applicable to antibiotics, this proliferation has also involved other antimicrobials, including antifungals, antimycobacterials, antivirals, and antiparasitic agents.

## Antibiotics

### Beta-lactam antibiotics

Beta-lactam (B-lactam) antibiotics constitute a large group, comprising the penicillins, cephalosporins, monobactams, and carbapenems (Table 152.1). All of these agents share the feature of the beta-lactam ring structure, and they inhibit bacterial growth through their action on cell wall synthesis (Table 152.2).

*Penicillins*

Despite the decline in the spectrum of activity of the natural penicillins (e.g., penicillin G) through decades of use, they are still the drug of choice for some streptococcal infections and are quite useful in other infections, including those by spirochetes and anaerobes. Through changes in various side chain structures, other types of penicillins have been developed with changed antimicrobial spectra, such as the penicillinase-resistant penicillins (e.g., methicillin or nafcillin, which have expanded coverage against *Staphylococcus aureus*) and the carboxypenicillins and ureidopenicillins (with broad spectrum gram-negative activity). Another way to overcome bacterial resistance and expand the antimicrobial spectrum of penicillins is to use a **beta-lactamase inhibitor** together with a penicillin (e.g., amoxicillin-clavulanic acid, ampicillin-sulbactam, piperacillin-tazobactam).

The most common side effects of the penicillins are hypersensitivity reactions. Fortunately, IgE–mediated anaphylactic reactions, the most serious of these, are uncommon. The more common morbilliform rashes are felt to be IgM-mediated or IgG-mediated.

*Cephalosporins*

Cephalosporins have been commonly categorized into four generations (see Table 152.1). **First-generation cephalosporins** are active primarily against gram-positive bacteria (*Staphylococcus aureus* and streptococci, but not enterococci). As a general rule, the later (more recent) generation cephalosporins cover gram-negative bacteria better, albeit at the loss of some of their gram-positive activity. Some of the **second-generation cephalosporins,** also called cefamycins (cefoxitin, cefotetan), also have enhanced activity against anaerobes. Ceftazidime, a **third-generation cephalosporin,** is particularly active against *Pseudomonas aeruginosa.*

Overall, these agents are well tolerated. Given the potential for cross-reactivity, patients with a history of an immediate hypersensitivity reaction to penicillin (or

**TABLE 152.1. Beta-lactam Antibiotics**

| | |
|---|---|
| **Penicillins** | |
| Natural penicillins | Penicillin G |
| Penicillinase-resistant penicillins | Methicillin, nafcillin |
| Aminopenicillins | Ampicillin, amoxicillin |
| Carboxypenicillins | Carbenicillin, ticarcillin |
| Ureidopenicillins | Mezlocillin, azlocillin, piperacillin |
| β-lactamase inhibitor combinations | Amoxicillin clavulanic acid, ticarcillin clavulanic acid, ampicillin sulbactam, piperacillin-tazobactam |
| **Cephalosporins** | |
| First generation | Cephalothin, cefazolin, cephalexin |
| Second generation | Cefamandole, cefuroxime, cefaclor, cefoxitin |
| Third generation | Cefotaxime, ceftizoxime, ceftriaxone, ceftazidime |
| Fourth generation | Cefpirome, cefepime |
| **Other β-lactams** | |
| Monobactams | Aztreonam |
| Carbapenems | Imipenem, meropenem |

those with skin reactivity to minor penicillin determinants) should avoid cephalosporins.

*Monobactams and carbapenems*

Other beta-lactam antibiotics include the monobactams **(aztreonam)** and carbapenems **(imipenem).** Although aztreonam is effective only against gram-negative organisms, imipenem covers gram-negative organisms and anaerobes. However, gram-positive bacteria, including *Corynebacterium bacillus (JK strain),* methicillin-resistant *Staphylococcus aureus,* and coagulase-negative staphylococci, should be considered as imipenem-resistant. Although imipenem is contraindicated in patients with a serious beta-lactam allergy, aztreonam is not. Seizures due to imipenem have been noted, especially in patients with underlying renal insufficiency or underlying CNS disease.

### Vancomycin, teicoplanin, and the streptogramins

Vancomycin, a glycopeptide antibiotic, is a cell-wall agent but acts at a different site from the beta-lactams. It has a narrow spectrum of activity, primarily against gram-positive bacteria. Susceptible organisms include streptococci, staphylococci (including methicillin-resistant *S. aureus*), enterococci (usually), and *Corynebacterium* JK bacillus. Among the anaerobes, most clostridia are sensitive.

**TABLE 152.2. Features of Commonly Used Antibiotics**

| Class of Drug | Site of Action | Major Side Effects | Major Activity or Spectrum of Organisms |
|---|---|---|---|
| β-lactams | Cell wall | Hypersensitivity, GI, hematologic, hepatotoxicity | Gram-positive (gram-negative with extended-spectrum agents) |
| Vancomycin | Cell wall | Infusion-related hypersensitivity, nephrotoxicity | Gram-positive (especially methicillin resistant *S. aureus*) |
| Aminoglycosides | Multiple ribosomal sites | Nephrotoxicity, ototoxicity | Gram-negative (synergistic for some gram-positive) |
| Macrolides (erythromycin) | 50S ribosomes | GI, hepatotoxicity | Gram-positive, *Mycoplasma, Chlamydia, Legionella, Campylobacter* |
| Clindamycin | 50S ribosomes | Hypersensitivity, GI | Gram-positive, anaerobes |
| Chloramphenicol | 50S ribosomes | Hematologic | Broad spectrum *Rickettsia, Salmonella* |
| Tetracycline | 30S ribosomes | Photosensitivity, GI | *Mycoplasma, Rickettsia, Chlamydia,* Lyme disease |
| Rifampin | RNA polymerase | GI, hepatotoxicity, hematologic | Gram-positive, *Neisseria, Legionella* |
| Trimethoprim-sulfamethoxazole | Nucleic acid synthesis | Hypersensitivity, hematologic, GI | *Nocardia, Listeria* |
| Quinolones (ciprofloxacin) | DNA gyrase | GI, hypersensitivity | Gram-negative |
| Nitroimidazoles (metronidazole) | DNA damage | CNS, GI | Anaerobes |

CNS = central nervous system; GI = gastrointestinal.

Vancomycin penetrates many tissues, but cerebrospinal fluid (CSF) levels are variable. Absorption after oral dosing is minimal. The most frequent adverse reaction is called the **"red man" syndrome.** It is due to histamine release from a rapid intravenous infusion and is reversible with slowing the infusion rate. The frequency of nephrotoxicity is low with vancomycin alone (5%) but increases (35%) with concomitant aminoglycoside use. Teicoplanin can be used as an alternative antibiotic in those patients with neutropenic or allergic reactions to vancomycin. Quinupristin-dalfopristin (Synercid), a streptogramin, is also effective for gram-positive bacteria, including VRE.

### Oxazolidinones

The oxazolidinones represent a newer class of antibiotics, and are represented by linezolid. They act at a unique early step in protein synthesis and are bacteriostatic. They have activity primarily against gram-positive bacteria, including MRSA, VRE, and penicillin-resistant *Streptococcus pneumoniae.*

### Aminoglycosides

Aminoglycosides, which contain an aminocyclitol ring linked to two or more amino sugar residues by glycosidic bonds, inhibit bacteria through their action on multiple ribosomal sites. Commonly used aminoglycosides include gentamicin, tobramycin, and amikacin. Although their spectrum covers primarily gram-negative organisms, they (mostly gentamicin) also act in synergy with a penicillin against enterococci, streptococci, and staphylococci (e.g., for endocarditis therapy). When used in serious gram-negative infections, they are usually combined with a beta-lactam antibiotic.

The volume of distribution of aminoglycosides is similar to extracellular fluid (due to low serum protein binding). They penetrate poorly into the CSF and are excreted renally. Primary toxicities include nephrotoxicity and ototoxicity, which can be cochlear or vestibular.

### Macrolides

Macrolides have macrocyclic ring structures and inhibit bacterial protein synthesis through 50S ribosomal binding. **Erythromycin** is the oldest macrolide, with clarithromycin and azithromycin being more recent additions. Erythromycin is active against gram-positive cocci (streptococci, *S. aureus*), certain gram-negative agents (e.g., *Neisseria gonorrhoeae, Campylobacter jejuni, Legionella pneumophila*), and others (e.g., *Chlamydia* and *Mycoplasma*). Newer macrolides have broader activity, particularly against *Haemophilus influenzae, Moraxella catarrhalis, Chlamydia trachomatis, Ureaplasma urealyticum* and some mycobacteria (e.g., *M. avium*).

Erythromycin toxicity commonly involves the gastrointestinal tract (vomiting, nausea, diarrhea) and hepatitis. These are less frequent with the newer agents.

### Clindamycin

Clindamycin is a lincosamide, similar to lincomycin. Its mechanism of action is similar to that of the macrolides. The spectrum of clindamycin includes gram-positive aerobes (streptococci, *S. aureus*), gram-positive and gram-negative anaerobes, and certain other agents (e.g., *Pneumocystis carinii*). It attains high concentrations in many tissues, including neutrophils, but does not cross the blood–brain barrier. Elimination is primarily by biliary excretion, and therefore, the dose is usually unaffected by renal failure.

Toxicity includes hypersensitivity reactions, hepatotoxicity, and colitis. Although pseudomembranous (*Clostridium difficile*) colitis was originally associated with clindamycin, other antibiotics also cause this complication.

### Chloramphenicol

Chloramphenicol is an older antibiotic that inhibits protein synthesis by binding to the 50S ribosome. Its spectrum of activity covers many aerobic gram-positive bacteria, some gram-negative bacteria (e.g., Enterobacteriaceae), anaerobes, rickettsiae, chlamydiae, and spirochetes. It is lipophilic and gains access into most body fluids, including CSF and the brain.

Chloramphenicol is primarily indicated for severe rickettsial disease, but may also be useful in severe salmonella or in CNS infections in patients with serious penicillin allergy, and may also be used in certain patients infected with VRE. Its hematologic toxicity relegates its use to these few indications. Bone marrow suppression is most commonly dose-dependent and reversible, but rarely is it idiosyncratic and irreversible.

### Tetracyclines

Tetracyclines are classified into three groups, short-acting (tetracycline, chlortetracycline, oxytetracycline), intermediate-acting (demeclocycline, methacycline), and long-acting (doxycycline, minocycline). They all inhibit protein synthesis through inhibition of the 30S ribosomal subunit.

The emergence of bacterial resistance has limited the use of tetracyclines to specified situations, which include spirochetal (drug of choice in early Lyme disease), rickettsial, ehrlichial, and chlamydial (genital) infections. Tetracyclines are considered alternate agents in atypical pneumonias (e.g., *Mycoplasma pneumoniae, Chlamydia* species, *Legionella pneumophila*) and are combined with other antibiotics for some less common infections (e.g., brucellosis, melioidosis, tularemia, and plague).

Tetracyclines accumulate in the skin and can cause phototoxicity; patients receiving them should therefore be warned to avoid direct sunlight. Because tetracyclines stain teeth, they should be avoided in children and pregnant women.

### Rifampin

Rifampin, a rifamycin, inhibits DNA-dependent RNA polymerase. Although its principal use has been against mycobacteria, rifampin's broader range of activity is not well emphasized. Among gram-positive organisms, rifampin is most active against staphylococci, regardless of coagulase status. Covered gram-negative bacteria include *Neisseria*, *Haemophilus*, and *Legionella* species. It is active against anaerobes (e.g., *Clostridium* species), *Chlamydia*, and some fungi.

Rifampin resistance develops rapidly, and therefore, it should never be used alone (except for short term prophylaxis). Orange-red discoloration of the urine is the most common side effect. Others include gastrointestinal upset, hepatitis, interstitial nephritis, and bone marrow toxicity.

### Trimethoprim-sulfamethoxazole

Trimethoprim-sulfamethoxazole (TMPSMX) is a drug combination that acts at sequential steps in folinic acid synthesis. The fixed 1:5 ratio of drugs in TMPSMX gives maximum synergistic inhibition.

TMPSMX covers numerous gram-positive and gram-negative organisms. Other susceptible organisms include *Nocardia asteroides, Chlamydia trachomatis, Listeria monocytogenes, Pneumocystis carinii,* and some mycobacteria. There are many clinical indications for TMPSMX, including treatment of infections of the respiratory and urinary tracts, sinusitis, and gastrointestinal infections (salmonellosis and traveler's diarrhea), as well as treatment and prevention of *Pneumocystis carinii* pneumonia in immunosuppressed patients. They also appear to reduce the relapses in Wegener granulomatosis. However, adverse reactions can be limiting and are particularly frequent in AIDS patients. Those most commonly seen include cutaneous, hematologic, and gastrointestinal reactions. Drug resistance to TMP-SMX is being encountered increasingly.

### Quinolones

The quinolones have been available for more than 30 years, but over the past several years, many new agents have been introduced. They inhibit DNA gyrases that are needed to supercoil bacterial DNA during replication. With a wide volume of distribution, they attain high concentrations in neutrophils; however, CSF levels are only low to negligible. Excretion is by renal and/or hepatic mechanisms.

The quinolones are particularly active against gram-negative bacteria. Evolving resistance and lack of reliability against gram-positives limited the early quinolones, such as ciprofloxacin. The newer fluoroquinolones, (e.g., levofloxacin, grepafloxacin, moxifloxacin, or gatifloxacin) have a better spectrum against these organisms, especially streptococci.

Quinolones are generally well tolerated. Toxicity includes cutaneous hypersensitivity, phototoxicity, gastrointestinal, and CNS reactions. Some quinolones (e.g., ciprofloxacin) prolong theophylline clearance. All quinolones are presently considered unsafe in pregnancy. Because of several instances of arthropathy among children treated with quinolones, their use in the pediatric age group is best avoided.

### Nitroimidazoles

**Metronidazole,** the most widely used nitroimidazole, undergoes intracellular reductive activation into reactive intermediates that interact with microbial DNA. The drug is widely distributed in tissues, including CSF, and is metabolized in the liver. It is primarily effective against anaerobes, especially *Bacteroides* species, and some parasites (e.g., *Entamoeba histolytica, Trichomonas vaginalis and Giardia lamblia*). Side effects are infrequent, but seizures, cerebellar ataxia, and peripheral neuropathy are the most serious.

## Antimycobacterial Agents

The most commonly prescribed agents against *Mycobacterium tuberculosis* are isoniazid, rifampin, pyrazinamide, and ethambutol (see Chapter 218 and Table 152.3). **Isoniazid** (INH) is believed to act on the cell wall (mycolic acid) or nucleic acids. **Pyrazinamide** has an unknown mechanism of action. It enters the CSF well and is active intracellularly, where mycobacteria reside. **Ethambutol** inhibits nucleic acid synthesis. Significant CSF levels are reached only with inflamed

**TABLE 152.3. Antimycobacterial Agents**

| Antituberculosis Agents | Drugs for Other Mycobacterial Diseases* |
|---|---|
| Isoniazid | Macrolides |
| Rifampin | Quinolones |
| Pyrazinamide | Rifamycins (Rifabutin) |
| Ethambutol | Clofazimine |
| Streptomycin | Amikacin |
| Capreomycin | |
| Ethionamide | |
| Cycloserine | |
| Thiacetazone | |
| Quinolones | |

*Primarily *M. avium* complex infections.

meninges. It is excreted solely through the kidneys, a matter of importance in renal failure. Drug resistance is an important problem in the therapy of tuberculosis (see Chapter 225).

The drugs used for **other mycobacterial diseases** are primarily the macrolides and quinolones, although many of the antituberculous agents are also useful (see Chapter 226). **Rifabutin** is more active than rifampin against strains of *M. avium* complex. **Clofazimine** directly binds to DNA, inhibiting transcription. It is lipophilic and does not enter the CSF. Originally an antileprosy drug, its primary use now is in *M. avium* infections.

## Antiviral Drugs

The features of commonly used antiviral agents are shown in Table 152.4. **Acyclovir** has a high affinity for herpesviruses and a low cellular toxicity. Epstein-Barr virus and cytomegalovirus (CMV) are affected somewhat (although minimally). **Foscarnet** inhibits DNA polymerase by a different mechanism and does not require activation, thus covering acyclovir-resistant, thymidine kinase mutants. Its advantage over **ganciclovir** is its lack of bone marrow toxicity; however, renal toxicity is observed with foscarnet.

**Amantadine** is useful both in preventing and treating influenza A infections. **Rimantadine** compares well in efficacy with amantidine but with fewer side effects. Newer agents, oseltamivir and zanamivir cover both influenza A and B. **Ribavirin,** a nucleoside analog, is used in aerosolized form.

Criteria for the appropriate use of the anti-HIV agents continue to evolve. Other anti-HIV agents are currently being developed and tested (see Chapter 165).

**TABLE 152.4. Features of Commonly Used Antiviral Agents**

| Agent/Class | Major Side Effects/Toxicity | Major Activity |
|---|---|---|
| **Guanosine analogs (inhibit DNA polymerase)** | | |
| Acyclovir | Crystallizes in renal tubules, GI | Herpes simplex, herpes zoster |
| Ganciclovir | Hematologic | CMV, herpes viruses |
| Foscarnet | Renal dysfunction | CMV, herpes viruses |
| Ribavirin | Bronchospasm | RSV |
| Valcyclovir | CNS, GI | Varicella zoster |
| Famcyclovir | CNS, GI | Varicella zoster |
| Cidofovir | Renal dysfunction | CMV |
| **Reverse transcriptase inhibitors (nucleoside)** | | |
| Zidovudine (AZT) | Headache, hematologic, nausea/vomiting | HIV |
| Didanosine (ddI) | Dermatologic, GI, peripheral neuropathy | HIV |
| Zalcitabine (ddC) | Dermatologic, GI, peripheral neuropathy | HIV |
| Stavudine (d4T) | Hepatitis, peripheral neuropathy | HIV |
| Lamivudine (3TC) | Hematologic, GI | HIV |
| Abacavir | Hypersensitivity reaction | HIV |
| **Reverse transcriptase inhibitors (nonnucleoside)** | | |
| Nevirapine | Dermatologic, GI | HIV |
| Delavirdine | Dermatologic, GI, CNS, hematologic | HIV |
| Efavirenz | Headache, rash | HIV |
| **Protease inhibitors** | | |
| Saquinavir | Nausea/vomiting, diarrhea, abdominal discomfort, rash, endocrine | HIV |
| Ritonavir | Nausea/vomiting, diarrhea, taste disturbance, paresthesia, hypertriglyceridemia, drug interactions | HIV |
| Indinavir | Nephrolithiasis, asymptomatic hyperbilirubinemia | HIV |
| Nelfinavir | Diarrhea | HIV |
| Amprenavir | Nausea, vomiting, rash | HIV |
| Lopinavir/ritonavir | Diarrhea | HIV |
| **Others (? inhibits viral uncoating/assembly)** | | |
| Amantadine | Confusion, hallucination | Influenza A |
| Rimantadine | Confusion, hallucination | Influenza A |
| Oseltamivir | Nausea | Influenza A & B |
| Zanamivir | Bronchospasm | Influenza A & B |

CMV = cytomegalovirus; CNS = central nervous system; GI = gastrointestinal; RSV = respiratory syncytial virus.

TABLE 152.5. Features of Commonly Used Antifungals

| | Site of Action | Major Side Effects | Major Activity |
|---|---|---|---|
| Amphotericin B | Binds ergosterol (disrupts fungal cytoplasmic membrane) | Azotemia, renal tubular acidosis, hypokalemia, hypomagnesemia | Serious or life-threatening fungal disease |
| Ketoconazole | Interacts with C14 alpha demethylase enzyme, affecting ergosterol synthesis<br>Absorption affected by gastric hypochlorhydria | GI, hepatotoxic depresses serum testosterone level and ACTH stimulated cortisol level | Mucocutaneous candidiasis<br>Nonmeningeal blastomycosis<br>Coccidioidomycosis<br>Cryptococcosis<br>Histoplasmosis |
| Miconazole | Same site of action as ketoconazole | Fever, GI, hematologic | *Pseudallescheria boydii* |
| Fluconazole | Same site of action as ketoconazole<br>Absorption less affected by gastric hypochlorhydria<br>Better CSF levels<br>Not metabolized<br>Renally excreted | GI, hepatotoxic | Oropharyngeal candidiasis<br>Hepatosplenic candidiasis<br>Cryptococcal meningitis (maintenance therapy) |
| Itraconazole | Same site of action as ketoconazole<br>Low CSF levels<br>Absorption needs gastric acidity | GI, hepatotoxic | Nonmeningeal histoplasmosis<br>Blastomycosis<br>Coccidioidomycosis |
| Caspofungin | Cell wall | GI, hepatotoxicity | Aspergillus |
| Vorconazole | Similar to fluconazole | GI, hepatotoxicity | Candida species, Aspergillus |
| Flucytosine | Cytosine analog (inhibits DNA and protein synthesis) | GI, hepatotoxic hematologic | Cryptococcal meningitis<br>Invasive candidiasis (with amphotericin B)<br>Monotherapy for candiduria |
| Pentamidine isethionate | ?Interferes with nuclear metabolism | Hypotension, renal insufficiency, hypoglycemia | *Pneumocystis carinii* |

ACTH = adrenocorticotropic hormone; CSF = cerebrospinal fluid; GI = gastrointestinal.

## Antifungal Agents

Features of commonly used antifungals are listed in Table 152.5. **Amphotericin B** and lipid-complexed **amphotericin B** are the drugs of choice for serious, life-threatening, invasive fungal infections, such as those caused by *Aspergillus* or *Mucorales* species (see Chapter 220). **Fluconazole** is better absorbed in the presence of gastric hypochlorhydria (a common problem in AIDS patients) than **ketoconazole.** In cryptococcal meningitis in AIDS, fluconazole should be used instead of amphotericin B only in less severe disease. **Itraconazole** is metabolized in the liver. Its bioavailability is improved when it is taken with food. Neither fluconazole or itraconazole adversely affects steroidogenesis. Toxicity of amphotericin B is discussed in Chapter 220.

## Antiparasitic Drugs

Commonly used antiparasitic drugs, including those used for protozoal and helminthic infections, are listed in Table 152.6. Most of these parasitic diseases are uncommon in the United States. However, protozoal infections (e.g., *Cryptosporidium*) are relatively frequent in AIDS patients.

## Principles of Antimicrobial Use

Considering the management of a febrile patient as an example, it is easy to see that the treatment of infectious diseases often poses problems. Although many diverse conditions may cause fever, it is a common symptom of infection. Often, these infections are viral and lack any specific therapy. Even if the infection causing fever is bacterial, the organism and its sensitivity are unknown. Thus, antibiotics are often chosen empirically initially. Associated symptoms and signs may offer clues to the underlying process, and the setting of the infection (hospital versus community-acquired) may help. The immunocompetence of the host adds another dimension. Because microbial resistance patterns vary, local patterns of antimicrobial susceptibility assume an important role.

An allergy or concomitant pregnancy may contrain-

TABLE 152.6. Features of Commonly Used Antiparasitic Drugs

| Drug | Site of Action | Major Side Effects | Major Activity |
|---|---|---|---|
| Metronidazole | ?DNA damage | CNS, GI | *Entamoeba histolytica, Giardia lamblia, Trichomonas vaginalis* |
| Paromomycin (Humatin) | ?Ribosomes | Possible renal toxicity if absorbed (with ulcerative bowel lesions) | *Cryptosporidium, Entamoeba histolytica, Dientamoeba fragilis* |
| Chloroquine phosphate | Asexual erythrocyte forms | GI<br>CNS | Malaria |
| Mefloquine (Lariam) | Blocks invasion of sporozoites into red blood cells | Vomiting<br>Dizziness | Drug resistant malaria |
| Primaquine phosphate | Acts on hyphozoites in the liver | GI<br>Headache<br>Hemolytic anemia (in G6PD deficiency) | Malaria *(Plasmodium vivax, Plasmodium ovale)* |
| Mebendazole (Vermox) | Blocks glucose uptake by helminths | GI | Trichuriasis<br>Ascariasis<br>Enterobiasis |
| Thiabendazole (Mintezol) | Interferes with micro-tubule aggregation<br>Inhibits fumarate reductase | GI<br>Headache<br>Dizziness | Strongyloidiasis<br>Cutaneous and visceral larvae migrans |
| Praziquantel (Biltricide) | | Dizziness<br>Drowsiness | Schistosomiasis |

CNS = central nervous system; GI = gastrointestinal.

dicate an otherwise sound choice of an antibiotic. Although age, underlying disease (e.g., renal insufficiency), and concurrent medications may influence the selection, their implications for dosing and monitoring are profound. Infection in a patient who was previously on antibiotics might suggest resistance or a nonbacterial etiology. Cost may simply preclude certain agents, despite their better side effect profile and dosing interval than those of the cheaper agents. If home-based outpatient parenteral therapy is chosen, the reliability and meticulousness of the patient become important considerations.

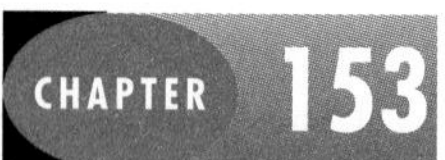


# FEVER AND FEVER OF UNKNOWN ORIGIN

## Body temperature homeostasis

### Normal body temperatures

Body temperature, normally set around 37°C (98.6°F), varies greatly. The **hypothalamus,** as the thermoregulatory center, maintains the temperature of internal organs and great vessels (aortic blood) between 37°C and 38°C. Esophageal and tympanic membrane temperatures are closest to that of aortic blood, but rectal and liver temperatures are about 0.5°C higher, ostensibly due to the high metabolism at both sites (fecal bacterial metabolism in the rectum). Oral and axillary temperatures are about 0.25°C and 1.0°C lower than core temperature, respectively. Skin temperature is even lower.

Body temperature is lowest in the early morning and highest in the late afternoon, with the amplitude of variation not usually exceeding 0.6°C (1°F). Individuals maintain body temperature at slightly above or below the so-called normal of 37°C (98.6°F). However, temperature exceeding 37.8°C (100.2°F) is considered abnormal.

### Normal temperature homeostasis

The normal body temperature is a balance between heat production and heat loss. The major source of heat is internal, from the body's basal metabolism. Digestion of food and muscular activity add to this basal heat generation. Under normal circumstances, radiant external heat is not a major source of heat, except in some tropical or industrial settings (e.g., working near a furnace). Heat loss, the other half of the equation, occurs primarily from the skin into the environment by radiative losses.

In order to maintain the most efficient temperature balance, the circulatory system must be intact and behavioral mechanisms and the autonomic nervous system must be functional. Behavioral mechanisms dictate how a person deals with ambient temperatures, both in terms of the clothing worn and the level of physical activity.

## Fever and Hyperthermia

**Mechanisms of fever and the body's response**

Fever is a body temperature above that seen in normal diurnal variation and is sustained by abnormal thermoregulatory mechanisms. The evolution of a febrile response is illustrated in Figure 153.1. The primary initiating event is the release of endogenous **pyrogens** (e.g., interleukins 1 and 6, interferon, tumor necrosis factor), which cause fever and a number of other systemic changes collectively called **acute phase responses.** These involve alterations in leukocytes, liver protein synthesis, serum iron, hormone metabolism, and other phenomena. These changes and the behavioral and autonomic responses are outlined in Table 153.1.

Fever has some beneficial effects, such as enhanced stress response modulated by glucocorticoids; increased neutrophil counts, opsonins, and complement components; as well as enhanced T-lymphocyte activation and expansion of lymphocyte clones.

**Hyperthermia**

Whereas fever is a regulated response, **hyperthermia** is dysregulated and caused by a dysfunction of excessive heat production, decreased heat loss, malfunction of the thermoregulatory center, or a combination of these. Several causes of hyperthermia are listed in Table 153.2.

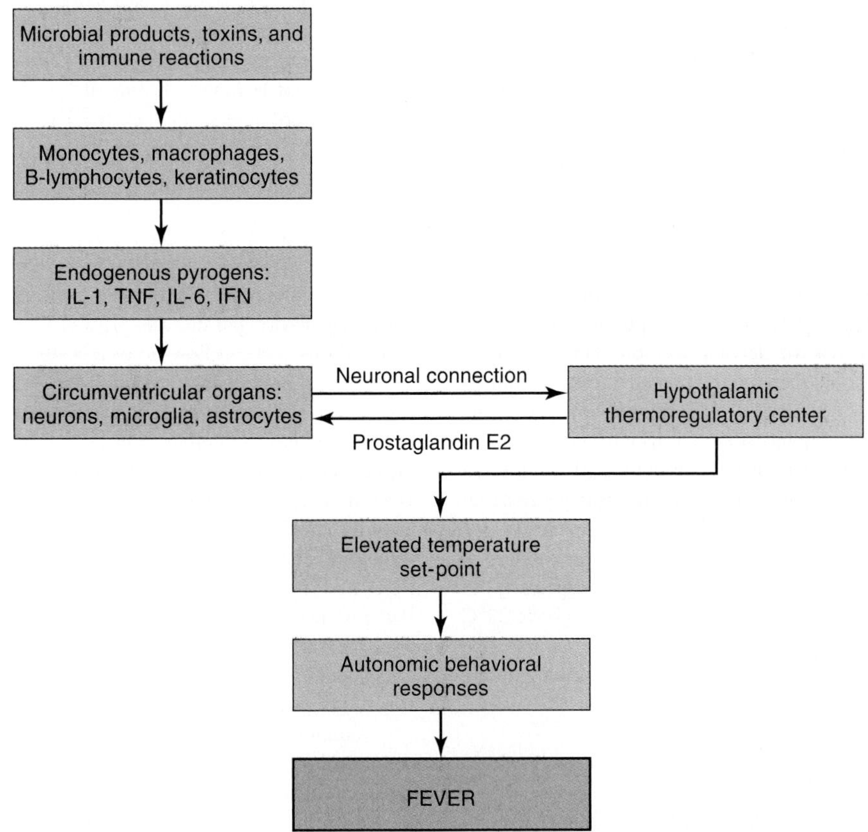


**FIGURE 153.1.** Pathogenesis of fever. Release of the endogenous pyrogens interleukin (IL), tumor necrosis factor (TNF), and interferon (IFN) is the primary initiating event, leading to the acute phase responses.

**TABLE 153.1. Systemic Aspects of Fever**

| Behavioral Responses | Acute Phase Responses | Autonomic |
|---|---|---|
| Seek warmth | ↑ WBC count | ↓ Skin blood flow |
| Anorexia | Liver protein changes | ↑ Pulse and blood pressure |
| Malaise | ↓ Serum iron | |
| | Altered hormone metabolism (glucocorticoids, aldosterone, vasopressin, growth hormone) | ↓ Sweating |

**TABLE 153.2. Causes of Hyperthermia**

| Excessive Heat Production | Diminished Heat Loss | Hypothalamic Dysfunction |
|---|---|---|
| Exertional hyperthermia | Heat stroke | Neuroleptic malignant syndrome |
| Status epilepticus | Neuroleptic malignant syndrome | Cerebrovascular accident |
| Thyrotoxicosis | Dehydration | Trauma |
| Pheochromocytoma | Autonomic dysfunction | Encephalitis |
| Malignant hyperthermia of anesthesia | | |
| Neuroleptic malignant syndrome | | |

### Management

Treatment of **fever** should focus more on the underlying cause and the effect(s) on the host rather than the temperature itself. For example, if a bacterial infection is the cause, the infection itself should be the focus of treatment. As antibiotics are given, the fever becomes the gauge of an appropriate response. Although fever may enhance the immunologic response, withholding antipyretics in viral respiratory infections has not yielded a clinical benefit.

Fever enhances oxygen consumption, and thus, persons with underlying cardiac or pulmonary diseases suffer a high risk of decompensation. Fever in these individuals should therefore be treated. **Acetaminophen** and **aspirin** are equally effective in lowering the hypothalamic set point. Although usually not a consideration in adults, aspirin is contraindicated in children with influenza and varicella because of the concern about Reye syndrome.

**Hyperthermia,** being an unregulated and abnormal response, generally requires treatment, especially in compromised individuals with temperatures above 39°C (102°F). The initiating event must, of course, be identified and reversed (e.g., discontinue exertion, initiate rehydration, etc.).

## ■ Fever of Unknown Origin

Whereas fever is a common manifestation of infection, sometimes the actual cause of the infection is difficult to identify. When this happens, the cause is often a transient viral illness. Occasionally, febrile states are more enduring and become difficult clinical problems. **Fever of unknown origin** (FUO) is defined as a prolonged febrile illness, lasting at least 3 weeks, with temperatures of at least 38.3°C (101°F) and no diagnosis after 1 week of evaluation in the hospital (or a similarly intensive outpatient workup).

### Etiology

In their classic 1961 article, Petersdorf and Beeson found that infections (36%), neoplastic disease (19%), and collagen-vascular diseases (13%) accounted for most cases of FUO. In a follow-up of this study, lasting from 1970–1980, infections accounted for 30%, neoplastic disease for 31%, and collagen-vascular diseases for 16% of cases. In these and other series, these three causes and miscellaneous entities account for 80–90% of FUO. In 10% of cases, no diagnosis is made.

Causes of FUO are listed in Table 153.3. Although **infections** continue to cause a substantial proportion of FUO, the types of infections have changed over the years. For instance, because blood cultures are commonly obtained early in a fever evaluation, bacterial endocarditis is currently a less common etiology of FUO than it was in the past.

Common infectious causes today include intra-abdominal (e.g., periappendiceal, hepatic, pericolic, perinephric, splenic) and pelvic abscesses. Dental or brain abscesses are less common. Tuberculosis is another common cause of FUO, particularly that involving extrapulmonary sites (e.g., renal, miliary, meningeal).

Less common infectious causes include enteric fever, HIV infection, osteomyelitis, toxoplasmosis, endocarditis due to fastidious or nonculturable organisms, relapsing fever, leptospirosis, malaria, and others.

Despite innovations in imaging, **neoplastic disease** remains a common cause of FUO. A number of primary or metastatic tumors cause fever, but some are more prone to do so than others. Occult lymphoma, particularly in the retroperitoneal area, may present with weight loss, anorexia, and fever, but usually without hepatosplenomegaly. Another common cause of FUO is renal cell carcinoma, which may be difficult to localize and diagnose because hematuria may be absent. Metastatic cancer to the liver is more common than primary liver tumors, but both may cause FUO. Usually, these pose no diagnostic problems unless liver function abnormalities are absent. Other neoplasms causing FUO include leukemias, pancreatic carcinoma, atrial myxoma, and CNS tumors.

Because of improved diagnostic techniques, certain **collagen vascular disorders** have become less common causes of FUO. For example, serologic testing has improved the detection of systemic lupus erythematosus (SLE) and rheumatoid arthritis (RA), reducing the likelihood of their presenting as an FUO. Both diseases, however, may still be rare causes of FUO. Many rheumatic and vasculitic diseases causing FUO lack specific diagnostic tests and thus require a diagnostic tissue biopsy. Examples include giant cell arteritis, periarteritis nodosa, and other vasculitides, such as Takayasu arteritis.

**TABLE 153.3. Causes of Fever of Unknown Origin**

| Common | Uncommon |
|---|---|
| **Infections** | **Collagen–Vascular Diseases** |
| Pelvic abscess | Giant cell arteritis |
| Intra-abdominal abscesses | Periarteritis nodosa |
| Extrapulmonary tuberculosis | Adult Still disease |
| **Miscellaneous** | Systemic lupus erythematosus |
| Drug fever | Rheumatoid arthritis |
| Alcoholic hepatitis | **Miscellaneous** |
| Cirrhosis | Familial Mediterranean fever |
| **Neoplastic diseases** | Hyperthyroidism |
| Renal cell carcinoma | Pheochromocytoma |
| Lymphoma | Subacute thyroiditis |
| Metastatic cancer to liver | Cyclic neutropenia |
| | Recurrent pulmonary embolism |
| | Factitious fever |

Drug fever tops the list of **miscellaneous causes** of FUO. Drugs usually cause fever by acting as a foreign antigen, sensitizing T cells, and leading to endogenous pyrogen release. Common offenders are antibiotics, particularly beta-lactams and sulfonamides, analgesics, diuretics, hypnotics, anticonvulsants, and antiarrhythmics. Intermittent eosinophilia and elevated liver enzyme levels may be associated. Some drugs (e.g., penicillin, isoniazid, salicylates, phenytoin, thiouracil, iodides, and methyldopa) are notable for causing fever without other clinical signs. Alcoholic and granulomatous hepatitis are liver diseases that cause FUO; these are confirmed by liver biopsy.

### Evaluation

Almost by definition, an FUO is a diagnostic challenge, even to an astute clinician. Close attention must be paid to the **history.** Recent abdominal or pelvic surgery (abscess), exposure to tuberculosis, history of a heart murmur (consideration of endocarditis), or history of high-risk behavior (unsuspected HIV infection) are examples of historical clues that require further exploration. In addition to an examination of specific complaints, contacts, or exposures, the patient's medications should be checked. Drug fever may follow even years of use, so that the diagnosis is usually made by exclusion (i.e., withdrawing the drug and observing).

A detailed **physical examination** should follow, especially pursuing clues from the history. Of particular importance are the cardiac, abdominal, lymph node, and musculoskeletal examinations. Useful findings are heart murmurs (endocarditis or atrial myxoma), hepatomegaly (some liver diseases require subsequent evaluation by liver biopsy), lymphadenopathy (infection or lymphoma), and spinal tenderness (vertebral osteomyelitis or epidural abscess).

Routine **laboratory studies,** such as a complete blood count, can give some clues. For instance, leukopenia might suggest lymphoma; eosinophilia may be consistent with lymphoma or drug fever; and a lymphocytosis might suggest infectious mononucleosis (especially if the peripheral smear shows atypical lymphocytes). Noninvasive **imaging tests** for FUO evaluation include ultrasound, computed tomography (CT), magnetic resonance imaging (MRI), and radionuclide scans. Abdominal or pelvic abscesses and retroperitoneal lymphoma are readily detected by CT or MRI.

In certain settings, **invasive tests** are required to make a specific diagnosis. Physical findings such as tenderness over the temporal arteries in the right clinical setting might suggest giant cell arteritis, but temporal artery biopsy is required for definitive diagnosis. In another setting, the finding of a liver mass on CT scan might indicate the need for a biopsy to direct definitive therapy.

# CHAPTER 154 UPPER RESPIRATORY TRACT INFECTIONS

## The Common Cold

The common cold is an extremely common, self-limited ailment, and is caused by several viruses, including rhinoviruses, coronaviruses, parainfluenza viruses, respiratory syncytial virus, and adenoviruses. Of these, the rhinoviruses (with 100 immunotypes) are the most frequent etiologic agents.

A year-round disease, the common cold is most frequent in the colder months of the year. Transmission, particularly with the rhinoviruses, is generally by close physical contact, and spread within families is common. Acquisition of new viral strains accounts for the frequency of repeat attacks (e.g., from the school or day-care setting into the family).

The incubation period of the common cold is generally 1–3 days. Usual symptoms are rhinorrhea (coryza), nasal stuffiness, sore throat, and cough. Adults are usually afebrile, but a slight fever may be present (fever is more frequent in children). Nasal discharge and glassy nasal membranes are the cardinal signs. The diagnosis is usually based on these symptoms and signs, although some confusion with allergic or vasomotor rhinitis is possible. Pharyngeal erythema and exudate are not associated with rhinovirus or coronavirus infections, and these signs may implicate other respiratory viruses (e.g., adenoviruses) or streptococcal pharyngitis.

Colds due to rhinoviruses do not involve destruction of nasal mucosal membranes. Instead, many inflammatory mediators are released (e.g., bradykinin, prostaglandin, histamine, interleukin1), and neurologic reflexes activated. Some of the other viruses may cause more destructive changes.

The common cold usually lasts about 1 week. Treatment is directed toward the control of symptoms, with decongestants, saline gargles, and cough suppressants being frequently used. Antibiotics should be avoided; however, because a small number of cases can lead to bacterial sinusitis or otitis media, the occurrence of either of these two entities after a cold will require appropriate antibiotics.

## Pharyngitis

Pharyngitis is an inflammation of the posterior pharyngeal membranes and their draining lymphatics, including the lymphatics of Waldeyer ring (adenoid, palatine, and lingual tonsils) and cervical lymph nodes. According to the extent of local inflammation, this condition is referred to by several terms, including **pharyngitis, tonsillitis,** or **pharyngotonsillitis.**

### Etiology

The etiology of pharyngitis is diverse, and infectious causes are listed in Table 154.1. Most common in the colder months of the year, pharyngitis is caused by infected aerosols or direct contact with infectious materials.

The most frequent infectious causes are group A streptococci *(Streptococcus pyogenes),* various respiratory viruses (e.g., adenoviruses, influenzaviruses, rhinoviruses), and Epstein-Barr virus. Whereas rhinoviruses have little cytopathic effect (sore throat associated with them appears to be through stimulation of nerve endings by inflammatory mediators), other respiratory viruses (adenoviruses and coxsackieviruses) and *S. pyogenes* do show evidence of invasion. *S. pyogenes* also produces a number of toxins and proteases that may be important pathologically.

### Clinical Features

Throat discomfort, variably described as irritation, scratchiness, or pain, is the cardinal symptom of pharyngitis. Pharyngeal mucosa and tonsils are usually hyperemic and edematous; there may or may not be a tonsillar exudate.

The major differential diagnosis of pharyngitis is between *S. pyogenes* and one of several other infectious causes (Table 154.2). In some of these illnesses (e.g., *S. pyogenes*), pharyngitis is the major pathologic process,

**TABLE 154.1. Infectious Causes of Pharyngotonsillitis**

| Bacteria | Viruses |
|---|---|
| Group A, B, C, and G streptococci | Rhinoviruses |
| *Neisseria gonorrhoeae* | Influenzaviruses |
| *Corynebacterium diphtheriae* | Adenoviruses |
| *Francisella tularensis* | Enteroviruses |
| Mixed anaerobes | Epstein-Barr virus |
| *Chlamydia trachomatis* | Herpes simplex virus |
| *Mycoplasma pneumoniae* | Human immunodeficiency virus |
| | **Fungi/Mycobacteria** |
| | *Candida* species |
| | *Mycobacterium tuberculosis* |

**TABLE 154.2. Clinical Features of Major Causes of Pharyngitis**

| Organism | Major Associated Clinical Symptoms | Clinical Syndrome or Associated Diseases |
|---|---|---|
| Group A streptococci (*S. pyogenes*) | Fever, tonsillar exudate, tender cervical nodes | May lead to rheumatic fever or glomerulonephritis |
| Rhinoviruses | Mild pharyngeal discomfort, rhinorrhea | Common cold |
| Influenzaviruses | Fever, myalgia, headache, cough | Influenza |
| Epstein-Barr virus | Fever, tonsillar exudate, tender cervical nodes, palatal petechiae, atypical lymphocytosis | Infectious mononucleosis |
| Coxsackie virus | Fever, soft palate vesicles | Herpangina |
| Adenoviruses | Fever, malaise, tonsillar exudate, conjunctivitis | Pharyngoconjunctival fever |
| Herpes simplex virus | Soft palate vesicles | Immunosuppression |
| *Candida albicans* | White plaquelike lesions | Predisposing factors include AIDS, corticosteroids, antibiotics |
| Mixed anaerobes and spirochetes | Membrane, tonsillar exudate, foul odor | Vincent's angina |

whereas in others (e.g., influenza and Epstein-Barr viruses), the pharyngitis is merely part of a more systemic illness. It is usually difficult to make an etiologic diagnosis of pharyngitis on clinical grounds alone. However, S. *pyogenes* is especially important to identify because of the potential sequelae of rheumatic fever or glomerulonephritis.

### Management

Because many of the viral causes of pharyngitis lack specific therapy, the primary diagnostic goal is to identify or exclude *S. pyogenes* through culture or a latex agglutination from a throat swab. The latex agglutination test will give results more quickly than culture; however, given its 5–30% false-negative rate, a negative latex agglutination result should be followed by a throat culture. Specific diagnostic tests for other treatable causes of pharyngitis (e.g., *Candida albicans,* herpes simplex virus) depend on the clinical setting.

Patients with a **group A streptococcal pharyngitis** should be given a 10 day course of oral penicillin or benzathine penicillin (1.2 million units intramuscularly). Penicillin-allergic patients may be given a macrolide. Depending on the circumstances, treatment may be given empirically while culture results are pending or may be started after the results are available; however, it should be instituted within 1 week of the onset of pharyngitis for effective prevention of rheumatic fever.

Treatment also prevents bacteremia and suppurative **complications,** which include peritonsillar abscess and, rarely, septic thrombophlebitis of the internal jugular vein with metastatic infection (postanginal sepsis). Suppurative complications feature prominent involvement by anaerobes.

In **recurrent tonsillitis,** poor compliance, microbial resistance, or reinfection are considerations. Amoxicillin-clavulanate, clindamycin, or metronidazole plus a macrolide may be tried.

## Laryngitis

Acute laryngitis, or inflammation of the vocal cords and surrounding structures, is manifested by hoarseness. **Infections** account for a significant number of cases, but an extremely common noninfectious disorder causing laryngitis is **gastroesophageal reflux disease.** Although all of the common respiratory viruses cause hoarseness, those most frequently associated are rhinoviruses, influenzaviruses, and adenoviruses.

Acute laryngitis is diagnosed when **dysphonia** (hoarseness) occurs in the setting of a respiratory viral illness. Laryngeal examination, if performed, reveals hyperemia and edema of the vocal cords.

**Treatment** consists of resting the voice and inhalation of cool, moistened air. Antibiotics are generally not beneficial, except in specific circumstances (e.g., group A streptococcal or *Corynebacterium diphtheriae* infections). Usually, the disease is mild and self-limited. If symptoms persist longer than 10–14 days, laryngoscopy should be performed to rule out a tumor, granulomatous process, or other chronic laryngeal pathology.

## Acute Bronchitis

### Etiology and Pathology

Acute bronchitis is due to inflammation of the tracheobronchial tree and is typically due to a viral infection (Table 154.3). With the viruses, bronchitis may be part of the clinical spectrum of both upper (e.g., rhinovirus) and lower (e.g., influenza) respiratory tract infections.

The degree of damage to the tracheobronchial tree varies with the agent involved; while usually minimal

**TABLE 154.3. Causes of Acute Bronchitis**

| Common | Uncommon |
|---|---|
| Influenzavirus | *Mycoplasma pneumoniae* |
| Adenovirus | *Bordetella pertussis* |
| Rhinovirus | *Chlamydia psittaci* |
| Coxsackie virus | *Chlamydia pneumoniae* |
| Respiratory syncytial virus | |
| Coronavirus | |
| Parainfluenza virus | |

with rhinovirus, it may be serious with influenzavirus. Hyperemia and excess bronchial secretions are generally present. Airway ciliary dysfunction and epithelial sloughing can occur in severe disease. Besides causing inflammation, some viruses (e.g., respiratory syncytial virus) may also enhance airway reactivity.

### Clinical Features and Management

Acute bronchitis is most common during the winter months. It is characterized by **dry cough** initially, but may become productive of purulent secretions later in the illness. Other symptoms, depending on the causative agent, include rhinorrhea and sore throat. Severe disease may be associated with substernal burning with breathing or with coughing (tracheitis). Fever is unusual with mild disease but is common with illness due to some viruses (influenzavirus, adenovirus) and *Mycoplasma pneumoniae.* Chest examination may reveal rhonchi. Signs of consolidation indicate progression to pneumonia.

Most individuals with acute bronchitis probably do not seek medical care. In more severe cases with persistent cough, other causes of a persistent cough such as pneumonia, congestive heart failure, asthma, and thromboembolic disease should be excluded. Cough may persist for several weeks, especially after respiratory syncytial virus or *M. pneumoniae* infection. Bacterial cultures of sputum are usually not helpful.

**Treatment** of acute bronchitis is generally symptomatic with over-the-counter cough remedies, although hospitalization may occasionally be needed in patients with underlying cardiac or respiratory disease. Antibiotics are not advocated routinely, as bronchitis is mostly a self-limited viral illness. However, some patients may benefit from them, particularly those with *M. pneumoniae* or *Bordetella pertussis.* In cases of influenza virus, there may be some benefit with early initiation of amantidine or rimantadine (influenza A); or newer agents, oseltamivir or zanamivir (influenza A or B).

In patients with underlying chronic obstructive lung disease, acute bronchitis may exacerbate the lung disease. Clinical features and treatment of such **acute exacerbations of chronic bronchitis** are discussed in Chapter 228.

# CHAPTER 155 PNEUMONIAS

### Pathogenesis and Pathology

Pneumonia is a common cause of morbidity and mortality among adults, particularly those with underlying diseases. It occurs by three possible routes: inhalation or aspiration of organisms, hematogenous spread, or contiguous spread of organisms.

Inhalation is by far the most common route. Whereas some inhaled organisms cause pneumonia because of their enhanced virulence (e.g., influenzavirus), others do so more easily after a breach in local host defenses. Aspiration pneumonia, an example of disrupted local defenses, is discussed in Chapter 246. Hematogenous pneumonia most typically follows right-sided *Staphylococcus aureus* endocarditis and, less commonly, complicated oral infections. Contiguous spread to the lungs may rarely follow peritonsillar abscess (with ensuing suppurative jugular venous thrombosis and septic pulmonary emboli), complicated oral or pharyngeal infections, or even intra-abdominal infection with spread across the diaphragm.

**Local mucosal defenses** (see Chapter 148) play a pivotal protective role against respiratory infections. Microbes are abundant in the mouth, but several local pulmonary defense mechanisms usually keep the lungs sterile below the carina. Corruption or transgression of these defenses causes pneumonia (Table 155.1).

Turbulent airflow through the nasal and oral passages traps larger particles (>10 μm), and the tracheobronchial mucociliary blanket traps most smaller ones (2 or 3 μm), which are then cleared from the airway by ciliary action and coughing. The smallest particles that penetrate into the alveoli are normally tackled by phagocytosis and humoral and cellular immune mechanisms.

When one or more of these defenses breaks down or becomes overwhelmed by a large load of organisms, it sets the stage for pneumonia (see Table 155.1). Such microbial invasion is met by release of inflammatory mediators (complement components and cytokines), which attract neutrophils for phagocytosis and killing of the invaders. Cell-mediated immune mechanisms play a

**TABLE 155.1. Pulmonary Defense Mechanisms and Pneumonia**

| Defense Mechanism | Examples of Breakdown |
|---|---|
| Trapping of particles in upper airway | Mechanical disruption (endotracheal intubation) |
| Mucociliary blanket | Hypoxia, cigarette smoke, viral infections, alcohol |
| Cough reflex and intact epiglottis | Drugs and alcohol, cerebrovascular accident, anesthesia, seizures |
| Phagocytic cells | Dysfunction (alcoholism), reduced numbers (neutropenia) |
| Humoral and cellular immunity | Hypogammaglobulinemia, multiple myeloma, AIDS |

prime role in the defense against certain organisms (e.g., *Legionella,* mycobacteria, viruses, *Cryptococcus neoformans,* and *Pneumocystis carinii*).

## Community-Acquired Pneumonia

### Etiology

Community-acquired pneumonia (CAP) is a common clinical entity that often presents difficulties with diagnosis and treatment. Frequently encountered pathogens in the immunocompetent host are listed in Table 155.2. Nosocomial (hospital-acquired) pneumonia and pneumonia in the immunocompromised patient are discussed subsequently.

A specific etiologic diagnosis of CAP is identified in only one half of cases. Some of these organisms (e.g., *Legionella pneumophila, Chlamydia pneumoniae*) are not easily isolated from sputum, which is an important reason that an etiologic diagnosis so often remains elusive. Other reasons contributing to the difficulty in isolating an etiology include the initiation of empiric antibiotics prior to culture, the inability to raise an adequate sputum sample (especially in the obtunded or elderly patient), and the difficulty in isolating organisms such as pneumococci even with an adequate sputum sample (i.e., containing abundant neutrophils).

In the preantibiotic era, most pneumonias (>80%) were due to ***Streptococcus pneumoniae***. Although *S. pneumoniae* remains an important cause of CAP (20–60%), its relative role has declined in recent years as newer pathogens have emerged.

### Clinical Features

Given the many etiologic agents in CAP, clues from the **medical and environmental history** and host factors (e.g., underlying disease) may be helpful in suggesting the potential causative agent (Table 155.3). **Symptoms** of

**TABLE 155.2. Causative Agents in Community-Acquired Pneumonia**

| Bacteria/bacteria-like Organisms | Viruses |
|---|---|
| *Streptococcus pneumoniae* | Influenzavirus |
| *Haemophilus influenzae* | Adenovirus |
| *Legionella pneumophila* | Respiratory syncytial virus |
| *Mycoplasma pneumoniae* | **Fungi** |
| *Chlamydia pneumoniae* | *Histoplasma capsulatum* |
| Anaerobes (oral) | *Coccidioides immitis* |
| *Moraxella catarrhalis* | *Blastomyces dermatitidis* |
| *Staphylococcus aureus* | *Cryptococcus neoformans* |
| Aerobic gram-negative Bacilli | |
| *Chlamydia psittaci* | |
| *Mycobacterium tuberculosis* | |

**TABLE 155.3. Environmental and Host Factors Suggesting a Microbial Etiology of Community-Acquired Pneumonia**

| Clinical Feature | Potential Etiology |
|---|---|
| **Environmental factors** | |
| Residence in or travel to: | |
| Southwestern United States | *Coccidioides immitis* |
| Mississippi, Ohio River Valleys | *Histoplasma capsulatum*<br>*Blastomyces dermatitidis* |
| Exposure to bat caves | *Histoplasma capsulatum* |
| Exposure to psittacine birds, turkeys | *Chlamydia psittaci* |
| Exposure to contaminated air-conditioning system | *Legionella pneumophila* |
| Prison, homeless shelter residence | *Streptococcus pneumoniae*<br>*Mycobacterium tuberculosis* |
| Outbreak in winter season | Influenza virus |
| Cluster cases | *Mycoplasma pneumoniae*<br>Influenza virus |
| **Host factors** | |
| Chronic obstructive lung disease | *Streptococcus pneumoniae*<br>*Haemophilus influenzae*<br>*Moraxella catarrhalis* |
| Diabetes mellitus | *Streptococcus pneumoniae*<br>*Staphylococcus aureus* |
| Alcoholism | *Streptococcus pneumoniae*<br>*Staphylococcus aureus*<br>*Klebsiella pneumoniae*<br>Oral anaerobes |
| Elderly age | *Streptococcus pneumoniae*<br>Influenza virus |
| Young, healthy adult | *Mycoplasma pneumoniae*<br>*Streptococcus pneumoniae*<br>Chlamydia |

pneumonia include fever, chills, pleuritic chest pain, and cough, which may or may not be productive. However, pneumonia presentations are protean. Confusion, gastrointestinal symptoms and hepatic dysfunction, once felt to be peculiar for *Legionella* pneumonia, are no longer considered unique to it.

Traditional teaching has held that pneumonias could be separated based on their presentation into "typical" and "atypical" types. **"Typical"** pneumonias resembled the classical presentation of pneumococcal pneumonia—acute onset, high fever, rigors, pleuritic chest pain, and productive cough. **"Atypical"** pneumonias exhibited a more subacute onset, generally nonproductive cough, and less ill-appearing patient, as exemplified by pneumonias due to *Mycoplasma pneumoniae, Legionella pneumophila,* and *Chlamydia pneumoniae.* More recent analysis has shown that an etiology for pneumonia cannot be reliably determined from the clinical presentation alone.

The **physical examination** is more useful in evaluating the extent of illness than in assessing an etiology. In some cases, lobar consolidation or diffuse disease may be predicted from the physical findings (see Table 215.5), whereas in other cases (e.g., *M. pneumoniae*), the physical findings underestimate the radiographic extent of illness ("x-ray looks worse than the patient"). Other helpful physical findings may include extrathoracic inflammation (e.g., meningitis associated with pneumococcal pneumonia) or skin rashes that may be consistent with a viral etiology.

## Diagnosis

Diagnostic evaluation beyond the history and physical examination includes a chest radiograph, analysis of pulmonary secretions (i.e., sputum), and other ancillary tests.

### Roentgenographic assessment

The **chest radiograph,** the gold standard for diagnosing pneumonia, must be interpreted in light of clinical findings. Other inflammatory conditions (e.g., connective tissue disorders), pulmonary edema and blood, and malignancy are often indistinguishable radiographically from pneumonia.

Common radiographic patterns in pneumonias by different etiologic agents are shown in Table 155.4. **Lobar consolidation** is classically due to bacterial pathogens such as *S. pneumoniae,* whereas **interstitial infiltrates** are due to viruses, *M. pneumoniae,* or *Pneumocystis carinii. P. carinii,* usually seen in profoundly immunosuppressed hosts, may present initially with interstitial infiltrates and without a prior diagnosis of HIV disease, thus generating diagnostic confusion with pneumonias due to other pathogens. **Cavitation** features prominently, but not invariably, in anaerobic, gram-negative, or tuberculous causes of pneumonia.

**TABLE 155.4. Community-Acquired Pneumonia: Chest X-ray Patterns**

| **Lobar consolidation** | **Interstitial** |
|---|---|
| *Streptococcus pneumoniae* | Viruses |
| *Haemophilus influenzae* | *Pneumocystis carinii* |
| *Moraxella catarrhalis* | *Mycoplasma pneumoniae* |
| *Mycoplasma pneumoniae* | *Chlamydia psittaci* |
| *Legionella pneumophila* | **Cavitation** |
| *Chlamydia pneumoniae* | Mixed aerobes/anaerobes |
| **Multifocal opacities** | Aerobic gram-negative bacilli |
| *Streptococcus pneumoniae* | *Mycobacterium tuberculosis* |
| *Legionella pneumophila* | |
| *Staphylococcus aureus* | |

Evaluation for **pleural fluid** is also important. Pneumonias usually associated with interstitial infiltrates (e.g., viruses, *M. pneumoniae*) rarely have significant pleural fluid. However, nearly 50% of patients with pneumococcal pneumonia show pleural effusions (frank empyema in only 1–5%).

### Examination of expectorated sputum

Pulmonary secretions can usually be analyzed noninvasively by examining expectorated sputum (see Chapter 216). Sputum Gram stain and culture pose many problems, despite their traditional role in the diagnosis of pneumonia. Patients may produce a poor sputum sample or none at all. Cultures take time and are therefore not helpful initially. Although *S. pneumoniae* and *Haemophilus influenzae* often can be pathogens, their presence on culture may reflect only oropharyngeal colonization.

**Sputum Gram stains** are most predictive when one adheres to strict criteria of acceptability. Only samples with over 25 neutrophils and less than 10 epithelial cells per low-power field are acceptable for analysis. On such samples, the finding of over 10 gram-positive, lancet-shaped diplococci is highly predictive of identifying pneumococci on culture (Figure 155.1). On the other hand, finding none or a few mixed organisms may suggest that organisms not easily identified on the Gram stain should be considered (e.g., *M. pneumoniae, L. pneumophila, Mycobacterium tuberculosis*).

Although the routine use of **sputum cultures** in the initial management of CAP has been questioned, cultures are helpful in certain situations. For example, cultures are necessary if antibiotic sensitivity needs to be determined or if unusual organisms (e.g., *L. pneumophila, Cryptococcus neoformans,* or *M. tuberculosis*) are suspected.

When sputum is not obtainable by expectoration or after induction, respiratory secretions may be obtained by invasive methods, such as by fiberoptic bronchoscopy using **bronchoalveolar lavage** (BAL, see Chapter 219). BAL, which has not been fully evaluated in CAP, is an expensive method and may be potentially compromised by contamination with oral flora. Samples obtained through a double-catheter brush system can be cultured quantitatively. Many consider bacterial growth exceeding $10^3$ organisms/ml to be significant. Quantitative cultures, however, are expensive and not provided by all laboratories.

### Other studies

Other potentially helpful diagnostic tests include a variety of blood tests, such as a complete blood count, blood chemistries, blood cultures, cold agglutinins, and antibody titers. Tests for *Legionella* involve a direct fluorescent antibody assay, which can be done on sputum, pleural fluid, or other pulmonary secretions, and an antigen assay performed on urine.

Currently, none of these tests is recommended in the initial management of patients with CAP, except the complete blood count, electrolyte determinations, and renal function tests, which can help assess the prognosis and determine the need for hospitalization. However, hospitalized patients with pneumonia should routinely have blood cultures (two sets) performed, as well as assessment of arterial oxygen saturation.

## Management

Only occasionally do all the pieces of the diagnostic puzzle fit together easily to yield an etiology of CAP, and thus therapy is necessarily empiric most of the time (Table 155.5). In most ordinary cases of CAP, a specific etiologic diagnosis, although worthwhile, is not crucial. A few agents—*Streptococcus pneumoniae, Haemophilus influenzae, Mycoplasma pneumoniae, Chlamydia pneumoniae, Legionella pneumophila,* or viruses—cause most cases.

For **empiric outpatient therapy,** a macrolide, beta-lactam agent (e.g., cefuroxime or amoxicillin-clavulanate or a newer quinolone would be appropriate. Erythromycin covers *S. pneumoniae, M. pneumoniae,* and *L. pneumophila* but not *H. influenzae.* It often causes gastrointestinal side effects. The newer macrolides, clarithromycin and azithromycin, albeit more expensive than erythromycin, can cover all four agents with fewer side effects. Penicillin is still an effective, inexpensive agent for pneumococcal pneumonia when resistance is not present. For strains that show an intermediate level of resistance, high dose penicillin or cefotaxime or ceftriaxone are appropriate; highly resistant strains mandate vancomycin.

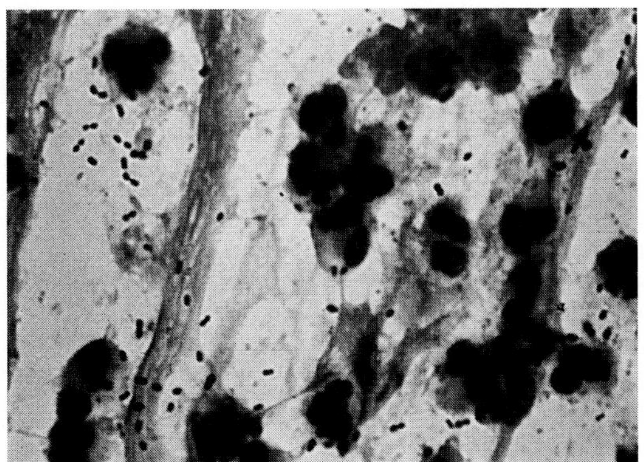

**FIGURE 155.1. Sputum Gram stain in pneumococcal pneumonia showing leukocytes and gram-positive diplococci.**

**TABLE 155.5. Antibiotic Treatment of Community-Acquired Pneumonia**

| Suspected Pathogen | Preferred Antibiotic(s) |
|---|---|
| *Streptococcus pneumoniae* | Penicillin, ceftriaxone, macrolide |
| *Haemophilus influenzae* | Amoxicillin, TMP/SMX, macrolide (not erythromycin), cefuroxime |
| *Mycoplasma pneumoniae* | Macrolide, tetracycline |
| *Legionella pneumophila* | Macrolide, TMP/SMX, ciprofloxacin |
| Mixed anaerobes | Clindamycin, penicillin |
| *Staphylococcus aureus* | Nafcillin, cefazolin |
| Aerobic gram-negative bacilli | Second- or third-generation cephalosporin |

TMP/SMX = trimethoprim/sulfamethoxazole.

The initial evaluation also entails determining the **need for hospitalization.** Mild pneumonias in patients without major debilitating conditions can be treated in the outpatient setting with oral antibiotics. If expectoration is problematic or intravenous therapy is necessary to cover more pathogens, hospitalization may be needed. Similarly, a significant abnormality in vital signs (hyperthermia, tachycardia, hypotension, extreme tachypnea), changes in mentation, respiratory failure, inability to take medications at home, or other risk factors for complications are indications for hospitalization.

For **inpatient therapy,** if the possible causes include *S. pneumoniae, H. influenzae, L. pneumophila,* and even aerobic gram-negative bacilli, often a second-generation or third-generation cephalosporin and a macrolide (or a newer quinolone) may suffice. Complicated pleural effusions (see Chapter 250) require chest tube drainage. Antibiotics can be given orally after fever is resolved and clinical response is evident; they should be continued for a total of 7–10 days. *Legionella* pneumonia, however, requires 21 days of therapy.

## Nosocomial Pneumonia

Nosocomial pneumonia is defined as pneumonia developing after a patient has been hospitalized, usually for an unrelated condition. It is a frequent problem, accounting for up to 15% of hospital-acquired infections, and ranks second only to nosocomial urinary tract infections. The most common microbial causes are listed in Table 155.6.

## Pathogenesis and Predisposing Factors

Pneumonia develops in the hospital setting due to either aspiration of oropharyngeal flora or bacteremia. Aspiration is the most frequent mechanism. Within 2 days after hospitalization, oropharyngeal colonization occurs with a high frequency, with organisms such as *Pseudomonas aeruginosa* and enteric, gram-negative, aerobic bacilli. Daily monitoring of cultures from various sites has shown that the enteric gram-negative organisms are primarily derived from the patient's own flora, whereas *P. aeruginosa* appears to be from an environmental source. Predisposing factors for nosocomial pneumonia are listed in Table 155.7.

**TABLE 155.6. Common Causative Microbes in Nosocomial Pneumonia**

| Agent | Approximate Frequency (%) |
|---|---|
| *Pseudomonas aeruginosa* | 17 |
| *Staphylococcus aureus* | 15 |
| *Klebsiella* spp. | 7 |
| *Escherichia coli* | 6 |
| *Haemophilus influenzae* | 6 |
| *Serratia marcescens* | 5 |
| *Proteus mirabilis* | |
| *Enterobacter* spp. | |
| *Acinetobacter* spp. | |
| *Legionella pneumophila* | |
| *Streptococcus pneumoniae* | <3 |

## Diagnosis

Fever, productive cough, elevated WBC count, hypoxemia, and a new infiltrate in chest radiographs of a hospitalized patient strongly suggest nosocomial pneumonia. However, the diagnosis is not always straightforward. Fever and cough may not always be present, or alternatively, fever and a high WBC count may be explainable by other entities, such as possible catheter-associated infections and antibiotic-associated colitis.

Pulmonary infiltrates in hospitalized persons are not specific for pneumonia, because other disease states also may cause a chest infiltrate and hypoxemia (e.g., a mucus plug with atelectasis, aspirated tube feeding, pulmonary embolus, congestive heart failure, pleural effusion, tumor, hemorrhage).

## Management and Prevention

Treatment of nosocomial pneumonia is usually empiric, but special attention should be paid to underlying host factors that may predispose to specific pathogens, prior antibiotic use, and pathogens unique to specific institutions or units.

Traditionally, broad-spectrum antibiotic combinations (e.g., an anti-pseudomonal penicillin or cephalosporin, combined with an aminoglycoside) are used to cover the common gram-negative pathogens. Single agents, especially those with anti-pseudomonal activity (e.g., aztreonam, quinolones, and anti-pseudomonal penicillins or cephalosporins), have demonstrated comparable efficacy. Combination therapy should be used, however, in certain circumstances, such as in neutropenic patients, in the presence of bacteremia, and with organisms at high risk for developing resistance.

Nosocomial pneumonia caused by some pathogens may be adequately treated with 10–14 days of therapy, but those due to gram-negative organisms (especially when associated with a necrotizing pneumonia) should be treated for 21 days. Pleural effusions meeting criteria for drainage should be drained as well.

**TABLE 155.7. Predisposing Factors Associated with Nosocomial Pneumonia**

| Predisposing Factor | Comment |
|---|---|
| Intubation, mechanical ventilation | Disruption of cough mechanism; damage to respiratory epithelium, equipment colonized by bacteria |
| Respiratory (aerosol-generating) equipment | Equipment colonized by bacteria; frequent handling of tubes |
| Advanced age | Poor cough, impaired local defenses |
| Underlying disease | Debilitation, increased aspiration risk |
| Prior antibiotics | Selection |
| Recent surgery | Aspiration |
| Antacids, $H_2$ blockers | Increased stomach colonization and subsequent aspiration |
| Poor infection control precautions (e.g., hand washing) | Enhanced risk of transmission of gram-negative organisms from patient to patient within the same units |

**TABLE 155.8. Pneumonia in the Immunocompromised Host**

| Immune Defect (Clinical Examples) | Common Microbes Causing Pneumonia | Usual Chest Radiographic Patterns |
|---|---|---|
| **Neutropenia** | | |
| Cancer chemotherapy | Gram-negative bacilli | No infiltrate/lobar |
| | *Staphylococcus aureus* | No infiltrate/lobar |
| | *Aspergillus* spp. | Cavitary/diffuse |
| **γ-Globulin deficiency/dysfunction** | | |
| Multiple myeloma | *Streptococcus pneumoniae* | Lobar |
| AIDS | *Haemophilus influenzae* | |
| Common variable hypogammaglobulinemia | | |
| Lymphoma | | |
| Cell-mediated deficiency | | |
| AIDS | *Pneumocystis carinii* | Diffuse |
| Transplant | *Cryptococcus neoformans* | Nodular/cavitary/diffuse |
| Corticosteroid therapy | *Aspergillus* spp. | Nodular/cavitary/diffuse |
| | *Mycobacterium* spp. | Diffuse |
| | *Legionella* spp. | Lobar/diffuse |
| | Herpes viruses | Diffuse |

Because nosocomial pneumonia often develops in the setting of prior gram-negative enteric colonization, the use of **prophylactic antibiotics** has received attention. Whereas antibiotic prophylaxis can decrease colonization of the oropharynx by gram-negative bacilli, it can also enhance selection of resistant organisms. Therefore, this approach does not merit widespread application. Other preventive measures include proper hand-washing, isolation, decreased manipulation of respiratory equipment, and preferential use of sucralfate for peptic ulcer prophylaxis.

## Pneumonia in the Immunocompromised Host

Analysis of pneumonia that develops in the immunocompromised host must be accomplished with an awareness of the likely unique pathogens responsible for pneumonia in specific immune defects. Infections in immunocompromised hosts in general, and those in AIDS in particular, are discussed in detail in Chapters 164 and 165. Common causes of pneumonia as associated with specific defects in systemic immune defenses are outlined in Table 155.8.

Pneumonias in these patients may be acquired either at home or in the hospital, and the clinician must be aware of the possibility of one of these immune defects when taking the patient's history. One must recognize that these patients are also prone to noninfectious causes of pulmonary infiltrates, such as pulmonary emboli, radiation pneumonitis, pulmonary hemorrhage, nonspecific interstitial pneumonitis, or drug reactions (e.g., bleomycin, methotrexate). Overall, immunocompromised patients need careful attention in this often difficult diagnostic and therapeutic entity.

# CHAPTER 156 URINARY TRACT INFECTIONS

## Definitions

Infections of the urinary tract are described by many terms (Table 156.1). Patients with **bacteriuria** may be asymptomatic or symptomatic. Individuals with symptomatic bacteriuria may be divided into those with infection in the lower **(cystitis)** or upper urinary tract **(pyelonephritis).** Some patients with lower urinary tract symptoms have less than $10^5$ bacteria/ml of urine, a symptom complex called the **acute urethral syndrome,** which includes early cystitis as well as other possibilities, such as nongonococcal urethritis.

Urinary tract infections (UTIs) may be **complicated** or **uncomplicated,** depending on whether or not the infection is accompanied by structural urinary tract

**TABLE 156.1. Urinary Tract Infections: A Glossary of Terms**

| | |
|---|---|
| *Bacteriuria* | Bacteria in the urine (usually ≥$10^5$ bacteria/ml) |
| *Cystitis* | Infection of the lower urinary tract |
| *Pyelonephritis* | Infection of the upper urinary tract |
| *Acute urethral syndrome* | Symptoms of UTI with <$10^5$ bacteria/ml |
| *Complicated UTI* | UTI in the presence of a structural abnormality |
| *Recurrent UTI* | Repeated UTI that may be either a relapse or reinfection |

abnormalities (e.g., congenital duplication of the collection system, vesicoureteral reflux, prostatic hypertrophy, tumors, calculi, and urinary catheterization).

Finally, UTIs may be sporadic (or infrequent) or **recurrent** events. Recurrent UTIs are further divided into relapsing infections or reinfections. **Relapsing** infections arise from a persistent focus of infection that is not eradicated, whereas **reinfections** are new infections that follow eradication of the previous episode.

## Etiology

Differentiating uncomplicated from complicated UTIs not only helps identify urinary tract abnormalities, but also helps determine the microbial etiology. Most uncomplicated episodes of either cystitis or pyelonephritis (>80%) are due to certain strains of *Escherichia coli.* Approximately 10% of cases of uncomplicated cystitis (but not pyelonephritis) result from a coagulase-negative staphylococci, *S. saprophyticus.*

Complicated UTIs, on the contrary, arise from a wider range of organisms (Table 156.2). Most are gram-negative, but gram-positive organisms and fungi are also frequent.

## Pathogenesis and Predisposing Factors

**Cystitis** usually occurs by ascent of pathogenic microorganisms from the urethra to the bladder. Whereas pyelonephritis can result from further ascent of these microbes, hematogenous spread may also be causative. As mentioned, acute, uncomplicated cystitis is usually caused by a few uropathogenic *E. coli* strains that normally colonize the bowel. The proximity of the female genitourinary tract to the anus predisposes to the **colonization** of the vagina and the urethral meatus. After such colonization, the shorter female urethra permits an easier ascent of organisms to the bladder, a process that is facilitated by sexual activity.

A prerequisite of colonization is attachment of organisms to mucosal epithelial cells. In women with recurrent UTIs, it has been shown that bacteria increasingly bind to uroepithelial cells. Genetic susceptibility (nonsecretors of blood group antigens), hormonal factors (estrogen), and other factors (spermicide use) may all increase the attachment process and subsequent susceptibility to infection.

**Protective mechanisms** against UTI include the normal systemic host defenses (see Table 148.4), but also local factors, including the act of micturition, high osmolality and urea content of urine, and possibly prostatic secretions in men. As sufficient bacteria overcome these barriers, an inflammatory response, primarily neutrophilic, develops. Infection of the bladder tends to be localized to the mucosa, without a prominent antibody response, whereas tissue invasion and a systemic antibody response characterize pyelonephritis.

## Epidemiology

The prevalence of UTI by age groups in women and men is shown in Table 156.3. Except during infancy, women have a life-long higher incidence of UTIs, which peaks between ages 16–35 due to sexual activity and diaphragm use. The increased incidence in older men is primarily due to prostatic hypertrophy; incontinence and long-term urinary catheterization are other factors.

## Clinical Features

The common "classic" symptoms of acute cystitis and pyelonephritis, as seen in young women, are shown in Table 156.4. People at the extremes of life, including catheterized patients, may have either nonspecific symptoms or no symptoms at all except fever. Whereas suprapubic tenderness and gross hematuria are seen in only 10% and 30% of cystitis cases, respectively, they are fairly specific findings for cystitis. As many as one third of patients with only symptoms of cystitis have unrecognized pyelonephritis.

Of the symptoms listed, fever and flank pain are the most specific for pyelonephritis; dysuria, frequency, and urgency may or may not be present. Clinical manifesta-

**TABLE 156.2. Common Microbes Causing Uncomplicated and Complicated Urinary Tract Infections**

| Uncomplicated | Complicated |
|---|---|
| *Escherichia coli* | *Escherichia coli* |
| *Staphylococcus saprophyticus* | *Klebsiella* spp. |
| | *Enterobacter* spp. |
| | *Proteus* spp. |
| | *Pseudomonas* spp. |
| | Enterococcus spp. |
| | *Staphylococcus epidermidis* |
| | Yeast (*Candida* spp.) |

TABLE 156.3. Epidemiology of UTI by Age

| Age Group (years) | Prevalence (%) | | Risk Factors |
|---|---|---|---|
| | Women | Men | |
| <1 | 1 | 1 | Anatomic or functional anomalies |
| 1–5 | 4–5 | 0.5 | Congenital anomalies, uncircumcised penis (M) |
| 6–15 | 4–5 | 0.5 | Vesicoureteral reflux (W) |
| 16–35 | 20 | 0.5 | Sexual intercourse, diaphragm use (W), homosexuality (M) |
| 36–65 | 35 | 20 | Gynecologic surgery (W), prostatic hypertrophy (M), catheterization |
| >65 | 40 | 35 | Catheterization, incontinence |

M = men; W = women.
(Adapted and reprinted with permission from: Stamm WE. In Gorbach SL, Bartlett JG, Blacklow NR (eds.): Infectious Diseases. Philadelphia, PA: Saunders, 1992, pp 788–798.)

TABLE 156.4. Differentiating Clinical Features of Cystitis and Pyelonephritis

| Cystitis | Pyelonephritis |
|---|---|
| Dysuria | Dysuria and frequency |
| Urinary frequency | Fever |
| Urgency | Flank pain |
| Suprapubic tenderness (10%) | Nausea and vomiting |
| Gross hematuria (30%) | Malaise |

tions vary widely, with an illness ranging from mild nausea, dysuria, fever, and flank pain to fever and septic shock. Presentation with septic shock, however, tends to occur in the elderly or those with underlying disease. Patients may report low back pain or abdominal pain as opposed to flank pain.

## Diagnosis

When UTI is clinically suspected, a urine sample should be obtained for confirmation. A **clean, midstream voided sample** is preferred in most patients, although urine can be obtained by suprapubic puncture or from a urethral catheter in those who are already catheterized. Inflammatory cells **(pyuria)** and erythrocytes **(hematuria)** in a clean-catch urine sample support the diagnosis of a UTI.

Although **pyuria** is universally present in clinically significant UTI, it also occurs in other conditions, such as gonococcal urethritis, reducing its specificity. The presence or number of leukocytes does not differentiate a lower from an upper UTI, but the presence of leukocyte casts is consistent with pyelonephritis. Some laboratories screen urine with a leukocyte esterase dipstick method, which is somewhat less sensitive than a microscopic examination for pyuria.

Erythrocytes **(hematuria)** are not as commonly seen as WBCs. Their presence may suggest additional diagnostic possibilities, such as urinary stones or tumor, and excludes urethritis, which is not normally associated with hematuria.

Finally, an uncentrifuged urine should be **Gram-stained** and examined for bacteria. The observation of *any* bacteria is consistent with a significant colony count of bacteria, but also the Gram stain findings may help guide therapy.

In patients treated as outpatients with suspected, uncomplicated, acute cystitis, a **urine culture** may not be practical or cost-effective because the typical treatment covers the usual narrow spectrum of organisms. However, any patient with suspected pyelonephritis or a complicated UTI, or any patient sick enough to require hospitalization for suspected UTI, needs to have a urine culture. To be significant, a urine culture must (classically) show $>10^5$ colony forming units (CFU) of an organism per milliliter of urine. More recently, though, it has been recognized that even $>10^2$ CFU/ml may be significant in acutely symptomatic patients.

## Management

Successful management of a UTI is based on a clinical estimation of the site of infection, coupled with knowledge of likely pathogens and pharmacokinetics of antibiotics in the urine.

### Cystitis

Because cystitis is a superficial bladder mucosal infection, choosing an antibiotic that attains good urinary concentrations against the usual pathogens is critical. A 3 day course of therapy with a variety of agents (Table 156.5) has been shown to attain a cure rate similar to that for more prolonged therapy (7–10 days). Prolonged therapy should be given to those with symptoms lasting for 7 days or more, diabetes, immunosuppression, pregnancy, or an anatomic urinary tract abnormality.

TABLE 156.5. Suggested Antibiotic Regimens for Urinary Tract Infections

| Cystitis | Pyelonephritis |
|---|---|
| Trimethoprim/sulfamethoxazole* | Trimethoprim/sulfamethoxazole* |
| Trimethoprim* | Third-generation cephalosporin‡ |
| Quinolone† | Quinolone† |
| Amoxicillin or amoxicillinclavulanic acid‡ | Aminoglycoside† plus antipseudomonal penicillin‡ |
| Cephalexin‡ | |

Fetal risk: Although all drugs carry some fetal risk, the following comments apply to use of these agents in pregnancy.
*Use with caution in early pregnancy.
†Unsafe.
‡Appears safe.

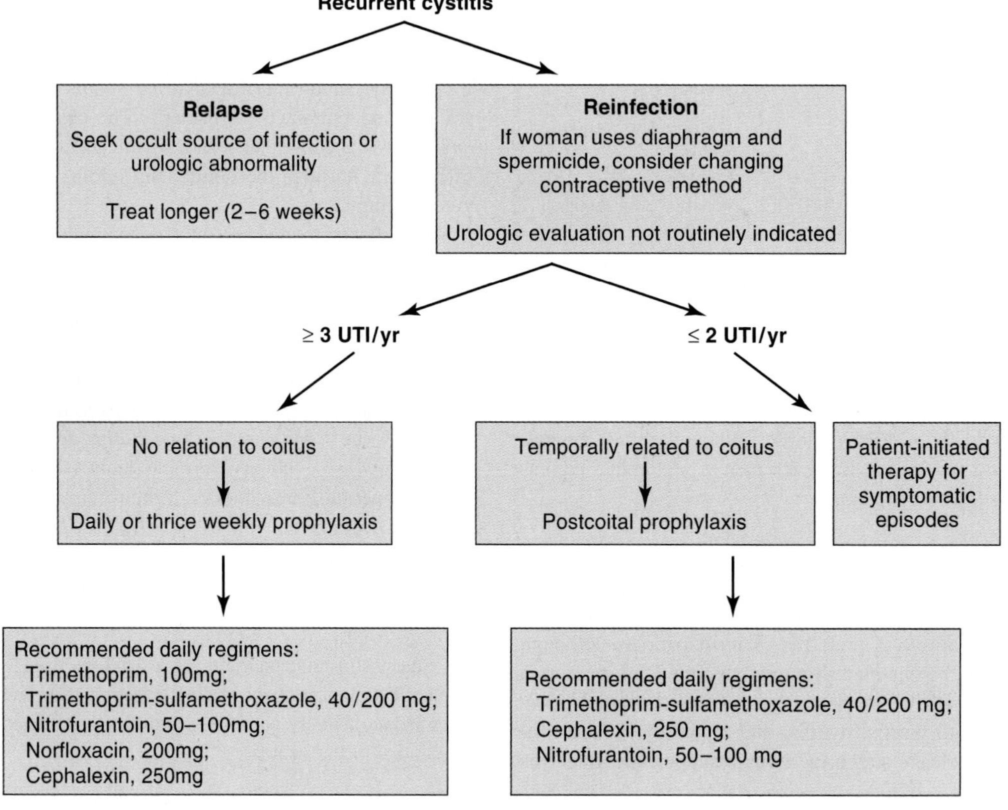


**FIGURE 156.1.** Strategies for managing recurrent cystitis in women.
(Reprinted with permission from: Stamm WE, Hooton TM. N Engl J Med 1993;329:1328–1334.)

Patients with **recurrent cystitis** are divided into those with a relapsing infection (usually due to an occult renal source) and those with reinfection. Relapsing infections are caused by the same organism as the primary infection and usually appear within 2 weeks of the primary episode, whereas reinfections usually occur after that time and are caused by a different species or strain. Management of recurrent cystitis is outlined in Figure 156.1.

### Pyelonephritis

Initial management of patients with pyelonephritis is based on the need for hospitalization and parenteral therapy. Some patients, particularly younger women with only a moderate illness, can be given outpatient oral therapy. All others should be given parenteral agents.

Because patients with pyelonephritis, especially those with complicated infections, have a wider range of pathogens, initial therapy should anticipate this possibility (see Table 156.5). Also, because gram-negative rods and enterococci are possibilities, the urine Gram stain can also help guide initial therapy. Further modifications can follow once the antibiotic sensitivity pattern is known. With clinical improvement and abatement of fever, one can substitute and continue a suitable oral agent for a total of 14 days.

If no improvement occurs within 48–72 hours on appropriate therapy, a urinary tract abnormality should be suspected. A urinary ultrasound or CT scan should be done, and possibly, a consultation with a urologist.

## Catheter-associated Urinary Tract Infections

In evaluating patients with urinary catheters, one must realize that bacteriuria is common and that most catheter-associated UTIs are asymptomatic. Catheterized patients with **asymptomatic bacteriuria** do not require therapy. Treatment does not reduce the chance of future infection and, in fact, may predispose to colonization with more resistant bacteria. Therefore, only symptomatic patients should be treated.

Symptoms may include fever or flank pain or patients may present more acutely with sepsis or septic shock. **Treatment** should include removal or replacement of the catheter, initiation of parenteral antibiotics, and fluid and/or pressor support as appropriate. Antibiotic selection is similar to that for complicated pyelonephritis (see Table 156.5), with special attention to the institutional nosocomial flora.

Reducing the risk for catheter-associated infections includes substitution of condom catheters, intermittent straight catheterization, and, if possible, removal of indwelling catheters.

## Asymptomatic Bacteriuria

As described in Table 156.1, asymptomatic bacteriuria is defined as $10^5$ or more bacteria per milliliter of urine in a patient who has no urinary symptoms. Asymptomatic bacteriuria is a common finding in certain populations, particularly catheterized patients, as described above. It is also fairly common in the elderly without catheters. In general, asymptomatic bacteriuria should not be treated in adults with or without catheters. Those populations in which asymptomatic bacteriuria should be treated, however, include children, pregnant women, and possibly certain high-risk immunosuppressed patients (e.g., neutropenic or renal transplantation patients).

## Prostatitis

Inflammation of the prostate gland occurs in a manner similar to cystitis, with the usual mechanism being ascent of pathogens via the urethral ducts into the proximal posterior urethra. Common pathogens are similar to those listed above for UTIs, with enteric gram-negative organisms (usually *Escherichia coli*) and enterococcal species predominating.

The usual types or classifications of prostatitis include **acute bacterial prostatitis, chronic bacterial prostatitis,** and **nonbacterial prostatitis.** The symptoms of acute bacterial prostatitis include dysuria, acute urinary retention, perineal and low back pain, and sudden fever and chills. The prostate is swollen and tender on examination.

Given the similar array of pathogens, therapy for prostatitis is the same as that for other UTIs, except that prolonged therapy is needed (usually 30 days). Nonbacterial prostatitis is a relatively common inflammatory disorder of the prostate with an undefined etiology. Although the role of chlamydiae or mycoplasmas is not well supported, a 2-week trial with a macrolide or a tetracycline may be utilized in these patients.

## Epididymitis

Epididymitis occurs by ascent of pathogenic bacteria through the urethra and vas deferens and into the epididymis. Symptoms are those of a UTI, including fever and urethral discharge. Examination reveals a unilateral, tender scrotal mass that is initially separable from the testis but may gradually involve the testis as well. Signs of prostatitis may also be noted. Conditions simulating acute epididymitis, for example, testicular torsion or tumor, can be differentiated on ultrasound.

Epididymitis may be sexually transmitted (usually due to *Chlamydia trachomatis* or *Neisseria gonorrhoeae*) or non–sexually transmitted (usually due to enteric gram-negative organisms). It may be treated as outlined in Figure 156.2.

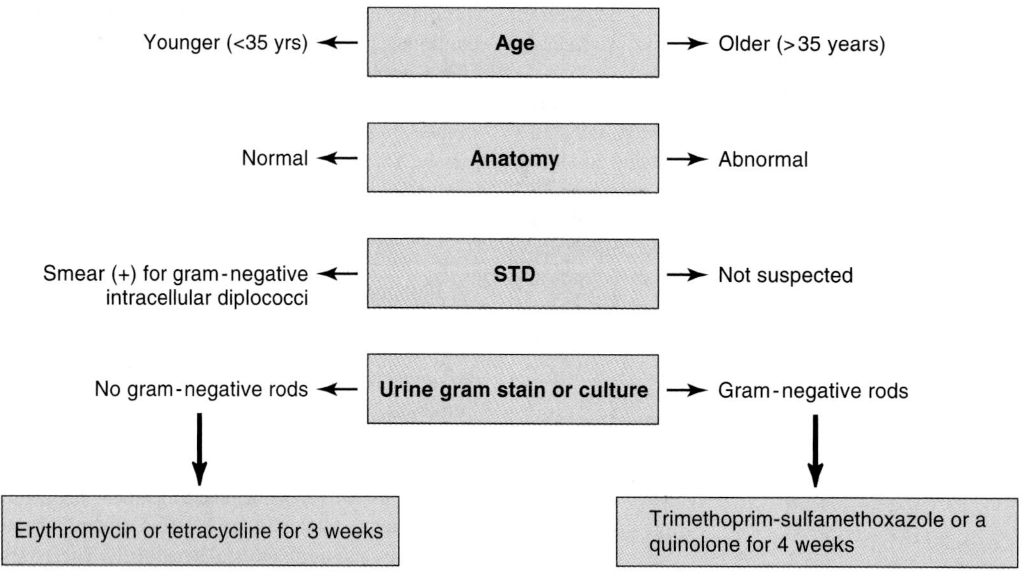


**FIGURE 156.2.** Therapy for epididymitis. STD = sexually transmitted disease.

# CHAPTER 157 SEXUALLY TRANSMITTED DISEASES

A list of sexually transmitted diseases (STDs) is provided in Table 157.1. In most industrialized nations, the incidence of syphilis, gonorrhea, and chancroid has steadily declined during the last 2 decades. However, in more recent times, the incidence of these disorders, particularly syphilis and chancroid, has risen strikingly in the United States.

It is common to be infected with more than one organism when a person acquires an STD. Thus, the individual found to have gonorrhea should be screened for incubating syphilis. Persons with syphilis should also be screened for HIV. STDs should be viewed as a reflection of "high risk" behavior, rather than a sporadic disease with which the individual presents.

**TABLE 157.1. Sexually Transmitted Diseases**

Syphilis
Gonorrhea
Chancroid
Granuloma inguinale (Donovanosis)
Nongonococcal urethritis
Acute pelvic inflammatory disease (PID)
Vaginitis
- *Trichomonas vaginalis*
- *Chlamydia trachomatis*

Lymphogranuloma venereum (LGV)
Herpes simplex virus (HSV)
Hepatitis B
HIV
Anorectal disease
Infections among homosexuals
- Herpes simplex, gonorrhea, syphilis
- Anorectal infection due to *Neisseria meningitidis*
- Ulcerative proctitis due to *Chlamydia*
- Epididymitis (from coliform organisms and *Haemophilus influenzae*)
- Enteric bacterial pathogens (*Shigella*, Salmonella, *Campylobacter jejuni, Entamoeba histolytica, Giardia*)
- Hepatitis
- Cytomegalovirus (CMV)

## General Overview of Genital Lesions

The hallmark of an STD is a **genital lesion** (except in those engaging in anal-receptive intercourse, who may harbor internal lesions). The morphology of genital lesions is an important clue in diagnosis. Causes of ulcerative lesions are shown in Table 157.2. In the United States, most (>50%) genital lesions are caused by herpes simplex virus (HSV). Syphilis follows as the second leading cause.

Although appearance, incubation period, travel history, or mode of onset may be helpful in evaluating

TABLE 157.2. Genital Lesions Due to Sexually Transmitted Diseases

| Diagnosis/Entity | Causative Organism | Clinical Feature(s) | Confirmatory Study | Treatment |
|---|---|---|---|---|
| Herpes genitalis | Herpes simplex virus | Grouped vesicles | Culture | Acyclovir |
| Syphilis | *Treponema pallidum* | Painless ulcer, adenopathy | Darkfield examination | Penicillin |
| Chancroid | *Haemophilus ducreyi* | Painful ulcer, adenopathy | Gram stain (?) | Erythromycin, ceftriaxone |
| Donovanosis (granuloma inguinale) | *Calymmatobacterium* | Heaped up tissue | Giemsa | Tetracycline, ampicillin, TMP/SMX |
| Lymphogranuloma venereum | *Chlamydia Trachomatis* | Inguinal adenopathy with bubo | Serology | Tetracycline |

TMPSMX = Trimethoprim/sulfamethoxazole.

genital lesions, **laboratory testing** is essential for specific diagnosis (except classic HSV with grouped vesicles). Essential laboratory studies for ulcerated lesions include culture for HSV, a dark-field examination for syphilis, and serologic tests for syphilis. Culture for *Haemophilus ducreyi* also may be done if chancroid is suspected.

## Herpes Simplex Virus

### Epidemiology

Genital HSV causes over 400,000 episodes of primary infection each year in the United States. Up to 90% of these infections are with HSV2, and the remainder are with HSV1. Infection is spread by contact with infected secretions. However, recent studies have shown that viral shedding may occur without apparent lesions (subclinical infection).

### Clinical Features and Diagnosis

The incubation period (time from infection to the first clinical manifestation) is usually 2–7 days. HSV usually starts as grouped, thin-walled vesicles that ulcerate. In heterosexual men, the vesicles present on the shaft of the penis or glans, whereas in homosexual men, they may occur perianally or present as proctitis. In women, lesions may occur on the vulva, vagina, or anus.

The lesions are usually painful. The primary infection lasts 2–3 weeks and may be accompanied by fever and tender adenopathy. Sacral radiculitis with urinary retention and aseptic meningitis are unusual presentations. Recurrent episodes are usually less severe without the systemic manifestations—fewer lesions are seen, and the duration is usually a few days. These episodes may have prodromal pain and burning. The organism lies latent within sensory ganglia between episodes.

For confirmation of the diagnosis, the base of the ulcer may be swabbed and sent for culture, direct immunofluorescence staining, antigen detection, or Tzanck preparation (Figure 49.2). The yield is highest (90%) when specimens are taken during the vesicular stage rather than the ulcerative stage (50%). There is little role for serologic diagnosis.

### Management

Acyclovir remains the drug of choice for HSV infection. A dose of 200 mg five times per day for 7–10 days is recommended for the immunocompetent host with genital lesions or 400 mg five times per day for persons with proctitis or HIV coinfection. There is no clinical role for topical acyclovir. Newer options with reduced dosing frequency include valacyclovir and famcyclovir.

Patients with primary infection benefit the most from acyclovir treatment, and those with relapses benefit only minimally. **Prophylaxis** of frequent, recurrent episodes can be done with acyclovir, 200 mg three times per day or 400 mg twice a day, which reduces the rate of recurrence in over 80% of patients. Acyclovir should be stopped after 1 year to assess further need for it; however, HIV patients usually require continuous therapy.

Acyclovir-resistant HSV has been seen among immunosuppressed persons. It should be suspected when a response is lacking, especially to intravenous therapy. Intravenous foscarnet is then indicated.

## Syphilis

### Etiology and Epidemiology

Syphilis is caused by a spirochete, *Treponema pallidum*. It is a slender, coiled organism that replicates slowly and cannot be cultivated in vitro. Syphilis is primarily acquired by sexual contact, but it may be transplacentally transmitted in congenital disease. Very rarely, it is transmitted by accidental inoculation or blood transfusion. An individual with a chancre (syphilitic ulcer) or condylomata lata (flat, wart-like plaques) is most infectious.

Although no age is exempt, most cases occur in sexually active persons aged 15–30 years. In the 1980s, the incidence of syphilis began to increase in the United States, which was primarily due to increased numbers of cases among homosexual men. However, in the 1990s, there has been a rapid increase in the number of heterosexual cases due to the trade of sex for drugs, especially involving crack cocaine.

## Pathogenesis

*T. pallidum* may penetrate intact mucous membranes or abrasions in the skin and thus enter the lymphatics and bloodstream, disseminating to almost any organ in the body. The incubation period is nearly 3 weeks, but can vary from a few days to 3 months depending on the size of the inoculum.

## Clinical Features

Syphilis is classified into the four categories of *primary, secondary, latent,* and *tertiary phases,* which differ in their clinical manifestations and treatment. It may also be divided into the two broad categories of *early* (primary and secondary stages) and *late* syphilis (tertiary stage). The skin manifestations are discussed in Chapter 59.

### Primary and secondary stages

The classic **primary** syphilitic lesion is the **chancre,** which begins as a single papule that erodes into a painless ulcer (Figure 157.1), along with painless inguinal lymphadenopathy. Spontaneous healing occurs in a few weeks. Multiple chancres may be seen in HIV patients.

**Secondary syphilis,** indicating acute dissemination, usually occurs 2–8 weeks after the chancre appears. Although there are no symptoms between the primary and the secondary stage, cutaneous findings are the most prominent feature in the secondary stage, occurring in 90% of cases. The classic **"coppery rash,"** that is, fleeting, rapidly progressive reddish-brown macules, precedes a generalized, symmetric polymorphous eruption of macules and papules. Involvement of the palms and soles is characteristic.

Systemic features—fever, anorexia, arthralgia, and generalized adenopathy (classically epitrochlear)—occur in 70% of patients with secondary syphilis. Infrequently, patients may have hepatitis, nephritis, or meningitis. Anemia, leukocytosis, significantly elevated alkaline phosphatase, and a high erythrocyte sedimentation rate are the notable laboratory findings.

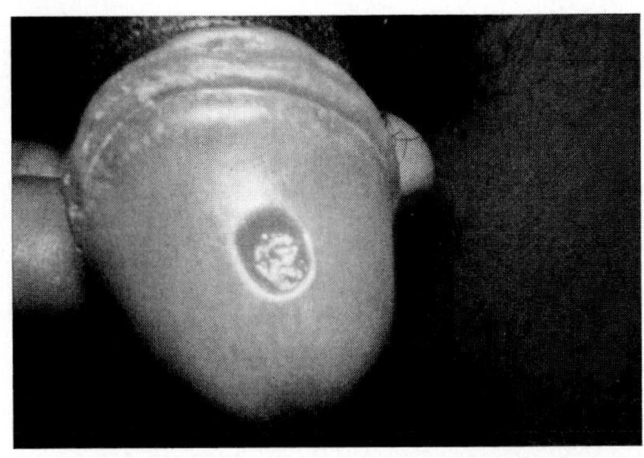

**FIGURE 157.1. Chancre of primary syphilis.**

### Latent and tertiary stages

Syphilis is considered **latent** when there is a positive test for syphilis without any manifestations of disease, including cerebrospinal fluid findings. Overall, 30% of untreated patients develop one of the forms of late-stage, **tertiary** syphilis: neurosyphilis, cardiovascular syphilis, or gumma (erosive lesions affecting organs or mucous membranes). Tertiary syphilis is now extremely rare in the United States, owing to early treatment.

## Diagnosis

**Dark-field examination** allows direct visualization of the spirochete and should be performed in patients with a chancre of primary syphilis or the condylomata lata of secondary syphilis. A scraping of the lesion is placed on a slide and viewed with a phase-contrast microscope. However, the necessary expertise may not be available in all facilities.

**Serologic tests for syphilis** include non-treponemal tests and a specific anti-treponemal antibody test. The former tests are nonspecific and include the Venereal Disease Research Laboratory (VDRL) or the rapid plasma reagin (RPR). These tests measure IgM and IgG antibodies directed against a lipid antigen formed by interaction of *T. pallidum* and the host and are used for screening or following up disease activity. A fourfold change (2 dilutions) is considered significant.

Because of frequent false positives (Table 157.3), a confirmatory test is usually done using treponemal tests, such as the fluorescent treponemal antibody absorption (FTAABS) or, the microhemagglutination assay for antibody to *T. pallidum* (MHATP).

## Management

**Penicillin** remains the drug of choice for all stages of syphilis (Table 157.4). For penicillin-allergic patients, oral doxycycline or erythromycin may be used, except in neurosyphilis because these drugs do not penetrate the

CSF. Penicillin desensitization should be strongly considered for penicillin-allergic patients with neurosyphilis, and in penicillin-allergic women regardless of the stage.

All patients with syphilis should be evaluated for HIV infection. Management of syphilis in patients with HIV is similar to that for the non-HIV patient, and close follow-up is necessary with serological examination at 1, 2, 3, 6, 9, and 12 months. Penicillin-allergic patients should be desensitized.

## Gonorrhea

### Epidemiology

Gonorrhea causes an estimated 1 million infections yearly in the United States. Infection may be readily recognized in symptomatic persons who seek medical attention, but a sizable number of infected men and women are asymptomatic; this reservoir may be responsible for the ongoing spread of this disease. Although no age is exempt, teenagers and young adults are most commonly infected. Its prevalence correlates with low socioeconomic status.

### Clinical Features

The incubation period is typically 3–4 days, but may be as long as 2 weeks.

**TABLE 157.3. Causes of False-Positive Results in Serologic Tests for Syphilis**

| Infectious Causes | Noninfectious Causes |
|---|---|
| Other spirochetes | Narcotic addicts |
| Tuberculosis | Connective tissue disorder |
| Leprosy | Pregnancy |
| Endocarditis | Old age |
| *Mycoplasma* infection | Chronic liver disease |
| Rickettsial infection | Laboratory error |
| Hepatitis | |
| Mononucleosis | |

In heterosexual men, dysuria and purulent urethral exudate are the most common presenting symptoms; pharyngitis is infrequent. Among homosexual men, besides urethritis, proctitis may be encountered in one third to one half of cases and pharyngitis in one fifth of cases.

Among symptomatic women, dysuria, urethritis, pyuria, vaginal discharge, menorrhagia or menometrorrhagia (bleeding between menses), and abdominal pain are the more common features. Pharyngitis is uncommon, and anal canal infection may sometimes lead to proctitis. Other presentations are acute pelvic inflammatory disease and Bartholin gland abscess. However, the disease may be asymptomatic, despite isolation of the organism from endocervical smears or the anal canal or the pharynx.

**Disseminated infection,** more common among women, results from bacteremia. Patients are febrile and generally toxic. A pustular distal skin rash, arthralgias, polyarthritis, tenosynovitis, or septic arthritis (gonococcus is the most common cause of septic arthritis in the sexually active age group) evolves as the illness progresses.

Skin lesions, more frequent in the extremities, are papular and erythematous and have a hemorrhagic or necrotic center. Typical urethral or cervical signs and symptoms may not be present. As the initial febrile episode resolves, a purulent mono or oligoarticular arthritis may develop (see Bacterial Arthritis in Chapter 263). In some, the initial febrile illness may be very transient or nonexistent, with the arthritis being the initial presentation. Endocarditis may develop as a complication.

### Diagnosis

In a person presenting with another STD (e.g., syphilis), coexistent gonorrhea may be diagnosed even when asymptomatic if the physician is careful enough to suspect it. In such individuals as well as in symptomatic

**TABLE 157.4. Treatment of Primary, Secondary, and Latent Syphilis**

| Stage | Treatment Regimen | Comments |
|---|---|---|
| Primary, secondary, and early latent | Benzathine penicillin 2.4 MU intramuscularly | If penicillin allergic, doxycycline 100 mg orally twice daily for 14 days for all stages; desensitize for syphilis complicating pregnancy |
| Late latent or unknown duration | As above, except benzathine penicillin weekly for 3 weeks and doxycycline 100 mg orally twice daily for 28 days | |
| Tertiary syphilis (excluding neurosyphilis) | As above | |

MU = million units

persons, urethral or endocervical smears should be submitted for Gram stain (intracellular gram-negative diplococci are diagnostic) and culture. Gram stain of the urethral discharge in men is highly sensitive (>95%) and specific. It is less sensitive in cervical (50%) and rectal infection (20%). The smears should be inoculated into selective (Thayer-Martin) medium for best results.

In patients with suspected disseminated gonorrhea, the urethra and cervix, if applicable, should be cultured. Joint fluid, if present, is often sterile initially, but with purulent arthritis, cultures are often positive. Skin lesions (sampled with a punch biopsy) and blood cultures are positive in about one half of cases.

### Management

Many therapeutic options exist for gonorrhea, including ceftriaxone (125 mg intramuscularly), cefixime (400 mg orally in a single dose), or ciprofloxacin (500 mg orally in a single dose). Treatment should always cover chlamydia. For penicillin-allergic patients, ciprofloxacin and ofloxacin are effective alternatives for uncomplicated anogenital gonorrhea in men and nonpregnant women. For disseminated gonococcal infection, hospitalization and intravenous antibiotics (ceftriaxone) are necessary. Purulent arthritis requires additional measures (see Chapter 266).

**Antibiotic resistance** among gonococci has been a vexing public health problem, with resistance to penicillin, ampicillin, and tetracycline being commonplace. Strains of penicillinase-producing *N. gonorrhoeae* (PPNG) account for 7–8% of all isolates, and tetracycline-resistant *N. gonorrhoeae* (TRNG) account for nearly 5%. The drug resistance develops through chromosomal mutations and plasmid-mediated penicillinase production. Whereas PPNG are encountered in high numbers on both the eastern and western U.S. coasts, TRNG are seen throughout the country. Spectinomycin-resistant gonococci are also penicillin-, cefoxitin-, and tetracycline-resistant. Fortunately, resistance has not been reported to **ceftriaxone,** making it the preferred agent for treatment of gonorrhea.

Follow-up examination is not necessary if a recommended regimen is used to treat gonorrhea. Persistent symptoms may suggest a resistant organism, associated nongonococcal urethritis, or reexposure to an infected partner. Clinical evaluation and reculturing are then necessary. Notification of public health personnel is essential for the control of gonorrhea.

## Urethritis, Cervicitis, and Vaginitis

Urethritis, or inflammation of the urethra, is characterized by discharge of mucopurulent material and dysuria. It is broadly classified as gonococcal or nongonococcal, according to the etiology. **Nongonococcal urethritis** is diagnosed when neutrophils exceed five per oil immersion field, devoid of any organism. *Chlamydia trachomatis* is responsible for nearly 50% of cases, *Ureaplasma urealyticum* for 20–40%, and *Trichomonas vaginalis* for 2–5%; the remainder are unidentified. Complications include epididymitis and Reiter syndrome.

Treatment of nongonococcal urethritis is **doxycycline,** 100 mg twice daily for 7 days. Failure to respond to doxycycline may indicate resistant ureaplasma, in which case erythromycin should be tried. Recently, azithromycin, 1.0 g as a single dose, has been approved as treatment for chlamydia. Sexual contacts should also be treated.

**Mucopurulent cervicitis** is characterized by a yellow cervical discharge. Microbiology is similar to urethritis and includes *N. gonorrhoeae* and *C. trachomatis.* In women, the two organisms often occur concurrently. Treatment includes both doxycycline and therapy for gonorrhea.

**Vaginitis,** characterized by vulvar irritation with itching and abnormal vaginal discharge, is due to local vulvovaginal infection or to bacterial vaginosis, in which the normal vaginal flora is replaced by an overgrowth of extraneous organisms. Vaginitis is commonly caused by *Trichomonas vaginalis* and *Candida albicans.*

Trichomonal vaginitis, although often asymptomatic, may cause pain on sexual intercourse (dyspareunia), dysuria, vaginal discharge, and/or vulvar pruritus, often occurring during or slightly after menstruation. Abundant, frothy, foul-smelling, vaginal discharge is common. *T. vaginalis* is readily seen on Papanicolaou stain and on urinalysis, and isolated on culture of vaginal secretions. *Candida* overgrowth, on the other hand, causes vulvar pruritus and a thick, whitish vaginal discharge that often precedes the menses. Dyspareunia is uncommon. Often, an underlying process such as diabetes mellitus, corticosteroid therapy, broad-spectrum antibiotic therapy, or pregnancy is readily identifiable in the background. Candidal vaginitis is not an STD.

Bacterial vaginosis follows replacement of the normal vaginal *Lactobacillus* flora with anaerobes (*Peptostreptococcus*, *Peptococcus*, and *Bacteroides*). Despite a correlation with heightened sexual activity and the number of sexual partners, not all forms of bacterial vaginosis are sexually transmitted. Patients report a fetid discharge, and occasionally pruritus. Dyspareunia is quite uncommon. The major diagnostic aids are the examination of the vaginal discharge for pH (>4.7) and KOH test. If either one of these studies does not confirm the diagnosis, then infection with *C. trachomatis* or *N. gonorrhoeae* should be pursued.

*T. vaginalis* is treated with metronidazole, given orally in a single 2.0-g dose or a multi-dose regimen (500 mg twice daily for 10 days). Failure of therapy is an indication for re-treatment with the longer regimen because of reported drug resistance of the organism. Patients should avoid alcohol because a disulfiram-like reaction can occur if alcohol is consumed while taking metronidazole. In order to reduce the reinfection rate, the male sexual partner should also be treated with one single 2.0-g dose of metronidazole; the importance of this cannot be overemphasized. Candidal vaginitis is treated with nystatin or one of the topical azoles. Bacterial vaginosis is treated with metronidazole, 2.0 g daily for 5 days, or clindamycin vaginal cream.

### Pelvic Inflammatory Disease

Pelvic inflammatory disease is an inflammatory disorder of the upper genital tract in women and includes endometritis, salpingitis, and tubo-ovarian abscess. The causative agents are *N. gonorrhoeae, C. trachomatis,* and the anaerobic-aerobic vaginal flora.

The clinical presentation may vary from subtle with mild abdominal pain to frank peritonitis. Regrettably, clinical diagnosis is unreliable, with laparoscopy confirming the diagnosis in only two thirds of suspected cases. Minimal diagnostic criteria include lower abdominal tenderness, adnexal tenderness, or cervical motion tenderness.

With uncertain diagnosis, abscess, pregnancy, or an HIV-positive patient, inpatient therapy is recommended, cefoxitin (or cefotetan) and doxycycline being appropriate agents. Outpatient regimens include cefoxitin intramuscularly (plus probenecid) or ceftriaxone (250 mg intramuscularly) and doxycycline (100 mg twice daily) for 10–14 days.

# CHAPTER 158 INFECTIOUS DIARRHEA

Infectious enteritis is discussed further in Chapter 79. The occurrence of infectious diarrhea depends strictly on the balance between the pathogenicity of the microbe (e.g., *Shigella* requires an infectious dose of only 100 organisms) and predisposition of the host (intactness of defenses).

## Etiology and Epidemiology

Agents causing infectious diarrhea are listed in Figures 86.1 and 86.2. Epidemiologic clues to the causative agent in infectious diarrhea are summarized in Table 158.1. **Noninvasive diarrhea** is enterotoxin-induced, often voluminous, and lacks inflammation. **Enterotoxigenic** *Escherichia coli,* which produces a heat-labile enterotoxin that activates mucosal adenylate cyclase, is the most common responsible organism worldwide; it also causes most instances of **traveler's diarrhea.**

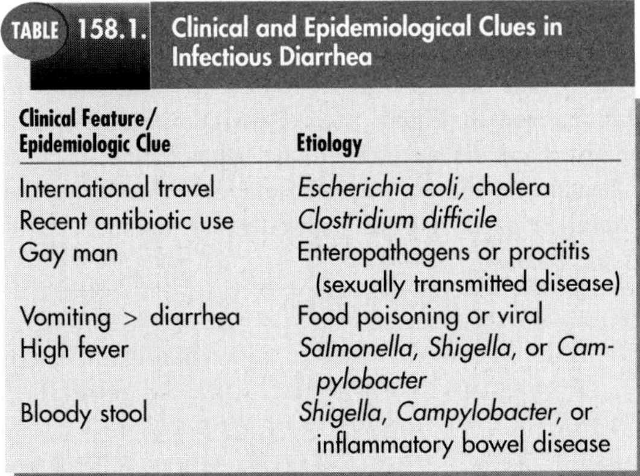

TABLE 158.1. Clinical and Epidemiological Clues in Infectious Diarrhea

| Clinical Feature/ Epidemiologic Clue | Etiology |
|---|---|
| International travel | *Escherichia coli,* cholera |
| Recent antibiotic use | *Clostridium difficile* |
| Gay man | Enteropathogens or proctitis (sexually transmitted disease) |
| Vomiting > diarrhea | Food poisoning or viral |
| High fever | *Salmonella, Shigella,* or *Campylobacter* |
| Bloody stool | *Shigella, Campylobacter,* or inflammatory bowel disease |

## Clinical Features

Primarily upper gastrointestinal symptoms (i.e., nausea and vomiting, or vomiting out of proportion to diarrhea) suggest a viral illness or a preformed toxin ingested in food. Such symptoms usually present within 6 hours after ingesting food that contains a preformed bacterial toxin, such as potato salad (*Staphylococcus aureus*) or improperly reheated fried rice (*Bacillus cereus*). Norwalk virus can cause epidemics in families and nursing homes.

Associated fever suggests **invasive organisms,** including *Shigella, Campylobacter,* or *Salmonella.* Bloody stools are more frequent with *Shigella* or *Campylobacter.*

Many parasites cause diarrhea, including *Giardia lamblia, Entamoeba histolytica* (more common in overseas travelers or travelers to Mexico), *Strongyloides stercoralis* (fulminant disease in the immunosuppressed), *Cryptosporidium* (recent water-borne outbreaks in several United States cities; also in AIDS), *Isospora belli* (acid-fast; seen in AIDS patients), and microsporidia (AIDS patients).

## Diagnosis

The history—especially of fever, bloody stools, or weight loss—dictates the need to pursue laboratory evaluation (Table 158.2). **Stool examination** for leukocytes is the first step, and if positive, is followed by culture. Bloody stool without leukocytes suggests ame-

**TABLE 158.2. Specific Organisms Causing Infectious Enteritis**

| Agent | Transmission | Features | Treatment |
|---|---|---|---|
| *Shigella* | Person-to-person | Inflammatory bloody diarrhea; bacteremia or dissemination rare; complications are HUS or Reiter syndrome | TMPSMX (resistant in developing countries) |
| *Salmonella* (nontyphoid) | Contaminated water or food, especially poultry | Nausea, vomiting, abdominal pain, fever | None unless severe |
| *Campylobacter jejuni* | Undercooked poultry | Prodrome of constitutional symptoms or a biphasic course (diarrhea-recovery-diarrhea); mimics IBD | Macrolides; quinolones (alternative) |
| *Yersinia enterocolitica* | Unknown | Infrequent; mesenteric adenitis or terminal ileitis may mimic appendicitis; may cause polyarthritis and erythema nodosum; patients with anemia, cirrhosis, or hemochromatosis may develop septicemia | TMPSMX, tetracycline, quinolones or third generation cephalosporins |
| *Escherichia coli* | Contaminated food/water<br>EH through poorly cooked ground beef | Travelers' diarrhea; hemorrhagic colitis occurs without fecal leukocytes; antibiotics may predispose to HUS; HUS more frequent at extremes of age | None |
| *Clostridium difficile* | | Trivial illness to toxic megacolon; prior antibiotic therapy is the predisposing factor; relapse occurs in 10% | Oral metronidazole; oral vancomycin for toxic patients |

EH = enterotoxigenic strains; HUS = hemolytic-uremic syndrome; TMPSMX = trimethoprim/sulfamethoxazole; IBD = inflammatory bowel disease.

**TABLE 158.3. Fecal Leukocytes in Intestinal Infections**

| Present | Variable | Absent |
|---|---|---|
| Shigella | *Salmonella* | *Vibrio cholera* |
| *Campylobacter* | *Vibrio parahaemolyticus* | Toxigenic *E. coli* |
| Invasive *Escherichia coli* | *Clostridium difficile* | Viral *Giardia* |
| | | *Entamoeba histolytica* |

biasis (the parasite destroys leukocytes) or enterohemorrhagic *E. coli* O157:H7. The finding of stool leukocytes indicates an inflammatory process (Table 158.3). However, their absence, although not excluding an inflammatory process, usually implies a self-limited, noninflammatory process.

HIV-positivity, weight loss, and diarrhea lasting for 10 days all indicate the need for further evaluation. Appropriate use of the laboratory in this setting is summarized in Figure 86.2. General management of diarrhea and the use of oral rehydration are discussed in Chapters 76 and 86. Antimicrobial agents that may be useful in acute diarrheal episodes are summarized in Table 86.3.

# CHAPTER 159 INTRA-ABDOMINAL INFECTIONS

Intra-abdominal infection can be divided into peritonitis, visceral abscesses, and extravisceral abscesses.

## Peritonitis

Patients with peritonitis usually present with steady abdominal pain that is worsened by any movement or respiration and that may be sudden if a viscus has ruptured. Fever is usually present. Tenderness with rebound, guarding, rigidity, and diminished or absent bowel sounds are characteristic.

Spontaneous (primary) peritonitis is discussed in Chapter 110. **Secondary peritonitis** arises from rupture of a part of the gastrointestinal tract (due to trauma, infarction, prior abdominal surgery, or simple perforation, such as a ruptured appendix) with leakage of its contents. The microbiology is dictated by the location of the leak. In most cases, multiple organisms are responsible. Enterobacteriaceae (*E. coli*), anaerobes (*Bacteroides fragilis,* other *Bacteroides* spp., clostridia) and enterococci constitute the most frequent pathogens. Because the colon has the largest population of microorganisms, sepsis is more likely after colon perforation.

Free air below the diaphragm on a plain chest radiograph is an excellent clue to the presence of peritonitis because it indicates the rupture of a large hollow viscus (stomach or colon). Treatment is surgical repair of the underlying defect.

Peritonitis may also be seen with peritoneal dialysis catheters. The etiology is usually *Staphylococcus aureus* or *S. epidermidis.* With antibiotic treatment, the catheter can usually be left in place unless there is a tunnel infection. Fungal infections and tuberculosis are other infrequent causes of peritonitis.

## Abscesses of Solid Organs

Thirty to 40% of **liver abscesses** are amebic due to *Entamoeba histolytica.* The remaining pyogenic liver abscesses are usually caused by other underlying conditions, including biliary disease, infections in the drainage area of the portal vein, systemic bacteremia, trauma, or contiguous infection. Among these, the most common condition (in 30% of cases) is ascending cholangitis from biliary obstruction or procedures involving the biliary tract.

The microbiology depends on the underlying cause. Anaerobes are increasingly implicated in liver abscesses, especially *Streptococcus milleri.* Patients with neutropenia are at increased risk for fungal abscesses.

The signs and symptoms of liver abscess usually include fever and abdominal pain. The liver may be enlarged, palpable, and tender. The most consistent laboratory abnormality is elevation of alkaline phosphatase levels, although other liver test results may also be abnormal. CT is the most sensitive and specific test. Finding *E. histolytica* in the stool in the United States is considered diagnostic, but in endemic areas, this may only represent a carrier state. In a high proportion of cases (>85%), the indirect hemagglutination test result is positive.

Percutaneous or open surgical drainage is usually needed. Initial antibiotic selection is guided by consideration of potential bowel pathogens until culture results become available. *E. histolytica* infection is treated with metronidazole.

## Extravisceral Abscess

Extravisceral abscesses usually arise from disruption of the gastrointestinal tract with loculation of fluid from peritoneal defenses, especially the omentum (without loculation, generalized peritonitis develops). Ruptured appendix is the leading etiology. The microbiology consists of colonic flora.

Clinical features include local symptoms with fever and leukocytosis. Subphrenic and pelvic abscesses may lack any local findings, a feature shared by immunosuppressed or debilitated patients. CT scan represents the best diagnostic study.

Once the abscess is localized, surgical or percutaneous drainage should follow. Percutaneous drainage is being applied increasingly, even for complex cases. The choice of antibiotics is guided initially by Gram stain results and later by culture. A lack of response to catheter drainage within 48 hours calls for open surgical drainage.

# CHAPTER 160 CENTRAL NERVOUS SYSTEM INFECTIONS

Meningitis, encephalitis, epidural abscess, subdural empyema, and brain abscess represent the spectrum of principal intracranial infections. A variety of organisms may cause these infections. The portal of entry of infections into the intracranial cavity is generally the blood or contiguous extension from adjacent structures (e.g., bacteria may spread from infected paranasal sinuses or neurotropic viruses may penetrate via exposed endings of olfactory nerves).

The blood vessels are often involved in the inflammation, and their resulting thrombosis or occlusion produces important clinical manifestations. Cytokine-induced vascular permeability and inflammation lead to increased intracranial pressure. In leptomeningeal infections, CSF, obtained by lumbar puncture, shows protein and cellular alterations and often contains the infecting organism. Antibiotics selectively cross the blood–brain barrier to penetrate the substance of the brain and meninges, which limits the choice of antibiotics in therapy for intracranial infections. Because all cranial nerves exit the skull at the base, cranial nerve involvement is an important aspect of chronic meningitis.

### General diagnosis and management

Depending on the process, fever, headache, confusion, seizure, nuchal rigidity, or focal neurologic deficit may occur in varying combinations. The axiom in managing intracranial infections is to decide clinically if acute bacterial meningitis is present and to proceed accordingly.

Intracranial abscesses are space-occupying and inevitably cause increased **intracranial pressure.** With such enlarging mass lesions, lumbar puncture carries a high risk of transtentorial herniation and death. Bacterial meningitis also raises intracranial pressure, but the increase is spread diffusely across the subarachnoid space. Thus, unless the meningitis is advanced, the risk for transtentorial herniation after lumbar puncture is negligible, if any. Obtaining a CT scan in every patient prior to lumbar puncture can avoid this risk, but it is expensive and inefficient.

The **acuteness of presentation** and findings vary according to the process. Fulminant symptoms with fever, lethargy, and nuchal rigidity make bacterial meningitis likely, which calls for immediate lumbar puncture and antibiotic therapy within 1 hour. A subacute history over weeks or months, especially with focal signs and symptoms, implies a mass effect. CT is indicated first because lumbar puncture is risky. When these distinctions are blurred and meningitis is still a consideration, blood cultures are drawn, antibiotics are given, and lumbar puncture is deferred until the CT scan is completed.

## Bacterial Meningitis

Meningitis, an inflammation of the meninges, may be acute (hours to several days) or chronic (weeks to months) according to its evolution. Acute meningitis has a variety of causes (Table 160.1).

### Epidemiology

Three organisms together cause 80% of all cases of community-acquired bacterial meningitis: *Streptococcus pneumoniae, Neisseria meningitidis,* and *Haemophilus influenzae.* A strong relationship with age is evident, in that *H. influenzae* is usually seen in children below 1 year of age and rarely in adults unless asplenia, sinusitis, or alcoholism is present. Meningococcus is usually seen in children under age 5 but may occur in young adults sporadically or during epidemics.

Pneumococcus is seen in all ages, but is the most common organism in the adult. Predisposing factors for pneumococcal meningitis include otitis media or mastoiditis (30%), pneumonia (20%), and head trauma (10%). The number of sporadic bacterial meningitis cases increases in the autumn and winter months and declines during the spring, reaching a nadir during summer.

Enteric gram-negative bacillary meningitis is seen primarily in trauma, neurosurgical, or hospitalized patients. Whereas coagulase-negative staphylococcus is seen in patients with CNS shunts, *S. aureus* is usually related to trauma or endocarditis. Among adults, *Listeria* meningitis may occur in the elderly or those with defective cell-mediated (T-cell) immunity.

### Pathogenesis and Pathophysiology

The portal of entry of pathogens into the meninges is not conclusively known, but mucosal colonization followed by bacteremia and penetration of the blood–brain barrier through the choroid plexus are believed to be important steps. Contiguous extension of an infected focus (sinusitis or otitis media) and entry through the cribriform plate are other possible mechanisms. The survival of the organisms in the CSF is related to the virulence of the organism (e.g., encapsuled bacteria are more virulent) and also to the general lack of defense mechanisms in the CSF (e.g., the CSF is deficient in complement concentration and immunoglobulins). To-

**TABLE 160.1. Causes of Acute Meningitis**

| Infectious | Noninfectious |
|---|---|
| Bacterial | Medications |
| *Streptococcus pneumoniae* | Nonsteroidal anti-inflammatory agents |
| *Neisseria meningitidis* | Azathioprine |
| *Haemophilus influenzae* | Carbamazepine |
| Group B streptococci | Connective tissue disease |
| Gram-negative bacilli | Systemic lupus erythematosus |
| Staphylococci | Miscellaneous |
| *Listeria monocytogenes* | Following seizures |
| | Migraine |
| Viral | |
| Enterovirus | |
| HIV | |
| Rickettsial | |
| *Rickettsia rickettsii* (Rocky Mountain spotted fever) | |
| Typhus *(R. prowazekii, R. tsutsugamushi, R. typhi)* | |
| Spirochetal | |
| *Treponema pallidum* (syphilis) | |
| *Borrelia burgdorferi* (Lyme disease) | |
| Protozoa | |
| *Naegleria fowleri* | |

gether, these two factors cause a compromised opsonizing ability.

In the subarachnoid space, the bacteria evoke an intense **leptomeningitis.** The permeability of the blood–brain barrier may increase with the evolving inflammation, causing cerebral edema. Other sequelae include increased intracranial pressure, CSF acidosis, and encephalopathy that accompanies meningitis. The subarachnoid space inflammation may also impede the CSF flow, causing hydrocephalus and increased intracranial pressure.

Thrombotic or vasculitic involvement of the blood vessels causes areas of cerebral infarction. Compromised blood supply and perhaps other factors cause the meningeal and cerebral glycolysis to shift to the anaerobic pathway, thus resulting in lactate accumulation. The resultant CSF acidosis may be partly responsible for the **encephalopathy.**

**TABLE 160.2. Clinical Features of Bacterial Meningitis**

| |
|---|
| Extremely common (80–100%) |
| Confusion |
| Fever |
| Headache |
| Neck pain and stiffness (meningismus) |
| Common (50–80%) |
| Kernig sign |
| Brudzinski sign |
| Sometimes (30–35%) |
| Seizures |
| Vomiting |
| Uncommon (<20%) |
| Lateralizing neurologic deficits |
| Rare (<1%) |
| Papilledema |

## Clinical Features

One fourth of patients have a rapid onset with headache, lethargy, and confusion within 24 hours (Table 160.2). In the others, symptoms evolve over 1–7 days. In some patients, the features of meningitis may develop as an aftermath of or in continuity with a pneumonic process.

Petechial and purpuric rash are a clue to meningococcal infection (Gram stain yields a positive result in 70% of cases) and indicate **meningococcemia.** Focal findings, consisting of cranial nerve deficits (especially cranial nerves 3, 6, and 8), may be noted in 10–20% of patients. Papilledema is rare.

## Laboratory Features

The CSF classically shows an elevated WBC count that exceeds 1000/mm$^3$ with a predominance of neutrophils, an elevated protein level above 150 mg/dl, and a decreased glucose level below 40 mg/dl (hypoglycorrhachia). On average, Gram stain of the CSF is positive in 80% (50% or so with *Listeria*) and has a 100%

specificity (Table 160.3). Whereas latex agglutination tests are available for *H. influenzae, S. pneumoniae,* and *N. meningitidis,* their contribution to diagnosis beyond Gram stain has been questioned. CSF cultures are reportedly positive in 80%, with blood cultures being positive in 40–80%.

## Differential Diagnosis

Occasionally, viral meningitis can resemble a bacterial process, with neutrophil counts as high as 500/$mm^3$.

Usually, on repeat lumbar puncture within 12–36 hours, the cellular response becomes mononuclear. In the elderly and neutropenic patients, the CSF leukocyte count may not be high, and Gram stain is essential in ascertaining the presence of meningitis. If the diagnosis is in doubt, the lumbar puncture should generally be repeated within 12–36 hours.

## Management

The initial approach to the patient with suspected meningitis is outlined in Figure 160.1. Increasing anti-

**TABLE 160.3. Diagnostic Value of CSF Studies in Bacterial Meningitis**

| Test | Sensitivity |
|---|---|
| ↑ CSF opening pressure | Universal |
| ↑ CSF protein | Universal |
| CSF latex agglutination | 80–95% |
| CSF Gram stain | 70–90% |
| CSF culture | 80% |
| Blood cultures | 40–80% |
| CSF glucose: serum glucose <0.31 | 70% |
| Gram stain of petechiae | 70% |
| ↓ CSF glucose | 60% |
| CSF glucose <34 mg/dl, glucose ratio <0.23, protein >220 mg/ml, CSF leukocytes >2000/$mm^3$ (or >1180/$mm^3$ of CSF polymorphs) | Each >99% |

CSF = Cerebrospinal fluid.

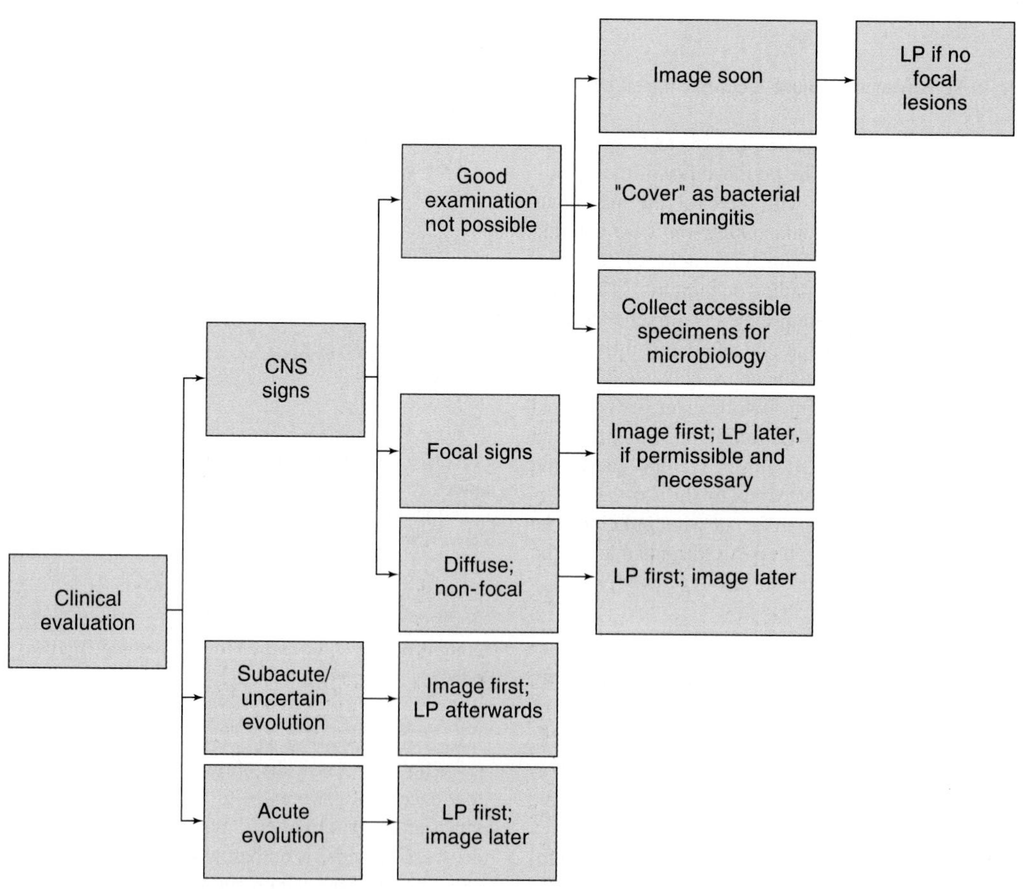


**FIGURE 160.1.** Initial management of suspected meningitis. The sequencing of lumbar puncture (LP) and imaging studies (CT scanning) for various presentations is outlined.

**TABLE 160.4. Bacterial Meningitis: Choice of Antibiotic Therapy**

| Age | Likely Microorganism | Empiric Initial Therapy | Alternative Therapy |
|---|---|---|---|
| Children <10 | *Haemophilus influenzae*, pneumococcus, meningococcus | Ceftriaxone and vancomycin until results of susceptibility testing are known | Chloramphenicol |
| Young adults | Meningococcus | Ceftriaxone/vancomycin | Chloramphenicol |
| Elderly | Pneumococcus, *Listeria*, and gram-negative bacilli | Ceftriaxone/vancomycin/ampicillin | |

biotic resistance among pneumococci has prompted changes in empiric antibiotics used in adults (Table 160.4). Presently, a third-generation cephalosporin is recommended for initial community-acquired bacterial meningitis, along with vancomycin until penicillin susceptibility is known; ampicillin should be added for individuals at risk for *Listeria* infection (elderly, alcoholic, or immunosuppressed patients). Penicillin G remains the drug of choice for penicillin-sensitive pneumococci, ensuring a MIC <0.1 mg/ml.

In general, 7 days of therapy is necessary for meningococci, 10 days for *H. influenzae,* and 14 days for pneumococci. Adjunctive **corticosteroid** use in children decreases hearing loss from *H. influenzae* meningitis. Its role in adults remains controversial. Complications of meningitis include cerebral edema, brain abscess, and residual neurologic deficit(s), particularly hearing deficit.

### Prevention

Close contacts of patients with meningococcal meningitis, defined as household members, day-care contacts, or medical personnel performing mouth-to-mouth resuscitation, are at a 500-fold to 800-fold increased risk of developing meningococcal meningitis. Rifampin, 600 mg every 12 hours for 2 days, or a single dose quinolone are effective prophylactic agents.

**TABLE 160.5. Causes of Aseptic Meningitis**

| Type | Specific Examples |
|---|---|
| Viral | Enterovirus or HIV |
| Bacterial | Listeria or parameningeal focus |
| Spirochete | Syphilis, Lyme, or Leptospirosis |
| Noninfectious | Vasculitis, sarcoid, drug, or tumor |

**TABLE 160.6. Causes of Chronic Meningitis by Cerebrospinal Fluid Cell Predominance**

| Lymphocytic | Neutrophilic |
|---|---|
| Tuberculosis | *Actinomyces* |
| Syphilis | *Nocardia* |
| Lyme disease | *Brucella* |
| *Cryptococcus* | *Candida* |
| *Coccidioides* | Aspergillosis |
| Histoplasmosis | Blastomycosis |
| Cysticercosis | Drug |
| Sarcoid | |
| Vasculitis | |
| Behçet syndrome | |
| Tumor | |
| Parameningeal | |

## Aseptic Meningitis

Aseptic meningitis is a misnomer because it denotes culture-negative meningitis (usually with lymphocytic predominance in the CSF), even though infectious agents are usually the cause (Table 160.5). In particular, viral agents are the most common cause, with enterovirus leading the list (coxsackie and ECHO virus).

The classic clinical presentation includes headache, fever, and neck pain and stiffness (meningismus) in children or young adults during the summer months. The CSF may be neutrophilic in two thirds of patients (usually <200 cells/mm$^3$), initially with mononuclear predominance occurring in 6–24 hours. The CSF glucose level is usually normal, and protein is below 100 mg/dl. Cultures of CSF and throat swabs may be positive.

## Subacute (Chronic) Meningitis

The classic definition of subacute or chronic meningitis is a meningitis exceeding 4 weeks' duration. The diagnosis can further be classified into **lymphocytic** or **neutrophilic** meningitis (Table 160.6).

Routine laboratory evaluation of the CSF may include the following tests: cryptococcal antigen, VDRL, complement fixation for *Coccidioides* and *Histoplasma*, Lyme index, cytology, *Brucella* and mycobacterial cultures. High-volume lumbar punctures with multiple cultures may be necessary. If no diagnosis is made and clinical status is worsening, then treatment for tuberculosis should be initiated.

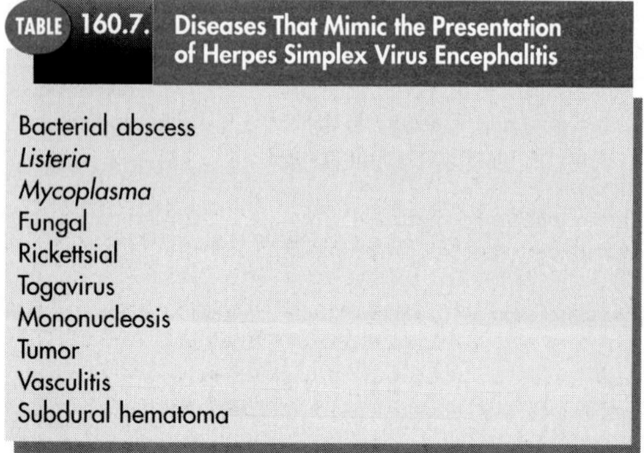

**TABLE 160.7. Diseases That Mimic the Presentation of Herpes Simplex Virus Encephalitis**

| |
|---|
| Bacterial abscess |
| *Listeria* |
| *Mycoplasma* |
| Fungal |
| Rickettsial |
| Togavirus |
| Mononucleosis |
| Tumor |
| Vasculitis |
| Subdural hematoma |

## Encephalitis

Encephalitis is characterized by fever, altered sensorium, seizures, and focal neurologic deficits. There may be evidence of meningeal irritation as well. Classically, encephalitis is viral in etiology, with **herpes simplex virus** (HSV) being the most common cause. However, nonviral causes may masquerade as herpes encephalitis (Table 160.7).

The pathogenesis usually involves viremia by neurotropic viruses with hematogenous seeding of the brain or ascent of viruses to the brain via peripheral nerves. In HSV, the transmission is slow. Invasion of the host cell is followed by viral replication and cessation of, or interference with, cellular function. In most cases, such infections are subclinical.

Encephalitis may be epidemic or nonepidemic. Epidemic forms include **mosquito-borne arborvirus encephalitides** including St. Louis, La Crosse, and eastern and western equine encephalitis in the United States and the flaviviral west nile virus; Japanese encephalitis is common in Southeast Asia. Rarely, enteroviruses or measles virus may cause an encephalitis. The nonepidemic form is most commonly HSV. Rabies is very uncommon in the United States.

### Clinical Features

The clinical presentation does not allow differentiation between the different causes. However, epidemiologic clues are useful. History of travel and contact with animals are important factors in the history. A history of animal bite is useful in the diagnosis of rabies.

At the onset, generally there is fever, altered sensorium, headache, vomiting, and confusion. Seizures may occur. Hyperpyrexia indicates involvement of the pontine temperature regulatory center. HSV encephalitis classically has bizarre behavior and hallucinations suggestive of a temporal lobe focus. There may be hydrophobia reported in rabies.

The course may be one of relentless progression, culminating in death (massive cortical destruction), or one of quick recovery with minimal or no sequelae (effective host response offsetting cellular damage). Progression followed by stability and slow recovery may also occur.

### Diagnostic Tests

Specific microbiological diagnosis is difficult in encephalitis. The CSF response is nonspecific and may be normal in HSV in 5–10% of cases. MRI and electroencephalography may be suggestive of HSV, but their specificity is unknown. **Polymerase chain reaction** of the CSF has become the best tool for diagnosing HSV, short of brain biopsy.

Acute and convalescent titers may be helpful, retrospectively, for the epidemic viruses only. Recently, an IgM antibody to the arborviruses has been developed and may be diagnostic upon presentation.

### Management

Management of encephalitis is complicated by the nonspecific clinical picture for individual causative agents. The difficulty in making a specific microbiological diagnosis and in ruling out HSV and the clinician's reluctance to perform a brain biopsy for HSV further compound the management dilemma. Because of these factors and because HSV is the only treatable cause, acyclovir is usually given at 10 mg/kg every 8 hours for 10–14 days whenever HSV is a possible cause. Patients whose condition progresses despite treatment should undergo brain biopsy.

# CHAPTER 161 BACTEREMIA, SEPSIS, AND SEPTIC SYNDROME

## Bacteremia

Bacteremia is defined as the invasion of blood by bacteria, as detected by blood cultures. Because blood circulates in a closed system, bacteremia always presupposes an infectious focus elsewhere in the body (the source), from which the blood becomes seeded. Bacteremia also forms the quintessential diagnostic feature of infective endocarditis.

For any infection, bacterial or otherwise, the development of bloodstream invasion portends a worse prognosis and a major threat to life. Bacteremic patients have a higher rate of complications, longer hospital stay, and higher mortality. Bacteremia carries an overall mortality of 30%, which is influenced by several factors, such as the source, identity, and virulence of the organism on one hand, and a number of host factors on the other, including the status of the specific defenses, functional status, underlying diseases, and the presence or absence of complications.

### Epidemiology

Bacteremias may be transient, intermittent, or continuous. **Transient** bacteremia may follow dental manipulations or instrumentation of infected areas, such as dental procedures or even brushing teeth. Bacteremia that complicates undrained abscesses is generally **intermittent.** In conditions characterized by endovascular infection (endocarditis, endarteritis, or septic thrombophlebitis), the bacteremia is **continuous.**

In general medical wards, bacteremia is much more prevalent among the elderly and those with diabetes mellitus, cerebrovascular accidents, underlying neoplastic disease, or chronic renal failure.

The prevalence of bacteremia may vary, depending on the amount of blood that is obtained for individual blood cultures, because it has been shown that use of a larger volume of blood (15 ml or more per culture) increases the rate of detection of bacteremia. The epidemiology of bacteremia differs, depending on whether it is community-acquired or nosocomial. By tradition, bacteremia detected within 72 hours of hospitalization is considered community-acquired (unless the patient was a resident of a long-term care facility). Although the use of 72 hours may seem arbitrary, the separation of bacteremias into community-acquired and nosocomial has clear implications in terms of the organism(s) involved, source of the bacteremia, complication rate, and mortality.

#### Community-acquired bacteremia

Community-acquired bacteremia is more frequent among the elderly. The most frequent sources and most common organisms are listed in Table 161.1. In some cases, more than one organism may be detected in blood cultures. Once contamination has been excluded, polymicrobial bacteremia suggests the biliary tract, intra-abdominal sepsis, or a UTI as a source.

Some organisms tend to be associated with specific underlying infections (e.g., pneumococcal bacteremia with pneumonia). It is also important to note that in some cases, the source may remain elusive after a diligent search, a feature most likely to occur with *E. coli,* Enterococcus, *Pseudomonas*, *Bacteroides*, and some polymicrobial bacteremias.

**TABLE 161.1. Community-Acquired Bacteremia: Most Frequent Source(s) and Common Organisms**

| Organism | Most Likely Primary Infectious Process/Source | Next Most Likely Source |
|---|---|---|
| *Escherichia coli* | Urinary tract infection | Biliary tract (unknown in some cases) |
| *Streptococcus pneumoniae* | Pneumonia | Meningitis |
| *Klebsiella species* | Biliary tract | Urinary tract/lower respiratory tract |
| *Staphylococcus aureus* | Lower respiratory tract | Endocarditis |
| Enterococcus | Urinary tract | |
| *Proteus* | Urinary tract | |
| *Pseudomonas* | Urinary tract | |
| *Streptococcus bovis* | Endocarditis | |
| *Streptococcus viridans* | Endocarditis | |

(Data from: Esposito AL, Gleckman RA, Cram S, et al. Community-acquired bacteremia in the elderly: analysis of one hundred consecutive episodes. J Am Geriatr Soc 1980;28:315–319.)

### Nosocomial bacteremia

Nosocomial bacteremias may be primary or secondary. A focus (source) is identifiable in the secondary and absent in the primary types. However, bacteremia occurring from an intravascular device in the absence of local purulent infection at the infusion site is also considered primary nosocomial bacteremia. Nosocomial bacteremia may also be endemic or epidemic.

Risk factors for nosocomial bacteremia are summarized in Table 161.2. Most endemic nosocomial bacteremias arise from skin (e.g., postoperative wound or intravenous catheter infections), intra-abdominal, urinary tract, pulmonary (pneumonias), or other focal infections. The most common organisms causing endemic nosocomial bacteremias are *Staphylococcus aureus, S. epidermidis, Klebsiella*, group D streptococcus, *S. pneumoniae,* and *Escherichia coli.*

## Clinical Features

Features of bacteremia are listed in Table 161.3. **Fever** and **shaking chills** are classic symptoms, but rigors may be absent in the debilitated patient. In a significant number of patients, the fever and chills are preceded by **hyperventilation** and **changes in mental status. Hypotension** is present in those who manifest septic shock. A **decline in urinary output** may also be noted. Patients with gram-positive bacteremias may show diffuse reddening of the skin (erythroderma), and those with *Pseudomonas* bacteremias may show a central vesicular lesion surrounded by a halo of erythema and induration, which becomes ulcerated **(ecthyma gangrenosum).** Hemodynamic compromise may develop when bacteremia evolves into septic shock or systemic inflammatory response syndrome (SIRS). Multiorgan failure may evolve.

**TABLE 161.2. Risk Factors for Nosocomial Bacteremia**

| |
|---|
| Host factors |
| Elderly patient |
| Systemic antimicrobial therapy |
| Multiple trauma or burns |
| Life-threatening underlying illness |
| Granulocytopenia |
| Immunosuppression (corticosteroids or cytotoxic agents) |
| Environmental factors |
| Intensive care unit |
| Vascular or nonvascular invasive device |
| Hemodialysis |
| Infusion of large volume of parenteral fluids or blood products |

(Adapted from: Maki DG. Am J Med 1981;70:724. Used with permission.)

**TABLE 161.3. Manifestations of Bacteremia**

| |
|---|
| Fever |
| Confusion, drowsiness, delirium |
| Lethargy |
| Tachycardia |
| Hyperventilation |
| Chills/rigors |
| Hypotension |
| Nausea/vomiting |
| Hypotension |
| Diarrhea |
| Falls† |
| Incontinence from altered mentation† |

†In the elderly.

Although fever is the general rule, bacteremia without fever has been well-documented. The elderly, especially those with associated renal failure or hypoalbuminemia, seem to exhibit this feature more frequently. Bacteremia may be detected incidentally in these persons from the blood cultures performed to elucidate some other disturbance. Whereas the lack of fever is a poor prognostic sign, the development of hypothermia is even more ominous.

Although further validation is necessary, five variables apparent within 24 hours of hospitalization have been proposed that may have a high predictive value for bacteremia: a low performance status prior to hospitalization, chills on admission, renal failure, low serum albumin, and presumptive admitting diagnosis of UTI.

## Management

Major problems related to blood cultures are the false-positive (positive blood culture with no bacteremia) and false-negative cultures. The frequency of false-positive blood cultures varies widely, and most are related to contamination from the skin flora. Clues for recognizing false-positive cultures are listed in Table 161.4. False-negative cultures may be due to an inadequate volume of blood sampled, an inadequate number of blood cultures obtained, or the low prevalence of the bacteremia in a given condition (low pre-test probability).

Guidelines for the use of blood cultures to diagnose bacteremia are shown in Table 161.5. Use of a larger volume of blood (>15 ml/culture) increases the rate of detection of bacteremia. An underlying issue in many false positive cultures is improper technique, which is remediable with proper education.

Patients who manifest symptoms suspicious for bacteremia should have a blood culture performed. A careful assessment is necessary to elucidate the source. Once the necessary laboratory material is obtained for examination, the patient should be started on appropriate **antibiotic therapy.** Because the exact organism is not known initially, treatment is empiric until culture results become available. The initial choice of antibiotics should cover the most likely organisms. Because gram-negative organisms are the most common in community-acquired bacteremia, an aminoglycoside and anti-pseudomonal penicillin would suffice. If *Staphylococcus aureus* bacteremia is suspected, nafcillin or vancomycin should be added.

### Catheter-related infections

The association of bacteremia with a catheter requires quantitative methods. In suspected cases of intravascular catheter-related infections, the catheter should be removed and the distal 2 inches of the catheter should be aseptically clipped into a sterile container and sent for quantitative cultures. In addition, blood cultures should also be obtained. Others have recommended obtaining two sets of blood cultures, one through the intravascular line and another from a peripheral vein. Because the catheters are often colonized, such colonizing organisms are isolated from the culture drawn through the catheter. Aerobic organisms (*S. aureus*, *S. epidermidis*, *Klebsiella,* etc) are usually responsible, and the initial antibiotic management should take into account these possibilities.

Intravenous hyperalimentation solutions are another potential source of nosocomial bacteremia, but with a dedicated team for initiating the catheter insertion and its follow-up care, this can be minimized.

**TABLE 161.4 Clues to False-Positive Blood Culture Results**

Isolation of the following organisms:
- Diphtheroids
- *Staphylococcus epidermidis*
- Bacillus species*

Inability to isolate same organisms in subsequent cultures
Isolation of multiple organisms in the same culture
Isolation of organism after delayed bacterial growth (broth only)
Same species, but with varying antibiotic sensitivity patterns
Lack of correlation with clinical course
- No identifiable primary infection by the same organism

Lack of identifiable predisposing factors, such as
- Prosthetic devices
- Intravenous drug abuse
- Recent hospitalization
- Immunosuppression

Lack of leukocytosis or left shift

*Isolation of enteric gram-negative aerobic organisms, *Streptococcus pyogenes*, or *Streptococcus pneumoniae* is seldom false-positive.
(Adapted and reprinted with permission from: Aronson MD, Bor DH. Ann Intern Med 1987;106:246–253.)

**TABLE 161.5. Guidelines for Blood Cultures**

1. Use strict asepsis (disinfect the skin).
2. Draw at least 10 ml of blood per culture, preferably more.
3. Draw blood through a closed collecting system or syringe and needle and transfer into the culture bottle. Disinfect the rubber stoppers of bottles before inoculating the medium.
4. Never draw blood for culture through an indwelling catheter.
5. Use universal precautions, as for handling all body fluids.
6. One blood culture is seldom enough; obtain multiple cultures.
7. If the anticipated organisms can be mistaken for a skin contaminant (e.g., *S. epidermidis* when a prosthetic valve endocarditis is suspected), then multiple sets of cultures should yield the same organism.
8. The number of cultures required depends on the anticipated organism (AO) and the pretest probability of bacteremia.
   a. If the AO is not usually a contaminant, and probability is moderate—obtain 2 sets.
   b. If continuous bacteremia is suspected—obtain 3 sets.
   c. If there has been prior antibiotic therapy—obtain 4 sets.

AO = anticipated organism.
(Adapted and reprinted with permission from: Aronson MD, Bor DH. Ann Intern Med 1987;106: 246–253.)

## Complications and Prognosis

Bacteremia carries a high overall mortality rate of 30%. The mortality increases with increasing age and with hospital-acquired bacteremias. The mortality from pneumococcal bacteremia seems to have changed little over the decades and stands at 20%, with most deaths occurring within the first 48 hours of hospitalization.

## ■ Sepsis and Sepsis Syndrome

The terminology and nomenclature of sepsis, as prepared by the Society of Critical Care Medicine, is shown in Table 161.6.

**TABLE 161.6. Terminology for "Sepsis"**

| Term | Definition |
|---|---|
| Sepsis | Evidence of infection plus ≥2 of the following:<br>Temperature >38°C or <36°C<br>Heart rate >90 bpm<br>Respiratory rate >20/min or $Paco_2$ <32 mm Hg<br>WBC >12,000/mm$^3$ or <4000/mm$^3$ |
| Sepsis syndrome | Sepsis plus organ hypoperfusion: hypoxemia, oliguria, altered mentation |
| Hypotension | BP <90 mm Hg or reduction >40 mm Hg from baseline |
| Severe sepsis | Sepsis with organ dysfunction, hypoperfusion or hypotension; including lactic acidosis, oliguria, or altered mental status |
| Septic shock | Sepsis with hypotension despite fluids, plus above criteria for severe sepsis |
| Refractory septic shock | Shock lasting >1 hr despite intervention |

**TABLE 161.7. Suggested Empiric Antibiotic Therapy for Sepsis Syndrome**

| Disease | | First Choices | Alternates |
|---|---|---|---|
| Nonneutropenic | Community-acquired UTI | Third-generation cephalosporin ± aminoglycoside | Piperacillin-tazobactam/ticarcillin/quinolones |
| | Community-acquired infection, not UTI | Third-generation cephalosporin/ampicillin-sulbactam ± aminoglycoside | Ticarcillin-clavulanic acid/ piperacillin-tazobactam ± aminoglycoside |
| | Hospital-acquired | Piperacillin-tazobactam ± aminoglycoside | Third-generation cephalosporin ± aminoglycoside or imipenem ± aminoglycoside |
| Neutropenic | | Piperacillin-tazobactam ± aminoglycoside | Imipenem ± aminoglycoside or piperacillin-tazobactam ± aminoglycoside |
| Intravenous catheter-related | | Same as neutropenic + vancomycin | Same as neutropenic + vancomycin |

UTI = urinary tract infection.

## Pathophysiology

Although any organism can cause sepsis, sepsis involving gram-negative organisms has been best studied. The bacterial **endotoxin,** which is responsible for initiating sepsis, is a lipopolysaccharide making up part of the cell wall. This lipid moiety is relatively conserved among all gram-negative bacteria and is responsible for triggering sepsis via cytokines.

The **cytokines,** especially tumor necrosis factor (TNF) and IL1, are macrophage-derived and are the primary mediators of sepsis. TNF causes the release of prostaglandins, platelet-activating factors, leukotrienes, and thromboxane, which results in excessive vascular permeability, activation of the clotting cascade, and endothelial damage. What results are the signs and symptoms identified with sepsis (see below). The irony is that in low doses, TNF and IL1 are protective, priming host defenses, but their massive production as in sepsis can be lethal.

## Clinical Features

The earliest manifestation of sepsis is **hyperventilation,** occurring even before fever. **Fever** is typical, but hypothermia may occur and portends a poor prognosis. Mental status changes, especially lethargy, and rarely agitation may occur. Further complications may include hypotension (initially; from vasodilation or "warm shock"), characterized by decreased peripheral and pulmonary vascular resistances. The cardiac index may be elevated.

Thrombocytopenia (with or without a coagulopathy) and organ failure, including respiratory failure (hypoxia, adult respiratory distress syndrome [ARDS]), renal failure (oliguria), or liver failure (jaundice, hepatic encephalopathy), may be associated or follow. Hypoperfusion may cause lactic acidosis. The picture at this point is one of systemic endothelial dysfunction, with enhanced capillary permeability affecting many organs, such as the gut, liver, and lungs.

### Management

A good **history** is a key component of the clinical evaluation. Attention to underlying diseases, travel, exposures, and other factors is essential. Signs and symptoms pointing to a nidus should be sought (e.g., headache, joint pain, or diarrhea may suggest the site of focal infection). Careful, thorough **physical examination** should be completed with the realization that in immunosuppressed hosts, disease manifestations may be blunted. Two sets of **blood cultures** should be taken.

**Further testing** is dictated by the clinical setting. Usually, complete blood counts, liver function tests, and coagulation studies are performed. If no nidus is apparent, a urinalysis and chest radiograph should be done. Abdominal pain should prompt surgical consultation. Obstructing hydronephrosis should be excluded if a UTI is the nidus. One should always consider diseases that require immediate surgical intervention.

Appropriate **antibiotic selection** is extremely important in the early phases of sepsis, because mortality is reduced as much as 50% when antibiotics are chosen properly. Because microbiological data are not available for 1–2 days, initial antibiotic selection is empiric. The clinical setting should dictate antibiotic selection (Table 161.7). The hospital's **antibiogram** (antibiotic resistance patterns) must also be considered, and recommendations may vary for individual institutions. If aminoglycosides are used, aggressive dosing is essential for sepsis because they have concentration-dependent killing.

# CHAPTER 162 NOSOCOMIAL INFECTIONS

Nosocomial infections are usually defined as infections acquired 48–72 hours after hospital admission. Approximately 5% of hospitalized patients develop a nosocomial infection, with UTI being the most common. Other sites include the respiratory tract, surgical wounds, intravascular catheters, nonvascular prostheses, and instrumentation (e.g., endoscopy).

The microbiology varies according to site (Table 162.1), and rates for nosocomial infection vary according to patient population. Hospital size influences nosocomial infection rates, with the highest incidence (8.5%) being in municipal teaching hospitals and the lowest (3.7%) in small nonteaching hospitals.

Nosocomial bacteremia is discussed in Chapter 161, and nosocomial pneumonia, in Chapter 148. Suggested

**TABLE 162.1. The Microbiology of Nosocomial Infections According to Site***

| Urinary tract infection | Pneumonia | Intravenous catheter–related |
|---|---|---|
| *Short-term catheterization* | *Frequent pathogens* | *Staphylococcus epidermidis* |
| *Escherichia coli* | *Pseudomonas aeruginosa* | *Staphylococcus aureus* |
| Yeast | *Staphylococcus aureus* | Gram-negative bacilli |
| *Pseudomonas aeruginosa* | *Enterobacter* spp | *Candida* spp. |
| *Klebsiella* spp. | *Klebsiella* spp. | |
| Coagulase negative staphylococci | *Escherichia coli* | |
| Other gram-negative bacilli | *Haemophilus influenzae* | |
| *Proteus* spp. | *Serratia marcescens* | |
| *Long-term catheterization* | *Streptococcus pneumoniae* | |
| *Providencia* spp. | *Infrequent pathogens* | |
| *Proteus* spp. | *Streptococcus pneumoniae* | |
| *Escherichia coli* | *Legionella* spp. | |
| *Pseudomonas aeruginosa* | Influenza | |
| Enterococcus spp. | Surgical wounds | |
| *Morganella morganii* | *Staphylococcus aureus* | |
| *Klebsiella* spp. | Enterococcus spp. | |
| | Coagulase-negative staphylococci | |
| | *Escherichia coli* | |
| | *Pseudomonas* spp. | |

*Causative organisms are arranged in the order of prevalence.

**TABLE 162.2. Suggested Antibiotic Selection for Nosocomial Infections**

| Site | Likely Organisms | Antibiotics |
|---|---|---|
| Urinary tract | Enterobacteriaceae | Third-generation cephalosporin, extended-spectrum penicillin, quinolone, or aminoglycoside |
| | Enterococcus | Ampicillin plus aminoglycoside |
| Intravenous catheter | Staphylococci | Nafcillin ± aminoglycoside (vancomycin if MRSA is endemic) |
| Pneumonia | *S. pneumoniae* | Penicillin G or vancomycin |
| | *S. aureus* | Nafcillin (vancomycin if MRSA is endemic) |
| | *P. aeruginosa* | Piperacillin-tazobactam ± aminoglycoside |
| | *H. influenzae* | Ampicillin or ceftriaxone |
| Site unknown | Organism unknown, urgent empiric therapy needed | See Table 161.7 |

MRSA = Methicillin-resistant *Staphylococcus aureus.*

antibiotic selection for nosocomial infections is provided in Table 162.2.

## Urinary Tract Infection

Most nosocomial UTIs (80%) are catheter-associated, with an additional 10% occurring after genitourinary manipulations. **Catheter-associated bacteremia** occurs at a rate of around 5% per day. Organisms from the patient's own colonic flora first colonize the urethra and then ascend the catheter's extraluminal surface. Intraluminal entry has been much less frequent since closed systems have become standard.

Certain independent factors have been associated with the risk for **bacteriuria,** especially length of catheterization, gender (female), diabetes, and periurethral colonization. The colonizing organism may change every 1–2 weeks. Long-term catheterized patients have complications with infected urinary stones (struvite) or periurinary infections.

Treatment is unnecessary for asymptomatic bacteriuria in catheterized patients. Bacteriuria persisting after removal of the catheter may indicate a higher likelihood of UTI and thus may warrant a short course of antibiotics. Changing of the catheter because of bacterial biofilm on catheters is also suggested.

Treatment of **candiduria** remains controversial. Possible treatment options include fluconazole or amphotericin bladder irrigation. Upper urinary tract disease should be a consideration (i.e., fungus ball) in difficult-to-treat patients and may require ultrasound or CT for evaluation.

Obviously, avoidance of catheterization is the best prevention. External devices (e.g., condom catheters or intermittent catheterization) are alternative solutions. Suprapubic catheters may have lower rates of bacteriuria (less colonization of abdominal skin) and may help avoid problems of urethral strictures. The role for catheters impregnated with antimicrobials (i.e., silver-impregnated catheters) for prevention of bacteriuria is unclear. Oral antibiotics may prevent bacteriuria for a few days but may lead to selection of resistant microbes.

# CHAPTER 163 SKIN, SOFT TISSUE, AND BONE INFECTIONS

## Cellulitis

Cellulitis is an acute infection involving the deeper dermis and subcutaneous fatty tissues. It is most commonly caused by *Streptococcus pyogenes* and *Staphylococcus aureus.* Factors predisposing to bacterial invasion are usually present (Table 163.1).

The involved area becomes warm, swollen, and erythematous, sometimes with lymphangitis, regional adenopathy, chills, and fever. Unlike **erysipelas,** the borders of the lesions lack distinct boundaries and are not elevated; however, like erysipelas, the diagnosis is usually clinical. Aspirating the leading edge of the cellulitis yields an etiologic diagnosis in only about 25% of cases. If the patient is febrile, blood cultures should be obtained.

Although most cases of cellulitis are due to *Streptococcus pyogenes, Staphylococcus aureus* is also covered by treatment with a penicillinase-resistant penicillin. Serious cases require parenteral therapy until clinical improvement occurs, when one may substitute oral therapy. Certain types of cellulitis with tissue necrosis (e.g., clostridial anaerobic cellulitis) require both antibiotics and surgical debridement.

## Necrotizing Fasciitis

Necrotizing fasciitis is an infrequent infection of subcutaneous and fascial tissues. There are two types: one is caused by *Streptococcus pyogenes,* and the other is caused by a mixture of anaerobes (e.g., *Bacteroides* or *Peptostreptococcus* species) and aerobes, including gram-positive cocci (e.g., staphylococci, streptococci, enterococci) and gram-negative bacilli (e.g., *Escherichia coli, Klebsiella, Enterobacter, Proteus* species). The first type tends to follow minor trauma in the extremities. Underlying diabetes mellitus, drug abuse, and alcoholism are generally present. The mixed infection tends to follow abdominal surgery or bowel perforation secondary to a gastrointestinal neoplasm or diverticulitis. In both types, patients have high fever and appear seriously ill.

A type of necrotizing fasciitis of the male genitalia, a mixed anaerobic and aerobic infection, is **Fournier gangrene.** The patient, generally a diabetic, has had a recent local skin, perianal, or urinary tract infection that rapidly spreads into the genital soft tissues, causing swelling, erythema, and crepitation.

In necrotizing fasciitis, the affected soft tissues display rapidly progressive and very painful erythema. Necrosis of underlying tissues and destruction of vessels and cutaneous nerves follow. Consequently, changes in the skin color, skin breakdown, and variable degrees of anesthesia result. In the mixed infection, tissue gas and a foul odor may be present, which are absent with streptococcal fasciitis. Therapy for necrotizing fasciitis includes immediate surgical debridement and antibiotics—a combination to cover the mixed flora—is appropriate before definite microbiological data are available.

## Myositis with Eosinophilia

Helminthic infections with muscle involvement often manifest eosinophilia, which helps distinguish these processes. Examples that may be seen in the United States include the nematode *Trichinella spiralis* and the cestode *Taenia solium.*

**Trichinosis** follows the ingestion of undercooked infected pork. By the second week of infection, Trichinella larvae enter the circulation and invade skeletal muscle, where they cause muscle pain, swelling, and weakness. Extraocular muscle involvement causes a prominent periorbital edema. The diagnosis is usually

**TABLE 163.1. Causes of Cellulitis and Associated Conditions**

| Etiologic Agents | Predisposing Conditions | Antimicrobial Agents |
|---|---|---|
| *Streptococcus pyogenes* (and other streptococci) | Trauma, puncture wound, tinea pedis | Penicillin, macrolide |
| *Staphylococcus aureus* | Trauma, puncture wound, tinea pedis | Penicillinase-resistant penicillin (e.g., nafcillin, vancomycin) |
| Gram-negative bacteria (e.g., Enterobacteriaceae, *Serratia, Pseudomonas, Proteus* spp.) | Granulocytopenia | Third-generation cephalosporins, extended spectrum penicillins, quinolones, aminoglycosides |
| *Vibrio* spp. (e.g., *Vibrio vulnificus, Vibrio parahaemolyticus*) | Traumatic wound in salt water or brackish inland water | Chloramphenicol, tetracycline, aminoglycosides |
| *Aeromonas hydrophila* | Traumatic wound in freshwater | Third-generation cephalosporins, quinolones, aztreonam, aminoglycosides |
| *Erysipelothrix rhusiopathiae* | Abrasion from handling saltwater fish, poultry, meat, hides | Penicillin |
| *Clostridium perfringens* | Contaminated traumatic or surgical wound | Penicillin |
| Nonclostridial anaerobic cellulitis (*Bacteroides, Peptostreptococcus, Peptococcus,* aerobic streptococci, gram-negative bacilli) | Diabetes mellitus, local trauma | Broad-spectrum therapy to cover the range of pathogens |

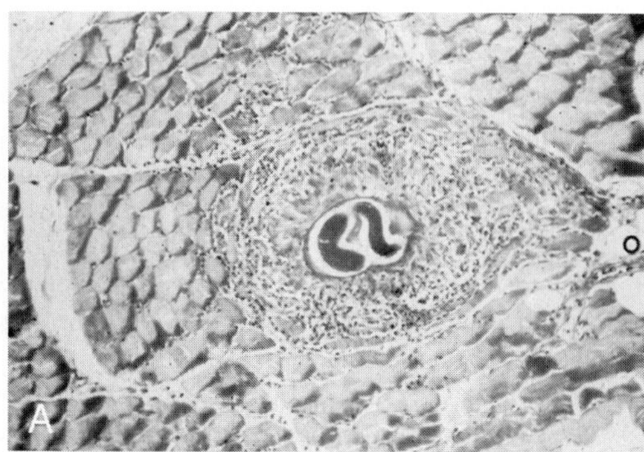


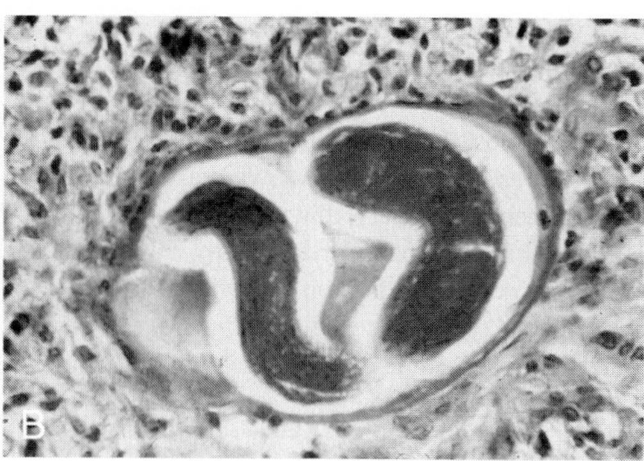


**FIGURE 163.1. Trichinosis. A, Muscle biopsy showing encysted larvae of *Trichinella spiralis*, with muscle necrosis and a predominantly eosinophilic infiltrate. B, Magnified view of encysted larva.** (Courtesy of Lawrence S. Hurwitz, MD, Milwaukee, Wisconsin.)

made serologically. Muscle biopsy, when performed, shows encysted larvae, with muscle necrosis and a predominantly eosinophilic infiltrate (Figure 163.1).

**Cysticercosis,** which occurs primarily in visitors or immigrants from endemic areas (e.g., Mexico, South America, Africa), is transmitted by ingestion of food contaminated with *Taenia solium* (pork tapeworm) eggs. Widespread systemic involvement follows, including the CNS, subcutaneous tissues, and muscle (Figure 163.2). Muscle involvement is usually asymptomatic and often detected by the appearance of calcified cysts on radiographs. The diagnosis, as with trichinosis, is usually made serologically.

## Infected Bite Wounds

Bite wounds are common from dogs, cats, and humans, and the likelihood of infection at the site depends on the degree of tissue injury and delay in obtaining appropriate wound care. Although there is usually a localized cellulitis, there may be a deeper soft-tissue infection (including abscesses), septic arthritis, or osteomyelitis or metastatic foci from bacteremia.

Common infecting organisms and the usual therapeutic options are listed in Table 163.2. Some patients with more severe infections may need equivalent types of parenteral antibiotics and surgical debridement. The need for tetanus and/or rabies vaccines should be assessed as well.

## Osteomyelitis

Osteomyelitis, or bone infection, is primarily bacterial, occurring either hematogenously or by contiguous extension from a soft-tissue focus of infection. Some clinical examples and typical organisms are

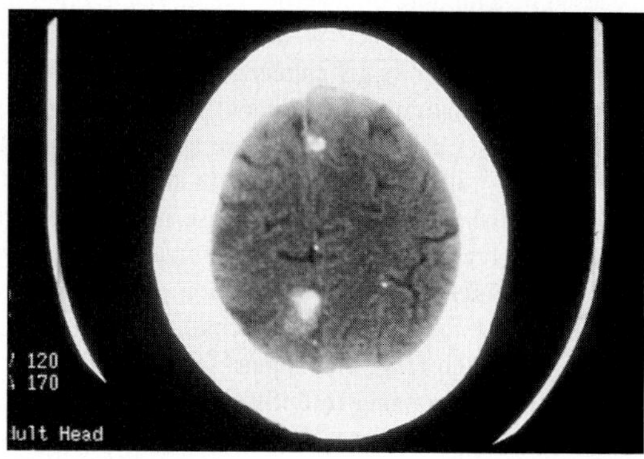


**FIGURE 163.2. Cerebral cysticercosis. A CT scan first suggested this diagnosis in this patient with seizures.** (Courtesy of Katherine Slattery, MD, Medical College of Wisconsin, Milwaukee, Wisconsin.)

outlined in Table 163.3. Bone infection is associated with tissue edema and vascular occlusion. With chronic infection, areas of bony necrosis, termed **sequestra,** develop.

Characteristically, the symptoms are subacute or chronic, despite the well-known acute presentation in adults with localized pain and fever (more common with the hematogenous type). Fever may or may not be present. The onset may be particularly insidious in the diabetic patient with peripheral neuropathy, owing to the lack of sensation in the extremity, and it may present with a nonhealing, chronically draining ulcer.

Bone **radiographs** may reveal nonspecific changes or the typical periosteal elevation and soft tissue swelling, but these changes lag behind the clinical disease process. Radionuclide studies or MRI can detect these inflammatory changes sooner and with more accuracy. Definitive diagnosis of osteomyelitis, however, is by culturing a biopsy or aspirate of affected bone. Except for infections involving *S. aureus,* culture of the sinus tract does not yield a good correlation with cultures of bone.

Osteomyelitis is treated using an antibiotic appropriate for the pathogen. **Antibiotics** are traditionally given parenterally for 4–6 weeks, although long-term oral antibiotics are appropriate in certain settings (e.g., oral quinolones for sensitive gram-negative organisms). Surgical debridement may be integral to successful therapy in selected cases, especially in chronic osteomyelitis, in which necrotic bone precludes proper penetration of antibiotics. With preexisting ulcers or prior debridement, tissue flaps may be necessary.

Recurrences are well known, particularly in the diabetic patient. In these patients, antibiotic therapy is termed **suppressive** and does not eradicate the infection. Over time, continued infection may necessitate an amputation.

## Infection in Orthopedic Prosthetic Devices

Orthopedic prosthetic devices have an infection rate of 1–5%. Infection, usually initiated at the bone–cement interface, occurs by local introduction of organisms or, less commonly, hematogenously. Staphylococci (both coagulase-negative and positive) are the most frequent pathogens, followed by streptococci and gram-negative bacilli.

Although an acute clinical presentation occurs with joint pain and fever in some patients, the typical onset is more insidious. Diagnosis rests on sampling joint fluid and isolating the pathogen. When the diagnosis is in question, more than one arthrocentesis should be performed to confirm the pathogen. Successful treatment usually involves removal of the prosthesis, followed by a 6-week course of appropriate antibiotics and then reimplantation.

**TABLE 163.2. Bite Wound Infections**

| Type of Bite | Usual Infecting Organisms | Antimicrobial Therapy |
|---|---|---|
| Dog or cat | *Pasteurella multocida*<br>*Staphylococcus aureus*<br>*Streptococcus* spp.<br>*Prevotella* spp.<br>*Fusobacterium* spp. | Amoxicillin-clavulanic acid, penicillin, or ampicillin |
| Human | *Streptococcus* spp.<br>*Staphylococcus aureus*<br>*Prevotella* spp.<br>*Peptostreptococcus* spp.<br>*Fusobacterium* spp. | Amoxicillin-clavulanic acid, penicillin, or ampicillin |

**TABLE 163.3. Categories and Etiology of Osteomyelitis**

| Underlying Disease | Typical Organisms |
|---|---|
| Hematogenous spread | |
| Endocarditis, infected intravascular catheter, urinary tract infection, intravenous drug use | *Staphylococcus aureus, Pseudomonas aeruginosa* (and other gram-negative bacilli), *Candida* spp. |
| Sickle cell disease | Salmonella spp., *Staphylococcus aureus* |
| Secondary to a contiguous focus | |
| Without vascular insufficiency | *Staphylococcus aureus*, gram-negative bacilli, anaerobes |
| Contamination from surgery or trauma, local soft tissue infection (e.g., decubitus ulcer) | |
| With vascular insufficiency | |
| Lower extremity soft tissue injury in a patient with diabetic neuropathy and vascular insufficiency | Staphylococci, streptococci, enterococci, gram-negative bacilli, anaerobes |

# CHAPTER 164 INFECTIONS IN THE IMMUNOCOMPROMISED HOST

This chapter explores infections in patients with relatively common acquired immunosuppressive conditions, such as trauma, cancer, and transplantation. Each of these conditions is associated with specific defects in host immunity (see Chapter 148), with an associated set of typical pathogens. Additional information about immunodeficiencies is also given in Chapter 21. Infection with HIV is discussed in Chapter 165.

## Infections in Patients with Trauma

Examples of physical injury with prominent infectious complications include major burns and trauma (e.g., multiple trauma, spinal cord injury).

Major blunt or penetrating trauma, such as that from an automobile accident, compromises the host defenses and increases risk of infection. Natural cutaneous barriers are violated, and injured tissues are made nonviable and ischemic; thus, the ability of the host to combat invading microbes is imperiled.

The nature and geographic location of the injury predisposes to certain types of microbes (e.g., injuries contaminated with freshwater may lead to wound infection with *Aeromonas hydrophila).* Although aggressive resuscitation enhances survival, it also contributes partly to the significantly increased infection-related mortality in this population. An overview of infections in trauma patients and their mechanisms is provided in Table 164.1.

## Infections in Spinal Cord Injury Patients

Spinal cord injury often follows traumatic injury and may occur with multiple trauma. However, the patient who is chronically or permanently disabled from spinal cord injury is also at risk for infectious complications, generally because of a breakdown of the natural defense barriers. Some of the more common causes or sites of infection, predisposing factors, and organisms are outlined in Table 164.2.

## Infections in Patients with Cancer

Patients with malignant disease may be at risk for infectious complications for a variety of reasons. Host defense defects in these patients may result from impaired clearance of microbes, destruction of normal defense barriers, and tumor or treatment-related effects. Major immunodeficient states common to cancer patients, including likely infecting organisms seen with each deficiency, are listed in Table 164.3. There is very little overlap in pathogenic organisms among these three immunodeficient states, and so, once the immune deficiency is recognized, it has profound implications for an empiric therapeutic approach. Multiple defects may

**TABLE 164.1. Infections in Patients with Severe Trauma**

| Site | Cause for Predisposition at This Site | Usual Organisms Involved |
|---|---|---|
| Wound | Blunt or penetrating trauma | *Staphylococcus aureus*, Streptococci<br>Possible mixed flora |
| Urinary tract | Urinary catheters | Gram-negative rods, *Enterococcus* spp. |
| Lower respiratory tract | Endotracheal intubation, sedation, aspiration, chest trauma | *Haemophilus influenzae*<br>*Staphylococcus aureus*<br>Gram-negative rods |
| Intravenous line–associated bacteremia | Nonsterile insertion, contamination from proximate wounds, frequent manipulation | *Staphylococcus aureus*<br>Coagulase-negative staphylococci |
| Gastrointestinal tract–associated sepsis | Penetrating trauma, shock, bacterial translocation | Gram-negative rods<br>*Enterococcus* spp.<br>Anaerobes |
| Central nervous system | Basilar skull fracture, cerebrospinal fluid leak, cerebrospinal fluid catheters | Gram-negative rods<br>*Staphylococcus aureus* |
| Pleural space | Chest tubes | *Staphylococcus aureus*<br>Gram-negative rods |

**TABLE 164.2. Causes of Infection in Patients With Spinal Cord Injury**

| Site | Cause for Predisposition at This Site | Usual Organisms Involved |
|---|---|---|
| Lower respiratory tract | Aspiration, poor cough causing inability to clear secretions | *Streptococcus pneumoniae*<br>*Haemophilus influenzae*<br>Gram-negative bacilli<br>*Staphylococcus aureus* |
| Urinary tract | Urinary stasis, catheterization | Gram-negative bacilli<br>*Enterococcus* spp. |
| Skin and soft tissue | Pressure sores, wound contamination | *Staphylococcus aureus*<br>*Streptococcus* spp.<br>Possible mixed flora |
| Bone | Pressure sores, wound contamination | *Staphylococcus aureus*<br>Streptococcal species<br>Gram-negative bacilli<br>Anaerobes |
| Intra-abdominal | | |
| Gallbladder, pancreas | Cholelithiasis | Gram-negative bacilli<br>*Enterococcus* spp. |
| Colon | Antibiotics | *Clostridium difficile* |

**TABLE 164.3. Organisms Commonly Involved With Immunodeficient States**

| Class of Organism | Neutropenia | Antibody Deficiency | Cell-Mediated Immunodeficiency |
|---|---|---|---|
| Bacteria | Enterobacteriaceae<br>*Pseudomonas aeruginosa*<br>*Staphylococcus aureus*<br>*Staphylococcus epidermidis* | *Streptococcus pneumoniae*<br>*Haemophilus influenzae* | Salmonella spp. *Listeria monocytogenes*, Legionella species, Mycobacteria *Nocardia asteroides* |
| Fungi | *Candida* spp.<br>*Aspergillus* spp.<br>*Mucor* spp. | | *Cryptococcus neoformans, Coccidioides immitis, Histoplasma capsulatum* |
| Viruses | | Enteroviruses | Herpesviridae Vaccinia virus Rubella virus |
| Parasites | | *Giardia lamblia*<br>*Pneumocystis carinii* | *Pneumocystis carinii, Toxoplasma gondii, Strongyloides stercoralis, Cryptosporidium parvum* |

occur in the same patient, however, leading to a wider array of pathogens.

## Neutropenia

Patients with hematologic malignancies such as acute myelogenous leukemia are especially likely to become neutropenic because the aggressive chemotherapy for these cancers is typically toxic to the bone marrow. Infection risk associated with neutropenia depends on the rapidity of the decline; it increases when the neutrophil count falls below 500/mm$^3$ and becomes especially prominent at counts <100/mm$^3$. The common bacteria leading to initial infection are listed in Table 164.3, with Enterobacteriaceae being the most prevalent. An approach to the febrile neutropenic patient is outlined in Figure 164.1.

## Humoral Immune Deficiencies

Hematologic malignancies, including multiple myeloma and chronic lymphocytic leukemia, may develop a malignancy-associated defect in normal immunoglobulin production. When serum gamma globulin levels are low, defense against encapsulated bacteria (e.g., *Streptococcus pneumoniae, Haemophilus influenzae*) is reduced, and these patients become especially prone to respiratory infections with these organisms. Clearing of encapsulated organisms is also diminished in patients with splenectomy, which may be done as therapy for advanced

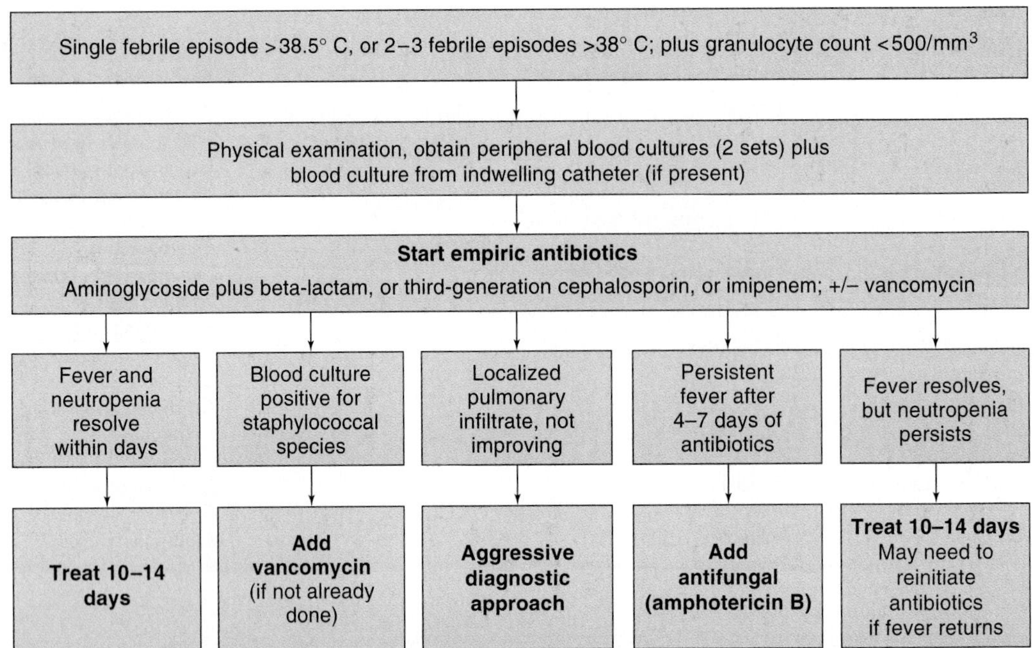

Single febrile episode >38.5° C, or 2–3 febrile episodes >38° C; plus granulocyte count <500/mm3
Physical examination, obtain peripheral blood cultures (2 sets) plus blood culture from indwelling catheter (if present)
Start empiric antibiotics
Aminoglycoside plus beta-lactam, or third-generation cephalosporin, or imipenem; +/– vancomycin
Fever and neutropenia resolve within days
Blood culture positive for staphylococcal species
Localized pulmonary infiltrate, not improving
Persistent fever after 4–7 days of antibiotics
Fever resolves, but neutropenia persists
Treat 10–14 days
Add vancomycin (if not already done)
Aggressive diagnostic approach
Add antifungal (amphotericin B)
Treat 10–14 days May need to reinitiate antibiotics if fever returns

**FIGURE 164.1.** Suggested approach to the febrile, neutropenic patient.

chronic lymphocytic leukemia. With aggressive chemotherapy, these patients also become at risk for neutropenia-related infection.

### Cellular Immune Dysfunction

Malignancy-associated cellular immune dysfunction generally occurs in lymphoreticular (lymphoma, Hodgkin disease) and hematologic (monocytic or lymphocytic leukemia) malignancies and is associated with defects along the pathway to the activated macrophage. Not only are these patients susceptible to many pathogens, based on their cellular immune dysfunction (see Table 164.3), but, with chemotherapy, they may also be at risk for neutropenia-associated infections.

Therapeutic decisions are helped by focusing more on pathogens that have affinity to a certain organ system—for instance, meningitis in a patient with lymphoma or Hodgkin disease is most likely due to *Listeria monocytogenes* or *Cryptococcus neoformans*. It is also helpful to know the association of pathogens with a particular malignancy—for example, patients with Hodgkin disease (especially those who have had irradiation therapy) are at high risk for herpes zoster, and patients under treatment for acute lymphocytic leukemia are particularly at risk for *Pneumocystis carinii* pneumonia. The many infectious possibilities in these patients generally require a search for a specific etiology. Empiric therapy is usually reserved for febrile and neutropenic patients.

## Infections in Transplant Recipients

An ever-increasing number of transplantations, including those of bone marrow and solid organs (kidney, liver, heart, lung, pancreas, and small bowel), are being done for a variety of medical conditions. Just as the patient's life expectancy may be enhanced by the transplantation, so is the risk of life-threatening infection (Table 164.4).

Bone marrow transplantation is performed primarily for severe aplastic anemia, certain hematologic or lymphoreticular malignancies, and some solid tumors. Infections in patients undergoing bone marrow transplantation occur during three fairly predictable periods following marrow infusion (Figure 164.2).

Like bone marrow transplantation, transplantation of solid organs also has been an expanding field, but the infectious complications differ. Overall, patients with transplantations involving the lung (heart–lung or lung) have the highest incidence of infection and infection-related mortality, whereas infections in renal transplant patients are least frequent. Despite these differences, some generalizations can be made regarding infections after solid organ transplantation. Table 164.5 shows a timetable of infection risk and associated types of infections in solid organ transplantation recipients.

Because of the predictability of certain types of infections, it is standard in the management of transplant recipients to use prophylactic regimens, including certain vaccines (e.g., pneumococcal and influenza vaccines) and various combinations of antibacterial, antifungal, and antiviral agents. Because prophylaxis may be difficult

**TABLE 164.4. Risk Factors for Infection and Associated Types of Infections in Transplant Recipients**

| Risk Factors for Infection | Types of Infections or Organisms Involved |
|---|---|
| **Host factors** | |
| Underlying medical conditions (e.g., diabetes mellitus, COPD) | Bacterial infections common to the underlying disease |
| Previous infection in latency | Altered host colonization and associated infection risk—infection by CMV, HSV, varicella-zoster virus, toxoplasmosis |
| **Factors at the time of transplantation** | |
| Length, location, and complexity of surgery | Bacterial or fungal infections at site of surgery |
| Infected donor organ | CMV, HSV, hepatitis bands |
| Infected blood products | Toxoplasmosis (cardiac), hepatitis C |
| **Therapy for graft survival or graft versus host disease** | |
| Use of immunosuppressive drugs e.g., corticosteroids, cyclosporin, OKT3 | Wide range of primarily cell-mediated pathogens (see Table 164.3) |
| **New exposures** | |
| Environmental pathogens | *Legionella*, *Aspergillus* spp. |

COPD = chronic obstructive pulmonary disease; CMV = cytomegalovirus; HSV = herpes simplex virus.
(Adapted and reprinted with permission from: Ho M, Dummer JS. In Mandell GL, Bennett JE, Dolin R (eds): Principles and Practice of Infectious Diseases. 4th ed. New York, NY: Churchill Livingstone, 1995, pp 2709–2717.)

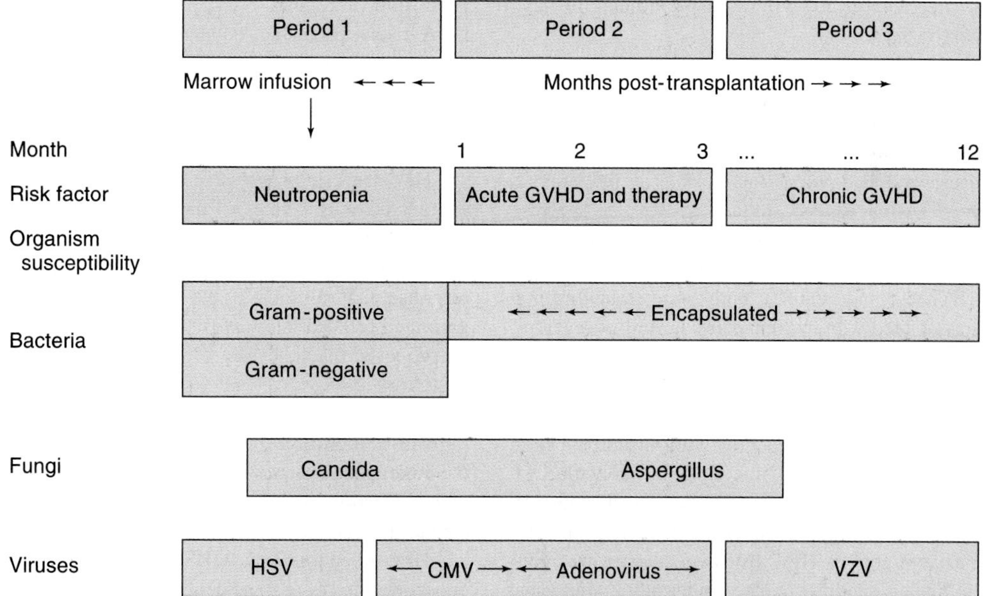


**FIGURE 164.2. Timetable of infection risk after bone marrow transplantation. GVHD = graft-vs-host disease; HSV = herpes simplex virus; CMV = cytomegalovirus; VZV = varicella-zoster virus.**

(Adapted and reprinted with permission from: Winston DJ. Chapter 292: Infections in bone marrow transplant recipients. In Mandell GL, Bennett JE, Dolin R, et al (eds). Principles and Practice of Infectious Diseases. 4th ed. New York, NY: Churchill Livingstone, 1995, p 2718, Figure 1.)

TABLE 164.5. Timetable of Infectious Risk and Associated Infections in Solid Organ Transplantation

| Time Period Post-Transplantation | Types of Infections Seen in Each Period |
|---|---|
| 0–1 mo | Wound infections, nosocomial infections |
| 1–6 mos | Infections due to cell-mediated immunosuppression (see Table 164.3)<br>Immunomodulating viruses (e.g., CMV, EBV) can worsen other infections |
| Over 6 mos | Graft infection; Later onset infections due to immunosuppression (e.g., cryptococcal meningitis, CMV retinitis)<br>Infections common to the community in patients with minimal immunosuppression (e.g., influenza) |

CMV = cytomegalovirus; EBV = Epstein-Barr virus.

due to side effects (e.g., use of ganciclovir for cytomegalovirus), the approach of **preemptive therapy**—starting therapy at the time of positive cultures to prevent clinical disease from developing—has shown some success. In established infections, empiric therapy is sometimes necessary, but the clinician should be prepared to pursue a specific etiologic diagnosis aggressively so that therapy can be optimized.

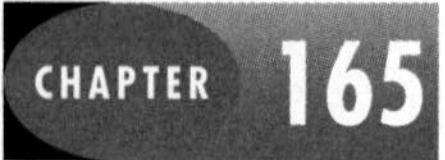

# CHAPTER 165 HUMAN IMMUNODEFICIENCY VIRUS INFECTION AND THE ACQUIRED IMMUNODEFICIENCY SYNDROME

Infection with HIV and the subsequent development of AIDS have become prevalent. Although the current understanding of the disease and its treatment are summarized here, ongoing studies (particularly clinical HIV treatment trials) will require continual medical education updates.

## Etiology

HIV, the etiologic agent for HIV infection and AIDS, is an RNA virus within the family of Retroviridae. Retroviruses have a wide distribution in the animal kingdom, causing related disease in several species. Retroviruses recognized to be associated with human disease include oncoviruses, human T-lymphocyte virus 1 (HTLV1) and HTLV2, both being transforming viruses associated with malignancies as well as myelopathies, and lentiviruses, HIV1 and HIV2. The lentiviruses are celiopathic, with destruction of a particular target cell being the usual pathology.

Viral infection of cells begins with attachment to a surface receptor. In HIV infection, it is the CD4 cell-surface molecule. Because **CD4 positive T cells** and **monocytes** express high levels of this receptor, they are the primary targets of HIV. However, numerous other cells (follicular dendritic cells, epidermal Langerhans cells, megakaryocytes, oligodendrocytes and epithelial or mucosal cells from the kidney, cervix, and rectum) can express the CD4 molecule, and these cells are infected as well.

The unique aspect of the retroviruses, as compared with other human RNA viruses, is the presence of the **reverse transcriptase** enzyme. After the virus enters the infected cell, the reverse transcriptase makes a DNA copy of the HIV RNA, which is then incorporated into the host DNA genome (Figure 165.1). This proviral DNA remains latent until a cellular activation event initiates proviral DNA transcription and sequential protein formation. The appropriate complement of viral genomic RNA, processed protein, and enzymes are then assembled at the cell surface and, subsequently, bud from the cell as mature virus particles.

HIV causes a progressive dysfunction and depletion of infected cells. The exact mechanisms are not entirely clear. Interference with the host cell's functions, a virally stimulated but host-mediated cytopathic T-cell immune response that eliminates the infected cells, and programmed cell death (apoptosis) activated by the virus are all proposed mechanisms.

## Epidemiology

The first clinical reports of AIDS were in 1981 from the east and west coasts of the United States, affecting mainly homosexual men. Since then, the disease has spread dramatically in the United States and the world.

HIV infection and AIDS occur with the highest concentration of cases being found in sub-Saharan Africa. However, in the United States, the highest concentrations are noted on the east and west coasts. It is estimated that approximately 33 million people are infected worldwide (1998 estimate), with about 260,000 being in the United States. These figures are ever-increasing, particularly in sub-Saharan Africa and Asia.

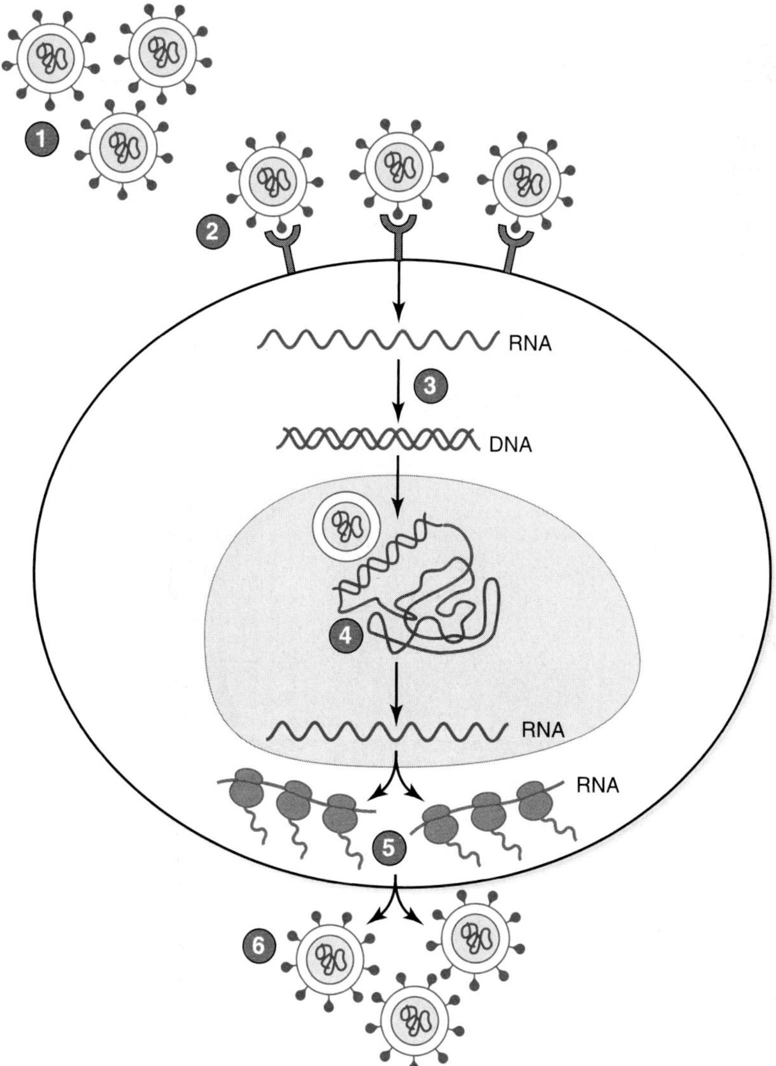


**FIGURE 165.1.** Life cycle of HIV virus. 1 = virions; 2 = attachment to CD4 receptor; 3 = reverse transcriptase; 4 = incorporation of provirus into the host genome; 5 = protein coating; 6 = mature viral particle.

Of the three modes of HIV spread (Table 165.1), sexual transmission is the most prevalent. In the United States, homosexual spread is the most common form, although heterosexually contracted HIV infection is increasing. Worldwide, heterosexually transmitted HIV infection is the most common.

**TABLE 165.1. Modes of HIV Transmission**

| Mode | Examples |
|---|---|
| Sexual | Homosexual<br>Heterosexual |
| Blood and blood products | Contaminated needles<br>Transfusions |
| Maternal fetal | Intrapartum<br>Perinatal<br>Postnatal (breast milk) |

## Natural History of HIV Infection

Currently, HIV infection can be divided into three general phases (Figure 165.2).

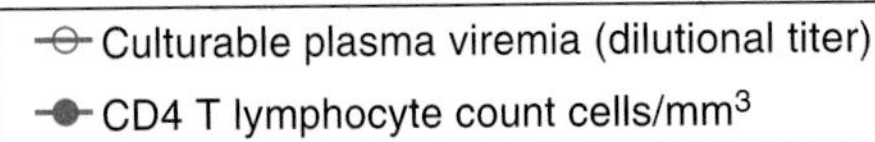


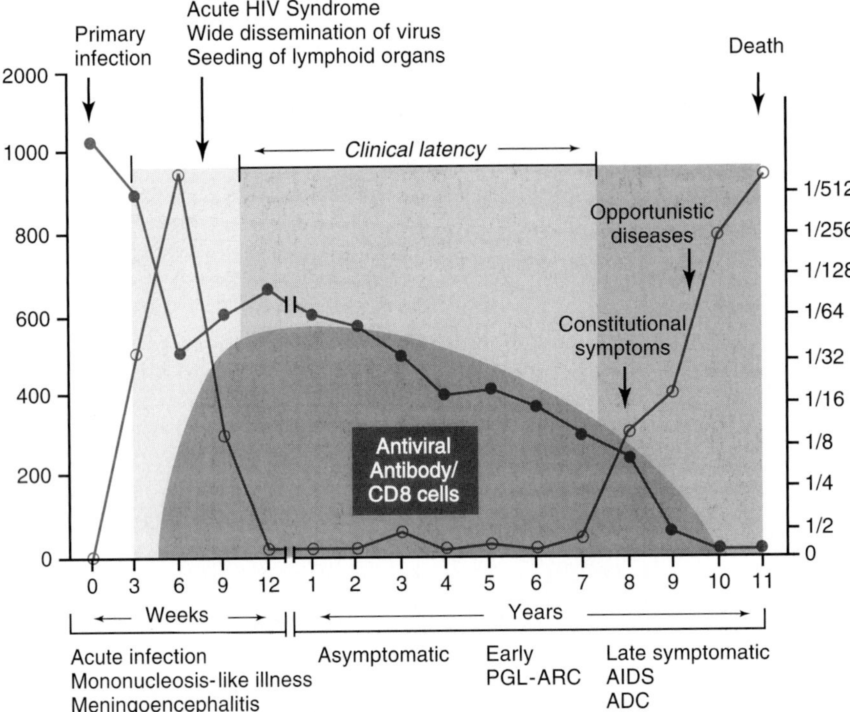


**FIGURE 165.2.** **Time course of typical HIV infection. Widespread viral dissemination occurs early in the primary infection and encompasses an abrupt decline in peripheral blood CD4+ T-cell number. The ensuing immune response is accompanied by a decrease in plasma viremia (culturable virus) and a lengthy period of clinical latency. However, the CD4+ T-cell count continues to decline during this period until a critical level is reached, where the risk of opportunistic infections is markedly increased. ADC = AIDS dementia complex; ARC = AIDS-related complex; PGL = persistent generalized lymphadenopathy.**

(Adapted and reprinted with permission from: Haase AT. Chapter 145: Lentiviruses: an overview. In: Mandell GL, Bennett JE, Dolin R (eds). Principles and Practice of Infectious Diseases. 4th ed. New York, NY: Churchill Livingstone, 1995, p 1585; and from: Pantaleo G, Graziosi C, Fauci AS. The Immunopathogenesis of human immunodeficiency virus infection. N Engl J Med 1993;328:329.)

### The acute retroviral syndrome

First described in 1985, the acute retroviral syndrome is believed to affect one half to two thirds or more of HIV-infected individuals. This syndrome, which occurs from 3–6 weeks after primary HIV infection, resembles mononucleosis and is characterized by fever, myalgias, arthralgias, malaise, nausea, vomiting, diarrhea, and headache. Frequent findings include adenopathy (usually cervical, axillary, or occipital), pharyngitis, a truncal rash (macular, papular, or urticarial), and, less commonly, hepatosplenomegaly.

Aseptic meningitis, encephalitis, peripheral neuropathy, or Guillain-Barré syndrome are less frequent neurologic manifestations. Abnormal blood counts (thrombocytopenia or leukopenia) or abnormal liver test results may be noted. The **differential diagnosis** of the acute retroviral syndrome includes infectious mononucleosis, other viral illness (e.g., influenza, herpes simplex, measles, rubella), and secondary syphilis.

During this symptomatic phase, there is a high level of HIV viremia (see Figure 165.2), and HIV core antigen (p24) is first detected. Immunologically, there is lymphocytopenia, including both CD4 and CD8 cell populations.

### The asymptomatic phase

Generally within 1 week to 3 months after the acute retroviral syndrome, there is an immune response to HIV (see Figure 165.2) involving both antiviral antibodies (e.g., neutralizing antibodies and antibodies involved in antibody-dependent cellular cytotoxicity) and components of the cellular immune system. Because of this host immune response and the trapping of virus particles in lymph node germinal centers, there is reduction of viremia and p24 antigen detection.

During this immune response, a period of clinical latency occurs. This asymptomatic period may last up to 10 years or more but may be shorter in individuals with a higher initial viral inoculum (e.g., blood transfusion recipients, intravenous drug users). Although it was originally believed that the virus was also latent during this time, recent studies indicate that active viral replication is ongoing within lymph node germinal centers.

Despite the lack of symptoms during this period, viral replication leads to destruction of the lymph node architecture, with a subsequent decline in overall immune status. There is a progressive reduction in both the number and function of CD4 cells. Other cell-mediated immune response impairments can be seen in monocytes and natural killer cells. In addition, B-cells are abnormally activated, likely by HIV itself. This increased B-cell proliferation and immunoglobulin secretion lead to hypergammaglobulinemia. B-cells also develop a reduced capacity to respond to mitogens or antigens.

### Symptomatic HIV infection

During clinical latency, HIV replication progresses and immune function worsens to the point at which individuals begin to manifest symptoms. Generally, these symptoms begin to appear as CD4 counts fall below 500/mm$^3$. These early symptoms of HIV disease include generalized lymphadenopathy, oral thrush (candidiasis), oral hairy leukoplakia, and herpes zoster (shingles). Thrombocytopenia, which is due to direct viral infection of megakaryocytes, can also manifest during this time.

As immune function progressively declines and CD4 counts drop below 200/mm$^3$, individuals enter a stage of **late symptomatic** disease. As this disease progresses, specific antiviral immunity also declines, and there is a renewed detection of viremia (see Figure 165.2). Patients become at risk for a range of opportunistic illnesses and direct effects of the virus itself.

One of the direct effects of the virus, which may occur throughout the stages of illness, is **neurologic disease.** After gaining access to the CNS possibly via infected monocytes, HIV evokes inflammatory changes (e.g., aseptic meningitis) or demyelinating or degenerative changes (myelopathy, AIDS–dementia complex). HIV may also cause CNS inflammation without obvious signs, because it has been shown that asymptomatic HIV-positive patients can have a CSF pleocytosis and positive HIV cultures.

## Diagnosis of HIV Disease and AIDS

Within 1–3 months after primary HIV infection, circulating specific anti-HIV antibodies are detected. Determination of the presence of these antibodies by an enzyme-linked immunosorbent assay (ELISA) has become the standard screening test for HIV infection.

### Serologic tests

The **ELISA test** result may be negative, indeterminate, or positive. Patients with a negative result and continued high-risk behavior may be retested at intervals. Because of the possibility of a false-positive result (particularly in low-risk individuals), patients with indeterminate or positive results should have the results confirmed with a western blot.

The **western blot,** although not a good screening test, requires the presence of antibody reactivity to several HIV-specific proteins. This reactivity is determined by a banding pattern on the blot. The presence of bands to at least two major HIV gene products (p24, gp41, and gp120–160) determines a positive result. Otherwise, the test is determined to be negative or indeterminate.

If the ELISA result is positive but the western blot result is negative, the ELISA is considered to be false-positive. If the ELISA result is positive and the western blot result is positive, the patient is confirmed to be HIV-positive. If, however, the blot result is indeterminate, patients may either have cross-reacting antibodies or the antibody response may be in evolution (less likely). Indeterminate western blot result should be repeated in about a month. A stable, indeterminate western blot result makes HIV infection less likely.

Other tests for HIV include a PCR test for HIV, p24 antigen assay, and culture of HIV.

### AIDS-indicator conditions

The diagnosis of AIDS has generally rested on indicator diseases, usually opportunistic infections that occur as HIV infection progresses and CD4 counts decrease. As experience with this disease has accumulated, the Centers for Disease Control (CDC) has revised their case definition several times to include an increasing range of indicator diseases (Table 165.2). The latest CDC AIDS definition, revised in 1993, expanded the surveillance case definition to include a CD4 count <200/mm$^3$ (<14%), pulmonary tuberculosis, recurrent pneumonia, or invasive cervical cancer (Table 165.3).

## Management of HIV Infection

Therapy for HIV infection has been an area of intense study over the past several years. Because of the unique life cycle of the retroviruses, there are several potential

**TABLE 165.2. Centers for Disease Control Case Definition for AIDS (1987 Revision)**

| |
|---|
| **Diseases diagnosed definitively without laboratory evidence of HIV infection (in the absence of other immunodeficiency states)** |
| Candidiasis of the esophagus, trachea, bronchi, or lungs |
| Cryptococcus, extrapulmonary |
| Cryptosporidiosis with diarrhea persisting >1 month |
| Cytomegalovirus disease of an organ other than liver, spleen, or lymph nodes in a patient older than 1 month of age |
| Herpes simplex virus infection causing a mucocutaneous ulcer that persists over 1 month; or bronchitis, pneumonitis, or esophagitis for any duration affecting a patient >1 month of age |
| Kaposi sarcoma affecting a patient below 60 years of age |
| Lymphoma of the brain (primary) affecting a patient <60 years of age |
| Lymphoid interstitial pneumonia and/or pulmonary lymphoid hyperplasia (LIP/PLH complex) affecting a child <13 years of age |
| *Mycobacterium avium complex* or *M. kansasii* disease, disseminated |
| *Pneumocystis carinii* pneumonia |
| Progressive multifocal leukoencephalopathy |
| Toxoplasmosis of the brain affecting a patient >1 month of age |
| **Diseases diagnosed definitively with laboratory evidence of HIV infection** |
| Any disease listed above in Section A |
| Recurrent or multiple pyogenic bacterial infections (<13 years of age) |
| Coccidioidomycosis, disseminated |
| AIDS dementia |
| Histoplasmosis, disseminated |
| Isosporiasis, with diarrhea exceeding 1 month in duration |
| Kaposi sarcoma, any age |
| Primary CNS lymphoma |
| Non-Hodgkin lymphoma, B-cell or unknown phenotype (small, noncleaved lymphoma or immunoblastic sarcoma) |
| Disseminated mycobacterial disease (other than *M. tuberculosis*) |
| *M. tuberculosis,* extrapulmonary |
| Recurrent nontyphoid *Salmonella* septicemia |
| HIV wasting syndrome |
| **Diseases diagnosed presumptively with laboratory evidence of HIV infection** |
| Esophageal candidiasis |
| Cytomegalovirus retinitis with loss of vision |
| Kaposi sarcoma |
| Lymphoid interstitial pneumonia and/or pulmonary lymphoid hyperplasia (<13 years of age) |
| Disseminated mycobacterial disease |
| *Pneumocystis carinii* pneumonia |
| Toxoplasmosis of the brain (>1 month of age) |
| **Diseases diagnosed definitively with negative laboratory test results for HIV (in the absence of other immunodeficiency states)** |
| *Pneumocystis carinii* pneumonia |
| Any other disease listed above in Section A and a CD4 count <400/mm$^3$ |

(Reprinted with permission from: Centers for Disease Control and Prevention. Revision of the CDC surveillance case definition for acquired immunodeficiency syndrome. MMWR. 1987;36:1S–15S.)

targets for therapy (Table 165.4). These inhibitors have been studied to various degrees; some only in vitro and others extensively in clinical trials.

Currently, the therapy for HIV consists of a combination of **nucleoside analogs** (nucleoside analogs plus nonnucleoside analogs), or nucleoside analogs plus a **protease inhibitor** (usually a total of three or more drugs). Results have been promising, but therapy may be limited by toxicity, cost, or the development of resistance.

## Recognition and Management of Opportunistic Infections

Most opportunistic infections or AIDS-defining illnesses occur in late-stage disease when the CD4 count is falling and the immune system is unable to provide adequate protection. Often, these illnesses can be fatal or become chronic and, ultimately, fatal.

The CD4 counts at which common opportunistic infections usually occur are shown in Figure 165.3.

**TABLE 165.3. Expanded CDC Case Definition for AIDS (1993 Revision)**

1. All HIV-infected individuals with a CD4 count <200/mm$^3$, or a CD4 percent of less than 14%
2. Pulmonary tuberculosis
3. Recurrent pneumonia (≥2 episodes within 1 year)
4. Invasive cervical cancer

(Reprinted with permission from: Centers for Disease Control and Prevention. 1993 revised classification system for HIV infection and expanded surveillance case definition for AIDS among adolescents and adults. MMWR. 1992;41:1–19.)

**TABLE 165.4. Potential Molecular Targets for HIV Therapy**

| Phase of HIV Replication Cycle | Examples of Types of Inhibitors |
|---|---|
| Viral binding and penetration | Soluble CD4 neutralizing antibodies |
| Reverse transcriptase | Nucleoside analogs<br>Nonnucleoside analogs |
| Integration | Anti-integrase |
| Transcription | Antisense oligonucleotides<br>tat antagonists<br>Interferons |
| Assembly | Protease inhibitors<br>Glycosylation inhibitors |
| Budding | Interferons |

Whereas tuberculosis usually occurs at a CD4 count >200/mm$^3$, most other infections occur <200/mm$^3$, and some, such as cytomegalovirus, occur at very low CD4 counts. Because of this observation, prophylaxis (as discussed below) is recommended for several of these diseases. However, because effective antiretroviral therapy is often associated with a significant CD4 count increase, prophylaxis can sometimes be discontinued. Common opportunistic infections seen in AIDS patients and the therapeutic options are shown in Table 165.5.

### Pulmonary infections

The most common opportunistic cause of pneumonia in AIDS patients is ***Pneumocystis carinii***. Unlike non-AIDS patients with *P. carinii* pneumonia, in whom respiratory symptoms are usually abrupt, AIDS patients have a more gradual onset of symptoms. The chest radiograph usually has an interstitial infiltrate (although it may be normal), and the differential diagnosis usually includes mycobacteria, fungi (i.e., *Cryptococcus*, *Histoplasma*, *Coccidioides*), cytomegalovirus, Kaposi sarcoma, non-Hodgkin lymphoma, and nonspecific interstitial pneumonitis. Bacterial pneumonia may also need to be considered, but symptoms are usually more acute, with a productive cough and a lobar infiltrate. Bronchoalveolar lavage is often needed to secure the diagnosis of *P. carinii* pneumonia.

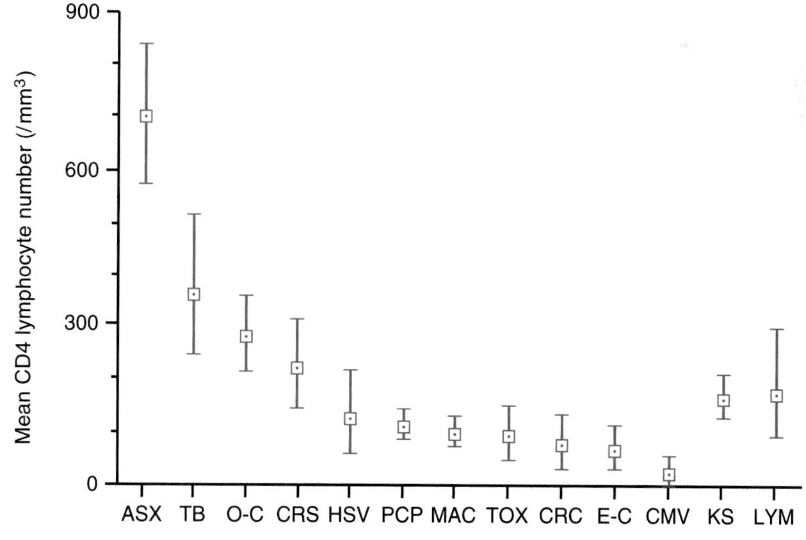


**FIGURE 165.3.** Mean CD4 cell levels with standard deviations (boxes) and 95% confidence intervals (bars) in 222 HIV-infected patients with opportunistic diseases and HIV-infected asymptomatic controls. ASX = asymptomatic; CMV = cytomegalovirus retinitis; CRC = cryptococcal meningitis; CRS = cryptosporidiosis; EC = esophageal candidiasis; HSV = recurrent herpes simplex virus; KS = Kaposi sarcoma; LYM = lymphoma; MAC = *Mycobacterium avium* complex; OC = oral candidiasis; PCP = *Pneumocystis carinii* pneumonia; TB = tuberculosis; TOX = toxoplasmosis.

(Redrawn and reprinted with permission from: Crowe SM, Elbeik T, Ulrich PP, et al. J AIDS 1991;4:770-776, Figure 2.)

TABLE 165.5. Common Opportunistic Infections in AIDS

| Organ or Organ System | Etiology or Type of Infection | Therapeutic Options |
|---|---|---|
| Pulmonary | *Pneumocystis carinii* | TMP/SMX, TMP/dapsone, clindamycin/ primaquine, pentamidine |
| | *Mycobacterium tuberculosis* | Isoniazid, rifampin, pyrazinamide, ± ethambutol (see text) |
| Esophagus | *Candida albicans*, Cytomegalovirus (CMV), Herpes simplex | Fluconazole, ganciclovir, foscarnet, acyclovir |
| GI | Cryptosporidiosis, Microsporidiosis | Paromomycin |
| | Isosporiasis | TMP/SMX |
| | CMV colitis | Ganciclovir, foscarnet |
| CNS | Cryptococcal meningitis | Amphotericin B, fluconazole |
| | Neurosyphilis | Penicillin |
| | Toxoplasma encephalitis | Sulfadiazine/pyrimethamine, clindamycin/pyrimethamine |
| Eye | CMV retinitis | Ganciclovir, foscarnet |
| Disseminated | *Mycobacterium avium* complex | Ciprofloxacin, macrolide, ethambutol, clofazimine, rifabutin (multidrug combination) |
| | Histoplasmosis | Amphotericin B, itraconazole |

TMP = Trimethoprim; SMX = sulfamethoxazole.

Of the treatment options for *P. carinii* pneumonia, **trimethoprim-sulfamethoxazole** is the first choice, but it may not always be tolerated. Treatment should continue for 21 days and, if the $Pao_2$ is below 70 mm Hg, **adjunctive steroids** should be used. **Prophylaxis** for *P. carinii* pneumonia may be done primarily (CD4 <200/$mm^3$) or secondarily (after the first pneumonia episode).

Pulmonary **tuberculosis,** unlike most other AIDS-defining illnesses, tends to occur before CD4 counts fall below 200/$mm^3$. It has been a particular problem because of the emergence of multidrug-resistant strains. In areas with this problem, a four-drug regimen should be used initially (see Table 165.5); if the strain is sensitive, three drugs are continued for 2 months, with isoniazid and rifampin then continued for a total of 9 months. Because of the high rate of tuberculosis reactivation, all AIDS patients with at least a 5mm reactive tuberculin (PPD) skin test result or those with a negative skin test result and a suspicious history (i.e., chest radiograph consistent with previous, untreated tuberculosis; close contact with active tuberculosis; or a history of a positive skin test result not adequately treated) should receive antituberculosis prophylaxis with 9 months of isoniazid.

### Esophageal infections

**Esophagitis** usually presents with symptoms of nausea, anorexia, dysphagia, or odynophagia and is most likely due to *Candida albicans,* particularly when there is the finding of oral thrush. A cobblestone appearance on an upper gastrointestinal tract radiograph (due to ulcerations and plaques) suggests the diagnosis, but most patients are treated empirically. Lacking a response to fluconazole, patients may require an upper gastrointestinal endoscopy to rule out the presence of other pathogens, such as cytomegalovirus or herpes simplex.

### Gastrointestinal infections (enterocolitis)

**Diarrhea** is a frequent problem in patients with AIDS and includes a number of bacteria, parasites, and viruses as causative agents. Common bacterial pathogens include *Salmonella*, *Shigella*, or *Campylobacter* species. Although these organisms, as a cause of enterocolitis, are not associated with an AIDS diagnosis, recurrent *Salmonella* (nontyphoid) bacteremia is an AIDS-defining illness. Mycobacteria also may cause diarrhea, and there should also be concern about *Clostridium difficile*-associated diarrhea because of the frequent use of antibiotics in these patients.

Of the parasitic causes, cryptosporidiosis and isosporiasis are AIDS-defining illnesses. Whereas numerous therapies have been tried for cryptosporidiosis, none has been particularly successful; transient benefit has been shown with paromomycin.

CMV is the most common viral etiology of enterocolitis in AIDS patients and is usually seen in late stage disease. Stool examinations should be performed to evaluate the other possibilities, but the definitive diagnosis of CMV colitis requires colonoscopy and biopsy. HIV enteropathy also may be a cause of diarrhea in AIDS patients, but all other causes should be ruled out before assuming this diagnosis.

**Central nervous system infections**

The most common infection of the CNS in HIV-infected individuals is HIV itself. HIV can cause asymptomatic inflammation, aseptic meningitis, or other destructive changes. **Aseptic meningitis** may be seen throughout the symptomatic phase but not in the late stages of illness, because it appears to be an immunologically mediated process.

Although there are a number of potential causes of meningitis in AIDS patients (e.g., fungal, tuberculosis, bacterial, syphilis, herpes, and other viruses), the most common opportunistic cause of meningitis is *Cryptococcus neoformans.* Most patients have nonspecific symptoms, including fever and headache, whereas a minority (≤20%) have more classic findings of meningitis (meningeal signs, photophobia, altered sensorium). CSF usually only has mild abnormalities. Tests supportive of the diagnosis include positive india ink (50–90%), cryptococcal antigen (90–95%), and culture results. Amphotericin B is the preferred treatment, particularly with severe disease, but fluconazole is the agent of choice for chronic suppression after initial therapy.

HIV disease has led to an increased recognition of **neurosyphilis** and has shortened the natural history of neurosyphilis manifestations after primary syphilis. Therefore, patients with positive serum syphilis titers and neurologic abnormalities should be considered for a spinal tap. An abnormal CSF (with or without a positive CSF VDRL) should lead to the consideration of treatment with parenteral penicillin.

With the presence of localizing neurologic findings (e.g., hemiparesis, ataxia, cranial neuropathies, seizure), intracranial mass lesions are likely, and imaging should be performed, preferably with magnetic resonance scanning. **Cerebral toxoplasmosis** is the most common cause of intracranial contrast-enhancing masses, whereas other less common causes include tuberculosis, bacterial abscesses, cryptococcosis, nocardiosis, and, possibly, lymphoma. Patients are usually treated presumptively and for life. If there is no response to treatment, brain biopsy should be considered to exclude other diagnoses.

**Eye infections (retinitis)**

CMV has an affinity for the retina and causes most of the cases of retinitis in AIDS patients. Visual symptoms include blurring, a painless vision loss, and increase in "floaters." The diagnosis is generally made by an ophthalmologist, and treatment usually initially (with ganciclovir) includes an induction of 14–21 days, followed by maintenance therapy.

**Disseminated infections**

*Mycobacterium avium* complex usually presents as a widely disseminated illness in late-stage disease, with fever, sweats, weight loss, fatigue, abdominal pain, and diarrhea. Patients have a continuous bacteremia, and the diagnosis is usually made by blood cultures. Whereas treatment often needs to be altered due to medication intolerance, it should be with a multidrug regimen and often needs to be life-long. Experts also recommend prophylaxis for this disease (e.g., rifabutin, newer macrolides) when CD4 counts fall lower than 100/mm$^3$.

Another common disseminated opportunistic infection is **histoplasmosis.** This illness, particularly seen in the Ohio and Mississippi River Valleys, has systemic symptoms similar to those seen in *M. avium* complex disease. The diagnosis is made by blood cultures or antigen testing (urine or blood). Treatment is with amphotericin B followed by itraconazole.

## Malignancies Complicating HIV Infection

Of the malignancies complicating AIDS (Table 165.6), Kaposi sarcoma and non-Hodgkin lymphoma are the most frequent. These malignancies, as well as cervical cancer, are currently recognized as AIDS-defining illnesses.

**Kaposi sarcoma,** a vascular (or lymphatic) endothelial neoplasm, commonly manifests as painless cutaneous lesions that appear as pigmented nodules. This clinical appearance is usually sufficient to suggest the diagnosis, but a biopsy may be required for definitive diagnosis. The disease typically is indolent but may become extensive or spread to visceral organs. Gastrointestinal Kaposi sarcoma, for instance, may present with bowel obstruction or gastrointestinal bleeding. Pulmonary Kaposi sarcoma may mimic *Pneumocystis carinii* pneumonia, but the chest radiograph has a more nodular pattern, often with bloody pleural effusions. Patients may also present with lymphedema (face or lower extremity), suggesting lymphatic obstruction with tumor.

Treatment of Kaposi sarcoma is individualized, depending on the location and extent. Localized lesions are treated if they are associated with significant pain or discomfort or if they present a cosmetic problem (e.g., facial lesions). Cryotherapy, localized radiation, or intralesional vinblastine are usually used when treatment of localized lesions is indicated. More extensive disease may require interferon or chemotherapy.

| TABLE 165.6. Malignancies Complicating HIV Infection |
| --- |
| Kaposi sarcoma |
| CNS non-Hodgkin lymphoma |
| Hodgkin disease |
| Cervical cancer |
| Squamous cancer of the anus |

The second most common malignancy seen in AIDS patients is **non-Hodgkin lymphoma.** Non-Hodgkin lymphomas are of B-cell origin and include peripheral lymphoma (including immunoblastic lymphoma or Burkitt lymphoma) or primary CNS lymphoma. Most cases (80%) are peripheral lymphomas. Presentations vary, and extranodal disease is common, as are systemic symptoms (fever, sweats, weight loss). CNS lymphoma usually presents with focal neurologic findings and is in the differential diagnosis of a space-occupying brain lesion. Chemotherapy is used for peripheral lymphoma, and radiation and/or corticosteroids have been used for primary CNS lymphoma.

## Questions

**Instructions:** For each question below, select only **one** lettered answer that is the **best** for that question.

1. A patient has had three documented episodes of pneumococcal pneumonia over the past 6 months. Possible underlying contributing diseases include all of the following except:
   A. Common variable hypogammaglobulinemia
   B. Multiple myeloma
   C. Chronic lymphocytic leukemia
   D. DiGeorge syndrome

2. Corticosteroids affect the host defenses through which of the following mechanisms?
   A. Affecting neutrophil kinetics
   B. Affecting antibody production
   C. Inhibiting lymphocyte and mononuclear cell function
   D. All of the above

3. *Chlamydia* organisms can cause which of the following illnesses?
   A. Pneumonia
   B. Keratoconjunctivitis
   C. Pelvic inflammatory disease
   D. All of the above

4. Tissue invasion by which of the following may cause eosinophilia?
   A. Nematodes
   B. Trematodes
   C. Cestodes
   D. All of the above

5. Of the following beta-lactam antibiotics, which is particularly noted to predispose to seizures?
   A. Cefoxitin
   B. Ceftazidime
   C. Imipenem
   D. Aztreonam

6. Of the following beta-lactam antibiotics, which can be used in a patient with a serious beta-lactam allergy?
   A. Cefoxitin
   B. Ceftazidime
   C. Imipenem
   D. Aztreonam

7. A patient is started on antituberculosis therapy with isoniazid, rifampin, ethambutol, and pyrazinamide. Several weeks later, the patient complains of a decrease in vision. Visual acuity is noted to be decreased. Which one of the following best explains the finding?
   A. Isoniazid
   B. Rifampin
   C. Ethambutol
   D. Pyrazinamide
   E. Cataract

8. After travel to the southwestern United States, a 52-year-old Hispanic man develops a pneumonia. Which of the following organisms is a potential cause?
   A. *Candida albicans*
   B. *Coccidioides immitis*
   C. *Histoplasma capsulatum*
   D. *Blastomyces dermatitidis*

9. In a patient presenting with pneumonia, a sputum Gram stain shows small coccobacillary gram-negative organisms. Appropriate initial choices for antibiotics include all of the following except:
   A. Amoxicillin-clavulanic acid
   B. Trimethoprim-sulfamethoxazole
   C. Erythromycin
   D. Cefuroxime

10. If a patient presents with a sore throat, a tonsillar exudate may be seen with all of the following except:
    A. Epstein-Barr virus
    B. Rhinovirus
    C. Group A streptococcus
    D. Adenovirus

11. Frequency, dysuria and/or urgency, and $<10^5$ bacteria/ml of urine (acute urethral syndrome) are caused by which of the following?
    A. Acute cystitis
    B. Nongonococcal urethritis
    C. Chemical sensitivity
    D. All of the above

12. In which of the following settings should asymptomatic bacteruria be treated?
    A. Elderly patient
    B. Catheterized patient

C. Pregnant patient
D. All of the above

13. A patient presents with a painless genital ulceration as shown in the following figure. Which of the following is the best test to determine the etiology?
A. Gram stain
B. Serology for herpes
C. Culture
D. Dark-field examination

14. One of the preceding tests is performed in the patient. Additional measures should include which of the following?
A. HIV test
B. VDRL
C. Urethral swab to be inoculated into Thayer-Martin medium
D. Benzathine penicillin 2.4 MU intramuscularly
E. All of the above

15. Close contacts of which of the following causes of meningitis should receive prophylaxis to prevent disease?
A. *Streptococcus pneumoniae*
B. *Neisseria meningitidis*
C. *Listeria monocytogenes*
D. ECHO virus

16. A cause of cellulitis associated with traumatic wounds in salt water is which of the following?
A. *Staphylococcus aureus*
B. *Pseudomonas aeruginosa*
C. *Vibrio vulnificus*
D. *Aeromonas hydrophila*

17. An organism that is prominent in cat or dog bites, as opposed to human bites, is:
A. *Streptococcus pyogenes*
B. *Staphylococcus aureus*
C. *Pasteurella multocida*
D. *Fusobacterium nucleatum*

18. A patient with Hodgkin disease is suspected of having meningitis. Of the etiologic agents listed, the most common bacterial cause is:
A. *Listeria monocytogenes*
B. *Staphylococcus aureus*
C. Group A streptococcus
D. *Pseudomonas aeruginosa*

## Answers

| | | | | |
|---|---|---|---|---|
| 1. D | 2. D | 3. D | 4. D | 5. C |
| 6. D | 7. C | 8. B | 9. C | 10. B |
| 11. D | 12. C | 13. D | 14. E | 15. B |
| 16. C | 17. C | 18. A | | |

## SUGGESTED READING

### *Textbooks and Monographs and Reviews*


Fauci AS, Lane HC. Human Immunodeficiency Virus (HIV) Disease. In: Braunwald E, Fauci AS, Kasper DL, et al (eds). AIDS and Related Disorders. New York, NY: McGrawHill, 2001, pp 1852-1913.

Mandell GL. Update in Infectious Diseases. Ann Intern Med 2001;135:897–905.

Mandell GL, Bennett JE, Dolin R (eds). Principles and Practice of Infectious Diseases. 5th ed. New York, NY: Churchill Livingstone, 2000.


### *Articles*

*Manifestations of Infection*


Norman DC, Yoshikawa TT. Fever in the elderly. Infect Dis Clin North Am 1996;10:93–99.


*Laboratory Diagnosis of Infectious Diseases*


Ma TS. Applications and limitations of polymerase chain reaction amplification. Chest 1995;108:1393–1404.

Whelen AC, Persing DH. The role of nucleic acid amplification and detection in the clinical microbiology laboratory. Ann Rev Microbiol 1996;50:349–373.

Wilson ML. General principles of specimen collection and transport. Clin Infect Dis 1996;22:766–777.


*Antimicrobial Agents*


Thompson LR, Wright AJ. General principles of Antimicrobial Therapy. Mayo Clin Proc 1998;73:995–1006.


*Fever and Fever of Unknown Origin*


Cunha BA. Fever of unknown origin. Infect Dis Clin North Am 1996;10:111–127.

Gordon SM. Recognizing and treating new and emerging infections encountered in everyday practice. Cleve Clin J Med 1996;63:172–178.

Konecny P, Davidson RN. Pyrexia of unknown origin in the 1990s: time to redefine. Br J Hosp Med 1996;56:21–24.

Larson EB, Featherstone HJ, Petersdorf RG. Fever of undetermined origin—Diagnosis and follow up of 105 cases, 1970–1980. Medicine 1982;61:269–292.

Simon HB. Hyperthermia. N Engl J Med 1993;329:483–487.


*Pneumonias*


American Thoracic Society Board of Directors. Guidelines for the Management of Adults with Community-acquired Pneumonia. Am J Respir Crit Care Med 2001;163:1730–1754.

Bartlett JG, Breiman RF, Mandell LA, et al. Community-acquired pneumonia in adults: guidelines for management. Clin Infect Dis 1998;26:811–838.

Bartlett JG, Mundy LM. Current concepts: community acquired pneumonia. N Engl J Med 1995;333:1618–1624.

Friedland IR, McCracken GH. Drug therapy: management of infections caused by antibiotic-resistant streptococcus pneumoniae. N Engl J Med 1994;331:377–382.


*Urinary Tract Infections*


Kunin CM. Urinary tract infections in females. Clin Infect Dis 1994;18:1–12.

Nicolle LE. Urinary tract infection: traditional pharmacologic therapies. American Journal of Medicine 2002;113 Suppl 1A:35S–44S.


*Sexually Transmitted Diseases*


Anonymous. Drugs for sexually transmitted diseases. Med Lett Drugs Ther 1995;37:117–122.

Levine WC, Brady WE, Schmid GP, et al. Sexually transmitted diseases treatment guidelines. Clin Infect Dis 1995;20: 1–109.

Workowski KA, Levine WC, Wasserheit JN. U.S. Centers for Disease Control and Prevention guidelines for the treatment of sexually transmitted diseases: an opportunity to unify clinical and public health practice. Annals of Internal Medicine 2002;137(4):255–262.

*Infectious Diarrhea*

Bartlett JG. Antibiotic-associated diarrhea. N Engl J Med 2002;346:334–339.

Farthing MJ. Travellers' diarrhea. Gut 1994;35:1–4.

Framm SR, Soave R. Agents of diarrhea. Med Clin North Am 1997;81:427–447.

Ryan ET, Wilson ME, Kain KC. Illness after international travel. New Engl J Med 2002;347:505–516.

*Intra-abdominal Infections*

Gilbert JA, Kamath PS. Spontaneous bacterial peritonitis: an update. Mayo Clin Proc 1995;70:365–370.

McClean KL, Sheehan GJ, Harding GKM. Intra-abdominal infection: a review. Clin Infect Dis 1994;19:100–116.

van den Hazel SJ, Speelman P, Tytgat GNJ, et al. Role of antibiotics in the treatment and prevention of acute and recurrent cholangitis. Clin Infect Dis 1994;19:279–286.

Wittmann DH, Schein M, Condon RE. Management of secondary peritonitis. Ann Surg 1996;224:10–18.

*Central Nervous System Infections*

Lipton JD, Schafermeyer RW. Central nervous system infections. The usual and the unusual. Emerg Med Clin North Am 1995;13:417–443.

Nelsen S, Sealy DP, Schneider EF. The aseptic meningitis syndrome. Am Fam Phys 1993;48:809–815.

Quagliarello VJ, Scheld WM. Treatment of bacterial meningitis. N Engl J Med 1997;336:708–716.

Segreti J, Harris AA. Acute bacterial meningitis. Infect Dis Clin North Am 1996;10:797–809.

Townsend GC, Scheld WM. The use of corticosteroids in the management of bacterial meningitis in adults. J Antimicrob Chemother 1996;37:1051–1061.

*Catheter-related Infections*

Brun-Buisson C. New Technologies and Infection Control Practices to Prevent Intravascular Catheter-related Infections. Am J Respir Crit Care Med 2001;164:1557–1558.

*Bacteremia, Sepsis, and Septic Syndrome*

Aronson MD, Bor DH. Blood cultures. Ann Intern Med 1987;106:246–253.

Esposito AL, Gleckman RA, Cram S, et al. Community-acquired bacteremia in the elderly: analysis of one hundred consecutive episodes. J Am Geriatr Soc 1980;28:315–319.

Leibovici L, Greenshtain S, Cohen O, et al. Bacteremia in febrile patients. A clinical model for diagnosis. Arch Intern Med 1991;151:1801–1806.

Lynn WA, Cohen J. Adjunctive therapy for septic shock: a review of experimental approaches. Clin Infect Dis 1995;20: 143–158.

Maki DG. Nosocomial bacteremia. An epidemiologic overview. Am J Med 1981;70:719–732.

Richardson JP. Bacteremia in the elderly. J Gen Intern Med 1993;8:89–92.

*Skin, Soft Tissue, and Bone Infections*

Bisno AL, Stevens DL. Streptococcal infections of skin and soft tissues. N Engl J Med 1996;334:240–245.

Carroll JA. Common bacterial pyodermas. Taking aim against the most likely pathogens. Postgrad Med 1996;100:311–313.

Chartier C, Grosshans E. Erysipelas: an update. Int J Dermatol 1996;35:779–781.

Hacker SM. Common infections of the skin. Characteristics, causes, and cures. Postgrad Med 1994;96:43–46.

Smith JW, Piercy EA. Infectious arthritis. Clin Infect Dis 1995;20:225–231.

*Infections in the Immunocompromised Host*

Rubin RH, Ferraro MJ. Understanding and diagnosing infectious complications in the immunocompromised host. Current issues and trends. Hematol Oncol Clin North Am 1993;7: 795–812.

Rubin RH, Fischman AJ. Radionuclide imaging of infection in the immunocompromised host. Clin Infect Dis 1996;22: 414–423.

Thomas Cr Jr, Wood LV, Douglas JG, et al. Common emergencies in cancer medicine: infectious and treatment-related syndromes, Part I. J Natl Med Assoc 1994;86: 765–774.

*Human Immunodeficiency Virus Infection and the Acquired Immunodeficiency Syndrome*

Deeks SG, Smith M, Holodniy M, et al. HIV1 protease inhibitors. A review for clinicians. JAMA 1997;277:145–158.

Dybul M, Fauci AS, Bartlett JG, et al. Guidelines for Using Antiretroviral Agents among HIV-Infected Adults and Adolescents. Ann Intern 2002;137:381–433.

Gallant JE, Moore RD, Chaisson RE. Prophylaxis for opportunistic infections in patients with HIV infection. Ann Intern Med 1994;120:932–944.

HIV/AIDS Treatment Information Service (http://www.hivatis.org)

Lipsky JJ. Antiretroviral drugs for AIDS. Lancet 1996;348: 800–803.

Polsky B. Treatment of HIV infection and its complications. Clin Chest Med 1996;17:647–663.

Sullivan M, Feinberg J, Bartlett JG. Fever in patients with HIV infection. Infect Dis Clin North Am 1996;10:149–165.

Yeni PG, Hammer SM, Carpenter CC, et al. Antiretroviral treatment for adult HIV infection in 2002: updated recommendations of the International AIDS Society-USA Panel. JAMA 2002;288(2):222–235.

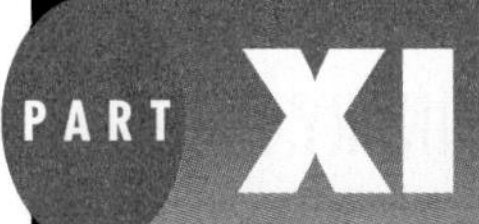

PART XI

Walter F. Piering
Eric P. Cohen
Mahendr S. Kochar

# KIDNEY DISEASES, ELECTROLYTE DISORDERS, AND HYPERTENSION

# CHAPTER 166 STRUCTURE AND FUNCTION OF THE KIDNEYS AND URINARY TRACT

The kidneys are located in the retroperitoneal space at a level between the 12th thoracic vertebra and the 2nd lumbar vertebra. Each kidney weighs about 150 g and measures about 12 × 6 × 3 cm. The functional unit of the kidney is called the nephron; there are approximately 1 million nephrons in each kidney. The fundamental structure of the nephron is illustrated in Figure 166.1.

## The Glomerulus

The glomerulus is about 200 μm in diameter and is formed by the invagination of a tuft of capillaries into the dilated blind end of the nephron (Bowman's capsule). The capillaries are supplied by an afferent arteriole and drained by a slightly smaller efferent arteriole. The two cell layers separating the blood from the glomerular ultrafiltrate, forming the urinary space in Bowman's capsule, are the capillary endothelium and the epithelium of Bowman's capsule, which becomes the epithelium of the tubule. The endothelial cells that line the capillary lumen are filled with pores covered by thin diaphragms. The glomerular basement membrane is a hydrated gel of glycoproteins containing interwoven collagen fibers. Foot processes extend from the epithelial cells over the basement membrane. Their lack of tight approximation allows for the formation of a filtration slit covered by a thin semipermeable membrane. The barrier formed by these three layers allows passive entry of water and low-molecular-weight solutes, but not cells and protein,

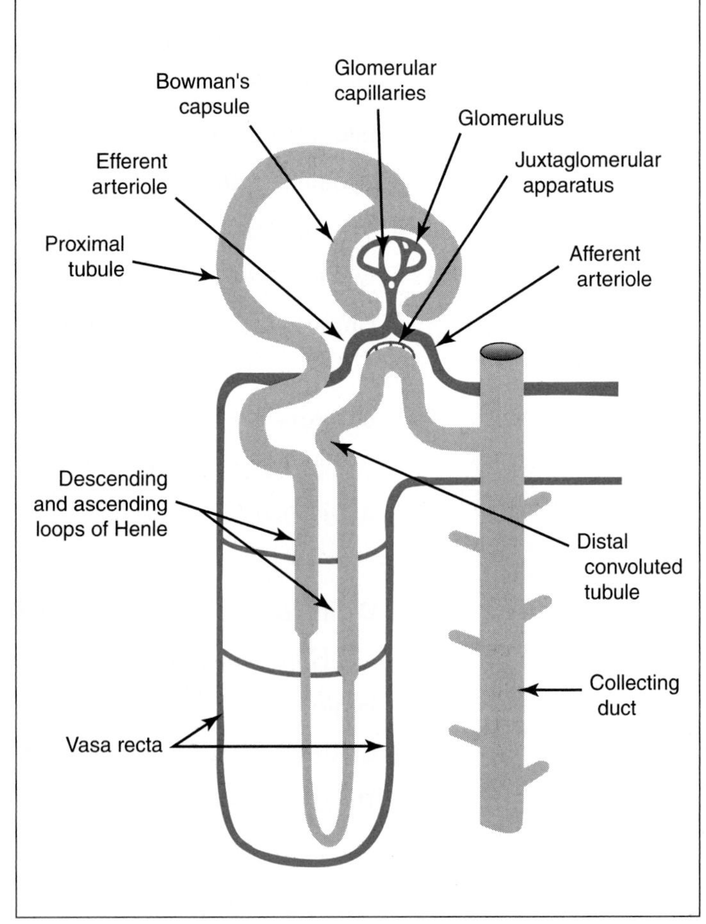


**FIGURE 166.1.** Functional unit of the kidney: the nephron.

into the urinary space. Moreover, clusters of anionic bridge macromolecules on the surface of these cells and within the glomerular basement membrane, further restrict filtration of large negatively charged serum proteins such as **albumin.**

An interwoven lattice known as the mesangium serves to suspend the glomerular tufts within the urinary space. Mesangial cells are enclosed by a matrix of homogeneous fibrillary material containing mucopolysaccharides and different glycoproteins. These cells are of a contractile nature and have many properties that affect the glomerular filtration rate (GFR).

## The Tubule

The tubule receives the glomerular filtrate and is composed primarily of four segments: the proximal convoluted tubule; the loop of Henle, with a thin descending limb and a thick ascending limb; the distal convoluted tubule; and the collecting duct.

The **proximal convoluted tubule** is the most metabolically active portion of the entire nephron, handling many substances, including creatinine, uric acid, albumin, and sodium. Over 75% of filtered sodium is reabsorbed in the proximal tubule; the remainder is absorbed distally. The convoluted portion of the proximal tubule drains into the straight portion. The proximal tubule terminates in the descending limb of the loop of Henle. This loop forms a hairpin turn in the medulla and returns forward to the cortex, forming the **distal tubule.** The tubule is finally directed again into the medullary tissues as the collecting duct empties into the renal pelvis at the ducts of Bellini, located at the tips of the renal papillae.

This interesting arrangement of the tubule allows the distal tubule to come in close approximation with the vascular pole of the glomerulus (Figure 166.2). The distal tubular cells in this area are taller and more numerous. This region, called the macula densa, together with cells originating from the adjacent afferent arteriole, creates a specialized structure called the **juxtaglomerular apparatus.** The juxtaglomerular apparatus is the site of renin formation as well as endothelial-derived relaxing factor or nitric oxide (NO).

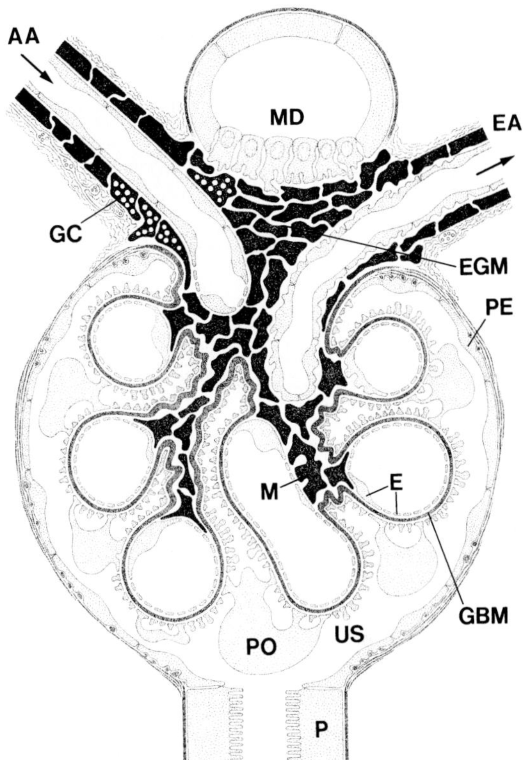


**FIGURE 166.2. Schematic diagram of a longitudinal section through a glomerulus and the juxtagomerular apparatus. At the vascular pole, an afferent arteriole (AA) enters and an efferent arteriole (EA) leaves the tuft. The glomerular capillary tuft is surrounded by Bowman's capsule. There are different epithelia. One is the visceral epithelium (podocytes; PO), which, at the vascular reflects onto Bowman's capsule at the parietal epithelium (PE). Between both epithelia lies the urinary space (US), which is continuous with the lumen of the proximal tubule (P). The endothelium (E) of the glomerular capillaries is fenestrated. Between the endothelial cells and the podocytes, the glomerular basement membrane (GBM) is found. At the vascular pole, the GBM continues as the basement membrane of Bowman's capsule. Mesangial cells (M) are situated in the axis of glomerular lobules. At the vascular pole, mesangial cells are continuous with extraglomerular mesangial cells (EGM); together with the granular cells (GC) and the macula densa (MD), they make up the JGA. (Modified from Kriz W, et al.: Morphological aspects of glomerular function. In Davison MA ed. Nephrology. London: Baillere Tindall, 1988, p 2. With permission.)** (Reprinted with permission from Jennette J, Olson J, and Schwartz M.: *Heptinstall's Pathology of the Kidney*, 5th ed. Philadelphia, Lippincott Williams & Wilkins, 1998, fig. 1.34.)

## Renal Physiology

The kidney not only ensures body fluid homeostasis by excreting excess solute and water in the urine, but also regulates a number of other bodily functions (Table 166.1).

### Renal Hemodynamics

The renal plasma flow (RPF) and glomerular filtration rate (GFR) maintain a ratio of 5:1. In a healthy person, the RPF is about 600 ml/min and the GFR is 120 ml/min. These rates are maintained over a wide range of mean arterial pressures, with autoregulation of renal function secondary to efferent and afferent arteriolar regulation of pressures within the glomerular capillaries.

**TABLE 166.1. Homeostatic Functions Performed by the Kidney**

| |
|---|
| Electrolyte maintenance ([$Na^+$], [$K^+$], [$Cl^+$], [$PO_4$], [$Ca^{2+}$]) |
| Urea clearance |
| Erythropoietin production for RBC maintenance |
| Acid–base balance |
| Vitamin D metabolism |

**TABLE 166.2. Factors Affecting Afferent and Efferent Arteriolar Tone**

| |
|---|
| Angiotensin II |
| Arginine vasopressin |
| Prostaglandins |
| Nitric oxide |
| Endothelium-derived relaxing factor |
| Catecholamines |
| Renal nerves |
| Endothelin |

The neurohumoral factors that influence this vascular tone are summarized in Table 166.2. Many factors affect GFR; they are listed in Table 166.3.

GFR may be expressed by the following equation:

$$GFR = kS\ [(P_{GC} \times P_T) \times (\Pi_{GC} \times \Pi_T)]$$

where k is the capillary permeability, S is the size of the capillary bed, $P_{GC}$ is the mean hydrostatic pressure in the glomerular capillaries, $P_T$ is the mean hydrostatic pressure in the tubules, $\Pi_{GC}$ is the colloid osmotic pressure of the plasma in the glomerular capillaries and $\Pi_T$ is the osmotic pressure of the filtrate in the tubule. Because serum creatinine, which is produced daily by muscle metabolism, is filtered by the kidney without major handling by the tubules, a 24-hour urinary creatinine clearance (Ccr) commonly is used to measure the GFR.

**TABLE 166.3. Factors That Affect the Glomerular Filtration Rate**

| |
|---|
| **Decrease GFR** |
| Decrease in renal blood flow |
| Decrease in glomerular capillary hydrostatic pressure |
| Reduction in systemic blood pressure |
| Afferent arteriolar constriction |
| Efferent arteriolar dilation |
| Increase in hydrostatic pressure in Bowman's capsule |
| Ureteral obstruction |
| Edema of kidney inside the tight renal capsule |
| Decrease in concentration of plasma proteins |
| Decrease in total area of glomerular capillary bed |
| Diseases that destroy glomeruli |
| Partial nephrectomy |
| **Increase GFR** |
| Opposite effects of factors that decrease GFR |

The endogenous Ccr is represented by the following formula:

$$GFR = Ccr = \frac{UcrV}{Pcr}$$

where Ucr is the urinary creatinine concentration, V is the volume of urine in a timed collection, and Pcr is the plasma creatinine concentration.

# CHAPTER 167 INITIAL EVALUATION OF KIDNEY DISEASE

The cornerstone of any evaluation is a detailed history and physical examination. In patients with renal disease, an additional vital element is to note the **time sequence** of changes in renal function. This can be done only by correlating the history with the laboratory data. The **basic laboratory tests** that should be performed on the **initial visit** in all patients with suspected renal dysfunction are summarized in Table 167.1. Urinalysis should be performed on a midstream collection in men and a "clean catch" sample in women to avoid contamination of the specimen by the external genitalia. The tests should be performed within 30 to 60 minutes after the specimen has been voided. Abnormal tests should be followed by additional studies, including measurement of creatinine clearance to assess GFR or diagnostic studies such as a renal ultrasound, radionuclide studies, arteriography, or renal biopsy.

A practical method used to assess renal function in clinical practice is measuring the creatinine clearance. However, because creatinine is secreted as well as filtered, it can serve only as a fair estimate of GFR. Moreover, this property of creatinine makes it vulnerable to influence by drugs (Table 167.2). It is vitally important to ensure an adequate urine collection when obtaining a 24-hour collection by calculating the anticipated amount of creatinine in the collection. Creatinine is directly

**TABLE 167.1. Initial Laboratory Screening of Renal Patients**

| Blood | Urine |
|---|---|
| Complete blood count | Specific gravity |
| Electrolytes, glucose, BUN, creatinine | Dipstick test for pH, protein, glucose, ketones, bilirubin, urobilinogen, blood, nitrate |
| Liver function studies | Sulfosalicylic acid test for protein |
| $Ca^{2+}$, $PO_4^{2-}$, albumin, cholesterol | Test for microalbuminuria (only if dipstick is negative for protein and patient has diabetes mellitus or hypertension) |
| | Microscopic analysis: urinary sediment (cells, casts, and crystals) |

**TABLE 167.2. Drugs That Affect Serum Creatinine**

Compounds that decrease creatinine excretion by altering secretion
- Cimetidine
- Trimethoprim

Compounds measured as creatinine in certain assays
- Acetoacetic acid in ketoacidosis
- Cefoxitin
- Flucytosine

reflective of muscle mass. The 24-hour urine collection should contain about 22 mg/kg of creatinine in men and 18 mg/kg of creatinine in women. Total urine volume should *not* be used to estimate whether the collection is adequate.

Loss of up to one half the nephron mass of both kidneys correlates with a reduction of 20% to 30%, not 50%, in GFR because of compensatory hyperfiltration by the remaining nephrons. The fluid and electrolyte balance may be maintained, and, depending on the kidney disease, urinalysis may be normal. Thus, serum creatinine and even creatinine clearance lack the sensitivity to detect an early decline in renal function.

Creatinine clearance also may be estimated using the Cockcroft and Gault equation:

$$\text{Creatinine clearance in ml/min} = \frac{(140 - \text{age}) \times \text{body weight (kg)}}{72 \times \text{serum creatinine (mg/dl)}}$$

For women, the result should be multiplied by 0.85. *These formulas are not accurate in patients whose body weight or muscle mass deviates markedly from normal, as in obesity, muscle wasting, and muscle denervation.*

Plotting the reciprocal serum creatinine (1/Scr), which roughly indicates the residual renal function, on the ordinate and the months of observation on the abscissa, yields useful predictive information on the progression of renal failure in chronic kidney diseases. Extending the regression or trend line obtained from such a plot can predict with reasonable accuracy when an individual patient is going to reach a level of renal failure requiring dialysis or transplantation. It also can be used to monitor improvement in renal function in response to therapy (Figure 167.1).

Recent studies suggest it may be more accurate to measure serum cystatin C levels than serum creatinine for the estimation of GFR. But this measurement is not routinely done, and it costs five times as much as a creatinine measurement.

## Hematuria

Hematuria is defined as the presence of more than 3 RBC per high-power field on microscopic examination of the urine sediment. Gross hematuria is an insensitive indicator of the degree of blood loss, because as little as 1 ml of blood is enough to change the color of 1 L of urine to red or brown. Hemoglobinuria caused by hemolysis and myoglobinuria caused by rhabdomyolysis also can cause a red or brown urine and yield a positive hemoglobin dipstick. However, in myoglobinuria, the spun specimen has a red supernatant and no red blood cells in the urine sediment. Thus, true hematuria can be diagnosed only by microscopic examination. Causes of hematuria are shown in Table 167.3.

### History

One should inquire regarding family and personal history of primary renal disease, hereditary nephropathies, polycystic kidney disease, sickle cell anemia, tuberculosis, or other related causes. In addition, recent infection of the upper respiratory tract should suggest the possibility of a postinfectious glomerulonephritis or IgA nephropathy. Intravenous drug use and AIDS also are associated with glomerular disease. Flank pain radiating to the groin may indicate a kidney stone. Fever and weight loss may suggest a vasculitis, tuberculosis, or renal cell carcinoma. Rheumatic symptoms such as joint pain and rash may be present in systemic lupus erythematosus (SLE), progressive systemic sclerosis, or vasculitis. Pulmonary complaints or hemoptysis may suggest

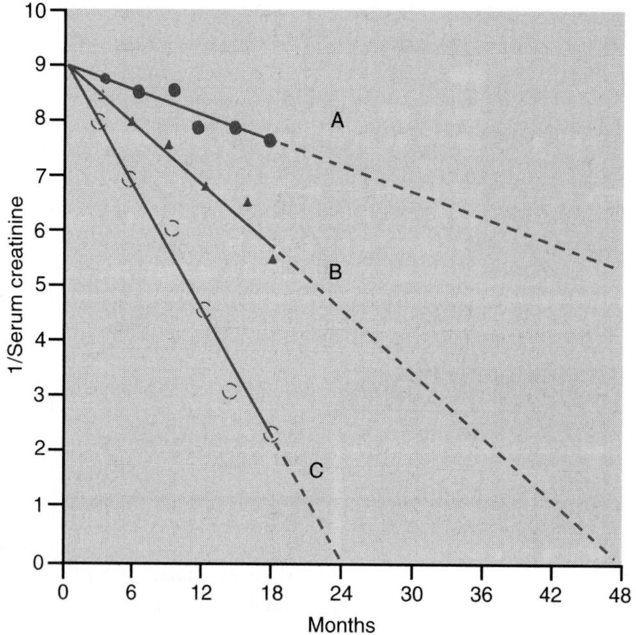


**FIGURE 167.1.** Plotting 1/serum creatinine against time can help predict the onset of end-stage renal disease (ESRD). Follow-up of three patients (A, B, and C) over an 18-month period is shown (*solid lines*). One can say with reasonable confidence that in the case of patient A, it would be several years before ESRD occurs; patient B will need dialysis in another 2 years; and patient C will require dialysis within the next 6 months.

**TABLE 167.3. Causes of Hematuria**

*Glomerular bleeding*
- Benign familial hematuria
- Progressive hereditary nephropathy (Alport syndrome)
- Mesangioproliferative glomerulonephritis
- IgA nephropathy (Berger's disease)*
- Henoch-Schönlein purpura
- Postinfectious glomerulonephritis
- Rapidly progressive glomerulonephritis
- Focal glomerular sclerosis
- Membranoproliferative glomerulonephritis
- Systemic diseases (e.g., systemic lupus erythematosus, Wegener's granulomatosis, Goodpasture syndrome, hemolytic-uremic syndrome, progressive systemic sclerosis, cryoglobulinemia, thrombotic thrombocytopenic purpura, polyarteritis nodosa)

*Nonglomerular bleeding*
- Renal tumors
- Polycystic disease
- Papillary necrosis (analgesic abuse, diabetes, sickle cell disease)
- Renal trauma
- Sickle cell disease or trait
- Renal tuberculosis
- Drugs (sulfonamides)
- Urolithiasis

*Most common etiology, worldwide

Goodpasture syndrome or Wegener's granulomatosis (Table 167.3). Passage of blood clots in the urine is not associated with glomerular disease and is seen more commonly with disorders that involve the urinary bladder. Specific risk factors for bladder cancer include heavy smoking, long-term administration of cyclophosphamide, prolonged heavy phenacetin use, radiation therapy, and exposure to some dyes. Use of medications (e.g., anticoagulants, cyclophosphamide) should be noted.

## Laboratory Tests

Routine evaluation may include measurement of the blood urea nitrogen (BUN), serum creatinine and tests for hepatitis B surface antigen, VDRL, streptococcal serologic test, antinuclear antibody (ANA), and a hemoglobin electrophoresis. Tests such as complement levels, cryoglobulins, and other related tests also should be considered. After the screening tests, additional studies should be guided by the history, physical examination, and clinical assessment. If renal tuberculosis is suspected, a PPD (tuberculin) skin test should be performed with anergy controls, and at least **three** first voided morning urine specimens should be sent for acid-fast smear and mycobacterial culture. Antiglomerular basement membrane (anti-GBM) antibody titers or antineutrophilic cytoplasmic antibody (ANCA) titers should be ordered if a vasculitis is suspected.

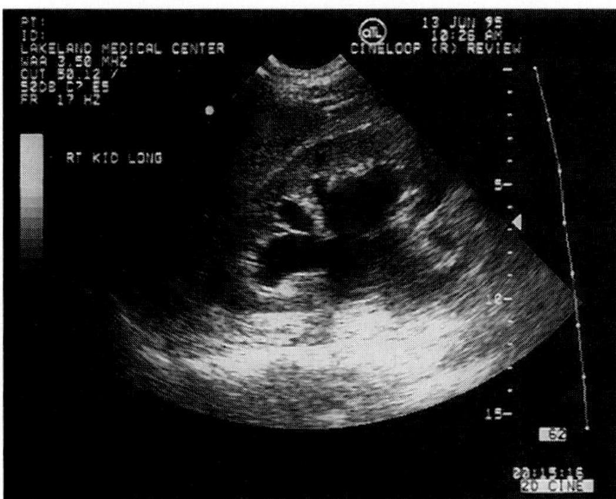


**FIGURE 167.2.** Hydronephrosis. The dark shadows in the center of the picture are dilated calyces.

Microscopic examination of the spun urine showing the presence of red blood cell casts is diagnostic of glomerular bleeding and disease (Figure 167.2). However, the absence of red blood cell casts does not rule out glomerular disease. Dysmorphic red cells correlate highly with glomerular bleeding. Dysmorphic red blood cells and acanthocytes result from cell membranes traumatized either by passage through the glomerular capillary or by osmotic trauma as they pass through the nephron. Finally, dipstick results indicating 4+ proteinuria are highly suggestive of glomerular disease.

### Imaging

If the cause of hematuria remains elusive, then imaging studies should be considered. Renal ultrasound is performed to evaluate renal size and calyces and to identify calculi, renal masses, and urinary tract obstruction. Figure 167.2 shows hydronephrosis as a result of a blocked ureter. Intravenous pyelogram requires injection of radiocontrast agents and is seldom used except for evaluation of nephrolithiasis. If these tests are negative, a cystoscopy is recommended for evaluation of the bladder and prostate, especially in men older than 50 years of age. If a renal tumor is suspected, a CT scan of the kidneys should be performed.

### Renal Biopsy

A renal biopsy is performed to diagnose suspected glomerular or tubulointerstitial disease. In some circumstances, biopsy results not only provide a diagnosis, but also help guide treatment. In advanced chronic renal failure, it is of limited value. The most common complication of renal biopsy is bleeding; it is usually self-limited, however, and requires no therapy. The presence of coagulopathies, poorly controlled blood pressure (>160/110 mm Hg), or a solitary kidney are relative contraindications to renal biopsy.

## Hematuria of Extrarenal Causes

Sixty-five percent of patients with hematuria have bleeding from extrarenal sites. Common causes of extrarenal bleeding include calculi or neoplasms in the renal pelvis, ureter, bladder, and prostate. Infectious causes such as tuberculosis and *Schistosoma hematobium* are common in certain parts of the world. Other causes such as trauma to the urinary tract and therapy with cyclophosphamide or anticoagulants also should be considered.

## Proteinuria

Proteinuria, the hallmark of renal parenchymal disease, is defined as a urinary protein excretion of 150 mg or more in 24 hours. Nephrotic range proteinuria is defined as a urinary protein excretion rate exceeding 3.5 g/day, and often is accompanied by hyperlipidemia and edema. In glomerular diseases resulting from excess glomerular capillary permeability, large amounts of albumin can leak into the urine. In tubulointerstitial diseases most of the urinary proteins are globulins. The normal glomerulus is permeable to the light chain globulins produced by plasma cells in conditions such as multiple myeloma. These can be identified on urinary electrophoresis as monoclonal globulin peaks. Thus, proteinuria should be viewed in the clinical context. Finally, proteinuria may be the only evidence of serious underlying disease, as exemplified by the discovery of an occult malignancy, most commonly lung, breast, or colon, in 10% to 15% of patients with membranous nephropathy.

The approach to the patient with proteinuria in the nonnephrotic range should include a careful history, including all medications used, and a thorough physical examination. Among the numerous causes of nonnephrotic-range proteinuria (Table 167.4), prolonged, poorly controlled **essential hypertension** probably is the most common. Renal function should be

| TABLE 167.4. Causes of Nonnephrotic-Range Proteinuria |
|---|
| Hypertension causing nephrosclerosis |
| Primary glomerular disease |
| Tubulointerstitial nephritis |
| Cystic kidney diseases |
| Fanconi syndrome |
| Obstructive nephropathy |
| Multiple myeloma |
| Benign proteinuria |

determined in these patients. The urine specimen should be carefully examined for casts, cells, crystals, and bacteria. If multiple myeloma is suspected, a serum and urine electrophoresis should be performed.

Several methods may be used to screen for urinary protein. The **dipstick method** detects albumin in the concentrations of 10 to 30 mg/L (trace) up to 2000 mg/L (4+). Highly alkaline urine (pH >8) may yield false-positive reactions. False-negative reactions also occur in very dilute urine or when urine globulins and light chain immunoglobulins are present. **Sulfosalicylic acid method** detects 40 to 50 mg/L of all proteins, including hemoglobin and immunoglobulin light chains. The test is performed by adding 8 drops of 20% sulfosalicylic acid to 2 ml of urine. Turbidity is proportional to the amount of protein present and ranges from visible turbidity to dense precipitation. False-positive reactions occur under the following conditions: alkaline urine; high concentrations of penicillin or cephalosporins; radiographic contrast media; administration of nonsteroidal anti-inflammatory agents; and presence of sulfonamide or tolbutamide metabolites. Benign forms of proteinuria require no treatment (Table 167.5).

A 24-hour urine collection for protein is commonly used to quantify proteinuria. Alternatively, a spot urine for protein and creatinine concentrations in mg/dl provide a protein:creatinine ratio that correlates well with the 24-hour protein quantification. With this method, a protein:creatinine ratio of 0.1 is equivalent to a normal daily protein excretion of 100 mg or less; a protein:creatinine ratio of 3 or greater is associated with a protein excretion of 3 g per day or more, consistent with nephrotic-range proteinuria.

**Microalbuminuria** refers to the excretion of albumin in the range of 30 to 300 mg per day (15–200 μg/min). Albumin excretion cannot be quantified accurately by the usual dipstick or quantitative protein methods; it requires sensitive immunoassay techniques.

**TABLE 167.5. Benign Forms of Proteinuria**

| |
|---|
| Functional proteinuria: Occurs in subjects with one of the following conditions: |
| High fever |
| Congestive heart failure |
| Strenuous exercise |
| Cold exposure |
| Idiopathic proteinuria: Occurs with normal renal function and is characterized by normal microscopic urinalysis. |
| Orthostatic proteinuria: most commonly occurs in adolescence and is detected only when the patient is in an upright position. Total urinary protein is generally <2 g/day. |

In a healthy person, urinary albumin excretion ranges from 2 to 31 mg/day. Screening for microalbuminuria is done by measuring the albumin:creatinine ratio in a first voided morning urine. Testing for microalbuminuria may have its greatest clinical value in detecting the earliest stages of diabetic nephropathy.

### Leukocyturia

Normally, the urine microscopic examination contains less than 3 to 5 white blood cells per high-power field (hpf). If clean voiding techniques are followed carefully, the number of white blood cells in the urine is the same for men and women. Polymorphonuclear leukocytes contain esterases. Reagent strips detect leukocytes by the action of these esterases which causes a color change in 1 to 2 minutes. The dipstick is able to detect leukocytes in excess of 3 to 4 WBCs/hpf with a sensitivity of 92%. Leukocyturia often is seen in urinary tract infections, but it also may occur in tubulointerstitial disease and in some patients with renal stones, even in the absence of infection.

# CHAPTER 168 NEPHROTIC SYNDROME

## Definition and Etiology

The basic definition of **nephrotic syndrome** includes proteinuria exceeding 3.5 g per day, with changes in serum lipids (increased serum cholesterol and triglycerides) and a reduced serum albumin. Edema and hypercoagulable state are its clinical accompaniments. The hypercoagulability stems largely from urinary losses of factors that maintain clotting homeostasis, such as antithrombin III. Lipiduria with epithelial cells containing fat droplets or "oval fat bodies" also is commonly seen, but usually with massive proteinuria exceeding 5 to 10 g/day. The causes of nephrotic-range proteinuria are listed in Table 168.1. The most common primary renal causes of nephrotic syndrome are **minimal change disease** in children and **membranous glomerulopathy** in adults. The most common systemic disease that causes nephrotic syndrome is **diabetes mellitus.**

The **hypoalbuminemia** that occurs with nephrotic syndrome is the result largely of the urinary loss of albumin, which is not compensated for by hepatic synthesis. A marked reduction in plasma oncotic pressure follows, with consequent edema, which can be generalized (generalized anasarca) and massive. Hypercholesterolemia and hypertriglyceridemia, the other components of nephrotic syndrome, occur because of increased hepatic cholesterol synthesis and decreased peripheral metabolism. Because of these changes and loss of anticlotting factors and immunoglobulins, patients become more susceptible to atherosclerosis, thrombotic processes, and infections by **encapsulated bacteria** with capsular antigens such as *Pneumococcus* spp, *Streptococcus* spp, *Staphylococcus* spp, and others.

**TABLE 168.1. Causes of Nephrotic Syndrome**

*Primary glomerular diseases*
- Minimal change disease
- Membranous nephropathy
- Focal glomerulosclerosis
- Membranoproliferative glomerulonephritis

*Secondary glomerular diseases*
- Postinfectious: poststreptococcal, endocarditis, syphilis, hepatitis B, cytomegalovirus, protozoa, parasitic
- Metabolic: diabetes mellitus, myxedema
- Connective tissue diseases and vasculitis: systemic lupus erythematosus, Sjögren syndrome, polyarteritis nodosa, Goodpasture syndrome, Henoch-Schönlein purpura, scleroderma, dermatomyositis
- Neoplastic: solid tumors, lymphoma, leukemia
- Drugs: gold, penicillamine, mercury, probenecid, NSAIDs, captopril
- Allergens: poison ivy, insect bites
- Systemic diseases: amyloidosis, malignant hypertension, sarcoidosis, severe congestive heart failure, constrictive pericarditis
- Inherited diseases: sickle cell disease, hereditary nephritis, congenital nephrotic syndrome, Fabry disease, nail-patella syndrome
- Miscellaneous: thrombotic thrombocytopenic purpura, hemolytic-uremic syndrome, preeclampsia

## Diagnosis

In the absence of an obvious cause such as diabetes mellitus, patients with acute or new-onset nephrotic syndrome within the preceding 6 months to 1 year should have a renal biopsy to diagnose the etiology. An acute increase in proteinuria, defined as an increase of more than 2 to 3 g/day in less than 1 year, may signify another glomerular disease or immunologic process. This is particularly important in people with diseases such as diabetes mellitus; as many as 20% may have another glomerular disease that accounts for the acute increase in proteinuria. Nonsteroidal anti-inflammatory agents may cause a tubulointerstitial nephritis and increased proteinuria. Hypertension, rash, lymphadenopathy, or diabetic retinopathy may be present on physical examination. Evidence for an occult malignancy (usually an adenocarcinoma) also should be sought if clinically suspected. Acute flank pain with a significant rise in proteinuria should alert one to the possibility of renal vein thrombosis, an entity which may complicate nephrotic syndrome. Venography or renal ultrasound with Doppler flow can be diagnostic.

## Management

Treatment of the nephrotic syndrome usually depends on the underlying etiology. General principles of management, however, include the following: a sodium-restricted (2–3 g/day), low fat, and 0.8–1.0 g/kg/day protein diet is recommended. Higher protein intake may actually exacerbate the nephrotic syndrome. Fluid intake also should be restricted if hyponatremia is present. Edema usually is managed through leg elevation and loop diuretics, although antihypertensive agents such as angiotensin-converting enzyme (ACE) inhibitors also are useful. ACE inhibitors reduce size selectivity and improve charge selectivity of the glomerular membrane to proteins, thereby helping to reduce the proteinuria in the nephrotic syndrome. These effects are independent of the drugs' hypotensive effects. Other drug therapies that should be considered are related to the primary etiology of disease: corticosteroids, cyclophosphamide, cyclosporine, and chlorambucil have all been found to reduce nephrotic-range proteinuria associated with membranous nephropathy. However, with the exception of diabetes mellitus, there are no data to suggest that reduction in proteinuria reduces mortality.

# CHAPTER 169 ACUTE RENAL FAILURE

Acute renal failure presents as a sudden and rapid decline in kidney function, with or without oliguria, and—depending on the underlying cause—hypovolemia or hypervolemia. Hyperkalemia and metabolic acidosis commonly are present, depending on the stage of evolution.

## Etiology and Classification

The causes of **rapidly progressive renal failure** are summarized in Table 169.1. The more common of these include volume depletion, acute tubulointerstitial nephritis, malignant hypertension, and atheroembolic renal disease. These should always be considered in situations in which renal function has changed acutely. Perhaps even as common is the initiation of treatment with an ACE inhibitor in patients with hypertension secondary to subtle and unrecognized bilateral renal artery stenosis. A decrease in the effective circulating blood volume, caused by volume depletion, a reduction in cardiovascular function (heart failure), or marked peripheral vasodilation, as in sepsis, probably is the most common etiology for acute renal failure in the United States. Renal underperfusion is detected by measuring the fractional excretion of sodium ($FE_{Na}$) in the urine. $FE_{Na}$ is the urinary sodium excretion as a percentage of filtered sodium or % excreted Na/filtered Na (% $E/F_{Na}$). It is calculated as follows:

$$FENa = \frac{UNa \times Pcr}{PNa \times UCr}$$

A random or "spot" urine specimen together with an accompanying blood sample is needed for the required measurements of plasma and urine Na and creatinine concentrations. When the kidney is underperfused, the $FE_{Na}$ usually is far below the normal value of about 1%. Treatment of such patients is aimed at restoring renal perfusion with volume repletion, treatment of heart failure, or blood pressure support. Prolonged periods of renal hypoperfusion may lead to acute tubular necrosis and a prolonged course of renal failure.

Acute tubular necrosis is secondary to renal ischemia or exposure to nephrotoxic drugs. Proximal renal tubular epithelial cell necrosis and sloughing of cells occur, with subsequent obstruction of the tubular lumen by casts.

**TABLE 169.1. Causes of Acute Renal Failure**

*Prerenal failure*

- *Volume depletion:* poor fluid intake, diuretics, gastrointestinal losses, hemorrhage, third spacing
- *Peripheral vasodilation:* sepsis, shock, liver failure, antihypertensive agents
- *Increased renal vascular resistance:* anesthesia, surgery, prostaglandin inhibitors, hepatorenal syndrome
- *Cardiovascular disease:* acute myocardial infarction, congestive heart failure, cardiac tamponade, arrhythmia, pulmonary embolism
- *Renal vascular occlusion:* renal artery stenosis, embolism, thrombosis, vasculitis

*Intrinsic renal failure*

- *Renal vascular disorders:* malignant hypertension, cholesterol emboli, vasculitis, thrombotic thrombocytopenic purpura, hemolytic-uremic syndrome, scleroderma renal crisis, toxemia of pregnancy
- *Glomerular diseases:* acute postinfectious, diffuse proliferative, and rapidly progressive glomerulonephritis, systemic lupus erythematosus, infective endocarditis, Goodpasture's syndrome, vasculitis
- *Acute tubular necrosis:* ischemia, nephrotoxic agents (aminoglycosides, cephalosporins, cyclosporine, amphotericin B, acyclovir, pentamidine, chemotherapeutic agents, radiographic contrast dye, heavy metals, hydrocarbons, anesthetics), rhabdomyolysis with myoglobinuria, hemolysis with hemoglobinuria, hypercalcemia, myeloma proteins, light-chain nephropathy
- *Tubulointerstitial diseases:* allergic tubulointerstitial nephritis (antibiotics, diuretics, allopurinol, rifampin, phenytoin, cimetidine, NSAIDs), infection (staphylococcus, gram-negative bacteria, leptospirosis, brucellosis, viruses, fungi, tuberculosis) infiltrative disease (leukemia, lymphoma, sarcoidosis)

*Postrenal failure*

- *Ureteral obstruction:* retroperitoneal fibrosis or tumor, bilateral strictures after surgery or radiation, bilateral ureteral calculi, bilateral papillary necrosis, bilateral fungus balls, benign prostatic hypertrophy, prostatic cancer, bladder cancer, cervical cancer, neurogenic bladder

TABLE 169.2. Urinary Characteristics in Acute Renal Failure

| | Prerenal Azotemia | Acute Tubular Necrosis (ATN) | Postrenal Azotemia |
|---|---|---|---|
| Urine volume (mL/d) | <500 | Oliguric <400 nonoliguric >400 | Variable, from anuria to polyuria |
| Urine osmolality (mOsm/kg $H_2O$) | >500 | <350 | Early, resembles prerenal failure; late, more resemblance to acute tubular necrosis |
| $U_{osm}/P_{osm}$ | >1.5 | ≤1 | |
| Urine Na+ (mEq/L) | <20 | >40 | |
| $FE_{Na}$ % | <1 | >2 | |
| Urine sediment | Benign; few granular or hyaline casts | Renal tubular epithelial cells; hyaline and granular casts, "muddy brown" casts of ATN | Normal; or hematuria pyuria, crystalluria |

Some of the more common causes of intrinsic renal failure in the hospital are antibiotics (e.g., aminoglycosides, cephalosporins) or radiocontrast media. The general urinary manifestations of acute renal failure are summarized in Table 169.2. A BUN:creatinine ratio exceeding 10:1 suggests a **prerenal** cause such as volume depletion. Hyponatremia and hyperkalemia usually accompany this process and are related to the inability of the damaged kidney to excrete water in the presence of ongoing water intake and inability to secrete potassium into the urine.

The most common cause of death from acute renal failure is infection. Gastrointestinal bleeding is noted in up to 30% of cases; cardiovascular events such as pulmonary edema and congestive heart failure also are quite common. Lastly, there is a critical need to reduce doses of drugs that normally are excreted by the kidneys.

## Diagnosis

The cause of acute renal failure can largely be determined by a history of recent exposure to nephrotoxic agents, hypotension during surgery, or any preceding symptoms of an illness. Physical examination is helpful in determining the volume status of a patient, but usually does not give clues to the etiology of acute renal failure. A search for urinary tract obstruction should be made in all patients with acute renal failure. This examination includes ultrasonography to examine the kidneys and ureters and a single straight catheterization of the bladder to detect urethral obstruction, especially in men. Laboratory tests begin with urinalysis. Heavy proteinuria with RBCs or hemoglobin casts is typical of severe acute glomerulonephritis. Proteinuria together with "muddy-brown" coarse granular casts is typical of tubular necrosis. Red-brown pigmented casts with no or few RBCs are typical of rhabdomyolysis. Other laboratory tests may reveal abnormalities of serum electrolytes, BUN, creatinine, calcium, phosphorus, and uric acid. Urine sodium and creatinine should be measured to estimate $FE_{Na,}$ and urine and plasma osmolality should be measured to estimate the U/P osmolality ratio.

Imaging of the kidney usually is unrewarding and does not aid in the diagnosis of acute renal failure except in the exclusion of obstruction as a cause. If the renal ultrasound is normal, no further imaging studies are warranted. The possible exception is arteriography for diagnosis of polyarteritis nodosa or assessment of renal trauma. Renal biopsy usually is not indicated in acute renal failure, unless the history and physical examination point to a glomerular process.

## Management

The general approach to treatment of acute renal failure is to address the primary etiology. If the patient is dehydrated, volume repletion is required to restore effective circulating volume. Loop diuretics also have a role in converting renal failure from oliguric to non-oliguric. Careful monitoring of serum electrolytes and acid-base status obviously are warranted. Care also should be taken to monitoring calcium and phosphate status, especially if acute renal failure is secondary to rhabdomyolysis, where hyperphosphatemia and hypocalcemia can occur quite rapidly. In these circumstances, intravenous calcium gluconate, oral calcium carbonate, or acetate should be administered, along with aluminum hydroxide, if necessary, to control hyperphosphatemia.

Nutrition in patients with renal failure should aim at minimizing negative nitrogen balance while avoiding volume overload. Enteral nutrition is preferred over hyperalimentation. Specific formulations exist for patients with renal failure. These formulations have low protein content and contain little to no potassium.

Calories are provided largely from carbohydrates. When enteral nutrition is not possible, hyperalimentation should be considered. Hyperalimentation should consist of 0.8–2 g/kg/day of amino acids in nondialyzed patients, plus an added 10–20 g/day of nonessential amino acids in the dialyzed patients.

The indications for dialysis in patients with acute renal failure are summarized in Table 169.3. Generally, uremia should be avoided and dialysis initiated before severe acidosis, mental changes, or seizures develop. In addition, patients who have acute renal failure with a high catabolic rate or who are hemodynamically unstable may benefit from continuous arteriovenous hemofiltration or hemodiafiltration. This form of modified dialysis is useful in removing large amounts of fluid from patients who require continuous parenteral hyperalimentation. Patients who are hypotensive (i.e., systolic pressures <100 mm Hg) usually cannot be hemodialyzed effectively and may require continuous arteriovenous or veno-venous hemofiltration, or, possibly, peritoneal dialysis.

**TABLE 169.3. Indications for Dialysis in Acute Renal Failure**

Inability to control volume status: failure to respond to maximal doses of diuretics
Inability to control acidosis with intravenous therapy: pH persistently < 7.2
Uremic symptoms (stupor, lethargy, pericarditis, nausea, vomiting, seizures)
Hyperkalemia: levels exceeding 6 mEq/L unresponsive to resin binders or with ECG changes

# CHAPTER 170 CHRONIC RENAL FAILURE

## Definition and Etiology

Chronic renal failure is defined as a progressive and irreversible deterioration of renal function caused by a variety of diseases. The underlying primary disease is often difficult to identify when advanced renal failure is established. The two most common causes of chronic renal failure in the United States are diabetes mellitus and hypertension.

Laboratory manifestations of chronic renal failure are not seen until over 40% of renal function is lost, and clinical manifestations usually do not occur until over 80% of GFR is lost. When GFR declines below 10% of the normal value, uremia ensues and dialysis is required. The major changes that occur in chronic renal failure are summarized in Table 170.1. Causes of chronic renal failure are summarized in Table 170.2.

**TABLE 170.1. Changes in Body Fluid Homeostasis in Chronic Renal Failure**

| Problem | Cause |
|---|---|
| Hyperkalemia | ↓ renal function (≥90%) and distal tubular function |
| Hyperchloremic acidosis (non-anion gap) | ↓ renal and tubular function |
| ↓ calcitriol synthesis | Parenchymal mass, then hyperphosphatemia |
| Normocytic normochromic anemia | ↓ Erythropoietin production (GFR <30 ml/min) |

↓ = Decreased.

## Clinical Features

Nearly all of the organ systems may be affected by chronic kidney failure, with resulting symptoms that include hypertension and congestive heart failure. A bleeding diathesis occurs secondary to platelet dysfunction in patients with chronic kidney failure, manifested by an increased bleeding time. **Gastrointestinal problems** such as bleeding are common secondary to **arteriovenous malformations** or **angiodysplasia.** In addition, gastric erosions are commonly seen in patients with chronic renal disease. Elevations in **amylase** to three times normal are common in dialyzed patients, but pancreatitis is uncommon. Dysfunction of many organ

**TABLE 170.2. Common Causes of Chronic Renal Failure**

Diabetic nephropathy (most common)
Hypertensive nephrosclerosis (second most common)
Primary glomerular disease
Renovascular disease
Glomerular diseases associated with systemic illness
Tubulointerstitial diseases
Polycystic disease and other hereditary diseases
Thromboembolic disease
Chronic urinary tract obstruction (reflux)

systems complicate chronic renal failure; the important dysfunctions are summarized in subsequent sections.

**Bone disorders**

**Secondary hyperparathyroidism** develops early during the course of progressive renal failure in most patients. The mechanisms that cause increasing parathyroid hyperplasia and increased parathyroid hormone (PTH) secretion as kidney failure worsens include: (1) an increase in the relative body burden of phosphate as functioning kidney mass decreases, leading to hyperphosphatemia as GFR falls below 30 ml/min, and (2) reduced renal synthesis of calcitriol, which leads to reduced intestinal absorption of calcium. The effect of PTH on stimulation of bone resorption sustains near-normal plasma calcium concentrations but at the price of hyperparathyroid bone disease, osteitis fibrosa cystica. Because plasma phosphate concentrations rise above normal while plasma calcium concentrations remain normal or are only slightly reduced, the product of the two concentrations may rise above 55, potentially leading to metastatic calcification of blood vessels and joints.

**Cardiovascular diseases**

The most common cause of death among patients with end-stage renal disease is cardiovascular disease. The incidence of coronary artery disease is affected by hypertension, abnormal lipid metabolism and elevated calcium-phosphorus product. Constrictive pericarditis and pericardial effusions occasionally are seen in dialyzed patients; however, they are confined to patients who do not receive adequate dialysis or are noncompliant with dialytic therapy. Pericardial effusions seen with uremia usually are hemorrhagic.

**Hematopoietic system**

The anemia seen in chronic renal failure results largely from a reduction in erythropoietin synthesis by interstitial cells in the area of the proximal tubule of the kidney. Erythropoietin is responsible for red blood cell differentiation from stem cells. Although the leukocyte count in dialysis patients usually is normal, the chemotactic mechanism usually is defective, resulting in atypical immune responses. The platelet count likewise is normal; however, platelet function may be defective.

## Management

The most important measure for slowing progression of chronic renal failure is to gain control of the blood pressure. There is ample evidence in humans that hypertension can accelerate renal damage, and control of blood pressure slows deterioration in a number of renal diseases. ACE inhibitors may have a selective advantage in preserving renal function in patients with diabetic glomerulosclerosis and IgA nephropathy. Although many patients do not adhere strictly to a protein-restricted diet, education about the potential value of such a diet and avoidance of excessive protein ingestion are recommended.

Management of patients with chronic renal failure should include: (1) sodium and visible water restriction to a maximum of 1.5 L/day; (2) potassium restriction by limiting fruits (especially dried fruits) and potatoes and other vegetables with a high potassium content; (3) daily calcitriol and calcium supplementation with each meal, not only to provide calcium but to bind phosphate; and (4) recombinant erythropoietin, if the hemoglobin is below 10 g/dl, and in those with angina if the hemoglobin is below 11 g/dl with the goal of raising the level to 11 to 12 g/dl. Erythropoietin administration may be followed, by unknown mechanisms, by clinically important hypertension in approximately 20% of patients. Modifications in drug therapy may be necessary in renal failure; the common drugs for which this may be necessary are summarized in Table 170.3.

## End-Stage Renal Disease

End-stage renal disease (ESRD) is defined as permanent and almost complete (>90%) loss of kidney function, when life can be sustained only by dialysis or kidney transplantation. The U.S. National Institutes of Health reported that, as of December 31, 2000, 350,000 people had ESRD, with an incidence of 311 per million population and a cost of almost $20 billion in 2000. The primary causes of ESRD are diabetes mellitus (40%), hypertension (27%), and glomerular diseases (13%), with various other causes accounting for the remaining 20%.

**TABLE 170.3. Dosage Adjustments of Commonly Used Medications in Renal Failure**

| Use With Major Reduction in Dose | Use With Minor or No Reduction in Dose | Avoid Altogether |
|---|---|---|
| *Antibiotics* | | |
| Aminoglycosides | Erythromycin | Tetracycline |
| Penicillin G | Nafcillin | Nitrofurantoin |
| Cephalosporins | Clindamycin | Nalidixic acid |
| Sulfonamides | Chloramphenicol | |
| Vancomycin | Isoniazid/rifampin | |
| Amphotericin B | | |
| *Other drugs* | | |
| Digoxin | Antihypertensives | Aspirin |
| Procainamide | Benzodiazepines | Sulfonylureas |
| $H_2$ antagonists | Quinidine | Lithium carbonate |
| | Lidocaine | Acetazolamide |
| | Codeine | Spironolactone |
| | Propoxyphene | Triamterene |

Early referral to a nephrologist is recommended when the serum creatinine is 2 mg/dl or greater or the creatinine clearance is less than 50 ml/min. The nephrologist, working with the primary care physician, can help detect and treat renal disease early and slow its progression, especially aiding with blood pressure control. Working together, they can prevent complications such as renal osteodystrophy by controlling calcium and phosphorus and improving nutrition. Treatment of anemia with erythropoietin requires close monitoring. The nephrologist can help prepare the patient for dialysis by arranging for access to proper dialysis when it is needed and by helping the patient with necessary social, financial, psychological, and dietary needs. It has been shown that morbidity and mortality are lower in the first year of dialysis when a nephrologist is involved early in the course of chronic renal failure. Dialysis is performed using hemodialysis or peritoneal dialysis. Cardiovascular disease is the primary cause of death.

Once the patient's condition is stabilized and there are no complications, kidney transplantation may be performed. The kidney may be harvested from a matched related or unrelated live donor or a cadaver. On occasion, renal transplantation may be performed even before the patient requires dialysis. The first successful kidney transplant was performed in 1954 between twins. For 3 decades azathioprine and prednisone were the main immunosuppressive agents. The introduction of cyclosporine and OKT3 in the 1980s and mycophenolate mofetil, tacrolimus, and rapamycin in the 1990s have reduced rejection rates and improved patient survival at 1 year to 97.3% for living-donor and 93.7% for cadaver-donor transplantation. The surgical techniques are well-defined, and the recent development of laparoscopic-assisted living donor nephrectomy has shortened recovery for the donor. Unfortunately, the supply of organs is less than the demand, and the number of patients on the waiting list continues to grow.

# CHAPTER 171 NEPHROLITHIASIS

Nephrolithiasis (kidney stones) is a common disorder. Two to three percent of the population suffer at least one episode of nephrolithiasis during a lifetime. The risk of recurrent stones averages about 35% during the decade following the first episode.

## Etiology

The diagnosis of nephrolithiasis depends on the history, laboratory tests, and stone analysis. The history should include a family and personal history of stone disease and dietary habits, including intake of food high in calcium or oxalate such as dairy products, nuts, rutabagas, spinach, beets, and chocolate. The initial evaluation of patients with this problem is summarized in Table 171.1. Laboratory tests should include serum electrolytes, calcium, phosphate, uric acid, urine pH, and microscopic examinations for crystals, as well as a urine culture. Passed stones should be saved for analysis. Metabolic evaluation of kidney stones should always be performed before starting on a therapeutic regimen. In general, metabolic abnormalities are found in patients with recurrent calcium stones, rather than a single episode of a calcium stone. Moreover, calcium oxalate stone formation, which is common, can be corrected largely by dietary modifications. Thus, calcium stones do not require a full work-up after the initial episode; however, noncalcium stones should be investigated completely after the first episode. The general workup should include two 24-hour urine collections for calcium, phosphate, uric acid, oxalate, citrate, creatinine, sodium, urea nitrogen, and cystine. If hypercalcemia is present, a

**TABLE 171.1. Evaluation of the Patient With Urolithiasis**

| Blood | Urine | Radiography |
|---|---|---|
| Calcium | pH | Plain film (KUB) |
| Uric acid | Crystals (oxalate, citrate) | Ultrasound |
| Phosphate | Gram stain (WBCs, bacteria) | IVP |
| Alkaline phosphatase | Culture | Serial KUBs |
| Parathyroid hormone | 24-hour urine calcium | |
| 1,25(OH)$_2$ vitamin D$_3$ | 24-hour urine uric acid | |

KUB = Kidney, ureter, bladder

PTH level should be obtained. Despite thorough evaluation, a correctable cause of stones can be found only in 20% of patients.

### Calcium stones

Calcium stones, which are radiopaque, constitute 80% of all kidney stones. If hypercalcemia is present, hyperparathyroidism is likely. However, other causes, such as sarcoidosis, hyperthyroidism, multiple myeloma, or malignancy, also should be considered. If hypercalciuria is present with normocalcemia, stones may be secondary to a distal renal tubular acidosis, renal calcium or phosphate leak, or hyperthyroidism. If hyperuricosuria is present, even with a normal urinary and serum calcium, uric acid crystals may serve as the nidus for calcium stone formation. In this case, correction of the uricosuria would be useful in that it would eliminate this focus of stone formation. Hyperoxaluria with normal serum and urinary calcium levels may also be the result of acquired hyperoxaluria secondary to vitamin C abuse, excessive dietary oxalate intake, ileal resection, or disease (see Chapters 87 and 91), or jejunoileal bypass surgery.

### Struvite stones

Struvite stones (also known as triple phosphate stones) are radiopaque and are composed of magnesium, ammonia, and phosphate hydroxyapatite. These stones are unique in that they form in high urinary pH that results from urea-splitting organisms such as *Proteus* spp. These stones must be surgically removed to treat the infection adequately. If stones are of the appropriate size and in the proper location, lithotripsy also is an option.

### Cystine stones

Cystine stones also are radiopaque, and are created by an inherited defect in the renal tubular absorption of cystine that results in cystinuria. The diagnosis is suggested by a positive urine nitroprusside test and confirmed by stone analysis. Urinalysis of cystine stones may show the characteristic hexagonal crystals of cystine.

### Uric acid stones

Uric acid stones are the only radiolucent stones, and account for 10% of the cases. Uric acid stones are formed in hyperuricosuric states, volume depletion, and acidic urine, which reduces the solubility of uric acid. Fifty percent of patients with uric acid stones also have gout.

## Clinical Features

Hematuria and severe colicky pain are two common presentations of kidney stones. Hematuria may be gross or microscopic, and the nature of pain depends on the location of the stone. Pelvic stones usually are painless unless an infection or obstruction is present. Ureteral stones, on the other hand, cause nausea, vomiting, and severe abdominal flank pain radiating into the groin, urethra, or genitalia, or the tip of the penis. Stones at the ureterovesical junction may result in dysuria, frequency, and urgency. Fever and pyuria suggest associated urinary tract infection, but if complete obstruction is present, pyuria may not occur. Chronic and complete obstruction can result in hydronephrosis.

## Management

### Acute episode

In an acute episode of nephrolithiasis, an effective analgesic must be given; opiates may be needed. A plain abdominal radiograph usually shows calcium-containing stones. The helical CT scan of the abdomen is replacing the time-honored intravenous pyelogram (IVP) in assessing the size and position of the stone. However, a non-contrast helical CT scan may be the quickest and most accurate test to locate urinary tract stones. A fine mesh straining device should be used to strain all urine to retrieve the stones. Water intake should be increased to maintain a daily urine output of 2 L or more. If this is not possible, intravenous fluids should be given to increase urinary output. If large ureteral or pelvic stones cause obstruction, extracorporeal shock wave lithotripsy or surgical removal may be necessary.

### Recurrent stones

For the more common type of stones, such as calcium oxalate stones, hydration of at least 2 to 3 L/day and increase in calcium and reduction in oxalate intake are quite useful in preventing recurrent stones. Thiazide diuretics, such as 12.5 mg of hydrochlorothiazide, reduce urinary calcium excretion and are effective when administered to hypercalciuric calcium stone formers. Potassium citrate (60 mEq/day) in divided doses also may help prevent recurrence. Citrate prevents calcium oxalate and phosphate crystallization in the urine. Patients with hyperuricosuria (≤1000 mg of uric acid/24 hrs) and normal serum calcium can be benefited by 100–200 mg/day of allopurinol to reduce uric acid synthesis. Patients with acquired hyperoxaluria secondary to disease, restriction, or bypass of the small intestine may benefit from oral calcium supplements to precipitate dietary oxalate within the intestine or from cholestyramine (4 g three times a day), which binds oxalate in the gut. Patients with primary hyperoxaluria may be helped by pyridoxine, which reduces endogenous oxalate synthesis.

Prevention of recurrent cystine stones is aimed at decreasing urinary concentration of cystine below the solubility limit of 200 to 300 mg/L. Besides the methods already described, alkalinization of the urine to a pH above 7.5 is critical. This usually can be achieved with

Shohl's solution, which contains sodium citrate. In recalcitrant cases, sulfhydryl-containing drugs such as D-penicillamine may be useful by increasing cystine solubility by forming mixed disulfide compounds of cystine.

Treatment of patients with uric acid stones includes increased water intake as above, and alkalinization of the urine to a pH of 7 or above with potassium citrate or potassium bicarbonate, or sodium bicarbonate in divided doses; both measures are aimed at increasing dissolution of uric acid. Additionally, acetazolamide may be used to alkalinize the nocturnal urine. Allopurinol should be given for hyperuricemia in doses of 200 to 300 mg/day to reduce the formation of uric acid. Purine-rich foods such as beef and liver should be avoided.

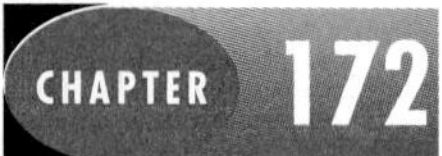

# CHAPTER 172 GLOMERULAR DISEASES

Most of the glomerular diseases have an immunologic basis. Discrete deposition of granular deposits of immunoglobulins and complement commonly is seen on the glomerular basement membranes of renal biopsy tissue. Alternatively, antigens can localize to this membrane and cause an antigen–antibody reaction, which then initiates a cascade of reactions that results in glomerular injury.

Other glomerular diseases such as minimal change disease also are thought to have an immunologic basis; however, no deposits are found on tissue examination. The terminology used in describing the pathology of the glomerular diseases is presented in Table 172.1. Some of the more common glomerular diseases are discussed in the following sections.

## Poststreptococcal Glomerulonephritis

Poststreptococcal glomerulonephritis is manifested by sudden onset of gross hematuria, RBC casts in the urine, and proteinuria that can occur 1 to 2 weeks after a pharyngeal or 3 to 6 weeks after a skin infection with group A β-hemolytic streptococci. Presenting symptoms include gross hematuria, edema, hypertension, back pain, oliguria, renal insufficiency, and, in some cases, symptoms of heart failure secondary to volume overload. Nephrotic syndrome, although rare, occurs in 5% of newly diagnosed patients. Throat and skin culture may yield β-hemolytic streptococci if no antibiotic therapy has been given. Serum complement levels are depressed for 8 weeks, and anti-DNase antibodies and ASO titers are elevated. Although antibiotics are advised to eliminate residual streptococci, no specific therapy is curative. Thus, treatment is supportive, with specific aims of reducing blood pressure and correcting volume overload. Diuretics are very useful in this context. It should be noted that in most cases of poststreptococcal glomerulonephritis the serum creatinine generally does not exceed 4 mg/dl. The prognosis for this condition is much better in children than adults. Less than 2% of all patients die or develop end-stage renal disease, and recovery usually is complete within 2 months. Patients over the age of 40 can develop a crescentic glomerulonephritis and usually have a poor prognosis.

## IgA Nephropathy

Worldwide, IgA nephropathy is the most common glomerular disease. The disease is characterized by recurrent attacks of gross hematuria, often following a nonspecific viral illness. Hypertension and nephrotic syndrome are uncommon and, if present, portend a poor prognosis. The disease shows a 6-fold greater predilection for men. Eighty percent of the patients with this disease are between the ages of 15 and 35 at the time of diagnosis. Although gross hematuria is the most common

**TABLE 172.1. Pathologic Features of Glomerular Disease**

| | |
|---|---|
| Focal | <50% of glomeruli contain the lesion |
| Diffuse (global) | Most glomeruli (>50%) contain the lesion |
| Segmental | Only a part of the glomerulus is affected by the lesion (most focal lesions are also segmental, e.g., focal segmental glomerulosclerosis) |
| Proliferation | An increase in cell number of one or more of the resident glomerular cells, with or without an inflammatory cell infiltration |
| Membranous changes | Capillary wall and matrix thickening |
| Crescent formation | Epithelial cell proliferation and mononuclear cell infiltration in Bowman's space |

**TABLE 172.2. Causes of Rapidly Progressive Glomerulonephritis**

Anti-GBM disease
- With lung hemorrhage (Goodpasture syndrome)
- Without hemorrhage (anti-GBM nephritis)
- Complicating membranous nephropathy

Immune complex–mediated glomerulonephritis
- Postinfectious glomerulonephritis
  - Poststreptococcal
  - Endocarditis
  - Visceral abscess
- Collagen-vascular disease
  - Systemic lupus erythematosus
  - Cryoglobulinemia
  - Henoch-Schönlein purpura
- Primary renal disease
  - Membranoproliferative glomerulonephritis
  - IgA nephropathy

ANCA-associated glomerulonephritis
- Polyarteritis nodosa (p-ANCA)
- Wegener granulomatosis (c-ANCA)

Idiopathic crescentic glomerulonephritis

laboratory finding, other abnormalities such as elevations in serum IgA level and skin biopsies showing deposits of IgA usually are positive. Serum complement levels are normal. Henoch-Schönlein purpura, a related disorder, may be present.

Treatment is generally supportive, and most patients have recurrent episodes. Only about 25% of all patients progress to end-stage renal disease. Poor prognostic indicators include male gender, older age, hypertension and proteinuria exceeding 2 g/day. Impaired renal function at the time of initial presentation is a poor prognostic sign.

## Rapidly Progressive Glomerulonephritis

Rapidly progressive glomerulonephritis (RPGN) is defined as loss of renal function exceeding 50% over a period of 3 months, associated with greater than 50% glomerular crescents on renal biopsy. This is not a specific disease but a syndrome that can occur with a severe form of primary or secondary glomerular disease, examples of which are listed in Table 172.2. One form of RPGN is anti-GBM disease. Anti-GBM antibody reacts with glomerular and alveolar basement membrane, causing nephritis and Goodpasture syndrome. This pulmonary–renal syndrome can present as an isolated pulmonary or renal disorder with the other organ affected later in the disease course. **Anti-GBM nephritis** may occur in the absence of pulmonary hemorrhage.

Clinically, anti-GBM disease accounts for 20% of all cases of rapidly progressive glomerulonephritis. Goodpasture disease often occurs in children and young adults and is eight times more common in men than women. In contrast, anti-GBM nephritis affects middle-aged adults and has relatively equal gender distribution. Presenting symptoms can include hemoptysis, dyspnea on exertion, volume overload, uremia, fever, arthritis, and abdominal pain. Nephrotic-range proteinuria is uncommon, and hypertension is present in one fifth of all patients. The treatment of choice is plasma exchange combined with steroids and immunosuppressive medications such as cyclophosphamide. Therapy is most effective when started early in the course of disease, specifically when creatinine is less than 6 mg/dl. Prognosis for recovery of renal function is poor when the disease is already in the advanced stage at the initial presentation.

### Immune-Complex Mediated Crescentic RPGN with Immune Deposits

Immune-complex mediated crescentic RPGN with immune deposits accounts for 30–50% of patients with RPGN. These patients usually are middle-aged and older and have symptoms of anti-GBM disease; they also usually have hypocomplementemia. Treatment for this disease includes pulse steroid therapy with gradual tapering. The prognosis is poor.

### Antineutrophilic Cytoplasmic Antibody Glomerulonephritis

Antineutrophilic cytoplasmic antibody (ANCA) glomerulonephritis is similar to RPGN, but no immune antibody deposits have ever been identified. The blood test for antibodies to neutrophils (ANCA) may be positive. Presenting features are those of systemic vasculitis and include fever, weight loss, arthritis, and abdominal pain. Therapy includes intravenous or oral cyclophosphamide, usually in combination with intravenous steroids. Therapy should be continued for a minimum of 1 year and at least 6 months after all clinical evidence of disease has disappeared.

## Minimal Change Disease

Minimal change disease accounts for 20% of all cases of nephrotic syndrome in adults and 75% to 80% of all cases in children. The peak age of onset is 2 to 6 years of age; however, it also may be seen as late as 15 to 18 years of age. A second peak occurs in adults around the age of 50. This disease is characterized by the absence of hypertension. It can occur, rarely, with malignancy (mainly lymphomas) as well as with medications such as nonsteroidal anti-inflammatory drugs. It is treated with oral corticosteroid therapy. In general, patients are responsive to oral prednisone in divided doses of 1 mg/kg for a period of 1 month or continued for 1 week after remission of nephrotic syndrome. Over 90% of these patients have remission; however, 50% have a recurrence or relapse, and when this occurs, low-dose alternate-day prednisone for 6 to 12 months is used. Unresponsive or "steroid-resistant" patients should be treated with oral cyclophosphamide 2 mg/kg per day for 2 months or oral chlorambucil 0.2 mg/kg/day for 3 months.

## Focal Segmental Glomerulosclerosis

Focal segmental glomerulosclerosis is present in about 15% to 20% of all patients with nephrotic syndrome. Patients usually present with nephrotic syndrome, hypertension, and renal insufficiency. This disease often is confused with minimal change disease, but minimal change disease does not cause hypertension. Focal glomerulosclerosis is more common in African Americans; in persons with intravenous heroin, analgesic, or other drug abuse; and in persons with AIDS. The etiology is unknown, and the prognosis is poor. There is no specific therapy, but some reports suggest that high-dose prednisone for 4 to 6 months may induce remission. Some of the small studies suggest that the addition of plasmapheresis to steroids may slow progression of the disease.

## Membranous Glomerular Disease

Membranous glomerular disease is the most common cause of nephrotic syndrome in adults, accounting for up to 50% of cases. Affected people usually are between the ages of 30 and 50 years, with men affected more commonly than women. The GFR usually is normal, or slightly decreased. If the history and physical examination are abnormal, malignancy should be sought, especially adenocarcinoma of the lung, colon, and breast. Other secondary causes of membranous nephropathy include hepatitis B, SLE, and drugs such as gold, penicillamine, captopril, and nonsteroidal anti-inflammatory drugs. No definitive therapy exists; however, high-dose, alternate-day steroids over a period of 2 months, with gradual tapering, may be beneficial. Cyclophosphamide and chlorambucil may induce remission in subjects with declining kidney function.

## Membranoproliferative Glomerulonephritis (MPGN)

Membranoproliferative glomerulonephritis accounts for about 10% of all cases of nephrotic syndrome in adults. It occurs with equal frequency between males and females in their teens and twenties often (40% cases) following an upper respiratory infection. The initial presentation includes acute glomerulonephritis, nephrotic syndrome, hematuria, hypertension, and decreased GFR associated with a low C3 level. There is no definitive therapy. Fifty percent of patients with MPGN progress to end-stage renal disease. Aspirin, 325 mg, plus dipyridamole 75 mg three times per day has been reported to slow progression of this disease in some patients.

## Glomerular Disorders Associated With Systemic Disease

Diabetes mellitus and SLE are the two systemic diseases most commonly associated with glomerular injury (Table 172.3). Renal disease due to SLE is also discussed in Chapter 275.

Almost 67% of all patients with SLE have renal disease based on biopsy findings. Nephrotic syndrome commonly occurs in up to 60% of patients with SLE. GFR is reduced in 15% to 20% of patients at the time of diagnosis. Renal biopsy is necessary to establish the diagnosis.

Patients with pathologic changes of lupus nephropathy of types 1, 2, and 5 are treated with oral prednisone, 1 mg/kg/day, for 2 months, with an 8-week tapering period. Fifty percent of these patients have proteinuria of less than 2 g, and their GFR and complement levels normalize. Those with class 3 and 4 lesions have much more extensive disease and require cyclophosphamide in addition to steroids.

### Diabetic Nephropathy

Diabetic nephropathy is the most common cause of end-stage renal disease in the United States. Microalbuminuria, defined as albumin excretion of 30–300 mg/24 hrs is the first indication of diabetic nephropathy. Urine should be monitored for microalbuminuria every 6 to 12 months in all diabetic patients, and those exhibiting it should be treated with an ACE inhibi-

| TABLE 172.3. Systemic Diseases With Renal Involvement |
|---|
| Diabetes mellitus (most common) |
| Systemic lupus erythematosus |
| Multiple myeloma |
| Polyarteritis nodosa |
| Wegener granulomatosis |
| Scleroderma |
| Hemolytic-uremic syndrome |
| Thrombotic thrombocytopenic purpura |
| Amyloidosis |
| Cryoglobulinemia |
| Postpartum renal failure |
| Disseminated intravascular coagulation |

tor, regardless of blood pressure, to forestall renal failure. Calcium channel blockers such as verapamil and diltiazem (but not dihydropyridines) and angiotensin receptor blockers (ARB) also reduce proteinuria. ACE inhibitors and calcium channel blockers, along with a diuretic, are the treatment of choice for controlling hypertension in the diabetic. When proteinuria appears and impaired renal function develops (serum creatinine ≥ 2 mg/dl), referral to a nephrologist is recommended to assist in preserving renal function and preparing the patient for end-stage renal disease care. Early and aggressive control of blood sugar and arterial pressure preserves renal function.

The hallmark morphologic change seen in diabetic nephropathy is mesangial matrix expansion; when nodular, it is called nodular sclerosis or **Kimmelstiel-Wilson lesion**. This is not seen in early stages of hypertension without diabetes.

# CHAPTER 173 TUBULOINTERSTITIAL NEPHROPATHY

Tubulointerstitial nephropathy refers to a group of clinical disorders that affects the renal tubules and interstitium, sparing the glomeruli and renal vasculature. Both acute and chronic forms of this disease exist, with the acute type resulting in a rapid decline in renal function over a period of days to weeks, and the chronic form resulting in progressive azotemia and histologic changes of interstitial scarring and fibrosis that evolve over a period of years.

## Acute Tubulointerstitial Nephritis

Acute tubulointerstitial nephritis is characterized by an acute decline in renal function associated with biopsy findings of inflammatory cell infiltrates within the renal interstitium. The two most common causes of acute tubulointerstitial nephritis are nonsteroidal anti-inflammatory drugs (NSAIDs) and antibiotics, specifically, sulfonamides or penicillins (Table 173.1). Acute pyelonephritis is classified histologically as a form of acute tubulointerstitial nephritis; however, the mechanism for nephritis is direct bacterial invasion of the renal medulla and not an allergic reaction, as is the case with other causes.

**TABLE 173.1. Causes of Acute Interstitial Nephritis**

| |
|---|
| *Drug-related* |
| Antimicrobial drugs |
| Penicillins (esp. methicillin) |
| Rifampin |
| Sulfonamides |
| Nonsteroidal anti-inflammatory drugs |
| Allopurinol |
| Loop diuretics |
| *Systemic infections* |
| Streptococcal infections |
| Cytomegalovirus |
| Infectious mononucleosis |
| Legionnaires' disease |
| Leptospirosis |
| *Primary renal infections* |
| Acute bacterial pyelonephritis |
| *Immune disorders* |
| Acute glomerulonephritis |
| Systemic lupus erythematosus |
| Transplant rejection |
| *Idiopathic* |

The major clinical finding in acute tubulointerstitial nephritis is the development of acute renal insufficiency. One third of patients develop the triad of fever, skin rash, and peripheral eosinophilia with arthralgias, whereas as many as 50% have peripheral eosinophilia alone. The absence of these features does not exclude the possibility of acute tubulointerstitial nephritis. Hypertension and edema are important features of acute glomerulonephritis but usually are not seen in acute tubulointerstitial nephritis.

The first clue to the diagnosis of acute tubulointerstitial nephritis usually is urinary abnormalities and a rise in serum creatinine. Hematuria, often microscopic, is common in cases with a drug-induced etiology. Sterile pyuria with leukocyte casts also may be seen. The presence of eosinophiluria as noted by Hansel stain or Wright stain may be helpful, but this usually is present only within the first 5 to 7 days of the disease. Eosinophiluria is not pathognomonic for tubulointerstitial nephritis—it is also seen in trauma and cystitis. Lastly, the presence of red blood cell casts indicates glomerulonephritis rather than tubulointerstitial nephritis.

It is important to distinguish between tubulointerstitial nephritis induced by antibiotics and that induced by NSAIDs. Corticosteroids may be effective in shortening the course of antibiotic-induced tubulointerstitial nephritis but confer no benefit in NSAID-induced type. Cessation of the offending drug is mandatory in both types.

**TABLE 173.2. Conditions Associated With Chronic Tubulointerstitial Nephropathy**

| |
|---|
| *Urinary tract obstruction* |
| Vesicoureteral reflux |
| Mechanical |
| *Drugs* |
| Analgesics |
| Nitrosurea |
| Cisplatin |
| Cyclosporine |
| *Vascular diseases* |
| Nephrosclerosis |
| Atheroembolic disease |
| Radiation nephritis |
| Sickle hemoglobinopathies |
| Vasculitis |
| *Heavy metals* |
| Lead |
| Cadmium |
| *Metabolic disorders* |
| Hyperuricemia/hyperuricosuria |
| Hypercalcemia/hypercalciuria |
| Hyperoxaluria |
| Potassium depletion |
| Cystinosis |
| *Hereditary diseases* |
| Medullary cystic disease |
| Hereditary nephritis |
| Polycystic kidney disease |
| *Malignancies* |
| Multiple myeloma |
| *Granulomatous diseases* |
| Sarcoidosis |
| Tuberculosis |
| Wegener granulomatosis |
| *Immunologic diseases* |
| Systemic lupus erythematosus |
| Sjögren syndrome |
| Cryoglobulinemia |
| *Endemic diseases* |
| Balkan nephropathy |

**TABLE 173.3. Findings Suggestive of Chronic Tubulointerstitial Diseases**

| |
|---|
| Hyperchloremic metabolic acidosis (out of proportion to the degree of renal insufficiency) |
| Hyperkalemia (out of proportion to the degree of renal insufficiency) |
| Reduced maximal urinary concentrating ability (polyuria, nocturia) |
| Partial or complete Fanconi syndrome: phosphaturia, bicarbonaturia, aminoaciduria, uricosuria, glycosuria |

## Chronic Tubulointerstitial Nephropathy

A wide variety of diseases may cause chronic tubulointerstitial nephritis (Table 173.2).

Chronic tubulointerstitial nephropathy is responsible for 25% to 30% of all cases of end-stage renal disease. Most patients with chronic tubulointerstitial nephritis have little to no clinical evidence of active renal inflammation. Lithium therapy and disorders such as analgesic toxicity, sickle cell disease, or polycystic disease affect the concentration mechanism of the kidney; polyuria is a common sequel. The urinalysis may show modest amounts of sterile pyuria and minimal hematuria, but in most cases, there are no cellular casts. Different diseases affect different portions of the tubule. Conditions such as multiple myeloma and heavy metal toxicity (e.g., lead) primarily affect the proximal tubule and usually result in proximal renal tubular acidosis, glycosuria, aminoaciduria, and uricosuria. Conversely, chronic obstruction of the urinary tract primarily affects the distal renal tubule and can present with distal tubular acidosis, salt wasting, and hyperkalemia. The clinical findings associated with chronic tubulointerstitial disease are summarized in Table 173.3.

# CHAPTER 174 VASCULAR DISEASES OF THE KIDNEY

## Arteriosclerosis

Disorders of the main renal vessels usually are unilateral and are discussed later in this chapter. The processes that involve the smaller vessels of the kidneys, however, are diffuse and usually affect both kidneys. These arterial disorders usually are associated with hypertension. Renal failure may occur acutely, but it is usually progressive over a period of weeks to months.

## Thromboembolic Disease

Thromboembolic disease, the most common form of arteriolar disease, is secondary to atheroembolism. This process usually is seen in people with severe atherosclerotic disease who have undergone an aortogram, cardiac catheterization, or other arterial manipulation. During or after the procedure, emboli of cholesterol crystals may shower the kidney. These subsequently occlude the peripheral capillary beds within the kidney and choke off circulation to that portion of the nephron. Hypertension and renal failure are the usual sequelae. Associated eosinophilia and eosinophiluria help establish the diagnosis of atheroembolic disease, but are present in only about 25% of patients. At times, peripheral extremity emboli with necrosis ("blue toe" syndrome) raise the suspicion of renal emboli.

## Scleroderma

Scleroderma is a progressive connective tissue disease of uncertain etiology (see Chapter 259). Renal arterioles usually demonstrate intimal proliferation with progressive luminal occlusion. The clinical course of renal involvement reflects these pathologic changes. However, the development of proteinuria or mild hypertension in this disease often heralds the onset of sclerodermal renal crisis and subsequent renal failure. This poorly understood process may be improved by antihypertensive therapy with angiotensin-converting enzyme inhibitors.

## Hemolytic-Uremic Syndrome and Thrombotic Thrombocytopenic Purpura

The hemolytic-uremic syndrome (HUS) and thrombotic thrombocytopenic purpura (TTP) are characterized by microangiopathy. The renal lesion is characterized by fibrin thrombi in the glomerular capillary loops. HUS usually is observed in children following a bout of gastroenteritis or a flu-like syndrome. Among adults, it is seen more often in young women, in association with the use of oral contraceptives. However, some antineoplastic agents and immunosuppressive drugs, such as cyclosporine, have been associated with its development. The clinical syndrome of TTP is dominated by neurologic features. The clinical course of renal involvement is acute and rapidly progressive. The prognosis is poor. Plasmapheresis is the treatment of choice for TTP.

## Renal Arterial Occlusion

Partial obstruction of the renal arterial system by atheromatous plaques or fibromuscular dysplasia is linked directly to renovascular hypertension. Thrombosis of the renal arteries most often is seen in cases of severe blunt abdominal trauma and rarely after surgical manipulation or during angiographic study of the renal artery. Thrombosis also can occur as an embolic phenomenon in patients with underlying atherosclerotic vascular disease; it also may occur following radiocontrast studies. Rarely, valvular vegetations of bacterial endocarditis embolize and obstruct renal arteries. Symptoms include severe, localized flank pain, nausea, vomiting, and oliguria. Nuclear renography is useful in diagnosis.

## Renal Vein Thrombosis

Renal vein thrombosis usually is seen in states of heavy proteinuria, with urinary loss of clotting factors and antithrombin III, such as occurs in membranous nephropathy or minimal change disease. It is associated with flank pain and, in rare cases, pulmonary embolism. Diagnosis can be made by Doppler renal ultrasound or renal venography. Anticoagulation is required, and renal function usually improves with resolution of the thrombus. Prophylactic anticoagulation is not recommended, however, for patients with nephrotic syndrome who are at risk for developing thrombosis.

# CHAPTER 175 CYSTIC DISEASES OF THE KIDNEY

Cysts are commonly found in the kidneys. They are characterized by epithelial-lined cavities filled with fluid or semi-solid debris. This chapter discusses the most commonly seen clinical entities associated with cystic disease.

The finding of a solitary cyst in a middle-aged person is most likely to be a simple cyst. However, the same finding in a neonate with an abdominal mass suggests the possibility of autosomal dominant polycystic kidney disease (ADPKD) or an autosomal recessive form of the disease (ARPKD).

## Simple Cysts

Simple renal cysts increase in frequency with age and are present in 50% of the population over the age of 50 and in more than 90% of the population over the age of 75. They usually are asymptomatic and do not increase the risk of neoplastic disease. They usually can be found on renal ultrasound examination.

## Polycystic Kidney Disease

### Clinical Features

There are both autosomal dominant and autosomal recessive forms of polycystic kidney disease (PKD). Autosomal dominant polycystic kidney disease (ADPKD), which is much more common, is carried on chromosome 16. It is the most common hereditary disease in the United States, affecting approximately half a million people. Clinical manifestations of this disease are rare prior to the age of 20. Patients usually present either for screening because of a family history of the disease or for evaluation of symptoms. Although pain and hematuria are the most common clinical manifestations, a number of patients present with vague urinary tract symptoms and new-onset hypertension. Thus, patients with hypertension and microscopic hematuria should receive a renal ultrasound to screen for cystic disease, especially if there is a family history of this disorder.

Hypertension can occur in up to 60% of patients before any findings of renal insufficiency are noted. Nocturia often is present at the time of diagnosis, due to a urinary concentrating defect. Urinary tract infection and pyelonephritis are common complications. Up to one-third of patients with PKD have multiple asymptomatic hepatic cysts, and 10% have cerebral "berry" aneurysms. Twenty-five percent also have mitral valve prolapse. The natural history of renal functional impairment from ADPKD is variable. The disease progresses to end-stage renal disease in about 25% of individuals by age 50 and 50% by age 70.

### Diagnosis and Management

The diagnosis is based on radiographic evidence of multiple cysts distributed throughout the kidney and is associated with renal enlargement, increased cortical thickening, and splaying of the renal calyces. A contrast CT in adults usually defines the anatomy well. Renal ultrasonography accurately determines whether a mass is cystic or solid. Two thirds of renal masses fulfill all ultrasound criteria for simple cysts and require no further work-up. However, when a mass is suspected, but not confirmed by ultrasound, a CT is required. If the mass on ultrasound is solid or complex, renal CT scanning, both with and without contrast, is the next diagnostic step. For indeterminate cases, arteriography, needle aspiration cytology, or both may be needed.

It is now possible to screen patients for polycystic disease through genetic linkage analysis. Although this can predict the likelihood with a 99% certainty, it is quite expensive and requires cooperation from family members. Moreover, because there is no definitive therapy for ADPKD, testing should be reserved for individuals who can afford it and have the desire to know. The employment and insurance implications should be fully considered prior to undertaking genetic linkage analysis.

There is no definitive therapy for polycystic kidney disease; however, the results of recent studies demonstrate that aggressive control of arterial blood pressure tends to slow the disease process. A low-protein diet does not influence its natural history. Patients with ESRD secondary to ADPKD are candidates for kidney transplantation. A unique feature of ADPKD is that the coexistent anemia may be less severe than the anemia of other forms of renal failure. This reflects the ability of the kidney to secrete some erythropoietin despite the end-stage nature of the renal disease.

### Acquired Cystic Disease

Cysts develop in large numbers of patients with end-stage renal disease who undergo dialysis. The risk of developing a renal carcinoma is heightened in these cysts.

### Medullary Sponge Kidney

Medullary sponge kidney is a benign disorder that often is detected incidentally on abdominal radiographs.

It is commonly associated with the development of renal stones, especially the calcium oxalate variety. It is estimated that 10% of patients who present with renal stones have medullary sponge kidney. Nephrocalcinosis occurs in about 50% of these patients, but it usually is asymptomatic and is noted as an incidental finding. Renal failure does not occur as part of this disease; nonetheless, aggressive treatment of any urinary tract infection or stone is similar to that previously presented in this chapter.

# CHAPTER 176 HUMAN IMMUNODEFICIENCY VIRUS NEPHROPATHY

Chapter 158 provides a full discussion of human immunodeficiency virus (HIV) infection and HIV disease. Because it is a systemic disease, HIV infection is associated with various forms of renal disease as well. The most common glomerular disease is a collapsing form of focal glomerular sclerosis. This process may be seen in people with active acquired immune deficiency syndrome (AIDS), or asymptomatic HIV infection. Besides this primary glomerular lesion, patients with HIV infection also can develop other forms of renal disease. These diseases may be due not only to HIV infection, but to associated infections involving cytomegalovirus (CMV), hepatitis B, syphilis, and other related infections seen in this population. Antiretroviral drug, indinavir, can precipitate in the renal tubules causing nephrolithiasis and renal failure and should be avoided in patients with elevated serum creatinine. Pentamidine, foscarnet and aminoglycoside antibiotics used to treat opportunistic infections can cause acute tubular necrosis.

Approximately 6% of patients with HIV infection develop a collapsing focal glomerular sclerosis. Interestingly, and for unknown reasons, most of these patients are black men. Clinically, their presentation is similar to that of idiopathic focal glomerulosclerosis: they present with hypertension, substantial peripheral edema, evidence of nephrotic syndrome, hypoalbuminemia, and occasional RBCs and WBCs in the urinary sediment without RBC or WBC casts. The laboratory examination usually reveals a significant reduction in renal function, as manifested by an abnormally high blood urea nitrogen (BUN) and creatinine. On ultrasound, the kidneys in these patients may be large and echogenic. Renal biopsy can distinguish the HIV form from that of idiopathic focal glomerulosclerosis. The distinguishing features of HIV renal disease are collapse and sclerosis of the entire glomerular tufts and microcyst formation in tubules with tubular degeneration.

Combination therapy, generally referred to as highly active antiretroviral therapy (HAART) (see Chapter 165) may prevent or slow the progression of renal disease. Therapy of established renal disease with glucocorticoids, cyclosporine and angiotensin-converting enzyme inhibitors (ACEI) has met with modest success. Long-term hemodialysis survival is possible. Initial CD4 count of <50 and albumin of < 2.5 g/dl predict poor survival. Some centers are now doing renal transplants in HIV positive individuals.

# CHAPTER 177 DISORDERS OF WATER BALANCE

In healthy persons, the plasma osmolality is maintained between 285 and 300 mOsm. This regulation depends on thirst, antidiuretic hormone secretion, and renal concentrating and diluting mechanisms. Antidiuretic hormone (ADH) is the nonapeptide arginine vasopressin. There are two feedback loops. The first relies on stimulation or suppression of ADH secretion because of, respectively, a rise or fall in osmolality of the extracellular fluid (ECF). A rise in ECF osmolality of less than 5% causes increased ADH secretion, which acts on the kidney to enhance water conservation, thereby tending to lower the ECF osmolality. The converse occurs when the ECF osmolality falls. Greater changes in osmolality bring the second loop into play, that of thirst. After an increase in ECF osmolality that is greater than that for the first feedback loop, thirst occurs, leading to water intake that tends to decrease the ECF osmolality. Conversely, suppression of thirst should occur when the ECF osmolality declines. A failure of these adaptive responses results in disturbances of water excretion.

Hyponatremia and hypernatremia are the major disorders of water balance. Plasma osmolality, in mOsm/kg $H_2O$, can be either measured directly or estimated using the following formula:

$$P_{osm} = 2 \times [Na^+] + BUN/2.8 + glucose/18.$$

In the formula $Na^+$ is in mEq/L, and BUN and glucose in mg/dl. From the formula, it is apparent that $Na^+$ and its accompanying anion, Cl-, are the most important determinants of plasma osmolality.

## Hyponatremia

Hyponatremia, defined as a plasma $Na^+$ below 135 mmol/L, is a common electrolyte abnormality in hospitalized patients. Usually hyponatremia is a hypo-osmolal state, and the low osmolality causes a shift of water into cells. Occasionally hyponatremia may be associated with a normal or elevated plasma osmolality. It is important to recognize such situations because they are not associated with the shift of water into cells that is seen with hypo-osmolal hyponatremia. Thus, the first step in the evaluation of hyponatremia should be a determination of plasma osmolality (Table 177.1). Hyponatremia associated with an elevated plasma osmolality usually is due to hyperglycemia but may be due to the infusion of mannitol or glycine. These solutes cause the osmotic shift of water out of cells, which can result in hyponatremia. Laboratory artifact or pseudohyponatremia should be suspected when hyponatremia is associated with a normal plasma osmolality. This can occur with extreme elevations of lipids (usually triglycerides increased by more than 500 mg/dl) or proteins (e.g., multiple myeloma or Waldenstrom macroglobulinemia, with increase in protein level of > 4 g/dl). In these settings, the increased quantity of lipid or protein occupies a larger portion of the plasma volume, and use of standard flame photometry yields a low $Na^+$ concentration because it measures the concentration of $Na^+$ per liter of plasma. However, under the same circumstances, a $Na^+$-selective electrode would detect a normal $Na^+$ concentration, because this method measures $Na^+$ concentration in the aqueous phase of plasma.

**TABLE 177.1. Types of Hyponatremia Based on Plasma Osmolality**

| |
|---|
| *Elevated osmolality (hypertonic hyponatremia)* |
| Hyperglycemia |
| Glycine infusion |
| Mannitol infusion |
| *Normal osmolality (pseudohyponatremia)* |
| Severe hyperlipidemia |
| Severe hyperproteinemia |
| *Low osmolality (true or hypotonic hyponatremia)* |

**TABLE 177.2. Causes of Hyponatremia**

| With Decreased ECV | Normal ECV | Increased ECV |
|---|---|---|
| Renal losses | SIADH (see Table 64.4) | Nephrotic syndrome |
| Diuretics | | Congestive heart failure |
| Salt-losing nephropathy | Hypothyroidism | Cirrhosis |
| Hypoaldosteronism | | |
| GI losses | | |
| Diarrhea | | |
| Vomiting | | |
| Skin losses | | |
| Fever, burns | | |

ECV = effective circulating volume; SIADH = syndrome of inappropriate antidiuretic hormone secretion.

### Classification and Etiology

Once hypotonic hyponatremia is found, an assessment of the volume status is essential to find the cause of hyponatremia and to choose the right therapy (Table 177.2).

Hypovolemic hyponatremia occurs when total body $Na^+$ is depleted in relation to total body water (TBW). This can occur with both renal and nonrenal $Na^+$ loss. Causes of renal $Na^+$ loss include diuretics and, rarely, salt-wasting nephropathy. Nonrenal $Na^+$ loss can occur with diarrhea or vomiting, or skin losses. In all of these settings, hypovolemia induces the release of ADH, which promotes the reabsorption of water. Hyponatremia then occurs as a result of the loss of $Na^+$ and the retention of water. Urinary electrolytes may be useful in distinguishing between renal and nonrenal losses. With renal losses, urinary $Na^+$ usually exceeds 20 mEq/L. In contrast, urinary $Na^+$ usually is below 20 mEq/L with nonrenal $Na^+$ loss.

In euvolemic hyponatremia, volume status is normal and hyponatremia is due to a relative excess of TBW. The most common cause of euvolemic hyponatremia is the syndrome of inappropriate ADH secretion (SIADH; see Chapter 64). As shown in Table 64.4, common causes of SIADH include cancers, pulmonary disease, intracranial disease, and medications. Urinary $Na^+$ typically exceeds 20 mEq/L, and the urine is inappropriately concentrated ($U_{osm}$ >100 mOsm/kg) for the degree of plasma hypoosmolality. Another cause of euvolemic hyponatremia is hypothyroidism (see Table 177.2).

Hyponatremia also may occur in congestive heart failure, cirrhosis, and nephrotic syndrome. These illnesses are characterized by decreased effective circulatory volume despite a higher-than-normal TBW. The decrease in effective circulatory volume results in a volume-mediated secretion of ADH, which, in turn, leads to water retention and dilutional hyponatremia. In these settings, hyponatremia usually serves as a marker of the severity of the underlying disease, because it tends to occur only when advanced disease is present. For example, the plasma sodium might fall to about 130 mEq/L when the cardiac index is 1.5 L/min/m$^2$ or less. In such conditions, urine $Na^+$ concentrations are below 20 mEq/L because of avid $Na^+$ reabsorption.

## Clinical Features

Symptoms of hyponatremia are primarily neurologic and can include lethargy, confusion, seizures, and coma. The severity of symptoms is related to the degree of hyponatremia and to the rate of development of hyponatremia. **Acute hyponatremia** is more likely to cause symptoms due to brain swelling. In contrast, symptoms may be mild or absent with **chronic hyponatremia** because adaptive processes (involving the cellular extrusion of electrolytes and "osmoles") minimize the degree of brain swelling.

## Management

In treatment of hyponatremia, the rate and magnitude of correction must be determined (Table 177.3). A consensus has emerged that acute hyponatremia should be corrected more rapidly than chronic hyponatremia. Acute as opposed to chronic hyponatremia usually can be differentiated on the basis of symptoms. With acute hyponatremia, rapid correction is necessary to decrease brain swelling. In chronic hyponatremia, in contrast, because adaptive processes have normalized brain water, slower correction is indicated to minimize the risk of **central pontine myelinolysis**. With rapid correction, the goal of therapy is to raise the plasma $Na^+$ 1 to 2 mEq/L/hour until the patient becomes asymptomatic, which generally corresponds to a plasma $Na^+$ of 120 to 125 mEq/L. The plasma $Na^+$ should not be raised more than 12 mEq/L over 24 hours, and overcorrection of plasma $Na^+$ (>135–140 mEq/L) should be avoided. Fluid restriction (1000–1500 ml/day) may be all that is needed to treat chronic hyponatremia. Correction should occur over 48 to 72 hours; the rate of correction should not exceed 0.5 to 1.0 mEq/L/hour. In all cases of hyponatremia, underlying diseases should be treated and offending medications stopped.

The specific mode of therapy to raise the plasma $Na^+$ is best determined by the type of hyponatremia (see Table 177.3). To correct hypovolemic hyponatremia, the $Na^+$ deficit must be calculated and replaced. The $Na^+$ deficit is calculated as follows:

$$Na^+\ deficit = (desired\ plasma\ Na^+ - actual\ plasma\ Na^+) \times TBW$$

Another approach is just to give intravenous saline to restore circulating volume. This raises the blood pressure, thereby turning off the volume-mediated stimulus to ADH secretion.

To correct euvolemic hyponatremia, it is useful to know the free water excess, which can be derived as follows:

$$Desired\ TBW = (actual\ plasma\ Na^+/desired\ plasma\ Na^+) \times actual\ TBW$$

$$Free\ water\ excess\ (in\ liters) = actual\ TBW - desired\ TBW$$

Restriction of water intake corrects the hyponatremia by a percentage, per day, equal to the net water balance divided by the total body water. A net negative water balance of 500 ml in a 60 kg woman, for example, raises the plasma sodium by 0.5/30, or 1.6%. If that subject's starting plasma sodium is 120 mEq/L, and no other change in water metabolism occurs, the next day's plasma sodium will be 122 mEq/L.

**TABLE 177.3. Treatment of Hyponatremia**

*I. Determine the rate of correction*
- Acute hyponatremia
  - Rapid correction at a rate of 1–2 mEq/L/hr until plasma $Na^+$ 120 mEq/L
- Chronic hyponatremia
  - Slow correction at a rate of 0.5 mEq/L/hr until plasma $Na^+$ 120 mEq/L

*II. Determine the mode of correction*
- Hypovolemic hyponatremia
  - Saline
- Euvolemic hyponatremia
  - Fluid restriction; furosemide alone or with saline to replace urine $Na^+$ losses
  - Demeclocycline in SIADH if above is insufficient
- Hypervolemic hyponatremia
  - Treat underlying disease
  - Fluid restriction
  - Furosemide alone or with saline to replace urine $Na^+$ losses if above is unsuccessful

## Hypernatremia

Hypernatremia is a plasma $Na^+$ above 150 mEq/L. It is relatively uncommon because the thirst mechanism protects against its development. As a result, most cases occur in individuals who lack access to water; hypernatremia is most likely to occur in very young, elderly, and comatose patients. Occasionally, hypernatremia can occur in patients with a defective thirst mechanism secondary to a central nervous system disease.

**TABLE 177.4. Causes of Hypernatremia**

| |
|---|
| *Hypervolemic* |
| Administration of sodium loads |
| *Euvolemic* |
| Diabetes insipidus |
| Nephrogenic |
| Central |
| *Hypovolemic* |
| GI losses (diarrhea) |
| Renal losses |
| Osmotic diuresis (glucose, mannitol) |
| Loop diuretics |
| Insensible losses (burns, fever) |

## Etiology

Hypernatremia, like hyponatremia, can be categorized according to the associated volume status (Table 177.4). Patients with hypervolemic hypernatremia have an increase in total body $Na^+$. This uncommon form of hypernatremia is caused by hypertonic saline, bicarbonate or hypertonic feedings.

Euvolemic hypernatremia is seen with diabetes insipidus (DI) and is the result of pure water loss. It is important to stress that in DI, hypernatremia is a complication seen only in patients with limited access to water or a thirst defect. That is, both the ADH feedback loop and the thirst feedback loop must fail for hypernatremia to develop in DI.

Diabetes insipidus may be central or nephrogenic. In central DI, ADH secretion by the posterior pituitary is absent or incomplete. Central DI may occur as a result of surgery, trauma, cancer, encephalitis, or granulomatous disease (such as sarcoidosis), or may be idiopathic. In nephrogenic DI, there is an impairment in the tubular response to ADH. Nephrogenic DI occurs rarely as a congenital disease due to a mutation of the gene for the ADH receptor. More commonly, it is an acquired disorder and may be due to tubulointerstitial diseases (e.g., sickle cell disease), metabolic disorders (hypokalemia, hypercalcemia), or drugs (lithium, demeclocycline). With both central and nephrogenic DI, urine osmolality is inappropriately low for the degree of hypernatremia. Water deprivation testing and the responsiveness to exogenously administered ADH is useful in distinguishing nephrogenic from central DI. If diagnostic uncertainty persists, serum ADH level should be measured.

Hypovolemic hypernatremia is due to hypotonic losses of $Na^+$ and water. These may be GI, renal, or insensible losses (see Table 177.4). With nonrenal losses, urine $Na^+$ is low (<20 mEq/L) and urine osmolality is high (>400 mOsm/kg).

## Clinical Features

As with hyponatremia, symptoms are mostly neurologic and are more severe when the disorder is acute than when it is chronic. Initially, the increase in plasma osmolality pulls water from the intracellular space and leads to cellular dehydration. Symptoms can include twitching, seizures, and coma. In infants, subdural hemorrhage may occur as a result of ruptured bridging veins. After 12 to 24 hours of hypernatremia, cerebral dehydration is counteracted by adaptive processes that involve the cellular uptake of electrolytes and amino acids. Nonetheless, the in-hospital mortality rate is greater than 50% for adults with plasma $Na^+$ above 160 mEq/L.

## Management

It is prudent to correct hypernatremia slowly at a rate no greater than 0.5 mEq/L/hour. Once the adaptive process has begun, overly rapid correction may lead to cerebral edema. In planning therapy, it is useful to estimate the free water deficit, which can be derived as follows:

$$\textit{Actual TBW} = \textit{body weight (kg)} \times 0.6\ (0.5 \textit{ for women})$$

$$\frac{\textit{Actual plasma Na+}}{\textit{Desired plasma Na}^+} \times \textit{actual TBW} = \textit{desired TBW}$$

$$\textit{Free water deficit (liters)} = \textit{desired TBW} - \textit{actual TBW}$$

Specific therapy for hypernatremia is dictated by the associated volume status and the underlying etiology (Table 177.5). With hypervolemic hypernatremia, administration of $Na^+$ should stop. If necessary, loop diuretics such as furosemide can be given and urinary water loss replaced with free water so that there is a net loss of $Na^+$. If renal failure is present, dialysis may be necessary to correct the hypernatremia.

Patients with central DI are best managed using the ADH analogue desmopressin acetate (DDAVP), which is administered by nasal insufflation (0.1–0.4 ml) once or twice daily. Nephrogenic DI is resistant to the use of ADH. If the cause of nephrogenic DI cannot be eliminated, and if polyuria is symptomatic, treatment

**TABLE 177.5. Treatment of Hypernatremia**

| | |
|---|---|
| Hypervolemic | Discontinue administration of hypertonic load; use loop diuretics if needed, replace water loss |
| Euvolemic | Free water replacement<br>Central DI: ADH analogue (DDAVP)<br>Nephrogenic DI: salt restriction, thiazide, +/− NSAIDs |
| Hypovolemic | Saline until euvolemic; then free water |

DI = diabetes insipidus; ADH = antidiuretic hormone; NSAID = nonsteroidal anti-inflammatory drugs.

may be needed. The goal of therapy is to induce a state of mild volume depletion, which limits the volume of filtrate delivered to the diluting segment (the thick ascending limb of Henle) and thus reduce the degree of polyuria. This can be accomplished using a low $Na^+$ diet, thiazide diuretics, and occasionally, nonsteroidal anti-inflammatory agents.

When hypovolemia is present, normal saline should be administered until euvolemia is restored and then fluids can be given to replace the free water deficit.

# CHAPTER 178 DISORDERS OF POTASSIUM BALANCE

Whereas $Na^+$ is the most important extracellular cation, $K^+$ is the most important intracellular cation, with an intracellular concentration of approximately 150 mEq/L. Extracellular $K^+$ accounts for only about 2% of total $K^+$ stores, and the plasma $K^+$ level does not always provide an accurate estimate of total $K^+$ stores. Potassium homeostasis is influenced by intake, excretion, and cross-membrane shifts. Daily intake of $K^+$ usually is 50 to 100 mEq/day. Approximately 90% of dietary $K^+$ is excreted in the urine as a result of the distal tubular secretion of $K^+$. The delivery of an adequate amount of $Na^+$ to the distal nephron and the actions of aldosterone are important in renal $K^+$ excretion. The distal delivery of $Na^+$ is important because $Na^+$ reabsorption by the distal nephron results in a negative luminal potential, which favors $K^+$ secretion. This distal sodium reabsorption is under the control of aldosterone, which thereby exerts its effect as a potassium-excreting agent. Potassium enters cells via $Na^+$-$K^+$ ATPase. Insulin, $\beta_2$ agonists, and aldosterone each enhance the activity of this enzyme system and thus can result in the cellular uptake of $K^+$.

## Hypokalemia

Hypokalemia is a plasma $K^+$ below 3.5 mEq/L.

### Etiology

Hypokalemia can be due to decreased $K^+$ intake, increased $K^+$ loss, and intracellular $K^+$ shifts (Table 178.1). Hypokalemia due to decreased intake is uncommon, because $K^+$ is present in many foods. In addition, gastrointestinal and renal $K^+$ losses are minimized when the intake of $K^+$ is low. Eventually, however, hypokalemia does develop if potassium intake is very low (<20–30 mEq/day) for a prolonged period. This can occur in malnourished alcoholics and in elderly patients consuming a "tea and toast" diet.

A common cause of hypokalemia is long-term use of diuretics, either thiazides or loop diuretics. These enhance distal nephron sodium delivery, which, in turn, enhances sodium–potassium exchange at that site and causes kaliuriesis.

**TABLE 178.1. Causes of Hypokalemia**

| |
|---|
| *Decreased potassium intake* |
| Alcoholism, "tea and toast" diet |
| *Potassium losses* |
| GI losses (diarrhea, villous adenoma) |
| Renal losses |
| Diuretics |
| Drugs (cisplatin, aminoglycosides, amphotericin) |
| Nonreabsorbed anions (ketone, carbenicillin) |
| Tubular disorders (RTA, Bartter syndrome) |
| *Intracellular potassium shifts* |
| Alkalosis |
| Insulin |
| $\beta_2$ agonist |
| Hypokalemic periodic paralysis |
| Following treatment of megaloblastic anemia |
| Thyrotoxicosis |

### Clinical Features

Symptoms of hypokalemia are related to changes in membrane polarization. Cardiac, neuromuscular, and renal manifestations dominate. Electrocardiographic changes of hypokalemia can include T-wave flattening, U-waves, ST segment depression, and PR prolongation. Hypokalemia can predispose patients to arrhythmias, which can include atrioventricular block, paroxysmal atrial tachycardia, and rarely, ventricular tachycardia. Hypokalemia also can predispose patients to digoxin toxicity.

Patients with hypokalemia may have muscle cramps and weakness. Leg weakness may occur first and then involve ascending muscle groups. In severe cases, weakness can progress to paralysis. Severe hypokalemia may even result in rhabdomyolysis. Effects on smooth muscle can lead to ileus. Hypokalemia also may evoke a resistance to the kidney tubular action of ADH and result in nephrogenic diabetes insipidus and associated polyuria and polydipsia.

### Management

Therapy must be directed at the underlying cause of hypokalemia and at replacing the $K^+$ deficit. A decrease in plasma $K^+$ from 4.0 to 3.0 mEq/L suggests a total body deficit of 200 to 400 mEq. Potassium levels below 2.0 mEq/L may represent a deficit exceeding 1000 mEq. Acidosis may influence the distribution of potassium across cell membranes, such that for every drop in pH of 0.1, the plasma $K^+$ may rise by 0.6 mEq/L. When acidosis is present and the plasma $K^+$ is low, it is important to provide $K^+$ replacement before correcting the acidosis, because the $K^+$ level will fall further as the pH rises. This effect is compounded by the effect of bicarbonate in enhancing urinary potassium excretion.

For most non-urgent situations, it is preferable to use oral $K^+$ replacement, because it is the safest route of therapy. Oral doses can vary from 20 to 120 mEq/day. Potassium usually is administered as potassium chloride. Other available forms include potassium bicarbonate, citrate, and gluconate. When life-threatening hypokalemia is present or if the patient cannot tolerate oral replacement, intravenous $K^+$ replacement may be necessary. Administration through a peripheral line should not exceed a rate of 10 mEq/hour, with a concentration no greater than 40 mEq/L of potassium in the infused fluid. If necessary, rates of up to 20 to 40 mEq/hour can be given via a central line with continuous cardiac monitoring.

## Hyperkalemia

Hyperkalemia is a plasma $K^+$ above 5.0 mEq/L. In the clinical approach to hyperkalemia, spurious or pseudohyperkalemia must first be excluded. Pseudohyperkalemia is defined as hyperkalemia that occurs after the blood is drawn. It usually is due to hemolysis resulting from improper venipuncture technique (prolonged tourniquet application or excessive fist clenching). In addition, marked leukocytosis (>70,000/μL) and thrombocytosis (>1 million/μL) can lead to pseudohyperkalemia, if a serum $K^+$ rather than a plasma $K^+$ level is measured. This occurs because the clot that is formed with serum may release intracellular $K^+$ into the serum, whereas plasma is collected in an anticoagulated tube and clotting will not occur.

### Classification and Etiology

Once pseudohyperkalemia is excluded, the etiology of hyperkalemia must be determined. Hyperkalemia can be due to increased $K^+$ intake, shifts of $K^+$ from the intercellular space, or decreased renal excretion of $K^+$ (Table 178.2). The presence of hyperkalemia usually points to renal impairment, because 90% of the daily $K^+$ load is excreted by the kidneys.

**TABLE 178.2. Causes of Hyperkalemia**

| |
|---|
| *Pseudohyperkalemia* |
| Improper venipuncture technique |
| Severe leukocytosis or thrombocytosis |
| *Reduced renal $K^+$ excretion* |
| *Decreased distal delivery of $Na^+$* |
| Volume depletion |
| Renal failure |
| *Aldosterone deficiency or resistance* |
| Hypoaldosteronism RTA |
| *Drug-related* |
| NSAIDs |
| Co-trimoxazole |
| $K^+$-sparing diuretics |
| Angiotensin-converting enzyme inhibitors |
| *Redistribution of $K^+$ from cells* |
| Insulin deficiency |
| Beta Blockers |
| Massive digoxin overdose |
| Succinylcholine |

Hyperkalemia can rarely occur with massive $K^+$ loads, even in individuals with normal renal function. This can be the result of exogenous loads (oral or intravenous) or endogenous loads (as can occur with tumor lysis, crush injuries, massive hemolysis, or burns).

Hyperkalemia may result from medications. Angiotensin-converting enzyme inhibitors or angiotensin II receptor blockers may cause hyperkalemia by blunting the synthesis of aldosterone, an effect that is compounded by the effect of these medicines to lower the GFR. Nonsteroidal arthritis medicines such as ibuprofen or naproxen inhibit prostaglandin synthesis, thus also reducing GFR as well as aldosterone synthesis. These effects are especially apt to occur in subjects with already reduced kidney function.

### Clinical Features

Symptoms of hyperkalemia usually develop when the plasma $K^+$ rises above 6.5 mEq/L. They are related to changes in membrane polarization. Cardiac manifestations are the most serious. On the electrocardiogram, peaked, symmetrical T-waves are seen earliest (see Figure 32.8). Later findings can include PR prolongation, QRS widening, ventricular fibrillation, complete heart block, and asystole. Weakness, paralysis, and respiratory failure also may occur because of hyperkalemia.

### Management

Therapy for mild hyperkalemia should include dietary $K^+$ restriction and cessation of any drugs that interfere with $K^+$ excretion. In addition, diuretics (loop diuretics or thiazides) may be used to increase renal $K^+$ excretion. In the treatment of hypoaldosteronism, mineralocorticoid replacement is useful.

Life-threatening hyperkalemia requires immediate attention. When ECG changes are present, calcium should be given to antagonize the effect of hyperkalemia on the cell membrane. It can be given intravenously as 10% calcium gluconate (10 ml over 15 minutes), and the dose can be repeated in 5 to 10 minutes. Calcium has a rapid onset, and the duration of action is about 30 minutes.

At the same time, $K^+$ must be shifted into the intracellular space. This can be accomplished with insulin. Typically, 25% to 50% dextrose and insulin (5–10 units) may be given together intravenously, and repeated in 15 minutes as required. Use of albuterol or other beta-mimetic inhaled drug may lower the plasma potassium by 0.5 mEq/L.

As a third component of therapy, $K^+$ removal can be facilitated with the use of the cation exchange resin sodium polystyrene sulfonate (Kayexalate). Orally, 30 to 50 g can be given in sorbitol (to prevent constipation), and repeated every 3 to 4 hours as needed. When the oral route is not feasible, it may be given as a retention enema. Sodium retention is a potential complication, because each gram of the resin releases 1 to 2 mEq of $Na^+$ for each 1 mEq of $K^+$ that is bound. Finally, hemodialysis may be needed when volume overload, severe acidosis, or uremia is present. Peritoneal dialysis is a far less efficient method of treating hyperkalemia.

# CHAPTER 179 ACID-BASE DISORDERS

In a healthy person, the arterial pH is maintained between 7.35 and 7.43. The following three mechanisms are important in the regulation of arterial pH: extracellular and intracellular buffering, pulmonary ventilatory exchange, and renal hydrogen ($H^+$) excretion. Bone, proteins, hemoglobin, and the bicarbonate–carbonic acid ($HCO_3$– $H_2CO_3$) system are the key elements in the buffer system. The importance of the renal and respiratory components is highlighted in the Henderson-Hasselbalch equation:

$$pH = 6.1 + \log \frac{[HCO_3]^-}{0.03\ PaCO_2}$$

A primary change in the $HCO_3$ is caused by a metabolic disorder, whereas a primary change in the $PaCO_2$ is caused by a respiratory disorder. These primary changes evoke secondary responses in the other member of the Henderson-Hasselbalch equation in order to restore the pH toward, but not completely to normal—the so-called compensation. For example, the $PaCO_2$ should fall in response to a drop in plasma $HCO_3$. For the clinician, it is useful to know the magnitude of compensation expected for a given acid–base disorder (Table 179.1). When the observed response differs from what is expected, then a mixed acid-base disorder is present.

## Metabolic Acidosis

Metabolic acidosis is a primary decrease in the plasma $HCO_3$ level. It is helpful to categorize metabolic acidosis according to the anion gap (Table 179.2). The anion gap is defined as follows:

$$AG = [Na^+] - [Cl^- + HCO_3^-]$$

The normal anion gap (unmeasured anion) is about 8 to 12 mEq/L. In general, in states of acidosis, a high anion

**TABLE 179.1. Simple Acid-Base Disorders**

| Acid-Base Disturbance | Primary Disorder | Compensatory Response | pH | Predicted Compensation | Limits of Compensation |
|---|---|---|---|---|---|
| Metabolic acidosis | ↓$HCO_3$ | ↓$PaCO_2$ | ↓ | $\Delta PaCO_2 = 1.0\text{-}1.5 \times \Delta HCO_3$ | 10 mmHg |
| Metabolic alkalosis | ↑$HCO_3$ | ↑$PaCO_2$ | ↑ | $\Delta PaCO_2 = 0.5\text{-}1.0 \times \Delta HCO_3$ | 60–70 mmHg |
| Respiratory acidosis | ↑$PaCO_2$ | ↑$HCO_3$ | ↓ | Acute: $\Delta HCO_3 = 0.1 \times \Delta PaCO_2$ | 32 mEq/L |
| | | | | Chronic: $\Delta HCO_3 = 0.4 \times \Delta PaCO_2$ | 45 mEq/L |
| Respiratory alkalosis | ↓$PaCO_2$ | ↓$HCO_3$ | ↑ | Acute: $\Delta HCO_3 = 0.2 \times PaCO_2$ | 18–20 mEq/L |
| | | | | Chronic: $\Delta HCO_3 = 0.5 \times \Delta PaCO_2$ | 12–15 mEq/L |

↓ = Decrease; ↑ = Increase; Δ = Change.

**TABLE 179.2. Metabolic Acidosis**

| |
|---|
| *Elevated anion gap* |
| Ketoacidosis |
| Diabetic ketoacidosis |
| Alcoholic ketoacidosis |
| Starvation ketosis |
| Renal failure |
| Lactic acidosis |
| Toxic ingestions |
| Alcohols: methanol, ethylene glycol |
| Salicylate |
| *Normal anion gap* |
| Gain of HCl |
| Hyperalimentation |
| Ammonium chloride, arginine hydrochloride |
| Bicarbonate loss |
| Gastrointestinal |
| Diarrhea |
| Urinary diversions (ureterosigmoidostomy) |
| Renal |
| Renal tubular acidosis (proximal and distal) |
| Carbonic anhydrase inhibitors |

HCl = Hydrochloric acid.

gap indicates gain of an acid, and a normal anion gap reflects loss of $HCO_3^-$.

## Elevated Anion Gap Acidosis

### Lactic acidosis

Lactic acidosis is a common problem in the critically ill patient. Usually, the rates of lactate synthesis and metabolism are closely matched, and, as a result, lactate levels normally are less than 2 mEq/L. Lactic acidosis occurs as a result of the overproduction or impaired metabolism of lactate (Table 179.3). Overproduction of lactate usually is due to inadequate oxygen delivery, such as occurs with shock (septic, hypovolemic, or cardiogenic). Rarer causes of lactate overproduction include certain malignancies, diabetes mellitus, or use of metformin. Impaired lactate metabolism usually is due to hepatic failure.

Lactic acidosis is associated with a poor prognosis. The underlying cause of the lactic acidosis must be identified and, whenever possible, corrected. Bicarbonate therapy may be used when acidosis is severe (pH <7.1). Potential complications of bicarbonate therapy include fluid overload, hypertonicity, and overshoot alkalosis.

### Ketoacidosis

Ketoacidosis may be seen in the settings of diabetic ketoacidosis (DKA), alcoholic ketoacidosis, and starvation ketoacidosis (see Table 179.2). The nitroprusside test is used to detect ketone bodies in the blood and is useful in diagnosing ketoacidosis. However, a negative test does not rule out the diagnosis, because it detects only acetoacetate and not beta-hydroxybutyrate, which is the predominant ketone in some cases of ketoacidosis. A simple way to detect ketoacidosis is to smell the odor of ketones on a patient's breath.

Treatment of DKA must include volume repletion and insulin. There is no evidence that bicarbonate therapy hastens recovery from DKA, and it should be used only if the pH is below 7.1. Therapy for alcoholic ketoacidosis includes feeding and fluid repletion.

### Renal failure

Acidosis develops when the GFR falls below 25% of normal because net acid excretion can no longer be maintained. In severe renal failure, the retention of phosphoric and sulfuric acids elevates the anion gap. It is important to correct the acidosis of chronic renal failure because acidosis may have long-term effects such as enhanced muscle catabolism and bone mineral loss.

### Toxic ingestions

The metabolism of "toxic" alcohols can lead to a high anion gap metabolic acidosis. Methanol (wood alcohol, often in windshield washer fluid) is first metabolized by alcohol dehydrogenase to formaldehyde and later to formic acid. Both of these metabolites have ocular toxicity; consequently, methanol ingestion may result in blindness. Ethylene glycol (antifreeze) is first metabolized to glyceraldehyde (again by alcohol dehydrogenase) and later to other metabolites. Besides metabolic acidosis, it may cause oliguric renal failure due to the precipitation of calcium oxalate in the tubules. In

**TABLE 179.3. Causes of Lactic Acidosis**

| |
|---|
| *Excessive lactate production* |
| Shock* |
| Hypovolemic, cardiogenic, septic |
| Toxins |
| Carbon monoxide, cyanide, salicylates, metformin |
| Enzyme deficiencies |
| Glucose 6-phosphatase, fructose 1,6- diphosphatase |
| Pyruvate carboxylase, pyruvate dehydrogenase |
| Sepsis |
| Hypoxemia (severe) |
| Anemia (severe) |
| Malignancy |
| Seizure, exertional heat stroke |
| D-lactic acidosis |
| Mitochondrial myopathies |
| *Impaired lactate metabolism* |
| Hepatic failure |

*A component of impaired metabolism often is present due to poor hepatic perfusion.

such cases, urinalysis shows abundant calcium oxalate monohydrate crystals. Ethanol is useful in the treatment of toxic alcohol ingestion because it is a substrate for alcohol dehydrogenase, and thus it can competitively inhibit the metabolism of both methanol and ethylene glycol. An alternative treatment is the use of fomepizole, an inhibitor of alcohol dehydrogenase. The loading dose of fomepizole is 15 mg/kg intravenously.

The presence of an elevated osmolar gap may be useful in diagnosing toxic alcohol ingestion. As stated previously osmolality is calculated as follows:

$$P_{osm} = 2 \times [Na^+] + glucose/18 + BUN/2.8$$

The osmolar gap is calculated by subtracting the calculated osmolality from the measured osmolality. A gap less than 10 mOsm/kg is normal. A significantly elevated osmolar gap (>25 mOsm/kg $H_2O$) has a high specificity for the diagnosis of toxic alcohol ingestion.

Salicylate (aspirin) intoxication also can be associated with a high anion gap acidosis, because it increases the production of lactic acid, ketoacids and other organic acids. In children, aspirin overdose results in metabolic acidosis, whereas a combination of metabolic acidosis and initial respiratory alkalosis is more common in adults. Alkalinization is an important part of therapy for aspirin overdose because it favors the ionized form of salicylate, which is trapped in the urine and maximally excreted.

## Hyperchloremic Metabolic Acidosis

Hyperchloremic metabolic acidosis may be due to either the gain of hydrochloric acid (HCl) or the loss of bicarbonate (see Table 179.2). HCl gain is far less common, but it may be seen with administration of hyperalimentation when cationic amino acids are metabolized to form $H^+$.

Bicarbonate can be lost from the kidneys or from the gastrointestinal (GI) tract. Renal loss of bicarbonate usually is due to renal tubular acidosis (RTA), whereas diarrhea is the most common cause of GI loss of bicarbonate. It usually is possible to distinguish between GI and renal losses on the basis of history. However, when the history is unclear, a determination of the urinary anion gap is useful in distinguishing between the two. The urinary anion gap is calculated as follows:

$$Urinary\ anion\ gap = Na^+ + K^+ - Cl$$

The urinary anion gap is an indirect gauge of ammonium excretion. Chloride is the anion that accompanies ammonium. When the urinary ammonium concentration is high, chloride concentration also is high and, consequently, the urinary anion gap is negative. When the urinary ammonium concentration is low, chloride concentration also is low and, consequently, the urinary anion gap is positive. A hallmark of renal disease is deficient ammonium excretion; therefore, renal disease is associated with a positive urinary anion gap (with an average value of +20 mmol/L). Normally, ammonium excretion is greatly augmented in response to acidosis and thus acidosis due to diarrhea is associated with a negative urinary anion gap (with an average value of −20 mmol/L).

**Renal tubular acidosis** can be either proximal or distal. **Proximal RTA** is less common and is characterized by a defect in the proximal reabsorption of bicarbonate. This defect may be isolated or associated with the defective proximal reabsorption of other substances (including glucose, amino acids, uric acid and phosphate) which is known as the Fanconi syndrome. The urine pH in proximal RTA is variable. At low plasma bicarbonate levels (<15 mEq/L), the distal nephron is able to reabsorb the filtered load of bicarbonate and, as a result, the urine pH is low (<5.5). At higher plasma bicarbonate levels the distal nephron is unable to reabsorb the filtered load. As a result, bicarbonaturia occurs and the urine pH becomes high.

There are hypokalemic and hyperkalemic **distal RTAs**. There are two kinds of hypokalemic distal RTA. A defect in the function of the distal $H^+$ pump (a so-called **secretory defect**) is one common type of distal RTA. It is associated with a low plasma $K^+$ and a urine pH above 5.5. This can occur in immune diseases such as Sjögren syndrome, or it may be inherited. With a **gradient defect,** there is an abnormal increase in the permeability in the lumen and secreted $H^+$ leaks back into the cell. This type of defect may be caused by amphotericin. It is associated with hypokalemia and a urine pH above 5.5. There are two kinds of hyperkalemic distal RTAs. **A voltage-dependent defect** occurs when distal $Na^+$ reabsorption is disrupted. Normally, the distal reabsorption of $Na^+$ leads to a negative luminal potential, which potentiates the secretion of $H^+$ and $K^+$. Trimethoprim and amiloride can cause a voltage dependent defect by blocking distal $Na^+$ reabsorption. This type of hyperkalemic RTA also may occur in urinary tract obstruction. Finally, aldosterone is an important factor in distal acidification because it enhances distal $Na^+$ reabsorption, stimulates the $H^+$ pump and increases the synthesis of ammonia. Thus, aldosterone deficiency or resistance is associated with a distal acidification defect. **Hyporeninemic hypoaldosteronism**, which may occur in diabetic nephropathy, interstitial nephritis, and other chronic kidney diseases, is characterized by hyperkalemia with intact ability to lower the urine pH, but low urinary ammonium excretion and thus a positive urine anion gap.

The cornerstone of therapy is treatment of the underlying cause and alkali replacement. Patients with proximal RTA require a much higher dosage of alkali (up to 10–15 mEq/kg). Therapy for hyperkalemic RTA includes a low $K^-$ diet, loop diuretics, and, if necessary, mineralocorticoid replacement.

## Metabolic Alkalosis

Metabolic alkalosis is a primary increase in the plasma bicarbonate. Clinically, it is important to recognize the factors which are responsible for the generation and maintenance of metabolic alkalosis. Metabolic alkalosis is generated by either **bicarbonate gain** or **HCl loss** (Table 179.4). Once metabolic alkalosis is generated, it is often maintained by the presence of volume depletion and/or hypokalemia since both of these may decrease the GFR and, thereby, limit bicarbonate excretion.

Kidneys have a high capacity to excrete bicarbonate so that metabolic alkalosis due to bicarbonate administration is uncommon. However, it can occur when there is a limitation in the ability to excrete bicarbonate (e.g., when bicarbonate is administered to a patient with renal insufficiency). More commonly, metabolic alkalosis is generated by gastrointestinal or urinary loss of acid. Vomiting is the most common cause of the former. Diuretics are a common cause of metabolic alkalosis. This occurs because diuretics increase distal $Na^+$ delivery and may also lead to secondary hyperaldosteronism (by inducing volume depletion). The combination of these two factors results in increased distal $H^+$ secretion.

In the differential diagnosis of metabolic alkalosis, it often is useful to measure the urine chloride concentration (Table 179.5). Metabolic alkalosis with a low urine chloride concentration (<15 mEq/L) is associated with volume contraction and is usually due to vomiting, nasogastric suction or diuretics. This type of alkalosis is called **"chloride-responsive"** because volume repletion with sodium chloride is an essential part of therapy. Metabolic alkalosis with a high urinary chloride usually is due to mineralocorticoid excess (as in Cushing or Conn syndrome), Bartter syndrome, or the ingestion of imported licorice (which can have mineralocorticoid activity). This type of alkalosis is called **"chloride resistant"** because the alkalosis cannot be corrected with sodium chloride.

**TABLE 179.4. Causes of Metabolic Alkalosis**

| Causes of Metabolic Alkalosis |
|---|
| *Bicarbonate gain* |
| Bicarbonate or citrate administration |
| Metabolism of ketoacids or lactate |
| Milk-alkali syndrome |
| *HCl loss* |
| Gastrointestinal |
| Vomiting |
| NG suction |
| Villous adenoma |
| Congenital chloride diarrhea |
| Renal |
| Diuretics |
| Mineralocorticoid excess (primary or secondary) |
| Non-reabsorbable anions (such as carbenicillin) |
| Post-hypercapnic metabolic alkalosis |
| Bartter syndrome |

HCl = Hydrochloric acid; NG = nasogastric.

**TABLE 179.5. Urine Chloride in Metabolic Alkalosis**

| Urine Chloride in Metabolic Alkalosis |
|---|
| *Low urine chloride = saline-responsive* |
| Vomiting |
| Nasogastric (NG) suction |
| Diuretics* |
| *High urine chloride = saline-resistant* |
| Mineralocorticoid excess (primary/secondary) |
| Bartter syndrome |
| Licorice (black) ingestion |

*Urine chloride may be high if diuretic use is recent.

Treatment must be directed toward the correction of factors that cause the generation of the alkalosis (for example, discontinuing diuretics or removing an adrenal adenoma). Therapy also must be directed toward the correction of volume depletion and hypokalemia, which can be responsible for the maintenance of the alkalosis.

## Respiratory Acidosis

Respiratory acidosis is a primary rise in $PaCO_2$ due to alveolar hypoventilation. This disorder can be due to diseases which affect the respiratory center, the chest wall muscles or the lung itself (see Chapter 254). Intracellular buffering constitutes the initial compensatory response. After several days, renal net acid excretion rises so compensation is more complete (see Table 179.1). Treatment of respiratory acidosis should be directed at the underlying cause of hypoventilation and must also include correcting hypoxia and improving pulmonary function.

## Respiratory Alkalosis

Respiratory alkalosis is a primary decrease in the $PaCO_2$ resulting from alveolar hyperventilation. This can be due to stimulation of the central respiratory center or peripheral and intrathoracic chemoreceptors (Table 179.6). Compensatory responses to acute and chronic respiratory alkalosis are as listed in Table 179.1. Again, treatment must be directed at the underlying cause.

The acid-base nomogram (Figure 179.1) is a useful and practical way to detect the type of acid-base disorder, including mixed acid-base disturbances. To use it, one finds the point on the nomogram corresponding to the subject's pH and plasma bicarbonate, or $pCO_2$.

TABLE 179.6. Causes of Respiratory Alkalosis

| Site | Mechanism | Specific Examples |
|---|---|---|
| Stimulation of respiratory center | ↑ ventilation | Salicylate intoxication<br>Hyperventilation<br>Psychogenic<br>Hepatic cirrhosis<br>Brain stem lesions<br>Encephalitis<br>Pregnancy<br>Sepsis |
| Stimulation of peripheral chemoreceptors | ↑ ventilation | Hypoxemia<br>Hypotension |
| Stimulation of intrathoracic chemoreceptors | ↑ ventilation | Restrictive lung disease<br>Pulmonary embolus<br>Pneumonia<br>Pneumothorax |

↑ = increase.

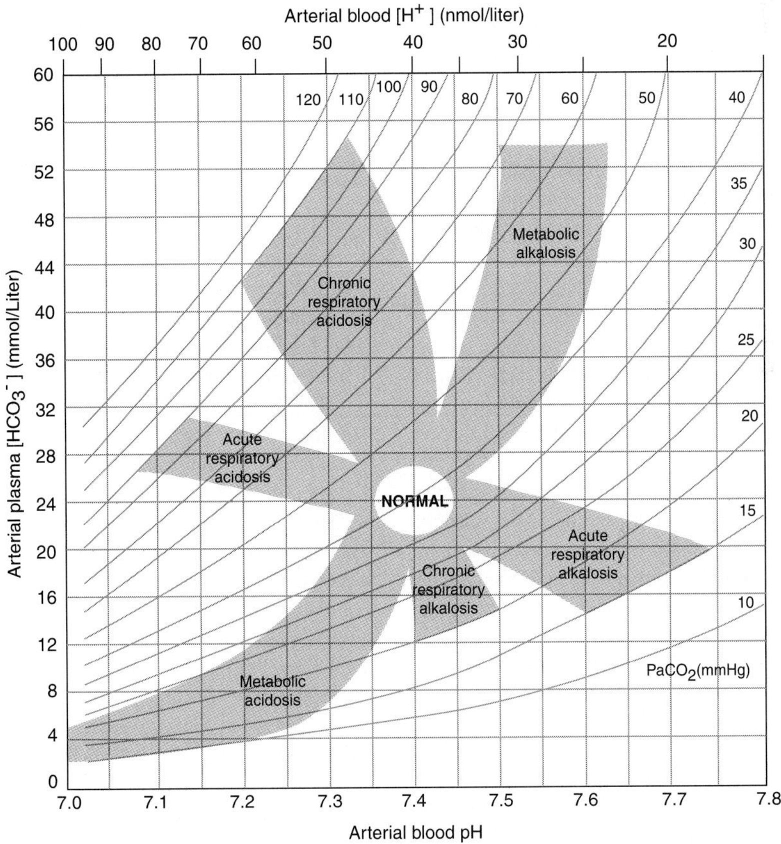


**FIGURE 179.1. Acid-base nomogram. The 95% confidence limits for the normal respiratory and metabolic compensations for primary acid-base disturbances are shown.** (Reproduced with permission from: Brenner BM, Rector FC [eds]. The Kidney. Philadelphia: WB Saunders Co., 1986.)

# CHAPTER 180 DEFINITION, EPIDEMIOLOGY, AND PATHOPHYSIOLOGY OF HYPERTENSION

## Definition

Blood pressure (BP) is a physiologic measurement, similar to body temperature, heart rate, respiratory rate, height, and weight. Elevated blood pressure often leads to complications and, therefore, must be lowered. Blood pressure in adults is based on the average of at least two readings on separate days, and is classified as shown in Table 180.1.

When the systolic and diastolic BP are elevated, the severity classification is based on which type is higher. Isolated systolic hypertension (ISH) is defined as systolic blood pressure (SBP) of 140 mm Hg or higher and diastolic blood pressure lower than 90 mm Hg, and should be staged appropriately (e.g., 178/85 mm Hg is stage 2 ISH). In more than 85% of cases, the systolic BP is in a higher category than the diastolic BP. Besides classifying stages of hypertension, the physician should also specify presence or absence of target organ disease (Table 180.2) and additional risk factors for cardiovascular disease.

**TABLE 180.2. Manifestations of Target-Organ Disease**

| Organ System | Manifestations |
|---|---|
| Cardiac | Clinical, electrocardiographic, or radiologic evidence of coronary artery disease<br>Left ventricular hypertrophy or "strain" by electrocardiography or left ventricular hypertrophy by echocardiography<br>Left ventricular dysfunction or cardiac failure |
| Cerebrovascular | Transient ischemic attack or stroke |
| Peripheral vascular | Absence of one or more major pulses in the extremities (except for dorsalis pedis) with or without intermittent claudication; aneurysm |
| Renal | Serum creatinine >1.5 mg/dl<br>Proteinuria (1+ or greater)<br>Microalbuminuria |
| Retinopathy | Hemorrhages or exudates, with or without papilledema |

## Epidemiology

Hypertension is the most common cardiovascular disease and one of the greatest public health problems of our time. In the United States, it is estimated that there are 60 million people with a systolic BP of 140 mm Hg or higher and/or a diastolic BP of 90 mm Hg or higher or who are taking medications for hypertension. Hypertension is more common in men than in women and in African Americans than Caucasians. Men and African Americans have greater hypertensive morbidity and mortality. Hypertension contributes to the deaths of at least 250,000 Americans each year.

There is now considerable evidence for genetic determination and control of blood pressure. Central obesity and higher body mass index are determined by major genes and strongly predispose an individual to hypertension. They are responsible for at least part of the familial aggregation of hypertension. Single-gene causes of hypertension also exist. Glucocorticoid-remediable aldosteronism is an autosomal disorder that causes early hypertension and strokes.

**TABLE 180.1. Classification of Blood Pressure for Adults**

| Category | Systolic (mm Hg) | | Diastolic (mm Hg) |
|---|---|---|---|
| Optimal | <120 | and | <80 |
| Normal | <130 | and | <85 |
| High normal | 130–139 | or | 85–89 |
| Hypertension | | | |
| Stage 1 (mild) | 140–159 | or | 90–99 |
| Stage 2 (moderate) | 160–179 | or | 100–109 |
| Stage 3 (severe) | ≥180 | or | ≥110 |

The major complications of hypertension include stroke, coronary artery disease, chronic renal failure, and peripheral vascular disease. Most strokes that occur between the ages of 35 and 65 result from hypertension. Although stroke deaths have been declining in recent years, largely because of early detection and better control of hypertension, it is still responsible for an estimated 150,000 deaths and 225,000 disabilities per year in the United States. Hypertension is the major risk factor for coronary artery disease, which is 3 to 5 times more common in hypertensives than in normotensives. Coronary artery disease and its complications are the most common causes of death in hypertensive patients. Target organ disease (see Table 180.2) increases the risk of cardiovascular events, even if BP is controlled. Concentric left ventricular hypertrophy (LVH), which occurs when the left heart constantly pumps blood against a high arterial blood pressure over a long period of time, regresses if hypertension is kept under control. Sometimes, LVH precedes hypertension and probably is due to increased sympathetic tone. LVH is a powerful predictor of sudden death and myocardial infarction in hypertensive persons. Echocardiography is more sensitive than electrocardiography in detecting LVH. Although the incidence of kidney failure due to hypertension has declined markedly in recent years, it remains an important cause of kidney failure among African Americans. Hypertension, diabetes, and increasing age lead to a higher probability of peripheral vascular disease.

For a long time, physicians focused their attention on the diastolic BP, because in the cardiac cycle the diastole is at least twice as long as the systole. It is now clear that the cardiovascular risk is greater for systolic than diastolic BP. Moreover, the higher the pulse pressure, the greater the risk; and the increased pulse pressure is primarily related to the increased systolic pressure. Intensive antihypertensive therapy reduces, but does not normalize, both morbidity and mortality from complications of hypertension. Attention is now being directed toward preventing hypertension. Although the role of excessive sodium intake in causing hypertension remains somewhat controversial, because the average daily sodium intake in the U.S. is 10 to 20 times the physiologic need, a lower sodium intake is recommended for most people. Obesity, particularly upper body obesity, also is a contributing factor to the development of hypertension. Every effort should be made to avoid childhood obesity, because obese children often develop into obese adults. Obese patients with hypertension should be encouraged to make a vigorous effort to lose weight. Reduction in alcohol consumption also can reduce blood pressure and forestall the development of hypertension. Regular dynamic exercise and increased dietary potassium intake are also helpful in preventing hypertension.

Severe hypertension among children usually is of the secondary form. However, mild to moderate hypertension usually is the essential type. Children 3 years of age and older should have their blood pressure measured annually as part of their continuing health care.

## Pathophysiology

### Normal Regulation of Blood Pressure

Under normal circumstances, blood pressure is maintained by the interplay of various mechanisms. It is primarily a function of cardiac output and peripheral resistance. This relationship is summarized by the following formula:

$$\textit{Blood pressure} = \textit{cardiac output} \times \textit{peripheral vascular resistance}$$

Cardiac output is the volume of blood ejected by the left ventricle into the aorta per minute. It, along with the elasticity of the aorta, is the major determinant of systolic blood pressure. Diastolic blood pressure is determined primarily by the resistance in the arterioles. Cardiac output and peripheral resistance are directly and indirectly affected by such factors as blood volume, blood viscosity, sympathetic nervous system activity, the renin-angiotensin-aldosterone system, arginine vasopressin (AVP), insulin, and vasodilator substances such as nitric oxide, prostaglandins, bradykinin, and atrial natriuretic peptide (ANP).

### Essential Hypertension

More than 95% of patients with elevated blood pressure have essential (idiopathic, primary) hypertension. These patients do not have an identifiable cause for their hypertension but have a disease of blood pressure regulation. In earlier stages with mild hypertension, the cardiac output is elevated. As the pressure rises further, cardiac output falls and the elevated blood pressure becomes a reflection of increased peripheral resistance. The state of vasoconstriction is maintained by excess sodium content of the arteriolar smooth muscle cells, increased sympathetic nervous system activity, imbalance between endogenous vasoconstrictors and vasodilators and other unknown mechanisms. Other factors associated with hypertension include heredity, obesity, alcohol consumption, sleep apnea, lack of regular physical activity, low dietary potassium and calcium intake, and increasing age. Significant factors involved in the regulation of blood pressure and possible mechanisms of hypertension are shown in Figure 180.1.

### Secondary Hypertension

A specific cause of high blood pressure can be identified in less than 5% of people with hypertension. This type of hypertension, with an identifiable cause, is called secondary hypertension. It is discussed in greater length in chapter 184.

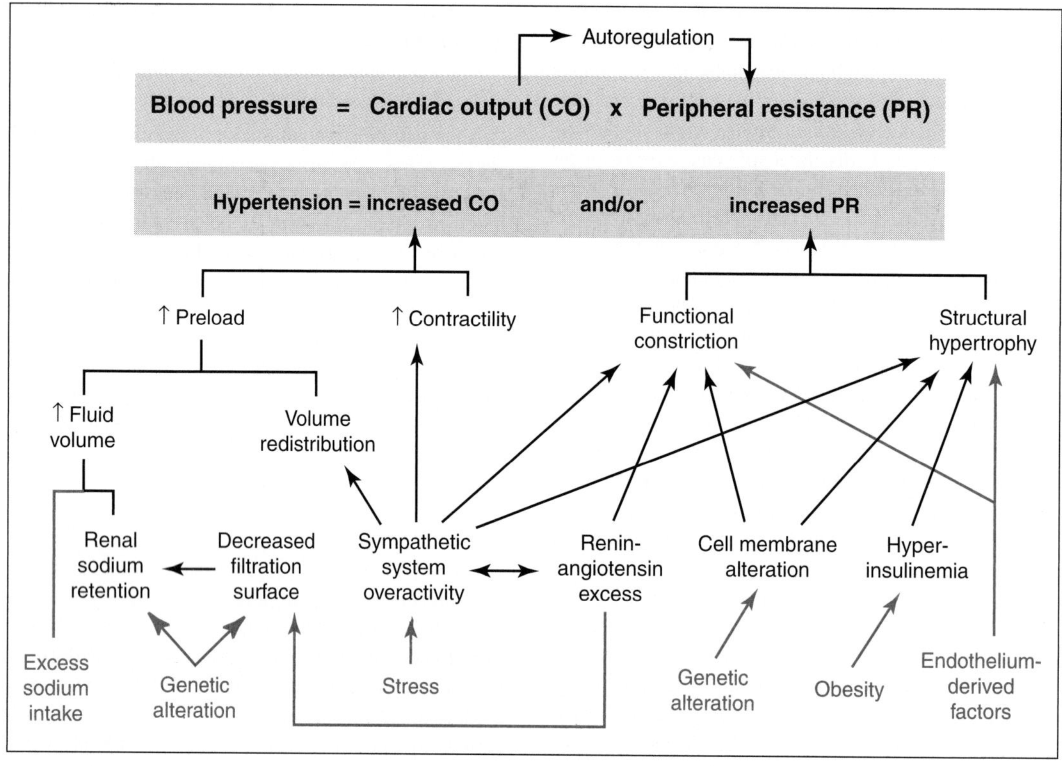


**FIGURE 180.1. Pathogenesis of essential hypertension.**
(From: Kaplan NM. Clinical Hypertension. 7th ed. Philadelphia: Lippincott Williams & Wilkins, 1998. Used with permission.)

# CHAPTER 181 EVALUATION OF THE HYPERTENSIVE PATIENT

## Purpose of the Evaluation

The purpose of the evaluation is to answer the following questions:

- Does the patient have hypertension? Before a patient is labeled hypertensive, at least three readings of blood pressure should be recorded. Two of the three readings and the average of the three should be elevated.
- Is it secondary hypertension?
- What is the extent of target organ damage?
- Are other cardiovascular risk factors and/or alcoholism present?
- Are certain antihypertensives contraindicated?
- How much does the patient know about hypertension? Because hypertension is a chronic disorder requiring lifelong treatment, it is imperative that the patient understand this and participate in the medical care as much as possible.
- Does the patient have sleep-disordered breathing? Hypoxemia and hypercapnia lead to increased sympathetic tone and can cause hypertension and, ultimately, heart failure.

## History

After the patient identification information is obtained, the duration of hypertension and previous therapy should be determined. Although most patients with mild to moderate hypertension are asymptomatic, the severely hypertensive patient may be quite symptomatic. The symptoms of hypertension are listed in Table 181.1. Review of systems may reveal symptoms suggestive of secondary hypertension. Family history in regard to hypertension, heart disease, diabetes, stroke, and kidney disease must be recorded. The personal history is an extremely important part of the evaluation and includes information on diet, smoking, alcohol consumption, drug abuse, exercise, sleep, and sexual function.

Several medications and herbs can raise blood pressure or interfere with the effectiveness of antihypertensive drugs (Table 181.2). A history of all prescribed and over-the-counter (OTC) medications and herbs should, therefore, be obtained.

## Physical Examination

The patient's general appearance is noted, particularly in relation to gait, coordination, and speech, the telltale signs of a past stroke. Hirsutism and truncal obesity are indicative of Cushing syndrome. Weight and height are recorded and compared with standard charts to see if and by how much the patient is overweight. Abdominal and hip girth are measured and waist to hip ratio is calculated. Pulse rate and regularity should then be noted. Peripheral pulses, i.e., the radial, carotid, femoral, dorsalis pedis and posterior tibial pulses, are palpated. A weak pulse or a bruit indicates the presence of arteriosclerosis.

**TABLE 181.1. Symptoms Associated With Hypertension**

- Occipital headache, worse on arising in the morning
- Epistaxis (nosebleeds)
- Cardiovascular symptoms
  - Angina
  - Dyspnea
  - Edema
  - Claudication
- Cerebrovascular symptoms
  - Dizziness
  - Blackouts
  - Numbness
  - Tingling
  - Unilateral weakness (may suggest impending stroke)

**TABLE 181.2. Drugs and Herbs that May Raise BP**

| Drugs | Herbs |
|---|---|
| Estrogen | Ephedra |
| Progesterone | Gentian |
| Steroids | Ginseng |
| NSAIDs | Golden seal |
| Nasal decongestants | Grindelia |
| Appetite suppressants | Licorice |
| Cyclosporine | |
| Erythropoietin | |
| Tricyclic antidepressants | |
| MAO inhibitors | |
| Cocaine | |

MAO = monoamine oxidase.

**TABLE 181.3. Grades of Hypertensive Retinopathy**

| Grade | Finding |
|---|---|
| i/iv | Arteriolar narrowing, spasm, copper wiring, or silver wiring |
| ii/iv | Same changes as for i/iv + arteriovenous (AV) nicking |
| iii/iv | Same changes as for i/iv and ii/iv + hemorrhages and exudates |
| iv/iv | Same changes as for i/iv, ii/iv, and iii/iv + papilledema (blurred optic disc margin) |

At the initial visit, the blood pressure should be recorded in both arms and a note made as to which side is higher. A discrepancy of up to 5 mm Hg is not unusual. However, a larger difference may indicate the narrowing of the axillary or brachial artery on the side in which blood pressure is lower. On follow-up visits, the blood pressure is always recorded on the side with the higher blood pressure.

For measurement of BP, the patient should be seated with arm bared, supported, and at heart level. He or she should not have smoked or ingested caffeine within 30 minutes and should have rested for 5 minutes prior to measurement. An appropriate cuff size, wherein the bladder encircles at least 80% of the arm and has width equal to one third to one half of the length of the upper arm, is necessary for accurate measurement of BP. Measurement should be taken with a mercury sphygmomanometer, a recently calibrated aneroid device, or a calibrated electronic device. Appearance of Korotkoff sounds is recorded as the systolic BP; disappearance of these sounds is recorded as the diastolic BP. Standing BP should also be recorded. Normally, the standing BP is a little higher than seated BP. If it is lower by more than 20 mm Hg systolic or 10 mm Hg diastolic, it signifies orthostatic hypotension. Patients should be informed and taught to measure their own BP and encouraged to do so periodically.

The fundi are examined in a dark room with the patient looking straight at a distant point. The hypertensive retinopathy is graded from I to IV, with increasing number reflecting increasing severity (Table 181.3).

The neck is examined for a carotid bruit, goiter, or any other swelling. A note is made if the jugular veins are prominent and distended.

The cardiac examination consists of palpating the point of maximal impulse (PMI, or apex beat), which is shifted downward and laterally as the left ventricle enlarges. A left ventricular heave signifies left ventricular hypertrophy. Auscultation is performed for rhythm, heart sounds, and the presence of murmurs. An S4 sound is produced by atrial contraction against a rigid left ventricle due to left ventricular hypertrophy. An S3 sound is due to rapid ventricular filling in a dilated ventricle and is a sign of heart failure.

The lungs are then auscultated for rales or wheezing. Basal rales are present in congestive heart failure. Wheezing may indicate heart failure, chronic bronchitis, or asthma.

The abdomen is inspected and palpated to detect kidney enlargement. Polycystic kidneys and grossly enlarged, hydronephrotic kidneys usually are easily palpable. Palpable aortic pulsations may indicate aortic aneurysm. Careful auscultation over the epigastrium usually reveals a continuous (systolic and diastolic) bruit in patients with renal artery stenosis. It is not uncommon to hear a systolic bruit in the epigastrium, particularly in older patients. This is produced by the flow of blood through the celiac or hepatic artery and is of no significance. A bruit produced by renal artery stenosis may lateralize to the side of the lesion.

The legs are examined for the presence of edema and signs of peripheral vascular disease such as discoloration of the skin, loss of temperature, or absence of arterial pulsations. The skin should be inspected closely for neurofibromatosis and café-au-lait spots, which may be seen in patients with pheochromocytoma.

A neurologic examination for muscle strength and deep tendon reflexes is performed to detect the presence of stroke, of which the patient may or may not be aware.

The prostate is examined in older men. An enlarged prostate and urinary retention may cause kidney damage, which can lead to or contribute to hypertension.

## Laboratory Studies

Certain laboratory investigations are performed routinely as part of the evaluation of a hypertensive patient (Table 181.4). Urinalysis is necessary, because proteinuria usually indicates renal disease, and hypertension may be secondary to renal parenchymal disease. However, long-standing hypertension can cause nephrosclerosis, ischemic glomerulopathy, and proteinuria. Glycosuria can be diagnosed easily with dipstick urinalysis. Almost 10% of hypertensive patients also have diabetes mellitus. The presence of occult blood may indicate a renal or urinary tract disorder. A microscopic examination of the urine always must be undertaken, if the dipstick urinalysis is abnormal (presence of protein or blood). This helps determine the nature of renal disease. Red blood cell casts are pathognomonic of glomerulonephritis; however, granular casts simply indicate the presence of a renal disease. In diabetics, if the dipstick is negative, the urine should be examined for microalbuminuria to detect early glomerulosclerosis. It is a good practice to record the patient's hematocrit routinely before undertaking treatment of hypertension. Many hypertensives tend to have a somewhat higher hematocrit. If the patient is anemic, dizziness may be from anemia rather than hypertension. Fasting blood glucose (FBS) or a 2-hour postprandial blood sugar (PPBS) measurement should be done for the diagnosis of diabetes. If the FBS is more than 125 mg/dl or PPBS is more than 139 mg/dl, glycosylated hemoglobin (HbA1c) should be measured. Elevation of blood urea nitrogen (BUN) or serum creatinine indicates renal insufficiency, which may be either the cause or the result of hypertension. Serum potassium measurement is an excellent screening measure for primary aldosteronism. A normal serum potassium (3.5–5 mEq/L) on a normal diet excludes primary aldosteronism for all practical purposes. Serum lipid measurements are done to detect other risk factors such as hypercholesterolemia or low levels of high-density lipoprotein (HDL) cholesterol. After diuretic therapy, serum lipids may rise slightly. Uric acid measurement is not essential for evaluation or to determine the presence of a risk factor; however, the uric acid level may rise with diuretic therapy, and some patients may develop clinical gout. Serum calcium measurement is useful in uncovering hyperparathyroidism, which can cause hypertension. Also, the serum calcium level may rise with thiazide therapy. Thyroid-stimulating hormone (TSH) can help diagnose hyper- or hypothyroidism, because both can cause hypertension.

**TABLE 181.4. Laboratory Tests in Evaluating Hypertension**

Urinalysis
Hematocrit
Serum chemistry
- Glucose
- Creatinine
- Potassium
- Lipids
- Uric acid
- Calcium

TSH
ECG or echocardiogram

An electrocardiogram (ECG) should be done routinely in patients 40 years of age or older and in younger patients with severe hypertension, cardiac symptoms, arrhythmias, or a strong family history of heart disease. Left ventricular hypertrophy (LVH) and myocardial ischemia are signs of hypertensive cardiovascular disease. Although echocardiogram is more sensitive, the expense precludes its routine use to diagnose LVH.

Chest x-ray examination is done primarily to determine the heart size and the presence of congestive heart failure, and it is not necessary for routine evaluation of hypertension.

### Special Studies

After the initial evaluation, if secondary hypertension is suspected, appropriate laboratory and radiologic studies are undertaken to prove or disprove the suspected diagnosis. It is fruitless to investigate a patient for all possible causes of secondary hypertension. Only those investigations need be carried out that would help in the diagnosis of a specific, suspected cause of secondary hypertension (discussed later in chapter 184).

# CHAPTER 182 CLINICAL PHARMACOLOGY OF ANTIHYPERTENSIVE DRUGS

The antihypertensive drugs can be classified in various ways (Table 182.1). The more important ones are discussed here based on their site of action.

## Diuretics

In many patients, particularly the elderly, diuretics are an appropriate first-line therapy for the treatment of essential hypertension.

**TABLE 182.1. Classification of Common Antihypertensive Drugs**

*Diuretics*
- Thiazides and related diuretics
- Loop diuretics: furosemide, bumetanide, torsemide, ethacrynic acid
- Potassium-sparing: spironolactone, triamterene, amiloride, eplerenone

*Sympathetic inhibitors*
- Centrally acting: methyldopa, clonidine, reserpine

*Adrenergic receptor blockers*
- Alpha blockers: prazosin, terazosin, doxazosin
- β-blockers
  - Nonselective: nadolol, pindolol, propranolol
  - Selective: acebutolol, atenolol, metoprolol
- Alpha and β blocker: labetalol, carvedilol

*Angiotensin-converting enzyme (ACE) inhibitors:* benazepril, captopril, enalapril, fosinopril, lisinopril, perindopril, quinapril, ramipril, etc.

*Angiotensin II receptor blockers (ARBs):* candesartan, eprosartan, irbesartan, losartan, telmisartan, valsartan, etc.

*Vasodilators:* hydralazine, minoxidil, diazoxide, sodium nitroprusside

*Calcium entry blockers:* verapamil, diltiazem, and dihydropyridines: amlodipine, felodipine, nicardipine, nifedipine, nitrendipine, etc.

### Thiazide Diuretics

Hydrochlorothiazide is the most commonly used thiazide diuretic in the United States. The early predominant action of thiazides is to enhance sodium and water excretion, producing a mild to moderate extracellular fluid volume depletion. In addition, they mobilize sodium and chloride ions from the arteriolar smooth muscle and decrease vascular reactivity, blunting the effects of sympathetic reflexes. This results in a blood pressure drop by an average of 10–20/5–10 mm Hg. Adverse reactions of clinical importance are hypokalemia, hyperuricemia, hyperglycemia, hypercalcemia, and hyperlipidemia. Hypokalemia is more common with long-acting diuretics such as chlorthalidone and metolazone, and may require potassium supplementation or the simultaneous use of potassium-sparing diuretics. Although hyperuricemia is not uncommon, it need not be treated unless clinical gout develops. Approximately 10% of patients develop hyperglycemia with chronic diuretic use. Hypercalcemia after thiazides is seldom of clinical importance. Fetal jaundice and thrombocytopenia have been reported after thiazide use in pregnancy. Indapamide has the same antihypertensive efficacy as hydrochlorothiazide but the biochemical alterations are somewhat less pronounced.

### Loop Diuretics

The loop diuretics, furosemide, bumetanide, and ethacrynic acid, constitute a pharmacologic rather than a chemical class. They produce diuresis far greater than thiazides over a short period of time but are not better than thiazides as antihypertensive drugs. They act at the loop of Henle. Their antihypertensive mode of action is similar to that of the thiazide diuretics. Their major use in the treatment of hypertension is in patients with renal insufficiency and fluid retention. Patients who develop hypercalcemia secondary to thiazides are candidates for a loop diuretic, because the latter increases calcium excretion. Hypokalemia can be a troublesome side effect in patients receiving loop diuretics.

### Potassium-Sparing Diuretics

These include spironolactone, triamterene, amiloride, and eplerenone. Spironolactone is a steroid compound with a structural formula similar to that of aldosterone; it is an aldosterone antagonist. It increases sodium and water excretion and diminishes potassium excretion. Gynecomastia in men and menstrual irregularities in women are important side effects. It should be avoided in pregnancy and during lactation. Aldactazide is a combination of hydrochlorothiazide and spironolactone in a single tablet. Eplerenone is similar to spironolactone but has minimal side effects. Triamterene is used primarily to conserve potassium and prevent hypokalemia in patients treated with thiazide or loop diuretics. It is contraindicated in patients with renal insufficiency, in whom it can cause fatal hyperkalemia. Dyazide and Maxzide are proprietary combinations of hydrochlorothiazide and triamterene. Amiloride is similar to triamterene as a potassium-retaining diuretic. Moduretic is a combination of hydrochlorothiazide and amiloride.

## Inhibitors of the Sympathetic Nervous System

This group includes drugs that interfere with sympathetic nerve impulses at different sites from the brain to target organs. The decreased arterial and venous constriction causes a fall in blood pressure. The adverse effects depend on the site of action and include orthostatic hypotension, nasal congestion, increased gastrointestinal motility, impotence, delayed ejaculation, and bradycardia.

### Centrally Acting Sympathetic Inhibitors

The centrally-acting sympathetic inhibitors include reserpine, methyldopa, clonidine, guanabenz and guanfacine. The β-adrenergic blocking agents also may have central action.

### Receptor Blockers

Antihypertensive agents, which block α and β receptors selectively, are available.

#### Alpha blockers

The α-adrenergic blocking agents include prazosin, terazosin, and doxazosin. They block postsynaptic α-adrenergic receptors, diminishing vascular constriction without affecting the α-adrenergic presynaptic negative feedback which inhibits norepinephrine release. When used alone, they are not as effective as diuretics in preventing congestive heart failure in hypertensive patients. They can cause postural syncope particularly after the first dose in a small percentage of patients. The therapy is initiated with 1 mg, usually given at bedtime, and the patient instructed not to stand up for several hours. Postural dizziness and drowsiness, lethargy, palpitations, and nausea are infrequent adverse effects. Terazosin and doxazosin have a longer duration of action. The α-blockers are also useful in treatment of prostate hypertrophy, because they relax the smooth muscle in the prostate and can increase the urine flow. For this reason, they can be doubly beneficial in treatment of hypertension in men with prostate hypertrophy.

#### Beta-blockers

Beta-adrenergic receptors are classified in two main groups: $\beta_1$ in the heart, and $\beta_2$ receptors in the bronchi and blood vessels. The chemical structures of β-blocking drugs have several features in common with the β-agonist isoproterenol. Most β-blockers such as propranolol and metoprolol are completely metabolized and are excreted by the liver. However, the longer-acting drugs, nadolol and atenolol, are poorly metabolized and are excreted by the kidney. All the β-blocking drugs are competitive antagonists of catecholamines at β-adrenergic receptor sites. They are classified as selective or nonselective according to their relative ability to antagonize the different classes of β-receptors. The selective $\beta_1$ receptor blockers, such as atenolol and metoprolol, when employed in low doses, do not affect the bronchial and vascular $\beta_2$ receptors; however, in higher doses, both $\beta_1$ and $\beta_2$ receptors are blocked. Labetalol is a nonselective β-blocker which is also an α-blocker and a weak vasodilator. β-blockers are contraindicated in patients with asthma, greater than first-degree heart block and bradycardia.

## Blockers of the Renin-Angiotensin System

Because the renin-angiotensin system often has an important role in the maintenance of hypertension, agents that inhibit the production or action of the pressor hormone angiotensin II are potentially useful hypotensive agents. Two classes of compounds are available: angiotensin I-converting enzyme (ACE) inhibitors, and angiotensin II receptor blockers (ARBs). They are particularly useful in renin-dependent forms of hypertension such as renovascular hypertension, malignant hypertension, and other conditions associated with elevated plasma renin levels. The β-receptor antagonists partially block the release of renin. Other sympatholytic agents such as methyldopa and clonidine also inhibit renin release.

### Converting Enzyme Inhibitors

Converting enzyme inhibitors competitively inhibit the angiotensin I-converting enzyme (ACE), which converts angiotensin I to angiotensin II. In addition, they inhibit the kininase enzyme responsible for the degradation of bradykinin. Thus, these drugs can lower blood pressure both by preventing the formation of the endogenous vasoconstrictor angiotensin II and by decreasing the metabolism of the endogenous vasodilator bradykinin. Captopril is a short-acting ACE inhibitor requiring 2 to 3 doses per day. Enalapril, lisinopril, quinapril, fosinopril, perindopril, and ramipril are longer-acting drugs requiring only a once-a-day dose. Side effects include cough, rash, and taste disturbance. Contraindications include pregnancy and bilateral renal artery stenosis.

### Angiotensin Blockers

Drugs such as losartan block the angiotensin II (A-II) receptors and are useful antihypertensive drugs that do not cause cough, a nagging side effect of ACE inhibitors. They work particularly well in combination with a diuretic.

## Calcium Entry Blockers

Verapamil, diltiazem, and dihydropyridines such as amlodipine, felodipine, isradipine, nifedipine, nitrendipine, and nicardipine are coronary and peripheral vasodilators that act by interfering with the excitation-contraction coupling of smooth muscle by blocking the entrance of calcium into the cell. They are indicated in the treatment of hypertension and angina. Severe adverse reactions are rare. Side effects include hypotension, peripheral edema, headache, and constipation. Asthma is not a contraindication to their use, because they have a weak bronchodilator effect and are ideal agents to use in asthmatic hypertensive patients. They are particularly effective in African American patients and are highly effective when used in combination with a diuretic. Short-acting dihydropyridines can cause myocardial infarction in patients with underlying coronary artery disease.

# CHAPTER 183 THERAPY OF ESSENTIAL HYPERTENSION

The goal of the treatment of hypertension in the adult is to reduce the blood pressure below 140 mm Hg systolic and below 90 mm Hg diastolic by the least intrusive means possible. In addition, other modifiable cardiovascular risk factors must be controlled to reduce morbidity and mortality from complications of hypertension. Further reduction of BP to 130/85 mm Hg may be pursued.

Lifestyle modifications, which include weight reduction, increased physical activity, and moderation of dietary sodium and alcohol intake, are useful in definitive or adjunctive therapy of hypertension. They not only help lower the blood pressure, but, by ameliorating diabetes and dyslipidemia, they help lower the risk of cardiovascular disease from these disorders. If BP remains at or above 140/90 mm Hg over a 3- to 6-month period, despite vigorous encouragement of lifestyle modifications, antihypertensive medications should be started.

Diuretics, β-blockers, and ACE inhibitors repeatedly have been proven to reduce cardiovascular morbidity and mortality in controlled clinical trials and are, therefore, recommended for initial drug therapy (Figure 183.1). Other drugs can be used when diuretics, β-blockers, and ACE inhibitors are unacceptable or ineffective.

Drug therapy is initiated in small doses, and the dose is increased gradually until the desired therapeutic effect is achieved, side effects develop, or the maximal

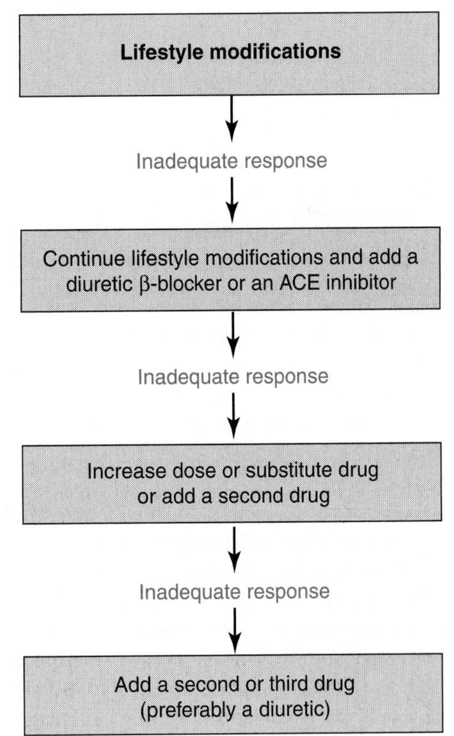


FIGURE 183.1. Algorithm for treatment of hypertension.

**TABLE 183.1. Choice of Initial Antihypertensive Drug Therapy**

| Associated Condition(s) | Drugs of Choice | Agents Not Recommended |
|---|---|---|
| Asthma, chronic obstructive pulmonary disease | Calcium channel blockers (CCBs), thiazides | β-blockers |
| Coronary disease | β-blockers | Vasodilators |
| Left ventricular failure (systolic) | Angiotensin converting enzyme inhibitors (ACEIs), thiazides, A-II receptor blockers (ARBs) | Most β-blockers, CCBs |
| Hypertrophic cardiomyopathy with severe diastolic dysfunction | β-blockers, CCBs (diltiazem, verapamil) | Diuretics, vasodilators, α–1 antagonists |
| Diabetes mellitus | ACEIs, ARBs | |
| Chronic renal failure (serum creatinine >3.0 mg/dl) | Loop diuretics, CCBs | |
| Preeclampsia | Methyldopa, hydralazine labetalol, nifedipine | ACEIs, ARBs |

recommended dose is attained. If the first drug does not control the blood pressure or is poorly tolerated, it is replaced by another drug. If a drug is well tolerated but proves inadequate, a second drug may be added. For the convenience of patients and to facilitate compliance, several combination preparations of antihypertensive drugs are available. Often, more than one drug is required for optimum control of BP.

## Special Situations and Coexisting Conditions

It is important to individualize the therapy of hypertension to maximize the benefit and minimize risks to the patient. Hypertension among African Americans usually responds well to diuretics, because these patients often have an expanded plasma volume and low renin levels. Treatment of hypertension in the elderly is best initiated with half the usual dose to avoid postural hypotension and syncope. Converting enzyme inhibitors are also useful in the treatment of congestive heart failure and are, therefore, preferable in hypertensive patients with heart failure. β-blockers are helpful in patients with angina or migraine and may be the antihypertensive agents of choice when those conditions coexist. β-blockers should be avoided in patients with asthma. Calcium channel blockers are particularly useful in asthmatics because of their mild bronchodilatory properties. Patients with peripheral vascular insufficiency may experience exacerbation of claudication if treated with nonselective β-blockers, which should be avoided in those individuals. In patients with severe Raynaud's disease associated with collagen vascular disease such as scleroderma, treatment with ACE inhibitors, with or without calcium antagonist, may ameliorate both Raynaud's disease and the hypertension.

Patients with hypertension and diabetes mellitus are vulnerable to cardiovascular complications and present a special challenge. Diuretics and β blockers may impair the control of diabetes. The nonselective β blockers also may interfere with catecholamine-mediated counterregulatory responses to insulin-induced hypoglycemia. Some patients with diabetes who also have renal insufficiency may have hyporeninemic hypoaldosteronism with resultant hyperkalemia. Potassium-sparing diuretics, ACE inhibitors, and β blockers can aggravate this hyperkalemia. It is, therefore, imperative to monitor serum potassium and creatinine along with blood glucose in these patients. ACE inhibitors have been shown to reduce albuminuria and are considered the antihypertensives of choice in diabetic, hypertensive patients. Diabetics with proteinuria of 1 g or more per day should have their BP reduced to 125/75 mm Hg. Calcium blockers such as verapamil and diltiazem, but not dihydropyridines (Table 183.1), also reduce albuminuria in patients with diabetes.

Diuretics can induce short-term increases in levels of total plasma cholesterol, triglycerides, and LDL cholesterol. β-blockers may increase levels of plasma triglycerides and reduce those of HDL cholesterol. The alpha blockers and central adrenergic agonists may decrease serum cholesterol concentration slightly, especially in the lipoprotein subfraction, and, therefore, may offer an advantage in managing hypertensive patients with hyperlipidemia. ACE inhibitors and calcium antagonists have no adverse effects on serum lipids and are appropriate for these patients. Table 183.1 summarizes the influence of some of the coexisting conditions on the choice of initial antihypertensive therapy.

# CHAPTER 184 SECONDARY HYPERTENSION

Although most hypertensive patients have essential hypertension, a significant number (approximately 5%) have secondary hypertension. In children, severe hypertension is almost always secondary to another process. In the evaluation of recent-onset hypertension in adults older than 50, one should seriously entertain the possibility of secondary hypertension. Table 184.1 lists the important causes of secondary hypertension. The following paragraphs discuss the major forms of secondary hypertension.

## Renal Hypertension

Kidney disease of almost any nature can cause hypertension; the more important ones are listed in Table 184.1. The exact mechanism of hypertension in these renal disorders is not always clear. Fluid retention may be responsible in patients with end-stage kidney disease, in which case the hypertension is called *renoprival* hypertension. In some patients with severe renal disease, plasma renin is elevated, and the renin-angiotensin-aldosterone system may be responsible for hypertension. In others with renal disease and normal plasma renin activity, hypertension is presumed either to be due to accumulation of certain vasopressor substances that normally are metabolized and excreted by the kidney, or to be a result of the inability of the diseased kidney to generate certain vasodilator substances such as prostaglandins and kinins.

**TABLE 184.1. Causes of Secondary Hypertension**

| |
|---|
| Renal diseases |
| Acute glomerulonephritis |
| Chronic glomerulonephritis |
| Polycystic kidney disease |
| Dysplastic kidney |
| Diabetic nephropathy |
| Hydronephrosis |
| Connective tissue disorders |
| Renin-producing tumors |
| Renal trauma |
| Analgesic nephropathy |
| Renal artery stenosis |
| Fibromuscular hyperplasia |
| Atherosclerosis |
| Adrenal disorders |
| Cortical |
| Primary aldosteronism |
| Glucocorticoid remediable aldosteronism |
| Cushing syndrome |
| Congenital adrenal hyperplasia |
| Medullary |
| Pheochromocytoma |
| Medications, OTC drugs, and herbs (see Table 181.2) |
| Coarctation of the aorta |
| Toxemia of pregnancy |
| CNS disorders |
| Other hormonal disorders |
| Hypo- and hyperthyroidism |
| Hyperparathyroidism |
| Acromegaly |
| Sleep-disordered breathing |

Laboratory investigations usually reveal albuminuria, with or without hematuria, and an elevated serum creatinine. Ultrasonography is used to detect kidney size, followed by intravenous pyelography, if better delineation of individual kidney function is desired. If one kidney is smaller (>2 cm) than the other, split renal vein renin studies, along with renal angiography in some cases, may be undertaken to confirm unilateral renal artery stenosis as the cause of secondary hypertension. In such cases, the renal vein renin on the abnormal side may be 1.5 to 2 times that of the opposite kidney. Prior administration of an ACE inhibitor augments this difference between the two kidneys in the presence of a unilateral stenosis. If parenchymal renal disease is suspected, kidney biopsy may be necessary for an accurate diagnosis.

When hypertension is a result of bilateral kidney disease, medical therapy as described for control of essential hypertension is indicated. When hypertension is due to unilateral kidney disease, such as a dysplastic or severely traumatized kidney, removal of the diseased kidney may cure hypertension. Removal of a kidney should never be undertaken lightly, and a prior trial of medical therapy is always indicated. A converting enzyme inhibitor, starting with one half the usual recommended dose, sometimes can control the blood pressure. Serum potassium and creatinine should be monitored closely. Verapamil or diltiazem may be added if ACE inhibitor alone fails to control BP. Minoxidil, when used in combination with furosemide and a β-blocker, also may control BP in patients with severe, intractable hypertension.

### Renal Artery Stenosis

Constriction of one or both renal arteries, such as may occur in congenital fibromuscular hyperplasia or atherosclerotic narrowing of the renal arteries, often results in hypertension. Fibromuscular hyperplasia, also called fibrous dysplasia, is more commonly encountered in white women under 50 years of age. In such cases, renal ischemia leading to excessive renin secretion and activation of the renin-angiotensin-aldosterone system causes elevated blood pressure. A continuous (systolic/diastolic) upper abdominal bruit that radiates to the side of the lesion often is present. Radionuclide renogram after 50 mg of oral captopril or 2.5 mg of IV enalapril shows a slower uptake and excretion of the radionuclide on the side of the lesion. The diagnosis is confirmed by MR angiography or contrast renal angiography. ACE inhibitors are particularly useful in controlling blood pressure in many patients. These drugs should be avoided, however, in the presence of bilateral renal arterial stenosis or in patients with one kidney and renal arterial stenosis. The reason for this is that these patients need a high tone in the efferent glomerular arterioles to maintain glomerular filtration, and the ACE inhibitors, by reducing the intrarenal synthesis of angiotensin II, lead to dilatation of the efferent arterioles, causing the glomerular filtration rate to drop and serum creatinine to rise. If blood pressure cannot be readily controlled with medical therapy, angioplasty or surgical treatment should be considered.

Angioplasty or dilatation of the narrowed segment by an inflatable balloon catheter and stent placement is the treatment of choice. Surgical treatment may be necessary to salvage the kidney, if medical therapy and angioplasty have failed or if angioplasty is deemed inappropriate. The surgery consists of resection of the stenotic lesion, bypass of the lesions using either a Dacron graft or a saphenous vein graft, or an endarterectomy, with or without patch plasty. Nephrectomy is considered only as a last resort if a revascularization procedure is technically impossible or has failed. Surgical treatment may cure hypertension in these patients. However, in some cases, fibromuscular hyperplasia is progressive and can recur after surgery.

Renal artery stenosis due to atherosclerosis usually occurs in patients over the age of 50. The atherosclerotic narrowing is most frequently present at the origin of the renal artery. In almost all cases, there is evidence of extensive atherosclerosis elsewhere. Most of these patients have a history of long-standing, untreated, essential hypertension. In most patients, blood pressure can be controlled on medical therapy with an ACE inhibitor. Selected patients can be treated with angioplasty. Surgical therapy should be undertaken only in patients with severe, uncontrolled hypertension or in those with inevitable risk of losing kidneys due to ischemia. Unilateral nephrectomy of an unsalvageable kidney, combined with contralateral revascularization, sometimes is lifesaving in properly selected patients. In those treated medically, serum creatinine and renal size, using ultrasonography, should be monitored every 3 to 6 months.

## Adrenal Disorders

Adrenal cortical and medullary disorders can cause hypertension (see Chapter 68).

## Coarctation of the Aorta

Coarctation of the aorta is a narrowing of the aortic lumen due to a localized deformity of the vascular media and a curtain-like infolding. It is characteristically located distal to the origin of the left subclavian artery, but it can, occasionally, occur proximal to it as well. Headache, spontaneous epistaxis, and leg fatigue are the usual symptoms. Bicuspid aortic valve and an aneurysm of the circle of Willis may be associated. The hallmark of the condition is hypertension in the upper extremities. The femoral pulses are feeble and delayed. Collateral arteries may be seen and felt on the patient's back. Chest radiographs may show rib notching due to enlarged intercostal–internal mammary collateral arteries and "3 sign" from dilation of the aorta above and below the constriction (see also Chapter 140). The diagnosis is confirmed by transesophageal echocardiography, MR angiography, or contrast aortography. Reduced blood supply to the kidney can stimulate renin secretion, thereby activating the renin-angiotensin-aldosterone system, which then leads to exacerbation of hypertension. Section of the narrowed segment with end-to-end anastomosis or bypass with a Dacron graft is the surgical procedure of choice. Postoperative hypertension requiring medical therapy is not uncommon. Angioplasty with stent placement is becoming increasingly popular and may become the treatment of choice.

## CNS Disorders

Disorders causing increased intracranial pressure, such as may occur in respiratory acidosis, encephalitis, brain tumor, and hemorrhagic stroke, can cause increased sympathetic outflow from the brain and hypertension that can be very severe and often labile. Reduction of intracranial pressure by reversal of the underlying cause usually leads to normalization of blood pressure.

## Sleep-Disordered Breathing

Most patients with sleep-disordered breathing are obese and snore habitually. These breathing problems are associated with daytime and nocturnal hypertension. Activation of the sympathetic nervous system by hypoxia or acidosis appears to be the physiologic cause of hypertensive episodes. Cardiovascular morbidity and mortality are increased in patients with sleep apnea. Further information on sleep- disordered breathing is provided in Chapter 257.

# CHAPTER 185 HYPERTENSIVE EMERGENCIES

A hypertensive emergency or crisis is a clinical situation in which the blood pressure is so elevated as to constitute a threat to life or certain organ systems. The diastolic BP usually is above 120 mm Hg. Conditions such as acute left ventricular failure and acute dissecting aneurysm of the aorta qualify as hypertensive emergencies, not so much because of the severity of hypertension but because there may be coexisting life-threatening complications. Some of the clinical situations that constitute hypertensive emergencies are listed in Table 185.1. Asymptomatic patients, despite a very high blood pressure, are in no immediate danger and should not be treated as hypertensive emergencies.

**TABLE 185.1. Hypertensive Emergencies**

Hypertensive encephalopathy
Acute dissecting aneurysm of the aorta
Acute pulmonary edema (hypertension with acute left ventricular failure)
Malignant or accelerated hypertension
Intracerebral or subarachnoid hemorrhage
Severe hypertension in a patient with acute coronary insufficiency or myocardial infarction
Diastolic blood pressure >130 mm Hg without symptoms
Hypertension associated with acute glomerulonephritis
Curable conditions that may require prompt reduction in blood pressure:
- Pheochromocytoma
- Toxemia of pregnancy
- Oral contraceptive-induced severe hypertension
- Renovascular hypertension

The use of sublingual or oral nifedipine is no longer recommended in the treatment of hypertensive emergencies because there may be serious adverse sequelae such as myocardial infarction and stroke. Intravenous administration of antihypertensive drugs often is necessary to achieve blood pressure control. The intravenous medications currently used include furosemide, sodium nitroprusside, diazoxide, labetalol, enalaprilat, and nitroglycerin. The dose and side effects of these drugs are summarized in Table 185.2. During administration of these potent antihypertensive agents, close monitoring of arterial blood pressure, preferably using an intraarterial line, is essential; these patients are, therefore, best treated in an intensive care unit. Oral antihypertensive medications should be started as soon as possible to keep hypertension under control as evaluation of the patient proceeds.

## Questions

**Instructions:** For each question below, select only **one** lettered answer that is the **best** for that question.

1. A 42-year-old woman has new-onset hypertension. Her review of systems is unremarkable. Urinalysis is normal except for microscopic hematuria. Serum chemistries and blood counts also are normal. An ultrasound of the kidneys demonstrates multiple fluid collections. The most likely diagnosis in this patient is which of the following?
   A. Medullary sponge kidney
   B. Bilateral renal carcinomas
   C. Polycystic kidney disease
   D. Toxoplasmosis
   E. Echinococcus cysts

**TABLE 185.2. Selected Intravenous Drugs for Hypertensive Emergencies**

| Drugs | Dose | Important side effects |
|---|---|---|
| Diazoxide (Hyperstat) | 50–100 mg bolus or 15–30 mg/min infusion | Hypotension, tachycardia, angina, vomiting, hyperglycemia |
| Enalaprilat (Vasotec) | 1.25–5 mg q 6 hrs | Hypotension, renal failure if bilateral renal artery stenosis is present |
| Fenoldopam (Carlopam) | 0.1–1 μg/kg/min | Myocardial infarction, CHF, hypokalemia, arrhythmias, leukocytosis |
| Furosemide (Lasix) | 40–160 mg q 4-6 hrs | Hypotension, hypokalemia, hyperglycemia on prolonged use |
| Labetalol (Normodyne, Trandate) | 20–80 mg by bolus q 10–15 min or 0.5–2 mg/min infusion | Hypotension, bronchoconstriction, heart block, bradycardia |
| Sodium nitroprusside (Nipride) | 0.25–10 μg/kg/min (Maximum dose for 10 min only) | Vomiting, twitching, thiocyanate intoxication, methemoglobinemia, cyanide poisoning |
| Nitroglycerin (Nitrobid IV) | 5–100 μg/min | Headache, vomiting, methemoglobinemia, tolerance |

2. A 24-year-old man has malaise, bilateral leg edema above the knees, and hypertension. His review of systems is otherwise unremarkable. Three of his six siblings have been placed on dialysis, but he does not know the etiology of their renal disease. Examination is otherwise normal. Serum creatinine is 2.4 mg/dl; BUN, 28 mg/dl; and 24-hr urine protein, 10 g, with a creatinine clearance of 60 ml/min. Urinalysis demonstrates 4+ protein and 5 to 10 RBCs. Three different antihypertensive medications in sufficient doses lower blood pressure only to 160/90 mm Hg. Which of the following conditions would be the most likely diagnosis on a renal biopsy?
   A. Acute glomerulonephritis
   B. Chronic interstitial nephritis
   C. Focal segmental glomerulosclerosis
   D. Membranous nephropathy
   E. Goodpasture syndrome

3. A 27-year-old woman reports left flank pain and hematuria. There is a history of frequent urinary tract infections with *Proteus mirabilis.* She is currently taking suppressive antibiotic therapy to prevent recurrence. A renal ultrasound shows a large stone in the left kidney. Her renal function is normal, and urinalysis shows hematuria and crystals. Urine shows: pH, 7.5; trace blood; and protein. Which of the following types of kidney stone is most likely in this patient?
   A. Calcium oxalate stones
   B. Calcium phosphate stones
   C. Cystine stones
   D. Struvite stones
   E. Uric acid stones

4. A 32-year-old man has recurrent attacks of gross hematuria, occurring after flu-like symptoms or colds. These bouts have been present only over the past year. His review of systems is otherwise normal. His laboratory studies are normal; urinalysis reveals only microscopic hematuria. The most likely diagnosis is which of the following?
   A. Alport's syndrome
   B. Anti-glomerular basement membrane disease
   C. IgA nephropathy
   D. Acute glomerulonephritis
   E. Crescentic glomerulonephritis

5. A 58-year-old woman with oat cell carcinoma of the lung is admitted for obtundation. Her weight is 60 kg; BP, 130/80 mm Hg with no orthostatic hypotension; and focal signs are absent. Serum sodium: 115 mEq/L; plasma osmolality: 240 mOsm/kg $H_2O$; urine osmolality: 680 mOsm/kg $H_2O$; normal renal function; other laboratory tests normal. Which of the following conditions is the most likely diagnosis?
   A. Hyponatremia due to decreased effective circulating volume
   B. Inappropriate ADH release
   C. Pseudohyponatremia
   D. Nephrogenic diabetes insipidus
   E. Central diabetes insipidus

6. A 31-year-old epileptic suffers a grand mal seizure. Laboratory tests taken immediately after the seizure reveal pH, 7.14; $PaCO_2$, 45 mm Hg; serum sodium, 140 mEq/L; potassium, 4 mEq/L; chloride, 98 mEq/L; and bicarbonate, 17 mEq/L. Which of the following best explains this acid-base disorder?
   A. Metabolic alkalosis
   B. Combined metabolic alkalosis and respiratory alkalosis
   C. Respiratory acidosis with normal anion gap metabolic acidosis
   D. Combined respiratory and high anion gap metabolic acidosis
   E. Metabolic acidosis alone

7. A 29-year-old woman with end-stage renal disease has become dyspneic in the previous 24 hours, with orthopnea. During the past 2 to 3 months, she has missed at least one dialysis treatment every week. Bibasilar rales and bilateral leg edema to hips are noted. Arterial pH is 7.45 and $PaO_2$ is 90 mm Hg. After being dialyzed for 5 minutes, she becomes severely hypotensive. Which of the following best explains her clinical picture?
   A. Myocardial infarction
   B. Pulmonary embolus
   C. Pericardial effusion
   D. Volume overload
   E. Dialyzer reaction

8. A 62-year-old man with chronic renal failure is started on a low-sodium diet for hypertension. Two weeks later he reports being unable to lift himself out of a chair. His skin turgor is slightly decreased, and there is marked proximal muscle weakness. The serum creatinine is 2.1 mg/dl; sodium, 130 mEq/L; potassium, 9.8 mEq/L; chloride, 98 mEq/L; bicarbonate, 17 mEq/L; and arterial pH, 7.32. Widened QRS complexes and peaked T waves are noted on ECG. Which of the following factors significantly contributed to the genesis of hyperkalemia in this patient?
   A. Renal insufficiency
   B. Superimposed volume depletion
   C. Metabolic acidosis

D. Dietary potassium intake
E. All of the above

9. A 64-year-old man undergoes a routine physical examination. Pedal edema and heme-positive stools are found. His laboratory chemistries and CBC are within normal limits, but 3+ proteinuria is found. A renal biopsy demonstrates membranous nephropathy. Given this clinical picture, what additional evaluation should be performed?
   A. Immunologic work-up to rule out collagen vascular disease
   B. Hematologic work-up to rule out a hemolytic process
   C. Gastrointestinal work-up to rule out malignancy
   D. Bronchoscopy to evaluate for pulmonary renal syndromes
   E. None of the above

10. A 65-year old man, a nursing home resident, is hospitalized for dehydration and a gram-negative urinary tract infection. He has been given ibuprofen three times daily over the past four days for his fever. Except for WBCs, his urinalysis is normal. In the hospital, he is started on gentamicin. Ten days later, at the time of discharge, his serum creatinine has doubled from his baseline value of 1.0 mg/dl. What is the most likely etiology for his acute renal insufficiency?
    A. NSAID-induced nephropathy
    B. Urinary tract obstruction
    C. Aminoglycoside nephropathy
    D. Volume depletion
    E. Dehydration and aminoglycoside nephropathy

11. A 42-year-old man with 4 months of progressive azotemia is now hospitalized for increasing low back pain, lethargy, and anorexia. Vital signs are normal, and pallor of mucous membranes and costovertebral angle tenderness are noted. Hemoglobin is 7 g/dl; BUN, 45 mg/dl; creatinine, 5 mg/dl; calcium, 12 mg/dl; $K^+$, 3.0 mEq/L; $HCO_3$, 18 mEq/L; and $PO_4^-$, 2.0 mg/dl; the blood sugar is normal. Urinalysis shows a pH of 6, no protein, glucose 2+, and occasional hyaline and granular casts. What is the most likely cause of this man's renal failure?
    A. Urinary tract obstruction
    B. Primary hyperparathyroidism
    C. Multiple myeloma with nephropathy
    D. Distal renal tubular acidosis
    E. Metastatic oat cell carcinoma

12. A 37-year-old woman complains of polyuria. Her physical examination is normal. Urinalysis, including microscopy, is normal. Urine osmolality is 80 mOsm/kg $H_2O$, rising to 120 after 12 hours of dehydration. Serum Na is 133 mEq/L, K, 3.9 mEq/L, $HCO_3$, 25 mEq/L, creatinine, 0.7 mg/dl, serum osmolality—268 mOsm/kg $H_2O$. What is the most likely diagnosis?
    A. Central diabetes insipidus
    B. Nephrogenic diabetes insipidus
    C. Diuretic abuse
    D. Psychogenic polydipsia
    E. Essential hyponatremia

13. Which of the following statements concerning the incidence and severity of hypertensive disease in the United Stages is false?
    A. The incidence of hypertension increases with age, regardless of race.
    B. The incidence of hypertension is higher in men than women.
    C. The incidence of systolic hypertension is higher in young blacks than whites.
    D. The incidence of diastolic hypertension is twice as high in blacks than whites.
    E. Blacks suffer more severe complications of hypertension.

14. Which of the following laboratory investigations does not need to be performed routinely in the evaluation of hypertension?
    A. Urinalysis
    B. Blood glucose
    C. Serum potassium
    D. Plasma renin
    E. Serum creatinine

15. If lifestyle modifications prove inadequate and there is no contraindication or coexisting diseases, the antihypertensive of choice is a:
    A. Calcium blocker
    B. Alpha blocker
    C. Sympathetic inhibitor
    D. Diuretic
    E. Vasodilator

16. Which of the following statements regarding diuretics is correct?
    A. Long-acting diuretics produce hypokalemia less often than short-acting diuretics.
    B. Loop diuretics are better antihypertensives than thiazides.
    C. Diuretic-induced hyperuricemia causes renal damage.
    D. Diuretics can cause hyperglycemia, hypercalcemia and hyperlipidemia.
    E. Diuretics should be avoided in diabetics.

17. Contraindications to β-blocker therapy include:
    A. Hepatic insufficiency.
    B. Asthma.
    C. First-degree heart block.
    D. Diastolic heart failure.
    E. Renal insufficiency.

18. When hypertension remains uncontrolled despite the combination of a diuretic and a sympathetic inhibitor, which of the following drugs should be tried in place of the previous therapy?
    A. An ACE inhibitor
    B. Minoxidil
    C. Hydralazine
    D. Diazoxide
    E. An alpha blocker

19. Which of the following is/are appropriate in the follow-up examination of a well-controlled hypertensive patient?
    A. Monthly serum potassium
    B. Annual general examination and laboratory tests of blood sugar, serum potassium, creatinine, uric acid, and lipids
    C. Annual rapid sequence IVP
    D. Annual plasma renin
    E. Annual chest x-ray

20. Drugs known to elevate arterial blood pressure include which of the following?
    A. Oral contraceptives
    B. Appetite suppressants
    C. Phenylephrine nose drops
    D. Indomethacin
    E. All of the above

## Answers

| | | | | |
|---|---|---|---|---|
| 1. C | 2. C | 3. D | 4. C | 5. B |
| 6. D | 7. C | 8. E | 9. C | 10. E |
| 11. C | 12. D | 13. C | 14. D | 15. D |
| 16. D | 17. B | 18. A | 19. B | 20. E |

## SUGGESTED READING


### *Textbooks*

Brenner BM. Brenner & Rector's The Kidney. 6th ed. Philadelphia: WB Saunders, 2000.

Greenberg A. Primer on Kidney Diseases. 3rd ed. San Diego: Academic Press, 2001.

Jennette JC, Heptinstall S. Pathology of the Kidney. 5th ed. Philadelphia: Lippincott Williams & Wilkins, 1999.

Izzo JL, Black HR, Taubert KA. Hypertension Primer. 2nd ed. Dallas: American Heart Association, 1997.

Kaplan NM, Lieberman E. Clinical Hypertension. 8th ed. Baltimore, Lippincott Williams & Wilkins, 2002.

### *Articles*

*Initial Evaluation of Kidney Disease*

Carroll MF, Temte JL. Proteinuria in adults: a diagnostic approach. Ame Fam Physician 2000;62:1333-40.

*Nephrotic Syndrome*

Fogo A. Nephrotic syndrome: molecular and genetic basis. Nephron 2000;8-13.

Orth SR, Ritz E. The nephrotic syndrome. N Engl J Med 1998;338:1202-11.

*Nephrolithiasis*

Pak CY. Kidney stones. Lancet 1998;351:1797-801.

*Glomerular Diseases*

Hricik DE, Chung-Park M, Sedor Jr. Glomerulonephritis. N Engl J Med 1998;339:888-99.

Couser W G. Glomerulonephritis. Lancet 1999;353(9163): 1509-15.

*Tubulointerstitial Nephropathy*

Rastegar A. Kashgarian M. The clinical spectrum of tubulointerstitial nephritis. Kidney International 1998;54:313-27.

*Vascular Diseases of the Kidney*

Bouyounes BT, Libertino JA. Renovascular hypertension. Curr Opin Urology 1999;9:111-4.

Vidt DG. Cholesterol emboli: a common cause of renal failure. Annu Rev Med 1997;48:375–385.

*Cystic Disorders of the Kidney*

Torres VE. New insights into polycystic kidney disease and its treatment. Curr Opin in Nephrol Hyperten 1998;7:159-69.

Hildebrandt F. Renal cystic disease. Curr Opin Peds 1999;11: 141-51.

*HIV Nephropathy*

Schwartz EJ, Klotman PE. Pathogenesis of human immunodeficiency virus (HIV)-associated nephropathy. Semin Nephrol 1998;18:436-45.

*Disorders of Water Balance*

Adrogue HJ, Madias NE. Hyponatremia. N Engl J Med 2000;342:1581-9.

Adrogue HJ, Madias NE. Hypernatremia. N Engl J Med 2000;342:1493-9.

*Disorders of Potassium Balance*

Halperin ML. Potassium. Lancet 1998;352:135-40.

Gannari FJ. Hypokalemia. N Engl J Med 1998;339:451-8.

*Hypertension*

Joint National Committee. The report of the Joint National Committee on detection, evaluation and treatment of high blood pressure (JNCVI). Arch Intern Med 1997;157:2413–2446.

Vaugh CJ, Delanty N. Hypertensive emergencies. Lancet 2000;356:411-7.

Whelton PK, He J, Appel LJ et al. Primary prevention of hypertension. JAMA 2002;288:1882–88.

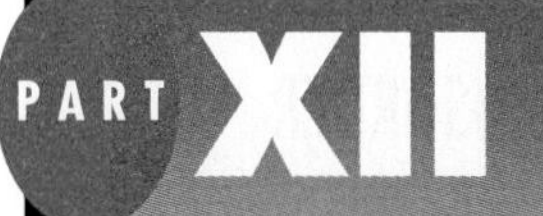

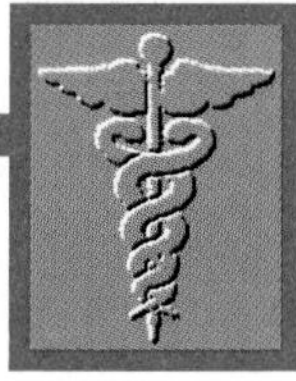

Safwan Jaradeh, MD

# PART XII NEUROLOGIC DISORDERS

# CHAPTER 186 APPROACH TO THE PATIENT WITH A NEUROLOGIC DISORDER

## History

After eliciting a detailed history, the physician should develop an initial working hypothesis that describes the location(s) and pathologic process that would explain the patient's symptoms. A neurologic examination should follow, which is meant to prove one's hypothesis or suggest another if the findings refute the first. As the site/level of lesion is more ascertained, one should outline the most likely (top three) pathologic processes. Then, one should select the most appropriate laboratory test(s) to confirm one's diagnosis. In most patients, the diagnosis is derived from the history, from an unexpected physical finding in some, and, occasionally, from a laboratory finding. The most important historical information concerns the onset and course of symptoms and signs (Figure 186.1). In diagnosing selected neurologic disorders (i.e., degenerative diseases), the family history may help significantly.

## Neurologic Examination

### Mental status examination

Level of consciousness and orientation to person, place, and time should be noted. Language function, attention, concentration, behavior, knowledge of current events, judgment, and mood can be assessed while taking the history. A mini-mental status examination is outlined in Table 121.1.

### Evaluation of speech and language

*Dysarthrias*

Dysarthrias are the product of neurologic disorders affecting the mechanisms that control and coordinate speech. This is reflected by changes in the acoustic quality of speech without alteration of language per se. Written language is always spared.

*Aphasias*

Aphasia is a disturbance of language expression, comprehension or both. The dysfunction involves both spoken and written language, albeit to a variable extent. The examination assesses fluency of language production, language comprehension, ability to repeat, and presence of word substitutions known as **"paraphasias."** Fluency is impaired if the patient produces speech slowly or laboriously, utters unusually brief sentences, pauses frequently to find a word, or uses only the most essential words ("telegraphic speech"). Comprehension is tested by requiring the patient to answer questions or carry out commands of varying complexity. Repetition of words and sentences measures the integrity of cortical regions surrounding the Sylvian fissure. Paraphasias usually indicate injury posterior to the peri-sylvian region. Patterns of aphasia are summarized in Table 186.1.

### Cranial Nerves

Assessment of **cranial nerve function** is summarized in Table 186.2.

### Evaluation of sensory function

The main sensory modalities are primary (light touch, pinprick, temperature, vibration, and joint position sensation) and complex (2-point discrimination, graphesthesia, and stereognosis). **Impairment of sensory function** usually presents with **numbness.** One should ask for a description of the feeling in the patient's own words. Paresthesia (tingling or prickling) or dysesthesia (disagreeable sensory symptoms) may be associated. The isolated feeling of heaviness or deadness may be due to either sensory or motor impairment. If the history suggests sensory impairment, the sensory functions should be tested first. The **Romberg procedure** tests the posterior column and vestibular (not cerebellar) function because it eliminates **visuo-spatial cues.** Cerebellar pathology is manifest with or without the eyes closed. Patterns of sensory loss in various disorders are shown in Table 186.3.

### Motor system

Besides gait, the motor system is most efficiently assessed by checking **fine and gross coordination** (i.e., **finger and toe tapping**), observation for wasting or fasciculations (lower motor neuron), muscle tone, and individual muscle strength. Neuromuscular junction defects (e.g., myasthenia gravis) more often present with fatigue on exertion, rather than primary weakness (Table 186.4).

Striated muscles are composed of multiple motor units. Each motor unit consists of a single motor neuron (called the **lower motor neuron**), its axon, and the muscle fibers it innervates. Various descending cerebral pathways (corticospinal tract being the most important) that control these units form the **upper motor neurons**. Diseases of either the upper or the lower motor neuron cause weakness, which may be partial (**paresis**), or complete (**paralysis**). Paralysis of one limb is **monoplegia**, and of both legs, **paraplegia**; paralysis of one side is **hemiplegia**, and of all limbs, **quadriplegia**. Weakness of muscles innervated by the brain stem, such as face,

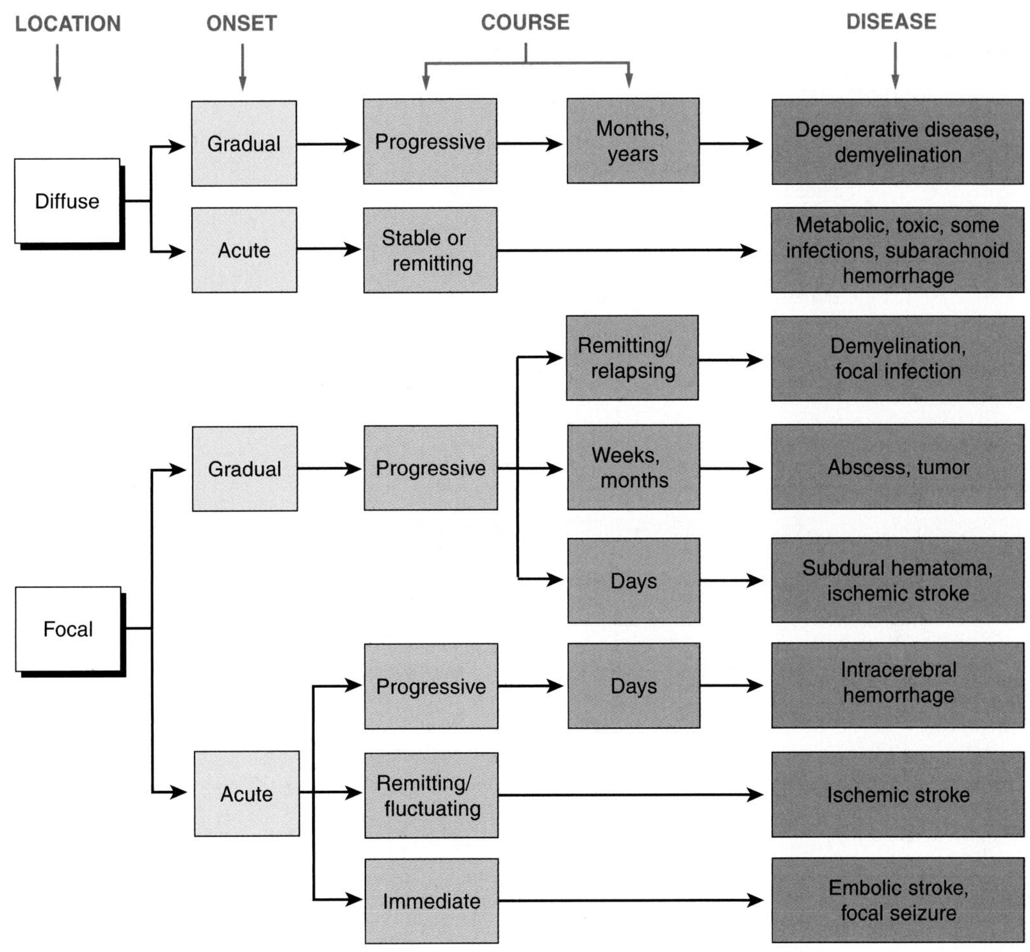


**FIGURE 186.1.** Examples of Symptom Onset and Course. (Adapted from: Caplan LR. The Effective Clinical Neurolologist. Cambridge: Blackwell Scientific Publishers, 1990; 45–52.)

**TABLE 186.1. Clinical Differentiation of Major Aphasias**

| Type | Fluency | Comprehension | Repetition | Lesion site |
|---|---|---|---|---|
| Broca | Impaired | Usually intact | Impaired | Usually left frontal, infero-posterior |
| Wernicke | Intact, paraphasic | Impaired | Impaired | Left temporal, supero-posterior |
| Global | Impaired | Impaired | Impaired | Left frontal and temporal |
| Conduction | Intact, paraphasic | Intact | Impaired | Left arcuate fasciculus, or left supra-marginal gyrus |
| Transcortical motor | Impaired | Usually intact | Intact | Antero-superior to Broca's |
| Transcortical-sensory | Intact, paraphasic | Impaired | Intact | Infero-posterior to Wernicke's |
| Anomic | Intact, naming difficulty | Intact | Intact | Left angular gyrus, or left posterior temporal |

(Adapted from: Damasio AR. N Engl J Med 1992; 326:531-539. Used with permission.)

TABLE 186.2. Cranial Nerve Examination

| Site to Examine | What to Look for: | Which Cranial Nerve Will This Examine? |
|---|---|---|
| Fundus | Optic disk, venous pulsations[a], visual fields | II |
| Pupils | Size, shape, symmetry, light reaction | III, cervical sympathetic[b] |
| Eye movements | Nystagmus, paralysis, dissociation, diplopia | III, IV, VI, VIII |
| Corneal reflex | Sensation[c], blink | V, VII |
| Facial symmetry | Upper versus lower motor weakness | VII |
| Gag reflex | Sensation (IX), motor | IX, X |
| Neck/shoulder | Turn neck from one side to the other; shrugging of shoulders; sternocleidomastoid/trapezius | XI |
| Tongue | Protrusion in midline | XII |

[a]The ability to detect venous pulsations is very important; when present bilaterally, the probability (approx. 95%) is that intracranial pressure is not elevated.
[b]The cervical sympathetic is not a cranial nerve.
[c]Tests only cranial nerve V.

TABLE 186.3. Patterns of Sensory Loss in Various Disorders

| Site/Disease | Pattern/Distribution of Sensory Loss |
|---|---|
| Thalamus or sensory cortex | Impaired complex sensory functions |
| Spinal cord lesion | Involves trunk plus upper and/or lower extremity |
| Root or peripheral nerve | Dermatome/peripheral nerve territory |
| Mononeuropathy | Territory of the involved nerve |
| Polyneuropathy | Symmetric, gradual transition from distal to proximal; stocking and glove distribution |
| Hysteria | None, sharp transition from anesthetic to normal areas |

TABLE 186.4. Motor System in Various Disorders

| Location | Tone | Bulk | Strength | Reflexes |
|---|---|---|---|---|
| Upper motor neuron | Spastic | +/– | Decreased | Increased, Babinski sign |
| Basal ganglia | Rigidity | No change | No change | No change |
| Cerebellar | Hypotonic | No change | No change | Pendular |
| Anterior horn cell | Decreased | Atrophy, fasciculations | Decreased | Decreased |
| Radiculopathy | +/– | +/– | Decreased | Decreased |
| Peripheral nerve (motor) | +/– | Decreased distally | Decreased distally | Decreased |
| Muscle | Decreased | Decreased | Decreased | Decreased |
| Neuromuscular junction | Variable | Variable | Fatigue | Variable |

+/– = may or may not be abnormal.

tongue, and pharynx is **bulbar palsy**. Differentiation between upper and lower motor neuron disorders is outlined in Table 186.4.

### Gait

One useful screening test is to observe a patient's gait, including standing, walking, stopping, turning, and associated arm swing movements. These maneuvers require integration of sensory, motor, basal ganglia, cerebellar, vestibular, and visual processing, and are, therefore, sensitive indicators of abnormal function of one or more systems. In a unilateral **upper motor neuron lesion**, the patient walks by circumducting the affected leg while keeping the affected arm close to the body in a mildly flexed position. In extrapyramidal disorders, particularly Parkinsonism, there is mild stooping of the body, with difficulty initiating gait or performing rapid turns. Initial shuffling is seen once walking begins, with a mild increase in the speed **("festinating" gait).** In mild disease, only reduced swinging of the arms may be noted. A **wide-based gait,** often with instability on turning, frequently follows cerebellar disorders. The patient is unable to perform a **heel-to-toe** tandem gait. The unsteady gait in vestibular or proprioceptive sensory deficits dramatically worsens when visual input is removed, such as walking in the dark. When joint position sense is severely impaired, patients lift their legs significantly before landing on the ground with their heels **("tabetic gait").** A unilateral vestibular lesion, particularly when associated with a cerebellar lesion, results in veering to the side of the lesion. Finally, proximal weakness, as in myopathies or spinal muscular atrophies, cause **"waddling"** due to pelvic tilting. However, foot and leg weakness from a neuropathy results in a gait with bilateral foot drop ("steppage gait").

#### Cerebellum

This system is most efficiently tested by observation of heel-to-toe tandem walking, and **finger-to-nose** and **heel-to-shin** movements. Slurred or dysarthric speech, clumsiness or **ataxia, hypotonia, nystagmus, dysarthria**, and **gait dysfunction** usually result from cerebellar dysfunction. Patients also usually have an abnormal finger-to-nose and/or heel-to-shin testing (dysmetria). With severe cerebellar disease, an intention tremor is commonly observed.

#### Reflexes

Deep tendon reflexes (DTRs) test both sensory and motor limbs of the spinal reflex arc, besides the degree of upper motor neuron input. One evaluates the amplitude, symmetry, proximal versus distal pattern, and the isolated diminution or absence of a single response. Most commonly tested reflexes are listed in Table 186.5. The plantar response, normally flexor, should be assessed in every patient. Extension of the great toe, with or without fanning of the other toes, is the Babinski sign and indicates upper motor neuron involvement.

#### Formulation

When assessing a neurologic problem, both the probability and "treatability" of the underlying neurologic disease should be considered. Even though a diagnosis may not be the most likely, one should pursue it, if it is possible and reversible (i.e., hypothyroidism, vitamin $B_{12}$ deficiency, subdural hematoma).

### Localization

The following principles are very useful in neurologic diagnosis: 1) one lesion or process can often explain the neurologic symptoms and signs; 2) abnormal neurologic function can usually be localized to regions, and 3) it is often helpful if one neurologic sign is longitudinal (corticospinal, spinothalamic, posterior column) and another is segmental (sensory level, reflexes, cranial nerves, cerebellum). For example, in paraplegia with a sensory level, one can localize the lesion within one to three spinal segments.

### Laboratory Studies

#### Lumbar puncture (LP)

LP is useful in diagnosing meningitis, encephalitis, encephalopathies, subarachnoid hemorrhage, inflammatory disorders, and multiple sclerosis. It is contraindicated if bleeding disorders are suspected, or with increased intracranial pressure, intracranial mass, and spinal cord mass. Often, it should be preceded by CT to exclude an intracranial mass. In the lateral decubitus position, normal cerebrospinal fluid (CSF) opening pressure is less than 200 mm water.

The CSF should be collected in 4 tubes. Tube 1 is usually for cell count, but if the fluid is bloody, cell counts should be done on tubes 1 and 4. Tube 2 is usually for glucose and protein; tube 3 for microbial stains, and tube 4 for cultures. Other tests include IgG and oligoclonal bands in suspected demyelination, and cytology for malignant cells. With a traumatic tap, the supernatant is

**TABLE 186.5. Clinical Manifestations of Common Radiculopathies**

| Root | Pain/Sensory Loss | Reflex Arc | Motor Deficit |
|---|---|---|---|
| C5 | Shoulder | Biceps | Shoulder abduction |
| C6 | Lateral arm, forearm, thumb | Biceps, brachioradialis | Elbow flexion |
| C7 | Dorsal arm and forearm, middle finger | Triceps | Elbow extension |
| C8 | Medial arm & forearm, little finger | Finger flexion | Finger flexion |
| L3 | Anterior and medial thigh | Adductor, patellar | Thigh adduction |
| L4 | Medial leg | Patellar | Leg extension |
| L5 | Lateral calf and leg, posterior thigh, dorsum of foot | Hamstring | Ankle dorsiflexion |
| S1 | Posterior calf and leg, plantar surface | Achilles | Ankle plantar flexion |

**TABLE 186.6. CSF Findings in Main Neurologic Conditions**

| Condition | Cell Type and Count | Protein | Glucose | IgG Index/Bands[a] |
|---|---|---|---|---|
| Acute meningitis: bacterial | PMN, elevated | Elevated | Decreased | Increased/none |
| viral | Lymph, elevated | Elevated | Normal | Increased/none |
| Chronic meningitis | Lymph, elevated | Elevated | Decreased | Increased/rare |
| Viral encephalitis | Lymph, elevated | Elevated | Normal | Increased/none |
| HIV | | | | |
| Aseptic meningitis | Lymph, elevated | Elevated | Normal | Increased/rare |
| AIDS-related dementia | Lymph, elevated | Elevated | Normal | Increased/often present[b] |
| Multiple sclerosis | Rarely elevated | Slightly elevated | Normal | Increased/present |
| Subarachnoid hemorrhage | RBC, abundant | Slightly elevated | Normal | Normal/none |
| Leptomeningeal tumor | Malignant cells | Slightly elevated | Decreased | Normal/none |

[a]Refers to oligoclonal bands.
[b]Depends on the stage of the disease; myelin basic protein is normal; β2 microglobulin in CSF is high.

**TABLE 186.7. Laboratory Testing and Imaging Studies in Neurological Diagnosis**

| Test | Indication/Comments |
|---|---|
| | **Electrophysiologic studies** |
| EEG | Suspected seizures, encephalopathies, changes in consciousness, and brain death |
| EP | Suspected multiple sclerosis, assess and prognosticate after brain trauma or hypoxia, evaluate spinal cord integrity after trauma or during spine surgery |
| EMG/NCV | Suspected motor neuron disease, radiculopathy, peripheral neuropathy, myasthenia gravis, and myopathy |
| | **Imaging studies** |
| **Cranial** | |
| Plain x-rays | Very limited |
| CT | Differentiate infarction from intracranial hemorrhage; evaluation of suspected subarachnoid hemorrhage, trauma, and tumor; good visualization of bony changes |
| MRI | Early (<48 hours) suspected non-hemorrhagic stroke, posterior fossa tumors, demyelination syndromes, and white matter edema associated with infections |
| Angiography | Intracranial aneurysms, AVMs, fistulae, TIA in surgical candidates, venous sinus thrombosis, meningiomas, dissecting aneurysms, and vasculitis |
| **Spinal** | |
| Plain x-rays | A good screening test for neck/low back pain since it shows congenital, traumatic, degenerative, and neoplastic bony abnormalities, as well as spinal stenosis |
| Myelography | Suspected spinal cord or nerve root compression; being supplanted considerably by MRI |
| CT | Lateral disk herniations (when combined with myelography); also helpful in evaluation of bony abnormalities |
| MRI | Visualize spinal cord, nerve roots, herniated disks, and spinal cord compression |
| Ultrasonography | |
| B-mode | Evaluation of extracranial carotid disease; screen for suspected ICA stenosis |
| Doppler | Measure velocity of carotid blood flow as a screening test |
| | **Biopsies** |
| Temporal artery | Suspected giant cell arteritis |
| Muscle/nerve | Suspected myopathies, polymyositis, vasculitides, and infectious and inflammatory disorders; not necessary for diagnosing peripheral neuropathy |

a-v m = arteriovenous malformations; CT = computed tomography; EEG = electroencephalography; EMG/NCV = electromyography and nerve conduction studies; EP = evoked potentials; ICA = internal carotid artery; MRI = magnetic resonance imaging; TIA = transient ischemic attack.

usually colorless, the cell count is significantly less in tube 4, and the WBC to RBC ratio is 1:1000, similar to peripheral blood. Following subarachnoid hemorrhage, CSF is usually pink. Xanthochromia (from conversion of hemoglobin to bilirubin) appears within 8–12 hours and lasts up to 3 eeks. CSF findings in major neurologic diseases are shown in Table 186.6.

The role of additional laboratory, imaging and electrophysiological testing in neurologic diagnosis is summarized in Table 186.7.

# CHAPTER 187 COMA

## Definition and Etiology

**Coma** is a medical emergency that requires simultaneous attention to treatment of life-threatening problems (e.g., ventilation, cardiovascular status, trauma, hypoglycemia) and evaluation to determine the cause, which may be apparent or elusive.

Defining coma and normal consciousness is not difficult. Disruptions of consciousness between these two extremes are variously described with confusing and often misapplied terminology. Consciousness has two facets: **arousal** and **content**. These are obviously codependent for normalcy but can be disrupted independently at variable intervals. For instance, a sedative overdose will acutely depress arousal with conscious content initially maintained. Conversely, **dementia of the Alzheimer type** disrupts memory and cognition with general sparing of arousal. Coma is a state of unarousable unresponsiveness. In practice, a statement recording the responses elicited with various stimuli should be used to define arousal states. Confusing terms may pose an impediment to the accurate portrayal of the clinical course. Nonetheless, certain terms deserve mention. **Lethargy** is simply a tendency toward **sleepiness—drowsiness**. The obvious presence of excessive amounts of sleep and inattention to the environment with the maintenance of spontaneous arousal may be described as **obtundation**. **Stupor** is a state where arousal is only maintained with constant vigorous stimulation.

Depression of arousal has an important neurologic localization, indicating impairment of the rostral brainstem (rostral pons and midbrain) or both cerebral hemispheres. If a comatose patient has a lesion that does not conform to this localization, then further investigation is necessary. A single, large, acute unilateral hemispheric lesion can depress arousal transiently. If the altered consciousness persists, then other pathology must be present. Diffuse processes such as metabolic encephalopathies or infection will, of course, disrupt both hemispheres and brainstem. The causes of coma are listed in Table 187.1.

## Initial Management of the Comatose Patient

Coma is a medical emergency and assessment of the airway, respiration (breathing), and circulation (ABCs) take precedence over all other issues. Head and neck trauma must always be considered and excluded using radiographic studies of skull and cervical spine before proceeding with manipulation during the examination. Periorbital ecchymosis, hemotympanum, or CSF rhinorrhea and otorrhea indicate skull fracture. Early funduscopy will detect papilledema or hemorrhage as evidence for increased intracranial pressure. Intravenous access should be established and blood collected for laboratory studies, including CBC with differential and platelet count, basic chemistries with immediate glucose determination, liver tests, TSH, blood culture, and toxicology screen. Urine should be sent for the additional toxicology tests as well as routine analysis and culture. Arterial blood gas analysis, chest x-ray, and ECG should be done as soon as possible (comatose patients will not report chest pain). Oxygen, thiamine, and 50 ml of 50% dextrose are given. **Naloxone** is administered if narcotic overdose is suspected, and **flumazenil**, if benzodiazepine overdose is suspected.

## Bedside Examination of the Comatose Patient

As the initial urgent management measures are deployed, a history is obtained from the patient's family, friends, and the medical record. Particular attention should be paid to the patient's recent health and behavior, medication changes, and the possibility of any recent trauma. The past medical history is of increased importance since little else may be known about the patient. Frequently, telephone calls to pertinent individuals may provide key information in diagnosing the cause of coma.

**TABLE 187.1. Causes of Coma**

| |
|---|
| Supratentorial lesions |
| Mass effect from edema, hemorrhage, infection or tumor |
| Posterior fossa lesions |
| Vertebrobasilar occlusion |
| Pontine or cerebellar hemorrhage |
| Other mass lesions (abscess or hemorrhage into a tumor) |
| Diffuse and multifocal causes |
| Hypoxic ischemic insult following cardiac arrest |
| Meningoencephalitis, carcinomatous meningitis |
| Drug intoxication |
| Renal or hepatic failure |
| Hypothyroidism, Addisonian crisis, hyperglycemia, hypoglycemia, acid-base disturbances |
| Nutritional deficiencies |
| Acute demyelination (disseminated encephalomyelitis, central pontine myelinolysis) |
| Seizures, especially nonconvulsive status epilepticus |

**TABLE 187.2. Principal Elements of Examination of the Comatose Patient**

Assessment of arousal
- Spontaneous movement
- Response to exogenous stimuli

Respiratory pattern
- Cheyne-Stokes respiration
- Irregular respirations

Pupil size, symmetry and reflexes

Ocular motility
- Spontaneous eye movements
- Oculocephalic reflex
- Oculovestibular reflex

Motor responses
- Spontaneous movement
- Abnormal posturing
- Response to pain
- Tone

*The five principal elements of the coma examination are assessment of arousal, respiratory pattern, pupils, ocular motility, and motor responses* (Table 187.2). Observation for any spontaneous movement or elements of arousal from internal or environmental stimuli is a useful, but often forgotten step. Next, the response to progressively increasing stimuli should be recorded. This begins with gentle verbal cues and progresses to more noxious stimuli by first calling the patient's name, then shouting or clapping, followed by perioral stimulation with a tongue blade and progressing to pressure in the supraorbital notch, over the sternum or to the nail beds. The patient should be uncovered so that any reactive movement can be observed. A one or two line statement describing the spontaneous and reflex responses is an accurate and useful way to record the state of arousal.

Spontaneous respiratory pattern is important. **Cheyne-Stokes respiration** is a pattern of periods of hyperpnea alternating with apnea. Bihemispheric lesions, congestive heart failure with cerebrovascular disease, and metabolic derangements (hepatic and renal failure and sedative intoxication) are causes. **Central neurogenic hyperventilation,** ascribed to lesions of the midbrain, is exceedingly rare, and a systemic cause for hyperventilation is invariably present. Cheyne-Stokes respiratory pattern may deteriorate into an irregular periodic pattern indicating progressive dysfunction, such as with rostral caudal deterioration due to an expanding supratentorial lesion.

*Pupillary size*, symmetry, and reflexes are an essential part of the coma examination. Metabolic and toxic disturbances generally do not cause abnormalities of pupillary size and reactivity. Asymmetry in size and reactivity are most pronounced with midbrain and third cranial nerve lesions. *Probably the most important pupillary abnormality to recognize is the presence or development of a unilateral dilated and unreactive pupil suggesting compression of the midbrain from the medial aspect of the temporal lobe due to expansion of a laterally placed supratentorial lesion.* The pupillary change alone may herald this uncal herniation syndrome. On occasion, a pontine lesion will cause very small and weakly reactive pupils, sometimes referred to as **"pinpoint pupils."** One should suspect narcotic overdose when this is seen with no other brainstem abnormalities.

*Ocular movements* provide important information about brainstem function. Spontaneous full eye movements, while commonly roving and slow in coma, nevertheless indicate integrity of the third, fourth, and sixth cranial nerves. Horizontal dysconjugate gaze is relatively common in coma, while vertical separation more often indicates brainstem or cerebellar pathology. Any persistent gaze deviation suggests a destructive lesion, either in the ipsilateral cerebral hemisphere or contralateral pons. Ocular oscillations may be present. When the eyes seem driven downward and medially, insult to the diencephalon should be suspected, particularly as part of increasing pressure from a more rostral supratentorial lesion.

*Assessment of oculocephalic* and **vestibulo-ocular** reflexes should follow next. The term **oculocephalic responses** should be used instead of "dolls eyes," since the latter term is ambiguous. Any cervical spine trauma must be excluded prior to this test. The head is turned rapidly from one side to the other and the eyes are observed for any slow phase movement in the opposite direction. If the oculocephalic response is inadequate, then caloric stimulation of the vestibular labyrinth should follow, but only after careful examination of the external auditory canal and tympanic membrane for impacted cerumen or other pathology that might contraindicate the test. The absence of any response to oculocephalic maneuver and properly performed caloric stimulation strongly suggests disruption of the vestibulo-ocular pathways between the rostral medulla up to the mid pons and midbrain.

The *motor examination* also begins with observation for any spontaneous movement. Any asymmetry in spontaneous movement is particularly important. Motor responses to noxious stimuli may be either purposeful and localizing, or abnormal posturing movements. It can be difficult to determine which, although if the movement is toward the noxious stimulus, then this might indicate posturing. Abnormal upper extremity posturing can be either in flexion or extension. The latter indicates injury progressing below the diencephalon and into the brainstem, whereas flexion response occurs with hemispheric lesions above this level. Lower extremity posturing is extensor with both hemispheric and brainstem lesions, although becomes weakly flexor or flaccid with lower brainstem injury. Muscle stretch reflexes and plantar responses are tested, particularly looking for asymmetry and pathologic responses.

### Laboratory Evaluation of Coma

A non-contrast CT scan of the head is needed in the acute stage to detect hemorrhage, mass lesion, or edema. Imaging should always be obtained prior to lumbar puncture. A CSF examination is required for suspected subarachnoid hemorrhage, acute demyelination, vasculitis, infection or if the etiology is elusive despite initial studies. Electroencephalography (EEG) is important for the diagnosis of nonconvulsive status epilepticus, metabolic encephalopathies, encephalitis, and psychogenic coma. EEG should also be performed whenever the cause of coma is elusive.

### Continued Management of the Comatose Patient

Continued management of the comatose patient depends upon careful recording of serial examinations as treatment of the underlying cause is initiated. Nutrition management and usual precautions against complications of chronic immobility must also be remembered. Patients do not remain in a coma for longer than days or weeks and either begin to show recovery or progress to death or a persistent vegetative state. The latter is a condition where arousal patterns normalize with development of a sleep-wake cycle and yet are without evidence of conscious content. Studies using serial examination protocols to predict prognosis for comatose patients who have suffered hypoxic injury have been published.

# CHAPTER 188 HEADACHES

### Epidemiology and Pathophysiology

Headache is an extremely common symptom, with an estimated 40% of Americans having suffered from severe headaches at some point in their lives. Headaches may signal the presence of life-threatening illness, or be a chronic, recurrent, life-long condition. **Migraine** and **cluster headache** cause significant disability and days lost from work for some patients.

Pain-sensitive structures of the head and neck include the scalp, head and neck muscles, cerebral venous sinuses, dura, dural arteries, intracerebral arteries; the third, fifth, sixth, and seventh cranial nerves; and cervical nerves. Irritation of any of these structures will produce pain referred to the head, felt as headache. The neurotransmitter serotonin appears to play a role in at least the recurrent headache syndromes, since drugs that alter serotonin levels in the central nervous system affect headache frequency. Since such response is not universal, it indicates a role for other transmitters also.

## Sudden, Severe Headache

Sudden, severe headache in a patient not otherwise prone to headache should not be attributed to migraine without careful evaluation. **Subarachnoid hemorrhage** (SAH) from ruptured **intracerebral aneurysm** or **arteriovenous malformation** (AVM) must be considered, particularly if there is neck stiffness. Headache, neck stiffness, and fever suggest meningitis. **Intracerebral hemorrhage** usually produces focal neurologic deficits. Seizures may accompany any of the foregoing. With chiefly retro-orbital pain, **acute glaucoma** should be considered. **Acute sinusitis** presents with sinus tenderness and fever. **Acute hydrocephalus** from tumor, hemorrhage, or meningitis (cancerous or infectious) may present with altered consciousness, nausea, vomiting, and headache.

### Emergency Approach to Headache

Neuro-imaging should be performed on any patient presenting with a first, sudden, severe headache. A non-contrast CT suffices to demonstrate an acute bleed in a subarachnoid, intraparenchymal, epidural, or subdural locus. If tumor is suggested, a follow-up CT with contrast or MRI can follow. If suspicion of SAH lingers despite a negative CT, a lumbar puncture (LP) should be done. Fever, headaches, and nuchal rigidity strongly suggest acute bacterial or viral meningitis. This mandates LP and antibiotic therapy within one hour to cover for possible bacterial meningitis until CSF results become available. Proper use of CT in this setting is discussed in Chapter 160. Evaluation for pseudotumor involves a similar workup, imaging, and LP; sedimentation rate (ESR) is necessary in persons older than 50 years to exclude temporal arteritis.

## New, Progressive Headache

Conditions with prominent, new, progressive headache and subacute presentation include brain tumor, pseudotumor cerebri, and temporal arteritis. Progressive neurologic signs evolving over days to weeks suggest a **brain tumor**; a history of a known primary malignancy is helpful, but a malignant tumor may present initially with cerebral metastasis. Papilledema implies raised intracranial pressure and may be seen in brain tumor or hydrocephalus. It should prompt urgent neuro-imaging. If these processes are excluded, **pseudotumor cerebri** (papilledema, normal neural imaging, and elevated CSF pressure on LP) should be considered. **Temporal arteritis** should be excluded in anyone over 50 years of age with new onset of headaches; jaw claudication, muscle aches (polymyalgia rheumatica), fever, anemia, and weight loss may be associated. ESR is typically markedly elevated. Left untreated, this entity can cause blindness. **Subdural hematomas** can cause progressive headache and confusion, with or without focal signs; the preceding trauma need not be severe, especially if there is concurrent anticoagulant therapy. Non-neurologic systemic febrile illness also commonly causes headaches.

## Recurrent Headache Syndromes

## *Migraine*

### Etiology

Migraine headaches, recognized since ancient times, more commonly affect women. They typically begin in young adulthood and have a familial tendency. Dietary migraine triggers include ingestion of caffeine, alcohol, and food such as chocolate or aged cheeses. Disordered regulation of serotonin systems in the CNS has been implicated.

### Clinical Features

Migraine has 2 broad categories, classic and common. **Classic migraine** begins with an aura, which is typically visual and often described as flashing lights in one visual field, with a jagged configuration, leading to the term "fortification spectrum." This spectrum may move slowly across the visual field, leaving in its wake, a hemianopia. This visual disturbance may last 20–60 minutes. Tingling or numbness may be reported in the hand or side of the face, which spreads slowly over minutes in contrast to the spread of a sensory seizure. As the aura subsides, the headache begins. Described as pounding or throbbing, it is often accompanied by photophobia, nausea, and vomiting. It typically peaks within minutes to an hour and lasts one to several hours. The patient usually seeks a dark, quiet place to lie down. Sleep may end the pain. In some, the pain may last a day or two. **Common migraine** lacks aura or neurologic symptoms; the pounding headache may be associated with nausea and vomiting.

The term **complicated migraine** is used when objective neurologic deficits accompany the headache. Aphasia, hemiparesis, or third nerve palsies may transiently follow migraine. However, other causes of headaches and focal deficits such as stroke, AVM, aneurysm, or tumor must first be excluded.

### Diagnosis

**Migraine headaches** should be differentiated from other causes of recurring headaches, such as cluster or muscular headaches, as well as AVM. AVM may present with a long history of recurring pounding headache with pain that is usually unilateral. **Cluster headaches** are primarily nocturnal and brief, associated with conjunctival injection and tearing. Features of cluster and migraine may overlap in some patients, and others may share features of migraine and muscle **contraction headache**. Diagnosing migraine requires an accurate headache history. With typical features, confusion seldom arises. Neurologic examination should be normal. Atypical features in history, complicated migraine, and abnormal examination call for neuro-imaging. Even in the migraine patient, a change in headache character or lack of response to therapy may necessitate imaging. Migraine with a third nerve palsy may require cerebral angiography to exclude a cerebral aneurysm.

### Management

#### Acute migraine

Although rest combined with acetaminophen or nonsteroidal anti-inflammatory agents (NSAIDs) suffice in some patients to abort a headache, for many others, these are inadequate. Analgesic combinations that contain codeine or barbiturates can help occasional headaches; however, for those patients with frequent migraines, these agents may entail both drug dependence and withdrawal headaches. Limitation of weekly and monthly use is important in the successful use of these agents. Ergotamine given by tablet or nasal aerosol can effectively abort migraine with aura. A dose taken at the onset of the aura can prevent the headache. Dihydroergotamine (DHE), given IM, can also help abort a refractory attack. Because it causes pronounced nausea, an antiemetic should be given simultaneously. A new class of 5-hydroxytryptamine-1 receptor agonists is very effective in abortive therapy. Sumatriptan, the first used agent, is currently the only one available in oral, nasal, and injectable forms. The injection acts rapidly, usually within a matter of minutes and is nonsedating. Its use must be limited to 2 injections per day. Several patients experience tightness and discomfort in the chest, the so-called "triptan syndrome," and these agents are contraindicated in patients with coronary artery disease and uncontrolled hypertension. Other oral agents (zolmitriptan, naratriptan, and rizatriptan) are sometimes better tolerated albeit slightly less potent.

### Prophylaxis

When the number of migraine episodes exceeds 3–4 per month, prophylactic therapy, combined with abortive therapy, is reasonable. With any prophylactic agent, a few weeks of therapy must elapse before changing the dose or ascertaining effectiveness. Amitriptyline, usually begun with 25 mg at bedtime and increased gradually, is effective for prophylaxis. Side effects include dry mouth, constipation, blurry vision, and sedation. Its sleep-promoting effect can be a plus when there is sleep disturbance. Calcium channel blockers, such as verapamil, or the beta-blocker, propranolol, in doses similar to that used for hypertension, can also be extremely effective for prophylaxis. Beta-blockers may cause fatigue, dizziness, and exercise intolerance. Use of both these agents has been simplified by sustained release formulations.

## Muscle Contraction Headaches

Muscle contraction headache is sometimes used as a nonspecific term for headaches that "do not fit the mold." Often referred to as tension headaches, the pain is reportedly steady, nonthrobbing, "band like" or "vise like," with no associated nausea, vomiting, or visual changes. Onset is typically gradual. They generally do not interfere with work. Their pathophysiology is unknown. Physical examination is normal. Neuro-imaging is often not required, although cervical spine films may be necessary to evaluate for degenerative disease. Treatment depends upon the frequency and severity of these headaches. Acetaminophen and NSAIDs, taken on a daily basis, may be helpful. A tricyclic agent (amitriptyline) can be beneficial in refractory cases. Biofeedback may similarly be successful in motivated patients. Some consider this headache to be a manifestation of depression, and an assessment for depression is reasonable.

## Cluster Headaches

Cluster headache is relatively uncommon but six times more prevalent in men. "Cluster" describes a tendency for recurrence over a period of a few to several weeks. These tend to occur at the same time of day and are particularly nocturnal, often waking the patient from sleep. Onset is usually between ages 20–50. The headache begins rapidly, without aura, peaks within minutes, and is intense and brief (30–120 min). It most often affects an eye and/or temple; face, neck, ear, or head may or may not be involved. During an attack, tearing of the eye, conjunctival injection or transient **Horner's syndrome** may occur. A pain-free interval lasting months to years commonly follows a cluster. Family history of recurrent headaches is usually absent. Neurologic examination and imaging studies are usually normal. Attacks may be aborted by inhaling 100% $O_2$ for 10–15 minutes, or aerosolized ergotamine or sumatriptan injection. Effective preventive agents include prednisone, lithium, cyproheptadine, methysergide (risk of retroperitoneal fibrosis), indomethacin, and calcium channel blockers.

# CHAPTER 189 DIZZINESS

## Evaluation of the Dizzy Patient

**Dizziness** is a common complaint, and a variety of disorders produce symptoms evoking this description. A reasonable diagnosis can be determined in the majority of cases through a careful clinical assessment and selected ancillary tests. The four principal symptom categories that present with the complaint of dizziness are vertigo, syncope, dysequilibrium, and lightheadedness. Syncope is discussed in Chapter 36.

The patient should describe the problem without using the word "dizziness;" the history is then refined with specific inquiries. An illusion of self motion or environmental motion—vertigo—or a sense of impending faint should be explicitly determined. Often, syncope is initially accompanied by a sense of floating, drifting, or moving, and, likewise, vertigo may evoke a fear of fainting. One of the two sensations will generally predominate. Precipitating, palliative and temporal features must be detailed. Particular attention is given to the effect of physical activity and postural changes, as well as accompanying cardiac and neurologic symptoms.

The "dizzy" patient should receive a general physical examination, a standard neurologic examination, and special or provocative tests. A careful cardiovascular examination should be done, searching for dysrhythmias, murmurs, cervical and supraclavicular bruits, and evidence of peripheral vascular disease, and recording postural changes in blood pressure and pulse. Coordination should be tested and special attention paid to vision, eye movements, hearing, and lower extremity sensory function. Natural and tandem gait should be observed for a good distance while ensuring the patient's safety.

Romberg sign, and finger-to-nose, heel-to-shin, and rapid alternating movements should be examined, and nystagmus (spontaneous or position-induced) elicited.

## Vertigo

Vertigo is an illusion of self motion or environmental motion. Most often rotational, this may also be a sensation of tilt or linear motion. Dysfunction of the vestibular system, either centrally (brainstem vestibular nuclei and vestibulocerebellar pathways) or peripherally (labyrinth and vestibular nerve) is responsible; the initial challenge is to determine which one of these is operative. Determination of the underlying cause should follow next.

Generally, peripheral vertigo is more severe; nausea and vomiting are prominent. Patients fall toward the side of the vestibular lesion and have a jerk nystagmus (direction of nystagmus is denoted by the direction of the fast phase movement) away from the lesion. Direction of peripheral nystagmus will not reverse with eye position, and the magnitude is more likely to dampen with fixation. Facial weakness might occur in both central and peripheral vertigo, but is most pronounced in conjunction with lesions of the eighth nerve, since the facial nerve runs directly proximate to it. Other features are shown in Table 187.1.

### Peripheral Disorders

Peripheral vestibular disorders cause vertigo in the majority of patients with dizziness. Patients with labyrinthine or vestibular nerve lesions usually report true rotational vertigo, often with a positional character. Common forms have distinguishing clinical features.

**Benign paroxysmal positional vertigo** (BPPV) is, perhaps, the most common form of peripheral vertigo; its incidence rises with age. The symptoms begin with a change in head position. Frequently, the patient notes the first attack when rolling over in bed. Hearing is usually not disturbed. A latency is present between the head rotation and the vertigo. Barany's maneuver (Figure 189.1) is important in eliciting the typical nystagmus of BPPV. In BPPV, there is a latency to the onset of nystagmus from 2–20 seconds. The nystagmus fatigues over a few seconds to a few minutes and may recur in the opposite direction on return to the sitting position. After repeating the maneuver a few times, there is habituation of the response. The nystagmus has a specific upward-rotatory character. Trauma and forms of labyrinthine inflammation or ischemia also manifest as BPPV. Most patients recover over days or weeks. A special exercise can hasten improvement (Figure 189.2). A few repetitions of this cycle are completed two or three times a day. Vestibular suppressants (meclizine, promethazine, diphenhydramine, astemizole, diazepam) may help in the acute phase. Any deviation from the typical character of symptoms, signs, positional nystagmus, or clinical course should raise concern for another etiology or central disturbance.

In **Meniere's disease**, sudden, severe attacks of disabling rotational vertigo of variable durations (minutes to 24 hours) occur, heralded by tinnitus and aural fullness or pain. Symptoms are worse with head motion but a definite postural precipitation is absent. The vertigo recurs at variable intervals from weeks to months. Documentation of sensorineural hearing loss is important to the diagnosis. Tinnitus varies in conjunction with the attacks and becomes more persistent as the disease progresses. Treatment consists of a sodium- and caffeine–restricted diet, diuretics and vestibular suppressants. The most disabling, refractory forms may require surgical intervention. Serial audiograms (it may progress to bilateral disease) and neuro-otologic consultation are essential.

**Labyrinthitis** and **vestibular neuronitis** may be due to viral infection or a postinfectious, immune-mediated inflammation. The pattern is one of nonrecurrent, acute or subacute peripheral type vertigo occurring within a few weeks of a viral illness. Symptoms usually last days to weeks, although milder symptoms may persist longer. The vertigo gradually resolves as the inflammation subsides and central compensatory mechanisms evolve. Treatment is supportive in the acute phase, with hospitalization being required for disabling nausea, vomiting, and ataxia. Short-term use of vestibular suppressants and a course of physical vestibular therapy help the recovery.

### Central Disorders

A central lesion is suggested when the vertigo and constitutional symptoms are less intense, despite significant ataxia and nystagmus. The presence of brainstem symptoms (diplopia, dysarthria, dysphagia, vision loss) and signs (facial or appendicular motor and sensory changes) clearly point to a central localization. Abnormalities of eye movement or pupil function (e.g., Horner's syndrome) often betray a brainstem lesion. Limitation of eye movement, especially internuclear ophthalmoplegia, skew deviation (vertical dysconjugate eye position), gaze paresis, or specific palsies of cranial nerves III, IV, or VI, implicates brainstem pathology. Cerebellar tremor and appendicular ataxia point to a direct lesion of the cerebellum or its pathways. Corticospinal tract dysfunction or hemisensory loss, which should be contralateral to brainstem findings, strongly support a central lesion. Neuro-otologic consultation and electronystagmography (ENG) may help distinguish between peripheral and central lesions.

Central lesions causing vertigo involve the vestibular nuclei, their projections to the ocular motor nuclei, and cerebellum or the cerebellum itself. Contrasting features of central vs. peripheral vertigo and nystagmus are mentioned above and summarized in Table 189.1. A few causes of central vertigo deserve specific mention.

**Brainstem ischemia** due to thromboembolic disease of the vertebrobasilar circulation may cause acute and recurrent central vertigo. Generally, there are cranial nerve, cerebellar, visual field, or long tract symptoms and signs. Transient ischemia, causing deficits lasting minutes, commonly precedes brainstem infarction and are often reported as "dizzy spells." Suspicion for such a vascular cause of vertigo increases when patients have risk factors for cardiac and cerebrovascular disease. These patients require a swift evaluation and initiation of stroke prevention therapy including antiplatelet aggregation agents or possible anticoagulation. Urgent hospitalization is necessary for presumed acute ischemia or if there is a history of increasing frequency and severity of transient vertigo with concern for progressive vertebrobasilar insufficiency.

In **multiple sclerosis** (MS) and other demyelinating disorders, vertigo is usually more subacute, worsening

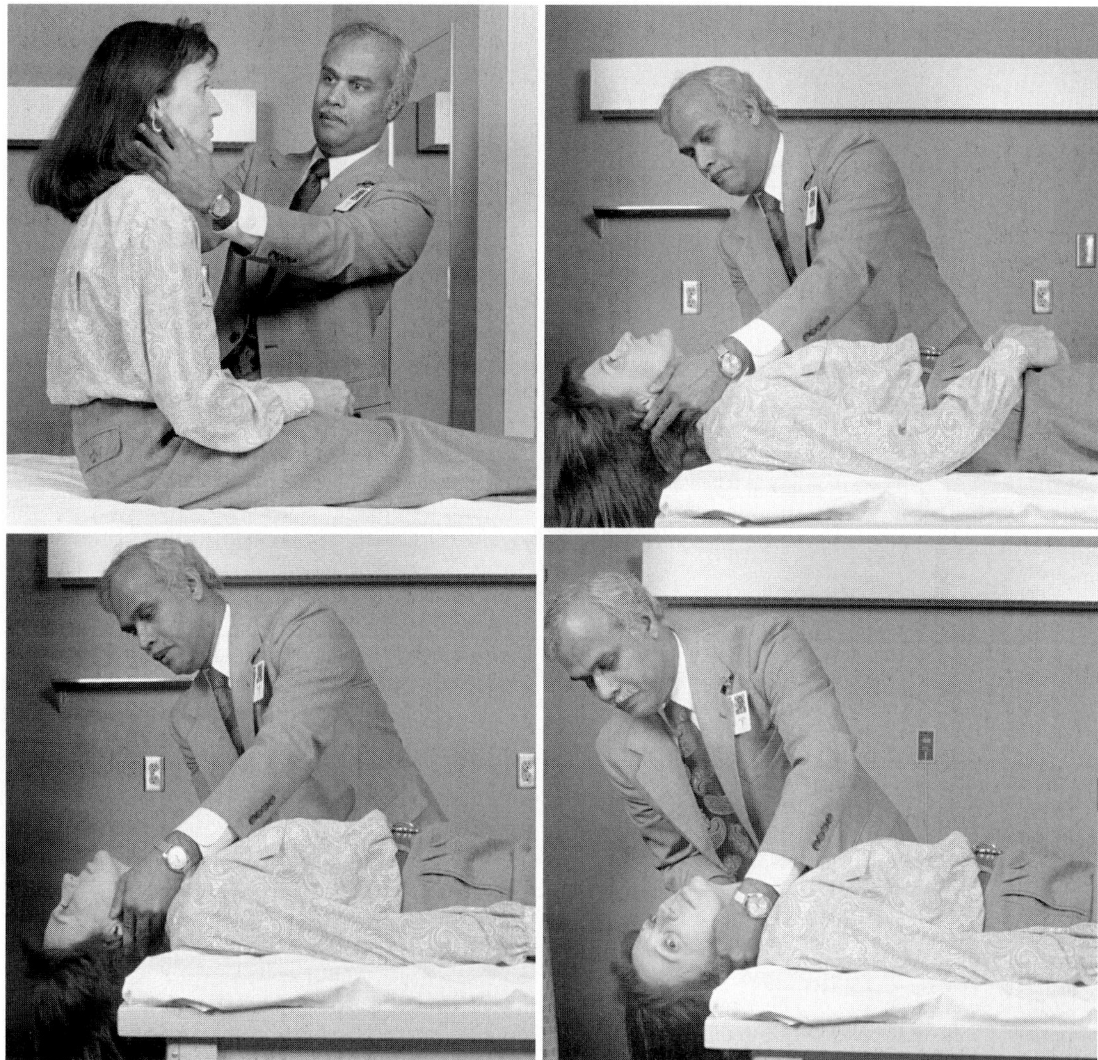

**FIGURE 189.1.** Barany's maneuver. The patient is positioned with the head hanging 30–45° over the table edge first in the midline, which is repeated with the head rotation to right and left. Frames 1 through 4 show the procedure in sequence.

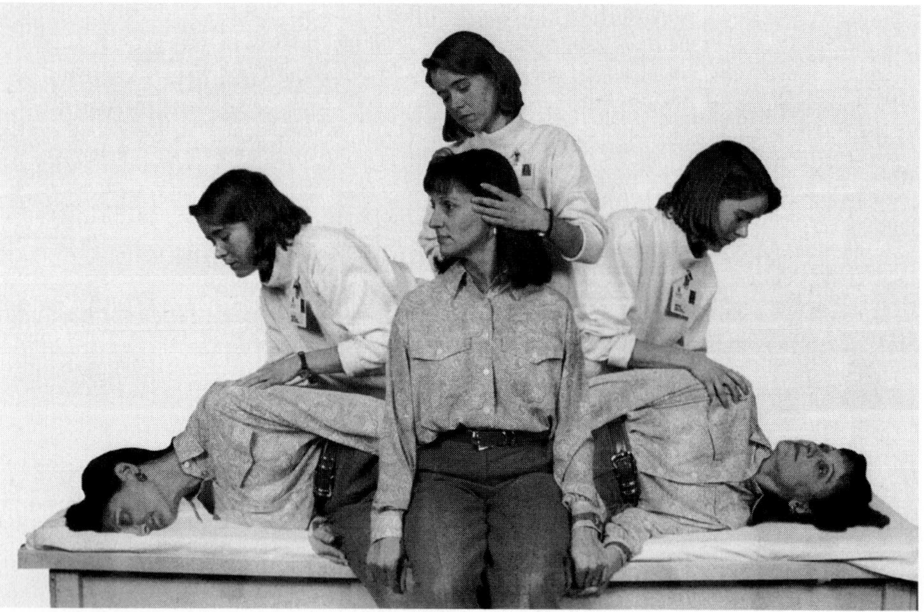

FIGURE 189.2. Special exercise to hasten improvement in BPPV, performed by sitting on the edge of a bed, turning head to one side by 45° and moving sequentially to the right or left and back to the sitting position, each time allowing the vertigo to nearly extinguish prior to making the next move. The entire sequence is shown with the motions superimposed.

TABLE 189.1. Differentiating Between Peripheral and Central Vertigo

| Criterion | Peripheral | Central |
|---|---|---|
| Direction of nystagmus | Unidirectional, fast phase away from lesion | Bi- or unidirectional; may change with direction of gaze |
| Pure vertical or rotary | Never | Possible |
| Pure horizontal without rotary | Uncommon; usually horizontal or vertical with rotary component | Common |
| Visual fixation | Inhibits nystagmus and vertigo | No inhibition |
| Intensity of vertigo and constitutional symptoms | Severe | Often mild to moderate; may be severe |
| Environmental movement | Toward fast phase of nystagmus | Variable |
| Romberg fall and past pointing | Toward slow phase of nystagmus | Variable |
| Tinnitus or deafness | Often present, unilateral; important clue | Usually absent |
| Latency to vertigo and nystagmus after position change, and habituation of response | Often present | Usually absent |

(From: Danoff RB. In Harrison's Principles of Internal Medicine. Isselbacher KJ et al. (ed.). 13th ed. New York: McGraw Hill, 1994. Used with permission.)

over hours to days, but can be rather rapid. Distinction from labyrinthitis and vestibular neuronitis rests on the central features and cranial nerve or long tract findings. Certainly, vertigo occurring in a patient with known MS is presumed to be from an acute demyelinating lesion, unless proof for a peripheral vestibular etiology is overwhelming. Patients with probable central vertigo having clinical features consistent with a demyelinating disorder should be referred to a neurologist for a more detailed examination. An MRI and CSF examination are often necessary.

**Acoustic neuromas** usually originate from Schwann cells in the vestibular portion of the eighth nerve at or near the internal auditory meatus. Their slow growth allows ample time for central compensation of the disordered vestibular input, making acute vertigo infrequent. However, when it occurs, it typically has more of a peripheral character. Progressive hearing loss with poor speech discrimination and tinnitus are typically the most prominent early symptoms. Enlargement of these tumors in the cerebellopontine angle causes compression of adjacent cranial nerves and brainstem, e.g., facial anesthesia and weakness. Ataxia and disequilibrium worsen and long tract signs begin to emerge. Early detection is paramount; surgical resection is the treatment. Brainstem auditory evoked responses are sensitive to changes early in the course.

### Disequilibrium

Another important category of dizziness, best termed disequilibrium, is really a sense of imbalance and unsteadiness, worsened by walking, turning, and in certain provocative situations. Postural stability depends on reliable sensory input from vision, vestibular function, joint position, skin pressure, and light touch sensation. A disturbance of any one of these systems will cause some element of instability, with compensation through undue dependence on the other sensory inputs. Dysfunction in multiple systems destroys this compensatory agility. For instance, an elderly diabetic patient with peripheral neuropathy and mild labyrinthine disease who develops a retinal artery occlusion may become severely impaired, since maintaining posture is critically dependent on normal vision and stereopsis. More commonly, the alterations are slow to develop and less dramatic, resulting in a complaint of increasing "dizziness." Abnormal muscle strength and tone, skeletal/joint deformity, and cervical spondylosis and myelopathy could compound the patient's difficulty.

Primary diseases of the cerebellum also lead to disequilibrium. Appendicular and gait ataxia, hypotonia, diminished reflexes, central nystagmus, and ocular dysmetria may be found. Alcoholic cerebellar degeneration affects the anterior vermis preferentially, and, therefore, the disturbance of axial stability and gait is much more pronounced than that of appendicular metrics.

### Lightheadedness

This category represents a wide variety of causes. These patients find it difficult to characterize the sensation any further than dizzy or lightheaded, and yet may affirm any other symptom description suggested. They are more likely to report the experience as being constant and daily. The largest subset in this group is psychogenic dizziness, with depression and anxiety disorders most commonly encountered. Panic attacks, phobic disorders—especially agoraphobia, and somatization often feature dizziness as one of the presenting complaints. It is also important to remember that patients with episodic vertigo develop varying degrees of anxiety regarding recurrent attacks, especially toward the possibility of incapacitation in public. They may report features that closely resemble a primary neurosis or phobic disorder. Additionally, the cardiovascular and extrapyramidal side effects of many psychiatric medications easily cause syncope and postural instability. Finally, patients with early dementia and confusional states may report their advancing cognitive disability as dizziness.

# CHAPTER 190 STROKE

Stroke is the third leading cause of death and the leading cause of adult disability in the United States. It is increasingly considered a serious neurologic emergency warranting expedient evaluation, acute treatment, and carefully considered preventive measures. Just as effective medical and surgical interventions for coronary artery disease have evolved over the past several decades, so has management of cerebrovascular disease evolved away from a nihilistic "watch and wait" attitude toward an increasingly interventional and analytical approach, bolstered by the results of several recent, successful clinical trials.

Stroke is a sudden neurologic deficit or symptom attributable to vascular disease of the central nervous system, encompassing many diverse entities, including transient brain ischemia, brain infarction, brain hemorrhage, subarachnoid hemorrhage, and vascular disease of the spinal cord. The most common of these by far is brain infarction. Brain infarction may follow embolism, large artery atheroma, and small vessel occlusion. The term "transient ischemic attack" (TIA) has traditionally been applied to clinical syndromes lasting less than 24 hours, however, many, if not most, "TIAs" lasting more than 1 hour are associated with some degree of brain infarction.

## Ischemic Stroke

### Pathophysiology

**Ischemic stroke** is caused by embolic occlusion in one-third or more of cases. Potential sources of emboli include the heart (atrial fibrillation, sick sinus syndrome, myocardial infarction with mural thrombus, dysfunctional or artificial valves, congestive cardiomyopathy, and infective endocarditis), the proximal internal carotid and vertebral arteries, the aortic arch, and the deep venous system. Patent foramen ovale (PFO) is increasingly recognized as a conduit for paradoxical embolism. Emboli from the aortic arch and cervical vessels may arise from the irregular surface of atherosclerotic lesions. Hypercoagulable states, including pregnancy, oral contraceptive therapy, and antiphospholipid syndrome may increase the likelihood of embolization by promoting thrombus formation at any of these sites. Emboli most typically cause large (>1 cm) infarcts involving the cortical surface, basal ganglia, or cerebellum.

The small vessel or "**lacunar**" stroke, seen in roughly 20% of ischemic strokes, arises from gradual occlusion of a small arteriole following hypertension-induced necrosis, atherosclerosis, and lipid deposition. Since the area supplied by the affected vessel is small, occlusion causes a small (<1 cm) infarct, located typically in the basal ganglia, internal capsule, thalamus, or pons. Ischemia may result, albeit less commonly, from occlusion or tight stenosis of a large artery (e.g., the carotid, vertebral, or basilar). In that case, infarction may be visible in the surface or deep white matter **"watershed"** areas (boundaries between main vascular territories). Uncommon causes of ischemic stroke include arterial dissection, vasospasm due to migraine, and cerebral vasculitis.

## Clinical Features

Neurologic symptoms of ischemic stroke begin suddenly, although patients may be unaware or only gradually aware of their own deficits. This unawareness (anosognosia) is particularly likely with right hemispheric lesions. Common features of brain ischemia include unilateral weakness (**hemiparesis** or **hemiplegia**), unilateral visual field deficit in both eyes (**hemianopia**), impaired speech production or comprehension (**aphasia**), and unilateral sensory deficit. Brainstem ischemia (vertebro-basilar system) may cause nausea and vomiting, vertigo, gait imbalance, diplopia, dysphagia, dysarthria, or ptosis. Ischemic stroke may impair alertness, or cause sudden disorientation, inability to remember new information, deviation of the eyes or head to one side, and inability to read. These features may be isolated or combined with other impairments. While not a stroke by definition, retinal ischemia (brief monocular blindness, or amaurosis fugax) may be associated. Lightheadedness is not a symptom of stroke, and is possibly due to anemia, hypovolemia, autonomic dysfunction, vasovagal phenomena, or cardiac arrhythmia.

## Management

Despite the highly promoted distinction between "completed stroke" and TIA, there is no reason to treat these syndromes differently from a management point of view. Patients with TIA might be considered more urgently in need of attention, given the potentially greater opportunity to prevent permanent deficits. Acute management of ischemic stroke includes airway protection as needed, ECG to exclude arrhythmia and myocardial infarction, correction of anemia, dehydration, and glucose abnormalities, neurology consultation and urgent CT to exclude hemorrhage. Most patients with acute stroke are hypertensive at presentation, which may in part be a normal physiological pressor response to ischemia. Antihypertensive medications should be avoided or used with great caution in these cases, and only if the systolic pressure persists above 220 mm Hg. A recent multicenter trial found that systemic tissue plasminogen activator (tPA) administered within three hours of a stroke improved patient outcomes significantly. Careful evaluation is necessary before this drug is administered, given the significant risk of cerebral hemorrhage. Other thrombolytic and neuroprotective agents are currently being evaluated for their ability to minimize brain injury.

Intravenous heparinization is recommended for patients with cardiogenic embolism devoid of very large brain lesions (i.e., half of a hemisphere or more). However, stroke complicating bacterial endocarditis should be treated with antibiotics without any heparin, given the inherent risk of mycotic aneurysmal rupture. Heparin is given to reduce the risk of early recurrence of embolism, which probably exceeds 10% during the first 2 weeks after cardiogenic stroke. The risk of fatal hemorrhage is higher with a very large infarct, which outweighs the benefit of heparin in such patients. Heparin is usually given as a constant infusion, beginning with 800–1000 units per hour depending on age and body mass. The author does not recommend an initial loading bolus. Heparin may also be used in patients with an unknown or uncertain mechanism of infarction, pending diagnostic tests to exclude a cardiac source. Heparin is often given to patients with TIAs in an attempt to prevent subsequent infarction and to help predict the response to oral anticoagulation. Heparin is indicated for cranial arterial dissection, as the usual mechanism of stroke in such patients is embolism from the dissection site.

An expedient evaluation should follow, to clarify the mechanism of ischemia. This determination is relatively straightforward, using lesion size and location information from a brain image. At present, brain imaging between 2–7 days after onset with either CT or MRI perhaps most reliably distinguishes embolic, lacunar, and watershed infarctions (Figure 190.1 and Figure 190.2).

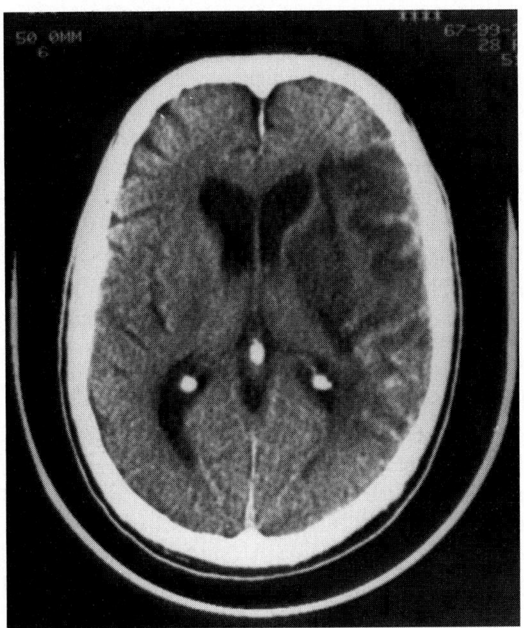

**FIGURE 190.1.** Head CT scan shows a hemorrhagic infarction of embolic origin involving the distribution of the left middle cerebral artery.

Carotid and vertebral duplex Doppler studies can adequately detect severe extracranial stenosis. Large stenoses in the distal internal carotid or basilar arteries, if suspected, can be detected noninvasively by transcranial Doppler or MR angiography. Echocardiography is necessary in those with a suspected cardiac embolic source. Transesophageal echocardiography is superior for detecting PFO and for visualizing the left atrium, atrial appendage, and aortic arch, and should be performed in patients with suspected embolism in whom the transthoracic echocardiogram is not revealing. Cardiac Holter monitoring or loop recording may occasionally detect paroxysmal atrial fibrillation. Catheter angiography is reserved for cases with suspected intracranial stenosis, dissection, or arteritis, in whom other tests have been not revealing. In young patients (<50 years) and older patients with no clear cause for stroke, a workup for occult hematologic abnormalities is recommended, including prothrombin time (PT), partial thromboplastin time (PTT), anti-nuclear antibodies (ANA), serum protein electrophoresis (SPEP), serological tests for syphilis (STS), sedimentation rate, lupus anticoagulant, anticardiolipin antibody, protein C, protein S, and antithrombin III.

Long-term warfarin therapy is generally recommended to prevent recurrence in patients with emboli of cardiac source. Aspirin has been suggested as a treatment for patients with noncardiogenic causes of ischemic stroke, although the risk reduction associated with aspirin, regardless of the dose, is only 20–25%. A recent trial found that a combination of low dose aspirin (50 mg) and sustained-release dipyridamole (400 mg; EPSP2 study) was significantly superior to aspirin alone in preventing future ischemic stroke. Cost of the drug and iatrogenic headaches are the major limiting factors. Another alternative in this group is ticlopidine, an antiplatelet agent that, in one controlled study, was significantly superior to aspirin for secondary prevention. Ticlopidine has some intolerable side effects; complete blood counts (CBC) must be monitored every 2 weeks during the first 3 months of therapy, given the risk of neutropenia during this interval. Clopidogrel is another useful antiplatelet, but is perhaps less effective than the latter two choices; its advantage is its high safety profile.

Patients who are good surgical risk with significant carotid disease demonstrated by duplex imaging should undergo carotid angiography. With high-grade (>70%) carotid stenosis, surgery is superior to aspirin in preventing stroke recurrence. In such cases, carotid endarterectomy should be performed by an experienced surgeon, whose documented perioperative stroke and mortality rates are low (i.e., total <5%). The benefit of surgery in moderate (40–69%) stenosis is possibly below that in severe stenosis, but studies are ongoing to assess this; the skill of the surgeon would perhaps be crucial in this setting.

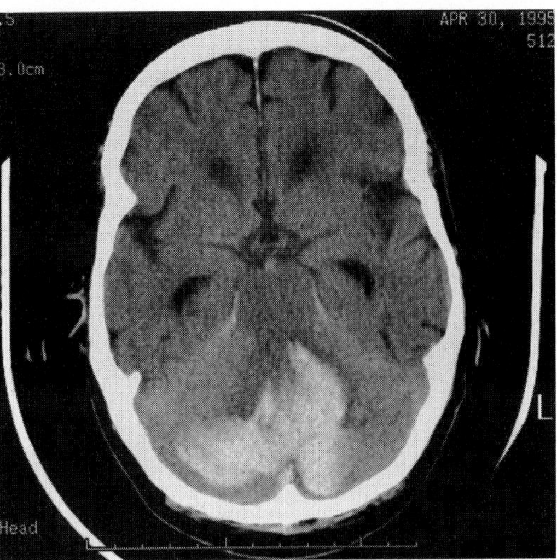


**FIGURE 190.2.** Head CT scan of a patient with cerebellar hemorrhage. This hypertensive woman developed dizziness and sudden inability to walk.

## Intracerebral Hemorrhage

### Etiology and Pathophysiology

The most common type of intracerebral hemorrhage is the "hypertensive" bleed, which occurs when a small, deep vessel weakened by chronic hypertension **(Bouchard's aneurysm)** ruptures. A large bleed may raise intracranial pressure sufficiently to impair consciousness, or cause brain herniation and death. Cerebellar hemorrhage is particularly ominous, given its proximity to the brainstem. Patients who survive the acute bleed, even a fairly large one, often recover remarkably well, because permanent damage is usually limited to the ischemic zone immediately surrounding the bleed. A bleed in the hemispheric white matter is not usually due to hypertension. Possible causes include vascular malformation, brain tumor, amyloid angiopathy, mycotic aneurysm, cerebral venous thrombosis, coagulopathy, anticoagulants, thrombolytic agents, vasculitis, and sympathomimetic drugs, including cocaine.

### Clinical Features

Clinical signs of intracerebral hemorrhage are the same as those listed for ischemic stroke. While patients with intracerebral hemorrhage tend to be somewhat younger, more hypertensive, more stuporous, and report headaches more than patients with ischemic stroke, hemorrhage should be differentiated from infarction by CT scan rather than by the clinical presentation.

### Management

Emergency evaluation includes airway management if needed, ECG, coagulation tests including PT, PTT, CBC, and platelet count, and emergent CT. Toxicology screen is useful in young patients. Blood pressure, if elevated, is reversed gently to maintain the systolic below 180 mm Hg. Urgent neurology or neurosurgery consultation should be obtained. Alert patients with small hemorrhages may be observed on a general inpatient ward with frequent monitoring of vital signs and mental status. Patients with impaired alertness or large hemorrhages, being at high risk for deterioration, brain herniation, and death from increased intracranial pressure, should be admitted to an intensive care unit experienced in cerebral hemorrhage management.

Surgical evacuation of intracerebral hemorrhage/hematoma, while controversial, is sometimes undertaken in patients who deteriorate despite intensive medical treatment for elevated intracranial pressure. However, surgical evacuation to prevent brainstem compression is usually recommended in cerebellar hemorrhage, if the hematoma exceeds 3 cm in diameter. For those with unexplained bleed and without hypertension, a search is made for the cause of bleeding. MR scan with gadolinium contrast will detect most vascular malformations and brain tumors. Catheter angiography is often necessary to detect or exclude aneurysm, vasculitis, venous thrombosis, and very small vascular malformations. Pressure effects during the acute period may obscure small aneurysms, tumors, and malformations. Definitive exclusion of these causes requires follow-up MRI and angiogram after resorption of the hematoma.

## Subarachnoid Hemorrhage

### Definition and Pathophysiology

Subarachnoid hemorrhage (SAH) results from rupture of an intracranial saccular aneurysm, most of which are located at the base of the brain near branch points of the major arteries. Bleeding into the subarachnoid space causes pain through elevation of intracranial pressure and meningeal irritation. Focal signs may occur from local pressure or ischemic effects on nearby brain tissue and exiting nerves. Recurrence of bleeding in the first few weeks after initial rupture is common (25%) and catastrophic. Vasospasm produces secondary infarction and is the most common cause of morbidity associated with SAH. It frequently occurs between 4–14 days after SAH and is due to irritation of blood vessels by subarachnoid blood. Other common complications of SAH are hydrocephalus, problems of antidiuretic hormone secretion (both inappropriate and deficiency), seizures, and brain injury from increased intracranial pressure.

### Clinical Features

The cardinal symptom is sudden, symmetric or asymmetric, severe pain in the head or neck. In nearly one-half of cases, consciousness is lost briefly or for days. Many patients present with drowsiness, while some experience primarily neck pain and stiffness due to meningeal irritation, as the blood settles in the cervical subarachnoid space. Nausea and vomiting are common; photophobia may occur. Focal neurologic signs, most commonly, hemiparesis, aphasia, and paralysis of 3rd and/or 6th cranial nerves, may be present.

The diagnosis of SAH is missed in roughly 25% of cases. Misdiagnosis is particularly common when symptoms are less severe. The combination of neck stiffness and nausea may resemble a viral syndrome, while that of headache, nausea, and photophobia may simulate migraine. One should consider SAH when there is abrupt neck pain or headache, particularly if the patient perceives the pain symptoms to be in any way different from past experience(s).

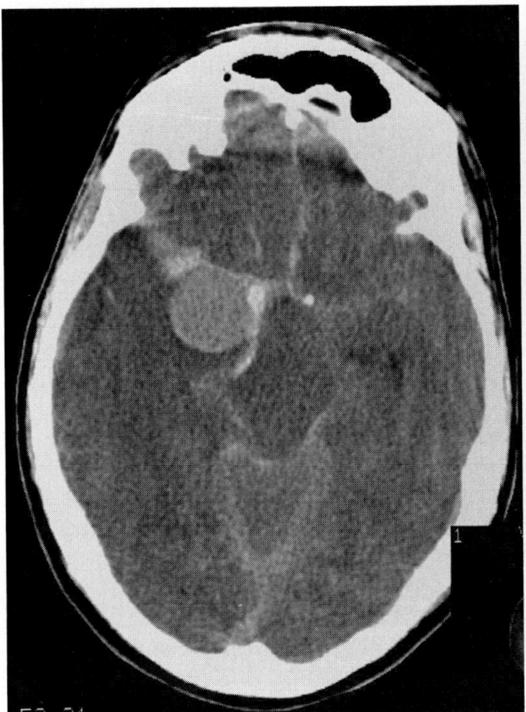


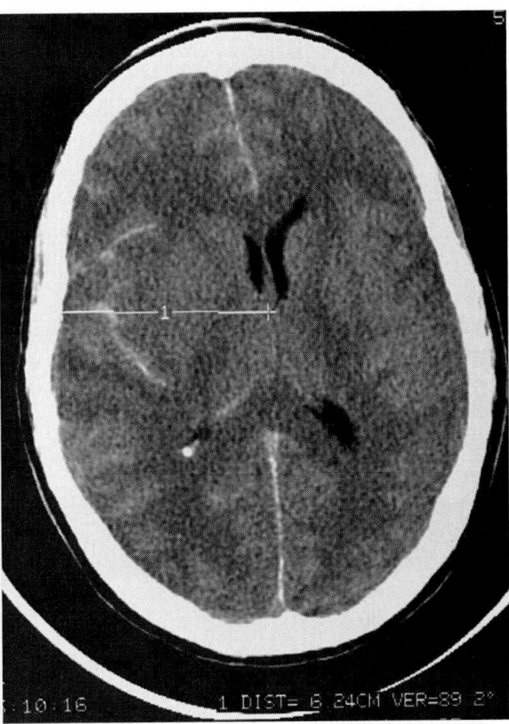


**FIGURE 190.3. A. Head CT scan shows subarachnoid hemorrhage secondary to aneurysmal rupture. Midline shift is evident. The scan also shows a large aneurysm, which was the source of the bleed. Aneurysms of this size are unusual. B. Same case as 190.3A, at a level above the aneurysm showing midline shift.**

### Management

Urgent CT must be done when SAH is suspected. It is positive in nearly 90% of cases, the subarachnoid blood appearing as a bright area surrounding the brain or settling within the ventricular system on noncontrast images (Figure 190.3). Because CT may miss a small bleed, the diagnosis should be pursued using lumbar puncture (LP) when CT is negative and the suspicion is strong. The cerebrospinal fluid (CSF) is sent for cell count and other tests; a centrifuged sample is examined for xanthochromia. Xanthochromia in the CSF may take 3–4 hours to appear after symptom onset, as it entails breakdown of red blood cells. Xanthochromia may persist for more than a week; thus, patients presenting many days after the onset of symptoms may still be reliably diagnosed by LP. Once SAH is diagnosed, patients should be transferred urgently to an intensive care unit (or one where expert SAH management is available). Bed rest, stool softeners, analgesia, and treatment of high blood pressure are undertaken to minimize the risk of recurrence of bleeding. Nimodipine, a lipophilic calcium channel blocker, is effective in reducing brain injury from vasospasm after SAH, in a dose of 60 mg q 4h, given for 14–21 days after onset.

Definitive treatment for SAH consists of surgical clipping of the aneurysm responsible. Catheter angiography is required to locate the aneurysm and for planning a surgical approach. Timing of angiography depends on the planned timing of surgery. With improvements in surgical technique and a growing recognition of the dangers of early recurrence of bleeding, the trend is for surgery to be performed at the earliest possible opportunity. Many experienced centers now recommend urgent angiography and surgery on the first day after bleeding. Besides protecting against recurrence of bleeding, early clipping also makes possible the use of intravascular volume expansion therapy, which may lower the risk of vasospasm-induced ischemia.

## Primary Prevention of Stroke

The physician has a key role in the primary prevention of strokes by identifying patients at high risk and deploying suitable risk reduction strategies.

Hypertension is most strongly associated with stroke. Modern therapy of hypertension has probably brought forth the modest decline in strokes observed over the last several decades. Hypertension is the major cause in lacunar stroke and deep intracerebral hemorrhage, and contributes to accelerated atherosclerosis in larger cerebral arteries. Early diagnosis and therapy of hypertension, particularly in younger persons, remains the simplest and most effective means of stroke prevention. Diabetes mellitus and cigarette smoking are also strongly associated with stroke. Uncontrolled diabetes greatly accelerates cerebral atherosclerosis, particularly in small and medium-sized arteries. Cigarette smoking is most closely linked to large vessel disease, particularly, carotid bifurcation stenosis. Other modifiable stroke risk factors include elevated cholesterol and/or triglycerides, alcohol abuse, and obesity.

Nonvalvular atrial fibrillation (AF) increases stroke risk nearly fivefold, and accounts for about 75,000 strokes per year in North America alone. Nearly 1 in 3 persons with AF will experience a stroke. Warfarin reduces stroke risk in AF by roughly 70% (reductions range from 55–86% in different trials), with a risk of serious bleeding below 1% per year. The benefit of aspirin is less clear, with risk reductions ranging from 0–42%. It is now generally recommended that patients with AF be treated chronically with warfarin, maintaining the international normalized ratio (INR) between 2.0 to 3.0. This must be weighed against the perceived risks of anticoagulation in individual patients, and against the inconvenience and cost of monitoring and maintaining anticoagulation. The risk of major bleeding in the elderly (>75 yrs) treated with warfarin was 4.2% per year compared to 1.6% per year for aspirin in one study, although this finding requires further confirmation. There may also be subgroups of patients—e.g., younger patients with "lone" atrial fibrillation—in whom the risk of stroke is low enough that treatment costs and risks of warfarin outweigh any real benefits.

### Asymptomatic Carotid Artery Stenosis

In the Asymptomatic Carotid Atherosclerosis Study (ACAS; random assignment of patients with carotid stenosis exceeding 60% to either aspirin or aspirin plus surgery), the combined incidence of stroke or death from angiography and surgery was 3.5%. Despite this surgical/angiographic risk, the total stroke incidence in the surgical group was 4.8% compared to 10.6% in the nonsurgical group, a relative risk reduction of 55%. Therefore, it appears reasonable to recommend carotid endarterectomy in asymptomatic patients with angiographically defined stenosis exceeding 60% to reduce the risk of subsequent stroke. Patients must be appropriate surgical candidates and must undergo aggressive risk factor management and aspirin therapy before and after surgery. The success of the operation depends on an experienced surgical team with documented perioperative stroke and mortality rates of <3%, and a low rate of angiographic complications.

# CHAPTER 191 SEIZURES

Seizure is a sudden excessive electrical discharge in the brain leading to abnormal movement, abnormal sensation, or alteration of consciousness. Causes are numerous, some are benign, while others are life-threatening. A seizure is a symptom, not a diagnosis. It is not synonymous with epilepsy, which refers to an underlying tendency toward having seizures, and may be an inherited tendency or due to trauma, malformation, tumor, surgery, cerebrovascular anomalies, or idiopathic. Epilepsy can also be called seizure disorder, a term many patients prefer.

## Generalized Motor Seizures

A generalized motor seizure may begin with sudden, tonic posturing, which usually leads to a fall. Tonic contraction of the diaphragm causes apnea. Tonic-clonic activity follows with flexion and extension of the limbs, as apnea continues. The pupils dilate; incontinence and tongue biting may occur. The clonic movements then subside and respiration resumes. The pupils begin to react to light. The patient is now typically limp and poorly responsive. Postictal confusion and depression of consciousness follow, as the patient awakens tired and disoriented. Typically, there is amnesia for the seizure, part of the events preceding the seizure, and part of the postictal state.

### Focal Seizures

A focal seizure, depending on its brain locus, may lead to motor activity (motor cortex, focal motor seizure), sensory phenomenon (sensory cortex, sensory seizure; medial temporal lobe, olfactory hallucination), or alteration of consciousness (temporal lobe, partial complex seizure). Focal phenomena typically spread quickly, affecting contiguous areas of brain rapidly. Movement may spread from mouth to arm to leg because of contiguous representation of these areas in the motor cortex. Sensory phenomenon such as tingling or other paresthesias may quickly spread in a similar distribution. Mesial temporal lobe discharges may lead to olfactory hallucinations where a smell, which is frequently unpleasant, is perceived, or a rising abdominal feeling is noted. Temporal lobe discharges may also alter consciousness; the patient may become out of touch with the environment or stare or fumble with the hands. Posture is typically maintained. While there is typically amnesia for these events, consciousness is not lost.

### Auras

Auras conscious are phenomena the patient experiences from a focal electrical discharge and are actually focal seizures. Because amnesia from a partial complex or generalized seizure may involve the events immediately preceding the seizure, the memory for the aura or onset may be lost. If there is a history of an aura, the seizure is most likely focal in onset. If none, the seizure may be focal or generalized in onset. EEG can distinguish between these possibilities and help in the choice of anticonvulsant.

## *Considerations in Emergent Care of Seizures*

Emergency considerations in seizures are numerous. Upon initial evaluation, besides the ABCs (airway, breathing, and circulation), one must determine if the seizure is ongoing or has stopped. Status epilepticus is defined as ongoing seizure activity without return to normal consciousness. This includes continuous convulsions, as well as intermittent seizures that are interspersed with postictal confusion not proceeding to normal consciousness. Status epilepticus is a life-threatening condition requiring aggressive treatment. Glucose and thiamine should be administered at the onset, and blood obtained for anticonvulsant levels (if the patient was previously receiving them), general chemistry and toxicology screen. Benzodiazepines such as lorazepam control convulsions but may produce respiratory depression. A long-acting anticonvulsant, usually phenytoin, should be administered concurrently in a typical loading dose of 20 mg/kg. If seizures persist, phenobarbital 20 mg/kg may be added; however, significant respiratory depression necessitates intubation. If seizures continue, general anesthesia is next pursued to produce a burst suppression pattern on EEG.

The emergency approach to a self-limited seizure depends upon the history and examination. Is this an unprecedented or a breakthrough seizure in a patient already on anticonvulsant therapy? An unprecedented seizure merits careful analysis with a long differential diagnosis (Table 191.1). Seizures occur in 10–26% of

**TABLE 191.1. Differential Diagnosis of New Onset Seizures**

| |
|---|
| Subarachnoid hemorrhage |
| Arteriovenous malformation |
| Subdural/epidural hematoma |
| Stroke |
| Meningitis/encephalitis |
| Abscess |
| Tumor |
| Primary brain tumor |
| Metastatic |
| Metabolic derangement |
| Calcium, magnesium, sodium, glucose, others |
| Drug intoxication |
| Theophylline |
| Cocaine |
| Drug withdrawal |
| Alcohol |
| Benzodiazepines |
| Barbiturates |
| Anticonvulsants |
| Non-compliance |
| Associated with degenerative disease |
| Cerebral malformation |
| Post-traumatic |
| Birth injury |
| Impact seizure |
| Idiopathic |

cases of subarachnoid hemorrhage; blood is demonstrated by CT or lumbar puncture (LP). In meningitis and encephalitis, besides fever, headache, and seizures, neck rigidity may be present. LP will demonstrate pleocytosis and other abnormalities, depending on etiology (viral versus bacterial). Drug intoxication should be considered and patient's medications reviewed; drug screen (both licit and illicit) is performed. Cocaine use and alcohol withdrawal are common causes of seizures at some medical centers. Brain tumors, both primary and secondary, are characterized by progressive neurologic dysfunction over a period of days to months. Papilledema from increased intracranial pressure, or focal motor signs may be noted.

Emergency evaluation of a first-time seizure should include evaluation for metabolic disturbance, a drug screen, and a neuro-imaging study, either CT or MRI. CT is the initial procedure of choice in trauma, status epilepticus, and suspected subarachnoid hemorrhage. MRI is otherwise preferable because it demonstrates certain tumors and reveals smaller lesions than CT. EEG is generally not required urgently.

The differential diagnosis of chronic seizure disorder includes numerous entities. Symptoms suggestive of a seizure disorder include episodic impairment or loss of consciousness. Witnessed generalized seizures usually leave little doubt. Complex partial seizures may present with memory lapses that may initially be confused with other medical or psychiatric conditions. Witnessed staring spells or automatisms (e.g., lip smacking or fumbling with the hands) suggest partial complex seizures. Olfactory hallucinations just prior to events are highly suggestive of complex partial seizures.

Syncope and episodic metabolic disturbances are other causes of episodic alteration of consciousness. Syncope due to cardiac arrhythmias may be accompanied by a few clonic jerks, which may mimic a seizure. Episodes of hyperglycemia or hypoglycemia may alter consciousness or cause actual convulsions. Cardiac evaluation including 24-hour cardiac monitoring and/or blood screening for glucose abnormalities may be needed, depending on the history. Further workup for seizures will usually include a neuro-imaging study (CT or MRI). MRI may reveal subtle abnormalities such as mesial temporal lobe sclerosis, or evidence of tumor, stroke, trauma, or vascular anomalies and is the test of choice, a contrast-enhanced CT being the next best. Commonly, the scan may be entirely normal. Further studies such as angiography usually depend on the CT or MR findings. Unless the seizures are extremely frequent, EEG usually does not capture an event itself. Thus, a normal EEG does not exclude seizure.

### Pseudoseizures

Pseudoseizures mimic seizures, but are psychologically based. Many patients with pseudoseizures also have electrical (real) seizures. Diagnosis can be very difficult, and may be suggested by witnessing events with phenomena atypical for seizures. These include out-of-phase (asynchronous) clonic jerks, lateral head movements, and pelvic thrusting. Pseudoseizures are not influenced by anticonvulsant medications. Video EEG monitoring may be confirmatory. Treatment is difficult; patients may accept neither a psychological basis for the events, nor counseling.

**TABLE 191.2. Medications for Seizures**

| Petit Mal | Primary Generalized | Focal Generalization (±) |
|---|---|---|
| Valproic acid | Phenytoin | Phenytoin |
| Ethosuximide | Valproic acid | Carbamazepine |
| Gabapentin | Lamotrigine | Vigabatrin |
| Topiramate | Carbamazepine | Valproic acid |
| | Phenobarbital | Primidone |
| | Clonazepam | |

### Medication Management

The initial choice of an anticonvulsant depends upon the seizure type (Table 191.2). In general, it is best to maximize one medication before adding a second. When seizures escape their previous control, the most common cause is medication noncompliance. Others include lowered blood medication level due to drug interaction, alcohol withdrawal, sleep deprivation, or progressive neurologic lesion, particularly when new symptoms and signs appear.

The management should also include patient education to avoid precipitating events, e.g., alcohol use or sleep deprivation, and to be informed of their obligation to notify the Department of Motor Vehicles in their state regarding temporary suspension of driving privileges. Similarly, occupational adjustments need to be made. Tapering anticonvulsant therapy over a few months can be discussed with individuals who were seizure-free for 2 or more years, provided their examination, contrast imaging (CT or MRI), and EEG studies are all normal.

Refractory epilepsy requires a thorough evaluation in an epilepsy center. Prolonged monitoring often leads to surgical management. The most common interventions are modified temporal lobectomy and vagal nerve stimulation implant.

# CHAPTER 192 NEUROLOGIC ASPECTS OF LOW BACK PAIN AND NECK PAIN

The rheumatologic aspects of low back and neck pain are reviewed in Chapter 259. Spinal pain can be classified into the following major categories: local, referred, and radicular.

### Etiology

The pain of **acute disk rupture** is acute and radiating, with muscle spasm and stiffness, and exacerbated by coughing and Valsalva. Neurologic examination is abnormal. Because the first cervical root exits above C1, herniated intervertebral cervical disk affects the root corresponding to the lower vertebrae. The process reverses in the thoracic spine because the C8 root exits above T1, and therefore, a herniated thoracic intervertebral disk will affect the root corresponding to the higher vertebrae. This continues into the T12-L1 space. In the lumbosacral spine, the cauda equina roots angle in such a way that they exit above their corresponding vertebrae, and a herniated intervertebral disk at any level usually results in compression of the root one level below, unless the disk is extruded or far lateral in which case it compresses the root at that level (see Table 186.5). Most herniations occur at the C5-C6, C6-C7, L4-L5, and L5-S1 levels.

Other causes of neck or low back pain can be compressive or noncompressive. The first category includes all spinal neoplasms, which can be intramedullary, extramedullary-intradural, or epidural. Early and severe spine pain, followed later by weakness, typifies an epidural spinal process (e.g., Schwannomas, meningiomas, and metastatic tumors) while early weakness and sensory symptoms in association with a mild and rather vague pain exemplifies an intramedullary spinal process (e.g., ependymomas, gliomas, and syringomyelic conditions). Vascular malformations may present in either form. Noncompressive etiologies are mainly comprised of infectious or inflammatory disorders of the spine. They are discussed in Chapter 259.

### Approach to the Patient

History should focus on the location of the pain, its radiation, exacerbating/alleviating factors, associated neurologic symptoms, history of trauma or work injury, litigation, drugs, and malignancy. The general examination should search for signs of systemic infection, occult malignancy, tenderness, muscle spasm, spine and hip range of motion, and straight leg raising. The neurologic part of the examination should focus on the patient's affect and mood, presence or absence of muscle weakness, muscle atrophy, sensory loss, changes in the reflexes, and rectal examination, if there are sphincter complaints.

### Management

If spinal bony pathology appears likely and further imaging is desired, CT scan of the cervical or lumbosacral spine would be helpful. However, the soft tissue images have a lower resolution than that obtained from MRI. Disk protrusions or herniations may be radiologically present in some healthy asymptomatic adults, and their importance should be weighed clinically. Patients with persistent neck or low back pain or abnormal neurologic findings should undergo electrodiagnostic testing. This helps differentiate between radiculopathies and neuropathies, confirms the presence of radicular involvement, evaluates its activity, and allows its accurate localization.

The management of neck and low back pain depends chiefly on the underlying etiology. Conservative treatment, as outlined in Chapter 259, is the main therapy. Definite indications for surgical treatment include severe or progressive neurologic deficits, sphincter changes, or the failure of conservative management with emphasis on spine rehabilitation for 6 weeks. Following surgery for spine pain, at least one-third of the patients will be left with persistent pain and one-fourth would not be able to return to their previous work.

# CHAPTER 193 DISORDERS OF SPINAL CORD, NERVES, AND MUSCLES

## ■ Spinal Cord Diseases

The level of a spinal cord lesion is determined by the pattern of sensory and motor abnormalities. Because the spinothalamic fibers cross the midline over one to two segments, the location of a lesion may be one to two levels higher than found by dermatomal sensory examination. Acute cord lesions cause areflexia and hypotonia at, and below, the level of the lesion. With time, upper motor neuron signs (spasticity, hyperreflexia, extensor plantar responses) are present below the level of the lesion while lower motor neuron signs (atrophy, hyporeflexia) persist at the level of the lesion. Bowel and bladder dysfunction are hallmarks of spinal cord lesions. Lesions of the conus medullaris and cauda equina may be difficult to distinguish but should be suspected with early sphincter dysfunction, saddle anesthesia, or radicular pain of the lower extremities. Compressive myelopathies require urgent evaluation. MRI is the procedure of choice as it is noninvasive and the entire cord can be viewed, if necessary, to exclude multiple lesions. Myelography should be used if MRI cannot be obtained, to prevent any delay in diagnosis. High-dose corticosteroids are indicated while definitive treatment is determined.

Compressive lesions may be extramedullary or intramedullary. **Extramedullary lesions**, which may be intradural or extradural, often begin as a radicular process with unilateral weakness and/or pain radiating into a limb. Upper motor neuron signs are present early with hyperreflexia, spasticity, and Babinski sign. Sphincter abnormalities occur later. **Metastatic tumors** are classic examples of extradural extramedullary compressive lesions that cause cord compression, either by bony destruction or as epidural masses. Most frequent primary cancer sites are breast, lung, or prostate; others include lymphoma, multiple myeloma, melanoma, renal cell carcinoma, or sarcoma. **Primary bone tumors** may also cause bony destruction, as can osteomyelitis or tuberculosis (Pott's disease), leading to cord compression. Epidural abscesses occur more often in the immunocompromised, IV drug abusers, or diabetics. Fever and leukocytosis may be present. **Cervical spondylitic myelopathy** from narrowing of the spinal canal usually occurs in older persons. **Meningiomas** or **neurofibromata** are examples of intradural extramedullary lesions; their slow growth allows the cord time to accommodate; even large masses may thus produce sparse signs.

Spinal cord infarction may follow dissection, surgery, or trauma of the descending aorta. Occlusion or narrowing of the anterior spinal artery, which supplies all areas of the cord except the posterior columns, leads to dysfunction of all modalities below the level of the lesion, except vibration and joint position sense. Infectious processes causing intrinsic cord damage include HIV vacuolar myelopathy or HTLV-1-associated myelopathy. HIV vacuolar myelopathy generally involves the posterior and lateral cords and occurs with other neurologic symptoms of AIDS. HTLV-1-associated myelopathy occurs in only a small subset of infected patients, suggesting the myelopathy may be immune-mediated. Vitamin $B_{12}$ deficiency, with or without megaloblastic anemia, causes posterior column and lateral corticospinal tract damage. Patients display hyperreflexia and Babinski signs; the associated peripheral neuropathy causes decreased ankle reflexes. Some intrinsic lesions (e.g., demyelinating disease) are well-visualized by MRI, whereas others (e.g., $B_{12}$ deficiency) require further laboratory testing.

## Neuromuscular Diseases

The disorders of the neuromuscular system may involve the motor neuron, the peripheral nerve, the neuromuscular junction, or the muscle, and all manifest weakness as their hallmark. Patterns of weakness and associated clinical features for each of these major components are shown in Table 193.1.

### Motor Neuron Disease

The most common motor neuron disease is **amyotrophic lateral sclerosis** (ALS, Lou Gehrig's disease). This rarely familial, idiopathic disorder usually begins after the fourth decade with often asymmetric weakness and wasting of the hands. Less frequently, the onset is with weakness and wasting in either one lower extremity or in the bulbar innervated muscles. Cramps and fatigue are other symptoms. In most patients, its relentless progression is usually fatal in less than 5 years. The neurologic findings include scattered fasciculations, wasting of the affected muscles, and hyperreflexia with or without Babinski sign(s). Even when the onset is in one extremity, patients frequently develop progressive spastic dysarthria, dysphagia, and dysphonia. The sparing of the extraocular muscles, sphincters, sensory perception, and cognitive functions is striking, and so is the unique and characteristic combination of upper and lower motor neuron dysfunction. The latter is due to degeneration of both motor neurons and corticospinal tracts. Electromyographic examination shows diffuse denervation and confirms the diagnosis. Symptomatic treatment, rehabilitation, and support to the patient and family are important; there is no cure. Death is usually due to respiratory failure and/or aspiration pneumonia.

**TABLE 193.1. Differential Diagnosis of Weakness**

| Sign | Motor Neuron | Peripheral Nerve | Neuro-Muscular Junction | Muscle |
|---|---|---|---|---|
| Wasting | Yes | Yes | Absent | Late |
| Distribution | Distal<br>Bulbar | Distal | Cranial<br>Proximal | Proximal |
| Reduced reflexes | Late | Early | Late | Late |
| Brisk reflexes | Yes | No | No | No |
| Fasciculations | Common | Rare | Absent | Absent |
| Sensory loss | Absent | Present | Absent | Absent |
| Elevated CK | Rare | Absent | Absent | Frequent |
| Elevated CSF Protein | No | Yes | No | No |
| Nerve conduction | Normal | Abnormal | Normal | Normal |
| Motor decrement | Rare | Absent | Present | Absent |
| Electromyography | Neurogenic | Neurogenic | Normal | Myopathic |
| Muscle biopsy | Neurogenic | Neurogenic | Endplate | Myopathic |

CK = creatinine kinase.

## *Peripheral Nerve Disease*

Nerve dysfunction involving the sensory fibers, motor fibers, autonomic fibers, or a combination of these may afflict the cranial nerves, spinal nerve roots, brachial and lumbosacral plexus, and peripheral nerves. Sensory fiber dysfunction results in sensory loss, paresthesias, and pain. Motor nerve involvement causes weakness, wasting, and hypo- or areflexia. The involvement of the autonomic systems leads to trophic changes involving the bone and skin, in addition to sweating and cardiovascular abnormalities.

The most important step in approaching peripheral nerve disease is to characterize the pattern of deficit. **Mononeuropathy** refers to dysfunction in the territory of a single nerve, and is most often due to an acute compression or chronic entrapment of that nerve, e.g., carpal tunnel syndrome, peroneal neuropathy at the fibular head, or ulnar neuropathy at the elbow. Asymmetric involvement of multiple nerves is usually termed **mononeuritis multiplex** and indicates an ischemic condition such as seen in diabetes or connective tissue disease. Proximal and distal weakness with hyporeflexia or areflexia indicates **polyradiculoneuropathy** or a polyradiculopathy, most of which are inflammatory in origin. Finally, bilateral symmetric involvement of the peripheral nerves, usually greater distally, indicates a polyneuropathy and is the most common but least specific presentation of the peripheral nerve diseases.

**Polyneuropathy** can be hereditary or acquired. Hereditary types include 1) motor and sensory (Charcot-Marie-Tooth, Dejerine-Sottas, Refsum, metachromatic leukodystrophy, and Krabbe disease); 2) sensory and autonomic; 3) porphyria; and 4) amyloidosis. Acquired causes can be remembered by the mnemonic "INDICATE," outlined in Table 193.2.

The approach to peripheral neuropathy begins by confirming the diagnosis, usually through nerve conduction studies (NCV) and electromyographic (EMG) examination. In addition, EMG-NCV may elucidate a certain pattern of neuropathy that was not apparent clinically, such as an asymmetry among limbs, or over various nerve trunks in one limb that could provide clues to the etiology. Once the diagnosis is confirmed, preliminary studies should include CBC with differential, sedimentation rate, fasting chemistry, serum $B_{12}$ and folate, thyroid function tests, and chest x-ray. If these tests are unrevealing, additional tests (antinuclear antibody, serum protein electrophoresis, urine protein electrophoresis, 24-hour urine for porphyrins and heavy metals) should follow. If the etiology is still elusive, it is important to again review the patient's family history, drug, and occupational exposures. Further diagnostic studies include CSF analysis before proceeding with a nerve biopsy.

**TABLE 193.2. Etiologic Diagnosis of Acquired Polyneuropathy**

| | |
|---|---|
| **I** | Immune: acute inflammatory demyelinating polyneuropathy or Guillain-Barré syndrome, chronic inflammatory demyelinating polyneuropathy, sarcoidosis, connective tissue disorders |
| **N** | Nutritional deficiencies and malabsorption: vitamins $B_1$, $B_6$, $B_{12}$, folate, and vitamin E |
| **D** | Diabetes mellitus |
| **I** | Infections: leprosy, Lyme disease, HIV, herpes zoster, diphtheria |
| **C** | Cancer and dysproteinemia |
| **A** | Alcoholism |
| **T** | Toxic-metabolic: pharmaceutical or environmental, renal- or hepatic failure |
| **E** | Endocrine causes: hypothyroidism, acromegaly |

### Carpal Tunnel Syndrome

Carpal tunnel syndrome (CTS) is the most common entrapment neuropathy. Besides its occurrence in a variety of occupations involving frequent use of wrists and hands, as well as many medical conditions, CTS may occur for the first time during pregnancy, most probably because of volume expansion and fluid shifts. The symptoms reflect dysfunction of the median nerve underneath the flexor retinaculum, characterized by dysesthesias, which are more severe at night and involve primarily the first three digits. Pain at rest that may radiate more proximally up to the shoulder is another symptom. As the condition worsens, hypesthesia develops over the first three digits, sparing the palm, along with weakness in several of the thumb muscles and partial atrophy of the thenar eminence. Tinel's sign (paresthesia radiating into the fingers provoked by gentle tapping over the median nerve at the wrist) is helpful if found. The diagnosis is confirmed by NCV. Symptomatic relief may be obtained by using wrist splints during repetitive manual activities and at night. Underlying causes such as diabetes mellitus, acromegaly, hypothyroidism, gout, or rheumatoid arthritis should be sought and corrected, if possible. However, the definitive treatment consists of surgical section of the transverse carpal ligament.

### Guillain-Barré Syndrome

Also known as acute inflammatory demyelinating polyneuropathy (AIDP), Guillain-Barré syndrome (GBS) is the most dramatic of polyneuropathies, featuring acute onset of peripheral and cranial nerve dysfunction. No age or gender predilection is seen. Triggered by a viral illness, immunization, or surgery within 1–3 weeks preceding symptoms, it usually presents with distal paresthesias that show proximal extension, along with rapidly evolving distal and proximal muscle weakness and symmetric areflexia. The deficit usually peaks 3 weeks after the onset. Unilateral or bilateral facial nerve paralysis occurs in approximately one-half of cases. Autonomic instability may occur, particularly in more severe cases. GBS can cause respiratory failure requiring mechanical ventilation. CSF examination is characteristic and shows significant elevation of the protein without pleocytosis, the so-called albumino-cytologic dissociation. NCV-EMG reveal demyelinating polyneuropathy and confirm the diagnosis. Management includes close observation, supportive care, physical therapy, and mechanical ventilation once the vital capacity falls below 15 ml/kg (see Chapter 254), and treatment of the autonomic instability syndrome when present. Plasmapheresis for 2 weeks lessens the duration and severity of the neurological deficit, and is indicated whenever ambulation becomes difficult. IV gamma globulin administered over 5 days can be substituted in children or in hemodynamically unstable patients. Their combined use has not proven significantly superior to either modality alone. The prognosis is relatively good, particularly when NCV show well-preserved distal responses.

## Neuromuscular Junction Diseases

### Myasthenia Gravis

Myasthenia gravis (MG) is a common autoimmune disorder in which a cell-mediated immune response leads to the formation of various antibodies directed against the acetylcholine receptors. The initial rapid turnover of these receptors is followed by their later, complete destruction. The hallmark of MG is fatigability of the involved muscles, with predilection for the extraocular, other cranial, and proximal limb muscle groups. The pupils are spared. Intermittent initially, the symptoms tend to follow exertion or occur at the end of the day. As the disease progresses, they become constant with superimposed fluctuations. The presence of acetylcholine receptor antibodies in the serum establishes the diagnosis. However, being highly sensitive for only generalized MG, these antibodies are not detectable in a significant number of patients with more focal forms of myasthenia. Such cases are diagnosed on EMG. Repetitive nerve stimulation produces a decrement of the motor evoked potential, at least in the weak muscles. When the disease is confined to the extraocular- or bulbar muscles, the EMG is negative. The diagnosis can then be made by single fiber EMG, which examines increased neuromuscular transmission time at individual end-plates. In the Edrophonium (Tensilon) test, the patient is given 2 mg of the drug, and if tolerated, an additional 8 mg; the test is positive if it reverses the patient's deficit within 1 minute, and if such reversal lasts 10 minutes. However, both false-positives and false-negatives occur. Atropine (0.4 mg) should be available to correct any muscarinic effects. The test is rapid and can be administered in the ER or office, but is not as reliable as electrophysiological testing.

Definitive diagnosis of MG should be followed by thyroid function tests to detect any thyroid dysfunction, antistriated muscle antibodies (association with thymomas), and chest CT scan or MRI (to rule out an enlarged thymus). Patients should be made aware of drugs that could worsen their condition, such as aminoglycoside antibiotics, certain antiarrhythmics, and sedatives.

Symptomatic management of MG is with anticholinesterase drugs. The prototype drug is pyridostigmine (Mestinon), in doses of 60–90 mg every 4–6 hours, depending upon the disease severity. Side effects include diarrhea, abdominal cramps and muscle twitching or fasciculations. Pyridostigmine overdose may result in paradoxical weakness of the muscles known as "cholinergic crisis."

Immunosuppressive treatment is also necessary, primarily with prednisone, with a low dose of 10 mg daily for several days begun in the outpatient setting. If no response occurs, the dose is gradually increased up to 1 mg/kg body weight; the dose is maintained for a few weeks, after which it can be tapered gradually, and an alternate day schedule adopted. An initial high dose may paradoxically worsen muscle weakness in a small subset of patients. Serum glucose, electrolytes, and blood pressure are monitored carefully. A tuberculin test is also done before instituting prednisone. Other immunosuppressive agents include Azathioprine (Imuran) and Cyclosporin. Thymectomy is indicated whenever chest imaging studies show thymic enlargement or a thymoma. When imaging is negative, thymectomy is indicated in generalized MG, and in localized myasthenia that has failed to respond to anticholinesterase agents and prednisone.

Occasionally, MG may present with a rapidly progressive weakness of all extremities along with respiratory difficulties and bulbar weakness. This condition, known as myasthenic crisis, constitutes a neuromuscular emergency. Hospitalization and temporarily withholding anticholinesterase agents are necessary to rule out a cholinergic crisis. If the patient's vital capacity is poor, endotracheal intubation and mechanical ventilation are required. Once myasthenic crisis is confirmed, anticholinesterase therapy must be resumed, and a trial of plasmapheresis begun, at the rate of 3 sessions for the first week, after which the frequency may be reduced. Pulmonary and supportive care are of prime importance. When recovered from the myasthenic crisis, the patient should undergo thymectomy.

### Eaton-Lambert Myasthenic Syndrome

This is an autoimmune disorder in which various antibodies bind to the calcium channels located on the presynaptic axonal end. This reduces the amount of acetylcholine released from the axonal end and thus, the activation of the muscle membrane. The disease has a strong association with malignancy, particularly small cell lung cancer, but an association with autoimmune disorders seems to be emerging. The usual clinical features are fatigability and weakness that improve with exercise. A greater involvement of the limb and respiratory muscles is noted, with less frequent involvement of the extraocular muscles. Distal paresthesias, dryness of the mouth, and orthostatic hypotension may be noted.

The diagnosis is confirmed by neurophysiologic testing. A single stimulus to a motor nerve evokes a low muscle action potential amplitude. A train of stimuli at low rate (2–3 Hz) results in a small decrement. Following brief exercise for 10 seconds, the motor evoked amplitude increases massively, usually by several fold; the decrement also improves. When the diagnosis is confirmed, work up for malignancy and connective tissue disease should follow.

Pharmacologic treatment with anticholinesterase agents may modestly benefit some patients. Presynaptic activating agents such as Guanidine and 4-aminopyridine do cause symptomatic relief, but with toxic side effects. A recent investigational drug, 3,4-diaminopyridine, has proven useful in the symptomatic management of the disorder. The underlying condition should be treated, if possible. Immunosuppression with prednisone alone, or together with Azathioprine, can result in improvement. Plasmapheresis is indicated in moderately severe cases or when there is rapid deterioration.

## *Muscle Diseases*

### Myotonic Dystrophy

The most common adulthood dystrophy is myotonic dystrophy, an autosomal dominant disorder, where a gene defect is located on chromosome 19, and with an anticipation phenomenon, i.e., an earlier phenotypic expression in subsequent generations. Quite uniquely the myopathy is predominantly distal. Besides weakness of hands and feet, there are thin facies, ptosis, wasting of temporalis and masseter muscles, and thinning of the sternomastoids. Other features are percussion myotonia, high arched palate, frontal baldness, cataracts, intellectual deficit, endocrine changes, and cardiac conduction abnormalities.

The clinical presentation, characteristic retrocapsular cataracts, and myotonic discharges on EMG form the basis for diagnosis. Confirmation is by DNA blood testing, which would also be useful in genetic testing and prenatal diagnosis. Serial electrocardiograms are necessary for early detection of conduction abnormalities. The treatment of muscular weakness is primarily supportive. Although myotonia responds to anticonvulsants (e.g., phenytoin) and Class Ia antiarrhythmics, the latter are generally contraindicated in this disease, because of the underlying cardiac conduction system involvement.

# CHAPTER 194 MULTIPLE SCLEROSIS

### Epidemiology

Multiple sclerosis (MS) is a relapsing-remitting, and sometimes progressive disease that affects roughly 350,000 persons in the United States. It is twice as common in women as in men. While it is most common in 20–40 year olds, no age is exempt. The disease may occur through genetic predisposition and subsequent environmental exposure to an as yet unknown, possible viral agent. Abnormal immune function is likely the underlying theme. In general, the prevalence of the disease increases at higher latitude. This risk is possibly acquired before age fifteen, as moving away from a higher prevalence area after this age does not seem to lower the risk of developing the disease. The high prevalence of disease in Italy and Sicily, but not in Spain, is an exception to this pattern. Multiple sclerosis is less common in African Americans than Caucasians, which raises the question of genetic influence. Further, the risk of developing the disease is increased in children or first-degree relatives of a patient afflicted by multiple sclerosis. The risk is even higher for dizygotic twins.

### Clinical Features

Patients most often present with sensory symptoms, which are varied, but a common symptom is an ascending abnormal sensation progressing from one foot to both lower extremities over several days. **Lhermitte's sign** is a brief but unpleasant electrical sensation passing down the back to the legs or arms when the patient flexes the neck. It is a common, but not exclusive symptom of MS. Frequent involvement of the posterior columns leads to balance or gait abnormalities. Weakness is characterized by upper motor neuron signs of spasticity and hyperreflexia. While spasticity may inhibit walking and be more disabling than actual weakness, it may also allow one to remain ambulatory if the spastic limb helps maintain an upright posture. Lesions of the pyramidal tract or cerebellum cause coordination difficulties. **Intention tremor** is unusual in early stages of the disease, but with progression, may prohibit use of the upper extremities.

**Optic neuritis**, manifest as loss of central vision or decreased visual acuity in one eye (rarely bilateral), poor color vision, and orbital pain, may occur at anytime during the disease. An afferent pupillary defect (decreased pupillary response to light) may persist indefinitely as a residuum of previous optic neuritis. Blurring of vision on exercise may be the only symptom, possibly disabling, of an optic nerve lesion. While most notable for visual symptoms, many patients with multiple sclerosis also report worsening of their other symptoms when their body temperature rises even a few tenths of a degree. This is an effect of increased temperature on action potential transmission and not a true exacerbation of the disease. Various ocular movement abnormalities may lead to diplopia, the most common of which is **internuclear ophthalmoplegia** (INO). In INO, difficulty with adduction of the eye is noted on the affected side with nystagmus in the abducting eye. The patient reports double vision when looking horizontally.

Vertigo, as an initial symptom in multiple sclerosis, may not be distinguishable from vestibular neuronitis unless other central nervous systems signs are evident. **Bladder dysfunction**, while rarely the sole presenting complaint, is very common. Most common is bladder dyssynergia where the detrusor contracts at the same time the sphincter closes, preventing expulsion of urine. Patients may also have incontinence, urgency, frequency, or nocturia. Fatigue is also very common. Depression occurs and the suicide rate for patients with multiple sclerosis is higher than the general population.

## Diagnosis

There is no clinical sign that is unique to multiple sclerosis. Nor is any one test diagnostic. MRI is a sensitive tool, positive in most cases of clinically definite multiple sclerosis. It is, however, not specific for MS. Demyelinating plaques appear in the white matter as hypointense lesions on T1 and hyperintense on T2 weighted images (Figure 194.1). Lesions may be confined to either the spinal cord or brain; thus, clinical localization is important. A lumbar puncture may help exclude other abnormalities. While CSF total protein is normal in 60% of cases, it rarely exceeds 70 mg/dl. The leukocyte count is normal in two-thirds of patients. When high, it is usually below 20 cells/mm$^3$. Oligoclonal bands, elevated IgG synthesis rate, and IgG index also help diagnostically, although they are not specific. Evoked potentials can document subclinical involvement of various areas of the central nervous system (e.g., abnormal visual evoked potentials in subclinical optic neuritis; somatosensory evoked potentials in subclinical spinal cord involvement).

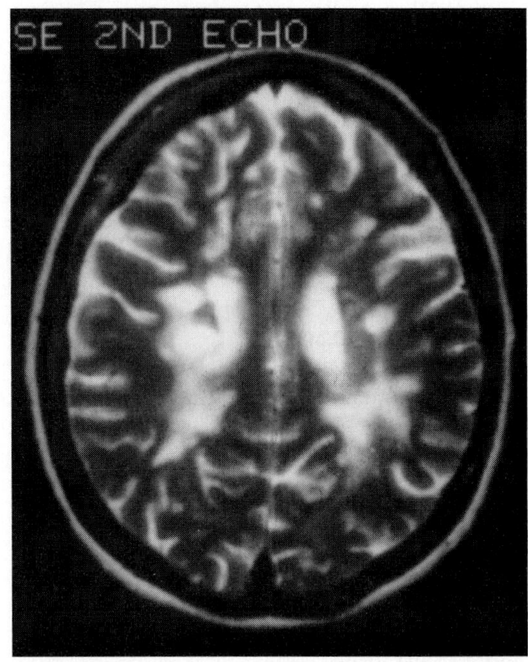


**FIGURE 194.1.** T2-weighted image of head MRI from a patient with multiple sclerosis, showing the presence of foci of hyperintense signal in the peri-ventricular white matter bilaterally ("Dawson fingers").

## Management

Symptomatic therapy is of utmost importance. Spasticity may respond to baclofen, diazepam, tizanidine, dantrolene, or intrathecal baclofen. Tremor is very resistant to therapy although propranolol, primidone, or benzodiazepines may provide partial relief. Urinary incontinence may respond to anticholinergic agents such as oxybutynin. Cholinergic agents such as bethanechol are used to stimulate bladder emptying although usually patients require intermittent self-catheterization. Erectile dysfunction is treated in several ways, including penile intracorporeal papaverine injections. Paroxysmal sensory and motor symptoms often respond to carbamazepine, other anticonvulsants, or baclofen. Treatment of chronic dysesthetic pain includes tricyclic antidepressants, carbamazepine, and clonazepam, to name a few. Fatigue may require adjustment of the patient's daily schedule. Amantadine, pemoline, fluoxetine, selegiline, or modafinil may provide some relief, but their mechanism of action is not well established. Finally, depression should be treated aggressively, along with monitoring for suicidal tendency. Acute exacerbations of multiple sclerosis may be treated with ACTH or methylprednisolone, but these agents do not affect the long-term prognosis, and are not indicated for chronic use. In a prospective study of optic neuritis, patients receiving IV methylprednisolone followed by oral steroids had more rapid recovery of vision than those on oral steroids alone. Those on oral steroids alone had higher risk of recurrence of optic neuritis. During the 2-year follow-up, fewer patients given methylprednisolone developed clinically definite multiple sclerosis. Thus, exacerbations of multiple sclerosis are not generally treated with oral steroids alone.

The mainstay of chronic maintenance therapy consists of either interferon alpha, interferon beta, or glatiramer acetate. All three agents are effective in reducing the rate of disability in relapsing-remitting MS, but long-term disability seems unaffected. These agents are being studied for chronic MS. The future seems optimistic for treatment and possibly, prevention of this disease.

# CHAPTER 195 MOVEMENT DISORDERS

Movement disorders may be **hypokinetic**, i.e., those lacking spontaneous movements, and **hyperkinetic**, i.e., those with excessive involuntary movements. Hypokinetic disorders feature slowness, muscular stiffness, postural instability, tremors, and a tendency for the handwriting to become small (micrographia). Muscular rigidity on passive manipulation of the limbs, or decreased associated movements in walking such as poor arm swing, retropulsion (the tendency to tip backwards, demonstrated by a backward pull on the shoulders), or shuffling gait may all be seen on examination. Such generalized hypokinesia may occur in Parkinson's disease, drug-induced parkinsonism, progressive supranuclear palsy, and multiple systems atrophy. Hyperkinetic disorders are mainly chorea, dystonia, or dyskinesia, tremor, and tic. Bedside differentiation of these movement disorders is shown in Table 195.1.

The extrapyramidal function is arranged in a series of closed loops. Cortical projections reach neostriatal small neurons, while neostriatal large neurons send efferents to the cortex via connections with the globus pallidus and thalamic nuclei. Acetylcholine and glutamate are important excitatory substances. The nigro-neostriatal system (dopaminergic) has inhibitory projections on neostriatal (cholinergic) neurons. The striatum and pallidum influence nigral dopaminergic neurons via GABA and substance P pathways. Reciprocal connections exist between striatum and subthalamus, and between red nucleus and mesencephalon (partly serotoninergic).

**TABLE 195.1. Differentiating Movement Disorders at the Bedside**

| Disorder | Features |
|---|---|
| Athetosis | Slow, writhing, flowing appearance |
| Ballismus | Rapid, flinging-like, non-repetitive |
| Chorea | Rapid, random, flowing, non-repetitive |
| Dystonia | Twisting, repetitive |
| Myoclonus | Rapid, non-twisting, stimulus-sensitive |
| Tic | Random, patterned, coordinated, "urge" |
| Tremor | Rhythmic, oscillatory, continuous |

## *Essential Tremor*

Essential tremor is probably the most common movement disorder. A postural and kinetic tremor may affect the hands most commonly but also can affect the head and the voice. Essential tremor is not associated with any other neurologic abnormalities. Its relationship to Parkinson's disease has been debated. No brain pathology has been found. Treatment depends upon symptoms; β-blockers (propranolol) or use of primidone can be effective.

### ■ Parkinson's Disease

Parkinson's disease is characterized by four cardinal features: **resting tremor, muscular rigidity, bradykinesia**, and **postural instability**. Its onset is gradual and progression insidious over many years. The loss of the pigmented, normally dopaminergic neurons in the substantia nigra leads to declining dopamine levels in the striatum. Over many years, 70–80% of the neurons are lost in the substantia nigra, when symptoms appear. No clear etiology for Parkinson's disease has yet been identified. Associated features may include depression and/or dementia. The diagnosis of Parkinson's disease is clinical. Some consider the resting tremor to be nearly pathognomonic.

The treatment of Parkinson's disease depends on the severity of symptoms. Several factors should be taken into account including quality of life, and function in both employment and daily activity as well as social embarrassment. Several medications are currently in use. Deprenyl (Eldepryl) has been studied extensively and has been felt to slow disease progression. Some patients note minimal improvement in symptoms with this agent. Anticholinergic agents may be helpful when tremor is the dominant symptom, but, cognitive side effects, especially decreased memory, may limit their use. Amantadine, which acts as an anticholinergic agent and promotes dopamine release from CNS stores, may improve all aspects of disease. When there is a threat to employability, activities of daily life, or balance, carbidopa/levodopa (Sinemet) is indicated. Initial improvements and smooth response to this drug tend to be followed in several years by the development of a fluctuating response, and drug-induced dyskinesias. The addition of a dopamine agonist may improve parkinsonian features as well as dyskinesias. Surgical procedures such as thalamotomy or pallidotomy improve the tremor significantly on the contralateral side of the procedure. However, bilateral thalamotomy leads to significant speech abnormalities. Pallidotomy appears promising for the control of motor symptoms. More recently, pallidal or subthalamic stimulation have been tried with success and lower morbidity, and may become the future surgical treatment of choice. Transplantation surgery continues to be evaluated, but its current role is only experimental.

Dopamine antagonists may produce secondary parkinsonism by blocking dopamine receptors in the striatum. Antipsychotic agents are most commonly associated with this syndrome; however, antiemetics such as prochlorperazine (Compazine) and metoclopramide (Reglan), also dopamine antagonists, may produce this syndrome. Withdrawal of the offending agent should alleviate the movement disorder. Debate continues as to whether those who develop drug-induced parkinsonism are at a higher risk of ultimately developing Parkinson's disease.

## Neuroleptic Malignant Syndrome

Neuroleptic malignant syndrome (NMS) is a life-threatening condition, which can present as an akinetic rigid state. This occurs typically in a patient on dopamine antagonists, usually after a dose increase. The patient develops fever, confusion, and muscular rigidity. Serum creatinine kinase is elevated. Treatment of NMS involves withdrawing the dopamine antagonist. For mild cases, this may suffice as treatment. In more severely affected patients, dantrolene and bromocriptine can improve rigidity, reduce fever, and improve mental status.

# CHAPTER 196 BRAIN DEATH

The advent of life saving and sustaining technologies lead to a re-appraisal of the concept of death. Respiratory and/or cardiac standstill leads to so-called somatic death. With severe brain injury including the brain stem, respiration and blood pressure control are lost. Such events also lead to somatic death, but artificial respiration and blood pressure support can maintain the vital signs in such a brain-injured patient for prolonged periods of time. When the severity of brain injury is such that there is irreversible loss of function of the brain and the brain stem, the patient is said to be brain dead.

Strict diagnostic criteria should be adhered to in confirming this diagnosis. The American Academy of Neurology has recently published a statement with recommended guidelines (*Neurology* 1995; 45:1012–1014). The coma must be of an established and irreversible cause. Drug intoxication and hypothermia both may mimic brain death, but are reversible and must be excluded. Most patients with brain death from a primary neurologic cause have suffered a head injury or subarachnoid hemorrhage; however, other etiologies occur, including large stroke with herniation and hypoxic ischemic injury.

On examination, the patient is comatose and unresponsive to any and all stimuli. Temperature must be greater than 32°C. All brain stem reflexes are abolished. Pupils show no light reaction. Oculocephalic maneuvers or caloric testing produce no eye movements. Corneal responses are absent. Gag and cough are absent. Spontaneous respiration is absent, but testing methods vary. Apneic oxygenation is best performed by delivery of 100% oxygen at the carina, removing ventilatory support until blood gases document $PaCO_2$ of >60 mm Hg. Posturing is not present. Muscle stretch reflexes may vary; diagnosis of brain death does not require their loss, as they reflect spinal cord function. CT is usually done to document the extent of cerebral injury, particularly with trauma.

Examination may be beset with some difficulties. Trauma with an unstable cervical spine makes oculocephalic maneuvers inadvisable. Preexisting pupillary abnormalities may be confounding. Chronic $CO_2$ retention may cloud interpretation of apnea testing. Spinal reflexes may produce movements difficult to distinguish from cortically based movement. With unambiguous features, two clinical evaluations performed 6–12 hours apart are widely accepted as conferring the diagnosis as brain death. Confirmatory testing may be desirable in difficult situations. EEG for 30 minutes should show no cerebral activity, or a cerebral angiogram should show no cerebral perfusion at the level of the carotid bifurcation or circle of Willis. Technetium[99] brain scan should show no parenchymal tracer uptake.

It must be emphasized that these guidelines are for adults. The diagnosis of pediatric and in particular, infant brain death, is best made in consultation with a pediatric neurologist.

## Questions

**Instructions**: For each question below, select only **one** lettered answer that is the best for that question.

1. A 36-year-old woman was found unconscious behind the steering wheel following a motor vehicle accident. Her neurologic examination in the ED showed mild drowsiness, normal oculocephalic reflexes and pupillary responses and a supple neck. She was moving all her extremities spontaneously and symmetrically. Her plantar response was extensor bilaterally. The most likely diagnosis is which of the following?
   A. Bilateral intracerebral hemorrhage
   B. Bilateral epidural hematoma
   C. Pontine stroke
   D. Post-ictal state
   E. Central cord syndrome

2. A 70-year-old man has progressive memory difficulties. The most important part of his neurologic examination would be which of the following?
   A. The mental status
   B. The cranial nerves
   C. The muscle strength
   D. The sensory examination
   E. The gait testing

3. A 65-year-old hypertensive man has intermittent cramping pain in the back of his thighs and legs after climbing steps or walking a variable distance. The lower extremity pulses are symmetrically reduced. The ankle jerks are absent on the left and slight on the right, while the right knee jerk is moderately decreased. Muscle strength is normal, and the sensory examination shows reduced pinprick over the dorsal aspect of both feet. The most likely diagnosis is which of the following?
   A. Arterial insufficiency with claudication
   B. Herniated L5-S1 disc
   C. Lumbar stenosis
   D. Buerger's disease
   E. Peripheral neuropathy

4. A 21-year-old woman complains of intermittent horizontal diplopia for the past 3 months. Her examination revealed mild bilateral weakness of her lateral rectus and her facial muscles. Her neck flexors were mildly weak. The rest of her neurologic examination was normal. The most likely diagnosis is which of the following?
   A. Lyme disease
   B. Pontine stroke
   C. Multiple sclerosis
   D. Myasthenia gravis
   E. Motor neuron disease

5. A 35-year-old man has intermittent horizontal diplopia and intermittent numbness of the right cheek for the past 2 months. During right lateral gaze, there is limited adduction of the left eye with nystagmus in the right. The right corneal reflex is mildly decreased. Rapid alternating movements are mildly decreased on the left. The rest of his neurologic examination was normal. The most likely diagnosis is which of the following?
   A. Lyme disease
   B. Pontine stroke
   C. Multiple sclerosis
   D. Myasthenia gravis
   E. Motor neuron disease

6. A 65-year-old man notes gradual weakness and numbness of the right hand and leg for the past 18 months. Mild wasting of his right hand muscles is evident with reduced vibration over both feet but greater on the right, and bilateral Babinski signs. The neurologic examination is otherwise normal. Useful diagnostic tests would be which of the following?
   A. Serum Folate and B12 levels
   B. Syphilis serology
   C. MRI of the cervical spine
   D. Nerve conduction and electromyography
   E. All of the above

7. A 31-year-old woman reports intermittent stiffness in her legs for the past 4 months, followed 2 months later by urinary urgency. There is mild bilateral horizontal nystagmus, bilateral Babinski, and decreased vibration sense over hands and feet. The

neurologic examination is otherwise normal. Which of the following tests will be useful?
A. Visual evoked responses
B. MRI of the brain
C. MRI of the cervical spine
D. CSF analysis
E. All of the above

8. A 27-year-old asthmatic woman was found by her husband to have episodes of brief staring followed by lip smacking, lasting less than 1 minute. Her only medication is theophylline. She does not remember the episodes. Her neurologic examination is normal. Which of the following would you do now?
A. Serum chemistry
B. Theophylline level
C. MRI of the brain
D. EEG
E. All of the above

9. A 21-year-old man was found unconscious by his parents. The paramedics noticed intermittent jerking of his arms and legs and twitching of his face during transport to the ED. While unresponsive to verbal stimuli, he was moving all his extremities symmetrically in response to pain, and had preserved oculocephalic reflexes and pupillary responses. The neck was supple. His plantar responses were extensor bilaterally. His vital signs are stable. Which of the following is/are indicated?
A. Serum chemistry and toxicology screen
B. One ampule of 50% dextrose and thiamine
C. Intravenous phenytoin 20 mg/kg
D. EEG
E. All of the above

10. A 60-year-old woman notes shaking in her hands, greater on the right side, whenever she carries weights. It disappears at rest. Her father had similar problems around the same age. Her symptom is likely to respond to which of the following?
A. Propranolol
B. Primidone
C. Methazolamide
D. Alcohol
E. All of the above

11. A 30-year-old man has had three episodes of loss of consciousness preceded by brief "metallic taste" in his mouth lasting less than 1 minute. The neurologic examination is normal. Which of the following is most appropriate for this patient?
A. Phenytoin
B. Carbamazepine
C. Valproic acid
D. All of the above
E. None of the above

12. A 39-year-old man came to the ED complaining of abrupt headache after lifting weights at the gymnasium. He noticed transient visual blurring at the peak of his headaches. In the ED, he vomited once. His examination is normal. A noncontrast head CT scan is negative. The next step is which of the following?
A. Send home with analgesics
B. Schedule a head MRI
C. Repeat the head CT with contrast
D. Perform a lumbar puncture
E. None of the above

13. A 60-year-old man reports progressive walking difficulties over 6 days, with "numb, tingly" feeling in his fingers and feet. Mild weakness of the face and hand intrinsics is noted, along with moderate weakness of the lower extremities, absent ankle jerks, and diminished vibration sense over fingers and feet. Which of the following best describes his condition?
A. Brainstem stroke
B. Brainstem abscess
C. Guillain-Barré syndrome
D. Myelitis, subacute
E. None of the above

14. A 46-year-old man presents with 6 months of unilateral rest tremor. Unilateral cog-wheeling of the upper limb is noted. The initial treatment of choice is which of the following?
A. Trihexyphenidyl
B. Amantadine
C. Bromocriptine
D. L-Dopa
E. None of the above

15. A 67-year-old hypertensive man had transient loss of vision in the right eye for 30 minutes. Other than a high-pitched bruit over the right carotid artery, examination is normal. The next step is which of the following?
A. Intravenous heparin
B. Carotid angiography
C. Surgical consultation
D. All of the above
E. None of the above

## ANSWERS

| | | | | |
|---|---|---|---|---|
| 1. D | 2. A | 3. C | 4. D | 5. C |
| 6. E | 7. E | 8. E | 9. E | 10. E |
| 11. D | 12. D | 13. C | 14. A | 15. D |

## SUGGESTED READING

*Approach to the Patient with a Neurologic Disorder*

Caplan LR. The effective clinical neurologist. Blackwell Scientific Publications, 1990.

Fishman RA. Cerebrospinal fluid in diseases of the nervous system. 2nd ed. Philadelphia: WB Saunders, 1992.

Mayo Clinic & Mayo Foundation Clinical Examinations in Neurology. 6th ed. St. Louis: Mosby Year Book, 1991.

*Disorders of Consciousness and Cognition*

Plum F, Posner JB. The diagnosis of stupor and coma. 3rd ed. Contemporary Neurology Series, Vol 19. Philadelphia: F.A. Davis Co., 1980.

*Headaches*

Dalessio DJ. Diagnosing the severe headache. Neurology 1994; 44 (5 Suppl 3):S6–S12.

Goadsby PJ, Olesen J. Diagnosis and management of migraine. Br Med J 1996; 312 (7041):1279–1283.

Kumar KL, Cooney TG. Headaches. Med Clin North Am 1995; 79(2):261–286.

Welch KM. Drug therapy of migraine. N Engl J Med 1993; 329(20):1476–1483.

*Dizziness and Syncope*

Baloh RW. Approach to the dizzy patient. Baillieres Clinical Neurology 1994; 3(3):453–465.

Brandt T. Vertigo and dizziness. In Asbury AK, McKhann GM, McDonald WI (eds.). Diseases of the Nervous System: Clinical Neurobiology. 2nd ed. Philadelphia: WB Saunders, 199:451–467.

McGee SR. Dizzy patients. Diagnosis and treatment. West J Med 1995; 162(1):37–42.

Sloane PD. Evaluation and management of dizziness in the older patient. Clin Geriatr Med 12(4):1996; 785–801.

*Stroke*

Adams HP Jr. Use of anticoagulants or antiplatelet aggregating drugs in the prevention of ischemic stroke. Adv Intern Med 1995; 40:503–531.

Barnett HJ, Meldrum HE, Eliasziw M. The dilemma of surgical treatment for patients with asymptomatic carotid disease. Ann Intern Med 1995; 123(9):723–725.

Brickner ME. Cardioembolic stroke. Am J Med 1997; 157(6): 605–617.

Broderick JP, Brott T, Tomsick T, et al. The risk of subarachnoid and intracerebral hemorrhage in blacks as compared with whites. N Engl J Med 1992; 326 (11):733–736.

Brott T, Toole JF. Medical compared with surgical treatment of asymptomatic carotid artery stenosis. Ann Intern Med 1995; 123 (9):720–722.

Gorelick PB. Stroke prevention. Arch Neurol 1995; 52(4):347–355.

The National Institute of Neurological Disorders and Stroke rt-PA stroke study group. Tissue plasminogen activator for acute ischemic stroke. N Engl J Med 1995; 333(241):1581–1587.

Raps EC, Galetta SL. Stroke prevention therapies and management of patient subgroups. Neurology 1995; 45(2 Suppl 1):S19–S24.

Sherman DG, Dyken ML, Gent M, et al. Antithrombotic therapy for cerebrovascular disorders. An update. Chest 1995; 108(4 Suppl):S444–S456.

*Seizure Disorders*

Engel J. Seizures and Epilepsy. Contemporary Neurology Series, Vol 31. Philadelphia: F.A. Davis Co., 1989.

So EL. Update on epilepsy. Med Clin North Am 1993; 77(1):203–214.

Thomas RJ. Seizures and epilepsy in the elderly. Arch Intern Med 1997; 157(6):605–617.

Wyllie E. The Treatment of Epilepsy: Principles and Practice. Philadelphia: Lea & Febiger, 1993.

*Disorders of Spinal Cord, Nerves, and Muscles*

Byrne TN, Waxman SG. Spinal Cord Compression: Diagnosis and Principles of Management. Contemporary Neurology Series, Vol 33. Philadelphia: F.A. Davis Co., 1990.

Griggs R, Mendell J, Miller R. Evaluation and Treatment of Myopathies. Contemporary Neurology Series, Vol 44. Philadelphia: F.A. Davis Co., 1995.

Schaumburg HH, Berger AR, Thomas PK. Disorders of Peripheral Nerves. 2nd ed. Contemporary Neurology Series, Vol 36. Philadelphia: F.A. Davis Co., 1992.

*Multiple Sclerosis*

Brod SA, Lindsey JW, Wolinsky JS. Multiple sclerosis: clinical presentation, diagnosis, and treatment. Am Fam Phys 1996; 54(4):1301–1306.

Lublin FD, Whitaker JN, Eidelman BH, et al. Management of patients receiving interferon beta-1b for multiple sclerosis: report of a consensus conference. Neurology 1996; 46(1):12–18.

McDonald WI. Diagnosis of multiple sclerosis. Br Med J 1989; 299(6700):635–637.

Tourtelotte WW, Pick PW. Current concepts about multiple sclerosis. Mayo Clin Proc 1989; 64(5):592–596.

*Movement Disorders and Parkinson's Disease*

Ahlskog JE. Treatment of early Parkinson's disease: are complicated strategies justified? Mayo Clin Proc 1996; 71(7):659–670.

Jankovic J, Brin MF. Therapeutic uses of botulinum toxin. N Engl J Med 1991; 324(17):1186–1194.

Krauss JK, Jankovic J. Surgical treatment of Parkinson's disease. Am Fam Phys 1996; 54(5):1621–1629.

Quinn N. Drug treatment of Parkinson's disease. Br Med J 1995; 310(6979):575–579.

Quinn N. Parkinsonism—recognition and differential diagnosis. Br Med J 1995; 310(6977):447–452.

Stacey M, Brownlee HJ. Treatment options for early Parkinson's disease. Am Fam Phys 1996; 53(4):1281–1287.

*Head Trauma*

White RJ, Likavec MJ. The diagnosis and initial management of head injury. N Engl J Med 1992; 327(21):1507–1511.

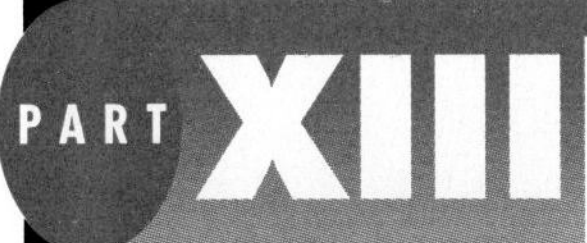


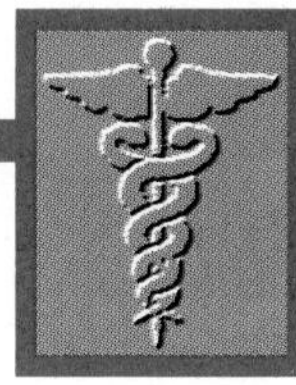

Tom Anderson
Janet R. Hosenpad
Christopher R. Chitambar

# ONCOLOGY

# CHAPTER 197 CANCER AND CARCINOGENESIS

Cancer ranks a close second to cardiovascular disease as the major cause of overall morbidity and mortality in the United States. With the continued aging of the population and recognition of the myriad genetic and environmental factors influencing carcinogenesis, cancer has profound implications for the 21st century. In 2002, an estimated 1,220,000 new cases of cancer will be diagnosed and 552,200 cancer deaths will occur in the United States. These figures are based on data from the National Cancer Institute Surveillance, Epidemiology and End Results (SEER) program as well as state cancer registries and the Bureau of Vital Statistics of the United States. Table 197.1 lists the sites where cancer most commonly occurs.

## Etiology of Cancer

### Age and heredity

Over 60% of all cancer deaths occur in persons over 65 years of age. The increased incidence of common cancers with age may reflect the duration of exposure to environmental carcinogens. Certain cancers do cluster in the young, however, including brain tumors, Hodgkin disease, bone sarcomas, testicular cancer, and some leukemias. Many common tumors have an increased genetic predisposition, including breast, colon, lung, ovary, and prostate cancers, which occur more commonly at an earlier age in those with first-degree relatives afflicted. Common neoplasms and inherited conditions that predispose a person to develop malignancies are shown in Table 197.2.

### Carcinogens

Carcinogenesis is a multistep process, with a latency period of varying length between initiation and the development of premalignant and, finally, malignant changes. Chemical carcinogens, ubiquitous in our society, include dietary, industrial, and medicinal products. Most are metabolically activated derivatives of parent compounds in the environment. The activated carcinogen forms DNA adducts; these in turn lead to DNA strand breaks or interstrand cross-linking events, which may cause mutations and deletions in growth-regulating genes or tumor- suppressor genes. In addition to these chemicals, physical (e.g., sunlight, ionizing radiation) and biological (e.g., viruses, helminths) agents also may have carcinogenic potential (Table 197.3).

**Promoting agents** are noncarcinogenic compounds that induce cell proliferation in tissues (e.g., estrogen in women). If a preexistent carcinogenic injury exists, promoting agents increase the likelihood of progression from hyperplasia to neoplasia.

## Molecular Genetics and Carcinogenesis

The discovery that certain viruses could induce neoplasia in infected animals, made by inserting a **viral oncogene** into normal host cells, unraveled many theories of the molecular events in carcinogenesis. Many oncogenes have been isolated; they have been named for the tumors they cause in animals (e.g., *ras* group for rat sarcoma viruses) or after their discoverers (e.g., v-*abl* for the Abelson leukemia virus).

**TABLE 197.1. Major Cancers in the United States by Site & Gender—2002**

| Site | Total | Men (%) | Women (%) |
|---|---|---|---|
| Lung | 169,400 | 90,200 (14) | 79,200 (12) |
| Prostate | 189,000 | 189,000 (29) | NA |
| Breast | 205,000 | 1,500 (0.2) | 203,500 (31) |
| Colorectal | 148,300 | 72,600 (10) | 75,700 (12) |
| Melanoma | 53,600 | 30,100 (4) | 23,500 (4) |
| Oropharynx | 37,800 | 25,800 (3) | 12,000 (2) |
| Pancreas | 30,300 | 14,700 (2) | 15,600 (2) |
| Stomach | 21,600 | 13,300 (1) | 8,300 (1) |
| Urinary tract | 90,700 | 62,200 (9) | 28,500 (4) |
| Ovary | 23,300 | NA | 23,300 (4) |
| Leukemia | 30,800 | 17,600 (3) | 13,200 (2) |
| Lymphoma | 60,900 | 31,900 (5) | 29,000 (4) |
| All other sites | 255,000 | 88,600 (14) | 135,600 (21) |
| Total | 1,284,900 | 637,500 (100) | 647,400 (100) |

(Adapted from: Greenlee RT, et al. Cancer statistics, CA - A Cancer Journal for Clinicians.)

The rapid development of molecular biology techniques made it possible to discover that viral oncogenes are homologous to a wide array of genes in normal cells (which are called **cellular oncogenes** or **proto-oncogenes**) that have been conserved through evolution in many classes and species of animals. Subsequent work showed the importance of these genes in normal growth and differentiation. Further laboratory studies uncovered a class of oncogenes called **tumor-suppressor genes** (anti-oncogenes or recessive oncogenes).

Figure 197.1 illustrates some of the mechanisms of oncogene activation in cancer. In dominant oncogenes, point mutations, translocations, or amplification of only one allele (gene copy) is sufficient to result in unregulated growth, which may result in malignant transformation. The tumor suppressor genes usually require a lesion in both alleles to alter the inherent growth-suppressive effect of the normal gene products. Dominant oncogenes and tumor-suppressor genes are listed in Tables 197.4 and 197.5, with the postulated function of their protein product. Whereas theoretically a single mutation creating a dominant gene should be capable of carcinogenesis, such single mutations rarely seem able to confer the malignant phenotype on a cell. At least two steps are required in autosomal dominant cancers such as retinoblastoma, and it is believed that carcinogenesis is a multistep process involving mutations in *several* regulatory and growth-promoting genes. There are hereditary cancers characterized by the loss of one allele in the **germline** [loss of heterozygosity (LOH)] wherein a second mutation, acquired due to some environmental insult, becomes the "triggering event" that causes cancer. Because **LOH** is transmitted genetically, certain families have an increased propensity for specific cancers.

**TABLE 197.2. Selected Inherited Cancers**

*Autosomal Dominant* (neoplastic and preneoplastic)
- Retinoblastoma
- Neurofibromatosis
- Von Hippel-Lindau syndrome
- Li-Fraumeni syndrome
- Dysplastic nevus syndrome

*Autosomal Recessive*
- Xeroderma pigmentosa
- Ataxia-telangiectasia

*X-Linked Recessive*
- X-linked agammaglobulinemia
- Wiskott-Aldrich syndrome
- Familial adenomatous polyposis
- Nonpolyposis colorectal cancer
- Hereditary breast cancer
- Hereditary breast/ovarian cancer

**TABLE 197.3. Chemical, Physical and Biological Agents Linked to Cancer**

| Agents | Principal Tumors |
|---|---|
| Tobacco | Lung, head/neck, esophagus, pancreas, bladder, kidney |
| Increased dietary fat | Colon, prostate, rectum, endometrium |
| Charred, smoked, salted, pickled foods | Esophagus, stomach |
| Low fiber diet | Colon |
| Alcohol | Oral cavity, esophagus (synergism with smoking) |
| Asbestos | Mesothelioma, lung (synergism with smoking), larynx |
| Benzene | Leukemia |
| Nickel, chloromethylether, arsenic, mustard gas | Lung |
| Aromatic amines | Bladder |
| Alkylating agents, nitrosoureas, etoposide | Leukemia |
| Estrogens | Breast, ovarian |
| Diethylstilbestrol | Vaginal adenocarcinoma; ingestion during pregnancy causes cancer in daughters |
| Androgens, oral contraceptives | Liver (?) |
| Immunosuppressives (azathioprine, cyclosporine) | Lymphoma, skin cancer |
| Sunlight (UV rays) | Basal and squamous cell cancers, melanoma |
| Radiation | Leukemia, lung |
| Epstein-Barr virus | Burkitt lymphoma, nasopharyngeal cancer |
| Hepatitis B and C | Hepatocellular carcinoma |
| Human papilloma virus (HPV 16, 18) | Cervix, anus, penis, oral cavity |
| Herpes virus | Kaposi sarcoma |
| *Clonorchis sinensis* | Cholangiocarcinoma |
| *Schistosoma haematobium* | Urinary bladder cancer |

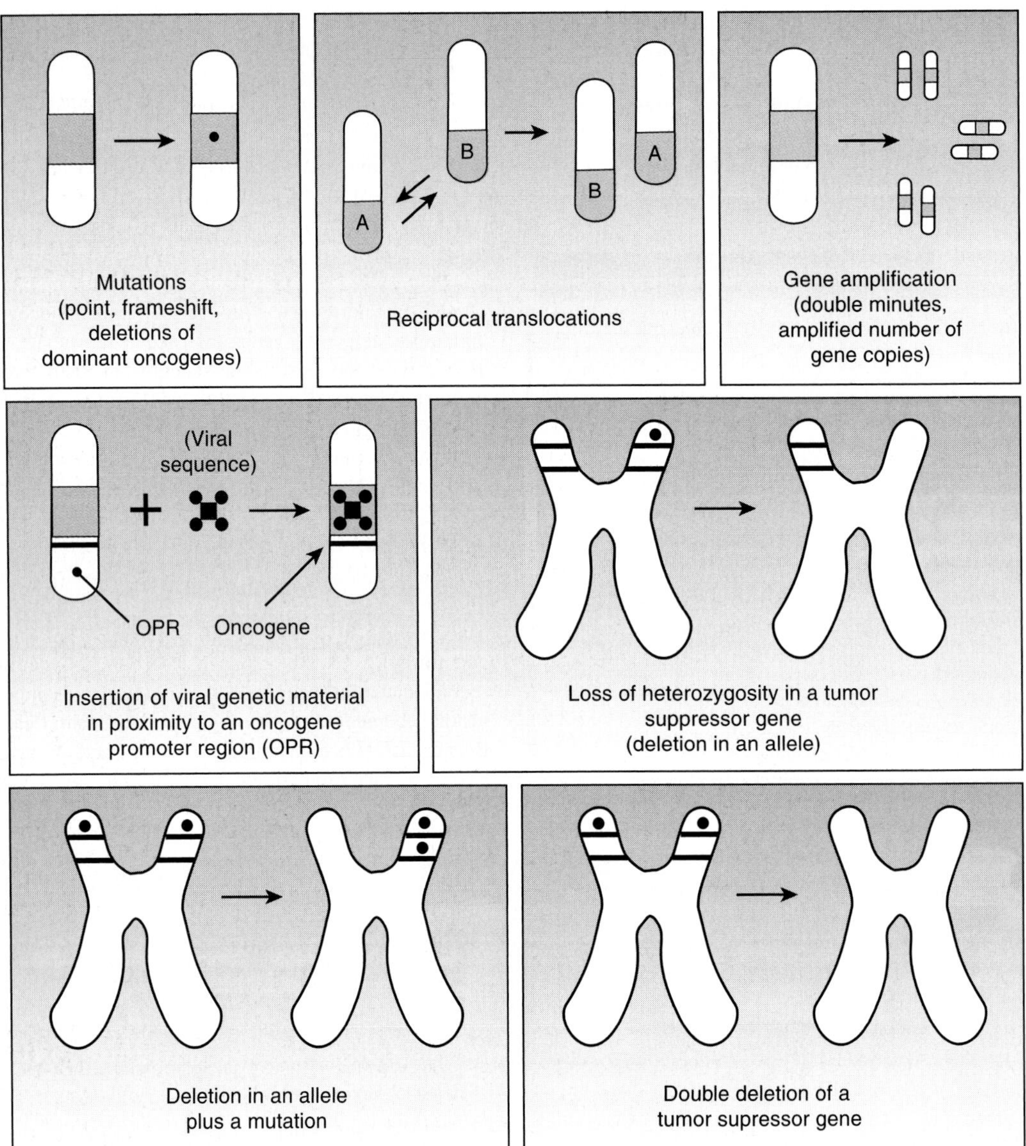


**FIGURE 197.1.** **Mechanisms of oncogene activation and inactivation of tumor-suppressor genes.**

Examples include retinoblastoma in children, familial polyposis coli and its resultant colon carcinoma, hereditary breast cancer, and **the multiple endocrine neoplasia (MEN)** syndrome. Such entities demonstrate that the neoplasia is genetically predisposed because of the transmission of the germ cell mutation, but is consistent with the "second hit" theory that requires another mutation, presumably induced by our environment, to cause the subsequent cancer. This explains why not everyone in a hereditary cancer family may suffer the disease; development of the cancer requires both the genetic predisposition and the environmental insult. In contrast, the concept of somatic mutations represents the observation of sporadic cancers, and implies that both mutations, on a random basis, were caused by separate environmental insults. Examples include the cancers commonly associated with smoking—e.g., lung, head and neck, esophagus, and bladder cancers.

## Cancer Invasion and Metastasis

The fully developed malignant tumor has a distinct pattern of cellular and subcellular processes referred to as its **phenotype,** due to the mutations that altered the cell's

**TABLE 197.4. Dominant Oncogenes in Human Cancer**

| Oncogene | Activation/Function | Tumors Associated |
|---|---|---|
| *ras* family | Point mutation signal transduction | Multiple human solid tumors and leukemias |
| *bcl*-2 inner mitochondrial (membrane protein) | Translocation prevents apoptosis | B cell lymphomas (follicular) |
| *abl* tyrosine protein kinase | Translocation | Chronic myelogenous leukemia (Philadelphia chromosome), ALL |
| *raf* serine threonine kinases | Rearrangement | Gastric |
| Growth factor receptors and growth factors (erbB2 [Her2/Neu] int2, C-sis) | Amplification homology with growth factors and receptors | Many tumors, including breast |
| Cyclins | Translocation, regulate cell cycle | B-cell lymphomas |
| MYC family (c-myc l-myc n-myc) | Translocation, amplification | Lymphomas, neuroblastoma, small cell lung carcinoma |

ALL, acute lymphoblastic leukemia.

**TABLE 197.5. Examples of Tumor Suppressor Genes**

| Gene | Chromosome | Tumors |
|---|---|---|
| rb1 | 13q | Retinoblastoma, osteosarcoma, small cell lung cancer, sarcomas, breast, genitourinary |
| wt1 | 11p | Wilms tumor |
| nf1 | 17q | Neurofibromatosis, type 1 |
| nf2 | 22q | Acoustic neuromas, neurofibromatosis type 2 |
| men1 | 11q | Adenomas of multiple endocrine organs |
| men2 | 10q | Pheochromocytomas, medullary carcinomas of thyroid, parathyroid hyperplasia |
| p53 | 17p | Li-Fraumeni syndrome, in many tumors as acquired mutations |
| BRCA1 | 17q | Hereditary breast, and breast-ovarian cancer as autosomal dominant |
| apc | 5q | Familial adenomatous polyposis, sporadic colon cancer |
| dcc | 18q | Sporadic and familial colon cancer |
| msh2 | 2p | Hereditary nonpolyposis colorectal cancer |
| Deletions | 3p | Renal cell carcinoma, Von Hippel-Lindau disease, lung cancer (most common in small cell) |

original genotype. Malignant cells often have decreased expression of cell surface adhesion molecules and loss of contact inhibition, which otherwise restrain the growth of normal cell populations; receptors target specific basement membrane proteins, and activation of proteolytic enzymes allows tissue invasion, with subsequent lymphatic and blood vessel invasion. The growth of cancer is clonal, but genetic instability leads to the development of subclones with variable metastatic potential and treatment susceptibilities.

# CHAPTER 198 PRINCIPLES OF CANCER THERAPY

## Surgical Therapy

Surgical therapy has been employed for cancer since antiquity and remains the treatment of choice for most cancers, provided early diagnosis allows curative intervention and minimizes the extent of surgery. In the first half of the 20th century, progressively more aggressive surgery was employed, based on the theory that cancers grow in an orderly sequence of contiguous spread, from local tumor, to lymphatic extension, to distant metastasis. This belief fostered the routine use of radical surgery for many cancers (e.g., radical mastectomy, radical head and neck resections, limb amputation). In general, it was believed that en bloc resection involving wide excision of the primary tumor and the first or second echelon of regional nodal metastases offered the best chance of local regional cure. The later realization that lymphatic involvement is in essence a metastasis, combined with the recognition that hematogenous metastases occur coincident with, but biologically independent of, lymphatic metastases has led to the modern approach of using less disfiguring surgical resection of the primary tumor (e.g., lumpectomy for breast cancer, limb preservation surgery for sarcomas involving the extremities).

Although surgery remains the major therapy option for most cancers, the current emphasis in clinical research is not how to perform more aggressive curative surgery for primary tumors, but rather how best to use additional therapeutic modalities, such as radiotherapy and chemotherapy, to augment the curative potential of currently available surgical techniques while producing less morbidity. With the use of other modalities of treatment as adjuncts to surgery, the current trend is toward surgery that is more selective and less radical and has better functional and cosmetic outcomes. Paradoxically, the selective use of aggressive surgical resection of liver, lung, and even brain metastases has become highly effective as palliation for certain patients whose primary tumor is under control.

## Radiotherapy

Remarkable innovations in ionizing radiation were made in the 20th century. Electromagnetic radiation and gamma rays exert their cytotoxic effects through free radical generation from intracellular water and molecular oxygen, leading to irreparable breaks in double-stranded DNA. Particulate radiation from subatomic particles also causes direct DNA damage (Table 198.1). Conventional radiotherapy uses a series of daily doses (fractions) administered over a period of weeks to achieve the optimum cumulative dosage for tumor control while minimizing side effects in normal tissues. Modern high-energy linear accelerators make it possible to penetrate tissues selectively and to triangulate on the tumor target ("conformal radiation"); with the ability to vary daily dose fractionations, the efficacy has increased steadily, and acute and—most importantly—late complication rates have decreased.

**Brachytherapy,** the implantation of radiation sources directly into the tumor bed, has the advantage of limiting radiation exposure to a relatively precise body region. Successful applications include intracavitary implants for cervical and endometrial cancers and interstitial treatments for oral cancers. The administration of intravenous radionuclides takes advantage of tumor or normal healing processes. Thus, iodine-131 is used to treat functioning thyroid cancers; similarly, strontium-89 and sumarium-153 can palliate bone metastases.

**TABLE 198.1. A Glossary of Terms in Radiation Oncology**

| Term | Definition |
|---|---|
| Type of radiation | |
| Electromagnetic | External beam. Produced by linear accelerator |
| Gamma rays | Decay of isotopes, e.g., cobalt$^{60}$ |
| Particulate | Decay-producing subatomic particles |
| Dose units | |
| Gray (Gy) | 1 Joule/kg tissue absorbed dose |
| Rad | Absorbed dose/g tissue = 0.01 Gy |
| Beam energy | |
| Orthovoltage | 100-400 KeV |
| Supervoltage | Usually 4–25 MeV; deeper penetration with higher energy units; less skin absorption |
| Means of administration | |
| Teletherapy | External beam therapy, e.g., linear accelerators, cobalt units. |
| Brachytherapy | Implanted in treatment area (interstitial, intracavitary) |

## Systemic Chemotherapy

Cytotoxic drugs were first used to treat cancer when, in 1945, the effect of the alkylating agent, nitrogen mustard (mechlorethamine) on Hodgkin disease and small cell lung cancer was discovered. In 1948, the anti-folate compounds aminopterin and methotrexate were demonstrated to produce temporary remissions in childhood leukemia. Combination chemotherapy programs evolved over the ensuing decades, leading to an increasing number of cures of childhood lymphoblastic leukemia, Hodgkin disease, aggressive intermediate-grade non-Hodgkin lymphoma, and germ cell tumors of the testes. Almost without exception, the advances made in chemotherapy have resulted from the successful integration of multiple drugs into a comprehensive, concomitant treatment program. The principles of such combination chemotherapy involve the design of regimens that have the following characteristics:

1. Each drug in the combination has demonstrably independent activity, or favorably affects the metabolism or binding of another drug in the program
2. Because multiple drugs are used simultaneously, it is more difficult for an individual tumor cell to express or acquire a resistance to that particular pharmacological challenge

3. Each drug can be given in a therapeutic dose approximating the one that can be used as a single agent when palliating the same disease
4. Each drug's dose-limiting toxicity profile allows it to be combined with other drugs in the regimen, such that the use of one drug does not adversely affect the ability to utilize others.

### Classes of chemotherapeutic agents and mechanisms

The major mechanisms of currently available antineoplastic drugs fall into several categories, with DNA damage being a common theme. These categories include alkylating agents, antimetabolites, antibiotics, plant alkaloids and miscellaneous agents (Table 198.2).

Alkylating agents, such as cyclophosphamide, cisplatin, chlorambucil, melphalan, and mechlorethamine, produce cross-links between guanine nucleotide base pairs on opposite DNA strands, preventing subsequent DNA repair and replication.

**Antimetabolites,** such as methotrexate, 6-mercaptopurine, and 5-fluorouracil, inhibit key enzymes in DNA synthesis, usually as competitive inhibitors.

**Tubulin inhibitors** interfere with normal microtubular activities necessary for subcellular function and cell division. Thus, the plant-derived **vinca alkaloids** vinblastine and vincristine disassemble microtubules, whereas the **taxanes** paclitaxel and docetaxel polymerize them, leading to excessive stabilization and functional incompetence.

**TABLE 198.2. Activity and Toxicity of Major Cytotoxic Agents**

| Drug | Activity | Toxicity |
|---|---|---|
| **Alkylating Agents** | | |
| Cyclophosphamide | Broad spectrum | N/V, My, cystitis, carcinogenic |
| Mechlorethamine | Hodgkin disease | N/V, My, carcinogenic, vesicant |
| Chlorambucil | CLL, lymphoma | My, carcinogenic |
| Busulfan | CML | My, carcinogenic, pulmonary fibrosis |
| Melphalan | Myeloma | My, carcinogenic |
| Ifosfamide | Testicular, sarcomas | N/V, My, carcinogenic, cystitis, acidosis, confusion |
| **Antimetabolites** | | |
| Methotrexate | Broad spectrum | N/V, M, My, renal failure, cirrhosis |
| 5-Fluorouracil | Adenocarcinoma | N/V, My, M, cardiac ischemia, cerebellar ataxia |
| 6-Mercaptopurine | Leukemia | My, hepatitis |
| Cytarabine | Leukemia | N/V, My, CNS, hepatic |
| Fludarabine, Cladribine | CLL, low grade lymphoma | My, immunosuppression |
| **Antibiotics** | | |
| Doxorubicin | Broad spectrum | My, M, N/V, alopecia, cardiotoxicity |
| Mitoxantrone | Lymphoma, breast | N/V, My, cardiomyopathy |
| Actinomycin D | Childhood tumors | N/V, M, My |
| Plicamycin | Hypercalcemia | N/V, My, hepatitis, coagulopathy |
| Bleomycin | Testicular, lymphoma | Dermatitis, fever, pulmonary fibrosis |
| Mitomycin C | Adenocarcinomas | My (delayed), hemolytic uremic syndrome |
| **Plant Alkaloids** | | |
| Vincristine | Leukemia, lymphoma, breast cancer | Neurotoxicity |
| Vinblastine | Germ cell, bladder | My, neurotoxicity, myalgia |
| Etoposide | Germ cell, broad spectrum | N/V, My, leukemogenesis |
| Paclitaxel (Taxol) | Ovary, breast | My, myalgia, neuropathy, anaphylaxis |
| **Miscellaneous** | | |
| Cisplatin | Broad spectrum | N/V, renal, otic, neuropathy, hypomagnesemia. |
| Carboplatin | Broad spectrum | My, esp. thrombocytopenia |
| Carmustine, Lomustine | Brain tumors | N/V, My (delayed), pulmonary fibrosis, leukemia |
| Hydroxyurea | CML | My, dermatitis |
| Streptozotocin | Endocrine tumors | N/V, renal failure, diabetes |
| L-Asparaginase | ALL | Anaphylaxis, pancreatitis, coagulopathy, thrombosis |

ALL = acute lymphoblastic leukemia; CLL = chronic lymphocytic leukemia; CML = chronic myelocytic leukemia; M = mucositis; My = myelosuppression; N/V = nausea, vomiting.

Epipodophylotoxins, another class of plant alkaloids, create DNA intercalation events similar to the anthracyclines and antibiotics noted in the preceding paragraphs.

**Topoisomerase inhibitors** are agents that disrupt the critical function of enzymes that prevent DNA tangling during replication. Topoisomerases in category I are enzymes which catalyze formation of single-strand DNA breaks; topoisomerases in category II catalyze both single- and double-strand breaks. These enzymes are critical for the faithful replication or transcription of DNA segments. Drugs that bind to these enzymes can lead to lethal damage by disruption of these critical replicative events. Camptothecin analogues are the only topoisomerase I inhibitors utilized as chemotherapy in human tumors; however, it is now known that many of the drugs originally developed because of their putative intercalating effects also depend on inhibition of topoisomerases II for their action. These include the anthracyclines (e.g., daunomycin and doxorubicin, the anthracenediones (e.g., mitoxantrone), Bleomycin, and the epipodophylotoxins (e.g., VP-16).

It has been postulated that some cancer chemotherapeutic agents and radiotherapy act in part by promoting **apoptosis** (programmed cell death). Apoptosis, a natural process, provides a mechanism for removal of cells with DNA damage or mutations and eliminates the cells made defective or potentially neoplastic by toxic agents or radiation. This recently discovered concept probably explains the antineoplastic activity of corticosteroids such as prednisone and dexamethasone.

### Drug resistance

Drug resistance may be intrinsic or acquired. Some tumors, such as renal cell and hepatocellular carcinoma, display a high degree of intrinsic resistance to virtually all chemotherapeutic agents. However, other cancers, such as malignant lymphomas and small cell lung cancer, initially are highly sensitive to many cytotoxic agents, but acquire resistance after exposure to them.

There are several well-defined mechanisms of resistance specific to particular drugs, including increased efficiency of DNA repair, gene overexpression (amplification) leading to increased production of the protein product, and production of enzyme with altered affinities. Of more clinical importance is the mechanism of resistance to a variety of naturally derived anticancer compounds mediated by the ***MDR-1* gene** (multidrug resistance), which encodes for a membrane–based efflux pump that ejects chemotherapeutic compounds from the cell. Sublethal exposure to any one compound of several classes of natural products, (e.g., doxorubicin of other anthracyclines) often results in induction, or amplification of this p170 glycoprotein, calcium channel-dependent pump, creating resistance to virtually all compounds in these classes.

### Toxicity of chemotherapeutic agents

The available cancer chemotherapeutic agents act principally on cycling cells (i.e., rapidly proliferating tissues) and therefore affect both tumors and normal tissues. The toxicity of chemotherapy is extremely pervasive and often is dose-limiting. Whereas some toxic effects are common to several agents, other effects are unique to or especially severe with particular chemotherapeutic compounds (see Table 191.2).

**Nausea and vomiting** depend on the agent and on the dose and schedule. Although nausea and vomiting were common with many chemotherapeutic drugs in the past, these side effects now are almost universally controllable with newer antiemetic agents, which selectively block the 5-HT receptors in the brain responsible for most chemotherapy-induced nausea. **Myelosuppression,** affecting principally leukocytes but, to a lesser extent, platelets and erythrocytes, is common to alkylating agents, antimetabolites, and the antibiotics. In general, transient leukopenia appears early after exposure to antimetabolites and most alkylating agents, with a nadir at 10 to 14 days and subsequent rapid recovery. Its severity can be abrogated by judicious dose scheduling. **Mucositis** and **enteritis** also are common, occurring most commonly with antimetabolites and antitumor antibiotics. Mucositis can be ameliorated by mouth-rinsing formulations used after the admnistration of chemotherapy.

Treatment schedules usually involve intermittent administration of drugs, with intervening rest periods to allow for recovery of normal tissue. Such schedules tend to maximize antitumor effects and minimize immunosuppression. Nevertheless, dose-limiting toxicity may disrupt the schedule. A variety of cloned growth factors and some chemical compounds may be used to alleviate chemotherapy-related toxicity and help maintain the dose and schedule (Table 198.3). For example the recent advent of granulocyte-colony stimulating factors (G-CSF) or granulocyte, monocyte-colony stimulating factors (GM-CSF) has made more aggressive chemotherapy regimens feasible because co-administration of such growth factors produces a more rapid neutrophil recovery from the cytotoxic effects of chemotherapy.

Supralethal doses of chemotherapy have been used in an effort to destroy widely metastatic cancers, with subsequent reconstitution of the bone marrow by **bone marrow** or **stem cell transplantation.** Allogeneic bone marrow transplantation (from haploidentical donors) has an established role in acute leukemia and chronic myelogenous leukemia. Autologous (self-donated) mar-

**TABLE 198.3. Agents to Modify Chemotherapy-related Toxicity**

| Agent | Mechanism of Action | Clinical Use |
|---|---|---|
| Interleukin-3 (IL-3) | Stimulates stem cells of WBC, RBC, and platelets | Investigational—shortens duration of neutropenia and thrombocytopenia after chemotherapy |
| Granulocyte-monocyte colony stimulating factor (GM-CSF) | Acts to stimulate granulocyte/monocyte precursors | Shortens duration of neutropenia after bone marrow transplantation |
| Granulocyte colony stimulating factor (G-CSF) | Stimulates proliferation of granulocyte precursors | Shortens neutropenia after chemotherapy; may reverse drug-induced neutropenia |
| Interleukin-6 (IL-6) | Stimulates platelet production | Investigational—reduces thrombocytopenia from chemotherapy |
| Erythropoietin | Stimulates red cell production | Reverses anemia of cancer and chemotherapy |
| MESNA | Binds toxic cyclophosphamide and ifosfamide metabolites in bladder urine | Prevents hemorrhagic cystitis |
| Amifostine | Scavenges free radicals | May prevent some radiation and alkylating agent toxicity |
| ICRF 187 | Chelates free radicals | Reduces risk of cardiotoxicity from large doses of doxorubicin and other anthracyclines |

**TABLE 198.4. Toxicity of Hormonal Therapy**

| Agent | Use In | Toxicity |
|---|---|---|
| Prednisone | Lymphoma, breast | Iatrogenic Cushing disease |
| Fluoxymesterone | Breast | Virilization, erythrocytosis, hepatic toxicity |
| Diethylstilbestrol | Prostate, breast | Nausea, gynecomastia, edema, cardiac failure |
| Megestrol | Breast, anorexia in AIDS | Weight gain, thromboembolism |
| Tamoxifen | Breast | Thrombosis, hot flashes, endometrial cancer |
| Leuprolide/Goserelin | Prostate | Hot flashes |
| Flutamide/Bicalutamide | Prostate | Diarrhea, hepatotoxicity |
| Aminoglutethimide | Breast, Cushing disease | Drowsiness, rash, leukopenia |

row or stem cell reconstitution is effective in otherwise refractory Hodgkin disease, non-Hodgkin lymphomas, and selected leukemias. Efficacy in traditional solid tumors is limited. Despite widespread initial enthusiasm, results in breast cancer have been uniformly disappointing.

## Hormonal Therapy

Because breast and prostate cancers proliferate on exposure to physiologic levels of hormones, initial hormonal therapies were ablative (e.g., oophorectomy, orchiectomy). Pharmacologic doses of estrogens, androgens, and progestins, given in the appropriate settings (e.g., androgens in women with breast cancer, estrogens in men with prostate cancer), also produce responses due to subsequent down-regulation of the endogenous hormone production (Table 198.4). More recently, the antiestrogen tamoxifen has emerged as the primary hormonal therapy in breast cancer. Tamoxifen, actually a weak estrogen agonist rather than a true biochemical antagonist, binds to the estrogen receptor but, contrary to endogenous estrogen, fails to stimulate cancer cell growth. Newer analogues with putatively better therapeutic indices, e.g., toremifene and raloxifene, have been made available or are undergoing extensive clinical trials. More recently aromatase inhibitors, which block residual endogenous estrogen synthesis, have been approved as alternative hormone treatments with some toxicity advantages, e.g., anastrozole, letrazole, gamestane, fulvestrant.

## Biologic Response Modifiers

The biotherapies include a heterogeneous group of compounds and natural agents that act by altering immunity or suppressing proliferative activity (Table 198.5). **Alpha-interferons,** expressed by a wide variety of cells, including leukocytes, up-regulate tumor-associated antigens and have antiproliferative activity.

**TABLE 198.5. Selected Biologic Response Modifiers in Clinical/Investigative Use**

| Agent | Mechanism of Action | Clinical Use |
|---|---|---|
| Bacille Calmette-Guerin (BCG) | Activation of macrophages, T and B cells | Intravesical therapy for superficial bladder cancer |
| Levamisole | Immunostimulatory | Modifies action of 5-fluorouracil in colon cancer |
| Interferons | Antiproliferative, enhance immune responses | Chronic myelocytic leukemia, other hematologic malignancies, carcinoid tumors |
| Interleukin-2 (IL-2) | Enhances cytotoxicity of natural killer cells and T cells | Renal carcinoma, melanoma |
| Tumor necrosis factor | Mediator of sepsis, acute phase reactions | Investigational |
| Monoclonal antibodies | Antibodies to tumor antigens, carriers for radioactive isotopes and cytotoxic compounds | Effective in breast cancer and lymphomas |

They are effective in hairy cell leukemia, chronic myelogenous leukemia, multiple myeloma, and Kaposi sarcoma (in AIDS). They result in toxicity at high doses, causing a flu-like syndrome, fever, myalgia, and malaise. **Interleukin-2** (IL-2) is a T-cell growth factor and is believed to stimulate the cytotoxic function of natural killer and cytotoxic T cells. High doses produce serious toxicity, including massive edema, hypotension, and respiratory failure.

## Monoclonal Antibodies

**Monoclonal antibody** technology has led to the exciting development of chimeric antibodies with demonstrable important clinical effects. By grafting a murine "antigen recognition site" fragment of antibody into an otherwise intact human monoclonal immunoglobulin, it is now possible to develop antibodies that are directed solely to those cells expressing membrane-bound antigens. Thus, one can semi-selectively target tumor-associated antigens and, via the endogenous immune system, produce tumor cell cytotoxicity. The "naked" antibodies currently available include rituximab (Rituxan) directed against the lymphoid antigen CD-20, which is overexpressed in many lymphomas, and transtuzimab (Herceptin), which targets the protein product of the oncogene Her-2/neu, which is over-expressed in breast cancer. The CAMPATH-1 monoclonal antibody, targeting yet another lymphocyte antigen (CD52), has demonstrated activity in chronic lymphocytic leukemia. A newer generation of monoclonal antibodies is designed to be conjugated with cytotoxic moieties to enhance efficacy. Thus $^{131}$I-Tositumoab (Bexxar) is another anti-CD-20 monoclonal antibody, which is conjugated to iodine-131, as is Ibritumomab tiuxten (Zevalin) while Denileukin diftitox (Ontak), conjugated to a plant toxin, targets the CD-25 antigen (interleukin-2 receptor) expressed on cutaneous T-cell lymphomas. Monoclonal antibodies also can be used ex vivo to purge bone marrow of malignant B and T cells to reduce graft rejection and graft-versus-host disease in allogeneic transplant recipients.

## Cancer Management

### Cancer diagnosis

The diagnosis of cancer requires tissue confirmation, done by surgical biopsy. Traditional surgical methods are still widely used, but use of fine-needle aspiration and cutting core needle biopsy (which provides a larger tissue sample for histologic analysis) is increasing. Many nonmalignant diseases mimic cancers, and a cytologic or histologic diagnosis is mandatory in virtually all suspected cancers.

### Cancer staging

In general, cancer stages range from I through IV, referring, in order, to early localized, regional, locally advanced, and metastatic cancers. The tumor-node-metastasis (TNM) classification is widely used to help determine the stage for prognostic and therapeutic decisions, particularly for solid tumors. Examples are included in the relevant disease sections.

Many additional variables are used to determine the prognosis of specific malignancies and supplement the prognostic determination from staging. **Performance status** (Table 198.6) is an assessment of the patient's degree of debility or overall functional level. The **histologic type** and **grade** of the tumor give an indication of its rate of growth and nuclear atypia. In addition, the presence of paraneoplastic syndromes, such as hypercalcemia, lymphoma-associated "B" symptoms, or weight loss, convey additional adverse prognostic information.

### Therapeutic approaches and goals

Following cancer diagnosis and staging, the clinician must design a therapeutic plan. Whenever possible, an initial strategy should be clearly defined: e.g., potentially curative; noncurative but prolonging life; or palliative.

Increasingly, tumors are treated with combined-modality therapy, either simultaneously or sequentially. When used sequentially, the primary curative modality of therapy is used first. Subsequent additional therapies are then used as "adjuncts" to reduce the risk of relapse. Traditionally, postoperative radiotherapy has been the modality most commonly applied to such clinical situations and is used in many disease sites. As the efficacy of chemotherapy has improved, the use of "adjuvant chemotherapy" has developed for those cancers responsive to chemotherapy in the relapsed setting. Use of such adjuvant chemotherapy has now been shown to significantly reduce the risk of relapse in colon, breast, esophageal, head and neck, stomach, and some lung cancers.

In some cancers (e.g., of the breast), adjuvant chemotherapy has replaced adjuvant radiotherapy for patients undergoing mastectomy; in patients undergoing breast lumpectomy and irradiation, the radiation becomes the primary modality of cure, and the chemotherapy assumes the adjuvant treatment role. For selected cancers such as that of the breast, such adjuvant therapy can be hormonal therapy. The term *neoadjuvant therapy* alludes to the use of such treatment before the application of the curative modality. The rationale for neoadjuvant chemotherapy is that it allows one to assess the efficacy (antitumor activity) of adjuvant chemotherapy prior to curative therapy. This information can then be used to determine whether it is efficacious and cost-effective to administer the same drugs as adjuvant chemotherapy after curative therapy. Neoadjuvant therapy also can produce significant regressions of the primary tumor, perhaps leading to more successful primary treatment by shrinking tumor masses for which surgical removal is compromised by such factors as tumor size and location. Neoadjuvant chemotherapy often is used in Hodgkin disease to shrink large bulky mediastinal lymph nodes to avoid subsequent radiation injury to adjacent lung tissue.

Consultation and close cooperation among the practitioners of the different modalities—surgery, radiation oncology, and medical oncology—are vital for the optimum treatment of most cancers. Chemotherapy is curative in a few tumors when used alone and contributes significantly to curability in many cancers when used in conjunction with other modalities (Table 198.7). However, several tumor types are virtually unresponsive to chemotherapy, and in advanced-stage cancers, chemotherapy is principally palliative, or may not be indicated. Several general factors are germane in deciding on the use of palliative chemotherapy: (1) the probability of therapeutic benefit; (2) the patient's general physical condition; and (3) the preferences of the patient and family after a candid discussion of the benefits and risks of treatment. Patients with poor performance status (ECOG 3 or 4) rarely benefit from chemotherapy unless their particular tumor is known to be highly responsive to such treatment.

### Outcome of treatment

To define a patient's disease status and the prognosis accurately, physicians have developed definitions based on identifiable responses to therapy. With response to

**TABLE 198.6. Performance Status Scales**

| ECOG | | Karnofsky | |
|---|---|---|---|
| **Score** | **Criteria** | **Score** | **Criteria** |
| 0 | Asymptomatic | 100 | Asymptomatic |
| 1 | Symptomatic, fully ambulatory | 90 | Normal activity, minor signs and symptoms |
| 2 | Less than fully ambulatory but in bed <50% of the day | 80 | Normal activity with effort |
| 3 | In bed >50% of the day | 70 | Cares for self, unable to carry on normal activity or work |
| 4 | Bedridden | 60 | Requires occasional assistance but self-cares for most needs |
| | | 50 | Requires considerable assistance |
| | | 40 | Disabled; requires special care and assistance |
| | | 30 | Severely disabled; hospitalization indicated |
| | | 20 | Very sick; hospitalization needed |
| | | 10 | Moribund |
| | | 0 | Dead |

ECOG = Eastern Cooperative Oncology Group.

**TABLE 198.7. Response of Adult Tumors to Systemic Therapy**

| |
|---|
| Frequent cures with chemotherapy |
| ALL |
| Gestational choriocarcinoma |
| Hodgkin disease |
| Intermediate/high grade non-Hodgkin lymphomas |
| Germ cell tumors |
| Highly responsive—cure in a minority |
| Adult AML |
| Small cell lung cancer |
| Ovarian cancer |
| Highly responsive and variably curable with combined modality therapy |
| Sarcomas of bone |
| Operable breast cancer |
| Cancer of esophagus |
| Bladder cancer |
| Head and neck cancer |
| Colon and rectal cancer |
| Responsive, but essentially noncurable |
| Metastatic breast cancer |
| Metastatic prostate cancer |
| Low-grade non-Hodgkin lymphomas |
| Chronic leukemias |
| Multiple myeloma |
| Endocrine tumors |
| Less responsive tumors |
| Adult soft tissue sarcomas |
| Gastrointestinal cancers (except operable colon and rectal cancer) |
| Metastatic non–small cell lung cancer; cancers of endometrial, cervical, head and neck origin; renal cell carcinoma and melanoma |
| Hepatocellular carcinoma |
| Primary brain tumors |

treatment, survival and, perhaps, quality of life are increased proportionately to the magnitude of response. The survival of patients whose treatment fails is analogous to the natural history of disease. Whenever the patient has one or more lesions, these allow reproducible measurements of the diameter of the lesion, usually in at least two dimensions over a period not less than 30 days. Patients with **stable disease** (or **no change**) are those whose tumors are unchanged. In patients with **progressive disease,** the lesions(s) increase over 25% in the product of bidimensional diameter, or new lesions develop. Patients with **partial response** are those whose tumor diameter (as previously defined) decreases over 50%. Such patients survive longer than those with progressive disease. Those patients in whom all evidence of disease disappears after therapy are said to have **complete response.** These responses often are described in clinical terms based on physical examination and radiographic studies. In selected situations, repeat biopsies allow the determination of progressively more sensitive probes of "minimal residual disease." Histologic reexamination is more accurate than clinical re-evaluation, but is less sensitive than cytogenetic or molecular reassessments. Patients who achieve a complete response live significantly longer than other patients; a subset of such patients is potentially cured of their disease. Patients with no detectable minimal residual disease have a better prognosis; thus, the more sensitive and accurate the reassessment, the more likely that the patient has truly been rendered disease-free.

Other definitions used in outcome analysis of cancer include **overall survival (OS),** in which all patients are followed from the time of diagnosis until death from any cause. **Disease-free survival (DFS)** denotes the time from initiation of adjuvant treatment until relapse or death from disease. **Event-free survival (EFS)** is the time from diagnosis until death either from disease or from therapy. Many research studies report multiple outcomes. Because allogeneic bone marrow transplantation has a 30% mortality rate, it is important to know whether the survival curves separate treatment mortality events from overall survival and relapse and death from the underlying disease. In prostate cancer, which affects an advanced-age population, deaths from comorbid diseases are so common that an analysis of disease-free survival can establish treatment efficacy, but overall survival may not be improved if there are too many intercurrent deaths from cardiovascular or other disease.

## Supportive Care of the Cancer Patient

Good medical care of the cancer patient requires more than simply treating the disease process. A general policy of honesty and open, compassionate communication with the patient and family results in better cooperation and serves to lessen the anxiety derived from common misconceptions about the disease or the proposed therapy. Complications of the various treatment modalities can result in multiple problems during therapy, all of which must be addressed. In the later stages of cancer, control of symptoms becomes paramount.

### Nutrition

Nutritional concerns and weight loss may be addressed by dietary modifications, feeding through nasogastric or gastrostomy tubes, or, at times, parenteral support. Such supportive measures must be implemented in the context of the patient's disease and treatment options. Intensive, expensive, complicated, and inherently risky forms of nutritional support should be offered only if a potential exists for long-term survival. Megestrol acetate (Megace), 800 mg/day, is an appetite stimulant with minimal side effects, allowing many patients with advanced cancer (and AIDS) to regain their appetite, gain weight, and enjoy eating again.

### Pain management

*Analgesics*

Pain accompanies advanced or metastatic cancer in at least 60% of cases. Cancer pain may result from the cancer itself, through direct pressure of the tumor on adjacent structures, infiltration of nerves and tissues, gastrointestinal tract infiltration or obstruction, or damage to bony structures. Pain also may arise as a treatment-related effect, as with mucositis, edema, or nerve damage. Specific treatment, such as palliative radiation, chemotherapy, hormonal therapy, nerve blocks, or neurosurgical procedures, may be designed to interrupt pain pathways.

Pain control must be individualized. A careful history and physical examination, a thorough evaluation of the intensity of the pain and its temporal relationships (preferably by using analog rating scales), and the development of a prospective management plan that seeks to minimize pain and cope with the frequent side effects of analgesic medications are necessary steps. In rating pain-control measures, the World Health Organization's "pain ladder" and similar schemata are useful. Each step is a response to increasing levels of pain and the need for increasing therapeutic intensity.

- **Step 1: Mild pain.** In many cases, the patient has already used nonprescription analgesics. For control of mild pain, acetaminophen, aspirin, or nonsteroidal anti-inflammatory agents (e.g., ibuprofen or naproxen) in effective, regularly scheduled doses is sufficient.
- **Step 2: Moderate pain.** Oral narcotic agents of moderate potency, usually in fixed dosages and combined with acetaminophen, are used for moderate pain. Examples include codeine, hydrocodone, or oxycodone, combined with acetaminophen. At higher doses, preparations such as oxycodone or codeine alone may better control pain without the potential for acetaminophen toxicity.
- **Step 3: More severe pain, uncontrolled by Step 2 agents.** Strong oral narcotics are used after Step 2 agents fail and work best when used on a regular schedule, with additional doses for "breakthrough" episodes of increased pain. Unless there are problems with absorption or gastrointestinal intolerance, oral administration is desirable.

  The prototypical agent is morphine, given at an initial oral dosage of about 30 mg every 3–4 hours. Sustained- release morphine preparations, administered every 8–12 hours, provide increasing flexibility because their dosage may be increased gradually to optimum levels, thus obviating interim dosing with immediate-release morphine for breakthrough pain. Alternatives to morphine include hydromorphone, levorphanol, oxycodone, and methadone. Transdermal fentanyl patches, which are changed every 3 days, should be reserved for those patients who are less compliant or who have gastrointestinal problems, making oral administration unreliable.
- **Step 4: Most severe pain.** Severe pain often requires parenteral narcotics when consciousness is altered, the gastrointestinal tract is dysfunctional, or pain intensity requires rapid relief. Examples include the immediate postoperative state, pathologic fracture, or intestinal obstruction.

Morphine can be administered every 3 hours around the clock, or by a programmable pump, which can deliver a constant or variable dose via IV or subcutaneous routes. **Patient-controlled analgesia** allows the patient to control the frequency of metered intravenous analgesic dosages, with additional boluses of drug for breakthrough pain, and provides an important physiologic and psychologic benefit to the patient and family. This or another version of continuous morphine infusion often is the preferred strategy for rapid control of severe pain because it can be "titrated" hourly until pain control is achieved.

*Nonanalgesic adjuncts to pain management*

Nonanalgesic adjuncts for enhancing pain relief come under several classes: tricyclic antidepressants, phenytoin, carbamazepine, and gabapentin for neuropathic pain; antiemetics with anxiolytic effect for controlling nausea; and short courses of corticosteroids to enhance feelings of well-being. As cancer progresses and disability increases, the dose of pain medication required may escalate. It must be emphasized that there is no ceiling dose; an adequate dose is the amount of the analgesic that ensures pain control, given regularly by whatever chosen route. The use of sedation at this time may be very important. Relatively short-acting benzodiazepines, barbiturates, or phenothiazines can be useful in this context.

### Managing gastrointestinal alterations

**Constipation** is universal with opioid use and is compounded by patient inactivity and dehydration. Adequate fluid intake and stool softeners should be supplemented with oral peristaltic stimulants, suppositories, and enemas. Regularly scheduled use of stool softeners or mild laxatives often is preferable to suppositories and enemas.

Another problem that plagues cancer patients is **nausea and vomiting.** If this is due to gastrointestinal obstruction, nasogastric suction may be the only effective measure for relief. Many chemotherapeutic agents and opiates are emetogenic, but effective antiemetics are available. For minor degrees of nausea, a phenothiazine antiemetic, such as prochlorperazine, given IV or orally, usually is effective and well-tolerated. If there is evidence of any dystonic complications, diphenhydramine or lorazepam may be coadministered. The prophylactic use of the new 5-HT serotonin-blocking agents ondansetron and granisetron represents a major breakthrough in the control of nausea and vomiting.

**Care of the terminal patient**

As cancer progresses and life is shortened, close communication among the primary physician, specialist consultants, the patient, and family members is essential. A realistic plan for further care, discussion concerning limiting or terminating specific anticancer treatment, discussion of artificial life support and cardiopulmonary resuscitation ("code" status), and issues of home or hospice care become paramount. Hospice programs center around home care, with hospitalization for brief periods for crises and respite for the caregivers.

# CHAPTER 199 HODGKIN'S DISEASE

Hodgkin's disease is a malignant lymphoma. Most of the tumor mass is composed of nonmalignant lymphocytes, histiocytes, granulocytes, plasma cells, eosinophils, and fibrosis, all apparently reactive (unlike non-Hodgkin's lymphomas). The characteristic **Reed-Sternberg cells** and their variants form only a minority of the cellular component of the lymph node.

## Incidence and Epidemiology

Hodgkin's disease is relatively uncommon, with 7000 cases expected in the U.S. in 2002. There is a striking bimodal age distribution, with the first peak occurring in young adulthood and a second peak after age 50. Slightly more men than women are affected (1.1 : 1). Rare geographic clusters in neighborhoods have been observed.

## Etiology and Pathogenesis

The disease is more common in upper socioeconomic groups and in persons with a prior history of infectious mononucleosis. Epstein-Barr viral DNA has been detected in the genome of Reed-Sternberg cells, suggesting an etiologic relationship to this agent. The origin of the Reed-Sternberg cell is unclear; it shows features of both B and T cells, varying with the histologic type of Hodgkin's disease, and may represent a malignancy of the antigen-processing cells known as dendritic cells.

## Pathology

There are four main histologic types of Hodgkin's disease. These include, in order of decreasingly favorable prognosis, lymphocyte predominant, nodular sclerosis, mixed cellularity, and lymphocyte depletion subtypes. The first three subtypes tend to present with more limited disease, whereas lymphocyte-depleted Hodgkin's disease often is widespread by the time of diagnosis. Nodular sclerosing Hodgkin's disease has a predilection for the mediastinum, especially in young women.

## Clinical Features

Most patients with Hodgkin's disease present with the complaint of a painless mass, usually in the neck but occasionally in the axilla or groin. On examination, rubbery, usually painless **lymphadenopathy** is noted. Occasionally, an **abdominal mass**, representing enlarged retroperitoneal nodes, or **splenomegaly** is the initial finding. Some patients are totally asymptomatic, and the physician may discover lymphadenopathy during the course of a routine physical examination or detect mediastinal adenopathy on a chest radiograph obtained for other indications (Figure 199.1). Gallium scans are helpful to confirm the biologic activity of disease. Sometimes after apparently curative therapy the patient has a residual mediastinal mass discernible by computed tomography (CT). If the mass was "gallium-positive" prior to therapy, and is "gallium-negative" after therapy it is most likely a residual fibrotic mass rather than residual active Hodgkin's tissue.

Occasionally, extensive lymphadenopathy causes symptoms by **compression of adjacent organs**, (e.g., venous obstruction in an extremity, hydronephrosis (and renal failure if both ureters are compressed), superior vena cava syndrome, tracheal compression, dysphagia due to esophageal compression, and spinal cord compression). With early recognition and prompt treatment, compression of the adjacent organs is potentially reversible, but they may be medical emergencies.

A minority of patients (about 25%) present with characteristic paraneoplastic **systemic "B" symptoms,** such as unexplained fever, weight loss, and night sweats. The presence of B symptoms implies a less favorable prognosis in any given stage. Another occasionally noted

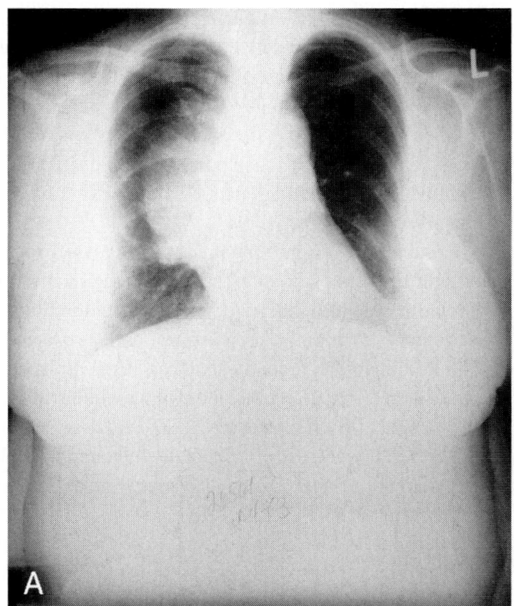


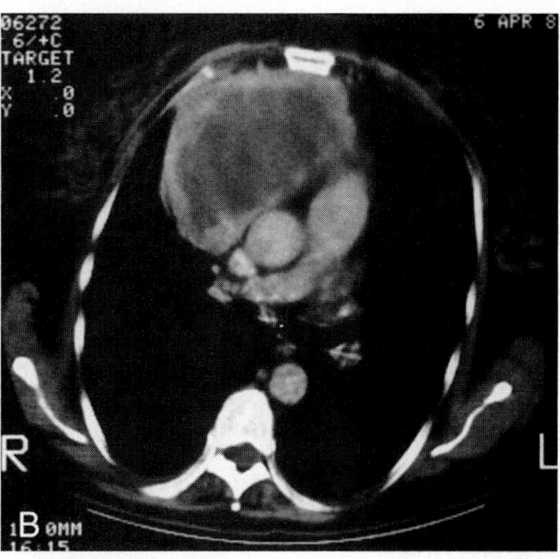


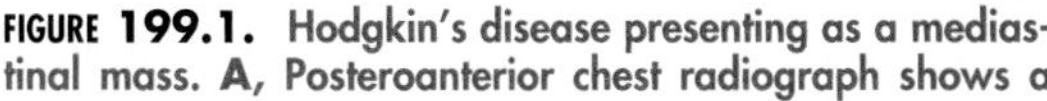
**FIGURE 199.1. Hodgkin's disease presenting as a mediastinal mass. A, Posteroanterior chest radiograph shows a large mass to the right of the ascending aorta. B, CT scan showed it was an anterior mediastinal mass.**

symptom is **pruritus**, which typically is intense and refractory to symptomatic treatment. Hodgkin's disease of unfavorable cell types (e.g., mixed cellularity and advanced stage) is commonly observed in HIV-infected patients.

## Diagnosis and Staging

The differential diagnosis of Hodgkin's disease consists primarily of infectious, inflammatory, autoimmune, or other neoplastic diseases. Reed-Sternberg cells are the hallmark of Hodgkin's disease, but their presence alone is insufficient for diagnosis, because similar cells may be seen in other conditions (e.g., lymphomas, carcinomas, infectious mononucleosis, and toxoplasmosis).

Even when Reed-Sternberg cells are observed in the appropriate cellular milieu, establishing the diagnosis of Hodgkin's disease is still arduous. Because careful tissue acquisition, preservation, and fixation, and expert pathologic examination are key elements in the diagnosis, all lymph node biopsy samples should be presumed to be positive for Hodgkin's disease until proven otherwise. The false presumption that a lymph node is "not lymphoma" often engenders inadequate tissue handling and, thus, renders diagnosis difficult. Newer immunologic markers are making the diagnosis somewhat more accurate.

**Staging** of Hodgkin's disease is facilitated by the knowledge that it spreads most commonly by contiguous extension to adjacent nodal groups and structures. The clinical stage is established by a careful history, physical examination, laboratory studies (complete blood count with differential, platelet count, erythrocyte sedimentation rate, and liver and renal function tests), and imaging studies (CT of the neck, chest, abdomen, and pelvis; Figure 199.2). In addition to determining the risk of extranodal disease in bone marrow or liver, laboratory studies help assess whether anemia of chronic disease, nephrotic syndrome, or other rare manifestations of Hodgkin's disease (or concomitant independent disease) are present. Bipedal lower extremity lymphangiography (Figure 199.3) shows nodal architecture and size, but it is technically difficult and uncomfortable, and thus is done only when critical to selecting between treatment modalities. With rare exceptions it has been replaced by computed tomography. The modified Ann Arbor staging system is shown in Table 199.1.

Bone marrow status is evaluated by iliac crest biopsy; such involvement is important to identify, but is rare without extensive, widespread adenopathy, "B" symptoms, a positive bone scan, or an elevated alkaline phosphatase. Staging **laparotomy** or laparoscopy may help clarify an otherwise ambiguous assignment of stage category. As with lymphangiography, these procedures are required only when precise staging would make a difference in selecting therapy or to perform a concomitant oophoropexy to avoid radiotherapeutic toxicity

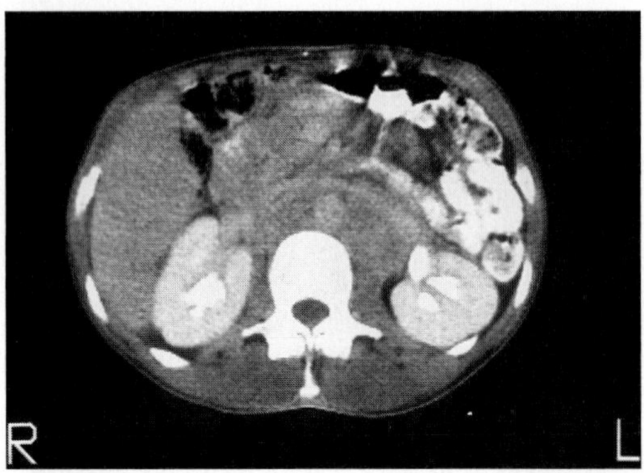


**FIGURE 199.2.** CT scan showing retroperitoneal lymphadenopathy.

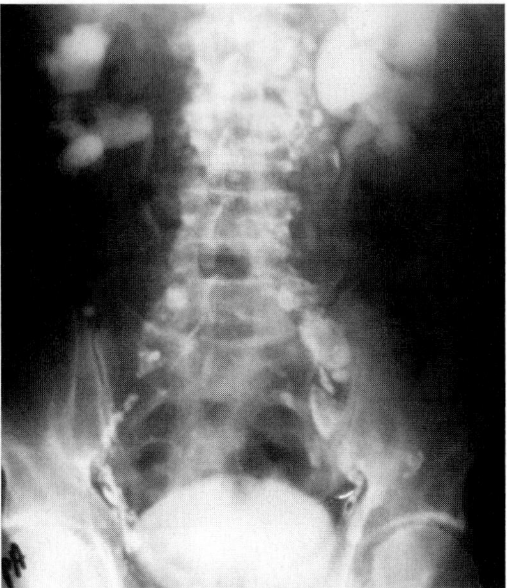

**FIGURE 199.3.** Bipedal lymphogram in Hodgkin's disease showing replaced lymph nodes and ureteral obstruction.

in a woman of childbearing age. The postsplenectomy state is a risk factor for lethal pneumococcal sepsis, and whenever possible, patients should receive the pneumococcal vaccine preoperatively.

## Management

The treatment options for Hodgkin's disease include radiation alone, radiation plus chemotherapy, and chemotherapy alone. Treatment decisions are based on stage more than histology. A simplified outline of treatment decisions by stage is shown in Table 199.2.

Definitive radiotherapy for early stage (stages I and IIA) Hodgkin's disease includes treatment of the upper mantle (cervical, mediastinal, and axillary nodes) and upper abdomen (celiac, portal, and splenic hilar nodes; the spleen, if present; and periaortic nodes to the aortic bifurcation). Stage III disease sometimes is classified further into subcategories to allow for less extensive radiotherapy when possible, while still treating all known involved nodal sites plus the next contiguous uninvolved nodal area.

Combination chemotherapy has been used to treat Hodgkin's disease since 1970. The first regimen to cure the majority of Hodgkin's patients was mechlorethamine, vincristine (Oncovin), prednisone, and procarbazine (MOPP), but more recently that has been replaced by doxorubicin (Adriamycin), bleomycin, vinblastine, and dacarbazine (ABVD) because of its equal or superior efficacy and lower toxicity, especially in gonadal and late bone marrow effects. There are many other effective regimens that can be used selectively if ABVD is contraindicated due to concomitant conditions (e.g., ischemic cardiac disease or pre-existing pulmonary fibrosis may result in enhanced cardiac or pulmonary toxicities from doxorubicin or bleomycin, respectively).

Chemotherapy is used in patients who have advanced disease (most stage III and all stage IV) or who have experienced relapses after previous radiotherapy. A subset of stage II patients also may receive neoadjuvant chemotherapy before definitive, curative radiotherapy is given: the chemotherapy reduces the size of large mediastinal masses, thereby making subsequent radiotherapy more effective and less toxic (as discussed in subsequent sections of this chapter).

## Prognosis

In contrast to the poor survivals seen in the 1960s, the overall survival rate today for patients with early-stage

**TABLE 199.1. Modified Ann Arbor Staging of Hodgkin's Disease and Non-Hodgkin's Lymphomas**

| Stage* | Definition |
|---|---|
| I | Involvement of a single node group |
| IE | Stage I, accompanied by a single extranodal site |
| II | Two or more involved nodal groups on the same side of the diaphragm |
| IIE | Stage II accompanied by a single extranodal site |
| III | Involved nodes on both sides of the diaphragm |
| $III_1$ | Upper abdominal nodes or spleen (S) involved |
| $III_2$ | Periaortic, iliac, or mesenteric nodes involved |
| IV | Extranodal disease beyond that indicated by E |

*The suffix A or B may be used with any stage. A indicates no systemic symptoms; B indicates documented fever, night sweats, or weight loss of >10% of body weight.

Hodgkin's disease is 75% to 90%, and for those with disseminated disease, it is 50% or greater. When patients experience relapses of Hodgkin's disease following radiotherapy, full-course chemotherapy results in a high percentage of complete remissions and a prolonged survival rate that approximates that of previously untreated patients with advanced disease. With modern radiotherapy techniques and better staging and therapy, such occurrences are less frequent. Failure to obtain a complete remission with chemotherapy or relapse within 1 to 2 years after achieving a remission predicts survival less than 3 years, although bone marrow or stem cell transplantation can extend survival for some patients.

## Complications

The complications of Hodgkin's disease are myriad (Table 199.3). **Infectious complications,** both acute and long-term, probably are more prevalent in Hodgkin's disease because of the inherent, and probably permanent, immunodeficiency in these patients, which is transiently worsened by the extensive radiotherapy and chemotherapy.

**Radiotherapy** causes early local complications such as sore throat, dysphagia, nausea and diarrhea as well as later complications such as radiation pneumonitis or fibrosis, pericardial effusion, pericardial constriction, coronary artery disease, radiation spinal cord

**TABLE 199.2. Treatment Regimens for Hodgkin's Disease**

| Stage | Treatment Alternatives | 5-Year Disease-Free Survival (%) |
|---|---|---|
| IA, IIA (includes E) | Extended-field radiotherapy | 80–90 |
| IB, IIB | Chemotherapy alone, or extended field radiotherapy if pathologically staged | 60–85 |
| IIA with bulky mediastinal disease | Combination chemotherapy plus mantle radiotherapy | 80 |
| $IIIA_1$ | Extended-field radiotherapy | 60–85 |
| $IIIA_2$ | Combination chemotherapy + total lymphoid radiotherapy | 70–85 |
| IIIB | Combination chemotherapy | 60–80 |
| IVA, IVB | Combination chemotherapy | 50–70 |

**TABLE 199.3. Complications of Hodgkin's Disease and Its Therapy**

- Infections
  - Complications of splenectomy
  - Infections with encapsulated bacteria (e.g., *S. pneumoniae*)
  - Other infections
    - Related to immunosuppressive therapy or corticosteroids
      - Reactivation of varicella/zoster
      - *Pneumocystis carinii* pneumonia (PCP)
      - *Cryptococcus neoformans* meningitis
- Thyroid dysfunction
  - Clinical hypothyroidism (6-25%)
  - Progressive elevation in TSH (31–53%)
- Cardiovascular (mostly related to mantle irradiation)
  - Accelerated coronary artery disease
  - Acute and chronic pericarditis
  - Pericardial effusion
  - Acute and chronic myocarditis
- Pulmonary
  - Acute radiation pneumonitis
  - Airway obstruction
  - Chronic pulmonary fibrosis
  - Interstitial lung disease (related to chemotherapy)
  - Opportunistic infection
- Gonadal dysfunction
  - Impaired spermatogenesis
  - Decreased testosterone levels
  - Transient amenorrhea
  - Permanent ovarian failure
  - Premature menopause
  - Spontaneous abortion (if therapy given in first trimester)
- Second neoplasms
  - Leukemia (acute non-lymphocytic leukemia)
  - Non-Hodgkin's lymphoma
  - Solid tumors (bone and soft tissue sarcoma, lung cancer, cancers of head and neck, melanoma, breast cancer)
- Hematologic
  - Reduced circulating T-cells
  - Secondary myelodysplasia
- Metabolic
  - Hypercalcemia
  - Lactic acidosis
- Neurologic
  - Paraneoplastic cerebellar degeneration
  - Neoplastic meningitis
  - Epidural compression

(Adapted from: Young RC, et al. Monogr Nat Cancer Inst 1990;10:55–60.)

damage, hypothyroidism, and late-onset solid tumors of the skin, lung, esophagus, and breast. Acute leukemia, although an extremely rare complication of radiotherapy alone, occurs more commonly when both radiotherapy and chemotherapy are given together, especially salvage chemotherapy with MOPP after failure of radiation. Careful lifelong follow-up is necessary to detect such complications in patients.

# CHAPTER 200 NON-HODGKIN'S LYMPHOMAS

The non-Hodgkin's lymphomas (NHL) are a heterogeneous group of malignant neoplasms of the immune system that, despite diverse origins, share a common link in the characteristic monoclonal proliferation of malignant B or T cells. In contrast to the predominantly reactive, polymorphic cells of Hodgkin's disease, those of the NHLs are monomorphic and monoclonal. Unlike Hodgkin's disease, which tends to spread by contiguity, NHL often spreads hematogenously to involve diverse sites important in immune regulation and lymphocyte proliferation. The bone marrow often is involved, although NHLs can arise in diverse extranodal sites. Thus, the site of presentation and spread of NHL are more unpredictable and widespread than in Hodgkin's disease. Most patients present with stage III or IV disease, thus rendering NHL somewhat less curable.

## Incidence and Epidemiology

Malignant lymphomas account for 6% to 7% of malignancies. It is estimated that 53,900 new cases will be diagnosed and 26,100 deaths from these lymphomas will occur in 2002. The incidence increases with age, although NHLs occur in all age groups. High-grade lymphomas are common in younger patients, with the frequency of indolent (low-grade) lymphomas increasing with age. States of immunosuppression—e.g., AIDS, rheumatoid arthritis, Sjögren syndrome, and a history of Hodgkin's disease—are all associated with an increased incidence of NHL, which shows a slight preponderance among men. It is one of the few cancers with a truly significantly increasing incidence in the United States: the frequency has doubled in less than a generation since the early 1970s.

## Etiology and Pathogenesis

The precise etiology of most cases of NHL is elusive. African Burkitt's lymphoma, the post-transplant lymphomas, and lymphomas associated with AIDS are strongly associated with **Epstein-Barr virus** (EBV) infections. The human T-cell leukemia virus 1 (HTLV-1) is implicated in adult T-cell leukemia and the lymphomas endemic in southwestern Japan and the Caribbean basin.

**Cytogenetic abnormalities** accompany several types of NHL. The 8;14 translocation in Burkitt's and other high-grade lymphomas and the 14;18 translocation in most follicular small cleaved lymphocytic lymphomas are the most striking findings. In the 8;14 translocation, the c-*myc* oncogene on chromosome 8 is translocated to the region of the immunoglobulin heavy-chain gene locus on chromosome 14. In the 14;18 translocation, the *bcl*-2 gene on chromosome 18 is translocated to the immunoglobulin heavy-chain promoter region on chromosome 14. The 8;14 abnormality seems to cause unregulated transcription and rapid growth, and the 14;18 translocation leads to increased cellular longevity, probably by retarding apoptosis.

## Pathology and Classification

The diagnosis of NHL is established by biopsy of an involved lymph node or other tissue, including bone marrow and the many extranodal sites where lymphomas may arise. The lymph node histology must be distinguished from that of infection (e.g., cytomegalovirus, mononucleosis, toxoplasmosis, HIV), Hodgkin's disease, and various reactive lymphadenopathies. The hallmark of malignancy, a clonal lymphocyte population, is established by immunohistochemical study, flow cytometry, or DNA analysis. Light microscopy can define the cell size and architecture.

Malignant lymphomas are classified according to either the Working Formulation or the Revised European-American Lymphoma (REAL) classification system (Table 200.1). Indolent lymphomas almost invariably arise from B cells, whereas a sizable portion of the intermediate and high-grade lymphomas are of T-cell origin.

## Clinical Features

The manifestations of NHL can best be described as protean. This group of diseases should always be included in the differential diagnosis of a patient with an unidentified organ disease process.

NHL commonly presents with lymphadenopathy similar to Hodgkin's disease, although hepatosplenomegaly and anatomically widespread, palpable adenopathy

**TABLE 200.1. Basic Classification of Lymphocytic Lymphomas**

| Working Formulation | REAL System | Cell of Origin |
|---|---|---|
| **Low-grade** | | |
| A. Small round lymphocytes, plasmacytic | B-CLL; small lymphocytic lymphoma<br>Lymphoplasmacytoid lymphoma | 98% B-cell; 2% T-cell |
| B. Follicular, predominantly small cleaved lymphocytes | Follicular center lymphomas | B-cell |
| C. Follicular mixed, small cleaved and large cells | Mantle cell lymphomas<br>Marginal zone lymphomas (MALT) | B-cell<br>B-cell |
| **Intermediate-grade** | | |
| D. Follicular, predominantly large cell | Follicular large B-cell lymphoma | B-cell |
| E. Diffuse small cleaved cell | Mantle cell lymphoma<br>MALT | 95% B-cell |
| F. Diffuse mixed small and large cell, including epithelioid component | Mantle cell lymphoma | 85% B-cell |
| G. Diffuse large cell, cleaved and non-cleaved | Diffuse large B-cell<br>Peripheral T-cell | 85% B-cell |
| **High-grade** | | |
| H. Large cell immunoblastic, including plasmacytoid, clear cell, polymorphous, lymphoblastic | Diffuse large B-cell lymphoma | 85% B-cell |
| I. Lymphoblastic, convoluted and nonconvoluted cells | Anaplastic large cell | 85% T-cell |
| J. Small non-cleaved cell, Burkitt and non-Burkitt | Burkitt's lymphoma | 100% B-cell |
| **Miscellaneous** | | |
| Cutaneous T-cell lymphoma | Mycosis fungoides;<br>Sezary syndrome | |
| Composite lymphomas | Miscellaneous | |
| Anaplastic large cell | Anaplastic large cell | |
| Unclassified | | |

REAL = Revised European American Lymphoma Classification System.

are more common. Conversely, clinically or radiographically significant mediastinal lymphadenopathy is less frequent. The adenopathy may be bulky, and large abdominal masses may be felt. Massively enlarged nodes may cause organ compression or obstruction. The nodes are usually described as discrete or rubbery, unlike the hard nodes of metastatic carcinoma. The bone marrow is commonly involved (20%–40% of cases), more frequently when hepatosplenomegaly or hematologic abnormalities are present and especially when the histology is low-grade.

Lymphomas with a large-cell component and a diffuse histologic growth pattern are known collectively as **high-grade,** or aggressive. They are more likely to be localized, limited-stage disease, but also are likely to show locally aggressive, invasive characteristics; hence, the historical term *reticulum cell sarcoma*. High-grade NHLs also may involve the central nervous system (CNS), manifesting as a parenchymal mass or lymphomatous infiltration of the meninges and cranial or spinal nerve roots, with resultant nerve dysfunction. Diplopia and facial weakness, myelopathy, or radiculopathy at any level may occur.

The presentations of **extranodal lymphomas** are legion, mimicking tumors of the brain, thyroid, gastrointestinal tract, lung, or genital tract of either gender. The B symptoms characteristic of Hodgkin's disease occur in NHL as well.

## Evaluation and Staging

The evaluation of patients with NHL is similar to that of Hodgkin's disease. Physical examination and CT scanning of the abdomen and occasionally the chest are useful to show enlarged nodes. The mediastinum is infrequently involved, except in high-grade lymphoblastic lymphomas.

Bone marrow biopsy is required. The marrow is involved in most disseminated low-grade lymphomas but is not as prognostically important. In intermediate and high-grade lymphomas, marrow involvement is less frequent, but, when present, it is more ominous. Additional investigation may be necessary, such as examination of the cerebrospinal fluid or GI tract.

The Ann Arbor staging system is shown in Table 199.1. The "E" category is used often in extranodal lymphomas. Indolent, low-grade lymphomas rarely present with localized disease (stages I or II), but intermediate and high-grade lymphomas are localized in up to 40% of cases.

## Management

Treatment of lymphomas is complex, because the biology of disease varies with the subtype. Unlike Hodgkin's disease, in which treatment decisions depend primarily on the stage of disease, in NHL, histologic features often are more important than stage in treatment strategies. Table 200.2. presents an overview of the treatment options.

### Low-grade lymphomas

Low-grade lymphomas, listed as subtypes A, B, or C in Table 193.1, are almost always stage III or IV disease. Initially, even patients with stage IV disease often can be observed without treatment. Palliative radiotherapy or oral-based chemotherapy may be used on disease progression. The rare patient with low-grade, low-stage lymphoma usually is curable with precise, comprehensive radiotherapy, but rarely, if ever, with chemotherapy.

Survival averages 7 to 10 years, with many patients living 10 to 20 years even if not treated to remission. This "watch and wait" approach has become the standard of care for such patients. However, such an approach requires regular, careful monitoring of disease status, and the more aggressive combination chemotherapy must be implemented if the indolent disease can no longer be managed conservatively. More aggressive intervention usually is used with younger patients, those with B symptoms, or those with symptoms due to bulky disease.

#### *Complications and prognosis*

About 5% of indolent lymphomas secrete a monoclonal immunoglobulin. Depending on the class of immunoglobulin secreted or the antigen it recognizes, patients may present with a syndrome of hyperviscosity (Waldenström's macroglobulinemia), renal failure, autoimmune hemolytic anemia, or autoimmune thrombocytopenia.

Complications of treatment include marrow failure from repetitive and prolonged radiotherapy or chemotherapy, increased susceptibility to infection, and occasional chemotherapy-induced leukemia.

Careful follow-up is necessary because of the propensity of low-grade diseases to transform into intermediate or high-grade, diffuse large-cell lymphomas. Such transformation markedly worsens the prognosis, and more aggressive therapy must be offered.

### Intermediate-grade lymphomas

Large-cell diffuse lymphoma is the most commonly diagnosed subgroup of intermediate-grade lymphomas. Localized disease is managed with excisional biopsy, followed by combination chemotherapy and consolidative radiation, an approach particularly suitable for

**TABLE 200.2. Treatment Options in Non-Hodgkin's Lymphoma**

| Histology/Stage | Options | Results |
|---|---|---|
| *Low grade* | Observation, local radiation, chemotherapy | Median survival 7–10 yrs<br>Few cures |
| I-II | Definitive radiation | ~80% 5-yr survival; finite cure rate |
| III-IV | Observation, single or combination chemotherapy | Median survival 5–10 yrs |
| *Intermediate* | Combination of radiotherapy + chemotherapy | 80% 5-yr survival; 30-65% only with radiation alone |
| I-II, including extranodal | | |
| III-IV | Combination chemotherapy; high-dose therapy in some cases with marrow transplantation | Complete response 50–70% with 30–40% 5-yr survival |
| *High-grade* | Chemotherapy + radiation; intrathecal chemotherapy with or without radiation; maintenance therapy for 2 yrs | 50–60% 5-yr survival |
| I-II, including extranodal (E) | | |
| III-IV | Combination chemotherapy; intrathecal chemotherapy with or without radiation; consider high-dose therapy with marrow transplantation | 20–30% 5-yr survival |

extranodal presentations (stages IE and IIE). Initial excision is especially important in primary gastrointestinal lymphomas, which may manifest rapid tumor lysis with combination chemotherapy, resulting in bleeding or perforation.

In stage III or IV disease, chemotherapy with cyclophosphamide, doxorubicin, vincristine (Oncovin), and prednisone (CHOP), given every 3 weeks for 6 to 8 cycles, results in a 50% to 60% rate of complete responses. Among these responses, 60% to 80% are durable, resulting in a 30% to 45% cure rate. Alternative dose-intensive regimens have now been proved to be no more effective and are reserved for the rare patient with high-grade lymphoma. Derivative regimens omitting doxorubicin are available for patients with pre-existing cardiac disease. High-dose consolidation therapy with autologous bone marrow or stem cell reconstitution is a promising approach for high-risk younger patients because of its proven ability to salvage a few such patients in relapse.

*Complications and prognosis*

Meninges and nerve roots are involved by lymphoma in 9% to 10% of patients with diffuse large-cell lymphomas, especially those with preexisting bone marrow infiltration. With suspected CNS involvement, cerebrospinal fluid should be analyzed.

Localized intermediate-grade lymphomas, whether nodal or extranodal in presentation, can be cured with combined modality therapy in 50% to 80% of cases. Stage III and IV disease poses more of a problem, with only about 45% of patients surviving disease-free for over 5 years. Failure to achieve a complete response to initial chemotherapy results in death within 1 to 2 years. Favorable prognostic factors include age less than 60 years, a normal lactate dehydrogenase level, stage III disease, stage IV disease without marrow or CNS involvement, and a rapid response to therapy (complete response in one to three cycles). One fourth or fewer of older patients and those with adverse prognostic factors are cured.

## High-grade Lymphomas, Including AIDS-associated Lymphomas

The high-grade lymphomas include three uncommon histologic types.

### Large-Cell Immunoblastic Lymphomas

Large-cell immunoblastic lymphoma is so named because the cells resemble the normal immunoblasts of the follicular centers. Lymphomas of this histology are more aggressive than those of the intermediate grades. They often are associated with the Epstein-Barr virus (EBV), organ transplantation, and HIV infection (where they are an AIDS-defining neoplasm).

These lymphomas are often extranodal in presentations, with a predilection for spread to the CNS when they present as widely disseminated disease. Combination chemotherapy is less successful than with the intermediate-grade lymphomas, and opportunistic infections and associated HIV-induced myelosuppression in persons with AIDS make aggressive chemotherapy hazardous. Lymphomas arising in the setting of iatrogenic immunosuppression (e.g., after solid organ transplantation) can represent polyclonal (post-transplant lymphoproliferative disease [PTLD]) as well as monoclonal B-cell proliferations. Conventional therapies in this latter setting almost always fail.

### Burkitt's Lymphoma

Burkitt's lymphoma, a diffuse B-cell lymphoma, has a distinctive histology, an aggressive course, and remarkable sensitivity to chemotherapy. In Africa, the EBV-associated form is endemic, but this lymphoma is rare in the United States. In the United States, it usually is seen in older children and young adults and presents with massive abdominal disease, with frequent bone marrow, peripheral blood, and meningeal involvement.

Whereas the African form of disease often is cured with single-agent chemotherapy, the American form requires more aggressive chemotherapy to achieve a respectable cure rate. With this intensive therapy, the prognosis for localized involvement is favorable (50%–80% cure). With dissemination and organ or meningeal involvement, however, the prognosis is guarded (20% long-term survival).

This tumor is so responsive to chemotherapy that massive **tumor lysis** may ensue with the first cycle. Pretreatment with allopurinol, vigorous hydration, and diuresis with meticulous monitoring and intervention for hyperkalemia are imperative during the first few days of the first treatment cycle.

### Adult Lymphoblastic Lymphomas

Adult lymphoblastic lymphomas are predominantly thymic T-cell lymphomas and are closely related to T-cell acute lymphoblastic leukemia. Their incidence clusters in the teen and young adult years, predominantly in men. They usually are associated with prominent mediastinal masses, one of the few NHLs to present this way. Treatment is identical to that of acute lymphoblastic leukemia, with CNS prophylaxis and prolonged maintenance therapy, in contrast to the more limited duration of treatment for other high-grade lymphomas.

## Angioimmunoblastic Lymphadenopathy

Angioimmunoblastic lymphadenopathy starts as a polyclonal, usually nonneoplastic, proliferation of immune cells with similarities to, and frequent evolution into, a peripheral T-cell lymphoma. This disorder presents in older persons as generalized lymphadenopathy, hepatosplenomegaly, skin rash, fever, weight loss, anemia (frequently autoimmune hemolytic anemia), and polyclonal hypergammaglobulinemia. A polymorphous cell population and capillary proliferation are seen in affected lymph nodes. Treatment is with corticosteroids or cautious combination chemotherapy, but survival is usually only 1 to 2 years.

# CHAPTER 201 MULTIPLE MYELOMA AND PLASMA CELL DYSCRASIAS

The plasma cell dyscrasias are a clonal proliferation of immunoglobulin-producing cells, including plasma cells and plasmacytoid lymphocytes. This proliferation leads to the production of a monoclonal immunoglobulin which may represent an intact antibody or just the light-chain component. The clinical manifestations depend on the proliferative and secretory characteristics of each patient's malignant clone of cells. The clonal proliferation and resultant diseases or syndromes can be classified into distinct syndromes, including the nonmalignant monoclonal gammopathy of unknown significance (MGUS), isolated plasmacytoma (essentially a malignant myeloma limited to a single osseous or extraosseous site), multiple myeloma, Waldenström macroglobulinemia, or systemic amyloidosis.

## Incidence and Epidemiology

The age distribution is similar for all the plasma cell disorders. MGUS is more common after the seventh decade of life, when approximately 2% of individuals over age 70 are thought to have this syndrome.

Multiple myeloma is an uncommon disease. Its incidence is 3 to 4 per 100,000 Caucasians and 6.7 to 9.6 per 100,000 African-Americans (for women and men, respectively), with 14,600 new cases predicted to be diagnosed in the U.S. in 2002. Less than 2% of cases occur in persons under age 40; the median age is 68 years for men and 70 for women.

## Etiology and Pathogenesis

The etiology of plasma cell tumors is elusive. Previous exposure to ionizing radiation may be a risk factor. The cell of origin is a precursor B cell. The clonal progeny (i.e., plasma cell or plasmacytoid lymphocytes) are terminally differentiated, usually functional cells, in that they can synthesize and secrete immunoglobulin molecules or fragments. This is in contrast to the malignant cells of most non-Hodgkin's lymphomas, which are arrested at intermediate stages of differentiation and do not routinely produce immunoglobulin.

Proliferation of myeloma cells is accompanied by secretion of **$\beta_2$-microglobulin** (the light chain of the major histocompatibility complex), which may be used as a marker of disease activity. The pathogenesis of **amyloidosis** involves the tissue deposition of light chains in a protein matrix secreted by a dysplastic clone of aberrant, albeit nonmalignant, plasma cells.

## Pathology

Gross pathologic findings in the plasma cell disorders include osteolytic bone lesions, and, in advanced cases, involvement of lymph nodes and other organs such as the kidneys. Light microscopy shows proliferation of plasma cells of variable phenotypic expression, with focal or diffuse infiltration of the bone marrow (Figure 201.1). The accompanying osteolysis seen on bone biopsies is caused by the proliferation of osteoclasts actively resorbing bone. Pathologic fractures may be seen.

The kidney may show amyloid deposition in the glomeruli. However, the most common lesion is **Bence-Jones kidney,** or light-chain nephropathy. Protein casts, degenerative changes, and inflammatory reactions in the renal tubules are characteristic and lead to renal failure.

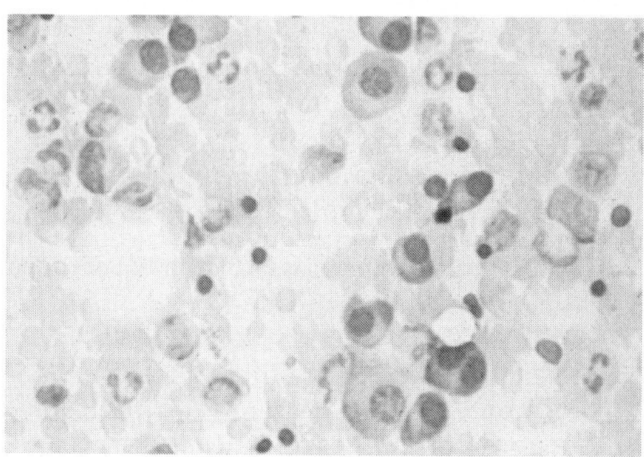

**FIGURE 201.1. Bone marrow in multiple myeloma showing a significant increase in plasma cells.**
(Courtesy of Lawrence S. Hurwitz, MD, Milwaukee, Wisconsin.)

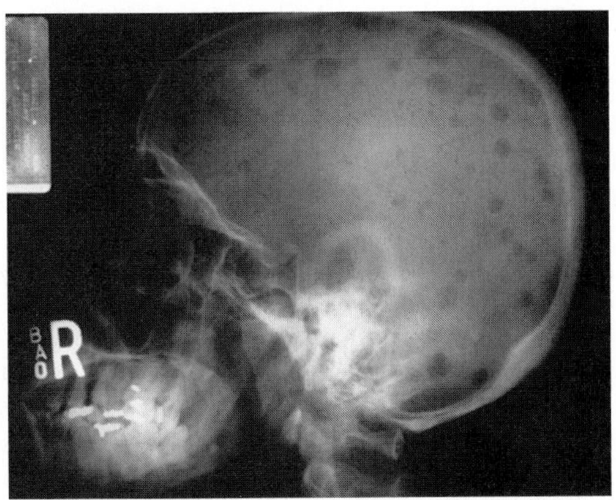

**FIGURE 201.2.** Lytic skull lesions with punched-out appearance in multiple myeloma.

## Clinical Features

Persons with MGUS are asymptomatic. Multiple myeloma sometimes is found in patients in an asymptomatic stage, when routine blood tests or urinalysis reveals an increased erythrocyte sedimentation rate (ESR), mild anemia, or unexplained proteinuria. Such patients have a better prognosis and tolerate therapy better than debilitated patients in a more advanced stage.

**Bone pain** is the most common presenting symptom of overt myeloma. The pain often is sudden and severe, due to an incidental pathologic fracture. Radiographs usually reveal widespread, multiple osteolytic or "punched-out" lesions throughout the skeleton (Figure 201.2). On occasion, diffuse osteoporosis is seen, rather than lytic lesions. Skeletal surveys are preferred to radionuclide bone scans in myeloma, because the lytic bone lesions in myeloma do not evoke an osteoblastic response. As the disease progresses, the lytic lesions increase in size and number; vertebral compression fractures follow, with resultant marked skeletal deformity and possible spinal cord compression. The patient may actually lose several inches in height.

Patients with myeloma have increased susceptibility to **bacterial infections,** particularly pneumococcal infections. Although 99% of patients with multiple myeloma secrete an aberrant antibody product, synthesis of functioning polyclonal antibody is routinely suppressed.

**Impaired kidney function** is found in up to 80% of patients and may be the presenting feature. Renal disease in myeloma most commonly results from tubular damage related to the reabsorption of large amounts of Bence-Jones proteins. Use of IV contrast media can exacerbate renal dysfunction and should be avoided if multiple myeloma is suspected or previously diagnosed. **Neurologic problems** develop in many myeloma patients and involve all levels of the nervous system, including peripheral neuropathies (from amyloid infiltration) and nerve root symptoms (from vertebral compression fractures). Spinal cord compression, due to vertebral involvement, is a medical emergency. Confusion and stupor may accompany azotemia, hypercalcemia, or hyperviscosity.

Certain patients present with solitary **plasmacytomas** of bone or soft tissue. Soft tissue plasmacytomas are most commonly located in the upper airway and progress to myeloma less commonly. However, myeloma develops within 5 years in many patients with a solitary plasmacytoma of bone.

## Laboratory Features

In multiple myeloma, peripheral blood almost invariably demonstrates **rouleaux** formation of the red cells and a markedly elevated ESR. Hypercalcemia, azotemia, and hyperuricemia also are common. Monoclonal immunoglobulin (Ig) composed of a single heavy-chain type and a single light-chain class (kappa or lambda) is characteristic of myeloma, MGUS, and Waldenström's macroglobulinemia, whereas secretion of light chains characterizes amyloidosis. The most common monoclonal myeloma protein type is IgG, followed by IgA or IgD. When associated with proven myeloma, these individual paraproteins are called myeloma proteins, or "M spikes," referring to their appearance on immunoglobulin electrophoresis. In about 25% of cases, Bence-Jones proteinuria (isolated light chains filtered so effectively by the glomeruli that they are absent in the serum) may be the sole evidence of a paraprotein secretion. Bone marrow examination in multiple myeloma usually reveals an excess of abnormal plasma cells, usually exceeding 30%, frequently in large coalescent masses that efface normal marrow architecture.

## Diagnosis and Evaluation

Diagnostic criteria for **MGUS** include a 24-hour urine showing a monoclonal Ig (<3.5 g/dl for IgG, <2 g/dl for IgA, or <1 g of light chains), with less than 5% plasma cells in the bone marrow aspirate and no bone lesions or extraskeletal tumors. Reactive plasmacytosis, as seen in chronic diseases such as rheumatoid arthritis, usually is less than 15% and is untenable with a diagnosis of myeloma unless other evidence is strong (e.g., lytic bone lesions). Monoclonal immunoglobulins are found in a few (<5%) patients with chronic lymphocytic leukemia, rarely in non-Hodgkin's lymphomas, and incidentally in some patients with a variety of chronic diseases.

**Multiple myeloma** is a fatal disease, and every effort must be made to avoid confusing MGUS and reactive states with myeloma. The diagnostic criteria of overt multiple myeloma (Table 201.1) include bone marrow plasmacytosis over 15%, presence of a serum or urine monoclonal Ig (0.5% of cases are nonsecretory), and lytic bone lesions or osteoporosis on skeletal survey. Those presenting with renal failure pose difficult diagnostic problems, especially if no serum paraprotein (M protein) is apparent; one must remember that renal failure due to secretion of only light chain (Bence-Jones nephropathy) or amyloid deposition might be present.

Once multiple myeloma is diagnosed, the tumor burden is determined, based on the number of bone lesions, the serum or urine levels of monoclonal Ig (M protein), and the presence or absence of hypercalcemia, anemia, or renal failure (Table 201.2).

**Amyloidosis** complicates multiple myeloma in about 15% of cases. It also may occur as a primary disorder with or without monoclonal immunoglobulin spikes on electrophoresis and significant marrow plasmacytosis. It is suggested by the presence of amyloid deposition in the tongue, peripheral nerves, kidney, heart, or gastrointestinal tract, leading to macroglossia, peripheral neuropathy, renal failure, cardiac failure, or intestinal malabsorption. The diagnosis is confirmed by amyloid staining of tissue sections of rectum, tongue, kidney, or aspirated abdominal fat.

**TABLE 201.1. Diagnostic Criteria for Multiple Myeloma**

*Major*

1. Biopsy-proven plasmacytoma
2. Marrow plasmacytosis (>30% plasma cells)
3. SPEP: M-spike with:
   IgG >3.5 g/dl, or
   IgA >2.0 g/dl
   UPEP: kappa or lambda light chains >1.0 g/24 h

*Minor*

A. Lytic bone lesions
B. Marrow plasmacytosis (plasma cells 10–30%)
C. M-spike present, but less than that needed to fulfill major criteria
D. IgM normal, IgG <600 mg/dl, or IgA <100 mg/dl

*Diagnosis confirmed when:*

One major (1) + minor A, C or D are present; or
One major (2) + Minor A, C or D are present; or
One major (3) + Minor B or A are present, or
Minor criteria A, B and C are present; or
Minor criteria B, C and D are present

SPEP = serum protein electrophoresis; UPEP = urine protein electrophoresis

## Management

No therapy is required for MGUS. About 10% to 25% of cases eventually evolve—over years to decades—into myeloma, macroglobulinemia, or systemic amyloidosis. This transformation can be detected through comprehensive follow-up. Most patients with this benign condition never develop a disease requiring therapy.

Occasionally a patient with myeloma will have an indolent course requiring little or no intervention for months or even years. These patients, classified as having **smoldering myeloma,** should be followed closely with

**TABLE 201.2. Staging of Multiple Myeloma**

| Stage* | Myeloma Cell Mass | Criteria |
|---|---|---|
| I | Low (0.6 × $10^{12}$ cells/$m^2$) | All of the following: Hemoglobin >10 g/dl<br>Serum calcium† ≤12 mg/dl *or*<br>Normal bone survey or solitary lesion only<br>M component production:<br>IgG <5 g/dl<br>IgA <3 g/dl<br>Urine light chain <4 g/24 hr |
| II | Intermediate (0.6-1.2 × $10^{12}$ cells/$m^2$) | Values intermediate between those for stages I and III |
| III | High (>1.2 × $10^{12}$ cells/$m^2$) | Any of the following: Hemoglobin <8.5 g/dl<br>Serum calcium† >12 mg/dl *or*<br>Advanced lytic lesions on bone survey<br>M component production:<br>IgG >7 g/dl<br>IgA >5 g/dl<br>Urine light chain excretion >12 g/24 hr |

*Stages subclassified according to serum creatinine (Scr) and blood urea nitrogen (BUN). Subtype A = Scr <2 mg/dl or BUN <30 mg/dl; B = Scr ≥2 mg/dl or BUN ≥30 mg/dl.
†Should be corrected for serum albumin level.
(Reprinted with permission from: Durie BG, Salmon SE. Cancer 1975;36:842.)

laboratory and radiologic monitoring. Solitary plasmacytomas should be treated with irradiation and closely followed.

### Chemotherapy

For overt, symptomatic **multiple myeloma,** chemotherapy is clearly indicated, with an alkylating agent (melphalan or cyclophosphamide) plus prednisone given intermittently every 3 to 6 weeks until maximum response, followed by observation until relapse. Subjective and objective responses occur in 50% to 70% of those treated, as manifested by a decline in the M protein levels and improvement in pain, anemia, and renal function. Combinations of multiple alkylating agents, nitrosoureas, vincristine, and doxorubicin usually lead to higher response rates, with some but not all studies showing an improvement in survival. Current research studies are focusing on the role of autologous or allogeneic bone marrow transplantation. Early analysis suggests that such therapies improve survival with acceptable degrees of toxicity. However, to date there is no evidence that this, or any other, treatment cures multiple myeloma.

Amyloidosis secondary to multiple myeloma may resolve with successful chemotherapy. However, primary amyloidosis treated with identical melphalan-prednisone regimens is more refractory, with the largest series reporting only an 18% response of limited duration.

### Other measures

General supportive measures play an important role in the management of patients with these disorders. Careful attention to proper hydration, caloric intake, regular ambulation, and adequate analgesia will enhance patient comfort and avoid hypercalcemia and renal failure. Palliative radiotherapy to specific, painful bone lesions, while highly effective, cannot substitute for systemic chemotherapy. Prophylactic orthopedic stabilization may be necessary for impending pathologic fracture. Despite a suboptimal immune response in these patients, pneumococcal vaccine is recommended.

## Complications

Table 201.3. lists the complications of plasma cell disorders. Anemia may respond to erythropoietin or androgens. Hypercalcemia has been successfully treated with corticosteroids or the new bisphosphonates, such as pamidronate, and hydration. Infectious complications are more common in the first few months of treatment, when chemotherapy-induced granulocytopenia and disease-related antibody deficiency coexist. Late complications of chemotherapy include acute nonlymphocytic leukemia in 5% to 10% of long-term survivors.

**TABLE 201.3. Complications of Multiple Myeloma**

| |
|---|
| Mechanical |
| Bone pain |
| Pathologic fractures |
| Epidural spinal cord compression |
| Infections |
| By viruses and encapsulated bacteria (e.g., *Streptococcus pneumoniae*) |
| Hypercalcemia |
| Due to osteolysis (IL-6, TNF-β, IL-1) |
| Marrow failure |
| Anemia, leukopenia |
| Thrombocytopenia |
| Plasma cell leukemia |
| Renal insufficiency |
| Light chain nephropathy |
| Amyloid |
| Hypercalcemia |
| Hyperuricemia |
| Renal failure due to IV contrast |
| Plasma cell infiltration |
| Hyperviscosity |
| With $IgG_3$ and IgM |
| Cryoglobulinemia |
| Amyloidosis |
| Malabsorption |
| Cardiomyopathy |
| Renal failure, nephrotic syndrome |
| Second malignancies |
| Acute nonlymphocytic leukemia |
| Myelodysplastic syndrome |
| Undifferentiated, large-cell, or immunoblastic lymphoma |

IL = interleukin; TNF = tumor necrosis factor.

Late in the course of disease, myeloma may transform into an aggressive form that resembles large-cell immunoblastic lymphoma or leukemia and is especially fulminant.

## Prognosis

Multiple myeloma is universally fatal. The prognosis varies with the stage of disease at presentation and the response to treatment. Median survival ranges from 2 to 3.5 years, with survival of 20% to 30% at 5 years and less than 10% at 10 years. Progressive drug resistance, renal failure, infection, and second malignancies are the usual causes of death. Coexisting amyloidosis further worsens the prognosis.

## Waldenström's Macroglobulinemia

Waldenström macroglobulinemia is a low-grade malignant lymphoma of plasmacytoid lymphocytes, which secrete excessive amounts of a monoclonal IgM paraprotein. Bone marrow, lymph node, liver, and spleen infiltrations are typical.

Most patients with macroglobulinemia present with symptoms related to anemia or the presence of the macroglobulin, such as cryoglobulinemia (e.g., Raynaud phenomenon), hyperviscosity (e.g., visual disturbances), and protein–protein interactions (e.g., platelet dysfunction with petechiae and ecchymoses). Unlike multiple myeloma, renal failure and lytic bone lesions are rare. The diagnosis requires the demonstration of a monoclonal IgM paraprotein in the serum and characteristic infiltration of plasmacytoid lymphocytes in the bone marrow or lymph nodes.

Because cell proliferation is low, this indolent lymphoma usually is treated with the same regimens used in multiple myeloma, although patients usually respond to any typical treatment regimens used for lymphoma. Plasmapheresis is used to control hyperviscosity emergently or prophylactically when the serum viscosity rises above 4 units while waiting for response to chemotherapy (which may require weeks to be effective). Overall, the median survival in Waldenström's macroglobulinemia is 5 years.

# CHAPTER 202 BREAST CANCER

Breast cancer is the most common cancer in women and the second leading cause (following lung cancer) of cancer-related death (in women). Its incidence has been slowly increasing over the past 30 years, with a marked increase in diagnoses since 1990 due to wider screening.

## Incidence and Epidemiology

In 2002, 205,000 new cases of breast cancer were diagnosed and 40,000 deaths from breast cancer occurred in the United States. The distribution of breast cancer shows striking international variations. It is most common in the northern latitudes, the Western world, and among Caucasians. Despite a low incidence in Asia and the tropics, Asian immigrants to Western areas gradually assume the incidence patterns of their adopted new homes.

Various factors can be used to estimate an individual's risk for developing breast cancer (Table 202.1). In large populations of breast cancer patients studied for these risk factors, 20% to 40% had one or more of the "high-risk" characteristics. However, most women who develop breast cancer are not of unusually high risk. The current estimate of an overall lifetime incidence is 10% to 12%, with the greatest risk concentrated in the sixth decade and beyond.

## Etiology and Pathogenesis

Hereditary susceptibility accounts for 5% to 20% of cases and is associated with recently discovered germline abnormalities on multiple chromosomes, including the *BRCA-1, BRCA-2,* and *p53* genes. Amplification of the *HER2/NEU* gene, which codes for the epidermal growth factor receptor, is a somatic mutation associated with cancer progression and a prognostic predictor of disease behavior, but is not a risk factor for disease development.

Hormonal factors appear to play an important role in disease development and progression (see Table 202.1). The effect of early menarche, delayed pregnancy, and late menopause is to prolong the cyclic stimulation. Diet and obesity may lead to a relative state of excess estrogens, and alcohol may alter estrogen metabolism. In these instances, prolonged estrogen stimulation probably acts as a promoter to more fundamental molecular perturbations. Prolonged estrogen therapy (e.g., hormonal replacement therapy), with or without progestins, is a minor risk factor.

## Pathology

Almost all breast cancers are **adenocarcinomas.** Cancer arising in ductal tissue, termed **infiltrating ductal carcinoma,** accounts for 60% to 80% of invasive breast cancer cases. Carcinoma arising from the secretory lobules is termed **infiltrating lobular carcinoma** and accounts for about 10% to 15% of cases. **Carcinoma in situ** is a tumor that has not broken through the basement membrane and invaded the surrounding stroma. It remains confined within the ducts or lobules. Whereas lobular carcinoma in situ (LCIS) is considered premalignant, with a 25% chance of progression into malignancy, ductal carcinoma in situ (DCIS) is considered a malignancy. DCIS is six times more common than LCIS, and is treated analogously to minimally invasive disease, with the caveat that lymph node sampling and systemic chemotherapy are not warranted.

Other rare forms of breast cancer include **Paget disease** of the nipple, which presents as an eczematoid dermatitis caused by infiltration of the nipple with an underlying carcinoma, and **inflammatory breast carci-**

**TABLE 202.1. Risk Factors for Breast Cancer**

| Risk Factor | Estimated Risk Magnitude |
|---|---|
| Feminine gender | Overwhelming |
| Age over 30 | Risk begins ~ age 30; escalates rapidly ~ age 50–60. |
| Obesity | Potentially a factor after menopause |
| Regular alcohol intake | A factor in case control studies |
| History of previous breast cancer | Risk is 1% annually in opposite breast |
| Previous premalignant breast disease | Relative risk: |
| Hyperplasia | 1.6 |
| Atypical hyperplasia | >4.0 |
| LCIS | 20–25% cancer risk in either breast over 2 decades |
| Heredity | |
| One affected first-degree relative | 1.5 |
| Two affected first-degree relatives | ≥3.0 |
| Premenopausal bilateral cancer in first-degree relatives | 8.0 |
| Hormonal factors | |
| Age at menarche <12 | 1.5–1.7 |
| Age at menopause >54 | 1.5–1.7 |
| First pregnancy after age 30–35 | 1.5–2.0 |
| Nulliparity | 1.5 |
| Early pregnancy, age <21 | ↓ risk by 60% |
| Early castration without hormone replacement | Marked reduction in risk |
| Prolonged hormone replacement | 1.3 |
| Prolonged oral contraceptives | Debatable effects; may be a risk factor when started at a very "young" age |

LCIS = lobular carcinoma in situ

**noma,** a distinct clinical entity presenting as erythema and edema of the overlying skin due to extensive involvement of the dermal lymphatics from an underlying aggressive ductal carcinoma.

The current understanding of breast cancer recognizes that there is the potential for occult hematogenous dissemination even in otherwise early presentations and that it may be systemic almost from inception. Involvement of the regional lymph nodes is a marker for likely metastasis to other sites, as are other prognostic features discussed in the following sections.

## Clinical Features

The usual clinical presentation is a painless lump or localized thickening (fibrosis) in the breast. The majority of breast lumps are discovered by the patient herself; most breast masses, however, are not cancer. Breast masses in premenopausal women usually are due to fibrocystic disease or fibroadenoma. Additional causes for masses in the postmenopausal age group are sclerosing adenosis, fibrocystic disease, fibroadenomas, or fat necrosis due to unappreciated trauma. Because age is the most important risk factor, suspicion should be adjusted accordingly.

With screening, early breast cancer may present as a mammographic abnormality, before it is detectable on breast examination. Typically, the physical examination reveals a localized, firm mass or thickening of the breast tissue. In more advanced cancer, there may be dimpling or puckering of the overlying skin, distortion of the breast or nipple, or palpable axillary or supraclavicular nodes. More locally advanced cancer is characterized by skin fixation, ulceration, adjacent skin nodules or inflammatory skin changes.

Pain or discomfort, while more common in nonmalignant breast conditions, may be a presenting symptom in breast cancer. Rarely, the patient will report an axillary mass with or without an evident breast abnormality. Nipple discharge most often is due to benign intraductal papillomas, but cancer must always be excluded.

Metastases cause symptoms related to the organ of involvement (e.g., bone pain, jaundice, cough, CNS symptoms).

## Diagnosis, Clinical Evaluation, and Staging

When a breast mass is discovered, either clinically or on mammography, the diagnosis must be established pathologically. In premenopausal women, a painful, cystic mass may be observed for resolution through one menstrual cycle to exclude the possibility of fibrocystic disease, but any persistent or suspicious mass must be biopsied promptly. **Mammography** is always done

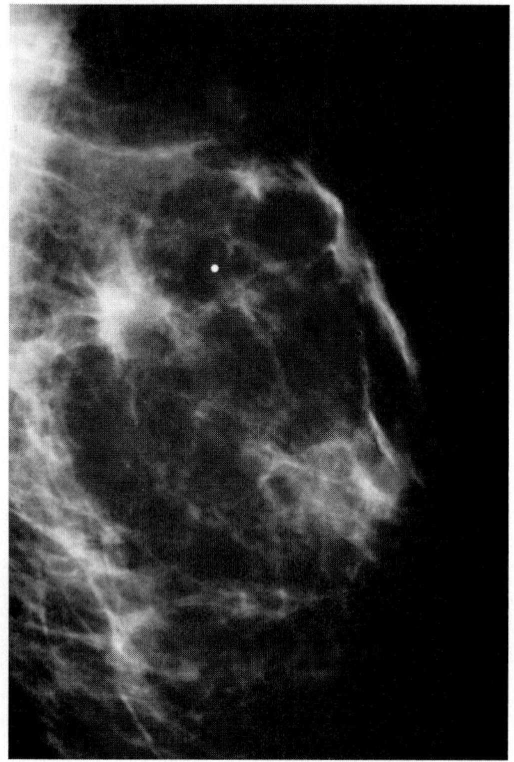

**FIGURE 202.1.** **Mammographic findings in breast cancer. The characteristic findings associated with cancer are a spiculated irregular mass or clustered microcalcification. Only a biopsy procedure can establish whether a mammographically detectable lesion is benign or malignant.**

before biopsy to evaluate the appearance of the mass and both breasts (Figure 202.1). **Ultrasonography** is now routinely incorporated into diagnostic evaluations, often distinguishing solid from cystic masses, showing satellite lesions, and so on. Palpable abnormalities may be biopsied by fine needle aspiration or direct excision. When mammography shows an abnormality but a mass is not palpable, radiologically guided fine-needle aspiration or excisional biopsy with needle or wire localization is necessary.

**Fine-needle aspiration** (FNA) of cystic lesions can exclude cancer accurately, but clinical and mammographic follow-up are necessary to ensure that the apparently benign disease process behaves as expected. FNA is about 90% sensitive in tumors presenting as solid masses. It is technically simple and, when positive for carcinoma, is reliable, with a false-positive rate of 1% to 2%. Because virtually all solid masses are subsequently excised for definitive diagnosis or therapy, the accuracy of FNA is acceptable and allows the patient and physician to plan subsequent treatment interventions. However, a negative or indeterminate cytologic result in a patient with a solid mass mandates subsequent excision and definitive histologic examination. Cytology from cystic lesions has true negative rate of about 95%. Again, postaspiration studies are mandatory, as is appropriate follow-up.

Further clinical evaluation after the diagnosis of cancer includes reevaluation of the physical examination, chest radiograph, and screening blood studies. Following primary surgery to remove the lump lymph node, sampling is indicated if the lesion is invasive. Over the past few decades the extent and concurrent morbidity of axillary node resection has decreased, culminating in the current technique of "sentinel node" biopsy, in which a radionuclide and visible blue dye are injected into the tumor bed; within about 10 minutes the surgeon can identify the lymph node or nodes draining the tumor site. With very careful histologic and immunohistochemical study of these nodes, it is possible, with about 95% accuracy, to rule out lymph node involvement. If the sentinel nodes are involved, the surgeon usually proceeds to remove the level I and sometimes level II nodes to understand the extent of nodal metastases, which guides staging and prognosis. **TNM staging** can be completed (Table 202.2) and a decision made regarding further staging procedures and subsequent treatment. Additional tests may include CT scans of chest, abdomen, and pelvis,

**TABLE 202.2. TNM Staging of Breast Cancer**

| | |
|---|---|
| *Tumor* | |
| T1s | Carcinoma in situ |
| T1 | Tumor <2 cm in diameter |
| T2 | Tumor >2 cm but <5 cm |
| T3 | Tumor >5 cm |
| T4 | Extension to chest wall; skin edema, ulceration, satellite nodules on breast; inflammatory carcinoma |
| *Nodes* | |
| N0 | No clinically palpable nodes |
| N1 | Movable ipsilateral axillary nodes |
| N2 | Nodes (ipsilateral) fixed to one another or to axillary structure |
| N3 | Internal mammary nodes |
| *Metastases* | |
| M0 | No metastases |
| M1 | Metastases, including ipsilateral supraclavicular node |

From the American Joint Committee on Cancer. Manual for Staging of Cancer. 4th ed. Philadelphia, JB Lippincott, 1992. Used with permission.)

TABLE 202.3. Prognostic Factors in Operable Breast Cancer

| Factor/Criterion | Favorable | Unfavorable |
|---|---|---|
| Nodal status | Histologically negative nodes | Increasing number of positive nodes |
| Tumor size | <1 cm | Increasing tumor size |
| Tumor grade | Well-differentiated | Poorly differentiated |
| Hormone receptors | ER+/PR+, ER–/PR+ | ER+/PR– esp.<br>ER–/PR– |
| DNA analysis | Diploid, low S phase (varies with laboratory) | Aneuploid, high S phase (usually >5) |
| Oncogene amplification | <5 copies HER2/NEU | >5 copies HER2/NEU |

ER = estrogen receptor; PR = progesterone receptor.

or a radionuclide bone scan to exclude metastases. These tests are not mandatory in low-stage disease (i.e., $T_1N_0M_0$)

The size of the tumor and the presence of involved axillary nodes remain the principal **prognostic factors.** The presence of estrogen receptor (ER) also is an important prognostic factor and is key in deciding whether to use adjuvant hormone therapy. Flow cytometric analysis gives information on DNA content (ploidy) and proliferative activity (S phase), which also are of prognostic significance, as is overexpression of the oncogene Her-2/neu. Table 202.3 lists the more important prognostic factors in the approximate order of relative importance.

## Management

### Management of noninvasive (in situ) carcinoma

**Lobular carcinoma in situ (LCIS)** rarely presents as a palpable mass or discrete mammographic findings but usually is discovered as an incidental histologic finding in biopsy specimens taken for other reasons. It signifies increased later cancer risk in either breast (20% to 30% incidence over 15 to 20 years). Careful annual screening for cancer is recommended. Prophylactic bilateral mastectomy is the only alternative for women unwilling to accept the risk of subsequent cancer, but this is still considered a drastic step. Use of tamoxifen prophylaxis has recently been demonstrated to be of benefit.

**Ductal carcinoma in situ (DCIS)** may present as a lump or mammographic abnormality. Tumor excision (lumpectomy) followed by radiotherapy reduces the risk of local relapse. Alternatively, a mastectomy usually is curative, but for most patients it is cosmetically less desirable than a "breast-sparing" lumpectomy and radiotherapy.

### Local therapy for invasive cancer

Surgery, radiotherapy, and systemic adjuvant therapy are all used in the treatment of localized invasive breast cancer. For local (primary) treatment, choices between lumpectomy plus radiotherapy, segmental resection plus radiotherapy, and total (modified radical) mastectomy depend on the disease stage and entail a thorough discussion between the patient and physician. Survival with **"breast-conserving" therapy** (lumpectomy with axillary sampling plus radiation) is comparable to that with a total mastectomy and axillary lymph node dissection for the treatment of most stage I and II cancers. Most women desire breast preservation for cosmetic reasons, but the higher risk of local recurrence must be thoroughly explained.

In general, the concept behind breast-conserving therapy is related to the understanding that the control of local disease depends first on adequate surgical resection of the primary tumor. Cosmetic results depend on the relative size of the tumor and breast. Thus, unless there are unusual biological issues such as nipple involvement or multicentric disease, patients have the choice of either mastectomy or lumpectomy plus radiation. Even if technically feasible, though, removal of a large tumor from a small breast results in an inferior cosmetic result. Such patients are better served with a mastectomy followed by reconstruction. As with all cancer operations, there must be clear postresection surgical margins. Thus, some tumors do not lend themselves to simple lumpectomy, because of the location of the tumor. Multiple tumors that are multifocal (i.e., more than one distinct tumor in the same quadrant of the breast) can be managed with breast-conserving surgery, whereas multiple tumors in different quadrants of the breast (multicentric tumors) require mastectomy. This latter recommendation relates not only to cosmetic issues but also to the principle of optimal anti-cancer therapy.

Treatment of breast cancer mandates either removal of all breast tissue (mastectomy) or radiation to residual breast tissue after lumpectomy not only to eradicate any residual disease, but also to deal with possible occult additional microscopic primary tumors in other areas of remaining breast tissue. Experience has shown that patients with multicentric disease have an unacceptable risk of relapse after breast-conserving therapy. When mastectomy is selected, the classic "Halstead mastectomy" is performed only rarely these days. This surgical technique evolved a century ago when the concept of an "en bloc" cancer operation was invented. The procedure involved removal not only of the breast, but also of the underlying pectoralis muscles and fascia. It included complete removal of all three levels of axillary nodes. Although it was definitive, it had excessive morbidity, and, most importantly, did not dramatically change the risk of relapse. Nowadays, a modified or simple mastectomy is performed to accomplish the goal of removing the tumor and remaining breast tissue and to sample the ipsilateral axillary lymph nodes to assess potential spread of disease. By omitting resection of the chest wall musculature, and only "sampling" the axillary nodes, morbidity is significantly reduced, disease control is unimpaired, and reconstructive surgery can be performed more easily. If lumpectomy is selected, adjuvant radiotherapy is usually initiated within 3 to 6 weeks of lumpectomy and administered over 6 to 7 weeks, unless there was evidence of lymph node involvement ($TxN_{1\text{-}2}M_0$) disease, in which case adjuvant chemotherapy usually is interposed between the lumpectomy and radiation.

#### Systemic adjuvant therapy for operable breast cancer

Relapse after primary locoregional therapy usually occurs in distant sites and is primarily the result of prior occult micrometastases. Recurrent breast cancer is, with rare exception, incurable. Adjuvant (prophylactic) therapy can reduce the risk of relapse in all patients; studies are underway to determine the most successful regimens and which patients benefit most from the various options noted in Table 202.4. Most patients with tumors larger than 1 cm or with evidence of metastasis in the lymph nodes (node-positive) are routinely given **combination chemotherapy** following surgery and radiotherapy; in patients with estrogen receptor (ER)–positive tumors, especially postmenopausal women, **hormonal treatment** with the estrogen agonist tamoxifen is now standard, and may be substituted for chemotherapy. Combination chemotherapy for 4 to 8 cycles is most effective for patients younger than 50 years of age (premenopausal); hormonal therapy is more effective in older patients (postmenopausal). Both significantly lower the risk of relapse. Current recommendations are listed in Table 202.5.

In contrast to the excellent prognosis in patients with minimal disease (i.e., a small primary lesion and no nodal involvement), the prognosis worsens in patients with positive axillary nodes; over 85% of patients with 10 or more positive nodes would eventually relapse if not treated with systemic adjuvant therapy. Fortunately, such treatment can reduce the risk of relapse by about 30% to 45%.

#### Management of locally advanced breast cancer

Locally advanced disease is defined as tumors or axillary lymph nodes with fixation to the chest wall, extensive ulceration or satellite cutaneous nodules, or inflammatory cancer with diffuse dermal involvement. In all these presentations, mastectomy alone rarely effects local control. However, combining initial or **neoadjuvant chemotherapy** with subsequent radiotherapy or surgery leads to control of disease in 30% to 40% of patients.

#### Follow-up after primary treatment

Long-term follow-up after primary treatment is essential. In asymptomatic patients, expensive complex surveillance tests—e.g., CT scans—should be performed only if the patient is symptomatic, the physician is concerned about persistent toxicities, or the patient is in an extremely high-risk group and would be a candidate for specific follow-up therapy if there were relapse. Continued vigilance and prompt investigation of symptoms remain the best policy. New cancers occur in the contralateral breast at the rate of 1% annually, a risk that can be reduced by the administration of tamoxifen. In patients who undergo a breast-sparing procedure, a relapse of the first cancer or a new cancer ultimately will develop in 5% to 20% of patients. Thus, previously treated patients must be followed carefully and screened with annual breast examinations and mammography. Historically, 5% to 30% of patients with negative axillary lymph nodes would relapse within 10 years, compared to 30% to 70% of those with positive nodes. Adjuvant chemotherapy or hormonal therapy (or a combination) has cut these relapse risks in half.

Being relapse-free for 5 years does not guarantee cure in breast cancer. Adjuvant therapy reduces the relative risk of recurrence by about 50%, so the absolute risk ranges from <5% to 50%, depending on initial risk factors, but the risk of metastasis is lifelong. The most common sites of metastatic spread are bone (40%–50%), soft tissue, regional lymph nodes (10%–30%), and lung or pleura (25%).

#### Management of metastases

The approach to metastatic disease is summarized in Table 202.6. In general, aggressive diagnostic evaluation is appropriate when relapse is suspected. In most instances, circumstantial evidence is convincing that newly discovered lesions are relapsed breast cancer, but many older women also are at risk for developing other cancers (e.g., colon, lung). Therefore, if possible, biopsy documentation is desirable at the apparent first relapse. With the advent of fine-needle aspirate (FNA) biopsies,

**TABLE 202.4. Adjuvant Systemic Therapies for Breast Cancer**

| Regimen | Agents/Dosage | Duration/Adjuvant | Comments |
|---|---|---|---|
| **Chemotherapy** | | | |
| CMF | Cyclophosphamide, 100 mg/m$^2$ orally on days 1–14<br>Methotrexate, 40 mg/m$^2$ IV on days 1 and 8<br>5FU, 600 mg/m$^2$ IV on days 1 and 8 | 6–12 cycles q 28 days | 40–50% response in metastatic disease |
| CAF | Same as CMF, except doxorubicin, 30 mg/m$^2$ IV instead of methotrexate on days 1 and 8 | 6 cycles q 28 days | 50–70% response rate in metastatic disease |
| FAC | Cyclophosphamide, 500 mg/m$^2$ and doxorubicin, 50 mg/m$^2$ on day 1<br>5FU, 500 mg/m$^2$ IV on days 1 and 8 | 6 cycles q 22 days | Similar activity to CAF |
| AC | Doxorubicin, 60 mg/m$^2$ IV<br>Cyclophosphamide, 600 mg/m$^2$ IV | 4 cycles q 21 days | Similar to CAF, FAC |
| AC + T | Same as above, with addition of 4 cycles of either Paclitaxel, 175 mg/m$^2$, or Docetaxel, 100 mg/m$^2$ | All 8 cycles q 21 days | Addition of Taxane further reduces relapse risk |
| **Hormonal Therapy** | | | |
| Oophorectomy | Surgical, radiation, or GnRH agonists | N/A | Used in premenopausal women; alternative to tamoxifen |
| "SERMS"—Tamoxifen | 10 mg BID | 5 years | ~45% RRR; current standard of care for estrogen receptor positive tumors |
| Toremifen | 60 mg qd | ?5 yrs | Comparable in metastatic disease; trials underway |
| Raloxifene | 60 mg qd | ?5 yrs | Approved for osteoporosis; trials underway in metastatic, adjuvant, and prophylaxis |
| **Aromatase Inhibitors** | | | Active in metastatic disease; trials underway |
| Anastrozole | 1 mg qd | ?5 yrs | |
| Letrozole | 2.5 mg qd | ?5 yrs | |
| Examestane | 25 mg qd | ?5 yrs | Active in metastatic ds; trials underway |
| GnRH agonists | | | |
| Goserilin | 10.8 mg q 3 mos | ?5 yrs | |
| Leuprolide | 22.5 mg q 3 mos | | |

SERMS = selective estrogen receptor modulators; 5FU = 5 fluorouracil; GnRH = gonadotropin-releasing hormone; RRR = relative reduction in recurrence.

most lesions can be successfully documented to be recurrent cancer. The diagnosis of metastatic disease has serious implications, because it is rarely curable. The median survival of patients with relapsed breast cancer is 2 to 3 years; 15% to 25% of patients will survive 5 years, and 5% to 10% of patients may survive for 10 years. Restaging is important once relapse has occurred. Patterns of involvement dictate specific interventions. Radiation with or without orthopedic stabilization of impending fractures can preserve mobility and prevent

**TABLE 202.5. Recommendations for Adjuvant Therapy of Operable Breast Cancer**

| Menopausal Status | Nodal Status | Hormone Receptor (ER/PR) | Therapy Options* |
|---|---|---|---|
| Premenopausal | – | + | Chemotherapy + Tamoxifen† |
| Premenopausal or postmenopausal | + | – | Chemotherapy |
| Postmenopausal | – | + | Tamoxifen ± chemotherapy‡ |
| Postmenopausal | + | + | Tamoxifen ± chemotherapy‡ |
| Elderly (>70–75 yrs) | Any | Any | Tamoxifen§ |
| Tumor <1 cm (pre- and postmenopausal) | – | Any | Usually no adjuvant therapy |

*Chemotherapy: 4–6 mo of standard combinations; tamoxifen for 5 years.
†Tamoxifen is an alternative in node-negative patients.
‡Chemotherapy may add benefit.
§Fit patients of high risk may receive chemotherapy.

**TABLE 202.6. Decisions in Managing Recurrent/Metastatic Breast Cancer**

- Confirm *first* apparent relapse by histology or cytology if feasible
- Re-stage using original spectrum of tests, including clinical, CT and bone scans, serum chemistries
- Select proper systemic therapy (See Table 202.7)
- Hormone-receptor–positive, long disease-free interval, few metastatic sites, soft tissue or bone → endocrine approach initially
  Hormone-receptor negative, multiple extensive metastases, symptomatic visceral metastases, failure of endocrine therapy → combination chemotherapy
  Radiation for palliation of locally refractory disease
  Supportive care
- Identify, and pre-emptively treat impending emergent conditions
  Brain, epidural metastases → steroids, radiation
  Impending pathologic fracture → fixation, radiation

**TABLE 202.7. Treatment Options in Recurrent or Metastatic Breast Cancer**

| Hormonal Therapy | Chemotherapy |
|---|---|
| First-line | First-line |
| Oophorectomy—surgical, radiation, or GnRH agonists | CMF |
| Tamoxifen | CAF |
| Megestrol acetate | CNF |
| Second-line | Second-line |
| Androgens | Paclitaxel (Taxol) |
| Estrogens (DES) | Docetaxel (Taxotere) |
| Aromatase inhibitors (aminoglutethimide) | Vinorelbine (Navelbine) |
| | Vinblastine (Velban) + Mitomycin-C |
| Prednisone | Methotrexate + calcium leucovoran |

paraplegia; brain metastases, which are relatively resistant to chemotherapy because of the blood-brain barrier, also can be palliated by radiation.

Patterns of disease recurrence are important determinants of subsequent therapy. Hormonal therapy often is successful in patients who have had a long interval between initial therapy and relapse. This is especially true in postmenopausal women with exclusively or predominantly osseous metastases whose tumors were originally ER-positive. Conversely, premenopausal women often have receptor-negative cancers. They are somewhat more likely to relapse earlier, and often have predominantly visceral disease such as liver or lung metastases. These patients rarely respond to hormonal therapies. Table 202.7 outlines treatment options in addition to emergent care. In general, the selection of treatment modalities is based on empiric knowledge, clinical trials, and hormonal status (positive estrogen or progesterone receptor analysis). The strategy in such patients is to maximize control of disease while minimizing morbidity of therapy. Thus, compared to initial adjuvant treatments, chemotherapy regimens are less intensive, utilize fewer drugs at any one time, and are given for more prolonged periods. In the case of hormonal treatments, response to one intervention often predicts the response to further hormonal treatment. Thus unless the pattern of disease changes, patients successfully treated with one hormonal program often benefit from further therapies (see Table 202.7). Supportive care with pain management, nutritional support, and psychological counseling are all important aspects of good medical care.

## Complications

**Surgery** with axillary dissection may result in postoperative lymphedema—swelling of the arm due to blockage of lymphatic vessels—which may develop months or even years later. **Radiotherapy** causes minor, transient, acute erythema and edema of the breast in most patients; later, scarring, shrinkage, and distortion of the breast, delayed lymphedema, radionecrosis of ribs or clavicle, and brachial plexus neuropathy may follow. **Chemotherapy** produces transient nausea or vomiting; anorexia; alopecia, fatigability, and myelosuppression are common in most patients (see Table 198.2). **Tamoxifen** therapy produces or worsens a hypoestrogenic state with menopausal-like symptoms and may, in rare cases, induce the development of endometrial cancer (although the reduction in risk of breast cancer relapse far outweighs the possible risk of inducing endometrial cancer). Leukemia is a rare late complication of chemotherapy.

### Prevention of Breast Cancer

Primary prevention by early pregnancy or dietary modification is neither feasible nor of proven value. Secondary prevention using tamoxifen has recently demonstrated about a 47% reduction in occurrence of breast cancer in postmenopausal and high-risk premenopausal patients. With the advent of genetic screening for high-risk patients based on the newly discovered BRCA-1 and BRCA-2 genes, the issue of prophylactic mastectomy has resurfaced, because it is not yet known whether tamoxifen prophylaxis is effective in these oncogene-positive patients. Although it is theoretically beneficial in selected patients, such drastic interventions impact significantly upon the patient's body image; besides, the exact risk of breast cancer in such genetically prone families is still controversial. Alternatively, prophylactic oophorectomy in oncogene-positive premenopausal patients may be effective prophylaxis.

### Screening and Case-Finding in Asymptomatic Persons

Screening of women at risk for breast cancer is key to its early detection. **Breast examination** is not easy, and the skill of the examiner is pivotal to avoid missing or overdiagnosing cancers. Although breast examinations by physicians and other health professionals are important and cause a significant number of the cancers to be diagnosed, the physician must realize that patients often can feel masses which the physician can not. **Breast self-examination** has been recommended for years and is widely taught, but many older patients are reluctant to practice it. The physician must always take the patient's report of a breast mass seriously; the report should either prompt immediate follow-up with mammography and consultation or initiate a careful follow-up at short intervals to determine whether it is related to cyclical hormonal changes, as may be the case in premenopausal patients. It should never be dismissed out of hand, since failure to diagnose an early breast cancer has serious medical (and legal) consequences.

Mammography has been used since the 1960s for screening asymptomatic women and evaluating palpable breast abnormalities. Screening asymptomatic women aged 50 years or more at intervals of 1 to 3 years has been widely accepted because of convincing data that breast cancer mortality can be lowered by 25% to 30%. Although similar data in younger women are less convincing, a recent consensus panel concluded that annual mammography should begin at age 40, or even earlier in high-risk cases based on family history or genetic predisposition. It remains uncertain whether women over 70 need mammograms annually as opposed to every 2 to 3 years.

### Breast Cancer in Men

Only 1500 cases of breast cancer are diagnosed annually in men in the United States. The biology and treatment of the disease are identical to those in women, with the paradoxical caveat that breast cancer typically is clinically more advanced at diagnosis in men.

# CHAPTER 203 CARCINOMA OF THE LUNG

### Incidence and Epidemiology

Lung cancer was rare until cigarette smoking became endemic. The age-adjusted lung cancer mortality in men has risen from 11 per 100,000 in 1940 to 73 per 100,000 today. In women, whose endemic smoking patterns began a generation later, the rate rose from 5 per 100,000 in 1960 to 32 per 100,000 today. With 164,900 new cases and 154,900 deaths yearly, lung cancer is by far the most important cancer in the United States. The incidence and mortality of these cancers has finally begun to decrease in men, although, unfortunately, they still are increasing in women.

### Etiology

Cigarette smoking continues to be the major cause of lung cancer. Lung cancer is more prevalent in urban populations. Certain occupational hazards predispose to lung cancer; these include asbestos exposure, uranium mining, and exposure to arsenic and nickel. Known or suspected cofactors include exposure to radon, beryllium, mustard gas, and various hydrocarbons. Concurrent cigarette smoke exposure exerts a synergistic role. Passive smoke inhalation by the spouses of heavy smokers may account for as many as 8000 cases annually.

Patients should be strongly encouraged and taught to stop smoking, because continued tobacco use results in an increased relative risk of >12. Smoking cessation lowers the risk after 5 to 10 years, but an increased relative risk, about 1.5 to 2.0 compared to nonsmokers, remains indefinitely.

## Pathogenesis

Tobacco smoke, ionizing radiation, and industrial carcinogens are believed to exert a multistep carcinogenic process in the bronchial epithelium, where areas of dysplasia and metaplasia progress to carcinoma in situ and then to invasive cancer. Molecular genetic studies show frequent loss of alleles on chromosome 3, especially in small cell carcinoma; mutations and deletions in the p53 gene in all cell types; and reported mutations in the *RB*, *ras*, and c-*myc* genes.

## Pathology

The four basic types of lung cancer are adenocarcinoma, small cell, epidermoid (squamous cell), and large cell (Figure 203.1). A simple, widely used classification divides lung cancers into **small cell** and **non-small cell** types, reflecting the generally systemic nature of small cell lung cancer, which entails a minor role for surgery. With the exception of adenocarcinomas, which often occur in peripheral lung zones, most lung cancers arise in proximal bronchi.

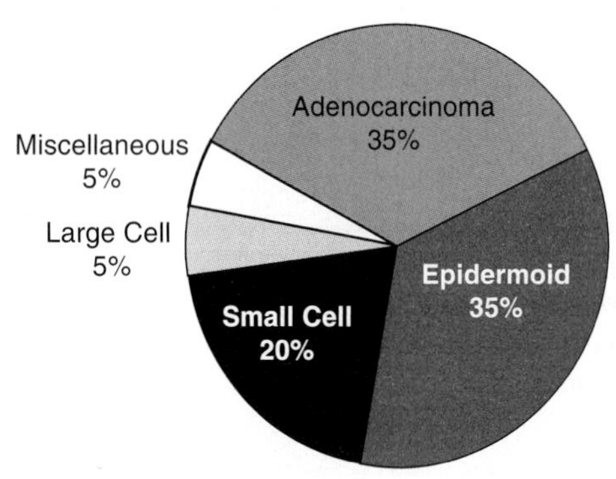


**FIGURE 203.1. Lung cancer cell types. Epidermoid and adenocarcinoma are the two frequent histologic types. The miscellaneous group includes bronchoalveolar, giant cell, and mucoepidermoid types.**

**TABLE 203.1. Clinical Features of Lung Cancer**

| Presentation | Features |
|---|---|
| Solitary pulmonary nodule | Asymptomatic |
| Primary symptoms | Cough, hemoptysis, dyspnea and wheezing, fever due to secondary infection |
| Regional effects | Hoarseness, superior vena cava syndrome, superior sulcus invasion, Horner syndrome, pleural and pericardial effusions, esophageal compression, phrenic nerve paralysis |
| Metastasis | Brain, bone, liver, adrenal |
| Systemic | Paraneoplastic endocrinopathy: SIADH, Cushing syndrome, hypertrophic pulmonary osteoarthropathy, gynecomastia, weight loss, Eaton-Lambert syndrome (see Chapter 206) |

SIADH = syndrome of inappropriate ADH secretion.

## Clinical Features

The usual presentations in patients with lung cancer are outlined in Table 203.1. Asymptomatic **solitary nodules** are important because of their potential for cure. The frequency of lung cancer among solitary pulmonary nodules is variable and depends on age, characteristics of the nodule, and smoking history (see chapter 249).

Primary symptoms with all cell types include cough and wheezing from bronchial irritation or obstruction, variable degrees of sputum production, and bloody expectoration varying from blood-streaked sputum to frank hemoptysis. A bout of pneumonitis or a lung abscess may be the initial clue to underlying bronchial obstruction from tumor. A pleural effusion is another manifestation.

Chest wall invasion ultimately causes pain. Mediastinal invasion causes dyspnea or entrapment of the recurrent laryngeal nerve(s), producing a voice change due to vocal cord paralysis. If right-sided, it can cause the superior vena cava syndrome, featuring pain and swelling in the face and upper extremities. Cancers arising from the apex of the lung may invade the brachial plexus, leading to shoulder and arm pain or weakness (Pancoast tumor, or superior sulcus tumor; Figure 203.2).

**Metastatic disease** is seen at presentation in most patients, justifying an extensive preoperative workup. Related paraneoplastic syndromes are listed in Table 203.1.

## Diagnosis, Clinical Evaluation, and Staging

Additional information on diagnosing and evaluating lung cancer appears in Chapter 248. Physical examination may detect supraclavicular adenopathy, pleural effusion or atelectasis, the localized wheeze of bronchial obstruction, weight loss, clubbing of the fingers (Figure 203.3), or signs of gross metastatic disease. Laboratory tests are designed to uncover anemia (complete blood count), hepatic dysfunction (alkaline phosphatase, serum albumin, lactate dehydrogenase), hypercalcemia, hyponatremia, and metabolic alkalosis.

Cytologic examination of sputum may provide a definitive, noninvasive clue, especially in central lesions arising from the bronchi; it is less accurate with peripheral nodules ("coin" lesions). Cytologic and histologic specimens are obtained from peripheral lesions

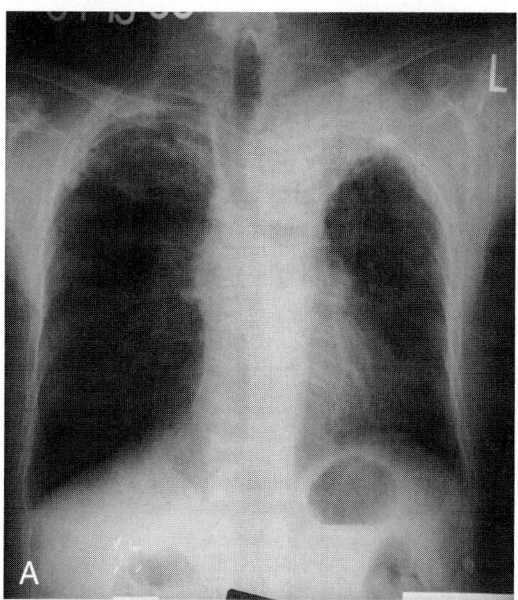


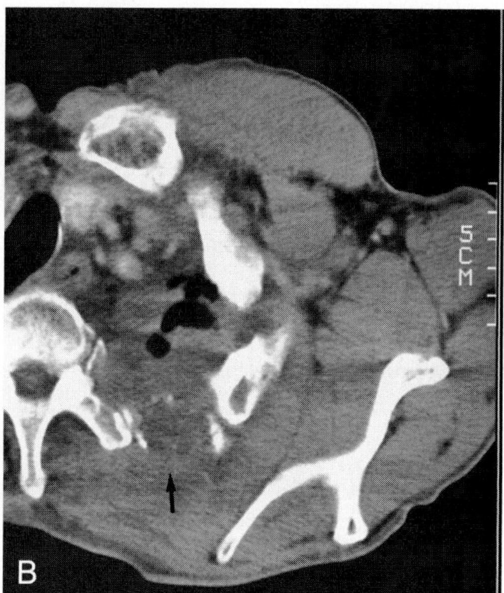


FIGURE 203.2. Pancoast's tumor (superior sulcus tumor) in lung cancer. A. Left shoulder pain and a new left apical lesion developed during long-term follow-up of this patient for previous tuberculosis. B. CT scan (magnified view) showed the lesion and associated destruction of the overlying rib (arrow).

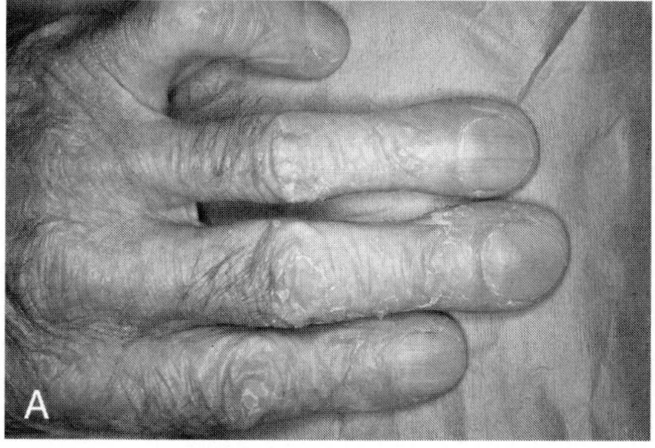


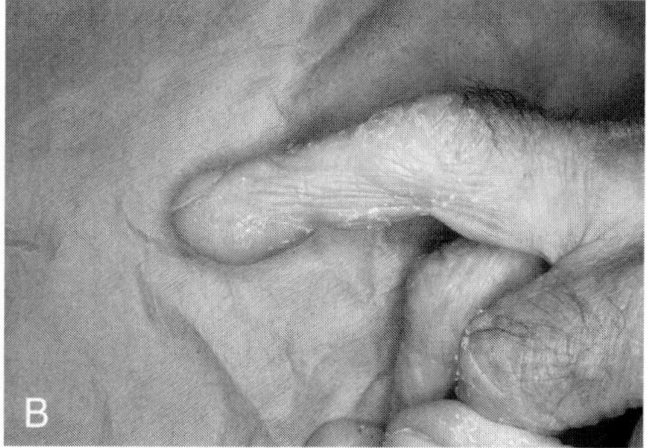


FIGURE 203.3. Finger clubbing in bronchogenic carcinoma. A. frontal view. B. profile.

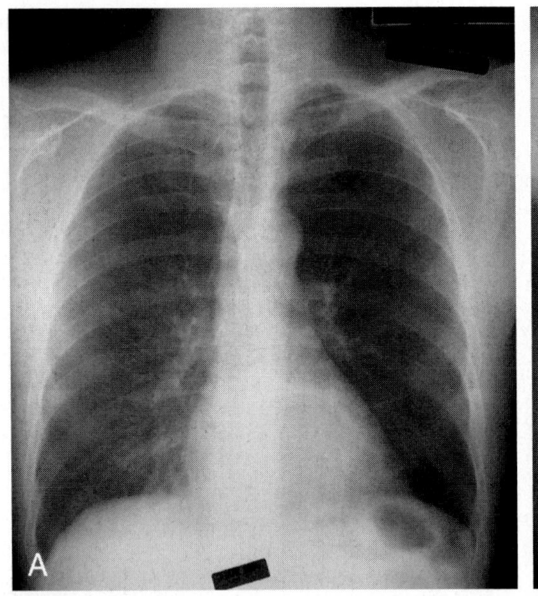


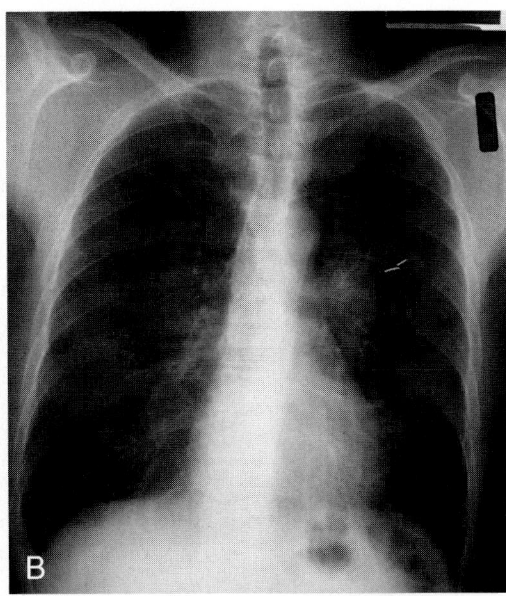


**FIGURE 203.4.** Chest radiographs in bronchogenic carcinoma. **A**, A prior chest radiograph was normal. **B**, Three years later, the chest film shows a left hilar mass (arrow). Adenocarcinoma was diagnosed by bronchoscopy.
(Courtesy of Jeffery Postles, MD, Wauwatosa, Wisconsin.)

**TABLE 203.2. Simplified Staging of Lung Cancer**

| Stage | Description |
|---|---|
| Small cell lung cancer | |
| Limited | Limited to one hemithorax |
| Extensive | Beyond one hemithorax |
| Non-small cell lung cancer | |
| TNM stage | |
| I | T1 (tumor <3 cm) or T2 (tumor >3 cm); N0 |
| II | T1 or T2 tumors; $N_1$ (positive peribronchial or hilar nodes) |
| IIIA | T3 (tumor invading chest wall, mediastinal pleura, or in main bronchus <2 cm from carina, or atelectasis of entire lung) N0-N1 T1-T3 with N2 (ipsilateral mediastinal lymph nodes) |
| IIIB | Any T with N3 nodes (contralateral or ipsilateral scalene, supraclavicular) |
| | $T_4$ (tumor invading deep mediastinal structures or malignant pleural effusion) with any N |
| IV | M1 (metastases) |

(Reprinted with permission from American Joint Committee on Cancer. Cancer Staging Manual. 5th ed. Philadelphia: JB Lippincott, 1997.)

through transthoracic fine needle aspiration or core biopsy, and centrally located tumors are usually accessed via bronchoscopy. Fiberoptic bronchoscopy is an essential tool in the diagnosis and staging of bronchogenic carcinoma. Imaging studies used during preinvasive diagnostic studies or as staging studies after diagnosis include chest radiographs (Figure 203.4); CT scans of the chest, abdomen, and pelvis; radionuclide bone scans; and a CT or magnetic resonance scan (MRI) of the brain.

**Small cell lung cancer** is not treated surgically. It is staged as **limited** (confined to the ipsilateral thorax and supraclavicular nodes) or **extensive,** based on the same tests used for all lung cancer patients. Regardless of the clinical stage, this disease nearly always is biologically disseminated. Thus, all patients undergoing treatment receive systemic chemotherapy. In contrast, **non-small cell lung cancer** disseminates only late in its course; thus, meticulous thoracic and mediastinal staging is required because of the potential for surgical cure (Table 203.2).

## Management

One cannot overemphasize the systemic nature of **small cell cancer** and the necessity of systemic chemotherapy, even in patients with **limited stage** disease. Untreated patients with this cancer have a median survival of only a few months. However, in most patients who undergo treatment, survival is meaningfully prolonged and the quality of life improved. Patients with disease limited to the ipsilateral thorax respond to chemotherapy with or without consolidation radiotherapy in almost 90% of cases. Instead of a median survival of only 2 to 4 months in untreated cases, average survival in treated patients exceeds 1 year; most importantly a small subset of patients (15%–30%) are alive and free of disease at 2 years, and are potentially cured. Patients with extensive disease also respond to therapy; about 80% of patients have a meaningful regression of disease, with improvement in their cancer symptoms. Their survival also is prolonged from 1 to 3 months to 8 to 12 months. However, because virtually all such patients are doomed to relapse, experienced oncologists treat them with less toxic regimens than the potentially curable patient with limited stage disease. A large number of chemotherapy regimens exist, usually based on the use of a platinum-containing compound (cis-platin or carboplatin), combined with either VP-16 or taxol. Treatment is given until best response is obtained, usually 4 to 6 cycles of treatment. Selected patients with limited stage disease are considered for thoracic radiation to areas of original involvement to maximize both local disease control and the chance of cure. In patients with advanced disease, radiation is reserved for palliation of lesions not responsive to chemotherapy.

**Non-small cell cancer** is treated surgically, if possible, with the magnitude of resection being determined by the extent of involvement. Unfortunately, the prognosis is still dismal for most patients. About 60% of patients have unresectable disease prior to thoracotomy; another 25% are found to be unresectable during surgery. Thus, fewer than 20% of all patients undergo a potentially curative procedure. Furthermore, only about 50% of patients successfully undergoing such surgery are truly cured. Thus, the overall survival of lung cancer patients is still dismal, and unlike breast cancer, the survival rate is only minimally affected by adjuvant radiotherapy or chemotherapy.

Patients believed to have unresectable tumors, due to extensive locoregional disease, or who have medical contraindications to surgery can be treated with radiotherapy. Long-term survival, and even a small chance of cure (<5%), can be obtained in selected patients. Chemotherapy has only modest palliative benefit in advanced stages of non-small cell lung cancer, with about 30% of patients alive at 1 year and more than 2% alive at 5 years.

## Complications

Surgical mortality is about 4%, depending on preoperative risk factors. Postoperative pulmonary compromise can be very limiting in patients with coexisting chronic obstructive lung disease. Radiation may cause transient esophagitis, bronchitis, and occasionally pneumonitis; delayed complications include constrictive pericarditis and small vessel myocardial disease. Toxicity from chemotherapeutic agents includes myelosuppression, renal dysfunction, and possible neurotoxicity.

A second lung cancer or a cancer of the head and neck region may develop in survivors of an initial lung cancer of any type. Depending on risk factors (with smoking the most important), new cancers occur at a rate of 1% to 5% annually for at least 10 years after successful treatment of the original cancer. (These rates are even higher with continued smoking).

## Prognosis

As noted, only the small subsets of patients with limited stage disease are potentially curable. Thus, the overall 5-year survival of lung cancer patients is only 14% (Figure 203.5). Persons with lung cancer presenting as a **solitary nodule** (<3 cm) and no lymph node involvement ($T_1N_0M_0$) may have a 5-year survival rate of 80%. **Small cell lung cancer,** when limited in extent, has a median survival of 12 to 18 months, a 2-year survival of 15% to 30%, and a 5-year survival of 10% to 15%. Death occurring after 2 years following treatment often is due to a new cancer. Patients with extensive disease have a median survival of 7 to 12 months and survival of 2% or less at 2 or more years.

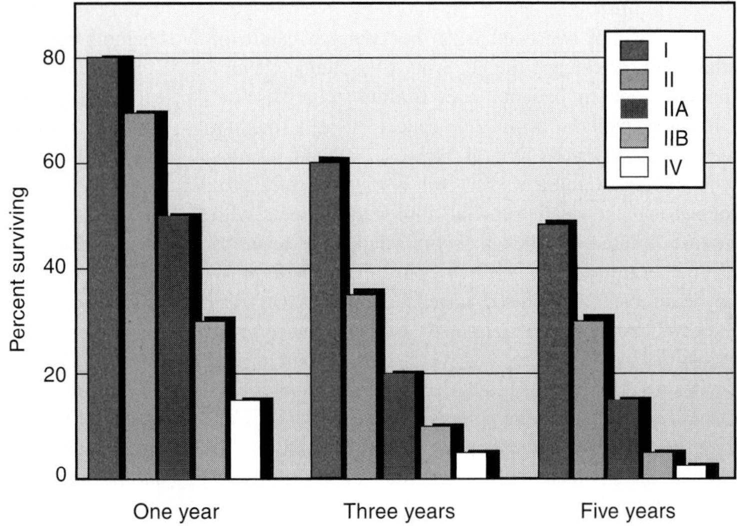


**FIGURE 203.5.** Survival in non-small cell lung cancer according to stage. Treatments for various stages included: stages I and II, surgery; stage IIIA, surgery and radiation; stage IIIB, radiation; stage IV, supportive care and chemotherapy.
(Adapted from: Mountain CF Semin Oncol 1988;15:2236–245.)

# CHAPTER 204 GASTROINTESTINAL CANCERS

Of the approximately 250,600 new cancers involving the gastrointestinal (GI) tract diagnosed annually, roughly two thirds (about 148,300) involve the colon and rectum. The other cancers are pancreatic (about 30,300), gastric (about 21,600), hepatobiliary (about 23,700), and esophageal (about 13,100). The incidence of gastric cancer continues to decline in the United States, and mortality from colorectal cancer, especially in women, has declined since 1940. The frequency of hepatobiliary cancer as a sequela of chronic active hepatitis induced by hepatitis C is increasing dramatically.

Esophageal cancer is discussed in Chapter 79, cancer of the stomach in Chapter 83, and pancreatic cancer in Chapter 104. Primary hepatocellular carcinoma is discussed in Chapter 113. This chapter discusses only colorectal cancers.

## Colorectal Cancer

### Epidemiology, Pathogenesis, and Pathology

The incidence and epidemiology of colorectal cancer (CRC) are reviewed in chapter 100; risk factors for CRC are shown in Table 204.1. The predominant histologic type in CRC is adenocarcinoma; sarcomas, lymphomas, and carcinoid tumors are very uncommon. Tumors are described as polypoid, flat, ulcerating, and constricting.

Regional lymph node **metastases** follow infiltration into the bowel wall, and the peritoneum also may be a major site of metastases, once transmural growth occurs. For colonic cancers, hematogenous spread occurs initially to the liver via the portal venous system. The rectal or anal areas drain via the inferior hemorrhoidal veins and thus bypass the hepatic capillary bed; cancers of these areas may present with pulmonary metastases.

Tumors in the cecum often are superficially ulcerated and bulky, are likely to bleed, but are less likely to infiltrate circumferentially within colonic musculature. These tumors usually are more advanced at the time of diagnosis. Conversely, most tumors of the descending colon or rectosigmoid tend to infiltrate the muscular layers, leading to concentric luminal narrowing and thus, a "napkin ring" (or apple-core) lesion on barium enema (Figure 204.1).

### Clinical Features

The primary symptoms and signs of colorectal cancer depend on the location of the tumor (see chapter 100). More often, right-sided lesions produce subtle alterations in bowel habits and iron-deficiency anemia; **rectal** cancer and **low sigmoid** cancers produce blood-streaked stools and obstructive symptoms. Weight loss, ascites, hepatomegaly, and multiple abdominal masses suggest metastases. More advanced lesions cause pain from nerve infiltration and invasion of neighboring structures. Lymphatic or venous obstruction may cause leg swelling.

TABLE 204.1. Risk Factors for Colorectal Carcinoma

| Risk Factor | Association |
|---|---|
| Age | >50 yrs |
| Diet | Increased incidence with high fat intake |
| Inflammatory bowel disease | Highest risk with ulcerative colitis of entire colon; less risk with Crohn's disease |
| Previous adenomatous polyps | Believed to be precursor lesions; increasing risk with size >1 cm and villous or tubulovillous histology |
| Hereditary | |
| Multiple polyposis/Gardner's syndrome | Autosomal dominant |
| Hereditary non-polyposis colon cancer | Autosomal dominant |
| Family history | 1.7- to 3.0-fold increase in first-degree relatives |
| Previous pelvic radiation | Rectal cancer |
| Ureterosigmoidostomy | Sigmoid cancer |
| History of breast, ovarian or endometrial cancer | Moderate risk factor |

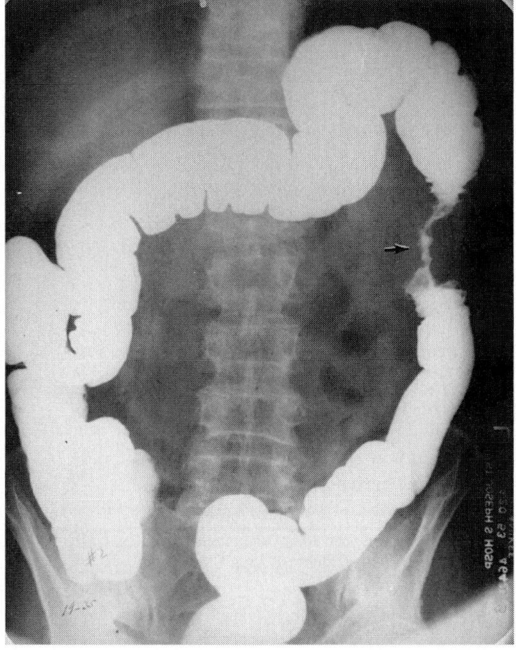

**FIGURE 204.1. Barium enema showing an applecore lesion (arrow) in the sigmoid colon, indicative of a colorectal tumor circumferentially infiltrating the muscular layers.**
(Courtesy of Radiology Museum, St. Joseph's Hospital, Milwaukee, Wisconsin.)

## Diagnosis, Clinical Evaluation, and Staging

Although many benign rectosigmoid lesions can bleed, any case of rectal bleeding should arouse a suspicion of cancer. The rectum extends to about 13 to 15 cm from the anal verge; thus, digital rectal examination, which is able to explore only 8 to 10 cm of the rectum, should always be followed by proctoscopy, unless the bleeding is fresh and hemorrhoids are obvious. Follow-up to rule out bleeding from other causes is mandatory in the absence of hemorrhoids or if bleeding persists.

The prolonged preclinical phase (8–10 years) of colorectal cancer and its association with adenomatous polyps have led to the recommendation of screening, case finding, and removal of any polyps encountered in asymptomatic persons. **Screening tools** include fecal occult blood testing (FOBT), digital rectal examination, proctoscopy, flexible sigmoidoscopy to 35–60 cm, and colonoscopy to examine the entire colon. Radiologic imaging consists of the **air-contrast barium enema**, which can augment colonoscopy in selected cases. Figure 204.2. shows the effectiveness of these screening tests in detecting colorectal neoplasms.

Suggestions for screening and surveillance are provided in Table 100.2 (see chapter 100). Logically, screening in patients known to be at higher risk because of a family history or known predisposing conditions (see Table 204.1) should begin at a younger age and be repeated frequently. All randomly occurring polyps should be removed if possible; hereditary polyposis patients must face the prospect of prophylactic colectomy. Because it takes years for transformation of a small precursor polyp into a malignant tumor, there are multiple opportunities to detect the disease before invasion occurs, as long as the patient and physician maintain a screening program. Colonoscopy has become the dominant screening tool because of superior accuracy; furthermore, cancer prevention, i.e. polypectomy, may be performed simultaneously.

Screening studies have shown that from 1% to 4% of FOBT will be positive. Most patients with a positive FOBT have hemorrhoids, anal fissures, or diverticula, not cancer. The incidence of polyps in this group is 30%; only

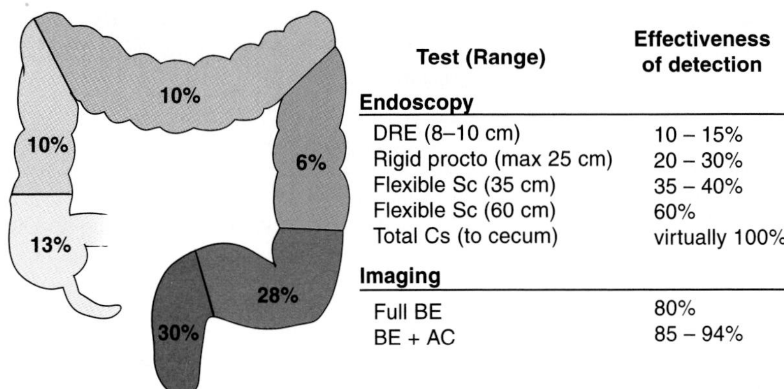


| Test (Range) | Effectiveness of detection |
|---|---|
| **Endoscopy** | |
| DRE (8–10 cm) | 10 – 15% |
| Rigid procto (max 25 cm) | 20 – 30% |
| Flexible Sc (35 cm) | 35 – 40% |
| Flexible Sc (60 cm) | 60% |
| Total Cs (to cecum) | virtually 100% |
| **Imaging** | |
| Full BE | 80% |
| BE + AC | 85 – 94% |

**FIGURE 204.2.** Distribution of large bowel cancers by anatomic site and their approximate rate of diagnosis by endoscopy and radiologic imaging. BE + AC = Air-contrast barium enema; Cs = colonoscopy; DRE = digital rectal examination; Procto = proctoscopy; Sc = sigmoidoscopy.

5% to 10% of patients with a positive FOBT will have cancer. Initial endoscopy or radiologic imaging detects about 95% of cancers. If bleeding persists, tests should be repeated at least once, and then diseases of the stomach and upper GI tract excluded by appropriate studies. In performing fecal occult blood tests, one must remember that even advanced cancers may bleed only intermittently. Symptoms such as abdominal pain, change in bowel habits, and occult or visible bleeding introduce an extensive differential diagnosis, including diverticular disease, inflammatory bowel disease, and enteric infection by bacteria, viruses, or parasites. Abdominal and bowel complaints without apparent bleeding are extremely common symptoms and are most often due to irritable bowel syndrome, not cancer.

When a lesion is identified, the diagnosis of cancer must be established by biopsy, usually of a specimen obtained by endoscopy. Subsequent **preoperative staging** is performed through abdominal and pelvic CT scans to evaluate the liver, kidneys, and ureters. The presence of iron deficiency anemia confirms a prior significant and repeated blood loss; an elevated alkaline phosphatase or γ-glutamyl transpeptidase level may reflect liver metastases. The serum level of carcinoembryonic antigen (CEA), a tumor marker, is high in one third of patients who have small, early-stage tumors and in 90% of patients with metastases. Knowledge that the CEA level was high prior to surgical resection of a primary tumor allows subsequent rational decisions about the timing and frequency of repeat tests postoperatively. A chest radiograph and a general medical evaluation complete the preoperative workup. A chest CT scan is not indicated in patients with a negative abdominal CT scan unless the tumor arises in the low rectal or anal area. The TNM and Dukes' staging systems are shown in Table 204.2.

**TABLE 204.2. Stage Classification of Colon Cancer**

| AJCC Stage | Dukes' Stage |
|---|---|
| I T1-2 N0 M0 | A, B1 |
| II T3, T4 N0 M0 | B2, B3 |
| III Any T, N1-3, M0 | C1, C2 |
| IV Any T, any N M1 | D |

T1 = tumor spread into submucosa
T2 = tumor spread into muscularis propria
T3 = tumor spread through muscularis propria
T4 = tumor spread through wall and visceral peritoneum or direct invasion of adjacent organs
N1 = 1-3 involved regional nodes
N2 = 4 or more involved nodes
N3 = second-echelon nodes along a vascular trunk
M0 = No distant metastasis
M1 = Distant metastasis

(Modified from American Joint Committee on Cancer. Cancer Staging Manual. 5th ed. Philadelphia: JB Lippincott, 1997.)

## Management of Colorectal Cancer

### Surgical treatment

Early detection of CRC not only increases the rate of survival but also improves the quality of life for patients. The type and extent of surgery depend on the location of the tumor. In general, a curative surgical operation includes removal of the involved bowel segment, with disease-free surgical margins at each end, and en bloc removal of the applicable blood vessels and lymphatics. Colostomy, if required, is only temporary. However, patients with extensive disease invading adjacent organs or with rectal tumors less than 5 cm from the anal verge do require permanent colostomy. When there is more than one primary tumor or associated multiple polyps, a subtotal or total colectomy may be required.

Palliative resections in the face of unresectable metastatic disease usually involve only resection of the colonic segment at risk of perforation or repeated hemorrhage. When the cancer cannot be resected because of adjacent organ infiltration, a "diverting" colostomy is constructed.

#### Adjuvant treatment of operable colorectal cancer

Postoperative radiotherapy is recommended for all Dukes' B2 or C patients with rectal cancers or colon cancers occurring below the peritoneal reflection (5–25 cm from the anal verge). Such therapy contributes slightly to overall survival, but, more importantly, reduces the risk of local recurrence. Lesions more than 25 cm from the anal verge are not amenable to radiotherapy and are less likely to produce debilitating morbidity from local relapse. Adjuvant chemotherapy decreases the risk of relapse, thus improving survival, especially when given concurrently with radiotherapy.

All patients who have colonic cancer with Dukes' C tumors (at high risk of relapse), and probably a subset of high-risk patients with Dukes' B tumors, benefit from postoperative adjuvant chemotherapy. Regimens consist of 5-fluorouracil, combined with either calcium leucovorin or levamisole, with or without CPT-11 (Irinotecan). Lower risk-Dukes' B patients are being enrolled in a trial using Panorex, a monoclonal antibody directed against a common colon cancer antigen.

#### Follow-up after initial therapy

Surveillance of the remaining colon is carried out with yearly fecal occult blood tests. Colonoscopy is required at 1 year to exclude recurrence, and if normal, every 3 to 5 years thereafter, because these patients are at a higher risk for development of a second cancer arising from new polyps as well as relapse of their first. Because of the nature of hematogenous spread via the portal circulation, it is important to identify metastases to the liver.

#### Management of recurrent and metastatic disease

Surgical resection or ablation is offered in selected patients for anastomotic recurrences, new primary tumors, and isolated metastases to lung or liver. Resection of hepatic metastases can significantly prolong patients' lives; 15% to 25% of patients may be cured by such "metastasectomies" if the number of lesions is limited (i.e., <5). Postoperative intra-arterial floxuridine, a 5-FU analogue, may reduce the risk of relapse. More extensive hepatic involvement can be palliated with cryosurgery, radiofrequency ablation, or intra-arterial chemoembolization. Radiotherapy can palliate local recurrence, pelvic masses, and bone metastases. Palliation with chemotherapy is feasible with reuse of the original adjuvant regimen, or its initial use if not previously administered.

### Complications

Diagnostic endoscopy is safe when done by experienced practitioners, and perforation or bleeding is rare. Surgical complications include wound disruption, anastomotic leak, and postoperative pulmonary complications common to older persons. Radiotherapy for rectal cancer can cause chronic cystitis, proctitis, or radionecrosis of pelvic bones (5%). If the small bowel cannot be excluded from the radiation field during the multiple treatments, late-onset adhesions or strictures may develop. Chemotherapy may cause reversible mucositis, enteritis, and leukopenia. Levamisole may cause reversible liver or CNS dysfunction.

### Prognosis

Lesions confined to the mucosa or submucosa (stage I, Dukes' A) carry an excellent prognosis; more than 90% are cured by initial surgical resection. Most (60%–85%) tumors penetrating the bowel wall (stage II, Dukes' B) are cured. In patients with stage III Dukes' C lesions with 1 to 3 positive lymph nodes, the 5-year survival is 56%; for those with 4 or more positive nodes, the survival is 30% or better. Adjuvant 5-FU–based chemotherapy reduces the relative risk of relapse by about 40%, and thereby improves the absolute survival in such patients by 15% to 20%; a lesser degree of improvement occurs in patients with high-risk stage II Dukes' B tumors. The same statistics apply to rectal cancers; postoperative radiotherapy in these patients further reduces local recurrence. Patients with advanced disease rarely survive beyond 2 years. Chemotherapy can improve the survival and quality of life for many patients; patients who respond to chemotherapy live longer than untreated patients (6–12 months), and about 5% live longer than 3 years.

# CHAPTER 205 CANCERS OF THE KIDNEY, URINARY BLADDER, AND PROSTATE

## Renal Cell Carcinoma

Renal cell carcinoma (hypernephroma) accounted for about 31,800 new cases in 2002, and is responsible for about 12,000 deaths annually in the United States. It is more prevalent among men by a 2:1 margin. With the exception of familial syndromes, the only established risk factors are age and probably cigarette smoking.

### Etiology, Pathogenesis and Pathology

Familial renal cell carcinoma occurs in 30% to 45% of patients with von Hippel-Lindau disease (syndrome of cerebellar hemangioblastoma and retinal angiomatosis with renal and pancreatic cysts), although clusters of disease occur in some families without this genetic disorder. A consistent deletion in chromosome 3p is seen in von Hippel-Lindau disease, and similar deletions are seen in sporadic renal cell carcinomas, indicating a probable tumor suppressor gene at that locus.

Ninety percent of renal cell carcinomas are adenocarcinomas of the tubular epithelium. The predominant types are clear cell (most common), granular cell, sarcomatoid, or papillary. Renal tumors are highly vascular—both the primary and metastatic tumors bleed with minimal trauma—and often have a necrotic, cystic appearance.

Limited early by Gerota's fascia, the tumor spreads by direct extension through the kidney and adjacent structures. Regional lymph node metastases and a high incidence of renal vein invasion are common. Renal vein invasion presents as a tumor thrombus, often extending into the inferior vena cava. Hematogenous metastases to the lung, liver, bone, and brain are common. Renal cell carcinomas, like melanomas, are notoriously unpredictable in their behavior.

### Clinical Features

Renal cell carcinomas have a variable, often lengthy, preclinical period and may be detected when unrelated conditions lead to abdominal CT or intravenous pyelography (IVP). Only 10% to 15% of patients exhibit the classic surgical triad of **hematuria, flank pain,** and a **palpable mass;** some patients present with one or more paraneoplastic signs or symptoms including fever, anemia, weight loss, hypercalcemia, or polycythemia (Table 205.1). Because of the tumor's location and frequent lack of symptoms, only 45% of patients have disease contained within the renal capsule; many patients have locally invasive cancer, and 30% have metastatic disease on presentation.

### Diagnosis, Clinical Evaluation, and Staging

Ultrasound or **IVP** may show a mass. However, IVP is neither very sensitive nor specific, and further workup is indicated if the patient has persistent hematuria or other signs or symptoms. **Ultrasound** can distinguish cysts from complex cystic and solid masses reliably. **CT** is best suited for diagnosis and staging, because it provides information (including vascularity) on the primary tumor, lymph nodes, renal vein, and inferior vena cava. Further information, including critical preoperative knowledge of vascular supply, is available by intra-arterial angiography or magnetic resonance angiography. The differential diagnosis of a renal mass with or without associated symptoms includes cysts, perinephric or renal abscess, renal lymphoma, renal tuberculosis, or benign tumor, as well as malignancy.

Patients are staged by the TNM classification or another simplified staging system. The latter system classifies stage I disease as tumor confined to the kidney; stage II, spread through the capsule; stage III, renal vein invasion or lymph node metastases; and stage IV, hematogenous metastases.

### Management

**Radical nephrectomy** is the standard surgical procedure. Tumor thrombi in the renal veins and vena cava may require extensive vascular resection and reconstruc-

**TABLE 205.1. Manifestations of Renal Cell Carcinoma**

| Manifestations | Incidence (%) |
|---|---|
| *Local* | |
| Hematuria | 60 |
| Flank pain | 40 |
| Mass | 40 |
| Surgical triad (hematuria, mass, and flank pain) | 10 |
| Varicocele | 2 |
| Metastasis as the initial presentation | 30 |
| Unexplained weight loss | Variable |
| *Systemic* | |
| Fever | 20 |
| Anemia | 20 |
| Hypercalcemia | 5 |
| Erythrocytosis | 3 |
| Amyloidosis | 1–2 |
| Hypertension | 20–30 |
| Hepatic dysfunction without metastasis | 10 |

tion. **Postoperative radiotherapy** can reduce the risk of local recurrence in Stage II or III disease but has not been shown to enhance survival. Neither adjuvant chemotherapy nor immunotherapy has yet been shown to be effective.

Metastases occasionally may appear as a solitary focus in brain, lung, thyroid, or liver and should be evaluated and considered for resection if the primary tumor has been resected. A 5-year survival of almost 35% has been reported after resection of solitary metastases. Nephrectomy in the presence of disseminated metastases, once disregarded as ineffective, has in a recent study, been shown to retard progression of metastatic disease in selected cases; further studies are underway to determine whether this should be routinely advocated. However, it may reasonably palliate pain or hematuria. Radiation is useful in palliating bone metastases.

Renal cell carcinomas are drug-resistant, and chemotherapy is rarely useful. Objective and, occasionally, durable responses occur in 15% to 20% of patients treated with aggressive regimes incorporating **recombinant interleukin-2** or **alpha-interferon.**

### Prognosis

Tumors confined within the kidney have a cure rate of 60% to 90%, depending on tumor size, although a minority of patients present with disease at this stage. Lymph node metastases, invasion of the inferior vena cava, and sarcomatoid histology are unfavorable prognostic factors. Survival in metastatic disease averages 8 to 10 months.

## Carcinoma of the Urinary Bladder

Bladder cancer is the most common malignancy of the urinary tract, afflicting about 41,500 men and 15,000 women annually in the United States. A disease of the urbanized, industrialized world, it is most prevalent in the fifth to seventh decades of life and is more common in Caucasians. In rural Egypt, chronic cystitis from bilharziasis (infection by *Schistosoma haematobium*) predisposes to a squamous cell variant of bladder cancer.

### Etiology and Pathogenesis

Cigarette smoking is the principal risk factor for bladder cancer, in addition to the well-documented occupational exposures to chemicals used in the rubber and aniline dye industries. Chronic cyclophosphamide use for cancer chemotherapy or immunosuppression and excessive phenacetin intake are causative in a few cases.

### Pathology

Ninety-five percent of bladder cancers arise from the transitional epithelium, the urothelium. Carcinoma in situ may be associated. Because the etiology involves carcinogenic chemicals excreted by the kidney, the entire urothelium is at risk for malignancy. Thus, patients with transitional cell carcinoma of the bladder have an increased risk of similar tumors involving the ureters and renal pelvis.

Bladder cancer spreads contiguously through the bladder wall into the adjacent structures; lymphatic spread is to pelvic and periaortic lymph nodes. Widespread hematogenous dissemination to lung, liver, and bone is common once the deep muscle and lymph nodes are involved. The grade of tumor directly relates to invasiveness. Patients with high-grade, low-stage disease have a prognosis as poor as that of some patients with lower-grade but higher-stage disease.

**TABLE 205.2. Marshall-Jewett Staging System for Transitional Cell Bladder Cancer**

| Stage | Description |
|---|---|
| 0 | Papillary noninvasive and carcinoma in situ |
| A | Invades submucosa |
| B1 | Invades superficial muscle |
| B2 | Invades deep muscle |
| C | Invades perivesical fat |
| D | Extension to adjacent organs, lymph nodes, or distant metastases |

### Clinical Features

Variable degrees of **hematuria** and **urinary frequency** are the most common presenting symptoms. Pain follows bladder wall invasion. Lymphatic obstruction can lead to lower extremity or genital swelling. Symptoms of distant metastases may coexist. The urinalysis reveals red blood cells, but hematuria may be intermittent and detected only through repeated urinalyses.

### Diagnosis, Clinical Evaluation, and Staging

The key step in the diagnosis of bladder cancer is the careful evaluation of any unexplained episodes of hematuria. Hematuria can be caused by infection or cancer anywhere in the urinary tract, glomerular disease, urolithiasis, and prostatitis.

Cytologic analysis of voided urine, cystoscopy, and IVP are appropriate diagnostic steps. At cystoscopy, suspicious areas should be biopsied and bladder washings obtained for cytologic examination. The IVP may show obstruction at the ureterovesical junction. CT or MRI can assess bladder wall thickness and detect invasion of contiguous structures, pelvic or periaortic lymphadenopathy, and possible concomitant renal tumors. The Marshall-Jewett staging system is commonly used (Table 205.2).

### Treatment

Carcinoma in situ may be benign but is often extensive, involving the entire bladder surface and producing intractable symptoms of dysuria, frequency, and incontinence. Treatment with the immunotherapeutic preparation bacille Calmette-Guérin (BCG), or the chemotherapeutic agent thio-tepa, may control some patients, but persistent disease, like frequent recurrence of invasive disease, mandates **cystourethrectomy.**

Low-stage, low-grade tumors are treated with limited **transurethral resection.** If the lesions recur or are high-grade, a chemotherapeutic agent or BCG, given intravesically, significantly reduces the risk of relapse. Up to 30% of patients so treated become permanently disease-free. About 30% develop multiple recurrences of low-grade, low-stage tumors requiring repeated therapy. The remainder ultimately develop invasive disease and require aggressive surgical intervention.

Most instances of invasive disease require **radical cystectomy** and urinary diversion. This procedure involves resection of the bladder, prostate, and seminal vesicles in men and the bladder, entire urethra, anterior wall of the vagina, uterus, and ovaries in women. This radical surgery allows for precise, pathologic staging.

Irradiation without cystectomy usually is reserved for patients whose comorbid conditions preclude radical surgery. Bladder sparing approaches are used in Europe, but surgery is preferred in the U.S. Transurethral resection may be employed for invasive disease in patients who are not surgical candidates. In only highly individualized circumstances, partial cystectomy may be considered for small localized lesions. In metastatic disease, combination chemotherapy with a cisplatin-based regimen produces effective short- term palliation.

### Prognosis

Recurrence after local treatment is frequent (40% to 80%), and patients must be followed for life. The 5-year disease-free survival for patients with localized, low-grade tumors (stage 0 or A) approaches 90%, but that for high-grade lesions is less favorable (60% to 80%). Patients with invasive cancer (stages B1, B2, and C) have 5-year survivals of 20% to 60%, whereas those with stage D disease rarely survive longer than 2 years.

## ■ Carcinoma of the Prostate

The recent introduction of serologic screening for prostate-specific antigen (PSA) has led to an artifactual explosive increase in the prevalence of prostate cancer. For example, earlier projections suggested that 340,000 new cases of prostate cancer would be diagnosed in 1997; however, revised estimates suggested 219,000 cases for 1997 and 184,000 cases for 1998. Even with these revisions, prostate cancer is the most frequently diagnosed cancer in the United States. In 2002 it is estimated that about 189,00 new cases would be diagnosed and that there would be about 30,200 deaths from prostate cancer. By identifying previously occult and asymptomatic disease, PSA testing has ushered in a vigorous debate regarding how, and even whether, to treat patients with newly diagnosed disease, given the typical indolent nature of the disease and the older patient population it affects.

### Incidence and Epidemiology

About 30% of men over age 50 have occult prostate cancer. Autopsy studies in men who died of cardiovascular or other disease have shown that almost all men over 90 years of age have one or more foci of prostate cancer on careful pathologic examination, raising the intriguing question of why the disease is clinically relevant in only a subset of patients. Clinically, less than 1% of prostate cancers occur in men under age 40. Most cases become clinically manifest over age 60, and death from prostate cancer is most common over age 75. The estimated lifetime risk of developing clinically significant prostate cancer is about 20%, and the lifetime risk of dying of the disease is 4%. Racial factors are important: African-American men have a 1.5-fold higher incidence than Caucasians, and Asians have one-half the incidence. The mortality from prostate cancer in African-American men is more than twice that of men of other racial groups.

### Etiology, Pathogenesis, and Pathology

Prostate carcinoma is not seen in castrated men, and androgens are believed to play a permissive role. The international variation in incidence positively correlates with fat intake. There are inherent racial variations in the prostatic tissue level of 5-$\alpha$ reductase, the enzyme that converts testosterone into its more potent derivative dihydrotestosterone. The highest values are found in African-American and white men, and lower values in Asians. Age is the most important additional risk factor; a positive family history doubles the patient's risk.

Virtually all prostate cancers are **acinar adenocarcinomas.** Rarely, there are small cell (neuroendocrine) carcinomas, squamous cell carcinomas, transitional cell carcinomas, or lymphomas. The **Gleason grading system,** which classifies prostate cancers into five grades, takes into account the two dominant histologic patterns, and sums them into a score: 2–4 = well-differentiated, 5–7 = moderately differentiated, and 8–10 = poorly differentiated. This system is universally used in assigning prognostic categories along with the anatomically staging information.

Unlike **benign prostatic hypertrophy** (BPH), which arises in the central periurethral zone, prostate cancers usually begin in the periphery of the gland, mainly the posterior lobe. Thus, obstructive urinary symptoms occur relatively late in the cancer's natural history; when manifest, the symptoms can mimic BPH, a disorder also common in this patient population.

As the disease progresses, local growth extends beyond the prostatic capsule to include the pelvic sidewalls and seminal vesicles. Regional pelvic lymph nodes are involved first, followed by the periaortic nodes. The pattern of hematogenous metastasis is unique, because almost all such patients have bone metastases. The axial skeleton is the most commonly involved, typically with new bone formation causing increased radiographic density (osteoblastic metastases). Distant metastases to the lungs, liver, and other locations usually occur late, signifying extensive metastatic disease.

## Clinical Features

Low-grade, low-stage prostate cancer may remain asymptomatic for the patient's life. In asymptomatic men, the initial evidence may be a high level of PSA on screening or a prostatic nodule noted on rectal examination. Locally advanced disease may cause urinary obstruction, hematuria, or hematospermia. Bone pain or stiffness may occur from metastatic disease. The differential diagnosis of urinary complaints includes infection, prostatitis, and BPH; skeletal complaints may simulate osteoarthritis, Paget disease, or degenerative disc disease.

Leukoerythroblastic anemia is typical of bone marrow involvement. High blood urea nitrogen and creatinine levels may indicate ureteral obstruction. Alkaline phosphatase elevation suggests osteoblastic bone metastases.

## Diagnosis, Clinical Evaluation, and Staging

Screening for the disease in asymptomatic patients can be done by **digital rectal examination (DRE)** or PSA. The DRE has been the historical test. It can be incorporated with a routine checkup and can also serve to investigate the patient's symptoms of dysuria, frequency, or hematuria. Its accuracy depends on physician experience, patient compliance, and whether there is co-existing benign prostatic hypertrophy. **Transrectal ultrasound (TRUS)** helps distinguish known or suspected foci of prostate cancer from areas of BPH, infection, or calcification and can guide the urologist in selecting areas within the prostate for **needle biopsy.** Typically, multiple biopsies are done from both prostatic lobes to facilitate staging and grading analysis. Even when the prostate is thought to be suspicious for cancers on TRUS, only 15% to 30% of patients have a positive biopsy.

The availability of the PSA test has revolutionized prostate cancer screening. Its better acceptance by patients has led to a dramatic increase in cases diagnosed within the last few years. PSA, a proteolytic enzyme from the prostatic acinar cells, serves to liquefy the seminal plasma coagulum. Cancer cells secrete PSA at about 3 times the rate of normal prostate cells. In healthy men, the PSA level is <4 ng/ml, and it may rise moderately in BPH and prostatitis (usually <10 ng/ml). Although prostate cancer may occur with normal PSA levels, higher PSA levels should raise the index of suspicion of prostate cancer. Thus, for a given volume of prostate tissue, the serum PSA value will be higher. The physician can then evaluate the PSA level, assess glandular size, and assess risk of early prostate cancer. In a man older than 70 years of age, the specificity of a PSA >10 ng/ml is more than 60% in the presence of palpable BPH, and more than 90% in its absence. Because the PSA level is related to the volume of cancer present, it not only can suggest the presence of prostate cancer, but also can roughly predict the stage of the disease. In general, the higher the PSA level the higher the risk of disease outside the prostatic capsule, and the lower the chances of cure. PSA levels of 4 to 10 ng/ml indicate a 20% to 25% risk of prostate cancer. Almost invariably, these patients have early-stage, highly treatable disease. When the PSA exceeds 10 ng/ml, the risk of cancer increases to about 60%, and the risk is more than 95% when the PSA is >20 ng/ml. Unfortunately almost all the latter patients have unresectable and/or metastatic disease.

Table 205.3 presents the staging of prostate cancer.

**Stage A disease** is clinically occult and is discovered incidentally, by histologic evaluation of tissue resected to relieve urethral obstruction from BPH or obtained by biopsy of all prostate quadrants to investigate an elevated PSA.

**Stage B disease** may be detected by DRE of the prostate. It is categorized as unilateral, bilateral, or diffuse in its involvement. The category has implications regarding curability and whether the "nerve-sparing"

**TABLE 205.3. Clinical Staging of Prostate Cancer**

| Stage | Description |
|---|---|
| A | No palpable disease (T1) |
| A1 | Well differentiated ≤3 foci |
| A2 | Poorly differentiated or disease in ≥4 foci |
| B | Clinically palpable, confined to prostate (T2) |
| B1 | One lobe, single nodule |
| B2 | Diffuse disease in one lobe |
| B3 | Bilateral, confined to prostate |
| C | Disease extending outside the prostate ($T_3$-$T_4$) |
| D | Metastases |
| D1 | Pelvic node metastases |
| D2 | Upper abdominal, osseous, or visceral metastases |

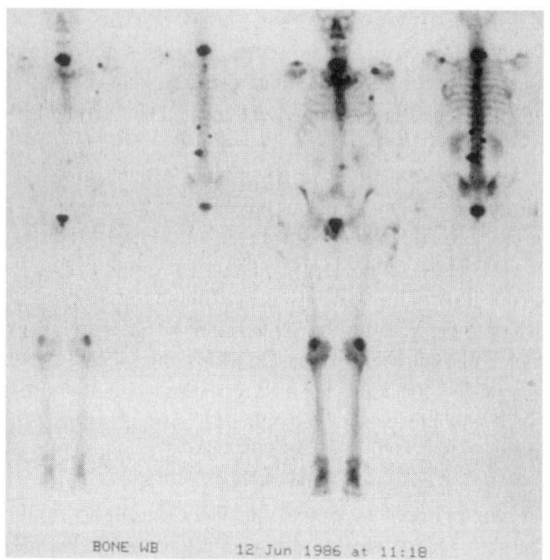


**FIGURE 205.1.** Radionuclide bone scan in prostate cancer showing scattered foci of uptake, which indicate metastases.

prostatectomy, designed to preserve sexual functioning, can be successfully performed.

**Stage C disease,** which signifies disease beyond the capsule, appears on DRE as an area of diffusely indurated enlargement, with loss of palpable landmarks of the prostate. This type of disease is not surgically curable; these patients are treated with radiotherapy.

In **Stage D,** in addition to local disease on DRE, distant metastases are apparent by bone scan, CT, and other imaging techniques (Figure 205.1).

## Screening for Prostate Cancer in Asymptomatic Men

The asymptomatic period of prostate cancer is probably more than 10 years, which makes screening attractive with the goal of reducing the mortality through early intervention. An annual DRE in addition to PSA testing is recommended for African-American men over age 45, for white men over 50, and for all men over 40 with an affected first-degree relative. Because of the long latency of the disease and the advanced age of the affected group, many patients will die of other diseases common to this age group; because of this, screening has not been adopted in Europe, where early stage patients are not routinely treated. In the United States there is a strong consensus that early-stage disease is curable, and that unless there are serious, active comorbidities (not just age alone), patients should be screened and usually treated. The currently accepted approach is that if the clinician feels that the patient's life expectancy exceeds 10 years, screening for prostate cancer probably is relevant.

## Management

Treatment options for localized prostate cancer include **prostatectomy** or **radiotherapy**. Although radiotherapy is comparably effective for 10 to 15 years, there is concern that late relapses may be more common than after a classical radical prostatectomy. Thus, radiotherapy is used selectively for older patients, those with higher operative risks, and those patients unwilling to suffer the unavoidable consequence of impotence attendant on a radical prostatectomy. "Watchful waiting" is reasonable in asymptomatic men with comorbidities or those unwilling to undergo curative surgery or radiotherapy.

Specifically, patients with stage A1 disease usually are observed, except for especially young men or those with intermediate or high-grade disease. Over a 10-year period, the disease will progress in approximately 15%.

Patients with disease of stages A2 and B1 to B3, if medically fit, normally are treated for cure with radical prostatectomy or radiotherapy. Treatment selection depends on the preference of the patient and physician and the complication rate. **Radical prostatectomy** entails 1% mortality, 1% to 5% incontinence, and 100% impotence. Recent "nerve-sparing" prostatectomy techniques for early-stage patients appear to reduce the postoperative impotence rate to less than 50%. High-risk surgical patients usually receive **radiotherapy,** the late complications of which are significant chronic radiation cystitis or proctitis in 2% to 5% of patients as well as impotence in about 50%. Brachytherapy is being implemented. As with the nerve-sparing prostatectomy it will require more than a decade of follow-up to determine whether these treatment modifications will maintain the same degree of efficacy while reducing morbidity. All patients should be counseled extensively about the risks and benefits of both treatment options, and older patients (>75 yrs) should have the option of watchful waiting.

With rare exceptions, patients with nonmetastatic disease extending beyond the prostatic capsule, stage C (T3), receive radiation. Symptomatic patients with stage D disease usually receive hormonal therapy, although a subset with positive pelvic nodes but no skeletal metastases (stage D1) sometimes are given radiotherapy as well. In patients with skeletal metastases (stage D2), hormonal therapy is the mainstay of treatment; temporary observation may be appropriate in asymptomatic persons wishing to avoid impotence or the hypoandrogenic consequences of antiandrogen therapy ("male menopause"). In hormone-refractory disease, radiation to painful bone metastases or strontium-90 for systemic metastases may help. Corticosteroids may give short-term relief. Chemotherapy is generally ineffective.

**TABLE 205.4. Options for Endocrine Therapy for Prostate Cancer**

| Treatment | Effect |
|---|---|
| Orchiectomy | Achieves rapid androgen control |
| LHRH agonists (leuprolide, goserelin) | Control takes an average of 3 weeks; symptoms may flare dangerously (from increased androgens) in the first 2 wks |
| LHRH agonists or orchiectomy plus the antiandrogen flutamide | Produces total androgen blockade; flutamide blocks dihydrotestosterone receptors and prevents the flare from excess androgens; combined therapy modestly improves disease-free survival and is widely used |
| Diethylstilbestrol | Decreases androgen secretion by feedback inhibition of hypothalamic-pituitary axis |

LHRH = luteinizing hormone-releasing hormone.

#### Hormonal therapies

Options in **hormonal therapy** for prostate cancer are summarized in Table 205.4. Patient and clinician preferences dictate the choice of approach. **Orchiectomy** is the simplest, cheapest, and most rapid in onset of effect but also the least popular.

Monthly or quarterly injections of **luteinizing hormone-releasing hormone** (LHRH) agonists have comparable effects and side effects but, in addition, have the theoretical advantage of reversibility and the psychological advantage of avoiding the patient's image of castration. Because a flare of the disease may occur from a transient rise of androgens soon after therapy starts, a short course of an antiandrogen preferably accompanies LHRH therapy, especially in those with impending spinal cord compression from extensive vertebral involvement. **Flutamide** and **Casodex** are nonsteroidal antiandrogens that are of limited value when used alone, but when used in conjunction with either orchiectomy or LHRH therapy produce "total androgen blockade." Although their contribution to longer-term control is controversial, their initial use to prevent a flare of disease is well-proven. All patients with symptomatic stage D disease should receive one of these agents with the initiation of LHRH therapy. After 30 days discontinuation can be considered.

Exogenous **estrogen** therapy, although it is cost-effective and avoids the hypoandrogenic syndrome ("male menopause"), is rarely used because of its risks of gynecomastia and thromboembolic disease. It is contraindicated in patients with known hypertensive or atherosclerotic cardiac disease.

Any of these hormonal interventions generally can produce clinical and biochemical responses in 60% to 80% of patients, typically lasting 18 to 36 months and occasionally more than 5 years. During this time, bone pain, obstructive urinary symptoms, and weight loss are under control. However, failure is inevitable, and secondary hormone therapy (with progestational agents, adrenal suppression with ketoconazole, or the anticancer agent aminoglutethimide) is successful in inducing further remission in 20% to 30% of cases.

### Prognosis

The prognosis depends on the stage and grade of tumor in localized disease. The 5-year survival is 88% to 95% for localized prostate cancer, 70% to 85% for locally advanced disease, and 20% to 30% for metastatic disease. Radical prostatectomy and radiation series achieve survival in the range of 70% to 75% at 10 years for stage A2 and B disease, but only 25% to 30% of patients with stage C disease survive 10 years (although a subset of patients with low-grade disease have prolonged survivals without active intervention). Fifty percent of patients with metastatic prostate cancer live 2 to 3 years, 20% survive 5 years, and only a few survive 10 years.

# CHAPTER 206 CANCER OF THE TESTIS

## Germ Cell Tumors

Nearly 7,500 new cases of germ cell testicular cancer occur annually in the United States. The peak age of incidence is 15 to 35 years. The only known risk factor is a history of cryptorchism. There is no convincing evidence that an orchiopexy, the surgical correction of this congenital problem, obviates the subsequent risk of testicular cancer.

### Pathology

The basic classification divides these tumors into **seminomas** and **nonseminomas** (Table 206.1). All arise

**TABLE 206.1. Germ Cell Testicular Tumors**

| Category | Frequency (%) |
|---|---|
| Seminoma | 40 |
| Embryonal carcinoma | 25 |
| Teratocarcinoma | 25 |
| Choriocarcinoma | <1 |
| Yolk sac tumor | <1 |
| Mixed histology | <10 |

from the germinal epithelium of the testis. Grossly, the tumors appear as firm nodules, often with areas of necrosis or hemorrhage. Because of their embryonic origin, lymphatic spread is via the spermatic cord to the perirenal and periaortic lymph nodes at the level of the renal vessels, not the anatomically adjacent pelvic or inguinal regions. Hematogenous metastases appear first in the lungs, with widespread dissemination following.

## Clinical Features

A painless or minimally painful testicular mass is the usual presenting complaint in patients with testicular cancer. Spontaneous hemorrhage may cause rapid testicular enlargement and pain. Painful masses may erroneously be diagnosed as epididymitis or orchitis; painless masses are often erroneously considered to be hydroceles.

On examination, the testicular mass may be firm and irregular. Metastatic disease may cause abdominal or back pain from enlarged retroperitoneal nodes, cough, pleuritic chest pain, hemoptysis from lung metastases, and even gynecomastia if the tumor cells secrete an excess of β-human chorionic gonadotropin (β-HCG).

Seminomas may be relatively indolent; often, the reported duration of symptoms is 1 to 2 years before diagnosis. Nonseminomas are often explosive in growth and dissemination and are diagnosed within months of onset of a testicular mass. Inguinal adenopathy is uncommon, unless antecedent scrotal surgery was performed, such as orchiopexy or a transscrotal biopsy.

## Diagnosis, Evaluation, and Staging

Testicular **ultrasonography** may be useful in diagnosing the tumor mass and making the distinction between a tumor and hydrocele. **Biopsy** should always be performed via a **high inguinal incision**, with immediate orchiectomy if cancer is diagnosed. **Serum marker** studies for β-HCG, alpha-fetoprotein (AFP), and lactate dehydrogenase (LDH) should be obtained before biopsy or orchiectomy.

Testicular neoplasms present the ideal paradigm for use of blood tests to monitor the status of the patient's disease. β-HCG is modestly elevated in 7.5% of seminomas and markedly elevated in all choriocarcinomas and 50% of embryonal carcinomas. AFP is elevated in more than 50% of embryonal and mixed histology tumors, but never in seminomas. Knowledge that such a marker was elevated before orchiectomy allows the physician to monitor effectively for relapse. Almost 80% of patients with advanced or recurrent nonseminomatous germ cell tumors have a high β-HCG or AFP level.

**Staging** should include CT of chest, abdomen, and pelvis, and, if the primary tumor demonstrates a significant component of choriocarcinoma, the brain. Stage I disease is confined to the testis; stage II disease includes the testis plus retroperitoneal nodes; stage III includes lymphatic extension above the diaphragm or hematogenous metastasis to the lung, liver, or brain.

## Management

### Seminomas

Seminomas are highly sensitive to **radiotherapy.** Cure rates following orchiectomy and radiotherapy approach 100% for stage I disease and 75% to 85% for stage II. Patients with high-risk stage II disease with bulky (>10 cm) retroperitoneal masses are best treated with **chemotherapy** alone or with 2–3 cycles of neoadjuvant combination chemotherapy preceding radiotherapy. About 90% of patients with stage III are curable with combination chemotherapy.

### Nonseminomas

In patients with nonseminomas, a baseline evaluation of β-HCG and AFP is crucial for following the disease. Stage I patients in whom previously elevated tumor markers have returned to normal after **orchiectomy** can be observed without systemic therapy, unless relapse occurs. This careful surveillance approach demonstrates that nearly 75% of such patients are cured by orchiectomy alone. Because the potential for chemotherapy-induced cure is so high, patients should have monthly monitoring of tumor markers, with CT scanning every 3 months for 2–3 years.

**Retroperitoneal lymph node dissection** is performed for selected patients with stage II disease. **Chemotherapy** is also used and can achieve cure in 80% to 90% of patients, whether used as primary treatment for stage II disease or as salvage treatment in patients relapsing after surgical treatment for stage I or II disease.

#### *Stage III disseminated disease*

The treatment of nonseminomatous germ cell tumors represents one of the major successes in medical oncology. Over 80% of patients are now cured. Patients are classified as good- or poor-risk depending on the number, size, and site of metastases. β-HCG, AFP, and LDH levels help assess the patient's "tumor burden."

Chemotherapy is based on cisplatin with bleomycin and etoposide (VP-16); additional agents can be used but are probably unnecessary except in unusually poor-risk patients. Good-risk patients have a 90% to 95% cure rate after 3 or 4 cycles of chemotherapy, whereas the cure rate for poor-risk patients is only 30% to 50%.

A significant number of patients with stage II or III disease have persistent retroperitoneal adenopathy after definitive chemotherapy. Persistent elevation of the tumor markers β-HCG and AFP confirm the presence of residual disease, necessitating further chemotherapy or surgery. Conversely, if the tumor markers have returned to normal levels, patients may be followed carefully, although ideally such patients should undergo retroperitoneal dissection to rule out residual microscopic disease. Such surgical resection or restaging detects residual cancer in about 15% of patients; an additional two cycles of chemotherapy after successful surgical removal enhances curability in this subset of patients.

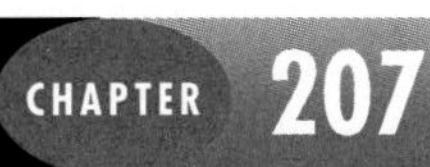

# CHAPTER 207 GYNECOLOGICAL NEOPLASMS

## Carcinoma of the Ovary

It is estimated that in 2002, about 23,300 new cases of ovarian cancer will be diagnosed, and there will be about 13,900 deaths from the disease. The incidence rises sharply after age 40, peaking at about 70 years. Hereditary ovarian cancer accounts for 5% of cases and may be associated with hereditary breast, ovarian, endometrial, or colon cancers. This previously puzzling spectrum of cancers is now better understood as the use of the BRCA-1 and BRCA-2 gene probes are applied to such patients. The chief endocrine risk is believed to be related to an abnormal repair mechanism after ovulation, so that the number of ovulatory cycles is a risk factor. Multiple births, prolonged lactation, and oral contraceptive use are partially protective.

### Pathology

Eighty percent of malignant ovarian tumors arise from the surface epithelium **(epithelial tumors).** Half of these are papillary serous cystadenocarcinomas; mucinous papillary cystadenocarcinomas and endometrioid or undifferentiated tumors each account for 10% to 15% of cases. **Stromal** and **germ cell** tumors are uncommon and include granulosa cell tumors and arrhenoblastomas. Germ cell tumors are responsible for only 1% to 2% and include dysgerminomas, malignant teratomas, embryonal carcinomas, and the rare choriocarcinoma. A few primary epithelial ovarian tumors, termed **borderline,** are very low grade and may have a prolonged clinical course of years or even decades, regardless of whether they are localized or metastatic.

### Clinical Features

Early ovarian cancer evokes few symptoms; as a result, most patients present with more advanced stage II or III disease. Early symptoms of lower abdominal pain or cramping may be confused with the irritable bowel syndrome, diverticular disease, or other nonmalignant abdominal discomfort. Advancing disease causes single or multiple mass effects. With spread to peritoneal and diaphragmatic serosal surfaces, ascites and pleural effusion develop. Ascites may be the presenting complaint and may be erroneously thought to be due to liver disease. Three fourths of patients have disease disseminated throughout the peritoneum at diagnosis (stage III or IV). Death usually results from bowel obstruction, often at multiple sites. Additional complications include cachexia, refractory ascites, or renal failure from ureteral obstruction.

Of laboratory features, the tumor marker **CA-125** is elevated in proportion to the tumor bulk of ovarian cancer. However, CA-125 is not specific for ovarian cancer; it is elevated in many other adenocarcinomas and benign diseases such as endometriosis, benign ovarian cysts, inflammatory peritonitis, and chronic liver disease. Nevertheless, it provides an index of disease activity in proven ovarian cancer and often is used to monitor the clinical course of therapy.

### Diagnosis, Clinical Evaluation, and Staging

There is no evidence that careful **screening** of asymptomatic women effectively detects early-stage disease. All tests, including pelvic examination, pelvic ultrasound, and CA-125 measurements, are limited by their lack of specificity or sensitivity for early ovarian cancer. Current screening methods, with the possible exception of transvaginal ultrasound in higher-risk women, probably are not cost-effective, given the relatively low prevalence of the disease and the limited sensitivity and specificity of current tests. However, patients with a history of breast or colon cancer or the familial ovarian cancer syndrome are at high risk. Evidence suggests that screening in this high-risk

**TABLE 207.1. FIGO Classification for Epithelial Ovarian Malignancy**

| Stage | Description |
|---|---|
| I | Growth limited to the ovaries |
| Ia | Single ovary involved |
| Ib | Both ovaries involved |
| Ic | Surface spread in one or both ovaries, rupture at surgery, ascites/peritoneal washing with positive cytology |
| II | Pelvic extension |
| IIa | Extension/metastasis to uterus or fallopian tubes |
| IIb | Extension to other pelvic structures |
| III | Spread outside the pelvis |
| IIIa | Microscopically confirmed seeding of abdominal peritoneum (micrometastases) |
| IIIb | Grossly apparent spread to serosal surfaces outside of the pelvis (maximum diameter <2 cm); retroperitoneal nodes negative |
| IIIc | Implants >2 cm or positive retroperitoneal nodes |
| IV | Confirmed distant metastasis; cytologically positive pleural effusion; parenchymal liver metastases |

FIGO = International Federation for Gynecology and Obstetrics.
(From: Richardson et al. N Engl J Med 1985;312–417. Used with permission.)

group may result in a survival benefit. Prophylactic **oophorectomy** is an option in patients with a strong family history, especially if they exhibit the BRCA-1 oncogene.

A pelvic (ovarian) mass in a **postmenopausal** woman requires open or laparoscopic biopsy. In **premenopausal** women, masses exceeding 8 cm should be diagnosed surgically promptly; most often, masses under 8 cm are functional cysts and, if confirmed by ultrasound, should be observed for regression over 2 to 3 menstrual cycles. In more advanced abdominal presentations, cytologic evaluation of ascitic fluid, laparoscopy, or direct laparotomy is indicated.

Staging procedures including serum CA-125, pelvic ultrasound, and abdominal CT scans are useful. Precise staging usually is accomplished by laparotomy or laparoscopy. Staging is commonly done by the International Federation for Gynecology and Obstetrics (FIGO) system (Table 207.1).

### Management

Surgical exploration is offered to most patients who have no contraindications to surgery. Localized disease is treated with total abdominal hysterectomy, bilateral salpingo-oophorectomy, and omentectomy. In more advanced disease, even when complete resection is not possible, meticulous tumor reduction (debulking), with excision of all apparent abdominal disease, results in a more favorable prognosis with subsequent chemotherapy. The few patients with borderline malignancy or stage I disease without penetration of the ovarian capsule usually are cured by surgery. With adjuvant chemotherapy, a group of stage II patients also can be cured.

Chemotherapy is the current principal treatment for advanced stages of ovarian carcinoma. Many chemotherapy regimens are moderately effective in this disease. Most recently, **Carboplatin** (or its parent compound cisplatin), combined with paclitaxel (Taxol) has become the treatment of choice, with higher overall response rates and occasional long-term survival.

### Prognosis

The overall 5-year survival is 60% to 85% for patients with stage I ovarian cancer, 40% to 70% for stage II, 15% to 35% for stage III, and up to 5% to 15% for stage IV. At 10 years, only about 10% of stage III patients are alive and disease-free. Because most long-term survivors have been given chemotherapy with alkylating agents (cisplatin or cyclophosphamide), there is a small but finite risk of leukemia.

## Endometrial Carcinoma

About 39,300 cases of endometrial cancer occur annually in the United States, mostly in women aged 55 to 70 years. Adenocarcinomas, including those with squamous elements, constitute 90% of tumors. Clear cell papillary variants, endometrial stromal sarcomas, carcinosarcoma and leiomyosarcoma constitute the remainder.

Endogenous risk factors include obesity, diabetes mellitus, hypertension, polycystic ovaries, and prior granulosa cell tumors. Exogenous risk factors include hormone replacement therapy with unopposed estrogen, which increases the risk 4- to 10-fold. The concomitant administration of progestins markedly reduces this risk. Prolonged treatment with the weak estrogen agonist tamoxifen in breast cancer appears to increase the risk of endometrial cancer by 2-4 fold.

### Clinical Features

Abnormal vaginal bleeding is the primary symptom, so that all women with postmenopausal bleeding require investigation. Advanced disease leads to pelvic and abdominal pain. Metastases may appear as supraclavicular adenopathy, hepatic metastases, or pulmonary nodules. Physical examination may reveal an enlarged uterus or pelvic masses.

### Diagnosis, Clinical Evaluation, and Staging

Cytologic assessments of the vaginal and cervical surfaces may be positive but are unreliable for screening. Although endometrial sampling is better, a thorough dilatation and curettage (D&C) is the most accurate test, and must be done if the disease is suspected.

Once cancer is diagnosed, preoperative sigmoidoscopy and cystoscopy help assess resectability, as do CT or magnetic resonance scans. Progesterone receptor determination and histologic grading provide additional prognostic data. Staging follows the anatomic spread of the disease: stage I, confined to the uterus; stage II, affecting the uterus and cervix; stage III, spread to the pelvic structures; and stage IV, local invasion of bladder, rectum, and areas outside the true pelvis (stage IVa) or distant spread (Stage IVb).

### Management

Surgical treatment is by total abdominal hysterectomy and bilateral salpingo-oophorectomy, with peritoneal washings and pelvic and periaortic node sampling. External beam and intracavitary radiation is an alternative to surgery in patients with poor surgical risks and as an adjunct to surgery in patients with high-risk stages I and II disease. Most patients with advanced stages III or IVA cancer are given radiotherapy. Patients with metastatic disease can be given medroxyprogesterone or megestrol (progestational agents) for palliation if their tumor expresses progesterone receptors. Systemic chemotherapy is much less effective in endometrial than in ovarian cancer.

### Prognosis

Localized stage I presentations are cured in 80% to 90% of patients, depending on the depth of myometrial invasion and tumor grade. The 5-year survival rate may reach 50% to 80% in stage II patients. Survival in stage III and IV is only 5% to 30%.

## Cervical Carcinoma

### Incidence and Etiology

In 2002, about 13,000 new cases of invasive cervical cancer and 55,000 cases of in situ cervical cancer were diagnosed in the United States. The earliest precancerous manifestation, cervical dysplasia, begins to appear in women in their 20s. Carcinoma in situ is prevalent in women in their 30s, and invasive carcinoma is seen in women beyond their 40s. Because of screening and improved medical care, the total rate of cervical cancer in the United States has decreased since the 1930s, but it has not decreased among African-American and Hispanic women.

The chief epidemiologic factors are age at first intercourse, socioeconomic status, and number of sexual partners. Cervical cancer is believed to result from a sexually transmitted infection: **human papilloma virus** (HPV) types 16 and 18 are strongly associated with premalignant lesions. Patients positive for HPV-16 or -18 at routine pelvic examination more often develop dysplasia or carcinoma in situ on follow-up, and are at increased risk for development of invasive disease between routine screening intervals. Such patients should be screened more frequently and taught to report any suspicious symptoms immediately. Cigarette smoking, HIV infection, and possibly herpes virus type 2 infection are cofactors.

### Pathology

Ninety-five percent of cervical carcinomas are **squamous cell,** typically arising from the squamocolumnar junction of the cervical epithelium. The uncommon adenocarcinoma also has an in situ counterpart. Unlike other disease sites, the influence of histologic grade in squamous cell carcinoma of the cervix is minimal; by far the most important prognostic factor is tumor stage.

Cervical cancer progressively invades the surface, then the base, of the cervix, followed by extension to the parametrium and pelvic sidewalls. Involvement of the regional lymphatics, including the obturator and iliac nodes, follows. Locally advanced disease invades the bladder and rectum.

### Clinical Features

Cervical dysplasia and carcinoma in situ usually are asymptomatic and are diagnosed incidentally during routine screening or during the evaluation of inflammatory or infectious diseases of the cervix. Until invasive tumors are well-established, there are no symptoms. Contact bleeding (postcoital) and discharge occur; these intensify with progression. Locally advanced disease causes pelvic pain, ureteral obstruction, and back pain. Edema of one or both lower extremities may occur. These symptoms of locally advanced disease portend a worse prognosis. Death results from infection, hemorrhage, or uremia due to ureteral obstruction. Distant metastases are a relatively uncommon cause of death.

### Diagnosis, Clinical Evaluation, and Staging

Because the premalignant phases of this disease normally span years, there is ample time for detection of premalignant changes, allowing successful treatment of dysplasia and carcinoma in situ before invasive disease develops. **Annual pelvic examinations** with a **Papanicolaou (Pap) smear** from the cervix should begin at the onset of sexual activity or at age 18. After 2 to 3 negative annual examinations, and if dysplasia and HPV infection are not present, the frequency of screening can be reduced to every 2 to 3 years. If premalignant changes have not developed on routine screening by age 65, invasive cancer is unlikely during remaining life. Conversely, patients with HPV-16 and -18 must be screened, often, indefinitely.

Occasionally, a Pap smear may be nondiagnostic or even normal in the face of cancer. Therefore, a normal Pap smear does not negate a prior positive test or suspicious finding at pelvic examination. Once suspicion is aroused by an abnormal Pap smear or visualized cervical abnormalities, colposcopy and biopsy should follow to obtain tissue from below the surface of the cervix. Staging and prognosis of cervical cancer are shown in Table 207.2.

**TABLE 207.2. Staging and Prognosis in Cervical Carcinoma**

| Stage | Description | 5-Year Survival (%) |
|---|---|---|
| I | Confined to cervix | |
| IA | Microscopic | 90 |
| IB | Gross invasion | 70–90 |
| IIA | Upper 1/3 of vagina invaded | 75–85 |
| IIB | Parametrium invaded | 60–65 |
| III | To pelvic side walls or to lower 1/3 of vagina | 30–50 |
| IVA | Mucosa of bladder or rectum | <20 |
| IVB | Distant metastases | <5 |

### Management and Prognosis

For premalignant lesions, local treatments are used. Dysplasia is treated with cryosurgery or conization of the cervix. Carcinoma in situ may be treated similarly or by hysterectomy. Microinvasive cancer is treated by radical hysterectomy. Higher stages of disease often are treated by external and intracavitary radiation. The prognosis depends exclusively on the stage of disease (see Table 200.2).

# CHAPTER 208 SELECTED ENDOCRINE GLAND TUMORS

Principal endocrine neoplasms represent a diverse group of malignancies (Table 208.1). Thyroid cancer is discussed in chapter 68; pheochromocytomas are discussed in chapter 184 (Adrenal Disorders) and chapter 177 (Secondary Hypertension).

## Adrenal Neoplasms

Adrenal carcinoma is rare and occurs most commonly in children, with a second peak of incidence occurring in the fourth and fifth decades. Functional (secreting) adrenal tumors are more common in women, whereas the nonfunctioning variant is more common in men. Hormonally nonfunctional tumors often are quite large at diagnosis, given their anatomical location.

Clinical presentations of adrenal tumors include those due to tumor bulk or endocrine syndromes (e.g., precocious puberty in children, feminization, virilization, or Cushing syndrome). Labeled iodocholesterol studies show uptake in benign adenoma, but only rarely in carcinoma. CT and magnetic resonance scans provide the best imaging of adrenal tumors. Any adrenal mass larger than 5 cm is presumed to be a primary or metastatic cancer and should be biopsied or resected, depending on the clinical situation. Adults usually present with more advanced disease, and only 20% to 25% are cured by surgery. Recurrent metastatic disease is treated with mitotane (*o',p'*-DDD), with partial responses in 60%. Nausea and CNS toxicity are dose-limiting effects. Chemotherapy is rarely effective.

## Multiple Endocrine Neoplasia

The rare but fascinating multiple endocrine neoplasia (MEN) syndromes have been recognized for over 80 years. **Type I MEN** (Wermer syndrome) involves the parathyroid and pituitary glands and pancreatic islet cells. Hyperparathyroidism is almost universal in these patients. The leading cause of death in MEN I is the Zollinger-Ellison syndrome, produced by a gastrin-secreting islet cell tumor causing intractable peptic ulcer disease. Less commonly, hyperparathyroidism-induced hypercalcemia or the complications of a space-occupying pituitary lesion result in death.

**MEN type IIa** consists of medullary carcinomas of the thyroid (MCT), pheochromocytomas, and hyperpara-

**TABLE 208.1. Endocrine and Neuroendocrine Tumors**

| | |
|---|---|
| Thyroid | Islet cell tumors |
| Well–differentiated | Insulinoma |
| Papillary, mixed | Gastrinoma |
| Follicular | Glucagonoma |
| Hurthle cell variant | VIPoma |
| Medullary | Somatostatinomas |
| Sporadic | MEN I |
| MEN IIa, IIb | Carcinoids |
| Undifferentiated (anaplastic) carcinoma | Bronchial (foregut) |
| Parathyroid | Gastric |
| Adenoma | Intestinal (midgut) |
| Carcinoma | Appendix, colon, rectum (hindgut) |
| Adrenal cortex | Extrapulmonary small cell carcinoma |
| Adrenal cortical carcinoma | Esophagus |
| Adrenal medulla | Cervix |
| Malignant pheochromocytoma | Prostate |
| | Many other viscera |

thyroidism (Sipple syndrome). Patients operated on for hyperparathyroidism or MCT may have unrecognized pheochromocytomas as part of MEN IIa and, thus, are at risk for hypertensive crises. Blood relatives of patients with this syndrome should be screened for MCT using stimulated calcitonin assays. A test for the responsible gene, known as the *RET* proto-oncogene, is now available to facilitate identification of family members at risk.

**MEN IIb** consists of the same triad of conditions, plus mucosal neuromas, a body habitus resembling Marfan syndrome, and a characteristic facies. Children and teenagers from families with either MEN II syndrome must be screened for MCT. Total thyroidectomy is curative in either premalignant hyperplasia or early malignancy; however, cases of MCT that are diagnosed after the development of clinical symptoms often are metastatic and almost invariably are fatal.

# CHAPTER 209 CANCER OF THE HEAD AND NECK

Squamous cancer of the head, neck, and laryngeal region accounts for about 37,800 cases and 11,100 deaths annually. These cancers have a predilection for men (3:1 for most sites, 5:1 for laryngeal tumors). The larynx is the site most commonly affected, followed by the oral cavity, pharynx, tongue, and lip. Nasopharyngeal cancer and carcinoma of the paranasal sinuses each account for less than 5% of cases.

## Etiology and Pathology

Tobacco smoke (cigarette and, to a lesser extent, pipe and cigar) and smokeless tobacco are the prime etiologic factors, with alcohol being a potent cofactor. The Epstein-Barr virus is convincingly associated with nasopharyngeal carcinoma, particularly in Eastern Asia, as well as oropharyngeal cancers in nonsmokers in the United States. Industrial exposure to wood dust and oils is implicated in the etiology of nasal and paranasal tumors.

Most tumors are **squamous** and arise from the surface epithelium of the oral, pharyngeal, and laryngeal mucosa. In the nasopharynx, dense lymphocytic infiltration often occurs; these tumors are termed **lymphoepitheliomas.** Rarely, adenocarcinoma (adenoid cystic carcinoma) arises from the major or minor salivary glands.

## Clinical Features

Symptoms depend on the site of origin. Leukoplakia, a premalignant lesion, usually is asymptomatic, and often identified during routine dental examinations. Symptoms and signs of malignancy include an oral ulcer or plaque, sore throat, trismus, or dysphagia. A neck mass due to metastatic adenopathy is a common presenting sign, especially in tumors arising from tonsillar, nasopharyngeal, or pharyngeal sites. Persistent serous otitis media and unilateral deafness are clues to nasopharyngeal cancer. Hoarseness is a cardinal feature of laryngeal cancers.

Local invasion and regional node metastases are more common than distant metastases, which occur late in the course of most of these cancers. Because of the underlying common risk factors, multiple primary tumors of the head, neck, lung, and esophagus are not unusual, either simultaneously or separated by months to years.

### Diagnosis, Evaluation, and Staging

Screening in high-risk persons can be done by the dentist or primary physician. Those with any suspicious symptoms and signs should be seen by an otolaryngologist for a more detailed evaluation using specialized techniques, such as nasopharyngoscopy and fiberoptic laryngoscopy.

Careful biopsy of suspected lesions is necessary to distinguish leukoplakia, the premalignant lesion, from early cancer. CT and magnetic resonance scans of the head and neck are helpful in defining the anatomic extent of disease and enlargement of lymph nodes not palpable on examination. There are peculiarities of staging in several sites, but the basic staging system illustrated in Table 209.1 provides a common basis for evaluation of treatment protocols.

**TABLE 209.1. Basic TNM Staging of Head and Neck Cancer**

| | |
|---|---|
| *Tumor* | |
| T1 | Maximum diameter <2 cm |
| T2 | Maximum diameter 2–4 cm |
| T3 | Maximum diameter >4 cm or extension to adjacent structures |
| T4 | Massive lesion with deep invasion |
| *Nodes* | |
| N0 | No cervical adenopathy |
| N1 | Single ipsilateral node <3 cm |
| N2 | One node >3 cm or multiple homolateral nodes, none >6 cm or bilateral nodes <6 cm |
| N3 | Ipsilateral node(s)>6 cm; bilateral nodes >6 cm |
| *Metastases (M)* | |
| M0 | No metastases |
| M1 | Metastases |
| Stage I | T1 N0 M0 |
| Stage II | T2 N0 M0 |
| Stage III | T3 N0 or T1-T3 N1 |
| Stage IV | T4 N0-2 M0; any T, N3 M0; any T, any N, M1 |

(Reprinted with permission from: American Joint Committee on Cancer. Cancer Staging Manual. 5th ed. Philadelphia: JB Lippincott, 1997.)

### Management

Because of the predominantly local nature of squamous cell cancers arising in the head and neck, **surgery** and **radiotherapy** are the primary modes of treatment. The size and location of the primary lesion and the presence or absence of regional nodal metastases determine the choice of initial therapy. The functional and cosmetic sequelae of both radical surgery and radiotherapy also are major considerations.

In stage I and II lesions of a number of sites, radiation and surgery yield similar long-term results, with cure rates of 70% to 85%. Lymph node involvement adversely affects the overall survival rate. Adjuvant chemotherapy further enhances cure rates. **Neoadjuvant chemotherapy** leads to rapid responses in stage III and IV disease, but does not appear to increase resectability or survival, except in nasopharyngeal cancer (in which chemotherapy and radiation lead to cure in 50% to 60%). Metastatic disease can be treated palliatively with several chemotherapy agents given either singly or in combination (e.g., methotrexate, cisplatin, 5-FU), but responses usually are incomplete and transient.

**Smoking cessation** is of paramount importance. Patients who continue to smoke respond less favorably to radiation. A second primary tumor of the head and neck region, esophagus, and lung occurs at a rate of 5% to 7% annually after treatment of the first tumor at one of these sites. Chemoprevention with 13-*cis* retinoic acid produces a 50% reduction in secondary primary tumors.

## Malignant Melanoma

The epidemiology, clinical features, and treatment of melanoma and nonmelanoma skin cancer are presented fully in Chapter 56. It was estimated that there would be about 53,600 new cases diagnosed in 2002; like non-Hodgkin's lymphoma, this is one of the few cancers with a truly dramatic increase in incidence over the past decades, undoubtedly due to changes in lifestyle.

### Diagnosis, Evaluation, and Staging

Ideally, all individuals should have a total skin inspection annually. Isolated dysplastic or suspicious lesions should be totally excised. Any excised lesion, no matter how innocuous it appears, should be sent for pathologic examination.

When melanoma is diagnosed, a careful comprehensive physical examination together with radiologic studies should be done to assess possible lymphatic spread or hematogenous dissemination. The most important assessment of melanoma is the careful evaluation of **depth of invasion,** using either the Clark or the Breslow system. Each is designed to allow for reproducible assessment of depth of invasion, which correlates with risk of relapse. The prognostic importance of depth of invasion is shown in Table 209.2. Survival is 60% to 70% for patients with localized disease, 15% to 40% with lymph node involvement, and less than 1% for distant disease. The prognosis is superior at all stages for women.

**TABLE 209.2. Level of Invasion and Prognosis in Localized Melanoma**

| Depth of Invasion | Class | 10-yr Survival (%) |
|---|---|---|
| *Clark classification* | | |
| Epidermis (in situ) | I | 100 |
| Invades papillary dermis | II | >90 |
| Invades junction of papillary dermis and reticular dermis | III | 75 |
| Invades reticular dermis | IV | 60 |
| Invades subcutaneous fat | V | 20–40 |
| *Breslow classification* | | |
| <0.76 mm | | 85–95 |
| 0.76–1.5 mm | | 75–95 |
| 1.51–2.5 mm | | 60 |
| 2.51–4.0 mm | | 45–55 |
| 4.1–8.0 mm | | 20–40 |
| >8.0 mm | | 20 |

(Adapted from: Balch CM, Houghton AN, Sober AJ and Soong SJ. (eds). Cutaneous Melanoma. St. Louis, Quality Medical Publishing, Inc., Third Edition, 1998, page 17. Used with permission.)

## Management

Initial therapy for malignant melanoma is **local excision.** For thin lesions (<1 mm depth of invasion), 2-cm lateral margins give equivalent outcome but better cosmetic results than the older, traditional 5-cm margin of resection. Wider excisions with 2- to 5-cm margins are done for lesions that invade more deeply. Skin grafting may be required. Lesions on fingers and toes require amputation. Routine prophylactic regional node dissections are not indicated. However, the sentinel node biopsy technique can identify subsets of patients who may benefit from adjuvant therapy. Adjuvant alpha-interferon reduces the risk of relapse in high-risk patients, defined as patients with deeply invasive tumors or occult lymph node metastases.

Metastatic melanoma shows an overall poor response to therapy; effective treatment regimens are lacking for this disease. **Radiotherapy** to the regional lymphatics may improve local control in head and neck melanomas. Many patients can benefit from resection of an isolated or limited metastasis. Isolated hyperthermic limb perfusion for extremity melanomas has led to a high rate of local control. **Combination chemotherapy** with cisplatin, carmustine, and dacarbazine, elicits a transient response rate of about 40%. For locally recurrent melanoma, intralesional BCG is effective. Interferons produce a response rate of 10% to 15%, and interleukin-2 (IL-2) produces a 15% to 20% response; however, these responses rarely are durable. Responses to IL-2, IFN, and combination chemotherapy product are now seen in >50% patients; some are durable.

# CHAPTER 210 MALIGNANT TUMORS OF THE CENTRAL NERVOUS SYSTEM

## Primary Brain Tumors

The incidence of brain tumors is bimodal, with an initial peak at age 4, a second rise after age 25 to 30, and then a plateau after age 65. Brain tumors in children differ from those of adults. The former are medulloblastomas, low-grade astrocytomas, and ependymomas, whereas the tumors affecting adults are predominantly high-grade astrocytomas, including grade III and IV lesions known as **glioblastoma multiforme**. In adults, benign meningioma is second to astrocytoma in incidence. The other malignant tumors shown in Table 210.1 are less common. There were an estimated 17,000 new cases and 13,100 deaths from brain tumors in 2002.

### Etiology

A number of hereditary disorders are associated with brain tumors. While uncommon, they include neurofibromatosis, tuberous sclerosis, the Li-Fraumeni syndrome (see Table 197.2), and Turcot syndrome, a rare entity in which patients with colonic polyposis and colonic cancer develop medulloblastomas or high-grade astrocytomas. Despite their obscure etiology, the incidence of astrocytomas has risen somewhat since 1973.

### Pathology

The principal brain tumors in adults are gliomas. More than one half of these are high-grade, highly

**TABLE 210.1. Malignant Brain Tumors**

| |
|---|
| Astrocytomas |
| Low grade (grade I-II) |
| Anaplastic (grade III) |
| Glioblastoma multiforme (grade IV) |
| Ependymoma |
| Oligodendroglioma |
| Medulloblastoma |
| Malignant meningioma |
| Primary CNS lymphoma |
| Pinealoma |
| Metastatic malignancies (breast, lung, colon, renal, melanoma) |

cellular, with new blood vessel formation, palisading of nuclei, and necrosis. Brain tumors rarely metastasize, but high-grade gliomas and medulloblastomas can seed the subarachnoid space along the spinal cord.

### Clinical Features

The brain, being enclosed in the rigid cranium, is subject to compression by space-occupying lesions, with elevation of intracranial pressure and cerebral edema. Because brain tumors often progress slowly, patients frequently do not seek medical attention until the disease is locally advanced. Progressive disease causes generalized headache, nausea, vomiting, and lethargy. Seizures occur in 20% to 50% of patients. Investigation of new onset of seizures in an adult rarely uncovers a latent brain tumor, but nevertheless, new-onset seizures should lead to appropriate diagnostic studies. Symptoms often are vague and include personality changes, depression, and fatigue. Primary or metastatic tumors may present with a hemispheric or cerebellar syndrome mimicking a vascular accident.

### Diagnosis and Evaluation

CT and MRI are highly effective diagnostic tools, and can delineate the extent of disease, concomitant edema, and distortion and shifting of vital brain structures. Biopsy is performed at the time of resection. Lesions in unresectable locations or in patients with comorbidities may undergo a stereotactic needle biopsy.

### Management and Prognosis

High-dose **dexamethasone,** to reduce edema and secondary symptoms, often is used to stabilize patients before and after initial surgery. Anatomy and limitations of surgery permitting, malignant brain tumors should be aggressively excised. Well-circumscribed, low-grade tumors (oligodendrogliomas, meningiomas, and low-grade astrocytomas) may do well for long periods. High-grade astrocytomas (anaplastic astrocytomas and glioblastoma multiforme) usually can be only subtotally resected. Prognosis improves in proportion to the extent of tumor resected.

Radiation is routinely given following surgery for anaplastic astrocytomas and glioblastoma multiforme. Nearly 50% of patients with astrocytomas survive 2 to 3 years after this regimen, compared to less than 5% for glioblastoma. Chemotherapy adds modest additional benefit. The newly received drug Temozolamide, designed to cross the blood-brain barrier, produces meaningful palliation with minimal toxicity. Precisely targeted radiation (gamma knife or stereotactic radiosurgery) or brachytherapy with iodine-125 or iridium-192 may further benefit localized tumors. Reoperation is attempted in localized recurrence or in post-radiation brain necrosis.

## Primary Central Nervous System Lymphomas

Primary CNS lymphomas are large-cell lymphomas formerly called **microgliomas** of the brain. They occur in near-epidemic proportions in immunosuppressed patients (e.g., AIDS patients, solid organ transplant recipients). The incidence also appears to be increasing in the normal population, predominantly in men in their sixth or seventh decade of life.

Multifocal presentations are common. Cerebrospinal fluid cytology may be positive. Patients respond dramatically and rapidly to steroid-based therapy with radiation, but control usually is only for a matter of months. Current studies are investigating the role of radiotherapy together with multidrug chemotherapy, including intraventricular and intravenous combination chemotherapy.

## Metastatic Brain Tumors

Cancers of the lung, breast, kidney, and large bowel, and melanoma together cause most brain metastases. Usually, uncontrolled tumor is obvious elsewhere, but melanoma and renal cell carcinoma are notorious for isolated cerebral metastases, even after a long, disease-free interval. Solitary or multiple brain metastases may be the harbinger of lung cancer.

Intracranial metastases cause symptoms similar to those of a primary brain tumor, and the diagnostic workup and therapeutic interventions are similar, especially for patients with an isolated metastasis. About 60% to 80% respond to treatment, with an average survival of 6 months, depending on the volume of tumor in the brain and the degree of control elsewhere. A patient with a solitary brain metastasis and minimal or no tumor burden elsewhere may survive months or even years following surgery or radiotherapy. This is especially true in patients with a long, disease-free period from primary therapy.

## Meningeal Carcinomatosis

Acute lymphocytic leukemia and intermediate and high-grade lymphomas may disseminate to the meninges, as may some solid tumors (e.g., breast and lung cancers, melanoma). A myriad of features result: confusion, headache, meningitis, back pain, and cranial or spinal neuropathies. Magnetic resonance imaging or CT may show paraventricular contrast enhancement.

The classic **cerebrospinal fluid (CSF)** findings include elevated pressure, elevated protein, and low glucose levels. Initially, the CSF may be nondiagnostic in 50% of patients, requiring multiple CSF examinations. Cytologic examination often (but not invariably) shows malignant cells.

Therapy may be considered in the appropriate clinical setting. Intrathecal methotrexate, cytarabine, or thiotepa is given twice weekly until the CSF clears, and then weekly for 6–8 weeks. A reservoir (Ommaya) providing intraventricular therapy is more convenient and safer than multiple lumbar installations, and the distribution of drug in the CSF is more uniform. Cranial irradiation usually is added. Intrathecal therapy can cause acute lethal demyelination, and chemotherapy plus radiation frequently elicits encephalopathy. Remissions are brief in carcinomatous and lymphomatous meningitis, but exceptions occur if the systemic disease is controlled.

# CHAPTER 211 SARCOMAS

Sarcomas, malignant tumors arising from multiple types of connective tissue, are uncommon (about 8,300 soft tissue sarcoma and 2,400 bone sarcoma cases are diagnosed annually). Bone sarcomas occur predominantly in childhood, whereas soft tissue sarcomas occur at all ages.

## Etiology and Pathology

Sarcomas may be inherited, as in the Li-Fraumeni syndrome. Previous radiation, neurofibromatosis, and Paget disease of bone are predisposing conditions for the development of **osteosarcoma.** Industrial exposure to vinyl chloride has been associated with hepatic **angiosarcomas.** Post-transplant immunosuppression and HIV infection are associated with **Kaposi's sarcoma,** which is an AIDS-defining malignancy. Sarcomas are defined by the tissue of origin (Table 211.1). Histologic grade and cell type are the most important features in establishing a prognosis.

## Management

Soft tissue masses should be biopsied by **core needle** or careful **incisional** technique to enhance subsequent resectability. **Surgery** of all soft tissue and bone sarcomas is designed to ensure totally clear margins. Because these tumors tend to extend along tissue planes, wide excisions are necessary. Modern reconstructive surgical techniques allow limb-sparing surgery, augmented by postoperative radiotherapy, to avoid amputation of tumor-bearing extremities. **Irradiation** is commonly employed postoperatively in adult sarcomas because a**djuvant chemotherapy** is of modest benefit. Conversely, pediatric sarcomas usually are quite sensitive to chemotherapy; therefore, chemotherapy is used preferentially as an adjunct to surgery, because radiation inhibits normal growth of skeletal structures.

**TABLE 211.1. Sarcomas of Bone and Connective Tissue**

| Bone or Tissue Affected | Type of Sarcoma |
|---|---|
| Bone | Osteosarcoma |
| | Periosteal osteogenic sarcoma |
| | Malignant giant cell tumor |
| | Ewing's sarcoma |
| | Primary lymphoma |
| | Fibrosarcoma |
| | Fibrous histiocytoma |
| Cartilage | Chondrosarcoma |
| Fat | Liposarcoma |
| Fibrous tissue | Fibrosarcoma |
| Smooth muscle | Leiomyosarcoma |
| Striated muscle | Rhabdomyosarcoma |
| Mesenchyme | Mesenchymoma |
| Synovia | Synovial cell sarcoma |
| Vascular/lymphatic system | Hemangiosarcoma |
| | Lymphangiosarcoma |
| | Hemangiopericytoma |
| | Kaposi's sarcoma |
| Nerve | Malignant schwannoma |
| | Malignant neurilemoma |
| Miscellaneous | Alveolar soft parts sarcoma |
| | Malignant fibrous histiocytoma |
| | Extraskeletal Ewing's sarcoma |
| | Primitive primary neuroectodermal tumors |
| | Clear cell sarcoma |

## Kaposi's Sarcoma

Kaposi's sarcoma (KS) deserves special mention because of its association with HIV infection and immunosuppression. It has three forms:

**Nonendemic KS** occurs among the elderly, chiefly men of Mediterranean or Ashkenazi Jewish extraction. It presents as nodules and plaques on the extremities, with an indolent course averaging 10 years.

**Endemic KS** occurs in young men in central Africa. It is manifested by frequent lymphadenopathy and spread to the lungs and gastrointestinal tract.

**Epidemic KS** especially affects homosexual men with HIV infection; whereas it is rarely seen in HIV-positive women in the United States. 1% of cases afflict recipients of solid-organ transplants. Because persons acquiring HIV through blood products or IV drug abuse rarely develop KS (unless sexual risk factors also are present), KS has long been suspected to have an infectious etiology. Recently, evidence of viral DNA in the tumor genome has pointed to a new virus of the herpes virus family (Human Herpes Virus-8).

Pathologically, the tumor nodules show spindle cells and endothelial cell proliferation with a marked proliferation of small blood vessels. The lesions are distributed in the skin, mucous membranes, lungs, trachea and bronchi, and GI tract.

The **endemic form** of KS in elderly men usually starts as purplish nodules on the lower extremities. The course is indolent: years may pass before progressive lymph node involvement and, ultimately, spread to the lungs and GI tract supervene. **KS in HIV-infected persons** more frequently involves the skin of the trunk, head and neck, or mucous membranes of the oral cavity. Lymph node involvement is universal, and dysphagia, GI hemorrhage, or hemoptysis is common, as are cough and dyspnea from pulmonary metastases. In HIV-infected patients, KS may be relatively indolent if the patient has a reasonably intact immune system, but with progressive immunosuppression, KS may progress parallel to the increasing risk of opportunistic infections.

### Management and Prognosis

Radiation is useful for local palliation. Alfa-interferon, in patients who are relatively immunocompetent, produces a 25% to 40% response, especially when combined with zidovudine. Single-agent chemotherapy with vinca alkaloids, etoposide, bleomycin, or anthracyclines achieves responses in at least 40% of patients, but combination chemotherapy is only marginally more beneficial.

The prognosis depends on the degree of immunosuppression. With associated opportunistic infections, survival beyond 2 years is unusual.

# CHAPTER 212 METASTATIC CANCER OF UNKNOWN PRIMARY SITE

Approximately 5% of cancer patients present initially with a metastasis, the origin of which remains elusive. When a careful history and physical examination fail to uncover a primary, a targeted work-up is undertaken, directed by anatomic site of presentation, symptoms, and histologic type of malignancy.

About 60% of patients with metastatic malignancies of unknown primary site have easily recognizable adenocarcinomas, and 30% have a poorly differentiated neoplasm or poorly differentiated carcinoma. About 5% have squamous cancers, and a lesser proportion represent metastatic melanoma or malignant lymphoma.

### Clinical Features

The features of malignancies with unknown primary sites are legion, but certain recurrent themes should lead to suspicion of particular sites of origin (Table 212.1). Combining these presentations with pathologic features and special examinations may disclose a treatable neoplasm. Consultation with a pathologist is especially helpful in the subset of patients with poorly differentiated neoplasms. In these patients, a battery of pathologic examinations, including immunohistochemical staining, may be employed (Table 212.2).

### Management

Metastatic squamous carcinoma of unknown primary that occurs in the neck region may be treated with radical neck dissection and radiation. In a considerable proportion of cases, long-term survival may follow. The same is true for cancer of unknown primary involving the inguinal lymph nodes.

Patients who have disease presenting in the lungs, liver, or peritoneal cavity represent difficult problems because these areas are common sites of metastases from many different tumors. In general, the emphasis is on the search for a primary tumor that is known to respond well to palliative therapy (e.g., breast or ovarian cancer in women, germ cell tumors in men). Serum tumor markers associated with these diseases sometimes can provide supportive evidence for a possible diagnosis or at least

**TABLE 212.1. Clinical Features Useful in Determining the Source of a Malignancy of Unknown Primary Site**

| Feature | Primary Tumors to be Suspected |
|---|---|
| Cervical lymphadenopathy | Lymphoma<br>Hodgkin's disease<br>Head and neck squamous carcinoma<br>Thyroid |
| Right supraclavicular node | Lung, mediastinum, lymphomas |
| Left supraclavicular node | Carcinoma originating below the diaphragm |
| Inguinal nodes | Cancer of the penis, vulva, anus, melanoma |
| Axillary nodes | Breast, melanoma |
| Brain tumor | Lung cancer |
| Pulmonary nodules | Many sites (kidney, melanoma, germ cell tumors) |
| Abdominal carcinomatosis | Ovary, pancreas, other GI tract |
| Undifferentiated cancer in young man | Germ cell tumor |
| Undifferentiated cancer in woman following pregnancy, abortion, or molar pregnancy | Choriocarcinoma |

**TABLE 212.2. Special Pathologic Stains and Markers in Carcinoma of Unknown Primary Site**

| Tumor | Immunostains and Serum Markers |
|---|---|
| Lymphoma | Leukocyte common antigen (LCA) |
| Carcinoma | Cytokeratin (epithelial membrane antigen) |
| Sarcoma | Vimentin, desmin, factor VIII antigen |
| Ovary | CA-125 (tumor and serum) |
| Breast | Hormone receptors |
| Prostate | Prostate-specific antigen (PSA) |
| Follicular thyroid | Thyroglobulin |
| Medullary thyroid | Calcitonin (tumor and serum) |
| Germ cell tumors | Human chorionic gonadotropin ($\beta$-HCG), alpha-fetoprotein (AFP) |
| Neuroendocrine tumors | Chromogranin A, neuron-specific enolase |
| Melanoma | S100, HMB-45 |

allow the treating physician to make reasonable treatment decisions.

**Patterns of disease** also may be helpful. In women with diffuse peritoneal carcinomatosis, ovarian cancer should be strongly considered. Malignant axillary adenopathy in women is considered to be breast cancer unless proven otherwise. In young men, the possibility of occult testicular tumor or extragonadal germ cell tumor must be considered; presentation with multiple pulmonary nodules or with mediastinal, retroperitoneal, or supraclavicular adenopathy mandate testing for serum AFP and $\beta$-HCG as well as an abdominal CT scan to look for retroperitoneal adenopathy, and a careful testicular examination and ultrasonography. In men with bone metastases, prostate cancer should always be suspected. Thyroid cancers are usually histologically apparent, but stains for thyroglobulin and calcitonin may provide further confirmation. Abdominal CT may be cost-effective, because pancreatic cancer is one of the most common primary sites for metastatic adenocarcinoma of unknown primary.

## Prognosis

Most patients whose tumor is suspected to be of lung, pancreatic, or other gastrointestinal origin tend to have a poor prognosis. Survival usually is brief. Palliative chemotherapy may be offered to patients with excellent performance status and minimal tumor burden, but its use should be discouraged in patients severely disabled by their disease, since it is normally of minimal benefit. Judicious radiotherapy to symptomatic sites of disease often is better therapy.

# CHAPTER 213 PARANEOPLASTIC SYNDROMES

The paraneoplastic syndromes encompass a diverse group of systemic disorders that represent the remote effects of cancer due to the action of ectopic hormones, antibodies, and various tumor products. Although not conceptualized as such, anemia, anorexia, weight loss, and fevers are in essence paraneoplastic signs or symptoms. The more classic syndromes are discussed in the following sections.

## Endocrine Syndromes

The endocrine syndromes (Table 213.1) include **Cushing's syndrome,** seen in 6% of small cell lung cancers and various other neuroendocrine tumors. **Ectopic secretion of antidiuretic hormone** (ADH) also is common in small cell lung cancer.

**Hypercalcemia** due to osseous involvement is encountered in lung, breast, and other solid tumors, multiple myeloma, and lymphomas. Tumor production of parathormone-related polypeptide (PTH-rp), with its partial homology to native parathormone, is a major cause of hypercalcemia in squamous cell carcinomas of the head and neck, esophagus, and lung, and in adenocarcinoma of the kidney. Calcitonin production in medullary carcinoma of the thyroid and small cell lung cancer usually is asymptomatic and serves as a marker for recurrent disease in both sporadic and familial types.

In contrast to hypercalcemia, **hypocalcemia** is quite rare and occurs occasionally in patients with osteoblastic bone metastases of breast and prostate cancer or in the syndrome of oncogenic osteomalacia in large mesenchymal tumors. **Hypoglycemia** also is rare and results from the secretion of insulin-like growth factors in massive retroperitoneal sarcomas or hepatoma; malignant insulinomas secrete endogenous insulin. **Gynecomastia** is seen occasionally in germ cell tumors in men and rarely in patients with large cell or adenocarcinoma of the lung.

## Hematologic Manifestations

Hematologic manifestations of malignancy are legion. **Anemia** can result from many mechanisms (Table 213.2). Besides chronic inflammation and blood loss from gastrointestinal cancers, immune hemolysis (Hodgkin's and non-Hodgkin's lymphoma, chronic lymphocytic leukemia, and ovarian teratomas), pure red cell aplasia (thymomas and chronic lymphocytic leukemia), and fragmentation (microangiopathy) hemolysis (disseminated intravascular coagulation [DIC] as seen in adenocarcinomas of diverse sites) are other mechanisms.

**Leukemoid reactions** and **eosinophilia** may occur in disseminated sarcomas, Hodgkin's disease, and some metastatic carcinomas. **Erythrocytosis** due to ectopic erythropoietin production is observed in about 3% of renal cell carcinoma patients, as well as in rare patients with hepatocellular carcinomas, cerebellar hemangioblastomas, and benign renal conditions. **Thrombocytopenia** is seen with marrow replacement or following the development of an autoimmune phenomenon or secondary to DIC.

The most common coagulation abnormality in cancer is activation of the coagulation system. Isolated **thrombophlebitis** of multifactorial origin is common in cancer patients, as is recurrent or **migratory thrombophlebitis**. In severe cases, there is life-threatening decompensated **disseminated intravascular coagulation** with hemorrhage and consumption of platelets, fibrinogen, and factors V and VIII. Nonbacterial thrombotic endocarditis

**TABLE 213.1. Paraneoplastic Endocrine Syndromes**

| Syndrome | Hormone | Associated Tumors |
|---|---|---|
| Cushing's syndrome | ACTH | Small cell lung cancer, other lung cancer, carcinoids |
| Syndrome of inappropriate ADH secretion (SIADH) | Arginine vasopressin | Lung cancer, mainly small cell |
| Hypercalcemia | PTH-rp, cytokines, vitamin D | Lung (squamous), renal, breast cancer, myeloma, lymphoma |
| Gynecomastia | Unknown and β-HCG | Germ cell—lung |
| Hyperthyroidism | β-HCG | Choriocarcinoma, germ cell tumors |
| Hypocalcemia | Unknown | Osteoblastic metastases |
| Hypoglycemia | Insulin-like growth factors | Sarcomas, esp. large fibrosarcomas |

HCG = human chorionic gonadotropin; PTH-rp = parathyroid-related peptide.

**TABLE 213.2. Hematologic Manifestations of Cancer**

| | |
|---|---|
| Anemia | Chronic disease<br>Blood loss<br>Marrow replacement<br>Microangiopathic (±DIC)<br>Pure red cell aplasia<br>Immune hemolysis |
| Leukocytosis | Leukopenia<br>Neutrophilic leukemoid reaction<br>Eosinophilia |
| Erythrocytosis | Due to ectopic erythropoietin production |
| Thrombocytopenia | Marrow replacement<br>Immune<br>DIC syndromes |

DIC = disseminated intravascular coagulation.

is due to fibrin deposition on the mitral or aortic valve, with systemic embolization to the brain, kidneys, and spleen or to the microcirculation of the extremities, leading to peripheral ischemia and gangrene.

## ■ Neurologic Syndromes

The remote effects of cancer on the nervous system are pervasive (Table 213.3) and include **cerebellar degeneration**, **dementia**, **limbic encephalitis**, and many other neurologic disorders. A syndrome of uncoordinated, spontaneous eye movements termed **opsoclonia** or opsoclonus has been reported in breast and lung cancer. **Necrotizing myelopathy** is seen in leukemia, and a variety of sensory, motor, and autonomic neuropathies are common in lung cancer. **Myasthenia gravis** is noted in association with thymomas (usually benign), and a myasthenic-like syndrome (**Eaton-Lambert syndrome**) is seen with small cell lung cancer.

## ■ Dermatologic Syndromes

A myriad of dermatologic syndromes exist. Most are associated with adenocarcinomas, especially of the gastrointestinal tract (e.g., syndrome of Laser-Trelat, which is the sudden appearance of large numbers of seborrheic keratoses). **Bowen's disease** is associated with internal malignancies of the lung, gastrointestinal tract, and genitourinary tract. Palmar and plantar **tylosis** is associated with cancer of the esophagus. **Acanthosis nigricans** (pigmentation involving the axillae and belt areas with a velvety appearance of the skin) is rare, but is striking in its appearance as well as relationship to (gastric) adenocarcinoma. The historically interesting Sister Mary Joseph's nodule, unlike the above-mentioned paraneoplastic syndromes, is the result of direct retrograde extension of cancer along the umbilical lymphatics, producing a periumbilical mass. Synopses of the myriad of such syndromes can be found in comprehensive oncology or dermatology textbooks.

**TABLE 213.3. Paraneoplastic Neurologic Syndromes**

| System Affected | Clinical Manifestation |
|---|---|
| Brain | Dementia<br>Subacute cerebellar degeneration<br>Limbic encephalitis<br>Optic neuritis<br>Opsoclonia<br>Progressive multifocal leukoencephalopathy |
| Spinal cord | Necrotizing myelopathy<br>Amyotrophic lateral sclerosis |
| Peripheral nerve | Sensory neuropathy<br>Sensory motor neuropathy<br>Autonomic neuropathy with orthostatic hypotension |
| Neuromuscular junction | Myasthenia gravis<br>Myasthenic (Eaton-Lambert) syndrome |
| Muscle | Dermatomyositis<br>Polymyositis |

# CHAPTER 214 ONCOLOGIC EMERGENCIES

A variety of cancer-related conditions may develop, typically as late complications, that require urgent or immediate treatment. The most common ones can be classified as mechanical, systemic, infectious, or iatrogenic complications (Table 214.1).

**TABLE 214.1. Cancer-Related Emergencies**

| |
|---|
| **Mechanical Complications** |
| Superior vena cava syndrome |
| Upper airway, esophageal, and bronchial obstruction |
| GI tract perforation and obstruction |
| Cardiac tamponade due to pericardial effusion |
| Increased intracranial pressure |
| Spinal cord compression |
| Pathologic fractures |
| **Coagulopathies** |
| Thrombocytopenia |
| Immune-mediated |
| Cancer treatment–related |
| Extensive marrow infiltration |
| Disseminated intravascular coagulation (DIC) |
| Life-threatening thrombosis or embolus |
| Possible severe anemia |
| **Renal Emergencies** |
| Obstruction of the urinary tract |
| Urinary hemorrhage |
| Tumors of bladder or prostate |
| Treatment-related: |
| Radiotherapy |
| Cyclophosphamide or ifosfamide therapy |
| **Metabolic Emergencies** |
| Hypercalcemia |
| Hyponatremia |
| SIADH |
| Small cell carcinoma of the lung |
| Nausea from cancer chemotherapy |
| Hypotonic fluid administration given with cancer chemotherapy |
| Adrenal insufficiency |
| Gastrointestinal fluid losses and dehydration |
| Cushing's syndrome |
| Small cell lung cancer |
| Carcinoids |
| Benign neuroendocrine tumors |
| **Emergencies Due to Cancer Treatment** |
| Neutropenia and sepsis |
| Tumor lysis syndrome |
| Initial treatment of acute lymphocytic leukemia, Burkitt or other undifferentiated lymphomas |

## Mechanical Complications

### Superior Vena Cava Syndrome

The superior vena cava (SVC) syndrome, although not always a medical emergency, occurs with primary tumors or adenopathy involving the right side of the mediastinum. Most cases are due to bronchogenic carcinoma, usually of the small cell type. The clinical syndrome results in edema of the upper extremity, thorax, neck, and face; neck vein distention; periorbital and conjunctival edema; and often headache, flushing, and cyanosis. Venous collaterals may be visible on the chest wall.

The clinical diagnosis is confirmed by a contrast-enhanced CT scan or radionuclide flow study. Other diagnostic studies include biopsy of superficial nodes or bronchoscopy, bearing in mind that excessive bleeding may follow. Transthoracic fine-needle biopsies probably are safer, if feasible. If at all possible, a histologic diagnosis should be made, because the underlying tumor often is a highly treatable, occasionally curable, neoplasm. Small cell lung cancer can be treated initially with radiotherapy or combination chemotherapy. Similar considerations may apply in germ cell tumors, Hodgkin's disease, and non-Hodgkin's lymphoma. In contrast, non-small cell carcinoma and adenocarcinomas metastatic to the mediastinum are best managed with radiotherapy, at least initially. SVC obstruction complicated by thrombosis is only marginally benefited by treatment with fibrinolytic agents, anticoagulants, and stenting.

### Upper Airway, Esophageal, and Bronchial Obstruction

Most airway obstruction syndromes are secondary to carcinoma of the lung and esophagus. Although chemotherapy and radiotherapy may be helpful in selected cases when a responsive tumor is known to be present, emergency management requires bronchoscopy and surgical creation of a lumen using a variety of techniques, including the neodymium-YAG laser. Esophageal obstruction may be treated by laser therapy, or by placing a bypassing gastrostomy tube or an indwelling endoprosthesis. Tracheoesophageal fistula, likewise, may require an emergency endoprosthesis.

### Perforation and Obstruction in the Gastrointestinal Tract

Gastrointestinal perforations and obstructions represent surgical emergencies. Before urgent surgical therapy or other maneuvers are undertaken (e.g., nasogastric suction, analgesia, and antibiotics), the patient's prognosis and fitness for surgery should be ascertained.

### Cardiac Tamponade due to Pericardial Effusion

Neoplastic pericardial effusion and tamponade occur most often with carcinoma of the lung or breast, melanoma, and lymphomas. It may also follow thoracic radiotherapy, infections of the pericardium, and conditions such as uremia and hypothyroidism, which may or may not be related to cancer. The diagnosis may be suggested by an enlarged cardiac shadow on chest radiograph and by weakness, fatigue, dyspnea, distended neck veins, and pulsus paradoxus (>12 mm Hg). In florid cases, prompt drainage may prevent death. Echocardiography, which shows the effusion as well as the signs of tamponade, is diagnostic.

### Increased Intracranial Pressure

Increased intracranial pressure usually is due to mass effects of primary or metastatic brain tumors. It presents with headache, nausea, vomiting, visual blurring, and a variety of neurologic signs with subsequent lethargy, somnolence, and coma. The diagnosis of a primary brain tumor or metastases is confirmed by CT scan or MRI of the brain. Some cases, especially with cranial neuropathies and negative CT or MRI, may be due to meningeal carcinomatosis.

Emergency treatment includes high-dose corticosteroids, usually dexamethasone, to control edema (10–20 mg initially followed by 4–10 mg q6h until maximal neurologic response is obtained). Emergent surgical resection should follow if feasible; radiotherapy is used for unresectable tumors, or patients with known active extraneurologic sites of disease. Meningeal disease usually is treated by intrathecal chemotherapy with methotrexate or cytarabine, accompanied in most cases by whole-brain radiotherapy.

### Spinal Cord Compression

Most cases of spinal cord compression are due to tumor extension into the epidural space from the vertebral body. On occasion, pathologic fracture of the involved vertebra can add the additional mechanical hazard of compression by bone. The diagnostic approach first involves a high index of suspicion. Increasing back pain and findings suggestive of metastatic tumor should lead to prompt MRI of the spine (Figure 214.1). When spinal cord compression is manifested by sensory or motor defects—decreased sensation, voluntary motor weakness (paraparesis or paraplegia), or involuntary motor dysfunction (e.g., bowel or bladder incontinence)—it is a true emergency. If an MRI scanning facility is not available, myelography is the alternative procedure. When combined with CT scanning, myelography with contrast provides useful information as to encroachment on the dural sac.

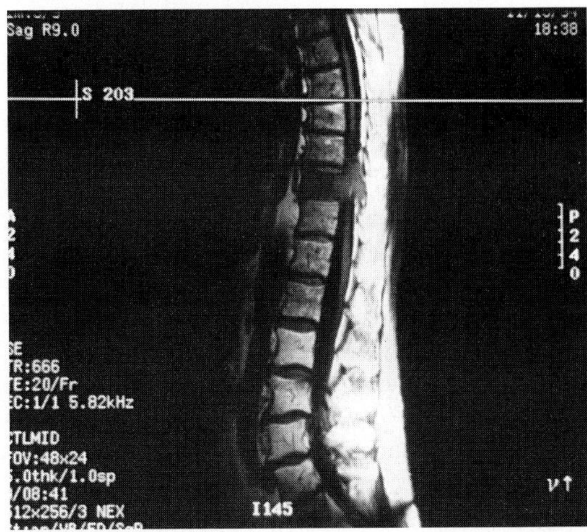


**FIGURE 214.1.** Magnetic resonance image of the thoracic spine showing metastatic prostate cancer invading the epidural space.

If the underlying tumor is known, or highly suspected, to be radioresponsive and the patient is neurologically stable, treatment with radiotherapy can be initiated. High-dose corticosteroids, similar to those used in patients with intracranial neoplasms, should be given concurrently. If there is a pathologic fracture with spinal instability and compression of the cord by bone, the tumor is radioresistant or accompanied by neurologic deterioration, or the cause of the spinal cord compression is unknown, one should proceed to surgery first. If the patient is ambulatory with minimal or no neurologic deficit, treatment by radiation or laminectomy followed by radiation permits continued ambulation in 60% to 80% of patients, which drops to 40% to 45% or less if the patient has paraparesis and to 3% to 10% with paraplegia or quadriplegia. In few other conditions is an early diagnosis more vital.

### Pathologic Fractures

Pathologic fractures of the femur and humerus, commonly from metastatic breast carcinoma, cause much disability. If a lesion is larger than about 3 cm or causes thinning of the cortex, prophylactic orthopedic fixation should be performed, followed by radiotherapy.

## Hematologic Emergencies

Many hematologic manifestations of cancer may present as emergencies. Severe anemia may require urgent transfusion. Thrombocytopenia and disseminated intravascular coagulation (DIC) may lead to bleeding, arterial emboli, and renal failure. Thrombocytopenia may be due to cancer treatment, extensive marrow infiltration, or immune-mediated mechanisms. After appropriate diagnostic studies, including bone marrow aspiration and biopsy, the etiology of the coagulopathy should be ascertained. The treatment of neoplastic DIC is difficult, because it involves the replacement of factors, cryoprecipitate, fresh frozen plasma, and platelets, and, ultimately, control of the underlying neoplasm. Occasionally, heparin therapy may reverse DIC and nonbacterial thrombotic endocarditis. Thrombosis or embolus can be a life-threatening emergency. As in consumptive coagulopathies, effective oral anticoagulation usually is ineffective, mandating long-term use of low-molecular-weight heparin. Recurrent, otherwise unexplained thrombosis or embolus should elicit a search for an occult malignancy.

## Renal Emergencies

Obstruction of the urinary tract and urinary hemorrhage are the most common renal emergencies. Obstruction can occur in the pelvis or higher in a wide variety of malignant neoplasms and, if bilateral, can lead to rapidly progressive uremia. Ureteral stenting through the bladder with a double J-stent or by percutaneous nephrostomy allows palliation of this complication. Hemorrhage from the bladder may occur with tumors of the bladder or prostate, following radiotherapy or therapy with cyclophosphamide or ifosfamide. The emergency treatment is urethral catheterization with continuous bladder irrigation to flush out clots.

## Metabolic Emergencies

### Hypercalcemia

The most common hormonal syndrome causing a metabolic emergency is hypercalcemia. Its principal features (see Table 66.1 and chapter 66) are CNS depression, urinary frequency, polyuria and resultant polydipsia, nausea, vomiting, dehydration, and severe constipation from gastrointestinal tract atony. Dehydration is universal in symptomatic hypercalcemia; nonzealous fluid replacement should be the initial therapy, followed by the judicious use of loop diuretics such as furosemide (thiazides must be avoided), which maximizes Na+-coupled calcium excretion. This regimen suffices for minimal elevations in serum calcium (i.e., <12 mg/dl). In patients with significant hypercalcemia (i.e., >14 mg/dl) or compromised neurologic states, bisphosphonates should be included, e.g., pamidronate. Medical therapy of hypercalcemic crisis is shown in Table 66.4. Hypercalcemia complicating multiple myeloma, some lymphomas, and breast cancer commonly responds to corticosteroids. Mithramycin and gallium nitrate are useful in treating refractory hypercalcemia. Specific antitumor treatment, appropriate to the type of neoplasm, may alleviate mild hypercalcemia and not require any specific calcium-lowering therapy.

A special case includes the hypercalcemic flare seen shortly after institution of **hormonal therapy in breast cancer** metastatic to bone. This effect had been encountered with estrogen and androgen therapy and now is seen with tamoxifen; paradoxically, it is a marker for a subsequent good response to hormonal therapy. Tamoxifen often can be continued while the hypercalcemia is being treated by specific measures.

### Hyponatremia

Euvolemic hyponatremia, resulting from the syndrome of inappropriate secretion of antidiuretic hormone (SIADH), may be seen in a variety of malignancies and nonneoplastic disorders. The chief cause is small cell lung cancer. Mild cases can be treated with water restriction and demeclocycline. This antibiotic is phototoxic, and sun exposure should be avoided to prevent severe sunburn.

Management of severe hyponatremia is shown in Figure 64.4 in Chapter 64. Emergencies can be managed by partial correction of the serum sodium with isotonic or hypertonic saline and administration of a loop diuretic to remove excess water. This must be done with care, correcting the serum sodium by no faster than 0.5 to1 mEq/hr to avoid central pontine myelinolysis.

### Cushing's Syndrome

Paraneoplastic Cushing's syndrome can lead to hypokalemia, muscle weakness, and acute psychosis. It is most common in small cell lung cancer, with more indolent types seen with carcinoids and benign neuroendocrine tumors. That seen with small cell carcinoma of the lung usually is associated with muscle wasting, hypokalemia, hypertension, and severe weakness and progresses rapidly to death. Treatment with high-dose ketoconazole, 1200–1800 mg/day, or aminoglutethimide and hydrocortisone is indicated. Acute Cushing's syndrome in small cell carcinoma of the lung portends a poor prognosis.

## Emergencies Associated With Cancer Treatment

### Neutropenia and Sepsis

Neutropenia and subsequent fever commonly follow chemotherapy. Sepsis, which is rare when neutrophil counts exceed 1500/mm$^3$, is increasingly common with falling counts, especially those below 500/mm$^3$. Fever above 38.3°C (101°F) with a neutrophil count below 500 mandates prompt examination, chest radiography, urinalysis, and cultures of blood, urine, and blood from venous access devices.

The most common causative organisms are gram-negative rods of the *Escherichia coli-Klebsiella* group, followed by *Pseudomonas* species. Gram-positive infections are becoming much more common. Empiric broad-spectrum antibiotics should be started immediately to cover gram-negative organisms.

When fever persists, vancomycin and subsequent antifungal therapy with amphotericin-B should be instituted. Cultures may be negative in more than one half of cases, and therapy is largely empirical. With positive cultures or identification of a specific infection site, therapy can be individualized. Prolonged, severe neutropenia, systemic fungal infections, and uncontrolled bacterial sepsis are unfavorable signs. Antibiotics can be discontinued in the culture-negative, afebrile patient when the absolute neutrophil count exceeds 500/mm$^3$. **Colony-stimulating factors** should be considered for prophylactic administration in subsequent courses of chemotherapy, but usually are ineffective in patients presenting with neutropenic fever due to their delayed onset of activity.

## Questions

**Instructions:** For each question below, select **one** lettered answer that is the **best** for each question.

1. In the past two decades, which cancer has increased in incidence?
   A. Carcinoma of the cervix
   B. Carcinoma of the breast
   C. Carcinoma of the stomach
   D. Carcinoma of the rectum

2. Tobacco-associated malignancies include:
   A. Head and neck cancer
   B. Bladder cancer
   C. Esophageal cancer
   D. Pancreatic cancer
   E. All of the above

3. A 30-year-old man has had daily fever for two months and has lost 25 lbs. The only positive physical finding is an enlarged right axillary lymph node. CT scanning shows periaortic adenopathy. Bone marrow biopsies show a hypercellular marrow. The node shows lymphocyte-depleted Hodgkin's disease on biopsy. The patient's stage and management should be:
   A. The stage is undefined; he should have a staging laparotomy.
   B. He has Stage IIIB disease and should have a staging laparotomy to determine treatment options.
   C. Stage IIIB or higher. He should receive at least six cycles of ABVD or similar chemotherapy.
   D. Stage IIIB. He should receive total lymphoid irradiation.

4. Drugs used in chemotherapy have myriad toxicities. Those that may cause lung injury include:
   A. Methotrexate
   B. Busulfan
   C. Bleomycin
   D. Mitomycin C
   E. All of the above

5. A 36-year-old woman presents with a 2.5 cm non-tender breast mass that fails to disappear after her subsequent menstrual period. There are no palpable axillary nodes. Mammography shows bilateral dense breast tissue without a dominant mass. Correct management now is:
   A. Reassure the patient because the mammogram is negative.
   B. Discontinue the oral contraceptives she is taking; observe at 3-month intervals.
   C. Magnetic resonance imaging of the breast.
   D. Ultrasonography and fine needle aspiration; if no fluid is obtained, proceed directly to surgical excision.

6. A 25-year-old man complains of cough and wheezing. A lymph node is palpable in the right lower neck. A chest radiograph shows a large superior mediastinal mass with tracheal deviation. The next step would be:
   A. Biopsy the lymph node.
   B. Proceed with radiation without histologic diagnosis.
   C. Start combination chemotherapy with MOPP without histologic diagnosis.
   D. Initiate a comprehensive workup for infectious diseases, including TB, infectious mononucleosis, fungal infections, and HIV.

7. A 40-year-old woman with a 2.5 cm breast cancer with three positive axillary nodes is treated with six cycles of CMF. She asks you what is the estimated absolute benefit in terms of 10-year mortality reduction. You answer:
   A. 5%
   B. 3-6%
   C. 10-12%
   D. 50%

8. A 75-year-old man with coronary heart disease and chronic obstructive lung disease has palpable adenopathy in the neck and inguinal regions. He feels

well and has normal blood counts. Lymph node biopsy shows follicular, small cleaved lymphocytic lymphoma. Bone marrow biopsy shows paratrabecular infiltrates of small cleaved lymphocytes. His lactate dehydrogenase is normal. The most reasonable management would be to:

A. Initiate comprehensive combination chemotherapy with doxorubicin, cyclophosphamide, vincristine, and prednisone (CHOP). Tell the patient he has a 50% chance of cure.
B. Discuss the potential indolent and incurable nature of this low-grade lymphoma; recommend close follow-up with palliative chemotherapy and/or radiotherapy only if/when progression is apparent.
C. Institute palliative radiation therapy to all the enlarged lymph nodes.
D. Institute non-toxic palliative chemotherapy using daily chlorambucil to be given indefinitely.

9. A 70-year-old man with known prostate cancer develops chronic back pain of two months' duration and is seen in the emergency department because of severe midthoracic pain with radiation to the left anterior chest. He reports difficulty in starting his urinary stream. Appropriate steps in this situation include:
   A. Tell the patient to use heat; prescribe an even stronger narcotic; encourage him to use stool softeners to avoid constipation since he may have this as well as urinary hesitancy due to narcotics.
   B. Refer the patient to see his urologist expeditiously.
   C. Obtain a CBC, ESR, and PSA.
   D. Obtain spine films and an MRI of the thoracic spine immediately.

10. A 68-year-old man has been diagnosed with pancreatic cancer. His wife reports he cannot sleep because of abdominal and back pain. He states his pain is mild, but he is visibly depressed and distressed. The best techniques for management are:
    A. Sustained-release morphine every 8-12 hours with oral immediate-release morphine as needed for breakthrough pain.
    B. Self-administration of meperidine (Demerol), 100 mg IM every three hours.
    C. Administer PRN oxycodone with acetaminophen.
    D. Prescribe ibuprofen, 800 mg orally every four hours.

11. A patient with known HIV infection develops a malignancy. Which of the following neoplasms are associated:
    A. Squamous anal cancer.
    B. Cervical cancer.
    C. High-grade non-Hodgkin's lymphoma.
    D. Kaposi's sarcoma.
    E. All of the above.

12. A 70-year-old woman with recently diagnosed metastatic breast cancer has generalized bone pain. She has widespread lytic bone metastases. Her original breast cancer was both estrogen- and progesterone-receptor-positive, but she has had no treatment since original surgery seven years ago. The best initial approach is:
    A. Endocrine manipulation; radiation to weight-bearing bones with large lytic lesions.
    B. Chemotherapy with cyclophosphamide and doxorubicin. Reserve radiation until pathologic fractures begin to develop.
    C. Radiation treatment to sites of most severe pain followed by radioactive strontium if her pain is not immediately relieved.
    D. Supportive care only.

13. A patient presents with sever hyponatremia and vomiting. Her serum sodium is 105 mEq/L; the blood urea nitrogen, 3 mg/ml; uric acid, 2.2 mg/ml. The most likely cause of a mediastinal mass in this setting is:
    A. Hodgkin's disease.
    B. Teratoma of the mediastinum.
    C. Small cell lung cancer.
    D. Mesothelioma.

14. Immediate and long-term management for the above patient includes:
    A. Correct serum sodium to 140 mEq/L in four hours.
    B. Correct serum sodium to 120 mEq/L in 10-15 hours with hypertonic saline and furosemide followed by fluid restriction and demeclocycline.
    C. Allow unrestricted fluid intake.
    D. Administer long-acting morphine sulfate.

15. In cancer of the colon, adjuvant chemotherapy using 5-flouracil and levamisole is beneficial in:
    A. Duke's A.
    B. Dukes B1
    C. Stage C
    D. Stage D

16. A 45-year-old man has carcinoma of the larynx (stage II). He is treated with laryngectomy. Three

years later, he develops a 2-cm module in the right upper lobe of his lung. The most likely etiology is:
A. Hamartoma
B. Metastasis of his laryngeal cancer
C. Granuloma
D. Primary lung cancer

17. Risk factors important in invasive cervical cancer include:
A. Early onset of sexual activity and multiple sex partners.
B. Smoking
C. HIV infection
D. Absence of prior screening in an elderly woman
E. All of the above.

## Answers

| | | | | |
|---|---|---|---|---|
| 1. B | 2. E | 3. C | 4. E | 5. D |
| 6. A | 7. C | 8. B | 9. D | 10. A |
| 11. E | 12. A | 13. C | 14. B | 15. C |
| 16. D | 17. E | | | |

## SUGGESTED READING

### *Books and Monographs*


Abeloff MD, Armitage JO, Lichter AS, et. al. Clinical Oncology. New York: Churchill Livingstone, 1995.

American Joint Committee on Cancer. Cancer Staging Manual. 5th ed. Philadelphia: JB Lippincott, 1997.

DeVita VT Jr, Hellman S, Rosenberg SA. Cancer: Principles and Practice of Oncology. 6th ed. Philadelphia: Lippincott-Williams & Wilkins, 2001.

Haskell CM, Berek JS. Cancer Treatment. 5th ed. Philadelphia: WB Saunders Co. 2001.

Holland JF, Frei E III, Bast RC, et.al. Cancer Medicine. 4th ed. Philadelphia: Lea & Febiger, 1997.

Lenhard RE Jr, Osteen RT, Gansler T. American Cancer Society's Clinical Oncology. Atlanta: The American Cancer Society, 2001.

US Preventive Services Task Force. Guide to Clinical Preventive Services. 2nd ed. Alexandria, VA: International Publishing, 1996.


### *Articles*


Jemal A, Thomas A, Murray T, Thun M. Cancer statistics, 2002. CA Cancer J Clin 2002; 52:23-47.

Levy MH. Pharmacologic treatment of cancer pain. N Engl J Med 1996; 335:1124-32.

Riparmonti C, Brucera E. Pain and symptom management in palliative care. Cancer Control 1996; 3:204-213.

Zech DF, Grond S, Lynch J, Hertel D, Lehmann KA. Validation of World Health Organization Guidelines for cancer pain relief: a 10-year prospective study. Pain 1995; 63:65-76.


### *Lymphomas and Plasma Cell Dyscrasias*


Aisenberg AC. Problems in Hodgkin's disease management. Blood 1999; 93:761-79.

Bataille R, Harousseau JL. Medical progress: multiple myeloma. N Engl J Med 1997; 336:1657-1664.

DeVita VT Jr. Canellos GP. The lymphomas. Sem Hematol 1999; 36:84-94.

Harris NL, Jaffe ES, Diebold J, Flandrin G, Muller-Hermelink HK, Vardiman J, et. al. World Health Organization classification of neoplastic diseases of the hematopoietic and lymphoid tissue: report of the Clinical Advisory Committee meeting—Arlie House, Virginia. J Clin Oncol 1997;17: 3835-49.

Hauke RJ. Armitage JO. Treatment of non-Hodgkin lymphoma. Curr Opin Oncol 2000;:412-8.

Josting A, Wolf J, Diehl V. Hodgkin disease: prognostic factors and treatment strategies. Curr Opin Oncol 2000; 12:403-11

Kyle RA. Mononclonal gammopathy of undetermined significance and solitary plasmacytoma. Implications for progression to overt multiple myeloma. Hematol Oncol Clin North Am 1997; 11:71-87.

Urba WJ, Longo DH. Hodgkin's disease. N Engl J Med 1992; 236:678-687.


### *Breast Cancer*


Burstein HJ. Winer EP. Primary care for survivors of breast cancer. N Engl J Med 2000; 343:1086-94.

Donegan WL. Evaluation of a palpable breast mass. N Engl J Med 1992; 327:937-942.

Goldhirsch A, Gelber RD. Endocrine therapies for breast cancer. Semin Oncol 1996; 23:494-505.

Hortobagyi GN. Treatment of breast cancer. N Engl J Med 1998; 339:974-84.

Kerlikowske K, Grady D, Rubin SM, Sandrock C, Ernster VL. Efficacy of screening mammography. A meta-analysis. JAMA 1995; 273:149-54.

Osborne CK. Tamoxifen in the treatment of breast cancer. N Engl J Med 1998; 339:1609-18.

Polychemotherapy for early breast cancer: an overview of the randomized trials. Early Breast Cancer Trialist's Collaborative Group. Lancet 1998; 352:930-42.

Sainsbury JR. Anderson TJ. Morgan DA. ABC of breast diseases: breast cancer. BMJ 2000;321:745-50.


### *Lung Cancer*


Chute JP, Chen T, Feigal E, Simon R, Johnson BE. Twenty years of phase III trials for patients with extensive-stage small-cell lung cancer: perceptible progress. J Clin Oncol. 1999; 17:1794-801.

Kunsel PR. Diagnostic tests for lung cancer. Mayo Clin Proc 1993; 68:288-296.

Mountain CF. Revisions in the international system for staging lung cancer. Chest 1997; 111:1710-7.

Patel AM, Peters SG. Clinical manifestations of lung cancer. Mayo Clin Proc 1993; 68:273-277.

Patz EF Jr., Goodman PC, Bepler G. Screening for lung cancer. N Engl J Med 2000; 343:1627-33.


### *Gastrointestinal Cancers*


Janne PA, Mayer RJ. Chemoprevention of colorectal cancer. N Engl J Med 2000; 342:1960-1968.

Winawer SJ, Fletcher RH, Miller L, Godlee F, Stolar MH, Mulrow CD, et.al. Colorectal cancer screening: clinical guidelines and rationale. Gastroenterology 1997; 112: 594-642.


### *Genitourinary Cancer*


Bosl GJ, Motzer RJ. Testicular germ-cell cancer. N Engl J Med 1997; 337:242-53.

Coley CM, Barry MJ, Fleming C, et.al. Clinical guidelines, part I. Early detection of prostate cancer: prior problility and effectiveness of tests. Ann Intern Med 1997;126:394-406.

Figlin RA, Belldegrun A. Renal cell carcinoma. Semin Oncol 1995; 22:1-91.

Frydenberg M, Stricker PD, Kaye KW. Prostate cancer diagnosis and management. Lancet 1997; 349:1681-1687.

Gurpeide DP. Endometrial cancer: biochemical and clinical correlates. JNCI 1991; 83:405-416.

Metts MC. Metts JC. Milito SJ. Thomas CR Jr. Bladder cancer: a review of diagnosis and management. J Natl Med Assoc 2000; 92:285-94.

Partridge EE. Barnes MN. Epithelial ovarian cancer: prevention, diagnosis, and treatment. CA Cancer J Clin 1999; 49:297-320.

### *Cancer of the Head and Neck*

Lang PG Jr. Malignant melanoma. Med Clin North Am 1998; 82:1325-58.

Papadimitrakopoulou VA. Carcinogenesis of head and neck cancer and the role of chemoprevention in its reversal. Curr Opin Oncol 2000; 12:240-5.

Vokes EE. Head and neck cancer. Semin Oncol 1994;21: 279-399.

### *Cancer of Unknown Primary Site*

Abbruzzese JL, Abruzzese MC, Lenzi R, Hess KR, Raber MN. Analysis of a diagnostic strategy for patients with suspected tumors of unknown origin. J Clin Oncol 1995; 13: 2094-103.

Greco FA. Burris HA 3rd. Erland JB. Gray JR. Kalman LA. Schreeder MT. Hainsworth JD. Carcinoma of unknown primary site. Cancer 2000; 89:2655-60, 2000

Hainsworth JD, Greco FA. Drug therapy: treatment of patients with cancer of an unknown primary site. Semin Oncol 1993;20:205-294.

### *Paraneoplastic Syndromes and Oncologic Emergencies*

American Society of Clinical Oncology Update of recommendations for the use of hematopoietic colony stimulating factors: evidence-based clinical practice guidelines. J Clin Oncol. 1996; 14:1957-61

Cascino TL. Medical complications of systemic cancer. Med Clin North Am 1993;77:265

Dalmau JO. Posner JB. Paraneoplastic syndromes. Arch Neurol 1999; 56:405-8.

Demetri GD, Kris M, Wade J, Degos L, Cella D. Quality-of-life benefit in chemotherapy patients treated with epoetin alfa is independent of disease response or tumor type: results from a prospective community oncology study. Procrit Study Group. J Clin Oncol. 1998;16:3412-25.

Paraneoplastic syndromes associated with lung cancer. Mayo Clin Proc 1993;68:278-287.

Pizzo PA. Fever in immunocompromised patients. N Engl J Med 1999; 341:893-900.

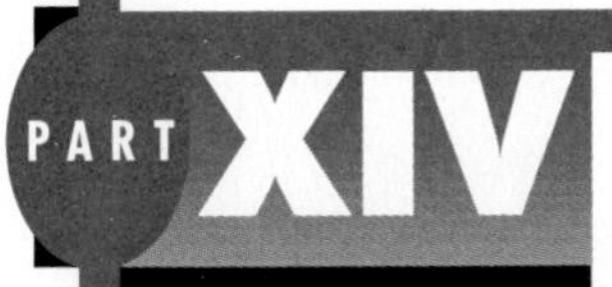

PART XIV

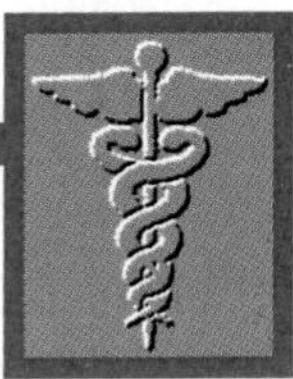

Ralph M. Schapira
Kesavan Kutty
Basil Varkey

# PULMONARY DISEASES

# CHAPTER 215 CLINICAL EVALUATION OF LUNG DISEASE

The prime function of the lungs is respiration, effecting oxygenation of blood and removal of carbon dioxide. Despite the recent advancement in diagnostic procedures (e.g., fiberoptic bronchoscopy, pleuroscopy and thoracoscopic surgery), the initial diagnostic approach for a patient with lung disease remains traditional: history, physical examination, the roentgenogram, and differential diagnosis, in that order.

## Presenting Complaints

### Cough

Cough, a very common symptom, generally implies airway disease. Its onset (acute or chronic) and the presence or absence of sputum should be noted. Associated fever suggests an infection. An acute cough of a few days is commonly caused by acute bronchitis. A cough lasting longer than 4 weeks is **chronic persistent cough** (Table 215.1). Rhinosinusitis with postnasal drip, asthma, and gastroesophageal reflux causes most instances of chronic persistent cough in nonsmokers; chronic bronchitis is the most common cause among smokers. Other causes in nonsmokers and smokers are left ventricular failure, interstitial lung disease, and viral infection (postviral cough). Combinations are not uncommon (e.g., postnasal drip in an asthmatic). While sinusitis and gastroesophgeal reflux can also cause a persistent cough in smokers, lung cancer should be excluded in this group.

**TABLE 215.1. Common Causes of Chronic Persistent Cough: Features, Diagnosis, and Therapy**

| Causes | | | |
|---|---|---|---|
| **Rhinosinusitis with Postnasal Drip** | **Asthma** | **GE Reflux** | **Chronic Bronchitis** |
| **Features** | | | |
| • "Tickle" in the throat<br>• Frequent throat clearing<br>• Nasal twang to voice<br>• Nasal discharge (±purulence), nasal stuffiness or sneezing<br>• Relation to supine posture<br>• Recent viral infection with sinusitis | • Cough may be the only symptom<br>• Cough may be productive<br>• Wheezing<br>• Relationship to cold air, exercise, or ingestion of cold liquids or ice cream<br>• Other atopic symptoms<br>• Relationship to supine posture<br>• Dyspnea on exertion<br>• Nocturnal periodicity | • Hoarseness<br>• Heartburn<br>• Chest pain<br>• Relation to supine posture<br>• Nocturnal periodicity | • Productive cough<br>• Smoking history<br>• Symptom diminishes or disappears after smoking cessation<br>• Wheezing<br>• Hemoptysis |
| **Diagnosis** | | | |
| Based on history and findings as above. | If spirometry is normal, perform methacholine bronchoprovocation test, which has a 100% sensitivity for asthma presenting as cough. | Causes 15–20% of chronic cough. Suspect if a basic evaluation reveals no cause. Ambulatory pH monitoring quite useful in diagnosis. | Essentially a clinical diagnosis. Pulmonary function tests commonly show airflow obstruction. High risk for lung cancer, which should be appropriately excluded. |
| **Therapy** | | | |
| Empiric therapy with antihistamines, decongestants. Others include intranasal corticosteroids; antibiotics for infection. | Inhaled corticosteroids and β2 agents (as needed). | H2-blocking agents. Proton pump inhibitors | Smoking cessation. |

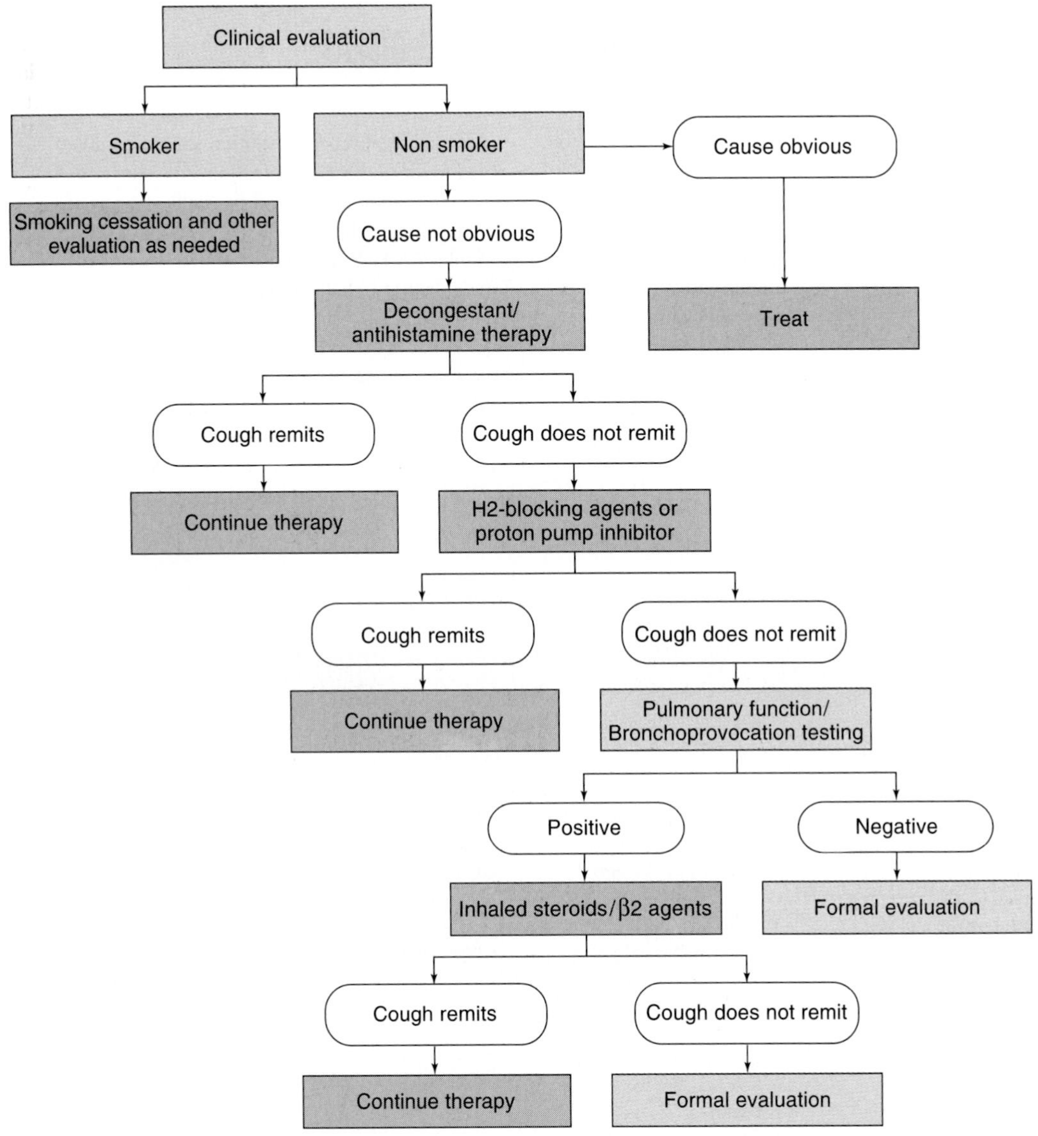


**FIGURE 215.1.** Approach to the nonsmoking patient with chronic persistent cough.

*Management of chronic cough*

A careful history and physical examination are key to an accurate diagnosis (see Table 215.1). Pulmonary function tests and a methacholine bronchoprovocation study may also be necessary. Chest x-ray is generally not useful unless considerations include heart failure (history of heart disease, edema, dyspnea, orthopnea, paroxysmal nocturnal dyspnea), interstitial lung disease (dry cough, dyspnea, finger clubbing, "Velcro" rales), or bronchogenic carcinoma (hemoptysis, weight loss, chest pain). Once a definite cause is obvious, treatment should follow (see Table 215.1). Among nonsmokers, a **stepwise management** is advocated (Figure 215.1), in which further treatment is recommended if the patient does not respond to the initial treatment and compliance by the patient is not in question. Cough may be due to multiple causes in the same patient, requiring multiple agents simultaneously. Medications (angiotensin-converting enzyme inhibitors and/or β-blocking agents) may need to be withdrawn if it appears that they are causing the cough. Generally, **fiberoptic bronchoscopy** is not very useful in the nonsmoker unless the chest x-ray (if taken) is abnormal or a foreign body is suspected. In most smokers, the cough disappears after smoking cessation; if it does not, other causes must be pursued. If the patient does not stop smoking, some evaluation (at a minimum, a chest x-ray) is necessary, depending on the likelihood of lung cancer.

### Sputum production

Sputum is mucus produced by mucin-secreting bronchial glands and cleared by the airway cilia. Expectoration of sputum is abnormal. Cough and sputum are integral features of **chronic bronchitis. Yellow sputum** is most commonly from bacterial bronchitis, stasis in the tracheobronchial tree, or asthma exacerbation when eosinophil-laden. **Abundant mucopurulent sputum** signifies bronchiectasis; **foul-smelling sputum** signifies anaerobic lung infection such as a necrotizing pneumonia or lung abscess.

### Dyspnea

Dyspnea is awareness of one's breathing. In clinical terms, **it means shortness of breath.** Dyspnea at rest is always abnormal, but during exercise it is contextual. If the patient previously tolerated similar levels of exertion well, then the dyspnea is significant. **Acute dyspnea** may be from acute airway obstruction, acute pulmonary edema, pneumothorax, or pulmonary embolism. Postoperative dyspnea is commonly from pulmonary embolism, massive atelectasis, or acute pulmonary edema from fluid overload. Associated cough, sputum production, or hemoptysis are useful clues in assessing **chronic dyspnea.** Orthopnea or paroxysmal nocturnal dyspnea suggests heart failure. With a normal chest x-ray, the causes are pulmonary embolism, interstitial lung disease, airway obstruction, chest wall or neuromuscular disorders, or anxiety. Abnormal chest x-rays accompany dyspnea due to heart failure, interstitial lung disease, large pleural effusion, or advanced emphysema. Worsening of pre-existent dyspnea in a smoker, whatever the chest x-ray results, should always alert the physician to possible bronchogenic carcinoma. In evaluating chronic dyspnea, an occupational history is also very important.

### Chest pain

Chest pain has varying patterns, among them angina (see chapter 30); pleural, muscular, and costochondral pain; and intercostal neuralgia. Pleuritic pain worsens upon inspiration, cough, or even movement of the chest wall. Commonly encountered in emergency departments, it is caused by pulmonary embolism in about one-fourth of the cases; other causes are pneumonia, or viral pleuritis.

Muscular pain is superficial and may follow strenuous movements of the chest wall muscles or trauma-induced muscle bruising. There may be rib fractures as well. Costochondral pain is typically along the costochondral articulations. **Tietze's syndrome** affects the upper costochondral joints. **Intercostal neuralgia** is a pain shooting from the back forward and characteristically worsened by movement but not generally by respiration. It is a pre-eruptive symptom of herpes zoster and occasionally persists after the eruptions have resolved.

### Hemoptysis

Hemoptysis—expectoration of frank blood—may signify a serious underlying disease (Table 215.2). (Patients with acute respiratory infections, acute bronchitis, or bacterial pneumonia may have minor hemoptysis—blood-streaked sputum, which is of lesser significance). The first step—distinguishing hemoptysis from hematemesis (vomiting of blood)—is generally easy with a history. The historical data that should be collected in hemoptysis, and their implications, are shown in Table 215.3. Clinical assessment includes examination of the ears, nose, and throat (epistaxis, lesions of Wegener's granulomatosis). Telangiectasia of

**TABLE 215.2. Common Causes of Hemoptysis**

| General Category | Specific Diseases/Causes |
|---|---|
| Infectious/inflammatory | Chronic bronchitis[a]<br>Mycobacterial diseases (tuberculosis and others)[b]<br>Bronchiectasis[a,b]<br>Lung abscess[b]<br>Blastomycosis |
| Cardiovascular diseases | Pulmonary thromboembolism<br>Mitral stenosis[a,b] |
| Neoplasms | Pulmonary<br>Primary: bronchogenic carcinoma,[b] bronchial carcinoid[a]<br>Metastatic<br>Extrapulmonary<br>Laryngeal carcinoma<br>Nasopharyngeal carcinoma |
| Autoimmune | Pulmonary hemorrhage syndromes<br>Wegener's granulomatosis<br>Lupus pneumonitis |
| Miscellaneous | Inhaled foreign body<br>Bleeding dyscrasias/anticoagulant ingestion[b]<br>Expectoration of aspirated blood (from vomiting/epistaxis) |

[a]May cause recurrent episodes.
[b]May cause massive hemoptysis.

**TABLE 215.3. Hemoptysis: Clinical Implications of Historical Data**

| Data | Implication |
|---|---|
| Amount | Massive hemoptysis can be lethal by asphyxiation. |
| Prior cough and sputum | Chronic bronchitis. |
| Prior episodes | Episodes of blood-streaked sputum common in chronic bronchitis. |
| Provocating factors | Repetitive, severe cough can cause hemoptysis, but is a diagnosis of exclusion. |
| Associated symptoms | |
| Chest pain | Complicates pulmonary embolism, tuberculosis. |
| Fever | Suggestive of infectious, inflammatory, or neoplastic process. |
| Weight loss | Suggestive of neoplasm or tuberculosis. |
| Leg pain/swelling | Suggestive of venous thromboembolism/heart failure. |
| Loss of consciousness | May have predisposed to a lung abscess. |
| History of smoking | Bronchogenic carcinoma; chronic bronchitis. |
| Prior recurrent pneumonia | Endobronchial obstruction or residual bronchiectasis. |

the lips may suggest a pulmonary arteriovenous fistula. Stridor, wheezing, clubbing (intrathoracic neoplasm or bronchiectasis), and mediastinal or tracheal shift indicating atelectasis are important findings that offer clues to a cause for hemoptysis.

Helpful laboratory studies include a complete blood count, platelet count, coagulation studies, oximetry or arterial blood gases, and sputum examination for cytology and fungi. A chest x-ray is pivotal. With a normal chest x-ray, likely causes include pulmonary embolism, acute exacerbation of chronic bronchitis, and bronchiectasis. If the x-ray suggests tuberculosis, the sputum should be examined for mycobacteria. Otherwise, a fiberoptic bronchoscopic examination is undertaken promptly to establish a site and cause of bleeding. Massive hemoptysis, defined as 600 ml of blood within 24 hours (prorated for smaller intervals of time), carries a 75% mortality. Rigid bronchoscopy under general anesthesia allows better control of the airway and suctioning of blood than does fiberoptic bronchoscopy and is the first step. Bronchial arteriography and embolization or surgical resection are options to control massive hemoptysis.

### Wheezing

Wheezing may be a symptom or physical finding; it is characterized by a high-pitched, whistling or squeaking continuous sound produced by the passage of air across a narrowed airway. Upper airway obstruction below the thoracic inlet causes wheezing rather than stridor, which is caused by airflow obstruction of extra-thoracic origin, such as laryngeal edema. Diffuse wheezing with a uniform pitch and intensity in both lungs suggests central obstruction; focal wheezing suggests localized bronchial obstruction. Since wheezing is a non-specific physical finding, the integration of clinical history, physical findings, and laboratory studies is essential. Asthma may occasionally appear for the first time after the age of 60, but unprecedented wheezing in someone of this age group more typically signifies left heart failure ("cardiac asthma"). Other causes of wheezing are listed in Table 215.4. Wheezing may be accompanied by an increase in the forced expiratory time (FET; the time from maximal inspiration to complete expiration), a bedside screening test for airways obstruction. A FET of ≥6 sec will correctly diagnose the greatest number of subjects with obstructive airways disease. Physical findings commonly found in pulmonary disorders are listed in Table 215.5.

## Bedside Clinical Assessment

The physical examination is crucial to assess lung disease. Besides a succinct history of present illness, a detailed history of all illnesses, particularly respiratory illnesses, should be obtained. It is important to inquire about past chest roentgenograms and their availability for review. All current and past use of drugs (legal and illicit), alcohol, and tobacco (expressed in "pack-years") should

**TABLE 215.4. Causes of Wheezing**

| Category | Specific Diseases/Causes |
|---|---|
| Upper airway obstruction (below the thoracic inlet) | Angioedema<br>Epiglottitis<br>Foreign body<br>Goiter<br>Tumor<br>Vocal cord paralysis |
| Lower airway obstruction | Asthma<br>Bronchiolitis<br>Left heart failure<br>Chronic obstructive pulmonary disease<br>Cystic fibrosis<br>Foreign body<br>Tumor<br>Tenacious secretions |
| Extrapulmonary disorders | Carcinoid syndrome |

TABLE 215.5. Typical Physical Findings in the Chest in Common Pulmonary Disorders

| Disorder | Mediastinal Shift | Percussion | Breath Sounds | Adventitious Sounds | Vocal Resonance | Other |
|---|---|---|---|---|---|---|
| Atelectasis | Present, toward side of lesion | Impaired over affected area | Reduced or absent | None | Reduced or absent | Diminished chest wall movement over affected side |
| Consolidation | None | Impaired over affected area | Bronchial | Mid to late inspiratory rales[a] | E to A changes, whispering pectoriloquy | Splinting from pain may reduce ipsilateral chest wall movement |
| Cavitation | May or may not occur, but if present, to side of lesion if there is fibrosis | Impaired | Bronchial | Rales | Increased<br>E to A changes | |
| Asthma | None | Normal | Normal with prolonged FET* | Wheeze, mostly expiratory | Normal | Accessory muscle use and pulsus paradoxus may be present |
| Emphysema | None | Increased | Reduced with prolonged FET* | Rhonchi ± | Reduced | Pursed-lip breathing; pink and cherubic |
| Chronic bronchitis | None | Normal | Normal with prolonged FET* | Expiratory rhonchi, rales throughout inspiration | Normal | Cyanosis ±, often obese |
| Pleural effusion | Present, to opposite side | Dull | Reduced or absent over the effusion | None | Reduced or absent | — |
| Pneumothorax | Present, to opposite side | Normal to hyperresonant | Normal to reduced | None | Reduced | Affected side may move less |

[a]Râles (crackles) are best classified according to their timing. Rales occurring in early and mid-inspiration suggest airway disease. Those in late inspiration are mostly representative of alveolar disease.
*FET is the forced expiratory time. See text and Schapira et. al JAMA 1993;270:731–736.

be reviewed. The patient's hobbies and the presence of household pets should also be recorded. Travel history is important, especially in endemic mycoses and some viral illnesses. One should ascertain all the jobs held, from the first one to the most recent. It is well known that some occupations may cause lung disease, but the long interval between exposure and manifest disease is not so readily appreciated.

# CHAPTER 216 BASIC LABORATORY TESTS

## Skin Tests

**Tuberculin skin testing** is used to diagnose latent tuberculosis infection, and is done using an intradermal injection of 0.1 ml (5 tuberculin units [TU]) of Tween-stabilized purified protein derivative (PPD). Skin testing is a key component of public health programs to identify individuals with latent tuberculosis infection and to identify (and potentially treat) such individuals who are at risk to progress to active tuberculosis. Tests for skin reactivity are also given (controls to identify anergy), using agents such as mumps and *Trichophyton* antigens. The extent of induration following tuberculin skin testing is carefully noted after 48–72 hours. Three cut-points (5 mm, 10 mm, and 15 mm of induration) have been defined to interpret skin test results based on the risk of the individual tested to develop active tuberculosis. Previous vaccination with BCG (bacille Calmette-Guérin; used in some countries to prevent tuberculosis infection) can be used to support the diagnosis of tuberculosis infection in patients so vaccinated. A positive reaction to tuberculin in a BCG-vaccinated person may indicate infection when the tested person is at increased risk for infection or has medical conditions that increase the risk of disease. Recommendations for the treatment of latent tuberculosis infection (formerly termed "chemoprophylaxis" or "preventative therapy") are based on age and the skin test interpretation. Revised criteria for tuberculin skin test interpretation are shown in Table 216.1; also see chapter 225 and Tables 225.1 and 225.3 (Tuberculosis).

## Sputum Examination

The sputum should be collected in a clean, sterile container. If the patient does not expectorate, induction may be needed. Gross characteristics such as viscidity, color, odor, and the presence of blood should be noted. Reliable results depend on prompt delivery of the specimen to the laboratory. A reliable sputum specimen will reveal several alveolar macrophages (round, large cells with granular inclusions and an oval, eccentric nucleus). Abundant squamous cells (large, flat cells, with a central nucleus) signify contamination with oral/pharyngeal secretions, making the sample unreliable. Many neutrophils (≥.25 at 10x power) signify infection, most often bacterial. More than 20% eosinophils means atopic disease.

### Staining procedures

Bacteriology is evaluated by a Gram stain. Acid-fast (Ziehl-Nielsen) staining is done for *Mycobacterium tuberculosis,* and pretreatment with 10% potassium hydroxide for visualizing fungi. Gram-positive cocci may be pneumococci (pairs or chains) or staphylococci (groups). Gram-negative bacilli may be *Haemophilus influenzae* (small, pleomorphic) or *Klebsiella pneumoniae* (large, often encapsulated). These results should be integrated with the clinical history and culture results; in the setting of a pulmonary infection, they provide a guideline for initial antibiotic therapy.

While a reliable microbiologic diagnosis of a pulmonary infection helps in determining effective treatment, routine sputum microbiologic tests are probably of

**TABLE 216.1. Tuberculin Skin Test: Interpretation of Skin Test Reactions**

| Tuberculin Test is Considered Positive with an Induration of: | Affected Population |
|---|---|
| ≥5 mm | • In recent contacts<br>• When fibrotic lesions in chest x-ray suggest old healed tuberculosis<br>• With co-existent HIV infection |
| ≥10 mm | • In medically underserved, economically disadvantaged minorities<br>• In those with<br>– other medical risks for tuberculosis<br>– residence in endemic areas or long-term care facility<br>– IV drug abuse<br>• All others with increased prevalence of tuberculosis |
| ≥15 mm | • All others |

See Diagnostic Standards and Classification of Tuberculosis in Adults and Children. Am J Respir Crit Care Med 161:1376–1395, 2000. Also see related Table 225.3.

limited use in community-acquired pneumonias (especially in an otherwise healthy, immunocompetent adult); also, the availability of broad-spectrum antibiotics that are effective against the majority of pathogens causing community-acquired pneumonias might preclude the need for a microbiologic diagnosis prior to therapy. However, in the hospitalized or immunocompromised adult, sputum should be examined if available, and if not, after induction. Cultures for fungi and mycobacteria are also useful.

**Cytologic examination**

The results of cytologic examination vary, depending on the number of sputum samples submitted and the proficiency of the cytopathologist. In bronchogenic carcinoma, sputum cytology has a high (69–80%) sensitivity, with a specificity of nearly 96%, particularly for centrally located lesions in the proximal airways.

## Arterial Blood Gas Analysis

Arterial blood gas analysis provides significant information about the gas-exchanging function of the lung. A sample of arterial blood is obtained in a heparinized syringe from the brachial or the radial artery. The syringe with the sample should be placed in ice immediately and the sample analyzed for the pH and the tensions of oxygen ($PaO_2$) and carbon dioxide ($PaCO_2$). The following stepwise approach is recommended for interpreting the data:

**Step 1.** Estimate the partial pressure of inhaled oxygen ($PIO_2$).

*Principle:* Atmospheric air, with water vapor removed, is essentially a mixture of oxygen ($O_2$) and nitrogen ($N_2$) in a ratio of 0.21 : 0.79. Their combined partial pressures make up the total pressure of the mixture—namely, barometric pressure ($P_B$)—with their individual partial pressures in this mixture bearing the same ratio (Dalton's law). At sea level, $P_B$ is 760 mm Hg and water vapor pressure ($PH_2O$) at body temperature is 47 mm Hg and the $FIO_2$ is 0.21.

*Formula:*

$$PIO_2 = (P_B - PH_2O) \times 0.21$$
$$= (760 - 47) \times 0.21$$
$$= 149.7 \text{ mm Hg}$$

Note: If the person is breathing supplemental oxygen, the appropriate $FIO_2$ should be substituted for 0.21.

**Step 2.** Estimate the alveolar oxygen tension ($PAO_2$).

*Principle:* The ratio of gases is altered in the alveoli because of the entry of $CO_2$ from the pulmonary capillaries. The rate at which $O_2$ is exchanged for $CO_2$ is determined by the respiratory exchange ratio, or R, which is usually 0.8. For purposes of calculation, the alveolar $PCO_2$ ($PACO_2$) is assumed to be equal to arterial $CO_2$ ($PaCO_2$).

*Formula:*

$$PAO2 = PIO_2 - (PACO_2/R)$$
$$\text{But } PACO_2 = PaCO_2$$

Therefore,

$$PAO_2 = PIO_2 - (PaCO_2 / 0.8)$$

or

$$PAO_2 = PIO_2 - (PaCO_2 \times 1.25)$$
$$\text{At sea level, with } PaCO_2 \text{ of 40 mm Hg,}$$
$$PAO_2 = 149.7 - (40 \times 1.25)$$
$$= 99.7 \text{ mm Hg}$$

**Step 3.** Estimate the alveolar-arterial (A-a) oxygen gradient.

*Principle:* The normally small difference between the $PAO_2$ and the $PaO_2$ is called the A-a gradient for oxygen, or $P(A\text{-}a)O_2$. It is age-dependent, rising from 10 mm Hg in a young adult to around 27–30 mm Hg in a nonagenarian. An abnormally widened age-adjusted gradient indicates lung disease.

*Formula:*

$$P(A\text{-}a)O_2 = PAO_2 - PaO_2$$

**Step 4.** Define the adequacy of ventilation.

*Principle:* $PaCO_2$, which maintains an inverse relationship to alveolar ventilation, is the sole harbinger of the adequacy of ventilation. A low value indicates hyperventilation and a high value reflects hypoventilation.

**Step 5.** Assess the hypoxemia.

*Principle:* Hypoxemia ($PaO_2$ below that predicted for the patient based on age) may be due to several mechanisms, the most common being a *mismatching of ventilation-perfusion (V/Q) relationships (also known as V/Q mismatch).* Hypoxemia due to V/Q mismatch readily improves with supplemental oxygen administration or induced hyperventilation. Another mechanism is *hypoventilation*, since $PaO_2$ and $PaCO_2$ maintain a reciprocal relationship. The sum of [$PaO_2$ + ($PACO_2 \times 1.25$) + the applicable gradient for age] approximates the calculated $PIO_2$ when hypoxemia is due to pure alveolar hypoventilation. A *shunt* (anatomic, as in a right-to-left intracardiac shunt) or *shunt effect* (as in various intrapulmonary processes, such as widespread atelectasis or adult respiratory distress syndrome) also causes hypoxemia, where the $PaO_2$ responds minimally to supplemental oxygen. *Diffusion defects*, by precluding equilibration of alveolar gas with the pulmonary end-capillary blood, can sometimes contribute, albeit trivially, to hypoxemia, although this mechanism is not usually of clinical importance. The final cause of hypoxemia is high altitude, such as occurs during mountain climbing or commercial aviation flights (airplane cabins are not pressurized to sea level).

**Step 6.** Estimate the arterial oxygen content.

*Principle:* Oxygen is transported in hemoglobin-bound and dissolved forms. Oxygen saturation ($SaO_2$), which represents the saturation of hemoglobin, may be determined by direct measurement as part of a blood gas analysis, or estimated from the oxyhemoglobin dissociation curves. Each gram of hemoglobin, upon full (100%) saturation, carries 1.34 ml of oxygen. Oxygen also dissolves in the plasma at a rate of 0.003 ml for every mm Hg of $PaO_2$.

*Formula:*

$$\text{Hb-bound oxygen} = 1.34 \times \text{Gm of Hb} \times SaO_2\%$$
$$\text{Dissolved oxygen} = 0.003 \times PaO_2$$

The sum of the above (Hb-bound oxygen + dissolved oxygen) represents the total oxygen transported by every 100 ml of arterial blood. Many blood gas laboratories automatically provide this information in the blood gas report.

**Step 7.** Assess the pH and acid-base status.

*Principle:* Normal pH varies from 7.35 to 7.45. A pH above 7.45 indicates **alkalosis,** and a pH below 7.35 indicates **acidosis.** (The range of acid-base disturbances is shown in Table 186.1.) Compensatory mechanisms that follow a primary disturbance bring the pH toward but not completely back to normal. The extent and effectiveness of such compensation varies with the primary disorder. Because renal $HCO_3$ retention takes several days, acute respiratory acidosis is least well compensated. Thus, the most effective therapy for acute respiratory acidosis is to increase alveolar ventilation, often through positive-pressure mechanical ventilation, if indicated.

# CHAPTER 217 IMAGING IN PULMONARY DIAGNOSIS

## Conventional and Special Studies

For most practical purposes, a posteroanterior (PA) chest x-ray is adequate. But unless supplemented by a lateral view, processes in the retrosternal and retrocardiac areas as well as a very small pleural effusion in the posterior costophrenic sulcus may be missed. Additional examinations may be dictated by circumstances (e.g., rib films in suspected rib fractures).

A small pleural effusion is most commonly manifested by a blunted costophrenic angle. An effusion that does not layer in the decubitus view is loculated. Loculations often portend an underlying infection in the pleural fluid. Ultrasongraphy can further define pleural processes (below). A comparison of **inspiration and end-expiration films** is most valuable for detecting a small pneumothorax. A **barium esophagogram** may also be helpful in investigating unexplained, recurrent lower lobe pneumonia that may be secondary to a Zenker's diverticulum esophageal stricture or achalasia. **Pulmonary arteriography** remains the criterion standard for the diagnosis of pulmonary embolism (chapter 233). It is also useful in diagnosing vascular anomalies such as pulmonary arteriovenous fistulae.

## Computed Tomography and Positron Emission Tomography

With computed tomography (CT), one can obtain an image of a transverse slice of the body. An x-ray beam, as it passes through organs of varying tissue density, gets variably attenuated. Computer analysis of such attenuations generates images of various organs, yielding valuable information about the density of a particular organ or tissue—for example, solid, cystic, and metallic (calcification). Using contrast media, vascular structures (arteries) can be distinguished from nonvascular ones (airways and lung parenchyma).

Chest CT overcomes the blind spots of the conventional radiographs and is, therefore, invaluable in evaluating mediastinal structures, lung masses, and pleural-based densities. It is essential in the preoperative staging of bronchogenic carcinoma. The technique of **spiral (helical) CT** in the diagnosis of pulmonary embolism has not been fully evaluated and its sensitivity varies from 53% to 100% in various studies (chapter 233). **Positron emission tomography (PET)** is a metabolic imaging technique that uses radioactive glucose as a tracer. Pulmonary tumors and other malignant cells actively metabolize this tracer. PET improves the detection of local and distant metastases in patients with lung cancer compared to CT and helps differentiate benign from malignant solitary pulmonary nodules.

## Magnetic Resonance Imaging

While very effective in detecting soft tissue contrast and visualizing in multiple planes, magnetic resonance imaging (MRI) requires no conventional contrast media and has no ionizing radiation. Its disadvantages are its high cost, lack of general availability, the hazard to individuals with various prosthetic devices, and the problems caused by air-containing lungs and their physiologic motion. MRI can diagnose central pulmonary emboli and venous thrombosis of the upper and lower extremities (chapter 233). While it can image hilar and mediastinal areas very well (e.g., evaluating mediastinal or neurovascular invasion by a neoplasm), it is unable to distinguish between reactive lymphadenopathy and malignant infiltration of lymph nodes. Its ability to image in multiple—especially coronal and sagittal—planes makes it an important tool in the management of **superior sulcus tumor.** Overall, technical shortcomings limit the role of MRI of the chest to one that is generally complementary to chest CT.

### Radionuclide Scans and Ultrasonography

**Perfusion, ventilation,** and **gallium scanning** are three categories of commonly performed radionuclide scans of the lung. Perfusion scans assess the vasculature of the lung. Intravenously administered $Tc^{99}$-labeled albumin microspheres enter the lung and become trapped in pulmonary capillaries. External imaging of the radioactivity of these trapped particles can assess the perfusion in each area. Areas devoid of perfusion are free of radioactivity. In pulmonary embolism, these defects usually have a lobar or segmental pattern. Ventilation scanning, performed by using a radioactive tracer gas (usually $133^{Xe}$), helps detect abnormal ventilation patterns such as air trapping. The gas is inhaled and equilibrated within the lung; during exhalation the washout is detected by imaging. In normally ventilated areas, the radioactivity clears in approximately 3 minutes. Gallium ($67^{Ga}$) has an affinity for leukocytes and when given parenterally it accumulates in inflammatory foci and tumor tissue. It is quite useful in detecting opportunistic infections in immunosuppressed patients and potentially useful in detecting other types of inflammatory lung or pleural disease.

Ultrasonography of the pleural space is used to detect pleural fluid and guide thoracentesis of small or loculated pleural effusions. It can also differentiate pleural fluid from pleural masses or thickening.

# CHAPTER 218 ANATOMY, PHYSIOLOGY, AND PULMONARY FUNCTION TESTING

## Segmental Anatomy

The lungs consist of two general components: **conducting airways** and the **terminal respiratory units.** Conducting airways (trachea, bronchi, and nonrespiratory bronchioles) transport air. Respiratory units (respiratory bronchioles, alveolar ducts, and alveoli) accomplish gas exchange. The trachea divides into right and left main bronchi at the carina. Because this angle of bifurcation is less acute on the right, gravitational (aspiration) processes occur more commonly in the right lung. Each lung has several bronchopulmonary segments, and each segment is supplied by a segmental bronchus and its corresponding segmental branch of the pulmonary artery. The right lung has 10 segments: three (apical, posterior, and anterior) in the right upper lobe, two (lateral and medial) in the middle lobe, and five (superior, medial basal, anterior basal, lateral basal, and posterior basal) in the right lower lobe. The left lung has 8 segments. The upper division bronchus of the left upper lobe has two segments, the apical-posterior and anterior. The lower division bronchus has two segments—namely, superior lingular and inferior lingular. The lower lobe has four segments: superior, anteromedial basal, lateral basal, and posterior basal (Figure 218.1).

Bronchopulmonary segmental anatomy is clinically relevant since certain disease processes tend to affect certain segments—for example, tuberculosis in apical and posterior segments of the upper lobes and gravitational pneumonia and lung abscess in posterior segments of the upper lobes and superior segments of the lower lobes.

## Physiology

**Ventilation** is the intake and distribution of air from the external environment to the alveolus and its return to the exterior. The process of gas exchange in the alveolus is **diffusion,** which involves the passive movement of gases based on concentration gradients. Gas exchange is facilitated by the maintenance of a constant blood flow—**perfusion**—through the pulmonary parenchyma. Optimal performance of the system requires careful matching of the body's metabolic needs with pulmonary ventilation and perfusion.

### Ventilation

Tissue oxygen demands increase substantially during exercise, febrile states, and other metabolic stresses. Impulses from the peripheral and central chemoreceptors as well as from the receptors in the lung are received in the medulla, where the information is assimilated and appropriate changes in ventilation initiated. These receptors are stimulated in pneumonia, asthma, various neurologic disorders, and following the ingestion of drugs (e.g., aspirin). Depression of these receptors leads

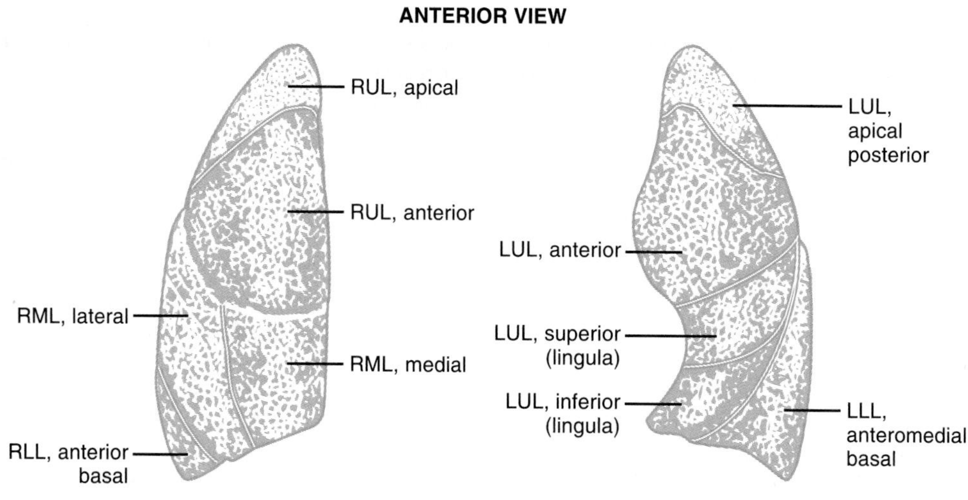


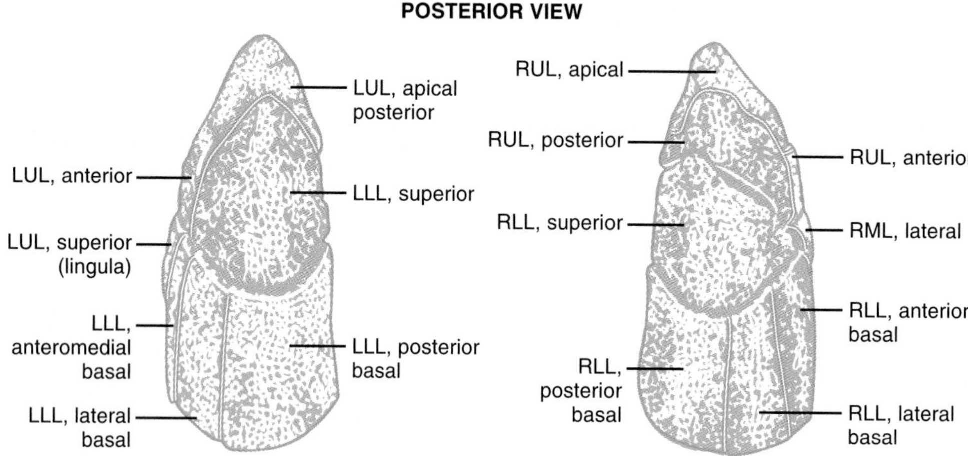


**FIGURE 218.1.** Bronchopulmonary segments.

to hypoventilation as seen in obesity, severe chronic bronchitis, severe metabolic alkalosis, and myxedema.

The various compartments of ventilation are represented in Figure 218.2. Even in healthy persons, the amount of inhaled air is distributed somewhat unevenly because of variations in intrapleural pressures. In an erect person, the intrapleural pressure tends to be maximally negative at the apices and less negative at the bases. This leads to more distention of the alveoli at the apex than at the bases and, thus, a slow breath from the functional residual capacity (FRC) level is distributed preferentially to the lower lobes. During rest, therefore, when the lower lobes get the maximal share of blood supply, ventilation is also preferentially distributed there. But with increasing breathing frequency and increasing rates of airflow, the distribution becomes more uniform. During exercise, a more equitable distribution of blood flow occurs; this is matched by a redistribution of ventilation.

### Diffusion

The quantity of a gas that diffuses across the alveolar-capillary membrane per unit time, based on gas-pressure gradients between the alveolus and the blood, is known as the **diffusing capacity of the lung** (DL) for that gas. The most common gas used for measuring DL is carbon monoxide (CO). The measurement ($DL_{CO}$) is expressed as ml/min/mmHg. It has a membrane ($D_m$) and capillary blood volume ($V_c$) components. The single-breath (SB) determination is easy to perform, although it involves breath-holding for about 8–10 seconds. $DL_{CO}$ is used clinically as an indirect measure of alveolar capillary surface area.

$DL_{CO}$ declines in diseases that destroy pulmonary alveolar-capillary units such as pulmonary vasculitis, interstitial lung diseases, and emphysema. Elevated values for $DL_{CO}$ may be seen in asthmatics (presumably from the augmented intrathoracic blood volume due to increased negative intrathoracic pressure) and in pulmonary hemorrhage where extravascular blood binds carbon monoxide.

### Perfusion

The distribution of blood flow in the lungs is uneven since the low-pressure circulation is vulnerable to gravity. Consequently, blood flow is relatively low at the apices and higher at the bases. In a normal person, this probably leads to very slight ventilation-perfusion mismatching, but its effects can be considerable in patients with underlying lung disease.

## Pulmonary Function Testing

Pulmonary function testing (PFT) evaluates the physiologic status of the lungs, which may be impaired to varying degrees and patterns by various diseases. Taken in conjunction with the clinical history and roentgenographic evaluation, PFT offers a strong clue to the underlying disease. Pulmonary function tests may be classified as **(1) commonly used tests**—spirometry, lung-volume studies, $DL_{CO}$, and arterial blood gases, **(2) those with special applications**—bronchoprovocation testing and body plethysmography, and **(3) those yet to gain clinical usefulness**—closing volume and frequency dependence of compliance. Some laboratories use body plethysmography for measuring lung volumes. PFT has many clinical applications (Table 218.1).

### Spirometry

This is the recording of a forced, rapid, and complete exhalation from a position of maximal inspiration. (Figure 218.3 shows a normal test.) The exhaled volume constitutes the **forced vital capacity (FVC),** and the volume of the FVC exhaled in the first second constitutes the **1-second forced expiratory volume ($FEV_{1.0}$).** Normally, the ratio of $FEV_{1.0}$ to FVC ($FEV_{1.0}$/FVC)

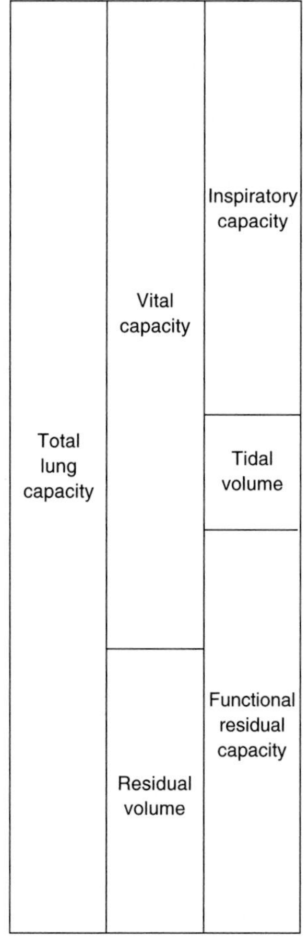


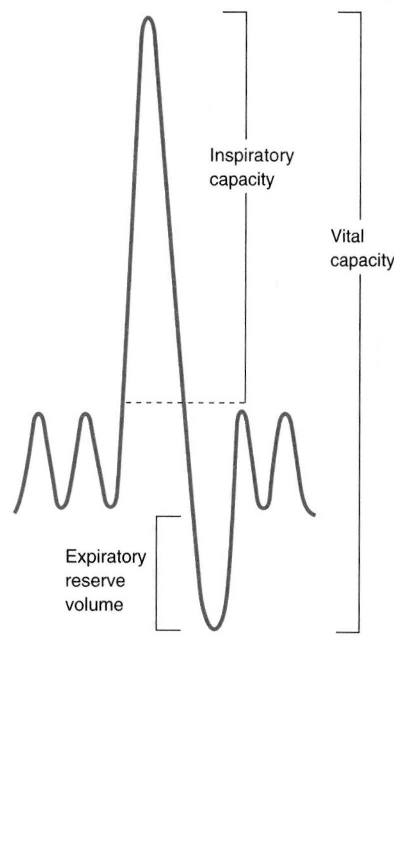


**FIGURE 218.2. Compartments of ventilation.**

expressed as % exceeds 70% in older adults and 85% in young adults. However, prediction formulas of $FEV_{1.0}$/FVC based on factors such as age and height are routinely used rather than general cutoff values. **There is only a single definition of airway obstruction: an $FEV_{1.0}$/FVC below that predicted for the individual.** If airway obstruction is found, an inhaled bronchodilator is administered and spirometry repeated to evaluate for a significant improvement in $FEV_{1.0}$ or FVC (so-called "significant bronchodilator response"). If airway obstruction completely reverses (the $FEV_{1.0}$/FVC normalizes with the bronchodilator), a diagnosis of asthma is supported.

**TABLE 218.1. Clinical Uses of Pulmonary Function Tests**

| Purpose | Identified Outcome |
|---|---|
| Detect | Lung disease early |
| Evaluate/ diagnose | Respiratory status prior to surgery |
| | Dyspneic states |
| | Severity and progression of lung disease, and response to specific therapy |
| | Extent of pulmonary disability |
| Screen | Patients being given medications with adverse pulmonary effects |
| | In epidemiologic surveys |
| | Persons working in environments hazardous to lung function |

**Restrictive impairments** are defined by a reduction in FVC. In the absence of airway obstruction (normal $FEV_{1.0}$/FVC), a reduction in the FVC noted by spirometry suggests a restrictive impairment, that is a reduction in the volume of gas in the lungs, usually due to lung diseases such as pulmonary fibrosis or non-pulmonary processes such as neuromuscular diseases. The confirmation of a restrictive impairment usually requires lung volume determination (below).

The rate of flow of the exhaled air is computed from the forced expiratory spirogram. The standard measurements are the forced expiratory flow between the initial 200 and 1,200 ml of the FVC ($FEF_{200-1,200}$), also known as the **peak expiratory flow rate** (PEFR), and that between 25% and 75% of the FVC ($FEF_{25\%-75\%}$). Reduction of the latter suggests the presence of airway obstruction. However, flow rates also may be reduced in restrictive lung disease secondary to a low vital capacity. Review of the spirograms, use of the $FEV_{1.0}$/FVC ratio, and clinical correlation are necessary under such circumstances. Most laboratories now perform spirometry and a **flow-volume curve**, in which a computer measures flow throughout inspiration and exhalation, and plots the flow against volume. Because instantaneous flows are measured throughout the vital capacity, they facilitate early diagnosis of upper-airway obstruction (chapter 231) and small airway dysfunction.

Lung volumes are determined using **helium dilution**, **nitrogen washout,** or **body plethysmography.** A

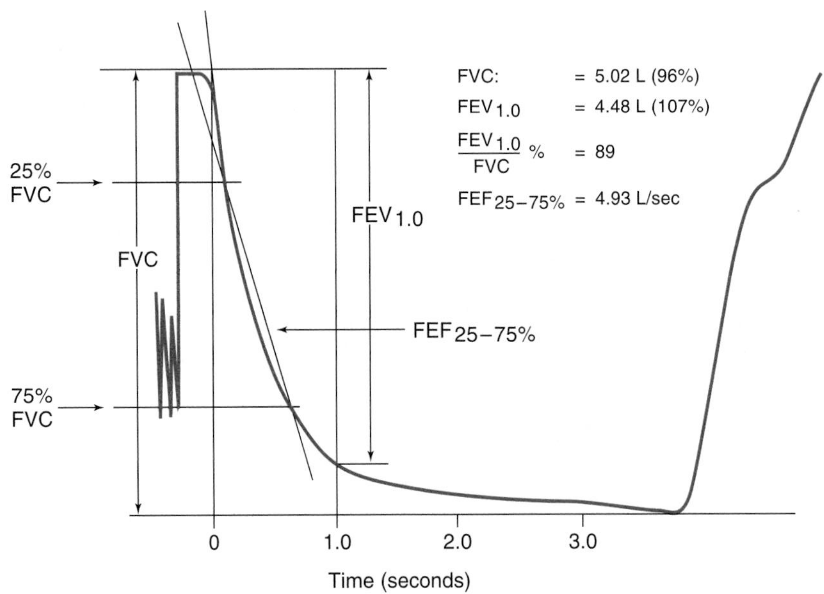


**FIGURE 218.3.** A normal forced expiratory spirometry. FVC = forced vital capacity; $FEV_{1.0}$ = 1-second forced expiratory volume; $FEF_{25-75\%}$ = forced expiratory flow between 25% and 75% of FVC.

**TABLE 218.2. Typical Pulmonary Function Abnormalities in Obstructive and Restrictive Ventilatory Impairments**

| Type of Impairment | VC | FVC | $FEV_{1.0}$ | *$FEV_{1.0}$/FVC (%) | $FEF_{25-75\%}$ | FRC and RV | TLC |
|---|---|---|---|---|---|---|---|
| Obstructive | May be normal | Usually reduced | Always reduced | < predicted | Reduced | High | Normal or high |
| Restrictive | Reduced | Reduced | May be normal or reduced | ≥ predicted | Normal | Normal or reduced | Always reduced |

VC = vital capicity; FVC = forced vital capacity; $FEV_{1.0}$ = 1-second forced expiratory volume; $FEF_{25-75\%}$ = forced expiratory flow between 25% and 75% of FVC; FRC = functional residual capacity; RV = residual volume; TLC = total lung capacity.
*obstructive impairment is defined as a $FEV_{1.0}$/FVC (%) less than that predicted for the subject using standard prediction formulas.

reduction in the total lung capacity (TLC) during the study of lung volume defines a **restrictive impairment.** Obstructive and restrictive abnormalities can co-exist. Patterns of ventilatory impairments as seen on clinical pulmonary function testing are outlined in Table 218.2.

### Bronchoprovocation testing

Bronchoprovocation testing (BPT) in the PFT laboratory using methacholine is used to detect airway reactivity. BPT is used principally to support the diagnosis of bronchial asthma, especially in atypical presentations (e.g., chronic cough with normal spirometry) or when episodic symptoms accompany normal spirometry. BPT is also quite useful in the diagnosis or exclusion of occupational asthma. BPT is never performed in the presence of established airway obstruction. The definition of a positive test is a 20% decline in $FEV_{1.0}$ from baseline. BPT helps only to determine the presence of nonspecific bronchial hyperreactivity (BHR). BHR is a prominent feature of asthma, correlating well with severity of symptoms, bronchodilator responsiveness, and medication requirements. However, BHR may also be seen in allergic rhinitis, cystic fibrosis, sarcoidosis, idiopathic pulmonary fibrosis, and even in the absence of apparent respiratory diseases. Thus, the presence of BHR must be correlated with the clinical findings before making the diagnosis of asthma.

# CHAPTER 219 BRONCHOSCOPY AND OTHER INTERVENTIONAL PROCEDURES

Bronchoscopy, performed using a fiberoptic or a rigid instrument, is indicated for the conditions shown in Table 219.1. **Rigid bronchoscopy** is the method of choice for foreign body retrieval, vascular tumors, massive hemoptysis, or upper airway obstruction. It requires general anesthesia, and the patient's neck must be extended, causing discomfort; only proximal (segmental) visualization is possible. **Fiberoptic bronchoscopy** (FOB) can be done transnasally or through an oral endotracheal tube and involves minimal discomfort; general anesthesia is generally not required and visualization to the sub-subsegmental level is easily accomplished. Bronchoalveolar lavage (BAL), brushings, and biopsies from abnormal areas can be performed during FOB. Brushings, biopsies, and needle aspirates can be fluoroscopically guided where appropriate. Postbronchoscopic sputa are collected when bronchogenic carcinoma is suspected.

## Bronchoalveolar Lavage

Bronchoalveolar lavage, performed by fiberoptic bronchoscopy, consists of segmental lavage with isotonic saline, which is suctioned back and examined by cytology and culture. BAL is particularly useful in evaluating lung cancer, diffuse lung infiltrates and/or opportunistic infections in the immunosuppressed. While it can diagnose 86–87% of cases of *Pneumocystis carinii* pneumonia complicating acquired immune deficiency syndrome (AIDS), the yield is appreciably lower for other infections and in immunosuppression from other causes. Normal cellular content is mostly macrophages (>90%) and lymphocytes (10%). A more lymphocytic response is seen in sarcoidosis and hypersensitivity pneumonitides and a more neutrophilic response in idiopathic pulmonary fibrosis. BAL can also be useful in the diagnosis of histiocytosis X and alveolar proteinosis.

TABLE 219.1. Indications for Bronchoscopy

| Purpose | Indication |
|---|---|
| Diagnostic | Hemoptysis, to determine cause and location of bleed |
| | Diagnosis of lung cancer |
| | Positive sputum cytology, with negative chest x-ray |
| | Paralysis of recurrent laryngeal nerve (hoarseness) |
| | Staging of known lung cancer |
| | Atelectasis from suspected endobronchial obstruction |
| | Cough of unclear etiology (see discussion in chapter 208) |
| | Acute inhalational injury |
| | Assessment of tracheal damage during mechanical ventilation with endotracheal tube |
| | Diagnosis of interstitial lung disease |
| | Diagnosis of pulmonary infections in both immunocompetent and immunosuppressed patients |
| Therapeutic | Foreign body in tracheobronchial tree |
| | Tracheobronchial toilet for excessive secretions |
| | Atelectasis (due to secretions) |
| | Aspiration |
| | Lavage |
| | Endobronchial brachytherapy |

## Biopsy Techniques

Tissue for diagnostic purposes may be obtained by use of interventional procedures involving the pleura (chapter 250), lung, mediastinal lymph nodes, and scalene nodes.

### Lung biopsy

Any persistent pulmonary lesion undiagnosed by conventional methods is an indication for lung biopsy, if a specific diagnosis would change management. Available methods are the **transbronchoscopic (via bronchoscopy) approach, transthoracic needle biopsy, open (thoracotomy) incision,** or **video-assisted thoracoscopic surgery (VATS).** The easiest and the least invasive approach should be tried first, unless circumstances dictate otherwise. The severity of the illness, urgency for treatment, x-ray appearance, expertise available, most likely diagnosis, and sample size the pathologist needs to provide a definite diagnosis should all be considered when selecting an approach. Transbronchoscopic lung biopsy is the preferred method to diagnose sarcoidosis. Open lung biopsy, performed through a 4"–6" thoracotomy, always provides a definite pathologic diagnosis, but a definitive etiologic diagnosis may still be elusive in about 20–30% of the cases, especially in the immunosuppressed. VATS is becoming more widely available and may avoid the need for an open thoracotomy. Finally, needle biopsy of the lung is often employed in the diagnosis of lung nodules, particularly those located peripherally.

### Mediastinal lymph node biopsy

Mediastinal node enlargement is the prime indication for mediastinal node biopsy, which is generally accomplished by a mediastinoscopy. The latter, performed through a suprasternal or anterior approach, is often used in the staging of bronchogenic carcinoma. However, its role in this setting compared with that of CT varies widely. For right-sided lesions, a suprasternal approach is appropriate; however, for left-sided lesions, an anterior approach is performed (Chamberlain procedure). Its yield in lung cancer varies with the histological type, the location and size of the tumor, the location of abnormal nodes within the mediastinum, and the presence or absence of abnormality detected in the mediastinal area by chest radiographs or computed tomography.

# CHAPTER 220 GENERAL ASPECTS OF ENDEMIC MYCOSES

Histoplasmosis, **coccidioidomycosis,** and **blastomycosis** are the most common endemic fungal infections in the United States, caused by *Histoplasma capsulatum*, *Coccidioides immitis*, and *Blastomyces dermatitidis*, respectively. *H. capsulatum* and *C. immitis* grow in the soil. Growth of *H. capsulatum* is favored by black bird, chicken, or bat droppings. When the soil or area of habitat is disturbed, the infecting conidia become airborne. The main endemic area for histoplasmosis in the United States is around the Mississippi and Ohio rivers; the disease is also common in Missouri, Tennessee, Kentucky, and Ohio. Coccidioidomycosis is seen mostly in the Southwestern United States and the lower Sonoran Life Zone. The major endemic areas for blastomycosis are the southeastern United States and the Mississippi Valley area including the Midwestern states. However, within these **endemic areas,** scattered foci of hyperendemicity occur, which share common characteristics of **acidic soil** with a **high organic content, abundant moisture,** and **proximity to waterways.**

## Pathogenesis and Pathology

Both *H. capsulatum* and *B. dermatitidis* occur in two forms (dimorphic fungi) — **a mold (mycelial) form** in the natural habitat and in artificial media, and as **yeast** in the human host. *C. immitis* is also dimorphic (grows and reproduces as mold and yeast), but the arthroconidia of the mycelia evolve into spherules (sac-like structures) containing endospores. Rupturing mature spherules release endospores, each forming another spherule and thus completing the cycle.

Pathogenetic processes common to these fungi include, in sequence, initial entry into the lungs by inhalation, conversion into yeast forms and multiplication, a host response that is initially by neutrophils and, later, macrophage-mediated, systemic dissemination to many organs, and finally, containment of infection once specific, cell-mediated immunity is acquired through T-cell proliferation. While mild infections resolve without significant pathologic residuals, more intense infections lead to caseating granulomas, which heal by fibrosis and calcification. Minor variations in this theme occur with specific entities. While the **portal of entry** is the respiratory tract, coccidioidomycosis and blastomycosis can be acquired, though rarely, through cutaneous inoculation. In histoplasmosis, a granulomatous change predominates, whereas in blastomycosis, the polymorphonuclear neutrophils remain in the area of inflammation, causing a picture of a mixed pyogranulomatous exudate. Both neutrophilic and granulomatous responses occur in coccidioidomycosis, but the neutrophilic response almost approximates that in blastomycosis.

While these mycoses have been increasingly recognized in immunocompromised patients who live in or travel to endemic areas, more often they occur in healthy persons. The shared common clinical characteristics are **asymptomatic** and **pneumonic forms** of the disease, **common drug therapy** and **diagnostic clues** (clustering of cases in family members or groups engaged in a common activity—e.g., camping, hiking, hunting, canoeing, excavating), a history of travel to an endemic area, failure to respond to antimicrobial treatment of a suspected bacterial pneumonia, and the presence of extrapulmonary disease, particularly involving the skin.

**Antifungal agents** used for treating deep mycoses are **Amphotericin B** (AmB) and the **azoles.** AmB may be infused intravenously (IV) in 60–90 minutes, thus obviating the traditional, longer infusion time. Infusion may cause fever and chills, which can be reduced by premedicating with aspirin and diphenylhydramine, although occasionally codeine or meperidine may be needed. If infused through a peripheral vein, adding a small dose of corticosteroids to the infusion can reduce the incidence of phlebitis. Drug toxicity due to AmB primarily affects the kidney. Renal tubular toxicity results in potassium wasting and progressive decline in renal function, which necessitates weekly or twice-weekly monitoring of renal function. The dose should be reduced when the serum creatinine level reaches 2 mg/dl, and the treatment should be stopped temporarily if it reaches 3 mg/dl. Saline loading before the infusion of AmB would reduce nephrotoxicity. Hypokalemic patients would need potassium supplementation. Liposomal preparations of amphotericin with reduced nephrotoxicity are now available.

Ketoconazole and itraconazole are orally administered and have gastrointestinal toxicity. Ketoconazole, in particular, may cause nausea, vomiting, and liver-function abnormalities. Because of its interference with testosterone biosynthesis, loss of libido may result. Both agents require gastric acidity for absorption; therefore, concurrent H2 blockers and antacids should be avoided. Ketoconazole (as well as erythromycin) blocks the metabolism of terfenadine, and polymorphic ventricular tachycardia (torsade de pointes) has followed the concurrent use of terfenadine with these agents. Itraconazole has emerged as a key drug and an intravenous preparation is now available but as yet there are no published studies comparing its efficacy with AmB. Newer drugs are undergoing trials or in early clinical use.

# CHAPTER 221 HISTOPLASMOSIS

Histoplasmosis is caused by *Histoplasma capsulatum.* Its epidemiology and pathogenesis are discussed in chapter 220. When the soil dries out or is disturbed, the infectious microconidia (<5%) of this fungus become airborne and may be inhaled.

## Clinical Features

The incubation period is 1–3 weeks (mean of 2 weeks). Inoculum size, the host's immunocompetence, and previous chronic lung disease may all change the clinical picture. Initial infection is most often asymptomatic. In others, the diagnosis may be missed because of trivial symptoms. **Acute histoplasmosis** in symptomatic, normal persons resembles influenza with abrupt fever, chills, chest pain, a nonproductive "brassy" cough, headaches, arthralgias, and body aches. Physical examination may be normal or reveal transient crackles, and skin lesions such as erythema nodosum and erythema multiforme. Hepatosplenomegaly is rare. Chest x-rays usually show single or multiple areas of infiltrates with lymphadenopathy (Figure 221.1). A parenchymal infiltrate with ipsilateral hilar adenopathy is a strong clue. Symptoms usually clear in 1–3 weeks. Most often, the x-ray changes also fully resolve; however, residual lesions include punctate parenchymal or hilar lymph node calcifications ("buckshot" and "mulberry" calcifications, respectively) or calcified or uncalcified parenchymal nodules (see Chapter 249).

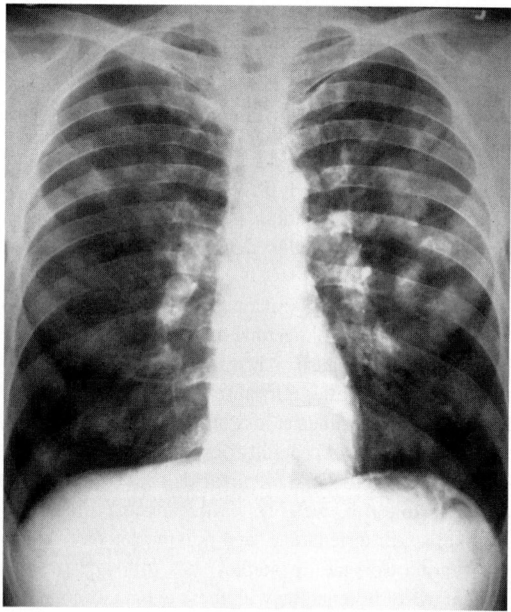

**FIGURE 221.1.** Primary histoplasmosis; multiple nodular infiltrates and hilar adenopathy.

Complications include pericarditis (not direct infection) and obstruction of adjacent mediastinal structures by adenopathy. In patients with emphysema, histoplasmosis infection may mimic tuberculosis in two ways: either during initial infection (apical cavities) or during progressive disease (apical cavities, low-grade fever, and weight loss). With a large infecting dose, a rapidly progressive illness may evolve with diffuse pulmonary infiltrates and severe hypoxemia, progressing to adult respiratory distress syndrome (ARDS), which may be lethal.

### Progressive Disseminated Histoplasmosis

**Progressive disseminated histoplasmosis** (PDH) is a progressive and often fatal systemic form of histoplasmosis in a host **immunocompromised** by medications (especially glucocorticoids), hematologic malignancies, or HIV infection. PDH may follow reactivation of a previously healed primary focus or an initial infection that the host cannot contain. High fever, weight loss, hepatosplenomegaly, and mucocutaneous ulcers are characteristic, with or without respiratory symptoms. Involvement and destruction of the adrenals may cause adrenal insufficiency. Rarely, other sites may be involved (e.g., the central nervous system, with mass lesions or meningitis). Abnormal liver function tests, pancytopenia, and, in some cases, disseminated intravascular coagulation may occur. Chest x-rays may be normal, or may show localized findings or a classic miliary pattern.

## Diagnosis and Management

In most cases, the diagnosis depends mainly on the clinical and x-ray findings. Other diagnostic tests in histoplasmosis are reviewed in Table 221.1. Diagnosis is confirmed by isolation of the organism from biologic material or tissue. All biopsied material should be examined with specific stains such as Giemsa, periodic acid Schiff (PAS stain), or Gomori methenamine silver stain. If characteristic yeast morphology is seen on microscopy, treatment could be started since the culture results may be delayed by weeks. Most cases of acute histoplasmosis do not require treatment. Indications for treatment and appropriate agents are shown in Table 221.2.

**TABLE 221.1. Histoplasmosis: Usefulness and Limitations of Diagnostic Studies**

| Test | Result/Usefulness | Comment |
| --- | --- | --- |
| Bone marrow biopsy | Good method in severely ill patients with PDH. | – |
| Blood cultures with lysis centrifugation | High diagnostic yield in immunocompromised patients with PDH. | Blood concentration of the organism is high in this population. |
| Sputum cultures for fungus | Should be performed in patients with cavitary disease. | If negative, bronchoscopy, lavage, brushings, and biopsies should follow. |
| Histoplasmin skin tests | Epidemiologic tool without clinical usefulness. | Avoid using this test. |
| Complement fixation (CF) test | Titer of 1:32 to the yeast phase antigen or a four-fold rise in the presence of consistent clinical disease strongly suggests diagnosis. | Becomes (+) 3–6 weeks after infection; remains (+) for a long time. Low sensitivity, especially in those with chronic cavitary disease and those with PDH. |
| Precipitating antibodies to H and M antigens of *Histoplasma capsulatum* | | – |
| Immunodiffusion | Low sensitivity. | – |
| RIA | High sensitivity but less specific than immunodiffusion or CF. | – |
| Urinary histoplasma antigen | Discoverable in most patients with PDH-complicating HIV infection. | HIV-infected patients have an increased density of organisms. |

PDH = progressive disseminated histoplasmosis; RIA = radioimmunoassay.

**TABLE 221.2. Histoplasmosis: Summary of Treatment Options**

| Indication | Agent | Dose/Duration | Comments |
| --- | --- | --- | --- |
| Severe illness (diffuse infiltrates, hypoxemia) | IV AmB (see chapter 213) | 35 mg/kg (some use 0.5–1.0 g as total dose) | AmB is the drug of choice |
| Massive adenopathy/ symptoms >1 week | IV AmB | Same as above | |
| PDH | IV AmB | Accelerate dose rapidly | Relapses uncommon after full AmB dose |
| PDH + HIV-infection | AmB full dose IV, plus weekly AmB or daily Itra | 1.0 g AmB + AmB (50 mg) weekly or Itra 200 mg/ daily | Long-term treatment necessary |
| Mild cases of PDH | Itra | 200–400 mg/daily for many months | May suffice as primary treatment |
| PCH | Itra | 200–400 mg/d × 6 mo. | Excellent results |

AmB = Amphotericin B; Itra = Itraconazole, PCH = progressive cavitary histoplasmosis; PDH = progressive disseminated histoplasmosis.

# CHAPTER 222 COCCIDIOIDOMYCOSIS

## Clinical Features

Acute coccidioidomycosis, caused by *Coccidioides immitis,* is a **mild respiratory illness** in most persons, but may become progressively worse. Fever, cough, headache, and pleuritic chest pain are the most common symptoms. Erythematous rash, erythema nodosum, and, less commonly, erythema multiforme are nonspecific features. Chest x-rays are abnormal in most cases, usually showing a pneumonitis with or without ipsilateral hilar lymphadenopathy. Isolated hilar adenopathy may also be seen. Spontaneous resolution occurs within 3 weeks.

In some patients, the symptoms and x-ray abnormalities persist beyond 6–8 weeks **(persistent pulmonary infection),** with the original pneumonia evolving radiographically into nodules and thin-walled cavities (Figure 222.1). Generally asymptomatic, these cavities can also cause hemoptysis or they can enlarge and rupture into the pleural space, causing a bronchopleural fistula. **Progressive primary coccidioidomycosis** (persistent symptoms of fever and cough with progressive radiographic worsening) is more likely among those with underlying immune defects and perhaps dark-skinned races. Rarely, pulmonary coccidioidomycosis may progress slowly with symptoms and x-rays that mimic pulmonary tuberculosis.

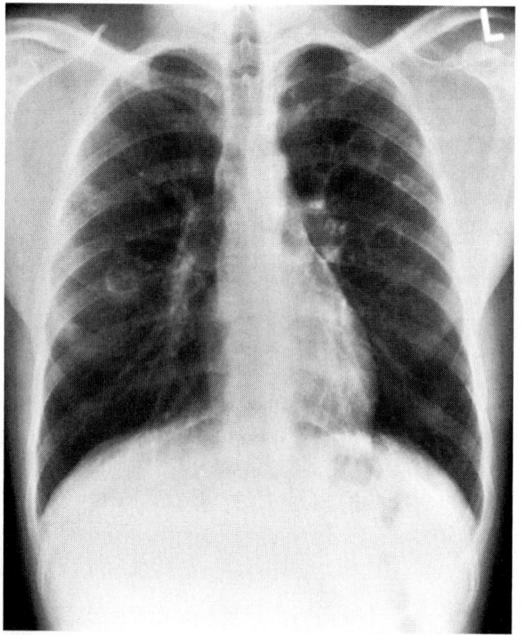


**FIGURE 222.1.** Coccidioidomycosis; multiple thin-walled cavities and nodules.

In a few patients, **systemic dissemination** follows. Patients at risk are the immunocompromised (patients receiving glucocorticoid or cytotoxic treatment patients, organ transplant recipients, and HIV-infected patients) and probably African Americans and Native Americans. Those at extremes of age and perhaps the pregnant are also at risk. Skin (draining pustules, ulcers, sinus tracts, and multiple abscesses), bones (vertebrae, skull and long bones, with osteomyelitis, large paraspinous abscesses), joints, and the genitourinary system may be involved. Meningitis occurs in about one-third of patients with disseminated disease; it may be present with no other evidence of the disease.

## Diagnosis

Given the nonspecific nature of the symptoms and x-ray findings, the diagnosis is confirmed by recovering the fungus from a **culture** of tissue or biologic fluids. However, with traditional methods for culture, accidental infection of laboratory personnel is a definite risk. **Serologic tests,** in the appropriate setting, are very helpful. Various available tests and their usefulness are summarized in Table 222.1.

**TABLE 222.1. Diagnostic Tests in Coccidioidomycosis**

| Test | Comment |
|---|---|
| Skin tests with coccidioidin or spherulin | Not diagnostic by themselves, but conversion from (–) to (+) in the setting of clinical infection strongly supports the diagnosis. False-negatives occur. |
| Tube precipitant test; latex particle agglutination (LPA) or immunodiffusion (ID) | LPA and ID detect IgM antibodies, which rise early; LPA is sensitive but not very specific. |
| Complement fixation (CF) or immunodiffusion (ID) | Detects IgG antibodies, which rise later. Rising CF titers may imply dissemination; serial titers can help assess treatment efficacy. Sensitivity and specificity of ID is similar to the CF test. |
| Microscopy of sputum, BAL, aspirated pus, or other body fluids | Best diagnostic method to detect spherules. Sputum and BAL Papanicolaou stains more sensitive than KOH digestion. |
| Tissue biopsy | H & E and special stains (i.e., silver stain or PAS) can detect both spherules and endospores. |

BAL = bronchoalveolar lavage; H & E = hematoxylin-eosin; KOH = potassium hydroxide; (–) = negative; (+) = positive; PAS = periodic acid Schiff stain.

## Management

Drug therapy is not required in most cases of acute coccidioidomycosis. Treatment with Amphotericin B (0.5–2.0 g) or oral fluconazole is indicated for immunosuppressed patients or those at risk for dissemination; symptomatic, persistent disease; progressive lung disease simulating tuberculosis; or persistent (>2 years), enlarging, or symptomatic cavities. Thin-walled cavities do not need treatment; small ones usually resolve. Disseminated disease or dissemination with AIDS requires aggressive therapy with Amphotericin B (2.0–3.0 g), given over several months, followed by suppressive fluconazole therapy. Disseminated disease with AIDS has a poor prognosis. Coccidioidal meningitis requires prolonged intrathecal or intracisternal Amphotericin B or oral fluconazole, because of relapses. Complications (subcutaneous abscesses, excision of cutaneous lesions, osteomyelitis, rapidly enlarging or hemorrhaging cavity) require surgery.

# CHAPTER 223 BLASTOMYCOSIS

Blastomycosis is caused by *Blastomyces dermatitidis,* which has a characteristic appearance (Figure 223.1): spherical, multinucleated, double-contoured, and refractile, displaying a single, broad-based bud of 5–15 microns. In the largest point source outbreak, reported in 1984 in Eagle River, Wisconsin, the organism was isolated from the soil. Its pathogenesis and pathology are discussed in Chapter 220.

## Clinical Features

Epidemiologic studies clearly identify a subclinical form of blastomycosis. In symptomatic patients, **acute blastomycosis** may be mild, simulating an upper respiratory viral infection, or severe, simulating a bacterial pneumonia, with productive cough, pleuritic pain, and fever. Extrapulmonary involvement is uncommon and skin lesions are very rare. Physical findings in mild, acute cases are unremarkable but if the disease mimics a bacterial pneumonia, signs of consolidation (shown in Table 215.5) may be noted. Other than leukocytosis and left shift in the pneumonic presentation, laboratory features are nonspecific. X-rays commonly show alveolar infiltrates, some with a typical consolidation pattern, solitary nodules, and nodules combined with infiltrates and cavitation. Lymphadenopathy and pleural effusions are uncommon. Acute blastomycosis may cause a rapidly progressive diffuse lung involvement, leading to acute respiratory distress syndrome (ARDS). Radiographically, this picture of ARDS is indistinguishable from ARDS due to other causes.

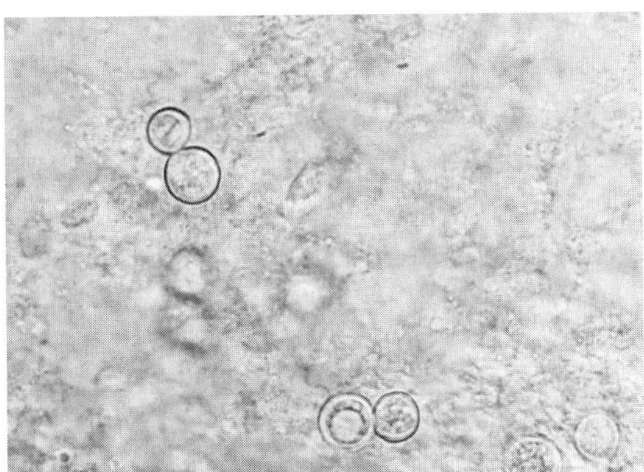

**FIGURE 223.1. Yeast forms of *Blastomyces dermatitidis.*** (From: Chest 1980;77:789. Reprinted with permission.)

Most cases of blastomycosis are sporadic in nature, with a **chronic** presentation. With low-grade fever, cough productive of mucopurulent sputum, weight loss, and hemoptysis in one-fifth of the cases, the resemblance to tuberculosis or bronchogenic carcinoma may be striking. With more chronicity, skin lesions are common, usually involving the face, hands, and legs. The lesions are characterized by an ulcerated center with heaped-up edges that contain microabscesses. With time, the ulcer enlarges and its edges become more verrucous. Chest x-rays show mass-like lesions, miliary and reticular nodular patterns, and/or cavitary disease. Less common extrapulmonary sites are genitourinary tract, bone and central nervous system.

Blastomycosis also occurs in patients who are immunocompromised from HIV disease, hematologic malignancy, long-term glucocorticoid use, and so forth. **Extrapulmonary dissemination** in such patients is common and the disease is rapidly progressive. The risk of mortality is high.

## Diagnosis

Skin tests are not useful. Blastomycosis is diagnosed by the isolation of the organism from **cultures** of biologic fluids or tissue. However, given the distinctive morphology of the fungus and the time lost in culture, all biologic material should be examined microscopically. This is best done by mixing a smear of the material (e.g., sputum) with an equal amount of 10% potassium hydroxide, and examining it as a wet mount. **Morphologic identification** is sufficient to institute treatment in symptomatic cases. Generally speaking, acute blastomycosis presenting as pneumonia can be diagnosed in this manner in over 75% of the cases.

Secretions and/or biologic materials may also be obtained by fiberoptic bronchoscopy, bronchial brushings, transbronchoscopic lung biopsy, and thoracentesis if a pleural effusion is present. Cytological preparations from these are a potentially reliable method to identify the organism. Involved extrapulmonary sites (e.g., skin lesions) should be biopsied. Microscopic examination of pus from the microabscesses around the edges of the lesion or biopsy of the lesion itself may be diagnostic. **Serological tests** have limitations in clinical practice. Complement fixation tests and immunodiffusion for antibody detection are not sensitive enough for diagnosis. Enzyme immunoassay to detect antibody against A antigen is more sensitive and the antibody is detected about 2 weeks after the onset of illness. Titers 1:32 or greater by this test strongly support the diagnosis. However, the time-delay factor limits its usefulness.

### Management

Symptomatic blastomycosis should be treated. Blastomycosis in the immunocompromised host, severe, life-threatening, or fast progressive disease and blastomycosis of the central nervous system should be aggressively and promptly treated with Amphotericin B (AmB), with a total dose of 2.0 g in adults. Another reasonable approach, although not rigorously studied, is to control the disease with AmB with a cumulative dose of 1.0 g, followed by itraconazole for several months. The severity of the illness, as in cases of ARDS, warrants aggressive treatment exceeding the usual recommended daily dose of AmB. In persons with mild to moderate nonmeningeal pulmonary disease, itraconazole is the drug of choice, as it is highly effective and is taken orally and does not have renal toxicity. The usual dose is 200 mg daily (400 mg daily, maximum), continued for 6 months. Good results have also been reported with ketoconazole. The use of AmB is preferred for any extrapulmonary involvement besides skin.

# CHAPTER 224 ASPERGILLOSIS

Aspergilli (*Aspergillus fumigatus* and many other species) are ubiquitous (soil, decaying organic matter, etc.) fungi responsible for a variety of human ailments. Infection is acquired through inhalation of *Aspergillus* spores (conidia). The development and form of the clinical disease depend on the intensity and frequency of exposure and on host factors (atopy, pre-existing cavitary disease, immunosuppressed state). The distinct clinical forms of the disease caused by aspergilli are summarized in Table 224.1. The three most commonly recognized forms of *Aspergillus* lung disease are **allergic bronchopulmonary aspergillosis** (ABPA), **aspergilloma,** and **invasive aspergillosis.**

**TABLE 224.1. Aspergillus-related Pulmonary Disorders**

| Syndrome/Disorder | Comment |
|---|---|
| Allergic bronchopulmonary aspergillosis, aspergilloma, and invasive aspergillosis | The three most commonly recognized forms of Aspergillus lung disease. |
| Extrinsic asthma | Aspergillus may act as a specific allergen; inhalation of spores cause mediator release from mast cells and bronchospasm. |
| Hypersensitivity pneumonitis | Result from inhalation of Aspergillus organisms present in moldy barley or moldy oats, corn, or hay. Occurs primarily in nonatopic individuals. |
| Chronic necrotizing pulmonary aspergillosis | Indolent, invasive infection affecting and limited to the lung, occurring in immunocompetent persons. |
| Aspergillus tracheobronchitis | Seen in immunocompromised patients; some have ulcers and pseudomembranes |

## Allergic Bronchopulmonary Aspergillosis

### Pathogenesis and Pathology

In atopic individuals, the inhaled *Aspergillus* may continue to reside in the bronchi; the host responds with both cell mediated and humoral immune reactions. Increased Th2 CD4 helper cell response is found locally and systemically. Cytokines appear to play an important role in increasing sensitivity of eosinophils and B cells. IgE and IgG antibodies against the fungus are produced, and immune reaction (type I and type III) of these antibodies against the fungal antigens cause **bronchospasm** and, probably, **immune complex injury** to the bronchi. **Proximal saccular bronchiectasis** is a serious complication of ABPA. Not all *Aspergillus*-sensitive asthmatic patients develop ABPA; therefore, genetically predetermined factors are involved. Abnormal mucus properties due to cystic fibrosis transmembrane regulator (CFTR) gene mutations are found in some patients with ABPA, and about 10% of patients with cystic fibrosis develop ABPA.

### Clinical Features

Wheezing, recurrent fever, cough productive of thick, brownish sputum, and sputum and blood eosinophilia are the common manifestations of ABPA. Roentgenographic findings are varied: transient pulmonary infiltrates, band-like densities, and atelectasis secondary to mucus plugging of bronchi. Contraction of lobes, pulmonary fibrosis, and extensive bronchiectasis may follow. Pulmonary function varies with the stage of the disease. Obstructive ventilatory impairment is common. In later stages, restrictive impairment and diminished diffusing capacity may result.

### Diagnosis and Management

The major criteria for the diagnosis of ABPA are asthma, blood and sputum eosinophilia, recurrent pulmonary infiltrates, and skin-test allergy to *Aspergillus* antigens (immediate wheal and flare reaction and late reaction). Virtually all patients with ABPA react to the skin test; therefore, immediate skin test (test) reactivity is useful as a screening test. Others include markedly elevated IgE, *Aspergillus* in sputum, *Aspergillus* precipitins in serum, a history of recurrent fever or pneumonia, and a history of coughing up sputum plugs. Specific IgE antibody to *A. fumigatus* (greater than 2 times the levels seen in asthmatics with *Aspergillus* skin reactivity, but without other criteria for ABPA) is considered a specific diagnostic finding of ABPA. CT finding of central bronchiectasis of a saccular type is highly specific for the diagnosis of ABPA in an asthmatic.

Glucocorticoids effectively reduce the symptoms, along with a decline in the serum IgE level, which is a useful index for adjusting the steroid dose. The usual starting dose of prednisone is 0.5mg/kg daily. After 2 weeks the dosing schedule can be changed to alternate days and after 3 months further tapering of the dose can be attempted. Long-term (> 6 months) treatment is usually necessary. Recent studies indicate that itraconazole at 200 mg twice daily for several months is a useful adjunctive treatment.

## Pulmonary Aspergilloma

### Pathogenesis and Pathology

Aspergilloma is a mycelial mass formed by colonization and growth of *Aspergilli* within an area of destroyed lung. Thus, diseases that cause parenchymal necrosis or bronchiectasis—namely, tuberculosis, sarcoidosis, pulmonary infarct, lung abscess, neoplasm, ankylosing spondylitis, and various pulmonary mycoses—predispose to the development of aspergilloma. Nearly 11% of patients with healed tuberculosis and residual cavities will develop aspergilloma in 3–4 years, the likelihood being higher in patients with a positive precipitin test by immunodiffusion. The cavitary wall and adjacent area may be highly vascular.

### Clinical Features

The most common symptom of a well-established aspergilloma is hemoptysis, which is usually minimal and recurrent and occurs in more than one-half of patients. However, severe, massive hemoptysis may occur, ostensibly from friction between the mycetoma and the cavitary wall, an endotoxin, and/or an anticoagulant liberated by *Aspergillus* and possible local vascular invasion. Other symptoms include chronic cough and shortness of breath. A minority of patients may get sensitized and develop asthmatic symptoms. A few cases of aspergilloma coexisting with ABPA have been reported. Aspergillomas have a very variable natural history, with stability, increase in size, and gradual or spontaneous lysis all possible.

### Diagnosis

Aspergilloma is mainly an x-ray diagnosis. It typically appears as an intracavitary oval, round, or irregular density surrounded by a crescent of air (Figure 224.1). It is usually solitary and located in the upper lobe. This typical x-ray appearance is not pathognomonic, since other processes (intracavitary hematoma, lung necrosis, neoplasm, and other mycoses) can mimic it. The absence of *Aspergillus* in the sputum does not exclude the diagnosis; however, a negative precipitin test virtually excludes it. A positive precipitin test with a typical x-ray appearance makes its diagnosis certain.

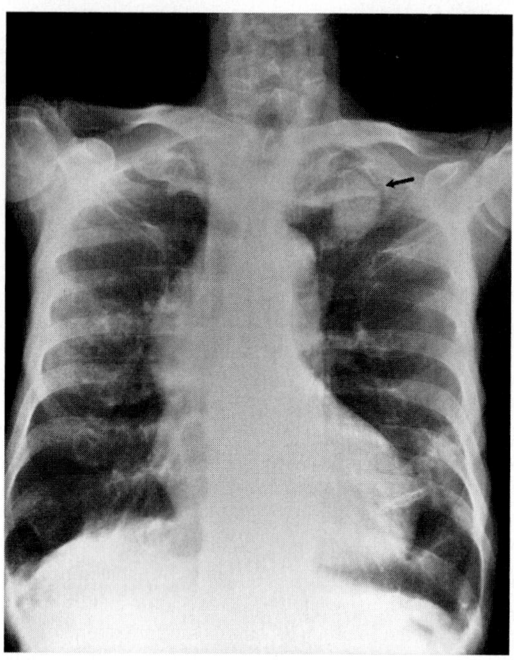

**FIGURE 224.1.** Aspergilloma; intracavitary density and typical crescent (arrow).

## Management

The prognosis and eventual outcome of aspergilloma depends on the severity of the underlying diseases rather than on the aspergilloma itself. Systemic antifungal therapy has not been shown to be effective. Routine surgical resection of an aspergilloma is not indicated. Patients with mild or intermittent hemoptysis should be carefully observed; usually these episodes are self-limiting. Surgical resection is an option in some as a recent series shows a postoperative mortality of about 6% that is considerably less than reported in the past decades. Massive or life-threatening hemoptysis calls for localization of the bleeding site followed by surgical resection or bronchial artery embolization. The latter is a particularly suitable option for those with severely compromised lung function.

# Invasive Aspergillosis

## Pathogenesis and Pathology

Invasive aspergillosis is an acute, severe, rapidly progressive infection of the lung with *Aspergillus*, with a tendency for systemic dissemination. The degree of immune suppression rather than the dose of the infecting agent determines the severity of infection. Prolonged and intense neutropenia is the most important predisposing factor. Invasive aspergillosis occurs in the immunosuppressed or myelosuppressed; the typical patient is **neutropenic,** with a **hematogenous malignancy** and undergoing **cytotoxic chemotherapy,** or an **organ transplant recipient.** Corticosteroids and immunosuppressive drugs are also predisposing factors.

Although invasion of the lung can occur through the walls of the trachea or main bronchi, more often the first infection is a distal pneumonia. Hyphae have a propensity to grow into blood vessels causing hemorrhagic infarction and cavitation of the lung. Aspergillomas may form within these cavities.

## Clinical Features

Abrupt fever, dyspnea, and cough are the most common symptoms. **Pleuritic chest pain** may be present, usually associated with a **pleural friction rub.** Hemoptysis, at times severe, may be a symptom. The x-ray features are usually those of a bronchopneumonia and the infiltrates may be miliary, patchy, or dense. Follow-up x-rays are likely to reveal progressive infiltrates and cavitation. Since *Aspergillus* has a **propensity for vascular invasion and thrombosis,** the clinical and x-ray features may mimic pulmonary embolism and infarction. Increasing size of a pneumonic consolidation toward the periphery, cavitation, and intracavitary density are roentgenographic clues to invasive *Aspergillosis*. CT of the chest and MRI can identify target-like lesions due to cavitation. Halo-sign and target sign by CT are strong clues to the diagnosis. MRI after gadolinium enhances the intensity of the rim of the cavity. The progressive worsening that follows is usually lethal within 1–2 weeks. Early therapy (medical and surgical) has been successful in some cases.

## Diagnosis

Correct diagnosis depends on a high index of suspicion. If an immunocompromised patient (especially one with a hematogenous malignancy) with bacterial pneumonia fails to respond to antibacterial therapy, the possibility of aspergillosis should be considered. However, proving this diagnosis is often difficult. Absence of aspergilli in the sputum does not exclude invasive aspergillosis. Lung tissue should be obtained promptly, preferably through an **open biopsy.** The finding of septate, acutely branching hyphae of aspergilli in tissue is diagnostic (Figure 224.2). If the patient's condition does not permit lung biopsy, presumptive treatment is justified when clinical and roentgenographic findings are consistent. In this context, the discovery of aspergilli in the sputum is sufficient reason to start Amphotericin B (AmB). Serologic tests for antibody detection are not very reliable for diagnosis and antigen detection is still not applicable for clinical use.

## Management

Untreated, invasive aspergillosis is lethal; even with treatment, only a minority survive. The drug of choice is AmB. Because the disease is life-threatening,

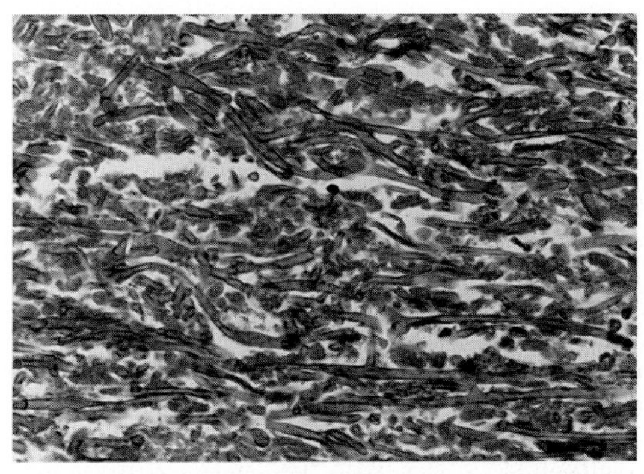

FIGURE 224.2. Aspergillus hyphae in tissue.

rapid increments of dose and larger doses are both necessary. In markedly neutropenic patients, 1.0–1.5 mg/kg of AmB is given daily until clinical improvement is noted. The latter is correlated with an increase in neutrophil count. Liposomal AmB is promising, as large doses can be delivered without the risk of significant nephrotoxicity. Itraconazole has also been used successfully, either as a sequel to AmB, or alone in less severe cases (300 mg twice daily, followed by 200 mg twice daily). Besides medical treatment, single localized pulmonary lesions may be excised to prevent complications of hemoptysis, pneumothorax, or relapse of aspergillosis.

Multiple prophylactic regimens are being studied in susceptible populations. Oral itraconazole, alone or together with intranasal AmB, appears to be effective prophylaxis.

# CHAPTER 225 TUBERCULOSIS

The term "tuberculosis" arises from "tubercle," which is its histopathological hallmark. A worldwide disease, it is caused by *Mycobacterium tuberculosis (ssp. hominis, africanum, and bovis).* Virtually all cases of tuberculosis in the United States are caused by *M. tuberculosis.*

## Epidemiology

Tuberculosis incidence in the United States has been declining since 1948. An intercurrent rise in the 1980s peaked in 1992 and was attributed to human immunodeficiency virus (HIV) infection and weakened tuberculosis control efforts owing to health care funding cuts. With a reported 16,377 cases in the year 2000 and a prevalence of 5.8 per 100,000 persons, urban populations, immigrants from endemic areas, and inmates of correctional institutions appear most vulnerable to tuberculosis. The 25–44-year age group is strikingly vulnerable, a group also most affected by HIV. Despite the declining incidence in the United States, more than one-third of the world's population remains infected by *M. tuberculosis.*

## Pathogenesis and Pathology

Tuberculosis is transmitted by infectious droplets from an active case of pulmonary tuberculosis. Normal respiratory aerodynamics generally carry inhaled droplets into the lower or middle lung zones. Phagocytosis by alveolar macrophages follows, but in the previously uninfected, the organism replicates unfettered within and outside the cell. The macrophage processes and presents mycobacterial antigens to the CD-4 lymphocytes, which generate lymphokines, thereby sensitizing the macrophage. Through cell-mediated immunity (CMI), granulomatous inflammation, and caseation, the initial infection is usually silent and contained. Although mycobacteria encased in the caseation remain dormant and fail to replicate, they may replicate later in the life of the infected individual, leading to **reactivation tuberculosis**. Contact of mycobacteria with the sensitized lymphocytes triggers immunologic memory, and tissue damage (necrosis, inflammation, and cavitation) follows through delayed type hypersensitivity. With mycobacterial replication, the host hypersensitivity to the tuberculoprotein generates a vicious cycle of tissue liquefaction, cavitation, and bacterial replication, all characteristic of reactivation tuberculosis.

A pneumonitis follows the initial infection. Multiplying bacilli spread into the lymphatics, causing hilar lymph node enlargement. The initial pneumonitis together with the lymphadenopathy characterize the primary (Ghon) focus. Hematogenous bacillary dissemination occurs next, causing formation of the secondary (Simon) foci. Generally, both Ghon and Simon foci resolve and heal; the organisms in most of these foci are killed. Residual organisms, contained by caseation, linger in these foci (latent infection). In some cases, Simon foci involving upper lobes of the lung, growing ends of bones, and renal cortices either progress immediately or, more commonly, reactivate after a period of latency. Bacterial replication, once begun, is perpetuated by a conducive local environment; a high local availability of oxygen is the alleged mechanism.

Primary infection with tubercle bacilli and the formation of Ghon foci and Simon foci are generally clinically silent events except for the development of a positive tuberculin skin test (PPD). Although the majority of clinical tuberculosis occur from endogenous reactivation of the dormant bacilli in the Simon foci, exogenous reinfection can also be responsible—as in areas with endemic tuberculosis, heavy exposure in overcrowded areas, and in severely immunocompromised persons. It is now clear that in some large urban areas of the United States, more than one-third of new cases of tuberculosis are due to recent transmission, and not reactivation. Among all those infected, roughly 10% will develop subsequent disease—5% within 2 years of infection and another 5% in the years following. Many factors and conditions (Table 225.1) increase this proclivity for endogenous reactivation.

Although the lung is the primary site of reactivation tuberculosis (84%), the early hematogenous dissemination predisposes to reactivation in other organs that lead to extrapulmonary tuberculosis. **Pleural tuberculosis** occurs from contiguous extension of a subpleural Ghon focus or when tuberculosis bacillemia spreads to the pleura. In either case, hypersensitivity to tuberculoprotein plays a role. Such effusions usually resolve spontaneously, only to be followed by frank cavitary pulmonary tuberculosis in over two-thirds of the cases within 2 years. A liquefying, cavitating caseous focus may erode a blood vessel, resulting in massive hematogenous dissemination and causing **miliary tuberculosis**, characterized by tiny lesions that mimic a spill of millet seeds.

**TABLE 225.1. Tuberculosis: Selected Factors that Favor Development of Active Disease Following Latent Infection**

| |
|---|
| Age (extremes of age, childhood) |
| Race |
| Impaired integrity of the cellular immune mechanisms |
| Human immunodeficiency virus (HIV) infection/ acquired immune deficiency syndrome (AIDS) |
| Corticosteroid, cytotoxic or other immunosuppressive therapy (including therapy with anti-TNF [infliximab] agents) |
| End-stage renal disease |
| Malnutrition |
| Hematological and reticuloendothelial malignancies |
| Associated diseases |
| Diabetes mellitus |
| Silicosis |
| Prior gastrectomy |
| Infection with measles virus |
| Alcoholism/drug addiction |
| Being underweight (≥10% below ideal body weight) |

TNF = tumor necrosis factor.

### Tuberculosis and HIV co-infection

In the United States, almost 6000 to 9000 of the newly diagnosed cases of tuberculosis in the year 2000 are expected to have afflicted patients with HIV. In a truly symbiotic way, HIV and *M. tuberculosis* increase the proliferation of each other. Interferon-$\gamma$ (IFN-$\gamma$), produced by T1 lymphocytes, is a key defense against mycobacteria; HIV infection impairs the IFN-$\gamma$ response, and thus, the host resistance to primary and reactivation tuberculosis. Also—perhaps by inducing the production of tumor necrosis factor-$\alpha$, interleukin (IL)-1, and IL-6 by host macrophages—*M. tuberculosis* boosts the host HIV replication. HIV infection is the strongest risk factor for endogenous reactivation of tuberculosis (reactivation of latent tuberculosis infection), with a risk of 10% per year in tuberculin skin test-positive HIV-infected individuals (compared with 10% per lifetime for tuberculin skin test-positive, HIV-negative persons). Also, a previously infected and immune individual is no longer protected against tuberculosis reinfection following HIV infection. Persons with HIV-infection and tuberculosis have twice the mortality of persons with HIV alone; this mortality is likely related to progressive HIV disease rather than tuberculosis. In a significant proportion of HIV-positive patients with proven tuberculosis infection, a tuberculin skin test often evokes little or no response (anergy). Granulomas are poorly formed and cavitation seldom occurs. Thus, the chest x-rays may be deceptively normal or reveal only minor abnormalities. However, the unfettered bacterial replication produces a large bacillary load, and the threat of transmission from these persons to others becomes a formidable public health issue.

## Clinical Features

Primary tuberculosis, which usually goes unnoticed or is mistaken for a viral illness, occurs most commonly in childhood and youth; however, 15% of primary tuberculosis in the United States occurs in the elderly. In all forms of tuberculosis, symptoms lag until the disease is moderately advanced. Weight loss, night sweats, and fever are general symptoms. **Pulmonary tuberculosis** is manifested by chest pain, cough, sputum, and hemoptysis, which is occasionally massive and life-threatening. A chronic unresolving or slowly resolving pneumonia is one of its infrequent but deceptive presentation in the elderly. It can mimic an acute bacterial pneumonia or present with catastrophic respiratory failure. Physical findings include fever and signs of inanition, and in pulmonary tuberculosis, signs of cavitation, consolidation, and/or pleural effusion. **Extrapulmonary tuberculosis** begins insidiously, often involving the kidneys, bones, and meninges. Fever, weight loss, progressive respiratory insufficiency, and prostration characterize miliary tuberculosis; **meningitis** is frequent. While miliary tuberculosis is sometimes the cause of a **fever of unknown origin** (FUO), this recognition is often delayed. The insidious presentation can delay the diagnosis.

## Ancillary Studies

**Anemia** and **hyponatremia** are common. **Abnormal liver function tests** may signify hepatic involvement. Acid-fast stains of sputum may show the organism, depending on the bacillary load and the extent of cavitation. The cerebrospinal fluid (CSF) in tuberculous meningitis is characteristically clear, with a high cell count that is neutrophilic initially and lymphocytic later. The protein is high; glucose is decreased to around 45 mg/dl. While the organism may be detected in the CSF, especially through polymerase chain reaction (PCR), the key feature that should arouse suspicion of tuberculous meningitis in most cases is the associated pulmonary or other extracranial disease. Tuberculous pleural effusion is discussed in chapter 250.

The slow growth of *M. tuberculosis* delays its identification. The **BACTEC-TB** system can detect mycobacterial growth in culture, reliably ascertain drug susceptibility, distinguish tubercle bacilli from atypical mycobacteria, and, in the febrile AIDS patient, help recover mycobacteria from the blood. Nucleic acid probes (nucleic acid sequences that hybridize with the counterparts of the mycobacterial DNA or RNA) hasten species recognition. The combination of nucleic acid probes and PCR can further hasten this process. PCR amplifies the *M. tuberculosis* DNA, making adequate nucleotide sequences available for testing with DNA probe. These nucleic acid probes were originally approved for use only in respiratory tract secretions obtained from patients who have received fewer than 7 days of antituberculous therapy, and are acid-fast smear positive. In such a setting, these expensive tests claim a sensitivity and specificity of 95%. More recently, based on a limited study, the FDA approved "enhanced" nucleic acid probe tests in both sputum smear-positive and -negative cases. When the clinician's suspicion of tuberculosis was high or intermediate, these tests were 70–88% sensitive, but maintained the same specificity. The use of nucleic acid tests should be individualized and not used to supplant culture techniques, because they lack the ability to obtain drug susceptibility tests at a later time, which culture techniques provide. Also, these highly sensitive, rapid, and specific tests may cause false-positive results by cross-contamination.

### Roentgenographic features

**Primary infection** generally appears as a hazy, unilateral, peripheral, middle, or lower lung infiltrate, with hilar lymphadenopathy and without cavitation. **Reactivation tuberculosis** manifests with generally bilateral, but not necessarily symmetrical upper-lobe infiltrates and typically involving the apical and/or posterior segments. Cavitation and fibrosis are common but hilar adenopathy is not (Figure 225.1). With HIV co-infection, atypical x-ray patterns are often seen. In general, the greater the immunosuppression (i.e., CD4 count <200/mm$^3$), the more the x-ray findings mimic primary infection. Further, with HIV infection, pulmonary tuberculosis may show no pulmonary infiltration.

## Diagnosis

A tuberculin skin test (PPD), chest x-ray, and sputum acid-fast smears should be done when pulmonary tuberculosis is suspected. PPD is positive in most cases (>85%) of active tuberculosis. A positive sputum smear does not necessarily mean tuberculosis, but is enough to initiate infection control (isolation) precautions and drug therapy if the clinical picture is compatible. When smears are negative, transbronchoscopic biopsy of the affected lung can rapidly and reliably provide a diagnosis, if caseating granuloma is seen. Bronchial brushing and lavage or transthoracic needle aspiration biopsy of pulmonary nodules may also provide material for microbiologic studies. Antimicrobial sensitivity testing should follow the identification of any positive cultures. In the acid-fast smear-negative patient, there are no reliable, rapid diagnostic tests that could supplant culture identification. However, culture is positive in most (75%) cases, making a presumptive diagnosis of tuberculosis inevitable in some. To diagnose extrapulmonary tuberculosis, pathologic material obtained from infected sites should be processed as described above. Presumptive treatment is not recommended in extrapulmonary tuberculosis.

## Management

Three groups of mycobacteria exist in tuberculous lesions: actively growing intracavitary ($10^8$), slow-growing intracellular ($<10^5$), and a very slowly or intermittently multiplying group inside caseous foci ($<10^5$). Mutants with primary resistance to one standard antituberculosis drug commonly occur in the larger groups ($>10^6$). With single drug therapy, mutants will selectively grow and replicate ("selection"). In the smaller ($<10^6$) groups, drug resistance and selection are not a problem. Their slow replication causes inadequate

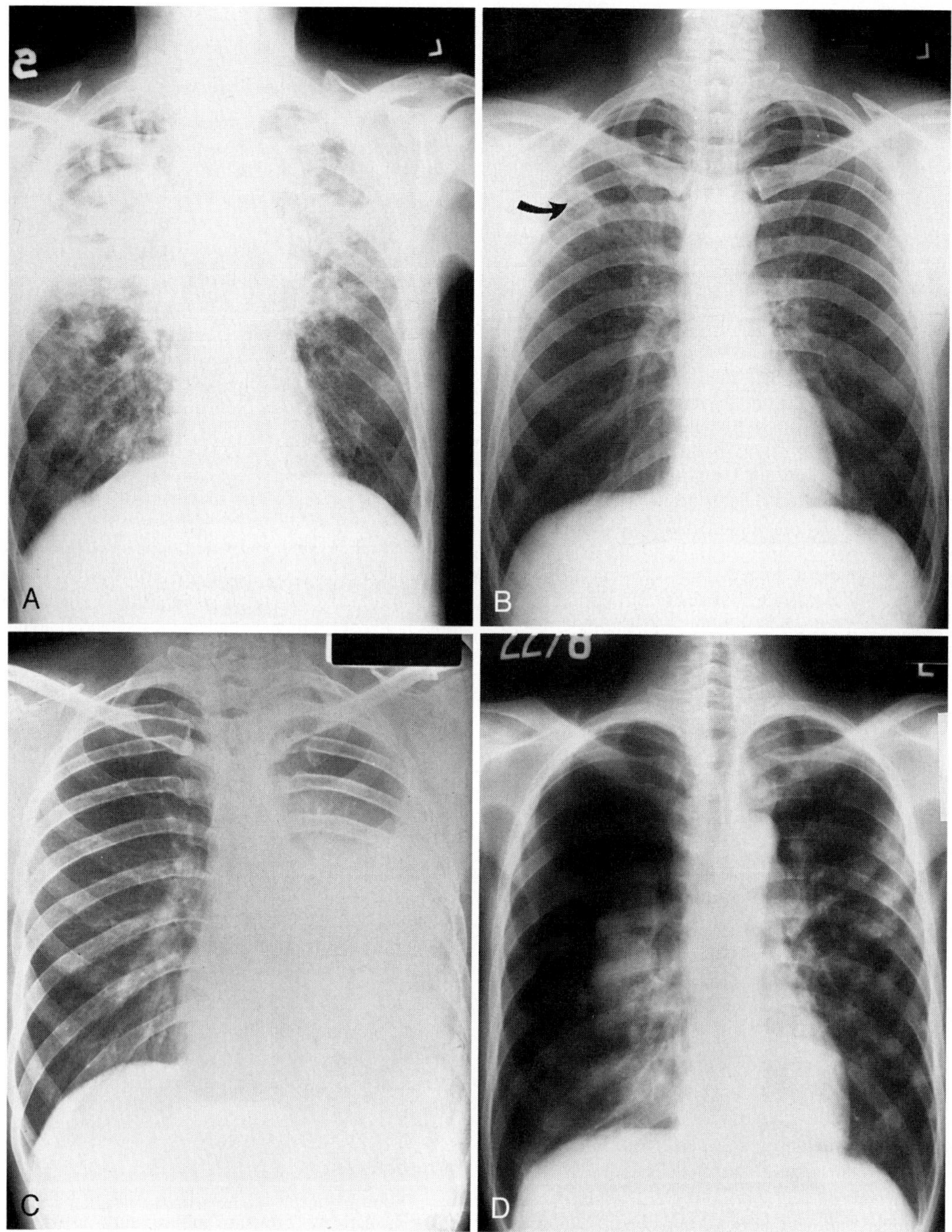

**FIGURE 225.1.** X-ray features of tuberculosis. **A.** Extensive bilateral upper lobe cavitary disease, most pronounced on the right side. **B.** Right upper lobe cavity (arrow). **C.** Pleural effusion. **D.** Right pneumothorax from rupture of one of the subpleural lesions into the pleural space; nodular infiltrates on the left side.

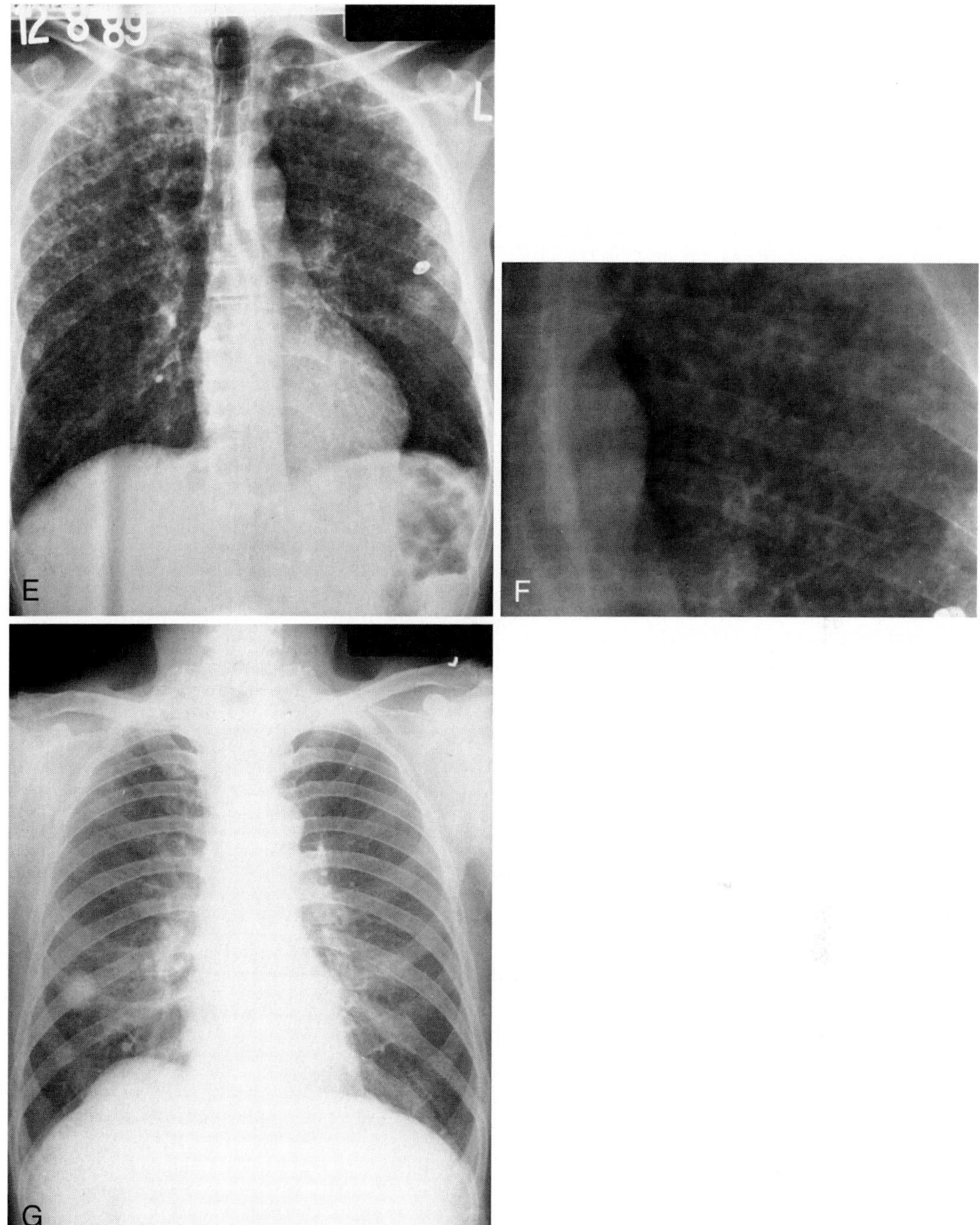


**FIGURE 225.1.**—*continued.* **E.** Extensive miliary tuberculosis. **F.** Magnified view of miliary nodules. **G.** Tuberculoma of the right lower lobe. Nodular lesions such as this may be confused for bronchogenic carcinoma. **A, B,** and **C** are more common and **D, E, F,** and **G** are unusual.

(Adapted from: Emergency Med 1983; 15:133. Used with permission.)

bacillary eradication and "relapse" on cessation of therapy. Thus, the treatment objectives are (1) to rapidly eliminate the first group, obviate selection, and make the patient rapidly noninfectious, and (2) to sterilize the tissues and prevent relapse. The first step involves simultaneous use of multiple drugs and the second one involves the extended use of agents to kill intracellular organisms.

Isoniazid (INH), rifampin (RFN), streptomycin (SM), and pyrazinamide (PZA) are mycobactericidal. Others, including ethambutol (EMB), are mycobacteriostatic (see also Table 152.3). Recent outbreaks of multidrug-resistant tuberculosis have necessitated several initial drug regimens (Table 225.2). Droplet spread is prevented by various isolation methods (mask, negative flow ventilation, etc.). Antituberculosis agents should be given in a single daily dose, since mycobacteria replicate only once per day. Baseline liver function studies are obtained before treatment. Treatment rapidly renders patients noninfectious, probably in about 2 weeks. Alcohol is best avoided during treatment. Isoniazid, RFN, SM, PZA, and EMB are considered first-line drugs. Directly observed therapy is of proven benefit to ensure compliance. Common side effects of antituberculous drugs are abnormal liver tests, hepatitis (INH, rifampin, pyrazinamide), peripheral neuropathy (INH), orange discoloration of secretions and urine (rifampin), hyperuricemia (pyrazinamide), vestibular toxicity, nephrotoxicity (streptomycin), and optic neuritis (ethambutol). INH is given with pyridoxine (50 mg daily) to prevent neurotoxicity. One-fifth of patients taking INH will show abnormal liver function tests (LFTs), which should be taken into account in the case of routine monitoring of LFTs. The exact LFT correlates of early hepatotoxicity are open to debate. When there is HIV co-infection, the treatment incorporates the same principles but for a minimum of 9 months.

Immediate contacts of a patient should be identified and given tuberculin skin testing and, if positive, a chest x-ray examination. All immediate contacts are given treatment for latent tuberculosis infection with INH and pyridoxine. Those with positive PPD are given this therapy for 6 months; those who are negative are retested 3 months later, and therapy is stopped if the PPD is unchanged. Revised criteria for positive tuberculin skin tests in various at-risk populations were provided in Table 216.1; indications for tuberculin skin testing and treatment of latent infections (formerly termed

**TABLE 225.2. Treatment Regimens for Active Tuberculosis, Incorporating HIV Status[#]**

| | HIV Status | | |
|---|---|---|---|
| **Drug Resistance** | **Negative** | **Positive** | **Concurrent Antiretroviral Therapy[**]** |
| None | INH, RFN, PZA, & EMB for 2 mo*; then INH & RFN for 4 mo | INH, RFN, PZA, & EMB for 2 mo; then INH & RFN for 7 mo<br>OR<br>INH, PZA, & EMB for 2 mo; then INH & RFBN[##] for 7 mo | No PI or NNRTI with RFN<br><br>RFBN may be used with indinavir or nelfinavir but not with saquinavir, ritonavir, or NNRTIs |
| Isoniazid | RFN, PZA, & EMB for 6 mo | RFN, PZA, & EMB for 9 mo<br>OR<br>PZA, EMB, and RFBN for 9 mo | No PI or NNRTI with RFN<br><br>RFBN may be used with indinavir or nelfinavir but not with saquinavir, ritonavir, or NNRTIs |
| Rifampin | INH, PZA, & EMB for 18–24 mo | INH, PZA, & EMB for 18–24 mo<br>OR<br>INH, PZA, SM, and EMB for 2 mo; then INH, PZA, and SM for 7–10 mo | All may be used<br><br>All may be used |

Adapted from Havlir DV, Barnes PF. N Engl J Med 1999; 340:369. Based on recommendations of the American Thoracic Society and the Centers for Disease Control (Sources: Bass JB Jr., Farer LS, Hopewell PC et al. Am J Respir Crit Care Med 1994; 149:1359–74 and MMWR Morb Mortal Wkly Rep 1998; 47 (RR:20):1–58.)

# = Regimens for pulmonary tuberculosis, for skeletal/miliary tuberculosis, recommended therapy is for 12months; * = streptomycin may be given in lieu of ethambutol; ** = if rifampin was being given, wait for at least 2 weeks after discontinuing it before protease inhibitors or non-nucleoside reverse transcriptase inhibitors are used; ## = increase dose of rifabutin to 450–600 mg if efavirenz is being used in antiretroviral therapy, reduce dose of rifabutin to 150 mg twice weekly if ritonavir is being used, and keep dose of rifabutin at 300 mg when being given bi- or tri-weekly with all protease inhibitors other than ritonavir and efavirenz. Rifabutin should not be given with delavirdine. EMB = ethambutol; INH = isoniazid; mo = months; NNRTI = non-nucleoside reverse transcriptase inhibitors; PI = protease inhibitors; PZA = pyrazinamide; RFBN = rifabutin; RFN = rifampin; SM = streptomycin.

**TABLE 225.3. Indications for Tuberculin (PPD) Skin Testing***

1. Suspected active tuberculosis
2. Targeted tuberculin testing**
   a. Close contacts (within 1–2 years) of active cases
   b. Associated medical or other conditions that increase risk of tuberculosis
      - Persons with HIV infection (or risk factors for and suspicion of HIV infection, but HIV status unknown)
      - Underlying silicosis, chronic renal failure, or diabetes mellitus
      - Persons significantly underweight (5% or more)
      - Immunosuppression (daily prednisone dose of 20 mg or more) or solid organ transplantation
      - Injection drug users
      - Cancer of head or neck
      - Homeless persons
      - Long-term institutional residence (nursing home, prisons, psychiatric institutions)
      - Otherwise low-risk persons who might engage in work that increases risk of exposure
   c. Persons whose chest radiographs are consistent with prior tuberculosis
   d. Health care workers with high risk of infection
   e. Recent immigrants from countries with a high prevalence of tuberculosis

*See chapter 216 and Table 216.1 for details on tuberculin skin testing and interpretation.
**The aim of PPD testing is to detect latent tuberculosis infection. The test is targeted to persons at high-risk for latent tuberculosis infection or high risk to develop active disease. Treatment for latent tuberculosis infection is indicated by a positive skin test regardless of age if risk factors exist such as HIV infection, close contacts, skin test conversion within a two year period, chest radiographs consistent with prior tuberculosis, IV drug use or predisposing medical conditions as indicated above. Otherwise, treatment should be considered for those with a positive skin test only if less than 35 years of age. (See Am J Resp Crit Care Med 2000; 161 (Suppl):S221–S247 for details.)

"chemoprophylaxis" or "preventative therapy") appear in Table 225.3.

Management of **HIV-related tuberculosis** entails some important considerations. When clinical suspicion of tuberculosis complicating HIV is high and the sputum acid-fast (AFB) smear is positive, using RNA or DNA probes for confirmation confers no additional benefit. The same is true when, in an HIV-positive person, clinical suspicion of tuberculosis is low and the sputum AFB smear is negative. Concurrent therapy with rifampin and protease inhibitors (PI) and/or non-nucleoside reverse transcriptase inhibitors (NNRTI) cause subtherapeutic levels of these antiretroviral agents; these agents in turn inhibit metabolism of rifampin, leading to toxic levels of rifampin. Thus, rifampin is not used with these agents. Rifabutin, the alternative, can be used with these agents, except for ritonavir (unless dose is significantly reduced) and delavirdine. Concurrent antituberculosis and antiretroviral therapy could evoke, after an initial improvement, a self-limited, **paradoxical worsening** of chest radiographs along with a marked augmentation of PPD reactivity. The reduced viral load and an enhanced immune status are said to be causative. The recommendation is to delay institution of antiretroviral therapy, if possible, when patient is begun on antituberculous drug therapy. **Latent tuberculosis infection** in HIV-infected persons is treated by INH given daily or twice weekly for 9 months along with pyridoxine 50 mg daily, or by daily PZA and RFN for two months. Also multi-drug resistance may often be seen in these patients (with 80% mortality in the 1980s; 44% in the mid-1990s). Finally, there is conflicting information as to whether malabsorption of antituberculosis drugs occurs in this population.

As the incidence of tuberculosis declines in the United States and becomes more confined to selected at-risk segments of the population—prisoners, HIV-infected, homeless, and recent immigrants, for example—complacency in tuberculosis control is likely to develop. Effective prevention of active tuberculosis depends on identification of those with latent tuberculosis infection, early case-finding of active tuberculosis, treating active cases, and environmental control so as to lower the pool of latent infections. Thus, screening these selected segments is essential to eliminate this pool, although the exact means to screen them is open to debate.

Targeted tuberculin skin testing using PPD, appropriate interpretation of the skin test, and administration of pharmacological therapy to treat latent tuberculosis infection are key public health efforts to decrease the incidence of active tuberculosis (see Chapter 216, Table 216.1; Tables 225.1 and 225.3).

Previous vaccination with BCG (used in some countries as a vaccine against tuberculosis) can be used to support the diagnosis of tuberculosis infection in patients so vaccinated. However, there is no reliable way to differentiate a skin reaction from BCG from that of tuberculosis (false-positive reaction). A positive reaction to tuberculin in a BCG-vaccinated person may indicate infection when the tested person is at increased risk for infection or has medical conditions that increase the risk of tuberculosis (see Table 216.1).

# CHAPTER 226 ATYPICAL MYCOBACTERIOSES

The phrase "atypical mycobacteria" (AM) rests on the premise that *Mycobacterium tuberculosis (ssp. hominis, africanum, and bovis)* produces the typical form of the disease and the other types of mycobacteria do not. **AM** causes a **range** of syndromes from colonization through clinically silent infection to frank disease.

## Clinical Features

Among the lung diseases caused by AM, the most frequent etiologic agents are *M. avium-intracellulare* complex (MAC) and *M. kansasii*. Compared to tuberculosis, pulmonary disease caused by these agents occurs more often in older, immunocompetent individuals. They frequently are asymptomatic and the disease is detected because of an abnormal chest x-ray (indolent or slowly progressive bilateral or unilateral upper lobe infiltrates) or because the organism is cultured from a resected, granulomatous pulmonary nodule. Symptoms, when present, and the chest x-ray appearances closely mimic those of *M. tuberculosis*. Localized pleural thickening adjacent to the area of infiltration is often found, but mediastinal disease and pleural effusions are unusual. Generally, systemic dissemination is uncommon in the immunocompetent host. Another common radiographic pattern, which is particularly common among women and best demonstrated by computed tomography, is bronchiectasis with small parenchymal nodules ("nodular bronchiectasis").

Disseminated (blood-borne) disease is a common problem among patients with AIDS, and as a general rule among those with more advanced immunosuppression. MAC infection in patients with AIDS is not a lung disease but a blood-borne infection affecting many organs. Although symptoms are numerous and nonspecific, intermittent fever, weight loss exceeding 20 pounds, anorexia, abdominal pain, and diarrhea are the most notable. Fever, hepatosplenomegaly, and generalized lymphadenopathy are the usual findings. Disseminated disease associated with AIDS is diagnosed by isolation of the organism from blood, stool, and/or bone marrow. In rare cases, biopsy and culture of other sites, such as the lymph nodes, liver, and small bowel, may be needed. Granulomas are usually absent, and abundant organisms are seen within foamy macrophages. HIV-associated AM presents almost invariably with systemic dissemination; localized pulmonary disease mimicking tuberculosis is rare.

## Diagnosis

Initially, when only the sputum acid-fast stain is positive, the patient must be presumed to have *M. tuberculosis*. However, when the sputum culture finally yields AM, diagnosis of disease must be made according to established criteria. This consideration arises from the ubiquitous nature of these organisms and their potential for contamination or transient infection. Newer macrolides have been found to be effective in the therapy of this disease. Practitioners should consult up-to-date journal articles that discuss the criteria for diagnosing AM-related diseases and their therapy.

# CHAPTER 227 OBSTRUCTIVE DISORDERS OF THE AIRWAYS

Airway obstruction, which is defined as limitation to expiratory airflow, occurs in many pulmonary disorders. In **chronic obstructive pulmonary disease** (COPD), the single, common feature is airway obstruction manifested by a permanent and progressive **reduction in the $FEV_{1.0}$/FVC below that predicted for the individual** (Chapter 218). The major types of COPD are chronic bronchitis and emphysema. The American Thoracic Society (ATS) considers **chronic bronchitis** to be "associated with prolonged exposure to non-specific bronchial irritants and accompanied by mucus hypersecretion and certain structural alterations in the bronchi." Some consider chronic bronchitis to be present when cough and sputum (productive cough) occur on most days for at least 3 months in a year for 2 successive years, after other causes of productive cough (e.g., tuberculosis and bronchiectasis) are excluded. Mucus hypersecretion without airway obstruction is termed **simple chronic bronchitis,** whereas mucus hypersecretion and airway obstruction sometimes complicated by significant hypoxemia and hypercarbia represent **chronic obstructive bronchitis. Asthmatic bronchitis** refers to a patient with chronic bronchitis who experience exacerbations characterized by dyspnea and prominent wheezing. In **emphysema**, according to the ATS, there is "abnormal, permanent enlargement of airspaces distal to the terminal bronchiole, accompanied by destruction of their walls, and without obvious fibrosis." Most patients with COPD clinically have a mixture of chronic bronchitis and emphysema. It is estimated that about 14 million people in the United States have COPD, and it is the fourth leading cause of death in the United States.

Asthma is also characterized by airway obstruction. In contrast to COPD, the airway obstruction of asthma is reversible, that is, there is normalization of the $FEV_{1.0}$/FVC between clinical episodes of asthma. However, some people with severe asthma develop irreversible airway obstruction (COPD) even in the absence of cigarette smoking.

# CHAPTER 228 CHRONIC BRONCHITIS AND EMPHYSEMA

## Chronic Bronchitis

### Etiology, Pathology, and Pathogenesis

Inhalation of tobacco smoke is the principal cause of chronic bronchitis, but exposure to environmental pollutants and irritants may also be causative. Chronic bronchitis is characterized by the hypersecretion of mucus. The subepithelial mucous glands and their acini hypertrophy and airway smooth muscles become hyperplastic. Goblet cell hyperplasia, intrabronchial mucous plugging, and distension of respiratory bronchioles with destruction of the wall (centrilobular emphysema) are other findings.

Tobacco smoke stimulates bronchial mucus secretion, impairs mucociliary clearance, and disrupts alveolar macrophage function. A vicious cycle of respiratory infections, bronchial damage, and further impairment of ciliary function follows. However, airflow obstruction develops in only about 15% of smokers, suggesting that host susceptibility is an important prerequisite. In this context, both smoking-related airway irritation and bronchial hyperreactivity (BHR) have been implicated in the genesis of airflow obstruction. Nonetheless, current evidence suggests that COPD evolves through smoking-induced BHR. Finally, cholinergic innervation is abundant (and sympathetic innervation sparse) in the large and medium airways. Vagal stimulation causes bronchospasm and bronchial gland secretion. Cholinergic airway tone increases significantly following airway damage. In susceptible persons, various provocative stimuli could thus produce bronchoconstriction through vagal reflex.

Airway obstruction produces unventilated or under ventilated alveoli; continued perfusion of these alveoli leads to hypoxemia (low $PaO_2$) from mismatching of ventilation and blood flow (V/Q mismatch). Hypoxemia occurs early in chronic obstructive bronchitis and when sustained leads to pulmonary hypertension. Ventilation of unperfused or poorly perfused alveoli increases dead space ($V_d$), causing inefficient $CO_2$ removal. Hyperventilation normally compensates for this, thus producing a normal $PaCO_2$. However, hyperventilation, which further increases the work required to overcome the already increased airway resistance, ultimately fails, resulting in $CO_2$ retention (hypercapnia).

### Clinical Features

The cardinal symptoms of established chronic bronchitis are cough and expectoration, which tend to be maximal in the morning and reflect pooling of secretions overnight. A productive cough, intermittent at first, becomes almost a daily occurrence with time. Sputum is clear and mucoid, but may become thick, tenacious, and yellow, and even blood-streaked during intercurrent bacterial respiratory infections. Blood-streaking may also be from repetitive coughing or intercurrent lung malignancy. Chronic bronchitis is the most frequent cause of hemoptysis. However, the amount of bleeding is generally modest and only infrequently life-threatening. Wheezing is generally present, especially during respiratory infections.

Dyspnea, usually absent in **simple chronic bronchitis,** is a feature of **chronic obstructive bronchitis,** which develops over many years. In addition to dyspnea, chronic obstructive bronchitis is characterized by cyanosis and marked wheezing, and is often complicated by heart failure. Physical examination is generally normal in simple chronic bronchitis, but reveals expiratory prolongation, rhonchi, and, less often, basilar crackles in obstructive bronchitis. Clubbing of the digits is not a feature of chronic bronchitis or COPD and when present should arouse suspicion of another disorder, especially bronchogenic carcinoma.

### Ancillary Studies

Sputum examination may show a mixed bacterial population. Erythrocytosis may occur in patients with significant hypoxemia, either at rest or with exercise. Roentgenograms may be normal or show increased lung markings, with or without cardiomegaly. Pulmonary function studies, while normal in chronic simple bronchitis, show airway obstruction in chronic obstructive bronchitis. Mild hypoxemia occurs early. However, significant hypoxemia and hypercapnia complicate ad-

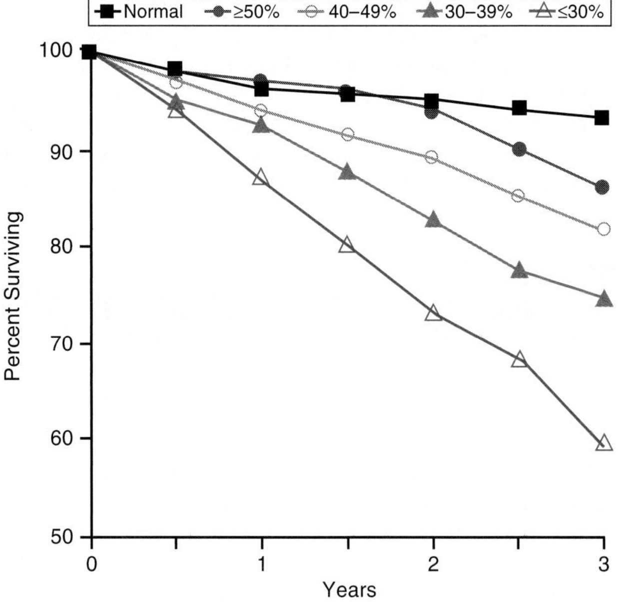


**FIGURE 228.1. Survival curves from the National Institutes of Health-Intermittent Positive Pressure Breathing Trial, based on baseline postbronchodilator $FEV_{1.0}$.**
(From: Anthonisen NR, et al. Am Rev Resp Dis 1986; 133: 14-20. Reprinted with permission.)

vanced airway obstruction usually when the $FEV_{1.0}$ falls below 1.0–1.25 L.

## Course, Complications, and Prognosis

Symptoms of chronic bronchitis persist with continued exposure to irritants, and generally improve with cessation of such exposure. The rate of decline in pulmonary function is less rapid in those who stop smoking. Expiratory flow rates may improve more rapidly following smoking cessation. Smoking cessation using behavioral modification, nicotine replacement, and buproprion is essential.

The complications of chronic obstructive bronchitis are bacterial colonization of the lower respiratory tract, respiratory infections, acute or chronic respiratory failure, and cor pulmonale. Most respiratory infections are initially viral, but also include acute bacterial bronchitis and pneumonia. Increased cough with thick, tenacious sputum along with a worsened respiratory status characterize these bacterial infections. Respiratory failure is usually caused by a respiratory infection; heart failure, sedation, chest trauma, pneumothorax, surgery under general anesthesia, and pulmonary thromboembolism are others. Hypoxemia, hypercarbia, increased blood viscosity from erythrocytosis, and the destruction of pulmonary vessels all contribute to pulmonary hypertension and cor pulmonale (chapter 234).

Pulmonary function generally declines progressively, and while less accurately predictable in a given patient, the average yearly loss in $FEV_{1.0}$ is 50–100 ml. Activity is markedly limited when the $FEV_{1.0}$ is about 1.0 liter. With lower values, dyspnea may even limit conversation. COPD shortens the life span, especially in persons younger than 65 years, but various investigators report highly variable survival statistics (Figure 228.1). Among the many variables that apparently influence survival (Table 228.1), the most important are age and the postbronchodilator $FEV_{1.0}$. The only intervention that improves survival in COPD, including chronic bronchitis, is supplemental oxygen, so-called long-term oxygen therapy (LTOT; chapter 239).

## Diagnosis and Differential Diagnosis

Chronic bronchitis (so-called blue bloater) is a clinical diagnosis, based on history; lung examination is generally abnormal. Chronic obstructive bronchitis is characterized by a relatively preserved diffusion capacity ($DL_{CO}$) in contrast to emphysema (so-called pink puffer), which usually has a significant decrease in $DL_{CO}$. Wheezing and dyspnea are symptoms common to chronic bronchitis, asthma, and emphysema; helpful distinguishing features are listed in Table 228.2.

## Management

### Bronchodilators

All patients with the diagnosis of COPD should be given a trial of inhaled bronchodilators (an anticholinergic or β-adrenergic agonist; Table 228.3), regardless of whether spirometry shows a significant bronchodilator response. Repeat spirometry after several weeks of treatment may help in providing objective evidence of

**TABLE 228.1. Factors of Prognostic Significance in Chronic Obstructive Pulmonary Disease (COPD)**

| Factors Correlating with Survival | |
|---|---|
| **Positively[a]** | **Negatively[b]** |
| Predominant chronic bronchitis | Age |
| $FEV_{1.0}$ | Progressive decrease in $FEV_{1.0}$ |
| $PaO_2$ | High resting heart rate |
| Reversibility of airflow obstruction | Increased $PaCO_2$ |
| Exercise capacity | Pulmonary hypertension/cor pulmonale |
| Diffusing capacity | Total lung capacity |
| Vital capacity | Continued smoking |
| Atopy | Malnutrition/weight loss |
| | α-1-antitrypsin deficiency |

[a]Presence of one of these or a higher value indicates a better prognosis.
[b]If present or high, the prognosis is worse.
(Adapted from: Hodgkin JE. Clin Chest Med 1990;11(3):556. Used with permission.)

**TABLE 228.2. Differentiating Between Asthma, Bronchitis, and Emphysema**

| Criterion | Asthma | Chronic bronchitis† | Emphysema |
|---|---|---|---|
| Principal symptom | Wheezing, paroxysmal dyspnea | Productive cough for many years | Progressive dyspnea for many years |
| Pattern of wheezing | Paroxysmal | Perennial | Perennial |
| Relationship of attacks to allergens | Temporal | None | None |
| Seasonal nature of symptoms | Seasonal; symptom-free intervals | None | None |
| Worsening/improvement over time with or without treatment | Characteristic | Not seen | Not seen |
| History of smoking | Variable | Integral part of history | Integral part of history |
| Personal/family history of asthma or atopy | Supports diagnosis | Incidental, not helpful in diagnosis | Incidental, not helpful in diagnosis |
| Exacerbations of the disease | Usually no purulent sputum; recovery from exacerbations generally rapid and nearly complete | Sputum ± purulent. Exacerbations from infection and/or heart failure. Recovery often prolonged. | Exacerbations from infection and/or heart failure. Recovery often prolonged. |
| Physical examination | Normal between paroxysms, ↑FET** | Rhonchi, râles, wheezing, cyanosis ±, ↑ FET.** | Barrel-shaped chest, breath sounds ↓, wheeze, ↑ FET.** |
| Laboratory | Blood and sputum eosinophilia. Atopy and high IgE levels helpful.[a] Reversibility of airflow obstruction >25%. DLCO nl, often ↑. CXR nl when stable. | Erythrocytosis. Atopy not a feature. $PaO_2$↓↓, $PaCO_2$ may rise. Reversibility of airflow obstruction minimal. DLCO nl or ↓. | Atopy not a feature. $PaO_2$ slightly ↓; $PaCO_2$ ↓. Reversibility of airflow obstruction minimal. DLCO ↓. Emphysematous changes in CXR (hyperinflation). |

†Refers to chronic obstructive bronchitis.
Note: Disorders are described here when they occur as "pure" entities. However, in clinical practice, chronic bronchitis and emphysema often co-exist.
[a]Atopy and high IgE levels are seen only in allergic asthma. Thus, the absence of these features does not exclude asthma.
↑ = increased; ↓ = decreased; ± = may be; CXR = chest x-ray; DLCO = diffusion capacity; nl = normal.
**FET = forced expiratory time. See Chapter 215 for explanation of the use of the FET.

TABLE 228.3. Commonly Used Bronchodilators

| Agent | Action | Dosage | Route |
|---|---|---|---|
| Ipratropium bromide *(Atrovent)*® | Anti cholinergic | 2 puffs qid<br>0.5 ml qid, diluted in 3 ml saline | MDI<br>Via nebulizer |
| Albuterol *(Proventil®; Ventolin®)* | β-2 adrenergic | 2 puffs q 4–6h;<br>2–4 mg[b] qid | MDI,<br>Tablets and syrup |
| Metaproterenol *Alupent®, Metaprel®* | β-2 adrenergic | 1–2 puffs q 4–6 h;<br>0.3 ml in 3 ml saline<br>q 4–6h 20 mg tid/qid. | MDI,[a]<br>Via nebulizer<br>Tablets and syrup |
| Salmeterol *Serevent®* | β-2 adrenergic | 1–2 puffs q 12 h. | MDI[a] |
| Ipratropium + albuterol *Combinent®* | Anti cholinergic + β-2 adrenergic | 2 puffs qid | MDI |
| Theophylline | See text. | See text. | Oral and intravenous |

[a]Preferably administered as two separate puffs with an interval of a minute between each.
[b]Sustained release (long-acting) preparation available with b.i.d. (twice daily) dosing.
MDI = Metered dose inhaler.

improvement in airway obstruction and in determining effectiveness of therapy. Education on the correct use of a metered dose inhaler (MDI) and the use of a spacer device with MDIs are essential in order to derive the greatest benefit from inhaled bronchodilators.

*Anticholinergic agents*

Anticholinergics are a common first-line agent recommended in COPD. **Ipratropium bromide,** a quaternary ammonium compound, is most widely used. When given as an aerosol, ipratropium is poorly absorbed from the airways, relatively nontoxic, and has little effect on mucociliary clearance. However, anticholinergics are not as effective in asthma as in COPD.

*β-Adrenergic agonists*

These agents mimic the effects of β-adrenergic receptor stimulation (see Table 228.3). Because the β receptors have both cardiovascular (β-1) and bronchodilatory (β-2) effects, β agonists with selective β-2 effects are highly desirable; such exclusive selectivity is unavailable at present. β agonists presumably stimulate adenyl cyclase, increasing intracellular cyclic adenosine monophosphate (c-AMP), thus causing bronchodilation. Both short-acting (i.e., albuterol) and long-acting β-2 agonists (i.e., salmeterol) are available.

The recommended therapy of COPD is shown in Figure 228.2. It is best to administer all inhaled bronchodilators with a metered dose inhaler (MDI) using a spacer device, providing fixed-dose, targeted delivery into the airway and thus minimizing systemic effects. Nebulizers deliver a larger dose, involve bulky equipment, and require skills in equipment care and medication dispensing. Thus, properly used MDIs attached to a spacer device are the most preferred method of delivery of inhaled medications.

*Theophylline*

Theophylline has a narrow therapeutic window. Its bronchodilatory action is serum level–dependent. It improves mucociliary clearance, reduces pulmonary hypertension, improves right ventricular performance in COPD, and augments diaphragmatic contractility by enhancing diaphragmatic blood flow. This beneficial effect on diaphragmatic function may help minimize or prevent diaphragm fatigue or respiratory failure in advanced COPD.

Theophylline metabolism, influenced by many factors, is 90% hepatic. For rapid dosing, IV loading is infused at 5–6 mg/kg, if the drug has not been recently used. Because maintenance dose regimens are not highly reliable, drug-level monitoring is critical. In nonsmoking adults, an acceptable dose is 0.5 mg/kg/hr, and in smokers it is 0.7 mg/kg/hr. The oral starting dose of anhydrous theophylline for adults is 400–600 mg daily in divided doses. Drug-level monitoring and dosage changes should follow until therapeutic levels are reached. Toxic side effects, uncommon with a therapeutic drug level (<20 mg/ml), include irritability, nausea, vomiting, diarrhea, palpitations, tachycardia, cardiac arrhythmias, confusion, agitation, and seizures. Regular drug-level monitoring is needed only for suspected toxicity, suboptimal response, or intercurrent factors that affect clearance of the drug. Many physicians target a theophyllline level of 8–10 μg/ml.

### Corticosteroids

Oral corticosteroids, despite their frequent adjunct use, are controversial in COPD. They might benefit a subset of COPD patients with a severe acute exacerbation of COPD, disabling dyspnea, or a progressive decline in $FEV_{1.0}$ exceeding 80 ml/year. Prednisone, initiated at

30–40 mg daily for 10–14 days, is continued at the minimum necessary dose to maintain objective improvement in spirometry (20% increase in $FEV_{1.0}$ or FVC). Spirometry is recommended immediately on initiation of prednisone and at the end of the trial. If no evidence of improvement is noted after 2–3 weeks, prednisone is tapered rapidly. The role and efficacy of inhaled steroids in classic, smoking-related COPD is controversial although these agents are clearly the first-line of therapy in persistent asthma.

**Control of secretions**

It is critical that patients stop smoking and avoid irritants. Avoiding passive smoke or pollutants may require a change in occupation, the use of filter masks, or modifications in the workplace and/or home. Increasing water intake is beneficial only when dehydration is present. Physical therapy with chest clapping and postural drainage is helpful for coexistent bronchiectasis or excess secretions. Expectorants have no proven benefit, but mucolytics (e.g., acetylcysteine by aerosol, 1–4 ml, q 4–6 h) may help liquefy tenacious secretions by breaking the sulfhydryl bonds in the mucus, usually in carefully selected hospitalized patients. Bronchospasm can result with administration of acetylcysteine, thus a concurrent bronchodilator aerosol should be given.

**Other ancillary measures**

Long-term oxygen theapy can prolong life in selected patients with COPD (Chapter 239). Vaccination against influenza should be given yearly, generally in early autumn. Pneumococcal vaccine is recommended, but the immunity wanes after about 5 years and revaccination may be required in patients at high risk of serious pneumococcal infection. Smoking cessation, using combinations of nicotine replacement therapy and bupropion, as well as behavior modification therapy is essential. While most patients with COPD are managed on an ambulatory basis, hospitalization may be required for significant exacerbations, for occurrence of serious

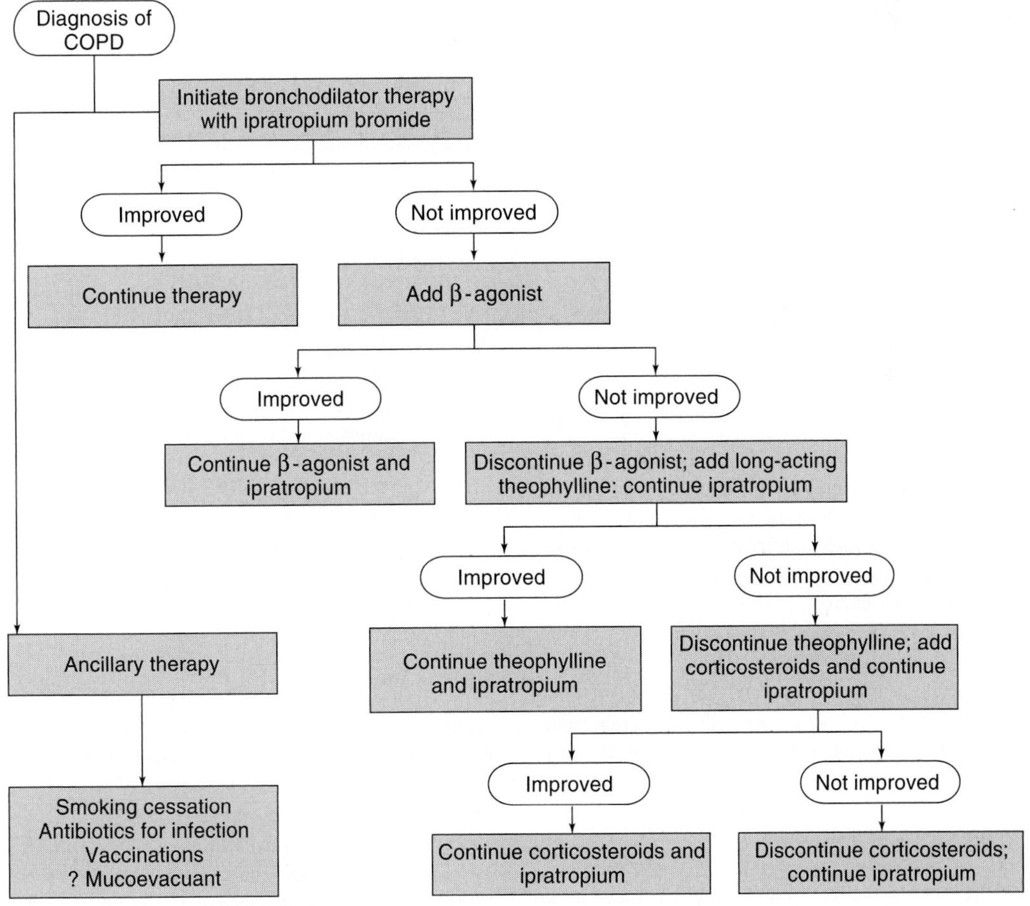


**FIGURE 228.2. Sequential application of drug therapy in COPD.**
(Adapted from: Ferguson JF, Cherniak RM. N Engl J Med 1993;328:1017. Used with permission.)

complications, and for operations or procedures that entail serious risk to the patient, significant analgesia, or anesthesia.

#### Treatment of exacerbations

Generally, 1–2 exacerbations occur yearly, precipitated by either respiratory infection or heart failure. It is critical to recognize and treat exacerbations, as they are notorious for precipitating respiratory failure. Usual features are increasing dyspnea, cough and sputum, and, when caused by infection, purulent sputum. Most infections are viral, generally caused by bacterial secondary infection resulting from *Haemophilus influenzae*, pneumococci, and *Moraxella catarrhalis*, in that order of frequency. When respiratory infection is suggested or when sputum becomes yellow, antibiotics should be started. Ampicillin (2.0 gm/d), doxycycline (200 mg/d), or sulfamethoxazole/trimethoprim (400/160 mg, respectively, twice daily), for 7–10 days, are all acceptable. Given the increase in β-lactamase–producing bacteria, the newer macrolides (e.g., clarithromycin) may have a role in these cases. Oral or intravenous corticosteroids are often used in severe COPD exacerbations or frank acute respiratory failure (methylprednisolone, 2.0 mg/kg initially, followed by 0.5 mg/kg q 6 h with a gradual taper over 14 days).

#### Pulmonary rehabilitation

When customized for the patient with COPD (or other debilitating respiratory disorders), a comprehensive program using bronchodilators, oxygen, exercise reconditioning, and psychosocial rehabilitation will be beneficial. These programs do not improve longevity or pulmonary function, but they enrich the quality of life and reduce hospitalizations.

## ■ Pulmonary Emphysema

### Etiology and Pathogenesis

Cigarette smoke is strongly implicated in the genesis of human emphysema. It is thought to result from an imbalance in the elastase-antielastase system. On exposure to tobacco smoke, alveolar macrophages secrete elastases and chemotactic factors for neutrophils, which in turn also release elastases. An anti-elastase system (e.g., α-1 antitrypsin) protects against elastase-induced lung injury. When anti-elastases are naturally defective or rendered ineffective by components of the smoke, lung injury follows. Collagen synthesis and repair are also impaired by the tobacco smoke.

### Pathology and Pathophysiology

The acinus distal to the terminal bronchiole enlarges and the alveolar septa are destroyed. Early ruptures in airway walls later become confluent, finally destroying the walls. Ultimately, the orderly appearance of the acinus and its components is disturbed and lost. Loss of elastic recoil and the resultant compressibility of large airways upon exhaling, as well as the loss of radial traction on the airways, all lead to expiratory obstruction and decreased expiratory airflow. As a result, α-1 antitrypsin, a normal element in the airway lining fluid, is damaged or destroyed; both emphysema and airway damage follow. Expiratory airflow obstruction compromises bronchial hygiene and lung defenses, causing chronic bronchitis to be associated.

### Clinical Features

The patient, generally an individual in the fifties, reports dyspnea and, if chronic bronchitis is associated, a productive cough. Findings include use of accessory muscles during inspiration, pursed lips on exhaling (which prevents premature airway collapse), barrel-shaped chest, hyperresonance to percussion, and obliteration of cardiac and hepatic dullnesses. Breath sounds are markedly diminished and forced expiratory time prolonged, often with a wheeze. The precordial heart sounds are distant, but generally well heard in the epigastrium.

### Ancillary Studies

Because chest x-rays are normal in early emphysema, they are unsuitable for screening. However, they are a good adjunct to the clinical evaluation of emphysema. The most accepted radiographic criteria for emphysema are over inflation of the lungs, low, flat diaphragms, and a large (>3.0 cm) retrosternal airspace. The heart is vertical and narrow. Lung vasculature is attenuated peripherally with prominent central pulmonary arteries (Figures 228.3 and 228.4). The chest x-ray can suggest the presence (but not severity) of emphysema. CT scan can show parenchymal destruction and bullae associated with emphysema. Spirometry remains the only diagnostic test for airway obstruction. The $DL_{CO}$ is decreased.

### Management

Respiratory function declines with age. However, the rate of decline is greater in those who continue to smoke than in those who cease smoking. Hypercapnia, resting tachycardia, and the presence of cor pulmonale indicate a poor prognosis. There is no specific therapy for emphysema, other than the management of associated chronic bronchitis—that is, relief of any reversible bronchospasm, oxygen therapy when appropriate, and prevention and treatment of bacterial pulmonary infections. In selected patients, the resection of bullous lesions using **lung volume reduction surgery (LVRS)** may improve symptoms and gas exchange, although it has not been known to influence survival. The pharmacological management of emphysema is similar to that of chronic bronchitis (above).

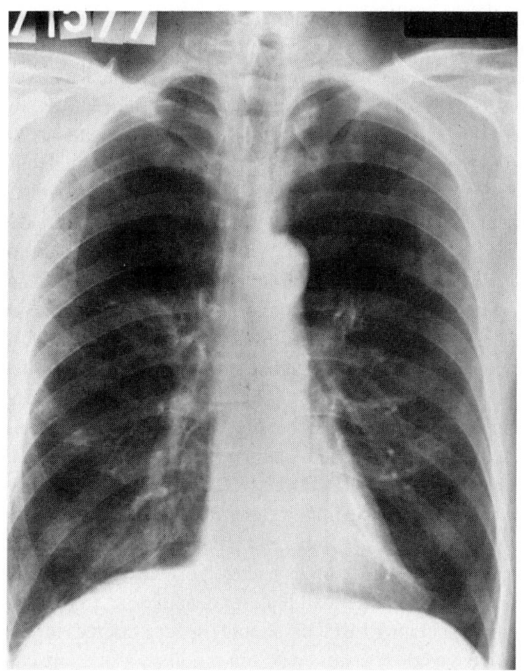

FIGURE 228.3. Pulmonary emphysema: note the hyperinflated lungs and flattened diaphragms.

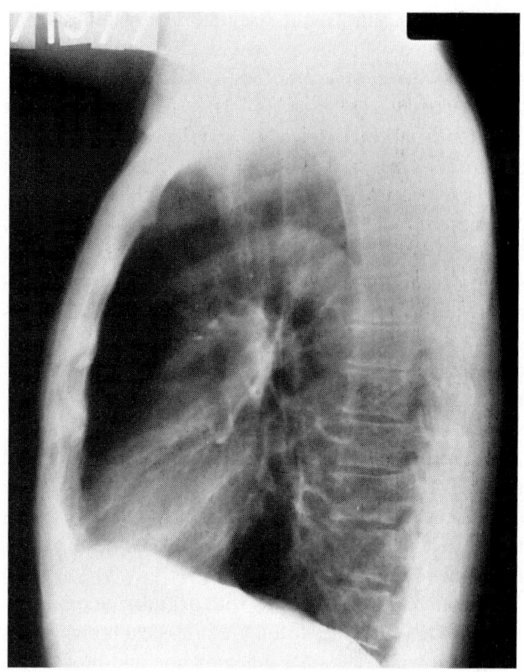

FIGURE 228.4. Pulmonary emphysema: note the attenuated vasculature, flattened diaphragms and increased restosternal airspace.

# CHAPTER 229 DISEASES OF THE BRONCHIOLES

First described in the 1960s, **bronchiolitis**—also known as small airways disease—consists of dyspnea, airflow obstruction, reticular changes in the chest x-rays, and pathological findings confined to the small airways. Bronchiolitis is an inflammatory process of the airways limited mainly to the bronchioles, airways 1–2 mm in diameter. The disease is heterogeneous, with several forms having since been described. **Diffuse panbronchiolitis,** primarily seen in Japan and predominantly involving middle-aged men, manifests with dyspnea, cough, purulent sputum, airflow obstruction, and sinusitis. Untreated, the 5-year mortality rate is about 40%. Long-term erythromycin, whose action is believed to be unrelated to antibacterial properties, can be beneficial. The epidemiology of **adult bronchiolitis** is not well known. Airflow obstruction develops over many years and without associated features of asthma, chronic bronchitis, or emphysema. Corticosteroid therapy has been found to be useful.

**Bronchiolitis obliterans** (BO) may be idiopathic or may have disparate causes, including viral infections, noxious dust and fume exposure, heart and/or lung transplants, bone marrow transplants, and connective tissue disorders (particularly rheumatoid arthritis treated with penicillamine). BO following heart/lung transplant occurs 3 or more months after the transplant, and represents chronic rejection. BO following bone marrow transplant develops within 6–12 months of the transplant and is associated with graft versus host disease. The features are relentlessly progressive dyspnea, dry or minimally productive cough, and evidence of airflow obstruction. Treatment options are augmentation of immunosuppression or retransplantation. Corticosteroid therapy produces equivocal results.

**Respiratory bronchiolitis (RB)** may follow inhalation of cigarette smoke and mineral dusts (asbestos, silica, etc.), viral infections, connective tissue disease, and exposure to drugs. The disease is characterized by submucosal mononuclear cell infiltration of the respiratory bronchioles, goblet cell hyperplasia, and airway epithelial metaplasia. Also, fibrosis and bronchiolar metaplasia may extend into immediately adjacent alveolar walls. Tan-brown–pigmented macrophages accumulate within and around the respiratory bronchioles, alveolar ducts, and alveoli. Respiratory bronchiolitis may be associated with an interstitial lung disease, which represents the most severe form of respiratory bronchiolitis. Cough and dyspnea are the most common symptoms of RB, followed by chest pain, weight loss, and fever. A history of current or past cigarette smoking is almost invariably present. Pan-inspiratory (lasting over the entire inspiration) rales are present at the lung bases. Finger clubbing is not a feature. Pulmonary function studies generally show a restrictive ventilatory impairment; airflow obstruction may co-exist. The $DL_{CO}$ is often reduced, and resting or exercise-induced arterial hypoxemia may be noted. The chest x-ray shows a fine, diffuse, reticulonodular infiltrate; peripheral ring-like shadows and bronchial wall thickening may be associated. Diffuse, patchy, "ground-glass" opacities or fine nodules may be seen on computed tomography. Given the significant relationship to smoking, smoking cessation is the most logical first step. Corticosteroids have reportedly been quite beneficial.

**Bronchiolotis obliterans with organizing pneumonia (BOOP)** combines features of classical bronchiolitis combined with interstitial inflammation and produces a restrictive impairment in contrast to pure bronchiolitis. Alveolar edema and inflammatory cellular infiltration follow a lung injury with necrosis of alveolar epithelia, alveolar ducts, and bronchioles. Fibroblasts and myofibroblasts then migrate into the alveoli, proliferate, and secrete type II collagen and fibronectin. Intraluminal fibroblastic plugs ("Masson bodies") form and foamy macrophages collect in the airspaces. Ultimately, proliferating bronchiolar cells and type 2 pneumocytes return these fibroblastic plugs to the lung interstitium, where they resolve by unknown mechanisms. While BOOP occurs in a variety of conditions (hypersensitivity pneumonitis, collagen-vascular disorders, vasculitis, infections, and drug exposure), the **essential aspects** of BOOP are **histology** (proliferative bronchiolitis), **exclusivity** (no other primary entity), and **intensity** (involvement of a majority of alveoli and bronchioles). The disease commonly occurs in the sixth or the seventh decade, with no apparent relationship to smoking. Symptoms often last longer than 2–3 months. An antecedent flu-like illness occurs in nearly one-third of the cases; the onset is subacute, with a dry, persistent cough and progressive dyspnea. Fever, malaise, and weight loss may each be noted in one-half of cases. Tachypnea and rales may be noted. Wheezing is rare and clubbing is absent. Pulmonary function tests commonly show a restrictive impairment with hypoxemia. Chest x-rays show diffuse, bilateral, patchy peripheral alveolar opacities while CT shows patchy, peripheral, lower-zone airspace shadows, small nodular densities, and bronchial wall thickening. BOOP should be considered in any patient who presents with an undiagnosed, subacute respiratory illness. An open lung biopsy is generally needed. Corticosteroids confer a 65–80% response with the best response seen in idiopathic BOOP. Prednisone (1–1.5 mg/kg) is started and continued for 2–3 months; whether smaller doses might suffice is not known. If the response is satisfactory, the dose is reduced over the next several months to 0.5–1 mg/kg and gradually tapered over a year. If the response is inadequate, cyclophosphamide may be added.

# CHAPTER 230 CYSTIC FIBROSIS AND BRONCHIECTASIS

## Cystic Fibrosis

Cystic fibrosis (CF) is a common, fatal genetic (autosomal recessive) disorder characterized by chronic sinopulmonary infection, exocrine pancreatic insufficiency, and airway obstruction. A heterozygous state for CF is said to be present among 2–5% of Caucasians. 70% of cases of CF are diagnosed by one year of age. Pulmonary problems in CF account for most of the morbidity and almost all the premature deaths. (Malabsorption and exocrine pancreatic deficiency are discussed in chapter 103.)

### Pathology and Pathogenesis

Approximately 70% of CF arises from a genetic mutation—deletion of three base pairs causing a phenylalanine deletion at F508 locus (ÄF508) on the CF gene, located in the long arm of chromosome 7. This gene encodes for a protein, **cystic fibrosis transmembrane conductance regulator** (CFTR). The defective gene produces a defective protein, which interferes with normal chloride ion permeability, causing intracellular entrapment of chloride ions. The chloride and sodium ions osmotically draw water from the airway mucus, causing its dehydration, inspissation, viscidity, and tenaciousness; glandular ducts are obstructed, bacteria are trapped, and infection results. Bacterial proteases and leukocyte elastases cause tissue injury, leading to bronchitis, bronchiolitis, and bronchiectasis, which perpetuate the infection; then the vicious cycle repeats itself. Pulmonary infection, especially by *Pseudomonas* strains, causes most of the morbidity and mortality in CF. The same genetic defect causes elevated sodium and chloride levels in the sweat and saliva. Pancreatic fibrosis is common.

## Clinical Features

The onset is usually in infancy or childhood—for example, intestinal obstruction from **meconium ileus in infancy, and pancreatic insufficiency** (see Chapter 103) by 2 years of age, with bulky, greasy, foul-smelling stools and failure to thrive. In others, **cough, sputum** production, repeated **respiratory infections,** and **asthmatic symptoms** develop and, as the severity of bronchiectasis increases, bloody sputum and frank hemoptysis become frequent. Finger clubbing and nasal polyps are common. Recurrent pneumothoraces or repeated respiratory infections with mucoid *Pseudomonas aeruginosa, Burkholderia cepacia,* or *Staphylococcus aureus* are clues to underlying CF. Infection with *B. cepacia* is a marker of CF severity and is associated with a poor prognosis. Cor pulmonale eventually develops and cardiac or respiratory failure is the usual cause of death. A list of complications of CF is provided in Table 230.1.

## Ancillary Studies

A sweat chloride level exceeding 60 mEq/L (>80 mEq/L in adults) after **pilocarpine iontophoresis** is diagnostic. False positive results can occur in hereditary nephrogenic diabetes insipidus and untreated adrenal insufficiency. Genetic testing can help confirm diagnosis or screen for carriers in first-degree relatives when CF is diagnosed. Pulmonary function testing shows airway obstruction in most cases. Sputum cultures may help antibiotic selection. Chest x-rays show peribronchial thickening, cystic and bullous lesions, and branching linear densities indicative of fluid-filled bronchi. Unresolved pneumonitis, atelectasis, and apical lesions mimicking tuberculosis are frequent.

**TABLE 230.1. Complications of Cystic Fibrosis and Their Frequency**

| Complication | Incidence (%) |
|---|---|
| Pneumothorax (adults) | 17–20 |
| Massive hemoptysis | 8 |
| Intestinal obstruction | 17 |
| Circulating immune complexes | 28–100 |
| Pancreatic insufficiency | 85–90 |
| Gallbladder disorders (stones, cholecystitis) | 50 |
| Biliary cirrhosis | 25 |
| Nasal polyps | 41 |
| Sinusitis | 90 |
| Azoospermia (men) | >95 |
| Systemic amyloidosis | Unknown |

## Prognosis and Management

The individual prognosis varies, but appears to be better for boys and with lack of respiratory symptoms on presentation, and residence in a temperate climate. Survival has been related to the abnormalities in the chest roentgenograms: the worse they are, the poorer the survival rate. However, with medical therapy at specialized centers, the median age of survival has reached 30 years. Thus, CF is no longer strictly a pediatric disease.

Pulmonary infection, airflow obstruction, nutritional failure, pancreatic insufficiency, and psychological issues need to be addressed. Segmental postural drainage with chest clapping should be performed about four times per day. Bronchodilators are indicated when airway obstruction is present. Antibiotics must be given for respiratory infections in full therapeutic doses for 3–4 weeks. Antibiotics and bronchial hygiene may help eradicate staphylococci, but *Pseudomonas aeruginosa* and *Burkholderia cepacia* generally persist. Prophylactic antibiotics are not recommended, however twice-daily aerosolized tobramycin (TOBI) can be used to treat colonization with *Pseudomonas aeruginosa* although the role in acute pneumonia is unclear. Aerosolized, recombinant DNAse I (dornase alfa) has been shown to reduce the number of infectious respiratory exacerbations requiring parenteral antibiotics, hospitalizations, and the frequency of CF-related symptoms.

# Bronchiectasis

Bronchiectasis is a permanent, abnormal dilatation of bronchi with destruction of elastic and muscular layers of their walls. Three varieties have been described: **saccular, tubular,** and **fusiform.** With the availability of antibiotics, its incidence has declined. However, it can be associated with hemoptysis, dyspnea, recurrent infection and airway obstruction.

## Pathology and Pathogenesis

Purulent secretions usually occupy the abnormal bronchial lumen. Dilated bronchial mucous glands, squamous metaplasia of the bronchial epithelium with ulcerations and fibrosis, and destruction of the elastic and muscular layers of the bronchus are the chief pathologic findings. The involved areas may contain extensive bronchial-pulmonary artery anastomoses.

Bronchiectasis may be acquired or congenital. Acquired bronchiectasis may follow an infectious process (*M. tuberculosis*, viruses or other pathogens) or mechanical bronchial obstruction (obstructive). Cystic fibrosis, rheumatoid arthritis, allergic bronchopulmonary aspergillosis and Mycobacterium avium complex (MAC) infection are also associated with bronchiectasis.

**Ciliary dysfunction** (primary ciliary dyskinesia) causes bronchiectasis. All cilia have the same architecture, whether they are in the respiratory epithelium or the flagella of the spermatozoa. Generalized ciliary dysfunction in immotile cilia syndrome (ICS) impairs airway mucus clearance and sperm motility, and bronchiectasis and male infertility follow. Bronchiectasis, infertility, sinusitis, and situs inversus constitute **Kartagener's syndrome.** Situs inversus presumably occurs when embryonic clockwise visceral rotation fails, as a result of the absence of ciliary activity within the archenteron. Bronchiectasis and male infertility also complicate **Young's syndrome** (the epididymal head becomes enlarged, palpable, and obstructed due to inspissated secretions) and cystic fibrosis. Immunodeficiencies, such as **IgG subclass deficiencies,** have also been found to cause bronchiectasis.

## Clinical Features

Cough and abundant mucopurulent or purulent sputum are principal symptoms. In severe cases, a collection of expectorated mucus may settle into three layers: a top mucoid, middle salivary, and bottom layer of purulent debris (Figure 230.1). Other symptoms are recurrent pneumonias involving localized areas and hemoptysis. Finger clubbing, wheezing, and rales that occur throughout inspiration are frequent findings. Lung abscess and empyema may arise as complications, although amyloidosis and brain abscesses are unusual. Sinusitis and otitis are important clues to ciliary disorders.

## Diagnosis

Clinical history and physical examination often suggest the diagnosis. Serum immunoglobulin levels may be low when immunodeficiencies are the underlying etiology. Arterial hypoxemia is common, from ventilation-perfusion mismatch. Chest x-rays are rarely normal; typical findings are increased bronchial markings, "tramline" shadows (parallel lines that resemble tracks of a tram), and cystic areas. High-resolution computed tomography is the best imaging study and has a high degree of sensitivity and specificity; "signet rings" are diagnostic (the hollow, dilated, thick-walled bronchus is the ring, and accompanying pulmonary artery is the signet). Spirometry often shows airways obstruction.

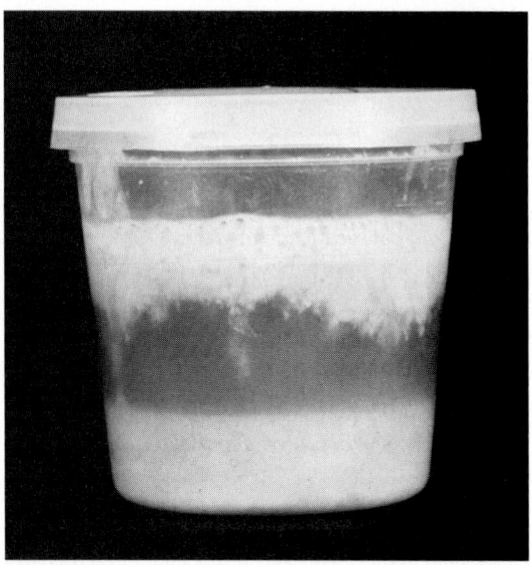

**FIGURE 230.1. Sputum from a patient with bronchiectasis showing the characteristic three layers.**

## Course and Complications

Repeated episodes of pneumonia lead to further worsening of bronchiectasis, creating a vicious cycle. Necrotizing infection may lead to a lung abscess. In the pre-antibiotic era, bronchiectasis often caused brain abscesses; although rare, they still represent a dreaded complication. Bronchial-pulmonary artery anastomoses, which line the bronchiectatic cavities may rupture, causing frequent (and occasionally massive) hemoptysis.

## Management

Dependent postural drainage and chest physiotherapy should be practiced daily, about three to four times if possible, preceding meals. Antibiotics are indicated for respiratory infection. The usual pathogens are *S. pneumoniae* or *Haemophilus influenzae.* Even though cultures may not yield these pathogens, empiric therapy is indicated, similar to that of bacterial infections in COPD (see Treatment of Exacerbations, chapter 228). Prompt therapy and bronchopulmonary hygiene together prevent further bronchial damage. Smoking cessation is essential. Yearly influenza vaccine and pneumococcal vaccine every 5 years are indicated. Severe, localized, disabling disease or severe hemoptysis may require surgery, although its role has dwindled due to the effectiveness of medical management.

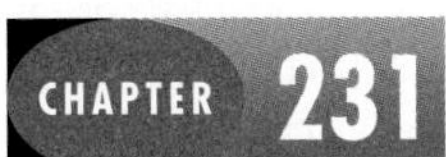

# BRONCHIAL OBSTRUCTION, ATELECTASIS, AND UPPER AIRWAY OBSTRUCTION

## Bronchial Obstruction

Bronchial obstruction may result from intraluminal lesions (e.g., a mucous plug, inhaled foreign body), mural lesions (e.g., benign and malignant neoplasms), and extrinsic compression (e.g., hilar or mediastinal lymph node enlargement, mediastinal tumors, and aortic aneurysms). In these, the manifestations arise from both the primary disease *and* the effects of the obstruction.

Bronchial obstruction most commonly results from a neoplasm, usually a lung cancer. Obstruction of a large bronchus may cause dyspnea, cough, hemoptysis, and focal wheezing. With significant atelectasis, there is ipsilateral mediastinal shift. Obstruction, regardless of cause, may produce localized hyperinflation from air trapping, distal atelectasis, bronchiectasis, and, with distal infection, pneumonia and/or lung abscess. Bronchial obstruction should be suspected when pneumonias resolve slowly or lung abscesses present without apparent risk factors. A cavitating lung cancer and abscess can co-exist. In suspected endobronchial obstruction, bronchoscopy is the most important diagnostic test. Computed tomography alone is not reliable in excluding an endobronchial obstruction. Sputum cytology may be diagnostic in the presence of a proximal endobronchial lung cancer.

## Atelectasis

With complete endobronchial obstruction, absorption of air from the lung distal to the obstruction causes a process known as **absorption atelectasis** (evidenced by ipsilateral mediastinal shifts). Likewise, a pneumothorax or large pleural effusion is called **compression atelectasis** (evidenced by contralateral mediastinal shift). Absorption atelectasis signifies bronchial obstruction and should be managed appropriately.

## Upper Airway Obstruction

### Tracheal Obstruction

Local extension of esophageal or bronchogenic carcinoma into the trachea, impaction of food in the esophagus with compression of the posterior tracheal wall (“cafe coronary”), and tracheal stricture following endotracheal intubation are the common causes of tracheal obstruction. Primary tracheal tumors are rare. Intrathoracic tracheal obstruction causes wheezing. Extrathoracic obstruction (outside the thoracic outlet) leads to stridor. Flow volume curve may be especially useful in identifying tracheal or upper airway disease as a cause of airway obstruction (Figure 231.1). Management of tracheal obstruction is dictated by the acuteness of onset and clinical circumstances. Emergency intubation, rigid

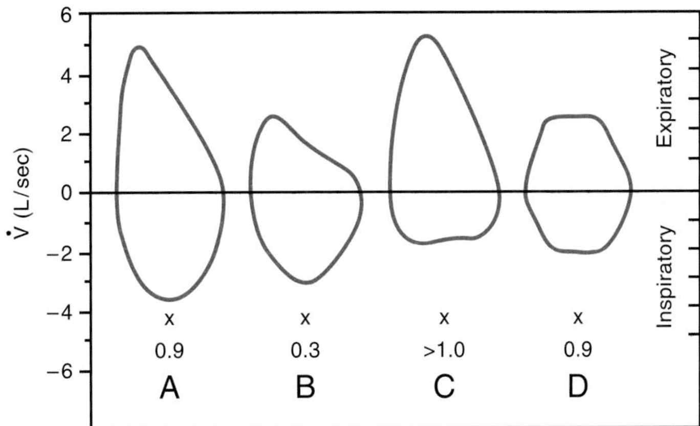


**FIGURE 231.1.** Flow volume loops in airway obstruction. V = flow rate. Numbers below each graph represent ratios of expiratory to inspiratory flow at the mid-vital capacity point (x). A = normal (ratio = 0.9); B = asthma or COPD; C = variable extrathoracic obstruction; D = fixed intrathoracic obstruction. (Note the plateau in the expiratory phase.)

bronchoscopy, tracheostomy, and tracheal stents are options. In suspected upper airway obstruction, fiberoptic bronchoscopy is best avoided. In selected cases, obstruction may be relieved by laser therapy.

### Laryngeal Obstruction

Laryngeal obstruction, characterized by stridor, characteristically occurs when a foreign body, usually food, is inhaled. Other causes are angioneurotic edema, croup, bilateral vocal cord paralysis, laryngeal tumors, laryngospasm, and edema following removal of an endotracheal tube. The victim with impaction of a foreign body in the larynx is unable to cough, speak, or breathe. Heimlich's maneuver (sudden, firm pressure with the fist in the area between the xiphoid and umbilicus) may dislodge the obstruction. Digital extraction of the foreign body may also be attempted. Emergency tracheostomy will be life-saving if other measures fail. In acute laryngeal obstruction due to hereditary angioedema, parenteral epinephrine is the treatment of choice.

# CHAPTER 232 PULMONARY EDEMA

### Definition and Pathogenesis

Pulmonary edema is a pathological state in which the extravascular lung water is increased. The normally small, constant egress of fluid from the microvasculature of the lung into the lung interstitium is removed by the lymphatics of the lung. Pulmonary edema is a dynamic extension of this process, where excessive filtration or excessive permeability of the microvasculature overwhelms the clearance capacity of the lymphatics.

Four major forces (also called **Starling's forces**) govern the transvascular fluid flow: a pair of hydrostatic forces (microvascular and perimicrovascular) and a pair of osmotic forces (microvascular and perimicrovascular). The components of each pair operate in opposite directions (Figure 232.1). Another determinant is the filtration coefficient of the capillary endothelium. The normal orientation of Starling's forces produces a net efflux of fluid from the capillary lumen into the pericapillary interstitial space, estimated to be about 10–20 ml/h, which is then cleared by the lymphatics. The pulmonary capillary endothelium is restrictive in its permeability for various molecules depending on their molecular weights. Its conductivity for fluid itself is low. The permeability of the alveolar epithelium is perhaps even more limited, mainly because of its intricate structure with tight intercellular junctions.

Thus, pulmonary edema may follow excessive fluid filtration (from increased hydrostatic pressure) or increased permeability of the capillary endothelium. Excessive fluid filtration, characterized by elevated left atrial pressures—pulmonary capillary wedge pressure (PCW)—and low protein levels in the edema fluid, is generally due to cardiogenic causes (left ventricular failure, arteriosclerotic heart disease, mitral stenosis, and fluid overload, discussed in chapter 37). Adult respiratory distress syndrome (chapter 256), drug-induced pulmonary edema, neurogenic pulmonary edema, and perhaps high altitude pulmonary edema all result from increased capillary permeability. Not only is the left atrial pressure normal or even low, but the edema fluid protein is high.

In early pulmonary edema, the excess fluid accumulates around the pulmonary capillaries accompanying the bronchiole, forming a perivascular and peribronchial fluid cuff. As the fluid accumulates, it raises the pressure in this cuff, and begins to leak into the alveoli at the bronchoalveolar junction. Lung compliance decreases

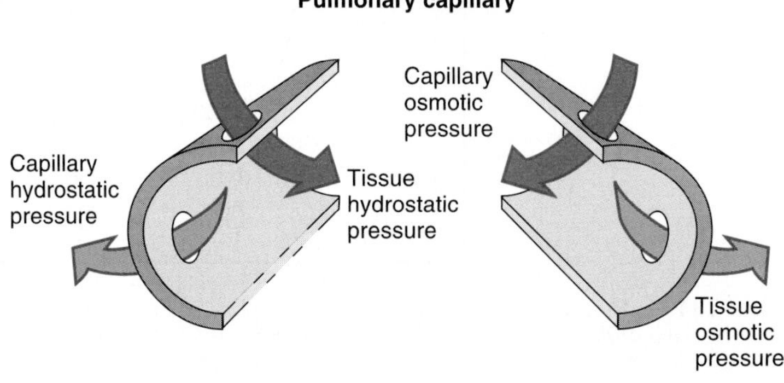


**FIGURE 232.1.** Starling's forces govern the transvascular fluid flow: the pair of hydrostatic forces (microvascular and perimicrovascular, operate against a pair of osmotic forces (microvascular and perimicrovascular). The hydrostatic and osmotic forces within the same compartment are also oriented in the opposite directions.

and, with the flooding of the alveoli, the work of breathing (i.e., the oxygen cost of breathing) rises profoundly; gas exchange is severely disturbed and respiratory distress becomes manifest.

### *Drug-induced Pulmonary Edema*

Opiates (most classically heroin) are the best-known drugs that cause pulmonary edema. Pulmonary edema with miotic pupils is typical, especially when the patient has a background of drug abuse. Enhanced capillary permeability from hypoxia, contaminants (in the heroin), or histamine released by opiates is the alleged mechanism. Naloxone (0.4 mg IV q 3–5 min) is the specific antidote for opiate intoxication. Respiratory failure and pulmonary edema may require endotracheal intubation. Drug screens of urine and blood are useful since multiple drug poisonings are quite common. Other less well-known drugs and chemicals that may cause pulmonary edema are salicylates, ethchlorvynol (refer to Figure 256.2), nitrofurantoin, propranolol, radiographic contrast media, paraquat, cyanide, and blood transfusions.

# CHAPTER 233 PULMONARY THROMBOEMBOLISM

Pulmonary embolism (PE) is not a disease in itself, but a complication of a thrombotic process elsewhere, usually a lower extremity **(ileofemoral)** deep vein thrombosis (DVT). Since PE and DVT are but two sides of the same coin, and the basic therapy for both are similar, they are jointly referred to as **venous thromboembolism** (VTE).

## Pathogenesis

The factors that predispose to VTE are summarized in Table 233.1. VTE without predisposing factors is considered idiopathic. In conditions with a proclivity for thrombosis—**thrombophilia**—examples of which include genetic mutations and deficiencies of anti-thrombin III, protein S, and protein C, the thrombotic process tends to be recurrent. Cancer has had an established relationship to VTE; in instances of cancer-related VTE, the thromboembolism might precede, accompany, or follow a neoplasm. Patients with idiopathic and recurrent VTE appear most likely to exemplify a risk of subsequent neoplasm. Cancer-related VTE is highly complex and is due to a hypercoagulable state (from products of cell-tumor cell interaction), from inadequate fibrinolysis (release of tumor-derived clotting factors), or from venous stasis (e.g., venous obstruction from a tumor).

## Pathophysiology

The sequelae of pulmonary embolism depend upon the extent of obstruction and the previous state of the cardiopulmonary system. Obstruction of the main pulmonary artery, generally at its bifurcation, may be lethal whether or not it is preceded by shock. In massive

**TABLE 233.1. Predisposing Factors for Venous Thromboembolism**

| Genetic (Inherited) Factors | Acquired Factors |
|---|---|
| • G1691A mutation in Factor V gene<br>• G20210A mutation in the Factor II gene<br>• Homozygous C677T mutation in the MTHFR gene<br>• Antithrombin III deficiency<br>• Protein C deficiency<br>• Protein S deficiency | • Immobilization (fracture with cast, prolonged travel, prolonged bed rest from stroke, respiratory failure, paraplegia, etc.)<br>• Postoperative states (hip, prostate, abdominal/thoracic surgery)<br>• Trauma<br>• Increasing age<br>• Malignancy<br>• Previous thrombosis<br>• Pregnancy and post-partum state<br>• Hormone therapy#<br>• Antiphospholipid antibodies<br>• Hyperhomocystinemia (e.g., due to cobalamin deficiency)<br>• Obesity<br>• Peripheral vascular disease (sluggish blood flow)<br>• Myocardial infarction* |

*Where anticoagulant therapy is not given; # = including oral contraceptives; MTHFR: methylenetetrahydrofolate reductase.

**TABLE 233.2. Pulmonary Embolism with Previously Normal Cardiopulmonary System: Classification of Severity**

| Extent of Occlusion | $\overline{PA}$ | RAP | CO | Clinical Correlates |
|---|---|---|---|---|
| <50% | <20 | <10 | Maintained | Usually not lethal if no other disease. |
| 50–75% | 25–40 | <10 | Usually maintained | Submassive embolism; clot fragments and migrates distally; reducing cross-sectional obstruction; survival depends on this |
| >75% | >40 | >10 | Decreased | Massive embolism; acute right ventricular failure; lethal unless treated; shock may or may not precede death |

$\overline{PA}$ = PA mean pressure; RAP = right atrial pressure; CO = cardiac output.

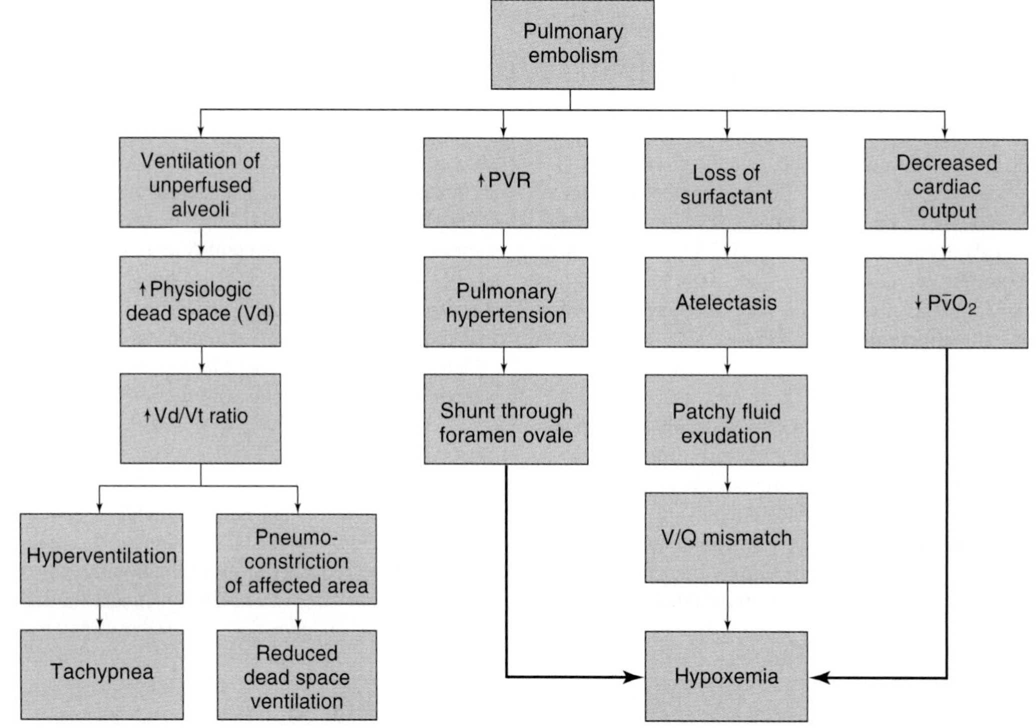


**FIGURE 233.1. Physiologic disturbances in pulmonary embolism. PVR = pulmonary vascular resistance; Vd = dead space; Vt = tidal volume; P$\bar{v}O_2$ = mixed venous oxygen tension.**

embolism the right ventricle must maintain a mean pressure above 40 mm Hg to sustain forward blood flow. A previously normal right ventricle (i.e., no cardiopulmonary disease) is not able to generate such levels of pressure and thus fails. Acute cor pulmonale and shock follow (Table 233.2).

The physiologic consequences of pulmonary embolism are shown in Figure 233.1. Pulmonary vascular resistance rises, with the extent of rise depending on the magnitude of vascular obstruction, vaso-active agents released from the clot itself, prior cardiopulmonary disease, and perhaps reflex events. Hypoxemia has many causes (atelectasis, shunting, perfusion of unventilated alveoli, the severe desaturation of mixed venous blood from decreased cardiac output, etc.). Fragmentation and mechanical reshaping of an embolized clot, and endogenous fibrinolysis help restore pulmonary blood flow; these bring forth the initial improvement seen in some cases of massive PE. Clot resolution is highly variable and totally fails in 0.5–12% of all cases. Large emboli (occlusion >35% on a perfusion lung scan), coexistent heart disease, and simultaneous, clinically apparent DVT all promote recurrent PE and predispose to poor clot resolution.

Pulmonary infarction (necrosis of lung tissue), an uncommon sequel of PE (5–10% of cases), results from peripheral, rather than central embolism. Because infarction requires total cessation of blood flow from both the bronchial and pulmonary artery circulations, pulmonary infarction generally indicates cardiopulmonary disease and/or diseased bronchial circulation. Congestive atelectasis mimics pulmonary infarction clinically and radiographically, except for the quick and complete resolution and the lack of tissue necrosis.

## Clinical Features

In many cases of PE, a predisposing factor to DVT is identifiable in the history. Despite the many symptoms and signs (Table 233.3), PE has three broad patterns of presentation: **acute cor pulmonale**, **unexplained dyspnea**, and **acute pulmonary infarction**. In acute cor pulmonale, which implies massive PE, acute dyspnea occurs with or without associated chest pain, and the patient's clinical status suddenly deteriorates, and sudden death may even result. Findings include hypotension, shock, pulmonary hypertension (right ventricular heave, loud $P_2$ [pulmonary valve closure], right-sided third or fourth heart sound), and significantly elevated right-sided pressures on cardiac catheterization. The second pattern (unexplained dyspnea) may be confused with worsening of pre-existent heart failure or lung disease in persons with these conditions. In contrast, hemoptysis and pleuritic chest pain herald the (more dramatic) presentation of pulmonary infarction. Physical examination discloses fever, splinting of the chest wall, ipsilateral consolidation, and pleural effusion. Pleural friction rub is often heard, at least early in the illness.

**TABLE 233.3. Symptoms and Signs of Pulmonary Embolism**

| Symptom | Incidence (%) |
|---|---|
| Pleuritic pain | 74 |
| Dyspnea | 85 |
| Apprehension | 59 |
| Cough | 53 |
| Hemoptysis | 30 |
| Chest pain | 14 |
| Syncope | 13 |
| **Sign** | **Incidence (%)** |
| Tachypnea | 92 |
| Rales | 58 |
| Increased $P_2$ | 53 |
| Tachycardia | 44 |
| Fever | 43 |
| Diaphoresis | 33 |
| Gallop | 34 |
| Phlebitis | 32 |
| Edema | 24 |
| Cyanosis | 19 |

(From Bell WR, Simon TL, DeMets DL. Am J Med 1977; 62:355–360.)

## Ancillary Studies

Leukocytosis is common, but it seldom exceeds 15,000/mm$^3$. In most cases, besides sinus tachycardia, an electrocardiogram (ECG) reveals no unique features and primarily helps exclude a myocardial infarction. Arrhythmias, such as atrial flutter and fibrillation, and varying degrees of A-V block, may be demonstrated. Massive embolism may be associated with P pulmonale, S in lead I, and a Q with T wave inversion in lead III (the so-called $S_1$–$Q_3$–$T_3$ pattern). Changes from the previous ECG (e.g., a change in axis) are more important. Hypoxemia and hyperventilation-induced hypocapnia are common, neither being specific for pulmonary embolism. In patients without prior cardiopulmonary disease, the extent of hypoxemia correlates well with the severity of embolism. $PaO_2$ above 85 mm Hg with the patient breathing room air makes pulmonary embolism less likely, but does not exclude it.

As thrombus formation continues, the cross-linked fibrin within the clot undergoes proteolysis by plasmin, thus leading to the release of **D-dimer** into the peripheral blood. This specific degradation product may be detected through various assays—latex agglutination, enzyme-linked immunosorbent assay (ELISA), or whole blood agglutination. ELISA assay has a high sensitivity, but low specificity for VTE. The latex test is much less sensitive than the ELISA. The whole blood agglutination method is easy, very rapid and reliable, can be performed at the bedside using a drop of whole blood, and depends on the use of a specific antibody with epitopes that are portions of D-dimer and red blood cells (RBC). With a high D-dimer level, the antibody agglutinates the patient's RBC. False positive tests follow recent surgery, trauma, stroke, acute myocardial infarction, disseminated intravascular coagulation, pregnancy or recent (10 days) delivery, metastatic cancer, or collagen vascular disease. These being common predisposing factors for VTE, they limit the potential usefulness of the test in confirming VTE; rather, the usefulness of the test lies in its high negative predictive value for VTE.

Pleural effusions accompanying pulmonary embolism show a wide range of features and may be transudates or exudates. In pulmonary infarction, the fluid is almost always an exudate and tends to be bloody or blood-stained, resolving with time. Lack of resolution or an intercurrent increase in size denotes coincident complications such as infection, reinfarction, or with other supporting evidence, heart failure.

**Imaging studies**

Chest roentgenograms, which are generally normal, primarily help exclude other conditions that can produce a similar picture (heart failure or pneumothorax). Pulmonary infarction classically shows a wedge-shaped opacity with ipsilateral pleural effusion. Effusions may occur without apparent infiltrate and are generally unilateral. The chest radiograph can also be very helpful in deciding on the exact imaging approach (see below).

Perfusion (Q) scanning using technetium macroaggregated ($^{99}$mTc) albumin is a very sensitive test and, thus, remains the mainstay of pulmonary embolism diagnosis. A normal six-view lung **perfusion** scan ("negative" scan) excludes clinically significant pulmonary embolism. However, not all positive scans indicate pulmonary emboli. In obstructive airway disease, atelectasis, bullae, heart failure, lung cancer, and respiratory failure, perfusion defects are usual. A ventilation (V) scanning can then augment the accuracy of perfusion scans. Perfusion defects with normal ventilation are **mismatched defects** and are the hallmark of pulmonary embolism (Figure 233.2). Perfusion defects with ventilation anomalies in the same area are **matched defects**, which portend a nonembolic disorder (e.g., heart failure, obstructive airway disease, etc). Large (segmental or larger), mismatched defects correlate well, and subsegmental defects, matched or mismatched, correlate poorly, with pulmonary embolism. The criteria for probability estimates of pulmonary embolism based on V/Q scanning vary, but a generally accepted set is shown in Table 233.4. V/Q scans are much more useful when integrated into the context of clinical probability of PE rather than interpreted on their own.

*Pulmonary Angiography*

Pulmonary angiography is the "gold standard" for the diagnosis of pulmonary embolism. It is invasive and may not be readily available in all institutions; even when available, its application may be precluded by several patient factors, or technical factors may severely limit the information it can provide. The indications for pulmonary angiography (arteriography) in the setting of pulmonary embolism are summarized in Table 233.5.

The diagnostic findings are intraluminal filling defects and vessel cut-offs (Figure 233.3). Other findings such as localized avascularity or sluggish blood flow are not diagnostic. In experienced hands, pulmonary angiography is safe, with a mortality and morbidity less than 0.5% and 1%, respectively.

*Computed Tomography and Magnetic Resonance Imaging*

Both helical (spiral) CT and MRI are sensitive imaging techniques that have a high specificity for VTE. CT scan requires iodinated contrast use (which places CT in a category similar to angiography); but the MRI does not; neither has the ability to measure pulmonary hemodynamic data. Both techniques are very reliable for diagnosing centrally located (proximal) pulmonary emboli (sensitivity and specificity of 94% or higher for proximal PE), but their ability to detect small, peripherally located emboli still remains a limitation (between 53% to 80% sensitive and about 95% specific). Artifacts related to motion of lungs and chest wall, and interobserver differences in interpretation could cause problems. Both CT and MRI offer the ability to image the lower extremity veins (see below) for DVT.

V/Q scans are most reliable when the chest radiograph shows normal lung fields, *and* when underlying lung disease is absent. If the radiograph shows significant abnormalities (infiltrate, pleural effusion, etc.), the reliability of the V/Q scan is significantly compromised. Helical CT or MRI become better diagnostic studies in such cases.

*Diagnosis of Deep Vein Thrombosis as a Surrogate Marker for Pulmonary Embolism*

PE is almost always a consequence of DVT, and treatments for isolated DVT and for PE without shock are generally identical. Thus, documented DVT in a patient with a compatible picture for PE supports the diagnosis of pulmonary embolism. Contrast venogram is the "gold standard," but other noninvasive tests such as impedance plethysmography (IPG) and B-mode (real-time) ultrasonography are excellent for diagnosing DVT (Table 233.6) in symptomatic patients. In most centers, B-mode ultrasonography has superseded IPG. The acoustic Doppler test is commonly combined with B-mode ultrasonography (duplex imaging). Lack of compressibility of the vein, and to a lesser extent, internal echoes from within it are diagnostic. The major drawback of duplex imaging is its less-than-ideal ability to detect small thrombi in the calf veins; also, conditions that preclude direct compression of the vein render it useless.

## Diagnosis

Many different algorithms are available for diagnosing or excluding pulmonary embolism, but none has universal appeal. Although the strength of clinical suspicion and the patient's condition dictate one's approach to suspected pulmonary embolism, the clinician must consider the following:

- What is the patient's condition (e.g., stable or life-threatening)?
- What is the clinical probability of pulmonary embolism (e.g., high, low, intermediate)?
- Is there underlying cardiopulmonary disease?
- Is the chest radiograph normal or abnormal?

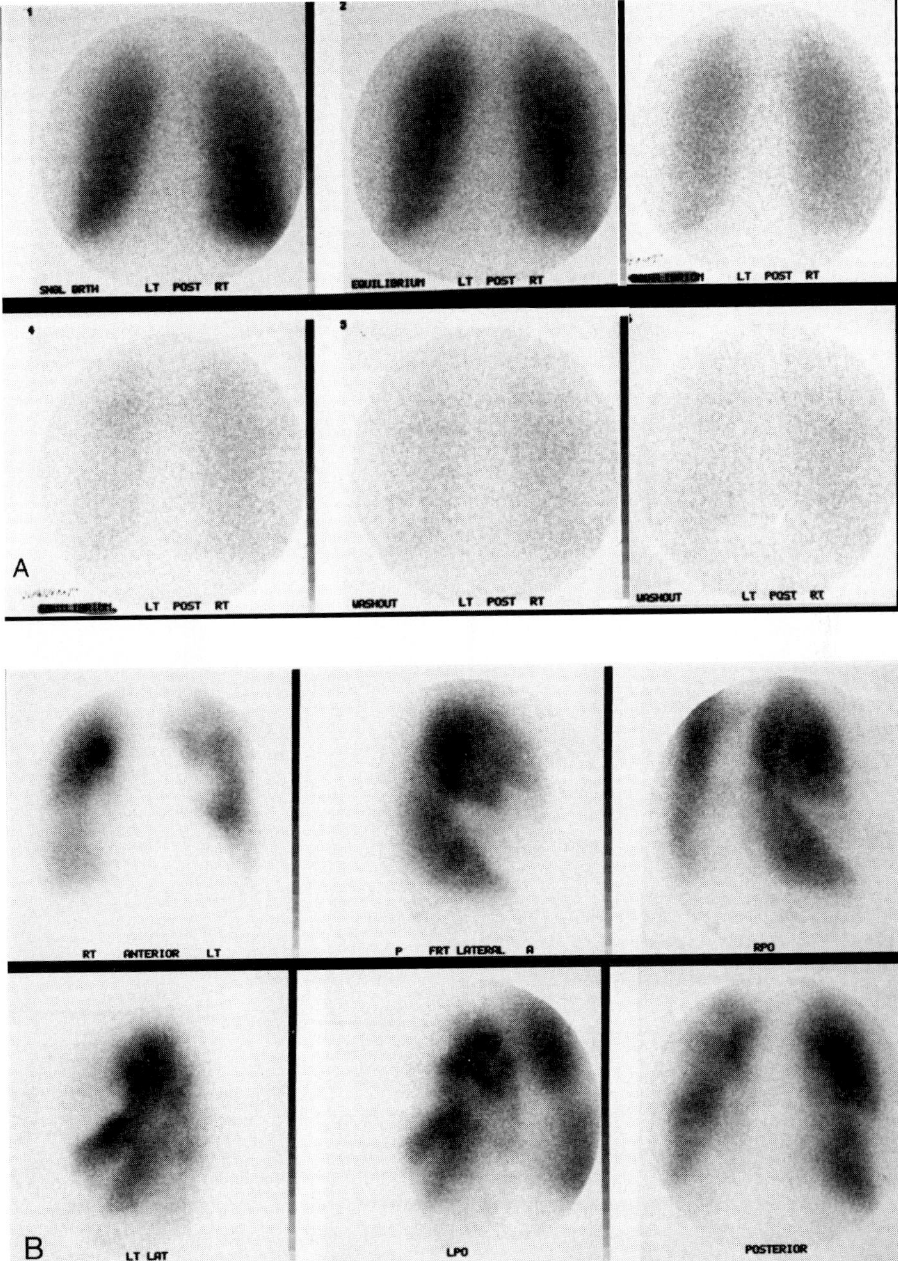


**FIGURE 233.2. A. Pulmonary embolism: normal ventilation scan. B. Pulmonary embolism: perfusion scan showing perfusion defects. These are mismatched defects, which together with A constitute a high-probability lung scan.**

- Are there barriers to effective imaging (e.g., morbid obesity and/or claustrophobia [affects CT/MRI], entire lower extremity in a cast [affects leg studies with ultrasound], contrast allergy [affects contrast CT], etc.)?
- What is the result of the ELISA D-dimer test (positive/negative if using SimplyRED)?
- Are there local conditions that compromise the diagnostic strategy (lack of access to various imaging techniques, tests etc.)?

**TABLE 233.4. Probability of Pulmonary Embolism Based on Ventilation-Perfusion Scan Patterns**

| Probability | Perfusion Scan Abnormality | Mismatch | Match | Frequency of Pulmonary Embolism (%) |
|---|---|---|---|---|
| High | One or more segmental or greater defects | + | | 86 |
| Intermediate | One or more segmental or greater defects | | + | 36 |
| | One or more subsegmental defects | + | | 40 |
| Low | One or more subsegmental defects | | + | 25 |
| Indeterminate | Perfusion defect with chest x-ray abnormality corresponding to the perfusion defect | | | 21 |

(Adapted from Hull RD et al: Chest 1985; 88:819–828.)

**TABLE 233.5. Indications for Pulmonary Angiography in Suspected Pulmonary Embolism (PE)**

Any of the following, where:
1. V/Q scans are unreliable for definitive diagnosis:
   - Co-existent lung disease
   - Heart failure
   - Respiratory failure
2. Diagnosis is emergent or where pulmonary embolectomy or fibrinolytic therapy or pulmonary endarterectomy are active considerations:
   - Shock with suspected massive pulmonary embolization
   - Chronic pulmonary embolism, prior to thromboendarterectomy
3. Substantial risk from anticoagulation obligates a positive diagnosis:
   - Bleeding diathesis
   - Recent stroke
   - Active/potential for active internal bleeding
4. One needs to differentiate PE from other conditions that cause similar picture:
   - Distinction between pneumonia and pulmonary infarction
5. Inferior vena caval interruption is being considered for recurrent PE.

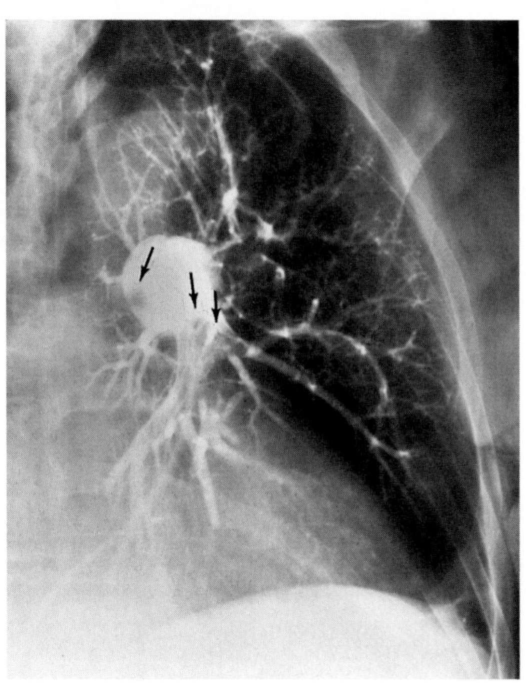

**FIGURE 233.3.** Pulmonary angiogram in a patient showing intraluminal filling defects (arrow).

- Are there contraindications to anticoagulation?
- Any previous episodes of documented venous thromboembolism?

Given the need for rapid and accurate diagnosis in hemodynamically unstable patients, pulmonary angiography or helical CT with contrast (CCT) should follow initial stabilization and, unless contraindicated, loading dose of IV heparin.

Using a point-scoring system (Table 233.7), Canadian investigators have designed a step-wise and simpler approach to diagnose PE in more stable patients: through a history, physical examination, chest radiography, oxygenation studies, and ECG, the pre-test probability of PE is assessed. PE is then confirmed or excluded by integrating results from whole blood D-dimer assay, V/Q scan, and real-time leg ultrasound, (Figure 233.4). For example, with a low clinical probability and non-detectable D-dimer, PE is excluded. Similarly, PE is diagnosed by a high probability V/Q scan in the setting of moderate or high clinical suspicion, or a non-high probability scan when the leg ultrasound is also positive. Between these two extremes, a myriad of possibilities is resolved by integrating the results of the D-dimer test, leg ultrasound, and pulmonary angiogram. As further clinical testing refines this algorithm, the exact roles of helical CT or MRI should become better defined. Helical CT or MRI appear to be maximally useful when

TABLE 233.6. Studies to Detect Deep Vein Thrombosis: Sensitivity, Specificity, Advantages, and Disadvantages

| Method | Sensitivity (%) | Specificity (%) | Advantages | Disadvantages |
|---|---|---|---|---|
| Contrast venogram | 90 | 100 | Visualizes the entire deep vein system and the pelvic and iliac veins and possibly, inferior vena cava; generally easily available; "gold standard" | Not well suited for repetitive use in the same patient<br>Dye allergy is a contraindication<br>Expensive |
| IPG | 95 (range, 87–100) | 95 (range, 92–100) | Noninvasive; highly reliable | Conditions with reduced arterial inflow or reduced venous outflow of blood cause false-positive tests<br>Facilities may not be available everywhere<br>Technical factors may cause false-positive and false-negative results |
| Venous (acoustic) Doppler | 77 | 50–60 for proximal DVT | More reliable than IPG in patients with peripheral vascular disease, congestive heart failure or limbs in plaster casts | Very operator dependent<br>Reliable graphic reproduction is not possible |
| Real time ultrasound (Duplex imaging) | 100 for proximal DVT | 99 for proximal DVT | Effective and accurate<br>Results most reliable for veins above the thigh<br>Can diagnose other conditions causing symptoms such as Baker's cyst | Results not reliable for isolated DVT in pelvic veins, or femoral vein in the adductor canal<br>Much less reliable for calf veins |

For helical CT and MRI, see text. DVT = deep vein thrombosis; IPG = impedance plethysmography.

TABLE 233.7. Estimating the Pre-Test Probability of Pulmonary Embolism

| Criteria | Points |
|---|---|
| Clinical signs/symptoms for DVT* | 3.0 |
| Heart rate >100/min | 1.5 |
| Immobilization# or surgery in the previous 4 weeks | 1.5 |
| Previous objectively diagnosed DVT/PE | 1.5 |
| Hemoptysis | 1.0 |
| Malignancy@ | 1.0 |
| Pulmonary embolism as likely or more likely than an alternative diagnosis† | 3.0 |

Total score <2 = low probability; 2–6 = intermediate probability; >6 = high probability.

(Adapted from: Wells, PS, et al. Ann Intern Med 2001; 135:99.)

*Objectively measured leg swelling and pain on palpation in the deep vein region

#Bedrest, except to access the bathroom for 3 or more consecutive days

@Cancer under therapy or palliative care, or treatment stopped within the past 6 months

†Using clinical information, chest x-ray and blood tests necessary to diagnose pulmonary embolism

the chest radiograph is abnormal or significant cardiopulmonary disease is present.

## Management

### Heparin and oral anticoagulants

Heparin, the mainstay of treatment of VTE, is available as unfractionated heparin (UFH) or as low molecular weight heparin (LMWH). Unless contraindicated, for suspected massive or submassive embolization a loading dose of 80units/kg units of heparin is given IV, followed by continuous IV infusion (15–20 units/kg/h) until and after the diagnosis is confirmed. Activated partial thromboplastin time (aPTT) is measured once before and repeated every 4–6 hours for the first 24 hours, the goal being its prolongation by two to two-and-a-half times above baseline (Table 233.8). Platelet count is measured initially and daily thereafter to detect any thrombocytopenia from heparin.

Although UFH is a very effective antithrombotic agent, it has many limitations: because of its binding to many different proteins, its bioavailability is low, and thus, it has to be administered continuously and intravenously, with frequent monitoring and adjustment of dose. Failure to achieve and maintain an adequate anticoagulation (aPTT of 55 sec) within the first 72 hours is followed by an enhanced risk of recurrence. UFH binds to platelet factor 4 (PF4) forming a UFH-PF4 complex, which leads to further release of PF4, and further binding of platelets to the UFH-PF4 complex leads to heparin-induced thrombocytopenia with thrombosis (HITT). LMWH, on the other hand, are 4000 to 6000 dalton molecules, synthesized by depolymerization of UFH. LMWH has a better bioavailability and longer half-life, and thus can be given by intermittent dosing. They are absorbed well after subcutaneous administration; thus IV route is not needed. They bind less to platelets and thus have less propensity for bleeding. Monitoring by aPTT is not required. Given their longer half-life, and absorption after subcutaneous administration, LMWH are well suited for outpatient therapy of DVT. The best known LMWH in the U.S. are enoxaparin and dalteparin. Both have been used in treating DVT; at present, only enoxaparin is FDA-approved for use in pulmonary embolism.

Regardless of whether one uses UFH or LMWH, warfarin, 5 mg, is begun on the first day of therapy, and its dose adjusted to produce an international normalized ratio (INR) of 2.0–3.0. Heparin is discontinued when satisfactory INR is reached; warfarin alone is then continued. Anticoagulant therapy merely inhibits further thrombosis; established clots or emboli are lysed by endogenous

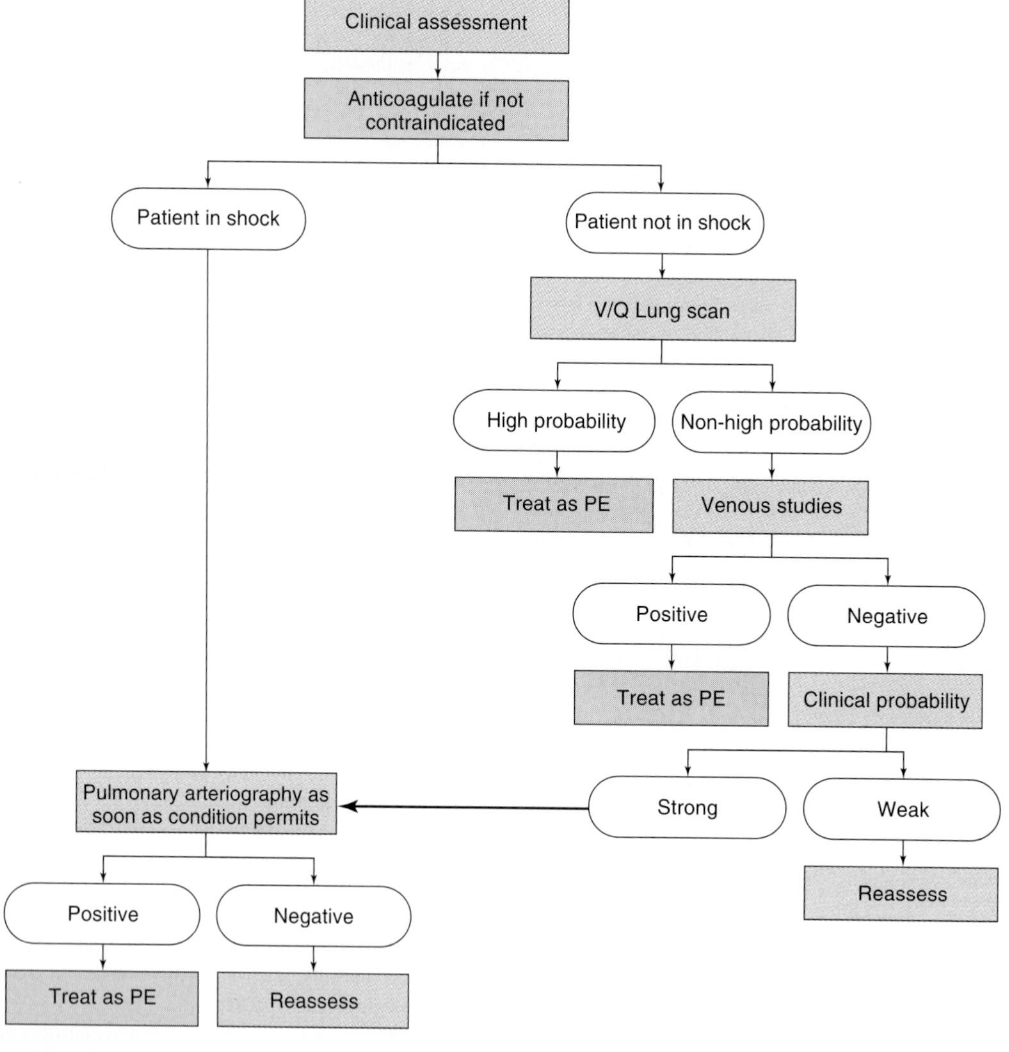


**FIGURE 233.4.** Suggested approach to the patient with suspected pulmonary embolism (PE). Rectangular boxes represent interventions/actions; boxes with rounded corners represent conditions.

TABLE 233.8. Weight-Based Nomogram for Heparin Therapy

**Unfractionated Heparin (UFH)**

| | APTT Sec/(x C*) | Bolus (U/Kg) | Basic Infusion Rate (U/Kg/h) | ↑ Basic by (U/Kg/h) | ↓ Basic by (U/Kg/h) |
|---|---|---|---|---|---|
| Initial | — | 80 | 18 | — | — |
| Subsequent | <35/<1.2 | 80 | Same | 4 | — |
| | 35–45/1.2–1.5 | 40 | Same | 2 | — |
| | 46–70/1.5–2.3 | — | Same | — | — |
| | 71–90/2.3–3.0 | — | Same | — | 2 |
| | >90/>3.0 | — | Hold 1h | | 3† |

**Low Molecular Weight Heparin (LMWH)**

| Agent | Dose/SD Max | Route | Frequency | Trade Name |
|---|---|---|---|---|
| Dalteparin sodium | 200 U **/Kg single dose NTE 8000 U | SC | qd | Fragmin |
| Enoxaparin sodium | 1 mg/kg/180 mg<br>1.5 mg/kg/180 mg | SC | q12h | Lovenox |
| Tinzaparin sodium | 175 U**/Kg | SC | qd | Innohep |
| Nadroparin calcium | 86 U/kg | SC | q12h/bid | Fraxiparine |

Bid = twice daily; *C = control APTT rate; SD Max = maximum single dose; † = when resumed; ** = anti-Xa units.
(Adapted from Hirsh J et al. Chest 1995; 108:262S. Used with permission.)

mechanisms. The exact duration of warfarin treatment, while subject to debate, generally is about 6 months following the initial episode of VTE (Table 233.9).

*Use of the International Normalized Ratio*

The prothrombin test (PT) reflects the level of factors II, VII, and X. The time taken to clot a citrated plasma sample using thromboplastins and calcium is measured (PT) and compared against a standard, yielding a PT ratio. PT depends on the intensity with which factor X activates factor VII, and the responsiveness of the thromboplastin. A sensitive thromboplastin causes less stimulation of factor X, and thus a lower PT; an unresponsive thromboplastin does the opposite. Because commercial thromboplastins vary in sensitivity, the same plasma sample may yield many PT values depending on the thromboplastin used. INR represents normalization of these values using an international reference. INR values may be calculated from a nomogram. The effective INR varies for different clinical conditions, but for VTE, the objective is an INR between 2.0 to 3.0.

TABLE 233.9. Duration of Oral Anticoagulation by Risk of Recurrence

| Risk Group | Duration |
|---|---|
| First event, reversible risk factor**, age ≤60 | 3–6 months |
| First event, reversible risk factor, age ≥60 or first event with idiopathic disease | 6–12 months |
| Recurrent event, or first event with a non-reversible risk factor, such as cancer, inhibitor deficiency, antiphospholipid syndrome, or homozygous activated protein C resistance | 12 months to lifetime |

** examples are surgery, trauma or transient immobility

**Thrombolytic therapy**

Emboli resolve faster and hemodynamic instability reverses quicker with thrombolytic agents in massive and submassive pulmonary embolism. It is uncertain whether they improve mortality. Early restoration of venous patency, early alleviation of the discomfort and pain, and, theoretically, less damage to the venous valves follow the use of thrombolytic agents in DVT. However, no evidence exists for long-term benefits or a reduction in the incidence of post-phlebitic syndrome (an indicator of venous valve damage) with these agents.Thrombolytic agents are mainly indicated in patients with no bleeding disturbance and an established diagnosis of either a large proximal DVT, or PE accompanied by shock. Active internal or intracranial bleeding, stroke within the preceding 2 months, or any other active intracranial process are absolute contraindications. Others include recent major surgery, recent gastrointestinal bleeding, and severe arterial hypertension. Careful dose monitoring and meticulous avoidance of any but absolutely essential invasive procedures are essential. If such procedures are performed, proper hemostasis should be secured. Available agents are streptokinase and recombinant tissue plasminogen activator.

**Embolectomy and inferior vena caval interruption**

If there is refractory shock, if massive or submassive emboli are angiographically demonstrable, and if proper facilities are available, emergency pulmonary embolectomy is an option. The procedure itself carries a high mortality. Clots may also be successfully removed using a specially devised suction catheter advanced into the pulmonary circulation. A variety of devices are available (Greenfield stainless steel vena caval filter, titanium Greenfield filter, and the bird's nest filter) to interrupt clots in the inferior vena cava (IVC), without affecting the blood flow. The indications for IVC interruption are listed in Table 233.9.

## Venous Thromboembolism and Pregnancy

Pregnancy is characterized by both hypercoagulability and venous stasis. Thus, VTE commonly complicates pregnancy, especially in the second trimester. The left leg has a severe susceptibility to DVT because of the longer couse of the left iliac vein. A clearly favored site is the ileofemoral vein. It appears that a significant number of patients who develop VTE during pregnancy and puerperium might harbor hereditary thrombophilias. It is uncertain whether women with VTE during one pregnancy have a higher risk of developing VTE during subsequent pregnancies. The risk to the mother continues postpartum, with the risk of VTE being higher after Caesarian section rather than after normal delivery. The accuracy of clinical diagnosis of VTE in pregnancy is low—only 10% for DVT in one study and 4% for PE. Thus, DVT during pregnancy should be unequivocally confirmed before treatment. The initial study may be duplex imaging or IPG. Anticoagulation can follow a positive study if the pregnancy is within the first or second trimester. A positive study during the third trimester should be confirmed by a limited venogram; if it is not confirmatory, then a complete study should follow. If IPG or duplex ultrasound is unavailable, a limited venogram will suffice; if it fails to confirm DVT, then a complete venogram should be performed.

For suspected PE during pregnancy, a chest x-ray and a V/Q scan are appropriate initial tests. A normal V/Q scan excludes PE. When clinical suspicion is strong, a high probability scan is sufficient indication for anticoagulation. A non-high probability scan requires additional studies, such as IPG or duplex imaging. When DVT is thus confirmed, anticoagulation can follow. With strong clinical suspicion, negative IPG/duplex imaging, and a non-high probability scan, a pulmonary angiogram with appropriate shielding of pelvis and abdomen is the next step.

Heparin is the drug of choice because it does not cross the placenta. Weight-adjusted full treatment doses of LMWH (e.g., dalteparin 200 U/kg/q24h or enoxaparin 1mg/kg/q12h) may be given subcutaneously throughout the pregnancy. LMWH is ideal for use during pregnancy; its longer half-life is conducive to intermittent dosing. Alternatively, weight-adjusted UFH may be given IV for 5 days (Table 233.10) followed by subcutaneous UFH for the rest of the pregnancy with the dose adjusted to keep aPTT at a therapeutic level. Postpartum anticoagulation is given for at least 6 weeks. Heparin may cause osteoporosis and thrombocytopenia, although preliminary data suggest that osteoporosis is less frequent with LMWH than UFH. Labor is induced electively, and subcutaneous heparin is stopped 24 hours before. Warfarin crosses the placenta, causing warfarin embryopathy—stippled epiphyses and nasal hypoplasia—when used between 6–12 weeks of gestation. Use of warfarin in pregnant women with artificial heart valves led to embryopathy in 6.4% live births. Although substituting warfarin at or before 6 weeks of gestation eliminated this risk, warfarin is best avoided during pregnancy altogether.

## Prognosis and Prevention

Appropriate and timely therapy reduces the high mortality from pulmonary embolism. Effective anticoagulation during the acute episode significantly decreases VTE recurrence. If the precipitating factor for the initial event is evanescent, the prognosis is good. Pre-existing left ventricular failure and coronary artery disease adversely affect long-term survival in pulmonary embolism. In a small minority (0.15–2%), a syndrome of postembolic pulmonary hypertension evolves insidiously, with progressive dyspnea and eventual severe disability. Pulmonary hypertension is detected clinically and confirmed on right heart catheterization. In a majority of these patients, a previous history of pulmonary embolism is not present and most do not have a detectable hypercoagulable state. Perfusion lung scans generally

**TABLE 233.10. Indications for Inferior Vena Caval Interruption**

| |
|---|
| Recurrent pulmonary embolism despite adequate anticoagulation |
| Documented VTE with any of the following: |
| Contraindication to anticoagulation |
| Necessity for premature discontinuation of anticoagulation |
| Chronic, recurrent pulmonary embolism in the setting of pulmonary hypertension and cor pulmonale |
| During pulmonary embolectomy |
| Septic pelvic thrombophlebitis |
| Paradoxical embolism |
| Residual, large, free-flowing ileofemoral thrombus in the setting of massive pulmonary embolism |

**TABLE 233.11. Guidelines for Venous Thromboembolism Prophylaxis**

| Clinical Situation | Level of Risk*/Type of Procedure and Recommended Prophylaxis† | | | |
|---|---|---|---|---|
| | **Low risk** | **Moderate risk** | **High bleeding risk** | **High risk** |
| General Surgery | 1 | LDUH<br>LMWH[††]<br>ES[#]<br>IPC[#]<br><br>LDUH<br>LMWH<br>IPC | ES<br>IPC | LDUH/LMWH<br>*plus*<br>ES/IPC |
| Gynecologic Surgery | **Brief procedure** | | **Major Gyn surgery, no risk factor** | **Extensive surgery for malignancy** |
| | 1 | | LDUH (2x) or<br>[LMWH + IPC] | LDUH (3x)<br>[LDUH + ES or IPC**] or<br>LMWH at ↑ dose ** |
| Urologic Surgery | **TURP or low risk** | **Major open proc** | **Highest risk** | |
| | 1 | LDUH, ES, IPC, or LMWH | ES ± IPC *plus* LDUH/LMWH | |
| Major Orthopedic Surgery | **Elective THR** | | **Elective TKR** | **Hip Fx surgery** |
| | LMWH or ADW | | LMWH or ADW or<br>Optimal use of IPC | LMWH or ADW or<br>optimal use of IPC<br>LDUH possible alternative |
| Neurosurgery | **Intracranial neurosurgery** | | **Trauma + identifiable VTE risk** | **Acute spinal cord injury** |
| | IPC ± ES<br>High risk patients:<br>ES/IPC *plus* LDUH or postop LMWH | | LMWH as soon as safe;<br>if not IPC and/or ES<br>(or duplex US screen;<br>IVC filter if DVT [+]) | LMWH<br>LMWH or full dose oral anticoagulation during rehab |
| Medical Conditions | **Acute myocardial infarction** | | **Ischemic stroke** | **General medical patients + VTE risk ##** |
| | Prophylactic LDUH or full IV heparin | | LDUH, LMWH, or<br>danaparoid; ES/IPC if contraindicated | LDUH or LMWH |

*Risk groups: 1 = low risk (minor procedure in patients ≤40 yrs, no additional risk factors); 2 = moderate risk (minor procedure with additional risk for thrombosis, or non-major surgery in patients 40–60 years with no additional risk factors, or major surgery in patients <40 yrs with no additional risk factors); 3 = higher risk (non-major surgery in patients >60 yrs, or with additional risk factors, or major surgery in patients >40 years, or with additional risk factors); 4 = higher risk, but greater-than-usual risk for bleeding; 5 = very high risk (multiple risk factors).

†Methods of prophylaxis: 1 = early mobilization; ADW = adjusted dose warfarin; start with 5–10 mg qd day of or the day after surgery, and adjust dose for an INR goal of 2.5 with range of 2.0–3.0. ES = elastic stockings; Fx = fracture; IPC = intermittent pneumatic compression (start immediately preoperatively and continue until fully ambulatory; LDUH = low dose unfractionated heparin (5000 U subcutaneously, given every 8–12 hours starting 1–2 h before surgery); LMWH = low molecular weight heparin (see dosing, below); ** = may provide additional protection; (2x) = twice daily; (3x) = three times a day; duplex US = duplex ultrasound; VTE = venous thromboembolism; [+] = positive; ± = with or without; # = IPC/ES; ## = cancer, bed rest, heart failure, severe lung disease.

††Low molecular weight heparin dosing (dose expressed as anti-Xa units [for enoxaparin, 1 mg = 100 anti-Xa units]): Moderate risk (surgical): dalteparin 2500 U subcutaneously (SC) 1–2 h preoperatively (preop) and once daily (qd) postoperatively (postop) OR enoxaparin 20 mg SC 1–2 h before surgery and qd postop, OR tinzaparin 3500 U SC qd starting 2 h preop. High risk (surgical): dalteparin 5000 U SC 8–12 h before surgery and qd postop OR enoxaparin 40 mg SC 1–2 h preop and qd postop. Orthopedic: dalteparin 5000 U SC 8–12 h before surgery and qd starting 12–24 h postop, OR enoxaparin 40 mg SC qd starting 10–12 hr preop, OR tinzaparin 75 U/Kg SC qd starting 12–24 h preop. Major trauma: enoxaparin 30 mg SC q12h starting 12–36 h postinjury if hemodynamically stable. Acute spinal cord injury: enoxaparin 30 mg SC q12h. Medical conditions: dalteparin 2500 U SC qd, OR danaparoid 750 U SC q12h, OR enoxaparin 40 mg SC qd. (Source: Geerts WH et al. Chest 2001; 119:133S–175S.)

show large, lobar, or segmental defects. Untreated, the mortality depends on the severity of pulmonary hypertension (90% 5-year mortality with mean pulmonary artery pressure exceeding 50 mm Hg). Gratifying results follow early diagnosis and timely surgery.

Prevention of DVT is the key component of reducing the risk of PE. Early ambulation following surgery, trauma, and other illnesses is key to reducing the incidence of DVT. The risk of VTE and the appropriate methods of prophylaxis are shown in Table 233.11.

Low-dose unfractionated heparin is not appropriate following surgery of the eye or central nervous system and in those with bleeding diathesis. Low-molecular weight heparin can effectively prevent VTE in susceptible populations; its efficacy is comparable to conventional heparin, but with a lower incidence of thrombocytopenia and with a comparable, if not lower risk of bleeding.

# CHAPTER 234 PULMONARY HYPERTENSION

## Physiologic Background

The pulmonary circulation system is a low-pressure system, with a normal resting pulmonary artery (PA) pressure of 25/10 mm Hg and a (resting) mean of about 15 mm Hg. The end-diastolic pulmonary artery pressure reflects the left ventricular end-diastolic pressure in persons without underlying lung disease. The pressure recorded after a catheter has been "wedged" into a small pulmonary artery to occlude its lumen is the pulmonary capillary wedge pressure (PCW), which is the left atrial pressure (normally 5–12 mm Hg). Exercise evokes little change in the systolic, whereas the diastolic may rise to 15 mm Hg and the mean to 20 mm Hg. A mean PA pressure exceeding 20 mm Hg or a systolic PA pressure higher than 30 mm Hg indicates definite pulmonary arterial hypertension ("pulmonary hypertension"). In early pulmonary hypertension, resting pressures are often normal and only exercise, by increasing flow, may unmask it.

## Pathogenesis

Although the entire cardiac output passes through the pulmonary circulation, it remains a low-pressure circuit, owing to the balance between various pressor influences (hypoxia, excessive blood flow) and the homeostatic dilatory mechanisms (ability to recruit blood vessels, distensibility of capillaries, the maintenance of vascular tone and patency by the endothelial cell, etc). The endothelial cell can modulate the pulmonary vascular tone, ward off in-situ thrombosis, and influence the migration and replication of vascular smooth muscle.

The pathogenesis of pulmonary hypertension is shown in Figure 234.1. Pulmonary hypertension is most often seen as secondary to another disease process. Primary or idiopathic pulmonary hypertension is uncommon. Abnormal pressor influences (hypoxia, shear stress, excessive blood flow) cause pulmonary vascular tone to rise. The endothelial cell normally responds to these influences through the release of endothelium-derived relaxing factor (EDRF), prostacyclin, and various agents that oppose platelet activation/adhesion and thrombin generation. EDRF might be nitric oxide (NO) or a nitroso-compound that releases NO. NO stimulates guanylate cyclase, which increases cyclic guanosine monophosphate in vascular smooth muscle; vasodilatation follows. However, the endothelial cell can be damaged and become dysfunctional; these homeostatic mechanisms then fail. Consequently, the pressor response evolves into sustained pulmonary hypertension. The damaged cell also releases various cytokines and growth factors, which cause cell proliferation and intimal thickening in the small precapillary pulmonary arterioles. In-situ thrombosis and proliferation and extension of smooth muscle in the vessel walls soon follow. These changes are collectively called vascular remodeling. Sustained pulmonary hypertension and vascular remodeling together lead to the syndrome of pulmonary hypertension.

### Secondary Pulmonary Hypertension

Common causes of secondary pulmonary hypertension are left-sided heart disease, pulmonary vasoconstriction (high altitude, COPD, massive obesity), excessive blood flow (congenital heart disease), sleep-disordered breathing, and obliteration of the pulmonary vasculature (pulmonary embolism). It has no unique symptoms. Physical signs include large "a" waves in the jugular venous pulse, a left parasternal heave due to a prominent right ventricular impulse, loud pulmonary valve closure ($P_2$), a right ventricular gallop, ankle edema, and pulsatile and often tender hepatomegaly if right ventricular dilatation has caused frank tricuspid insufficiency. The most reliable way to diagnose pulmonary hypertension is right heart catheterization. Useful measurements include PA pressures (PAP), PCW and cardiac output during rest, oxygen, and exercise. Doppler echocardiography can noninvasively estimate pulmonary artery pressures. With the integration of clinical evidence, it is usually possible to ascertain the cause of secondary pulmonary hypertension. For example, since the mean PAP seldom exceeds 40 mm Hg even in massive, acute pulmonary embolism, a mean PAP of 50 mm Hg during acute pulmonary embolism indicates prior pulmonary vascular disease or prior thromboembolism with incomplete resolution.

Hypoxia-mediated pulmonary hypertension responds well to oxygen therapy. Pulmonary hypertension due to left-sided valvular heart disease often abates after replacement of the diseased valve. Some pulmonary

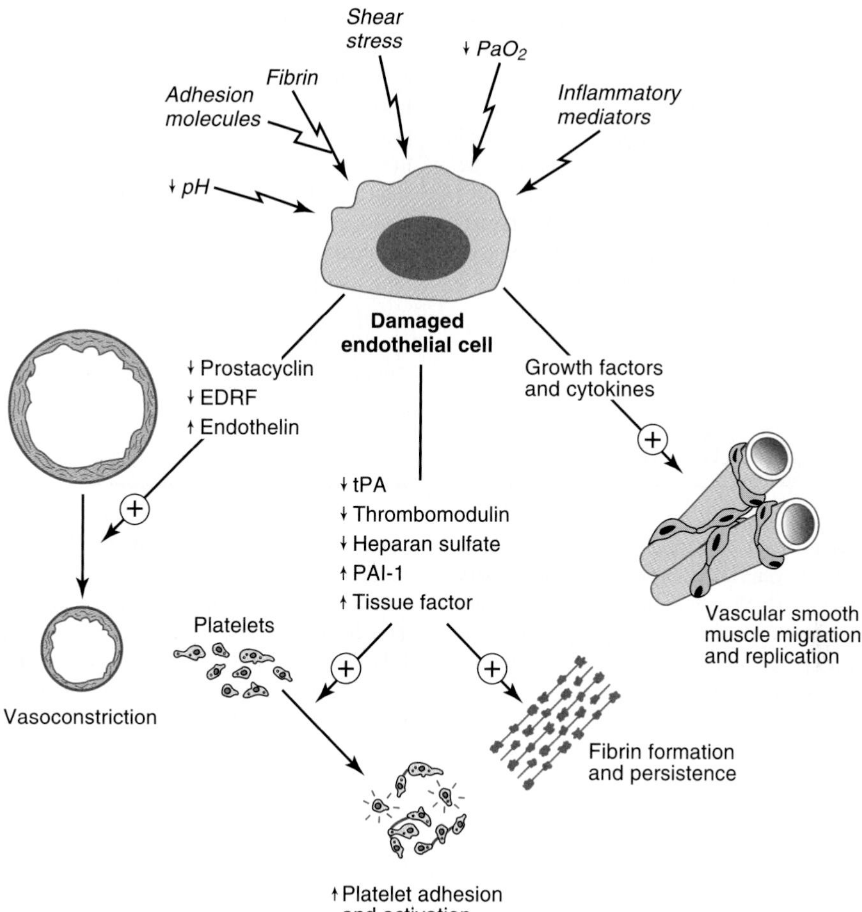


**FIGURE 234.1. Pathogenesis of pulmonary hypertension following damage and/or dysfunction of the pulmonary vascular endothelial cell. Abbreviations: EDRF = endothelium dependent relaxing factor; PAI-1 = plasminogen activator inhibitor 1; tPA = tissue plasminogen activator; + = stimulation or permissive action.**

hypertension will persist if the vasculature has undergone remodeling. The course of postembolic pulmonary hypertension is improved by early diagnosis and pulmonary endarterectomy. Pulmonary hypertension due to sleep-disordered breathing responds well to therapy of sleep apnea (see Chapter 257).

## Primary Pulmonary Hypertension

Primary pulmonary hypertension (PPH) occurs predominantly in women in their thirties or forties. Pathological findings include organized microemboli, intimal fibrosis, and medial hypertrophy with well-developed and hypertrophied longitudinal muscles. Intraluminal angiomatoid changes, adventitial vascularization, and perivascular lymphocytic collections are other changes. Whether recurrent thromboembolism causes or affects these changes is uncertain.

Exertional dyspnea, lasting months to years, effort syncope (the right ventricle is unable to increase pulmonary blood flow against a fixed, high pulmonary vascular resistance), and chest pain (which often mimics angina) are common symptoms. Raynaud's phenomenon (a triphasic color reaction on exposure to cold, consisting of *pallor*, followed by *cyanosis*, and further followed by a *red color*) may occur. (Inquiries about Raynaud's phenomenon should be discrete, since leading questions generally produce positive answers, indicating the susceptibility of the complaint to suggestion.) Signs of pulmonary hypertension may be evident. A tender, pulsatile liver, ascites, and edema (signs of right-sided heart failure) represent advanced disease. Chest x-rays may show right ventricular enlargement, a prominent central pulmonary artery, and even dilatation of the main pulmonary artery. On occasion, pulmonary angiography and, to a lesser extent, perfusion lung scans, have been lethal in these patients.

### Management and Prognosis

Despite occasional cases of prolonged survival and spontaneous remissions, the prognosis is poor. The response of pulmonary vascular resistance to prostacyclin (epoprostenol, $PGI_2$) during right-heart catheterization is used to select patients for high-dose nifedipine or diltiazem therapy. Intravenous infusions of Iloprost, a prostacyclin analog, have also produced more sustained reductions in pulmonary artery pressures. Another new agent is bosentan (an endothelin-receptor antagonist). Inhaled NO has some significant advantages in that it produces pulmonary vasodilation without significant lowering of systemic blood pressure. In selected instances, **sildenafil** has led to improvement, presumably by local release of nitric oxide. For those with more advanced disease, heart-lung transplantation and single-lung transplantation offer additional avenues of therapy.

# CHAPTER 235 COR PULMONALE

Cor pulmonale is any structural or functional change in the right ventricle imposed by pulmonary hypertension, which, in turn, results from a disease process (or processes) primarily involving the lungs, pulmonary vasculature, chest wall, or respiratory gas exchange; congenital or left-sided heart disease is excluded. Cor pulmonale may be acute, (e.g., massive pulmonary embolism) or chronic (e.g., COPD).

### Etiology and Pathogenesis

**Pulmonary vasoconstriction** is the initial event, usually brought about by hypoxemia, hypercarbia, and/or obliteration of the pulmonary vascular bed. Hypoxemia is the mechanism in early COPD and in residents of high altitudes, whereas hypoxemia and hypercarbia are responsible in patients with **alveolar hypoventilation** (chest wall abnormalities, neuromuscular respiratory failure, or sleep-disordered breathing). Obliteration of the pulmonary vasculature (recurrent pulmonary thromboembolism, advanced pulmonary emphysema, interstitial lung disease, schistosomiasis, and sickle cell disease) and hypoxemia may operate together in some cases.

The pathogenesis of cor pulmonale in COPD, from which it most commonly results, is shown in Figure 235.1. Obliteration of the vascular bed, increased blood flow brought about by exercise, hypoxemia, compression of resistance vessels from increased alveolar pressure, vasoconstriction from hyperventilation in advanced COPD, hypercapnia, and acidemia are the major contributors to pulmonary hypertension. Acidemia enhances the pulmonary vasoconstriction for any given level of arterial hypoxemia.

**Arterial hypoxemia** is compensated by an excess peripheral extraction of oxygen and, over time, **erythrocytosis**. Arterial hypoxemia lowers mixed venous oxygen saturation, and erythrocytosis raises blood viscosity; both exacerbate pulmonary hypertension. Heart failure as traditionally implied is absent; however, the cardiac output is inadequate for the extent of hypoxemia. This inadequate rise in cardiac output shortens survival. Oxygen therapy, by correcting hypoxemia, might be expected to improve the cardiac output but not completely. Finally, coronary artery disease, hypoxemia, and erythrocytosis with increasing blood viscosity may all evoke left ventricular dysfunction, which may follow as a secondary event.

### Clinical Features and Diagnosis

Cor pulmonale has no unique symptoms. Dyspnea, weakness, and changes in cerebral function, despite being frequently reported, most likely are due to the underlying disease and the attendant hypoxemia. Pulmonary hypertension may cause chest pain. Symptoms of the underlying lung disease also may be evident. Physical findings are the same as those of pulmonary hypertension (chapter 234).

The diagnosis of cor pulmonale depends on determining the presence of a disease that can cause cor pulmonale and the clinical features described above. ECG and x-ray criteria of cor pulmonale are listed in Table 235.1. Erythrocytosis may be evident. Distinguishing cor pulmonale from pulmonary hypertension due to left heart failure caused by disease is important, but could be difficult. Unless the patient has pulmonary edema or congestion, significant arterial hypoxemia ($PaO_2$ <60 mm Hg) and hypercapnia favor the diagnosis of cor pulmonale. Pulmonary function tests (PFT) generally reflect the underlying lung disease, but if PFT are normal in the presence of cor pulmonale, **sleep-related hypoxemia** should be suspected. However, even in those with underlying lung disease, sleep-related hypoxemia contributes on its own to cor pulmonale.

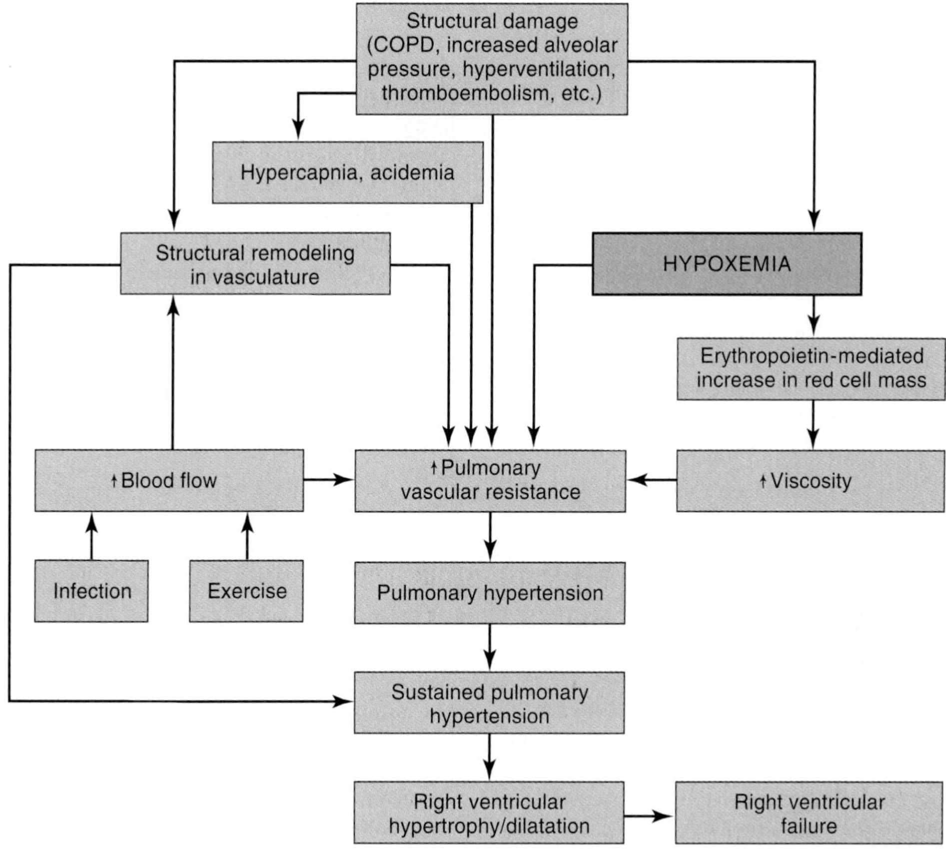


**FIGURE 235.1.** The pathogenesis of cor pulmonale.

**TABLE 235.1. Electrocardiographic and Radiographic Manifestations of Cor Pulmonale**

| Measure | Manifestations |
|---|---|
| Electrocardiographic[a] | Right axis deviation of QRS complex, +110 or greater |
| | R wave to S wave ratio >1 in $V_1$[b] |
| | R wave to S wave ratio <1 in $V_6$ |
| | P pulmonale |
| | $S_1$ $S_2$ $S_3$ or $S_1$, Q3 pattern |
| | Clockwise rotation of electrical axis[b] |
| | Incomplete right bundle branch block pattern[b] |
| Radiographic | Cardiomegaly with right ventricular and often right atrial enlargement |
| | Prominent central pulmonary artery with attenuated peripheral branches |
| | Features of the associated lung disease that leads to cor pulmonale[b] |

[a]Any two of first six would confirm presence of cor pulmonale.
[b]Most characteristic when associated airway obstruction is present.

### Management and Prognosis

Besides appropriate treatment of the underlying disease, the following agents are important in cor pulmonale: oxygen, phlebotomy, digitalis, diuretics, and theophylline.

Long-term oxygen therapy (LTOT) in significantly hypoxemic patients with COPD lowers pulmonary artery pressures and improves survival (see chapter 239 for a detailed discussion of LTOT and how it is prescribed).

Digitalis might improve right ventricular ejection fraction in only those who have a concomitant decline in the left ventricular ejection fraction. Digoxin may increase the risk of arrhythmias in the presence of hypoxemia. Fluid overload often complicates cor pulmonale, especially with frank right ventricular failure. However, the line between excessive volume and that needed to maintain adequate right ventricular filling is a thin one. Bed rest and oxygen therapy in most cases cause prompt diuresis. Diuretics, if needed, should be used judiciously, because of their propensity to reduce circulating volume, and therefore, venous return and cardiac output. By causing hypokalemic metabolic alkalosis they might also promote $CO_2$ retention. Electrolytes and volume should be closely monitored if diuretics are used. Theophylline, specifically in cor pulmonale due to COPD, reduces pulmonary artery pressure, improves right ventricular performance and pulmonary vascular resistance, and prevents diaphragm fatigue. A serum level of 8–10 μg/ml should be the goal.

The prognosis in cor pulmonale is essentially dependent on the underlying lung disease and how effectively it is being managed.

# CHAPTER 236 INTERSTITIAL LUNG DISEASE

### Definition, Etiology, and Classification

The **lung interstitium** is a layer of connective tissue between the epithelial layers of the alveoli and the endothelial layer of the capillaries. The interstitium is normally composed of connective tissue, macrophages, and fibroblasts. The lung interstitium may be involved by a wide array of disorders that primarily affect the lungs or by systemic diseases such as collagen-vascular disorders. Regardless of the underlying cause, the pulmonary process is called interstitial lung disease (ILD). If there is no identifiable cause, it falls within the broad category of **idiopathic interstitial pneumonia** of which **idiopathic pulmonary fibrosis (IPF)** is a major form (chapter 244). The more common entities are shown in Table 236.1.

### Pathogenesis and Pathology

Regardless of etiology, interstitial lung diseases share a common pathway and some common clinical features. An initial **alveolar epithelial injury** leads to an **alveolitis;** changes in the lung interstitium and collagen along with infiltration by inflammatory and immune effector cells follow. Fibrosis and destruction of the alveolar-capillary units culminate in **"end-stage lung" and chronic respiratory failure.** In any tissue injury, a balance ordinarily prevails between inflammation and repair. This balance is disturbed in ILD, and the inflammation is perpetuated. The type, route, and duration of the injury, the genetic predisposition of the host, and co-morbid factors all determine the severity and rate of progression of the lung disease.

### Clinical Features

Because ILD often is associated with a systemic disorder, the manifestations of the primary disease may overshadow the pulmonary symptoms. Symptoms of ILD are often chronic, but an acute onset with rapid progression is well known. The usual symptoms are gradually progressive dyspnea, dry cough, and chest

**TABLE 236.1. Classification of Interstitial Lung Diseases (ILD)**

I. Rheumatic disorders (e.g., rheumatoid arthritis)
II. Granulomatous disorders
    sarcoidosis
    pulmonary histiocytosis X
    drug-induced (e.g., amiodarone)
    organic agents (hypersensitivity pneumonitis)
III. Hereditary disorders
    tuberous sclerosis
    neurofibromatosis
    metabolic storage disorders
IV. ILD from inorganic dusts (pneumoconioses)
    silicosis, asbestosis, coal
V. *Idiopathic pulmonary fibrosis (IPF)
VI. Miscellaneous
    eosinophilic pneumonia
    radiation pneumonitis
    lymphangioleiomyomatosis
VII. Infectious disorders in the immunocompromised host

*IPF (a form of idiopathic interstitial pneumonia) is a diagnosis of exclusion (Chapter 244)

pain, which may be pleuritic. Hemoptysis may follow severe cough or signify pulmonary hemorrhage syndromes that manifest as ILD. Pulmonary histiocytosis X and lymphangioleiomyomatosis may present with recurrent pneumothoraces. In diagnosing occupational pneumoconioses, hypersensitivity pneumonitis (HP), and drug-induced ILD, it is critical to obtain a history of exposure to possible offending agents (e.g., silica, asbestos, inorganic dusts, or cytotoxic drugs). While smokers do not seem to develop HP, they are singled out in histiocytosis X and Goodpasture's syndrome. Tachypnea is an early and constant feature of ILD. Finger clubbing and/or end-inspiratory rales vary, depending on the disease entity. Because the rales simulate the tearing apart of Velcro, some use the term **"Velcro rales."** A distinct feature of idiopathic pulmonary fibrosis, they are less commonly heard in granulomatous ILD (sarcoidosis, HP, silicosis, and histiocytosis X).

## Ancillary Studies

Chest x-rays are abnormal in 90% of ILD cases. Besides the features of the primary disease, other findings include low lung volumes or diffuse interstitial (nodular, reticular, or reticulo-nodular) abnormalities. High resolution computed tomography (HRCT) has a higher sensitivity than specificity in diagnosing ILD and in determining the underlying process.

Pulmonary infection in the immunocompromised patient often presents with interstitial infiltrates. Thus, human immunodeficiency virus (HIV) infection should be excluded if risk factors exist. Because of the autoimmune basis of many of these disorders associated with ILD, laboratory studies addressing them are quite useful. Some disorders have characteristic laboratory abnormalities that foster their diagnosis—for example, elevated creatinine kinase in polymyositis, specific antinuclear antibody patterns in scleroderma and lupus erythematosus, or rheumatoid factor in rheumatoid arthritis. ILD occurring in these settings may be attributed to these specific disorders without resorting to lung biopsy.

Pulmonary function studies show a restrictive impairment in ILD (as was shown in Table 218.2). The $DL_{CO}$ is typically reduced. The $PaO_2$ and $PaCO_2$ are low. The $PaO_2$ declines further with exercise compared to that at rest. In the absence of such signs, clinically significant interstitial lung disease is unlikely.

## Diagnosis

Diagnosis involves two steps: the first confirms an interstitial disease, and the second determines its etiology (Figure 236.1). A clinical assessment (focused history and examination) is the first step. Specific inquiries should be made about the following:

- symptoms, their progression, and how they alter work and daily activities,
- the presence or absence of underlying heart disease,
- the presence of immunosuppression,
- exposure to tobacco smoke, various noxious agents, or organic matter in the workplace and/or through hobbies, and the temporal relationship of such exposure to symptoms (especially important in diagnosing hypersensitivity pneumonitis),
- medication use (e.g., amiodarone, nitrofurantoin)
- radiation therapy
- family history of pulmonary disease (familial pulmonary fibrosis and sarcoidosis).

Pulmonary function tests, current chest x-rays, and review of old x-rays to determine progression should be reviewed. Heart disease should be excluded, since chronic left ventricular failure may mimic ILD. If a potentially reversible cause is found, it should be eliminated. If clinical recovery follows, no further work-up may be needed.

If no reversible process is identified, an attempt should be made to exclude a connective tissue disease or vasculitis by appropriately directed biopsies, if indicated (muscle for polymyositis, skin for vasculitis, etc.). If none is identified—and sarcoidosis, alveolar proteinosis, eosinophilic pneumonia, or lymphangitis carcinomatosa merit serious consideration—a fiberoptic transbronchoscopic lung biopsy is undertaken. Bronchoalveolar lavage (BAL) specimens obtained during bronchoscopy help in obtaining samples for microbiological studies (mycobacteria and fungi). If no specific diagnosis is established, a lung biopsy is performed, usually by video-assisted thoracoscopic surgery or by open thoracotomy. Most disorders that cause ILD, including idiopathic pulmonary fibrosis, will ultimately require this step to establish a specific diagnosis and determine the prognosis. Pathological findings of a cellular (inflammatory) process generally respond better to therapy than findings of primarily fibrosis. IPF is a diagnosis of exclusion.

## Management

There is no uniformly successful or satisfactory therapy for ILD that tends to be progressive and disabling. If an offending agent (especially medication or inhaled organic antigens) is identified, removal might stop further progression and even result in some improvement. Treatment also depends on the type of ILD diagnosed. In general, corticosteroids may produce

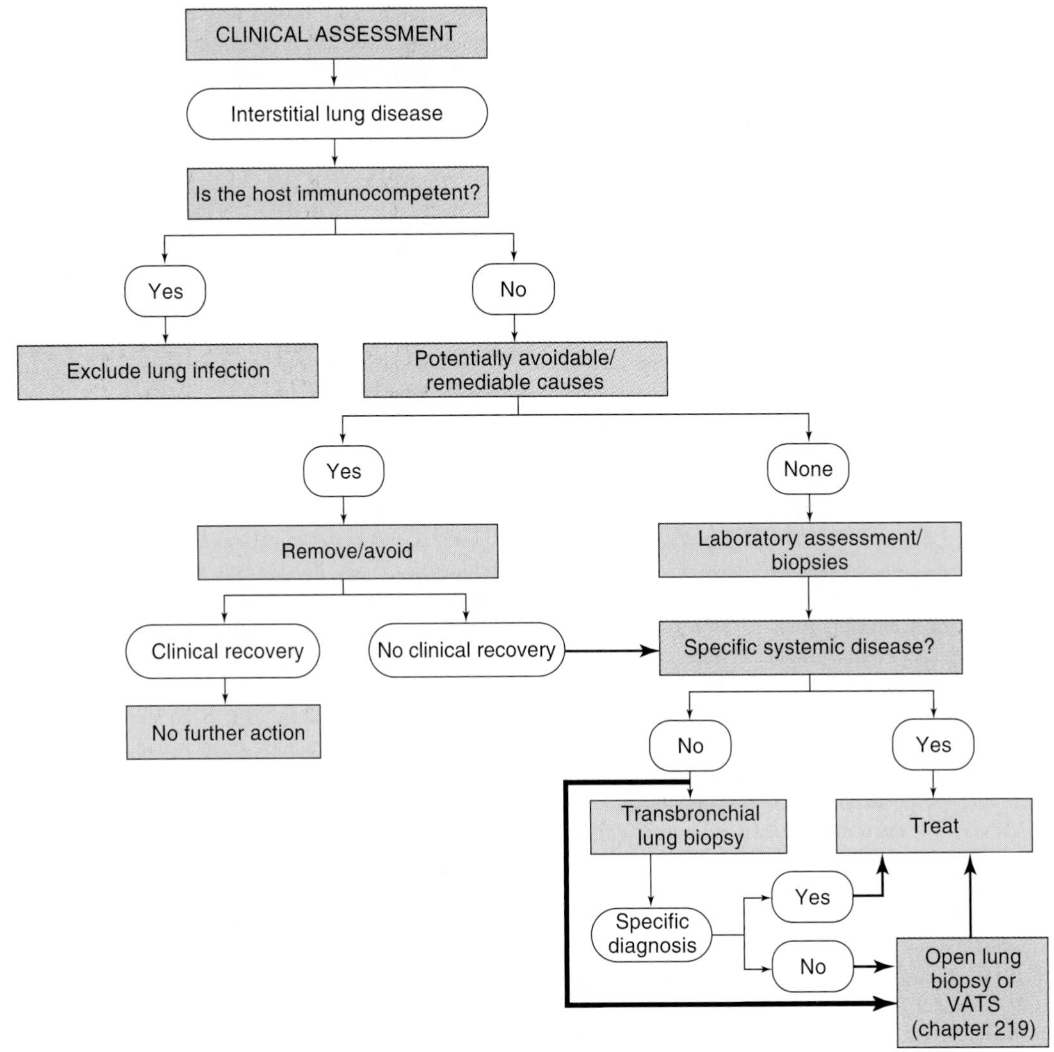


FIGURE **236.1.** **Suggested general approach to the diagnosis of intersitial lung disease.**

improvement or stabilization in less than 10%-20% of patients. The generally recommended dose of prednisone (1–2 mg/kg) can produce serious side effects (e.g., hypertension, hyperglycemia, osteoperosis). Prednisone is gradually tapered over three to six months, using clinical and physiological markers (chest x-rays, pulmonary function tests) of effectiveness. However, there are no *reliable* and uniformly accepted markers to measure disease activity. Immunosuppressive agents or interferon gamma-1b may be combined with prednisone in the treatment of IPF. Supportive care using long-term oxygen therapy and pulmonary rehabilitation may be beneficial. The age and the medical condition of the patient permitting, and depending upon the diagnosis, single- or double-lung transplantation offers the best hope for some.

## Prognosis

The prognosis varies depending on the underlying condition or process. Spirometric values, $DL_{CO}$, and gas exchange progressively decline, and eventually pulmonary hypertension and cor pulmonale supervene. Survival is shortest in lymphangitis carcinomatosa and in some very acute and relentlessly progressive forms of ILD. Long-term survivals, however, do occur in idiopathic pulmonary fibrosis. Many instances of drug-induced interstitial lung disease, sarcoidosis, and hypersensitivity pneumonitis have a favorable prognosis.

# CHAPTER 237 SARCOIDOSIS

## Definition and Epidemiology

Sarcoidosis is a systemic disease of unknown etiology. Its essential features are a compatible clinical picture along with noncaseating epithelioid cell granulomas in several affected organs and tissues that either resolve or become featureless hyaline connective tissue. Ninety percent of the patients with sarcoidosis are between 20 and 40 years of age with a higher prevalence in the United States among African Americans and women. The predilection for race, certain HLA types, and family clustering indicates a genetic basis.

## Etiology, Pathogenesis, and Immunology

The noncaseating granuloma, which is a reaction against an unidentified antigenic stimulus, contains epithelioid cells, giant cells, lymphocytes, and plasma cells with variable fibrosis and hyalinization. The $CD_4$ T-cells are increased in all affected tissues and decreased in the peripheral blood, which indicates their redistribution. Mononuclear phagocytes, epithelioid cells, and giant cells are transformed monocytes, which are attracted into the lung by monocyte chemotaxis, initiated by sarcoid lung T-lymphocytes. Proliferation of all these cells perpetuates the granuloma. The products of the accumulated cells (i.e., proteases, elastase, myeloperoxidase cationic proteins and oxidants from neutrophils and type IV collagenase, tumor necrosis factor [TNFα], and oxidants from macrophages) cause lung injury (alveolitis). Macrophages and epithelioid cells promote in-situ proliferation of fibroblasts, and fibrosis follows.

## Clinical Features

Sarcoidosis is often detected initially by an **abnormal chest x-ray,** obtained generally while evaluating another illness or, less commonly, during a pre-employment physical examination. Symptoms of sarcoidosis (Table 237.1) arise from the granulomatous involvement of various organs. The lungs are affected in more than 90% of patients with sarcoidosis; thus, pulmonary symptoms predominate. **Cough** is generally dry, and sputum and hemoptysis are infrequent. Physical examination findings of rales over the lung fields and clubbing of fingers are rarely noted. The reported extent of **extrapulmonary involvement** (Figure 237.1 and Table 237.2) varies depending on the histologic versus clinical criteria and the specialty of the investigator (pathologist, dermatologist, etc). Such extrapulmonary involvement is suggested by signs and symptoms of respective organ dysfunction, especially with an established diagnosis.

## Laboratory Features

Cutaneous anergy and leukopenia reflect T-cell kinetics, and serum immunoglobulins rise due to the B-cell overactivity. Hypercalcemia is from calcitriol (1,25 dihydroxycholecalciferol), one of the many biologically active agents secreted by activated macrophages. Other important anomalies are hypercalciuria, hyperuricemia, elevated serum angiotensin converting enzyme (SACE), and lysozyme. SACE is elevated in nearly 80% of sarcoidosis patients. Elevated SACE may be seen in many other diseases, but elevations greater than two times the upper limits of normal are less common and seen in tuberculosis, other granulomatous diseases, Gaucher's disease and hyperthyroidism.

## Roentgenographic Features

Based on characteristic chest x-ray findings sarcoidosis can be grouped in 5 stages. Stare 0—no chest x-ray abnormality; Stage 1—bilateral hilar lymphadenopathy (BHL) with or without paratracheal adenopathy (Figure 237.2); Stage 2—BHL with parenchymal infiltrate(s); (Figure 237.3); Stage 3—Parenchymal infiltrates without

**TABLE 237.1. Presenting Symptoms in Sarcoidosis**

| Symptom | Frequency (%, Range) |
|---|---|
| None | 12–34 |
| Constitutional | |
| Weight loss | 20–28 |
| Fatigue | 20–27 |
| Fever | 17–22 |
| Malaise | 0–15 |
| Night sweats | 0–14 |
| Chills | 0–13 |
| Pulmonary | |
| Cough | 30–32 |
| Dyspnea | 28 |
| Chest pain | 15–24 |
| Sputum | 11–12 |
| Miscellaneous | |
| Skin lesions | 14–32 |
| Visual complaints | 10–21 |
| Lymph node enlargement | 8–73 |
| Joint symptoms | 5–12 |

(Adapted from: Thrasher DR, Briggs DD Jr. Clin Chest Med 1982; 3:546. Used with permission.)

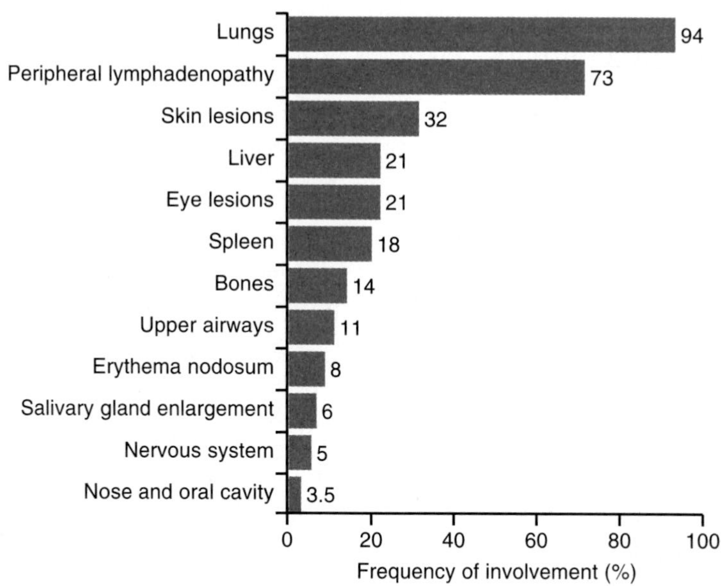


**FIGURE 237.1. Involvement of selected organ systems in sarcoidosis and the frequency of involvement.** (Data from: Maylock RL et al. Am J Med 1963;35:67-89.)

**TABLE 237.2. Extrapulmonary Involvement in Sarcoidosis: Frequency and Patterns of Cutaneous, Ocular, and Neurologic Lesions in Sarcoidosis**

| Cutaneous Lesions (32%) | | Ocular Lesions (21%) | | Neurologic Lesions (5%) | |
|---|---|---|---|---|---|
| Maculopapular lesions | 46% | Uveitis | 37% | Extremity paresis | 16% |
| Subcutaneous nodules | 14% | Blindness | 8% | Facial paralysis | 12% |
| Hypopigmentation or depigmentation | 12% | Blurred vision | 3% | Paresthesias | 12% |
| Alopecia | 7% | Scotoma | 3% | | |
| E. nodosum | 6% | Conjunctivitis | 3% | | |
| Lupus pernio | ≤1% | | | | |

(Adapted from: Mayock RL et al. Am J Med 1963;35:67–89. Used with permission.)

BHL (Figure 237.4); Stage 4—fibrosis with hilar retraction, honeycombing and bullae.

## Diagnosis

Differentiation is mainly from lymphomas (Hodgkin's disease; Table 237.3) and other causes of mediastinal adenopathy such as mycobacterial and fungal infections, toxoplasmosis, berylliosis and metastatic renal cell carcinoma. Tissue confirmation is recommended in all cases; transbronchoscopic lung biopsy is the recommended initial procedure. It is a simple, safe, low-morbidity procedure with a high diagnostic yield. The yield depends on the stage of the disease and the experience of the operator and is more than 90% in Stage 2 and 3 disease when at least 4 lung biopsies are done. Even in Stage 1 disease the yield is good (40 to 90%) reflecting microscopic lung involvement despite normal lung fields on chest x-ray. Other possible biopsy sites are skin or palpable lymph nodes. Biopsy of erythema nodosum is not recommended as they do not show granulomas. Liver biopsy is not indicated even in the presence of hepatomegaly and abnormal liver function tests. Mediastinoscopy may be needed in some instances when bronchoscopic biopsy is non diagnostic. Thoracoscopic or open lung biopsy is seldom indicated.

## Management

Our suggested management approach to pulmonary sarcoidosis is shown in Figure 237.5. Spontaneous resolution is so frequent in stage 1 that all that is needed is observation until resolution or progression into another group. Corticosteroids are the major drugs available for treatment of sarcoidosis. Vital organ involvement (e.g., eye, heart, kidney), hypercalcemia and disfiguring skin

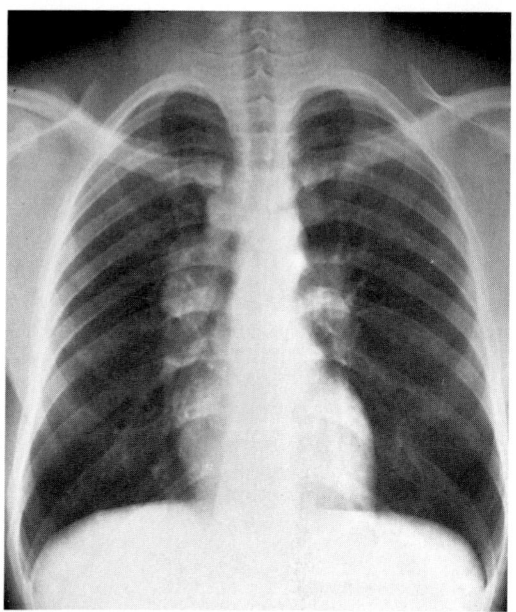

FIGURE 237.2. Sarcoidosis with bilateral hilar and paratracheal adenopathy (stage 1).

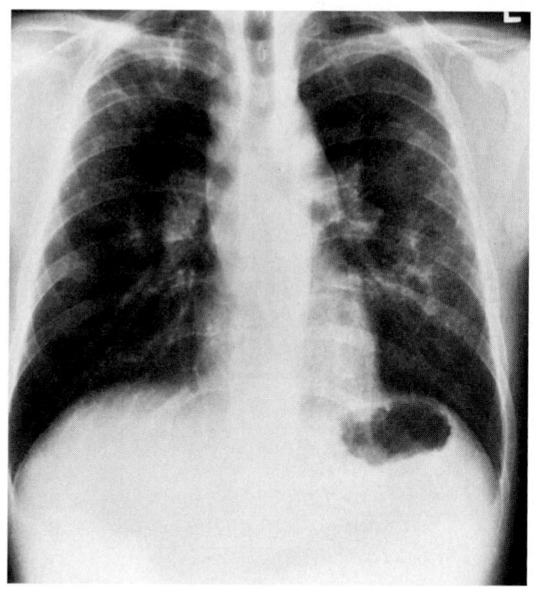

FIGURE 237.3. Sarcoidosis with BHL and parenchymal infiltrates (stage 2).

lesions, and progressive pulmonary disease (best indicated by worsening pulmonary function tests) are indications for corticosteroid treatment. The optimal dose and duration of treatment with corticosteroids has not been established by randomized prospective studies.

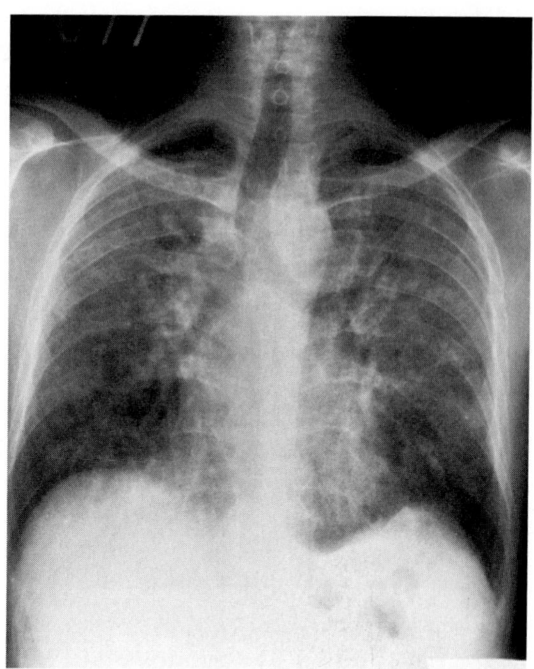

FIGURE 237.4. Sarcoidosis with parenchymal infiltrates alone (stages 3-4). Upward displacement of minor fissure and buckling of the trachea indicated volume loss (stage 4 features).

Initial treatment is with prednisone usually a dose of 20 to 40 mg daily or its equivalent on alternate days (q.o.d.) for 8-12 weeks. If improvement follows or if worsening has been halted, then the dose is tapered by 5 to 10 mg every 8–12 weeks with clinical, physiologic, and x-ray monitoring. The minimum steroid dose needed to maintain the improvement is then given q.o.d. Therapy is discontinued after two years; observation is continued for possible relapse. Higher dosage of corticosteroids may be needed for cardiac and neurosarcoidosis. Topical corticosteroid therapy may be used in some patients with skin lesions, iritis/ureitis and nasal polyps. Nonsteroidal anti-inflammatory drugs are useful in treating musculoskeletal pain and erythema nodosum. In selected patients including those refractory to prednisone cytotoxic agents (methotrexate, azathioprine, cyclophosphamide) can be used. Antimalarial agents (chloroquine and hydrocycholoroquine) have also been used to treat pulmonary sarcoidosis, skin lesions and hypercalcemia.

## Prognosis

Patients with Lofgren's syndrome (acute onset, arthralgia, erythema nodosum and BHL) has an excellent prognosis as spontaneous resolution occurs in nearly all. Spontaneous remission happens in 55 to 90% of patients with stage 1 disease; in 40 to 70% of patients with Stage

**TABLE 237.3. Differentiating Sarcoidosis from Hodgkin's Disease**

| Criterion | Sarcoidosis | Hodgkin's Disease |
|---|---|---|
| Symptoms | | |
| Fever | May occur | Common |
| Pruritus | Not seen | Common |
| Weight loss | Uncommon | Common |
| Findings | | |
| Erythema nodosum | Frequent | Exceptional |
| Pleural effusion | Rare | Frequent |
| Enlarged spleen | Uncommon | Frequent |
| Skin lesions | Common, show NCG | ±, characteristic histopathology |
| Intrathoracic-lymphadenopathy | Bilateral hilar and paratracheal | Bilateral or unilateral; isolated paratracheal adenopathy |
| Eosinophilia | Not a feature | May occur |

NCG = noncaseating granuloma; ± = may or may not occur.

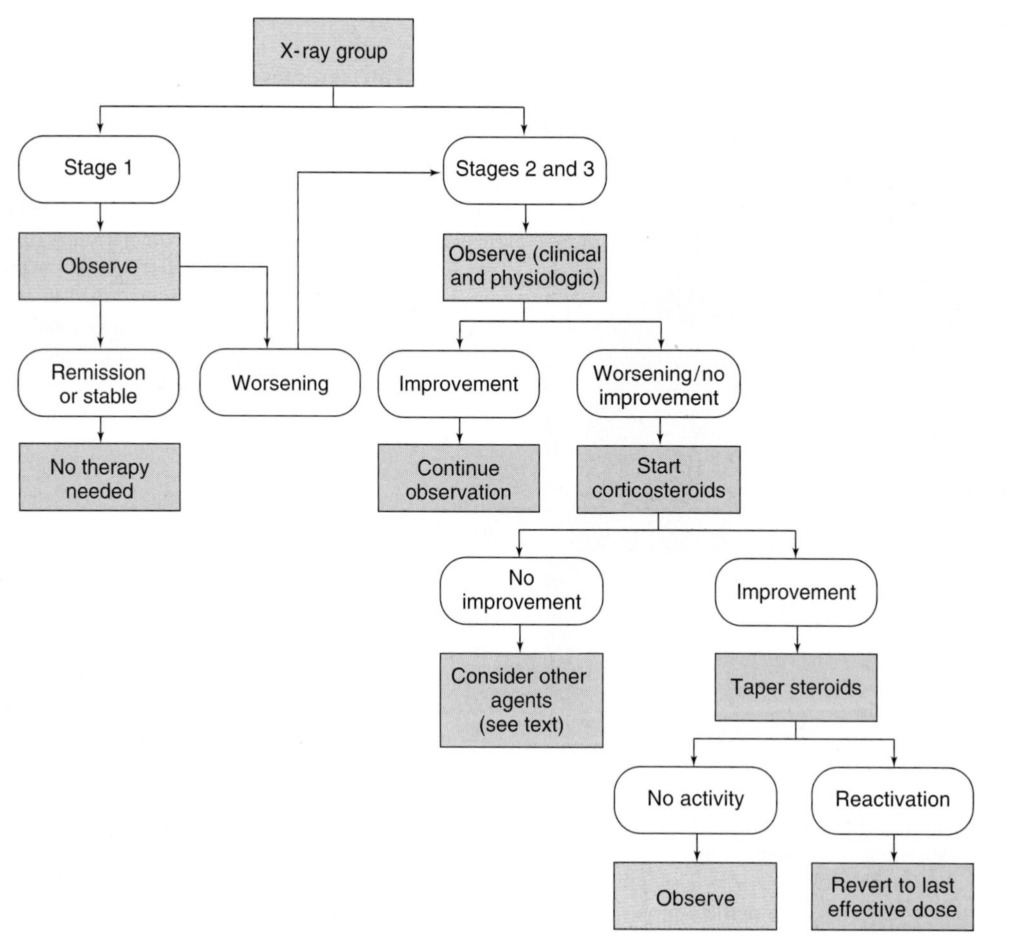


**FIGURE 237.5.** Suggested management of sarcoidosis.

2 disease; in 10 to 20% of patients with Stage 3 disease and 0% in Stage 4 disease. More than 85% of remissions are noted within 2 years of diagnosis, and late relapses after remission are infrequent (2 to 8%). A number of features are associated with chronicity or progression. These adverse prognostic factors include black race, age at onset greater than 40 years, lupus pernio, chronic uveitis, chronic hypercalcemia, nephrocalcinosis, nasal mucosal involvement, cystic bone lesions, neurosarcoidosis, myocardial involvement, progressive pulmonary sarcoidosis and chronic respiratory insufficiency. Reported mortality rate of sarcoidosis is 1 to 5% and deaths are attributed to progressive respiratory insufficiency or central nervous system or myocardial involvement.

# CHAPTER 238 PLEURO-PULMONARY MANIFESTATIONS OF RHEUMATIC DISORDERS AND VASCULITIDES

The abundance of vasculature and connective tissue in the lungs makes them vulnerable for involvement in many collagen-vascular disorders and vasculitides. The patterns and predominant sites of involvement vary depending on the primary disease and the incidence vary depending on the method of detection (clinical, roentgenographic, pulmonary function tests, histopathologic). Since connective tissue and blood vessels may be diffusely affected in these disorders, dysfunction of other organ systems might precede lung dysfunction and dominate the clinical picture. Depending on the type of disease, pleura and less commonly airway and vasculature may also be involved (Table 238.1). Despite the representation of various disorders here as pure entities, overlaps in their clinical picture do occur.

## Rheumatoid Disease

More common patterns of pleuropulmonary involvement in rheumatoid arthritis (RA) include diffuse interstitial fibrosis, pleurisy, and lung nodules. **Diffuse interstitial fibrosis** is characterized by a histologic picture similar to that of idiopathic pulmonary fibrosis (IPF). However prominent lymphocytic infiltrates and

**TABLE 238.1. Patterns of Pleuropulmonary Involvement in Connective Tissue Disorders**

| Disorders | Involvement |
|---|---|
| Rheumatoid arthritis and systemic lupus erythematosus | See text |
| Polymyositis-dermatomyositis | Interstitial fibrosis, aspiration pneumonia from pharyngeal muscle weakness, bronchiolitis obliterans, respiratory failure due to muscle weakness |
| Progressive systemic sclerosis | Interstitial fibrosis, pneumothorax, basilar pleural thickening, aspiration pneumonia, increased risk of broncho-alveolar cell carcinoma, pulmonary hypertension |
| Sjögren's syndrome | Interstitial fibrosis, pleural effusions, pseudolymphomas, lymphocytic interstitial pneumonia, amyloidosis, pulmonary hypertension |
| Ankylosing spondylitis | Apical fibrobullous disease, diffuse pleural thickening, aspergilloma formation in apical bullae |
| Goodpasture's syndrome | Hemoptysis |
| Necrotizing vasculitis of the polyarteritis nodosa type | Allergic angiitis with granulomatosis |
| Wegener's granulomatosis | Sinusitis and upper airway involvement, nodular infiltrates, cavitation, airway obstruction |
| Lymphomatoid granulomatosis | Bilateral, multiple pulmonary densities, pleural effusion |

concomitant findings of rheumatoid nodules, bronchiolitis obliterans organizing pneumonia (BOOP), or pleural fibrosis when present differentiate interstitial disease due to RA from IPF. Clinical manifestations are exertional dyspnea, cough, pleuritic pain, clubbing, end-inspiratory rales, and, in advanced stages, cor pulmonale. It is more frequent with subcutaneous nodules or when RA is more advanced. Restrictive ventilatory impairment and resting or exercise-induced hypoxemia may be present. The chest x-ray shows small nodular or punctate lesions in the early stages and medium to coarse reticulation and progressive loss of lung volume in the later stages. Computed tomography is more sensitive in detecting interstitial changes. Pleural effusion or pleural thickening may coexist. Mild disease needs only observation. There is no effective treatment for interstitial fibrosis, although corticosteroids may be tried. BOOP is often responsive to corticosteroid treatment.

**Pleuritis** *with or without effusion* is found in 20% or more patients with RA. It is more common in men and may rarely antedate RA. Often an asymptomatic and incidental finding, the effusion is exudative, generally unilateral with low glucose and high neutrophils, and may remain stable for months to years. There is no specific treatment. Repeated thoracentesis, corticosteroids, and decortication have all been tried. Pleuritis without effusion may cause a restrictive ventilatory impairment.

**Rheumatoid nodules** may be *nonpneumoconiotic* or *pneumoconiotic*. Nonpneumoconiotic rheumatoid nodules show a central zone of fibrinoid necrosis surrounded by a palisading layer of fibroblasts arranged perpendicular to the area of necrosis, and a layer of cellular or sclerotic granulation tissue surrounding the palisading layer. They are relatively uncommon and asymptomatic unless they enlarge or cavitate or become infected. Rheumatoid nodules may be present elsewhere and eosinophilia may be noted. X-rays show the nodules to be well-circumscribed, multiple, 2–7 cm in diameter, and generally peripheral. They often cavitate, leaving thick walls. Nodules may resolve or progress. Pleural effusion and **spontaneous pneumothorax** may coexist. Restrictive ventilatory impairment may be found. Unless complications occur, no treatment is necessary.

**Caplan's syndrome** refers to a (pneumoconiotic) rheumatoid nodule occurring in coal miners or those who have been exposed to silica or asbestos. The syndrome involves a central necrosis with peripheral fibroblasts arranged perpendicular to the necrotic zone containing the inorganic dust, with mononuclear, polymorphonuclear, or giant cell infiltration. A dark, concentric ring surrounds the central core. Other clinical features are the same as those in a nonpneumoconiotic rheumatoid nodule. On x-ray, the nodules are well circumscribed, round, 0.5–5.0 cm peripheral densities; they may cavitate, calcify, and become fibrotic. They may appear rapidly in "crops." No definite treatment is necessary.

Other patterns of respiratory involvement from RA include bronchiolitis and BOOP, apical fibrobullous disease mimicking tuberculosis, upper airway obstruction from vocal cord dysfunction caused by arthritis of the crico-arytenoid joints, and respiratory paralysis from atlanto-axial dislocation and vascular disease (pulmonary hypertension, vasculitis).

## Systemic Lupus Erythematosus

The extent of lung and pleural involvement may vary from 50–70% in systemic lupus erythematosus (SLE). The kidneys and central nervous system may also be involved.

**Pleurisy with or without effusion** is the most common manifestation of SLE. Pleuritic pain may be an early symptom. Effusions are frequently small and bilateral or may be massive. They are exudative and typically have a normal glucose level. Pleural fluid to serum ratio of antinuclear antibody (ANA) titer >1 confirms the diagnosis. LE cells may be seen in effusion. Pericardial effusion and cardiomegaly may coexist. Treatment is corticosteroid therapy. **Acute lupus pneumonitis** presents with dyspnea, fever, cough, and tachypena and may be the initial manifestation of the disease. The patients are severely ill. **Pulmonary infection** should be excluded first, since infectious complications are far more frequent than lung involvement by lupus. On x-ray, infiltrates are non homogenous and may be localized or diffuse. Cardiomegaly may be seen. Diagnosis is one of exclusion. Biopsy may show alveolar wall thickening and mononuclear cell infiltration. Evidence of vasculitis may be seen. Immunologic studies show granular IgG and C3 immunofluorescence. Treatment is corticosteroids with or without azathioprine. **Acute pulmonary hemorrhage** is a rare but serious manifestation of SLE.

**Diaphragmatic dysfunction** presents with dyspnea, striking orthopnea, and, characteristically, restrictive ventilatory impairment. Chest x-ray shows elevated diaphragms, which show very little movement on fluoroscopy. Lungs appear small as a consequence. There is no specific therapy. BOOP and vascular disease may also be seen. Vascular disease in SLE may manifest as pulmonary hypertension with Raynauds, vasculitis due to necrosis and initial fibrosis or pulmonary emboli caused by lupus anticoagulant.

## Polymyositis-dermatomyositis

**Polymyositis-dermatomyositis (PM-DM)** are inflammatory disorders that are associated with the development of interstitial lung disease. As many as one-third of patients develop this pulmonary complication which may precede the development of PM-DM.

## Vasculitis

In vasculitis, the lung may be the major site of involvement in Wegener's granulomatosis, allergic angiitis (Churg-Strauss syndrome), and lymphocytic angiitis. In many other vasculitic disorders, the lung may be involved either as part of a systemic process or in a minor way. Only Wegener's granulomatosis will be considered here.

### *Wegener's Granulomatosis*

This disorder, characterized by necrotizing granulomatous vasculitis of the respiratory tract, glomerulonephritis, and small vessel vasculitis, involves the upper and/or lower respiratory tract and/or kidneys (see Chapter 266).

The extent of lung involvement approaches 95%, followed by paranasal sinuses (90%), kidneys (85%), nasopharynx (70%), and eyes (60%). A limited form involving only the lungs is well known. Symptoms include nasal discharge, sinusitis, otitis media, and nasal ulcerative lesions. Cough, hemoptysis, and chest pain signify lung involvement. Wegener's granulomatosis may present as a pulmonary-renal syndrome with alveolar hemorrhage and nephritis or, less commonly, as diffuse capillaritis. Chest x-ray shows bilateral nodular infiltrative lesions that cavitate (Figure 238.1). Mass densities, airway obstruction from endobronchial lesions, and pleural thickening or effusions are uncommon.

In those without renal failure, cyclophosphamide is started at 1–2 mg/kg and continued for two weeks. If needed, the dose may be raised by 25 mg increments, keeping the WBC count over 3,000/mm$^3$. The duration of treatment is generally 12–18 months after a complete remission. When renal failure is associated, cyclophosphamide is started IV in 4 mg/kg for three days with a reduction in the dose thereafter to 1–2 mg/kg per day. Associated corticosteroid therapy is needed in both instances.

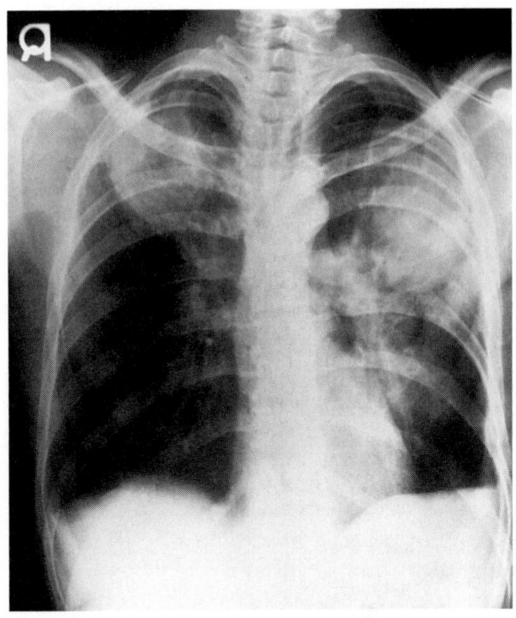

**FIGURE 238.1.** **Wegener's granulomatosis. Bilateral opacities are present. Right upper-zone density is cavitated.**

# CHAPTER 239 LONG-TERM OXYGEN THERAPY

Oxygen ($O_2$), an inhaled medication, is the only medication that has been shown to prolong survival in a subset of patients with chronic obstructive pulmonary disease (COPD). Oxygen prescribed to patients for use in an ambulatory setting is commonly termed long-term oxygen therapy (LTOT) or home oxygen therapy.

The two major clinical studies from the early 1980s that demonstrated the benefits of LTOT in patients with COPD still remain the scientific foundation on which the use of LTOT is based. In addition, oxygen has other established beneficial effects in patients with COPD, including a decrease in erythrocytosis and an improvement in exercise tolerance and neuropsychological functioning. Pulmonary arterial hypertension (PAH) commonly accompanies advanced COPD, and it is believed that oxygen, a potent pulmonary arterial vasodilator, prevents the progression of PAH, right-sided heart failure, and death, accounting for one of the mechanisms by which LTOT may prolong survival. Smoking-related COPD is by far the most common lung disease in patients prescribed LTOT.

There are several widely accepted indications to initiate the prescription of LTOT at rest (Table 239.1). The best initial determination for the need for LTOT is made on the basis of a resting, room-air arterial blood gas (ABG) analysis. The identification of patients with hypercapnia is important since LTOT may aggravate hypercapnia in some patients. Most patients prescribed for LTOT meet the indications for LTOT at rest, and these

TABLE 239.1. Indications for Long-term Oxygen ($O_2$) Therapy at Rest

1. Arterial partial pressure of oxygen ($PaO_2$) ≤ 55 mm Hg or arterial oxygen saturation ($SaO_2$) ≤ 88%
2. $PaO_2$ 56–59 mm Hg or $SaO_2$ ≤ 89% with the following conditions:
   Electrocardiographic evidence of cor pulmonale, or
   Erythrocythemia with hemocrit ≤ 56%, or
   Edema due to congestive heart failure

TABLE 239.2. *Indications for Long-term Oxygen ($O_2$) Therapy during Exercise and Sleep

| | |
|---|---|
| Exercise: | $PaO_2$ ≤ 55 mm Hg or $SaO_2$ ≤ 88% |
| Sleep: | $PaO_2$ ≤ 55 mm Hg or $SaO_2$ ≤ 88% during sleep or<br>$PaO_2$ drop of >10 mm Hg or $SaO_2$ > 5% with signs and symptoms of hypoxemia (e.g., diminished cognitive process, restlessness, or insomnia) |

*The need for long-term oxygen therapy (LTOT) during exercise or sleep is usually determined by a 6-minute walk test or sleep study, respectively.

patients should receive LTOT continuously, 24 hours per day. Dyspnea alone is not an accepted indication for initiation of LTOT without the demonstration of hypoxemia meeting the established criteria.

A subset of patients who do not meet the indications for LTOT at rest (see Table 239.1) experience oxyhemoglobin desaturation only with exercise or sleep (Table 239.2). The benefits of prescribing LTOT to these two groups of patients have not been established, although it has become common clinical practice to do so. The need for LTOT during exercise can be established by a 6-minute standardized walk test. Characteristics predicting desaturation with sleep have been even less well characterized. Patients with COPD who do not meet indications for LTOT at rest should be considered for a sleep study to assess for sleep-related desaturation if clinical evidence of right-sided heart failure is present.

Ideally, an evaluation for LTOT should take place with the patient under optimal management while in a chronic, stable state. Practically, however, many patients are evaluated for LTOT during a hospitalization or an acute illness, before reaching a chronic stable condition. If a patient has not reached a stable clinical condition at the time of evaluation for LTOT and meets the established criteria (see Tables 239.1 and 239.2), $O_2$ therapy should still be prescribed and the patient re-evaluated in 1–3 months. Titration of $O_2$ should be performed to maintain the $SpO_2$ > 92% at rest. In most cases, measurement by pulse oximetry is adequate for titration. In cases of hypercapnia, an ABG analysis after the initiation of $O_2$ is recommended to measure the $PaCO_2$.

The goal of evaluating patients for exercise-related hypoxemia is 2-fold: to identify patients who do not meet the requirements for LTOT at rest but may qualify with exercise and to determine whether patients who qualify at rest require an augmentation of $O_2$ flow with exercise above that prescribed at rest. To assess for exercise desaturation, a standardized 6-minute walk distance test should be performed. The flow of $O_2$ is titrated to maintain an $SpO_2$ level > 92% during exertion. Although some clinicians empirically prescribe an increase in the resting flow by 1 L/min during exercise, some patients require no increase in flow whereas some require a greater increase than 1 L/min.

Patients who meet the medical criteria for LTOT at rest should be instructed to use the $O_2$ during sleep. Similar to the practice with exercise, some clinicians empirically increase the $O_2$ flow during sleep by 1 L/min above that prescribed at rest, however there is no evidence to support this practice. If clinical symptoms exist to suggest sleep related hypoxemia such as daytime somnolence or coexisting obstructive sleep apnea, then a sleep study can determine the presence of desaturation and guide LTOT requirements during sleep. There are three types of $O_2$ delivery systems: stationary, portable and ambulatory (Table 239.3 and Figure 239.1). The most commonly used oxygen delivery device for LTOT is the nasal cannula. It is easy for patients to use and has few side effects (dryness of the nasal membranes, facial irritation). A disadvantage of the nasal cannula is that the amount of oxygen inspired is variable due to variations in the breathing pattern, including breathing through the mouth. LTOT can be delivered through a tracheostomy mask in patients with a tracheostomy. Humidfication should be provided with a tracheostomy mask. However,

TABLE 239.3. Long-term Oxygen Therapy Delivery Systems (see Figure 239.1)

Stationary: Oxygen concentrators, liquid oxygen reservoirs, or large, compressed oxygen cylinders such as "H" or "K" tanks
Portable: Systems that weigh 10 lb or more and are designed to be rolled and not carried ("E" tank in a stroller)
Ambulatory: Systems that weigh less than 10 lb when filled with oxygen and are carried and not rolled, e.g., portable liquid systems or fiber-wrapped lightweight cylinders with or without conserving device

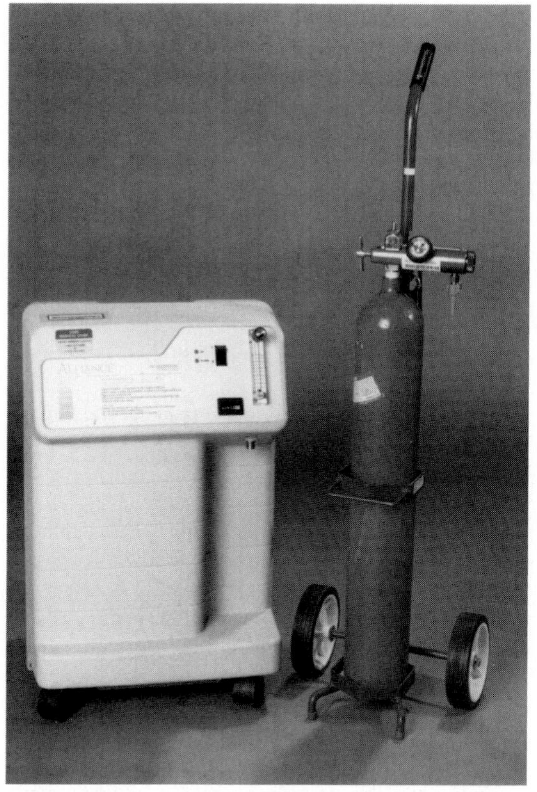

**FIGURE 239.1. An oxgen concentrator (left) and "E" tank (on right). The concentrator is a stationary source of oxygen used in the home. The "E" tank is designed to be rolled.**

standard use of humidification with flow rates < 4 L/min with a nasal cannula has not demonstrated any benefit.

Most clinicians retest patients within 1–3 months after the initiation of LTOT. If the patient no longer meets the criteria for LTOT, discontinuation of LTOT should be carefully considered. If LTOT is discontinued, it is recommended that an ABG or pulse oximetry be obtained 1 to 2 weeks later to verify that the patient continues to no longer meet the indications for LTOT. It is also common practice to conduct follow-up clinical evaluations to confirm an adequate prescription of $O_2$ every 6 months to one year.

There are serious potential dangers of smoking while using LTOT. Despite educating patients of the dangers of smoking, a considerable number of individuals continue this practice while using LTOT. The spark of a cigarette can ignite the cannula, a polyvinyl chloride product, particularly in the oxygen rich perioral region, with the process being sustained by the oxygen flowing through the nasal cannula. The practice of initiating LTOT to patients who smoke is quite controversial in the U.S. Although a policy of withholding LTOT to patients who smoke does not exist, some clinicians will not initiate LTOT to patients who continue to smoke. Clinicians must instruct patients who need LTOT to quit smoking for both medical and safety reasons. Smoking cessation programs should be offered to all LTOT patients.

# CHAPTER 240 PULMONARY HISTIOCYTOSIS X

Langerhans cells are a type of histiocyte derived from marrow stem cells that present antigen. Their proliferation is a shared feature of eosinophilic granuloma, Letterer-Siwe disease, and Hand-Schuller-Christian disease, collectively called histiocytosis X. The pathogenesis of pulmonary histiocytosis X (also known as pulmonary eosinophilic granuloma) is unknown. Smokers and patients with histiocytosis X share an excess of Langerhans cells in BAL fluid and an increased number of pulmonary neuroendocrine cells. The preponderance (>90%) of histiocytosis X patients are smokers. Pulmonary histiocytosis X may occur as isolated lung disease or as part of a systemic disease. Pathologically, there is severe interstitial fibrosis with nodular collections of histiocytes, lymphocytes, and eosinophils.

## Clinical Features and Diagnosis

Pulmonary histiocytosis X occurs mostly among young adults. Cough, sputum, dyspnea, chest pain, recurrent pneumothorax, hemoptysis, weight loss, and fever herald lung involvement. Extrapulmonary disease, splenomegaly, lymphadenopathy, and diabetes insipidus may occur. Peripheral eosinophilia is absent. X-rays most commonly show miliary nodules with a reticular pattern; cystic lesions and "honeycombing" are less frequent. There is generally a restrictive abnormality on pulmonary function testing, but airway obstruction is not uncommon. Diagnosis is generally made by open lung biopsy.

## Management

Spontaneous improvement may occur, but with extremes of age or with diffuse extrapulmonary or pulmonary disease, a poor outcome is likely. Thoracotomy and pleurodesis may be needed for recurrent pneumothoraces. No treatment regimen, including corticosteroids and vinblastine, has been found to be consistently effective, but several promising agents remain—for example, thalidomide, 2-chlorodeoxyadenosine and cyclosporin—or procedures such as allogenic bone marrow transplantation.

# CHAPTER 241 HYPERSENSITIVITY PNEUMONITIDES

## Definition

Hypersensitivity pneumonitis (HP), an immunologically mediated lung inflammation, follows inhalation of a variety of organic antigens, many of them fungal. Selected causative agents and the occupations that predispose to them are shown in Table 241.1. The immunologic reactivity and atopic status of the host are key factors, since HP develops only in a minority of those who are exposed. Atopic persons show airway obstruction immediately, followed later by a parenchymal reaction, whereas nonatopic persons generally show only the late reaction.

## Pathogenesis and Pathology

The basic mechanism of HP is an Arthus (type III) reaction in the lung. Cell-mediated immune mechanisms may also be involved. Lymphocytes and plasma cells infiltrate the lung interstitium and alveolar walls in a bronchocentric distribution. Granuloma formation, necrosis, Langhan's giant cells, epithelioid cells, and foreign body giant cells are also noted. The alveoli may contain foamy histiocytes and plasma cells. In chronic HP, there is interstitial and focal peribronchial fibrosis with alveolar septal thickening and lymphocytic infiltration.

## Clinical Features

In acute HP, myalgia, fever, chills, chest tightness, cough, and dyspnea occur 4–6 hours following exposure to the offending organic dust. The patient is acutely ill with tachypnea, tachycardia, and late inspiratory, basilar rales. Symptoms subside in 12–18 hours, with spontaneous recovery, but recur on re-exposure. Wheezing is conspicuously absent. Leukocytosis and elevated serum IgG, IgM, and IgA are generally present. IgE is elevated only with concomitant atopy (asthma or rhinitis). Serum precipitins to the offending organic antigen, while frequent, only indicate exposure. Chest x-rays may be normal or may show a patchy, diffuse infiltrate or a fine, symmetrical, nodular pattern. Pulmonary function studies show a restrictive impairment with diminished $DL_{CO}$.

Prolonged and recurrent organic antigen exposure may cause chronic HP, manifested by progressive dyspnea and diffuse interstitial fibrosis, often with "honeycombing," similar to that of idiopathic pulmonary

**TABLE 241.1. The Hypersensitivity Pneumonitides: Selected Sources of Exposure and Causative Agents**

| Disease | Source of Exposure | Specific Agent |
|---|---|---|
| Cheesewasher's lung | Moldy cheese | *Penicillium casei* |
| Malt worker's lung | Moldy barley | *Aspergillus clavatus* and *Aspergillus fumigatus* |
| Maple bark stripper's lung | Moldy maple bark | *Cryptostroma corticale* |
| Pigeon breeder's lung | Avian protein | None known |
| Ventilation pneumonitis | Humidifier water | *Acanthamoeba castellani* and *Acanthamoeba polyphaga* |
| Wheat weevil disease | Wheat flour | *Sitophilus granarius* |
| Wood pulp worker's disease | Moldy wood pulp | Alternaria |
| Isocyanate HP† | Resins | Toluene diisocyanate, diphenylmethane diisocyanate |
| Trimellitic anhydride (TMA)† | Paints, resins, plastics | Trimellitic anhydride |

† = More often produces occupational asthma; HP is less frequent.

fibrosis. A progressive restrictive abnormality, hypoxemia, and low $DL_{CO}$ are common.

### Diagnosis and Management

HP should be suspected when recurrent, self-limited respiratory and constitutional symptoms consistent with HP develop on exposure to specific environments or agents. A thorough history and pulmonary function test following careful challenge (controlled exposure) can be diagnostic although is rarely required. Serum precipitins and chest x-rays are only supportive. A search of the patient's work environment or home may help identify exposure to antigenic material from dusts or molds. Lung biopsy may be useful in helping to diagnose and differentiate HP from other interstitial lung diseases.

Identification and avoidance of the offending antigen are key factors in management, these alone being sufficient in the acute phase. In selected cases, corticosteroids may hasten the recovery. In chronic HP, corticosteroids may be useful, but once irreversible fibrosis has occurred they may confer only minimal benefit.

# CHAPTER 242 SILICOSIS

Silicosis, the interstitial lung disease caused by inhalation of silicon dioxide (silica), is associated with many occupations (e.g., mining or tunneling, quarrying, chipping, grinding, sandblasting, grinding or polishing in pottery and in foundry work, and cutting or manufacturing heat-resistant bricks). Silicosis is the most common occupational lung disease worldwide. Based on the x-ray, silicosis may be **simple** (small nodules throughout the lungs) or **complicated** (large, confluent masses). **Acute silicosis** follows a relatively brief exposure (several months to 3 years). A subset of acute silicosis is **silicoproteinosis,** which appears in an x-ray as homogenous alveolar infiltrates simulating pulmonary alveolar proteinosis.

### Pathogenesis and Pathology

Inhaled silica particles of 1–5 μ in size reach the respiratory units of the lung. They are ingested by the alveolar macrophages, some of which become activated. Activated macrophages release interleukin (IL)-1, which activates T-lymphocytes, which, by releasing cytokines (e.g., macrophage activating factor), further increase the number of activated macrophages. Chemoattractants released by macrophages attract blood monocytes, which are macrophage precursors. These amplification loops maintain an increased number of macrophages. The products of activated macrophages, IL-1 and macrophage-derived growth factor for fibroblasts, cause inflammation and fibrosis.

**Silicotic nodules,** the characteristic histopathologic finding, are mostly seen close to the respiratory bronchiole. Each nodule comprises refractile particles of silica, surrounded by whorled collagen centrally and in concentric layers, surrounded by macrophages, fibroblasts, and lymphocytes. Emphysematous blebs (large flaccid vesicles) surround the silicotic nodules, especially in the subpleural areas. Pulmonary infection may complicate silicosis. The morbidity of complicated silicosis is increased by associated collagen vascular disease (rheumatoid arthritis, scleroderma, and lupus erythematosus). Finer particle size and intense exposure are critical to the pathogenesis of silicoproteinosis.

### Clinical Features

Simple silicosis may be asymptomatic. It is recognized by its roentgenographic manifestations, which usually follow about 20 years after initial exposure. Exertional dyspnea, cough, and sputum production are frequent but concomitant cigarette smoking often makes their evaluation difficult. In complicated silicosis, besides dyspnea and cough, constitutional symptoms (malaise, weight loss) are also usually present. Physical findings vary with the extent of the disease. Expiratory prolongation, rales, and rhonchi may be present. Clubbing is unusual. Features of complicating infection or collagen vascular disease may be noted if complicated silicosis is present. Pulmonary function tests may reveal airflow obstruction; restriction or a combined impairment is less frequent. Lung compliance and diffusing capacity may be decreased and hypoxemia may be noted at rest or on exercise.

### Roentgenographic Features

Clinically significant disease does not arise without roentgenographic abnormalities. Simple silicosis manifests as multiple nodules of several millimeters each, scattered throughout but more noticeable in the upper lung fields. The nodules may calcify infrequently; associated hilar node enlargement and **"egg shell" calcification** may occur (Figure 242.1). Complicated silicosis manifests as bilateral, confluent, upper-lobe masses that may be necrotic in the center. As these masses

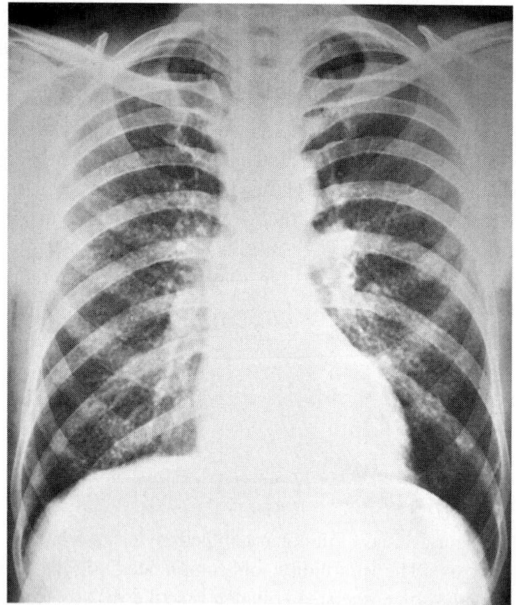

**FIGURE 242.1.** Simple silicosis; diffuse calcified nodules and prominent calcified (eggshell) hilar nodes.

retract toward the hilum because of the fibrosis, the nodules present in the lower lung fields become less obvious because of overinflation (Figure 242.2). Caplan's syndrome represents rheumatoid pulmonary nodules (0.5–5.0 cm) complicating pneumoconioses (silicosis, coal workers' pneumoconiosis).

### Diagnosis and Management

Diagnosis of silicosis depends on history of exposure and the chest x-ray findings. With discordant clinical or x-ray features, an open lung biopsy may be necessary for diagnosis. The excised lung tissue is examined for silica through microscopy with polarized light, scanning electron microscopy, or energy-dispersive x-ray analysis.

There is no specific treatment for silicosis. The main **complications** are infections (including *Mycobacterium tuberculosis*), progressive interstitial fibrosis, cor pulmonale, and respiratory failure. Efforts should be aimed at preventing the disease (use of respiratory protection in susceptible occupations) and preventing and treating the complications. Evidence of latent mycobacterial infection should be sought by tuberculin skin testing and treated appropriately (chapters 216 and 225). Silicosis can progress even in the absence of continued exposure.

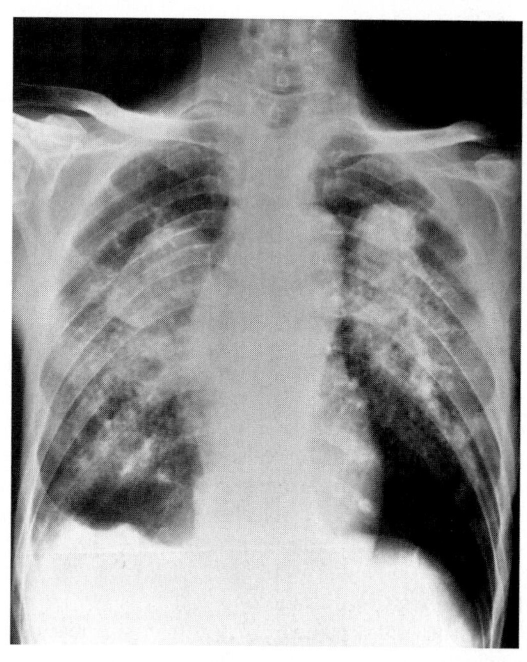

**FIGURE 242.2.** Complicated silicosis. Note the bilateral upper- and middle-zone confluent masses.

# CHAPTER 243 ASBESTOSIS

Pulmonary fibrosis caused by asbestos inhalation is called asbestosis. Asbestosis is one of several pleuro-pulmonary diseases caused by asbestos exposure (in addition to calcified and noncalcified pleural plaques, pleural effusion, rounded atelectasis, malignant mesothelioma, and bronchogenic carcinoma). Asbestos describes a group of heat-resistant fibrous minerals. Chrysotile, crocidolite, amosite, and anthophyllite are four of the more important forms. Because asbestos has thousands of industrial uses, occupational asbestos exposure is common (among, e.g., boiler makers, brake lining makers or workers, construction workers, dock workers, filter workers, insulation workers, gasket makers, pipe coverers or cutters, plumbers, rock miners, ship builders, and steam fitters). The use of asbestos has been banned in the United States because of the adverse health effects of exposure.

A latent period of 20 years or more usually follows exposure before clinical or x-ray manifestations appear. Because the development of asbestosis is dose-dependent, this latent period may be shorter with more intense exposure.

## Pathogenesis and Pathology

Chemoattractants are released when the inhaled asbestos activates both macrophages and dual complement pathways. Chemoattractants recruit neutrophils (PMN), which interact with asbestos to produce oxygen radicals (superoxide anion, hydrogen peroxide, and hydroxy radicals) that damage proteins and lipid membranes. Lipid peroxides may autocatalyze and perpetuate damage even without further asbestos exposure. Pathologic findings include both diffuse interstitial fibrosis and asbestos bodies (asbestos fibers coated with protein and iron). The respiratory bronchioles are thickened with connective tissue and fibrosis proceeds centrifugally. Macrophages accumulate, but granuloma or nodules (similar to silicosis) are absent. In advanced asbestosis, extensive fibrosis causes airspace distortion and a honeycomb pattern with cyst-like spaces.

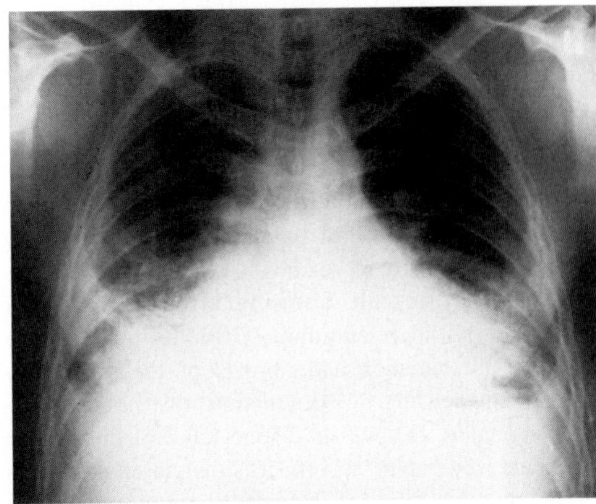

**FIGURE 243.1.** Asbestosis.
(From: Varkey B. Postgrad Med 1978;64:48. Reprinted with permission.)

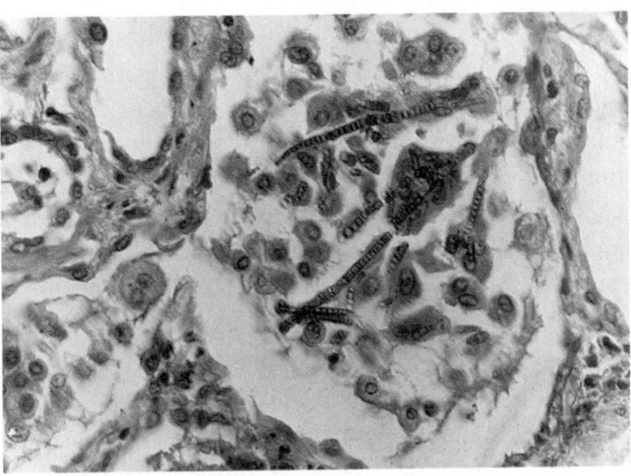

**FIGURE 243.2.** Asbestos bodies: asbestos fibers with an acid mucopolysaccharide and iron coating seen as elongated beaded bodies with clubbed ends.
(From: Varkey B. Postgrad Med 1978;64:48. Reprinted with permission.)

## Clinical Features

**Dyspnea on exertion** is the most common symptom, usually manifesting after 20 or more years of asbestos exposure. **Cough,** usually dry, may also be present. Tightness or pain in the chest may be reported, especially in advanced cases. Basilar **rales** and **finger clubbing** are the most important findings.

## Ancillary Studies

Pulmonary function shows a restrictive impairment, with reduced $DL_{CO}$; hypoxemia is present at rest or on exercise. Chest x-rays show interstitial, predominantly lower-zone infiltrates. Pleural thickening and pleural plaques may be present seen along the lateral chest wall and calcified pleural plaques may also be present (Figure 243.1). Hilar node enlargement or calcification is rare.

## Diagnosis and Management

Diagnosis depends on obtaining a history of significant occupational exposure, clinical features, typical x-ray findings, and the restrictive abnormality. A clinical diagnosis is usually sufficient and lung biopsy is only occasionally needed. Both asbestos bodies (Figure 243.2) and interstitial fibrosis, the hallmarks of asbestosis, are essential if a pathologic diagnosis is needed.

No specific treatment exists for asbestosis. Asbestosis may progress even in the absence of continued exposure. Besides efforts directed at prevention (i.e., avoiding exposure to asbestos), prompt treatment of respiratory infections is necessary because infections may accelerate the fibrosis. Complications of asbestosis are progressive fibrosis leading to cor pulmonale and respiratory failure. The risk of bronchogenic carcinoma of all cell types may be higher in persons exposed to asbestos even in the absence of cigarette smoking. Clearly, asbestos-exposed smokers are at particularly higher risk, as smoking and asbestos are synergistic co-carcinogens.

# CHAPTER 244 IDIOPATHIC PULMONARY FIBROSIS

Idiopathic pulmonary fibrosis (IPF) is one of the several forms (and the most important form) of the **idiopathic interstitial pneumonias.** IPF is a progressive disease of unknown etiology and is also known as **cryptogenic fibrosing alveolitis** (CFA) or **usual interstitial pneumonia** (UIP). Its pathogenesis includes inflammation and fibrosis of the pulmonary interstitium leading to destruction of the alveolar-capillary units. Despite its distinct clinical, histologic, and roentgenographic aspects, it is diagnosed only after excluding other forms of interstitial lung disease (ILD). The diagnosis of IPF is only made when there is no other identifiable cause of ILD.

## Pathogenesis

Idiopathic pulmonary fibrosis (IPF) is one of the several subsets of the **idiopathic interstitial pneumonias.** IPF, an elusive **alveolar epithelial injury** (a viral infection in some cases) initiates a cascade of events that culminate in **chronic alveolitis.** The initial injury causes immune complexes to develop locally; neutrophils and macrophages are brought in by chemotaxis. Activated macrophages release cytokines, which attract lymphocytes and more neutrophils. Neutrophil collagenase destroys lung collagen, which is replenished preferentially with type I collagen by fibroblasts. This process alters the normal (2:1) ratio of type I to type III lung collagen, but the total collagen remains the same. Thus, the lung collagen undergoes **sustained lysis and disordered resynthesis;** the process, with abundant scar tissue, has been compared to "excessive" wound healing.

## Pathology

In early IPF, alveolar walls and alveolar ducts show hyaline membrane formation and fibrin deposition. Alveolar walls, thickened with inflammatory cell infiltration, collapse from adhesions. Desquamated cells occupy the alveoli. Granulomas, arteritis, and mineral deposits are absent. As the disease progresses, peribronchiolar fibrosis, lymphoid hyperplasia, and hypertrophy of the media become noticeable, with intimal proliferation of the muscular pulmonary arteries. The lung architecture is grossly disturbed, with injury and repair seen simultaneously in different areas of the lung. In later stages, little inflammatory activity is evident and extensive widespread fibrosis supervenes.

## Clinical Features

The incidence of IPF peaks in the fifth and sixth decades of life, without apparent gender preference. It is known to run in families. The onset is often with a flu-like illness. Exertional dyspnea and nonproductive cough are common; weight loss, fever, myalgias, and arthralgias are other symptoms. With significant hypoxemia, central cyanosis may appear. Clubbing occurs in the majority and in virtually all of the familial cases. Tachypnea occurs early. Rales may be audible. Cardiac examination is normal, but pulmonic valve closure ($P_2$) may be loud, indicating pulmonary hypertension.

## Ancillary Studies

The erythrocyte sedimentation rate may be high. Immunologic abnormalities—including cryoglobulins, rheumatoid factor, antinuclear antibodies, and elevated serum immunoglobulins—are frequent. Circulating immune complexes correlate well with cellular infiltration in the biopsied lung specimen. Arterial hypoxemia is present at rest or on exercise, and is mostly due to ventilation-perfusion mismatching. Pulmonary function studies show a restrictive ventilatory impairment. The $DL_{CO}$ is reduced. Chest roentgenograms may be normal in about 10–15% of the cases. In the remainder, the roentgenogram may reveal (1) low lung volumes, (2) ground glass opacities, or (3) reticular, reticulonodular, or nodular infiltrates. Honeycombing signifies advanced disease (Figure 244.1).

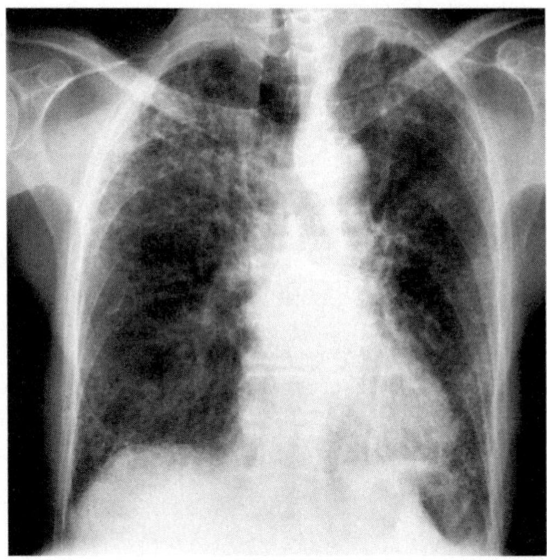

**FIGURE 244.1.** Idiopathic pulmonary fibrosis: widespread intersitial infiltration with honeycombing.

## Diagnosis

A general approach to the diagnosis of ILD is presented in chapter 236. A definitive diagnosis of IPF depends on a lung biopsy. However, a constellation of findings including rales, finger clubbing, and altered immune activity may suggest IPF, sometimes so strikingly that a biopsy is not essential (e.g., in an elderly person with no noxious dust exposure, rales, clubbing, and honeycombing on x-ray). Biopsy, however, makes it possible to reliably differentiate IPF from other forms of ILD and to differentiate the subtypes of IPF, each of which has a different prognosis. Because the minuscule tissue obtained by transbronchoscopic biopsy is inadequate for diagnosis, an open lung biopsy is the recommended method to obtain tissue.

## Management

Treatment of IPF is similar to that of ILD (chapter 236) and aims to prevent its progression by suppressing the inflammation. Treatment has generally been unsatisfactory and no drug regimen has been proven to prolong survival. About 40% of patients die of respiratory failure although the tempo of progression can be hard to predict. In general, the shorter the duration of illness and the more cellular and less fibrotic the findings on lung biopsy, the greater is the likelihood of corticosteroid-responsiveness. The duration of steroid therapy is indeterminate and only 10%-20% of patients respond. Azathioprine and other cytotoxic agents as well as colchicine may be beneficial when combined with corticosteroids. Recently, interferon gamma-1b has been found to be an effective agent when added to corticosteroids. Oxygen therapy is indicated for resting- or exercise-induced hypoxemia. Consideration for lung transplant is appropriate for some patients. The average survival in IPF is 47 months from the onset of the symptoms.

# CHAPTER 245 RADIATION PNEUMONITIS AND RADIATION FIBROSIS

Radiation-induced lung damage manifests in two syndromes, radiation pneumonitis and radiation fibrosis. Radiation toxicity is potentiated by some chemotherapeutic agents (e.g., dactinomycin [actinomycin-D], cyclophosphamide, bleomycin, and vincristine), previous radiation therapy, withdrawal of corticosteroid therapy, and infection.

## Pathogenesis and Pathology

An early dose-related effect of radiation is the formation of free radical -OH, which damages structural macromolecules, resulting in leaky cell membranes. The free radicals also directly damage DNA, and the broken DNA strands are incorrectly repaired or form cross-links. In severe cases, the cell dies. The surviving cells may divide abnormally, resulting in asymmetric mitosis or anaphase arrest. Inflammation, initiated and continued by unknown mechanisms, and mediated by neutrophils, lymphocytes, and alveolar macrophages through mediator release, causes tissue damage.

How radiation pneumonitis progresses to fibrosis is unknown. Irradiation alters the normal balance between synthesis and lysis of collagen. The connective tissue matrix may be damaged by the radiation or inflammatory mediators, and cytokines may alter the repair process.

In animal models, vascular permeability increases within 24 hours. Swelling of endothelial cells, alveolar capillary congestion, neutrophil accumulation, and focal alveolar hemorrhage occur in 2 months. In animals surviving a lethal radiation dose, leukocytes infiltrate gas-exchanging units and blood vessels. Vascular inflammatory infiltration, intimal thickening, and thrombi may cause obliteration of the vessel lumen. Animals surviving for 6 months after exposure develop a focal or diffuse interstitial pulmonary fibrosis. The exact onset of fibrosis following radiation is unknown.

## Clinical Features

Clinical **radiation pneumonitis** (RP) usually develops **2–6 months after** and occasionally as early as 2 weeks after the completion of radiation therapy. **Progressive exertional dyspnea** and a **dry cough** are the cardinal symptoms. **Fever** is common and usually low-grade; occasionally, it is high and intermittent. **Pleuritic chest pain** may be reported. **Tachypnea** is common. Auscultation is normal; occasionally, basilar rales and friction rub are present. RP may spontaneously resolve or may progress to acute hypoxemic respiratory failure and cor pulmonale. There are no characteristic laboratory findings, besides an increased sedimentation rate and neutrophilic leukocytosis. Restrictive ventilatory impairment and a decreased $DL_{CO}$ are typical; hypoxemia and widened $P(A\text{-}a\ O_2)$ are common.

Early x-rays show a **ground-glass appearance** in the area of irradiation. Patchy alveolar infiltrates with air bronchograms may follow. One important diagnostic clue is a **"straight-edge effect"**—that is, an infiltrate with sharp boundaries that correspond to the radiation field (port) but not to anatomic lung boundaries. However, in RP, infiltrates do occur outside the radiation field and even in the contralateral lung. Possible mechanisms for the latter include obstruction to the pulmonary lymphatic flow, absorption of radiation by lungs outside of the field, and inflammatory mediator release.

**Radiation fibrosis** (interstitial infiltrates radiating from the area of previous RP and often extending beyond the radiation field) becomes noticeable in x-rays about 1 year after the completion of treatment. Exertional dyspnea is common, but some persons may be asymptomatic. Progressive radiation fibrosis causes worsening dyspnea and orthopnea. Cyanosis and cor pulmonale may develop.

### Diagnosis

RP is diagnosed when its characteristic clinical picture occurs at least 2 weeks after the completion of radiation therapy. Differential diagnosis includes an infectious pneumonia and lymphangitis carcinomatosa. It is useful to compare previous x-rays with current ones and to compare the areas of x-ray abnormalities with the radiation port. Nonpurulent sputum and negative microbiologic studies are also helpful. Lymphangitis carcinomatosa involves the lung bases more with prominent septal lines and pleural effusions. Mediastinal or hilar adenopathy may be present. When differentiating these entities is difficult, bronchoscopy with bronchoalveolar lavage, quantitative bacterial cultures, and transbronchoscopic lung biopsy are helpful.

### Management

In symptomatic RP, **prednisone** therapy (60 mg/day) is recommended. However, there are no controlled human clinical trials of corticosteroids in RP, nor have the available studies shown uniform results. The steroids should be tapered slowly after a complete response, as pneumonitis may worsen markedly upon steroid withdrawal. Whether corticosteroids given before and during irradiation will prevent RP remains unknown. Supportive therapy includes supplemental oxygen, analgesics, antipyretics, and cough suppressants.

# CHAPTER 246 PULMONARY ASPIRATION SYNDROMES

The clinical syndromes caused by aspiration are variable and depend on the quantity and nature of the aspirated material, the frequency of aspiration, and the host response. The major aspiration syndromes are described in Table 246.1.

## Acute Aspiration Pneumonia

In 1946 Mendelson described the clinical syndrome caused by the aspiration of gastric contents. Risk factors for aspirating gastric contents are shown in Table 246.2. Radionuclide studies have shown occult aspiration occurring even in normal sleeping subjects. However, in normal persons, significant parenchymal lung disease does not follow these episodes.

**TABLE 246.1. Pulmonary Aspiration Syndromes**

| Aspirated Material | Manifestation |
|---|---|
| Irritant liquids | Acute aspiration of gastric contents (acute aspiration pneumonia) |
| Bacterial pathogens | Gastric contents contaminated with pharyngeal organisms<br>Gravitation of gingival secretions and saliva |
| Inert substances | Airway obstruction ("cafe coronary") |

### Pathogenesis

Animal studies show that lung injury due to aspiration depends on several characteristics of the aspirate, including the pH, volume, presence of food, particulate antacid, inert foreign body, bile, tube feeding formula, fecal contamination, and bacterial concentrations. Host factors such as alveolar macrophage function, nutritional status, functional status, structural lung disease, and the ability to cough are also important. Gastric juice with a pH of 2.4 in rabbits produces chemical injury; the severity correlates inversely with the pH. Increasing the aspirate volume from 0.5 to 4 ml/kg causes injury independent of pH. Both pH and volume are important; a **25 ml of aspirate with a pH <2.5 is critical** to produce a chemical pneumonitis in humans. Infection plays no role in the early chemical pneumonitis of acute aspiration pneumonia.

### Clinical Features and Diagnosis

Cough, dyspnea, and **acute respiratory distress** immediately follow an aspiration event. Tachypnea, tachycardia, râles hypotension, and shock are other

**TABLE 246.2. Aspiration of Gastric Contents: Predisposing Factors**

| Involved Organ | Problem | Predisposing Factors |
|---|---|---|
| Larynx and pharynx | Impaired function | Decreased level of consciousness (sleep, anesthesia, shock, drug overdose, ethanol, seizures, stroke) |
| | | Extremes of age |
| | | Postextubation, endotracheal or nasoenteric tube |
| | | Tracheostomy |
| | | Structural lesions (tumor, polyp) |
| | | Neuromuscular disease (myasthenia gravis, poliomyelitis, amyotrophic lateral sclerosis, Guillain-Barré syndrome, myopathies) |
| Esophagus | Decreased antegrade propulsion | Esophageal dysmotility (scleroderma, achalasia, presbyesophagus, gastroesophageal reflux disease) |
| | | Structural lesions (tumor, stricture, web, fistula) |
| | Decreased lower sphincter pressure | Increased gastric acidity (stress, anesthesia, peptic ulcer) |
| | | Ethanol, caffeine, tobacco, fatty foods, drugs, nasoenteric tube |
| Stomach | Increased volume | Gastric tube |
| | | Delayed gastric emptying (diabetes, outlet obstruction, ileus, drugs, pregnancy, trauma) |
| | | Food ingestion, tube feedings |
| | Increased pressure | Nausea and vomiting |
| | | Upper abdominal surgery |
| | | Pregnancy, labor |
| | | Obesity, ascites |

features. Apnea may be noted, and wheezing occurs in about one-third of the cases. Low-grade fever and rales are almost always present. Sputum initially may be scant and the initial Gram stain may show neutrophils without predominant bacteria. Chest x-ray findings are variable and may follow the clinical syndrome, without specific diagnostic patterns. Alveolar infiltrates, unilateral or bilateral, may occupy any lung zone, but the right lower lobe is commonly affected. In the early phases, pleural effusion or cavitation is very uncommon. An isolated area of atelectasis is rare, but when present suggests solid particle aspiration. Hypoxemia, often quite severe, starts early, caused by ventilation-perfusion mismatching and **intrapulmonary shunting.** Inflammation leads to capillary **endothelial damage;** as edema fluid leaks into the alveoli, the shunt increases and hypoxemia worsens further. In severe cases, the fluid shift leads to **hemoconcentration,** low pulmonary artery wedge pressure, and decreased cardiac output. Pulmonary artery pressures may increase.

The clinical course depends on the nature and volume of the aspirate, and the severity of underlying diseases. In one-third of high-risk patients who aspirate, acute respiratory distress syndrome (ARDS) follows. Some of these patients rapidly deteriorate and die within days. Others stabilize or improve initially, only to develop a bacterial superinfection or ARDS. A third group that ostensibly aspirate a small volume or less acidic material rapidly improve within a week, even radiographically and physiologically. Given the variability in its clinical features and its severity, acute aspiration pneumonia has a **wide range of mortality risk.** Aspiration of highly acidic material, multilobar involvement, initial shock or apnea, and development of ARDS or bacterial pneumonia indicate a poor prognosis.

**Bacterial infection** that develops in a significant proportion of patients after days of stability or improvement is usually accompanied by a new fever or worsening radiographic infiltrates, leukocytosis, and purulent sputum. In the hospitalized patient, the likely pathogens are gram-negative bacilli, but others include *Staphylococcus aureus* as well as mixed aerobic and anaerobic bacteria. Anaerobic infection is more likely in those who have gingivitis.

## Management

The initial step is to provide **adequate airway;** a bronchoscopy should be performed, if needed, to remove any solid material, but large-volume bronchial lavage is unnecessary. Intravascular volume needs to be maintained with a crystalloid. Hypoxemia should be corrected by supplemental oxygen. Ventilation should be ensured, if necessary, by mechanical ventilation and positive end-expiratory pressure (PEEP). Corticosteroids have no therapeutic role in acute aspiration pneumonia. Given the lack of controlled studies on empiric antibiotic therapy in this disorder, they are best withheld unless clinical, microbiologic, or radiographic features suggest a need.

Unwitnessed aspiration may mimic an atypical pneumonia. Clues to diagnosis include the clinical presentation (wheezing, sudden onset of respiratory distress that is disproportionate to the level of fever or radiographic infiltrates, etc.), predisposing factors, and sputum Gram stain (more neutrophils and few organisms). In mechanically ventilated patients, a low-grade fever, shifting rales or rhonchi, diffuse and/or migratory infiltrates, and increasing amounts of (purulent) tracheobronchial secretions are potential clues.

### Prevention

Preventive measures (Table 246.3) should be considered in patients predisposed to aspiration (those undergoing general anesthesia or enteral alimentation with feeding formula, and those with impaired pharyngeal and laryngeal function). Neither a gastrostomy tube nor a jejunostomy tube is totally protective; those with gastroesophgeal reflux may still aspirate.

## Aspiration of Pathogenic Bacteria

Pathogenic bacteria aspirated along with gastric contents may cause a bacterial pneumonia. A different mechanism is pneumonia caused by a gravitational process that transports bacteria—predominantly anaerobes—from the mouth into the dependent segments of the lung (most classically the superior segments of the lower lobe and posterior segments of the upper lobe). The predisposing factors are gingivitis and states of altered consciousness brought on by alcoholism, central nervous system diseases, drug overdoses, and seizures, among others.

**TABLE 246.3. Prevention of Aspiration Pneumonia in High-Risk Patients**

1. Use nonparticulate antacids and H2 blockers to reduce acidity and the residual gastric volume.
2. Use antiemetics selectively to increase lower esophageal sphincter pressure.
3. Confirm tube tip location radiographically prior to initiation of enteral tube feeding.
4. Elevate the head of the bed to 30 degrees.
5. Check residual gastric volume regularly. Residual should be <150 ml before the next feeding for those on bolus tube feeding.

### Pathogenesis

The aspirated material is largely oropharyngeal secretions, containing bacteria that are pooled on the tongue, gingiva, buccal mucosa, and pharynx. Oral anaerobes predominate, outnumbering aerobes by 5 : 1. In persons with poor oral hygiene and gingivitis, anaerobe concentrations may rise to $10^{11}$/ml. The most important pathogens are anaerobic streptococci, *Fusobacterium*, and *Bacteroides*. The lesion, initially a pneumonitis, evolves into an abscess.

### Clinical Features and Diagnosis

Typically, symptoms occur 1–2 weeks following the gravitational event. An indolent presentation with symptoms lasting several weeks or even months is not uncommon. The initial symptom is a productive cough with purulent sputum; the sputum infrequently has a putrid odor. Dyspnea and chest pain may be present, especially if an abscess or empyema has formed. Most patients are febrile, with low-grade fever. Auscultatory findings (bronchial breath sounds occasionally and rales) are localized, predominantly in the involved areas. Finger clubbing occurs in chronic cases.

The Gram stain of sputum shows multiple organisms; a culture is not helpful, as the predominant causative organisms are anaerobes (which the laboratory reports as "oral flora"). Cavitation often complicates the pneumonia, which involves the dependent segments (see Figure 218.1). Parapneumonic effusions are common and most evolve into an empyema. Diagnosis is by clinical, roentgenographic, and laboratory features, taken together with the circumstances. Complications are lung abscess (single or dominant cavity with an air-fluid level in a dependent lung segment, as shown in Figure 246.1) and empyema.

### Management

Antibiotics effective against anaerobic organisms are used to treat aspiration of pathogenic bacteria. Clindamycin (600 mg t.i.d.) is the antibiotic of choice. Treatment duration depends on the resolution of symptoms as well as the radiographic findings. Patients with a lung abscess will require many weeks of treatment, until the symptoms resolve x-rays resolve or stabilize. A concomitant pleural effusion calls for a diagnostic thoracentesis and, if an empyema is found, intercostal closed chest tube drainage.

## Aspiration of Inert Substances

Aspiration of foreign bodies into the tracheobronchial tree is the leading cause of accidental death at home for children under 1 year of age. Most of the patients with aspirated foreign bodies are below 12 years of age. In

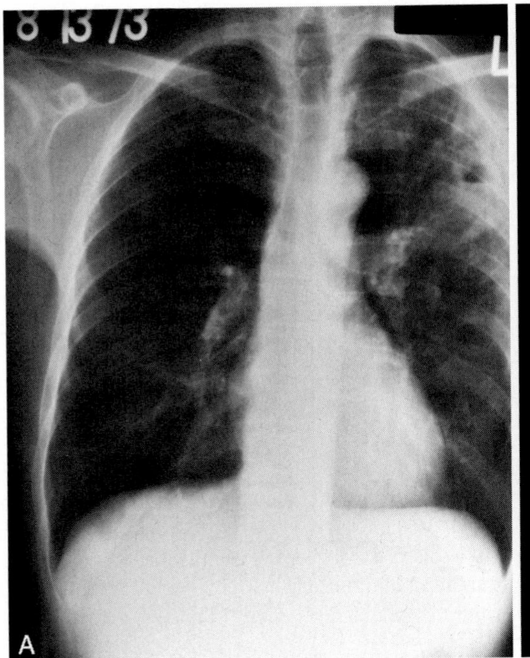


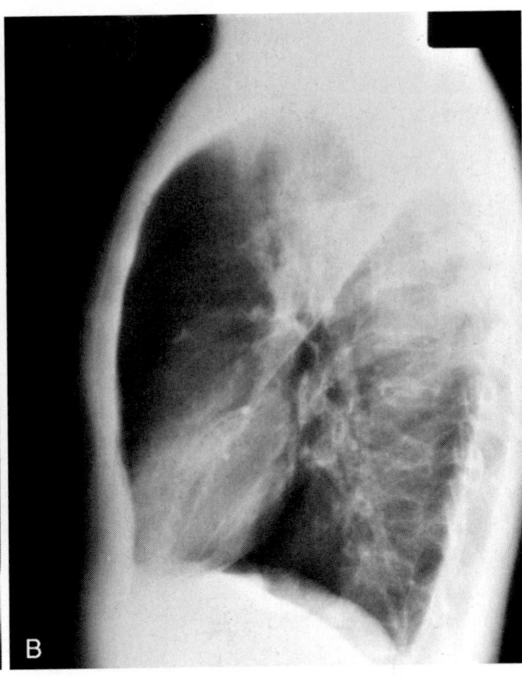


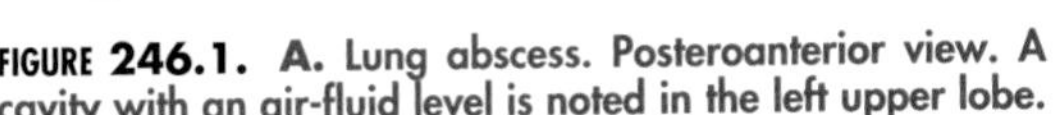

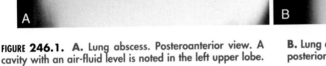

**FIGURE 246.1. A. Lung abscess. Posteroanterior view. A cavity with an air-fluid level is noted in the left upper lobe. B. Lung abscess. Lateral view showing lesion in the apical-posterior segment of the left upper lobe.**

adults, sudden, unexpected obstruction of the upper airway (**cafe coronary**) is not uncommon and could be lethal. Meat is the most commonly aspirated solid that causes a cafe coronary. Older age, poor dentition, alcohol consumption, and use of sedative drugs are all predisposing factors.

## Clinical Features and Diagnosis

The initial symptoms depend on the degree of obstruction, which depends on the size of the particle. Larger objects, such as poorly chewed meat, usually lodge in the larynx or trachea and cause **abrupt respiratory distress, inability to speak,** and **cyanosis.** Unrelieved, the obstruction is lethal. With significant, but incomplete tracheal obstruction by a foreign body, **stridor** and **intercostal retractions** may be noted. Obstruction in the distal trachea or in a mainstem bronchus may cause coughing and wheezing. Asymmetric breath sounds, unilateral wheeze, and unilateral decrease in air entry are clues. In general, the right lower lobe is more commonly affected than the left. Expiratory x-rays are useful to reveal air trapping on the affected side, manifested by a shift of the mediastinum to the opposite side. In difficult cases, endoscopy is the final arbiter. Smaller particles cause partial or distal obstruction in the tracheobronchial tree. Cough is the usual initial symptom, followed by shortness of breath, wheezing, chest pain, fever, nausea, and vomiting.

## Management

In foreign body–related upper airway obstruction, immediate **Heimlich maneuver** is indicated, with the rescuer performing abdominal thrusts between the xiphoid process and the umbilicus. This elevates the diaphragm and expels enough air from the lungs to expel the foreign body. For **nonemergent foreign body removal,** a **rigid bronchoscope** is preferable to a fiberoptic bronchoscope. Fiberoptic bronchoscopy is suitable for a peripheral foreign body or when rigid bronchoscopy is inadvisable because of neck or face injury. Occasionally, bronchoscopy may fail, necessitating a **thoracotomy.** Long-term sequelae of chronic foreign body impaction are **bronchial stenosis** and **bronchiectasis.**

# CHAPTER 247 DRUG-INDUCED PULMONARY DISEASE

More than one hundred drugs are associated with adverse affects on the lungs or pleura. Drug-induced pulmonary disease has a very wide spectrum (e.g., the life-threatening anaphylaxis due to penicillin, heroin-induced acute pulmonary edema, pulmonary fibrosis from amiodarone and bleomycin, and chronic cough from angiotensin-converting enzyme inhibitors). Table 247.1 will be helpful in approaching this important clinical problem. A number of drugs not listed in the table cause pleural or mediastinal disorders. For example, **nitrofurantoin** can cause **pleural effusion; procainamide, hydralazine, diphenylhydantoin,** and **isoniazid** can cause **pleural effusions** through **drug-induced lupus erythematosus** mechanism; and corticosteroids or phenytoin cause mediastinal and hilar prominences on x-rays (mediastinal lipomatosis and lymphadenopathy, respectively).

Because there are **no specific diagnostic** tests, a comprehensive history, supplemented by an assessment of the time from exposure to the development of symptoms and roentgenographic findings, is critical to diagnosis. The physical findings and x-ray findings vary, depending on the types of pulmonary reactions and sites of injury. In selected situations and under physician supervision, a **challenge with the suspected drug** may prove the diagnosis. An open lung biopsy is helpful in selected situations (e.g., newly developing infiltrates in a leukemic patient receiving cytotoxic therapy). A biopsy in these situations helps exclude infections or other causes and might possibly find a characteristic histologic picture to confirm the diagnosis of drug-induced pulmonary disease. The general principle of treatment is **further avoidance of the drug;** specific treatments vary with the type and severity of the disease.

**TABLE 247.1. Drug-Induced Pulmonary Disease***

| Type/Location of Reaction | Class of Drug | Specific Drugs (Partial List) |
|---|---|---|
| Pulmonary edema (noncardiac) | Narcotics | Heroin, methadone, morphine |
| | Analgesics | Aspirin, D-propoxyphene |
| | Others | Ethchlorvynol, hydrochlorothiazide |
| Pulmonary infiltrate with eosinophilia | Antibiotics and chemotherapeutic agents | Nitrofurantoin, penicillin, sulfonamides, methotrexate, procarbazine |
| | Others | Imipramine, cromolyn sodium |
| Diffuse alveolar/interstitial infiltrates | Chemotherapeutic agents | Bleomycin, busulfan, nitrofurantoin, cyclophosphamide, methotrexate, chlorambucil, azathioprine, gold, chloroquine |
| | Miscellaneous agents | Methysergide, oxygen, marijuana smoke, mineral oil, amiodarone, talc, tocainide |
| Pulmonary thromboembolism | Estrogens | Diethylstilbestrol, progesterone |
| Bronchospasm | Antibiotics | Penicillin, ampicillin |
| | Cholinergic agents | Mecholyl, neostigmine |
| | β-adrenergic blocker | Propranolol |
| | Analgesics | Ethyl ether |
| | Others | Piperazine, tartrazine |
| Respiratory muscle weakness | Antibiotics | Aminoglycosides, Polymyxin B |
| | Neuromuscular blockers | Tubocurarine, succinylcholine |
| Respiratory depression/acute respiratory failure | Narcotics | Heroin, methadone, morphine, cocaine |
| | Sedatives | Barbiturates |
| | Tranquilizers | Diazepam, chlordiazepoxide |

*Not a complete list.

# CHAPTER 248 BRONCHOGENIC CARCINOMA

Lung cancer, the most important malignant neoplasm in the United States, may be symptomatic on presentation, with cough, wheezing, new onset or worsening of sputum production, and bloody expectoration varying from blood-streaking of sputum to frank hemoptysis. Other well-known patterns of presentation of symptomatic lung cancer include post-obstructive pneumonia, lung abscess, pleural effusion, or an extrathoracic metastasis. Asymptomatic lung cancer classically presents as a solitary pulmonary nodule.

## Diagnosis

Given the high rate of metastases (80%) even at initial presentation, the goal of diagnostic evaluation is to establish an unequivocal diagnosis of lung cancer, including identification of the cell type and to stage the disease. The staging determined by all studies up to the time of surgery and lymph node dissection represents the **clinical staging;** clinical staging duly modified by operative and histological findings constitutes **pathological staging.** Tumor-node metastasis (TNM) staging for lung cancer is shown in Table 203.2.

The yield from cytological examination of sputum varies from less than 50% in peripheral lesions to almost 90% for lesions involving the central (proximal) lesions; the yield is higher with repeated samples or if hemoptysis is present, since hemoptysis suggests a tumor within the lumen of the airway. If small cell carcinoma is thus unequivocally diagnosed and the chest x-ray shows a central lesion, further surgical therapy or staging mediastinoscopy are not indicated since chemotherapy and radiation therapy are the main therapies for small cell carcinoma. However, staging procedures should follow for peripheral lesions; mediastinal nodal involvement ($N_2$) may preclude successful surgery.

Flexible fiberoptic bronchoscopy (FFB) is indicated (1) when lung cancer is suspected with normal or equivocal sputum cytological examination and (2) to assess resectability when sputum examination discloses malignant cells other than the small cell type. With visible endobronchial lesions, FFB makes a specific diagnosis in over 95% of cases. However, the yield of FFB drops to between 30% and 60% when no endobronchial lesions are visible and fluoroscopy is used to guide biopsies. If paratracheal and subcranial nodes are enlarged on CT scan, FFB may facilitate their transbronchoscopic aspiration for cytology.

If the foregoing methods are unrevealing, the clinical settings should dictate the diagnostic approach. Palpable lymph nodes should be biopsied. If the chest CT scan shows no significant mediastinal adenopathy or involvement by direct tumor extension, thoracotomy is the next step unless other medical problems, such as limited pulmonary reserve precludes resection. Positron-emission tomography (PET) is a new metabolic imaging technique used to detect local and distant metastases in patients with lung cancer (chapter 217). In general, mediastinal abnormalties on CT need confirmation with biopsy by mediastinoscopy or mediastinotomy before the tumor is deemed unresectable. Metastatic involvement of scalene nodes, contralateral mediastinal nodes (Stage IIIB), or ipsilateral mediastinal node involvement (Stage IIIA) with non-small cell lung cancer (NSCLC), or poor pulmonary reserve minimize surgical resection as an option. CT-guided transthoracic needle aspiration (TNA) is another approach used to diagnose lung cancer, especially in peripheral lesions (pleural-based). Pneumothorax from this procedure occurs in 20–30% of the cases, and bleeding occurs in about 20%. A definitive diagnosis may be obtained in over 90% of the cases.

## Management and Prognosis

Unless contraindicated (Table 248.1), surgical resection is the mainstay of therapy for NSCLC bronchogenic carcinoma. Neo-adjuvant therapy (chemotherapy and radiation therapy prior to surgery) or adjuvant therapy (chemotherapy or radiation therapy immediately following surgery) are being increasingly utilized. The entire neoplasm should be removed using a lobectomy or pneumonectomy depending on the individual situation. Surgical procedures carry a 30-day overall mortality of 3.7% (pneumonectomy, 6.2%; lobectomy, 2.9%). The age-related mortality in the eighth decade and beyond exceeds 7.1%. Prognosis depends on the staging (Figure 248.1) and other factors (Table 248.2). Chemotherapy and radiation therapy are the treatment modalities for small cell lung cancer.

*(Additional information on bronchogenic carcinoma appears in chapter 203.)*

**TABLE 248.1. Contraindications to Thoracotomy and Resection in Bronchogenic Carcinoma**

| | |
|---|---|
| **Operability** | Poor cardiac reserve (uncontrolled heart failure, uncontrollable arrhythmias, recent myocardial infarction, etc.)[a] |
| | Poor pulmonary reserve[a] |
| | Resting $PaO_2$ <50 mm |
| | Resting $PaCO_2$ >45 mm Hg |
| | Age over 70[b] |
| | Small cell carcinoma, unless it is a localized pulmonary nodule[a] |
| **Resectability** | Any disease beyond Stage IIIA |
| | Distant metastases[a] |
| | Malignant pleural effusion[a] |
| | Contralateral mediastinal lymph node involvement[a] |
| | Superior vena caval obstruction[a] |
| | Esophageal/phrenic nerve involvement[a] |
| | Recurrent laryngeal nerve involvement[a] |
| | Involvement of trachea, carina or lesion within 2.0 cm of carina[a] |

[a] = absolute.
[b] = relative.

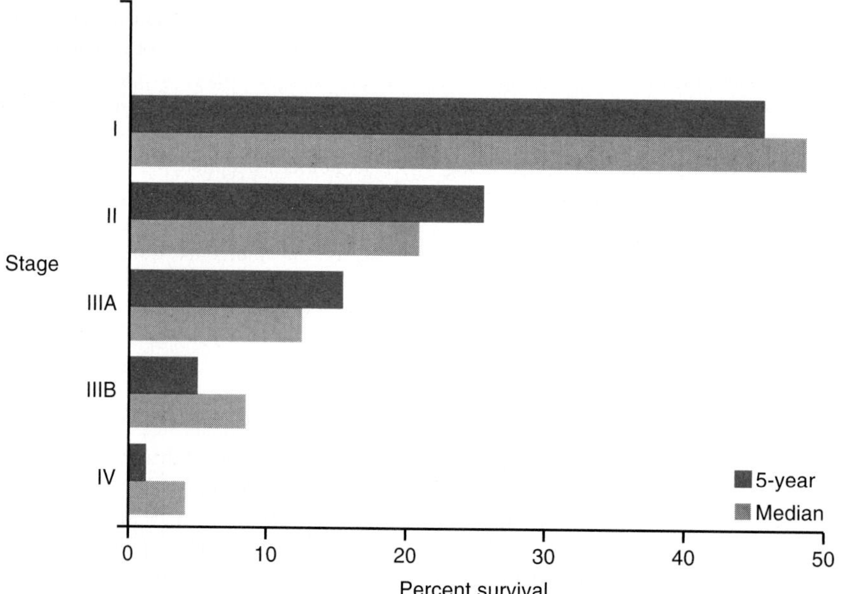


**FIGURE 248.1. Prognosis in nonsmall cell lung cancer. Estimated survival by stage with current optimal therapy.** (Data from: Briggs DD et al. MKSAP in the Subspecialty of Pulmonary and Critical Care. Philadelphia: American College of Physicians, 1994, p. 136. Used with permission.)

**TABLE 248.2. Prognostic Factors in Non-Small-Cell Lung Cancer**

| Factor | Favorable | Unfavorable |
|---|---|---|
| Age (operative cases) | Younger | Older |
| Gender | Women | Men |
| Histology (operative cases) | Squamous | Nonsquamous |
| LDH (inoperable cases) | Elevated | Normal |
| Liver/bone/brain metastases | None | Present |
| Mediastinal nodes (surgically resected) | Negative | Positive |
| Performance status | Fully ambulatory | Not fully ambulatory |
| TNM stage | See Figure 241.1 | See Figure 241.1 |
| Tumor-related symptoms | None | From metastases |

(Adapted from: Ihde DC, Minna JD. Curr Prob Cancer 1991; 15:91. Used with permission.)

# CHAPTER 249 THE SOLITARY PULMONARY NODULE

## Definition and Etiology

Solitary pulmonary nodule (SPN), a roentgenographic diagnosis, is a single, well-circumscribed (surrounded by aerated lung tissue), spherical pulmonary density. By convention, it is 3.0 cm or less in diameter (> 3.0 cm in diameter are designated as "masses"). SPNs are not accompanied by chest x-ray evidence of atelectasis, pleural effusion, or hilar or mediastinal adenopathy. SPNs may be either calcified or uncalcified. **The importance of the concept of an SPN is that it represents potentially the most curable stage of lung cancer.** Thus, it is essential to estimate the probability of malignancy of an SPN in order to decide on an appropriate approach.

A significant proportion of SPNs is malignant, from 10–68% depending on the series and patient population. Bronchogenic carcinoma tops the list of malignant SPNs. The incidence of bronchogenic cancer varies with advancing age and smoking history. SPNs can be benign, the vast majority being infectious granulomas (predominantly mycotic and mycobacterial), and also hamartomas, and miscellaneous entities including intrapulmonary lymph nodes, pulmonary infarction.

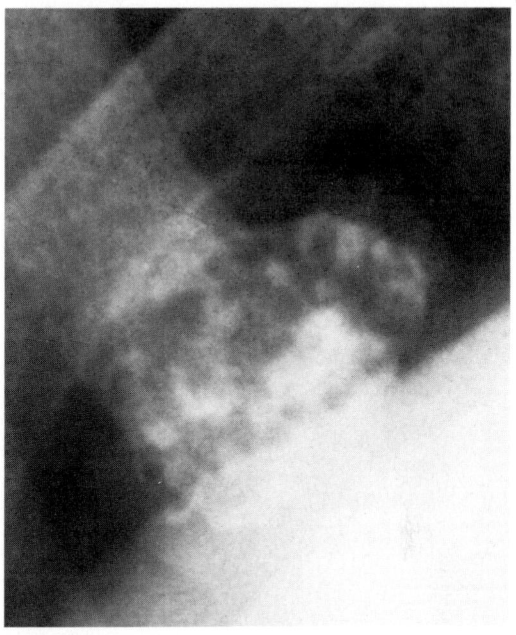

**FIGURE 249.1. Solitary pulmonary nodule. "Popcorn" calcification in a benign long nodule.**

## Management

The potential of lung cancer and the highly favorable prognosis (5-year survival rate in 50–80% of all cases) for lung cancer presenting as an SPN necessitate an organized and rapid approach to assessment and management of all SPNs. CT and the application of probabilistic reasoning (a high pre-test probability of a lesion being benign or malignant) are important components of the decision-making process. The essentials in decision-making include a thorough clinical history, physical examination, and review of current and old roentgenograms if available. Age, history of smoking, presence of coexistent lung disease, and roentgenographic (and, if available, CT) appearances of the nodule are important considerations. PET scanning can also help differentiate benign from malignant SPNs (chapter 217).

The **emphasis** in managing SPN continues to be **surgical resection of the SPN,** unless a specific benign lesion can be established with a high degree of accuracy. The two generally accepted criteria of benignity are **1) radiographic stability of the lesion** as evidenced by no change in size for at least 2 years and **2) characteristic patterns of calcification** (usually requiring CT), which include "popcorn" (Figure 249.1) or concentric (Figure 249.2) or central, "bull's eye" patterns. Younger age (<35

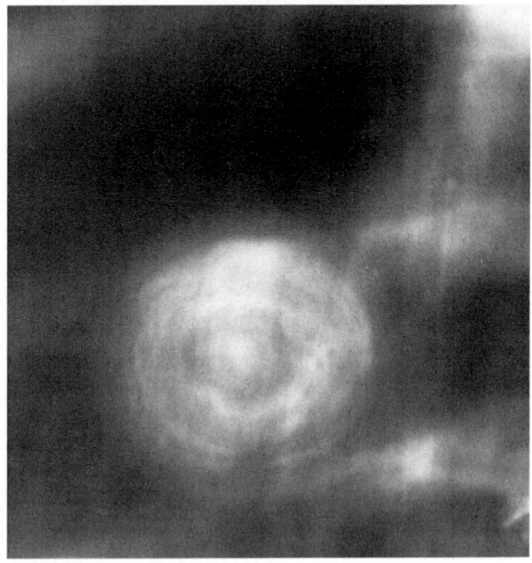

**FIGURE 249.2. Solitary pulmonary nodule: benign concentric calcification in a histoplasmosa.**

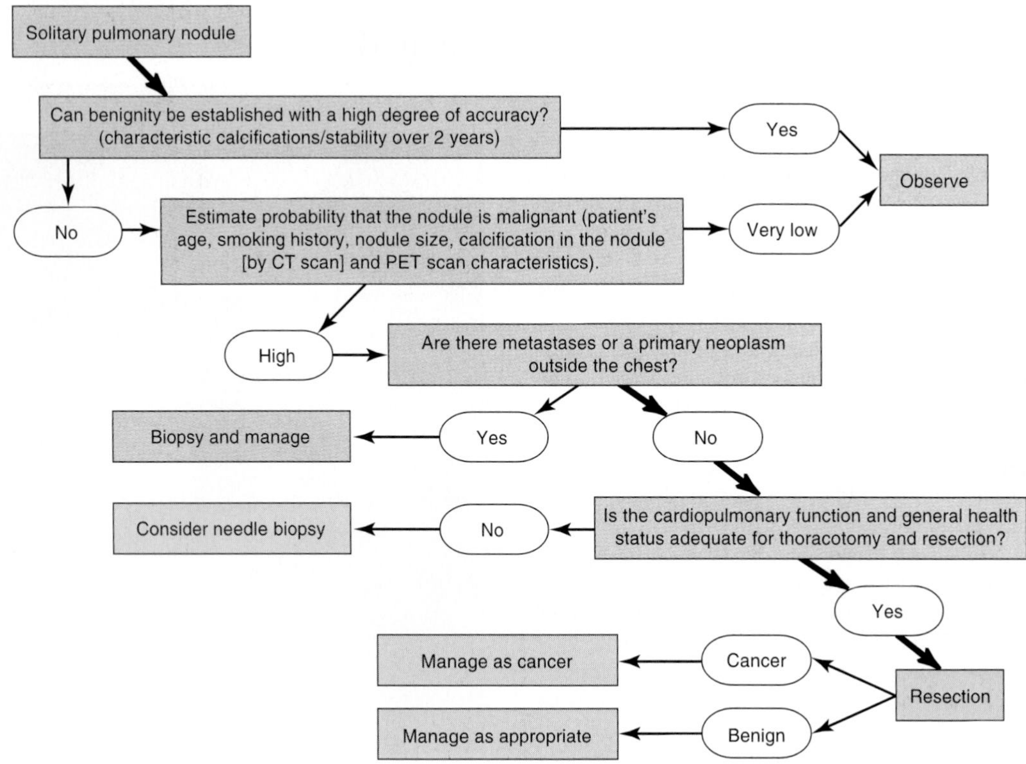


**FIGURE 249.3.** Suggested approach to managing solitary pulmonary nodule.

years) and an absence of smoking history also support a benign etiology. The management of SPN is outlined in Figure 249.3. "Watchful waiting" of a lesion that might be malignant is not acceptable medical practice. Note that video-assisted thoracoscopic surgery (VATS) is a technique that is also used to resect SPNs.

The **search for an extrapulmonary neoplasm** producing a metastatic SPN is indicated only when a previous history of neoplastic disease exists or when a review of systems or clinical examination suggests that possibility (e.g., a change in bowel habits or the presence of occult blood in the stools). Similarly, a search for metastases from a malignant SPN is indicated only if clinical features (pain and tenderness in long bones, enlarged nodular liver, localizing neurological findings, etc.) or basic laboratory studies (complete blood counts, urinalysis, liver function tests, and serum calcium) suggest that possibility. Bronchoscopy and brushing have no routine use. Mediastinoscopy is utilized if a CT scan shows significant mediastinal pathology. Fine-needle aspiration biopsy (FNAB) of SPN yields a positive result for malignancy in up to 90% of the cases when the nodule is malignant. These results vary widely. However, the diagnosis of a specific benign disease is definitively made by FNAB much less frequently (30–40%) and unless a specific benign diagnosis is made, the SPN can not be assumed to be benign. FNAB is indicated when resection is not feasible and a pre-operative diagnosis is essential. Other possible indications include a patient with borderline pulmonary function, in whom a definitive diagnosis of malignancy could lead to surgical resection. Video-assisted thorascopic surgery and open thoracotomy are utilized to make a definitive diagnosis and for complete resection.

# CHAPTER 250 PLEURAL EFFUSION

Pleural disease most commonly presents as a pleural effusion. It is an abnormal accumulation of fluid in the pleural space, caused by an imbalance in oncotic or hydrostatic pressures (transudate) or by an intrinsic abnormality of the pleura (exudate). Causes of pleural effusion are listed in Table 250.1.

## Pathogenesis

The pleural space, the vacuum between the parietal and the visceral pleura, contains a small amount (approximately 10 ml) of clear fluid with a low-protein content. Fluid enters and exits the space through capillaries or the lymphatics in the parietal or visceral pleura. Because an equilibrium prevails between the physiologic formation and removal of pleural fluid, a pleural effusion results from an increase in the formation or a decrease in the lymphatic removal of fluid or a combination of the two.

## Clinical Features

The symptoms of pleural effusion include dyspnea, pleuritic or nonpleuritic chest pain, and nonproductive cough. Sometimes it may be asymptomatic. Both a mechanical disadvantage of the diaphragm and restrictive ventilatory impairment resulting from the effusion cause the dyspnea. In addition, the underlying disease that caused the effusion may also cause symptoms and signs. Some of the historical clues to the etiology of the pleural effusion are listed in Table 250.2. Physical findings of pleural effusion are decreased tactile fremitus, dullness to percussion, and decreased breath sounds on auscultation. Large effusions (>1,000 ml) may cause contralateral mediastinal shift.

## Roentgenographic Features

Free pleural fluid has a characteristic x-ray appearance: a meniscus in the costophrenic angle in the posteroanterior (PA) view (Figure 225.1c) and blunting of the posterior gutter in the lateral view (Figure 250.1). The former requires at least 500 ml fluid. Free fluid layers out on a lateral decubitus view. Pleural fluid may assume other appearances, including that of a pseudotumor or tumors (Figure 250.2). Absence of contralateral mediastinal shift with a massive effusion suggests prior mediastinal fixation due to malignancy. Loculated pleural effusions may be detected using ultrasonography.

## Differential Diagnosis and Diagnosis

Sometimes, the cause is evident (e.g., bilateral effusions in clinically obvious congestive heart failure or asymptomatic, small effusions within 48 hours of

**TABLE 250.1. Causes of Pleural Effusions**

| Frequency | Transudates | Exudates |
|---|---|---|
| Common | Congestive heart failure<br>Cirrhosis of liver | Parapneumonic<br>Malignant neoplasm<br>Pulmonary embolism |
| Less common | Nephrotic syndrome<br>Pulmonary embolism | Tuberculosis<br>Nonbacterial infections<br>Collagen vascular diseases<br>Dressler's syndrome<br>Drugs<br>Pancreatitis<br>Iatrogenic trauma<br>endoscopic sclerotherapy, subclavian vein catheters |
| Rare | Peritoneal dialysis<br>Urinothorax<br>Atelectasis<br>Superior vena caval obstruction | Subphrenic/liver abscess<br>Esophageal rupture<br>Chylothorax<br>Benign asbestos effusion<br>Uremia<br>Sarcoidosis<br>Meig's syndrome<br>Yellow nail syndrome |

**TABLE 250.2. Diagnosing Etiology of Pleural Fluid: Clues from History**

| History/Feature | Diagnosis Suggested by History/Feature |
|---|---|
| Asbestos exposure | Benign asbestos pleural effusion, malignant mesothelioma |
| Smoking with or without asbestos exposure | Malignant effusion due to bronchogenic carcinoma |
| Drugs (see text) | Drug-induced pleural effusion |
| Exposure to tuberculosis; positive tuberculin skin test | Tuberculous pleural effusion |
| Cough with purulent sputum, chills, fever | Parapneumonic effusion |
| Immobilization, postoperative states, obesity, cardiac failure, past or present deep venous thrombosis | Pulmonary embolism |
| Joint pains, swelling, stiffness | Rheumatoid effusion |
| Chest trauma | Hemothorax |
| Recent subclavian venous line insertion | Hemothorax or infusion into pleural space |
| Urinary obstruction | Urinothorax |
| Abdominal pain, alcoholism | Pancreatic effusion |
| Vomiting, upper G.I. endoscopy, sclerotherapy | Esophageal rupture/post-sclerotherapy |
| Parturition, upper abdominal surgery | Self-limited pleural effusion |
| Cirrhosis, ascites | Transudative effusion due to cirrhosis |
| Orthopnea, paroxysmal nocturnal dyspnea, pedal edema | Congestive heart failure |

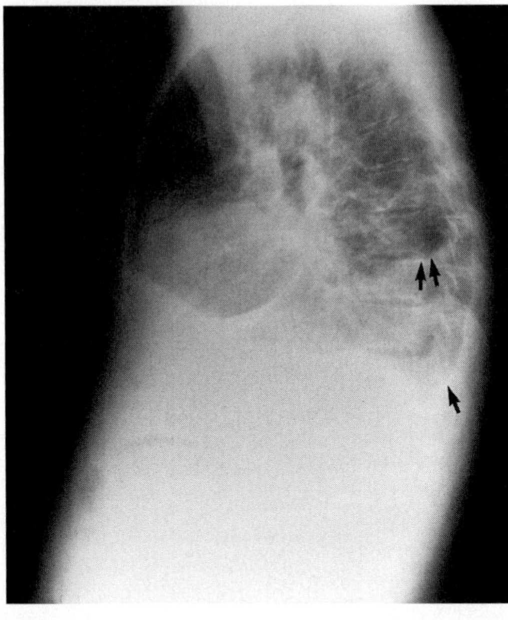

**FIGURE 250.1. Lateral view of a patient with bilateral effusions showing blunting of the posterior costophrenic sulcus (single arrow) representing one side and a posteriorly located meniscus (double arrows) representing the other.**

abdominal surgery or parturition). A repeat chest roentgenogram in a few days after appropriate treatment or observation will suffice. When the cause of the effusion is unknown, an evaluation is necessary to ascertain it. The physician must formulate a clinical diagnosis first, then obtain a pleural fluid sample by thoracentesis and determine whether it is a transudate or an exudate, and finally determine the exact cause by additional tests or invasive procedures.

To safely perform a thoracentesis, a lateral decubitus roentgenogram is helpful, but not essential. If the fluid layers along the inner chest wall and the "layer" is at least 10 mm thick, then one may proceed with thoracentesis. If the pleural effusion does not layer, it may be loculated and must be differentiated from pleural thickening or a pleural neoplasm, perhaps through an ultrasound. While computed tomography (CT) is not generally necessary, in select cases it gives useful information about the underlying lung and mediastinum and defines pleural loculations. An expiration chest x-ray is advisable after thoracentesis to detect a pneumothorax. Other complications are bleeding and infection.

The gross characteristics of the fluid should be noted. Yellow-green thick fluid is pus—that is, bacterial empyema. Foul-smelling fluid implies anaerobic empyema. Milky white fluid is either a chylous or a chyliform effusion; a grossly bloody fluid is likely a hemothorax. Protein and lactate dehydrogenase (LDH) of the pleural fluid along with simultaneous serum values can differentiate exudate from a transudate (Table 250.3). Exudates fulfill at least one of the following criteria: (1) pleural fluid: serum protein ratio >0.5; (2) pleural fluid: serum LDH ratio >0.6, or (3) an absolute LDH exceeding two-thirds of the upper limits of "normal" for the serum LDH. Transudative effusions meet none of these criteria.

## Transudative Pleural Effusions

Congestive heart failure is the most common cause of a transudate. Effusions are typically bilateral, but if unilateral, they are generally right-sided. The notion that diuresis converts a transudate into an exudate is unproven. Associated pleuritic pain or unilateral left-sided effusion should arouse the suspicion of pulmonary embolism. Liver cirrhosis is another cause of transudates, due to the egress of ascites from the peritoneal cavity into the pleural space through diaphragmatic defects and through the diaphragmatic lymphatics. Ascites and stigmata of chronic liver disease are found in such cases. Typically, the effusion is right-sided; less commonly, it is bilateral. Other causes are listed in Table 250.1.

## Exudative Pleural Effusions

The most common cause of an exudative pleural effusion is parapneumonic—that is, an ipsilateral effusion associated with a bacterial pneumonia. Such effusions complicate 40% of bacterial pneumonias and typically contain >10,000/μl of WBCs with a predominance of neutrophils. Most are uncomplicated and resolve with appropriate antibiotics alone. Others are an empyema (gross pus or bacteria seen on microscopy or culture) or a "complicated" effusion (a transitional fluid between uncomplicated parapneumonic effusion and an empyema), which requires chest tube drainage to avoid persistent infection, bronchopleural fistula, or adhesions. Conditions that impair local or systemic defenses such as bronchiectasis, chronic obstructive pulmonary disease, alcoholism, diabetes mellitus and rheumatoid arthritis increase the risk of empyema. In such high-risk patients, parapneumonic effusions with a pH ≤7.30 (if pH is unavailable glucose ≤100 mg/dl or LDH ≥600 IU/L) should be treated as empyema. In low-risk patients, a pH ≤7.20 or glucose ≤80 mg/dl or LDH ≥2000 IU/L are appropriate threshold values. These thresholds have a high negative predictive value in that patients with pleural fluid values not meeting the thresholds would not require chest tube drainage. Patients who do not fall in these categories should be monitored clinically and radiographically for resolution of the effusion. Although heavy reliance is placed on pH, glucose and LDH, other factors such as the size of the effusion and the presence of loculations should also be considered in making the decision as to whether to drain the effusion.

Malignant effusion, a common cause of exudative effusion, results from pleural invasion by the malignancy. Cancers of the lung and breast are the leading causes and, along with lymphomas, constitute 75% of the cases of malignant effusions. Pleural fluid cytology is diagnostic in 60–80% of malignant effusions. Pleural effusions may occur in malignancy without actual malignant pleural involvement. These cytology-negative effusions, best designated as **paramalignant effusions,** result from tumor invasion of mediastinal lymph nodes, atelectasis, or pneumonia.

A pleural effusion occurs in approximately one-half of patients with pulmonary embolism; about 80% of these effusions are exudative. It is usually unilateral and

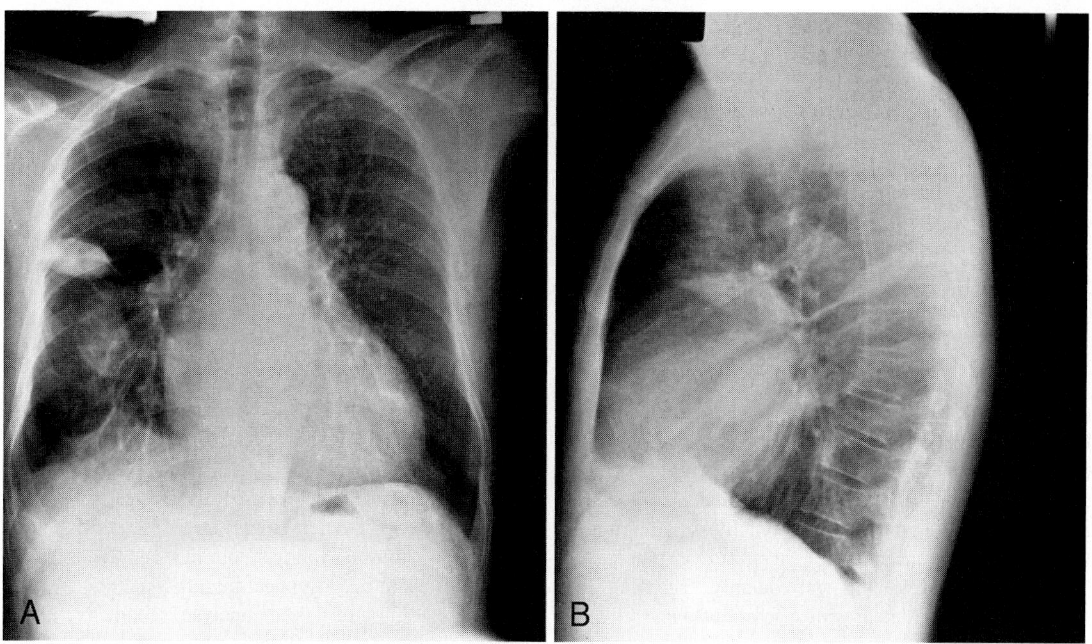


**FIGURE 250.2. A. Interlobar effusion (pseudotumor). Posteroanterior view. B. Interlobar effusion, lateral view. Figures A and B show accumulation of fluid in the major and minor fissures.**
(Courtesy of Lawrence R. Goodman, MD, Medical College of Wisconsin, Milwaukee.)

**TABLE 250.3. Pleural Fluid Tests and Their Usefulness**

| Tests | Usefulness | Comments |
|---|---|---|
| LDH | Separates transudates and exudates. | Useful in all. |
| Protein | Separates transudates and exudates. | Simultaneously obtain serum LDH and protein. |
| Gram stain, cultures | If positive, diagnostic of empyema. | Useful in all exudates. |
| Glucose | ↓ compared to a serum value in complicated parapneumonic effusions and empyema, rheumatoid pleural effusion, some malignancies, and TB. | Generally useful in all exudates. |
| Cytology | If positive, diagnostic of malignant effusion. | |
| Stains, cultures for mycobacteria, fungi | If positive, diagnostic. | |
| Antinuclear antibody (ANA) | ANA titer ≥1 : 160 and pleural fluid to serum ANA ratio ≥1 are highly suggestive of SLE pleuritis. | Only selective use (rarity of the diagnoses). However, diagnostic if clinical suspicion is high. |
| LE cells | Diagnostic of SLE pleuritis. | Same as ANA. |
| Amylase | ↑ and exceeds serum level in pancreatic effusion. Increased amylase of salivary origin in esophageal rupture, malignancies. | |
| Triglycerides | >110 mg/ml indicates chylothorax. | Selective use only. |
| Chylomicrons | Presence diagnostic of chylothorax. | |
| Hematocrit | ↑, approaching that of blood diagnostic of hemothorax. ≥1%, but not hemothorax, suggests malignancy, trauma or tuberculosis. | Useful only if combined with a strong pre-thoracentesis clinical diagnosis. |
| Red cell count | >100,000/mm$^3$ suggest same diagnoses as hematocrit >1%. | Same as hematocrit. |
| White cell count | >10,000/mm$^3$ in parapneumonic effusion, pulmonary embolism, malignancy, tuberculosis, Dressler's syndrome, lupus pleural effusion. | |
| Differential count | ↑ Neutrophils: indicates acute inflammation. ↑ Lymphocytic: malignancy or tuberculosis. | |
| pH | <6.0 accompanied by elevated amylase strongly suggests esophageal rupture. <7.20 due to a variety of causes. ≤7.30 in parapneumonic effusion in high-risk patients or ≤7.20 in low risk patients is indication for chest tube drainage (see text). | Useful in suspected esophageal rupture and parapneumonic effusions only. |

↑ = elevated; ↓ = decreased; cytology = for malignancy; LDH = lactate dehydrogenase; LE = lupus erythematosus; SLE = systemic lupus erythematosus; TB = tuberculosis.

may be bloody and associated with a pulmonary infiltrate. Bloody pleural fluid in pulmonary embolism does not contraindicate anticoagulation. Pleural tuberculosis often causes a unilateral, exudative pleural effusion (see chapter 225 for pathogenesis). Parenchymal abnormalities are generally absent in the chest x-ray. A tuberculin skin test is positive only infrequently. The fluid is lymphocyte-preponderant with sparse (<5%) mesothelial cells. Fluid culture alone has a low diagnostic yield (<25%) but percutaneous pleural biopsy showing granulomas markedly increases the diagnostic yield. Although the effusion resolves spontaneously, if untreated, most of these patients develop active tuberculosis within 5 years.

Acute and chronic pancreatitis can cause a high-amylase, generally left-sided, exudative effusion. A pleural effusion that follows vomiting and is associated with chest pain and dyspnea, might signal spontaneous esophageal rupture; fluid analysis characteristically shows high (salivary) amylase, a low pH, and, on Gram stain, a polymicrobial flora; ingested food particles are often seen. Finally, some medications cause exudative pleural effusions—for example, agents used in chemotherapy (methotrexate, procarbazine) and esophageal sclerotherapy, tocolytics (used in premature labor), bromocriptine, dantrolene, methysergide, L-tryptophan, nitrofurantoin, and amiodarone. Hydralazine, phenytoin, isoniazid, and procainamide can induce a lupus syndrome, an integral feature of which is a pleural effusion. Exudative pleural effusions may also occur in rheumatoid arthritis (RA), systemic lupus erythematosus (SLE), and Dressler's syndrome, also known as **postcardiac injury syndrome** (PCIS). The glucose in RA pleural effusions is typically low.

### Indications and Utility of Procedures

To fully and cost-effectively utilize the diagnostic potential of pleural fluid tests (see Table 250.3), all clinical information should be integrated and a pretest clinical diagnosis formed. Appropriate tests can then follow. Tuberculosis can be diagnosed in about 90% of the cases by combining percutaneous pleural biopsy (PPB) and pleural fluid smears and cultures. Pleural fluid cytology is superior to PPB in diagnosing malignancy. However, diagnostic yield improves by about 7% when PPB is added to a negative cytological study.

When a PPB is nondiagnostic, the options are clinical follow-up or thoracoscopy/fiberoptic bronchoscopy. Thoracoscopy with biopsy is particularly useful in the diagnosis of suspected tuberculous and malignant effusions and malignant mesothelioma. Fiberoptic bronchoscopy has a low yield in pleural effusion, unless there is hemoptysis, or a mass or complete or partial atelectasis is seen in the chest x-ray or CT scan. Even with an extensive work-up, a cause for pleural effusion may be elusive in 15–20% of the cases. However, the course and outcome of these patients are often favorable and the majority of such effusions resolve spontaneously.

### Management

The management of pleural effusion depends on the cause of effusion. Pleural fluid drainage is necessary in some cases for therapy or palliation. Empyema and complicated parapneumonic effusions require closed chest tube drainage. Complicated parapneumonic effusions can also be managed by combining percutaneous image-guided catheter drainage with intrapleural fibrinolytic therapy. Delay in establishing effective drainage increases morbidity and likely increases mortality. Inadequate drainage might necessitate drainage using a surgical procedure. An undiagnosed lymphocytic effusion and a positive PPD skin test is tuberculosis unless proven otherwise. Pleural effusion and pleuritis due to PCIS respond to nonsteroidal anti-inflammatory agents or corticosteroids. Effusions due to esophageal rupture or pancreatic pseudocyst require prompt surgical consultation. Pleural fluid drainage followed by chemical pleurodesis with talc slurry frequently relieves dyspnea from a recurrent malignant effusion. Chemical pleurodesis is also effective in recurrent or refractory nonmalignant or undiagnosed effusions.

# CHAPTER 251 PNEUMOTHORAX

Pneumothorax, or air in the pleural space, may be classified as traumatic, iatrogenic, or spontaneous. **Traumatic pneumothorax** results from penetrating or blunt injury to the chest. **Iatrogenic pneumothorax** results from surgical procedures (e.g., thoracentesis, subclavian vein catheterization, needle biopsy of lung) or therapeutic interventions (e.g., mechanical ventilation with or without positive end expiratory pressure). **Spontaneous pneumothorax** may be either primary occurring in persons without apparent lung disease or secondary in persons who have a preexisting lung disease. Primary spontaneous pneumothorax occurs more commonly in men (typically tall, thin, and young) than in women. Cigarette smokers are at increased risk. Its pathogenesis is elusive, but rupture of subpleurally located blebs is one proposed theory. The configuration of the thoracic cage and traction pressures exerted onto the alveolar walls are presumed predisposing factors. Causes of secondary spontaneous pneumothorax are shown in Table 251.1.

### Pathogenesis

The pressure in the normal pleural space is negative with reference to atmospheric and alveolar pressures. A communication between pleura and the atmosphere (as in penetrating trauma), or between the pleura and the lung (as in a ruptured bulla), causes air to enter the pleural space until the pleural and atmospheric pressures equalize. This increased pleural pressure causes the lung to collapse. In some instances, air that enters pleural space cannot leave it because of a "ball valve" mechanism. Intrapleural pressure then exceeds atmospheric pressure throughout expiration and often during inspiration also. The resulting "tension pneumothorax" is life-threatening

TABLE 251.1. Causes of Secondary Spontaneous Pneumothorax

| | |
|---|---|
| Common | Obstructive disorders |
| | Emphysema |
| | Bronchial asthma |
| | Cystic Fibrosis |
| | Infections |
| | Tuberculosis |
| | Necrotizing pneumonia |
| | Lung abscess |
| | Diffuse Infiltrative diseases |
| | Histiocytosis X |
| | Sarcoidosis |
| | Complicating ventilator management |
| | Associated with PEEP |
| | High airway pressures |
| | Airway obstruction |
| Rare | Malignant neoplasm of lung or pleura |
| | Pulmonary infarction |
| | Marfan's syndrome |
| | Ehlers-Danlos syndrome |
| | Tuberous sclerosis |
| | Catamenial (associated with menstrual periods) |

because it compromises ventilation via mediastinal shift and diminishes cardiac output by impairing venous return. Tension pneumothorax is more likely to occur with traumatic, iatrogenic or secondary spontaneous pneumothorax than with primary spontaneous pneumothorax.

## Clinical Features and Diagnosis

The clinical features depend on the volume of air in the pleural cavity and the nature and degree of the underlying lung disease. Most patients have some dyspnea; a few may be asymptomatic. The degree of dyspnea depends on the severity of the pneumothorax and the underlying disease. Chest pain is usually sudden. Physical findings include hyperresonance on percussion and diminished to absent tactile fremitus and breath sounds on the affected side. Underlying severe emphysema, particularly bullous emphysema, could make the diagnosis of pneumothorax by physical examination very difficult.

Tension pneumothorax is a respiratory emergency, manifested by respiratory distress, tachypnea, and tachycardia often accompanied by distended veins, thready pulse, and hypotension. Bulging of the ipsilateral intercostal spaces and mediastinal shift to the contralateral side may be detected.

The chest x-ray is diagnostic. The air separates the margin of the collapsed lung from the parietal pleura (Figure 251.1); mediastinal shift is present in tension pneumothorax. Occasionally, there is an air-fluid level in the pleural cavity. An expiratory chest roentgenogram is helpful in delineating a pneumothorax after procedures (e.g., following thoracentesis, transbronchial lung biopsy) that can cause this complication.

## Management

A variety of treatment options are available and the choice clearly depends on the severity of the pneumothorax, predisposing state, and underlying disease. Most asymptomatic or mildly symptomatic patients with unilateral and small (approximately 10–20% of lung volume) primary spontaneous pneumothorax can be observed without hospitalization as they resolve within a week. A chest x-ray should be repeated in 6–12 hours to detect any progression. Supplemental oxygen administration speeds the resorption of air in the pleural cavity. Evacuation of intrapleural air is recommended in primary spontaneous pneumothorax that is large or symptomatic or is increasing in size. Simple aspiration with small-bore (14 French) catheter is successful in most cases. If expansion of the lung does not occur, the catheter can be attached to a one-way Heimlich valve or to a water-seal device. Additional application of suction is rarely needed. Chest tube (>16F) drainage attached to a water-seal device is the preferred method for unstable large primary spontaneous pneumothorax, large secondary spontane-

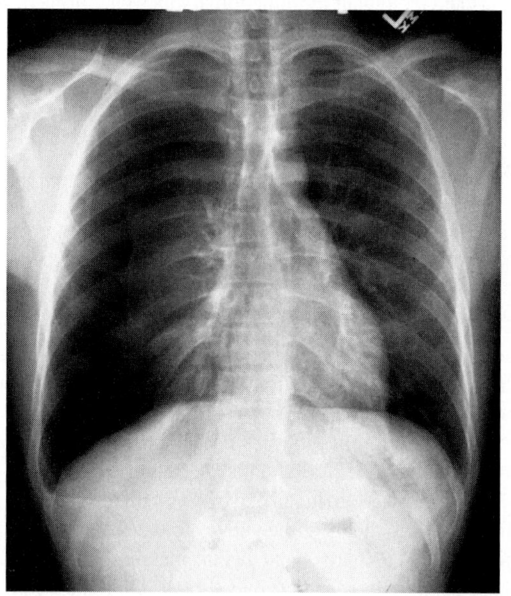

**FIGURE 251.1. Spontaneous pneumothorax: entire right lung is collapsed.**
(Courtesy of Lawrence R. Goodman, MD, Medical College of Wisconsin, Milwaukee.)

ous pneumothorax, tension pneumothorax, and hydropneumothorax. Tension pneumothorax is a medical emergency and, if the diagnosis is suspected, a large-bore needle should be immediately inserted into the second anterior intercostal space of the affected side to evacuate the air. Large amounts of air coming through the needle with relief of symptoms confirms the diagnosis. The needle should be left in place until a chest tube is inserted and the air drained under water seal. Primary spontaneous pneumothorax recurs in about one-half of all cases in 2 years. Chest tube drainage and chemical pleurodesis are recommended for ipsilateral recurrence. Any further occurrence is best treated by thoracotomy or thoracoscopy with resection of blebs and pleural abrasion. Persistent air leaks in spontaneous secondary pneumothorax most often resolve in 1 week. In unresolved cases, thoracoscopic procedure to repair the leak and prevent recurrence of pneumothorax is needed.

# CHAPTER 252 ASBESTOS PLEURAL DISEASE, FIBROTHORAX, AND PLEURAL TUMORS

## Asbestos Pleural Disease

Owing to their size and shape, asbestos fibers that enter the lungs are only minimally cleared. The retained fibers generate a chronic inflammatory response that causes both parenchymal and pleural injury. Five pleural disorders are associated with asbestos exposure: benign asbestos pleural effusion, pleural plaque, pleural fibrosis, rounded atelectasis, and malignant mesothelioma.

## Pleural Effusion and Pleural Plaques

**Benign asbestos pleural effusion** (BAPE) is the most common asbestos-related disorder that occurs within 10 years of asbestos exposure. It may be incidentally discovered on chest x-ray or may simulate a pneumonia with pleuritic pain and fever. The effusion is often unilateral and generally self-limited, but tends to recur. The fluid usually is blood-tinged and may be eosinophilic. The diagnosis depends on a history of asbestos exposure, a consistent clinical presentation, and an otherwise unexplained exudative effusion.

**Pleural plaques** commonly occur in the lateral areas and in the diaphragmatic pleura, and may be calcified. They occur at least 20 years after asbestos exposure and are the most common sequel thereof. Bilateral diaphragmatic pleural calcification is nearly pathognomonic of asbestos-induced pleural disease (Figure 252.1). Pleural plaques alone cause neither symptoms nor pulmonary function abnormalities; nor do they undergo malignant transformation. No therapy is needed. However, diffuse pleural fibrosis, which involves both the visceral and parietal pleura, commonly causes restrictive ventilatory impairment.

## Fibrothorax

Fibrothorax results from the deposition of fibrous tissue, causing a thick fibrotic visceral pleura, which limits the expansion of the underlying lung. It is a late complication of empyema, hemothorax, or pleural tuberculosis. Conditions causing chronic pleuritis (uremia, collagen vascular disease, pancreatitis, and asbestos pleural disease) may cause fibrothorax. Patients present with exertional dyspnea. Findings include decreased expansion and narrowed intercostal spaces on the affected side with ipsilateral mediastinal shift. Chest x-rays show the ipsilateral mediastinal shift and dense pleural fibrosis, often calcified, surrounding the lung. Pulmonary function tests show restrictive ventilatory impairment. Decortication—removal of the fibrous pleural peel—is the only effective treatment.

## Pleural Tumors

Primary tumors of the pleura are usually mesotheliomas that arise from mesothelial lining cells. They may be local or diffuse, benign or malignant. In histology, they

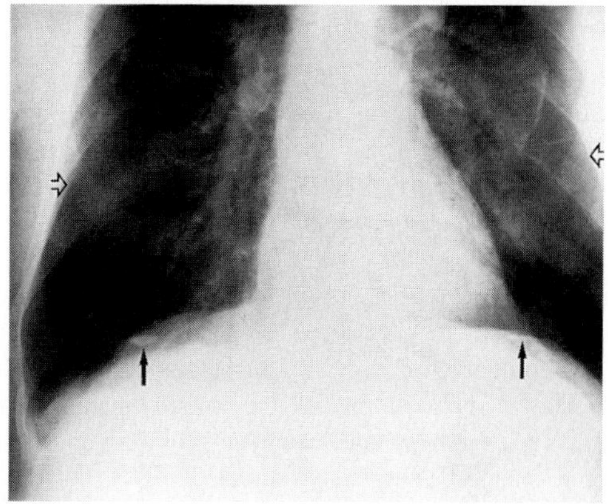

**FIGURE 252.1.** Chest x-ray of a patient showing several features of asbestos-related pleuropulmonary disease, including calcified pleural plaques (open arrows) and diaphragmatic calcification (solid arrows).

may appear as epithelial, fibrous, or mixed types. However, the vast majority of pleural malignancies are metastatic, the most common sources being cancers of the breast and lung. Hodgkin's and non-Hodgkin's lymphoma, and carcinomas of the ovary, stomach, and colon may also metastasize to the pleura. However, a pleural effusion in conjunction with a past history of one of these neoplasms need not necessarily mean that the effusion is malignant; it may well be due to other causes. (See "Exudative Pleural Effusions" in chapter 250.)

# CHAPTER 253 DISORDERS OF THE MEDIASTINUM

## Pneumomediastinum

Pneumomediastinum means the presence of air in the mediastinum. This may be of no clinical consequence or could indicate a serious disease (e.g., rupture of the esophagus or bronchus). The causes are many: coughing, straining, traumatic compression of the chest, asthma, pneumonia, miliary tuberculosis, diabetic ketoacidosis, abuse of inhaled illicit drugs such as marijuana and crack cocaine, and mechanical ventilation, particularly with positive end-expiratory pressure. All these share an abrupt change in the pressure gradient between alveoli and interstitium, resulting in shearing of alveolar walls. The free air moves along the perivascular sheaths into the mediastinum and then along the great vessels and vascular sheaths into the subcutaneous tissues of the neck.

### Clinical Features, Diagnosis, and Management

Typically, sudden substernal chest pain, radiating to the neck or arm, follows an episode of coughing or straining. Dyspnea is often present and may be aggravated by swallowing. Diagnosis is made by the feel of crepitus in the subcutaneous tissues of the neck. Roentgenographic demonstration of air in the mediastinal tissues is characteristic. The mediastinal structures, particularly the heart border and the aortic knob, are often outlined with unusual clarity. The lateral view shows free air anterior to the cardiac shadow.

No treatment is necessary in most cases since decompression occurs by the dissection of air in the subcutaneous tissues and the air is absorbed eventually. However, if large amounts of air progressively accumulate, venous return to the heart may be diminished. Treatment then would be a subcutaneous incision in the neck or a tracheostomy. If the pneumomediastinum follows a rupture of the esophagus or bronchus, the rupture should be surgically corrected.

## Mediastinal Masses

Primary neoplasms and cysts of the mediastinum may occur at any age. Their manifestations vary from no symptoms to nonspecific symptoms to chronic symptoms and even to acute, life-threatening cardiorespiratory emergencies.

The mediastinum may be divided into anterior, middle, and posterior compartments. This division, based on anatomic landmarks, is useful in the roentgenographic localization of mediastinal masses. Besides, certain masses have a predilection to be localized in certain compartments. The anterior mediastinum, which lies between the sternum anteriorly and the pericardium and brachiocephalic vessels posteriorly, shows a predilection for thymomas (see below). Other important tumors in this compartment are germ cell neoplasms, thyroid, parathyroid adenoma, malignant lymphoma (see Figure 199.1), primary carcinoma, and mesenchymal tumors. The middle mediastinum, which is between the anterior compartment and the anterior spinal ligament, has a predilection for congenital cystic lesions (pericardial, bronchogenic, enteric, thymic, etc.). The posterior mediastinum extends from the anterior spinal ligament to the posterior chest wall, medial to the pulmonary sulci. Neurogenic tumors are the most common (>90%) masses arising in this compartment.

Approximately 75% of all mediastinal masses are benign. The most common tumor in adults is **thymoma,** which represents 21% of all lesions. The frequency of other tumors is shown in Figure 253.1.

### Clinical Features

In adults, most mediastinal masses and cysts are asymptomatic and are unexpectedly discovered on chest x-ray. The presence of symptoms increases the probability of malignancy from 50% to approximately 95%. Symptoms (chest pain, cough, dyspnea, dysphagia, hoarseness, stridor, respiratory infections, and hemoptysis) result from direct invasion or compression of adjacent mediastinal structures by the mass. Other manifestations include obstruction to pulmonary outflow tract, pericardial effusion, cardiac tamponade, superior vena caval syndrome, vocal cord paralysis, Horner's syndrome, chylothorax, and chylopericardium. Prominent systemic manifestations may occur from hormonal

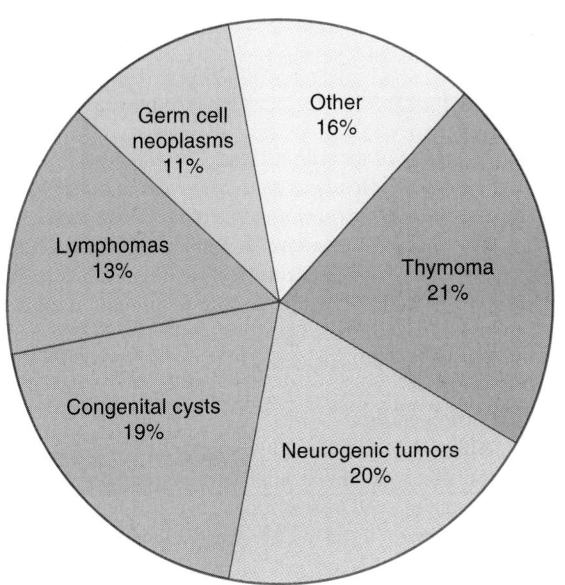


**FIGURE 253.1.** The etiology of mediastinal masses and their relative frequencies.

products of the mediastinal tumors (e.g., hypercalcemia from a parathyroid adenoma, thyrotoxicosis from an intrathoracic goiter, and hypertension due to a pheochromocytoma). Other notable associations are thymoma and myasthenia gravis, neurogenic tumors and osteoarthropathy, and Hodgkin's disease and Pel-Ebstein fever.

## Diagnosis and Management

Rarely does a clinical assessment provide a definitive diagnosis in a mediastinal mass. However, it provides a framework for an orderly diagnostic evaluation. The major steps in the correct diagnosis of a mediastinal mass are localization, excluding a mass of vascular origin, and obtaining a definitive histologic diagnosis. Chest x-rays, particularly a lateral view, help in localization. Comparison with previous roentgenograms, if available, is very helpful. Increasing size of the mass is more indicative of a neoplasm. Computed tomography with contrast injection can localize and define the mass, its vascular origin, density (cystic, solid, or calcified), relationship to adjacent structures, and any local invasion. Myelography or MRI can detect invasion of the intervertebral foramina by a posterior mediastinal lesion. Other tests include serum parathyroid hormone level in suspected parathyroid adenoma and measurement of α-fetoprotein and carcino-embryonic antigen in suspected germ cell neoplasms and primary carcinomas.

While many procedures are available, they should be used selectively, depending on the localization, presentation, and, most importantly, the probable diagnosis in a given patient. Anterior mediastinoscopy and mediastinotomy are the most useful procedures for a histologic diagnosis, followed by exploratory thoracotomy in some cases.

Specific treatment depends on the nature of the mediastinal neoplasm or cyst. Surgical treatment—that is, excision of the mass—is recommended in many; the operative mortality for all mediastinal tumors ranges from 0% to 4%. Complications such as infections, hemorrhage, and injury to the phrenic or recurrent laryngeal nerve may occur in 4–11% of patients. The extent of the disease plays a large role in determining the type of treatment. Radiation therapy is useful in certain situations. Chemotherapy, either alone or combined with other modalities, is used in the treatment of some neoplasms.

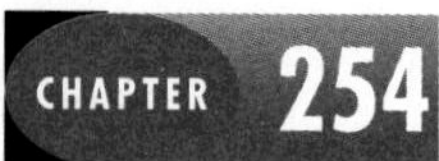

# ACUTE RESPIRATORY FAILURE

## Definition

The components of normal respiration include arterial oxygenation (represented by $PaO_2$, hemoglobin, and hemoglobin binding of $O_2$), alveolar ventilation (represented by $PaCO_2$), and tissue oxygenation (represented by arterial $O_2$ content [$CaO_2$] and cardiac output). In broad terms, acute respiratory failure (ARF) indicates a failure of one or more of these components. (A comprehensive definition characterizes ARF as "a state in which the $PaO_2$ is below the predicted normal range for the patient's age at the prevalent barometric pressure [in the absence of intracardiac right-to-left shunting], or the arterial $CO_2$ tension [$PaCO_2$] is above 50 mm Hg [not due to respiratory compensation for metabolic alkalemia]." Narrowly defined, respiratory failure is the inability of the lungs and heart to maintain adequate arterial oxygenation and/or adequate $CO_2$ elimination. Finally, a more practical and simple definition is the sudden decline of $PaO_2$ below 50 mm Hg with or without $CO_2$ retention.) Depending on its evolution, respiratory failure may be acute or chronic. Causes of ARF are listed in Table 254.1.

Clinical methods and oximetry are absolutely inadequate for diagnosing ARF, although they are commonly used for that purpose, and often without a thorough understanding of their limitations. *The diagnosis of ARF rests on arterial blood gas analysis, which measures both the adequacy of oxygenation and $CO_2$ elimination.* An acute rise in $PaCO_2$ to above 50 mm Hg represents **acute ventilatory failure**; an acute decline in $PaO_2$ below 50 mm Hg without $CO_2$ retention (hypercapnia) is **acute oxygenation failure**. This distinction has important pathogenetic and therapeutic implications.

## Clinical Features

Although symptoms of hypoxemia have been likened to those of alcohol intoxication (restlessness, combativeness, agitation, and loss of judgment), and symptoms of hypercapnia to those of an anesthetic administration (headache, vasodilation, gradual onset of drowsiness, and coma), this correlation mainly emphasizes the nonspecific nature of the symptoms of respiratory failure and the circumstances in which one needs to be vigilant for its appearance. Vasodilation, very often seen in the patient presenting with respiratory failure complicating chronic obstructive pulmonary disease (COPD), is accompanied by conjunctival injection and redness, sometimes with chemosis. Besides these "manifestations" of hypoxemia and hypercapnia, features of the causative disorders would also be present.

**TABLE 254.1. Respiratory Failure: Classification and Some Causes**

| Classification/General Cause | Specific Causes |
|---|---|
| **Ventilatory Failure** | |
| Thoracic diseases | • Lung and airway diseases: chronic obstructive pulmonary disease, asthma, bronchiolitis, epiglottitis, laryngeal edema, foreign body,<br>• Pleural diseases: pleural effusion, pneumothorax, fibrothorax<br>• Chest wall disorders: kyphoscoliosis, thoracoplasty, flail chest |
| Neuromuscular diseases | • Brain disorders: infections, cerebrovascular disease, drugs (sedatives, tranquilizers, analgesics, anesthetic agents), myxedema, primary alveolar hypoventilation<br>• Muscular and myoneural junction disorders: muscular dystrophy, myotonia, drugs (curariform drugs, aminoglycosides), myasthenia gravis, tetanus<br>• Neural and spinal cord disorders: Guillain-Barré syndrome, poliomyelitis, amyotrophic lateral sclerosis, peripheral neuritis, cervical cord transection |
| **Oxygenation Failure** | |
| Diffuse interstitial diseases | • Interstitial pneumonitis, fibrosis, sarcoidosis, pneumoconioses, lymphangitis carcinomatosa, interstitial pulmonary edema |
| Alveolar diseases | • Pneumonias, pulmonary edema, diseases with increased alveolar capillary permeability (see ARDS) |
| Vascular diseases | • Pulmonary embolism, fat embolism, vasculitis |
| Adult respiratory distress syndrome | • (see Table 249.1) |

## Diagnosis and Management

At one extreme, the onset of ARF may be dramatic (e.g., respiratory arrest or cyanosis) and at the other, subtle (e.g., acute ventilatory failure superimposed on chronic respiratory failure due to COPD). A lack of pathognomonic clinical features often makes the clinical diagnosis of ARF difficult. Thus, the first prerequisite for diagnosis is an awareness of the conditions that may lead to respiratory failure. Blood gas analysis, which should follow, must be interpreted in the light of clinical circumstances and in comparison to previous results, if available. Finally, the clinician should also assess the underlying disease and precipitating cause(s) of the acute respiratory failure.

The treatment of acute respiratory failure differs little from that of acute failure of other systems—that is, to support the failed system while maintaining the functioning of all other systems until the failure is corrected or returns to stability. The treatment can be considered in two phases: (1) support of respiration and circulation, and (2) treatment of precipitating factors and complications. Respiratory failure complicating various clinical disorders is further discussed in chapters 255 and 256.

# CHAPTER 255 ACUTE VENTILATORY FAILURE IN CHRONIC OBSTRUCTIVE PULMONARY DISEASE AND NEUROMUSCULAR DISEASES

## Ventilatory Failure in Chronic Obstructive Pulmonary Disease

Patients with COPD generally live precariously balanced between deteriorated muscle function and an altered mechanical load. Muscle dysfunction results from alterations in the chest configuration and shortening and flattening of the diaphragm. A shortened diaphragm cannot generate a good contractile force, a problem only worsened by its loss of curvature. The mechanical load comprises the airway characteristics (resistance) and characteristics of the lung parenchyma and chest wall (elastance).

Airway and parenchymal alterations in COPD lead to ventilation-perfusion (V/Q) mismatching. Perfusion of unventilated alveoli leads to hypoxemia. Ventilation of unperfused or underperfused alveoli increases dead space ($V_d$). As disease worsens, $V_d$ increases and a higher proportion of the tidal volume ($V_t$) ventilates the $V_d$; alveolar ventilation ($V_A$) falls (since $V_A = V_t - V_d$). A rise in total ventilation ($V_E$) can compensate for a declining $V_A$, provided the mechanical load can be overcome by increased respiratory muscle work. Normal resting humans devote roughly 1% of the cardiac output to supply working respiratory muscles; the energy equivalent of this is called "**work of breathing.**" With advancing COPD, work of breathing rises several-fold to overcome the increased mechanical load. Increased work of breathing diverts the cerebral and/or coronary blood supply to the respiratory muscles. In the patient with COPD, increased muscle work often precipitates respiratory muscle fatigue or worsens it if it is already present. If, however, the $V_E$ cannot increase, the abnormal $V_d/V_t$ ratio causes hypercapnia **(respiratory acidosis).**

The hypercapnia triggers **renal** retention of bicarbonate as **compensation for the respiratory acidosis.** Hypoxemia triggers tissue as well as other adaptive mechanisms to improve the oxygen delivery. When hypoxemia and hypercapnia evolve insidiously and fulfill the criteria for respiratory failure, a state of chronic respiratory failure prevails. Acute ventilatory failure in COPD often represents a **worsening of chronic failure**, but not invariably so. While the mechanical load and the muscle function are liable to many influences, the most important precipitating condition is airway infection, followed by congestive cardiac failure, bronchospasm (often from medication noncompliance), pulmonary embolism, and pneumothorax. The typical manifestations are increasing dyspnea, worsening exercise intolerance, and, as the gas exchange worsens, changes in mental status. Besides tachypnea, cyanosis, respiratory distress, and depressed sensorium, signs of right-sided heart failure may also be present.

### Management

Acute ventilatory failure is a progressive process where the body's compensatory mechanisms may prove ineffective in the available time. Therefore, the first priority is to decide if urgent invasive intervention—immediate endotracheal intubation and/or cardiopulmonary resuscitation—is needed. The following considerations apply: the condition of the patient, the rapidity of onset of the respiratory failure, the physician's estimate of (a) the probability/imminence of cardiovascular collapse or cardiac arrest or respiratory arrest, and (b) the reversibility of the etiology of the respiratory failure, the severity of hypoxemia, the severity of hypercapnia taken in conjunction with the extent of acidosis, and the presence or absence of associated terminal illness and/or advance directives from the patient. When these call for immediate invasive intervention, endotracheal intubation and mechanical ventilation are indicated. If not, a conservative approach using low flow oxygen, bronchodilators, corticosteroids (unless contraindicated), and specific management of the precipitating condition (e.g., antibiotics for respiratory infection, diuretics and/or angiotensin converting enzyme inhibitors for heart failure, etc.) constitute the essentials of the overall approach. A middle ground is also possible where endotracheal intubation is supplanted by non-invasive mechanical ventilation using a face mask and pressure-cycled ventilator.

### Oxygen therapy

The priorities are to assure adequate oxygenation and ventilation. Controlled oxygen therapy is the cornerstone of managing ventilatory failure in COPD. Oxygen should be used as a drug in the appropriate dose. The correct dose of oxygen is the dose that satisfies the oxygen needs of the tissues. Too little oxygen places the patient at risk for vital organ dysfunction, damage, and death while too much oxygen may cause progressive hypercapnia, $CO_2$ narcosis, and acidosis. Because tissue oxygenation is not directly measurable, the $PaO_2$ remains the most useful measure.

Because of the shape of the **oxyhemoglobin dissociation curve**—that is, the oxygen tension/saturation relationship—relatively small rises in $PaO_2$ evoke a substantial increase in oxygen saturation and, thus, $CaO_2$. An acceptable $PaO_2$ to aim for in this context is one between 50 and 60 mm Hg, achieved by using a Venturi mask or a nasal cannula. Venturi masks can deliver oxygen at precise inspired concentrations of 24–35% ($fiO_2$, 0.24–0.35). Oxygen can also be given using nasal cannula at a low flow of 1–2 L/minute, each liter of supplemental oxygen raising the $fiO_2$ by nearly 0.04 points (4%). Compared with the mask, a nasal cannula delivers oxygen uninterruptedly even when the patient is eating or talking; however, the $fiO_2$ cannot be adjusted as precisely with cannula as it can with a Venturi mask. A modest hypercapnia (10–12 mm Hg) often follows oxygen treatment, which in itself is neither a cause for discontinuing oxygen nor a cause for initiating mechanical ventilation.

If possible, endotracheal intubation and mechanical ventilation should be avoided in COPD patients because of the associated complications and because of the difficulty in liberating the patient from the ventilator. However, with uncontrolled oxygen therapy, or in some cases even with controlled oxygen therapy, hypercapnia and acidosis may escalate ("**$CO_2$ narcosis**"). Despite the established notion that $CO_2$ narcosis follows "suppression of respiratory drive" by oxygen use, it appears that changes in ventilation/perfusion induced by oxygen therapy, and not suppression of respiratory drive, are causative. Controlled oxygen therapy may also fail in initially severely hypoxemic and acidotic patients or when ventilatory drive is depressed (e.g., central nervous system [CNS] depressants). Although many criteria have been proposed for intubation and mechanical ventilation (Table 255.1), evaluation over a period of time of changes in mental status (confusion, restlessness), effectiveness of cough mechanism, and changes in arterial blood gases is more helpful than any particular criterion in making a decision.

For mechanical ventilatory assistance, a volume-cycled ventilator is used to deliver a tidal volume of 6–8 ml/kg and an inspiratory/expiratory (I/E) time ratio of 1 : 3 or greater. The respiratory rate (RR) should be adjusted to maintain an appropriate I/E ratio. In making any adjustment in the ventilator setting ($fiO_2$, $V_t$, RR), the goal of mechanical ventilation is to maintain arterial blood gas tensions that existed at a previous stable state, if known, but certainly not to normalize them. Although the availability of low-pressure cuffed endotracheal tubes has helped ease the strict deadlines for tracheostomy, it is appropriate to consider it if prolonged (>1–2 weeks) mechanical ventilation is anticipated. A list of monitoring aids in respiratory failure is shown in Table 255.2.

Any precipitating factors should be treated and all reversible elements corrected. The role of bronchodilators, corticosteroids, and antibiotics is discussed in the treatment of exacerbations of COPD in chapter 228. Optimal tracheobronchial secretion clearance should be achieved with inhaled bronchodilators; the patient should then assume a sitting posture, and coughing should be encouraged. This approach could be supplemented by nasotracheal suctioning. The role of proper nutritional support, incremental use of sitting periods, prevention of venous thromboembolism (Table 233.11) and early ambulation cannot be overemphasized.

Bedside assessment is necessary to determine when to initiate weaning. In general, a period of 24 to 48 hours

**TABLE 255.1. Criteria for Mechanical Ventilatory Assistance**

| | |
|---|---|
| Respiratory rate | >35 |
| Vital capacity (ml/kg) | <10 |
| Inspiratory force (cm $H_2O$) | −25 or less |
| $PaO_2$ (mm Hg) | <50 on room air<br><70 on mask oxygen |
| $P(A\text{-}a)O_2$ (mm Hg) | >450 on 100% oxygen |
| $PaCO_2$ (mm Hg) | >55 (with acidosis) |
| $V_d/V_t$ | >0.60 |

Note: Reverse of these criteria may be used for eligibility for weaning.

**TABLE 255.2. Monitoring Aids in Respiratory Failure**

- Arterial blood gases: $PaO_2$, $PaCO_2$, $P(A\text{-}a)O_2$
- Mixed venous oxygen tension ($P\bar{v}O_2$)
- Hematocrit and hemoglobin
- Electrolyte status, intake and output, daily weight
- Tidal volume, minute ventilation
- Endotracheal tube cuff pressure
- Vital capacity
- Maximum static inspiratory pressure ($P_iMax$)[a]
- Chest x-rays
- Bedside pulmonary artery catheterization
- Electrocardiogram
- Lung compliance
- Shunt fraction (Qs/Qt)

[a]Synonymous with inspiratory force, negative inspiratory force, or maximum inspiratory force, etc.

of ventilatory assistance is necessary to "rest" the fatigued respiratory muscles. Premature discontinuation could easily reinstate muscle fatigue. Many criteria for weaning are suggested (see Table 255.1), but none is appropriate for all instances. The patient should be alert and responsive, with an improved and stabilized clinical condition, and oxygenation should be adequate at an $fiO_2$ of <0.4 (40%). A trial of intermittent mandatory ventilation or pressure support or even "T-piece" may be used for weaning. Despite the fervor with which physicians embrace one measure or other, these are only measures to transition the patient over to spontaneous unassisted ventilation and not an end in themselves; *none can supplant careful clinical observation during this transition.* Several hours of this trial should precede the extubation. Rapid, shallow respirations that develop during this transition are an ominous sign that predicts failure of weaning. If weaning is successful, the patient may be extubated. In the immediate postextubation period, eating and drinking should be avoided to obviate the danger of aspiration. Intensive respiratory care, including cough and postural drainage to enhance secretion clearance, are critical in the first 24–48 hours after extubation. Some patients may require long-term oxygen therapy, at least temporarily, after hospital discharge (Chapter 239).

## Acute Ventilatory Failure in Neuromuscular Diseases

The common causes of neuromuscular respiratory failure are Guillain-Barre syndrome, myasthenia gravis, and demyelinating, degenerative, or infectious neuromuscular diseases. Ventilatory failure may occur even despite normal lungs and airways in these disorders. Often, weakness of inspiratory muscles and a poor cough mechanism are responsible. Unless associated with other disorders capable of producing them, chronic hypoxemia and cor pulmonale are generally absent in neuromuscular respiratory failure. Acute, chronic, or periodic bouts of ventilatory failure may be seen in spinal cord and myoneural junction diseases.

### Management

Respiratory muscle paralysis may be very subtle, yet has the potential to progress rapidly and culminate in a respiratory arrest. For this reason, clinical assessment and blood gas studies alone are unreliable; measurements that can assess respiratory muscle function—for example, vital capacity (VC) and maximum inspiratory pressure ($P_i$max, measured by an aneroid pressure manometer) should be regularly monitored. Intubation and mechanical ventilation are indicated when the VC falls to twice the predicted tidal volume or $P_i$max falls below –20 cm $H_2O$. Dysphagia, maximum expiratory pressure ($P_e$max) of <40 cm $H_2O$, and hypercapnia are also indications for mechanical ventilatory support. Ventilator management is similar to that used for a COPD patient in ventilatory failure, except that ventilation is more easily achieved, complications are less common, and tracheostomy is more often necessary. Physical therapy also plays a critical role in the management of these patients. Workup for and management of the underlying process is also critical. Non-invasive positive pressure ventilation (NPPV) through a face mask has significant utility in patients with neuromuscular respiratory failure, potentially avoiding intubation.

# CHAPTER 256 ACUTE RESPIRATORY DISTRESS SYNDROME

### Definition

**Acute lung injury** (**ALI**) is a term that describes a syndrome of severe, acute respiratory failure, featuring respiratory distress, severely impaired oxygenation, and noncardiogenic pulmonary edema. **Acute respiratory distress syndrome** (**ARDS**), on the other hand, describes a subset of severe ALI. Progressive respiratory distress, severe refractory hypoxemia, and often, an antecedent major medical or surgical illness or trauma characterize ARDS. The normal left ventricular filling pressures measured by PA catheter confirm noncardiogenic pulmonary edema. In contrast to respiratory failure in COPD, oxygenation failure generally requiring mechanical ventilation is a key feature of ARDS.

## Pathogenesis and Pathology

Diverse clinical states (Table 256.1, Figure 256.1) predispose to ARDS. In addition, many conditions either singly or in combination—including old age, feminine gender, severity of illness, cigarette smoking, and chronic alcohol abuse—enhance the risk of ARDS in these clinical states. The lung is injured directly or indirectly; indirect lung injury arises from the activation of systemic inflammation by an extrapulmonary process. Following a systemic or pulmonary injury, leukocytes and macrophages are activated. Pulmonary capillary endothelial cells are injured by the inflammatory cell mediators (tumor necrosis factor, proteases, prostaglandins, oxygen radicals, leukotrienes, platelet activating factor, and interleukin [IL]-1). **Pulmonary** capillary **structure** is damaged and its permeability enhanced. This excessive capillary permeability is widespread—thus the notion of ARDS as a "pan-endothelial" disease. Type I alveolar pneumocytes are **also injured**. During this process, the **surfactant mechanism is lost,** with resultant widespread atelectasis from alveolar instability. Interstitial and alveolar pulmonary edema follows. Lung compliance and volume decline. The lung pathology includes edema, congestion, hemorrhage, microatelectasis, and microvascular thromboses. In later stages, alveoli fill with granulation tissue. With recovery, **Type II pneumocytes re-epithelialize** the alveoli and differentiate into Type I pneumocytes. Capillaries and myofibroblasts migrate into the alveoli, causing **intra-alveolar fibrosis.**

**TABLE 256.1. Clinical States Predisposing to ARDS**

| General | Specific |
|---|---|
| Infections | Pneumonias from viral, bacterial or fungal agents<br>Miliary tuberculosis |
| Inhalation injury | Smoke inhalation<br>Oxygen toxicity<br>Hydrocarbon ingestion<br>Aspiration of gastric acid<br>Near drowning |
| Trauma | |
| Shock | Hemorrhagic or septic |
| Fat embolism | |
| Narcotic and illicit drug overdose | |
| Pancreatitis | |
| Neurogenic pulmonary edema | |
| Postcardiopulmonary bypass | |

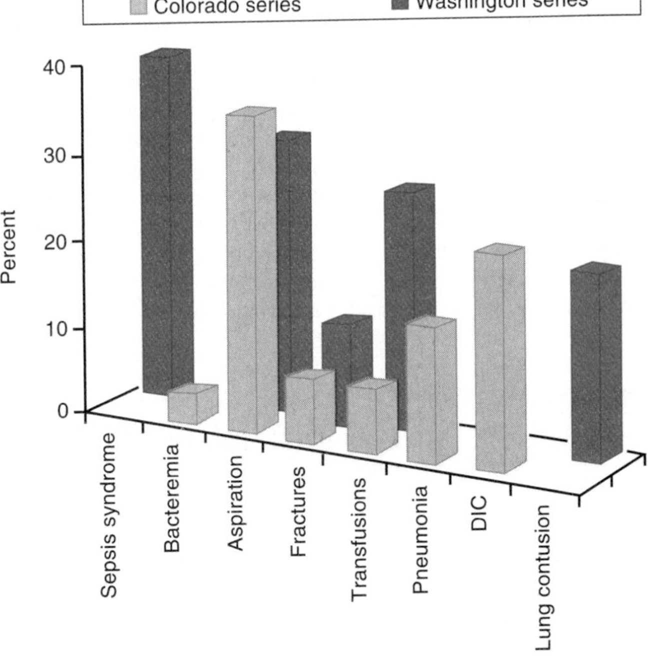


**FIGURE 256.1. The risk of acute respiratory distress syndrome (ARDS) in various predisposing conditions from two large series. Aspiration: aspiration of gastric acid. Pneumonia: pneumonia developing in the intensive care unit. Transfusions: defined as multiple (hyper) transfusions ≥10 units in 24 hours in Colorado series and ≥10 units in 6 hours in Washington series.**
(Modified from: Fowler AA et al. Ann Intern Med 1983;99:593–598, Colorado series; Pepe PE et al. Am J Surg 1982;144:124-130, Washington series. Used with permission.)

Bronchoalveolar lavage (BAL) fluid studies in patients with ARDS provide insights into the pathogenesis and resolution of ARDS. Neutrophils preponderate in the BAL fluid in patients at risk for early ARDS and ARDS; this neutrophilia is replaced by macrophages as the ARDS resolves, suggesting the resolution of the lung injury is macrophage-mediated. Also, in early ARDS, procollagen peptide-III (PCP-III) is elevated in the BAL fluid. Activated lung fibroblasts secrete procollagen, which yields Type III collagen; PCP-III, a residuum of this process, subsides as ARDS resolves. Thus, the usual response in these limited studies is a resolution of the BAL neutrophilia and declining levels of PCP-III in those that survive ARDS. Consequently, both neutrophilia and elevated PCP-III in the BAL fluid have been suggested as harbingers of high mortality and poor outcome.

## Clinical Features

The onset of ARDS is usually rapid, commonly within 12–24 hours of the predisposing event. Sepsis syndrome is the most frequent predisposing illness (see Figure 256.1). If the predisposing illness is trauma, the initial shock and resuscitation may be followed by a slightly longer latent period of stability before the dramatic onset of acute lung injury. This stability is more apparent than real, because fever, tachypnea, respiratory alkalosis, a widened alveolar-arterial oxygen gradient $P(A\text{-}aO_2)$, and often hypoxemia, are usually present during this period, despite the generally normal chest x-rays. As ARDS develops, progressive dyspnea, intercostal retractions, rhonchi, and crackles develop, along with progressive, diffuse pulmonary infiltration on x-rays (Figure 256.2). Hypocapnia and refractory hypoxemia develop. As ARDS progresses, $CO_2$ retention and a metabolic acidosis may develop.

## Diagnosis

Clinical suspicion is critical to the diagnosis of ARDS. The presence of a disease that predisposes to ARDS (see Table 256.1) should make one watchful for the development of ARDS. Frank hypoxemia and/or widening of the $P(A\text{-}aO_2)$ during an acute severe medical or surgical illness often herald early ARDS, and should be pursued with serial blood gas analysis, chest x-rays, and oxygen therapy.

Rather than depend on an arbitrary $PaO_2$ value, the ratio of $PaO_2$ to $fiO_2$ ($PaO_2/fiO_2$) has been advanced as a diagnostic criterion. This ratio is ≤200 in ARDS. Definitive diagnosis of ARDS depends on an acute onset, diffuse bilateral opacities consistent with pulmonary edema on chest radiographs, and severe hypoxemia ($PaO_2/fiO_2$ criterion). Left-sided heart failure, demonstrated by a pulmonary capillary wedge pressure above 18 mm Hg or clinical evidence of left atrial hypertension or left ventricular failure as a cause of pulmonary edema, must be excluded.

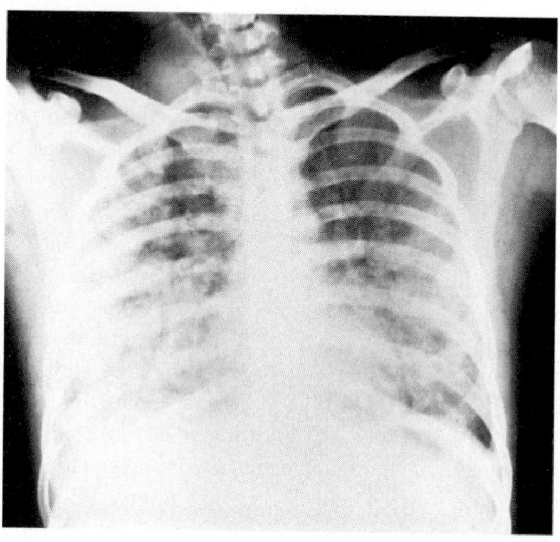

**FIGURE 256.2.** ARDS: chest x-ray showing diffuse pulmonary opacification. ARDS followed IV abuse of ethchlorvynol (Placidyl).

## Management

There is no specific therapy for ARDS, other than supportive care and a careful and appropriate search for an initiating cause. The major objectives are to stabilize the patient, adequately treat the underlying process, ensure adequate tissue oxygenation, and recognize and manage complication(s)—i.e., drainage of abscesses, fixation of long bone fractures, and so forth. Progressively increasing inhaled oxygen concentration ($fiO_2$) is needed to achieve acceptable oxygenation. All but the mildest cases will require mechanical ventilatory support; the general indications for which are shown in Table 256.1. Early anticipation and "elective" endotracheal intubation are appropriate when mental status and/or gas exchange progressively decline. For alert and cooperative patients, at least initially, noninvasive positive pressure ventilation (NIPPV) may be appropriate. NIPPV uses a tight-fitting face mask, which is connected to a pressure-cycled ventilator, without endotracheal intubation. In studies of limited numbers of patients with ARDS, NIPPV has been shown to postpone or avoid endotracheal intubation, although the proper indications for the use of NIPPV in ARDS are still controversial.

Mechanical ventilation is only supportive; although no specific type or mode (the usual modes are shown in Table 256.2) is superior, recent studies show that using a lower-than-traditional tidal volume (6 ml/kg of predicted body weight) leads to less mortality and lesser duration of mechanical ventilatory assistance.

Patients with ARDS usually require sedation and perhaps muscle relaxants (paralytic agents) during mechanical ventilation. Paralytic agents should never be used in lieu of sedation but rather to decrease the oxygen consumption of skeletal muscle, preserving oxygen for vital organs. One should aim for a satisfactory oxygenation—that is, a $PaO_2$ of 60–65 mm Hg (corresponding to a SaO2 of > 90%), using the lowest possible $fiO_2$ to avoid oxygen toxicity. Varying criteria exist for the application of positive end-expiratory pressure (PEEP). PEEP redistributes intra-alveolar fluid and improves gas exchange, allowing a decrease in $fiO_2$ requirements and minimizing the risk of oxygen toxicity, which can worsen underlying lung injury. PEEP decreases venous return and can cause hypotension, especially at levels above 10–15 cm $H_2O$. PEEP, started at an initial level of 5 cm $H_2O$, is increased in increments of 3–5 cm $H_2O$ until a desired response is obtained. With improving lung function—that is, steady $PaO_2$, decreasing $fiO_2$, P(A-a $O_2$), and shunt fraction—weaning may be considered.

Other important objectives in ARDS management are meticulous control of fluid and electrolytes, skilled nursing care, nutrition, control of infection, and prophylaxis against stress ulcer bleeding from the gastrointestinal tract and the formation of DVT. Careful diuresis to reduce extravascular lung water should be balanced against the need for fluid to counteract the hypotension from shock or PEEP. The lung injury in ARDS is a part of diffuse endothelial injury, the extent and severity of which vary. Such failing organs should be properly supported. When the gut fails, its compromised mucosal integrity predisposes to bacteremia. Preventing further episodes of sepsis, drainage of any localized abscesses, and, in the case of the trauma patient, definitive treatment of long bone fractures are all important goals.

**TABLE 256.2. Commonly Applied Ventilator Settings in ARDS**

| | |
|---|---|
| Tidal volume ($V_t$) | 4–6 ml/kg |
| Setting | Assist-Control |
| Resp. rate | 12–20 (highly variable) |
| $fiO_2$ | 1.0 initially, titrated along with PEEP to keep $PaO_2$ between 60 and 65 mm Hg |
| I:E ratio | 1:2 to 1:4 |
| PEEP | 5–15 cm $H_2O$ |

PEEP = positive end-expiratory pressure; $fiO_2$ = fraction of inspired oxygen; I:E ratio = inspiratory:expiratory ratio.

## Prognosis

The outcomes of ARDS range from complete recovery to severe disability to death (Table 256.3). Prognosis varies with the cause of ARDS (e.g., ARDS from fat embolism carries a relatively good prognosis compared with that from sepsis syndrome), which underscores the importance of identifying and treating the underlying cause. The number of failing organ systems significantly and adversely affects outcome (99% mortality with ≥3 organ failures). Nevertheless, the experience in a large medical center in Seattle indicates a declining overall mortality in ARDS (from 65% in early 1980s to 30–40% in the late 1990s). Patients with ARDS are more likely to die in the first 2 weeks of onset of ARDS; therefore, survival beyond 2 weeks usually indicates a better prognosis. Among those who recover, 50–75% suffer residual pulmonary dysfunction. Pulmonary function improves more rapidly during the first 3–6 months after recovery and more gradually in the next 6 months; the outlook for recovery is, therefore, better in the first year than thereafter. Residual impairments, in the order of frequency, are a reduced $DL_{CO}$, airflow obstruction, and a restrictive ventilatory impairment. Tracheal stenosis related to endotracheal intubation may also cause symptoms. Patients who recover from ARDS should have ongoing, regular follow-up.

**TABLE 256.3. Prognostic Factors in ARDS**

| Criterion | Favorable | Unfavorable |
|---|---|---|
| Age | <40 | >40 |
| Nonpulmonary organ failure | None | One or more |
| Etiology | Postoperative state<br>Transfusion-related<br>Fat embolism | Sepsis syndrome<br>Trauma |
| $C_{-stat}$ on day 3[a] | >50 | <25 |
| $PaO_2/fiO_2$ on day 3 | >250 | <150 |
| Secondary bactermia/sepsis | None | Present |

[a]$C_{stat}$ = static compliance.

# CHAPTER 257 SELECTED SLEEP DISORDERS

The conscious human being spends his/her time among recurring cycles of wakefulness and sleep, the latter comprised of rapid-eye movement (REM) and non-REM phases. Non-REM sleep is further divided into 4 stages, whereas stage 5 represents REM sleep. These sleep phases are determined via a polysomnogram (PSG), using EEG, OCG, and EMG (Table 257.1).

Sleep disorders generally assume the following patterns: excessive daytime somnolence (EDS), insomnia, parasomnias, and circadian rhythm abnormalities. The most important source of information in patients

**TABLE 257.1. Sleepiness and Sleep-Disordered Breathing: A Glossary of Terms**

| Term | Meaning |
|---|---|
| Apnea | Cessation of airflow for ≥10 sec |
| Apnea-hypopnea index (AHI) | See respiratory disturbance index (RDI) |
| Cataplexy | Loss of postural muscle tone (falling attacks) while emotional (laughing or crying) |
| Central sleep apnea | No airflow and no respiratory effort. A condition where most episodes of apnea are central in origin; generally in association with some neurologic disorder |
| Cheyne-Stokes' respiration | Crescendo increase in amplitude and rate of respiration (hyperpnea) followed by the reverse that alternates with periods of apnea; generally indicative of central nervous system disease or left ventricular failure associated with cerebrovascular disease |
| Excessive somnolence | Excessive sleepiness (excessive daytime somnolence, EDS) |
| Hypnagogic hallucinations | Vivid dreams or hallucinations during sleep-wake transition. |
| Hypopnea | Airflow decrease by ≥50% plus ≥4% drop in $O_2$ saturation or arousal on EEG |
| Insomnia | Inability to fall or stay asleep |
| Maintenance of wakefulness test (MWT) | Measures amount of time a person is able to stay awake in an environment conducive to sleep |
| Mixed apnea | Begins as central apnea but becomes obstructive in the same cycle |
| Multiple sleep latency test (MSLT) | Measures time to sleep onset, as measured by EEG, in an environment conducive to sleep; the test has the advantage of being able to overcome the motivation to stay awake |
| Obesity-hypoventilation syndrome | Morbid obesity, obstructive sleep apnea syndrome, and daytime hypercapnia (>45 mm Hg); pulmonary hypertension, right heart failure, and hypoventilation (i.e., hypercapnia) |
| Obstructive apnea | Apnea with continued respiratory effort |
| Obstructive sleep apnea syndrome | RDI >15 events per hour of sleep. |
| Overjet | Maxilla extrudes forward as compared to the mandible |
| Parasomnias | Abnormal behavior/activity during sleep (e.g., sleep walking, nocturnal seizures, enuresis, etc.) |
| Polysomnogram (PSG) | A recording of sleep events, typically during a night of sleep, using many sources: electro-oculography (OCG), electroencephalography (EEG), electromyography (EMG), electrocardiogram (ECG), oximetry, and recording of snoring, nasal and oral airflow measurements, and abdominal and chest wall movement |
| Respiratory disturbance index (RDI) | Sum of all apneas and hypopneas divided by number of hours of sleep (i.e., number of apneas and hypopnea events per hour of sleep) |
| Retrognathia | Gnathion is posteriorly displaced compared to the nasion |
| Sleep paralysis | Inability to move during the transition of sleep-wake states |
| Upper airway resistance syndrome | Increased upper airway resistance that manifests by progressively louder (crescendo) snoring that ends in an arousal with sudden decrease in upper airway resistance and cessation of snoring; generally no disturbances in oxygenation; repeated arousals fragment sleep, leading to daytime somnolence |

**TABLE 257.2. Essentials of a Sleep History**

| | |
|---|---|
| Sleep onset<br>• Time of sleep<br>• Use of bed for anything other than sleep and sex<br>• Time taken to fall off to sleep<br>• Sleep paralysis/hypnagogic hallucinations<br>• Achiness/crampy pain/creeping or crawling feelings in extremities | • Fear of falling asleep<br>• Fear of not being able to sleep after awakening<br>• Use of hypnotics<br>• Use of sleep medications<br>• Use of alcohol/caffeine or fluids before bedtime |
| Sleep maintenance<br>Awakenings<br>• Reasons for awakening (e.g., urination)<br>• Duration of awakenings<br>• Duration of sleep<br>• Snoring<br>Relationship to position<br>Snorting<br>Crescendo snoring<br>Seasonal nature, if any | • Witnessed episodes of apnea<br>• Awakenings with confusion/disorientation<br>• Limb movements<br>• Abnormal movements<br>• Restless sleep<br>• Diaphoresis (night sweats)<br>• Sleep walking<br>• Violent behavior |
| Awakening<br>• Time of awakening<br>• Difficulty awakening<br>• Muscle weakness, confusion or headache on awakening | • Mode of awakening (alarm, etc)<br>• Nature of bed on awakening (disheveled) |
| Daytime naps<br>• Number and duration | • Refreshing or not |
| Other<br>• Sleepiness scale (ESS, KSS, SSS,* etc)<br>• Automobile accidents<br>• Changes in/constancy of sleep patterns between weekdays and weekends<br>• Work hours<br>• Changes in body weight | • Difficulty staying awake<br>• Profession (airline pilot, truck driver, etc)<br>• Vegetative symptoms of depression<br>• Personality changes<br>• Use of alcohol, caffeine, antidepressants, hypnotics, sedatives, and illicit drugs |

*ESS = Epworth Sleepiness Scale; KSS = Karolinska Sleepiness Scale; SSS = Stanford Sleepiness Scale.

with all sleep disorders and especially those with EDS is the history (Table 257.2); it is important to interview not only the patient, but also the spouse or bed partner, as applicable. However, because the sleep history obtained in most medical encounters is at best brief, the true frequency of sleep disorders—thought to be considerable—remains elusive.

## Excessive Daytime Sleepiness

EDS is a common symptom that generally follows sleep deprivation or sleep restriction, and results from a complex interplay between the presence of environmental or other stimuli that help maintain wakefulness and those that promote sleep with the resultant lack of restorative sleep. Sleepiness can be observed directly, as for example, when an individual tends to "nod off" or exhibits a blank, sleepy look with droopy eyelids. Sleepiness may also be measured semi-objectively using questionnaires or rating scales, such as the Epworth Sleepiness Scale (ESS), Stanford Sleepiness Scale (SSS), or Karolinska Sleepiness Scale (KSS), and objectively using multiple sleep latency test (MSLT, see Table 257.1). EDS results from several causes, as listed in Table 257.3. In North America, inadequate hours of sleep and sleep apnea are common causes of excessive daytime somnolence.

Besides a thorough sleep history, a physical examination should focus on vital signs, including weight, the nasal passages, abnormalities of the face and jaw, size of the tongue, ease of visualizing the oropharynx, soft palate, uvula, and neck circumference. Unless the history indicates truncated sleep hours or disordered sleep hygiene or drug use, these patients generally require a PSG for confirmation of diagnosis. PSG findings of a short sleep latency corroborates EDS. A subset of these patients might require an MSLT or even an MWT (see Table 257.1).

## Sleep-Disordered Breathing

Sleep-disordered breathing (SDB) includes a variety of breathing disturbances that occur during sleep, exemplified by snoring, increased upper airway resistance, hypoventilation, apnea, Cheyne-Stokes' breathing and obesity-hypoventilation syndrome, best viewed as a spectrum of disorders rather than individual entities.

### Obstructive Sleep Apnea

SDB may be clinically expressed as central and obstructive sleep apneas. Central apneas arise from disturbances in central ventilatory control and obstructive apneas, from upper airway obstruction during sleep. Distinction between obstructive sleep apnea in the obese patient and obesity-hypoventilation syndrome is worth emphasizing: while both entities share SDB, the $PaCO_2$ is normal during wakefulness in the former, whereas it is elevated in the latter.

**TABLE 257.3. Common Causes of Excessive Sleepiness (Somnolence)**

| |
|---|
| Inadequate sleep (often a problem in adolescents) |
| Sleep-disordered breathing |
| Depression |
| Movement disorders related to sleep (e.g., bruxism, periodic limb movements of sleep) |
| Drug-induced (both legal and illicit) |
| Narcolepsy |
| Metabolic/toxic causes |
| Circadian rhythm disorders |
| Idiopathic hypersomnia |

#### Pathogenesis

Because sleep leads to loss or diminution of some of the protective mechanisms that lead to upper airway patency, ventilation during sleep is largely dependent on chemical stimuli. In general, SDB seems to arise from a variable combination of disturbances in ventilatory control during sleep and difficulty maintaining upper airway patency during sleep. A person with one of these disturbances may be shifted from one entity to the other as a result of use of alcohol, general anesthesia, and weight gain or weight loss.

Conceptually, the pharyngeal airway is a collapsible tube, the patency and dimensions of which depend on several influences, one of which is the transmural pressure, i.e., the difference between intraluminal pressure (which is negative during inspiration) and the extraluminal pressure (which is atmospheric). During early inspiration, and directly as a result of the respiratory thoracic muscle action (the "pump"), the pharyngeal airway intraluminal pressure is transiently lowered, thus transiently decreasing the pharyngeal airway diameter. Sleep, underlying sleep apnea, and obesity magnify this normal response, whereas the "stiffness" (compliance) of the pharyngeal wall, and the action of the upper airway dilating muscles counteract it (Figure 257.2).

The closure of the upper airway, the critical event in obstructive sleep apnea (OSA), is a complex process, and therefore, not eventuated by a single mechanism. The upper airway in OSA, either as a result of being significantly narrowed or being subject to an unduly high

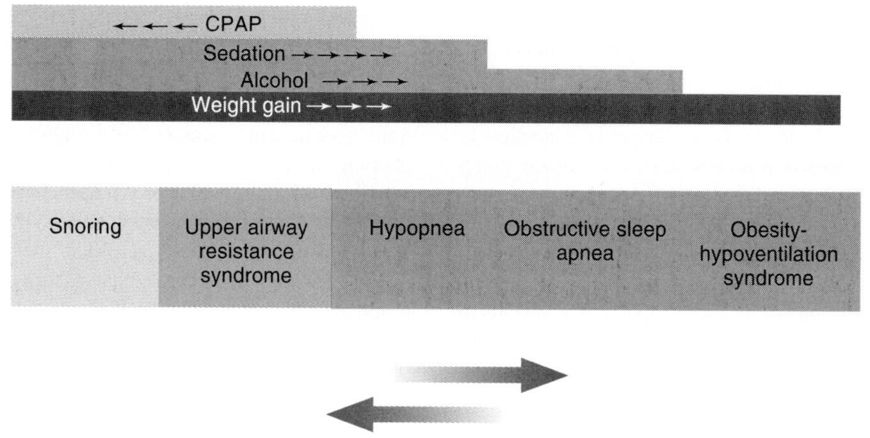


**FIGURE 257.1.** The clinical spectrum of sleep-disordered breathing from snoring through hypopnea into obesity-hypoventilation syndrome. Alcohol, sedation, general anesthesia, may all transiently shift a susceptible person from one category to the next, whereas weight gain shifts persons more gradually from one category to the next more severe category.

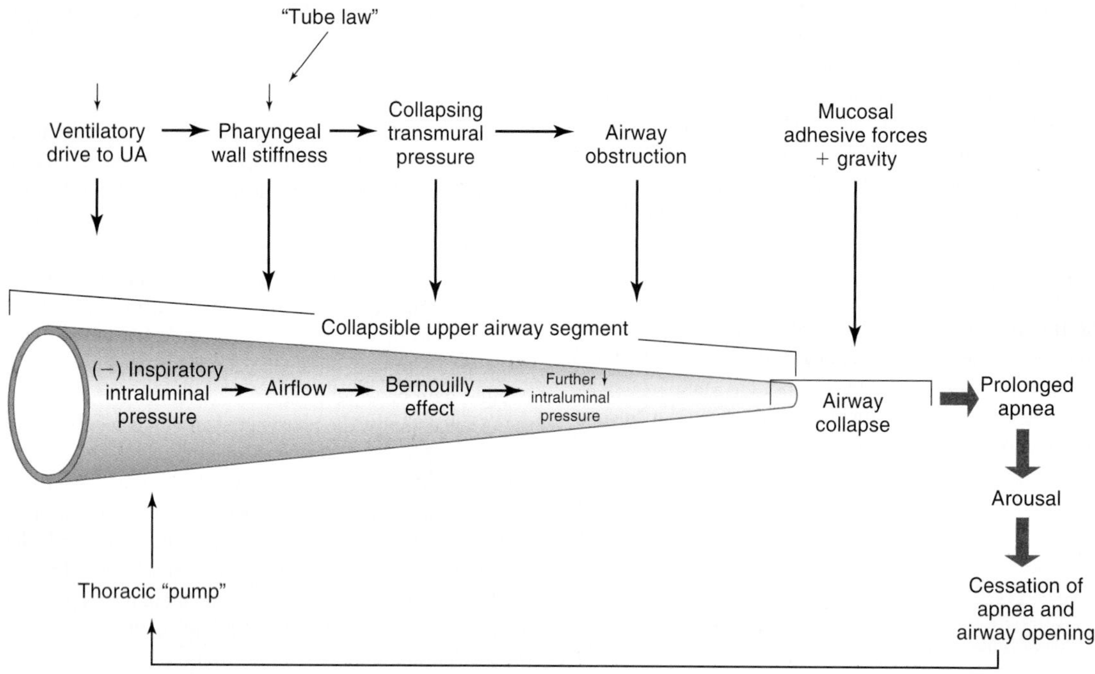


**FIGURE 257.2. Mechanism(s) of upper airway obstruction in obstructive sleep apnea (see text for details).**

external pressure on its collapsible portion, is highly susceptible to collapse. A reduced ventilatory motor output to the upper airway dilators has been theorized as the primary event, which implies that a problem in the central control of ventilation is an essential co-factor in the development of obstructive sleep apnea, along with an abnormally collapsible upper airway segment.

As the lumen of a collapsible tube narrows progressively, the stiffness of its walls continually diminish, and the lumen collapses altogether. Some experts invoke this "Tube Law" to explain the progressive loss of pharyngeal wall stiffness that follows progressive decline in lumen. As the airflow proceeds under the thoracic pump action, the decline in the airway intraluminal pressure perpetuates a further decrease in the intraluminal pressure (Bernoulli principle). As these forces bring the airway to closure, the adhesive forces in the mucosal surfaces and gravity together lead to prolonged apnea, which leads to arousal, and respiratory center stimulation. The latter resumes breathing and the cycle repeats as the depth of sleep progresses. These recurrent arousals fragment sleep architecture, and generate a "sleep debt," which generally expresses itself as daytime or inappropriate somnolence.

Apneic spells cause hypoxemia and desaturation of hemoglobin, and elevate pulmonary and systemic arterial pressures. In some cases, there is left ventricular dysfunction, causing elevation of pulmonary capillary wedge pressures and pulmonary congestion, thus aggravating the hypoxemia. Cardiac arrhythmias are quite common during these sleep-wake cycles, with bradycardia during apnea and tachycardia on resumption of ventilation.

## Clinical Features and Diagnosis

OSA is very common. Despite its distinct clinical features (Table 257.4), it might merely be a harbinger of many other clinical disorders including nasal obstruction, tongue enlargement (macroglossia), jaw and pharyngeal abnormalities, laryngeal obstruction, acromegaly, Cushing's disease or syndrome, goiter, hypothyroidism, and obesity. A thorough general medical history and sleep history are critical. Loud snoring of many, many years often underlies marital discord or other social problems. The severity of EDS may vary. Whereas the "fat boy" from Charles Dickens' *Pickwick Papers* represents obesity-hypoventilation syndrome (**an extreme subset** of OSA), the proxy for less severe forms may merely be accidents at work or while operating an automobile. On the deceptively benign side is the person who falls asleep while watching a (favorite) television show or movie. Sometimes, sleep fragmentation is misinterpreted as insomnia and the self-administration of ethanol by the patient or prescription of an hypnotic by the physician merely worsens the obstruction. Occasionally, arousals are reported as gasping or choking. The intellectual decline, personality changes, and headache may simulate an intracranial tumor and/or space-occupying lesion. Impotence is another symptom with an unclear pathogenesis.

Physical examination is sometimes normal, and consequently, a normal physical examination does not exclude OSA. Generally, an overweight state or obesity, a short, fat neck, or jowls around the jaw and upper neck are present. Besides congestion, edema and swelling of the uvula, and a small, narrow throat, specific findings include lateral narrowing of the pharynx (bands of tissue impinging into the observable posterior pharyngeal space), and enlarged tongue (upper surface above the level of the mandibular occlusal plane) with lateral ridging caused by pressure by teeth on tongue margins. The clinician should look carefully for anatomic abnormalities (especially retrognathia and overjet), since their correction may elicit cure or clinical improvement. A neck circumference of 17" or higher in men and 16" or higher in women are highly predictive of OSA. Arterial hypertension, drowsiness, pulmonary hypertension, and in advanced cases, cor pulmonale may also be noted. Erythrocytosis may be present; the $PaCO_2$ is normal unless complicated by obesity-hypoventilation syndrome. While OSA due to acromegaly is self-evident at presentation, hypothyroidism causing OSA may be clinically silent; thus, thyroid function should be evaluated in all cases of OSA.

**TABLE 257.4. Clinical Features of Obstructive Sleep Apnea**

| |
|---|
| Excessive daytime sleepiness |
| Obesity (not invariable) |
| Loud snoring or apnea (usually reported by spouse/bed partner) |
| Nocturnal or morning headaches |
| Impotence |
| Nocturnal enuresis |
| Violent movements, mistaken for seizures |
| Personality changes |
| Changes in mental status |
| Hypertension |
| Pulmonary hypertension and cor pulmonale |
| Dementia |
| Postanesthetic respiratory failure |
| Inability to wean from a mechanical ventilator |
| Laboratory abnormalities |
| Erythrocytosis |
| Proteinuria, rarely in the nephrotic range |

## Central Sleep Apnea

True, isolated central sleep apnea (CSA) is uncommon. It may especially follow encephalitis, poliomyelitis, and head trauma. In contrast to OSA patients, those with CSA usually perceive awakenings from sleep. Apneic events may be reported by the spouse or the bed partner. The patient may complain of an inability to fall off to sleep. Fatigue, depression, and sexual dysfunction may occur; however, the extent of daytime somnolence, SDB-related hypoxemia, and pulmonary hypertension are less clinically intense. Physical examination is also generally normal.

### Diagnosis

Although the clinical history may strongly suggest SDB, confirmation and classification of its type require PSG. Both types of SDB involve cessation of airflow at the mouth and nostrils. However, diaphragmatic and intercostal muscle activity, which are absent in CSA, are noted in OSA. PSG allows a determination of the respiratory disturbance index (RDI; see Table 257.1) and the extent of desaturation. The current practice entails the split of PSG into two parts: the first (half) enables a diagnosis and assessment of the disease severity; the second allows application of continuous positive airway pressure (CPAP) and titration of the dose thereof for suppression of snoring and 95% of all episodes of SDB.

### Management and Prognosis

Untreated OSA, especially with a high RDI, carries a high mortality. The patient should stop using alcohol, smoking materials, and/or hypnosedatives. In obese patients, weight reduction is a useful general measure, but it is difficult to accomplish, arduous to sustain, and not immediately useful. Certain tasks, such as driving, may be impaired when OSA is left untreated. Statutes regarding the reporting requirements for driver impairments vary from state to state; physicians should contact their respective state motor vehicle departments to ascertain which impairments require reporting.

Application of CPAP through the nose (NCPAP) or via a tight-fitting face mask is effective, and is the initial therapy for all patients with OSA with an RDI of 20 or greater (Figure 257.3). CPAP presumably acts as a splint for the upper airway. Some patients may not tolerate CPAP, but patient tolerance and acceptance may be improved by desensitization, reassurance, and education as well as follow-up within a week of institution of CPAP. Consultation is appropriate with a physician with experience and training in managing SDB.

OSA due to hypothyroidism responds well to thyroxine. Other approaches to treating OSA are removal of redundant palatal and pharyngeal tissue (uvulo-

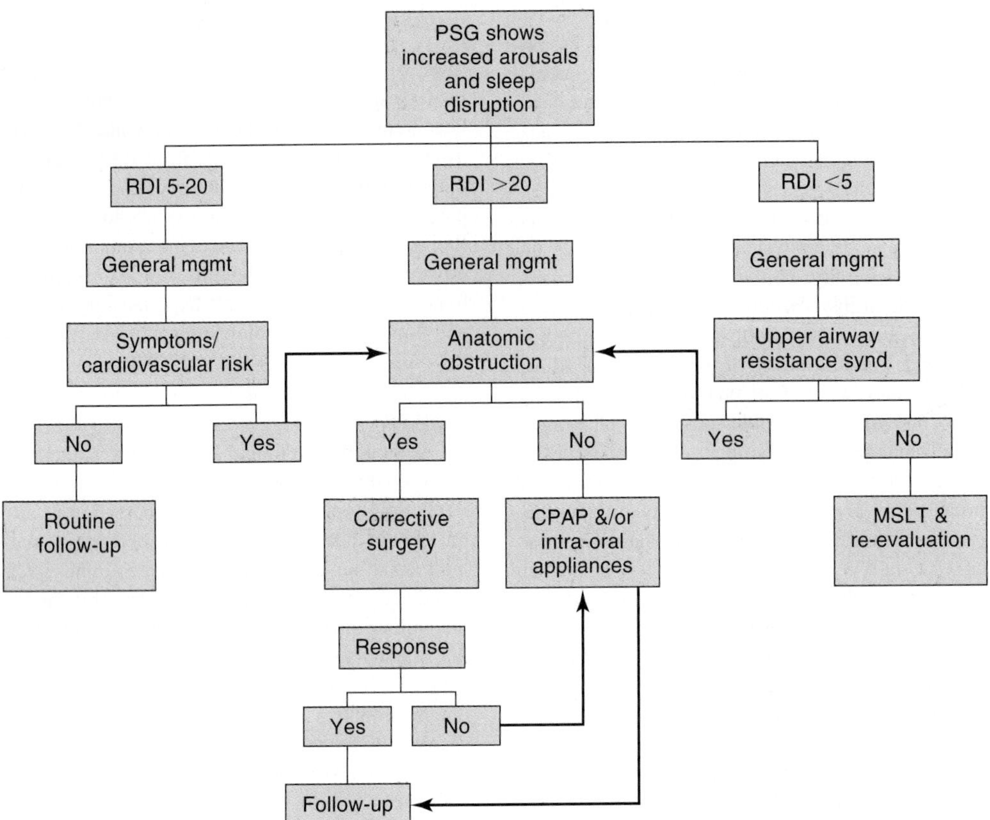


**FIGURE 257.3. Management of obstructive sleep apnea. CPAP = continuous positive airway pressure; General mgmt = General management, consisting of weight loss, avoidance of alcohol, smoking and sedatives, and sleep position modifications; MSLT = multiple sleep latency test; PSG = polysomnogram; RDI = respiratory disturbance index.**

palatopharyngoplasty [UPPP]), midline glossectomy, oral appliances, use of CPAP or non-invasive mechanical ventilation, tricyclic antidepressants, and—rarely, if ever—tracheostomy. Radiofrequency volumetric reduction of the tongue is effective in snoring.

Treatment of CSA is primarily with the use of CPAP, although non-invasive mechanical ventilation may be better tolerated in these patients. For the patient with obesity-hypoventilation syndrome or the CSA patient with awake hypercapnia, intermittent positive pressure ventilation administered through a tight-fitting nasal mask may be useful at night.

## Narcolepsy

Narcolepsy, first described in 1880 as a disease with episodes of irresistible sleep induced by strong emotions, is now recognized as a disease of disordered REM-sleep regulation.

### Pathogenesis

In the majority of patients with narcolepsy, an organic etiology is absent (primary narcolepsy). However, suprasellar lesions, cranial irradiation, and head injury may impair REM-sleep regulation and evoke features of narcolepsy (secondary narcolepsy). The primary type has an estimated prevalence in the general population of nearly 0.05% (1 in 2000 persons). Nearly 1–2% of affected persons have a first-degree relative with the disease. There is a very high prevalence of HLA-DQB1-0602 allele in patients with the disease. Curiously, 85–95% of persons with severe cataplexy (see below) and only 40% of those without cataplexy have this allele. Because HLA-associated disorders are commonly autoimmune and because most cases of narcolepsy now do not appear to be familial, an autoimmune mechanism is now favored.

An abnormal hypocretin (synonym: orexin) system was recently linked to narcolepsy. Hypocretin 1 and 2 (*hypo*thalamic factors of the in*cretin* family) are neurotransmitters released from the hypothalamus. The detection of hypocretin-containing neurons in the hypothalamic areas involved in the sleep-wake cycle suggested a role for hypocretin in sleep regulation. In 1999, a hypocretin-2 receptor gene mutation was found in canine narcolepsy. In hypocretin-knockout mice, features simulating narcolepsy were shown, i.e., behavioral arrest along with sleep-onset REM on EEG. These findings, a shared phenotype for canine and human narcolepsy, and undetectable hypocretin levels in the cerebrospinal fluid of a majority of cataplectic narcoleptics in one small study, all suggest a hypocretin-related pathogenesis for human narcolepsy; consequently, an HLA-mediated damage to the hypocretin mechanism is now theorized to cause human narcolepsy.

Accentuated brain stem cholinergic activity and decreased discharge of monoaminergic neurons in the locus ceruleus and raphe nuclei appear to play a role in initiating normal REM sleep. Excitatory axons from pontine-tegmental pedunculopontine nuclei project to ventromedial medullary neurons, whose axons, through inhibitory synapses, terminate in the anterior horn cells of the spinal cord, which provides a mechanism for muscle paralysis, which is an integral aspect of REM sleep. It is possible that a significantly impaired hypocretin mechanism might inappropriately provoke REM sleep; these neural connections merely evoke a normal skeletal muscle response to REM sleep—with resulting cataplexy.

### Clinical Features

Narcolepsy features a tetrad of symptoms, including EDS, sleep paralysis, hypnagogic hallucinations, and cataplexy. Only a majority—but not all—of patients with this disorder manifest the tetrad. Although not unique to narcolepsy, the initial symptom in the majority of patients with narcolepsy is excessive sleepiness (EDS) that affects their day-to-day activities. This sleepiness may cause accidents at work and while driving, and impaired work performance. Most patients report "compensatory" naps that, unlike those taken by sleep apnea subjects, are refreshing. Paradoxically, some patients may report insomnia, which arises from disturbed nocturnal sleep and many awakenings. Thus, the diagnosis of narcolepsy may be overlooked. Cataplexy, the most specific feature of narcolepsy, results in bouts of transient muscle weakness triggered by strong emotion. Functionally, cataplexy is an inappropriate intrusion of normal REM-sleep into wakefulness, although why it is triggered by emotion remains unknown. Only about 75% of subjects with narcolepsy exhibit cataplexy. Sleep paralysis and hypnagogic hallucinations, albeit very stressful for patients, lack specificity for narcolepsy. Narcolepsy may be associated with other conditions that cause EDS (e.g., sleep apnea).

### Diagnosis

Unambiguous cataplexy and EDS together make diagnosis of narcolepsy clinically certain. However, confirmation of the diagnosis is necessary, especially when cataplexy is absent or equivocal. Cataplexy being totally subjective, attempts to make its diagnosis more objective have involved telling jokes to the patients or having them watch a humorous videotape. Use of an ESS may help estimate EDS semi-objectively. The most commonly used methods of documenting narcolepsy are (a) by excluding other conditions that cause EDS via a nocturnal PSG, which also confirms a short sleep latency, and (b) an MSLT (see Table 257.1) on the next day to document occurrence of REM sleep on at least two naps on MSLT. Prior to MSLT, adequate sleep must be ensured on the night preceding the study (a PSG accomplishes this), and medications that affect REM sleep must be avoided. Use of illicit drugs should be excluded. Because untreated sleep apnea diminishes the specificity of an otherwise positive MSLT, sleep apnea must be adequately treated before MSLT is undertaken. Finally, idiopathic hypersomnia remains the only other condition from which separating narcolepsy may be difficult.

### Management

The importance of ensuring adequate sleep and sleep hygiene, and avoiding shift work cannot be overemphasized. Drug therapy involves stimulant medications, the most commonly used being methylphenidate, amphetamines, and pemoline. Severe fluctuations in drug levels and the consequent "up-and-down" feeling as well as other side effects severely limit the use of these agents, although most are inexpensive. Modafinil, albeit expensive, is an effective and well-tolerated agent for narcolepsy. Cataplexy responds to tricyclic antidepressants (protryptiline, imipramine, and clomipramine) or serotonin-reuptake inhibitors (fluoxetine and paroxetine). Insomnia may be treated with triazolam, whereas tricyclic antidepressants are effective for hypnagogic hallucinations and sleep paralysis.

## Insomnia

Insomnia may be defined as the inability to fall asleep or stay asleep. Because sleep needs are highly variable, the adequacy of sleep cannot be determined by the number of hours slept by an individual. Based on the duration of symptoms (≥ or < 3 weeks), insomnia may be divided into acute and chronic types.

**TABLE 257.5. Pharmacologic Therapy of Insomnia**

| Agent | Trade Name | Half-life (hrs) | Dose* | Comments |
|---|---|---|---|---|
| **Benzodiazepines** | | | | |
| Flurazepam | Dalmane | >24 | 15–30 mg | General side effects of benzodiazepines include tolerance, habituation, potential for abuse, daytime sedation, rebound insomnia |
| Temazepam | Restoril | 8–10 | 7.5–30 mg | |
| Triazolam | Halcion | 1.5–5.5 | 0.125–0.25mg | |
| **Non-benzodiazepine** | | | | |
| Zolpidem | Ambien | 2 | 5–10 mg | Abuse potential and risk of withdrawal symptoms appear low |
| Zaleplon | Sonata | 1 | 5–10 mg | |
| **Antidepressants** | | | | |
| Amitriptyline | Elavil | 24 | 10–50 mg | Constipation, dry mouth, daytime drowsiness, cardiac toxicity, urinary retention, and orthostatic hypotension; may worsen PLMS and restless legs |
| Trazodone | Desyrel | 7 | 25–100 mg | Same side effects as amitriptyline, but does not worsen PLMS and restless legs; may cause priapism |

*Use lower dose in elderly persons. Dosing regimens of most hypnotics are derived from therapeutic trials in persons with severe insomnia; thus, pronounced drowsiness is more liable to occur when these doses are used in the general population. PLMS = periodic limb movements of sleep.

Insomnia shows a higher predilection for women and older individuals. It is a risk factor for suboptimal job performance, depression, alcohol and other over-the-counter hypnotic use, and among the elderly, for admission to nursing homes. Many insomniacs may also suffer from sleep-state misperception, i.e., underestimation of their own sleep because of a perception that they were awake when they were actually sleeping.

## Etiology

More than 50% of all cases of insomnia are due to **psychiatric or psychological** causes. These include anxiety, depression, and significant stress. **Medical conditions** that lead to insomnia include restless leg syndrome (RLS), periodic limb movements of sleep (PLMS), pain, and asthma. **Psychophysiologic insomnia** refers to bad habits acquired when insomnia was first acquired due to other conditions (e.g., trying too hard to sleep). Stimulant **medications** (e.g., prednisone, theophylline, caffeine) may cause insomnia. Although alcohol may help initiate sleep, as its influence wears off, arousals develop that promote wakefulness. Withdrawal of chronic hypnotic therapy acts like a stimulant. **Poor sleep hygiene** (highly irregular sleeping and waking hours and lack of exercise) and **sleep state misperception** are other causes of insomnia. **Circadian rhythm abnormalities** that cause insomnia are often the cause of insomnia in adolescents, young adults, and the elderly. Here, the timing of sleep does not coincide with socially acceptable times. In some situations, the insomnia is **idiopathic**.

## Management

The importance of a thorough sleep history in managing insomnia cannot be overemphasized. Unless one is dealing with RLS or PLMS, or an occasional case of sleep apnea that masquerades as insomnia, PSG plays no role in diagnosis or management of insomnia. The type of insomnia (acute vs. chronic) and the segment of sleep where insomnia occurs (initiation or maintenance insomnia or early awakening) should be noted. In acute insomnia, where an identifiable cause is generally present, elimination of the cause and short-term therapy with hypnotics (Table 257.5) are effective strategies. Preventing evolution of acute insomnia into the chronic type is a fundamental goal of therapy. The emphasis in treating chronic insomnia is more on behavioral therapy (Table 257.5) rather than pharmacological therapy. Bright light therapy and relaxation therapy are useful in some instances. Insomnia and depression aggravate each other; therefore, careful evaluation for depression is important. Consultation with a physician experienced in managing sleep disorders is recommended in this setting.

# ■ Questions

**Instructions:** For each question below, select **one** lettered answer that is the **best** for each question.

1. A 60-year-old man has recently worsening dyspnea and a along history of productive cough, sputum production, frequent weheezing, and a 55-pack-year smoking history. He is on no medications. He is alert

and in moderate respiratory distress. The pulse is 100/min; respirations, 29/m; and BP 190/95 mm Hg. Diffuse wheezing and mild lower-extremity edema are noted. Hemoglobin is 18.0g and hematocrit is 53%. The initial $PaO_2$ is 35 mm Hg; $PaCO_2$, 85 mm Hg; and pH, 7.28. One hour after oxygen and bronchodilator, he is alert and responsive. Pulse is 95/min; BP, 170/92 mm Hg; and respiration, 26/min. The pH is 7.26; $PaCO_2$, 90 mm Hg; and $PaO_2$, 54 mm Hg. Which one of the following will you do now?

A. Increase the oxygen dose and repeat blood gases in 1 hour.
B. Administer aerosolized albuterol now; repeat blood gases in 1 hour.
C. Arrange for endotracheal intubation because of the rise in $PaCO_2$.
D. Continue present management.

2. On the night of an elective cholecystectomy and common blie duct exploration, a 68-year-old woman develops respiratory distress. She had quit chronic, heavy smoking 2 weeks previously. Her pulse is 120/min; BP, 169/90 mm Hg, respirations, 34/min, and temperature 99° F. Breath sounds are normal and symmetrical, with diffuse end-inspiratory crackles. Heart sounds are distant but otherwise normal. Her pH is 7.32; $PaCO_2$, 32 mm Hg; and $PaO_2$, 46 mm Hg. No preoperative blood gas results are available. Which of the following entities is MOST likely now?
A. Acute exacerbation of chronic obstructive pulmonary disease.
B. Atelectasis due to pain and secretions.
C. Acute pulmonary edema.
D. Acute respiratory failure from massive pleural effusion
E. Acute, submassive pulmonary embolism.

3. Besides administering oxygen, which of the following will you do now?
A. Give analgesia to control pain and take measures to effect lung expansion.
B. Perform an immediate ventilation-perfusion lung scan.
C. Get consent for and proceed to thoracentesis.
D. Give morphine sulfate and furosemide; perform 12-lead ECG.
E. Give ipratropium bromide by hand-held nebulizer and IV corticosteroids.

4. A 25-year-old man is found comatose. His pulse rate is 130/min; respiratory rate, 28/min; BP 100/50 mm Hg; and temperature, 103° F. Trachea is deviated to the left. Movement and percussion note are diminished and breath sounds are absent in the left lower chest posteriorly. The entire lower half of the left chest is opacified on chest x-ray. His arterial blood gases initially are as follows: pH, 7.35; $PaO_2$, 48; $PaCO_2$, 50. After oxygen (15L/min by non-rebreathing mask) his arterial blood gases are: pH, 7.36; $PaO_2$, 56; $PaCO_2$, 50. Which ONE of the following best represents your assessment?
A. Acute ventilatory and oxygenation failure related to ARDS.
B. He has acute, predominantly oxygenation failure due to left lower lobe atelectasis.
C. Acute, predominantly oxygenation failure due to a large left pleural effusion, which is very likely an empyema.
D. Acute, predominantly oxygenation failure due to pneumonia.

5. Which one of the following best explains the hypoxemia in the patient described in question 4?
A. It is caused by ventilation-perfusion abnormalities.
B. It is entirely explanined by the hypoventilation.
C. It is caused by left-to-right shunting.
D. It is related to a severe diffusion abnormality.
E. It is caused by right-to-left shunting.

6. A 58-year-old man has had productive cough, almost daily wheezing, and progressive exertional dyspnea for the last 5 years. He is a smoker. Which ONE of the following sets of tests best fits his condition?

| | FVC (L) | $FEV_{1.0}$ (L) | $DL_{CO}$ (observed/ predicted) | PaO2 | PaCO2 |
|---|---|---|---|---|---|
| A | 3.5 | 2.95 | 12/24 | 55 | 35 |
| B | 3.75 | 3.50 | 14/24 | 65 | 28 |
| C | 3.1 | 1.01 | 15/24 | 58 | 49 |
| D | 3.8 | 3.5 | 22/24 | 79 | 44 |

7. Which of the following will you now recommend for management of the patient described in question 6?
A. Long-term, low-flow oxygen; ipratropium bromide (2 puffs every 4-6 hours); smoking cessation.
B. Long-term, low-flow oxygen; sustained release theophylline (300 mg b.i.d.), and albuterol by metered dose inhaler (2 puffs q.i.d.).
C. All items in (B) above plus cessation of smoking and avoidance of atmospheric irritants.
D. All items in (C) above plus antibiotics when sputum changes in color or when symptoms indicate respiratory infection.

8. A businessman has a hematocrit of 61% and hemoglobin of 20.0 g. He has noted morning headaches, but no cough, sputum or wheezing. He is a nonsmoker. Obesity, swelling, and redness of uvula

and mild lower-extremity edema are noted. Which of the following data would match his clinical situation?

| | PA pressure | PCW | $PaO_2$ | $PaCO_2$ | pH |
|---|---|---|---|---|---|
| A | 48/30 | 20 | 76 | 38 | 7.48 |
| B | 58/30 | 12 | 70 | 35 | 7.39 |
| C | 52/28 | 22 | 55 | 44 | 7.34 |
| D | 50/28 | 8 | 50 | 48 | 7.34 |

(PA = pulmonary artery; PCW = pulmonary capillary wedge pressure)

9. What would you recommend now for managing the patient described in question 8?
   A. Furosemide, 40 mg; digoxin, 0.25 mg; theophylline, 600 mg; all daily.
   B. Furosemide, 40 mg, and digoxin, 0.25 mg daily; albuterol metered dose inhaler, 2 puffs q.i.d.
   C. Evaluation through a polysomnogram.
   D. Captopril, 12.5 mg q 6h; and oxygen, 2 L/min.

10. A 20-year-old student has had episodic wheezing, productive cough, and febrile episodes for the last 18 months. He does not smoke. A family history of atopic disease is noted. His symptoms improved briefly after a course of tetracycline. Chest x-ray shows a left upper-lobe infiltrate with cystic lucencies and a non-homogeneous right lower-zone infiltrate. Which ONE of the following studies would be most helpful?
    A. Tuberculin skin test.
    B. A histoplasmin skin test.
    C. Sweat chloride level.
    D. Serum $\alpha$-1 antitrypsin level.

11. In which of the following situations will you prescribe mini (low-dose) heparin therapy to prevent development of deep venous thrombosis?
    A. Elderly man with a prior history of DVT having a cataract surgery.
    B. Elderly woman undergoing a colectomy for cancer.
    C. Middle-aged woman having a craniotomy for meningioma extraction.
    D. All of the above.
    E. None of the above.

12. A 55-year-old asymptomatic steam fitter has a new, uncalcified 2-cm left upper lobe solitary nodule. He has a 50 pack-year history of smoking. Review of systems is normal. A PPD skin test shows 13 mm induration at 48 hours. Urinalysis, liver function tests, and complete blood counts are normal. The MOST appropriate management for the patient is:
    A. Abdominal CT, barium enema, and upper GI series, in that order.
    B. Careful follow-up every 3 months with chest x-rays.
    C. Six months of isoniazid with pyridoxine.
    D. Thoracotomy and resection of nodule.

13. A 25-year-old African American man has redness and swelling involving the shins bilaterally, fever, dry cough, and arthralgias. A chest x-ray shows bilateral hilar and paratracheal lymphadenopathy. Which of the following abnormalities is most compatible with his diagnosis?
    A. Increased sedimentation rate and increased peripheral T-lymphocytes.
    B. Increased B-lymphocytes and decreased T-lymphocytes (both in the lung).
    C. Serum calcium of 12.5 mg/dl.
    D. Positive tuberculin skin test.

14. What is the most appropriate management for the patient in question 13?
    A. Bronchoscopy, transbronchial lung biopsy; no corticosteroids.
    B. Bronchoscopy, transbronchial lung biopsy and corticosteroids.
    C. Lymph node biopsy through mediastinoscopy.
    D. Open lung biopsy.

15. A reduced pleural fluid glucose of 30 mg/100 ml (simultaneous plasma glucose 105 mg/100 ml) is consistent with a diagnosis of effusion caused by:
    A. Pancreatitis.
    B. Rheumatoid arthritis.
    C. Nephrotic syndrome.
    D. Hepatic cirrhosis.

16. In a patient with myasthenia gravis, which of the following can help the physician decide whether to use mechanical ventilatory assistance?
    A. Forced vital capacity and maximum inspiratory pressure.
    B. Arterial blood gases.
    C. $FEV_{1.0}$.
    D. Lung compliance.

## Answers

| | | | | |
|---|---|---|---|---|
| 1. D | 2. C | 3. D | 4. B | 5. E |
| 6. C | 7. A | 8. B | 9. C | 10. C |
| 11. B | 12. D | 13. C | 14. A | 15. B |
| 16. A | | | | |

## SUGGESTED READING

### *Books and Monographs*

Fishman AP, Elias JA et al (eds.). Fishman's Pulmonary Diseases and Disorders. 3rd edition. New York: McGraw-Hill Professional Publishing, 1999.

Murray JF, Nadel JA et al (eds.). Textbook of Respiratory Medicine. 3rd edition. Philadelphia: Saunders, 2000.

Schwarz MI, King Jr, TE (eds.). Interstitial Lung Disease. 3rd edition. Hamilton, London. B.C. Decker, 1998.

Sarosi GA, Davies SF (eds). Fungal Diseases of the Lung. 3rd edition. Philadelphia: Lippincott Williams & Wilkins, 2000.

### *Articles*

#### *Clinical Evaluation of Lung Disease*

American Thoracic Society: Guidelines for Methacholine and Exercise Challenge Testing. Am J Respir Crit Care Med 2000; 161:309–329.

Baughman RP, Conrado CE. Diagnosis of lower respiratory tract infections: what we have and what would be nice. Chest 1998; 113(3 Suppl):219S–223S.

Etinger NA. Invasive diagnostic approaches to pulmonary infiltrates. Semin Resp Infect 1993; 8:168–176.

Irwin RS, Madison JM. Symptom research on chronic cough: a historical pespective. Ann Intern Med 2001; 134 (9 (Part2)) supplement:809–814.

Schapira RM, Schapira MM, Funahashi A, McAuliffe TL, Varkey B. The value of the forced expiratory time in the diagnosis of obstructive airways disease. JAMA 1993; 270:731–736.

Seijo LM, Sterman DH. Interventional pulmonology. N Engl J Med 2001; 344:740–749.

#### *Pulmonary Mycoses and Mycobacterial Diseases*

American Thoracic Society: Diagnostic standards and classification of tuberculosis in adults and children. Am J Respir Crit Care Med 2000; 161:1376–1395.

American Thoracic Society: Diagnosis and treatment of disease caused by nontuberculous mycobacteria. Am J Respir Crit Care Med 1997; 156:S1–S25.

Burman WJ, Jones BE. Treatment of HIV-related tuberculosis in the era of effective antiretroviral therapy. Am J Respir Crit Care Med 2001; 164:7–12.

Havlir DV, Barnes PF. Tuberculosis in patients with human immunodeficiency virus infection. N Engl J Med 1999; 340:367–373.

Small PM, Fujiwara PI. Management of tuberculosis in the United States. N Engl J Med 2001; 345:189–200.

#### *Chronic Obstructive Pulmonary Disease, Cystic Fibrosis, and Bronchiectasis*

Bach PB, Brown C, Gelfand SE, McCrory DC. Management of acute exacerbations of chronic obstructive pulmonary disease: A summary and appraisal of published literature. Ann Intern Med 2001; 134:600–620.

Barnes PJ. Chronic obstructive pulmonary disease. N Engl J Med 2000; 343:269–280.

Niewoehner DE, Erbland ML, Deupree RH, Collins D, et al. Effect of systemic glucocorticoids on exacerbations of chronic obstructive pulmonary disease. N Engl J Med 1999; 340:1941–1947.

Stoller JK. Acute exacerbations of chronic obstructive pulmonary disease. N Engl J Med 2002; 346:988–994.

Barker AF. Bronchiectasis. N Engl J Med 2002; 346:1383–1393.

Pasteur MC, Helliwell SM, Houghton SJ, Webb SC, et al. An investigation into causative factors in patients with bronchiectasis. Am J Respir Crit Care Med 2000; 162:1277–1284.

Plant PK, Own JL, Elliott MW. Non-invasive ventilation in acute exacerbations of chronic obstructive pulmonary disease: long term survival and predictors of in-hospital outcome. Thorax 2001; 56:708–712.

Schapira RM, Reike LF. Supplemental (home) oxygen therapy: a comprehensive review of clinical and economic issues. Clin Pulmonary Med 2000; 7:69–75.

Snow V, Lascher S, Mottur-Pilson C, et al. Evidence base for management of acute exacerbations of chronic obstructive pulmonary disease. Ann Intern Med 2001; 134:595–599.

#### *Pulmonary Thromboembolism and Pulmonary Hypertension*

Hoeper MM, Galie N, Simonneau G, et al. New treatments for pulmonary arterial hypertension. Am J Respir Crit Care Med 2002; 165:1209–1216.

Fedullo PF, Auger WR, Kerr KM, Rubin LJ. Chronic Thromboembolic Pulmonary Hypertension. N Engl J Med 2001; 345:1465–1472.

Geerts WH, Heit JA, Claggett GP, et al. Prevention of venous thromboembolism. Chest 2001; 119:133S–175S.

Ginsberg JS, Greer I, Hirsh J. Use of Antithrombotic Agents During Pregnancy. Chest 2001; 119: 122S–131S.

Goldhaber SZ. Pulmonary Embolism. N Engl J Med 1998; 339:93–104.

Wells PS, Anderson DR, Rodger M, et al. Excluding Pulmonary Embolism at the Bedside Without Diagnostic Imaging: Management of Patients with Suspected Pulmonary Embolism Presenting to the Emergency Department by Using a Simple Clinical Model and D-Dimer. Ann Intern Med 1998; 135:98–103.

#### *Interstitial Lung Disease, Idiopathic Pulmonary Fibrosis, Sarcoidosis and Pleuro-Pulmonary Manifestations of Rheumatic Disorders*

DeRemee RA. Sarcoidosis. Mayo Cin Proc 1995; 70:177–181.

American Thoracic Society. Statement on Sarcoidosis. Am J Respir Crit Care Med 1999; 160:736–755.

American Thoracic Society/European Respiratory Society international multdisciplinary consensus classification of the idiopathic interstitial pneumonias. Am J Respir Crit Care Med 2002; 165:277–304.

King Jr. TE, Schwarz MI, Brown K, Tooze JA, et al. Idiopathic pulmonary fibrosis. Am J Respir Crit Care Med 2001; 164:1025–1032.

Wiedemann HP, Matthay RA. Pulmonary manifestations of the collagen vascular diseases. Clin Chest Med 1989; 10:677–722.

Douglas WW, Tazellar HD, Hartman TE, et al. Polymyosisits-dermatomyositis-associated interstitial lung disease. Am J Respir Crit Care Med 2001; 164:1182–1185.

Ziesche R, Hofbauer E, Wittmann K, Petkov V, Block L-H. A preliminary study of long-term treatment with interferon gamma-1b and low dose prednisolone in patients with idiopathic pulmonary fibrosis. N Engl J Med 1999; 341:1264–1269.

#### *Pulmonary Aspiration Syndromes*

Bartlett JG. Anaerobic bacterial infections of the lung and pleural space. Clin Infect Dis 1993; 16 Suppl4:S248–555.

Tiejen PA, Kaner RJ, Quinn CE. Aspiration emergencies. Clin Chest Med 1994; 15:117–35.

#### *Drug-Induced Lung Disease*

Ben-Noun L. Drug-Induced Respiratory Disorders: Incidence, Prevention and Management. Drug Safety 2000; 23:143–164.

Morelock SY, Sahn SA. Drugs and the Pleura. Chest 1999; 116:212–221.

Rosenow ECIII. Drug-induced pulmonary disease. Dis Mon 1994; 40:253–310.

### *Pleural Disease*

Glazer M, Berkman N, Lafair JS, Kramer MR. Successful talc slurry pleurodesis in patients with nonmalignant pleural effusion. Chest 2000;117:1404–1409.

Heffner JE. Infection of the pleural space. Clin Chest Med 1999;20:607–622.

Sahn SA, Heffner JE. Spontaneous pneumothorax. N Engl J Med 2000;342:868–874.

### *Lung Cancer*

Matthay RA. Lung Cancer. Clin Chest Med 1993; 14: 1–200.

Nesbitt JC, Putnam Jr JB, Walsh GL, Roth JA, Mountain CV. Survival in early-stage non-small cell lung cancer. Ann Thorac Surg 1995; 60:466–472.

Ost D, Fein A. Evaluation and management of the solitary pulmonary nodule. Am J Respir Crit Care Med 2000; 162:782–787.

Sazon DA, Santiago GW, Hoo S, Khonsary A, Brown C, et al. Fluorodeoxyglucose-positron emission tomography in the detection and staging of lung cancer. Am J Respir Crit Care Med 1996; 153:417–421.

### *Pulmonary Disease Due To Inorganic Dusts*

Banks DE, Cheng YH, Weber SL, Ma JK. Strategies for the treatment of pneumoconiosis. Occup Med 1993; 8: 205–32.

Begin R. Detailed occupational history. Am J Respir Crit Care Med 2001; 163:598–599.

Beckett WS. Occupational respiratory diseases. N Engl J Med 2000; 342:406–413.

### *Respiratory Failure and Acute Respiratory Distress Syndrome*

Bernard GR, Artigas A, Brigham KL et al.: The American-European Consensus Conference on ARDS. Definitions, Mechanisms, Relevant Outcomes, and Clinical Trial Coordination. Am J Respir Crit Care Med 1994; 149: 818–824.

Hilbert G, Gruson D, Vargas F, Valentino R, Gbikpi-Benissan G, Dupon M, Reiffers J, Cardinaud JP. Noninvasive Ventilation in Immunosuppressed Patients With Pulmonary Infiltrates, Fever and Acute Respiratory Failure. N Engl J Med 2001; 344:481–487.

Steinberg KP, Hudson LD. Acute Lung Injury and Acute Respiratory Distress Syndrome. Clin Chest Med 2000; 21:403–417.

The Acute Respiratory Distress Syndrome Network: Ventilation With Lower Tidal Volumes as Compared With Traditional Tidal Volumes for Acute Lung Injury and the Acute Respiratory Distress Syndrome. N Engl J Med 2000; 342:1301–1308.

Tobin MJ. Advances in Mechanical Ventilation. N Engl J Med 2001; 344:1986–1996.

### *Sleep and Its Disorders*

Badr SM. Pathophysiology of Upper Airway Obstruction During Sleep. Clin Chest Med 1998; 19:21–32.

Bahammam A, Kryger M. Decision-Making in Obstructive Sleep-Disordered Breathing: Putting it All Together. Clin Chest Med 1998; 19:87–97.

Hauri PJ. Insomnia. Clin Chest Med 1998; 19:157–168.

Krahn LE, Black JL, Silber MH. Narcolepsy: New Understanding of Irresistible Sleep. Mayo Clin Proc 2001; 76: 185–194.

Schellenberg JB, Maislin G, Schwab RJ. Physical Findings and the Risk for Obstructive Sleep Apnea. Am J Resp Crit Care Med 2000; 162:740–748.

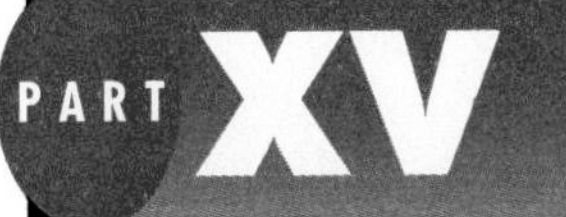


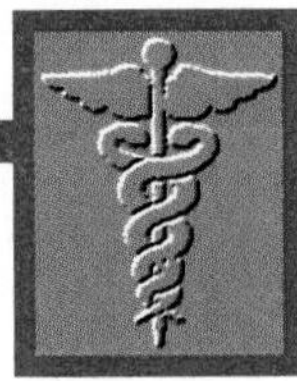

Paul B. Halverson

# RHEUMATIC DISEASES

# CHAPTER 258 EVALUATION OF JOINT DISEASES

## History

Rheumatic diseases usually are managed in the outpatient setting. Pain is the complaint that most commonly brings the patient to the doctor, but other complaints include joint swelling or enlargement, stiffness, loss of joint mobility, weakness, and, occasionally, numbness or tingling.

**Pain** may vary from mild and aching to severe and disabling. Its pattern (e.g., intermittent, chronic low-grade, progressive worsening), location, and evolution over time should be determined and may suggest a diagnosis. Some patients may report episodes of arthritis, but then have none seen on examination. A history of intermittent pain, swelling, and erythema in the great toe may suggest gout.

Sometimes, the main concern is **joint enlargement,** often noticed in the proximal interphalangeal (PIP) and distal interphalangeal (DIP) joints of the hands as osteoarthritis develops. Joint symptoms and the physical abnormalities of the joints may be discordant, and, thus, some joints with advanced joint damage manifest surprisingly little pain. Patients also may report **joint swelling,** which women may perceive as difficulty in removing rings. Because patients sometimes confuse fluid retention or edema with actual joint swelling, joint swelling must be confirmed by physical examination.

**Stiffness,** defined as discomfort in attempting to move joints after a period of inactivity, is common to most forms of arthritis. It may provide some clues about the type and severity of arthritis. Morning stiffness lasting for more than 30 minutes (What time do you get up? When are you as good or as loose as you're going to be?) suggests an inflammatory process. While morning stiffness lasting at least 1 hour (but often much longer) is one of the diagnostic criteria for rheumatoid arthritis, it also occurs in most other forms of "inflammatory" arthritis. However, in "noninflammatory" conditions such as osteoarthritis, morning stiffness usually is brief (30 min). Persons with osteoarthritis also report recurrent stiffness during the day following periods of inactivity **(gelling).** New-onset, severe morning stiffness in an older individual, even to the point of causing difficulty in getting out of bed, may suggest polymyalgia rheumatica.

**Loss of joint motion** is likely to be noticed in the shoulders or hands. Impaired glenohumeral motion often results in reduced shoulder abduction and rotation, thus making combing one's hair or dressing difficult. Similarly, making a fist or fully extending the fingers may not be possible.

Although **numbness** and **tingling** suggest a neurologic disorder, they also may reflect musculoskeletal disease. Hand numbness and tingling are common and most often are related to compression of either the median nerve at the wrist or the ulnar nerve at the elbow, or to cervical spine disease. Sciatic pain and tingling or numbness may reflect a **radiculopathy** (disease of the spinal nerve roots), such as may occur with a herniated disc. Buttock pain with radiation down the leg or sensory symptoms associated with walking or standing may suggest neurogenic claudication from spinal stenosis (usually in elderly persons). Sometimes, the cause of numbness and tingling in the extremities may be elusive if nerve conduction testing and imaging studies do not correlate.

A feeling of **weakness** is another common complaint that may be difficult to relate to physical findings. Proximal muscle weakness that is greater than distal weakness usually is due to a myopathic process (e.g., polymyositis), whereas the reverse usually is true in neurologic diseases.

Although nonspecific, **fatigue** often is a component of systemic rheumatic diseases. This fatigue follows activity and does not resolve after rest; the time for its onset after arising correlates inversely with the extent of inflammation. Fatigue on arising is more compatible with fibromyalgia or many nonrheumatic disorders (e.g., anemia, cancer, metabolic disorders, sleep apnea, insomnia, or a psychogenic problem).

The physician should assess the patient's reaction to a symptom by exploring its impact on his or her ability to perform activities of daily living, on sleep, employment, mental status, and family relationships. A family history of "arthritis" or "rheumatism" should be clarified to determine the type, disability or deformity, and treatment. A review of systems may provide clues to specific rheumatic syndromes (Table 258.1).

## Physical Examination

Because rheumatic diseases can affect multiple organs, the physical examination must be thorough. The skin should be examined for rashes (e.g., purpura seen in vasculitis; psoriatic plaques which may be hidden in the hair, umbilicus, or gluteal folds), thickening or tightness, erythema, ulceration or scarring in the fingertips or on the forearms and lower extremities, nail pitting, subcutaneous nodules, or calcifications. The nail folds should be examined, preferably with an ophthalmoscope for mag-

**TABLE 258.1. Review of Systems for Clues to Specific Rheumatic Diseases**

| | |
|---|---|
| Systemic | Fever, weight loss |
| Mucocutaneous | Rash, ulcers, nodules, sun sensitivity, alopecia, oral or genital sores |
| Head and neck area | Red painful eyes, dry eyes or mouth, jaw claudication |
| Cardiopulmonary | Pleurisy, cough, dyspnea, Raynaud's phenomenon, edema, claudication |
| Gastrointestinal | Dysphagia, abdominal pain, diarrhea, bloody stools |
| Genitourinary | Dysuria, bloody or cloudy urine, urethral discharge |
| Musculoskeletal | Weakness, myalgias, arthralgias; joint swelling, pain, warmth, redness, or decreased motion |
| Neurologic | Numbness, paraesthesias, urinary or fecal incontinence, radicular pain, weakness, exercise-induced pain or weakness, seizures, cranial or peripheral nerve abnormalities, visual disturbance, headache, vertigo |

nification, for capillary abnormalities (e.g., giant loops and reduced numbers of nail fold vessels in scleroderma).

A red eye or ciliary flush suggests conjunctivitis or iritis, respectively. Ulcerations of the nose or mouth and lymphadenopathy should be sought. Pericardial or pleural friction rubs suggest serositis. Dullness to percussion (pleural effusion) and crackles on auscultation (interstitial fibrosis) are important findings in the chest.

All joints and surrounding structures should be examined for tenderness (joints should be squeezed firmly, just enough to blanch the examiner's fingernail). Identification of tenderness at specific sites is critical to making diagnoses of tendinitis, bursitis, and fibromyalgia. Joints should also be examined for swelling, warmth, erythema, limitation of motion, and flexion contractures. Moving the joints actively and passively through a range of motion can detect pain and crepitus (audible or palpable grating or crunching occurring during joint movement). Loss of joint integrity is suggested by instability and deformity. Joint enlargement may result from several processes: joint effusion (most easily assessed in the knee); synovial thickening (spongy enlargement, as in rheumatoid arthritis); and bony enlargement (osteophytes). Periarticular tissues also should be palpated firmly to localize sites of tenderness, which may help identify either tendinitis or bursitis. A common mistake occurs when the palpating pressure on the joint, periarticular tissue, or muscle is insufficient to elicit pain in the abnormal site. The examiner should ask the patient to report what areas are painful on palpation, but also observe the patient for nonverbal cues of discomfort. If only one side of the body is involved, it is helpful to compare the involved joint(s) to their unaffected counterparts on the other side.

Muscle strength should be tested and muscle atrophy noted, as should motor and sensory deficits and reflexes. Tapping over a nerve at the site of compression may elicit tingling (e.g., Tinel sign at the wrist in carpal tunnel syndrome).

## Laboratory Tests

Laboratory testing, by itself, is rarely definitive for the diagnosis of rheumatic disorders. In most cases, diagnosis depends on a combination of history and physical and laboratory findings. The history and physical examination remain more essential tools for diagnosis than in most other specialties of medicine. Rheumatologic testing includes synovianalysis, serologic tests, imaging, and miscellaneous tests (Table 258.2).

### Synovianalysis

**Arthrocentesis** is the process of aspirating synovial fluid from effused joints for analysis **(synovianalysis).** Synovial fluid analysis should be performed whenever synovial fluid is obtainable (Table 258.3). The **gross appearance** of synovial fluid can provide important clues about etiology. Clear fluid is noninflammatory and is typical of osteoarthritis or a mechanical derangement such as a meniscal tear, whereas slightly cloudy or translucent fluid with increased cellularity suggests an inflammatory condition (gout or rheumatoid arthritis). Bloody fluid (hemarthrosis) suggests traumatic arthritis, whereas purulent (opaque) fluid suggests septic arthritis.

The synovial fluid **leukocyte count** reflects the degree of inflammation (see Table 258.2). Counts exceeding 2,000/mm$^3$ are considered inflammatory, but there are no "diagnostic" cell counts. As the leukocyte count increases, so does the proportion of polymorphonuclear leukocytes (PMN). Synovial fluid from patients with active rheumatoid arthritis, Reiter's syndrome, or gout often contain 30,000 or more cells/mm$^3$, whereas only 5,000 to 10,000 cells/mm$^3$ may be seen in gonococcal arthritis. Very high cell counts are more likely to occur with infection.

The **mucin clot** and **viscosity** tests reflect the intactness of polymeric hyaluronic acid, which gives "noninflammatory" synovial fluid its syrupy consistency. Low viscosity leading to a watery consistency and a poor mucin clot result when hyaluronic acid has

**TABLE 258.2. Common Laboratory Tests in Rheumatic Diseases**

| Synovianalysis | Result |
|---|---|
| Appearance | Clear, cloudy |
| Mucin clot | Intactness of hyaluronic acid |
| Leukocyte count | >2000 cells/cmm suggests inflammatory arthritis |
| Polarized light | Monosodium urate, calcium pyrophosphate |
| Gram stain, culture, glucose | Suspected infection |
| **Serum Tests** | **Result** |
| Rheumatoid factor | Present in 80% of patients with RA; 5% false positives |
| Anti-nuclear antibody | Screening test for autoimmune disease<br>Present in:<br>>95% of patients with SLE<br>>95% of patients with scleroderma<br>15–50% of patients with RA<br>15–50% of patients with inflammatory myositis |
| Complements | |
| $C_3$, $C_4$ | Reduced levels in some patients with SLE, cryoglobulinemia, and some cases of vasculitis |
| $CH_{50}$ | Same as C3,C4. Also reduced in inherited complement deficiency states |

RA = rheumatoid arthritis; SLE = systemic lupus erythematosus.

**TABLE 258.3. Synovial Fluid Analysis**

| | Group 1 (Noninflammatory) | Group 2 (Inflammatory) | Group 3 (Purulent) |
|---|---|---|---|
| **Gross examination** | | | |
| Color | Yellow | Pink to yellow to white (red if traumatic) | Purulent |
| Clarity | Transparent | Translucent to opaque | Purulent |
| Viscosity | High | Medium to low | Low |
| Mucin clot | Good | Fair | Poor |
| **Microscopic examination** | | | |
| WBC/$mm^3$ | <2000 | 5,000–50,000 | >50,000 |
| Neutrophils | <25% | <25-90% | >90% |

WBC = white blood cells.

been digested by inflammatory enzymes, as in rheumatoid arthritis.

In cases of suspected joint sepsis, useful tests include simultaneous serum and joint fluid glucose levels, Gram stain, and culture. Synovianalysis is definitive when a Gram stain shows microorganisms or compensated **polarized light microscopy** shows crystals. Negatively birefringent crystals of **monosodium urate** indicate gout (see Color Plate 32). In acute gout, these needle-shaped crystals often are found inside PMNs. When aligned with the direction of the red compensator, the crystals appear yellow, and when rotated 90 degrees, they appear blue. Although highly sensitive and specific for gout, gout crystals may coexist only rarely with septic or other arthritides. **Calcium pyrophosphate** crystals, in contrast, are positively birefringent, rhomboidal crystals found in pseudogout; they appear blue when aligned with the compensator and yellow when rotated 90 degrees (see Color Plate 33).

### Serologic Studies

The two serologic tests most often ordered in the investigation of rheumatic diseases are the serum rheumatoid factor and antinuclear antibody. These tests usually are ordered when symmetrical joint swelling is suggested by history or observed on examination.

**Rheumatoid factor** (RF), antibody to the Fc portion of immunoglobulin G, occurs in approximately 80% of rheumatoid arthritis patients (seropositive). Absence of RF, however, does not rule out rheumatoid arthritis, because nearly 20% of patients with the disease are seronegative. Rheumatoid factor also may occur in some other types of arthritis and in some chronic inflammatory states (Table 258.4). Rheumatoid factors may consist of any immunoglobulin class, but the agglutination methods used in most diagnostic laboratories detect essentially only pentameric IgM-RF.

The **antinuclear antibody** (ANA) test is a screening test for the connective tissue diseases (Table 258.5). Few tests engender more confusion, because of the notion that a positive ANA may signify systemic lupus erythematosus (SLE). Five percent to 15% of normal people have a positive ANA, or the ANA may be induced by drugs (e.g., procainamide, hydralazine). A negative ANA essentially excludes SLE, because more than 95% of SLE patients have a positive ANA; however, a positive ANA by itself does not strongly suggest SLE. Thus, the ANA is sensitive but not specific for SLE. The ANA is seen commonly in other autoimmune diseases (see Table 258.5). A positive ANA test becomes significant only when other features of SLE or other autoimmune disease are found by history, physical examination, or other routine laboratory testing or with more specific serologic testing (e.g., antibodies to native DNA or to Smith antigen, which are rare in other conditions). In evaluating a positive ANA, tests for antibodies to other nuclear antigens may help either to confirm or refute diagnoses of other connective tissue diseases.

**TABLE 258.4. Rheumatoid Factor: Frequency of Occurrence in Various Conditions**

| Disease | % Positive |
|---|---|
| Rheumatoid arthritis | 80 |
| Systemic lupus erythematosus, scleroderma, polymyositis | 30 |
| Bacterial endocarditis | 70 |
| Sarcoidosis | 10 |
| Aging (age >60 yrs) | 15–50 |
| Syphilis | 10 |
| Tuberculosis | 15 |
| Leprosy | 25 |
| Chronic liver disease | 25 |

### Other Blood Tests

The **erythrocyte sedimentation rate** (ESR) has very limited diagnostic value, especially in a patient with nonspecific symptoms. However, a markedly elevated ESR may be the sole laboratory finding in polymyalgia rheumatica or temporal arteritis. As a test of inflammation, some use the ESR to monitor response to therapy in chronic inflammatory arthritides (e.g., rheumatoid arthritis).

The serum **creatine kinase** (CK) may rise in many congenital and acquired inflammatory muscle disorders and may aid in evaluating patients with muscle pain or weakness. Hypothyroidism may also manifest myalgias, arthralgias, weakness, and, in some, an elevated CK.

Serum **complement** may be consumed in immune complex diseases (e.g., lupus nephritis), bacterial endocarditis, mixed or monoclonal cryoglobulinemia, vasculitis, or severe sepsis. Quantitative measurement of C3 and C4 proteins, while readily available, does not distinguish the activated from the unactivated components. Because levels of C3 in closed spaces, such as pleura or joints, and in some sera may represent already activated protein, the **hemolytic assay (CH50)** may be preferred, because it assesses the function of the entire complement cascade. Individual complement components may be congenitally low, the most common being the C2 heterozygous deficiency. Search for a complement

**TABLE 258.5. Antinuclear Antibodies: Frequency of Positive Finding in Various Rheumatic Diseases (%)**

| Antibody | SLE | Scl | CREST | PM/DM | RA | DLE | MCTD | SS |
|---|---|---|---|---|---|---|---|---|
| ANA | >95 | 95 | 95 | 20–50 | 15–35 | >95 | >95 | 75 |
| Anti-native DNA | 50 | | | | | | | |
| Sm | 40 | | | | | | | |
| RNP | 40 | 15 | 10 | 15 | | | >95 | 15 |
| Centromere | | | 50 | | | | | |
| Histones | 30 | | | | 20 | >95 | | |
| Scl-70 | | 40 | 15 | | | | | |
| SS-A/Ro | 25* | | | 10 | 10† | | | 50 |
| SS-B/La | 15 | | | | | | | 25 |
| PM-1 | | | | 30–50 | | | | |

*Positive in subacute cutaneous lupus, in which ANA may be negative.
†SS-A/Ro positive patients usually have secondary Sjögren syndrome.
ANA = antinuclear antibody; CREST = *c*alcinosis, *R*aynaud syndrome, *e*sophageal dysmotility, *s*clerodactyly, *t*elangiectasia; DLE = drug-induced lupus; DM = dermatomyositis; MCTD = mixed connective tissue disease; PM = polymyositis; RA = rheumatoid arthritis; RNP = ribonucleoprotein; Scl = diffuse scleroderma; SLE = systemic lupus erythematosus; Sm = Smith; SS = Sjögren's syndrome.

component deficiency may be prompted by an absent CH50 with normal or near-normal C3 and C4 levels.

Cryoglobulins (serum proteins which precipitate at 4°C) may be found in some patients with rheumatoid arthritis or SLE. Occasionally, they may be the sole serologic anomaly, as in infective endocarditis or essential cryoglobulinemia.

### Imaging in Joint Disease

Joint radiographs rarely are diagnostic in acute arthritis with several exceptions. Radiographs showing cartilage calcification (chondrocalcinosis, see Figure 260.2) or tendon calcification may suggest pseudogout or calcific tendinitis respectively. Radiographs also may detect stress fractures or tumors. Early radiographs in septic arthritis, osteomyelitis, SLE, rheumatoid arthritis, and other inflammatory arthritides typically show only nonspecific soft tissue swelling. In more chronic arthritis, radiographs may document the extent (i.e., progression) and severity of the disease process. Other imaging techniques, including magnetic resonance imaging, computed tomography, diagnostic ultrasound, and nuclear medicine bone scanning, may provide additional diagnostic information in specific clinical situations.

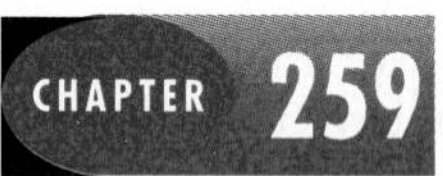

# CHAPTER 259 CLINICAL PRESENTATIONS OF RHEUMATIC CONDITIONS AND PRINCIPLES OF THERAPY

### Clinical Approach to Diagnosis

Diagnosis of rheumatic diseases may be facilitated by a stepwise approach, in which responses to a series of questions gradually limit the diagnostic possibilities (Figure 259.1).

*What is the source of pain?* The examiner should determine, through clinical assessment, whether the pain is based in joint, tendon, ligament, bursa, or nonarticular tissues.

*Is there evidence of a joint abnormality?* Tenderness, bony enlargement, intra-articular fluid, thickening of joint tissues (capsule and synovium), loss of joint motion, and joint instability are all signs of an abnormal joint.

*Is inflammation present?* The cardinal signs of inflammation are pain, warmth, swelling, erythema, and loss of function. The presence of all of these is most likely in gout or septic arthritis, but even without erythema or warmth, inflammation is still possible. Many persons with rheumatoid arthritis may have joint thickening and tenderness without significant warmth or erythema.

*Is the inflammatory arthritis monoarticular, oligoarticular, or polyarticular?* Monoarticular indicates that a *single* joint is affected; oligoarticular indicates that *several* (4 or fewer) joints are affected; and polyarticular indicates involvement of 5 or more joints (Table 259.1). Descriptions of specific syndromes follow; a glossary of definitions is provided in Table 259.2.

### Monoarthritis and Oligoarthritis

A **monoarthritis** in which the joint examination and synovial fluid show little or no signs of inflammation should suggest osteoarthritis, internal derangement of the knee (e.g., meniscal tear), or a traumatic arthritis.

In **inflammatory monoarthritis** (warm, red, swollen, painful *single* joint), the two primary considerations are **septic arthritis** and **crystal-induced synovitis.** Any inflammatory monoarthritis should be considered septic (i.e., infectious arthritis) until proven otherwise. The patient's age or immune status may suggest a responsible organism (e.g., gonococci in a young, sexually active patient, or gram-negative rods in a nursing home resident with an indwelling catheter). Crystal-induced synovitises include gout and pseudogout.

**Synovianalysis** is critical to the initial evaluation and management of a monoarthritis. If only a single drop of fluid is obtained, it should be cultured and examined for crystals; any remaining fluid should be sent for Gram stain and full synovianalysis. If crystals are found, therapy with a nonsteroidal anti-inflammatory drug (NSAID) or colchicine should be initiated unless contraindicated. With suspected infection, antibiotics should be started and the clinical response monitored for the first 24 to 72 hours; anti-inflammatory or antipyretic drugs should be avoided. Lack of a response requires reevaluation of the suspected diagnosis.

If, after 72 hours, a crystal arthritis has been ruled out and cultures (including blood and genital cultures for gonococci) are negative, therapy with an NSAID or, possibly, an intra-articular corticosteroid injection may be started. When the monoarthritis is proven nonbacterial and there has been no diagnosis or response to treatment for more than 2 months, alternative diagnoses should be considered, such as **spondyloarthropathies** (see Table 259.2), atypical presentations of polyarthritis, osteone-

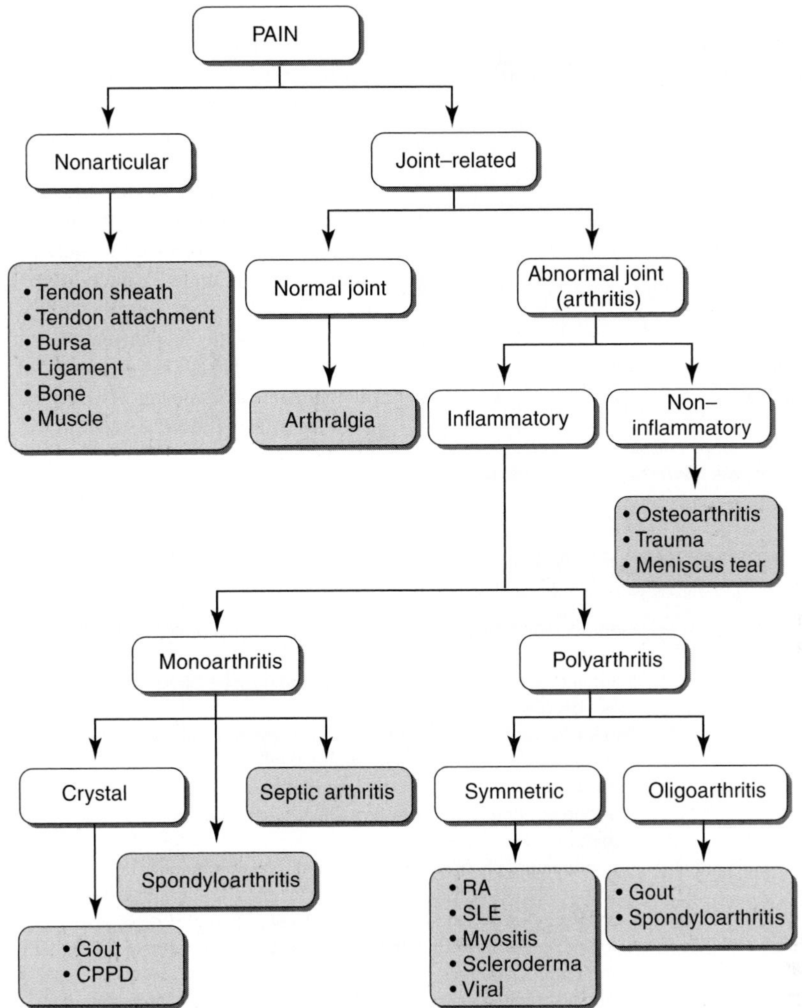


**FIGURE 259.1. Classification and diagnostic algorithm of rheumatic diseases. CPPD = calcium pyrophosphate dihydrate crystal deposition disease; RA = rheumatoid arthritis; SLE = systemic lupus erythematosus.** (Adapted from Lawrence M. Ryan, MD, Medical College of Wisconsin, Milwaukee, Wisconsin.)

crosis, articular neoplasm, or mycobacterial or fungal arthritis. A **synovial biopsy** may be helpful, particularly if cultures for these organisms are negative.

**Oligoarthritis** involves four or fewer joints, but may present initially as a monoarthritis. One or several joints, usually in the lower extremity, may be involved in spondyloarthropathies (e.g., Reiter's syndrome or psoriatic arthritis); skin and nail lesions may be a clue. Polyarticular gout usually follows gout that has been monoarticular. Systemic lupus erythematosus or rheumatoid arthritis may present atypically in up to 20% of patients with mono- or oligoarthritis.

## Polyarthritis

The etiology of **inflammatory polyarthritis** is broader (Figure 259.2). The presence or absence of inflammation and the pattern of joint involvement are useful clues. For instance, the metacarpophalangeal (MCP) and proximal interphalangeal (PIP) joints tend to be involved in a symmetric pattern in rheumatoid arthritis or systemic lupus erythematosus, whereas the weight-bearing joints, proximal interphalangeal (PIP), distal interphalangeal (DIP), and first carpometacarpal joints are affected, but not inflamed, in osteoarthritis. Associated clinical features, synovianalysis, and serum tests

**TABLE 259.1. Differential Diagnosis of Mono- and Oligoarticular Arthritis**

**Non-inflammatory**
- Trauma
- Osteoarthritis
- Meniscus/ligament tear

**Inflammatory**
- Gout
- Pseudogout
- Septic joint
- Spondyloarthritis
  - Reactive arthritis
    - Reiter's syndrome
  - Psoriatic arthritis
- Rheumatoid arthritis, lupus (unusual)

often are helpful in diagnosis. Sometimes the initial diagnosis is presumptive only until the evolving course verifies or alters the original diagnosis.

**Inflammatory spondyloarthropathies** include ankylosing spondylitis, reactive arthritis such as Reiter's syndrome, and spondylitis, seen in inflammatory bowel disease and psoriasis. Reiter's disease is more likely to involve the large joints of the lower extremities. Both Reiter's and psoriatic arthritis may present with one or more "sausage digits" **(dactylitis).** Psoriatic arthritis may present as oligoarthritis (70%) or as symmetric polyarthritis with a distribution similar to that of rheumatoid arthritis (15%); the remainder present with predominant involvement of DIP joints and nail lesions (5%), as arthritis mutilans (osteolysis of the phalanges and metacarpal joints, 5%), or as ankylosing spondylitis

**TABLE 259.2. A Glossary of Rheumatic Disorders**

| | |
|---|---|
| Osteoarthritis | Arthritis featuring cartilage degeneration in weight bearing joints and small joints of the hands |
| Gout | Inflammatory arthritis, usually mono- but may be oligo- or polyarticular, mediated by monosodium urate crystals |
| Pseudogout | Similar to gout but mediated by calcium pyrophosphate crystals |
| Spondyloarthropathy | A group of diseases with frequent back inflammation, peripheral joint arthritis, common extra-articular features, and increased frequency of HLA-B27 |
| Ankylosing spondylitis | A spondyloarthropathy with prominent back pain, stiffness, and progressive fusion of spinal joints |
| Reactive arthritis | A spondyloarthropathy associated with infection by enteric pathogens |
| Reiter's syndrome | A form of reactive arthritis, usually associated with genitourinary infection, and characterized by lower extremity arthritis, uveitis, skin and mucous membrane lesions |
| Rheumatoid arthritis | Inflammatory arthritis in which the synovial lining becomes thickened and causes damage to joints |
| Systemic lupus erythematosus | Multisystem inflammatory disorder mediated by autoantibodies |

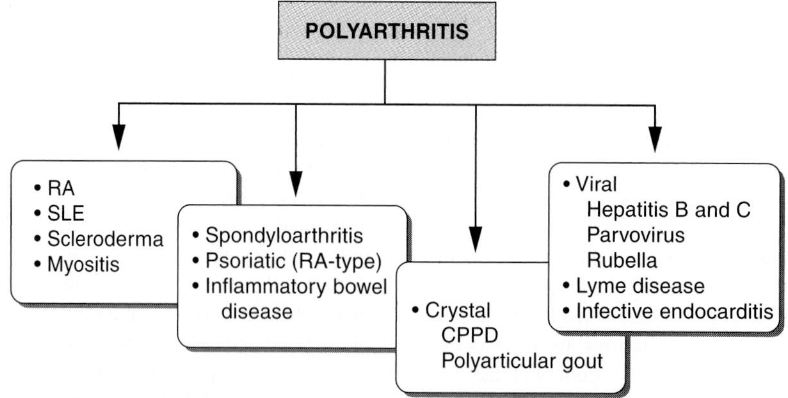


**FIGURE 259.2.** Possible causes of polyarthritis. CPPD = calcium pyrophosphate dihydrate crystal deposition disease; RA = rheumatoid arthritis; SLE = systemic lupus erythematosus.

(5%). Inflammatory bowel disease also may present or be associated with an inflammatory peripheral oligoarthritis, primarily in the lower extremities.

**Infectious arthritis** occasionally presents as acute polyarthritis. Lyme disease and viral infections (e.g., polyarthritis of rubella, either primary infection or vaccine-related; pre-icteric phase of hepatitis B and hepatitis C; and human parvovirus B19) are examples. Gonococcal arthritis, acute rheumatic fever, and bacterial endocarditis may be associated with a migratory polyarthritis (arthritis which moves from joint to joint).

## Muscle Weakness or Pain

To assess a patient's complaint of muscle weakness, it is necessary to grade muscle strength with a scale, albeit such scales are necessarily arbitrary. Early in their course, primary myopathies present almost entirely as **proximal weakness.** Altered functional capacity may be a clue: difficulty in combing hair suggests a proximal upper extremity myopathy, and trouble climbing stairs or getting out of a chair or tub suggests proximal lower extremity myopathy. Muscle pain may or may not accompany weakness.

A variety of conditions must be considered in a patient with true muscle weakness (Table 259.3). Polymyositis, dermatomyositis, and inclusion body myositis are the predominant rheumatic diseases that present with proximal weakness (Table 259.4). Although patients with polymyalgia rheumatica may report weakness because of trouble getting out of bed, this difficulty is due to pain and stiffness, mostly in the neck, shoulder, and pelvic girdle, rather than to true weakness.

The physician also must consider **neurologic causes** of muscle pain and weakness. Upper or lower motor neuron diseases, nerve root disease, or peripheral nerve disease usually displays altered reflexes and sensation. Myoneural junction disease may be confused with a primary myopathy, because muscle weakness in these disorders may be proximal. Myasthenia gravis is associated with muscle weakness that increases with exertion and decreases with rest. Eaton-Lambert syndrome is readily differentiated from myasthenia gravis by electromyography.

Drugs (e.g., corticosteroids, potassium-depleting agents such as diuretics or cathartics), toxins (e.g., alcohol), and rhabdomyolysis (e.g., from heroin or cocaine use, exertion, or crush injury) may cause muscle weakness or pain. Although any endocrinopathy (hyper- or hypofunction) may cause a proximal myopathy, the most common is hypothyroidism.

The **muscular dystrophies** are a group of primary muscle diseases with onset usually before the third decade; however, both limb-girdle and myotonic dystrophy present in early adult life. In limb-girdle dystrophy, shoulder or pelvic girdle muscles are involved initially, and serum muscle enzymes are slightly increased. In myotonic dystrophy, weakness is distal and serum muscle enzymes usually are normal. Diagnosis of these dystrophies and the rare congenital myopathies rests on associated symptoms and signs, family history, and

**TABLE 259.3. Differential Diagnosis of Weakness**

- Inflammatory myositis
  - Polymyositis
  - Dermatomyositis
  - Inclusion body myositis
- Drugs
  - Alcohol
  - Corticosteroids
  - Cocaine
- Endocrinopathies
  - Glucocorticoid excess
  - Glucocorticoid deficiency
  - Hyperthyroidism
  - Hypothyroidism
- Electrolyte abnormalities
  - Hypokalemia
- Neurologic disorders
  - Upper motor neuron (e.g., amyotrophic lateral sclerosis)
  - Lower motor neuron (e.g., Guillain-Barré syndrome)
  - Myasthenia gravis, Eaton-Lambert syndrome
- Muscular dystrophy
- Congenital myopathies
  - Glycogen storage disease, others
- Viral infection

**TABLE 259.4. Myositis: A Glossary**

| | |
|---|---|
| Polymyositis | Inflammation of muscle resulting in progressive muscle weakness and muscle enzyme elevation |
| Dermatomyositis | Similar to polymyositis with characteristic facial (heliotrope) rash and rash on knuckles (Gottron's sign) |
| Inclusion body myositis | Similar to polymyositis but more insidious in onset; biopsy shows inclusion bodies in muscle fibers by light and electron microscopy |

TABLE 259.5. Medications Used in the Treatment of Musculoskeletal Diseases

| Class | Examples |
|---|---|
| Non-steroidal anti-inflammatory drugs | Indomethacin, ibuprofen, naproxen |
| Analgesics | Acetaminophen, tramadol, narcotics |
| Corticosteroids | |
| Oral | Prednisone, methylprednisolone |
| Injectable | Methylprednisolone acetate, triamcinolone hexacetonide |
| Anti-malarial | Hydroxychloroquine |
| Gold | |
| Oral | Auranofin |
| Injectable | Aurothioglucose (IM), etanercept, infliximab, anakinra |
| Biologics | |
| Immunomodulators | Azathioprine, methotrexate, cyclophosphamide |
| Tricyclic antidepressants | Amitriptyline |

muscle biopsy (including special stains for carbohydrates and lipids). Less common causes of myopathy include disorders of glycogen, purine, and lipid metabolism and infectious myositis.

## General Principles of Therapy

The principles of management of rheumatic diseases are similar to those employed in other illnesses. They differ, however, in that response often is measured over weeks or months instead of days and is based more often on clinical response than on changes in laboratory measurements. Response time, quantification of response, and the decision whether to continue the current regimen as a more advanced drug is started all need assessment.

Rheumatic diseases are predominantly chronic, outpatient problems, with only a minority requiring hospitalization. Conditions requiring hospitalization include septic arthritis or bacteremia, visceral involvement (e.g., pericardial tamponade, neural vasculitis, or nephritis), or severe inflammation that renders the patient unable to care for oneself.

A variety of medications are employed in the treatment of musculoskeletal diseases (Table 259.5). Patients with joint inflammation commonly receive initial treatment with nonsteroidal anti-inflammatory drugs (NSAIDs) or aspirin, unless the patient has a suspected septic joint because NSAIDs may mask fever. In such instances, it is preferable to use analgesics such as codeine or propoxyphene until the diagnosis is clearer. Some cases of osteoarthritis may require only analgesics. Control of rheumatoid arthritis often requires additional medications (e.g., hydroxychloroquine, immunomodulating agents, anticytokines). Acute gout is treated with NSAIDs or colchicine. Recurrent attacks of gout are prevented by probenecid or allopurinol. Patients with arthritis may require several medications to control their disease, but polypharmacy does expose patients, particularly the elderly, to increased risks of drug side effects, greater likelihood of drug interactions, and also high costs from multiple medications.

### Aspirin and Other Nonsteroidal Anti-inflammatory Drugs

A wide variety of NSAIDs and aspirin, in dosages designed to attain a serum salicylate level of 20–25 mg/dl, provide a certain degree of anti-inflammatory effect. Traditional NSAIDs are safer than aspirin, although gastrointestinal bleeding remains a serious, potentially lethal complication. NSAIDs that are selective for the enzyme cyclooxygenase (COX-2), mostly induced at sites of inflammation, have reduced the risk of ulcer formation as compared to traditional NSAIDs, which block both COX-1 (normally present in gastric lining and platelets) and COX-2. COX-2—selective NSAIDs do not inhibit platelet aggregation. All NSAIDs, including COX-2—selective NSAIDs, may impair renal function in patients with underlying renal disease. The indole-pyrrole derivatives (e.g., indomethacin, sulindac, tolmetin) are more effective in acute gout and most spondyloarthropathies. Long-acting preparations requiring only once- or twice-daily dosing offer the advantage of better patient compliance; however, compounds that have a longer duration of action typically take longer to achieve steady-state therapeutic levels.

### Physical and Occupational Therapy

In musculoskeletal diseases, the goals of physical and occupational therapy are to reduce pain, maintain proper joint alignment and function, preserve range of motion, maintain muscle strength, minimize joint trauma, and maximize the ability to carry out activities of daily living. In general, extremely inflamed joints (such as those in septic arthritis) should be rested, preferably in the anatomic position, often using resting splints. As inflammation abates, gentle, assisted range-of-motion exercises may be started to help prevent loss of motion. At a later stage, muscle-strengthening exercises may be begun, initially as isometric exercises to minimize joint trauma. Later, when the inflammation has been suppressed sufficiently, active resistive muscle strengthening may be started. Stiff joints and painful muscles may respond to heat (hydrocollator packs), massage, or ultrasound treatments. Neck or back pain may respond to cervical or lumbar traction, respectively.

A complete discussion of the surgical management of arthritis is beyond the scope of this discussion. Severe arthritic damage of hips and knees usually is managed with total joint arthroplasty. Total joint arthroplasty is available but less commonly employed for other joints because of less favorable outcomes. Arthroscopic surgical procedures increasingly are being used for soft tissue repairs in the knee, shoulder, and ankle.

# CHAPTER 260 CRYSTAL-INDUCED SYNOVITIS

Crystals associated with synovial inflammation include monosodium urate, calcium pyrophosphate dihydrate (CPPD), and, less often, hydroxyapatite, oxalate, and adrenocorticosteroid esters. The cholesterol crystals that occasionally are found in chronic joint effusions probably are inert.

The pathophysiology of crystal-induced synovitis is incompletely understood. Although crystals certainly are causative in acute gout and pseudogout, crystals occasionally may be seen in quiescent joints as well. The precise inciting event in vivo is unknown but may involve crystal shedding from preformed cartilaginous or synovial deposits. Crystal phagocytosis by neutrophils in vitro induces release of lysosomal enzymes, humoral mediators, and chemotactic factors associated with acute inflammation.

Monosodium urate and CPPD crystals commonly cause acute synovitis and, and in some cases, chronic joint damage. Acute crystal-induced arthritis is rapid in onset and self-limited. Differences in crystal morphology and clinical features are helpful in diagnosis.

## Gout

Gout is a metabolic disease in which hyperuricemia and arthritis are variably expressed. Three possible stages exist: acute gouty arthritis, intercritical gout, and tophaceous gout. Urolithiasis (renal calculi) or other renal disease may also be associated with hyperuricemia.

### *Hyperuricemia*

Hyperuricemia, a biochemical abnormality defined solely by the serum urate concentration, results from increased production of urate, decreased excretion, or both (Table 260.1). Decreased renal clearance is responsible for most cases of hyperuricemia. By the uricase method, the upper limit of normal for serum urate is 7.0 mg/dl in men and 6.0 mg/dl in premenopausal women. Plasma is saturated with urate at 6.4–6.8 mg/dl at 37°C. Most clinical laboratories, however, use a colorimetric method and may report higher normal levels than the uricase method.

Normal urinary uric acid excretion is <600 mg/24 hr on a purine-free diet and <800 mg/24 hr on a regular diet. Approximately 150 mg of urate is secreted into the normal intestinal tract every 24 hours, but this rate is increased in hyperuricemia.

### *Acute Gout*

Acute gout features acute inflammatory arthritis, which usually is **monoarticular** and most often involves **lower extremity joints.** Acute gout may be triggered by trauma, alcohol ingestion, acute medical illness, surgical procedures, and certain drugs (see Table 260.1). Not all factors

**TABLE 260.1. Conditions Associated With Hyperuricemia**

| Urate Overproduction | Urate Renal Underexcretion |
|---|---|
| Idiopathic (primary) gout | Idiopathic (primary) gout |
| Inherited enzymatic defects | Clinical disorders |
| Polycythemia vera | Hypertension |
| (Paget's) | Dehydration |
| Hemolytic diseases | Obesity |
| Psoriasis | Sarcoidosis |
| Obesity | Renal insufficiency |
| Myelo- and lymphoproliferative diseases | Lead toxicity |
| Drugs | Starvation |
| Cytotoxic agents | Acidosis |
| High-dose salicylates | Toxemia of pregnancy |
| Ethanol | Salt restriction |
| Warfarin | Drugs |
| | Ethanol |
| | Diuretics |
| | Low-dose salicylates |
| | Cyclosporine |
| | Levodopa |

responsible for the precipitation of urate crystals are known, however, because hyperuricemia does occur without urolithiasis or gout. Gout occurs primarily in men, with onset usually in the 4th through 6th decades; in women, it is more likely to follow menopause.

An acute gouty attack is very painful. In 60% of cases, the first attack involves the first metatarsophalangeal (MTP) joint **(podagra)** or other joints in the foot. Acute gout also may occur in the ankle, the prepatellar or olecranon bursae, and midfoot, in which location it may resemble cellulitis (gouty cellulitis). Within a few hours, the affected joint becomes red, swollen, warm, and tender, but usually the attack resolves on its own within a few days to a few weeks without leaving apparent sequelae. Fever may be present. In a minority, the initial episode may be polyarticular. **Tophi** (discussed later in this chapter) usually follow years of gout; they are rare in conjunction with the first attack.

Although hyperuricemia is characteristic of gout, normal serum urate values may be seen during the acute attack. Synovial effusions in acute gout typically are inflammatory (5,000–50,000 leukocytes/$mm^3$, mostly neutrophils). Characteristic **needle-shaped, strongly negatively birefringent** crystals of monosodium urate crystals are seen either intra- or extracellularly on synovial fluid examination with a compensated polarizing microscope (see Color Plate 32).

## Intercritical Gout and Polyarticular Gout

As the acute gouty attack subsides, the patient becomes asymptomatic ***(intercritical gout).*** In most patients a second attack occurs within 6 months to 2 years. Ensuing attacks may become polyarticular and may last longer, yielding a different clinical picture from early gout. In this later phase, gout is suggested by prior hyperuricemia, history of gout, tophi, and acute arthritis, with clinical response to **colchicine;** but definitive diagnosis requires identification of monosodium urate crystals from a tophus or even from an asymptomatic (e.g., seemingly unaffected first MTP) joint.

## Chronic Tophaceous Gout

If recurrent gout is untreated, tophi can develop on the extensor surfaces of the elbows, in joints, and in surrounding tissues, especially the interphalangeal joints of the hands or feet and the helix of the ear. **Tophi** usually are firm, and, when aspirated, yield a chalky white material containing monosodium urate crystals.

***Chronic tophaceous gout*** may mimic rheumatoid arthritis, with arthralgias, progressive stiffness, nodules, joint swelling, and deformity (Figure 260.1), and even a high erythrocyte sedimentation rate and positive rheumatoid factor. Acute attacks manifest only soft tissue swelling on radiographs, but chronic gout manifests punched-out erosions at the ends of phalanges, most commonly at the medial aspects of the head of the first MTP joint. These are highly typical of tophaceous gout. Tophi may be detected first on radiographs, before they are clinically recognized.

## Renal Disease Associated With Hyperuricemia

Hyperuricemia is associated with several renal diseases: renal stones (see Chapter 171), urate nephropathy, and uric acid nephropathy. **Uric acid renal stones** occur in 10% to 25% of patients with gout but actually occur more often without gout or hyperuricemia. **Urate nephropathy** results from deposition of sodium urate crystals in the renal tubular epithelium and adjacent interstitium. It is rare in the absence of gout and is a late event in the natural history of gout, with very high serum urate levels. Aging and coexistent diseases, especially hypertension (rather than hyperuricemia), correlate with decreased renal function. The risk of renal failure from hyperuricemia alone is low. **Uric acid nephropathy** is a rare, reversible form of acute renal failure due to uric acid crystal precipitation in collecting ducts and ureters. It most often occurs in patients with leukemia or lymphoma who are receiving chemotherapy (tumor lysis syndrome).

### Management

**Symptomatic hyperuricemia**

NSAIDs or colchicine is the usual first line of treatment for acute gout. Oral **colchicine** is given in doses of 0.5–0.6 mg every 1–2 hours until either gout improves, gastrointestinal side effects (nausea, vomiting, or diarrhea) occur, or a total of 3.0–4.0 mg has been given. Intravenous colchicine, 1-2 mg, one or two doses, avoids gastrointestinal side effects. Colchicine should be used in lesser doses or not at all in elderly persons or patients with impaired renal function because of the increased risks of bone marrow suppression. A clinical response is not specific for gout because other crystal arthropathies, such as acute pseudogout or calcific tendinitis, also may respond.

**Indomethacin,** up to 200 mg/day in divided doses, usually for 4–5 days, is effective and more convenient than colchicine, but the maximal dosage often produces central nervous system and gastrointestinal side effects. Other NSAIDs may be similarly effective but have been used less commonly in acute gout. In the unusual instances when oral therapy is not possible, alternatives include local intra-articular corticosteroid injection, intravenous (IV) methylprednisolone (20–50 mg/day),

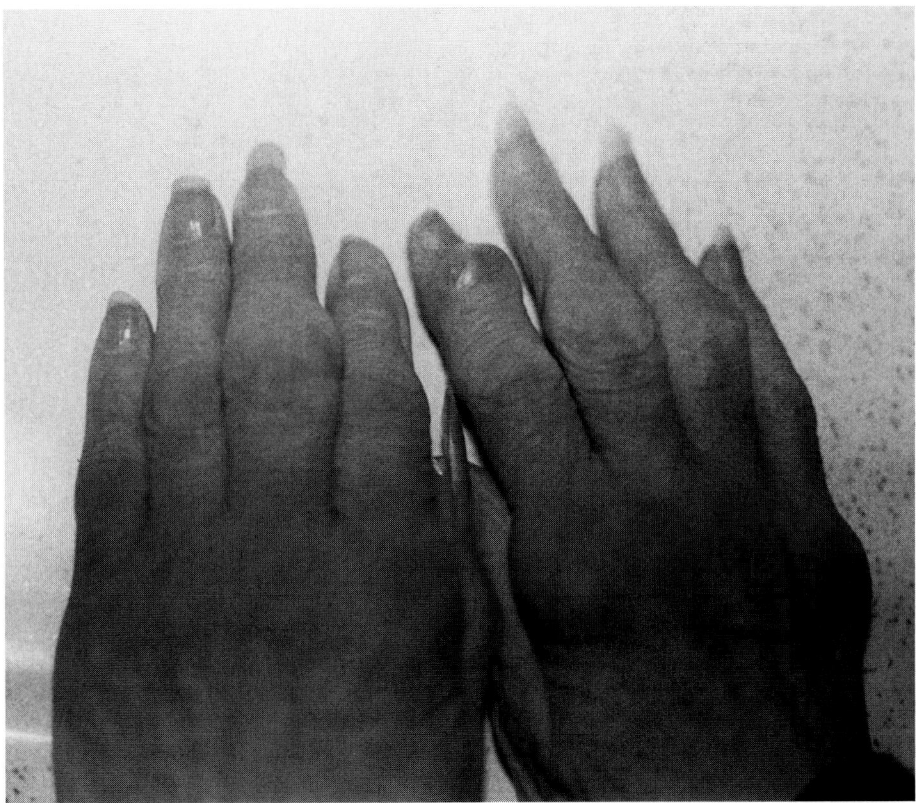

**FIGURE 260.1.** Hands of an elderly woman with chronic tophaceous gout. Some of the tophi appear to have formed in joints with previous osteoarthritic changes.

adrenocorticotropic hormone (40–80 U/day), or IV colchicine.

Small doses of colchicine (0.6 mg once or twice daily) or another NSAID may be prescribed as **prophylaxis** against recurrent attacks, but this prophylaxis does not prevent crystal deposition and possible joint destruction. Instead, after acute gout resolves, chronic hypouricemic therapy is begun using **probenecid** or **allopurinol.** Such therapy is indicated in patients with frequent recurrent attacks, tophi (clinically or radiographically manifest), or nephrolithiasis. A dosage that achieves a serum urate concentration below 6.4 mg/dl prevents further monosodium urate crystal deposition (although some patients may require even further lowering of the serum urate). Noncompliance is the usual reason for ineffective control of hyperuricemia.

Decreased uric acid excretion accounts for hyperuricemia in at least 90% of cases. A 24-hour urinary uric acid estimation should differentiate the overproducer from the underexcretor. The uricosuric drug **probenecid** may be used if the daily uric acid excretion is <800 mg/24 hr on a regular diet or when allergy to allopurinol is present; it is contraindicated with creatinine clearance below 60 ml/min or nephrolithiasis. **Allopurinol** and its metabolite **oxypurinol** inhibit xanthine oxidase to decrease uric acid synthesis. It is used in patients who excrete in excess of 800 mg uric acid per 24 hours on a regular diet and in those with severe tophaceous gout, chronic renal insufficiency, or allergy to uricosurics. Probenecid should be avoided in the overproducer because of the risk of nephrolithiasis. Allopurinol also may be used in underexcretors because of its ease of administration (once-daily dosing).

Toxic reactions to allopurinol occur in about 5% of patients, usually manifesting as skin rashes or gastrointestinal complaints; serious side effects such as vasculitis, granulomatous hepatitis, or agranulocytosis are rare. The dose should be reduced in patients with chronic renal failure or on azathioprine therapy.

### Asymptomatic hyperuricemia

Asymptomatic hyperuricemia need not be treated, because the incidence of gout is low and the first attack is easily managed. The only exception is the patient with very high levels of serum urate (>10.5 mg/dl), which may cause **urate nephropathy.** Patients with uric acid nephrolithiasis should increase their fluid intake to increase urine volume, maintain alkaline urine to decrease urate precipitation, and reduce total uric acid excretion, usually by using allopurinol.

## *Calcium Pyrophosphate Dihydrate Crystal Deposition Disease*

Calcium pyrophosphate dihydrate (CPPD) crystal deposition in hyaline cartilage and fibrocartilage is associated with several different patterns of arthritis. The incidence of CPPD deposition increases with age (5% at age 70; >40% at age 90). In most cases CPPD crystal deposition is idiopathic, but it may occur in hyperparathyroidism, hemochromatosis, hypomagnesemia, hypophosphatasia, and hypothyroidism. Younger patients should be screened for these disorders. Diagnosis is based on the demonstration of characteristic **positive, birefringent rhomboid or rod-like crystals** by compensated polarized light microscopy in synovial fluid (see Color Plate 32).

### Clinical and Laboratory Features

The most common form of CPPD deposition probably is asymptomatic radiographic **chondrocalcinosis,** consisting of punctate and linear radiodensities in cartilage (Figure 260.2) with minimal or no joint symptoms. Nearly 25% of patients have ***pseudogout,*** which mimics gout with self-limited, often monoarticular attacks that may last from 1 day to 4 weeks without treatment. Severe medical illness, surgical procedures, and trauma may precipitate attacks, although the mechanism of release of crystals from cartilaginous deposits remains elusive. Pseudogout more commonly involves large joints, especially the knees and wrists, and may coexist with gout (5%) and hyperuricemia (20%).

Synovial fluid during the acute attack typically is inflammatory (4,000–20,000 leukocytes/mm$^3$, with mostly neutrophils). The leukocytes show ingested CPPD crystals during acute attacks (see Color Plate 32). The crystals also may persist in joint fluid even after the attack has resolved. Radiographs in most cases show chondrocalcinosis.

Nearly 50% of patients present with a picture simulating **osteoarthritis,** most commonly in the knees, followed by the wrist, metacarpophalangeal (MCP) joints, hip, spine, shoulder, elbow, and ankle. Within this subgroup, one-half have a history of episodic acute attacks. In patients with "osteoarthritis" affecting joints not usually involved in osteoarthritis, radiographs of the knees, hands, wrists and pelvis are useful to detect CPPD deposition.

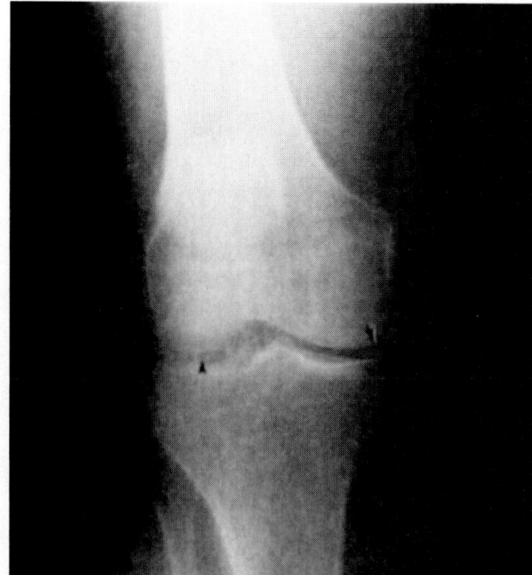

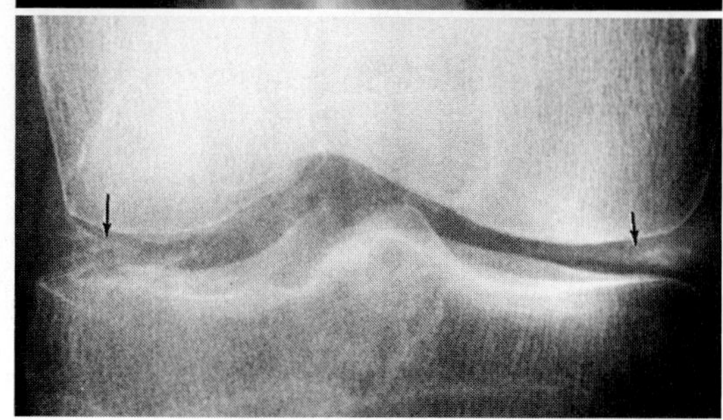

**FIGURE 260.2. Radiograph of a knee and a magnified view of the joint space (*inset*) showing chondrocalcinosis in the hyaline articular cartilage and meniscus fibrocartilage (*arrows*), suggesting calcium pyrophosphate crystal deposition.**

Another 5% of patients present with polyarthritis resembling rheumatoid arthritis. In almost 10% of this subset, the rheumatoid factor is positive in low titers. The inflamed joints tend to be more asymmetric than those in rheumatoid arthritis and, radiographically, have CPPD deposition and osteophytes without erosive disease typical of RA.

### Management

Treatment may be with **colchicine** (IV or oral), NSAIDs, joint aspiration alone, or intra-articular corticosteroid injection (similar to that of symptomatic hyperuricemia).

## *Hydroxyapatite-Associated Synovitis*

Hydroxyapatite (HA) crystals refer to a group of crystals called basic calcium phosphates and include hydroxyapatite, octacalcium phosphate, and tricalcium phosphate. (For simplicity, they are referred to as HA in this chapter.) These crystals have been detected by electron microscopy in **acute calcific periarthritis** (most commonly of the shoulder), **tendinitis,** and **bursitis.** More recently, HA crystals have been found in synovial fluids of patients with several forms of arthritis, including osteoarthritis.

In one form of HA-induced disease, the **Milwaukee shoulder/knee syndrome,** elderly patients, usually women, present with shoulder joint pain and stiffness, decreased motion, and, often, a large effusion. Bilateral disease often is noted clinically. One-half also have knee instability and pain with ambulation, but other joints may be affected, although this is uncommon. Radiographs show severe glenohumeral joint degeneration with small osteophytes and bony destruction of the humeral head. Soft tissue calcifications occur in 40% of patients. Rotator cuff lysis is evident by upward subluxation of the humeral head or by arthrogram or MRI.

Synovial fluids from affected joints have low leukocyte counts (<1000/mm$^3$, usually mononuclear). HA crystals are not birefringent and thus, usually are not detectable by polarized light microscopy; scanning or transmission electron microscopy or x-ray diffraction are required for crystal identification. In some synovial fluids, both HA and CPPD coexist. **Treatment** is unsatisfactory but includes NSAIDs, reduced shoulder use, and joint aspiration.

### *Steroid Crystal-Induced Synovitis*

In about 2% of patients receiving intra-articular crystalline corticosteroid injections, a brief (1–3 days) acute synovitis occurs several hours afterward. Its early occurrence after injection helps distinguish it from the extremely rare infection caused by the injection itself. On compensated polarized light microscopy, the crystals appear as positive and negative birefringent chunks, rods, or globular material.

# CHAPTER 261 OSTEOARTHRITIS

Osteoarthritis (OA), which affects approximately 12% of the population, is the commonest form of arthritis. The prevalence of OA rises with age, and most people exhibit some roentgenographic evidence of OA after age 60. Its etiology is unknown. Osteoarthritis may best be viewed as the final common pathway for many pathologic articular processes (Table 261.1).

Osteoarthritis that occurs in patients without known predisposing factors is termed **primary OA.** These usually are women with a history of similar disease in female kindreds, suggesting possible genetic or hormonal factors. Recent reports of inherited biochemical defects in type II collagen account for some families with premature OA.

**TABLE 261.1. Conditions Predisposing to Osteoarthritis**

| |
|---|
| Mechanical trauma |
| Weight-bearing joints in obese persons |
| Prior joint trauma |
| Excessive joint use (occupational) |
| Previous inflammatory arthritis |
| Congenital joint dysplasias |
| Avascular necrosis of bone |
| Metabolic diseases affecting cartilage |
| Hemochromatosis |
| Ochronosis |
| Calcium pyrophosphate crystal deposition |
| Neurologic disorders |
| Diminished pain perception |

## Pathogenesis

In the earliest stage of OA, chondrocytes, activated by unknown means, begin remodeling cartilage. Synthesis of proteoglycans is increased but so also is secretion of proteases which disrupt the cartilage matrix.

Osteoarthritis occurs in cartilage that has lost a significant portion of its glycosaminoglycan content. The surface cartilage initially shows microscopic fibrillation; deep fissuring follows, as shear forces disrupt the cartilage. Chondrocytes replicate within lacunae but eventually die. Underlying bone becomes sclerotic, and new bone growth occurs as a ridge around the margin of the joint **(osteophytes).** Ultimately, the cartilage fragments and disappears completely, leaving a bare surface of eburnated bone. Unlike rheumatoid arthritis, in which the cartilage thins diffusely as a result of more uniform damage, cartilage loss in the OA joint tends to be more asymmetric and confined to the area of greatest mechanical stress. Histologic examination of synovial tissues shows patchy hyperplasia.

## Clinical Features

Osteoarthritis most commonly manifests with pain, usually made worse by activity and relieved by rest. Morning stiffness, if present, usually is short (<30 min). **Gelling** is stiffness that occurs after 1 or more hours of rest and is relieved by stretching and resumption of activity. Primary OA most often involves the proximal (PIP) and distal (DIP) interphalangeal and first carpometacarpal (CMC) joints of the hand, the hips, the knees, first metatarsal joints, and apophyseal joints of the spine. It is useful to remember that knee pain can be referred from the hip and vice versa.

Patients may report periods of increased pain, sometimes with swelling, which leave bony enlargement in their wake. A few patients may have more persistent inflammation with synovial thickening and increased pain in one or a few of the small hand joints ("erosive osteoarthritis"). Some elderly women with underlying renal disease who are receiving thiazides may have gouty, tophaceous deposits with inflammation in osteoarthritic hand joints.

On examination, the involved joints exhibit variable pain and tenderness. Surprisingly, pain often is minimal, despite markedly abnormal finger joints. Enlargement in OA joints reflects underlying joint soft tissue thickening, effusion, or formation of osteophytes. Osteophyte formation of the DIP and PIP joints of the hands are called Heberden's and Bouchard's nodes, respectively. Wearing away of cartilage on one side of the joint leads to bony crepitus and malalignment (Table 261.2). Together, the bony enlargement and malalignment cause loss of motion (Figure 261.1).

Osteoarthritis of the spine occurs as the nucleus pulposus begins to liquefy in young adulthood, and the annulus fibrosus begins to desiccate and split. Disc collapse and extrusion follow, causing instability of the posterior (facet) joints, which later develop OA. The resultant vertebral and facet osteophytes and disc space narrowing can impinge on nerve roots and cause radiculopathy or spinal stenosis (see Chapter 259).

**TABLE 261.2. Common Deformities in Osteoarthritis**

| Joint | Deformity |
|---|---|
| Distal interphalangeal | Heberden's node |
| Proximal interphalangeal | Bouchard's node |
| First carpometacarpal | Squaring (shelf sign) |
| First metatarsophalangeal | Hallux valgus (bunion) |
| Knee, medial femorotibial compartment | Genu varus (bow legs) |
| Knee, lateral femorotibial compartment | Genu valgus (knock knees) |

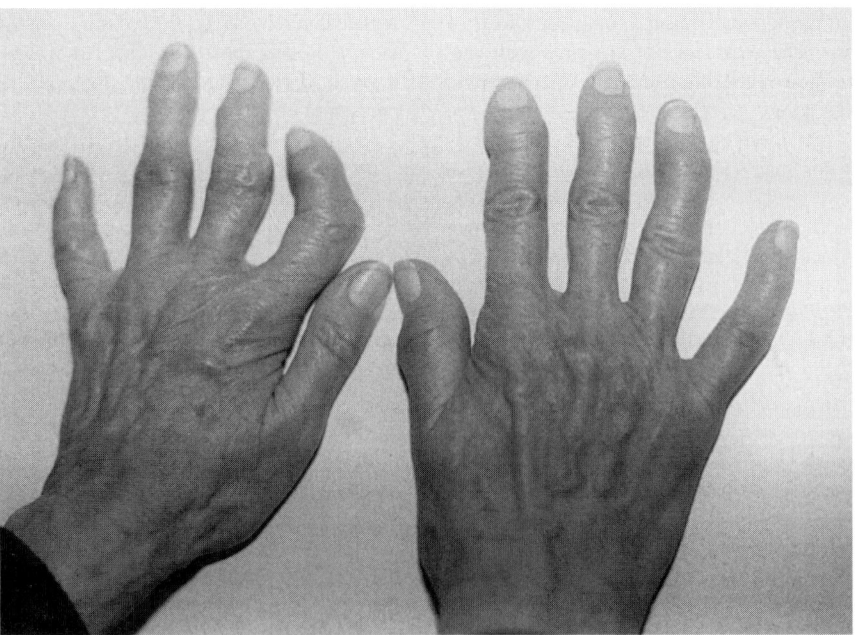

**FIGURE 261.1.** Hands of an elderly woman with osteoarthritis showing osteophytic enlargement of the proximal interphalangeal joint (Bouchard nodes) and distal interphalangeal joints (Heberden nodes), as well as angulation deformity in some joints.

### Ancillary Studies

Routine laboratory studies are normal in otherwise uncomplicated OA. Synovianalysis can help exclude crystal-induced and other inflammatory diseases. Joint fluid in OA has less than 1500 leukocytes/mm$^3$, predominantly mononuclear. Radiographs eventually show regional (asymmetric) thinning of the joint space, osteophytes, subchondral sclerosis, and cyst formation; however, symptoms correlate only weakly with radiographic severity (Figure 261.2). Such findings are very common in elderly persons and may conincidentally be present along with other forms of arthritis.

### Management

Therapy for OA is directed at relieving pain, minimizing further joint trauma, and preserving motion, alignment, and muscle strength. Treatment is started with mild analgesics (e.g., acetaminophen) and progresses to low-dose NSAIDs. In elderly patients with multiple medical problems, a COX-2–selective NSAID may be a safer alternative to the traditional NSAIDs, which are not COX–selective, if high-dose NSAIDs are needed. In general, the response correlates inversely with the severity of joint damage. Topical therapy (e.g., capsaicin cream) is useful in some instances.

Physical and occupational therapy can provide instruction in ways to protect the joints to minimize additional joint trauma and exercises to preserve or increase range of motion and maintain muscle strength. Intra-articular corticosteroid injections may provide temporary relief. Viscosupplementation therapy involves a series of injections with either hylan gf-40 or hyaluronan. The joint with severe destructive change often can be helped only by reconstructive surgery, which may include realignment of weight-bearing to a less involved area of the joint surface (e.g., tibial osteotomy), joint arthroplasty (e.g., first carpometacarpal joint), prosthetic joint replacement (e.g., total hip or knee replacement arthroplasty), or fusion to relieve pain in some joints where motion is not crucial to function (e.g., ankle, lumbar spine).

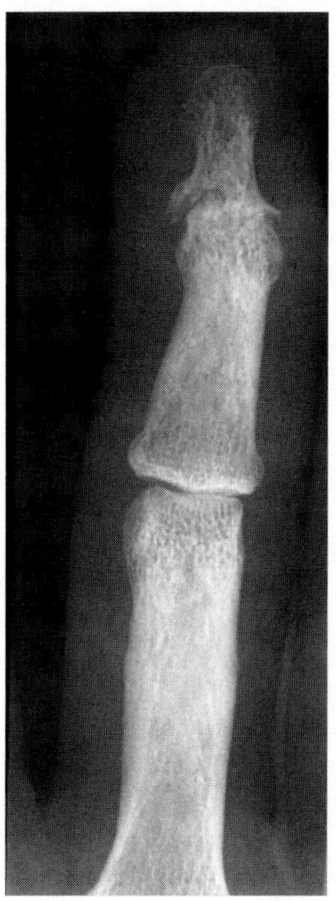

**FIGURE 261.2.** Radiograph of the third digit of a patient with osteoarthritis (erosive type) showing osteophyte formation, joint erosion, and mild sclerosis.

# CHAPTER 262 RHEUMATOID ARTHRITIS

### Etiology and Pathogenesis

Rheumatoid arthritis (RA), a systemic disorder of unknown etiology, afflicts approximately 1% of the population. Eighty percent of patients with RA are seropositive for **rheumatoid factor** (RF), which consists of autoantibodies of the IgG, IgM, or IgA classes that react with antigenic determinants on the Fc portion of IgG. In the 80% of patients with RA who have RF, the disease usually is more sustained, more systemic, and more destructive. About 70% of seropositive Caucasian patients are positive for HLA type DR4, which occurs in only 16% of the normal population and in a similar proportion of patients with seronegative RA. Patients with severely reduced functional capacities resulting from RA have shortened life expectancies.

In RA, the synovium is infiltrated with T lymphocytes, plasma cells, and macrophages, which may be attracted to the synovium by expression of **intercellular adhesion molecules (ICAM)** in synovial venules. Within the synovium, immunoglobulins (including RF) are actively synthesized. Formation of RF–IgG complexes and perhaps other immune complexes locally activate the complement, **kinin,** and other inflammatory cascades. Thus, complement levels in synovial fluid may be low.

Neutrophils predominate in RA joint fluid. As they phagocytize immune complexes, they release lysosomal enzymes locally and generate reactive oxygen species. Both these enzymes and the reactive oxygen species may cause cartilage destruction. Prostaglandins are elevated in such joint fluids. Cytokines, including interleukins 1 and 6, tumor necrosis factor, and probably other growth factors, activate synovial fibroblasts and possibly chondrocytes.

Proliferation of synovial fibroblasts causes expansion of the synovial membrane, demonstrating functional properties of a benign tumor, the so-called **pannus.** Collagenase from dendritic cells in the pannus destroys their collagen framework on contact with bone, cartilage, and ligaments. Large synovial effusions reduce synovial blood flow, causing ischemia of the joint tissues. Unchecked rheumatoid synovitis causes sustained inflammation with eventual thinning of cartilage, erosion of bone, and weakening of ligamentous structures, resulting in joint instability.

## Clinical Features

Rheumatoid arthritis has a variable natural history. Most patients experience recurrent and protracted exacerbations with gradual, cumulative, and irreversible tissue destruction. Less commonly, a single episode may be followed by lasting remission. Rare patients have progressive unremitting systemic disease, causing crippling disability and death.

The musculoskeletal system is the most commonly and the most visibly afflicted. Virtually any **diarthrodial (synovial) joint** may be involved, including the cricoarytenoid. The onset of systemic and musculoskeletal symptoms is insidious over weeks to months in most (55%–70%) patients, but more rapid (and sometimes acute) in the remainder.

**Symmetric involvement** is more common, but even if the initial presentation is asymmetric, with time, symmetry usually prevails. **Morning stiffness** may last for 1 hour or longer. Muscle atrophy may occur around involved joints, so that activities of daily living (e.g., household and self-care activities) become difficult. In some patients, there may be severe flares in one or a few joints or periarticular structures that last only a few days (palindromic rheumatism).

The joints most commonly involved are the proximal interphalangeal (PIP), metacarpophalangeal (MCP), and wrist, followed by the knee, ankle, metatarsophalangeal (MTP), shoulder, and elbow. Joint enlargement results from soft tissue swelling **(synovitis)** or synovial fluid accumulation (Figure 262.1). With time, joint deformities may occur (see Figures 262.2 and 265.1, and Table 262.1).

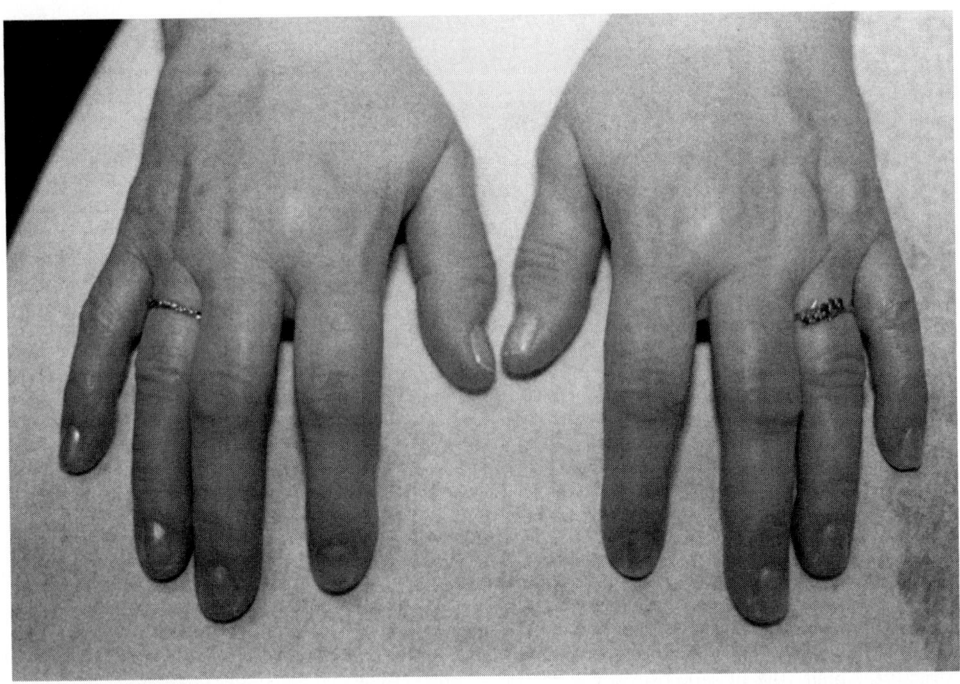

**FIGURE 262.1.** Hands of a woman with early rheumatoid arthritis showing synovial thickening of the metacarpophalangeal and proximal interphalangeal joints.

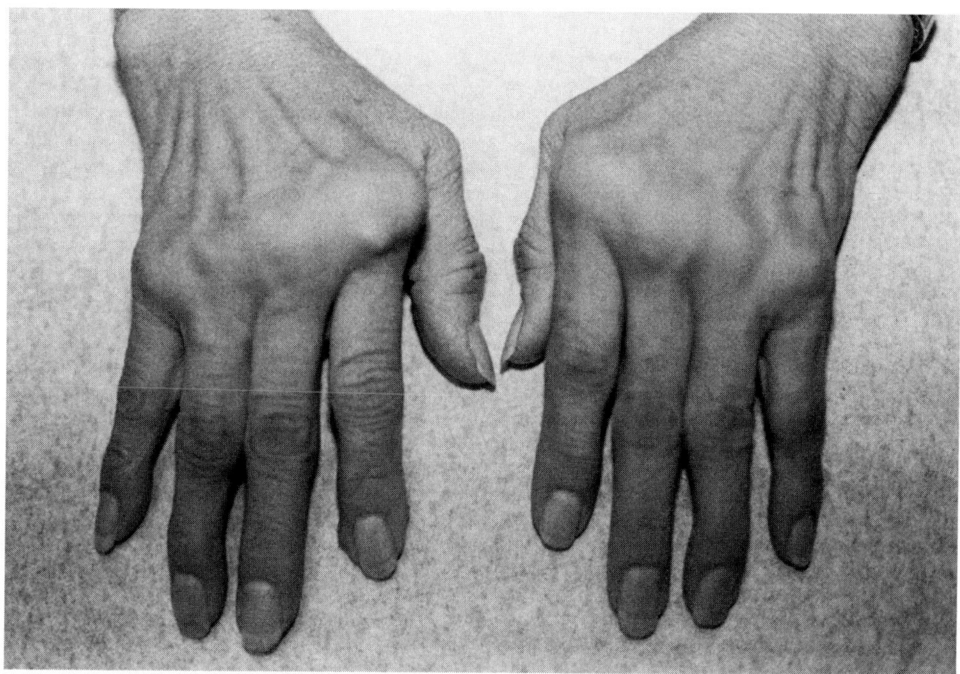

FIGURE 262.2. Hands of a woman with chronic rheumatoid arthritis showing ulnar deviation, metacarpophalangeal subluxation, and swan neck deformities.

TABLE 262.1. Common Joint Deformities in Rheumatoid Arthritis

| Deformity | Joint Involvement |
|---|---|
| Swan-neck | Hyperextension of PIP and flexion of DIP |
| Boutonniere | Flexion of PIP and extension of DIP |
| Ulnar deviation of fingers | Radial deviation of carpal bones |
| Cock-up toes | Metatarsal head subluxation |
| Hammer toes | Metatarsal head subluxation leading to pressure necrosis of dorsal PIPs |
| Bunion (hallux valgus) | First MTP |

DIP = distal interphalangeal; MTP = metatarsophalangeal; PIP = proximal interphalangeal.

Tenosynovitis at the wrist may produce carpal tunnel syndrome or cystic enlargement around the extensor tendons. Prolonged tenosynovitis may cause attrition and, eventually, rupture of extensor tendons, usually the fourth and fifth, resulting in inability to actively extend those digits. At the knee, expansion of the gastrocnemius-semimembranosus bursa by one-way flow of synovial fluid may produce a **Baker's cyst** in the popliteal space. This cyst usually is asymptomatic but may cause pain behind the knee or may rupture into the calf, simulating a deep vein thrombosis (pseudothrombophlebitis).

Neck pain in a patient with long-standing RA should prompt an evaluation of the cervical spine for C1-C2 subluxation. Cervical spine radiographs in flexion and extension may reveal widening of the space between the odontoid process and anterior arch of C1, suggesting laxity of supporting ligaments. This type of cervical instability as well as vertical subluxation of the odontoid into the foramen magnum may cause impingement on the spinal cord, with paralysis and respiratory failure. (It is important for an anesthesiologist to be aware of any cervical spine abnormalities prior to any contemplated surgery and intubation.)

## Extra-articular Manifestations and Associated Disorders

Although the joints are the most visibly afflicted parts, the systemic nature of RA produces prolific extra-articular manifestations (Table 262.2). About 60% of patients have at some time either pleuritis or pericarditis (usually asymptomatic). With active disease, anemia of chronic disease usually is present. Serious forms of pulmonary disease include interstitial pneumonitis producing restrictive lung disease and bronchiolitis obliterans.

**Granulomatous rheumatoid nodules** occur in 20% of patients, virtually all of whom are seropositive for RF. These nodules can occur in any organ, but the most common are, in diminishing order, subcutaneous, pulmonary (Figure 262.3), and myopericardial. Interestingly, the kidneys are virtually never affected in RA, and the appearance of significant proteinuria should prompt a search for other causes (e.g., amyloid, medication-induced).

**Sjögren's syndrome** (sicca complex) is found in RA, systemic lupus erythematosus, or other connective tissue diseases or by itself, without another associated disease. Lymphocytic infiltration of lacrimal and salivary glands produces dysfunction and damage, followed by reduced formation of tears and saliva. Prominent symptoms include dry eyes as well as burning, matter formation, and dryness of the mouth. Patients require frequent instillation of artificial tears or gels to prevent symptoms and corneal ulcers. Cholinergic agents (e.g., oral pilocarpine, cevimeline) or artifical saliva may reduce mouth dryness. In some patients, lymphocytic infiltration of lungs, kidneys, or other sites may evoke organ dysfunction. The risk of lymphoma is higher in patients with primary Sjögren's syndrome.

**Felty's syndrome,** affecting 1% of patients, is a triad of RA, splenomegaly, and cytopenia, usually leukopenia. Nearly all such patients are seropositive for RF in high titers, with more erosive, destructive arthritis than the average patient with RA. Such patients are at high risk for life-threatening pyogenic infections, although the actual peripheral blood leukocyte count and risk for infection are poorly correlated. Many RA patients have significant leukopenia without splenomegaly.

Signs of **vasculitis** occur in 8% of RA patients. In most, this includes minor digital infarcts (brown spots). In 1%, nearly all of whom are RF-seropositive in high titers, a severe systemic vasculitic syndrome occurs, with fever, skin ulcers, digital gangrene (Figure 262.4), and organ infarction.

Whereas nodules, Felty's syndrome, and vasculitis occur predominantly in those with more severe joint disease, they often flare asynchronously with the joint disease. Severe Felty's syndrome or vasculitis also may be seen in patients whose joint disease seems quiescent.

**TABLE 262.2. Extra-Articular Manifestations of Rheumatoid Arthritis**

| |
|---|
| Skin |
| Rheumatoid nodules |
| Vasculitic lesions |
| Mucous membranes |
| Sjögren's syndrome (20%) |
| Eyes |
| Sjögren's syndrome |
| Episcleritis |
| Scleromalacia perforans |
| Heart |
| Pericarditis (usually asymptomatic) |
| Lungs (see Chapter 231) |
| Pleurisy |
| Pulmonary rheumatoid nodules |
| Interstitial pneumonitis |
| Bronchiolitis obliterans |
| Pneumoconiosis (Caplan's syndrome) |
| Nervous system |
| Compression neuropathy |
| Median nerve |
| Posterior interosseous syndrome |
| Peripheral neuropathy |
| Mononeuritis multiplex (in vasculitis) |
| Cervical cord compression (C1-2 subluxation) |
| Hematologic |
| Anemia |
| Leukopenia |
| Felty's syndrome |
| Leukocytosis |
| Thrombocytosis |
| Vascular |
| Rheumatoid vasculitis |

## Diagnosis

A committee of the American College of Rheumatology developed a set of seven clinical criteria for epidemiologic and demographic use. These criteria, because they are nonspecific, usually indicate only that an inflammatory arthritis is present (Table 262.3).

## Ancillary Studies

Almost 80% of patients are seropositive for RF. The erythrocyte sedimentation rate may be high, but thrombocytosis and anemia of chronic disease also indicate active inflammation. Initially, radiographs may show only soft tissue swelling. Classically, periarticular demineralization, symmetric joint space narrowing, and marginal articular erosions are seen. In severe cases, marked bony destruction due to bony resorption, and malalignment due to weakened capsular, tendinous, and ligamentous structures, may occur (Figure 262.5). Joint ankylosis is unusual in RA.

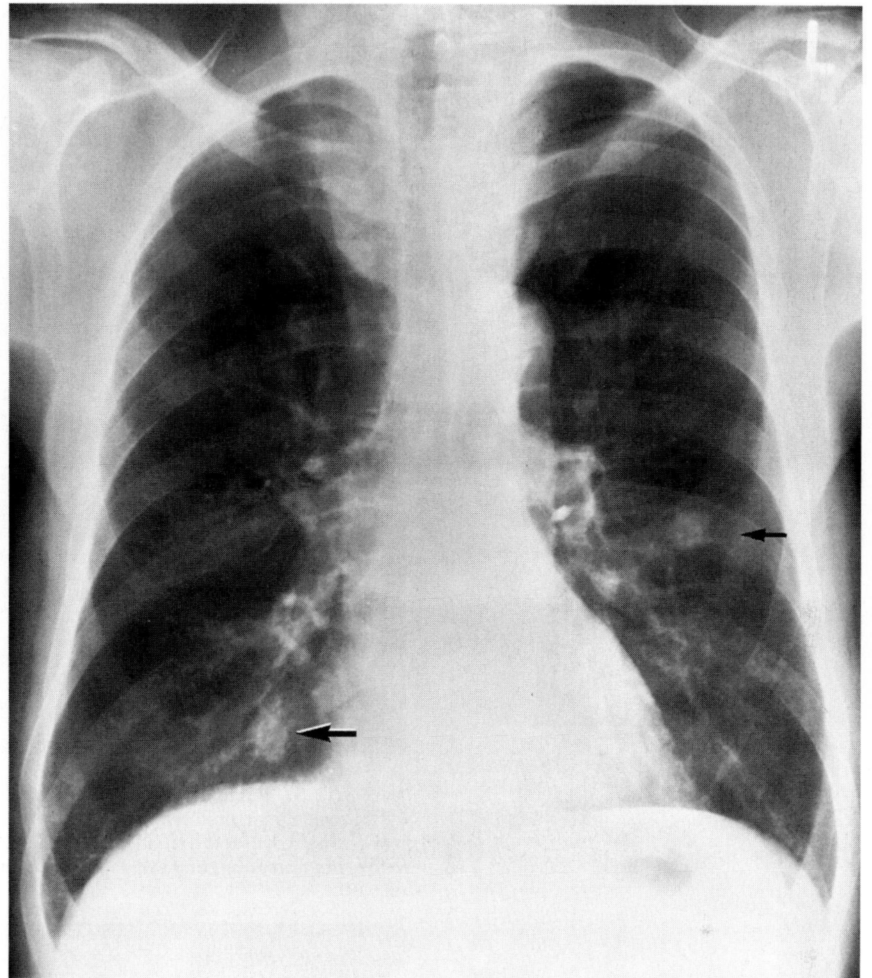

**FIGURE 262.3.** Chest radiograph of a patient with chronic rheumatoid arthritis showing rheumatoid lung nodules.

## Management

Therapy for RA is directed at reducing inflammation, controlling pain, halting progressive joint erosion, interrupting visceral involvement, and maintaining muscle strength, joint alignment, and joint mobility while awaiting remission. Because the disease course varies widely, medical therapy should be tailored to suppress synovitis or extra-articular manifestations of RA, if feasible, without exposing the patient to excessive risks of drug therapy. Considerable debate continues as to what represents optimal therapy. The consensus is that **early aggressive treatment** is warranted, given the serious disability and premature mortality due to RA.

Therapy is begun with a full dose of **NSAIDs** or high-dose **salicylates** (aspirin, 4 g/d usually) to attain a serum salicylate level of 20–25 mg/dl. Response is graded in terms of relief of pain, morning stiffness, and joint swelling and tenderness. Patients also should be questioned regarding potential side effects of NSAIDs including headache, rash, weight gain, dyspepsia, abdominal pain, or any other gastrointestinal symptoms. Many RA patients report some response to NSAIDs or aspirin but continue to have pain, morning stiffness, and joint swelling. If NSAIDs or aspirin fail to control pain and joint swelling adequately after 2 months, second-line drug therapy should be initiated.

The second-line agents, sometimes called **disease-modifying antirheumatic drugs (DMARDs)** are listed in Table 262.4. Of these, methotrexate is the most commonly used. Combinations of drugs are being prescribed increasingly, usually with methotrexate,

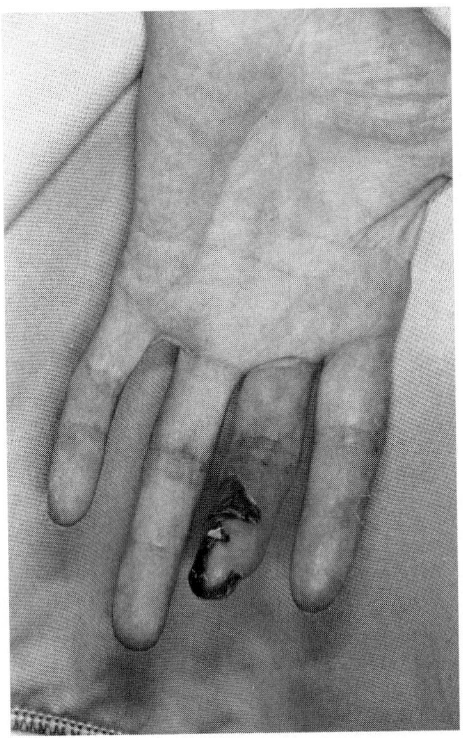

**FIGURE 262.4.** Digital infarction in a patient with rheumatoid vasculitis.

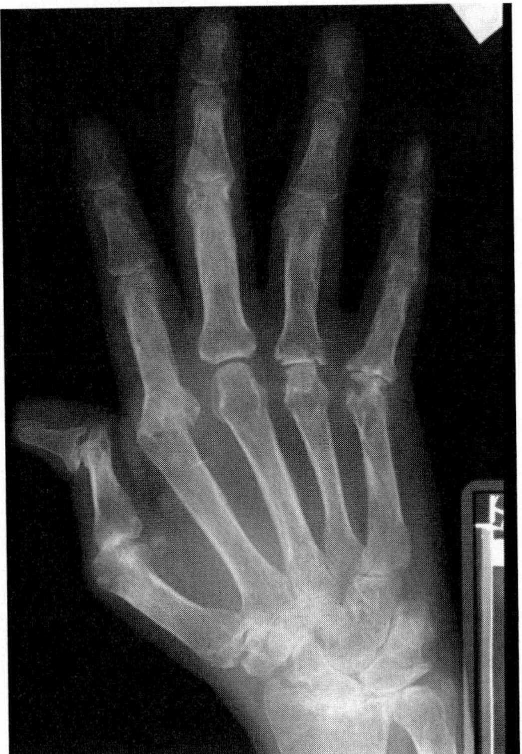

**FIGURE 262.5.** Radiograph of the right hand of a woman with chronic rheumatoid arthritis. Joint erosions are present in the carpal bones and second metacarpophalangeal joint. Joint space narrowing and subluxation also are present.

**TABLE 262.3. Revised American College of Rheumatology Criteria for Rheumatoid Arthritis (1987)***

1. Morning stiffness for at least one hour and present for at least six weeks
2. Swelling of three or more joints for at least six weeks
3. Swelling of wrist, metacarpophalangeal or proximal interphalangeal joints for six or more weeks
4. Symmetric joint swelling
5. Hand roentgenogram changes typical of rheumatoid arthritis that must include erosion or unequivocal bony decalcification
6. Rheumatoid nodules
7. Serum rheumatoid factor by a method that yields positive results in less than 5% of normals

*With exclusion of other joint disorders and fulfillment of 4 or more criteria, the diagnosis of RA is likely.
Reprinted with permission from Arnett et al. Arthritis Rheum 1988; 31:315–324.

**TABLE 262.4. Second-Line Drugs Used for Rheumatoid Disease PBH**

| Agent | Usual Dose |
|---|---|
| Intramuscular gold | 50 mg weekly during induction, less frequently later |
| Oral gold (Auranofin) | 3 mg bid |
| Hydroxychloroquine | 200 mg bid initially, once daily later |
| Methotrexate | 5.0–7.5 mg initially orally, subcutaneously or IM weekly, progressing to 15 mg weekly |
| Azathioprine | 50 mg once daily, progressing slowly to 150–200 mg daily |
| Leflunamide | 100 mg daily for 3 days, then 20 mg daily |
| Etanercept | 25 mg subcutaneously twice a week |
| Infliximab | 3 mg/kg IV every 2 months (after accelerated initiation schedule) |
| Anakinra | 100 mg subcutaneously daily |
| Sulfasalazine | 2000–3000 mg daily |

which has been referred to as an "anchor drug." Single drugs such as hydroxychloroquine, minocycline, auranofin (oral gold), or sulfasalazine may be adequate in milder cases. Other drugs less often used are intramuscular gold, azathioprine, and penicillamine. Each of these agents has its own unique, and in some cases potentially severe, toxicity that requires monitoring. One drawback of these drugs is their delayed onset of action. New agents including the pyrimidine pathway antagonist, leflunomide, and the biological agents, active against tumor necrosis factor (e.g., etanercept, infliximab), and anti-interleukin-1 receptor antagonist (anakinra) have provided more potent treatments that have significantly altered the treatment of rheumatoid arthritis.

Although cyclophosphamide and other alkylating agents clearly suppress RA, there is an increased risk of malignancy, which is an important consideration, relegating them to use for serious complications of RA, such as rheumatoid vasculitis.

**Systemic corticosteroid** therapy has an immediate ameliorative effect on inflammation. However, the long- and short-term side effects of high, or even moderate, doses of steroids argue against their use except in limited situations, including life-threatening visceral disease (e.g., pericardial tamponade, systemic vasculitis). Low-dose steroids, usually prednisone (5 mg/ day), sometimes are used in patients with more severe RA who are beginning a remittive regimen in order to maintain function and employability while awaiting a therapeutic response. The long-term goal is always to discontinue steroids, although a few patients with the most severe RA may require low-dose treatment for years.

**Intra-articular steroids** are of value when the clinical picture is dominated by one or two joints, and this approach may control the local inflammatory response for months. It is inadvisable to inject a given joint any more than 3 or 4 times per year, because excess exposure to intra-articular steroids has been reported to result in a Charcot-like arthropathy.

# CHAPTER 263 INFECTIOUS ARTHRITIS

Infectious arthritis is curable if appropriate therapy is initiated promptly to prevent joint destruction. Synovial fluid culture, Gram stain, and synovianalysis are mandatory when infection is suspected.

## Bacterial Arthritis (Septic Arthritis)

Among the 3 million cases of gonococcal (GC) infection that occur annually in the United States, nearly 1% of patients become bacteremic and develop arthritis, making GC infection the most common cause of joint sepsis (see Chapter 156 for more information on septic arthritis). The septic joint usually is inflamed, with marked redness, heat, swelling, tenderness, and limited motion. Usually monoarticular, the disease may be polyarticular in up to 10% of patients. Polyarticular septic arthritis is more likely to occur in immunosuppressed patients. Although any joint may become septic, large joints, especially the knees and hips, are the most vulnerable.

Most septic arthritides evolve hematogenously. Rarely, they originate by contiguous spread. Predisposing factors are extra-articular infection, a previously damaged joint, coexistent arthritis, chronic medical illness (e.g., malignancy, cirrhosis, diabetes mellitus, and IV drug use), and immunosuppression from any cause.

### Clinical Assessment and Diagnosis

Clinical assessment and directed studies may reveal a nidus of infection. Patients often are febrile and may report rigors.

**Disseminated gonococcal** infection (see Chapter 157) may present uniquely as a polyarthritis. Most patients with gonococcal arthritis have no genitourinary symptoms, despite positive cultures at these sites. They may report migratory or additive polyarthralgias. Patients with gonococcal infection tend to have tenosynovitis at multiple sites and multiple skin lesions, which usually are painless, hemorrhagic macules that may evolve into vesicles or pustules. Patients with monoarthritis have the dermatitis less often (40%).

Peripheral leukocytosis is common, and acute phase reactants are elevated in septic arthritis. At least two blood cultures should be drawn, and cultures obtained of any suspected portal of entry (e.g., skin lesion, urine, sputum). When gonococcal arthritis is suspected, rectal, urethral, cervical, and possibly pharyngeal cultures are mandatory. Gram stains of the urethral swabs are a useful initial screen in men, but the finding of gram-negative diplococci in cervical smears is nonspecific in women. In gonococcal arthritis, genitourinary cultures provide the best yield (>70% of cases); cultures of skin lesion and joint fluid often are unrevealing. In contrast, in more than two thirds of cases of nongonococcal bacterial arthritis, Gram stain and culture of joint fluid yield an organism. Radiographs show only soft tissue swelling initially, but may be of use in follow-up if osteomyelitis or joint damage is suspected.

**Synovianalysis** is mandatory when a septic joint is suspected. The fluid usually is cloudy, with decreased viscosity and poor mucin clot, and contains 5,000 to 250,000 leukocytes/mm$^3$ (mostly neutrophils). The fluid glucose often is 50% or less of a simultaneous serum level.

## Management

Although Gram stain and culture are essential for a correct diagnosis and to guide appropriate therapy (Table 263.1), therapy sometimes must begin despite a negative Gram stain (Table 263.2). For gram-positive cocci, a penicillinase-resistant penicillin or vancomycin should be begun; for gram-negative cocci, an extended spectrum cephalosporin is selected.

When no organisms are seen, treatment should be further individualized, keeping the clinical setting in mind (e.g., immunosuppression enhancing the risk for gram-negative rods or IV drug use increasing the risk of *Pseudomonas* infection). Cultures should be plated on blood agar routinely and on chocolate agar if *Neisseria gonorrhoeae* or *Haemophilus influenzae* is suspected. When indicated, fungal, mycobacterial, and anaerobic cultures also must be done. When the organism is identified, therapy should be modified accordingly and continued for at least 7 to 10 days after the inflammation abates. For *Staphylococcus aureus* and gram-negative bacilli, 3 to 4 weeks of parenteral therapy is recommended, followed by 2 to 4 weeks of oral therapy.

Initially, the joint should be immobilized to relieve pain, but passive range-of-motion exercises should be added gradually to prevent joint contracture (reduced range of motion of the joint). Until a microbe is identified or a clinical response is apparent, analgesics without antipyretic effect should be used. Joint effusions should be drained by simple aspiration, usually daily at first and then, later, as often as necessary. Synovial fluid volume, cell count, and cultures should be monitored.

If needle aspiration cannot accomplish adequate drainage, early orthopedic consultation should be sought for arthroscopic or open drainage. Prompt surgical

**TABLE 263.1. Intravenous Antibiotic Therapy Based on Culture Results**

| Organism | Antibiotic | Alternate |
|---|---|---|
| *Staphylococcus*† | Nafcillin | Vancomycin |
| *Streptococcus*† | Penicillin G | Vancomycin, cefazolin, clindamycin |
| *Neisseria gonorrhoeae*† | Ceftriaxone | Spectinomycin |
| *Haemophilus* | 3rd-generation cephalosporin | Chloramphenicol |
| Enterobacteriaceae | | |
| *Escherichia coli, Salmonella, Klebsiella, Enterobacter, Proteus* | Gentamicin | Tobramycin, amikacin |
| *Pseudomonas* | Antipseudomonal penicillin + gentamicin | |

†Common organisms

**TABLE 263.2. Initial Antibiotic Therapy for Suspected Septic Arthritis With a Negative Gram Stain, Based on Patient's Age**

| Age | Suggested regimen | Alternate | Coverage |
|---|---|---|---|
| <3 mos | Penicillinase-resistant penicillin + third-generation cephalosporin | | Gram-positive cocci, coliforms |
| 3 mos-14 yrs | Penicillinase-resistant penicillin, third-generation cephalosporin | Vancomycin | Staphylococci, Streptococci, *H. influenzae* |
| 15–40 yrs | Third-generation cephalosporin | Nafcillin (if Gram stain Shows gram-positive cocci in clusters) | *Neisseria gonorrhoeae*, Staphylococci |
| >40 | Penicillinase-resistant penicillin, third-generation cephalosporin | Vancomycin + third-generation cephalosporin | Staphylococci, coliforms |

drainage is required if the hip is infected, pus is loculated, or the arthritis does not respond to treatment after 3 or 4 days.

## Tuberculous Arthritis

Diagnosis of tuberculous arthritis often is delayed because its symptoms are generally less severe and indolent. Furthermore, skeletal tuberculosis is uncommon, and tuberculosis itself is nonendemic in the United States. Mycobacteria enter the joint hematogenously or from an adjacent osseous focus. Active pulmonary tuberculosis usually is absent, and constitutional symptoms usually are lacking.

One half of all skeletal tuberculosis occurs in the spine **(Pott's disease),** followed by weight-bearing joints (hip and knee, 15% each; ankle and wrist, 5%–10%). Back pain and muscle spasm are usual symptoms of spinal tuberculosis, and findings include local tenderness, kyphosis, and referred pain from root compression. Radiographs show disc space narrowing and vertebral collapse; a paraspinous abscess may be seen.

Articular tuberculosis usually presents insidiously with chronic low-grade monoarthralgia; swelling and stiffness are less frequent. Most patients have both osseous and synovial infection. Initially, radiographs show soft tissue swelling and osteopenia. Later, subchondral marginal erosions appear and eventually joint space narrowing and bony destruction occur without osteophyte formation.

Diagnosis depends on a high index of suspicion. The tuberculin skin test (PPD) is positive in 90% of cases, but older or very ill patients may be anergic. Synovial fluid shows leukocytosis (10,000–20,000 cells/mm$^3$, mostly neutrophils), elevated protein, and usually low glucose. Acid-fast smear is positive in 20%, and culture is positive in 80%. **Synovial biopsy** provides the quickest and most reliable diagnosis. Biopsy, culture, and DNA probe techniques (see chapter 218) can provide the diagnosis in over 90% of cases.

**Treatment** is similar to that of pulmonary tuberculosis, using 3 or 4 mycobactericidal drugs for 6 to 9 months. Surgical drainage is reserved for cases with severe joint destruction or, in spinal tuberculosis, patients with paraparesis.

## Lyme Disease

Lyme disease, a systemic illness, is caused by the spirochete *Borrelia burgdorferi.* Initial infection produces flulike symptoms, followed in 70% of cases by a characteristic rash, **erythema migrans** (EM), at the site of an *Ixodid* (deer) tick bite. A secondary phase leading to cardiac conduction defects or neurologic abnormalities (e.g., Bell's palsy) develops weeks to months later in some patients. A tertiary phase accompanied by intermittent or chronic arthritis appears months to years later in untreated patients. Most cases of Lyme disease in the United States occur in the summer and in three locations (Northeast, upper Midwest, and the Pacific coast).

Erythema migrans is a rapidly expanding annular erythematous rash that usually develops at the site of the tick bite. About 50% of patients develop multiple annular secondary lesions. Intermittent symptoms that often accompany the rash include malaise, fatigue, headache, fever, chills, stiff neck, myalgias, and arthralgias. Initially, **migratory arthralgias** occur; a large-joint **oligoarthritis** (60%) evolves later. Recurrences follow without sequelae for several years, but a chronic destructive oligoarthritis occurs in 10%.

Special spirochetal culture techniques are not routinely available. Specific IgM antibody titers or rising titers suggest a recent infection. False-positive tests and background positivity in endemic areas render diagnosis and evaluation of level of activity difficult. Western blot testing provides more specific evidence of infection. Polymerase chain reaction (PCR) on synovial fluid and cerebrospinal fluid may be employed when other testing is inconclusive.

Oral doxycycline or penicillin shortens the early stages and can prevent later major multisystem disease, although 50% still have recurrent bouts of headache or musculoskeletal pain. High-dose IV penicillin or ceftriaxone for 2 to 3 weeks is used to treat the later neurologic, musculoskeletal, and cardiac involvement.

## Viral Arthritis

Viral arthritis usually is accompanied by nonspecific symptoms related to the systemic viral infection, such as lymphadenopathy and rash. Arthritis often is **symmetric** with varying signs of inflammation. Rubella, human parvovirus B19, and hepatitis B and C are the common viral pathogens. Hepatitis B may present with polyarthritis, low serum complement, and urticaria that clear as jaundice appears.

Laboratory abnormalities are nonspecific. Most commonly, the erythrocyte sedimentation rate is high, and synovial fluid is inflammatory. The patient's history (rubella immunization, exposure to sick contacts, IV drug use for hepatitis B and C) and serologic tests provide the diagnosis. The course usually is short and uneventful. Treatment is symptomatic.

**Human immunodeficiency virus** (HIV) infection has been associated with a severe form of Reiter's syndrome, manifested as widespread joint involvement and a generalized rash resembling pustular psoriasis. Disease associations with HIV infection include polymyositis, dermatomyositis, vasculitis, and "diffuse infiltrative lymphocytosis syndrome," with some similarity to Sjögren's syndrome.

# CHAPTER 264 SERONEGATIVE SPONDYLOARTHROPATHIES

The seronegative (rheumatoid factor–negative) spondyloarthropathies are a group of disorders that often include back involvement (sacroiliitis or spondylitis), enthesopathy (inflammation at ligamentous or tendon insertions onto bone), and peripheral arthritis. They include ankylosing spondylitis, reactive arthritis and Reiter's syndrome, psoriatic spondyloarthropathy, and the spondyloarthropathy of inflammatory bowel disease (Table 264.1).

The peripheral arthritis typically is **oligoarticular** and **asymmetric.** Involvement of the metacarpophalangeal (MCP), proximal interphalangeal (PIP), and distal interphalangeal (DIP) joints on a single digit with sparing of adjacent digits leads to a **"sausage digit"** (dactylitis), which is typical of these diseases. On radiographs, juxta-articular osteoporosis is lacking, and entheses may show periostitis (new bone formation in the periosteum), erosions, and fluffy whiskering (small spicules of new bone formation). On presentation, radiographs in most patients show erosive **sacroiliitis**, which often is asymptomatic (Figure 264.1). Thus, a pelvis radiograph is more likely to yield an abnormal result than lumbar spine radiographs.

Patients with these diseases show an unusually high frequency of HLA-B27 (Table 264.2). HLA-B27 is noted in 8% of normal whites and even fewer blacks. Epidemiologic data suggest that the HLA-B27–positive person is susceptible to the development of a spondyloarthropathy following an infection or exposure to an antigen. For example, bacillary dysentery or nongonococcal urethritis often precedes reactive arthritis and Reiter's syndrome. A large proportion of patients with these diseases have incomplete or overlapping presentations of disease, which preclude formation of acceptable classification criteria.

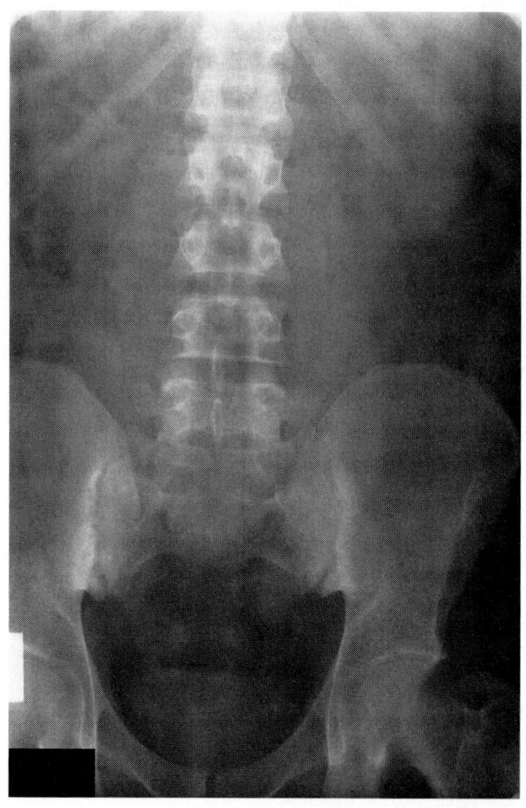

**FIGURE 264.1.** Roentgenogram of the pelvis showing bilateral sacroiliitis with sclerosis and irregularity of the joint margins in a young man with Reiter's syndrome. The sacroiliitis was asymptomatic.

**TABLE 264.1. Spondyloarthropathies: A Glossary of Conditions**

| | |
|---|---|
| Ankylosing spondylitis | Inflammation of spinal joints resulting in back pain, stiffness, and progressive fusion of the spine |
| Reactive arthritis | Usually oligoarticular lower extremity large joint arthritis following bowel infection by enteric pathogens. |
| Reiter's syndrome | A form of reactive arthritis, usually associated with genitourinary infection (e.g., *Chlamydia*), and characterized by arthritis, uveitis, urethritis, and skin and mucous membrane lesions. |
| Psoriatic arthritis | Arthritis affecting peripheral joints or spinal joints in association with psoriasis |
| Colitic arthritis | Arthritis affecting peripheral joints or spinal joints in association with ulcerative colitis or Crohn's disease |

## Ankylosing Spondylitis

The prevalence of ankylosing spondylitis in the U.S. is about 0.1 to 0.2%. Symptomatic ankylosing spondylitis usually begins before age 40, with a male-to-female ratio of 9 : 1. The most common symptom is **low back pain,** which differs from the common discogenic or mechanical causes of back pain in that it is worse on arising, is associated with morning stiffness, improves with light exercise, interferes with sleep, and infrequently causes radicular or neurologic deficits. In late cases, the cauda equina syndrome may occur, rarely.

Physical findings in early cases can be normal. About one third of patients develop peripheral joint disease at some time (Table 264.3), with ankylosing (causing progressive fusion) arthritis of the hips and shoulders being the most common nonaxial involvement.

**TABLE 264.2. Frequency of HLA-B27 in Spondyloarthropathies**

| Disease | Frequency (%) |
|---|---|
| Ankylosing spondylitis | 85–90 |
| Reiter's syndrome | |
| All patients | 60–75 |
| With sacroiliitis | 90–100 |
| Inflammatory bowel disease | |
| Peripheral arthritis | No increase |
| Spondylitis | 30–50 |
| Psoriasis | |
| Peripheral arthritis | No increase |
| Spondylitis | 40–50 |
| Normal Caucasian men | 8–9 |

Although most cases probably are not progressive, a minority of patients develop **ascending spinal inflammation.** Roentgenograms may progress from normal initially to sacroiliitis, followed by squaring of the vertebral bodies, and later ligamentous ossification **(syndesmophytes)** and joint fusion **("bamboo spine").** Involvement of the costovertebral joints can cause pleuritic pain and immobility of the rib cage which limits chest expansion. Eventually, fusion of the entire spine may occur.

Iritis occurs in 20% and may be the presenting complaint. In 5% of patients, inflammation of the aortic root causes aortic insufficiency or atrioventricular conduction disturbances.

Early diagnosis of ankylosing spondylitis can be difficult. Testing for HLA-B27 in persons with back pain offers minimal diagnostic help, because back pain is a very common disorder. **Treatment** consists of physical therapy to maintain mobility and posture, sleeping on a flat, firm surface, and NSAIDs. Indomethacin probably is the most effective NSAID; it may be used in divided doses up to 150 to 200 mg/day. Sulfasalazine or methotrexate may confer some benefit, but medications do not seem to halt progression of the disease. Etanercept has been shown to benefit some cases.

## Reiter's Syndrome and Reactive Arthritis

The classic triad of Reiter's syndrome consists of arthritis, conjunctivitis, and nongonococcal urethritis. The arthritis usually is oligoarticular, affecting joints in the lower extremity more than the upper extremity. The enthesitis most often is detected at the insertion sites of the plantar fascia and the Achilles tendon. Other features include spondylitis, shallow and usually asymptomatic ulcers on the tongue and palate, circinate balanitis of the

**TABLE 264.3. Features of Spondyloarthropathies**

| | Sacroiliitis | Spine | Peripheral Arthritis | Iritis | Aortitis | Cutaneous | Gastrointestinal | Genitourinary |
|---|---|---|---|---|---|---|---|---|
| Ankylosing spondylitis | +++[1] | +++[2] | + | + | ++ | – | – | – |
| Reiter's syndrome | +++[3] | +++[4] | +++[5] | ++[6] | + | +++ | ++ | +++ |
| Psoriatic arthritis | ++[3] | ++[3] | + | + | + | +++ | – | – |
| Inflammatory bowel disease | +++[1] | +++[2] | | + | + | – | ++++ | – |

[1] Bilateral involvement
[2] Ascending pattern
[3] Can be asymmetric, i.e., unilateral syndesmophyte or one side larger than the other
[4] Tendency toward "skip pattern," i.e., skips vertebral segments
[5] Usually in lower extremity
[6] Conjunctivitis is the first manifestation in most patients.

penis, and a characteristic desquamative rash on the soles or palms termed **keratoderma blenorrhagicum.** Spondylitis may involve the sacroiliac joints and vertebral column asymmetrically and may skip to the dorsal or cervical spine rather than ascending contiguously.

Acute attacks subside in several weeks to a few months in 95% of cases, with the remainder of patients becoming chronic. Remissions carry a 10% annual risk of recurrence, with recurrences occurring in half the cases.

One half of patients with Reiter's syndrome have evidence of *Chlamydia* infection, seen as antichlamydial antibodies, synovial biopsies showing chlamydial antigens and organism fragments, or isolation of chlamydia from the urethra. Urethritis also may be due to *Ureaplasma urealyticum.* Epidemics of Reiter's-like illness, nearly all in HLA-B27-positive persons, have followed outbreaks of *Shigella flexneri* dysentery. Similar illnesses that have followed *Salmonella, Campylobacter, Yersinia enterocolitica,* and *Clostridium difficile* infection are termed **reactive arthritis** because the arthritis is in some way occurring as a reaction to the infection.

There is no specific laboratory test for Reiter's syndrome, and the diagnosis is made on the constellation of clinical features. Initial **treatment** is similar to that for ankylosing spondylitis. Sulfasalazine, methotrexate, and azathioprine have been successful in controlling persistent synovitis in many of these patients.

### Psoriatic Arthritis

Arthropathy occurs in 6% of patients with psoriasis. In about 75%, the skin disease precedes the arthritis, and in 15%, the arthritis precedes the dermatitis; in the remainder, the two manifestations begin concurrently. There is poor correlation between the severity of the skin disease and joint involvement, and in some patients, nail pitting (see Figure 51.2) may be the only clue to the diagnosis.

An asymmetric oligoarthritis occurs in 70% of patients. In 5% to 15%, the peripheral arthritis involves the DIP joints almost exclusively. In about 15%, the arthritis is symmetric and mimics rheumatoid arthritis, with some cases even being RF-seropositive. (Some of these may represent the incidental occurrence of both diseases.) Severe, osteolytic, disfiguring arthritis of the hands, termed **arthritis mutilans,** occurs in 5%. Inflammatory spondylitis of the lumbar or cervical spine with a tendency to spare the sacroiliac joints occurs in 40% of patients; men are predisposed 6:1 over women.

**Treatment** is similar to that for rheumatoid arthritis, although the role of gold therapy is less well established. Although antimalarials have led to improvement in the arthritis, they can cause a severe flare of the skin disease and should be used with caution. Methotrexate, azathioprine, and sulfasalazine have proven effective. Cyclosporine and etanercept have been shown to be useful in resistant cases. Psoralen ultraviolet A (PUVA) therapy given to control skin symptoms may improve the peripheral joint disease. Remission of spinal disease remains undocumented.

### Arthritis and Inflammatory Bowel Disease

Peripheral arthritis occurs in 12% of patients with ulcerative colitis and 20% of those with Crohn disease, typically with symmetrical, large-joint arthritis in the lower extremities (colitic arthritis). The activity and severity of the arthritis usually parallel that of the bowel disease. About 7% of patients with inflammatory bowel disease have ankylosing spondylitis, the majority of whom are positive for HLA-B27 (see Table 264.1); however, little correlation is seen between the spondylitis symptoms and activity of the bowel disease.

Therapy for the joint disease should be directed at the underlying bowel disease. The spine disease is treated similarly to ankylosing spondylitis and the peripheral arthritis similarly to psoriatic arthritis. Treatment with infliximab for inflammatory bowel disease may also benefit active arthritis.

# CHAPTER 265 SYSTEMIC LUPUS ERYTHEMATOSUS

Systemic lupus erythematosus (SLE), first described in 1905 by Sir William Osler, predominantly affects women (90%) and usually begins between the ages of 15 and 40. It afflicts about 0.1% of the general population but appears to be slightly more common and more severe in nonwhites.

## Etiology and Pathogenesis

The cause of SLE is unknown. Its predilection for women suggests the influence of estrogen on the immunologic abnormalities. An increased frequency of HLA-B8, HLA-DR2, and HLA-DR3, as well as the occurrence of disease in monozygotic but not dizygotic twins strongly suggest a genetic predisposition. Environmental factors, such as exposure to ultraviolet light, may activate not only skin disease but also systemic disease. A panoply of antibodies against various tissue antigens may be found in the sera of such patients.

Elevated immunoglobulin levels reflect B-cell stimulation. However, specific autoantibodies that are antigenically driven cause disease by direct reaction with a target tissue (e.g., immune thrombocytopenia) or by tissue deposition of the resulting immune complex (e.g., SLE nephritis, immune complex vasculitis). These immune complexes are poorly cleared by the reticuloendothelial system, perhaps due to inherited deficiency of one of several complement components.

Some **drugs** can induce antinuclear antibody (ANA) and, occasionally, overt clinical symptoms of SLE. Procainamide, hydralazine, isoniazid, diphenylhydantoin, and **penicillamine** are the most common offenders. Over 60% of patients taking procainamide develop ANAs with time, but only 5% of these develop symptoms of SLE. Most often, such patients have only fever, serositis, and arthritis. Cessation of the drug usually leads to alleviation of symptoms over several weeks to months, although the serologic changes may persist for years.

## Clinical Features

Systemic lupus erythematosus potentially involves every body system (Table 265.1). However, not all systems are affected in any given case, so that insufficient criteria may be present to make a definitive diagnosis of SLE at initial presentation. Over time, other features appear that confirm the diagnosis.

The integument is commonly affected in SLE. A faint, relatively nonspecific **malar rash** is seen in 25% of patients, but the classic, **florid butterfly rash** is seen in only about 5%. Discoid lesions occur in about 10%. Other skin lesions include photosensitive skin eruptions, urticaria, macular or papular eruptions, bullae, and panniculitis. Livedo reticularis, Raynaud's phenomenon, nailbed telangiectasia, splinter hemorrhages, and Osler's nodes (tender, erythematous thickenings in the finger pads) reflect the underlying vasculitis. Oral mucosal or nasal septal ulcerations are often painless and, therefore, frequently missed. Patchy alopecia or brittle hair ("lupus hair") is seen in about 15% of cases and reflects involvement of the skin appendages.

**Joint pain** and **swelling** together represent the most frequent manifestation of SLE, and are seen in 95% of patients. Typically, the arthritis is nondeforming and nonerosive, unlike that in rheumatoid arthritis. However, a minority of patients can develop rheumatoid arthritis-like ulnar deviation and swan-neck deformities secondary to periarticular soft tissue changes (Figure 265.1). Aseptic necrosis of bone, most often involving the femoral or humeral heads, can follow steroid therapy or vasculitis.

Serositis may occur as pericarditis, pleuritis, or peritoneal inflammation. Pericarditis occurs in 25% of patients with SLE but rarely causes cardiac malfunction. Angina or myocardial infarction can result from vasculitis of the small coronary vessels or from coronary atherosclerosis as a result of corticosteroid therapy. Aortic or mitral valve insufficiency is seen in the rare patient with valvulitis. Libman-Sacks (verrucous) endo-

**TABLE 265.1. 1982 Revised American College of Rheumatology Criteria for the Diagnosis of Systemic Lupus Erythematosus***

| Criterion | Comment |
|---|---|
| Malar (butterfly) rash | Spares nasolabial folds |
| Discoid skin lesions | Atrophic scarring may occur in older lesions |
| Photosensitivity | Unusual reaction to sunlight |
| Oral ulcers | Usually painless; may be nasopharyngeal |
| Nonerosive arthritis | Involves >2 peripheral joints |
| Serositis | Pleuritis (pleurisy, pleural rub, or effusion) or pericarditis (abnormal ECG, rub, or pericardial effusion) |
| Renal disorder | Persistent proteinuria >0.5 g/24 hr, or >3% proteinuria on dipstick, or cellular casts |
| Neurologic disorder | Seizures or psychosis in the absence of offending drugs or metabolic derangements |
| Hematologic disorder | Cytopenias on >2 occasions: hemolytic anemia with reticulocytosis, leukopenia <4000/mm$^3$, or lymphopenia <1500/mm$^3$, or thrombocytopenia <100,000/mm$^3$ |
| Immunologic disorder | Anti-native DNA or anti-Smith (Sm) antibodies or positive anticardiolipin antibody, or false-positive VDRL |
| Antinuclear antibody | Abnormal ANA titer in the absence of drugs associated with drug-induced lupus |

*For the purposes of case definition, diagnosis of SLE requires the presence of 4 of these 11 criteria, either serially or simultaneously. (Adapted from Tan et al. Arthritis Rheum 1982; 25:1271-1277 and Hochberg ML. Arthritis Rheum 1997;40:1725.)

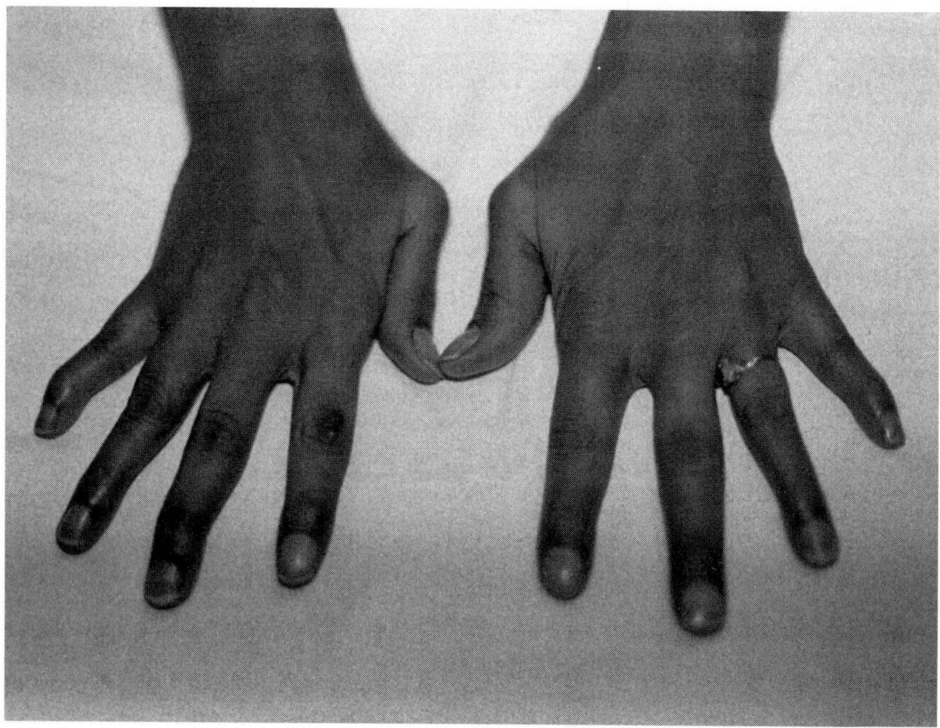

**FIGURE 265.1. Hands of a woman with systemic lupus erythematosus, showing synovitis in several proximal interphalangeal joints and swan-neck deformities.**

carditis typically is asymptomatic but may predispose to bacterial endocarditis.

Pleuritis, the most common pleuropulmonary manifestation, is seen in 30% of cases. Lupus pneumonitis is uncommon. Thus, a pulmonary infiltrate in SLE is more apt to be infectious than a result of the underlying pulmonary disease (see Chapter 238).

About 25% of patients exhibit some form of neurologic involvement. Virtually any central or peripheral neurologic structure can be affected, although seizures, cerebrovascular accidents, and organic mental syndromes predominate. Lupus cerebritis leading to diffuse cortical atrophy, irreversible dementia, and organic brain syndrome is especially ominous.

Another pathogenetic mechanism for CNS lupus is vaso-occlusive stroke. These patients usually present with physical signs of one or more specific ablative neurologic defects, which may be detectable on computed tomography, magnetic resonance imaging, or arteriography. Vascular occlusion in these patients is due to vasculitis or thromboembolism, the latter of which is related to hypercoagulability from antiphospholipid antibodies or lupus anticoagulant.

Proximal muscle weakness may reflect myositis with elevation of muscle enzymes and other features of myositis (see Chapter 259).

About one half of patients with SLE develop clinically apparent **renal disease** suggested by hematuria or proteinuria (see Chapter 165). In general, the more diffuse the glomerulitis, the worse the prognosis. Patients with minimal or focal change on light microscopy have a generally benign prognosis, and those with pure membranous change have an intermediate prognosis. About one third of patients with focal or membranous change, however, can progress in time to diffuse **lupus glomerulonephritis.** Thus, it is likely that every patient with clinically apparent renal involvement warrants treatment. Renal biopsy plays an important role in the management of lupus nephritis. Evidence suggests that a higher degree of chronic change on biopsy (e.g., scarring, crescents) identifies patients who do less well over several years.

Most patients with SLE have anemia of chronic disease. In 5% or less, the anemia is an autoimmune hemolytic type. Granulocytopenia or lymphopenia also can occur. Although mild thrombocytopenia occurs in one third of patients, severe autoimmune thrombocytopenia develops in 5%.

## Laboratory Features

Antinuclear, anti-DNA, and the variety of other autoantibodies possible in SLE are listed in Table 251.5. A peripheral (rim) pattern of nuclear staining on the ANA strongly suggests SLE. Whereas the presence of anti-Smith or high titers of antinative DNA antibodies are virtually diagnostic, they are only 40–50% sensitive. Conversely, a negative ANA virtually excludes SLE, except in the unusual subgroup of "subacute cutaneous lupus," in which the ANA is negative but anti-Ro (SSA) antibodies are present. This subgroup of SLE patients features primarily photosensitivity, causing annular skin lesions and arthritis.

Depressions of serum hemolytic complement correlate with immune complex nephritis or, alternatively, may reflect congenital absence of one of the complement components (C2 deficiency is the most common). The latter patients are significantly more likely than the general population to develop SLE, polymyositis, or another autoimmune disease.

Twenty percent of SLE patients have a false-positive VDRL test, which may antedate full-fledged SLE by decades. Among these, 5% have a prolonged partial thromboplastin time, attributable to an antibody against the platelet factor III–factor X–factor V complex **(lupus anticoagulant).**

Up to 50% of patients may have **anticardiolipin antibodies** or **lupus anticoagulant,** or both. Hemorrhagic problems are rare in such patients. Instead, about one third are at risk for thromboembolic disease, which may take the form of venous thromboembolism, stroke, or other vascular occlusive syndromes. Anticardiolipin antibody also identifies a group with recurrent spontaneous abortions, some of whom have no evidence of SLE.

The **antiphospholipid syndrome** should be considered in women with recurrent spontaneous abortions or persons with a hypercoagulable state (younger persons or those with recurrent thrombotic episodes without other risk factors). A prolonged partial thromboplastin time or thrombocytopenia may be the tip-off.

Synovianalysis in active arthritis reveals 2000 to 5000 leukocytes/mm$^3$. In patients with renal disease, a nephritic picture (microscopic hematuria or red cell casts), serum creatinine, blood pressure and serologic changes, and the degree of proteinuria can predict quite accurately the changes on biopsy. The closest correlate of lupus glomerulonephritis is a low serum complement, and the second is a high level of anti-native DNA.

## Diagnosis

The American College of Rheumatology criteria for diagnosis of SLE are useful in illustrating the protean clinical and serologic features of SLE (see Table 265.1). For the purpose of clinical studies, the case definition requires that four or more criteria be met serially or simultaneously for an unequivocal diagnosis of SLE. Many patients with SLE acquire four criteria only after some years.

## Management and Prognosis

Treatment of SLE is based on its severity. Rapid onset and the presence of both anti-DNA antibodies and low serum complement suggest more severe disease. Arthritis and, often, serositis respond to aspirin or other NSAIDs. Both arthritis and dermatologic manifestations can be treated with antimalarial agents, but ophthalmologic monitoring is required to detect early toxicity.

Indications for high-dose corticosteroid therapy (prednisone, 60–100 mg/day or equivalent, in divided doses) include severe multisystem disease, serositis unresponsive to NSAIDs, central or peripheral nervous system disease, vasculitis, hemolytic anemia, immune thrombocytopenia, and glomerulonephritis. Controlling blood pressure in hypertensive lupus patients is critical to prevent further renal deterioration. If an excessive dose of corticosteroid is required to suppress disease activity, azathioprine, mycophenolate mofetil, or methotrexate may effect disease control and be steroid-sparing. Cytotoxic drugs (e.g., cyclophosphamide) are indicated primarily for active renal disease.

Drug-induced lupus is treated by withdrawal of the offending agent, which leads to the gradual disappearance of symptoms and eventually of the ANA.

The prognosis for SLE patients has improved. Since the introduction of corticosteroids, 5-year survival rates of 93% to 94% are reported. The use of cytotoxic agents delays the onset of renal failure requiring dialysis. Infection is the most common cause of death, and those with renal and CNS disease have the worst 5-year survival rate.

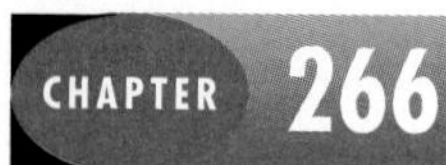

# OTHER CONNECTIVE TISSUE DISEASES

## ■ Myositis

Polymyositis (PM), dermatomyositis (DM), and inclusion body myositis are inflammatory disorders of the skeletal muscle, typically featuring symmetric proximal muscle weakness. These disorders are distinguished from each other by the presence of a rash in DM or by muscle biopsy findings. They may be associated with malignancy and may overlap with other connective tissue disorders, such as systemic sclerosis, systemic lupus erythematosus, mixed connective tissue disease, rheumatoid arthritis, and polyarteritis nodosa.

### Clinical Features

The incidence of the muscle disorders is about 1 : 100,000. Most cases develop in the 5th or 6th decade, predominantly in women (2 : 1). Cases associated with neoplasia have no gender predilection and usually present in the 7th decade.

The presenting symptom in most patients (70–95%) is insidious **proximal muscle weakness** (e.g., difficulty in arising from a low chair, going up steps, combing hair, or placing dishes in upper cupboards); others develop a waddling gait with severe weakness. Muscle pain and tenderness, which are not always prominent, occur at some time in two thirds of patients.

Although proximal muscles are weaker than distal muscles, distal muscle weakness occurs in 20%. Profound muscle atrophy and joint contractures may develop as the disease progresses. More severe cases (15%) develop dysphagia due to skeletal muscle weakness in the posterior pharynx and proximal third of the esophagus; the consequences are regurgitation and aspiration pneumonia. Although distal esophageal hypomotility may be seen in 50% on careful search, it usually is clinically insignificant. Interstitial lung disease is seen in 5 to 10%, but in a minority, dyspnea is due to intercostal muscle weakness. The ECG is abnormal, usually showing conduction defects in one half of patients, but without symptoms. Arthralgias without synovitis are common (25%), but these are more likely to have an associated connective tissue disease. Myocarditis is rare.

The classic rash of DM—a **dusky-red facial eruption** commonly affecting the malar and periorbital areas but also the neck, shoulders, and upper chest—occurs in 30% of adults and 7% of children with myositis. The eyelids may be lilac-colored (heliotrope rash), which is highly suggestive of DM, and these patients also may have periorbital edema and telangiectasia. A second rash is a deep red papular plaque, usually involving extensor surfaces, especially the knuckles, followed by elbows, knees, and medial malleoli **(Gottron's sign).** Whitish scaling may be noted. Nailfold capillaries may be dilated, with hyperemia and telangiectasia in the periungual area. Cutaneous vasculitis, with tender nodules, periungual infarctions, and digital ulcerations, is seen more commonly in adults with neoplasia or in children.

**Inclusion body myositis** is a more recently described form of myositis with a more subtle presentation. Inclusion bodies are seen as basophilic, rimmed vacuoles on light microscopy and as masses of filamentous material on electron microscopy. Inclusion body myositis tends to develop insidiously in older persons, affecting men more frequently and being less responsive to conventional agents. Thus, apparently ineffective therapy should be withdrawn so as to avoid needless risks from medications.

A **malignancy** is associated with myositis in about 5 to 20% of cases, with cancers of the lung, ovary, breast, and stomach being the most common. Myositis precedes the clinical appearance of cancer by 1 to 2 years in about two thirds of cases. Patients over 40 years of age, particularly those with diabetes mellitus (DM), are at a higher risk for a cancer, and a careful search for neoplasia is warranted in such patients.

### Laboratory Features

Elevated serum **muscle enzyme** levels from active muscle damage are a typical feature. Creatine kinase (CK) is the most sensitive, but aldolase, aspartate aminotransferase, glutamic pyruvic transaminase, and lactic dehydrogenase levels also may rise. Occasionally, elevations of ALT and AST (from a comprehensive metabolic panel) have been presumed to be of hepatic origin, resulting in delayed diagnosis of the underlying muscle disease. The CK is high initially in 70% and eventually in 95% of patients. Rheumatoid factor occurs in 40%, and ANA in 20% to 60%. Antiaminoacyl tRNA synthetases and anti-signal recognition particle may define subsets. The anti-Jo 1 (histadyl tRNA synthetase) is associated with interstitial lung disease, Raynaud's phenomenon, and arthritis.

The **electromyogram** (EMG) is abnormal in 70% to 90% of patients. The most typical EMG feature is a short-duration, low-amplitude, polyphasic action potential with voluntary contraction. Spontaneous fibrillations, positive sawtooth potentials (denervation pattern), and insertional irritability are other patterns.

The muscle biopsy is abnormal in 75% to 90% of affected persons. It is important to biopsy a muscle that is weakened but not atrophied. The quadriceps and deltoid muscles are biopsied most frequently. The EMG also may help select a biopsy site; however, because of electrode-induced changes, the biopsy should then be done on the opposite side. Biopsy findings include inflammation in 65% (fiber destruction and regeneration, inflammatory infiltrates); the predominantly lymphocytic infiltrate is seen between muscle fibers or around blood vessels. Muscle fibers may show necrosis and phagocytic invasion. Biopsy may be normal in 17%, given the patchy nature of the disease. Myositis associated with other connective tissue diseases or childhood more often shows vasculitis.

### Diagnosis and Differential Diagnosis

The following criteria are useful in diagnosis: symmetric proximal muscle weakness; characteristic EMG patterns; elevated muscle enzymes; abnormal muscle biopsy; and typical skin rash.

Polymyositis is definite if the first four criteria are met, and probable if three of the first four are present. Dermatomyositis is definite when the skin rash occurs with three of the other four criteria, and probable with two.

Patients with polymyalgia rheumatica have pain in proximal extremities that may be perceived as weakness, but muscle strength, CK, EMG, and biopsy are normal. Endocrinopathies (Addison's disease, Cushing's disease, thyrotoxicosis, and hypothyroidism) may mimic an inflammatory myopathy, but CK usually is normal (although it may rise in hypothyroidism). Drugs such as HMG-CoA reductase inhibitors, penicillamine, clofibrate, hydroxychloroquine, ipecac, and especially ethanol and cocaine may cause a toxic myopathy. Myositis related to sarcoidosis is distinguished by a compatible clinical picture and noncaseating granuloma on biopsy.

### Management

Initial therapy consists of prednisone, 50–100 mg/d, continued for 1 to 3 months. The dosage is then gradually reduced as muscle strength improves. The CK level is the most useful biochemical index to follow; its decline often precedes improved muscle strength, and its elevation signals a relapse.

Approximately 75% of patients can discontinue steroids eventually, but relapses are common. Some require maintenance steroids, either daily or every other day. Immunosuppressive therapy (with methotrexate, azathioprine, cyclosporine and, less often, Leukeran or cyclophosphamide) is employed commonly for steroid sparing or when steroids have been ineffective. Although they can control most cases of PM or DM, their onset of action is somewhat slower. Etanrecept also has proven useful in cases that are difficult to control.

### Prognosis

About 73% of patients will be alive after 8 years of disease. Younger age confers a better prognosis. Associated malignancy or profound weakness, especially of pharyngeal muscles, worsen the outlook. If myositis occurs as part of an overlap syndrome, the prognosis may be determined by the associated connective tissue disease. Death most commonly ensues from a malignancy or sepsis.

## Systemic Sclerosis

Systemic sclerosis is characterized by hardening, thickening, or tightening of the skin **(scleroderma)** and vascular changes. It may present as **diffuse scleroderma** (proximal and distal extremity, facial and truncal skin involvement, and early onset of visceral manifestations) or as limited scleroderma (also called **CREST syndrome:** *c*alcinosis, ***R***aynaud's phenomenon, *e*sophageal dysmotility, *s*clerodactyly with skin involvement usually limited to the fingers and face, and *t*elangiectasia, with delayed visceral manifestations). Other scleroderma syndromes are described subsequently. Overlaps occur with other connective tissue diseases.

Systemic sclerosis affects the skin, esophagus, and lungs and, less often, the joints, heart, small and large intestines, and kidneys. Its etiology is unknown. It features inflammation in tissues that evokes fibrosis. Vascular endothelial injury may be the primary abnormality, and the frequency of immunologic abnormalities supports an autoimmune etiology. The enhanced collagen synthesis seen in skin fibroblasts may be due to inflammation or locally released growth factors.

The disease affects 4–12 persons per million, usually between 30 and 50 years of age. There is a 3:1 predilection for women. Although the course may be variable, most persons have visceral involvement. Spontaneous remissions are rare.

### Clinical Features

The skin is almost always involved, although in a few patients, visceral lesions develop without skin changes. The earliest skin changes are edema and taut hands and feet. In the next, indurated stage, the skin becomes shiny, taut, and hidebound, limiting joint motion (Figure 266.1). Skin creases and hair follicles disappear. In the atrophic phase, tight skin over joints, particularly the hands, causes contractures with ulcerations over bony prominences.

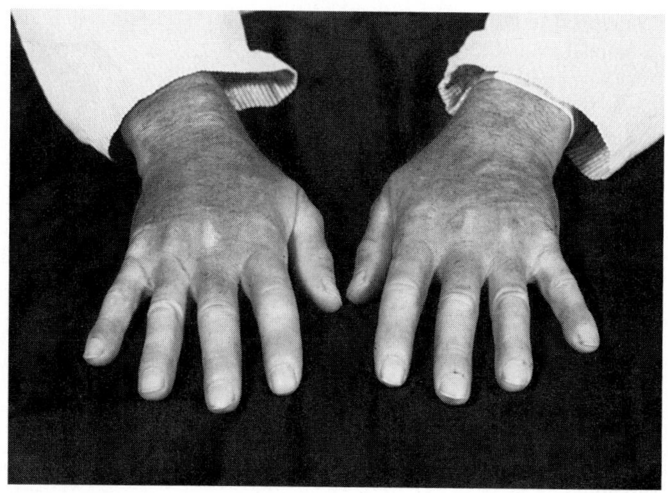

**FIGURE 266.1. Sclerodactyly in systemic sclerosis. Note the shiny skin, which is taut, hidebound and without skin creases.**

In **diffuse scleroderma,** the skin changes are most prominent in the distal extremities and spread gradually to the upper arms and legs, face, upper anterior chest, and abdomen. Hypo- or hyperpigmentation and telangiectasia may occur. Facial changes may narrow the oral aperture. In 3 to 15 years, the skin may enter the late phase of spontaneous softening. Skin biopsy in the classic and late stages shows increased subcutaneous collagen, epidermal thinning, and loss of rete pegs and sebaceous and sweat glands.

In **CREST syndrome,** the skin involvement usually is limited to the fingers and face. Subcutaneous calcifications of the digital pulp (Figure 266.2), extensor aspects of the forearm and olecranon, and prepatellar bursae may erode through the skin. Hand radiographs may show diffuse osteoporosis, resorption of the distal phalangeal tufts, and soft tissue calcifications.

**Vascular abnormalities** are a hallmark of scleroderma. Wide-field capillary microscopy of the nailfold edge shows giant capillary loops in areas rendered avascular by loss of blood vessels. **Raynaud's phenomenon,** producing a classic triphasic color change, is virtually universal: on exposure to cold or emotional stress, the hands may first turn white or ashen (tissue anoxia), then blue (cyanosis), and finally red with rewarming (increased blood flow). Pain, numbness, paresthesias, or a feeling of swelling as blood flow returns may be associated. Not all patients report all three phases. Raynaud's phenomenon has an extensive etiology, including mechanical injury (e.g., vibrating tool use), chemical exposure (e.g., vinyl chloride), certain drugs (e.g., ergot, β-blockers, bleomycin), paraproteinemias, fibromyalgia, carpal tunnel syndrome, and thoracic outlet syndrome, but often it is idiopathic and unrelated to a connective tissue disease.

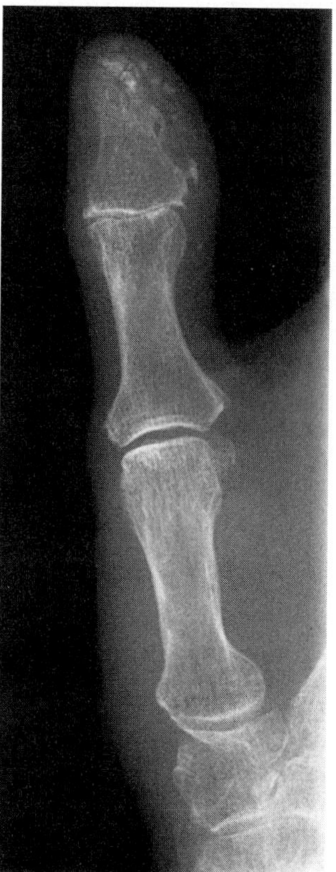

**FIGURE 266.2. Roentgenogram of the thumb of a woman with limited scleroderma (CREST syndrome) demonstrating soft tissue calcinosis.**

The **esophagus** is involved in 90% of cases. Reflux symptoms are the most frequent complaints; dysphagia occurs in 50%. Stricture formation and esophageal dilatation with nearly complete loss of peristalsis are seen in later stages of the disease. The small intestine often is involved, with bloating, cramping, intermittent diarrhea, constipation, and adynamic ileus suggesting bowel obstruction (pseudo-obstruction). Hypomotility may cause bacterial overgrowth with subsequent malabsorption, profound weight loss, and diarrhea alternating with constipation. Radiographic studies may show delayed transit with retention in the second and third portions of the duodenum which may be widely dilated. Asymptomatic large-mouth sacculations of the large and small bowel due to atrophy of the muscularis, while rare, are distinctive. Primary biliary cirrhosis develops in some patients with CREST. Patients are at risk for severe cachexia late in the disease.

Symmetric polyarthralgia or polyarthritis and stiffness are the presenting complaints in approximately one third, and eventually develop in most patients.

**Pulmonary involvement** is quite common. Diffuse interstitial lung disease most often is manifested by exertional dyspnea and, less commonly, a chronic dry cough. Functional abnormalities often antedate symptoms, possibly because of decreased physical activity. Physical findings consist of tachypnea and early basilar rales. Radiographs show diffuse reticular changes, predominantly involving the lower lung fields (Figure 266.3). Pulmonary function tests often show a restrictive impairment, with a low carbon monoxide diffusing capacity ($DL_{CO}$). Pulmonary hypertension may occur with or without interstitial disease, or as a late visceral manifestation of CREST (10%). Histologically, the major findings are interstitial and alveolar fibrosis. Patients with severe fibrotic lung disease may develop alveolar cell or other pulmonary neoplasm, the only malignancies with a greater frequency in this disease than in the general population.

The **kidneys** are involved in 50% of cases of diffuse scleroderma, and rarely in CREST. The lesions are slowly progressive arterial fibrinoid necrosis and intimal hyperplasia. Proteinuria, hypertension, azotemia, or low glomerular filtration rate are the features. Malignant hypertension may occur.

Congestive heart failure occurs in a few patients due to myocardial disease (contraction band necrosis) and malignant or pulmonary hypertension. Pericarditis may occur acutely or, more often, as an asymptomatic effusion. Arrhythmias and conduction defects are common.

Approximately 20% of patients with systemic sclerosis have myopathy with mild muscle weakness and mild or no elevation of muscle enzymes. A few have polymyositis with more marked weakness and abnormal biopsy and EMG. Systemic sclerosis also may be associated with Sjögren's syndrome and subclinical hypothyroidism.

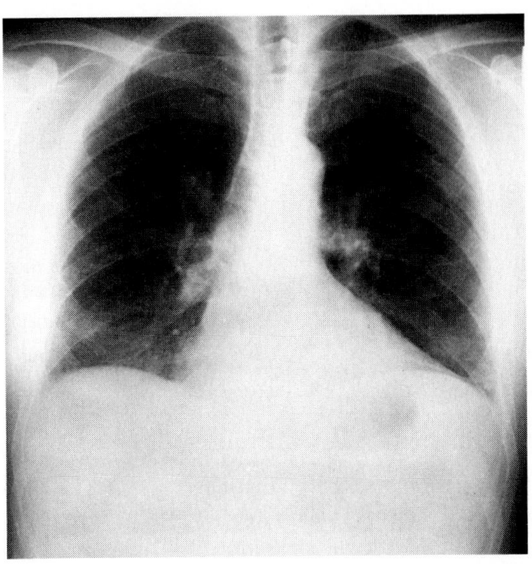

**FIGURE 266.3. Chest roentgenogram of the patient in Figure 266.1 with progressive systemic sclerosis, showing the characteristic bilateral, predominantly lower-zone interstitial infiltration.**

## Laboratory Features

About 50% of patients have a high erythrocyte sedimentation rate and polyclonal hypergammaglobulinemia. Rheumatoid factor is seen in 25%, and ANAs (usually speckled pattern) in 75% to 90%. Antinuclear antibodies with a nucleolar pattern and antibody to the Scl-70 nuclear antigen are very suggestive of systemic sclerosis. Anticentromere antibodies occur more often in CREST.

## Diagnosis, Management, and Prognosis

The diagnosis of systemic sclerosis can be made when the typical skin changes occur proximal to the digits. The diagnosis also can be made if two of the following are present: sclerodactyly; digital pitting scars; or typical lung disease.

The course of this disease does not appear to be altered by any treatment. General measures include avoidance of trauma (particularly to the hands) and severe cold. Tobacco smoke and vasoconstrictors such as beta-blockers should be eliminated. Vasodilators (nifedipine, phenoxybenzamine, guanethidine, methyldopa, reserpine, and prazosin) may help decrease the frequency of Raynaud's phenomenon in some patients. NSAIDs may alleviate joint symptoms. Aggressive blood pressure control and dialysis or transplantation have been used for patients with renal involvement. Although penicillamine and colchicine have been used to treat skin and visceral involvement, their efficacy is uncertain. Some patients with rapidly progressive disease appear to respond to intravenous cyclophosphamide. Gastroesophageal reflux is treated with elevation of the head of the bed, H2 blockers, and proton-pump inhibitors. Treatment for most other manifestations is symptomatic.

The 10-year survival ranges from 35% to 70%. Involvement of the kidneys, heart, and lungs, masculine gender, and older age imply a much worse prognosis.

## Other Scleroderma Syndromes

**Localized scleroderma** without systemic features has two forms. **Morphea** consists of waxy, ivory-colored, sclerotic plaques surrounded by a violaceous halo of inflammation; it occurs at any age. The lesions may be multiple and span several centimeters, and they usually heal over months to years, leaving atrophic areas of hyper- or hypopigmentation. The second form, **linear scleroderma,** usually occurs in children.

**Eosinophilic fasciitis,** another scleroderma syndrome, starts in the hands and feet. The extremities become swollen, painful, and tender, but induration of the skin and subcutaneous tissues follows, giving an orange peel-like, puckered appearance. The trunk and face occasionally are affected. Eosinophilia and hyperglobulinemia usually are present early. Full-thickness skin biopsy down to the muscle shows inflammation and fibrosis in all layers. Response to corticosteroids is good.

The **eosinophilia-myalgia syndrome** has developed following use of L-tryptophan, with a contaminant in its manufacturing process implicated. The syndrome has eosinophilia and many features of scleroderma. Other diseases, most commonly diabetic cheirarthropathy (skin thickening of the hands with flexion contractures of the proximal and distal interphalangeal joints), may mimic the skin changes of scleroderma.

## Undifferentiated Connective Tissue and Overlap Syndromes

Some patients do not develop a defined disorder ("undifferentiated connective tissue disease") or develop an **overlap syndrome** with features that satisfy the diagnostic criteria for two or more defined disorders (e.g., "sclerodermatomyositis" or "rhupus"). **Mixed connective tissue disease,** although its existence as a clinical entity is controversial, combines symptoms usually seen individually in systemic sclerosis, systemic lupus erythematosus, and polymyositis and is serologically defined by very high titers of antibodies to ribonucleoprotein.

# CHAPTER 267 VASCULITIS

The vasculitides are a group of heterogeneous conditions, which have in common inflammation and necrosis within the blood vessel walls. Although their etiology remains unknown, the similarity of vasculitis to lesions in acute experimental serum sickness suggests an immune complex pathogenesis in some of the vasculitides. The vasculitides show features of **systemic inflammation** (e.g., weight loss, fever) and manifestations due to **vasculitic occlusion** of specific vessels (e.g., stroke, intestinal infarction, renal impairment).

Many classification schemes have been proposed, but none is entirely satisfactory. One method bases the classification on the size of the vessel involved (large-, medium-, or small-vessel vasculitis), although this schema does not seem very logical (Table 267.1). In fact, many of the vasculitides bear no clinical, histologic, or serologic resemblance to each other.

## Polyarteritis Nodosa

Polyarteritis nodosa (PAN), a prototypic vasculitic syndrome seen predominantly in middle-aged men, usually involves the medium-sized and small muscular arteries. Histologic examination shows lesions of varying age, suggesting an evolving process. In some series, as many as 50% of patients have evidence of persistent hepatitis B antigenemia, and antigen, immunoglobulin, and complement have been shown in involved vessels, suggesting a true immune-complex-mediated process.

### Clinical Features

The onset of PAN is with systemic symptoms (e.g., fever, malaise, or weight loss), and the multisystem involvement often suggests the diagnosis. Coronary, renal, and mesenteric arteritis causes symptoms referable to the respective viscera and serious and potentially

**TABLE 267.1. Types and Features of Vasculitis Based on Blood Vessel Size**

| | |
|---|---|
| **Medium to large arteries** | |
| Temporal arteritis | Giant cell arteritis, affects mostly cranial arteries in the elderly |
| Takayasu arteritis | Aortic arch involvement in young, usually Asian women |
| **Small to medium arteries** | |
| Polyarteritis group | |
| Polyarteritis nodosa | Necrotizing vasculitis with renal, abdominal, coronary, CNS and peripheral nerve involvement |
| Churg-Strauss vasculitis | Similar to above with pulmonary involvement and eosinophilia |
| Overlap syndrome | Features of several types of vasculitis |
| **Small to medium arteries, veins** | |
| Wegener's granulomatosis | Granulomatous vasculitis, involves upper and/or lower respiratory tract, eyes, ears, kidneys, skin |
| **Arterioles, capillaries, venules** | |
| Hypersensitivity vasculitis | Leukocytoclastic vasculitis (often with "palpable" purpura) |
| Rheumatoid vasculitis | |
| Lupus vasculitis | |
| Drug-induced vasculitis | |
| Essential mixed cryoglobulinemia | |
| Malignancy | |
| Henoch-Schönlein purpura | Purpura, joint pain, abdominal pain, glomerulitis |

life-threatening complications (e.g., myocardial infarction, hypertension, abdominal pain, gastrointestinal hemorrhage, or bowel infarction). Involvement of the vasa nervorum and cranial vessels causes peripheral (e.g., mononeuritis multiplex) or central nervous system signs. Some refute pulmonary involvement, but this opinion may simply reflect problems in distinguishing it from Churg-Strauss disease (allergic granulomatosis), a granulomatous arteritis with lung involvement and eosinophilia in asthmatics or atopic persons.

### Laboratory Features

Leukocytosis, anemia of chronic disease, hypergammaglobulinemia, and an elevated erythrocyte sedimentation rate are common. An active urine sediment and azotemia reflect renal involvement. Cryoglobulinemia or hypocomplementemia occurs in 20% to 25% of cases. Diagnosis is by demonstration of the classic lesions by histologic examination or arteriography.

### Management

Polyarteritis nodosa is classically a catastrophic, often fatal, illness. Despite a lack of carefully controlled studies, it is likely that **corticosteroids** and **immunosuppressive** agents (e.g., cyclophosphamide) have improved the prognosis. High-dose corticosteroids (e.g., prednisone, 80 mg/d) should be used in severely ill patients, although steroids may aggravate hypertension and compromise serosal integrity in the involved bowel.

## Wegener's Granulomatosis

Wegener's granulomatosis features sinusitis, otitis, laryngitis and lung involvement (see Chapter 238), involvement of the eyes, and nephritis (Table 267.2), any or all of which may be seen at presentation. The antineutrophil cytoplasmic antibody with a cytoplasmic pattern of staining (c-ANCA) is positive in most cases. Because c-ANCA is not completely specific, biopsy confirmation is essential. Another staining pattern, the perinuclear or p-ANCA, is seen in other forms of vasculitis, particularly with renal involvement.

Cyclophosphamide, usually given orally, often results in cures in this otherwise fatal disease. In some, the disease may be relapsing or chronic.

A trimethoprim-sulfamethoxazole regimen reduces relapses.

## Hypersensitivity Angiitis (Leukocytoclastic Vasculitis)

Hypersensitivity angiitis (leukocytoclastic vasculitis) affects primarily small vessels, including arterioles and postcapillary venules. It often presents clinically as **palpable purpura.** Many of the original cases followed medication use, leading to the term "hypersensitivity." The histologic finding is hematoxyphilic debris resembling nuclear dust, predominantly in postcapillary venules. This vasculitis may be seen in association with connective tissue diseases such as systemic lupus erythematosus (see Figure 53.2), rheumatoid arthritis, and

**TABLE 267.2. System Involvement and Symptoms in Wegener's Granulomatosis**

| |
|---|
| General |
| Fever |
| Weight loss |
| Cranial |
| Headache |
| Ophthalmic |
| Inflammation-conjunctiva, sclera, uvea |
| Proptosis |
| Otologic |
| Otitis |
| Hearing loss |
| Upper respiratory |
| Epistaxis |
| Rhinitis/obstruction |
| Sinusitis |
| Oral ulcers |
| Lower respiratory |
| Cough |
| Hemoptysis |
| Dyspnea |
| Pleuritis/pleural effusion |
| Renal |
| Glomerulonephritis |
| Interstitial nephritis |
| Skin |
| Purpura |
| Nodules |
| Joints |
| Arthralgia |
| Arthritis |

cryoglobulinemia, or with other infectious or neoplastic syndromes.

Another example is **Henoch-Schönlein purpura,** which classically has glomerulitis with hematuria, arthritis, fever, and gastrointestinal involvement. Circulating IgA levels may be high, and immunofluorescence of biopsy tissue usually shows IgA deposition.

## Giant Cell (Temporal) Arteritis and Polymyalgia Rheumatica

Giant cell (temporal) arteritis and polymyalgia rheumatica are related and sometimes present with overlapping features. **Giant cell arteritis** involves larger vessels, typically from the cranium to the aortic arch, although any portion of the aorta and its major branches may be involved. The typical presentation is a new-onset temporal headache in an older person, but other symptoms may include jaw or tongue claudication and, rarely, ulcers of the scalp or tongue. Although the physical examination can reveal entirely normal findings, thickening and tenderness of the temporal arteries, as well as decreased or absent pulses, suggest temporal arteritis. Blindness and stroke are the most common complications, with the former occurring in 25% of the untreated.

No specific laboratory test exists for identifying temporal arteritis, although the erythrocyte sedimentation rate (ESR) is typically elevated above 50 and often exceeds 90 mm/hr. Diagnosis usually is by temporal artery biopsy. Because the lesions are segmental, a 2- to 3-cm section of temporal artery should be biopsied and multiple areas sampled to avoid missing the lesions. Some favor obtaining bilateral temporal artery biopsies. Treatment with steroids (prednisone, 60 mg/d) can deter blindness.

**Polymyalgia rheumatica** also is predominantly a disease of elderly persons and is unlikely in persons under age 50. A diagnosis of exclusion, it features neck, shoulder, and hip girdle pain, severe morning stiffness (with difficulty getting out of bed), and myalgias without atrophy or true weakness. These patients also may have fever, sweats, and weight loss.

The laboratory findings are nonspecific and include anemia of chronic disease and elevated serum $\alpha_2$-globulin and fibrinogen. The ESR is high (at least 40 and often >90 mm/hr). Rarely, the ESR may be normal, but the C-reactive protein or fibrinogen may be high. Serum muscle enzyme levels, electromyography, and muscle biopsy findings are normal. Random temporal artery biopsy reveals giant cell arteritis in 20% to 30% of patients.

The risk of blindness is less than 1% if cranial vessel symptoms are absent. Any cranial symptoms, (e.g., headaches, jaw claudication, or visual changes) in a patient with polymyalgia rheumatica should prompt a temporal artery biopsy. The myalgias respond dramatically to prednisone in doses as low as 15 mg/day. Both temporal arteritis and polymyalgia rheumatica run a course of 2 to 3 years before remitting, usually permanently.

# CHAPTER 268 REGIONAL (NONARTICULAR) MUSCULOSKELETAL PAIN

A glossary of key regional musculoskeletal disorders is provided in Table 268.1. Diagnosis of specific conditions is based mostly on the history and physical findings. Although trauma may play a causative role in some of these disorders, in many cases, no specific etiology is found.

## Neck and Shoulder Pain

### Neck Pain

Neck and shoulder pain are common symptoms, due to intrinsic lesions at either site or referred pain from one site to the other.

The neck consists of vertebrae, soft tissues (ligaments, paracervical muscles), neurovascular structures (vertebral arteries, spinal cord, nerve roots), and joints (apophyseal and lateral interbody joints and fibrocartilaginous discs). Acute neck pain, often with muscle spasm, can be triggered by ligamentous sprain (e.g., whiplash secondary to motor vehicle accidents, falls, or athletic injuries), prolonged cold exposure, tension, activities involving repetitive neck movement, or nerve root irritation.

Disc disintegration occurs as a result of aging and, probably, previous cervical sprain injuries. The physical examination often reveals limitation of neck motion, tenderness to palpation, and spasm. Cervical nerve root irritation usually is attributable to ligamentous sprains but occasionally is due to a herniated cervical disc. Radiographs of the cervical spine may show disc space narrowing, osteophyte formation (bony overgrowth at the margin of a joint), and sometimes abnormalities of vertebral alignment, but these types of changes are common (seen in 50% of persons older than 45 years of age) and correlate poorly with specific pain complaints.

Radicular pain and neurologic signs may accompany root irritation, which may be suggested by electrodiagnostic studies. Magnetic resonance imaging (MRI) can provide more definitive anatomic information. Occasionally, posterior osteophytes may form large bars, which impinge on the spinal cord, causing cervical myelopathy with weakness and alteration in deep tendon reflexes. Whereas chronic neck pain often is related to a myofascial pain syndrome, fibromyalgia, or degenerative disc disease, **referred neck pain** may be due to thoracic outlet syndrome, brachial plexus injury or compression, intrathoracic lesions (Pancoast tumor), diaphragmatic irritation (subphrenic abscess, splenic or gallbladder disease), temporomandibular joint disorders, and coronary disease.

Initial **treatment** consists of rest (avoidance of exacerbating activities, soft cervical collar), moist heat, a nonsteroidal anti-inflammatory agent for both analgesic and anti-inflammatory properties, and physical therapy (traction, deep heat, massage, exercises). Therapy for referred pain should be directed at the cause.

### Shoulder Pain

The shoulder consists of three joints—the glenohumeral, acromioclavicular, and sternoclavicular—and various soft tissues (tendons, capsules, ligaments, and bursae). Shoulder pain of various types often is lumped into the category of **"bursitis,"** thus rendering this term largely meaningless (Table 268.2).

**Tendinitis** most commonly involves the supraspinatus; tenderness is noted on shoulder palpation along with some loss of motion. **Calcific tendinitis,** occurring beyond the 4th decade, appears radiographically as a rounded or fluffy calcific deposit of hydroxyapatite within the tendon. Most of these deposits are asymptomatic, but acute calcific tendonitis with severe, disabling pain may reflect enlargement of the calcific deposit or rupture into the subacromial bursa. Persistent or recurrent cases may require needling or surgical removal of the calcific deposit.

**TABLE 268.1. A Glossary of Key Regional Musculoskeletal Disorders**

| | |
|---|---|
| Tendinitis | Inflammation of a tendon attachment point or another site of tendon friction |
| Bursitis | Inflammation of a bursa, a sac-like structure which facilitates sliding of one tissue over another |
| Enthesitis | Inflammation of an enthesis, a tendon attachment point |
| Reflex sympathetic dystrophy | Presumptively, a disorder of sympathetic nerve function causing chronic pain in an extremity, usually following some injury |
| Myofascial pain | Localized pain and tenderness in a muscle or group of muscles |
| Fibromyalgia | Chronic condition of widespread pain and tenderness in characteristic trigger points |

**TABLE 268.2. Regional Musculoskeletal Disorders**

| Disorder | Findings |
|---|---|
| **Shoulder** | |
| Calcific tendinitis | Found on radiograph, usually asymptomatic, most often supraspinatus, occasional severe pain |
| Rotator cuff | |
| Tendinitis | Aching shoulder pain, tenderness to palpation, may have reduced ROM |
| Tear | Variable pain, difficulty with active shoulder abduction and resisted abduction |
| Adhesive capsulitis | Markedly reduced glenohumeral motion (frozen shoulder) |
| Primary | Usually middle-aged women, no apparent cause |
| Secondary | Severe loss of motion related to another shoulder problem and failure to maintain ROM (e.g., prolonged use of shoulder splint) |
| Bicipital tendinitis | Tenderness over biceps tendon, clicking with shoulder rotation |
| **Elbow** | |
| Lateral epicondylitis | Lateral elbow and forearm pain, increased with arm use ("tennis elbow"), tenderness over the lateral epicondyle |
| Medial epicondylitis | Medial elbow and forearm pain, increased with use, tenderness over the medial epicondyle |
| **Wrist** | |
| DeQuervain's tenosynovitis | Radial wrist pain; tenderness over the distal radius; pain near base of thumb (over abductor pollicis longus, extensor pollicis brevis tendons) |
| **Hand** | |
| Flexor tendinitis | May affect any of the flexor tendons, finger may "lock" in flexion and snap with extension ("trigger finger"), flexor tendon may be tender in distal palm, may click with finger movement |
| **Ankle** | |
| Achilles' tendinitis | Tenderness at the insertion of the Achilles' tendon on the calcaneous |
| **Bursitis** | |
| Subdeltoid | Aching shoulder pain, similar to rotator cuff tendinitis |
| Olecranon | Usually caused by pressure or trauma, may have fluid accumulation over olecranon |
| Ischial tuberosity | Pain with sitting on hard surface, tenderness over the ischial tuberosity |
| Greater trochanter | Patients often complain of "hip" pain, especially when lying on that side, radiation of pain down the lateral thigh, tender over the greater trochanter |
| Prepatellar | Tenderness and swelling anterior to the patella, may ("housemaid's knee") have fluid accumulation |
| Anserine | Pain in medial knee, tenderness over proximal medial tibia |
| Achilles' | Swelling anterior to the Achilles' tendon |
| Bunion | Pain and swelling over medial distal first metatarsal, usually with hallux valgus deformity |

ROM = range of motion.

Most shoulder problems involve the **rotator cuff,** composed of the supraspinatus, infraspinatus, teres minor, and subscapularis tendons (see Table 268.2). The impingement syndrome or rotator cuff tendinitis represents a continuum of symptoms initiated by excessive overhead arm use that permits impingement of the cuff against the coracoacromial arch. Such activities may include tennis, baseball, swimming, painting, and paperhanging. In middle age, the cuff may fray (partial tear), eventually tearing completely.

Rotator cuff tears may be spontaneous or may follow trauma. They also may result from various types of arthritis (e.g., rheumatoid arthritis, systemic lupus erythematosus, hydroxyapatite-associated arthropathy), metabolic conditions (e.g., renal osteodystrophy, diabetes), or repeated local injections of corticosteroid.

A tear may be suspected by the patient's inability to abduct the affected arm or by weakness of resisted abduction. Diagnosis is confirmed by arthrography or MRI. Treatment is conservative. Pain and loss of function often necessitate surgical repair of acute tears in younger patients. Occasionally, elderly patients experiencing severe pain from a rotator cuff tear may benefit from surgery.

**Adhesive capsulitis** ("frozen shoulder") often follows established tendinitis or glenohumeral arthritis, with failure to maintain shoulder range of motion. It may also be idiopathic in middle-aged women with no predisposing disorders. Patients report generalized shoulder and upper arm pain and worsening limitation of motion. Arthrography shows a small joint volume. In the absence of an underlying condition, the process tends to be self-limiting, with symptoms resolving in about a year. Physical therapy may help restore motion.

In addition to pain from primary shoulder disease, pain from neurologic conditions, such as a cervical radiculopathy (specifically C5-6), and occasionally from carpal tunnel syndrome, can be referred to the shoulder. The exact cause of shoulder pain often remains elusive. Because radiographs of the most common conditions causing shoulder pain generally are unrevealing, radiography should be reserved for those patients who fail a month of conservative management.

The initial **treatment** of most shoulder disorders is conservative, including NSAIDs and physical therapy. One or two local corticosteroid injections may be attempted. Surgical resection of the anterior third of the acromion (acromioplasty) and coracoacromial ligament may provide relief for impingement symptoms.

## Reflex Sympathetic Dystrophy Syndrome

Reflex sympathetic dystrophy syndrome, seen most commonly in patients over age 50, typically features burning pain, tenderness, and swelling in a distal extremity. Predisposing conditions are trauma, fracture, cervical spine disease, hemiplegia, and myocardial infarction. Vasomotor instability (vasoconstriction or vasodilation, Raynaud's phenomenon, hyperhidrosis), tenderness and edema, altered sensation, and, in more long-standing cases, dystrophic skin changes (e.g., atrophy, scaling, increased or decreased hair, nail changes) may occur. Although bilateral involvement was noted in 18 to 50% of patients in older series, detailed analysis of a small cohort found it to be universal. Patchy osteopenia and heterogeneously increased radionuclide uptake may be seen on plain radiographs and bone scans, respectively.

Treatment is most effective when applied early, before atrophy and contractures develop. Basic therapy includes analgesics, local heat or cold, and therapeutic exercise to improve motion; when these therapies fail, systemic corticosteroids or sympathetic blockade is necessary.

## Low Back Pain

The lumbosacral region consists of vertebrae, soft tissues (ligaments, paraspinal and abdominal muscles), nerve roots and spinal cord, and joints (apophyseal or facet joints, sacroiliac, fibrocartilaginous intervertebral disc). Low back pain may be caused by disorders involving one or more of these structures. Its neurologic aspects are discussed in chapter 185. Low back pain affects nearly 80% of the population at some time in their lives and takes a toll on worker productivity as well as health care and legal expenses.

Low back pain may begin at any age but the peak onset is in the 5$^{th}$ decade. Patients should be asked about trauma and repetitive movements related to their occupation or hobbies (especially heavy lifting). It is important to determine if the pain is local, radicular, or referred. Pain referred from pelvic and abdominal viscera (e.g., pancreas, uterus, retroperitoneum, prostate, abdominal aorta) is deep and aching, but other identifying symptoms are usually present as well.

The exact cause of back pain is often elusive. Spinal pain may be sharp or dull and localized to the affected part (e.g., ligament, muscle) but may be referred to the sacroiliac and gluteal areas and posterior thigh. It may be positional, with associated reflex paravertebral muscle spasm.

**Acute sprain** is self-limited and responds to rest on a firm surface, a pillow behind the knees, hot packs, NSAIDs, and antispasmodics. Early mobilization is encouraged within a few days, as outcomes are better than with prolonged bedrest. Therapeutic exercises such as Williams' flexion exercises (knees brought up to chest) may help reduce muscle tightness and spasm. After recovery, work modifications (especially of lifting or prolonged sitting), weight loss, and exercises should be initiated.

**Chronic lumbosacral pain** usually worsens on activity and decreases with rest. Findings include tenderness of the spine and muscles, muscle spasm, abnormal posture, and partially restricted straight leg raise and back motion.

**Radicular pain** arises from nerve root compression or irritation and is suggested by radiation of pain into the buttock or down the lower extremity, with or without numbness or tingling. Root compression commonly follows degenerative disc disease with herniation or lumbar spinal stenosis. The deep aching pain of disc herniation (usually L5-S1 or L4-5) is worsened by maneuvers that increase intradiscal pressure (bending, sitting, coughing) and decreased with a standing or supine position. Neurologic signs, particularly loss of a reflex or sensory loss, may help determine the level of involvement. The crossed straight leg–raising test (root stretching) is nearly pathognomonic for herniation.

Root compression responds to conservative therapy, such as bedrest for 2 to 3 weeks and medications to relieve pain, inflammation, and muscle spasm. Thus, diagnostic tests are reserved for patients whose symptoms are atypical, persistent, or severe enough that

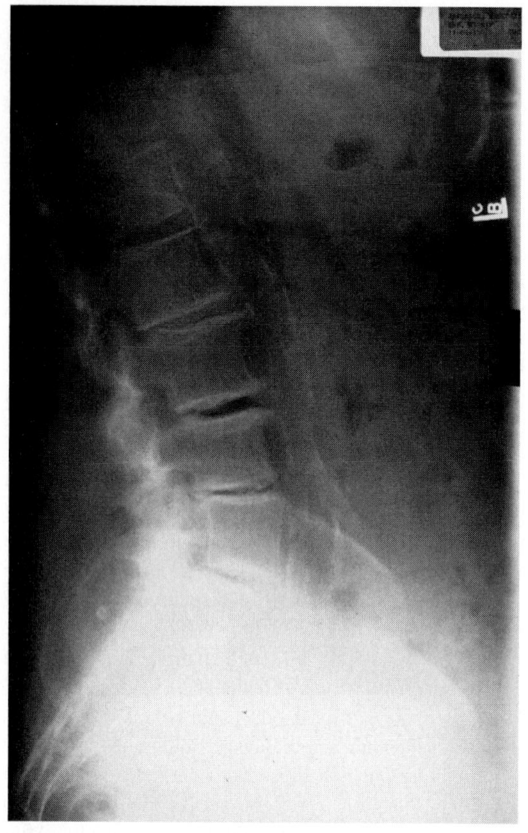

**FIGURE 268.1.** Lateral lumbar spine radiograph demonstrating disc space narrowing with vacuum disc phenomena, osteophyte formation, and facet joint sclerosis. Incidentally, the aorta is heavily calcified.

surgery is considered. Electrodiagnostic studies may be negative in the first several weeks but may help locate the site in 80% of cases. Plain radiographs may be normal or show only nonspecific, age-related osteoarthritic changes that correlate poorly with symptoms (Figure 268.1). Computed tomography (CT), MRI, or myelography are diagnostic in 90–95% of cases.

With midline herniation, bladder, bowel, or sexual dysfunction (cauda equina syndrome) may develop. Epidural corticosteroid injection may be tried in refractory cases before surgical intervention. Surgery is indicated for patients with unremitting pain, cauda equina syndrome, or progressive muscle weakness and neurologic deficits.

Bony entrapment of nerve roots or narrowing of the spinal canal occurs in **lumbar spinal stenosis.** Most cases of spinal stenosis occur in elderly persons in the setting of degenerative disc disease, osteoarthritis and subluxation of the facet joints, ligamentous thickening, or spondylolisthesis (slippage of one vertebra in relation to another). In contrast to discogenic pain, the pain of lumbar spinal stenosis is more diffuse; it typically worsens on standing or walking (neurogenic claudication) or hyperextension of the back, radiates to the buttocks or down the legs, and decreases on sitting or with supine position. Occasionally, it presents with cauda equina syndrome. Straight-leg raise usually is not markedly abnormal, and one or more dermatomal levels may be involved. CT, MRI, or myelography shows a narrowed spinal canal or nerve root entrapment. Initial therapy is conservative (back protection, NSAID, exercises). Epidural corticosteroids may be useful, but severe symptoms warrant surgery.

Other causes of low back pain are systemic inflammatory disease (spondyloarthropathy), metabolic bone disease (Paget's), infection (tuberculosis, pyogenic vertebral osteomyelitis, disc space infection), fracture, or tumor. **Diffuse idiopathic skeletal hyperostosis** (DISH, ankylosing hyperostosis, Forestier's disease) is a condition of new bone formation anterior to the vertebrae and spanning multiple vertebral levels, which causes a "flowing wax" appearance on lateral spine radiographs. Disc height is normal. Most patients are older, and many have glucose intolerance. Occasionally, dysphagia may result from esophageal compression. Spinal stiffness and restricted motion are more notable than pain.

## ■ Other Regional Pain Disorders

### Tenosynovitis

Tenosynovitis is inflammation of a tendon sheath, often at the site where a tendon passes through a fibrous ring or narrow bony canal. Its most common cause is injury or overuse, usually **cumulative trauma** from repetitive activity. Infection (gonococcal) or synovitis (rheumatoid arthritis, gout) are other causes.

Commonly involved sites are listed in Table 268.2. Therapy consists of cessation or modification of exacerbating repetitive activities (particularly important in work-related cases), treatment of the underlying disease, immobilization with splints, and NSAIDs. Recurrences are common. In selected cases, local corticosteroid injection and occasionally surgical excision of the fibrous constriction are indicated.

### Tendinitis

Tendon inflammation, or tendinitis, is usually due to strain or injury (see Table 268.2). Tendinitis commonly occurs at entheses (tendon attachment to bone) such as the medial ("tennis elbow") and lateral epicondyles of the elbow, but less often at the Achilles tendon. Therapy is similar to that for tenosynovitis, although surgery is rarely indicated. Local corticosteroid injection may be used at the elbow but is more risky at the Achilles' tendon because of possible subsequent tears and severe disability.

## Bursitis

A bursa is a sac-like structure that facilitates sliding of one tissue over another. Bursitis, or inflammation of a bursa with pain and sometimes swelling, may follow unusual use of an extremity or direct trauma. Common sites are listed in Table 268.2. Bursitis usually is recognized by tenderness to palpation over the respective bursa. Fluid accumulation may be noted in the olecranon and prepatellar bursae (Figure 268.2), but in others, there may be little to no swelling or other inflammatory signs. Calcific bursitis tends to be of more abrupt onset. Treatment consists of modification of the inciting activity or disease, NSAIDs, local application of heat or cold, or ultrasound. Local corticosteroid injection is often helpful.

Septic bursitis, which usually involves the olecranon or prepatellar bursa, is recognized by swelling, erythema and tenderness; often, the swelling is fluctuant on palpation. It is nearly always due to staphylococcal or streptococcal penetration through skin abrasion. Treatment requires bursal aspiration (daily if needed) and antibiotics.

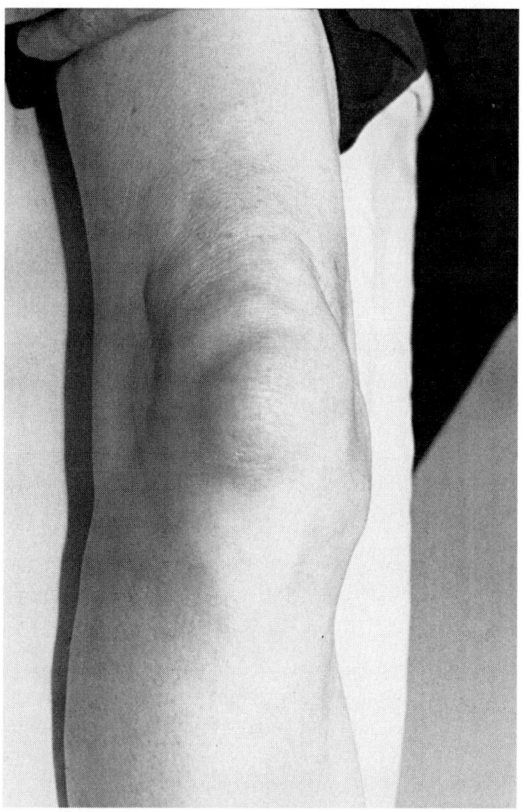

**FIGURE 268.2. Prepatellar bursitis of the knee. Note the circumscribed area of swelling anterior to the patella.**

## Fibromyalgia

Fibromyalgia (fibrositis) is a common musculoskeletal condition, second only to osteoarthritis in frequency. Patients report stiffness, weakness, and diffuse, poorly localized pain involving the neck, back, and extremities. Swelling or numbness also is reported, although objective evidence often is lacking. Symptoms are worse in the morning and with weather changes, stress, fatigue, or cold, and improve with heat, massage, or a vacation. Patients are chronically exhausted because of waking frequently, often due to pain, and characteristically awaken feeling unrefreshed.

Fibromyalgia is a generalized, pain-and-symptom-amplification syndrome so that its coexistence with irritable bowel syndrome and spastic bladder and its overlap with chronic fatigue syndrome are not uncommon. On physical examination, patients have a remarkably similar distribution of **tender points,** which are sites exquisitely sensitive on palpation; some of these tender points may not correlate with described areas of pain and thus may surprise the patient.

The American College of Rheumatology criteria for the classification of fibromyalgia identifies 18 tender points. The diagnosis of fibromyalgia rests on finding 11 of these 18 tender points, both above and below the waist and on both sides of the body, which have been present for at least 3 months (Figure 268.3). Pain in only one or a few localized areas is termed **myofascial pain,** and this is more likely to resolve over time.

Physical and laboratory studies should exclude rheumatic, endocrine, hematologic, musculoskeletal, and neurologic disorders. Although clinical data should guide laboratory tests, the complete blood count, erythrocyte sedimentation rate, and thyroid function should be examined.

Treatment often is frustrating. Patients may be defensive because they feel threatened by their symptoms and by physicians who dismiss their nonspecific symptoms as psychogenic or emotional.

Explanation of a "vicious cycle" of sleep deprivation and pain magnification is the first step. Drug therapy is controversial. Many patients respond to tricyclic antidepressants (e.g., amitriptyline) taken at bedtime to improve sleep, although side effects may limit their use. Exercise, particularly aerobics (e.g., swimming or bicycling 4–6 days a week), should be started gradually and increased as tolerated. Stress management and other relaxation techniques may be important for some pa-

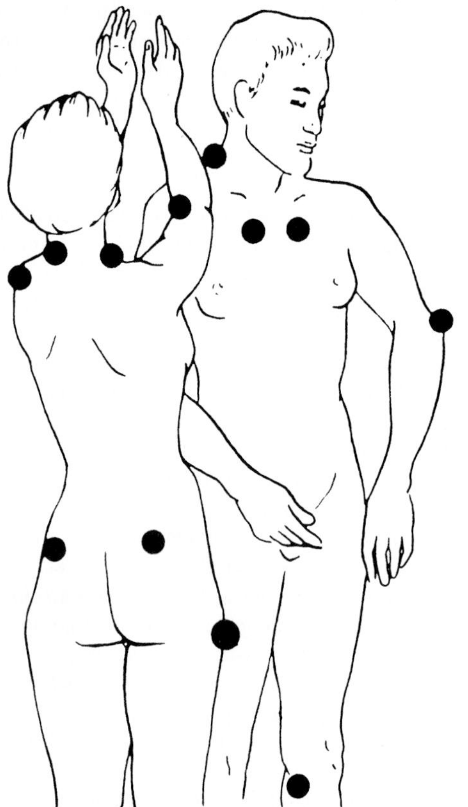

**FIGURE 268.3.** Location of 18 typical tender points in fibromyalgia. Tender points appear symmetrically in the body. The suboccipital muscle insertions onto the base of the skull; the lower lateral neck muscles; the midpoint of the trapezii; the medial supraspinatii; the second costochondral junctions; 2 cm distal to the lateral epicondyles; the upper outer glutei; the posterior aspect of the greater trochanters of the femur; and the medial proximal tibiae.

tients. Presented in a positive, concerned manner, these measures may alleviate the patient's fears and make symptoms more tolerable.

## Questions

**Instructions:** For each question below, select only **one** lettered answer that is the **best** for that question.

1. In a 27-year-old man with back pain and limited forward spinal flexion, which of the following tests best supports the diagnosis of ankylosing spondylitis?
   A. Radiograph of the pelvis
   B. Radiograph of the lumbar spine
   C. HLA-B27 typing
   D. Erythrocyte sedimentation rate
   E. Family history of back pain

2. A 60-year-old man has worsening back pain with no history of injury, mild paraspinal muscle tenderness, and extensive osteophyte formation with disc space narrowing on radiographs. Initial approach should include which of the following?
   A. Bed rest for 2 weeks followed by gradually increasing activity
   B. One month trial of back exercises and an NSAID
   C. Referral to an orthopedic surgeon
   D. Epidural steroid injection
   E. CT of the lumbar spine

3. A swollen right knee in a 45-year-old man is warm, red, and tender with a large effusion. The synovial fluid leukocyte count is 100,000/mm$^3$ with 95% PMNs and extracellular monosodium urate crystals. What would you do next?
   A. Inject the joint with a corticosteroid.
   B. Start the patient on an NSAID.
   C. Start IV colchicine.
   D. Obtain Gram stain and culture the synovial fluid.
   E. Start allopurinol

4. An 80-year-old woman reports pain in the right second DIP joint, which is very tender with synovial thickening and mild erythema. She has osteoarthritis of most PIP and DIP joints. Which of the following is most likely?
   A. Inflammatory osteoarthritis
   B. Rheumatoid arthritis
   C. Septic joint
   D. Pseudogout
   E. Psoriatic arthritis

5. The patient described in question 4 improves after treatment with an NSAID. One month later, the right third DIP and left fourth PIP become inflamed. Her RF is 1:32; ANA, 1:80; ESR, 30 mm/hr; creatinine, 1.9 mg/dl; uric acid, 8 mg/dl. What is the most likely diagnosis now?
   A. Inflammatory osteoarthritis
   B. Rheumatoid arthritis
   C. Systemic lupus erythematosus
   D. Gout
   E. Pseudogout

6. A 25-year-old woman reports blanching and pain of her fingers on cold exposure. Arterial pulses are normal. Which of the following is possible?
   A. Idiopathic Raynaud's phenomenon
   B. Carpal tunnel syndrome
   C. Fibromyalgia

D. History of vibrating tool use
E. All of the above

7. A 60-year-old man with scleroderma has had a 10-pound weight loss over the last 6 months. He has constipation and occasionally, diarrhea, but now has abdominal distention. What test is most likely to define his disorder?
   A. Esophagogram
   B. Upper gastrointestinal series with small bowel follow-through
   C. Barium enema
   D. CT scan of the abdomen
   E. Stool collection for fecal fat

8. Systemic lupus erythematosus (SLE) is diagnosed in a 24-year-old woman. Prednisone therapy is begun at 60 mg/day for 1 month. After 2 weeks, she has right hip pain. Limping and mildly reduced right hip motion are noted. Which of the following is most likely?
   A. Recurrence of active SLE
   B. Septic arthritis
   C. Osteonecrosis of the hip
   D. Muscle atrophy
   E. Greater trochanter bursitis

9. A 70-year-old woman with a 20-year history of rheumatoid arthritis had an auto accident. For her upper extremity pain and a sprained neck, rest, analgesics, and a cervical collar were given. Six days later, she notes leg weakness. Mild synovitis of her hands and wrists is noted, with small knee effusions, generalized weakness, brisk reflexes, and normal sensations. What is her diagnosis?
   A. Reactivation of rheumatoid arthritis
   B. Cervical myelopathy
   C. Subdural hematoma
   D. Disuse atrophy of muscles
   E. Myofascial pain

10. A 40-year-old woman with chest pain has a normal ECG, a high creatine kinase (all MM fraction), mildly enlarged thyroid, normal muscle strength, and no evidence of trauma, murmurs, or gallops. What is the most likely cause of the high CK?
    A. Heart attack
    B. Anxiety reaction
    C. Polymyositis
    D. Hypothyroidism
    E. Viral myopathy

11. A 35-year-old woman reports fatigue and widespread aching pain that disrupts sleep. She has, on palpation, 14 of 18 possible tender points. Fibromyalgia is suspected. What laboratory test is most likely to be abnormal?
    A. Increased ESR
    B. Normochromic, normocytic anemia
    C. Increased C-reactive protein
    D. Elevated CK
    E. None of the above

12. All of the following radiographic findings are typical of osteoarthritis EXCEPT:
    A. Periarticular osteoporosis
    B. Osteophytosis
    C. Sclerosis
    D. Geodes (subchondral cysts)
    E. Joint space narrowing

13. A 77-year-old woman has weakness with neck and shoulder stiffness. Tenderness is found in the neck and shoulder area, but no definite weakness. Her ESR is 75 mm/hr, hematocrit 33%, and hemoglobin 11 g/dl. Which ONE of the following is indicated now?
    A. Surgical consult for a temporal artery biopsy
    B. Start prednisone, 15 mg/day
    C. Start prednisone, 60 mg/day
    D. Start ferrous sulfate, 325 mg tid
    E. Start methotrexate 7.5 mg per week

14. A 68-year-old woman with a new-onset headache is febrile (100° F). She has normal temporal artery pulses and an ESR of 81 mm/hr. What would you do now?
    A. Spinal tap
    B. Blood cultures
    C. CT of the head
    D. CT of sinuses
    E. Temporal artery biopsy

## Answers

| | | | | |
|---|---|---|---|---|
| 1. A | 2. B | 3. D | 4. A | 5. D |
| 6. E | 7. B | 8. C | 9. B | 10. D |
| 11. E | 12. A | 13. B | 14. E | |

## SUGGESTED READING

### *Textbooks and Monographs*

Klippel JH (ed), Crossford LJ, Stone JH, Weyand CM (assoc. eds). *Primer on the Rheumatic Diseases,* 12th ed. Atlanta: Arthritis Foundation, 2001.

Koopman WJ (ed). *Arthritis and Allied Conditions,* 13th ed. Baltimore: Williams & Wilkins, 1997.

Polley HF, Hunder GG. *Rheumatologic Interviewing and Physical Examination of the Joints,* 2nd ed. Philadelphia: WB Saunders Co, 1978.

Ruddy S, Harris ED, Sledge CB (eds), Budd RC & Sergent JS (associate eds). *Textbook of Rheumatology,* 6th ed. Philadelphia: WB Saunders, 2001.

Samter M (ed). *Immunological Diseases,* 3rd ed. Boston: Little, Brown & Co, 1978.

### *Evaluation of Joint Diseases*

Dearborn JT, Jergesen HE. The evaluation and initial management of arthritis. Primary Care 1996;23:215–240.

Ostezan LB, Callen JP. Cutaneous manifestations of selected rheumatologic diseases. Am Fam Phys 1996;53:1625–1636.

Shmerling RH. Synovial fluid analysis. A critical reappraisal. Rheum Dis Clin North Am 1994;20:503–512.

Totemchokchyakarn K, Ball GV. Arthritis of systemic disease. Am J Med 1996;101:642–647.

Towheed TE, Hochberg MC. Acute monoarthritis: a practical approach to assessment and treatment. Am Fam Phys 1996;54:2239–2243.

von Muhlen CA, Tan EM. Autoantibodies in the diagnosis of systemic rheumatic diseases. Semin Arthritis Rheum 1995; 24:323–358.

### *Clinical Presentations of Rheumatic Conditions and Principles of Therapy*

Baker DG, Schumacher HR Jr. Acute monoarthritis. N Engl J Med 1993;329:1013–1020.

Crofferd LJ, Lipsky PE, Brooks P, Abramson SB, Simon LS, van de Putte LBA. Basic biology and clinical application of specific cyclooxygenase-2 inhibitors. Arthritis Rheum 2000; 43:4-13.

### *Crystal-Induced Synovitis*

Doherty M. Calcium pyrophosphate in joint disease. Hosp Pract 1994;29:93–96.

Schumacher HR. Crystal-induced arthritis: an overview. Am J Med 1996;100:46S–56S.

### *Osteoarthritis*

Altman RD, Hochberg MC, Moskowitz RW, Schnitzer TJ: American College of Rheumatology Subcommittee on Osteoarthritis Guidelines. Recommendations for the medical management of osteoarthritis of the hip and knee – 2000 Update. Arthritis Rheum 2000;43:1905-1915.

Block JA, Schnitzer TJ. Therapeutic approaches to osteoarthritis. Hosp Pract 1997;32:159–164.

Kraus VB. Pathogenesis and treatment of osteoarthritis. Med Clin North Am 1997;81:85–112.

### *Rheumatoid Arthritis*

Elliott MJ, Maini RN, Feldmann M, et al. Randomised double-blind comparison of chimeric monoclonal antibody to tumour necrosis factor alpha (cA2) versus placebo in rheumatoid arthritis. Lancet 1994;344:1105-1110.

Jain R, Lipsky PE. Treatment of rheumatoid arthritis. Med Clin North Am 1997;81:57–84.

Pope RM. Rheumatoid arthritis: pathogenesis and early recognition. Am J Med 1996;100:3S–9S.

Strand V, Cohen S, Schiff M, et al. Treatment of active rheumatoid arthritis with leflunomide compared with placebo or methotrexate. Arch Intern Med 1999;159:2542-2550.

Weinblatt ME, Kremer JM, Bankhurst AD, et al. A trial of etanercept, a recombinant tumor necrosis factor:Fc fusion protein in patients with rheumatoid arthritis receiving methotrexate. N Engl J Med 1999;340:253-259.

Youinou P, Moutsopoulos HM, Pennec YL. Clinical features of Sjögren's syndrome. Curr Opin Rheumatol 1990;2:687–693.

### *Infectious Arthritis*

Brower AC. Septic arthritis. Radiol Clin North Am 1996;34: 293–309.

Kramer N, Rosenstein ED. Rheumatologic manifestations of tuberculosis. Bull Rheumatic Dis 1997;46:5–8.

Mikhail IS, Alarcon GS. Nongonococcal bacterial arthritis. Rheum Dis Clin North Am 1993;19:311–331.

Norman DC, Yoshikawa TT. Infections of the bone, joint, and bursa. Clin Geriatr Med 1994;10:703–718.

Scopelitis E, Martinez-Osuna P. Gonococcal arthritis. Rheum Dis Clin North Am 1993;19:363–377.

Smith JW, Piercy EA. Infectious arthritis. Clin Infect Dis 1995;20:225–230.

Steere AC. Diagnosis and treatment of Lyme arthritis. Med Clin North Am 1997;81:179–194.

### *Seronegative Spondyloarthropathies*

D'Cruz D, Ross E, Morrow J. Psoriatic arthritis: identifying and controlling an insidious disease. J Musculoskel Med 1998; 15:17–35.

Khan MA. An overview of clinical spectrum and heterogeneity of spondyloarthropathies. Rheum Dis Clin North Am 1992; 18:1–10.

Underwood MR, Dawes P. Inflammatory back pain in primary care. Br J Rheumatol 1995;34:1074–1077.

### *Systemic Lupus Erythematosus*

Belmont HM, Abramson SB, Lie JT. Pathology and pathogenesis of vascular injury in systemic lupus erythematosus. Interactions of inflammatory cells and activated endothelium. Arthritis Rheum 1996;39:9–22.

Lehman TJ. A practical guide to systemic lupus erythematosus. Pediatr Clin North Am 1995;42:1223–1238.

Mills JA. Systemic lupus erythematosus. N Engl J Med 1871;330:1871–1879.

Pisetsky DS, Gilkeson G, Clair EW. Systemic lupus erythematosus. Diagnosis and treatment. Med Clin North Am 1997; 81:113–128.

Von Feldt JM. Systemic lupus erythematosus. Recognizing its various presentations. Postgrad Med 1995;97:79,83,86 passim.

### *Other Connective Tissue Diseases*

Anonymous. Systemic sclerosis: current pathogenetic concepts and future prospects for targeted therapy. Lancet 1996;347: 1453–1458.

Callen JP. Relationship of cancer to inflammatory muscle diseases. Dermatomyositis, polymyositis, and inclusion body myositis. Rheum Dis Clin North Am 1994;20:943–953.

Mastaglia FL, Phillips BA, Zilko P. Treatment of inflammatory myopathies. Muscle Nerve 1997;20:651–664.

Medsger TA Jr, Oddis CV. Classification and diagnostic criteria for polymyositis and dermatomyositis. J Rheumatol 1995;22: 581–585.

### *Vasculitis*

Allen NB, Bressler PB. Diagnosis and treatment of the systemic and cutaneous necrotizing vasculitis syndromes. Med Clin North Am 1997;81:243–259.

Bahlas S, Ramos-Remus C, Davis P. Clinical outcome of 149 patients with polymyalgia rheumatica and giant cell arteritis. J Rheumatol 1998;25:99–104.

Gross WL, Schmitt WH, Csernok E. Antineutrophil cytoplasmic autoantibody-associated diseases: a rheumatologist's perspective. Am J Kidney Dis 1991;18:175–179.

Hoffman GS, Kerr GS, Leavitt RY, et al. Wegener's granulomatosis: An analysis of 158 patients. Ann Intern Med 1992;116:488–498.

Hunder G. Vasculitis: diagnosis and therapy. Am J Med 1996;100:37S–45S.

Isenberg DA, Black C. ABC of rheumatology. Raynaud's phenomenon, scleroderma, and overlap syndromes. BMJ 1995;310:795–798.

Savage CO, Harper L, Adu D. Primary systemic vasculitis. Lancet 1997;349:553–558.

Sneller MC, Fauci AS. Pathogenesis of vasculitis syndromes. Med Clin North Am 1997;81:221–242.

Watts RA, Scott DG. ABC of rheumatology. Rashes and vasculitis. BMJ 1995;310:1128–1132.

### *Regional (Nonarticular) Musculoskeletal Pain*

Doherty M, Jones A. ABC of rheumatology. Fibromyalgia syndrome. BMJ 1995;310:386–389.

Evans PJ, Miniaci A. Rotator cuff tendinopathy: many causes, many solutions. J Musculoskel Med 1998;15:32–36.

McClaflin RR. Myofascial pain syndrome. Primary care strategies for early intervention. Postgrad Med 1994;96:56–59.

Reiffenberger DH, Amundson LH. Fibromyalgia syndrome: a review. Am Fam Phys 1996;53:1698–1712.

# Index

Page numbers in *italics* denote figures; those followed by "t" denote tables.